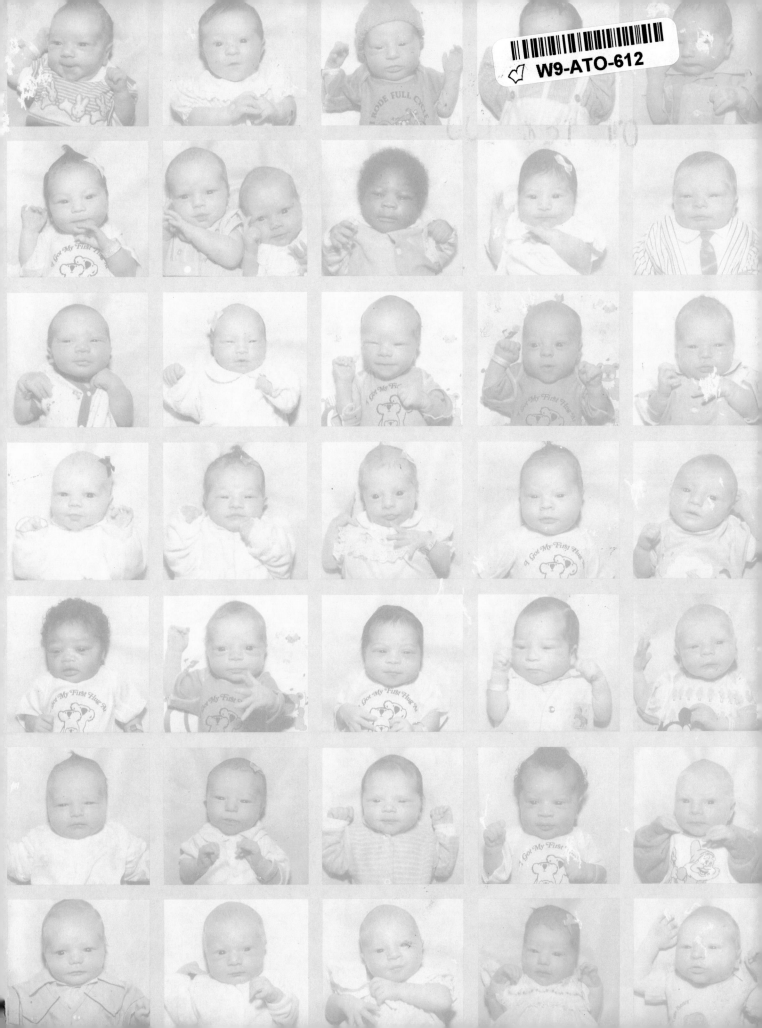

Maternal-Newborn Nursing

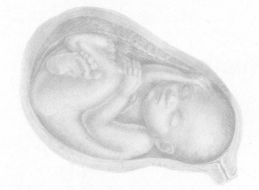

Third Edition

Maternal-Newborn

A Family-Centered Approach

Photographs by
Suzanne Arms Wimberley

 ADDISON-WESLEY PUBLISHING COMPANY

Health Sciences Division, Menlo Park, California
Reading, Massachusetts • Menlo Park, California • New York
Don Mills, Ontario • Wokingham, England • Amsterdam • Bonn
Sydney • Singapore • Tokyo • Madrid • Bogota • Santiago • San Juan

Nursing

Sally B. Olds, RNC, MS

Marcia L. London, RNC, MSN, NNP

Patricia A. Ladewig, RNC, MSN, NP

Third Edition

Sponsoring editor: *Nancy Evans*
Production supervisor: *Judith Johnstone*
Production assistant: *Brian Jones*
Book designer: *Detta Penna*
Cover designer: *Rudy Zehntner*
Designer, color chart: *Rudy Zehntner*
Illustrator, color chart: *Charles W. Hoffman III*
Photographer: *Suzanne Arms Wimberley (photos from earlier editions by
   William Thompson and George B. Fry III)*
Photographer, endsheets: *Barbara Miller, Cradle Pictures*
Illustrators: *Jack P. Tandy (line) and Charles W. Hoffman III (tonal)*
Developmental editor: *Deborah Gale*
Copyeditor: *Loralee Windsor*
Proofreader: *Melissa Moore*
Indexer: *Steven Sorensen*

ABCDEFGHIJ—RN—8910987

Addison-Wesley Publishing Company
Health Sciences Division
2725 Sand Hill Road
Menlo Park, California 94025

Library of Congress Cataloging in Publication Data
Maternal-newborn nursing : a family-centered approach / [edited by]
Sally B. Olds, Marcia L. London, Patricia A. Ladewig.
   p. cm.
   Includes bibliographies and index.
   ISBN 0-201-12818-7
   1. Obstetrical nursing. 2. Neonatology. I. Olds, Sally B., 1940-
II. London, Marcia L. III. Ladewig, Patricia A
   [DNLM: 1. Neonatology—nurses' instruction. 2. Obstetrical Nursing.
WY 157.3 M4258]
RG951.M3145 1987
610.73'678—dc19
DNLM/DLC   87-27310
for Library of Congress   CIP

The authors and publishers have exerted every effort to ensure that
drug selections and dosages set forth in this text are in accord with
current recommendations and practice at the time of publication.
However, in view of ongoing research, changes in government
regulations, and the constant flow of information relating to drug
therapy and drug reactions, the reader is urged to check the package
insert for each drug for any change in indications of dosage and for
added warnings and precautions. This is particularly important where
the recommended agent is a new and/or infrequently employed drug.

ISBN 0-201-12818-7

To women of the world
for the life they give, nurture, and sustain—sometimes at the cost of their own life,
sometimes when they are too young or too old or too sick or too poor
for the exquisite joy or despair their life brings them
and to a special woman, my daughter Allison Olds

To men
for their willingness to take an active part in the childbearing experience and to father
and to some special young men, our sons: Scott Olds, Craig and Matthew London, and Ryan and Erik Ladewig

To love
and the sense of wonder it gives to the world
and to those who love us: Joe Olds, David London, and Tim Ladewig

To students
who have the courage and energy to learn
and who touch our lives

To us
three rugged individualists who are bound together in our love for childbearing families
and who have been given this wonderful opportunity to grow together

We raise our cup to life.

SBO, MLL, PAL

Contributors

Authors

Sally B. Olds, RNC, MS
Associate Professor
Beth-El College of Nursing
Colorado Springs, Colorado

Marcia L. London, RNC, MSN, NNP
Associate Professor and
Director of Neonatal Nurse Practitioner Program
Beth-El College of Nursing
Colorado Springs, Colorado

Patricia A. Ladewig, RNC, MSN, NP
Director, Program in Nursing
Loretto Heights College
Denver, Colorado
and
Doctoral Candidate
University of Denver
Denver, Colorado

Joyce Boles, RN, MN, CPNP
Assistant Professor, Lansing School of Nursing
Bellarmine College
Louisville, Kentucky
Contributed to Chapter 29

Rena Brescia, RNC, MS
Coordinator of Practice Activities
Nurses' Association of the
American College of Obstetricians and Gynecologists
Washington, DC
Contributed to Chapter 26

Sharon Glass, RN, BS, NNP
Neonatal Nurse Clinician
Eastern Oklahoma Perinatal Center
Tulsa, Oklahoma
Contributed to Chapters 31, 32

Effie A. Graham, RN, PhD
Associate Professor, School of Nursing
University of Alaska
Anchorage, Alaska
Contributed to Chapter 7

Janet Griffith-Kenney, RN, PhD
formerly Associate Professor
School of Nursing
College of New Rochelle
New Rochelle, NY
Contributed to Chapter 5

Louise Westberg Hedstrom, RN, CNM, MSN
Assistant Professor, Department of Nursing
North Park College
Chicago, Illinois
Contributed to Chapter 19

Patricia Hemak, RN, MS
Assistant Professor
Loretto Heights College
Denver, Colorado
Contributed to Chapter 36

E. JoAnne Jones, RN, MEd, MSN
Doctoral Candidate
Associate Professor, School of Nursing
Norfolk State University
Norfolk, Virginia
Contributed to Chapter 24

Lynette Karls, BS, MS
Assistant Professor, Department of Nutrition
University of Wisconsin
Madison, Wisconsin
Contributed to Chapters 17, 30

JoAnn Kilb, RN, MSN, NNP
St. Joseph Hospital
Tucson, Arizona
Contributed to Chapter 32

Stephen Kilb, RN, NNP
University Medical Center
University of Arizona
Tucson, Arizona
Contributed to Chapter 32

Virginia Gramzow Kinnick, RN, CNM, MSN
Assistant Professor, School of Nursing
University of Northern Colorado
Greeley, Colorado
Contributed to Chapters 16, 23

Kathleen Knafl, RN, PhD
Professor, School of Nursing
University of Illinois
Chicago, Illinois
Contributed Chapter 3

Dietra Lowdermilk, RN, MEd
Assistant Professor, School of Nursing
University of North Carolina
Chapel Hill, North Carolina
Contributed to Chapter 11

Nancy McCluggage, RN, CNM, MA
Program Instructor
Maternal-Newborn (Nurse Midwifery) Program
Yale University School of Nursing
New Haven, Connecticut
Contributed Chapter 20 and to Chapter 22

Mary Ann Neihaus, RN, MSN, CEN, EMT-A
Flight Nurse, Critical Care Team
University of Cincinnati Hospital
Cincinnati, Ohio
Contributed to Chapter 12

Shannon Perry, RN, PhD
Department of Nursing
San Francisco State University
San Francisco, California
Contributed to Chapter 1, 35

Lovena L. Porter, RN, MS
Ob/Gyn Nurse Clinician
Colorado Springs Medical Center
Colorado Springs, Colorado
Contributed to Chapters 8, 9, 14

Carol Hawthorne Rumpler, RN, MS
Chairperson, Psychiatric/Mental Health Nursing
Franklin University
Columbus, Ohio
Contributed to Chapter 10

Madrean Schober, RNC, BGS
Ob-Gyn Nurse Practitioner
Bloomington Obstetrics and Gynecology, Inc.
Bloomington, Indiana
Contributed to Chapter 10

Constance Lawrenz Slaughter, RN, BSN
Assistant Professor, Maternal-Child Nursing
University of Portland
Portland, Oregon
and
Staff Nurse
Bess Kaiser Hospital
Portland, Oregon
Contributed to Chapters 25, 27

Deborah Sweeney, RN, CNM, MS
Instructor, School of Nursing
Medical College of Georgia
Athens, Georgia
Contributed Nursing Research Notes

Linda Ungerleider, RN, MSN
Assistant Professor
North Park College
Chicago, Illinois
Contributed to Chapter 19

First and Second Edition Contributors

Martha Cox Baily, RN
Elizabeth M. Bear, CNM, MS
Irene Bobak, RN, CNP, MN, MSN
Sallye P. Brown, RN, MN
Penelope Childress, RN
Pamela Crispin, RN
Marilyn Doenges, RN, MA
Nancy Donaldson, RN, MSN
Joan Edelstein, RN, PNP, MSN, MPH
Mildred R. (Holly) Emrick, RN, MSN
Jack Ford, MD, FACOG
Laurel Freed, RN, PNP, MN
Sandra L. Gardner, RN, PNP, MS
Pauline Goolkasian, RN, MSN
Ann Kelley Havenhill, RN, MN
Linda Andrist Hereford, RN, MSN, NP
Loretta C. Cermely Ivory, RN, CNM, MS
L. Jean Johns, RN, MS
E. JoAnne Jones, RN, MEd, MSN
Emma K. Kamm, RN
Janet Kennedy, DN, DNSc
Joy M. Khader, RN, MSN
Jean Theirl King, RD, BS
Virginia Gramzow Kinnick, RN, CNM, MSN
Nancy Ellen Krauss, RN, MS

Joan Kub, RN, MS
Eleanor Latterell, RD, MS
Eileen Leaphart, RNC, MN
Mary Ann Leppink, RN, MS
Anne L. Matthews, RN, MS
Mary Ann McClees, RN, MS
Nancy McCluggage, RN, CNM, MA
Cynthia A. McMahon, RN, MSN
Anne Garrard McMath, RN, MSN, PNP
Caryl E. Mobley, RN, MSN
Donna Rae Meirath Moriarty, RN, MSN
Karen Rooks Nauer, RN, BS
Sally J. Phillips, RN, MSN
Lovena L. Porter, RN, MS
Carol Freeman Rosenkranz, RN, MN
Joanne F. Ruth, RN, MS
M. Carole Schoffstall, RN, MS
Paula Shearer, RN, MSN
Mari Lou Steffen, RN, EdD
Marie Swigert, RN, MSN
Elvira Szigeti, RN, MN
Janel N. Timmins, RN, MA
Marcia Vavich, RN, MA
Janet Veatch, RN, MN
Betty Blome Winyall, RN, MSN

Preface

Today more than ever before nurses play a central role in the planning for and experience of birth, and in how families feel about the experience afterwards. As client educators and advocates, nurses have helped women and their families regain a strong voice in their health care decisions. Women now have choices about how and where they give birth and, in some cases, about whether their caregiver will be a physician or a nurse-midwife.

Preparing nurses to assume this increasingly important role in family-oriented maternity care continues in this third edition to be the primary goal. Designed for use in undergraduate nursing programs, this text encompasses the entire childbearing process, from preconception planning through pregnancy, birth, and the postpartum period. Content progresses from normal to at-risk information within each phase: pregnancy, labor and delivery, care of the newborn, and the postpartum period. Cultural aspects of childbearing and material on the childbearing adolescent are integrated appropriately throughout.

● New Content

In response to comments from many instructors, five new chapters on women's health have been added to this edition. Carefully integrated to provide a lifespan approach to women's health, the new material goes beyond gynecologic issues to include chapters on family violence and rape. The new chapters are: From Menarche to Menopause, The Woman's Experience; Disorders of the Female Reproductive System; Gynecologic Surgery; Family Violence; Rape. Because the content is organized in discrete chapters, any portion can be omitted without interfering with the student's understanding of subsequent information, thus making the text flexible enough to be used in any maternity nursing course.

A new chapter on Social Issues and the Childbearing Woman examines such issues as women and poverty, wage discrimination and environmental hazards in the workplace, maternity leaves and child-care benefits, and abortion. Within this chapter, students learn not only what the issues are but also what actions they can take to make a difference—personal actions, client actions, community actions, political actions, and research actions. Maternal Nutrition and Newborn Nutrition are the subjects of two separate new chapters. Other chapters new to this edition include Sexuality and Reproductive Choices, Special Reproductive Concerns, and Preparation for Parenthood.

Throughout the text, special boxes on **Contemporary Dilemmas** highlight the legal and ethical issues surrounding pregnancy, birth, and parenting. One such discussion explores the issues related to the decision about circumcision (page 914); another looks at the difficult questions surrounding surrogate parenting (page 18).

● Expanded and Updated Throughout

This new edition emphasizes the roles of the nurse as client advocate, client/family teacher, change agent, and researcher. In addition, the scope of the book has been expanded to include women's health, both physiologic and psychosocial.

Every page of this new edition has been updated to reflect the most current research and technology. The underlying philosophy of the text, however, remains unchanged: that pregnancy and birth are normal life processes, that members of the family are co-participants in care, and that the nursing process provides the nursing diagnoses. Each of these learning aids has been reflected in this new edition are grounded in that philosophy and in our commitment to a family-centered approach.

● Enhanced Visual Appeal

Today's visually oriented student will find that a new two-color design helps highlight key information and commands greater interest. Students are brought close to the childbearing experience through the use of dramatic photographs and the poignant personal reflections of childbearing women and their nurses. The photographs by Suzanne Arms Wimberley, internationally known author and childbirth educator, reveal an extraordinary sensitivity to the needs, desires, and customs of many women and cultures.

● New Full-Color Insert

Noting the popularity of the color photographs in the second edition, *we have expanded the color insert to eight pages.* **A new color chart, enhanced by the superb illustrations of Charles W. Hoffman III, depicts Maternal-Fetal Development month by month** (foldout in color insert). Client teaching and anticipatory guidance are noted below each developmental phase, giving the student an excellent learning tool and a ready reference.

● Increased Emphasis on Self-Care

From its inception, this text has recognized the importance of education for self-care. This edition highlights the topic with a special heading, "Education for Self-Care." As further support for the nurse's role as a client/family teacher, a complete Blue Pages listing of client/family resources is located following the Glossary at the end of the book.

● New Learning Aids

Since the first edition of this text, instructors and students have praised the wealth of learning aids provided. **Chapter Outlines** and clear, measurable **Objectives** open each chapter; a summary of **Key Concepts** conclud·s each chapter. Throughout the text, nursing **Research Notes**— brief summaries of current nursing research studies— heighten students' awareness of the relevance of research to nursing practice.

We have retained the popular **Nursing Assessment Guides, Drug Guides, Procedures,** and many summary tables. The **Nursing Care Plans** have been modified to focus on a specific family situation and to emphasize

framework necessary for optimal care. The many changes updated throughout; all reflect the 1986 NANDA nursing diagnoses.

● Complete New Teaching/Learning Package

To assist faculty in enriching their teaching presentation, this new edition offers the following supplements:

- **1000-item Test Bank**   Available in booklet form or as computer software for IBM or Apple, this totally new test bank helps faculty quickly and easily create numerous unique examinations. Test items are classified by cognitive level and nursing process step.
- **Student Workbook**   Written by the authors, this popular workbook has been revised and updated in keeping with the changes made in this revision. It incorporates strategies for students to increase synthesis of their knowledge.
- **Instructor's Manual**   Written by Virginia Gramzow Kinnick, RN, MSN, this timesaving aid has been thoroughly revised and now includes blackline transparency masters.
- **Transparency Resource Kit**   Forty-two two-color transparencies present enlarged versions of important text figures.

● Acknowledgments

Our goal with every revision of the text is to incorporate the newest research, the most up-to-date techniques, and the latest information from the literature of nursing and the other health care professions. We want to give a clear picture of current trends and practices in nursing, and to choose each word carefully to reflect the dynamic changes within the profession and society as a whole. This would not be possible without the support of our contributors. The volume and complexity of knowledge within maternal-newborn nursing demand that any state-of-the-art textbook reflect the collaboration of experts in each area of this practice discipline. Thus we are indebted to all our contributors for bringing their special knowledge and expertise to this revision.

We are particularly grateful to **Janet Griffith-Kenney** for granting permission to adapt material from *Contemporary Women's Health: A Nursing Advocacy Approach* for the women's health chapters in this new edition, and to her contributors: *Effie Graham, Dietra Lowdermilk, Mary Ann Niehaus, Carol Rumpler,* and *Madrean Schober.* In adapting and updating this material, we have continued their emphasis on nursing advocacy in the care of women.

We also owe special thanks to **Deborah Sweeney** for her contribution of the Nursing Research Notes in this edition. She identified and summarized relevant nursing research studies, heightening students' appreciation of the importance of research as a basis for nursing practice.

We are grateful to **Pamela Swearingen**, who generously gave her permission for the use of fourteen photographs from *The Addison-Wesley Photo-Atlas of Nursing Procedures*.

In publishing, as in health care, quality assurance is an essential part of the process; that is the dimension our reviewers have added. Some reviewers assist us by validating the accuracy of the content, some by their attention to detail, and some by challenging us to examine our present way of thinking and develop new awareness. Thus we extend a sincere word of thanks to the following reviewers:

- Bernadine Adams, Northeast Louisiana University, Monroe, Louisiana
- Verna Carson, University of Maryland, Baltimore, Maryland
- Margaret A. Cooper, University of Colorado, Denver, Colorado
- Dorothy Crowder, Virginia Commonwealth University, Medical College of Virginia, Richmond, Virginia
- Barbara Gilman, University of Cincinnati, Cincinnati, Ohio
- Karen Haller, Loyola University, Chicago, Illinois
- Jeanette Hines, San Diego State University, San Diego, California
- Helen Jacobson, Hunter College, New York, New York
- Jill Jaeckle, Healthworks, Haverhill, Massachusetts
- Diane Kruse, Arizona State University, Tempe, Arizona
- Wendy La Fage, Southeastern Louisiana University, Baton Rouge, Louisiana
- Susan Marchessault, Northeastern University, Boston, Massachusetts
- Michelle Gruen Noble, University of Kansas, Kansas City, Kansas
- Charlotte Patrick, Texas Woman's University, Denton, Texas
- Deborah Sweeney, Medical College of Georgia, Athens, Georgia
- Debbie Ulrich, Wright State University, Dayton, Ohio
- Joyce Vogler, Loma Linda University, Loma Linda, California

These women are both clinicians and scholars. They draw on their knowledge from clinical experience and from scrupulous research to revise and update the material. We are indebted to them for the care and expertise they bring to the project.

We also deeply appreciate the comments and suggestions from nurse educators and practitioners around the country who have used the earlier editions. Whenever a nurse takes the time to write or stops to speak when our paths cross at professional meetings, we realize again the intense commitment of nurses to excellence in practice. And so we thank our peers.

In addition, we want to thank nursing students everywhere. When we experience the wonder of a birth through the eyes of a student, or feel vicarious pleasure when a student provides exceptional nursing care, we are assured that the future is in good hands. Their questions challenge us to stretch and grow professionally. Their presence in our daily lives sets the standard of excellence for this text.

Pat and Steve Waldo have been close friends for years. We are honored and delighted that they were willing to share their family's experience of the birth of twins **Hilary** and **Rebecca**, as depicted in the birth sequence on pages 672–673.

The illustrations throughout this edition are the work of some very special people. **Suzanne Arms Wimberley**'s moving photographs never fail to capture the essence of a moment in the life of a childbearing family. We are also thrilled with the newborn photographs contributed by **Barbara Miller** of Cradle Pictures, Detroit, Michigan, for the very special endsheets of this book.

Jack Tandy, another good friend, has updated much of the line art throughout the text. The simple clarity of his drawings has great educational value.

Charles W. Hoffman III, a tremendously talented illustrator, has joined us for the first time in this edition. His remarkable style and meticulous research bring new beauty and depth to the text. We think his work for the maternal-fetal development chart conveys the miracle of the developing child exceptionally well.

Detta Penna joins us for this edition, bringing her special sensitivity and talent to a book design that is as warm and appealing as the newborns we celebrate here. Our hats are off to **Rudy Zehntner**, another newcomer to our team, whose design savvy has contributed so much to the new look of this edition.

Loralee Windsor brought us her professional skills as copyeditor, and **Melissa Moore** proofread the galleys skillfully; to both we say thank you. **Steve Sorensen** not only provided this new edition with an index of high professional caliber, but also checked the page proofs fastidiously.

Deborah Gale has lent her many-faceted talents to all three editions of this text. In the development of this edition, she acted as a catalyst, guide, and contributor. We think she is magical!

We want to acknowledge once again the talent and hard work of the people at Addison-Wesley. We are grateful to those beyond the scenes and to those who manage. We must single out a few people for special praise.

Judy Johnstone is responsible for conceptualizing the marvelous new look of this edition, and it is she who conceived and orchestrated the color chart. All aspects of production were in her capable hands. **Brian Jones** made a valued contribution by coordinating the art program. They are both very special people.

Nancy Evans, our editor and friend, never fails to give us the support, guidance, and encouragement that sustains us through the long process of birthing a book. Her creativity and firm sense of the marketplace are invaluable to us, and her natural wit makes problems seem to vanish. Her caring about women and her knowledge about women's issues help keep us at the cutting edge.

During the years the three of us have worked together to develop and refine this book, we've shared with each other both happiness and sorrow as we watched our own families grow and evolve. Our children are maturing, becoming their own unique selves—supportive, loving, and challenging! Our husbands remain steadfast and caring. We are grateful for their willingness to accept the unpredictable with generosity and humor. We are truly fortunate to be members of families that nurture our growth.

Reception of our first and second editions has been most gratifying. The comments from those who have used the book have helped to shape its continuing development. We hope this third edition will prove even more useful to faculty and to students in communicating the power and wonder of the miracle that is birth.

Sally B. Olds
Marcia L. London
Patricia A. Ladewig

Contents in Brief

Special Features

Contents in Detail

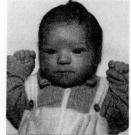

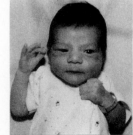

Part Five

Labor and Delivery   569

Chapter Twenty-One   570

Processes and Stages of Labor and Delivery

Chapter Twenty-Two   607

Intrapartal Nursing Assessment

Chapter Twenty-Three   645

The Family in Childbirth: Needs and Care

Chapter Twenty-Four   690

Maternal Analgesia and Anesthesia

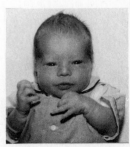

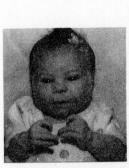

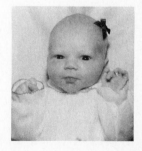

Contemporary Maternity Nursing

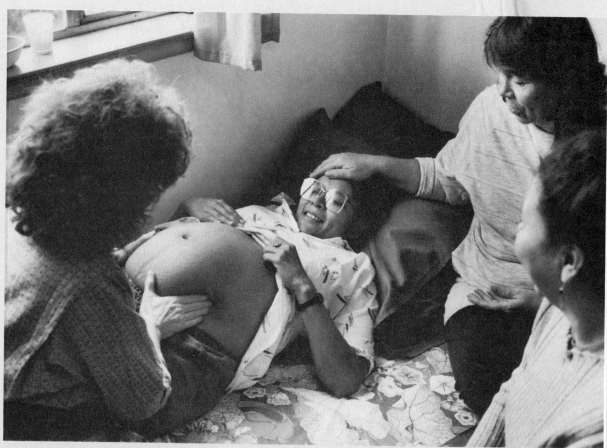

Women friends accompany this young Native American to her prenatal visit.

Part One

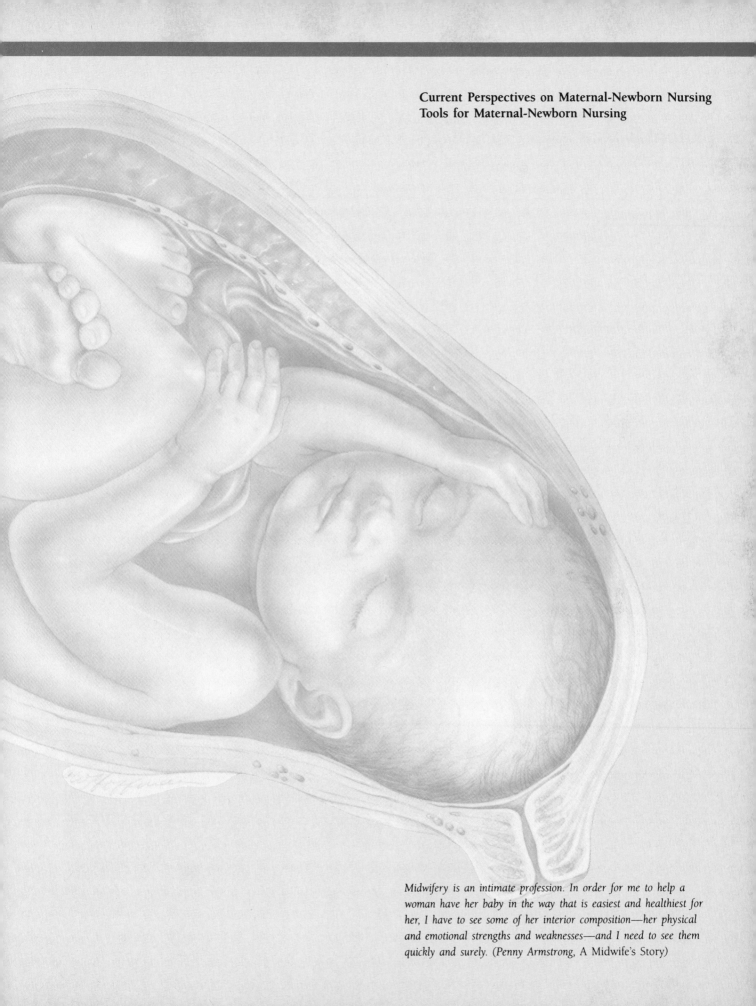

Midwifery is an intimate profession. In order for me to help a woman have her baby in the way that is easiest and healthiest for her, I have to see some of her interior composition—her physical and emotional strengths and weaknesses—and I need to see them quickly and surely. (Penny Armstrong, A Midwife's Story)

Current Perspectives on Maternal-Newborn Nursing

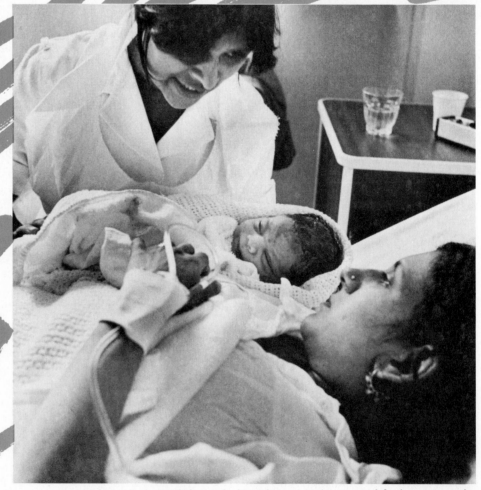

In a British hospital, this Pakistani mother is cared for by a nurse who speaks the same language.

Chapter One

OBJECTIVES

- **Relate the concept of the expert nurse to nurses caring for childbearing families.**
- **Discuss the impact of the self-care movement on contemporary childbirth.**
- **Compare the nursing roles available to the maternal-newborn nurse.**
- **Summarize the similarities and differences between certified nurse-midwives (CNMs) and lay midwives.**
- **Discuss the concept of childbirth as a business.**
- **Describe significant legal issues for nurses caring for childbearing families.**
- **Evaluate the potential impact of some of the special situations in contemporary maternity care.**

I've worked labor and delivery, helping families have their children, for 18 years now. My friends ask me how it is that I seem to know as soon as I see a woman get off the elevator whether I have time for a slow, low-key admission with lots of teaching and support, or whether I had better take care of the essentials first. It's not just how a woman's acting, although behavior is certainly a useful cue. I seem to have a sense of what is to come and the actions I need to take.

I like what I do. I like working with couples, involving them in the decision making and working with them for the kind of experience they planned for. I recall one birth experience vividly. I was working nights. The elevator door opened, and two ambulance attendants rushed out pushing a stretcher and calling for help. The woman on the cart was wearing a blue parka and pushing. The ambulance attendants were so scared they had trouble getting the stretcher into the room and kept bumping into things. Then they were all concerned about getting her into bed and doing paperwork. I could see there was no time for moving her to the bed or anything. I had to take over. I told them to wait outside for a little bit and told her I would take care of things. She had looked frightened, but when everyone left she calmed down. I think she knew it was safe with me. I pulled back the cover and found her naked from the waist down. The parka on top and nothing else. I wanted to laugh but there was no time. The head was coming. She did really well—pushed when I asked and then panted—and that baby just eased into the world. We were both thrilled. We'd shared something special. We didn't get that parka messy either!

A minute or so later her husband rushed in. He had followed the ambulance to the hospital. She looked up at him, smiled, and said, "Look, Dad, at what we've got!"

The nurse in the preceding anecdote will probably always remember the woman in the blue parka. Why? Because this nurse made a difference in the woman's life. Many nurses can recall special moments, shared experiences, in which they felt that they practiced the essence of nursing and, in so doing, touched a life.

What is the essence of nursing? It can be stated simply: Nurses care for people, care about people, and use their expertise to help people help themselves.

All nurses who provide care and support to childbearing women, their infants, and their families can make a difference. But how does this happen? How do nurses develop expertise in nursing and become skilled, caring practitioners?

Benner (1984) suggests that as nurses develop their skills in making clinical judgments and intervening appropriately, they progress through five levels of competence. Beginning as a novice, the new nurse progresses to advanced beginner and then to competent, proficient, and, finally, expert nurse.

The novice, lacking in experience, relies on rules to guide actions. As a nurse gains experience, he or she begins to draw on that experience to view situations more holistically. The nurse becomes increasingly aware of subtle cues that indicate physiologic or psychologic changes. The expert nurse has a clear vision of what is possible in a given situation. This holistic perspective is based on a wealth of knowledge bred of experience and enables the nurse to act "intuitively" to provide effective care.

In nursing practice, intuition is "the ability to experience the elements of a clinical situation as a whole, to solve a problem or reach a decision with limited concrete information. It is not the guessing of the beginning practitioner" (Schraeder & Fischer 1986, p 161). The use of intuitive perception is an important part of the "art of nursing," especially in areas such as maternal-newborn nursing, where change occurs quickly and families look to the nurse for help and guidance. Labor nurses become attuned to a woman's progress or lack of progress; nursery nurses detect subtle changes in their small charges; antepartal and postpartal nurses become adept at assessing and teaching: The list goes on and on.

In studying the expert nurse, Benner identified 31 competencies, which she grouped into seven domains of nursing practice. These domains of nursing practice are (Benner 1984, p 46):

The Helping Role

The Teaching-Coaching Function

The Diagnostic and Patient-Monitoring Function

Effective Management of Rapidly Changing Situations

Administering and Monitoring Therapeutic Interventions and Regimens

Monitoring and Ensuring the Quality of Health Care Practices

Organizational and Work-Role Competencies

The nurse in the introductory anecdote demonstrated expertise in at least three domains:

1. In describing her ability to sense how a woman is progressing in labor, she demonstrated expertise in the diagnostic and patient-monitoring domain.

2. Her interventions with the woman in the parka showed expert functioning in the helping role.

3. Her actions clearly demonstrated effective management in a rapidly changing situation.

The following situation provides another example of an expert nurse performing in the helping domain.

My first pregnancy ended in spontaneous abortion at eight weeks, so this time I decided not to tell anyone I was pregnant until I was three months along. We had just told both families the news the preceding day when it happened again. I began bleeding heavily and we rushed to the ER. Here I was, a maternal-newborn nursing instructor, and I couldn't seem to handle a pregnancy. I was in the bathroom when I passed the fetus into the johnny cap. My poor baby—so small, maybe 3 or 4 inches long. I began to sob uncontrollably as I rang for the nurse. I told her what happened and she helped me to bed. My husband sat with his arm around me as I cried while the nurse took our baby out. A few minutes later she came back and said, "I saw on your record that you are Catholic. Would you like me to baptize your baby?" I said "Oh, yes, please," and she left. I've never forgotten how that made me feel. She saw me as a total person. I'm still teaching, although now I have two children. Whenever I teach high-risk pregnancy I tell that story to the students. I want them to know what a difference a nurse can make.

We believe that many nurses who work with childbearing families are experts: They are sensitive, intuitive, and technically skilled. Such nurses do make a difference in the quality of care childbearing families receive.

● Contemporary Childbirth

As any nurse who has practiced in maternal or newborn areas for several years will tell you, the field has changed dramatically. Today's maternal-newborn nurse has far broader responsibilities than the nurse of 25 years ago. Today's nurses are less task oriented; they focus more on the specific goals of the individual childbearing woman or family. The use of the nursing process has helped bring this about.

Maternal-newborn nursing has changed. But then so has the whole experience of childbirth. No longer do laboring women leave their partners and family at the labor room door while they work to give birth without a family's loving presence; newborns are not routinely whisked away for a prescribed period, to reappear magically for feedings every four hours and then return to the safe atmosphere of a central nursery; no longer are young siblings treated like walking sources of infection that threaten every infant. Today fathers are active participants in the birth experience. Families and friends are included. Siblings are no longer separated from their mothers for extended periods but are encouraged to visit and meet their newest family member and may even attend the birth, although this practice is controversial. The concept of "family-centered childbirth" is accepted and encouraged.

Childbearing women today have many choices, including the place in which they will give birth. They can choose to give birth in hospital labor rooms, birthing rooms, or birthing centers (attached to the hospital or freestanding) or even at home. The primary caregiver may be a physician, a nurse-midwife, or even a lay midwife. Choices are available with regard to use of analgesia, position for labor, and even position for delivery. Women may elect to give birth sitting, squatting, on hands and knees, sidelying, standing, or in the more traditional position. Even practitioners who still prefer the lithotomy position have recognized the value of elevating the woman's head so that she can see better and push more effectively.

Unfortunately some of the choices of educated consumers may have a negative side. This is especially true with regard to the concept of early discharge. Until a few years ago even women with uncomplicated deliveries were required to stay in the hospital for several days after their babies were born. However, many women who had supportive families were eager to return home as soon as possible following delivery. They had the time and resources to return to the hospital or clinic for any necessary follow-up care and were well-prepared to care for themselves and their newborns. In a somewhat unanticipated development, as hospitals attempt to control costs, early discharge became the norm, and women with little knowledge, experience, or support find themselves discharged 24 to 48 hours after delivery. To compensate, nurses work hard to do necessary teaching and discharge preparation while the woman is in the birthing facility. In this early postpartal period, however, women are often not emotionally ready to learn.

In some areas follow-up care is provided to women discharged early. Nurses visit the women at home to assess their health and that of their infants and do any necessary teaching. This trend toward home care is a positive one, and we hope that this method of meeting the needs of families becomes standard practice.

● The Self-Care Movement

At the end of the 19th century most individuals were self-reliant consumers. No standardization of medical education existed, and *M.D.* following the name gave no guarantee of the nature of the education, if any, or experience and background of the practitioner. Numerous syrups and nostrums—Mrs Winslow's Soothing Syrup to Dr Walter's Eye Water—were available for self-treatment, including many products that contained opium or morphine. Home doctor books were available and even the Sears Roebuck catalog of 1897 contained 16 pages of medical instruments and drugs for both humans and animals. It was called the "Consumers Guide" (Mumford 1983). By the 1920s this had changed significantly. Medical education reform resulted in well-trained physicians with far more scientific knowledge than the average layperson. The more powerful medications were no longer readily available but were attainable only through a physician. Thus the age of the physician-reliant consumer began. The increasing specialization and evolving technology also contributed to the trend. Phrases such as "whatever the doctor says" or "I just need to see the doctor and get a shot to fix it" characterized the prevailing attitude. The health care provider assumed the major portion of responsibility for health maintenance (Hill & Smith 1985).

The self-care movement began to emerge again in the late 1960s as new consumers sought to understand technology and take an interest in their health and basic self-care skills. Toffler (1980) refers to these new consumers as "prosumers of medicine" because they are "people who are at the same time producers and consumers of health benefits." These prosumers exercise, control their diet, monitor their psychologic and physiologic status, and, in some cases, even do their own diagnostic tests. Thus they assume many primary care functions.

In evaluating this trend Naisbitt (1982) refers to it as a move toward self-help and away from institutional help (medicine). He stresses the return to self-reliance, with a focus on holistic care, wellness, and preventive medicine.

Today's nurses are being educated to recognize and value this self-help approach. It is more than patient teaching, which focuses on a specific condition and works to meet goals set by the provider. Self-care education is ed-ucation designed to help individuals attain their own health goals. Patient education and self-care education are different. In self-care education, the goals are based on the preferences and needs of the individual; no assumption of illness is made. In fact the individual is often well. Self-care education is aimed at reducing the individual's dependence on the health care provider; it may or may not generate income for the health care provider, depending on the preference of the individual (Hill & Smith 1985).

Practicing self-care—assuming responsibility for one's own health—often requires assertiveness as an individual actively seeks necessary information. This assertiveness is sometimes difficult for women. Abrums (1986) points out that health care providers develop their role expectations of women from previous experiences with women. If most of a health care provider's experience is with women who approach their health care passively, the provider may be disconcerted by an assertive woman who seeks to assume responsibility for her own health. Such a care giver may penalize assertive behaviors and reward more passive attitudes. Abrums suggests that nurses can play an important role in bringing about change in this area. As nurses grow to value self-care, they will also begin to reward assertive behavior in women. This will, in turn, encourage women to continue such behavior. Thus physicians and other providers will become more familiar with assertive women who seek to be active participants in their own health care and will eventually consider such behavior the norm.

Maternal-newborn care offers a special opportunity to promote active participation in health care and to foster a self-care "mind set" for several reasons:

1. It is essentially health focused, because childbirth is a healthy process.

2. In most cases clients are well when they enter the system.

3. The consumer movement that has already influenced childbirth encourages people to speak up for preferences in dealing with health care providers.

Self-care has gained an even broader appeal in recent years because literature suggests that it can significantly reduce health care costs. We believe that self-care will be a vital part of health care for years to come. Obviously self-care is not always realistic or appropriate, especially in acute emergencies, but in many situations self-care is appropriate. With this in mind, we have attempted throughout this book to suggest ways in which nurses might offer health information that would enable the childbearing woman or the parents of a newborn to meet their own health care needs. We see this as one of nursing's most important functions and one that nurses are especially well qualified to perform.

Because of our support of self-care we have used the term *client* rather than *patient* when referring to the childbearing woman. The term *client* implies an active role, not passive. The client seeks assistance from individuals who have special skills and knowledge that the client does not. Information and suggestions for a plan of action regarding the client's particular problem are offered to the client by the health care professional. The client can choose not to accept the professional's advice. Furthermore, the health care professional cannot proceed with the plan of action without the client's consent. In this relationship the client assumes responsibility for his or her decisions.

The nursing profession has been at the forefront in its recognition that people who are able to should take an active role in their health care, and the term *client* best fits this concept. Nurses involved in a maternity client–health care professional relationship must understand that it is their professional expertise and skill that is being sought. Any attempt to make decisions for the client is inappropriate.

● Nursing Roles

The contemporary maternal-newborn nurse has a variety of roles. In our opinion the most important roles are care giver, advocate, educator, researcher, change agent, and political activist.

Care Giver

The nurse uses professional expertise to help maintain and, when possible, maximize the health of the childbearing woman and her family. The nurse accomplishes this by making assessments, formulating nursing diagnoses, planning and providing care, and providing comfort and support when necessary. This may involve direct physical and emotional care of the childbearing woman or aid to the family caring for the mother.

Advocate

As a client advocate, the nurse supports the client's rights and assists him or her in making informed judgments.

The maternity nurse advocate informs clients by clearly identifying all the options available, as well as the risks of each one; by explaining simply but completely the nursing actions; and by answering all questions with facts and not personal opinions. The maternity nurse advocate then supports the client's decision by adhering to it and ensuring that others do the same.

The nurse advocate can enhance the consumer–health care provider relationship by providing individuals with complete information about the services desired so that the consumer's expectations are realistic. The client–health care professional relationship can also be enhanced by helping individuals understand that their participation in their health care is desired and indeed necessary.

Educator

As discussed in the preceding section on self-care, the nurse has an important role as educator. The nurse assesses the need for education and information based on personal observation and input from the woman or her family. The nurse provides information at the woman's level of understanding and confirms with the woman that the information is understood. The nurse then provides any additional information necessary based on the woman's goals for learning. Nurses in maternity settings are especially active in client education. Nurses on many postpartum units, mother-baby units, and newborn nurseries have developed teaching checklists, a variety of handouts and literature, and teaching programs. However, individualized teaching between nurse and client is still the cornerstone of education for the maternal-newborn nurse.

Researcher

More and more often nurses in clinical settings are becoming involved in nursing research. Some agencies hire doctorally prepared nurses to work with staff nurses and assist them in developing research proposals and implementing the planned research. Barnard (1985) states that the challenge for the next decade in nursing lies in developing research to evaluate the effectiveness of nursing interventions that are sometimes taken for granted. Barnard suggests that a "sense of inquiry must become a dominant characteristic of each practitioner" (p 63). Because of our belief in the value of nursing research we have incorporated research boxes into most of the chapters throughout this text.

Change Agent

Today's nurse works within the health care setting to effect change that will ensure safe, satisfying childbirth experiences for families and guarantee competent care for women and their babies. Nurses accomplish this change in a variety of ways: by working on utilization, quality assurance, peer review, and protocols and procedures committees; by becoming active in a professional organization; and, informally, by sharing pertinent articles and workshop information with colleagues to help them become more aware and concerned. Recently a group of Oregon nurses organized to obtain the statewide data necessary to convince their legislators that the state faced a serious problem because of inadequate access to care for childbearing families. Their research and organized efforts culminated in authorization by the state legislature of two large appropriations for perinatal care. Curry and Howe (1985) state,

> We were especially pleased that data from our study were used in oral and written testimony on behalf of the Medically Needy Bill and were considered pivotal in its passage. We hope our success will encourage nurses everywhere to try to effect change when they see problems that need correcting (p 228).

Political Activist

Nurses must become more involved in the political arena. This may begin simply with becoming active in one's professional organization and keeping abreast of political issues that affect nursing. Some nurses find a broader base for expressing concerns when they become members of their party caucuses and are elected as delegates to their party conventions. Some nurses find that they can be most effective by writing logical, factual, and concerned letters to legislators about important health care issues. Nurses can also take action by contributing to the campaigns of representatives who are attuned to health care issues. The contributions should be accompanied by a letter specifying why the support was given. Political representatives are always eager to know which of their actions gained them constituent support. Some nurses can best serve nursing by running for political office. This provides visibility and, more importantly, opportunities to make a difference through the laws of the country.

● Nurse-Physician Relationships

Today's professional nurse is being taught to function with physicians and other members of the health care team as a peer, not the passive handmaiden of the past. Nursing students are learning to view their relationships as collegial rather than dependent and to deal more assertively with difficult situations by establishing limits when the behavior of others is unacceptable. The following vignette describes an encounter between an irate obstetrician and a senior nursing student during her leadership rotation on a labor and delivery unit at a private hospital. The senior was also taking a course on nursing roles and issues.

I was sitting at the nurses' station doing some charting when Dr S came storming up to the desk. I was in scrubs so I don't think he knew I was a student, but it was quite obvious that he was very angry. He began berating me about a situation with another nurse. He was angry with her and seemed to include me even though I had no knowledge of the situation. When he finally stopped to catch his breath, I looked directly at him and said, "I cannot help you when you are yelling at me." He began heaping abuse again while I stood quietly until he paused. I then said, "I told you I cannot help you when you are yelling, and what's more, I think it would be more

appropriate to discuss this with the individuals involved." At that he stopped, appeared stunned, and then turned and walked away. Later that afternoon he sought me out to apologize for his behavior. I was amazed at his behavior and more amazed that I was actually able to deal with it effectively.

Relationships between nurses and physicians vary widely. In situations in which there is a high level of mutual confidence and respect, nurses find their work especially satisfying, and clients benefit from the high quality of the rapport.

A labor and delivery nurse recalls a situation in which she worked closely with a caring physician for the good of a childbearing woman and her family.

This happened several years ago before it was common to have families attend cesarean deliveries. I was working evenings and was caring for a woman—I'll call her Mrs V. She was 39 weeks along and her membranes had been ruptured for 26 hours. We tried to induce labor but it wasn't working. In those days the rule was that membranes should never be ruptured for more than 24 hours, so we were stretching it already. Finally her doctor decided that due to her failure to progress a cesarean was necessary. He went in to discuss it with Mrs V and her husband and to get the permit signed. Dr Waters was a really caring doctor and he spent a long time explaining, but she became terribly upset and just sobbed. He came out to the desk and said, "Mrs King, I need help. I can't seem to reach Mrs V. You have a good relationship with her. Will you please try?" I went in, let her cry for awhile, and then talked to her about her feelings. She said that she had taken childbirth classes with her husband and they had planned how they would share the birth of their baby. He even had a camera for pictures. She couldn't stand the thought of facing surgery alone. I remembered reading that several hospitals throughout the country had started letting fathers attend nonemergency cesareans, but we had never done it at our hospital. I went out and told Dr Waters about her feelings and about the literature I had read on the subject. He had done some reading on it too and said, "I'm willing to try it if you are and if you feel you can support Mr V." The evening supervisor agreed to circulate so I could stay near Mr V. Dr Waters and I talked to the family together, explaining what would happen and giving them the choice. They were so excited; Mrs V was like a new woman. She had an epidural so she would be awake, and her husband sat at the head of the table near her. When their daughter was born, he took pictures, held her for a while as he sat near his wife, and then carried the baby to the nursery while Dr Waters finished the surgery. I'm not a big trend setter or nursing leader, but that night Dr Waters and I took a risk together and we made a difference. Afterward we sat in the nurses' station, had a cup of coffee, and just grinned at each other. I'll never forget it.

As this vignette shows, nurses and physicians can work together as equals, and many changes have occurred to facilitate such a working relationship. However, nurses still have a long way to go in helping the less supportive physicians realize that as medicine becomes demystified, as consumers become active participants in their care, and as financial constraints demand cooperation, a collegial relationship between nurses and physicians will benefit everyone.

● Professional Options in Maternal-Newborn Nursing Practice

Nursing is unique in its adaptability and flexibility in providing maternity care in various settings. Maternity nurses are found in the obstetric departments of acute care facilities, in physicians' offices, in public health department clinics, in college health services, in family planning clinics, in school nursing programs dealing with sex education or adolescent pregnancies, in volunteer community health services, in abortion clinics, and in any other setting where a client has a need for maternity care. The depth of nursing involvement in various settings is determined by the qualifications and role/function of the nurse employed. Many different titles have evolved to describe the professional requirements of the nurse in various maternity care roles.

- *Professional nurses* are graduates of an accredited basic program in nursing who have successfully completed the nursing examination (NCLEX) and are currently licensed as registered nurses. Professional nurses use the nursing process and employ their clinical skills in a variety of settings to provide basic nursing care. Today's nurse assumes a collaborative role with the physician and other members of the health care team and is competent, assertive, and willing to take risks in the role of client advocate.

- *Nurse practitioners* are professional nurses who have received specialized education in either a master's degree program or a continuing education program. They function in a newer, expanded role, most often as providers of ambulatory care services. They focus on physical and psychosocial assessment, including health history, physical examination, and certain diagnostic tests and procedures. The nurse practitioner makes clinical judgments and begins appropriate treatments, seeking physician consultation when necessary. Within the scope of his or her clinical practice and expertise, the nurse practitioner is well qualified to clinically manage a client whose illness has stabilized.

- *Clinical nurse specialists* are master's degree prepared professional nurses, with additional specialized knowledge and competence in a specific clinical area. They assume a leadership role within their specialty and work to improve client care both directly and indirectly.

- *Certified nurse-midwives* (CNMs) are educated in the two disciplines of nursing and midwifery and possess evidence of certification according to the require-

ments of the American College of Nurse-Midwives (ACNM). Nurse-midwifery practice is the independent management of care of essentially normal women and newborns, antepartally, intrapartally, postpartally, and/or gynecologically. The nurse-midwife works within a health care system that provides for medical consultation, collaborative management, or referral in accord with the *Functions, Standards, Qualifications* for nurse-midwifery practice as defined by the American College of Nurse-Midwives (1979).

The nurse-midwife practices within the framework of a medically directed health service. The CNM functions in private practice or as a member of the obstetric team in medical centers, institutions, universities, and community health projects with active programs of nurse-midwifery.

CNMs and Lay Midwives

When nurse-midwifery began in the United States it provided quality maternity care to those unable to afford physicians. Time and again CNMs demonstrated that the care they provided significantly lowered perinatal mortality. Today, as consumers of health care seek more involvement in decisions about their birth experience, an exciting trend is evolving: Women who can afford a choice of health care

---

Research Note

Nurse-midwives assume both the role of a nurse and the role of a nurse-midwife. There is a potential for conflict both within the nurse (intrarole conflict) and between the obstetric nurse and the nurse-midwife (interrole conflict). This descriptive study examines these potential conflicts.

A questionnaire was mailed to 100 certified nurse-midwives and 100 OB nurses to explore the value differences between the two groups and the perception of content of care for CNMs by both groups and to investigate intrarole conflict within the CNM.

The data from the returned questionnaires showed that CNMs and OB nurses have basically positive views of one another. A few areas of interrole conflict were revealed, centering on intrapartum management. Some OB nurses felt that there was a confusion about expectations. Lack of communication seemed to be the major factor provoking conflict.

The researcher recommends clear communication to negotiate assignment of responsibilities and to discover how nurse-midwives and OB nurses can best work as a team.

Hazle R: Perceptions of role conflict between obstetric nurses and nurse midwives. *J Nurse Midwifery* 1985;30(May/June:166–173.

provider are choosing nurse-midwives. These women believe that the care provided by CNMs recognizes the dignity and individuality of each childbearing couple. The CNM recognizes that the childbearing family wants to share an experience, to feel close and supported, and to control the birth experience.

Although CNMs have established a positive reputation with consumers, their relationship with lay midwives is characterized by some uncertainty. Lay midwives accuse CNMs of being elitist, of treating lay midwives with the same condescension and discrimination that physicians have shown toward CNMs in the past. Lay midwives as a group strongly believe in the value and importance of their work. They believe they serve their communities by enabling families to share in a safe, rewarding experience that promotes family closeness and bonding (Weitz & Sullivan 1984).

Lay midwives and nurse-midwives share many values: Both have a philosophy of nonintervention; both value a family-centered birth experience. However, the CNM worries about the level of education of the lay midwife and about the quality of care provided (Weitz & Sullivan 1984). Judith Rooks, a CNM, suggests that "the problem with lay midwives, for themselves, for us, and for consumers, is that they lack the structure, standards, and all of the paraphernalia of a profession" (1983, p 6). The standards for competency and education established by the ACNM provide the public some reassurance about the qualifications of a CNM. In the many states where lay midwives are not licensed, no such guarantee exists. Some states have begun licensing lay midwives. In Arizona, for example, each applicant must show evidence of training and must have ob-

served a specified number of deliveries. In addition, the lay midwife must have performed a specified number of supervised deliveries (Weitz & Sullivan 1984).

Many CNMs believe that the education they received as nurses enhances their ability to function as midwives. Their nursing background helps CNMs function effectively in an emergency situation; it helps them deal with some of the broader health problems of the families they serve; it helps them understand how and when to collaborate with health professionals from other specialties; and it enables them to negotiate the health care system on behalf of their clients (Rooks 1983).

Many CNMs believe that the public would be best served if the ACNM developed more cordial relationships with the Midwives Alliance of North America (MANA), which is the association of lay midwives. Many CNMs also support the idea of sharing continuing education offerings because it is the childbearing woman who ultimately will benefit. Is there a place for a limited focus care giver such as the lay midwife in this country? There has been in the past, and many states seem to be saying that a place exists today. Regardless of the outcome, there is a place for the CNM in today's process of childbirth. Midwifery helps provide balance, a recognition of the magic of a process that has become increasingly technical. Flanagan (1986) sums it up well: "It is the humanity tempering the science of obstetrics" (p 198).

● The Business of Childbirth

As the consumer movement has gained momentum, hospitals have become aware that the revenue generated from maternity units is a significant factor in a hospital's success and stability. Childbirth represents profit, and that piques the interest of many agencies. In fact childbirth has become big business. Peruse any large city newspaper and note the number of hospitals marketing their "wares" (Figure 1–1). Hospitals proudly proclaim their commitment to women's health and boast of their women's "center," "hospital," "pavilion," or "core." Mention is made of the availability of Jacuzzis to labor in, tape decks to provide soothing music, double beds or birthing chairs for delivery, and celebration steak dinners for the woman and her partner.

This advertising has both positive and negative effects. On the positive side it is exciting to see the changes in care for the childbearing family. Women who previously were "only patients" are now recognized as consumers of a service and, as such, have clout. It is far less common for childbearing couples to feel they have to "fight the system" to have the birth experience for which they planned. The system wants childbirth to be satisfying, and health care agencies are more willing to work with the couples within the boundaries of good health care.

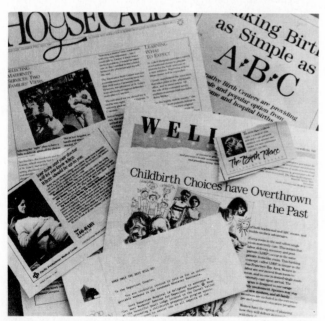

Figure 1–1 A variety of advertisements focus on programs and facilities geared toward women.

However, Nathan Boring (1986) raises an important question about the trend toward hospital advertising: Who pays for health care ads? Initially the costs of advertising are borne by the hospital but the costs eventually filter down to consumers of that care. The inescapable question is whether all the advertising is really necessary. Are the differences between accredited hospitals as great as their advertising suggests? Is the advertising that accurate? It is not unusual to learn that a hospital that proudly advertises its birthing room still does most deliveries in the delivery room because the birthing room is "dirty" or the woman is "too high risk," when in reality the physician or the nurses prefer the more traditional approach.

Physicians are also facing the rising specter of competition. A *Business Week* article (July 16, 1984) reported that physicians are enrolling in marketing and practice management classes, hiring consultants, and taking major steps to restructure their practices. These changes are related to an overall decline in physician income; a more-than-adequate supply of physicians, especially in specialty areas like obstetrics/gynecology; a decrease in demand for health care services as employers and insurance companies limit medical services; and a change in client attitudes with regard to satisfaction. This may represent an advantage to the financially solvent consumer who can enjoy the additional service engendered by competition but may interfere with adequate access to health care for the uninsured and those unable to bear the expense.

Health maintenance organizations (HMOs) are proclaimed by some as the way to provide high-quality care while containing rising health care costs. Others suggest that the structure of HMOs may lead to economizing at the client's expense. Since a member of an HMO pays an annual fee and sees group doctors, choice of care giver may be limited, especially in a smaller organization (Stickney 1985). Because of the wide range of quality possible among different HMOs and the doctors within the group, it certainly behooves the consumer to investigate an organization carefully before joining. An alternative, related approach is the preferred provider organization (PPO). In a PPO the health care provider has an agreement or contract with a purchaser (often an insurance company) to provide services at an agreed, generally discounted, charge. This guarantees a portion of the health care market for the provider and helps contain costs (Griffith 1985).

Nurses are playing a role in both kinds of organizations for two reasons:

1. Their services are less expensive than a physician's.

2. Nursing services often decrease the need for other, more costly services, including hospitalization (Griffith 1985).

Thus nurses often provide prenatal care, staff well-baby clinics, and do counseling in family planning.

Malpractice and the Cost of Insurance

One of the most significant influences on current maternity care involves the ever-increasing specter of litigation and the rising cost of malpractice insurance, especially in specialties such as obstetrics. In February 1986 in Massachusetts, hundreds of physicians refused to treat clients to protest a 68 percent rate increase that would result in malpractice insurance premiums of nearly $30,000 a year for some physicians, with the increase to be retroactive over the past two years (Boring 1986). In Georgia more than 1500 physicians gathered at the state capitol to urge the legislature to change the rules concerning malpractice suits. They were met by a contingent of attorneys and a group of people, many in wheelchairs, who said they were victims of malpractice (Newsweek Feb 17, 1986). The increases in rates have also affected many communities as more and more physicians drop the obstetrics portion of their practices or refuse to take new clients. In many areas family practitioners have given up obstetrics completely. Thus communities find themselves with no physician willing to perform deliveries. In some cases women must drive 100 miles or more to receive qualified obstetric care. The implications for the high-risk woman are profound and frightening.

What factors have contributed to this problem? Lander (1978) stated that three conditions are necessary for a malpractice action to occur: (1) an angry client, (2) an error by the physician or the hospital, and (3) injury to the client as the result of the medical intervention. Today's physicians suggest that a fourth factor must also be considered: the desire for money on the part of an attorney or a patient. Physicians suggest that careful doctors must bear the financial burden for the mistakes of careless or negligent colleagues. However, physicians do relatively little to police their ranks and remove the incompetent or impaired. Attorneys suggest that physicians should pay for their mistakes because these mistakes have such a lasting impact. The phrase "doctors bury their mistakes" has become their battle cry. Although lawsuits can force physicians to pay for serious errors, one can also argue that many frivolous lawsuits are filed that waste the courts' time and cost the physician and insurance company time and money in preparation.

It is easy to focus on the physicians and attorneys and lose sight of the insurance companies. These companies claim their rate increases are financially necessary because of the large financial awards made to victims by the courts. However, outspoken critics of the insurance industry suggest the increases are necessary because of poor financial management. Thomas G. Goddard, a former official with the Association of Trial Lawyers, suggests that the cause is even more devious: Insurance companies claim financial necessity while spiriting profits away in tax write-offs and reserve funds (Newsweek Feb 17, 1986).

The problem has become so visible that many state legislatures are considering legislation to attempt to control the problem. It seems obvious that something must be done to keep the many people who need skilled medical care from being penalized because of the malpractice crisis that has developed.

Nurse-midwives also face a serious malpractice insurance crisis, not because of poor performance, but because of the general problem facing many health care providers. From 1975 to 1985 more than 60 percent of obstetricians and gynecologists had a suit filed against them. Although fewer than 6 percent of the members of the American College of Nurse-Midwives have ever had a claim filed against them, and less than 1 percent have lost suits, in May 1985 the ACNM was notified that their group policy would not be renewed (*Am J Nurs* 1986). The American Nurses' Association attempted to help by offering coverage to nurse-midwives through its own policy. Unfortunately the ANA's insurer also revised its coverage to exclude CNMs. The very existence of nurse-midwifery as a profession in this country was threatened. Fortunately in the fall of 1986 Congress passed the Risk Retention Act. This enabled special groups to band together to self-insure. Although the cost will be far higher than previously (approximately $2500 to $3600 per year), it does permit CNMs to practice. In the future the cost of insurance will be influenced by claims lost data. Because of this, CNMs as a group must "give a high priority to the development of and adherence to standards for midwifery practice" (Sinquefield 1986, p 67). Sinquefield (1986) suggests that nurse-midwives are especially vulnerable in this insurance crisis because:

1. Nurse midwives are few in number and have rather limited assets.

2. Because most midwives attend deliveries, they are affected by the long-term disabilities that are often tied to childbirth. (Suits may be brought years after birth.)

3. As a profession CNMs are committed to cost-effective care. Thus CNMs find it difficult to justify passing on to clients as professional expenses the increases that occur.

Despite this vulnerability, some good for nurse-midwifery has come from the crisis. Nurse-midwives recognize the impact that each has on other CNMs. They have recognized anew the importance of maintaining positive, open relations with clients; of involving clients in decision making; of obtaining informed consent; and of carefully documenting their actions. In addition the ACNM has learned that the group can be a force; the members can mobilize, present a positive image to the public and to legislators, and make a difference politically (Sinquefield 1986).

● Legal Aspects of Maternal-Newborn Nursing

The maternal-newborn nurse must be aware of the many legal issues that affect nursing practice today. These issues are important and cannot be ignored, because ignorance is not considered adequate justification for failure to comply with current standards of care.

Scope of Practice

The scope of practice is the limits of nursing practice as defined by state statutes. Nurse practice acts broadly describe the practice of professional nursing. The practice of nursing includes such activities as observing, recording, and administering medications and therapeutic agents. Many nurse practice acts identify functions and actions that are appropriate for nurses functioning in expanded roles such as nurse-midwife and OB/GYN or neonatal nurse practitioner. Such actions may include diagnosis and prenatal management of uncomplicated pregnancies (nurse-midwives may also manage deliveries), and prescribing and dispensing medications under protocols in specified circumstances. A nurse must function within the scope of practice or run the risk of being accused of practicing medicine without a license.

Standard of Care

A minimum standard of care is required of all professional nurses. The standard against which practice is compared is the care that a reasonably prudent nurse would provide under the same or similar circumstances.

There are a number of examples of written standards of practice. The American Nurses' Association (ANA) has published standards of professional practice written by the ANA Congress for Nursing Practice. In addition, Divisions of Practice of the ANA have published standards including the standards of practice for maternal-child health. The Council of Perinatal Nurses has published standards for perinatal nursing. Specialty organizations, such as the Nurses' Association of the American College of Obstetricians and Gynecologists (NAACOG) and the Association of Operating Room Nurses (AORN), have developed standards for specialty practice. Agencies have policy and procedure books. Other guidelines for care include standardized procedures, that is, policies and protocols—developed through collaboration among administrators, physicians, and nurses within health care facilities—that cover overlapping functions of nurses and physicians. Nurses on units may develop standard care plans (Figure 1–2). Books and articles are another source of standards, as are common practice and those functions that have common acceptance. The identified standards range from those having the force of law to those that are suggestions or guidelines for care.

Patient Care Plan: Vaginal Delivery

Long Term Goals

Successful birthing experience, able to care for self and infant; avoidance of postpartum complications.

Date/Nursing Problem	Expected Outcome	Frequency of Evaluation	Nursing Action	M.D. Orders
Possible excessive blood loss due to: -delivery -or	Early detection of increased bleeding	q shift	1. B/P · 2. Position & firmness of fundus 3. Amount of lochia	
Possible alteration in comfort due to: -episiotomy -hemorrhoids	Relief of discomfort	prn	1. Positioning/pain meds as ordered	
Possible retention of urine	Voiding sufficient quantity q shift	Till voiding qs	1. Measure urine output	Straight Cath: Foley Cath: D/C: U/A: UC/S:
Potential constipation	Adequate bowel elimination	q shift	1. Note BM	
Potential for infection, due to: -delivery -or	Prevention &/or early detection of infection	q shift	1. TPR 2. Good hygiene/pericare 3. Note condition of epis	
Potential inflammation of veins	Early detection	BID	1. Check Homan's sign	
Potential deficit of knowledge related to: -infant feeding bottle/breast	Demonstrates ability to care for self and baby		1. Teaching guide at bedside ☐ 2. Instruction given ☐ 3. Breast care	
G P -infant care -self-care			1. Baby bath class ☐ 2. Postpartum class ☐	
Potential concern related to infant's condition: -NBICU: -Regular nursery:	Confident in care of baby	prn	1. Mother to NBICU ASAP 2. Assess family support systems	
Potential inadequate coping (individual or family) related to: -demands of new role -increased responsibility -disturbance of sleep/ rest	Verbalizes an adequate level of understanding of new role(s)	On adm	1. Discharge plan and coping mechanisms discussed ☐ 2. CHSF Social Services ☐	

Referrals - - - - - - - - - -

Figure 1–2   Sample care plan used postpartally following a vaginal delivery (Courtesy of Children's Hospital of San Francisco)

Some standards may be goals to strive for; others may define minimums, violations of which may provide grounds for accusations of nursing negligence. Nurse managers have a responsibility to keep the policy and procedure books on their units up to date so that the written standards are consistent with current practice in their agency. By the same token practicing nurses must follow the established policies and procedures. When a nurse acts outside the guidelines, he or she invites litigation and faces the difficult task of convincing a jury he or she was practicing competently.

Right to Privacy

The right to privacy is the right of a person to keep her or his person and property free from public scrutiny. Maternity nurses must remember that this includes avoiding unnecessary exposure of the childbearing woman's body. To protect the woman only those responsible for her care should examine her or discuss her case.

The right to privacy is protected by state constitutions, statutes, and common law (Baer 1985). Professional standards protecting the privacy of clients have been adopted by the American Nurses' Association (ANA), the National League for Nursing (NLN), and the Joint Commission on Accreditation of Hospitals (JCAH). Each health care agency should also have a written policy dealing with the privacy of its clients.

These laws, standards, and policies specify that information about the treatment, condition, and prognosis of a client can be shared only by health professionals responsible for his or her care. Information that is considered "vital statistics" (name, age, occupation, and so on) may be revealed legally but often is withheld because of ethical considerations. For example, revealing information about the admission of a single or divorced woman to the maternity unit may be legal but not in the best interests of the woman. Problems can be prevented by talking with the client to learn what information may be released and to whom. When the client is a celebrity or one who is considered newsworthy, inquiries by the media are best handled by the public relations department of the agency.

There are some instances when the public good takes precedence over the right to privacy. For example, state laws require the reporting of gunshot wounds, child abuse, animal bites, and communicable diseases.

Confidentiality

Confidential communications exist between persons in a trusting relationship, and such persons cannot be forced to divulge the information even in a court of law. Privileged communications exist between attorney and client, husband and wife, and clergy and those who seek their counsel. In many states physician-client privilege is also protected by law. Privilege is predicated on the idea that it is necessary for the client to disclose personal information for the physician to provide adequate care. Nurses are protected by laws of privilege in only a few states.

A client may waive his or her right to confidentiality of the medical record by action or by words. For example, if a childbearing woman sues a physician or hospital for negligence, she waives the right to confidentiality of the medical record because the medical record is an important source of evidence of the quality of care. In addition, clients commonly consent to disclose information to insurance companies or employers.

Informed Consent

Informed consent is consent given by a competent person who is of age and has had an explanation of the treatment or procedure. A person must give informed consent prior to receiving any medications or treatments. An individual should not even be touched unless permission to do so has been given.

The explanation of the treatment or procedure must include a description of the procedure, a statement of the benefits and risks associated with the procedure, and a discussion of the alternatives (including no treatment). Sufficient time must be provided for client questions. Some balance is necessary between too little information and an excessively detailed description of a treatment including all possible risks no matter how remote. Omitting necessary information may induce a person to give consent that might not be given if the risks were known. On the other hand, graphic details may so frighten the person that consent cannot be given.

How much information is enough to enable a person to make an informed decision is not clear. In some jurisdictions medical custom dictates the amount of information; in other jurisdictions the person is entitled to the information needed by a reasonable person to make the decision.

The physician is responsible for obtaining informed consent; the nurse may witness the signature on the consent form. If the nurse determines that the client does not understand the procedure or the risks, she or he must notify the physician, who must then provide additional information in order that the consent be informed. Anxiety, fear, pain, and medications that alter consciousness may influence a client's ability to give informed consent. An oral consent is legal, but a written consent is easier to defend in court.

Parents have the authority and responsibility to give consent for their minor children. Since the age of majority varies from state to state, nurses must be aware of the law in the state where they practice. Special problems can occur in maternity nursing when a minor gives birth. The minor may be able to consent to treatment for her infant but not for herself. In many states a pregnant teenager is considered an "emancipated minor." Emancipated minors and married minors are usually able to give consent for themselves.

A married woman may give consent for her own treatment; however, when the procedure involves sterilization or threatens the life of a fetus, it is customary in some areas also to secure the consent of her spouse.

The childbearing woman usually signs a general consent form on admission to an agency. This consent covers ordinary obstetric and nursing care, treatments, laboratory tests, and medications. Separate informed consent must be obtained for surgery, for unusual or experimental treatments, or for participation as a subject in research. Common situations in maternity nursing in which separate consent is necessary include administration of anesthesia, cesarean delivery, and tubal ligation.

A procedure that is not routine may be performed without informed consent in special instances:

1. There is a threat to life or limb if the procedure is not performed immediately.

2. The mental health of the client would be damaged by the explanation.

3. The client refuses to listen to the explanation.

4. The client is incompetent. In this case the information must be given to the next of kin (Rabinow 1983).

When a medication or procedure is indicated and the client makes an informed choice to refuse the medication or treatment, the client is usually required to sign a form to release the doctor and hospital from liability resulting from the effects of such refusal. For example, Jehovah's Witnesses commonly refuse blood transfusions or Rho (D) immune globulin. An example of such a release form is presented in Figure 1–3.

Reporting and Recording

The medical record (1) provides a basis for client care planning and for continuity in evaluation of the condition and treatment of the client; (2) provides written evidence of the client's course of evaluation, treatment, and changes in condition; (3) documents communications among the care givers; (4) protects the legal interest of the client, care giver, and hospital; and (5) furnishes data for research and continuing education (Joint Commission 1985).

Documentation should be viewed as an integral part of quality care. It is a clinical responsibility not just a clerical one. Nurses' notes are important because, unlike other parts of the client's record, they are in chronological order and document the medications and treatments that are given and how the woman or infant responded. Chagnon

and Easterwood (1986) point out that five types of nursing error frequently appear in maternity charts that come to litigation. These errors are (p 303):

● Incomplete initial history and physical

● Failure to observe and take appropriate action

● Failure to communicate changes in a client's condition

● Incomplete and/or inadequate documentation

● Failure to use or interpret fetal monitoring appropriately

The chart offers the only evidence that a nurse made appropriate assessments, provided quality care, took necessary action, notified physicians as quickly and clearly as necessary, and met the standards of care.

Good nurses' notes are clear, concise, and legible. They document what the nurse did, saw, heard, felt, and smelled. They contain objective descriptions rather than subjective labels. For example, it is far more effective to chart "Fundus firm, in the midline, 1 fingerbreadth below the umbilicus. No clots expressed." than to chart "Fundus normal." In addition to describing what the nurse observed, nurses' notes should describe interventions provided, responses to the interventions, safety measures, and when the physician was notified about the woman's condition or change in condition. When a treatment or medication is omitted, the reason should be charted.

Only acceptable abbreviations should be used. Errors should be corrected in an acceptable manner (by drawing a line through the error and writing *error* and the initials of the one who made and recorded the error). Correct grammar and spelling are important.

When a nurse forgets to record some information, the information can be recorded later as a *late entry* and identified as such. For example,

> 3/12/88, 3:20PM. Late entry. On 3/11/88 at 4:05PM cesarean incision dressing removed per Dr's order. Scant amount serosanguinous drainage present. Incision clean, dry. Edges well approximated. No redness or edema noted. S. Perry, RN.

Nursing Negligence

Negligence is defined as negligent conduct, that is, omitting or committing an act that a reasonably prudent person would not omit or commit under the same or similar circumstances. Malpractice is negligent action of a professional person. The elements of negligence are that there was a duty to provide care, the duty was breached, injury occurred, and the breach of duty caused the injury (proximate cause).

Hospital of San Francisco

REFUSAL TO PERMIT Rho (D) IMMUNE GLOBULIN ADMINISTRATION

Date _____

Time _____ _____ M.

    I hereby acknowledge that my attending physician, Dr. _____
has informed me of the availability of a drug for the prevention of Rh disease in newborn, has explained to me that the drug is
medically indicated in my case, and has described the potentially dangerous result of my failure to receive the drug at this time.

    Notwithstanding the advice of my attending physician, I hereby request that this drug not be administered to me during
my stay at   Hospital of San Francisco and hereby release the Hospital, its employees, and my attending physician
from any responsibility whatsoever for unfavorable or untoward results caused by my refusal to permit the use of this drug.

Patient's Signature _____

Witness _____

Witness _____

Figure 1–3   Sample release form (Courtesy of the California Hospital Association)

    The duty to provide care arises when the client arrives at the agency. By virtue of their employment at the agency nurses have a duty to provide care. Duty may be breached by omission—failing to give a medication, failing to assess properly, failing to notify a physician of a change in a laboring woman's condition, and so on—or by commission—giving the wrong medication, giving a medication incorrectly, placing the wrong infant in a crib, and so on. The injury that results may be physical—for example, an eclamptic woman who is left unattended and with the siderails down falls and breaks a leg during a convulsion—or mental—the injury causes pain and suffering. Finally, the breach of duty must cause the injury: If a client falls, for example, it must be proved that negligence, such as failure to take seizure precautions, was directly responsible for the fall.

    There are some exceptions to the definition of negligence. For example, leaving a sponge in a cesarean delivery client is negligent; cutting the ureters instead of the fallopian tubes is negligent. Such incidents are covered by the doctrine of *res ipsa loquitur:* The thing speaks for itself.

    In determining whether nursing negligence occurred, the care that was given is compared to the standard of care. If the standard was not met, negligence occurred. Birth injuries are common situations in which accusations of medical malpractice or nursing negligence are made. Because anoxia in the fetus can have such serious and long-lasting effects (death, cerebral palsy, mental retardation, and so on), judgments against defendants have run into the millions of dollars, contributing to the high cost of malpractice insurance, the practice of defensive medicine, and the rise in the rate of cesarean deliveries.

There have been many suits involving childbearing families. For example, a nurse in Utah did not do a vaginal examination on a woman admitted for induction of labor (*Nelson v Peterson,* 542 P2d 1075 [Utah 1975]). The nurse did an external examination and listened to fetal heart tones. She left to assist with another delivery. When she returned, she proceeded with the induction procedure. When the doctor examined the woman, he noted the umbilical cord was protruding from the vagina and the fetus was dead. If the nurse had examined the woman vaginally, the tragedy might have been avoided.

Another instance involved a woman who was admitted to a hospital for the birth of her second child (*Hiatt v Groce,* 215 Kans 14, 523 P2d 320 [1974]). The cervix was dilated to 7 cm. Her first child was born shortly after reaching 8 cm dilatation. The husband urged the nurse to call the physician. The nurse said she would decide when to call the physician. The infant was born a few minutes later and the mother had several lacerations. To compound the problems for the defense, the nurse inaccurately recorded that a physician delivered the baby since she had been instructed never to chart that she had delivered a baby. The jury determined that the nurse acted negligently and awarded damages to the woman.

Failure to call a physician in time can be considered negligence. A woman was in strong labor for seven hours with no documented progress (*Samii v Baystate Medical Center, Inc.,* 395 NE2d 455 [1979]). The woman started vomiting and had other signs of distress. At this point the nurse had difficulty hearing the fetal heartbeat. She did not call the physician until she was unable to hear the heartbeat. An emergency cesarean was performed at that time, but the baby died. The parents won the lawsuit.

In other cases, nurses and/or hospitals have been found liable when equipment failed (oxygen did not work during a resuscitation effort), was missing (no bulb syringe on delivery tray), or was used improperly (steam from a vaporizer too close to the infant caused burns). Many problems can be prevented if the nurse makes proper assessments, anticipates problems, calls for help when necessary, and ensures that equipment is available, in working order, and used properly.

Risk Management

Effective management of risks of liability includes recognizing the occurrence of incidents and promptly taking action to prevent recurrence. Many hospitals employ a risk manager, often an attorney, who examines incident reports and records of problems for trends and recommends changes in policy or procedure to reduce such occurrences. The risk manager may work with managers in high-risk areas, such as the emergency department, operating rooms, and critical care units, to plan programs of prevention. In the obstetrics area effectively reducing risks includes being aware of the woman's history, taking time to record findings on the physical examination, keeping good records, giving medications accurately and noting the woman's response, accurately interpreting fetal monitor tracings, recording descent of the presenting part as well as dilation, noting the date and time the physician was notified, recording teaching provided, and recording telephone calls and the advice given (Cohn 1984). The essence of risk management is anticipating problems and taking steps to prevent the problem from occurring.

Special Situations in Maternity Care

FETAL RESEARCH

Research with fetuses has been responsible for remarkable advances in the care and treatment of fetuses with problems. For example, treatment of Rh-sensitized infants and the evaluation of lung maturity by the lecithin/sphingomyelin ratio has been developed through such research (Committee on Research 1984). Federal regulations currently specify that experimentation is limited to meeting the health needs of an individual fetus. In nontherapeutic research there must be minimal risk to the fetus, and the knowledge must be important and not obtainable by other means (Elias & Annas 1983). Consent must be obtained from both parents, and an institutional review board must review the protocol.

The federal regulations also require that proposals involving fetal research and in vitro fertilization be reviewed by the National Ethics Advisory Board. Funding for the board expired in 1980 and, since no national review can be done, research has been severely restricted (Fletcher & Schulman 1985).

State laws may be more restrictive than the federal regulations. Some states have outlawed fetal research altogether while in other states therapeutic research may be permissible.

INTRAUTERINE FETAL SURGERY

Intrauterine fetal surgery, an example of therapeutic research, is a therapy for anatomic lesions that can be corrected surgically but are incompatible with life if not treated (Inturrisi et al 1985). Examples of such lesions are bilateral hydronephrosis due to obstruction, congenital diaphragmatic hernia, and obstructive hydrocephalus. The surgery involves opening the uterus during the second trimester (before viability), treating the fetus, and replacing it in the uterus. The risks to the fetus are substantial, and the mother is committed to cesarean deliveries for this and subsequent pregnancies (because the upper, active segment of the uterus is entered). The parents must be informed of the experimental nature of the treatment, the risks of the surgery, the commitment to cesarean delivery, and alternatives to the treatment. The parents must have the opportunity to ask questions and time to make a considered choice.

The question has been raised about the situation in which surgery is indicated and the mother refuses the procedure. Can she be forced to undergo the therapy? Currently the autonomy of the mother is the first consideration; she cannot be forced to submit to the surgery.

ABORTION

Since the 1973 Supreme Court decision in *Roe v Wade,* abortion has been legal in the United States. Abortion can be performed until the period of viability. After that time abortion is permissible only when the life or health of the mother is threatened. Before viability the rights of the mother are paramount; after viability the rights of the fetus take precedence. There are continuing efforts by individuals and states to limit or abolish abortion by prohibiting Medicaid funding of abortions and putting other restrictions on the procedure. These include restricting abortions to hospitals (which significantly increases the cost of the procedure) and requiring agencies to provide graphic details of the procedure, ostensibly to provide informed consent (Annas 1983). At present the decision for abortion is to be made by the woman and her physician. Care givers have the right to refuse to perform an abortion or to assist with the procedure if abortion is contrary to their moral and ethical beliefs.

ARTIFICIAL INSEMINATION

Artificial insemination (AI) is accomplished by depositing into a woman sperm obtained from the husband or a donor. The sperm can be deposited into the vagina, the cervical canal, or the uterus. Homologous insemination involves the husband's (or partner's) sperm (AIH); donor insemination (AID) involves a donor other than the husband (or partner). No states prohibit AIH. There is no question of adultery by the wife, and the child is legitimate. Legal problems may occur with AID, however. Since the child is a biologic child of the mother, legal concerns center around the donor. A donor must sign a form waiving all parental rights. The donor must also furnish accurate health information, particularly about genetic traits or diseases. The husband often also signs a form agreeing to the insemination. The husband must agree to assume parental responsibility for the child. Some men may legally adopt the child so there is no question of parental rights and responsibilities. Several states have legislation regarding paternity of the child conceived by AID.

SURROGATE CHILDBEARING

Surrogate childbearing is one example of "collaborative reproduction" (Robertson 1983). In this instance a woman agrees to bear a child for a couple who are unable to have a child of their own. The child is conceived by artificial insemination with sperm from the husband in the couple desiring the child and thus will be his biologic child. The biologic mother agrees to relinquish the child at birth, the wife of the father of the child agrees to adopt the child, and the biologic mother receives payment for the expenses associated with the pregnancy and birth and, usually, a lump sum payment of approximately $10,000 for her participation.

There are many arguments for and against surrogate childbearing. Those in favor of it recount the biologic

CONTEMPORARY DILEMMA

Whose Baby Is It?

Recently the issue of parenthood has been raised in surrogate contracts. Although more than 500 surrogate contracts have been fulfilled without problems, a few surrogate mothers have decided to keep their baby after birth. In these cases questions are raised regarding the rights of each parent. Biologically, the baby belongs to both the contractual father and the surrogate mother and it is the contract between them that stipulates the baby will be given to the father after birth.

The problems and concerns being raised are numerous:

- Should the practice of surrogate mothering be continued as an answer to childlessness for some couples?

- Should it be done for profit or should it be done out of compassion?

- Is the contract valid? Can it be rescinded, and for what reasons?

- If the baby is born with congenital problems, does it affect the contract?

- Is the concept of contracting for "production" of a child different from "baby selling" (treating the child as a commodity that may be sold)?

- Are government regulations regarding the surrogate contract needed to protect the "best interest" of the child?

mother's altruism in providing a couple who desperately want a child with the opportunity to be parents, the benefits and joys to the couple who receive the child, and the birth of a child who would otherwise not be born. They suggest that the problems and risks are no different from other instances of artificial insemination by donor (AID) and the emotional trauma of separating an infant from a birth mother for adoption.

Those who are against surrogate childbearing cite the possibility of the birth of a defective newborn that no one wants, a biologic mother who refuses to relinquish the newborn, the risks of a pregnancy to the biologic mother with no benefits, the appearance of buying a child (which is illegal in all states), and the identity problems when the child discovers she or he is adopted and wonders why he or she was relinquished by the birth mother. Others oppose surrogate childbearing on moral, ethical, and legal grounds and assert that questions of heritage and the legality of AID have not been resolved. In 1987 the case of Baby M received worldwide attention when the court ruled that the surrogate mother contract signed by Baby M's mother was valid and awarded sole custody of the baby to her father. The case is now to be considered by the New Jersey Supreme Court. The outcome has led to increased legislative activity in many states regarding regulation or even banning of surrogate motherhood.

IN VITRO FERTILIZATION AND EMBRYO TRANSFER

In vitro fertilization (IVF) and embryo transfer (ET) is a therapy offered to selected infertile couples. In this process ovulation is induced, one or more ova are retrieved by laparoscopy and fertilized with sperm from the husband or a donor, and the embryos are transferred to the wife when they reach the two- to six-cell stage. Often more than one embryo is transferred in order to enhance the probability of implantation. The success rate of the procedure is low; only 10 to 20 percent of the embryos implant in the uterus (Pace-Owens 1985). Legal issues associated with this procedure include questions of paternity if donor sperm is used, what to do with embryos that are not implanted, and what to do when a multiple pregnancy occurs.

SURROGATE EMBRYO TRANSFER

The procedure for surrogate embryo transfer (SET) consists of five steps (Annas 1984b):

1. The ovulation times of the donor and recipient are synchronized.

2. The donor is inseminated with sperm from the husband of the recipient.

3. The donor's uterus is washed out about five days after fertilization.

4. The embryo is recovered.

5. The embryo is transferred to the uterus of the recipient.

The procedure is subject to all the legal and ethical questions raised by surrogate childbearing and in vitro fertilization. The one difference from surrogate childbearing is that the development of a mother-child relationship is not an issue in SET.

Legal issues of IVF-ET, SET, and AID are similar in relation to determining who the legal parents are. Annas (1984a) recommends that current presumptions of the law be retained; that is, the birth mother is the legal mother, and the mother's husband is the legal father. When embryos are frozen for later use, either for implantation or research, legal protection becomes an issue. Annas recommends that embryos be frozen with the parent's consent for a designated period of time. If they are not used by that time or if both parents die, he suggests they should be destroyed. Others have suggested that such destruction is murder. Further deliberation must occur before such issues are resolved.

Freezing of embryos opens the possibility of sale of embryos. At present there is almost universal consensus against the sale of body parts. The case against the sale of human embryos is even stronger than that against the sale of body parts (Annas 1984a).

KEY CONCEPTS

Many nurses working with childbearing families are expert practitioners who are able to serve as role models for nurses who have not yet attained the same level of competence.

Contemporary childbirth is family centered, offers choices about delivery, and recognizes the needs of siblings and grandparents.

The self-care movement, which emerged in the late 1960s, emphasizes personal health goals, a holistic approach, and an emphasis on preventive care.

Nurses function in a variety of roles, including care giver, advocate, educator, researcher, change agent, and political activist.

Nurses are assuming a more collegial role in their dealings with physicians and other health care providers.

Nurses in maternity care may function in a variety of roles and settings.

In many ways childbirth has become big business.

A nurse must practice within the scope of practice or be open to the accusation of practicing medicine without a license.

The standard of care is that of a reasonably prudent nurse.

The right to privacy is protected by state constitutions, statutes, and common law.

Confidential communications exist between persons in a trusting relationship.

Informed consent—based on knowledge of a procedure and its benefits, risks, and alternatives—must be secured prior to providing treatment.

Documentation is an integral part of providing quality care.

Nursing negligence is omitting or committing something that a reasonable, prudent nurse would not omit or commit.

Risk management involves anticipating problems and taking steps to prevent them from occurring.

Fetal research is limited to meeting the health needs of an individual fetus.

Intrauterine fetal surgery is a therapy for anatomic lesions that can be corrected surgically and are incompatible with life if left untreated.

Abortion can be performed until the age of viability. There are continuing efforts to restrict or abolish abortion. Care givers have the right to refuse to perform an abortion or assist with the procedure.

Collaborative reproduction requires cooperation among health professionals, surrogate mother and adoptive mother, and fathers and donors of sperm.

REFERENCES

Abrums M: Health care for women. *J Obstet Gynecol Neonat Nurs* 1986;15(May/June):250.

American College of Nurse Midwives. *What Is a Nurse Midwife?* Washington DC, The College, 1979.

Annas GJ: Redefining parenthood and protecting embryos: Why we need new laws. *Hastings Cent Rep* 1984a;14:25.

Annas GJ: Roe VS Wade reaffirmed. *Hastings Cent Rep* 1983;13:21.

Annas GJ: Surrogate embryo transfer: The perils of parenting. *Hastings Cent Rep* 1984b;14:50.

Baer OJ: Protecting your patient's privacy. *Nurs Life* 1985;5(3):50.

Barnard KE: MCN keys to research: Blending the art and science of nursing. *Am J Mat Child Nurs* 1985;10(January/February):63.

Benner P: *From Novice to Expert.* Menlo Park, Calif, Addison-Wesley, 1984.

Boring NL: Health care ads—who pays? *US News & World Report,* February 17, 1986, p 73.

Chagnon L, **Easterwood** B: Managing the risks of obstetrical nursing. *Am J Mat Child Nurs* 1986;11(September/October):303.

Cohn SD: The nurse midwife: Malpractice and risk management. *J Nurse-Midwife* 1984;24:316.

Committee on Research: Fetal research. *Pediatr* 1984;74:440.

Curry MA, **Howe** CL: Nurses made a difference. *Am J Mat Child Nurs* 1985;10:(July/August)225.

Doctors are entering a brave new world of competition. *Business Week,* July 16, 1984, p 56.

Elias S, **Annas** GJ: Perspectives on fetal surgery. *Am J Obstet Gynecol* 1983;145:807

Flanagan JA: Childbirth in the eighties: What next? *J Nurse-Midwife* 1986;31(July/August):194.

Fletcher JC, **Schulman** JD: Fetal research: The state of the question. *Hastings Cent Rep* 1985;15:6.

Griffith H: Who will become the preferred providers? *Am J Nurs* 1985;85(May):538.

Hill L, **Smith** N: *Self Care Nursing.* Norwalk, Conn, Appleton-Century-Crofts, 1985.

Inturrisi M, **Perry** SE, **May** KA: Fetal surgery for congenital hydronephrosis. *J Obstet Gynecol Neonat Nurs* 1985;14:271.

Joint Commission on Accreditation of Hospitals: Medical Record Services. *Accreditation Manual for Hospitals.* Chicago, Joint Commission on Accreditation of Hospitals, 1985.

Lander L: *Defective Medicine: Risks, Anger and the Malpractice Crisis.* New York, Farrar, Straus, and Giroux, 1978.

The malpractice mess. *Newsweek,* February 17, 1986, p 74.

Mumford E: *Medical Sociology.* New York, Random House, 1983.

Naisbitt J: *Megatrends.* New York, Warner Books, 1982.

New insurers' consortium will cover nurse-midwives' practice. *Am J Nurs* 1986;86(September):1051.

Pace-Owens S: In vitro fertilization and embryo transfer. *J Obstet Gynecol Neonat Nurs* 1985;14(suppl):44s.

Rabinow J: Some legal precautions to keep in mind. *Nurs Life* 1983;3(6):28.

Robertson JA: Surrogate mothers: Not so novel after all. *Hastings Cent Rep* 1983;13:28.

Rooks JP: The context of nurse-midwifery in the 1980s: Our relationship with medicine, nursing, lay-midwives, consumers and health care economist. *J Nurse-Midwife* 1983;28(September/October):3.

Schraeder BD, **Fischer** DK: Using intuitive knowledge to make clinical decisions. *Am J Mat Child Nurs* 1986;11(May/June):161.

Sinquefield G: The medical malpractice insurance crisis: Implications for future practice. *J Nurse-Midwife* 1986;31(March/April):65.

Stickney J: Two cheers for HMOs. *Money,* May 1985, p 155.

Toffler A: *The Third Wave.* New York: Morrow, 1980.

Weitz R, **Sullivan** DA: Licensed lay midwifery in Arizona. *J Nurse-Midwife* 1984;29(January/February):21.

ADDITIONAL READINGS

Courtemanche JB: Powernomics: A concept every nurse should know! *Nurs Manage* 1986;17(July):39.

Creighton H: The nurse and artificial insemination. *Nurs Manage* 1985;16(May):18.

Curtin LL: Nursing in the year 2000: Learning from the future, editorial. *Nurs Manage* 1986;17(June):7.

Ellis JR, **Hartley** CL: 5 ways to prevent malpractice claims. *Nurs 87* 1987;17(1):97.

Elsea SB: Ethics in maternal-child nursing. *Am J Mat Child Nurs* 1985;10(September/October):303.

Graham P et al: Operationalizing a nursing philosophy. *J Nurs Admin* 1987;17(3):14.

Gustaitis R: *A Time to Be Born, A Time to Die: Conflicts and Ethics in an Intensive Care Nursery.* Reading, Mass, Addison-Wesley, 1986.

Hazle NR: Perceptions of role conflict between obstetric nurses and nurse-midwives. *J Nurse-Midwife* 1985;30 (May/June):166.

Hobson CJ, **Blaney** DR: Techniques that cut cost, not care. *Am J Nurs* 1987;87(February):185

Kendellan R: The medical malpractice insurance crisis: An overview of the issues. *J Nurse-Midwife* 1987;32(1):4.

Lyon J: *Playing God in the Nursery.* New York, WW Norton, 1985.

Mahowald MB, **Silver** J, **Ratcheson** RA: The ethical options in transplanting fetal tissue. *Hastings Cent Rep* 1987;17(1):9.

Mason DJ, **Talbott** SW: *Political Action Handbook for Nurses: Changing the Workplace, Government, Organizations and Community.* Menlo Park, Calif, Addison-Wesley, 1985.

Pagana KD: Let's stop calling ourselves "patient advocates." *Nurs 87* 1987;17(2):51.

Rhodes AM: Consent for medical treatment. *Am J Mat Child Nurs* 1987;12(March/April):133.

Thompson HO, **Thompson** JE: Toward a professional ethic. *J Nurse-Midwife* 1987;32(2):105.

Weiss SJ: The influence of discourse on collaboration among nurses, physicians, and consumers. *Res Nurs Health* 1985;8:49.

When I started out in practice by myself, I didn't fully appreciate that when I went single-handedly to deliver babies at home—one midwife in the midst of at least three generations of a family—that I would be, in many respects, at their mercy. The qualities of their lives and relationships crowded in on the relatively simple act of birth, making it rich with possibilities, some beneficial, some not. (A Midwife's Story)

Tools for Maternal-Newborn Nursing

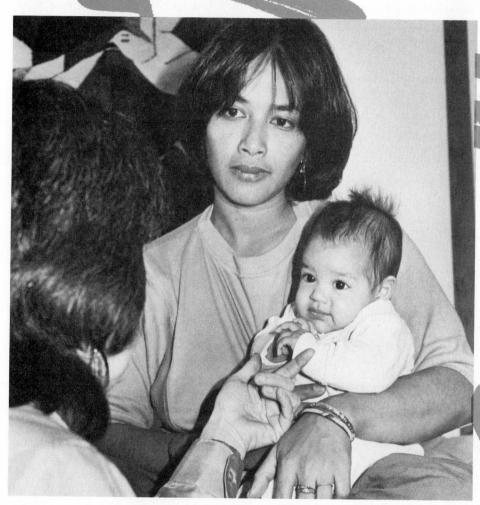

By engaging the baby's attention, this pediatric nurse allows the mother to concentrate more fully on their discussion.

Chapter Two

OBJECTIVES

- Discuss selected tools and the implications of each for maternity nursing practice.
- Describe the application of the nursing process in the maternity setting.
- Compare descriptive and inferential statistics.
- Relate the availability of statistical data to the formulation of further research questions.
- Discuss the application of nursing research in the maternity clinical setting.

Professional maternal-newborn nurses use a variety of "tools" in everyday practice that enable them to deliver high-quality nursing care. Some of the tools that are pertinent in the everyday practice of maternal-newborn nursing are:

- A comprehensive knowledge base that incorporates information from a variety of disciplines. With a firmly established knowledge base, the nurse is able to use the nursing process in planning and providing care to clients in a variety of settings.

- The nursing process, which provides a systematic way of organizing nursing care and becomes a framework for practice that moves the nurse through a process from assessment to evaluation of each client situation.

- Selected communication techniques. Knowledge about the client and care provided must be accurately documented to validate nursing care and also to share with other health team members. The problem-oriented medical record (POMR) and SOAP charting system are two methods to communicate health care data.

- Nursing standards, which guide the expectations and identify the standard of care that all should be following.

- Statistics. Descriptive statistics provide key factual data designed to answer a specific question. Inferential statistics explore possible causes and ramifications of the information obtained.

- Nursing research, which is essential to provide a scientific basis for nursing practice and to ensure the recognition of nursing as a respected profession. Whether this research is theoretical or conducted in

a clinical setting, it must be relevant to the practice of nursing.

This chapter presents selected tools of nursing practice and briefly discusses the use of each tool in the maternal-newborn nursing practice setting. The chapter is not designed to give a complete explanation of nursing tools but to highlight them and explore ways in which the maternal-newborn nurse may use them in providing high-quality care.

● Knowledge Base

The maternal-newborn nurse founds her practice on a comprehensive knowledge base that includes information regarding pregnancy, labor and delivery, postpartal period, and the newborn period. Information includes normal anatomical, physiological, and psychological processes; factors that place the woman at risk; and complications that may occur in the childbearing period. In addition to the maternal-newborn knowledge base, the maternity nurse uses information from other fields. Knowledge of family development is obtained from sociology and psychology. The sciences offer new ways of understanding, new theories, and a basis of theoretical knowledge. Anthropology provides insights into other cultural patterns, which increases understanding of the various women who come into the childbearing health care setting.

New technology is discovered and implemented at a rapid rate in our society; change is inevitable. Maternal-newborn nurses, and nurses in other fields, find it a challenge to keep their knowledge base current with this information explosion; therefore specialization has become prevalent. Specialization does not decrease the need to continue to acquire more knowledge, but it provides more of a focus for the learning process. Nurses in a specialty area find it a continuing challenge to update their knowledge and remain current. It is a lifelong learning process.

● Nursing Process

The nursing process, built on a comprehensive knowledge base, represents a logical approach to problem identification and resolution, and serves as the framework for nursing. Whether it consists of four or five steps (some authors combine the analysis/nursing diagnosis and planning phases), the nursing process is an analog of the problem-solving process used by nurses since Florence Nightingale.

Assessment

The maternal-newborn nurse gathers both subjective and objective data about the health status of the childbearing woman. Subjective information may be obtained from the woman and family members and includes their perception of the health impairment or problem and its management. Objective data are measurable and include physical assessment findings and laboratory test results.

Analysis and Nursing Diagnosis

The second step in the process is the analysis, assimilation, and clustering of assessment data into relevant categories from which *nursing diagnoses* are derived. Each nursing diagnosis describes a specific health problem, either actual or potential; its etiology; and the associated signs and symptoms. The formulation of a nursing diagnosis is the crucial step in the process, for the resulting plan of care is based on the problems as the nurse perceives them. In contrast to the medical diagnosis, which generally remains the same throughout the woman's health problem, the nursing diagnosis will reflect the changing *response* of the woman as her condition improves or worsens, and as she and her family adjust to those changes.

The term *nursing diagnosis* represents both a process and an outcome. The process is the analysis, assimilation, and clustering of data just described. It is a problem-solving technique. The outcome is a classification system of diagnostic labels (Carpenito 1983). The nursing diagnosis is a two-part statement that includes the health problem and related etiology (Gordon 1987). The North American Nursing Diagnosis Association (NANDA) has developed a list of acceptable nursing diagnoses.

Consider the following nursing diagnosis: Knowledge deficit related to inadequate knowledge of normal anatomic, physiologic, and psychologic changes in pregnancy. The health problem, knowledge deficit, is presented with specific knowledge deficit areas. Knowledge deficit is a client health problem that nurses clearly deal with, and it does not belong to the medical diagnosis realm.

Once established, nursing diagnoses serve to direct the nursing plan of care. Expected outcomes (goals) and priorities of care are identified. Nursing interventions necessary to achieve the specified goals are also identified. Nursing interventions are directed at altering or eliminating the etiological and/or contributing factors of the health problem, and the related signs and symptoms serve as a baseline for evaluation of the effectiveness of care.

Nursing diagnoses are incorporated in this text in various ways. In most chapters nursing diagnosis appears clearly as a part of the nursing process. The chapters devoted to high-risk situations present examples of nursing diagnoses that may apply to the specific problems being discussed. In addition, nursing diagnoses are emphasized in the nursing care plans, which focus on selected conditions or situations. These nursing diagnoses are used as the basis for organizing and directing nursing care.

Plan

Once the analysis is completed and nursing diagnoses are formulated, the nurse establishes outcome goals. The nurse identifies interventions that will help the client meet the established goals and develops outcome criteria that will signify that the goals have been met. Lastly the nurse prioritizes the care needed. The beginning nurse usually works through this process step by step, while the more experienced nurse is frequently able to develop an intricate plan of care covering all the steps simultaneously.

Implementation

In the fourth step of the nursing process, the identified plan of care and specific nursing interventions are implemented by the maternal-newborn nurse. The nurse uses many skills that are common to other areas of nursing, as well as many skills specific to the maternal-newborn setting. Common interventions include auscultation of fetal heart rate, Leopold maneuvers to determine fetal position in the uterus, measurement of the uterus to determine growth, sterile vaginal examinations to determine the woman's labor progress, and use of electronic monitors that provide continuous data regarding the fetal heart rate and uterine contractions.

Evaluation

The woman's progress or lack of progress toward the identified expected outcomes (goals) is evaluated by the woman and the nurse. These questions are asked: Have expected outcomes been met? Is reassessment needed? Are new problems present? Are changes in any part of the process necessary? Do new priorities need to be identified? Is revision of the plan of care required?

Evaluation is a logical end step, but it is also a continuous process throughout the whole nursing process. The nurse continually evaluates the assessments that have been made, the priorities of care, and the effectiveness of the nursing interventions as nursing care is delivered.

Application of the Nursing Process

The following brief example illustrates the application of the nursing process.

Sarah, a 16-year-old adolescent, comes to the school nurse's office and asks why she seems to be having trouble with her pregnancy. She states she doesn't have any energy and can't keep her weight down. She is in her sixth month of pregnancy and has gained 3 pounds. She exercises every day for one hour, smokes one pack of cigarettes a day, and has trouble sleeping because of the pressure of homework and a part-time job each evening.

The nurse applies the nursing process as follows:

Assessment: Subjective data—Sarah states "I have trouble with my pregnancy; I have no energy, have trouble keeping my weight down, and lots of trouble sleeping." Objective data—3-pound weight gain in six months of pregnancy (below recommended rate). Sarah appears underweight for her height, pale with dark circles under her eyes.

Analysis/nursing diagnosis: The objective and subjective data support problems with adequate nutrition and the statements regarding her weight suggest the need for information regarding nutritional needs during pregnancy. Sarah also needs to understand the need to obtain adequate rest and to clarify her perception of the role of exercise in pregnancy. The nurse ascertains that Sarah is going to the prenatal clinic on a fairly regular basis. The nurse decides the highest priority nursing diagnosis is knowledge deficit related to adequate nutritional needs during pregnancy. The nurse could have selected a nursing diagnosis directed toward the sleep disturbance or the potential for alterations in nutrition related to inadequate intake for pregnancy needs. But overall she decided that giving Sarah complete information about her pregnancy would address a number of problems.

Planning: The goals of care include: Client will be able to verbalize the nutritional requirements in pregnancy, will not lose any further weight, and will begin gaining at least 3 pounds per month.

Implementation: The nurse and Sarah plan sessions for the next few weeks during which there will be time for discussion and information to be shared. She gives Sarah some booklets designed for pregnant adolescents regarding nutritional and general care needs. The nurse obtains a current weight, and together they create a graph to record her weight each week. Sarah's interest in cartooning makes this a fun and creative project. The nurse asks her to keep a food intake record for three days and to drop it off at the end of the week.

Evaluation: As the relationship builds and they work together, the success of the interventions will be measured by Sarah's ability to verbalize nutritional needs and the objective data provided by her weight each week. The food intake record provides specific data to work with to encourage a diet to meet pregnancy needs.

The preceding example indicates the application of the nursing process. The nursing process can be used to provide logical, systematic care in any situation encountered in maternity nursing practice.

● Communication

The problem-oriented medical record (POMR) system allows for the systematic documentation and retrieval of information about the client's care and progress. Although originally intended for use with medical diagnoses, POMR can be adapted for documentation of nursing care using nursing diagnoses. POMR is a system of charting observations and interventions using the SOAP format. The acronym SOAP stands for the four components of each charting entry: subjective data, objective data, analysis (sometimes called assessment), and plan. The subjective and objective data come from the nursing assessment (the first step in the nursing process) and are recorded under the appropriate problem number (each nursing diagnosis is listed numerically on a problem sheet kept on the chart). The analysis entry represents the nurse's conclusions about the client's progress based on the data collected. Finally, the plan of care is continued or changed in accordance with the data analysis.

The importance of the POMR system for nursing is that the SOAP format, when used correctly, provides readily accessible data and ongoing evaluation of the effects of nursing care. The response to treatment can be evaluated regularly and as frequently as the client's condition dictates, and the plan for nursing care can be altered as necessary.

The POMR system and SOAP format for documenting information can be applied in the example just mentioned as follows:

After assessment of Sarah's situation, the nurse would analyze the data and determine a problem list that would include:

Inadequate weight gain

Insufficient information regarding nutritional needs of pregnancy

Inadequate rest

Presence of risk factors—age, inadequate weight gain, smokes one pack of cigarettes a day

A SOAP entry regarding the problem of inadequate weight gain would appear as follows:

S: Sarah states she is just not hungry and if she cuts down on exercise she feels like she has no energy.

O: Three-day food intake reveals diet is below RDA in calories, calcium, iron, and folic acid. One pound weight gain this week.

A: Although Sarah does not feel hungry, she has been trying to improve the quality and quantity of foods each day. She is willing to continue the food intake record and is incorporating suggestions and ideas from counselor and nutrition booklets. One pound weight gain is a positive sign even though diet is still inadequate in RDA requirements. Sarah has not been willing to cut down on exercise to date.

P: Supplement information she is gaining on nutrition and support her efforts to improve her diet. Work with her in interpreting and evaluating her food intake records. Continue to offer support and praise for gaining weight. Continue one-on-one conferences to share information and provide support.

Provide additional booklets on nutrition for Sarah. Use booklets specific for adolescents.

Have Sarah weigh herself and help her develop a weight graph to record and follow weights over the next few weeks.

Encourage Sarah to modify her exercise program. Perhaps cut her exercise by five minutes each session, and substitute some low-impact movements for some of the high-impact movements.

The nurse has used the SOAP format to record assessment of subjective and objective data and analysis of the present situation, and to formulate a plan that identifies interventions to address the problem of inadequate weight gain. At each visit the nurse may record new information using the same format. Other identified problems may be SOAP charted at the same time.

● **Nursing Standards**

In the midst of a rapidly changing health care system and widely divergent approaches to basic nursing education, nursing standards provide direction and information for the practicing nurse. Nursing standards identify basic expectations and functions of a particular role and therefore provide a framework for accountability in nursing practice. In addition they provide a basis for identifying quality in particular health care settings. The Nurses' Association of the American College of Obstetricians and Gynecologists (NAACOG) has been involved in the development of comprehensive obstetric, gynecological, and neonatal standards since 1974. These standards have played an integral part in providing direction for the development of high-quality maternity services in the United States. Because the health care setting may vary from one region to another, the standards are used as a basis for developing individualized policies and protocols. An example of the use of nursing standards follows.

See Appendix E for a complete listing of the NAACOG Standards for Obstetric, Gynecologic, and Neonatal Nursing.

Application of Nursing Standards

NAACOG NURSING STANDARD: NURSING CARE

○ *STANDARD* Comprehensive obstetric, gynecologic, and neonatal (OGN) nursing care shall be provided to the patient and her family and shall utilize all components of the nursing process, including assessment, nursing diagnosis, planning, implementation, and evaluation; it shall reflect informed consent and respect for the rights of the patient and her family.

○ *INTERPRETATION* The nurse has the responsibility for collecting pertinent data and assessing the patient's needs in order to determine the nursing intervention necessary to assist the patient and her family. The care plan should take into consideration psychosocial as well as physical aspects of the patient's history and should include active involvement of the patient and her family.

The OGN nurse should support the patient's and family members' desires to participate in the nursing process as appropriate. In addition, the patient and her family should be supported throughout the nursing process by assessing the potential for individual or family crisis and evaluating their resources for coping, by use of supportive services, and by family interaction.

The OGN nurse should be familiar with the type of patient records required and should share the responsibility for accurate and complete record keeping, maintaining appropriate confidentiality, to provide for continuity and coordination of nursing care, medical treatment, and patient progress. The documentation of nursing care given should reflect the achievement or nonachievement of predetermined goals. Records should be retained for the appropriate interval of time as governed by law and local regulations (NAACOG 1981).

○ *APPLICATION* Ms Gayle works in the mother-baby unit in a local hospital and has been participating on a committee to revise the chart forms. In reviewing the standards, the committee found the forms reflected the standards in using and documenting the nursing process and client care goals. The one area not clearly reflected involved documentation of informed consent and client/family wishes for the birth experience. A place was added to the Kardex, and each nurse was instructed to ask and record specific client/family wishes.

● **Statistics**

Evaluation of the health care system relies on *statistics,* the collection and analysis of pertinent numerical data.

Health-related statistics provide an objective basis for projecting client needs, allocating resources, and analyzing new data for evaluation of effectiveness of treatment.

There are two major types of statistics—descriptive and inferential. Descriptive statistics describe or summarize a set of data: they report the facts—what *is*—in a concise and easily retrievable way (an example is the birth rate in the United States). How the data are compiled and presented is determined by the question being asked. Although no conclusion about *why* some phenomenon has occurred may be drawn from these "vital" statistics, certain trends can be identified, high-risk "target groups" delineated, and research questions generated that will provoke further investigation using more sophisticated statistical testing.

Inferential statistics allow the investigator to draw conclusions or inferences about what is happening between two or more variables in a population and to establish or refute causal relationships between them. For example, descriptive statistics show that the infant mortality rate in the United States has declined over the past decade. Exactly *why* that trend has occurred cannot be answered by simply looking at these data, however. More data and inferential statistics, using smaller samples of the population of pregnant women, are needed to determine whether this finding is due to earlier prenatal care, improved maternal nutrition, use of electronic fetal monitoring during labor, and/or any number of factors potentially associated with maternal-fetal survival.

Descriptive statistics are the starting point that allows the formulation of research questions. Inferential statistics answer specific questions and generate theories to explain relationships between variables. Theory applied in nursing practice can help make changes in the specific variables that may be causing or contributing to certain health problems. The following section deals primarily with descriptive statistics, although inferential considerations are addressed through the use of possible research questions that may assist in identifying relevant variables.

Descriptive Statistics

BIRTH RATE

Birth rate refers to the number of live births per 1000 population. A related statistic, the *fertility rate*, is the number of births per 1000 women aged 15–44 years in a given population.

Table 2–1 compares live births, birth rates, and fertility rates by race for 1970–1984. After a peak of the birth rate for all races of 25.0 in 1955, there has been a decline until the rate remained constant in 1975 and 1976—14.6 live births per 1000 population. This is the lowest recorded birth rate in the history of the United States. Beginning in 1975–1976 there was a small yearly increase through 1982 and then another decrease was recorded in 1983–1984. Provisional data for 1985 indicates a 2 percent increase in the birth rate in 1985 (US Dept of Health and Human Services 1986).

Comparison of live birth rate between white and black populations in the United States reveals a decrease until 1975, when it was 13.6 for white women and 20.7 for black women. There was an increase through 1980, but

Table 2–1 Live Births, Birth Rates, and Fertility Rates, by Race of Child: United States, 1970–1984*

	NUMBER	BIRTH RATE[†]		All other		FERTILITY RATE[†]		All other	
Year	All races	All races	White	Total	Black	All races	White	Total	Black
REGISTERED BIRTHS									
1984	3,669,141	15.5	14.5	21.2	20.8	65.4	62.2	82.5	81.4
1983	3,638,933	15.5	14.6	21.3	20.9	65.8	62.4	83.2	81.7
1982	3,680,537	15.9	14.9	21.9	21.4	67.3	63.9	85.5	85.1
1981	3,629,238	15.8	14.8	22.0	21.6	67.4	63.9	86.4	85.4
1980[†]	3,612,258	15.9	14.9	22.5	22.1	68.4	64.7	88.6	88.1
1975[†]	3,144,198	14.6	13.6	21.0	20.7	66.0	62.5	87.7	87.9
1970[§]	3,731,386	18.4	17.4	25.1	25.3	87.9	84.1	113.0	115.4

[†]*Birth rates per 1000 population in specified group. Fertility rates per 1000 women aged 15 to 44 years in specified group. Population enumerated as of April 1 for census years and estimated as of July 1 for all other years. Beginning 1970 excludes births to nonresidents of the United States.*
[†]*Based on 100% of births in selected states and on a 50% sample of births in all other states.*
[§]*Based on a 50% sample of births.*

*Modified from National Center for Health Statistics: Advance report of final natality statistics, 1984. Monthly Vital Statistics Report. Vol. 35. No. 4, Supp. DHHS Pub. No. (PHS) 86–1120. Public Health Service, Hyattsville, Md. July 18, 1986.

Table 2–2 Live Births and Birth Rates, Canada, 1980–1985*

Year	Live births†	Birth rate†
1985	375,727	14.8
1984	377,031	15.0
1980	370,709	15.5

†Live births = per 1000 population
‡Live birth rate = per 1000 population

*Modified from Vital Statistics. Vol. I. Births and deaths. 1985. Canada Health Division Vital Statistics and Disease Registry. Cat. 84–204. Minister of Supply and Services. November 1986. Table 1, p. 2.

since then there has been a slight decrease each year in both groups.

Live births and birth rate for Canada are presented in Table 2–2. The birth rate remains lower than in the United States.

○ *INFERENTIAL CONSIDERATIONS* The "postwar baby boom" which followed World War II and resulted in a marked increase in the birth rate, has been in evidence for several years. The impact of this larger number of babies had implications for the number of maternity care facilities needed in the middle to late 1940s; for public school sys-

tems as the children entered and progressed through school; and again for maternity care as the postwar babies reached childbearing age.

Additional inferences about birth rates may be identified by posing some of the following research questions:

● Is there an association with changing societal values?

● Is the difference in birth rate between various age groups reflective of education? Does it represent availability of contraceptive information?

● Since women are averaging 1.8 children apiece and the replacement rate is 2.1/couple, what are the future implications of the declining rate?

AGE OF MOTHER

In the United States in 1984 the highest birth rate (108.3) for the first child was in women 25 to 29 years of age, followed by a birth rate of 107.3 for women 20 to 24 years of age. The next highest rate was for 18- to 19-year-olds (78.3) and then for 30- to 34-year-olds (66.5) (Table 2–3).

A decrease in birth rates has occurred in the 15–19, 20–24, and 25–29 age spans (Figure 2–1). The rates for women 15 to 19 were the lowest since 1950, and the rate for women 20 to 24 was the lowest on record.

Table 2–3 Birth Rates by Age of Mother, Live-Birth Order, and Race of Child: United States, 1984*

Live-birth order and race of child	15–44 years†	10–14 years	15–19 years Total	15–17 years	18–19 years	20–24 years	25–29 years	30–34 years	35–39 years	40–44 years	45–49 years
ALL RACES											
Total	65.4	1.2	50.9	31.1	78.3	107.3	108.3	66.5	22.8	3.9	0.2
First child	27.4	1.1	39.4	27.1	56.4	52.4	38.0	16.2	4.1	0.5	0.0
Second child	21.7	0.0	9.6	3.7	17.8	37.4	40.4	23.8	6.3	0.6	0.0
WHITE											
Total	62.2	0.6	42.5	23.9	68.1	101.4	107.7	66.1	21.7	3.5	0.2
First child	26.4	0.6	33.9	21.4	51.1	51.7	39.2	16.6	4.0	0.5	0.0
Second child	21.1	0.0	7.4	2.4	14.4	35.6	41.1	24.3	6.1	0.6	0.0
ALL OTHER											
Total	82.5	3.7	89.0	63.3	124.8	136.4	111.5	68.5	29.2	6.0	0.4
First child	32.8	3.6	64.2	52.5	80.5	55.6	31.8	13.9	4.4	0.6	0.0
Second child	24.7	0.1	19.5	9.6	33.4	46.0	36.9	21.3	7.2	0.9	0.0
BLACK											
Total	81.4	4.3	95.7	69.7	132.0	137.9	103.2	59.5	24.8	5.1	0.2
First child	32.2	4.2	68.7	57.7	84.2	54.5	25.5	9.9	3.1	0.5	0.0
Second child	24.1	0.1	21.2	10.7	35.8	46.9	34.5	17.2	5.4	0.7	0.0

*Based on 100% of births in selected states and on a 50% sample of births in all states. Rates are live births per 1000 women in specified age and racial groups. Live-birth order refers to number of children born alive to mother. Modified from National Center for Health Statistics: Advance report of final natality statistics, 1984. Monthly Vital Statistics Report. Vol 35, No. 4, Supp. DHHS Pub. No. (PHS) 86–1120. Public Health Service, Hyattsville, Md. July 18, 1986.
†Rates computed by relating total births, regardless of age of mother, to women aged 15–44 years.

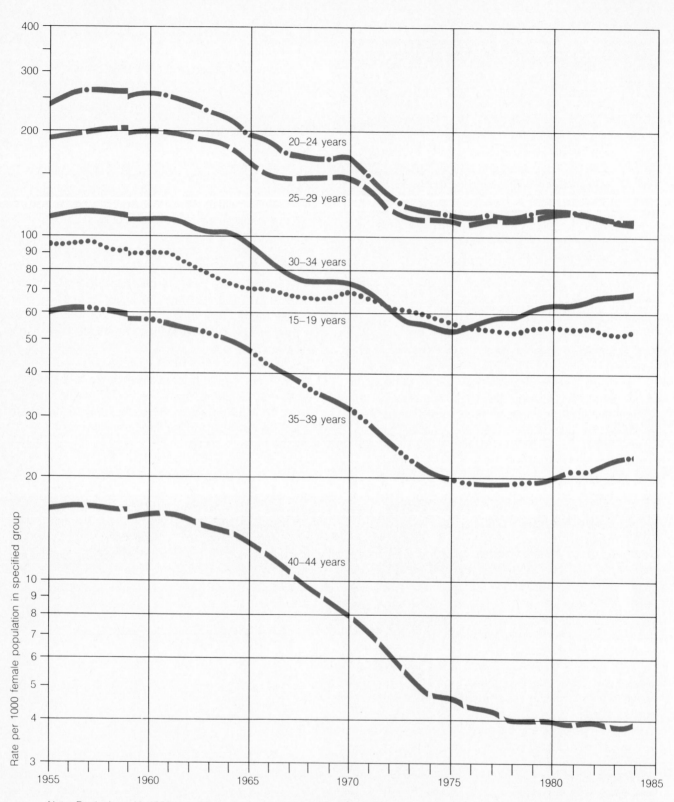

Figure 2–1 Birth rates by age of mother: United States, 1955–1984

Note: Beginning with 1959, trend lines are based on registered live births; trend lines for 1955–59 are based on live births adjusted for underregistration.

National Center for Health Statistics: Advance report of final natality statistics, 1984. Monthly Vital Statistics Report. Vol. 35, No. 4, Supp. DHHS Pub. No. (PHS) 86-1120. Public Health Service, Hyattsville, Md. July 18, 1986.

An increase in birth rate is observed in women in their thirties and forties, and this increase has been consistent since the early 1970s. Another interesting trend is that the percentage of women 30 to 34 who have yet to have their first child has increased from 14 in 1974 to 25 in 1984. It is not possible to predict what percentage of these women will remain permanently childless.

○ *INFERENTIAL CONSIDERATIONS* The identification of variables that affect the birth rate of different age groups and races may be addressed by posing the following research questions:

● Is there an association with changing societal values? With changing roles of women? With changing national economic conditions and financial status?

● Is there a correlation between years of education? Availability of contraceptive information for different age groups and races?

WEIGHT AT BIRTH

In 1984 the median birth weight of infants was 3420 grams (7 pounds, 9 ounces) for white babies and 3180 grams (7 pounds) for black babies. Both of these weights have shown a slight increase in the past five years. The median weight for all babies was 3360 grams (7 pounds, 7 ounces). The newborn posing the most concern to health professionals is the low-birth-weight (less than 2500 grams) infant. In the United States in 1984 low-birth-weight infants comprised 6.7 percent of all births. This rate is a slight decrease from the 1976 rate of 6.9 percent. However, as in previous years, a substantial racial difference persists, with 5.6 percent for white births, 12.4 percent for black births, and 11.1 percent for all other races. Teenagers and women between 40 and 49 years of age are likely to bear low-birth-weight infants. In 1984 the rate of low-birth-weight infants to teenagers under 15 years of age was more than 2.5 times the number born to women aged 25 to 29 and 30 to 34 years (Table 2–4).

Canadian statistics for 1980, presented in Table 2–5, reveal that the highest percentage of low-birth-weight infants occurs in women in the under 20 and 40 to 44 age ranges.

○ *INFERENTIAL CONSIDERATIONS* The review of the descriptive statistical data reveals discrepancies between differing age ranges and between races. To gain further data the following research questions may be addressed:

● Are there factors that affect different age and racial groups?

● Nutritional status before and during pregnancy?

● Educational level?

● Length of time between pregnancies?

● Availability of prenatal care?

● Desire and ability to seek prenatal care?

● Physical health of the mother?

● Presence of environmental factors such as high pollution levels or high altitude?

INFANT MORTALITY

The *infant death rate* is the number of deaths of infants under one year of age per 1000 live births in a given population. *Neonatal mortality* is the number of deaths of infants less than 28 days of age per 1000 live births. *Perinatal mortality* encompasses both neonatal deaths and fetal deaths per 1000 live births. (Fetal death is death in utero at 20 weeks or more gestation.) For statistical purposes the period from 28 days to 11 months of age is designated the *postneonatal period*. Table 2–6 delineates infant mortality by age.

The 1984 rate of 10.8 was the lowest rate ever recorded. The 1984 rate reflects a 4 percent decline from the 1983 rate of 11.2 percent. The infant mortality rate in blacks was approximately two times the rate for whites. This difference has persisted for years. The overall decline in infant mortality has slowed and in 1986 showed a slight rise.

Infant mortality for 1979 and 1980 in Canada is presented in Table 2–7. Comparison of Canadian and U.S. infant mortality reveals a lower rate for Canada.

The four leading causes of infant death in the U.S. are causes originating in the perinatal period: congenital anomalies, sudden infant death syndrome, respiratory distress syndrome, and disorders relating to preterm and low-birth-weight infants.

○ *INFERENTIAL CONSIDERATIONS* Some researchers currently predict that infant mortality may rise due to worsening economic situations, the increasing rate of poverty, cuts in federal programs affecting women and children, and decreased access to health care (Mundinger 1986).

Additional factors may be identified by considering the following research questions:

● Does infant mortality correlate with a specific maternal age?

● Is it associated with the time in pregnancy that the woman seeks prenatal care? Number of prenatal visits?

● Is there a difference between racial groups? If so, is it associated with educational level? Availability of prenatal care?

Table 2–4 Number and Percent Low Birth Weight and Live Births by Birth Weight, by Age of Mother, and Race of Child: United States, 1984*

Age of mother and race of child	LOW BIRTH WEIGHT Percent	Total	BIRTH WEIGHT† Less than 500 grams	500–999 grams	1000–1499 grams	1500–1999 grams	2000–2499 grams
ALL RACES							
All ages..........	6.7	3,669,141	4,444	16,794	22,261	47,059	155,547
Under 15 years.....	13.6	9,965	28	138	159	264	761
15–19 years.......	9.3	469,682	734	3,055	4,315	8,541	27,172
15 years.........	11.4	24,142	61	248	311	561	1,563
16 years.........	10.9	53,178	104	410	617	1,122	3,536
17 years.........	9.8	89,424	146	610	913	1,711	5,339
18 years.........	9.3	130,159	190	828	1,154	2,367	7,548
19 years.........	8.4	172,779	233	959	1,320	2,780	9,186
20–24 years.......	6.9	1,141,578	1,358	5,087	6,789	14,658	50,552
25–29 years.......	5.9	1,165,711	1,248	4,717	5,984	12,937	43,338
30–34 years.......	5.9	658,496	776	2,786	3,541	7,517	24,142
35–49 years.......	6.7	195,755	260	875	1,223	2,665	8,157
40–44 years.......	8.3	26,846	36	134	236	460	1,354
45–49 years........	9.8	1,108	4	2	14	17	71
WHITE							
All ages..........	5.6	2,923,502	2,541	10,093	14,281	31,168	105,034
Under 15 years.....	10.8	3,959	7	32	61	99	229
15–19 years.......	7.6	320,953	347	1,572	2,394	4,771	15,419
15 years.........	9.2	12,869	26	99	149	253	660
16 years.........	9.2	32,529	36	220	320	586	1,819
17 years.........	8.1	59,618	76	300	521	947	2,950
18 years.........	7.7	90,470	95	430	663	1,374	4,406
19 years.........	6.8	125,467	114	523	741	1,611	5,584
20–24 years.......	5.7	898,919	720	2,991	4,331	9,481	33,599
25–29 years.......	5.0	969,061	771	2,999	4,070	9,166	31,132
30–34 years.......	5.1	549,595	501	1,849	2,448	5,447	17,768
35–39 years.......	5.9	159,246	163	554	812	1,872	5,901
40–44 years.......	7.4	20,974	30	94	156	322	938
45–49 years........	9.0	795	2	2	9	10	48
ALL OTHER							
All ages..........	11.1	745,639	1,903	6,701	7,980	15,891	50,513
Under 15 years.....	15.4	6,006	21	106	98	165	532
15–19 years.......	13.0	148,729	387	1,483	1,921	3,770	11,753
15 years.........	13.8	11,273	35	149	162	308	903
16 years.........	13.6	20,649	68	190	297	536	1,717
17 years.........	13.2	29,806	70	310	392	764	2,389
18 years.........	12.9	39,689	95	398	491	993	3,142
19 years.........	12.5	47,312	119	436	579	1,169	3,602
20–24 years.......	11.3	242,659	638	2,096	2,458	5,177	16,953
25–29 years.......	10.2	196,650	477	1,718	1,914	3,771	12,206
30–34 years.......	9.9	108,901	275	937	1,093	2,070	6,374
35–39 years.......	10.6	36,509	97	321	411	793	2,256

†Equivalents of the gram weight in terms of pounds and ounces are as follows:
Under 500 g = 1 lb, 1 oz or less
500–999 g = 1 lb, 2 oz–2 lb, 3 oz
1000–1499 g = 2 lb, 4 oz–3 lb, 4 oz
1500–1999 g = 3 lb, 5 oz–4 lb, 6 oz
2000–2499 g = 4 lb, 7 oz–5 lb, 8 oz

*Based on 100% of births in selected states and on a 50% sample of births in all other states. Modified from National Center for Health Statistics: Advance report of final natality statistics, 1984. Monthly Vital Statistics Report. Vol. 35, No. 4, Supp. DHHS Pub. No. (PHS) 86–1120. Public Health Service, Hyattsville, Md. July 18, 1986.

Table 2–5 Live Births by Birth Weight, Sex, and Age of Mother: Canada (Excluding Newfoundland), 1985*

Age of mother		% 2500 g or less†
Under 20	Males	6.7
	Females	7.6
20–24	Males	5.4
	Females	6.6
25–29	Males	4.9
	Females	5.9
30–34	Males	4.9
	Females	6.0
35–39	Males	5.8
	Females	6.5
40–44	Males	6.4
	Females	8.0

†Based on stated birth weights

*Modified from Vital Statistics. Vol. I. Births and deaths. 1985. Canada Health Division Vital Statistics and Disease Registry. Cat. 84–204. Minister of Supply and Services. November 1986. Table 13, p 20–21.

Table 2–6 Infant Mortality Rates by Age: United States, 1950, 1960, 1965, and 1970–1985*

Year	Under 1 year	Under 28 days	28 days–11 months
1985 provisional†	10.6	...	...
1984 provisional†	10.8	7.0	2.8
1980 provisional†	12.6	8.4	4.1
1975	16.1	11.6	4.5
1970	20.0	15.1	4.9
1965	24.7	17.7	7.0
1960	26.0	18.7	7.3
1950	29.2	20.5	8.7

*For 1980, 1984, and 1985 based on a 10% sample of deaths; for all other years based on final data. Rates per 1000 live births.

†National Center for Health Statistics: Annual summary of births, marriages, divorces, and deaths, United States, 1985. Monthly Vital Statistics Report. Vol. 34, No. 13. DHHS Pub. No. (PHS) 86–1120. Public Health Service, Hyattsville, Md. September 19, 1986.
‡National Center for Health Statistics: Advance report of final mortality statistics, 1984. Monthly Vital Statistics Report. Vol. 35, No. 6 Supp. (2). DHHS Pub. No. (PHS) 86–1120. Public Health Service, Hyattsville, Md. September 26, 1986.

MATERNAL MORTALITY

Maternal mortality rate is the number of deaths from any cause during the pregnancy cycle (including the 42-day postpartal period) per 100,000 live births.

The maternal death rate in the United States has decreased steadily in the last 25 years (Table 2–8). The 1984 estimated maternal mortality of 7.8 is almost two-thirds less than the 1970 rate of 21.5. In 1984, 285 women died of causes listed as complications of pregnancy, childbirth,

Table 2–7 Infant Mortality (Total Infant Death Rate per 1000 Live Births): Canada, 1980, 1985*

Year	Under 1 year (infant)	Under 28 days (neonatal)	28 days–11 months (postneonatal)
1985	8.0	5.2	2.7
1980	10.4	6.7	3.8

*Modified from Vital Statistics. Vol. I. Births and deaths. 1985. Canada Health Division Vital Statistics and Disease Registry. Cat. 84–204. Minister of Supply and Services. November 1986. Table 22, p 54.

Table 2–8 Maternal Mortality Rate per 100,000 Live Births: United States, 1950–1984*

Year	Rate
1984	7.8
1983	8.0
1980	9.2
1975	12.8
1970	21.5
1965	31.6
1960	37.1
1950	83.3

*National Center for Health Statistics: Advance report of final mortality statistics, 1984. Monthly Vital Statistics Report. Vol. 35, No. 6, Supp. (2). DHHS Pub. No. (PHS) 86–1120. Public Health Service, Hyattsville, Md. September 26, 1986.

and puerperium. Black women were 3.6 times more likely than white women to die from these complications.

○ *INFERENTIAL CONSIDERATIONS* Factors influencing the decrease in maternal mortality include development of obstetrics and gynecology as a recognized medical specialty; the increased use of hospitals and specialized health care personnel for antepartal, intrapartal, and postpartal care of the maternity client; the establishment of high-risk centers for mother and infant care; the prevention and control of infection with antibiotics and improved techniques; the availability of blood and blood products for transfusions; lowered rates of anesthesia-related deaths; and the application of research for the prevention of maternal deaths (Danforth & Scott 1986).

Additional data may be identified by asking:

● Is there a correlation with age? Availability of health care? Economic status? Access to health care?

● Is there adequate federal funding to reach women in need?

Implications for Nursing

The successful implementation of the nursing process depends on the appropriate application of statistics. Nurses can make use of statistics in a number of ways. For example, statistical data may be used to:

- Determine populations at risk
- Assess the relationship between specific factors
- Help establish a data base for different client populations
- Determine the levels of care needed by particular client populations
- Evaluate the success of specific nursing interventions
- Determine priorities in case loads
- Estimate staffing and equipment needs of hospital units and clinics

Descriptive statistics may also be used to help decide whether a problem actually exists. For example, a nurse working in a large maternity center that has 6,000 births per year (500 births per month) notes that 2 babies with diaphragmatic hernia have been born in the last year. She wonders whether this number reflects the projected incidence and whether the rate is higher than normal.

A method of obtaining an answer has been illustrated by Layde and Rubin (1982). The rate of the defect would be determined by dividing the number of cases by the number of births.

$$\frac{2 \text{ (number of cases)}}{6,000 \text{ (number of births)}} = 0.0003 \text{ (rate)}$$

By calculating the hospital's rate, the nurse can demonstrate that although the number of cases has seemed excessive, it is within the "normal" rate of incidence, which is 1:3000 live births (rate 0.0003).

If the rate had been higher than normal, then additional questions would need to be asked. Is there a correlation with a particular maternal age? Diet? Illness during pregnancy? Place of residence? Treatment during pregnancy? Exposure to toxic materials?

Statistical information is available through many sources, including professional literature; state and city health departments; vital statistics sections of private, county, state, and federal agencies; special programs or agencies (family-planning agencies); demographic profiles of specific geographic areas. Nurses who make use of this information will find themselves well prepared to protect the health needs of maternity clients and their families.

● Nursing Research

Research is a vital step toward establishing a science of nursing. It is also a means to improve client care and to establish nursing as a true profession with its own unique knowledge base. Many nursing leaders have voiced the same sentiments as Wilson (1985):

> If nursing is to build a scientific body of knowledge and if nursing practice is to be shaped by research findings rather than tradition, intuition, or habit then the investigative skills of all nurses, regardless of their educational level, must be as integral to their repertoire as communication skills and sterile technique.

Once research is accomplished it must be translated into the clinical practice setting, that is, it must be made useful to nurses taking care of clients.

Success in this effort ultimately depends on the willingness and ability of practitioners to transfer research-generated knowledge into practical nursing interventions. How is this done? By taking completed research studies of relevance to the specific health problem or need, and trying out methods that worked for the investigator. Of course this is a gross oversimplification, but the process of applying research findings to improve client care should be made a relatively simple exercise in problem solving; otherwise the gap between research and action will remain wide.

Application of Research

The best way to begin the application of research to daily practice is to read research studies relevant to the practice setting. The following two brief examples specific to maternal-child nursing help illustrate how the findings of a research study might be applied to improve client care.

EXAMPLE 1

The benefits of breast-feeding have been known for quite some time, and increasing numbers of women are choosing this method of infant feeding. Without support and encouragement, however, many women breast-feed for only a short period of time.

One research team (Chapman et al 1985) investigated the concerns of breast-feeding mothers for four months after birth. They found that the concerns focused on breast condition, infant nutrition, and postpartum changes, and their findings are consistent with other studies. Women who successfully continued to breast-feed had a good information base and continued support and encouragement.

This finding implies that there is a need for continued care and pertinent usable information for successful breast-feeding. Furthermore the results of this study also support the need for nurses to teach in the birth setting and to establish a supportive relationship with the new mother. It stimulates questions about the effects of decreased postpartal stays on breast-feeding success. If the mother's postpartum stay is only a few hours, how can nurses provide the information and encouragement needed to begin successful breast-feeding? The implications for nursing practice may include the development of a postpartum home visitation program, a telephone follow-up program for the first few months, a telephone hot line that is available 24 hours a day, or a breast-feeding clinic where mothers can drop in for help or come to scheduled programs and support groups.

The study also opens up other questions. What will the long-term costs of short postpartum stay really be? Can a postpartum stay be too brief in terms of the mother obtaining sufficient information to care successfully for herself and her infant? If more and more information is packed into the few hours after delivery when the mother is in a dependent mode and her task is to regain her sense of integrity and self, how effective will the teaching be? These are a few of the questions to consider.

EXAMPLE 2

Over half of pregnant women experience nausea and vomiting during pregnancy, and the causes of this have been attributed to various physiological and psychological factors. DiIorio (1985) investigated the incidence and characteristics of nausea and vomiting in pregnant teenagers, the methods the teenagers used to relieve nausea and vomiting, and the effectiveness of the methods. The results of the study identified some areas of particular interest. There seemed to be a difference between the number of white and black teens who experienced nausea (95 percent white and 42 percent black). Girls who wanted the pregnancy were more likely to experience nausea, and, although the teens tried a number of relief measures, the most common measure was to lie down during an episode of nausea and vomiting. Earlier research has suggested that the nausea and vomiting of pregnancy may be associated with orthostatic hypotension, which may be an explanation for the relief measure the teens choose.

There are numerous implications for nursing from this particular study. Although the author suggests that more study is needed, the practicing nurse could begin to suggest to clients that lying down during an episode of nausea may be helpful. It provides another intervention that may also be helpful. As a matter of curiosity a woman's blood pressure may be recorded and compared with blood pressure during episodes of nausea. If lying down helps, then perhaps other information regarding prevention of orthostatic hypotension may be useful (rising slowly to a sitting position, then sitting on the side of the bed for a few minutes before standing, and so on).

These examples are meant to illustrate how a practitioner may begin to think about using nursing research to improve maternal care. There is, of course, much time and work between an idea and its implementation. Change must be regarded in terms of the costs and benefits before old ways are discarded for new.

● Application of Tools for Nursing Practice

Each of the tools—knowledge, nursing process, communication, statistics, nursing standards, and nursing research—can exist separately, but in practice they overlap and build upon each other. For example, the maternity nurse needs a knowledge base to use the nursing process, yet as one proceeds through the nursing process and evaluates the client response, one's knowledge base is affected.

Each of these tools for practice may be implemented in a variety of ways as the maternity nurse provides care for the childbearing family. An example of just one possible situation is presented in the following case study.

Two birthing unit nurses express concerns to each other about the seemingly high numbers of adolescents who have been delivering in their unit.

At the next staff meeting they voice their concerns and raise questions about whether the number of teenage mothers seen in their unit is higher than normal. After discussion the nurses decide that they need to formulate a plan to gather more information. Each nurse volunteers to pursue a particular aspect of a plan of action. Their plan includes contacting the local public health department for local and national statistics on this age group; looking at the availability of health care for adolescents in their community; investigating the particular health problems of the pregnant teenager and risks to their infants; checking the availability of prenatal education groups for adolescents; finding out whether their community has school health programs and what the program content is; looking at national statistics regarding when adolescents seek prenatal care; talking with community nurse-midwives, physicians, and prenatal clinic personnel to see if the national statistics apply to their community; collecting information about current legislative issues affecting adolescent health care; seeking further information about the needs of adolescents during pregnancy and delivery by doing a library search; and looking for continuing education programs dealing with the pregnant adolescent client.

At subsequent staff meetings each nurse shares information, and other areas are investigated as the need is identified. How they evaluate the data and apply them will depend on the requirements of their maternity unit and the unique needs of their community.

Possible outcomes may include developing a research study; volunteering in local adolescent clinics; developing and teaching prenatal classes for adolescents; volunteering to teach in community school health programs; organizing a continuing education program on the adolescent mother for community hospitals; and forming a network within their professional nursing organizations to stay informed about legislative issues pertaining to adolescents.

As the case study demonstrates, the application of tools for nursing practice helps define a problem, guides the collection of data, and provides a framework for intervention.

KEY CONCEPTS

Today's contemporary nurse uses a variety of tools in everyday practice.

A comprehensive nursing knowledge base forms the basis for nursing activities.

The nursing process, composed of assessment, analysis and nursing diagnosis, plan, implementation, and evaluation, provides a systematic method of approaching nursing practice.

Communication of nursing problems and care provided is an important aspect of nursing practice. Two methods to communicate client care data are POMR and SOAP.

Nursing standards provide information and guidelines for nurses in their own practice, in developing policies and protocols in health care settings, in directing the development of quality care, and in promoting the accountability of nursing practice.

Descriptive statistics describe or summarize a set of data. Inferential statistics allow the investigator to draw conclusions about what is happening between two or more variables in a population and to establish or refute causal relationships between them.

Nursing research is vital to add to the nursing knowledge base, expand clinical practice, and expand nursing theory.

REFERENCES

Carpenito LJ: *Nursing Diagnosis: Application to Clinical Practice.* New York, Lippincott, 1983.

Chapman JJ, Macey MJ, Keegan M, et al: Concerns of breast-feeding mothers from birth to 4 months. *Nurs Res* 1985;34(November/December):374.

Danforth DN and Scott JR: *Obstetrics and Gynecology,* ed 5. Philadelphia, Harper & Row, 1986.

DiIorio C: First trimester nausea in pregnant teenagers: Incidence, characteristics, interventions. *Nurs Res* 1985;34(November/December):372.

Gordon M: *Nursing Diagnosis: Process and Application.* New York: McGraw-Hill, 1987.

Kim MJ, McFarland GK, McLane AM: *Classification of Nursing Diagnoses: Proceedings of the Fifth National Conference.* St. Louis, Mosby, 1984.

Layde PM, Rubin GL: Counting diseases and deaths meaningfully. *Contemp OB/GYN* 1982;20(December):87.

Mundinger MO: Health service funding cuts and the declining health of the poor. *N Engl J Med* 1986;313(July):44. Public Health Service implementation plans for attaining the objectives for the nation. *Pub Health Rep* 1983;98 (September/October):suppl.

NAACOG: *Standards for Obstetric, Gynecologic and Neonatal Nursing,* ed 2. Washington, DC, Nurses Association of the American College of Obstetricians and Gynecologists, 1981.

North American Nursing Diagnosis Association: *Classification of Nursing Diagnoses: Proceedings of the Seventh Conference.* St. Louis, Mosby, 1987.

US Department of Health and Human Services: *NCHS Monthly Vital Statistics Report,* vol 35 (6) September 15, 1986.

Wilson HS: *Research in Nursing.* Menlo Park, Calif, Addison-Wesley, 1985.

ADDITIONAL READINGS

Baird D: Changing problems and priorities in obstetrics. *Br J Obstet Gynaecol* 1985;92:115.

Connolly K: Poverty and human development in the Third World. *Arch Dis Child* 1985;60:880.

Fortney JA, Susanti I, Gadally S, et al: Reproductive mortality in two developing countries. *Am J Pub Health* 1986;76(February):134.

Ingram DD, Makuc D, Kleinman JC: National and state trends in use of prenatal care, 1970–1983. *Am J Pub Health* 1986;76(April):415.

Moore TR, Origel W, Key TC, Resnik R: The perinatal and economic impact of prenatal care in a low-socioeconomic population. *Am J Obstet Gynecol* 1986;154:29.

NAACOG: Electronic fetal monitoring: Nursing practice competencies and educational guidelines. Washington, DC, NAACOG, 1986.

NAACOG: Nurse providers of neonatal care: Guidelines for educational development and practice. Washington, DC, NAACOG, nd.

Simmons JB: Reproductive mortality in developing countries. *AM J Pub Health* 1986;76(February):131.

Strobino DM, **Chase** GA, **Kim** YJ, et al: The impact of the Mississippi improved child health project on prenatal care and low birthweight. *Am J Pub Health* 1986;76(March):274.

UNICEF: *The State of the World's Children 1986.* Oxford, Oxford University Press, 1986.

Statistics have never been so real for me as when I used them to prepare my speech to prospective legislators on "Meet the Candidates" night. I wanted them to acknowledge prevention of preterm birth as an important area that deserved funding. When I told them how many preterm babies were born in our state—and how much it cost taxpayers—the candidates listened and asked how they could help.

The Contemporary Family: Trends, Issues, and Concerns

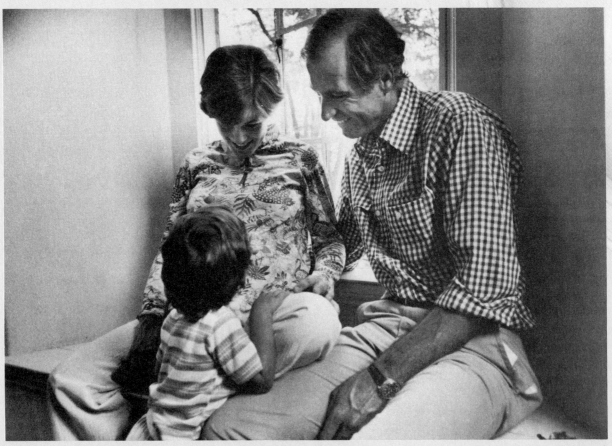

An American family in the last weeks of pregnancy talks about the arrival of a sibling.

Part Two

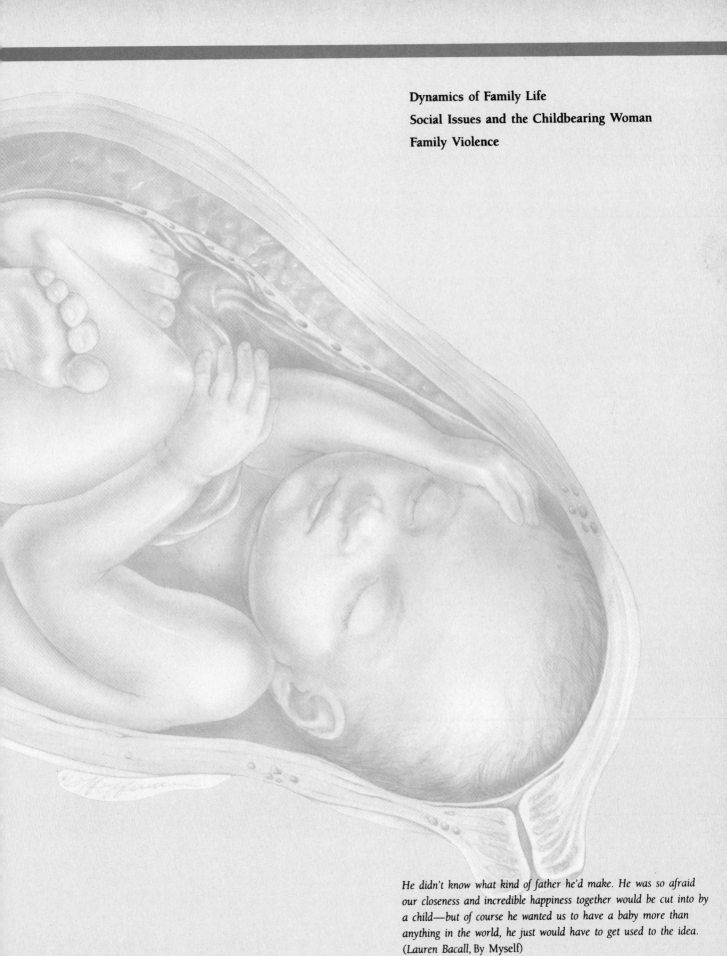

Dynamics of Family Life

Social Issues and the Childbearing Woman

Family Violence

He didn't know what kind of father he'd make. He was so afraid our closeness and incredible happiness together would be cut into by a child—but of course he wanted us to have a baby more than anything in the world, he just would have to get used to the idea. (Lauren Bacall, By Myself)

Dynamics of Family Life

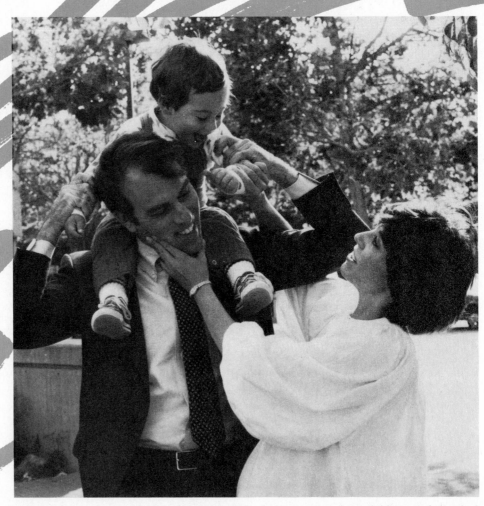

This professional couple chose to wait to have children until they had established their careers.

Chapter Three

OBJECTIVES

● **Discuss the status of the family in today's society.**

● **Describe major variations in family structure and function.**

● **Compare different approaches of conceptualizing family life as it relates to the childbearing family.**

● **Develop an overview of instruments for assessing family functioning.**

● **Discuss the implications for nursing practice of treating the family as a unit of care.**

Family health, long the domain of public health professionals, is becoming a primary concern of all health care professionals. Consumer pressures, professional initiatives, and research on the family-illness relationship have increased the emphasis on family-centered health care. As people become better educated, they want to know more not only about themselves but also about the purpose and consequences of health care services for themselves and their families. Changing value systems and escalating health care costs have created considerable consumer demand for alternative services and personnel. Growing awareness of the interdependence of stress and illness, as well as of physical fitness and health, has heightened interest in individual and family self-care.

Family-centered care is also widely endorsed by health care professionals, who recognize the family as the primary source of physical and emotional support for its members and the primary influence on its children's development. Research on childbearing families has shown that family involvement during pregnancy and birth can enhance the delivery experience, attachment between parents and infants, and parenting skills.

Many hospitals have responded to these forces by modifying the hospital environment and procedures. For example, many hospitals provide alternative birth rooms for couples who wish to be in a more homelike setting. Nurse-midwives on the staffs of many hospitals offer an alternative to physician-managed birth. Single-unit mother-baby care and early discharge for mothers are common.

Acknowledging that effective health care of individuals requires the involvement of their support network has necessitated an expanded role for the nurse. Including the family in health teaching, explanations of medical and surgical interventions, and coordination of health care activities has become the responsibility of the nurse. In addition, the family can provide important information about the client that affects the nurse's plan of care.

The ability to work effectively with a variety of families requires both understanding of how families function and willingness to consider the difficult issues inherent in achieving family-centered care. This chapter provides an introduction to varying family forms and functions and acquaints the reader with major conceptualizations of family life and instruments used to assess family functioning. It also discusses issues pertinent to considering the family (rather than the individual) as a unit of care. Because families are extremely diverse and complex entities, prescriptions for the "best" way to approach, interact, and intervene with them simply do not exist; nor would such prescriptions be appropriate. This chapter focuses on understanding families and the major issues the nurse is likely to encounter in working with them.

● **The Contemporary Family**

What is "the typical family?" In the 1950s and early 1960s, that phrase evoked an image of a happily married couple with their two or three children. As portrayed on television, this family was white and middle class, with the man as breadwinner and the woman as housewife. The children were fairly well behaved and well adjusted. The teenagers danced and drank soda pop at parties. Divorce was infrequent because it was socially unacceptable. An aura of stability, contentment, and complacency surrounded the family.

The political and social upheaval of the late 1960s and the 1970s drastically altered the image of the typical family. Civil rights demonstrations, antiwar protests, and the women's movement revealed that many people were not content but extremely dissatisfied and angry. Long-held values, traditions, and assumptions about social, racial, political, and gender matters became subjects for debate. Self-examination and personal development became important and accepted activities among the youth of that time, resulting in the label the "Me Generation."

Families responded to the political and social movements of the 1960s and 1970s in different ways. Some families remained virtually untouched by all that was going on around them; others responded by rethinking the values and assumptions underlying their views of family life. They questioned long-standing beliefs about what it meant to be a parent, a spouse, or a child and explored new forms of family grouping and being a family.

People have learned valuable lessons from this chaotic time. A great difference clearly exists between real families and the "typical" family created from statistical information (or wishful thinking). Real families are dynamic and unique. Many families do indeed consist of two adults and two or three children. However, the couple may not necessarily be married, or white, or middle class, or even of opposite sexes. A woman may be the breadwinner; a man, the "househusband." It is not unlikely that one or both adults have been or will be divorced. The children may be siblings by marriage (that is, stepsiblings), not by blood ties. The children may also be far less childlike than their counterparts of 20 years ago, due to their early and continued exposure (via television) to world events, technology, and varied life-styles. This phenomenon is sometimes referred to as "accelerated" childhood.

Contemporary family life is complex, with little room for complacency. What is typical about the typical family is that its members are faced with the difficult but usually gratifying task of coexisting with one another and their environment. In order to do this, each family must maintain itself as a functioning unit in the face of an everchanging situation. Hill (1974) captured the essence of the demands most families confront when he noted:

> The family is perhaps more subject to disturbance than any other organization because of its rapidly changing age composition and frequently changing plurality patterns. Its curious age and sex composition make it an inefficient work group, a poor planning committee, an unwieldy play group, and a group of uncertain congeniality. Its leadership is shared by two relatively inexperienced amateurs for most of their incumbency, new to the role of spouse and parent. They must work with a succession of disciples having few skills and lacking in judgment under conditions which never seem to remain stable long enough to bring about a settled organization (p 374).

A logical place to begin an exploration of this complex, changing entity called the family is with a definition. Not surprisingly, there is no single, generally accepted definition of *family*. Some authors focus on family structure or the configuration of actors and roles comprising the family. Others emphasize the activities or functions in which family members are engaged. The recent increase in nontraditional family forms has fostered a trend toward defining families in terms of the members' emotional ties to one another. Friedman (1986), for example, defined the family as two or more individuals who are emotionally involved and live in geographical proximity. None of these ways of

defining the family is inherently right or wrong, better or worse. Each does, however, direct one's attention to a different aspect of family life (composition, activities, emotional bonds). Moreover, the definitions have practical as well as academic implications. For example, hospital visiting policies based on a structural definition emphasizing kinship ties would be more restrictive than policies grounded in a definition emphasizing emotional bonds.

Childbearing is considered a major family event. The maternity nurse must consider the woman's definition of the family and acknowledge that her family is most often her primary support during the childbearing period. This family environment has a direct influence on the woman's emotional and physical health and is most likely the environment in which the baby will be nurtured and raised. The nurse must, therefore, have some understanding of common variations in family structure and function in our contemporary pluralistic society. The concepts of family structure and function are discussed in more detail in the following section.

Family Structure

Many trends and changes in attitudes have contributed to the increase in the kinds of family configurations. These configurations represent an array of family structures (Figure 3–1). Aldous (1978) defines *family structure* as the

> elements in the family system that are its positions. Positions specific to the family are husband-father, wife-mother, son-brother, and daughter-sister. These positions are filled by individuals who in their interaction with other family members create the structure that makes the family a system (p 26).

Thus a family's structure comprises its positional membership (relation of each family member to the others) and the kinds of patterned interactions arising among members in their respective positions. Family interactions are complex because of the various interpersonal relationships within a family. Much of the debate over what constitutes a family relates to the absence of one or more of the positions noted by Aldous or with the addition of other positions such as a live-in grandparent or friend. For example, when a graduate student studied lesbian couples who were rearing one or both partners' children (Levy 1984), even deciding on labels for the positions within the family was difficult since there was no generally accepted term to refer to the nonbiological relationships involved.

One of the primary reasons for the growing number of different family forms is our truly pluralistic, highly differentiated, and specialized society. A society such as ours needs to realize that any of the currently existing family forms may be suited to certain individuals in their search for fulfillment or to make ends meet. According to Hy-

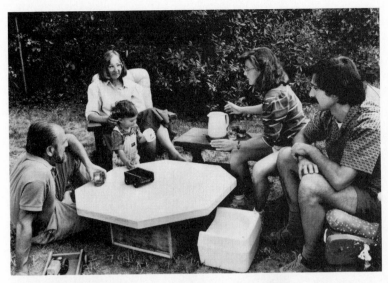

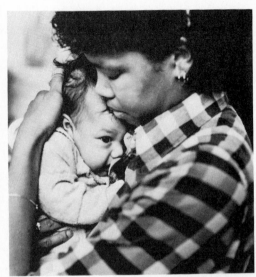

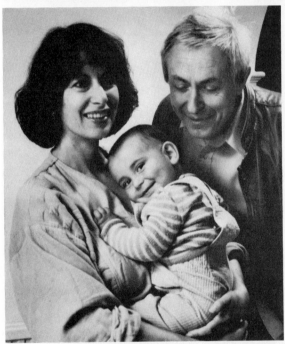

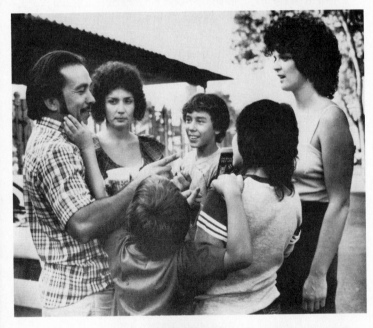

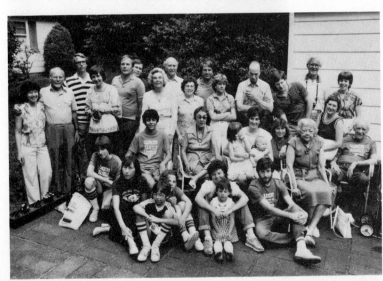

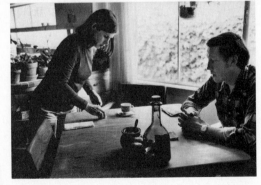

Figure 3–1 Different kinds of family configurations: (clockwise from upper left) a three-generation family, a single-parent family, a nuclear family with four children, a nuclear dyad, a kin network, and a nuclear family with one child

movich (1980) and Friedman (1986) most families belong to one of the following types of family configurations:

Single adult. According to Friedman's definition, the unmarried adult living alone is not considered to be a family configuration because the proximity, interaction, and support that are part of family life are not present. The person living alone must perform functions typically ascribed to the family, however, such as finding suitable housing and income and organizing relationships with the extended family and community.

A variation of the single-adult family configuration that the maternal-newborn nurse may encounter is the unmarried-parent family, usually consisting of a mother and a child. These parents either do not desire marriage at all or do not desire it in the near future. With society's increasingly liberal attitudes toward sexuality, a large number of unmarried women are choosing to keep a child rather than giving it up for adoption. In addition, an increasing number of single adults are adopting children. This family configuration is the same as that of the single-parent family, discussed later, with the important exception that the latter involves a disrupted family, in which one of the parents is no longer living in the immediate household.

Nuclear dyad. Frequently referred to as the *beginning family,* the nuclear dyad consists of a husband and wife living in a single-family residence. One or both partners are employed outside the home, and there are either no children or, in the case of an older couple, no children at home.

Single parent. One-parent families are becoming far more prevalent as the rate of divorce and separation is beginning to stabilize at a relatively high rate. One adult is left alone (by separation, divorce, or death) to raise minor children in a separate household with no other adults. If no other source of family income exists, or if the adult prefers, he or she may seek outside employment, adding even more responsibilities to family life. Many single parents eventually remarry, creating a need for additional role changes for both the former and the new family units.

Nuclear family. The traditional family structure in our society is the nuclear family. It includes husband, wife, and all minor children living together in a single household. Dual employment may or may not be a component of this family. In this chapter the nuclear family is generally the unit referred to, although many of the concepts discussed can be applied to other family types. Lamb (1980) found that nuclear families were more effective and reliable socializing

situations than single-parent families, but only when the nuclear families' marital relationships and overall emotional environments were harmonious.

Three-generation family. In the three-generation structure, one or more dependent grandparents live in a household with either a single-parent family or a nuclear family. The parents have authority over the household and care for the grandparents. Caring for grandparents usually falls to the oldest grown child or the female child of a family. The family can benefit from the grandparents' wisdom and experience, and the grandmother's role may also include responsibility for assisting with child care. This arrangement frees the mother to seek employment and is a feature of many Asian families.

Kin network (or extended family). The extended family includes two or more nuclear or unmarried households or any of the previously described configurations living in proximity, exchanging goods, and looking to each other for interaction and support. Although the parents have authority within their single households, the other adults are often consulted for advice, support, and authority in intrafamily affairs. A newly formed nuclear family may in fact be part of a kin network if relatives by blood or marriage are nearby and are part of the family's social group. For some families, the trend for mothers to return to work has revived the need to depend on relatives living in separate households to care for children while parents are working. Over 30 percent of child care in the United States is provided by relatives (Fantini & Rossi 1980). Many families are rediscovering the advantages of a well-maintained kinship system.

Reconstituted (blended, stepparent) families. Recent years have seen the nuclear family rocked by an increasing number of marital separations and divorces, which have often resulted in a variation of the nuclear family known as the reconstituted family (Fantini & Rossi 1980). This trend has been accompanied by a high rate of remarriage. Reconstituted or blended families are established through remarriage, raise children from previous marriages and/or from the current marriage, and in many instances create larger kinship systems for the child. According to McCubbin and Dahl (1985), the most common issues facing reconstituted families include winning acceptance, integrating the stepparent into an established family, and resolving the mixed allegiance that the biologic parent has toward the new mate and existing children.

In addition to the more common forms outlined above, the nurse may encounter clients who are members of other types of family structures. Hymovich (1980) described communal, common-law, and homosexual (gay) forms, all characterized by comparatively atypical configurations of positions and patterned relationships. Jane Howard's book *Families* (1978) provides an excellent indepth account of the composition and internal dynamics of a wide variety of family forms. Based on interviews and participant observation with a wide array of families, Howard concluded, "What families are doing, in flamboyant and dumbfounding ways, is changing their size and their shape and their purpose" (p 13). While it is impossible to identify and describe all the new sizes and shapes in which families now come, it is important to recognize the extent to which such variation exists and to be open to family structures that differ radically from one's own.

Family Function

The concept of family function focuses on the family as a task performance group. By accomplishing certain goals, the family contributes to the survival of the wider social system of which it is a part, the family unit as a whole, and the individual members of that unit. In a broader sense, *function* refers to the consequences that family's interrelated motives and subsequent behavior have for the family as a unit (Ritzer 1983). While there is some variation among authors regarding specific family functions, the following are often cited as important goals that families must achieve to continue functioning (Aldous 1978, Duvall 1977, Friedman 1986):

1. *Care and rearing of children.* Although childrearing functions have become less important in some families as a result of population control and individual desire not to have children, procreation remains a vital family function. Many young couples bear children and rear them in the traditions and with the values of their parent cultures.

2. *Socialization and social placement, including transmission of cultural values or rituals from one generation to another.* Primary socialization, which is frequently shared with outside institutions (such as schools), is directed toward making family members productive members of society as well as conferring social status. As children are told about and participate in cultural activities, traditions are passed from generation to generation. Children learn much of their behavior, including the values of right and wrong, by imitating parents or significant others. The desired outcome is "an adult whose personality characteristics are compatible with the demands and expectations of the society of which he is a member" (Kenkel 1977).

3. *Provision for physiologic needs.* The family meets its members' basic physical needs by providing sufficient food, shelter, clothing, comfort, and health care. The family has the additional responsibilities of allocating its economic resources appropriately and promoting the safety of its members.

4. *Affective function (personality maintenance).* The family provides for the psychologic needs of the family members according to the requirements of the individual or the unit.

5. *Family coping.* The family is continually confronted with internal and external demands and expectations that it is supposed to fulfill. To ensure family survival, stability, and growth, the family must use effective problem-solving mechanisms to cope with environmental requirements.

Given a particular configuration of members and a set of general tasks or goals that must be accomplished if the family is to survive, families develop rules and roles that characterize their day-to-day functioning. This means that much of family life has a taken-for-granted quality about it. Over time and through countless interactions, family members negotiate their ongoing roles and operating rules. Describing this process, Miller and Janosik (1980) note that a "normative system develops out of family rules and roles, becoming in effect a network of duties and expectations that support family functioning. Through the normative system, agreement concerning the obligations and rights of family members is sustained" (p 137).

A *role* is a cluster of interpersonal behaviors, attitudes, and activities associated with an individual in a certain situation or position. The behaviors tend to be learned through interactions with parents and siblings. *Attitudes* are the expectations of the society in which the child is raised; they affect and can be modified by the individuals' behaviors. Role activities are governed by expectations and behavior patterns of friends, relatives, and others outside the individual. Role behaviors, attitudes, and activities are learned to a large extent through the process of socialization.

Each family must define its role in the community and the roles of its individual members within the family unit. These roles are learned through interaction and imitation. Children learn the roles of their parents while learning their own roles and form their self-concepts on the basis of how well they execute their own roles. The roles that children assume affect their psychosocial development into adulthood.

Once the roles of family members are developed, family processes usually continue in a predictable pattern. When interruptions occur in the expected personal roles, family processes will also be interrupted. In most cases, one person will assume the other's role. For example, when the wage earner is disabled for a period, the spouse may need to find a job to replace the lost income, and the children may have to add more household duties and responsibilities to their roles.

Theoretical Frameworks for Understanding the Family

By defining and interrelating concepts, theoretical frameworks provide a tool for understanding and analyzing families. Nye and Berardo (1981) presented numerous different frameworks for viewing family life, including the structural, functional, interactional, psychoanalytic, anthropological, and developmental frameworks. Although varied, the purpose of these frameworks is essentially the same: each provides the reader with a lens for viewing the family. Depending on which lens is selected, the reader sees a somewhat different entity. Just as certain definitions of family focus attention on composition of the family, and others focus on function, theoretical frameworks shape our understanding of family life.

Overview of Frameworks

Three frameworks have been especially popular in nursing's study of the family: the interactional framework, the systems framework, and the developmental framework. The latter has been especially influential in family nursing. The interactional framework looks at family members' subjective views of their situation, emphasizing internal family dynamics. In contrast, the systems view of family is directed toward the relationship between the family and the larger social system. It is also concerned with how families maintain stability within an everchanging environment. The developmental framework emphasizes changing family structures and functions across the various stages of the family life cycle. Following a brief introduction to the interactionist and systems frameworks, the remainder of this section focuses on a more detailed presentation of the developmental framework.

Interactional Framework

In the interactional framework, the family is defined as a "unity of interacting personalities" (Burgess 1926). This framework centers on understanding interaction within the family by discovering how individual members define their situation (internal dynamics). Interactionists concentrate on subjective meaning as indicated by the three basic premises on which the framework is grounded:

1. Human beings act toward things on the basis of the meaning these things have for them.

2. The meaning of such things is derived from or arises out of the social interaction one has with others.

3. Meanings are modified through an interpretive process used by the person in dealing with the things he/she encounters (Blumer 1969).

The concepts of self, interaction, and role are central to the framework. The self is viewed as a constantly changing process that arises from interaction with others. Roles are seen as emergent rather than static entities. Interactionists direct their attention to understanding how individuals define their roles and the implications of these definitions for how they enact them.

Knafl (1985) used an interactional perspective to study how families responded to a child's routine hospitalization. Consistent with the interactional orientation, one aspect of the study was to discover how families defined the child's hospitalization and their parenting role within the hospital setting. The data revealed wide variations in parents' views of the hospitalization with some describing it as a "normal," expectable part of childhood, and others depicting it as a full-scale family crisis. Moreover, parents held quite differing views of what their parenting role should be in the hospital. Some preferred to delegate all caretaking and decision making to the professional staff, while others actively negotiated with staff to remain involved in caretaking and decision making.

The interactional framework is an appropriate lens for viewing families from the family's point of view. One can use data on these subjective views to identify and conceptualize common processes that family members use to define and manage various family life situations. It is helpful in isolating specific potential sources of difficulties as family members relate to one another and their community.

Systems Framework

The systems framework emphasizes the concepts of structure, function, boundary maintenance, and change. Aldous (1978, p 26) identified four fundamental characteristics of the family as a social system.

1. The positions occupied by family members are interdependent.

2. The family maintains boundaries and therein constitutes an identifiable unit.

3. The family performs certain tasks both for the larger social system and for family members.

4. The family as a unit is capable of change.

As noted before, family structure is defined by the patterned interactions that develop over time among individuals occupying the various positions in the family. The positions (such as wife-mother and husband-father) that comprise the family are viewed as interdependent, although the degree of interdependence may vary both across families and within a single family over time. For example, children typically become less dependent on their parents as they grow older, while parents may become increasingly dependent on their children.

Regarding the concept of boundaries, Hill (1974) conceptualized the family as a semiclosed system, maintaining links to other social systems and exercising control over the nature and frequency of those links. The family's ability to maintain control over its boundaries is linked to the previously described family functions. For example, if a family is unable to control a certain member's behavior, it may have to open its boundaries to law enforcement officials whether it wants to or not.

Regarding the family's ability to change, Aldous (1978) maintains that the family both reacts to and initiates change. In systems terminology, these two processes are referred to as *positive* and *negative* feedback respectively. Following a systems perspective, change is conceptualized in terms of goal attainment and information exchange. Families exchange information and receive feedback from their environment. Such feedback is processed by family members who interpret it in terms of the family's goals and tasks. Depending on the "fit" between the feedback and the intended goal, the family may respond by altering either its behaviors or its goals. In a negative feedback situation, the family takes a reactive stance and alters its behavior in response to outside input. In a positive feedback situation, the family takes a proactive stance and initiates change in response to an anticipated situation. For example, a couple changes their usual division of labor after their first child is born when they realize their former way of dividing household chores is no longer suitable. The change occurs only after a series of disruptive arguments in which each partner vehemently argues a different point of view. Such a change is reactive since it follows the birth of the baby and is made in the context of threatened family stability due to increased conflict between husband and wife. In a proactive situation, a couple anticipates that the birth of a baby will require a change in their established division of labor, and therefore they negotiate and try out several different arrangements before the baby is born.

The systems perspective is ideally suited to exploring family goal orientations, boundary maintenance, patterns of communication, and exchanges between the family and other social systems. It provides one with a framework for understanding these aspects of family life.

Developmental Framework

The developmental framework approach focuses on an analysis of the family as a small group progressing and changing as it goes through the life cycle from its beginning stages to its termination by the death of one or both spouses or by divorce if no children are involved. The developmental pattern is not rigid. For example, some families may decide not to have children, thus skipping those stages that involve childbearing and childrearing; in other families, adoption of older children may result in omission of particular steps in the developmental process.

The following is a summary of the principles governing family development (Duvall 1977):

1. Development is orderly, sequential, and predictable. Life in the traditional family usually follows a regular pattern from marriage to bearing children, raising children, and having them establish their own homes and eventually to death. Crises may alter this pattern, but in most instances family development continues.

2. Developmental stage time periods vary within certain stages according to the individual family's needs. Family members determine the duration of developmental stages. Generally a family moves through the early stages in a few years, with each successive stage becoming longer.

3. Socially prescribed expectations order the major events of development. Although marriage is certainly not a biological prerequisite for bearing and rearing children, it is expected in society that a couple will have a courtship period followed by a period of adjustment to marriage before bringing children into the world.

4. Family development proceeds in a specific direction from a known beginning to an expected end, with the anticipated endpoint of each developmental stage serving as family goals. Attainment of short-term and long-term family goals brings a sense of fulfillment and success to members.

5. When certain developmental tasks are successfully accomplished, further tasks evolve. For example, following the birth of a child, the couple prepares for the task of rearing the child.

6. Only the family can complete the developmental tasks it faces. The family relies on social interaction and internal resources and knowledge to direct the achievement of its goals.

Duvall (1977) has identified stages in the family life cycle. The two major phases in the family life cycle are the *expanding family,* from the beginning of the marriage until the children leave home, and the *contracting family,* from the launching of the children to the death of one or both spouses. These two major stages are further divided into the following eight stages, which are based on plurality patterns, the age of the eldest child, school placement of the eldest child, and the function and status of the family before children are born and after they leave home:

1. Married couples/beginning families (without children)

2. Childbearing families (eldest child 30 months)

3. Families with preschool children (eldest child 2½ to 6 years)

4. Families with schoolchildren (eldest child 6 to 13 years)

5. Families with teenagers (eldest child 13 to 20 years)

6. Families launching young adults (first child gone from home to the last child leaving home)

7. Middle-aged parent families ("empty nest" to retirement)

8. Aging family members (retirement to the death of both spouses)

The first two stages, married couples/beginning families and childbearing families, are discussed in the next sections (see Figure 3–2).

MARRIED COUPLE STAGE

The first stage of Duvall's developmental family life cycle is the married couple/beginning family stage, which starts when the couple enters marriage and ends with the birth or adoption of the first child. Prior to marriage each

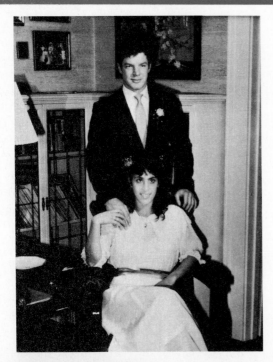

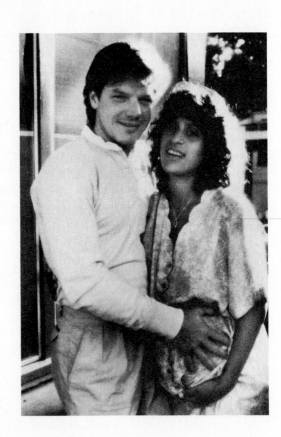

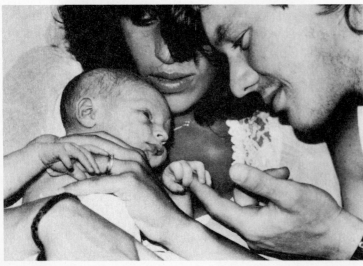

Figure 3–2 The developing family

couple has started to work on the tasks involved in the first stage; however, the intimate relationship of marriage accentuates the importance of these tasks and their evolution. The transition from single to married life involves a variety of changes including new roles to learn, new situations to deal with, and new relationships with people.

The primary family tasks of the married couple/beginning family are establishing a mutually satisfying marriage relationship, forming a new household, and deciding whether to become parents. For the remarried, an additional critical task is acceptance of the termination of the previous marriage in order to establish a healthy conjugal relationship with a new mate.

Open, honest communication on both intellectual and emotional levels provides a basis for mutually satisfying marriage. When conflict results, the couple must find appropriate methods to deal with the situations before they interfere with the marriage relationship. Successful conflict resolution and decision making are more likely if both partners display reciprocal respect, acknowledge individual differences, and are empathetic and mutually supportive.

A couple may experience difficulty in sexual adjustment because of inaccurate or incomplete information resulting in unrealistic expectations of each other. The degree of sexual experience, particularly the amount of factual knowledge the partners bring to the marriage, affects their adaptation to the relationship. If a couple brings their own unresolved needs and desires into the relationship, it can have an adverse effect on the sexual relationship (Goldenberg & Goldenberg 1985). Marriage partners who recognize each other's varying needs and expectations are able to cooperate to achieve a mutually fulfilling sexual relationship.

The formation of a new household occurs in conjunction with the couple's combining resources, altering roles, and assuming new family functions. These circumstances may be stressful unless the partners are willing to make mutually agreeable decisions about the home and the social responsibilities they will accept. With the selection of a home, the critical issues for the couple become financial planning, including budgeting, and the division of household and other duties.

The couple must establish patterns of social communication with friends and others in the community. They may find that they have more in common with other couples than with single people. Demands of work or other concerns may arise. Whatever the pressures, each couple needs to agree on ways to cope.

The couple's families of origin continue to be important, but relationships with them change. No longer is each partner a member of one family; each now has relationships with three families—the family of origin of each partner and the couple's own developing family. The young couple may maintain close ties with their original families, choose to keep distant from their families for fear of in-

terference, or establish a satisfying degree of involvement with both families.

Couples today face a decision about bearing children. Family planning and the use of contraceptives have received widespread acceptance in our society. Many couples are choosing not to have children; many more are limiting the size of their families because of economic concerns or the woman's desire to pursue a career or other interests. Some couples are unable to conceive a child despite their desire to have one and may seek medical help for a solution to their reproduction problem. (See Chapter 9 for discussion of special reproductive concerns).

Couples must also negotiate a philosophy of life as a couple. Optimally, each individual enters marriage with a philosophy of life, which must be correlated with that of the partner. They may disagree on particular issues, but they must be able to live with or accept these differences with compromises. The philosophy they develop will identify them and reflect their attitudes and priorities. In addition, it will provide a framework for later decision making.

The early stage of the married couple phase is a precarious period; the marriage is vulnerable to many stresses that could destroy it. The tasks just described may not be completed within the first few years of marriage or indeed may never be completed. However, the greater the success in meeting the demands of these tasks, the more likely the marriage is to be mutually satisfying to both partners.

BEGINNING FAMILY STAGE

In the latter part of the first stage in the family life cycle, a couple's expectations of having their own child may be fulfilled. This marks the *beginning family stage*. Although this stage may cover the shortest time span in the cycle, this period is filled with many intense and diverse feelings. When the couple is told that conception has occurred, they may either accept or reject the pregnancy. Some pregnancies are unplanned, although either partner may subconsciously desire it. Others are planned and may even have been anticipated for months or years before conception actually takes place.

After their initial reactions to the fact that the wife is pregnant, the couple must accomplish certain tasks that are an offshoot of those from the earlier part of the married couple phase. For example, arrangements must be made for the physical care of the baby. These arrangements may mean drastic changes for the family if they have to move into larger quarters or to a place where children are accepted.

In the beginning family period, the couple must make adjustments in patterns of earning and spending. Generally, the man is in the early phase of his career, and his salary may be low. The woman's salary, which may be a necessary part of the family income, may come to an end during the pregnancy. Many women who have worked during the early part of their marriage stop work during pregnancy or when the baby is born—a time when there are greater costs for shelter, food, clothing, and other supplies for the baby. Even if the mother chooses to return to work after the baby is born, child care is a costly item in the budget. Health care during the pregnancy and birth also requires large amounts of money, especially with rising medical costs.

Work loads and designation of authority in the household also change out of necessity during pregnancy. The man may assume more of the heavy household chores, as it is difficult for the woman to bend and move about. At the same time, pregnant women do not find that their physical state prohibits them from pursuing many of the activities they enjoy, such as working, entertaining, or even participating in sports.

Sexual activities must also be altered to accommodate the physical and emotional changes of pregnancy. The pregnancy may have positive, negative, or no effects on the couple's sexual relationship. Husbands are as likely to feel changes in their sexual responses as their wives are. Because of changes in breast and abdominal size, the couple will need to reorient their normal sexual activities.

As soon as the couple knows they are expecting a child, a new focus of interaction becomes evident, enlarging their need for and use of communication. Most couples feel a sense of fulfillment as they feel pride in their ability to conceive a child, as the wife begins to show signs of pregnancy, and as they make plans for the child's arrival. Husband and wife undergo changes in self-concepts in terms of masculinity, femininity, and parenthood. All of these tasks are accomplished with greater ease if the husband and wife develop communication patterns that help them cope with new responsibilities.

Communication with significant others also takes on a new perspective. Relatives and close friends may have a prominent role in helping the young couple with their baby after birth; they can give physical and emotional support to the wife as she undertakes the new tasks of child care. On the other hand, significant others can interfere with the couple's adjustment to pregnancy and childbirth by telling "old wives' tales" and frightening myths. Reorienting relatives and friends to the kind of relationship that is most desirable for new parents and their child is a major task of the beginning expectant family.

Reorientation must also occur in relationships with friends and in community activities. Recreational and social activities can continue to be a major part of the couple's life, curtailed only to the extent that the pregnancy decreases the woman's ability to participate. The mother-to-be may be more sensitive to her partner's activities because his mobility is not affected. She may believe that he is seeking outside interests as she becomes more introspective about the birth of the child. The man may feel left out of

many of the woman's activities as she visits the physician and attends groups to discuss the care and rearing of children. Planning joint activities while continuing to respect each other's needs for autonomy can help the couple make a comfortable transition to the complementary relationship that will be needed in future years.

An expectant couple is open to and eager for knowledge about pregnancy, labor and delivery, and child care. Their background knowledge may be based more on hearsay than fact. They may have had little or no experience with infants and small children.

The couple must also deal with the questions whether they are prepared to bring a child into their lives, how the baby will fit into their pattern of living, and how they will alter their life-style for their child. As mentioned earlier, both partners feel emotions that are new to them and seek understanding from each other. The more one partner is able to meet the other's emotional needs, the more love each will be able to give to their child.

CHILDBEARING FAMILY STAGE

The arrival of the first child marks a time of both crisis and great joy for the young family. Again the family faces a period of reorganization. During the *childbearing family stage* (from the birth of the first child until that child is 30 months old), the baby and family become stabilized in their schedules and relationships with each other. The parents feel great joy about the birth of their first child and share their joy with their family and friends; the new mother feels a sense of accomplishment and is ready to relax and let others care for her and her baby for a few days. At the same time, the young couple has a feeling of great responsibility for their child's growth and development.

The first task of the childbearing family is to arrange the home to meet the needs of the newborn infant. The primary responsibility of the parents is to provide a safe, comfortable environment for the infant. A primary need of the newborn is a quiet, clean place to sleep. As children grow and become more mobile, their immediate environment enlarges even though they are still unable to protect themselves from many of its dangers. Eventually curiosity leads them to explore, and their parents have to "childproof" the home, setting limits within which the child can function safely.

Costs of raising a child are drastically increasing, creating additional problems for a couple already dealing with the increased costs of daily living. Even in the United States, where prosperity is relatively common, many families are below poverty level and children are raised with a minimum of economic expenditure.

The birth of the first child requires a reworking of responsibility and accountability patterns. A baby requires round-the-clock care, much of which is assumed by the mother, particularly if she is breast-feeding the child. The father may assume more of the household tasks, such as shopping and running errands outside the home. The partners share in seeking solutions to problems that arise during the day. The child also has accountability to parents as he or she grows older. The approval or disapproval of parents teaches him or her what parents consider good and bad, and he or she recognizes good acts as pleasing ones.

Reestablishing a satisfying sexual relationship with one's partner is another task of the childbearing family stage. Sexual activity usually decreases or ceases during the postnatal period. The new mother becomes absorbed in her child, and her close physical relationship with the baby may decrease her sexual needs. The responsibilities of caring for a newborn may leave her physically exhausted. Her partner may feel rejected as the new mother focuses on the baby's needs instead of his. Much mutual patience and understanding is necessary as the couple strives to reunite to meet each other's needs.

Two stresses occur in the childbearing family period that can hinder or further the development of effective communication: the newborn's crying and the decreased sharing between the parents. Crying, the newborn's only means of communication, can be extremely disconcerting until the new parents are able to interpret what the various types of cries mean and until they learn to anticipate their infant's needs. When the parents believe they have met the needs of their child and the crying continues for no apparent reason, their frustration increases. However, as the parents attempt to meet the baby's needs lovingly, the baby's trust in them increases, and other methods of communication emerge such as smiling, cooing, and eventually talking.

The other strain on effective communication is decreased sharing between the parents. Their tasks may be more separately defined as the father works outside the home while the mother remains busy caring for their new baby and the house. They participate in different activities and have less time to be alone together. Instead of the one relationship of the couple, three relationships have developed to include the infant in the family circle. However, even though the parents may have distinct tasks, they can share more as they watch their baby grow.

Relationships with relatives are also a facet of the development of the childbearing family. The new parents will receive much advice on how to care for the child. If they are mature and have successfully completed their previous developmental tasks, they are able to sift through this information and use what is most meaningful to them. The greater the difference between the two parental families, the greater the likelihood of conflicting advice, because each set of grandparents will want the child to be raised according to the traditions of their family. And, of course, the parental families can also supply a great deal of support

and comfort to the new parents, who are trying to establish their own traditions.

The young family must participate in community activities to establish relationships outside the home. They are more involved in their home life than they were before their baby's birth and must find suitable babysitting arrangements if they desire to go out together. Their interests may change as they seek out congenial couples with young children who can share similar experiences.

A further responsibility of the childbearing family is to decide whether or when to have more children and to take appropriate measures. Having children in quick succession may prove to be a tremendous strain for both parents although some couples choose to have their children close together. If the first child has a defect or dies shortly after birth, the decision about whether or when to have another child becomes paramount.

Maintenance of motivation and morale in the childbearing family may become difficult. The repetitious tasks of everyday child care may overshadow the basic satisfactions of parenthood. Values placed on material objects may need to be changed, becoming dependent on what is good for the young child. The parents need to continue their independence as a couple while recognizing the child's dependence on them. The developmental needs of the child and those of the parents may be in conflict, so priorities must be set. The young family may need to accept assistance from relatives and friends at a time when they are still striving to be a separate unit.

The early childbearing and childrearing years have a significant influence on the ultimate strength of the family unit. Many crises occur that can either divide or unite the family. A division or conflict may not be evident while the children are still dependent but may manifest itself after the children have left home and there is little else to hold the parents together. Yet these same stresses can unite the family more solidly if they are faced as mutual problems and if individual needs and priorities are taken into account in family interrelationships.

● Factors Affecting Family Structures and Functions

Regardless of its structure, the family does not function in isolation. The well-being of a family can be promoted or hindered by the acts or policies of other persons or institutions. Inherent characteristics such as race and ethnicity or a less common family configuration may affect the family's social status, income level, and community acceptance.

Religion often has a strong influence on the values, beliefs, and moral concepts of the family. Many religions also dictate behavioral codes, rituals, traditions of family life, and childrearing practices.

The implications of these and other factors differ for each family. Members within each family can also be affected to varying degrees. The following sections explore the concepts of and factors affecting family life-style.

Family Life-Style

Families are characterized by diversity more than anything else. As mentioned earlier, families come in widely varying sizes and behave in widely varying ways. While every family is unique, certain factors, such as socioeconomic status, race, and ethnicity, can have an important impact on the family's life-style. Levin and Idler (1981) describe life-style as "this webbing material of values, beliefs, expectations, criteria of choice, problem solving, communication, and commitment that is unique to the family" (p 68).

Traditionally a family's socioeconomic status was determined by certain characteristics of the husband-father, including his occupation, education, and income. A more recent trend has been to include information from both parents in determining the family's socioeconomic status. (See Chapter 4 for discussion of the socioeconomic problems faced by single-parent families headed by women.) Social scientists consider education and occupational position to be the two main components of social class. Income is also a factor but is of less importance. According to Kohn (1979), four relatively distinct classes exist in American society: a small "lower class" of unskilled manual workers, a larger "working class" of manual workers in semiskilled and skilled occupations, a large "middle class" of white collar workers and professionals, and a small "elite" class differentiated from the middle class by wealth and lineage rather than occupation.

According to Kohn (1979), social class is important because

> Members of different social classes, by virtue of enjoying (or suffering) different conditions of life, come to see the world differently; they develop different conceptions of social reality, different aspirations and hopes and fears, different conceptions of the desirable (p 48).

Family life across social classes has been shown to vary with regard to both structural and functional characteristics. There is an inverse relationship between social class and family size: The more affluent the family, the smaller it is. Differences have been noted in such things as communication style and childrearing practices in families of differing social classes. For example, Kohn (1979) states that working class parents tend to punish their child based on their perception of the extent to which the child's behavior deviates from an established rule. Middle class parents are more concerned about the intent or motivation of the child's behavior. Kohn (1979) points out that working class and middle class parents usually differ in their

values, and they view their children's misbehavior differently, so that what is intolerable to parents in one social class can be taken in stride by parents of another. His conclusion speaks to the importance of discerning the values on which parents' interactions with their children are based. Health care professionals cannot understand the dynamics of family life unless they are willing to learn how families and their individual members subjectively define their situations.

Ethnic identity also influences family life. Mindel and Habenstein (1976) defined *ethnicity* as patterned differences based on the national, cultural, religious, or racial identification of a group of people. They described 15 different ethnic groups subdivided into early ethnic minorities (such as Irish and German), recent and continuing ethnic minorities (such as Vietnamese and Cuban), historically subjugated ethnic minorities (such as black and native American), and socioreligious ethnic minorities (such as Mormon and Greek Orthodox). They also identified some of the structural and functional differences often associated with families of varying ethnic backgrounds.

Nurse anthropologists and ethnographers such as Tripp-Reimer (1983), Leininger (1978), and Raggucci (1972) have provided valuable insights into the family life and health care beliefs and practices of various ethnic groups. Speaking to the importance of understanding ethnomedical practices, Tripp-Reimer (1983) said: "While it is crucial to be sensitive to cultural beliefs and practices, it is just as essential not to overgeneralize and assume that all members of the subculture hold to a particular belief or practice" (p 101). In a similar vein, Levin and Idler (1981) stressed the need for health care professionals to recognize the health care functions of the family in general.

> Many indigenous practices have emerged from historical test and may depend for their effectiveness on an integrated, interacting set of values and beliefs. It may well be that their effective power lies in the family's commitment to them and their symbolic contribution to family identity (p 66).

It is virtually impossible to describe in a meaningful way the socioeconomic and ethnic variations that exist in American families. However, such differences do exist. It is reasonable to expect that the "Yuppie" couple will have a different way of being a family than their working or lower class counterparts. Likewise it is reasonable to expect a recent Cuban immigrant to differ in her ideas about parenting from a third-generation Mormon from Salt Lake City. However, there is an important difference between "reasonable expectation" and stereotyping. On the one hand, professionals want to be sensitive to clients' diverse needs and expectations; on the other hand, they don't want to impute needs or expectations based on preconceived notions of what families in a given socioeconomic or ethnic group membership are like. In keeping with those words of caution, the reader is directed to the Additional Readings section at the end of this chapter for sources of information on different family types.

Societal Trends

STATUS OF WOMEN

The traditional role for a woman in our society gave her dominance in the home. Her role had value for the family but did not have prestige. The lack of prestige made it a safe role for women, one in which their men would not intervene. Thus the home became the stronghold for women.

Similarly, the man has traditionally been considered the head of the household, and the status and life-style of those within the home have depended to a large extent on him. But now more women are becoming part of the work force to supplement family income, to satisfy chosen career goals, or to work voluntarily in charitable organizations. As women move out into the working world, in addition to contributing income so that their families can enjoy a higher standard of living, they are gaining more status for themselves within their families and in the community.

In recent years, women have moved into the labor force in increasing numbers. Goode (1982) summarizes women's participation in the workforce:

> In the United States in 1981, women made up 43 percent of the civilian workforce. This participation changes with age, but has been moving toward a pattern much like that of men, which means that women's part in the labor force has been increasing at all ages beyond 20 years. Two-thirds of all divorced women with children under five are in the labor force, and the rate for mothers has been rising faster than other segments of the labor force (pp 131–132).

Goode (1982) identifies three areas of family life that the wife-mother's participation in the labor force is likely to influence: division of labor within the home, marital adjustment, and parenting. According to Goode, research conducted between 1962 and 1977 generally reported that the wife-mother's employment has little impact on household division of labor. In short the wife's employment had little influence on the husband's contribution to household tasks. However, Goode concluded that attitudes regarding the traditional division of labor within the family are changing.

> By 1977, attitudes *against* a traditional division of labor, with respect to household work, major decisions, and which kinds of jobs or tasks men and women should have, formed a majority of the total. In addition, as an apparent harbinger of the future, younger women, women with more education, wives with better-educated husbands, black women, and those who had held jobs for many years were more likely than others to move toward egalitarian sex role attitudes (pp 134–135).

It is difficult to determine how the wife's employment affects marital satisfaction. Of the many variables likely to influence the relationship, two of the most important are the family's financial situation and each partner's values or beliefs regarding the woman's participation in the labor force. Dissatisfaction is most likely when partners hold conflicting beliefs in this area.

Women's increased labor force participation has raised questions about how this affects their children. Based on review of the research in this area, Goode (1982) concluded that

> perhaps the most important finding is that it has not been possible to demonstrate that children who grow up in households with working mothers develop psychological problems or are more prone to various kinds of deviance than children whose mothers stay at home to supervise them (p 137).

VALUE OF CHILDREN

The value of children varies greatly, depending on the meaning each society attaches to children. In addition, the reaction of individual family members to a child is personalized and subjective. Historically the motivations for having children have been religious, political, and cultural. Some individuals want children for their own gratification—to have someone to guide and control, to reap economic gains, to improve one's status, to ensure one is cared for in old age, to satisfy cultural requirements, or to provide a means of personal immortality (Berelson 1976).

In industrial societies the degree to which children are wanted seems to depend somewhat on the state of the economy. For example, during the economic recession of the 1970s, the birth rate in the United States dropped and continued to decline until zero population growth was reached in 1976. This trend can be contrasted to the post–World War II "baby boom," which occurred in a thriving economy.

Many historical changes have influenced the importance of children in society. In agrarian societies, children are valued for the economic gain they bring to their family and society. Industrialization and urbanization in North America have reduced the economic necessity of having children. As a result, children have become less "valuable" and more valued.

Environmental Factors

Environmental factors influencing the family are closely interrelated with the cultural and socioeconomic factors discussed previously. The environment includes outside forces that may alter the behaviors and activities of the family member and family group. Forces such as relatives, friends, and significant others; home, neighborhood, and community settings; and social, religious, and governmental institutions within the community all have impact.

In childbearing families, environmental factors are most significant in terms of their effects on parents. Parents, based on their experience and background, interpret to their children the meaning of the interaction between environmental forces and the family. If their explanations are positive, they transmit to their children feelings of security, stability, and well-being. However, if the parents feel negative toward or threatened by their surroundings, they impart feelings of danger, hostility, and anger to their children. The nature of the family's interaction with its milieu is likely to have a direct effect on its ability to meet members' needs, individually and collectively.

The physical setting in which the family resides has a pronounced effect on family functioning. Poor housing may adversely influence family and member attitudes, behaviors, motivational levels, and self-esteem, which in turn increases stress and the risk of illness and accidents. The physical design of a home may interfere with privacy and result in unfavorable childrearing and housekeeping practices. Chaotic, disorganized homes may produce children with developmental delays or deviancies, which may be permanent. If family functioning continues to be impaired as the child's environment expands to settings outside the home, problems may become evident in the child's ability to communicate, solve problems, and form relationships.

Within the neighborhood and community, families tend to associate freely with community groups and institutions to identify resources and receive services as needed. The family's ability to seek help through contact with others appears related in part to the family's perception of itself as a part of a whole and to its successful dealings with the larger community in meeting physical, psychologic, and social requirements.

● Nursing Implications

There are no simple "recipes" for working with families. The information in the earlier sections of this chapter was meant to be sensitizing rather than prescriptive. Theories and research provide a basis for understanding families and suggest important areas of concern, typical patterns of behavior, and the range of variation surrounding the typical. Theories and research, however, do not prescribe what the nurse should do in a given situation. These decisions emanate from thoughtful interactions with family members in which the nurse interprets the family's definition of the situation in light of his or her own knowledge.

A major goal of family-centered maternity care is to help each member of an expectant family achieve optimal health by preventive, maintenance, and restorative measures. Nurses have the additional role of assisting families to accomplish appropriate developmental tasks at each family stage.

The success of the family depends on the achievement of these tasks. At times the family may find that success comes easily; at other times, they must overcome delay or failure. Since failure tends to follow failure just as success follows success, the nurse may need to intervene to break a family's cycle of failures in performing tasks and to guide them toward success.

When giving care to a client, the nurse should keep in mind the long-term, intimate relationships among family members. The person receiving care has performed a unique role within the family group that must be acknowledged if the family is to function optimally. Thus families have the right to examine the kind of care and service a family member is receiving, to complain when the service is unsatisfactory, and to seek other sources of services when they are dissatisfied.

To ensure the provision of appropriate individualized care, the maternity nurse uses the nursing process as the framework for planning and implementing responsible health care.

The Family as Client

Because the individual develops as a member of a family unit, the nurse must acquire understanding of the family to understand the individual. This is especially important in the maternity setting because the nurse is directly responsible for the well-being of two members of the same family—mother and child.

The concept of the family as a client is one of the most important components of family-centered maternity nursing. Ideally the family gives each member love, trust, and response consistently so that he or she may mature into an individual who is able to give these qualities to others.

Friedman (1986) identifies the family unit as being the critical resource for the delivery and success of health care services for the following reasons:

1. In a family unit a dysfunction of one or more family members generally affects each individual as well as the family unit. If the nurse considers only the individual, the nursing assessment is fragmented rather than complete and holistic.

2. Assessing the family helps the nurse understand the individual functioning within his or her primary social context. With the expectant and childbearing family, the nurse is able to assist the prospective parents to prepare for the new family member.

3. A strong interrelationship exists between the health status of a family as a unit and that of the individuals who constitute the family. By emphasizing health

promotion and maintenance in the family, the nurse should have a positive effect not only on the individuals in the family but also on the family unit. Health education becomes a primary learning modality for families.

4. In considering the family as a whole, the nurse identifies potential risk factors, thereby facilitating the nurse's role in illness prevention.

5. When illness occurs, the family is instrumental in seeking health care and in determining members' sick-role behaviors.

Levin and Idler (1981) emphasized that "self-care by individuals and families is a substantial proportion of all health care activity, is characteristic of many cultures, and appears to meet standards of efficacy as defined by expected benefits, safety, efficiency, and costs" (p 79).

In family-centered maternity nursing, the nurse generally focuses on health promotion and maintenance and prevention of illness, primarily with the beginning or childbearing family. In order to interact effectively with the wide variety of families she or he is likely to encounter, the nurse needs to:

● Reevaluate personal cultural beliefs and values.

● Recognize personal biases and beliefs about a particular culture (stereotyping).

● Assess the individual/family carefully and openly without judgment.

● Avoid generalizations and assumptions based on personal ideas and knowledge about a particular culture. There is diversity *within* every culture.

In view of these suggestions, it is a good idea to validate any inferences made regarding the particular culture or group by speaking tactfully with the individual or family. To do otherwise might compromise the nurse's goal of giving excellent care based on a complete biopsychosocial assessment that has included a cultural component.

Through the assessment process (discussed next), the nurse identifies risk factors that may precipitate health problems. Planning with the family determines health goals that may necessitate the involvement of other health team members. Assessment, intervention, and evaluation should be viewed as negotiative, interactive processes. Nurses and family members each bring unique knowledge and skills to a given health care situation. Ideally, they work together to achieve acceptable goals mutually.

Family Assessment

Assessment of the beginning or childbearing family's status is the first step in determining the family's level of functioning. Data may be gathered in a variety of settings, including the home, clinic, and hospital. When assessing the family of a maternity client, the nurse should be comprehensive but focused on areas of particular relevance to the family. In-depth data collection is necessary in those areas that pose a problem for the family or are of concern to the nurse.

To collect valid, pertinent data, the nurse must establish a positive relationship with the client, a family member, and/or the family group. The use of empathy, positive regard, and active listening enables the nurse to gather complete, yet selective, information about the family. The nurse should obtain:

● Basic identifying information, including the names, ages, gender, and relationships of all family members

● Religious and cultural associations

● Type of family configuration

● Data about the members of the extended family who are closest to the nuclear family, especially if they reside nearby and form a strong support group for each other

● Individual and family developmental history

HEALTH HISTORY

The nurse records a health history of the entire family since family health problems have potential effects on children born or unborn. The nurse gathers information about the extended and nuclear family regarding past acute and chronic illnesses, congenital defects, mental health, and such alterations as obesity or the occurrence of accidents. A family pedigree may be helpful in summarizing this information visually (see Chapter 9 on genetic counseling). With the beginning expectant family or the childbearing family, data about all pregnancies become significant. Knowledge of experiences of family members with health care delivery systems or hospitalization helps in deciding which approach to the family will be most helpful.

The nurse must also obtain data about the current health status of each family member. With the beginning and childbearing family, the nurse assesses the family's strengths and limitations in promoting and maintaining health by eliciting such information as the family's definitions of health and illness, their nutritional status, attitudes toward medicine use (prescription and nonprescription), recreational and exercise activities, exposure to environmental hazards, and sleep and rest practices. When a client is pregnant, prenatal assessment is essential (Chapter 15). Other important information includes data on each member's allergies, health problems requiring prescription medications, environmentally and genetically related illnesses, the family's knowledge about these disorders, and treatments recommended and implemented.

HEALTH PRACTICES

Assessing the competency of the family to promote and maintain health, care for ill members, and carry out health care instructions is vital in determining the nurse's interaction with the family. Many families use preventive health measures such as obtaining routine medical, dental, hearing, and ophthalmic examinations and immunizations and participating in other screening programs. If the family does not use such preventive measures, questions should arise about their availability or the family's knowledge about them. The nurse may find it necessary to identify health care facilities that are accessible to the family and how they are used.

HOME ENVIRONMENT

A valid assessment of the family may require several home visits. Some families feel that a home visit by a nurse is an invasion of privacy but most become more amenable as rapport is established. When assessing the characteristics of a home, the nurse must make objective observations; personal standards and values should not be allowed to distort evaluation of the living conditions. Living space that provides all family members with privacy and comfortable sleeping arrangements and permits each person to pursue interests and needs is important. If an additional family member is expected, preparation for arrival should be evident. Facilities for ill and convalescent family members should also be evaluated. Adequate heat, light, cooking facilities, water, storage facilities, and hygienic equipment are necessary for maintaining the well-being of all family members. Toys, books, and other recreational and educational equipment should be available for the children. Play areas should be away from safety hazards and should be adequately supervised. Safety hazards such as peeling paint, exposed electrical wiring, loose rugs, and exposed heating equipment can be of great danger, particularly to small children and the elderly. The distance of the home from health care facilities and the availability of transportation to them should also be investigated.

Appraisal of the home environment gives only some indication of the economic status of the family. Knowledge about the sources and amounts of family income and about the work skills of individual members aids in assessing health behavior and needs. Information about the allocation of income to shelter, clothing, food, savings, insurance, education, recreation, and health care reveals the family's economic priorities and its ability to meet the needs of all family members.

The assessment may also include observations of the population characteristics and resources of the neighborhood and the larger community in which the family resides, taking into account the family's associations and transactions within the community. How parents view their interaction with their neighborhood and community is significant in that their children tend to relate in a similar fashion. Certain health problems can also affect many within a community; for example, diseases can be transmitted by children to other children in schools and from them to the rest of the family. After identifying such situations, a nurse can make recommendations to help families cope with such problems.

ASSESSMENT TOOLS

In addition to the sources of information just described, several objective data collection instruments measure various aspects of family functioning. Some assessment tools concentrate on mother-infant interactions and needs for teaching and support. The Neonatal Perception Inventory evaluates parents' expectations and the discrepancies between their actual and imagined newborns. It identifies areas on which the nurse needs to focus in providing teaching, support, counseling, anticipatory guidance, and other interventions such as encouraging attendance at parent groups or referrals to enhance parental skills (Broussard & Hartner 1971). The Maternal Attachment Assessment Strategy provides a system of observing maternal-child behavior and establishing a profile of the mother's attachment behaviors (Avant 1982). The Mother-Infant Play Interaction Scale (MIPIS) is another tool that measures response reciprocity between mother and infant during unstructured play (Walker 1982).

The Feetham Family Functioning Scale (Roberts & Feetham 1982) assesses parents' views of relationships among family members and between the family and other social systems. It is a systematic method of assessing family functioning under stress. By identifying specific stressors, the maternal-newborn nurse can proceed to identify sources of support that will help diminish the stress. The Family APGAR test (Smilkstein 1978) assesses family functioning in the areas of adaptability, partnership, growth, affection, and resolve. The Family Environment Scale (Moos & Moos 1976) measures three components of family life: relationships, personal growth, and family system maintenance. The tool provides data that help the nurse compare parent and child perceptions and actual and preferred family milieus and assess and facilitate change in family environments. Speer and Sachs (1985) provide an excellent overview and evaluation of nine family assessment tools. Their evaluation is based on the following criteria: understandable, easily administered and scored, reliable and valid, appropriate for all types of families, and clinically relevant. Such tools can facilitate the nurse's assessment of the family.

Nursing Diagnosis and Planning

After completing the assessment of the family, the nurse analyzes the data to formulate nursing diagnoses. Goals based on each nursing diagnosis are then established for the family. These are divided into short- and long-range goals and should be a joint enterprise between the family and the nurse. Without this cooperative interaction, the goals may not meet the needs that the family believes are important, may not be realistic for the family, or may not be accepted by the family as its responsibility.

The priority of these goals must then be determined. This is a highly individualized process; input from the family continues to have great importance. A severe illness, an unplanned child, and lack of funds for a needed purchase can all be crucial matters. However, the family may consider obtaining funds to be the most pressing goal, the nurse may believe that accepting the child should receive immediate attention, and the physician may think that the treatment of the illness should be given top priority. Factors that affect priorities include the family's perceptions of its needs, the number of problems that require attention, the feasibility of goals set, the readiness of the family to meet the goals, and the amount of preparation or education necessary before the goals can be met (Sobol and Robischon 1970). Working with the family, the nurse must validate the goals and their importance to gain the family's support in achieving them.

Planning interventions is the next step in the nursing process. The nursing care plan must be based on the goals set in consultation with the family. There are generally many approaches to every problem, and the nurse must identify the one that seems most likely to work in the family's particular framework of attitudes, beliefs, and values. Family participation in the decision about the approach can be valuable, because the family is aware of its ability to deal with the situation. In any event, the nursing plan must be accepted by the family prior to putting it into action.

During the planning stage, decisions must be made about those health care workers, other professionals, and community agencies that will be of greatest value to the family. The nurse can explain the services available from these agencies. The family's needs may be best satisfied by several agencies, which will require interagency cooperation and coordination of efforts. The nurse may serve as the coordinator of these activities, assuring continuity of services to the family. One long-range goal for the family should be to strengthen its knowledge of community resources to meet its own health needs.

Intervention

In implementing a care plan, the nurse must constantly keep in mind the short- and long-range goals that have been set for the family. Therapeutic interaction continues to be of primary importance. Changes in family needs often produce stress on some or all members. The recommendations and teaching of the nurse or other professionals may cause more stress, as any change always causes some tension and anxiety. Family members may feel guilty about having certain needs and may be concerned about how these needs will be accepted by others. Any serious difficulties have probably already disrupted the family, and its members may have had to take on roles and responsibilities with which they are unfamiliar; this can modify the family's life-style.

The nurse must be aware not only of the family's changing situation but also of its members' changing views regarding their situation. In this sense, assessment is ongoing and cuts across the intervention and assessment stages of the nursing process. Further resources may need to be consulted to help in dealing with any problems.

When working with beginning and childbearing families, the nurse assumes many roles, including teacher, counselor, coordinator, researcher, and advocate. In these roles, the nurse is careful to communicate in a manner that is understandable and meaningful to the family. Knowledge of the family's developmental level, internal processes, socioeconomic status, and cultural background helps in determining the most effective method to use. A collaborative effort is necessary for learning to occur. The nurse assists the family to define change strategies and the family decides how to apply the learning primarily through their own resources. In some circumstances the nurse supports the family's position or initiates plans to foster further development, thus ensuring continued learning on the part of the family.

The nurse acts primarily as a teacher, counselor, and advocate in helping a couple determine their family-planning needs. The nurse offers information in a manner that the family can understand and use, demonstrating understanding and respect for needs and belief systems. Some families hesitate to use family-planning techniques because of fears or dislike of, or misunderstanding about, contraception; because of worries that they cannot afford family planning; or because of beliefs that others are trying to limit the size of their ethnic group.

The nurse's responsibilities to the beginning expectant family include preparing the couple for the woman's physical and emotional condition and needs, and planning for the man's desires for involvement. Teaching expectant couples about pregnancy, labor, and delivery and counseling them about child care and the parental role are important nursing responsibilities.

After the child is born, a primary concern of the nurse is to make sure that the family can meet the needs of the newborn infant. The nurse assumes the roles of teacher and counselor when discussing the needs of the infant and demonstrating infant care to the parents. In addition, the nurse acts as the family advocate by giving emotional support to new parents and by providing guidance on effective use of health care professionals.

Evaluation

To interpret the success or failure of the nursing care plan, the nurse must take into account the goals set for the family and the effects produced. Again, the family should play an important part in this evaluation, as it has in other steps of the nursing process. Members must be encouraged to respond freely and openly.

If a goal has been fully achieved, the nursing interventions have been successful. If a goal has not been attained, the nurse should explore the reasons for the failure and devise a new plan that might meet with greater success. If a goal has been partially achieved, the nurse and family determine whether the plan is realistic and simply needs more time or whether modifications are necessary. The nurse may find that changes in the family necessitate adjustments and adaptations in the nursing care plan at any point during its implementation. Even when all goals appear to have been attained, periodic reevaluation and encouragement are necessary for the family to continue to function at the best level.

Application of the Nursing Process: A Case Example

The following example illustrates the integration of theory and research in an application of the nursing process.

SITUATION

Mr and Mrs Hunter, both in their early thirties, have been married for seven years. They have a three-year-old son, Brian, and Mrs Hunter is in her second trimester of pregnancy. In the 12 months preceding the pregnancy, she experienced two spontaneous abortions, both during the first eight weeks of pregnancy. Mr Hunter is a mechanic for a local car dealer, and Mrs Hunter works three mornings a week as a receptionist in a real estate office. Her work schedule coincides with Brian's nursery school schedule. Since becoming pregnant, Mrs Hunter has been seen by a nurse-midwife at the HMO to which the family belongs. She and Mr Hunter plan to attend the HMO's childbirth and parenting classes during her last trimester. Mrs Hunter is in excellent physical health and has had a prob-

lem-free pregnancy. Nonetheless, during her last checkup with the nurse-midwife, she indicated two major areas of concern: (1) pressure from her husband and close relatives to quit her job and (2) negative comments from Brian about having a new family member. Mrs Hunter reported that she and her husband had had several "blowups" over her desire to continue working. In addition, both Mr and Mrs Hunter felt Brian should share their excitement about the new baby and were concerned about his "bad" behavior whenever they encouraged him to show enthusiasm about the baby.

NURSING ASSESSMENT

Working from an interactionist perspective, the nurse-midwife decided to elicit more detailed information from family members regarding their "definition of the situation." She suggested that Mrs Hunter schedule an appointment in the next two weeks for her and Mr Hunter to talk to the nurse-midwife about "plans for the new baby." During this family session, the nurse-midwife learned that Mr and Mrs Hunter viewed Mrs Hunter's working quite differently. For Mrs Hunter, work was a social outlet and source of income. She said she had always worked and felt proud to contribute to the family income even though it wasn't absolutely necessary. She hoped to move back into full-time employment as her children got older. Moreover Mrs Hunter identified physical benefits because she walked the half mile to and from work every day. Mrs Hunter resented her husband's efforts to "control her life" and noted that this was an aspect of his personality she had not experienced before.

In contrast Mr Hunter cited his wife's two previous spontaneous abortions as evidence that she should "take care of herself." He felt he had a responsibility to both his wife and the unborn child to make sure his wife took care of herself. He was confused by his wife's anger about what he saw as "good intentions."

With regard to Brian's behavior, Mr and Mrs Hunter feared that his negative outbursts probably were a prelude to even worse behavior after the baby was born. They described how they had intensified their efforts to convince Brian that having a new baby in their home would be wonderful. They mentioned that Brian's grandfather liked to tease him about having to cook his own meals after the baby was born since his mother would be too busy to prepare meals.

ANALYSIS AND NURSING DIAGNOSIS

The nurse-midwife concluded that the Hunter's did not have a shared definition of Mrs Hunter's work and that their discrepant views were the source of escalating conflict as the pregnancy progressed. While the couple had a shared view of their son's behavior, the nurse-midwife concluded that their definition of that situation and subsequent actions probably were contributing to Brian's negative feelings about the pregnancy.

Based on her interactions with the Hunters, the nurse-midwife identified two tentative nursing diagnoses: (1) altered family coping related to increased family conflict over Mrs Hunter's desire to continue working outside the home and (2) knowledge deficit about parenting of siblings related to inexperience with normal sibling responses to birth of a baby and anxiety over the son's reaction to the pregnancy.

INTERVENTIONS

The nurse-midwife pointed out to Mr and Mrs Hunter that they viewed Mrs Hunter's job in quite different ways although both believed that they were doing what was best for both Mrs Hunter and the baby. The HMO had several family therapists on staff and the Hunters agreed with the nurse-midwife that it would be a good idea to get some help on resolving any conflicts between them prior to the baby's birth.

The nurse-midwife was knowledgeable in the area of child development and sibling behavior. Through teaching and discussion, she was able to begin to alter the Hunters' definition of Brian's behavior. She provided them with several articles on sibling relationships from popular magazines and assured them that Brian's behavior was quite normal even if it seemed "bad" to them. She suggested that they deemphasize talk about the baby around Brian and that they gently encourage Brian's grandfather to stop teasing him.

At a subsequent prenatal checkup, Mrs Hunter reported that she and her husband still disagreed about her working, but the therapist had helped them to appreciate each other's viewpoint. She indicated that they no longer had "big battles," only "minor skirmishes" over the issue. She also indicated that the therapist had been helpful in getting them to anticipate possible issues regarding Mrs Hunter's return to work.

Mrs Hunter said she and her husband had been skeptical about the advice regarding Brian but had been desperate enough to try anything. While still not overjoyed at the thought of a new brother or sister, Brian was described as considerably less negative than he had been. Mrs Hunter laughingly reported that he had volunteered to "lend" the baby some of his old stuffed toys.

KEY CONCEPTS

The evolution of today's family is a result of social, political, economic, and philosophical changes.

Family structure describes the number of family members and the relation of each family member to the others; family function describes the effects of the family behaviors on the family unit.

The development of the family is defined by a set of developmental tasks that the family undertakes at various times during its life cycle.

Common types of families include nuclear, single-parent, reconstituted (blended), and extended families.

Family assessment is the process of gathering and analyzing data about a family and its members. During the process the nurse collects data about the family structure, function, roles, and knowledge about infant-child care.

Family assessment draws on a variety of disciplines and theories, which provide the nurse with a frame of reference to analyze the data obtained about the family.

Some assessment tools are the Family APGAR test, the Family Environment Scale, the Feetham Family Functioning Survey, and the Neonatal Perception Inventory. Other tools helpful for the maternal-newborn nurse are the Mother-Infant Play Interaction Scale and the Maternal Attachment Assessment Strategy.

The overall goal of family assessment is to promote family growth by identifying teaching and referral needs.

REFERENCES

Aldous J: *Family Careers.* New York, John Wiley, 1978.
Avant P: A maternal attachment assessment strategy, in **Humenick** S (ed): *Analysis of Current Assessment Strategies in the Health Care of Young Children and Childbearing Families.* New York, Appleton-Century-Crofts, 1982.
Berelson BB: The value of children: a taxonomical essay, in **Talbot** ND (ed): *Raising Children in America: Problems and Prospective Solutions.* Boston, Little, Brown, 1976.
Blumer H: *Symbolic Interactionism.* Englewood Cliffs, NJ, Prentice Hall, 1969.
Broussard ER, **Hartner** MS: Further considerations regarding maternal perception of the first born, in **Hellmuth** J (ed): *Exceptional Infant: Studies in Abnormalities,* Vol 2. New York, Brunner/Mazel, 1971.
Burgess EW: The family as a unity of interacting personalities. *The Family* 1926;7:3.
Duvall EM: *Marriage and Family Development,* ed 5. Philadelphia, Lippincott, 1977.
Fantini MD, **Rossi** A: Parenting in a pluralistic society: Toward a policy of options and choices, in **Fantini** MD,

Cardenas R (eds): *Parenting in a Multicultural Society.* White Plains, NY, Longman, 1980.

Friedman MM: *Family Nursing Theory and Assessment,* ed 2. New York, Appleton-Century-Crofts, 1986.

Goldenberg I, Goldenberg H: *Family Therapy, an Overview,* ed 2. Monterey, Calif, Brooks/Cole, 1985.

Goode WJ: *The Family,* ed 2. Englewood Cliffs, NJ, Prentice-Hall, 1982.

Hill RL: Modern systems theory and the family: A confrontation, in Sussman MB (ed): *Sourcebook of Marriage and the Family,* ed 4. Boston, Houghton Mifflin, 1974.

Howard J: *Families.* New York, Simon & Schuster, 1978.

Hymovich DP: *Child and Family Development: Implications for Primary Health Care.* New York, McGraw-Hill, 1980.

Kenkel WF: *The Family in Perspective,* ed 4. New York, Appleton-Century-Crofts, 1977.

Knafl KA: How families manage a pediatric hospitalization. *W J Nurs Res* 1985;7:151.

Kohn ML: The effects of social class on parental values and practices, in Reiss D, Hoffman H (eds): *The American Family: Dying or Developing.* New York, Plenum, 1979.

Lamb M: What can research experts tell parents about effective socialization? in Fantini MD, Cardenas A (eds): *Parenting in a Multicultural Society.* White Plains, NY, Longman, 1980.

Leininger M: *Transcultural Nursing: Concepts, Theories, and Practices.* New York, John Wiley, 1978.

Leslie GR: *The Family in Social Context,* ed 3. New York, Oxford University Press, 1976.

Levin S, Idler E: *The Hidden Health Care System.* Cambridge, Ballinger, 1981.

Levy ST: *Parenting in Lesbian Couples,* thesis. University of Illinois, Chicago, 1984.

McCubbin H, Dahl B: *Marriage and Family: Individuals and Life Cycles.* New York, Wiley, 1985.

Miller JR, Janosik EH: *Family Focused Care.* New York, McGraw-Hill, 1980.

Mindel CH, Habenstein RW: *Ethnic Families in America.* New York, Elsevier, 1976.

Moos RW, Moos BS: A typology of family social environments. *Family Process* 1976;15:357.

Nye FI, Berardo FM (eds): *Emerging Conceptual Frameworks in Family Analysis.* New York, Praeger, 1981.

Raggucci AT: The ethnographic approach and nursing research. *Nurs Res* 1972;21:485.

Ritzer G: *Contemporary Sociological Theory.* New York, Knopf, 1983.

Roberts C, Feetham S: Assessing family functioning across three areas of relationships. *Nurs Res* 1982;31:231.

Smilkstein G: The family APGAR: A proposal for a family function test and its use by physicians. *J Fam Pract* 1978;6:1231.

Sobol EG, Robischon P: *Family Nursing: A Study Guide.* St. Louis, Mosby, 1970.

Speer J, Sachs B: Selecting the appropriate family assessment tool. *Pediatr Nurs* 1985;11:349.

Stern PN: Affiliating in stepfather families: Teachable strategies leading to stepfather-child friendships. *W J Nurs Res* 1982;4:75.

Tripp-Reimer T: Retention of a folk health practice among four generations of urban Greek immigrants. *Nurs Res* 1983;32:97.

Turner R: Role-taking: Process versus conformity, in Rose A (ed): *Human Behavior and Social Processes.* Boston, Houghton-Mifflin, 1962.

Walker T: Mother-infant play, in Humenick S (ed): *Analysis of Current Assessment Strategies in the Health Care of Young Children and Childbearing Families.* New York, Appleton-Century-Crofts, 1982.

ADDITIONAL READINGS

Allan H: *Ethnicity and Medical Care.* Cambridge, Mass, Harvard University Press, 1981.

Beale E: Separation, divorce and single-parent families, in Carter E, McGoldrick M (eds): *The Family Cycle: A Framework for Family Therapy.* New York, Gardner Press, 1980.

Bernstein JL, Kidd YA: Childbearing in Japan, in Kay MA (ed): *Anthropology of Human Birth.* Philadelphia, Davis, 1982.

Davies M, Yoshida M: A model for cultural assessment. *Can Nurse* 1981;77(March):22

Enriquez MG: Studying maternal-infant attachment: A Mexican-American example, in Kay MA (ed): *Anthropology of Human Birth.* Philadelphia, Davis, 1982.

Griffith S: Childbearing and the concept of culture. *J Obstet Gynecol Neonat Nurs* 1982;11:181.

Harris M: *America Now: The Anthropology of a Changing Culture.* New York, Simon & Schuster, 1982.

Keshet H, Rosenthal K: Single-parent fathers: A new study, in Mussen P et al (eds): *Child and adolescent psychology.* New York, Harper & Row, 1980.

Lovell M, Fiorino DL: Combating myth: a conceptual framework for analyzing the stress of motherhood. *Adv Nurs Sci* 1979;1(July):75.

McGoldrick M: Normal families: An ethnic perspective, in Walsh F (eds): *Normal Family Processes.* New York, Guilford Press, 1982.

O'Brien ME: Pragmatic survivalism: Behavior patterns affect low-level wellness among minority group members. *Nurs Sci* 1982;4:13.

Olness K: Cultural aspects in working with Lao refugees. *Minn Med* 1979;62:871.

Orque MS et al: *Ethnic Nursing Care: A Multicultural Approach.* St. Louis, Mosby, 1983.

Overfield T: *Biologic Variation in Health and Illness*. Menlo Park, Calif, Addison-Wesley, 1985.

Robbins M, **Schacht** T: Family hierarchies. *Am J Nurs* 1982;82:284.

Rosenblum EH: Conversation with a Navajo nurse. *Am J Nurs* 1980;80:1459.

Sowell T: *Ethnic America: A History*. New York, Basic Books, 1981.

Terkelson K: Toward a theory of the family life cycle, in **Carter** E, **McGoldrick** M (eds): *The Family Life Cycle: A Framework for Family Therapy*. New York, Gardner Press, 1980.

U.S. Bureau of the Census: *Household and Family Characteristics,* Current Population Reports Series P-20 no. 366. Government Printing Office, September 1981.

U.S. Bureau of the Census: *Marital Status and Living Arrangements,* Current Population Reports Series P-20 no. 365. Government Printing Office, October 1981.

U.S. Bureau of the Census: *Money Income and Poverty Status of Families and Persons,* Current Population Reports Series P-60 no. 127. Government Printing Office, August 1981.

Whall AL: Congruence between existing theories of family functioning and nursing theories. *ANS* 1980;3 (October):59.

Wright LM, **Leahey** M: *Nurses and Families: A Guide to Family Assessment and Intervention*. Philadelphia, Davis, 1984.

On the eve before our first child was born, we were out for a ride. Just the two of us, wandering through the evening. As we returned home it suddenly hit both of us at the same time, that this may well be the last time we would be alone for the next twenty years! It was at this moment that the romantic fantasy of parenthood was replaced with a real sense of parenthood. We've never been sorry.

Social Issues and the Childbearing Woman

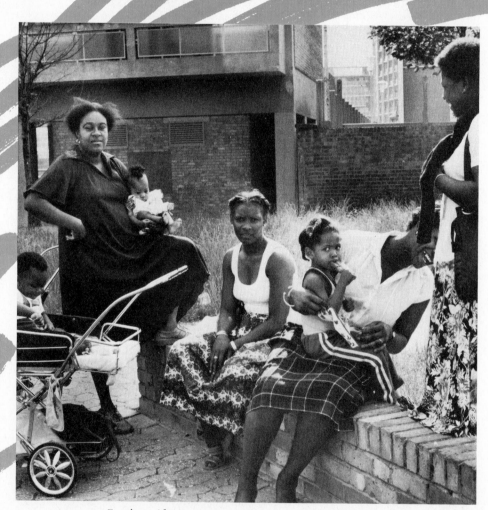

For these African immigrants living in a London housing project, pregnancy and parenthood cannot be divorced from the larger issues of race, class, and culture.

Chapter Four

OBJECTIVES

- Describe the concept of feminization of poverty.
- Discuss the current work environment and the factors that affect women's wages.
- Discuss work benefits that affect the childbearing woman.
- Describe environmental hazards present in the childbearing woman's work setting.
- Discuss briefly the philosophical differences in the question of abortion.

The woman of today has the opportunity to be a dynamic, challenging, and challenged individual. She has opportunities for personal and professional growth that did not exist 20 years ago.

Because of political and social changes that have occurred in this country within the past two decades, women's options have expanded dramatically. Although many women still choose the traditional "women's" careers and become nurses, teachers, and mothers, others are entering occupations that until recently were filled almost exclusively by men. More women than ever have joined the ranks of lawyers and judges, managers and corporate heads, scientists, journalists, legislators, construction workers, plumbers, and other laborers. Women can be found in almost all occupations and thus are sharing in many of the benefits that come with these positions.

Progress has its costs, however. For example, the woman with a career and a family may have difficulty maintaining both. The woman who would like nothing more than to be a wife and mother may be forced by the high cost of living to work outside the home and entrust the care of her children to others. The woman who has devoted her prime childbearing years to establishing a career rather than a family may find herself feeling pressure to find a partner and have children before it is too late.

Nurses must deal with many of the issues facing women, if not personally, then in their dealings with women as they come into the health care setting for maternal-newborn care. To help nurses better understand their clients' concerns and problems, this chapter addresses a few of the more serious issues facing women today

● Women and Poverty

The economic plight of many women is reflected in the phenomenon referred to as the *feminization of poverty,* a term suggested by Diana Pearce (1983). Simply stated, a growing number of women live on incomes below the poverty level, which in 1986 was $11,000 for a family of four (Colorado DHHS Income Poverty Guidelines effective 7/1/85–6/30/86). The extent of this problem is enormous and increasing at a rapid rate. Two-thirds of all poor people in this country are women and children, and it is projected that by the year 2000, nearly all people living in poverty will be women and children (see Box 4–1).

Single women with children make up the largest group of people living below the poverty level, and the number is increasing. This increase is happening at a time when many male-headed families who have been living at the poverty level are increasing their financial resources and moving out of the poverty range (Cahan 1985).

The statistics on the poverty of children are even more shocking. It is estimated that one in four preschoolers in our country lives in poverty (Sidel 1986). More than 53.9 percent of children living in female-headed families are below the poverty level (Sidel 1986). Some sources

Box 4–1 Some Facts about Poverty in the United States

The rate of poverty in the general population is 15.2 percent.

78 percent of all the poor are women.

5 percent of male-headed couple households live at or below the level of poverty.

36 percent of female-headed households live at or below the level of poverty.

21 percent of white female-headed households live at or below the level of poverty.

51.7 percent of black female-headed households live at or below the level of poverty.

53.4 percent of Hispanic female-headed households live at or below the level of poverty.

Source: Leslie & Swider 1986, Sidel 1986.

suggest that the children of female-headed families may be destined for persistent poverty in adulthood. A study of 5000 families (McLanahan 1985) revealed that there may be an increased risk of poverty in adulthood for children who grow up in poverty.

Although the statistics on poverty may be shocking, they reveal little about what living with poverty is like. It is a day-by-day experience fraught with struggle and hardship:

I thought this would never happen to me. Things were so good for us and our daughter that I thought we would not be another one of those divorced families. Two months after I became pregnant with our second child, it was over. My husband left us. Suddenly, I am the sole support of myself and my children. It's like I'm dreaming, like a nightmare. I'm a teacher, and I've always had a good job, but I have taken time off to stay with our first child and haven't worked for the last two years. I thought it was important to stay at home and take care of our baby, and Jim felt that way too. Since he left I haven't been able to get a teaching position or any job. So now I don't have medical insurance or any benefits to help with this pregnancy. Applying for Medicaid has to be one of the most humiliating experiences I have ever had. I'm an intelligent woman with a college degree and I couldn't figure out the forms. I'm smart really, surely I am, but I felt so dumb. The lines and the impersonal treatment that I had heard about but never believed in was there. I was a number and felt shuttled from one place to the next. You know, they don't do it on purpose. I know they have heard so many awful stories, but you know it hurt. It will take six weeks to qualify, and that means I will be more than halfway through the pregnancy. I've called and no one will accept me now, without paying money I don't have. I feel really caught. I know I should be getting prenatal care, I had problems with the last pregnancy and I know care is important. I'm caught. I can't get care without money, and I'm afraid when I start care they will be angry with me because I waited so long. It seems there is no way to win. There are only two doctors in our town that will accept Medicaid and they are clear across town. It's all right. I'm thankful that I can get some help now when I need it, but it is so hard. I never dreamed I'd be in this position. I just never dreamed.

Contributing Factors

The feminization of poverty has occurred as a result of three major factors:

- The increase of families headed by females (Leslie & Swider 1986) and the fact that women bear almost all the economic burden of raising the children (Pearce 1983)

- A labor market in which the largest percentage of women work in low-paying, low-status occupations with few benefits and little chance of advancement (Leslie & Swider 1986) and the sex discrimination

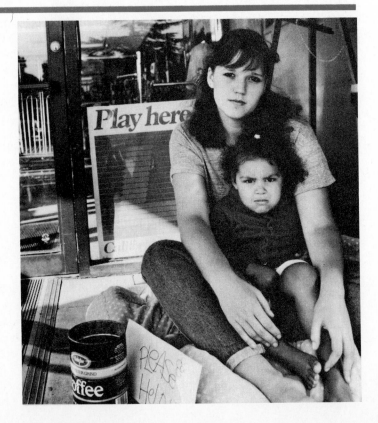

Figure 4–1 Two-thirds of all those Americans living in poverty are women and children.

and occupational segregation that occur in these positions (Pearce 1983)

- The welfare system

Abowitz (1986) has identified similar reasons for the feminization of poverty in Canada.

INCREASE IN FEMALE-HEADED HOUSEHOLDS

The increase in the number of female-headed families is closely associated with divorce. Almost one out of every two marriages end in divorce (Sidel 1986). As a result of divorce the woman's standard of living generally decreases approximately 73 percent and the male's increases by 41 percent (Leslie & Swider 1986). This dramatic change in the standard of living is usually associated with the lower earning capacity of women and the fact that the children remain with the woman. Women receive custody of the children in 90 percent of the cases (Enrenreich & Piven 1984), and the economic assistance provided by the father is minimal. Approximately 4 percent of women receive alimony; only 35 percent of women receive child support; and only half of those who are granted child support actually receive the total amount (Pearce 1983).

LABOR MARKET

The dual labor market is also associated with the prevalence of poverty in women. There are two sectors in the labor market (Pearce 1983). The primary sector is characterized by good pay and fringe benefits, job security, and a large number of union groups. The secondary sector has lower paying jobs, less unionization, and fewer benefits. Women are concentrated in the secondary sector, and the characteristics of this sector tend to keep the women in poverty even with full-time employment (Pearce 1983; Leslie & Swider 1986; Enrenreich & Piven 1984).

WELFARE SYSTEM

The welfare system provides much-needed assistance to many women. The amount of assistance, however, does not even raise the family to the poverty level. The elimination of work incentives and the incorporation of an earnings cap for Aid to Families with Dependent Children (AFDC) make it difficult to make ends meet (Zinn & Sarri 1984).

Effects on Health Care

The effects of poverty on health care are extensive. Since 1981, many funding cuts have directly affected programs that benefited those living in poverty. Funding cuts to Aid to Families with Dependent Children and Medicaid have resulted in more than 500,000 people losing their eligibility. The food stamp program has lost 1,000,000 due to decreased funding. The Women, Infants and Children nutrition program (WIC) is currently providing assistance to only one-third of the people who are eligible. These cuts come at a time when the benefits of adequate nutrition and prenatal care have been documented to save $2 to $11 for each $1 spent (Mundinger 1986).

Women living in poverty are also frequently without any kind of health insurance. Overall, 15 percent of the population is without any type of health insurance, which is a 25 percent increase since 1977. Since health insurance is used to obtain care and for preventive health measures, the implication is that the health of the general population will decline (Andersen et al 1986, Mundinger 1986).

Statistical data already is beginning to reflect the change in health insurance coverage and funding cuts. Women who do not receive prenatal care are three times more likely to have low-birth-weight babies, and the incidence of low-birth-weight babies is increasing. The decline of infant mortality rate has slowed since 1982, and in selected poor areas of 20 states there was even an increase in infant mortality (Mundinger 1986).

The effects of poverty on women's health care will require continued investigation. Currently the status of the mothers and babies is being studied by the Public Health Service Task Force on women's health issues, which is considering not only childbearing but also other factors that affect women's health. They have identified general recommendations such as promoting a safe, healthful, physical and social environment; providing services for the prevention and treatment of illness; coordinating research and evaluation; educating and informing the public; disseminating research information; and designing guidance for legislative and regulatory measures (see Box 4–2).

Suggestions for Nursing Action

The issue of women and poverty is critical, and the implications for childbearing care are very real. A pregnant woman who is suffering economically may also suffer physically. The physical and psychological states of the woman depend on her access to health care and her financial ability to act on her health care providers' recommendations. In the end, it is often the children who suffer the most, bearing the physical and psychological scars of their mothers' struggles.

Nurses should be concerned about the issue of women and poverty for two primary reasons. One reason is related to the nurse's professional role. The health care system and thus nursing is intricately woven into the political and social structures of society. Nurses often work with women on welfare; they *see* the effects of poverty on childbearing families and the pain and struggles of these families. Because of the limited resources of these women, nurses' efforts to provide quality care may be stymied.

Box 4–2   Objectives for the Nation

The United States Public Health Service has identified national objectives to improve the status of maternal-child health. The objectives address the following areas:

- The reduction of infant, neonatal, and maternal mortality rates.
- The reduction of low-birth-weight babies.
- Increased usage of car safety carriers, especially for infants leaving hospitals.
- Increased public and professional awareness of pregnancy risk factors and the need of adequate nutrition during pregnancy.
- The improvement of maternal services and well-child care.

Specific objectives that have been identified include the following:

	Status in 1984†
OBJECTIVE: Reduce the following mortality rates by 1990*	
Infant mortality to no more than 9 deaths per 1000 live births	10.8 per 1000
Neonatal death rate to no more than 6.5 deaths per 1000 live births	7 per 1000
Low birth weight to no more than 5 percent of all live births (or 9 percent for any specific county, racial, or ethnic group)	6.7 percent

*Promoting Health/Preventing Disease. Public Health Service Implementation Plans for Attaining the Objectives for the Nation. Pub Health Rep 1983;98(September/October Suppl):1.

†National Center for Health Statistics: Advance Report of Final Mortality Statistics. 1984. Monthly Vital Statistics Report. Vol 35, No 6 Suppl(2). DHHS Pub No (PHS) 86-1120. Hyattsville, Md, Public Health Service, 1986.

Source: Pub Health Rep 1985.

Box 4–3   Myths About Poverty

Myth	Reality
People living in poverty are black urban females who have been on welfare for many years.	Approximately two-thirds of the people on welfare are white (Sidel 1986).
Poverty is perpetuated from parents to children to grandchildren in a never-ending cycle.	Slightly over half of the individuals living in poverty do so from one year to the next. In a study from 1968 to 1978 only 2.6 percent of the population was persistently poor—at the poverty level for 8 of the 10 years (Sidel 1986). Recurrent poverty is rare and is generally not passed from one generation to the next (Hill 1985).
People in poverty are a different breed from the rest of us.	People who are temporarily poor are not different from the population as a whole (Sidel 1986).
People on welfare programs do not try to get off the programs and get a job.	The majority of women living in poverty sought employment even when the employment meant they lost benefits and were at an even lower economic level (Zinn & Sarri 1984).

PERSONAL ACTION

Be aware of your own beliefs about poverty and the women who need public assistance.

Explore your feelings regarding the myths of poverty (see Box 4–3).

Remain knowledgeable about the impact of poverty on the childbearing woman and her family.

CLIENT ACTION

Be sensitive in assessing a woman's economic status during intake interviews. Use the knowledge of the current extent of this problem to predict women who may be at risk.

Provide supportive counseling and determine the woman's ability to follow a treatment plan, especially when extra expenditure of funds is required.

Be alert for women who are not able to follow a treatment plan or accomplish self-care measures due to economic problems.

The other reason for concern is largely personal. The majority of nurses are women, and like the teacher on p. 62, some nurses may find themselves in financial difficulty, frequently due to circumstances beyond their control.

What can nurses do about the growing problem of female poverty? The following sections include suggestions for action that nurses can take to ease this crisis.

Stay knowledgeable about community resources to assist the woman with financial need and be prepared to offer suggestions and counseling regarding possible resources. It is much more helpful to give a group name and a phone number than to send the woman out to search on her own.

COMMUNITY ACTION

Identify resources in your community that are pertinent to the needs of the childbearing woman.

When possible, work with community organizations and planners to identify financial needs of childbearing women in the community.

Offer your nursing knowledge expertise to community groups to help them meet the financial and health needs of childbearing women and their families.

POLITICAL ACTION

Know your legislators and their views. Be available to discuss issues and act as a resource for them as they become more knowledgeable about issues that affect childbearing women.

Make your opinions and ideas known to your legislator.

Support programs that benefit childbearing women and help identify areas that need to be addressed.

Educate the legislators about the alarming increase of poverty among women.

RESEARCH ACTION

Investigate the impact of poverty on the health and welfare of childbearing women and their families. When women are unable to obtain adequate care, document it so it will be available for future use.

Conduct research projects to dispel myths associated with poverty.

● Wage Discrimination in the Workplace

Women are entering the work force in increasing numbers. In 1984 more than two-thirds of women between the ages of 25 and 54 were employed (Sidel 1986). In the past ten years, two-thirds of all newly created jobs have gone to women (Pennar & Merrosh 1985).

Despite the increase in new jobs, 80 percent of women are clustered in 20 of the 420 occupations listed by the Bureau of Labor Statistics (Sidel 1986; Enrenreich & Piven 1984). Table 4–1 lists these 20 occupations, ranking them according to the number of women in each. Most of these jobs are considered low-level occupations and are not highly paid.

The number of women in higher-ranking professions is changing slowly. Women represented 4 percent of the total number of lawyers and judges in 1971 and 14 percent in 1981. The percentage of female physicians rose from 9 percent in 1971 to 22 percent in 1981. Women engineers increased from 1 percent of the total number of engineers in 1971 to 4 percent in 1981 (Enrenreich & Piven 1984).

There has been a discrepancy between men's and women's wages since women first entered the work force in the mid-1800s. For more than 100 years, women's wages have been approximately 50 percent to 60 percent of men's wages. This situation has improved in the past 15 years. In the 1970s, with the rapid influx of women into the work force, women's wages were about 57 percent of men's. Since 1980, women's wages have risen to 64 percent of men's, and by the year 2000, women's wages are projected to be about 74 percent of men's (Pennar & Merrosh 1985).

The discrepancy between men's and women's wages is caused by many factors. From the beginning, women's wages were purposely set lower than men's, simply because it was a woman doing the job (Sidel 1986). The work of men and women was not valued equally. Unfortunately, this belief still affects women in the workplace.

Another factor is that women's education and experience have not generally been equal to men's, and this has affected women's ability to draw comparable salaries (Pennar & Merrosh 1985). This discrepancy in education and experience has its origins in the socialization process of girls and boys.

Young women traditionally have been socialized in ways that affect their opportunities and expectations. Girls

Table 4–1 Rank of Top 20 Occupations for Woman

1. Secretary	11. Sewer and stitcher
2. Bookkeeper	12. Cook
3. Sales clerk	13. Receptionist
4. Cashier	14. Secondary schoolteacher
5. Registered nurse	15. Assembler
6. Waitress	16. Building interior cleaner
7. Elementary school teacher	17. Bank teller
8. Private household worker	18. Hairdresser/cosmetologist
9. Nursing aide	19. Accountant
10. Typist	20. Child-care worker

Source: U.S. Department of Labor, Bureau of Labor Statistics: Employment and Earnings. Washington D.C.: U.S. Government Printing Office, Jan 1984.

are not expected to do as well as boys in technological fields such as the sciences (Eccles & Jacobs 1986), so they may not be encouraged to enter these fields. Boys are encouraged to develop a competitive spirit first in sports and then in other areas of their lives. They learn that "being a winner" and "knowing how to play the game" are valued qualities. Girls, on the other hand, are usually not encouraged to develop a competitive spirit; many cultures do not view competitiveness as an important or desirable trait for a girl to have. Girls learn from parents, the media, their peers, and others that physical attractiveness is the key to success since it is more likely to earn popularity than being smart (Pogrebin 1980, Muff 1982, Rubin 1976, Weitzman & Rizzo 1974, Maccoby 1966, Pierce 1961). Fearing loss of femininity, girls pull back from intellectual endeavors beginning at the secondary level and continuing into the college years (Pogrebin 1980, Scanzoni & Scanzoni 1976, Mednick et al 1975, Horner 1972). By the time these girls are women and ready to enter the work force, most do not have the educational training or the competitive skills to "play the game" that men of equal age and intelligence have.

Although women have received most of the newly created jobs, these jobs are frequently nonunion. This may adversely affect the pay scale and benefit package. In addition, the majority of the traditional women's occupations are low paying and are also not usually protected by a union.

Certainly all these factors have contributed to the wage discrepancy between men and women. But the *major* factor contributing to this problem is sex discrimination, usually manifested by wage discrimination, discriminatory job promotion policies, and inaccessibility of higher-paying jobs to women (Feldberg 1984). In a study on the wage discrepancy between men and women, the National Academy of Sciences found that only half of the wage discrepancy is caused by differences in age, experience, or education. The remainder is caused by gender differences, or, more plainly, sex discrimination (*Business Week,* 1983).

Currently, there are several factors exerting a positive force on the issue of wage discrimination.

- The number of women obtaining a college education continues to increase, and these women influence the work environment as they enter the work force. "In 1983, 86 percent of the female workers aged 20–24 who were college graduates were in the work force, while only 55 percent of females aged 55–64 who had the same amount of schooling were working" (Pennar & Merrosh 1985, p 81). The effect of this trend is a positive one as the younger, more educated women assume the positions of the older retiring women.

- Many working women are holding their jobs for extended periods and are not as likely to work for short

periods. They are gaining more experience in performing their jobs, and this has a positive effect on their productivity. As productivity rises, wages generally rise.

- Women have become more involved in the political arena and are raising the issue of comparable worth.

The basic premise of comparable worth is that the same wages should be paid for work that requires comparable skills, responsibility, education, and experience. This issue has created much controversy. The National Committee on Pay Equity believes that work can be equated based on evaluative studies. They agree that the Equal Pay Act has ended blatant discrimination but indirect discrimination continues (Arnold 1985). The National Association of Manufacturers, on the other hand, believes that instituting comparable worth standards would raise costs excessively. The projections of the resulting cost to manufacturers and business and individuals vary. Some believe that the increased financial burden would close businesses (Arnold 1985), and others believe that all women would lose because there would be fewer jobs available for women (Chavez 1985).

In some companies, comparable worth is a reality. Major companies such as IBM, AT&T, and Bank of America have instituted some forms of comparable worth. At least 30 states have comparable worth legislation pending or have commissions studying the issue.

NURSES' PAY

Nurses as a group experience many of the same problems that confront women in the general work force. The average salary of a staff nurse in 1985 was approximately $22,000, which is well below what other professionals with similar education and responsibilities were paid. There are a variety of reasons for the continuing low wages for nurses (Wright 1986):

- 97 percent of nurses are women and as with other professions or job categories that are held mainly by women, wages stay in the low range.

- The majority of nurses are employed in hospitals, and in many communities there is only one hospital. Because of this lack of competition the hospitals are in a position to keep wages low.

- There are only a few organized collective-bargaining groups for nurses.

- The recent federal, state, and local efforts to cut and contain health care costs have created a climate in which jobs are eliminated and pay increases are delayed.

What can nurses do about wage discrimination in the health care system? What can nurses do to help clients who are suffering financially because of wage discrimination? The following sections include suggestions for actions nurses can take.

Suggestions for Nursing Action

PERSONAL ACTION

Seek information regarding the wages for nurses in your community.

Share wage information with other nurses so more people will be informed. When wages are kept secret, disparities are more likely to exist.

Validate what it is that you do as a nurse and why you are cost efficient so you will know your own worth and will be better able to discuss wages.

Help other nurses maintain their self-esteem and feelings of worth.

CLIENT ACTION

Encourage women to push for wage equity.

Encourage women to talk together about wages so inequities can be identified.

COMMUNITY ACTION

Work with community leaders and groups to identify the lack of adequate jobs and wage inequity in your community.

POLITICAL ACTION

Educate legislators about the status of womens' wages and the impact low wages have on health care for the childbearing woman and her family.

Support programs that enhance employment opportunities and fair wages for women.

● Maternity Leaves and Child-Care Benefits

Maternity Leaves

Combining a career with childbearing can be a challenging task. However, leaving a job to have a child results at the very least in lost experience, most commonly in lost benefits, perhaps a lost opportunity for promotion, and sometimes loss of the job completely.

Parental leave for childbearing has been a national issue for a number of years. At this time, "only 40 percent of working women are allowed as much as six weeks of paid disability leave after childbirth . . ." (Brophy 1986 p. 57). Business, child development, and labor experts have recommended that some form of uniform parental leave be established in our country. Some type of child care is guaranteed by many other countries and at least 75 other industrialized countries provide some kind of parental leave (Lamm 1986). The United States is the only industrialized country that does not provide some statutory maternity leave or parental benefit (Sidel 1986). European countries offer six months leave as a standard (Brophy 1986). In most countries the woman's wage continues during the leave. For instance, Sweden grants a 52-week leave for either parent with 100 percent of wages for 38 weeks; Canada grants a maternal leave for 37 weeks with 60 percent of wages for 15 weeks; and Chile allows either parent an 18-week leave at 100 percent of wages (Brophy 1986).

Representative Patricia Schroeder of Colorado introduced a bill in 1986 to provide a minimum of 18 weeks of unpaid leave for parents. This leave could be used with the birth or adoption of a newborn or in the event of a child's serious illness (Kantrowitz et al 1986).

Although there is no standard national leave policy, women need to be aware of their rights, which were established by The Pregnancy Discrimination Act of 1978. This act provides guidelines regarding pregnancy, including the following (Brophy 1986):

● A pregnant woman cannot be denied a job if she is able to perform major job functions.

● The same procedure for using sick-leave pay or disability benefits must be used for the pregnant woman as for other employees.

● Employee medical coverage must include pregnancy benefits.

● The mother can use all her maternity benefits without penalty.

When a woman is planning a pregnancy, it would be wise to acquire information regarding pregnancy benefits in her work setting. The state in which she lives will also have guidelines or regulations regarding pregnancy. Questions that the woman may need to address include (California Department of Justice 1983):

Can I be forced to go on leave because I am pregnant?

What are my rights to sick leave or disability leave with my pregnancy?

Can I lose my job for taking disability leave associated with pregnancy?

Do I have any rights concerning infant care?

Is my employer required to provide maternity benefits and insurance coverage?

Recently the Supreme Court upheld the Pregnancy Discrimination Act by determining that a woman is guaranteed her job after returning from maternity leave (Court guarantees job . . . 1987).

Child-Care Benefits

Child care has been a working woman's problem for years. In our country, less than 10 percent of infants and about 24 percent of children under 3 are in licensed day-care centers (Belsky 1986). Almost half (45 percent) of the care of children under 3 is by a relative (Belsky 1986). In France, however, 95 percent of 3- to 6-year-olds are taken care of in free public schools (Kantrowitz et al 1986).

Some women work out arrangements for combining their careers with childbearing by taking a creative approach to hours and tasks. A full-time job may be shared by two women, with each one working 2½ days, or one working mornings and the other afternoons. At times, a work schedule can be temporarily reduced to two or three days a week for a few months. In one business, a "mother's shift" was instituted. It consists of working three-quarters of the day so that the mother can leave early to meet children after school (Kantrowitz et al 1986). To avoid losing valued executives, corporations with executive mothers may be more willing to implement creative planning in order to accommodate the woman's need (Companies start . . . 1983).

Given increased attention from citizens, legislators, and business, a uniform policy may not be far away. Until that occurs, women need to know their rights in the workplace. As women continue to remain in the work force, continued attention will be focused on the needs of parents for child care.

Suggestions for Nursing Action

PERSONAL ACTION

Examine the benefits in your own work environment. When questions arise or unmet needs are identified, follow the guidelines in your facility to suggest changes or additions in benefit policies.

Be knowledgeable about the current status of wage inequity and the effect this has on the childbearing woman's ability to afford adequate child care.

Once prepared with accurate knowledge, speak out when needed to provide information and correct inaccurate information about women's wages.

CLIENT ACTION

Talk with women to identify whether their benefit packages are useful.

Encourage women to investigate the benefits in their own work setting.

Provide resources that can be used to learn about regulations regarding benefits on the community, state, and national levels.

Encourage women to pursue their questions regarding benefits until they are answered satisfactorily.

COMMUNITY ACTION

Provide community leaders with information about the need for comprehensive maternal and child-care benefits for childbearing women and their families.

Work within the community to identify benefits for the nursing profession.

Work with community and professional nursing groups to enhance the status of nursing.

Work with your professional nursing organizations to improve benefits for nursing.

POLITICAL ACTION

Write your legislator and support legislation that addresses and corrects wage inequities. Let your legislator know if you do not support legislation and why. Educate legislators about the importance of a national policy on parental leaves and child care.

● Environmental Hazards in the Workplace

As more women enter the work force they are exposed to an ever-increasing number of chemicals and environmental pollutants (Figure 4–2). In 1977 there were 1,000,000 chemicals in common use, and more than 1000 new compounds are added yearly (Hill 1984). A number of substances have been identified as potential dangers to childbearing women.

1. *Hazards of the microelectronic industry.* Study of the microelectronic industry has indicated that there is a link between the various substances used in this field and birth defects, spontaneous abortions, and other reproductive problems. Among the "high-tech" hazards are glycol ethers, arsenic, lead, and radiation (Hembree 1986).

2. *Heavy metals (lead and mercury).* Lead was one of the first agents found to cause adverse reproductive effects. Lead contamination causes an increased rate of spontaneous abortions, stillbirths, and prematurity; surviving children are more likely to have impaired growth and neurological damage (Bang et al 1983).

These adverse effects have been found both in women who work in the lead industry and in wives of male workers (Hill 1984). A study of 35,000 female factory workers in Finland (Hembree 1986) demonstrated an increased spontaneous abortion rate in women who worked in electronics and with lead soldering. In addition, there is an increased level of lead in the blood of women who live near heavily traveled roads (Hill 1984).

Mercury was associated with an increased incidence of cerebral palsy when there was consumption of contaminated fish and shellfish in Japan from 1953 to 1960. The effects of occupational exposure are not yet clear, but mercury has been found to accumulate in the placentas of pregnant dental workers (Bang et al 1983).

3. *Vinyl chloride.* There is an increased incidence of spontaneous abortion and stillbirth in wives of workers exposed to vinyl chloride. Studies indicate that the fetal death may be caused by chromosomal changes in the male germ cell (Bang et al 1983).

4. *Chloroprene.* Chloroprene is a liquid used to manufacture neoprene rubber. A study of wives of chloroprene-exposed males indicated a threefold increase in the spontaneous abortion rate (Bang et al 1983). Direct effects on the exposed female worker are not known at this time.

5. *Halogenated hydrocarbons.* Halogenated hydrocarbons are associated with a twofold increase in births of children with malignancies (Bang et al 1983). Polychlorinated biphenyls (PCB) are the most widely known halogenated hydrocarbons and are used in the manufacture of plastics, and as heat-exchange fluids in the electrical industry (Hill 1984). PCBs have been associated with the birth of babies who are smaller than expected and have cola-colored skin, premature tooth eruption (Bang et al 1983), and eye defects (Hill 1984).

6. *Pesticides.* Women who are exposed to pesticides through employment with tobacco or as cotton pickers are at increased risk for spontaneous abortion, stillbirths, premature birth, and some degree of mental retardation in their children (Bang et al 1983).

7. *Anesthetic gases.* Women who work in operating rooms are exposed to anesthetic gases. This exposure is associated with lowered fertility (Hemminki et al 1985), a threefold increase in spontaneous abortion, and low-birth-weight babies (Bang et al 1983).

8. *Antineoplastic drugs.* Nurses who administer antineoplastic drugs may have some increased risk during the childbearing years. A study of Finnish nurses exposed to antineoplastic drugs revealed an increase in spontaneous abortions and fetal anomalies (Selevan et al 1985).

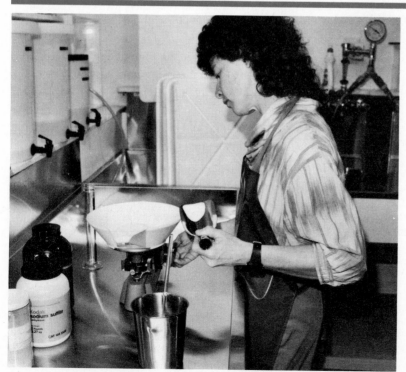

Figure 4–2 Women may be exposed to dangerous substances in the workplace.

9. Nurses have an occupational hazard in the exposure inherent in providing care for sick people.

Environmental hazards are increasing with the discovery and development of new products, and they exert their effect on all in that environment. Women are at particular risk while they are in the childbearing years. While no work environment is without risks, it is becoming more important for each woman to become knowledgeable about her own work environment. Information can be obtained from libraries, the Public Health Department, and special agencies that collect data regarding environmental hazards. The Resource Guide, found in the blue pages at the end of the book, contains references to a few of these agencies.

Suggestions for Nursing Action

Environmental hazards are an area of particular interest and importance to maternal-newborn nurses. Not only does the health care environment carry some risk to each nurse, but also the nurse needs to be knowledgeable about the possible risks to which childbearing women are exposed. Nurses can be influential in encouraging more investigation of chemical substances and environmental hazards so that work environments will be safer for all.

PERSONAL ACTION

Be knowledgeable about hazards in your own work environment.

Collect information regarding the effects of various environmental hazards on the childbearing woman and her family.

Follow guidelines and procedures in the work setting to decrease your risk.

CLIENT ACTION

Obtain information about environmental hazards in the woman's work environment.

Suggest resources to the woman to enhance her knowledge.

Recommend resource groups to obtain more information.

COMMUNITY ACTION

Work with community leaders and groups to identify environmental hazards in your community.

Provide education regarding the hazards to childbearing women.

POLITICAL ACTION

Provide information about environmental hazards in your community to your legislator.

Educate your legislator regarding the special effects of environmental hazards on the childbearing woman and her family.

Support legislation that addresses and solves problems involving environmental hazards.

RESEARCH ACTION

Document problems that are observed during your care of clients.

● Abortion

Abortion is a highly charged issue, and people both for and against legalized abortion are known for their heated confrontations. Even the terms used to refer to those with differing philosophical opinions about abortion are cause for argument. The antiabortion philosophy is dubbed "prolife" and the proabortion philosophy is called "prochoice." This seems to suggest that the prochoice philosophy would not be in favor of life. It is partly this politicized terminology that works to polarize opposing viewpoints.

The abortion issue is one that different factions have dealt with in one way or another for centuries. For the past 200 years the policies and philosophies in this country have been directed primarily by the medical community. Through the beginning half of the 1900s, abortion was a topic not to be discussed; it was a private matter. An important result of this privacy was that even though people held many divergent opinions about abortion, each philosophical position believed that its opinions were those of the majority. In the 1960s an effort to clarify laws and philosophies made the issue of abortion an open one; it was no longer a private issue that one could quietly hope that others would solve in the "right way." More importantly, people discovered that their opinion was not necessarily that of the majority.

There are many different opinions and many issues associated with abortion. One study on abortion (Luker 1984) identified four major arguments that are the basis of differing feelings about the rightness or wrongness of abortion:

1. The moral status of the embryo. Historically, the status of the embryo has been ambiguous from philosophical, religious, and moral viewpoints. Questions of the legal status of the fetus, the use of medical technology, and the value of children are central to this argument.

2. The moment that life begins. The fact that the heartbeat of a developing embryo can be observed by the end of the first month of gestation is accepted by both sides. However, there is no agreement on what this fact means. A heartbeat is necessary for life but the ability to breathe is also critical to maintain life. Does the fact that there is a heartbeat prove that life exists, or does life require a heartbeat and the ability to breathe?

3. The personhood of the embryo. Personhood carries with it inalienable rights to due process in our society. The question, then, is whether the embryo is a person. An additional issue is the allocation of scarce resources, which also involves the worth and value of an individual person but in a different way. If an embryo can be destroyed and denied care, what is to stop our society from deciding that another should not receive care?

4. The woman's role in our society. The ability to have an abortion gives the woman control over her reproductive life. But in establishing this control, the role of motherhood becomes just one role that women might choose. Some opponents fear that legal abortion devalues the role of motherhood and remaining in the home to raise children.

The abortion issue is clearly a complex one involving many philosophical points, values, and opinions. Table 4–2 presents some of the basic differences between those who support abortion and those who are against it. The belief systems are the result of extensive research (Luker 1984) and are characteristics identified by the majority of people on both sides of this issue. The differences are presented in general and may not be pertinent for individuals. A person who feels he or she is prolife may think the items listed are too narrow and may find items in both columns appropriate to their personal beliefs; a prochoice person may also identify with items from both lists.

The implications of abortion for maternal-newborn nurses are also complex. Each nurse will have many opportunities over the course of a professional nursing career to examine her or his personal feelings and opinions, and there is a good chance that these opinions will change over time as the nurse has new experiences and insights.

The philosophies of nurses mirror the society at large and it may be difficult to provide care for an individual who is participating in a procedure with which the nurse disagrees. If a client is having an abortion, the nurse who does not support abortion may be faced with a decision about whether to provide care. In some settings, nurses do not have to provide care for women having an abortion if it is against their own personal philosophy. The nurse with a prochoice philosophy may have difficulty understanding how a professional colleague could possibly choose not to

Table 4–2 Belief Systems Associated with Abortion

For Abortion as a Choice	Against Abortion
ROLE: Men and women are essentially equal. Women's reproductive and family roles are not "natural" or required. The reproductive function can be a barrier to full equality.	ROLE: Men and women are intrinsically different and have distinctly different roles in life. Abortion devalues the traditional roles of men and women.
ABORTION: Control over reproduction is essential to full equality.	ABORTION: Abortion is intrinsically wrong because it takes a human life. If a woman has control over her fertility it upsets basic social relationships between men and women.
CONTRACEPTIVES: Contraceptives should be very safe, effective, and readily available and preferably should not interfere with the spontaneity of sexual relations.	CONTRACEPTIVES: Contraceptives interfere with the potential to become pregnant, which disturbs the true meaning of sexual relations. The use of natural family-planning methods is preferred in that the potential for procreation exists.
SEX: Sex is natural and positive.	SEX: Sex is serious and filled with responsibility.
PARENTING: People should plan for beginning a family and fit children into family and life goals. They should attend parenting seminars and classes and seek information about effective parenting styles. The parent's duty is to prepare the child for the future. Optional parenting enhances the quality of parents. It is important for a child to be wanted.	PARENTING: Parenting is a natural role and does not need to be studied. The goal of marriage is to have children, not material things. Setting goals disturbs the reason for marriage. If a couple have financial and educational preparation it distorts the values. There is an antichild sentiment in the world today.

Note: The views delineated in this table are general and not meant to categorize individuals in either group. Each individual will probably find that his or her personal beliefs and philosophies are a blend of both groups.

Source: From Luker K, *Abortion and the Politics of Motherhood,* Berkeley, University of California Press, 1984.

care for a client based on the client's personal beliefs. If a nurse can choose not to care for a woman having an abortion, can the nurse also choose not to provide care for an alcoholic? A drug addict? A person of another race or religion? The questions facing nurses about the abortion issue have implications for other areas of nursing.

Suggestions for Nursing Action

PERSONAL ACTION

Explore your own feelings and beliefs regarding abortion.

Talk with others and gather information about abortion.

Be knowledgeable about the issues involved.

CLIENT ACTION

If your beliefs allow you to care for women considering abortion, provide counseling and support to women as they seek information. If your beliefs do not allow you to care for women who choose abortion, avoid imposing your opinions on them. Provide factual information.

Be nonjudgmental when working with women who have abortions.

COMMUNITY ACTION

Work with community groups that support your views.

Support adequate health care for women regardless of the option that the woman chooses (to seek an abortion or to continue with the pregnancy).

POLITICAL ACTION

Provide education, support, and assistance to legislators in order to attain legislation that promotes your philosophy and assures safe care for women.

KEY CONCEPTS

The number of women living in poverty is increasing at a rapid rate. Childbearing women seem to be at particular risk due to current trends in the divorce rate, the frequency with which the mother gains custody of children, and factors in the work environment that make it difficult for women to earn a good wage.

Women's wages have always been less than men's because of demand, education, skills, discrimination, and underlying philosophies that deem women's work as less valuable. Women are pushing to change the wage system especially with comparable worth legislation.

Work benefits that affect women pertain especially to maternity leave and child care. The United States does not have a standard policy regarding maternity benefits and leave at this time.

The chemical compounds present in the workplace are numerous and are increasing by 1000 each year. The implications of exposure during the childbearing years

are known in some instances, and others are currently being investigated.

The belief systems and philosophies regarding abortion are complex. Some general characteristics can be identified in people for and against abortion.

Nurses need to be aware of some of the current issues affecting the childbearing woman so they can better understand the client as she comes to the maternal-newborn health care setting.

REFERENCES

Abowitz DA: Data indicate the feminization of poverty in Canada, too. *Sociol Social Res* 1986;70(April):209.

Andersen RM, **Giachella** AL, **Aday** LA: Access of Hispanics to health care and cuts in services: A state-of-the-art overview. *Pub Health Rep* 1986;101(May/June):238.

Arnold B: Why can't a woman's pay be more like a man's? *Business Week,* January 28, 1985, p 83.

Bang KM, **Lockey** JM, **Keye** W: Reproductive hazards in the work place. *Fam Commun Health* 1983;6(May):44.

Belsky J: Infant day care: A cause for concern? *Zero to Three* 1986;6(September):1.

Bernstein A: Comparable worth: It's already happening. *Business Week,* July 18, 1983, p 170.

Brophy B: Expectant moms, office dilemma. *U.S. News and World Report,* March 10, 1986, p 57.

Cahan V: The feminization of poverty: More women are getting poorer. *Business Week,* January 28, 1985, p 84.

California Department of Justice: *Women's Rights.* Sacramento, Calif, 1983.

Chavez L: Pay equity is unfair to women. *Fortune* 1985;111(March):161.

Companies start to meet executive mothers halfway. *Business Week,* October 17, 1983, p 170.

Court guarantees job in maternity leave. *Denver Post,* January 14, 1987, p 1.

Eccles JS, **Jacobs** JE: Social forces shape math attitudes and performances. *Signs* 1986;11:367.

Enrenreich B, **Piven** FF: The feminization of poverty. *Dissent* 1984;31(Spring):162.

Feldberg RL: Comparable worth: Toward theory and practice in the United States. *Signs* 1984;10:311.

Hembree D: High-tech hazards. *Ms* 1986;14(March):79.

Hemminki K, **Kyyr** P, **Lindbohm** L: Spontaneous abortions and malformations in the offspring of nurses exposed to anaesthetic gases, cytostatic drugs, and other potential hazards in hospitals, based on registered information of outcome. *J Epidemiol Commun Health* 1985;39(June):141.

Hill LM: Effects of drugs and chemicals on the fetus and newborn. *Mayo Clin Proc* 1984;59(pt 2):755.

Hill MS: The changing nature of poverty. *Ann Am Acad Polit Social Sci* 1985;497(May):31.

Horner MS: Toward an understanding of achievement-related conflicts in women. *J Social Issues* 1972;28:157.

Kantrowitz B, et al: Changes in the workplace. *Newsweek,* March 31, 1986, p 57.

Lamm D: Best and brightest: They should be encouraged to have children. *Denver Post, Contemporary,* June 29, 1986.

Leslie LA, **Swider** SM: Changing factors and changing needs in women's health care. *Nurs Clin North Am* 1986;21(March):111.

Luker K: *Abortion and the Politics of Motherhood.* Berkeley, University of California Press, 1984.

Maccoby EE: Sex differences in intellectual functioning, in Maccoby E (ed): *The Development of Sex Differences.* Stanford, Stanford University Press, 1966.

McLanahan S: Family structure and the reproduction of poverty. *Am J Sociol* 1985;90(January):873.

Mednick M, et al: *Women and Achievement.* New York, John Wiley, 1975.

Muff J: *Socialization, Sexism and Stereotyping.* St. Louis, Mosby, 1982.

Mundinger MO: Health service funding cuts and the declining health of the poor. *N Engl J Med* 1986;313(July):44.

NAACOG. *Reproductive health hazards: Women in the workplace.* OGN nursing practice resource. February 1985.

Pearce DM: The feminization of ghetto poverty. *Society* 1983;21(November/December):70.

Pennar K, **Merrosh** E: Women at work. *Business Week,* January 28, 1985, p 80.

Pierce JV: *Sex Differences in Achievement Motivation of Able High School Students.* Cooperative research project No. 1097. University of Chicago, 1961.

Pogrebin LC: *Growing Up Free.* New York, McGraw-Hill, 1980.

Report of the Public Health Service Task Force on Women's Health Issues. *Pub Health Rep* 1985;100(January/February):73.

Rubin L: *Worlds of pain: Life in the working class family.* New York, Basic Books, 1976.

Scanzoni L, **Scanzoni** J: *Men, Women, and Change: A Sociology of Marriage and Family.* New York, McGraw-Hill, 1976.

Seixus NS, **Rosenman** KD: Voluntary reporting system for occupational disease: Pilot project, evaluation. *Pub Health Rep* 1986;101(May/June):278.

Selevan SG, et al: A study of occupational exposure to antineoplastic drugs and fetal loss in nurses. *N Engl J Med* 1985;313(November):1173.

Sidel R: *Women and Children Last.* New York, Viking, 1986.

Weitzman LJ, **Rizzo** D: *Images of Males and Females in Elementary School Textbooks.* New York, National Organization for Women's Legal Defense Fund, 1974.

Wright BW: Nurses' pay: Why so low? *U.S. News and World Report,* March 17, 1986, p 72.

Zinn DK, **Sarri** RC: Turning back the clock on public welfare. *Signs* 1984;10(Winter):355.

ADDITIONAL READINGS

Berger B: At odds with American reality. *Society* 1985;22(July/August):75.

Browner CH: Job stress and health: The role of social support at work. *Res Nurs Health* 1987;10(April):93.

Cartoof VG: Parental consent for abortion: Impact of the Massachusetts law. *Am J Pub Health* 1986;76(April):397.

Chatham L: The PHS task force on women's health issues. *Natl Inst Drug Abuse Res Monogr Ser* 1986;65:1.

Clark WAV, et al: The influence of domestic position on health status. *Soc Sci Med* 1987;24(6):501.

England P: The sex gap in work and wages. *Society* 1985;22(July/August):68.

England P, **Norris** B: Comparable worth: A new doctrine of sex discrimination. *Soc Sci Q* 1985;66(September):629.

Gray MW: Legal perspectives on sex equity in faculty employment. *J Soc Issues* 1985;41(Winter):121.

Holtzman NA, **Koury** MJ: Monitoring for congenital malformations. *Annu Rev Pub Health* 1986;7:237.

Jacobson AK: Sex role identity and depression in nurses. *Health Care Women Int* 1985;6(5/6):353.

Koszuta, et al: A women's place is . . . beside men? *Female EMT Emerg* 1985;17(December):36.

Long SO: Roles, careers and femininity in biomedicine: Women physicians and nurses in Japan. *Soc Sci Med* 1986;22(1):81.

Macinick CG, **Macinsk** JW: Toxic new world: What nurses can do to cope with a polluted environment. *Int Nurs Rev* 1987;34(March):40.

Majors BP: Comparable worth: The new feminist demand. *J Soc Polit Econ Stud* 1985;10(Spring):55.

May B: Comparable worth . . . an issue whose time has come? *Imprint* 1986;33(April/May):14.

McElveen JC: Reproductive hazards in the workplace: Some legal considerations. *J Occup Med* 1986;28 (February):103.

Robertson MJ, **Cousineau** MR: Health status and access to health services among the urban homeless. *Am J Pub Health* 1986;76(May):561.

Taube CA, **Rupp** A: The effect of Medicaid on access to ambulatory mental health care for the poor and near-poor under 65. *Med Care* 1986;24(August):677.

Walker LO, et al: Maternal role attainment and identity in the postpartum period: Stability and change. *Nurs Res* 1986;35(March/April):68.

Wood JL: Cover story: Right to know laws maintaining compliance. *Occup Health Safety* 1987;56(3):20.

Family Violence

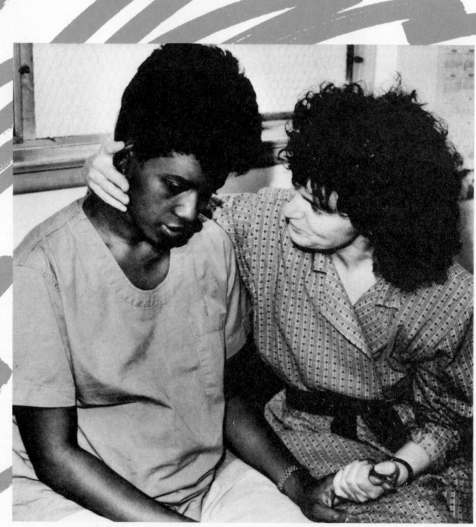

Sensing the degree of intimacy the client needs is a crucial skill for the nurse.

Chapter Five

OBJECTIVES

- Describe the types and extent of family violence.
- List the social, psychologic, political, and cultural factors that contribute to the occurrence of spouse abuse.
- Identify and refute the myths about spouse abuse.
- Discuss the role of the nurse who cares for battered women.
- Summarize the risk factors that place parents at risk for child abuse.
- Describe the short- and long-term effects of child abuse on the child and other members of the family.
- Identify the responsibilities of the nurse who suspects child abuse.
- Describe the community resources available to violence-prone families.

In the ideal family, every family member is kind and considerate toward the others in the family. Everyone acts in loving ways toward each other. The parents respect, nurture, and support each other and each of their children. In times of crisis, the family members work together to resolve the difficulty. Everyone in the ideal family flourishes because his or her physical and emotional needs are met.

Although many families try, it is very difficult to be an ideal family. This is not an ideal world, and the stresses and worries of daily living can provoke even the best intentioned person to behave toward others in less-than-loving ways. Moreover, families are made up of all kinds of people. Some of these individuals have physical and emotional problems that can impair their ability to interact with others in positive and adaptive ways.

Possibly the most serious result of unhealthy interpersonal interactions within a family is family violence—the threatened or actual use of physical force by one family member against another. In a violence-prone family, anyone can be the target: a spouse, a child, a grandparent. But in the end the entire family is the victim.

Family violence has serious immediate and long-term effects on all members of the family. The individual who is abused suffers mental and physical injury, possibly death. Children who witness violence often come to accept its use and often perpetuate it in their adult relationships. If the abuse comes to the attention of the legal system, the abuser may face charges of criminal assault and a jail sentence. In cases of child abuse, the children may be removed from their parents' care and placed in foster homes.

Family violence occurs in some form in more than half of the households in the United States (Mott et al 1985). It occurs in families of all races, religions, and socioeconomic and educational levels. The family may be loosely structured with unclear role differentiation, or it may be highly structured, with rigid, traditional, patriarchal roles. The adults in these families seldom share power or make decisions jointly or equally. Communication is poor, and partners often send hidden or double messages. Children may be overprotected and treated with extreme attention and love by one partner or neglected by both parents. Children may become the parents' scapegoats and may be subjected to harsh discipline and abuse.

Types of Family Violence

The most common types of family violence are spouse abuse and child abuse. Spouse abuse is the physical and/or emotional battering of one partner, typically the woman, by the other. The exact incidence of wife abuse and battering in North America is unknown. Official statistics indicate that one out of ten women is abused by the man with whom she lives, but experts believe this figure underestimates the problem. The actual ratio may be closer to one in five. One study estimated that one of every six couples engages in violence at least once a year, and that over the course of a marriage, the chances that a couple will come to blows are greater than one in four (Straus et al 1980).

Child abuse refers to physical, emotional, or sexual harm done to a child either by the child's parents or caretakers or by older siblings. As with spouse abuse, the exact incidence of child abuse is unknown. Estimates range as high as six cases per 1000 live births (Heins 1984). The incidence of sexual abuse is estimated to be between 100,000 and 360,000 cases each year (Ledray 1986).

Historical Factors Contributing to Family Violence

Family violence is not new. Wife battering is as old as the institution of marriage. Child abuse, ranging from neglect to infanticide, has occurred in almost every society.

Throughout history, both wives and children were considered "property." A woman was the property of her husband; he had the "right"—even the duty—to "keep her in line," even to kill her. Outsiders "kept out of it"; battering was a family matter.

Children were the property of their parents. Parents had the right to send their children to work in unsafe conditions, to transfer ownership to others as in child slavery or arranged marriages, even to dispose of them if they wished (Mott et al 1985). Severe disciplinary measures used by parents were acceptable and considered family business.

The legal status of women and children has improved over the years. Even so, in some states it is still legal to administer corporal punishment to children in school. And many people still hold on to the traditional views of male dominance in marriage, which can contribute to the occurrence of spouse abuse (Gelles & Cornell 1985).

Spouse Abuse

Spouse abuse, particularly wife battering, is the most common form of violence in the United States but the least reported serious crime (Mahon 1981). The women's movement and heightened public sensitivity to violence against women have stimulated recognition of the extent of this problem.

Spouse abuse may take many forms:

- Verbal attacks and insults
- Emotional deprivation and aggravation
- Social isolation and economic deprivation
- Intellectual derision and ridicule
- Sexual demands or deprivation
- Physical pain and injury

According to Walker (1979, p xv), a battered woman is one who

> is repeatedly subjected to any physical or psychological behavior by a man . . . without any concern for her rights. Battered women include wives or women in any form of intimate relationships with men [and] the couple must go through the battering cycle at least twice.

Wife abuse and battering occur in all ages, races, lifestyles, socioeconomic groups, educational levels, and occupations. One study (Straus et al 1980), however, found that battering is more prevalent among lower income groups, urban families, blue-collar workers, minority racial groups, people who have not completed high school, families in which the husband is unemployed, families with more than three children, and individuals with no religious affiliation. It is likely that the problem of battering is simply better hidden among the middle- and higher-income groups, where women have access to private health care providers, psychiatrists, and attorneys.

Contributing Factors

Spouse abuse is a result of the complex and dynamic interaction of social, cultural, political, and psychologic factors. Mahon (1981) identified these factors as follows:

- *Childhood experiences.* Children who witness or experience abuse and battering are more likely to become batterers (males) or to be abused (females) in their own marriages.

- *Sex role conditioning.* Females are socialized to believe they are inferior, inadequate, and dependent on males for approval. Women are expected to seek male approval by being nurturing and submissive. Males are socialized to expect this of females and to be financially successful, aggressive, and independent.

- *Economic insecurity of women.* Women receive less education and fewer job skills than men. Those with children are financially dependent on their husbands because their own earning power is limited.

- *Fear of humiliation.* Family members, friends, and neighbors may think the woman brought this on herself or may not understand why she does not leave the batterer. These personal supports may desert the battered woman in fear of their own safety.

- *Ages of children.* Families with young children are subject to more stress and demands; mothers depend on their husbands for economic and emotional support for themselves and their children.

- *Institutional indifference.* Law enforcement personnel, social service agencies, and the judicial system do not understand. They feel frustrated and impotent when battered women repeatedly return to their husbands.

- *Sociocultural tolerance of family violence.* Belief in the sacredness and privacy of the family has contributed to the lack of intervention by legal, social, and medical agencies (Lichtenstein 1981).

- *Malperception of inequity of power.* Men who perceive they lack power or resources in their homes or jobs may feel the need to prove themselves and resort to violence against those they perceive as less powerful to assert their superiority.

- *Religious traditions.* Most religions support the inferiority of women and believe that women should be dependent on their husbands. Laws and statutes based on these doctrines protect battering husbands from prosecution. Religion supports patriarchy, which is written into the laws and economic system to enforce the order of society.

Common Myths About Battering and Battered Women

Numerous myths about battering and battered women are believed by both professionals and the public. These myths often reinforce misunderstanding of battering and perpetuate the problem by keeping battered women silent. Myths range from the belief that the battered woman is a passive, innocent victim to the belief that she asked for and desires the beating. Professionals who provide services for battered women need to recognize and counteract these myths. Some commonly accepted myths are discussed here.

Battering occurs in a small percentage of the population. The statistics on reported cases underrepresent the true incidence. Battering is a seriously underreported crime: It generally occurs at night, in the home, and without witnesses. It is estimated that only one in ten women report battering assaults.

Battering is a lower-class problem. It is true that lower-class families have a higher incidence of battering (Gelles 1979) and are more likely to have contact with community agencies concerning this problem, but wife abuse also occurs in middle- and upper-income families. Lower-class families have more unemployment and less education and may have a tradition of expressing anger physically rather than verbally. Middle- and upper-class women may hide their batterings.

Battered women are masochistic. The myth that only women who "like it and deserve it" are beaten has been perpetuated by studies with erroneous conclusions. For example, Gelles (1974) reported that abuse frequently occurs when the woman provokes the man through verbal attacks, name-calling, and/or physical attack. An older study of 12 families that had been in court on wife abuse charges reported that wife abuse was related to the woman's masochistic needs and her aggressive, efficient, masculine, sexually frigid behavior, which triggered role reversal and the wife's need to be punished for her castrating activity (Snell et al 1964). This study suggested that women should try to change their behavior; be less provocative, aggressive, and frigid; and try to please their men.

These conclusions have perpetuated myths that cloud the issues. Since the women in the study had been subjected to years of abuse, the researchers might instead have concluded that women may provoke their husbands to release tension that, if left unchecked, might lead to a more severe beating and possibly death. A minor beating as the tension builds up is less damaging. The aggressiveness of the women might be interpreted as an attempt to ward off further assaults. "Frigidity" is hardly an unlikely response to years of severe beatings, psychologic abuse, and sexual injury. Unfortunately, some women believe that they are solely responsible for their marriages, their spouse's happiness, and their children. When their husbands repeatedly tell them they are failing in these roles, the women believe them and think they deserve to be punished and beaten.

Battered women provoke males to beat them; women push men beyond the breaking point and incite physical violence. As noted previously, some women who have been through the cycle of violence may provoke their husbands to relieve the tension and prevent a more severe beating if the tension escalates unchecked (Walker 1979). In other cases, Mahon (1981) observed that battered women blamed their husbands for their beatings and tried to distance themselves from them and others. These women had difficulty understanding that their silence and distancing maneuvers were part of the interplay that may have led to violent behavior; they tended to blame outside sources such as alcohol or their husband's unemployment. These blaming but aloof patterns of battered women can also contribute to violent scenes and continued battering.

It must be recognized that people are individually responsible for their behavior: Batterers lose self-control because of their own internal inadequacies and not because of what the women did or did not do. To accept responsibility for another's actions or to place the blame entirely on another person negates each individual's responsibility in an interaction.

Alcohol and drug abuse cause battering. Studies do show a relationship between battering incidents and alcohol use by batterers. In many cases alcohol is viewed as the primary trigger precipitating the battering. However, alcohol use may be an underlying problem in the relationship. Gelles (1976) proposed that batterers use alcohol as an excuse to carry out a violent act and shift the blame from themselves to the alcohol. Others suggest that alcohol reduces the batterers' inhibitions, increasing the likelihood of violent acts. Battered women often blame the violence on the batterer's drunkenness and think that the abuse will stop if their husbands stop drinking. Unfortunately, this usually does not happen.

Battered women were battered children. This myth holds true in only a few cases. Most women report that their husbands were the first person to beat them. Many battered women, however, were exposed to sex-role stereotyping that reinforced their own belief in their inability to take care of themselves. Consequently, they assumed a dependent role with men.

Battered women can easily leave the situation. Leaving is easier said than done. Women assume they are responsible for their marriages and children; they may still love their husbands, rely on them for financial support, and feel their children need a father. Usually battered women have been psychologically abused and have come to believe that family problems are their fault. They usually have isolated themselves from family, friends, and agencies that could assist them. They may fear retaliation and more severe beatings from their husbands if they leave. Many women with children have no place to go, and shelters have long waiting lists.

Batterers and battered women cannot change. If psychosocial learning theory is accurate, both batterers and battered women can be resocialized and can learn more effective ways of relating and interacting. Batterers can learn to verbalize their feelings, rechannel their aggressions, and accept the fact that women are not their property to punish or beat. Battered women can be resocialized to recognize their self-worth and develop assertive skills. They can learn to relate with men in more productive ways.

Characteristics of Battered Women

Battered women have similar histories of sex-role stereotyping in childhood. Many were raised to be submissive, passive, and dependent and to seek approval from male figures. Whereas some battered women were exposed to domestic violence between their parents, others first experience it from their husbands. Battered women are likely to accept the traditional female role in their marriage and believe their husbands will love and protect them. As traditionalists, they believe in family unity and accept prescribed female sex-role stereotypes, believing it is a woman's responsibility to keep her man happy. They believe that they are responsible for the marriage; they have an investment in it and want to make it work. If the marriage fails, they think they have failed as women, that it is their fault, and that their "punishment" is justified. This sex-role conditioning leads women to accept anything, even physical abuse, to keep their marriages intact.

Battered women typically attribute their beatings to some personal shortcoming or inadequacy. Battered women report that they believed their partners' insults and accusations of being bad wives and negligent mothers. As these women become more isolated, it becomes harder for them to judge who is right. Convinced that they are to blame, they find it easier to admit their guilt than to confront their husbands. For years the men they love and trust have been telling them how bad or incompetent they are. Eventually they fully believe in their inadequacy; they are psychologically destroyed. They feel worthless. Their low self-esteem reinforces their belief that they deserve to be beaten.

Many battered women do not work outside the home. They are isolated from their families, friends, and neighbors and totally dependent on their husbands for financial and emotional needs. Their extreme dependency makes them their husbands' victims. They do not believe they can be independent or self-sufficient.

After repeated beatings, a woman's self-esteem is virtually nonexistent. She feels depressed and guilty about the situation over which she has no control. Her sense of hopelessness and helplessness reduces her problem-solving ability. Women who have depended on others most of their lives often feel incapable of handling their abusive situation. Ignorance of available resources and personal despondency further contribute to their sense of powerlessness. Mahon (1981) found that battered women have a low tolerance for frustration, are easily upset, critical, aloof, and reserved. Although their intellectual functioning is diminished, they prefer to make their own decisions. Years of beatings contribute to a form of psychologic paralysis—an inability to see any options of escape.

Battered women often feel a pervasive, undefined guilt. They may internalize their anger at their husbands and the situation into depression or may express it indirectly with severe stress reactions and psychophysiologic symptoms. Some women live in constant fear that their husbands will strike again more severely than the last time or that they will strike the children. Fear permeates the woman's every action; she feels she cannot trust anyone because she no longer can trust the man who supposedly loves and protects her. Fear becomes part of her daily life because she knows that the slightest provocation, suspicion, or jealousy may incite another attack. Caught between their terror of remaining in the home and fear of the unknown if they leave, trapped by psychologic paralysis and complete dependency on their husbands, some women attempt suicide. Of all family conflicts, battering is the most frequent cause of female suicide attempts (Sherman 1983).

Characteristics of Batterers

Men who beat women may have been raised in families where beating and violence were commonly accepted, males reigned supreme, and the mother and sisters were treated as inferior. As children these batterers may have used violence to solve problems.

Batterers come from any profession, occupation, or socioeconomic group. One study (Stark et al 1981) showed a relatively high incidence of batterers among truck drivers but also among policemen and doctors—the very professionals to whom battered women turn for assistance (MacLeod 1980). Batterers often have lower educational and occupational levels than their wives, which may contribute to their feelings of inadequacy, inferiority, and insecurity. Battering is also more common in families where the husband is experiencing difficulty at work or is unemployed.

Many of the frustrations that abusive men cannot handle are related to their jobs, their perceptions of themselves and their wives, and their inability to achieve their goals. Their feelings of socioeconomic inferiority, powerlessness, and helplessness conflict with their assumptions of male supremacy. Emotionally immature or aggressive men may express these overwhelming feelings of inadequacy through violence.

Many batterers feel undeserving of their wives, yet they blame and punish the very person they value. They characteristically express their ambivalence by alternating episodes of unmerciful beatings with periods of remorse and loving attention. Extremes in behavior and overreacting are typical patterns.

Battered women often describe their husbands as lacking respect toward women in general, having come from broken homes or an unhappy childhood, and having a hidden rage that erupts into anger occasionally. Batterers accept conventional "macho" values, yet when they are not angry or aggressive, they appear childlike, dependent, and in need of nurturing. This dual personality of batterers reflects the conflict between their belief that they must live up to their macho image and their feelings of inadequacy and insecurity in the role of husband or provider. Combined with their immature personality and poor impulse control, their pervasive sense of powerlessness leads them to strike out at life's inequities by abusing women.

The Battered Woman and the Role of the Nurse

Increased publicity and public sensitivity and heightened awareness of women's rights are encouraging battered women to leave their homes and seek shelter and community assistance. During the 1970s, many cities in the United States developed programs, shelters, and resources for battered women. State and federal funds have assisted these efforts, but the needs of battered women and their children are insufficiently met in most communities.

Battered women enter the health care system in many different settings. Nurses may see these women in the phy-

sician's office with minor trauma or in the emergency room with multiple severe injuries. Battered women are frequently seen in obstetric services since battering often begins and occurs more frequently during a woman's pregnancy. Nurses in psychiatric–mental health services frequently counsel women who have been battered, and community health nurses may find battered women during home visits (Tilden & Shepherd 1987). Unfortunately, emergency rooms, hospitals, and social service agencies do not routinely recognize and report battering cases to the legal authorities for action and followup, although some states are initiating this policy.

Wife abuse is a major social problem that ignorance and lack of resources allow to continue. Society and health professionals must move beyond mere recognition of the problem to develop a better understanding of the dynamics of battering. Nurses can intervene in the cycle of violence by helping battered women recognize their options and take appropriate action.

THE NURSE'S ATTITUDES AND CHARACTERISTICS

Nurses in many different health care settings often come in contact with battered and abused women but fail to recognize them, especially if their bruises are not visible. Nurses who wish to help battered women need advanced knowledge of the dynamics of battered women, assessment skills for recognizing subtle cues of battering, and appropriate intervention skills in counseling and referral. Nurses should be sensitive to battered women's problems and able to tolerate their own empathic feelings of fear and terror as battered women describe their violent experiences and abusive situations. Finley (1981, p 12) stated that "if the nurse cannot tolerate the feelings of terror . . . [in] the empathic process, the nurse-client interaction will be counterproductive." Other skills required by the nurse include compassion, a sense of reality, and a sense of humor, along with the ability to set limits in decision making. Lichtenstein (1981, p 243) suggested that nurses assess their feelings about helping battered women cope by asking themselves:

1. To what extent am I meeting my own personal needs rather than those of the client?

2. Do my feelings include inappropriate ones such as pity and a sense of helplessness?

3. Am I inadvertently attempting to cope with my feelings about a person's level of progress by withdrawing, blaming her, prematurely confronting her, or prematurely pressuring her to make a decision?

4. Do I believe that she has the resources, strength, interests, and abilities to mobilize herself sufficiently to cope constructively with her difficulties?

Working with battered women is often frustrating, and many health care providers feel impotent when these women repeatedly return to their abusive situations without developing sufficient ego strength or coping abilities. Many health care workers are reluctant to become involved, knowing that battered women require long-term assistance and counseling, often for many years, before they are able to change or leave the situation. They become frustrated by spending their time and energy assisting women who remain in a violent situation and then return to the agency in a few months in worse condition than before. Nurses must realize that they cannot rescue battered women; these women must decide on their own how to handle the situation. The effective nurse provides battered women with information that may assist them in decision making and supports their decision, knowing that incremental assistance over the years may be the only alternative until they are ready to explore other options.

NURSING ASSESSMENT

Victims of family violence may be clients in any setting, yet they are difficult to identify because they rarely admit their problems. Women who are at high risk of battering often have a history of alcohol or drug abuse, child abuse, or abuse in the previous or present marriage. Other signs of possible abuse include:

- Unequal power in decision making between husband and wife (the authoritarian male)

- Expressions of helplessness and powerlessness: an attitude that the woman lacks control over her life

- Low self-esteem, as seen in the woman's dress, her appearance, and the way she relates to health care providers

- Signs of depression in remarks about fatigue, hopelessness, and somatic problems

During the assessment of female clients, the nurse should be alert to the following cues of abuse:

- *Hesitancy in providing detailed information about the injury and how it occurred.* The woman may appear timid and evasive and may avoid eye contact; she may seem embarrassed about having been injured.

- *Inappropriate affect for the situation.* The woman may appear overly frightened, disoriented, or depressed over minor injuries. She may display extremes in behavior by minimizing the importance of significant injuries or appearing fragile with minor injuries.

- *Delayed reporting of symptoms.* Considerable time may elapse between the injury and the woman's seeking treatment. She may have waited until the batterer left home to come in for treatment, or she may have hoped that her symptoms would disappear.

- *Types and sites of injuries.* The usual injuries are bruises, abrasions, or contusions to the head (eyes and back of neck), throat, chest, breast, abdomen, or genitals. Usually there are multiple injury sites. Nonbattered women's injuries are usually located at one or two sites and on the extremities such as sprains and strains.

- *Inappropriate explanation.* The woman's account of the cause does not fit the type and location of the injuries; the story just does not fit the injury. She may state she fell down the stairs or walked into a door, although she has abrasions and contusions around her eyes and throat.

- *Increased anxiety in the presence of the possible batterer.* The woman may look to him for approval before answering questions about her injury and its cause. He may hang around her, appear reluctant to leave her alone for fear she will talk, or demand to be present during the examination.

The nurse who suspects a woman has been abused or beaten should try to interview and counsel her in a quiet, safe place, away from the man or anyone else who brought her in. Different approaches to verify battering can be used by the nurse. Lichtenstein (1981) suggested obtaining an extensive history of family communication patterns, arguments, and conflict resolution; her article provides an excellent list of history questions. Other nurses prefer to share their observations concerning the inconsistency of the injuries with the nature of the cause, hoping the woman will change her story and admit to being beaten. Some nurses wait until the woman is willing to say she has been beaten, whereas others prefer direct confrontation and may ask, "Have you ever been physically hurt by anyone?" Nurses can analyze the woman's behavior and their own feelings to determine the most appropriate and effective approach.

The assessment of the woman should include information about her strengths and support system. Strengths may include education, employment history, activities in the home, community involvement, and her ability to cope or handle past problems. The woman's support system may include her family, friends, neighbors, and community agencies or organizations.

During the assessment phase, the nurse begins building a relationship with the woman based on trust, understanding, and advocacy. A woman may feel ashamed and embarrassed about her injuries and situation. She must be assured that all information she provides will be kept confidential. Trust begins as the nurse conveys an attitude of unconditional acceptance, empathy, and positive regard for the woman's worth and dignity. The woman may need to be asked or given permission to discuss her problems before she shares them. Asking questions with sensitivity is better than avoiding the issues. A gentle, firm approach is useful. Nurses should show that they recognize the woman's feelings and that they accept her right to feel as she does. If and when a woman reveals that she has been beaten, she may begin crying and pouring out details of her years of abuse. Empathic listening, support, and possibly some light nourishment, such as coffee, tea, or a soft drink with crackers, may be helpful.

NURSING DIAGNOSIS

Analysis of the woman's history and physical examination reveals patterns that may lead the nurse to suspect abuse and battering. If the woman's story of how she received her injuries is inconsistent with her symptoms, the nurse should record the woman's statements and the evidence, noting that the inconsistency suggests *possible* abuse and that further follow-up is recommended. The nurse can write in the chart, "injuries are inconsistent with her account of the accident" or "injuries are consistent with assault" if that is the case or "She denies being beaten" if the woman was asked directly and so responded.

In cases where the woman states she has been beaten, kicked, punched, or attacked but does not identify the assailant, the nurse should record the extent of injuries, note the woman's exact words, and describe the incident with a diagnosis of *probable* battering. Those cases in which the woman states she was beaten by a husband or mate may be diagnosed as *battering* with all evidence recorded, including the woman's statements.

When abuse or battering is suspected or determined, the nurse should formulate nursing diagnoses based on the assessment findings. Nursing diagnoses related to non-physical components of abuse or battering may be:

● Disturbance in self-concept related to feelings of worthlessness and powerlessness

● Knowledge deficit related to available community resources secondary to social isolation

NURSING GOAL: TO PROVIDE PSYCHOLOGIC AND EMOTIONAL SUPPORT

When a battered woman comes in for treatment, she needs to feel safe physically and safe in talking about her injuries and problems. If a man is with her, ask or tell him to wait in the waiting room while you examine the woman. This may reduce her fear, help establishing trust, and facilitate her expressions of guilt, shame, and embarrassment, along with pent-up anger, rage, and terror about her battering situation. Anger may be directed toward herself, the batterer, or health professionals.

A battered woman also needs to reestablish a feeling of control over her world. She needs to regain a sense of predictability by knowing what to expect and how she can interact. The nurse should provide sufficient information about what to expect in terms the woman can understand and assimilate. Simple explanations about how long she will stay, whom she will see, and what will be done are important. Some women ask no questions, whereas others produce a barrage of questions. Giving the woman control can be accomplished by asking her permission to do simple tasks and providing her with choices whenever possible. Inform her that her record will be kept confidential and not released or seen by anyone outside the hospital or agency without her permission.

The nurse encourages the woman to talk about her injuries and home situation by asking, "How did this happen to you?" or saying, "We often see injuries like yours when a woman has been beaten. Has this happened to you?" Directly confronting the injuries and possible battering may provide the opening for the woman who is trying to cope in private; she may feel less ashamed and frightened when offered this lead in a relaxed, supportive, and nonjudgmental manner. A woman may continue to deny her battering if she has resigned herself to living with the situation.

Supportive counseling and reassurance are professional skills nurses use throughout each phase of the nursing process with a battered woman. The nurse:

● Lets the woman work through her story, problems, and situation at her own pace

● Anticipates her ambivalence in the love-hate relationship with the batterer; after all, she knows he may be loving and contrite after the incident if she has been through the cycle of violence before

● Respects the woman's capacity to change and grow when she is ready

● Assists her in identifying specific problems and supports realistic ideas for reducing or eliminating those problems

● Helps clarify her beliefs and myths and provides information to change her false beliefs

For example, if the woman feels that she is responsible for or deserves the beating, the nurse assures her that her husband or male friend is totally responsible for his own actions and that she cannot be held responsible for another person's behavior. If the woman thinks that all men beat their women and that there is no way to avoid this problem, the nurse explains that this is not so and that both people in a relationship can change. If the woman thinks that she is the only one who is beaten, the nurse tells her that many women are battered and that until recently their problems were ignored, but that now various community agencies are available to assist battered women. If, having been through the cycle of violence, a woman thinks her husband will change, the nurse tells her that the abuse and beatings usually continue to get worse over time until the woman takes the initiative and changes the situation with the help of community resources. If a woman continues to see the positive side of the family situation, such as that the marriage is still intact; the children have a father, home, and food; and she loves the man, she needs to examine the benefits and consequences of remaining in the situation. The appropriate intervention is not to tell her what to do but to help her recognize her options and resources and exercise her own decisions. Advising or encouraging a woman to leave an abusive situation is not always in the woman's best interest; leaving the home is a major decision with long-lasting consequences. The woman may be economically unable to leave the situation, especially if she has young children. If the woman leaves prematurely and subsequently returns home, both husband and wife may become more frustrated, increasing the possibility of further beatings and even homicide. The most acceptable course of action is the one that woman freely chooses.

NURSING GOAL: TO PROVIDE INFORMATION ABOUT COMMUNITY RESOURCES

Besides offering emotional support, medical treatment, and counseling, the nurse should inform any woman she suspects may be in an abusive situation of the services available in the hospital, agency, and community. Battered women have many needs that require the assistance and coordination of different community agencies. Unfortunately, many battered women are unaware of community agencies that can assist them.

Battered woman may need:

● Medical treatment for injuries

● Temporary shelter to provide a safe environment for themselves and their children

● Counseling to raise their self-esteem and assist them in understanding the dynamics of family violence

● Legal assistance for protection and/or prosecution

● Financial assistance to provide shelter, food, and clothing

● Job training or employment counseling

● An ongoing support group with counseling on relationships with males and children

A network of community agencies can meet these numerous, varied needs of women, children, and batterers. Employees in these agencies must understand the complex dynamics of family violence and wife battering as well as how their services and those of other agencies can assist these families.

○ **EMERGENCY ROOM SERVICES** Many battered women are first seen and diagnosed in the emergency rooms of their neighborhood hospitals. One study (Stark et al 1981) reported that 21 percent of all women seen in the surgical emergency service were battered, yet medical personnel correctly diagnosed only 4 percent of those as battered women.

Emergency room nurses and personnel need to be alert to symptoms of battering, recognize these cues, and encourage women to seek assistance from community agencies. Some states require that suspected cases of abuse and battering be reported to the legal authorities or social service agencies.

○ **SHELTER AND HOUSING** Since family violence has been recognized as a major social problem, many community agencies have sought federal and state funds to provide needed services and shelters. Most shelters have a long waiting list, however, and many women must remain in an abusive situation until there is room for them and their children.

Shelters differ in the services they provide, depending on the governing body, financial resources and funding agencies, organizational structure, staff qualifications, and range of available community services. Typical shelters provide battered women and their children with a room, beds, food, clothing, and other basic necessities. If professional staff are available, the shelter may offer crisis counseling, individual and group counseling or therapy, and information about and networking with community agencies such as legal aid, welfare, job training, financial and employment agencies, and women's counseling or support groups.

For safety reasons, the location of most shelters is undisclosed, but they can be contacted through a community crisis line. Unfortunately, admission requirements usually state that the woman must have been beaten in the past; this eliminates those women in potentially violent situations until they have been beaten.

○ **LEGAL SERVICES AND OPTIONS** During incidents of domestic violence, the police are frequently called by the victim or neighbors. Family violence typically occurs on the weekend or in late evening when most social service agencies are closed; therefore the police department is often the first major agency involved. Few police officers are trained to intervene in domestic violence disputes, and many dislike responding to these calls, which are extremely dangerous and often result in death or injury to police officers (Sherman 1983). Many police officers do not understand the complex dynamics of family violence. They may fear for their own safety, believe that they should only go in and defuse the situation, and feel that these calls are not important because they seldom arrest anyone and most women do not press charges. Because an officer must see the crime committed before arresting anyone on misdemeanor charges and wife beating occurs in the privacy of the home before the police arrive, the police usually just warn the batterer to cool down. This leaves the woman in a more vulnerable position for having sought outside assistance.

Legal options for battered women vary according to state laws and services. In some states a woman may seek a restraining order from the family court or a domestic relations court to protect herself from the batterer. This restraining order specifies that the man may not physically abuse his wife or other family members but does not give the man a criminal record. If the battered woman decides to prosecute, the case is usually heard in criminal court, which handles crimes of assault, harassment, and battery. Criminal court hearings may result in a fine, probation, and/or a jail sentence if the batterer is convicted; then the male would have a criminal record. The prosecution process is often lengthy and may last more than a year. Some state judicial systems are introducing more lenient options such as mandatory counseling for batterers in lieu of prosecution. Divorce is another legal recourse a woman may choose, but divorce may take several months to a year. Although alimony and child support may be awarded, there is no guarantee that the woman will receive either. National statistics report that less than 25 percent of mothers receive full child support payments.

Most battered women are unaware of their legal options. They fear further beatings if they prosecute the batterer. Limited financial resources may also keep them from seeking legal assistance. Some women do not understand the complex judicial process and their options within it. Therefore, few battered women press charges against the batterer, so their fear and vulnerability to repeated beatings continue, with minimal assistance from the police and legal system. Some communities provide legal advocacy services to help battered women understand the judicial process and its consequences to the woman, children, and batterer.

○ *FINANCIAL SERVICES* Once battered women leave their homes or seek legal assistance, they usually receive no financial support from the batterer. Without funds, battered women and their children are at the mercy of community social service agencies, and it usually takes weeks for papers to be processed before any money is forthcoming. Agencies that may provide financial assistance to battered women include welfare, Aid to Dependent Children, United Way, women's support groups, religious organizations, and possibly the Salvation Army. There may be other local groups to assist these women in various ways such as providing food or clothing.

○ *EMPLOYMENT TRAINING OR PLACEMENT* Many battered women are full-time mothers who lack advanced education, training, and job experience. High unemployment rates, minimal skills, and inadequate transportation make it difficult for these women to obtain employment with an adequate salary. Women who have children must consider where to place them during working hours as well as the added cost of child care. Often the woman's choice is restricted to accepting welfare or taking a low-paying job. Either choice usually means lowering the standard of living to subsistence. Avoiding beatings at such a cost may not seem like a viable option.

Some women do seek job training if the opportunities are available, but training provides no guarantee of future job placement. A woman may still have to arrange for financial support and child care while obtaining advanced employment skills or an education.

○ *COUNSELING* Battered women may need a variety of counseling services, such as crisis intervention, short-term individual therapy, group therapy, or peer support groups, over an extended period. Counseling and therapy may be provided by nurses, social workers, psychologists, mental health specialists, or clergy with special training.

EVALUATION

After interacting with a battered woman, the nurse may wonder how to judge the effectiveness of her actions. It is helpful to remember that the average battered woman endures the situation for years before seeking meaningful assistance. The nurse may see the woman at the beginning of this long process when she is not yet ready to change her situation. Most women return home in resignation after each battering. Some seek temporary shelter several times before taking final steps to change their situation.

It takes a long time for a woman to concede that life may be better outside the battering situation and that there are effective ways to change the situation. Each woman must plan her own life when she has sufficient strength and knowledge of her options and consequences. The nurse should remember that if the woman decides to return home, it is the woman's decision and not the nurse's problem. Having recognized the battered woman, provided counsel, and properly referred her, the nurse has planted the seed for release from the cycle of violence. The seed may lie dormant for years; at a critical moment in the woman's life, it may sprout and change her life.

● Child Abuse

One of the most disastrous results of dysfunctional parenting is child abuse. Child abuse arises in part from the cultural sanctioning of physical discipline of children by their parents. Among the many serious effects of child abuse are physical handicaps, poor self-image, inability to love others, antisocial or violent behavior in later life, and death.

A small number of abusing parents are mentally ill, but most abusing parents have less serious problems that respond to intervention. Parents at risk for abusive behavior may manifest one or more of the risk factors identified in Table 5–1.

Patterns of Abuse

Child abusers are found among all socioeconomic, religious, and ethnic groups. Some child abusers are irrational or even psychotic, but most are ordinary people who feel trapped in stressful life situations with which they cannot cope satisfactorily. Many abusive parents are simply confused and overwhelmed by parenthood or by life in general and vent their frustrations on their children. Because all parents have negative feelings about their children at one time or another, the difference between parents who abuse and those who do not is often only a matter

of degree. All parents are at risk occasionally, but most parents are able to channel their frustrations and anger appropriately.

The parent with a potential for abuse is one who feels isolated, is unable to trust others, has no spouse, is too passive to be able to give, or has very unrealistic expectations for children. Parents at risk for abuse tend to expect their children to perform for their gratification, and they tend to use severe physical punishment to ensure a child's proper behavior (Kempe and Helfer 1972). As mentioned earlier, parents who abuse their children are likely to have been abused as children. This multigenerational pattern of child abuse, although disturbing, does help in identifying families in need of prevention.

Many abusive parents also have unrealistic expectations for themselves and unknowingly contribute to their problems. For example, one parent waxed the kitchen floor during a snowstorm and then abused the child who tracked mud into the house. The parent's behavior and expectations for the child clearly contributed to the problem.

Parents with a potential for abuse often expect their children to meet their needs and therefore are most likely to abuse a child who is viewed as "different." Young chil-

Table 5–1   Parental Risk Factors for Child Abuse

Risk Factor	Assessment Findings
Lack of nurturing experience	Inadequate experience with parenting (eg, multiple foster homes) Neglect or abuse as a child High demands of parents as a child
Lack of knowledge of normal growth and development	Inability to read "cues" of child Impatience when child does not respond as expected; unreasonable discipline Unrealistically high expectations for the child
Isolation	Inadequate use of supports Inability to identify resources Lack of acquaintance in community
Low self-esteem	Lack of trust, particularly of authority figures Expectations of rejection
High vulnerability to criticism	History of family violence in family of origin or in current family system (eg, spouse abuse) Low tolerance for frustration Impulsiveness
Many unmet needs	Feelings of being unloved or having unresponsive spouse, unstable marriage, or no marriage at all Youthful marriage, forced marriage, unwanted pregnancy
Multiple stressors	Poverty, unemployment, substandard housing, lack of job opportunities Inadequate clothing and insufficient food
Substance abuse	Abuse of alcohol or drugs
Role reversal	Emotional immaturity, lack of patience, inability to make judgments Preoccupation with self Depression Dependence on others

Source: Adapted from Mott SR, Fazekas NF, and James SR, *Nursing Care of Children and Families*, Menlo Park, Calif, Addison-Wesley, 1985.

dren are sometimes targets for abuse, as are high-risk infants, who are often unresponsive to parental attention.

Other children most at risk of abuse might be the result of difficult pregnancies or deliveries, born at inconvenient times, born out of wedlock, the "wrong" sex, or too active or too passive. Some children are abused because they are the result of a forced pregnancy with an unloved partner or the result of rape or incest. Others have characteristics, such as looks and mannerisms, that evoke negative associations in the abusing parent. Children who have been separated from their families because of prematurity or neonatal disease are more likely to be at risk for abuse. Children with congenital anomalies, mental retardation, hyperactivity, or chronic illness are also at risk. Children with abnormal sleep-wake patterns or feeding difficulties and those who are unresponsive to caregiving might also be at risk if they are living in a family with other risk factors (Steele 1980). Only a small percentage of premature or difficult children, however, are abused, and for all abused children, it is the combination of parental deficiencies and characteristics of the child that create the problems leading to abuse.

Child abuse is most likely to occur during times of crisis. The parent's loss of a job, for example, might be just enough to make the crying of a fretful infant unbearable. Some families hover on the brink of perpetual crisis, living with constant changes that contribute to feelings of inadequacy. The magnitude of the crisis is not always in proportion to the abuse. A relatively minor crisis might be viewed as the "last straw" in an unhappy situation.

Solving a crisis for troubled families is not enough if new crises and stressors merely reestablish dysfunctional patterns. Instead, the nurse teaches parents to develop their own coping strategies and to identify when and how to seek help. Parents who learn the problems inherent in isolation, for example, will then seek assistance when under stress and will avoid the patterns of behavior that cause them to abuse their children.

Types of Abuse

PHYSICAL ABUSE

Physical injuries might resemble those caused by accidents, but child abuse should be suspected whenever a child's injury has no explanation or plausible reason. Children who sustain many injuries should be considered possible victims of abuse. The presence of fresh and old injuries suggest a series of traumatic events rather than a single accident. Another important clue is the distance from the child's home to the treatment facility because parents may go to distant facilities to escape detection.

Physical abuse might be obvious if marks on the child's body are inconsistent with a traumatic injury. Some of the more common injuries include localized burns on the buttocks caused by placing the child on a stove or radiator and circular extremity burns from immersion in hot water. The child might have slap marks resembling a handprint; welts from beatings with coat hangers, belts, or buckles; or circular abrasions on the wrists and ankles from being tied down. A particularly harmful practice is shaking the child vigorously, which can lead to a whiplash injury and even cause brain damage, especially in the young infant who has not developed good head control. Children who are thrown into a crib or against a wall might have signs of both fractures and dislocations. During infancy, the periosteum is less securely attached to the bone, which allows it to be stripped from the shaft by hemorrhage. Sometimes the abused child has a "paradox of clothing," which is the parent's attempt to hide the abuse by dressing the child in clothing such as a baptismal dress.

Physical abuse might result from overdiscipline or from punishment that is too severe. Some children are punished for behavior that is perfectly appropriate for the child's developmental stage but is not perceived as appropriate by the parent. For example, crying in the infant or toilet training in the toddler might precipitate abuse. Most parents who abuse their children have good intentions and really care about the welfare of their children. They might be trying to change the behavior of the child but overreact to stressors. Many abusive parents know that they need help but are afraid to ask for fear of losing their children to foster care.

EMOTIONAL ABUSE

Emotional abuse is most difficult to define and diagnose because its scars are hidden and because both the victim and abuser might not recognize the behavior as dysfunctional. Variations in parenting styles and cultural norms compound the problem of defining and documenting the abuse. In most instances the child is called foul names, ridiculed, and made to feel stupid, hated, ugly, unlovable, or unwanted. The parent might blatantly reject the child and demonstrate a consistent lack of concern for the child's welfare. Sometimes siblings or other family members are invited to join in the abuse, and the abused child becomes the family scapegoat.

Emotional abuse causes suffering and lasting effects on the development of the child's self-concept. Emotional abuse ultimately affects the child's future relationships with others, but because the scars are not obvious, its effects tend to be diagnosed only years after the event.

Most physical abuse is accompanied by some degree of emotional abuse, but the reverse is not always true. Some children receive only verbal abuse, but the sequelae can have far-reaching effects, especially if these children repeat the pattern when they become parents. The manifested results of emotional abuse typically are speech disorders, developmental delays, apathetic or hostile behaviors, and depression. Sucking, biting, rocking, or enuresis are common behaviors; also common are sleep disorders, unusual fearfulness, and play disturbances.

SEXUAL ABUSE

Sexual abuse is the exploitation of a child for the sexual gratification of an adult. Statistics reflecting its incidence are not available. Because secrecy and social taboos prevent cases from being reported and recorded, a "conspiracy of silence" often keeps victimized children from telling adults about the abuse, and the denial of some adults further contributes to the secrecy. Sexual abuse of children is essentially a crime of power in which an adult exploits the child's vulnerability. The behaviors are sexual, but the intent is domination rather than intimacy.

Sexual offenses against children fall into two general categories: (1) nontouching offenses and (2) touching offenses. Nontouching offenses include verbal sexual stimulation, obscene telephone calls, exhibitionism, voyeurism, and violations of privacy in which the child watches or hears an act of sexual intercourse. Touching offenses include fondling; vaginal, oral, or anal intercourse or attempted intercourse; touching of the genitals; incest; prostitution; and rape (Gorline & Ray 1979). Some forms of sexual exploitation use children to enhance adult sexual pleasures for profit. "Kiddie pornography," for instance, is a lucrative though illegal business.

Incest is a form of sexual abuse of a child by a family member. The adult might be a parent, stepparent, extended family member (such as a grandparent, aunt, or uncle), or surrogate parent figure (such as a foster parent or common-law spouse). Incest always occurs within the family system, but the presence or absence of a blood relationship is far less important than the parental role of the adult (Sgroi 1982). Most victims of incest are girls who are abused by older male relatives. Adults who commit incest often are family members in whom children have placed trust, and the power of the adult over the child contributes to the enforced secrecy.

Incest can have serious, long-term consequences for the child. The child usually feels guilty for participating and is afraid of disrupting the family by revealing the incestuous relationship, which further contributes to the child's anxiety (Meiselman 1978). Incest contributes to delinquency, substance abuse, prostitution, sexually transmitted disease, and unwanted pregnancies. Among runaway children 75 percent are said to be running from incest, and research suggests that 60 percent to 90 percent of prostitutes claim to have been sexually abused as children (Densen-Gerber & Hutchinson 1978).

Legal Aspects of Child Abuse

Child abuse is against the law, and the reporting of child abuse and neglect is governed by federal standards and regulations, state laws, and local policies and procedures. Most state statutes define child abuse and neglect and specify who must report, the form and content of the report, and to whom the report is sent. Because of the diversity in laws and state statutes, the nurse needs a copy of the applicable reporting form, laws, or position papers. Many states do not record sexual abuse as a separate offense. Some state statutes do not cover sexual abuse, and definitions of terms vary from state to state.

The purpose of all child abuse legislation is not to punish parents but to protect children and prevent further abuse or maltreatment. Inherent in all laws is the assumption that the best way to help most children is to help their families. In essence, everyone is a mandated reporter. State laws mandate that suspicions of abuse and neglect be reported. No state requires the reporter to have proof of neglect or abuse, but incidents must be reported as soon as they are noticed. Sound nursing practice therefore means being honest with the family and reporting findings promptly. It is not wise to attempt to work with the family independently or to give family members a warning or second chance (McKittrick 1981) because this might cause valuable time to be lost and contribute to additional risks. There are times when the second chance results in multiple severe injuries to or even the death of the child.

A report is not an accusation but a request for investigation. All persons who report suspected abuse or neglect are given immunity from criminal prosecution and civil liability if the report is made in good faith. Mandated reporters who fail to report can be fined as much as $1000. At issue, however, is the cost of failing to protect children. Because anonymous reports are not as valuable as those that are signed, a reporter should give name, title, and reason for the report.

If a report is made to a social work supervisor or school principal, the nurse verifies that an official report was made and not lost. The nurse can also ask for an update on the progress of the case and will want to do so in anticipation of future dealings with the family or child. The report cannot, however, violate family confidentiality. The only information needed is whether the family is receiving assistance and attempting to learn alternative methods of coping with stress. Personal or family problems revealed during counseling are not shared without the family's permission.

Despite all the publicity and concern, many cases of child abuse or neglect still go unreported. The reasons for not reporting abuse or neglect include the following:

1. Professional denial because the child or parent looks well or the nurse has known the family for a long

time and refuses to believe abuse and neglect could happen

2. Professional doubt about the nurse's role

3. Fear of retribution, perhaps because of a history of violence in the family

4. Lack of "belief in the system," especially if the family was previously reported with no subsequent improvement

5. Professional neglect or failure to understand that the risk to the child is increased when abuse or neglect is not reported

6. Conflict between professionals over the importance of reporting

DOCUMENTATION

In situations of child abuse and neglect, documentation of evidence is vital. Records provide the legal basis for intervening on behalf of the child. Nursing history and daily notes need to be accurate, timely, and objective. The goal of documentation is to provide a written account of each visit or contact. If the nursing records become part of a court proceeding, they need to portray a family by specifying behaviors that indicate progress or failure in providing a safe, nurturing environment for the child. In some neglect cases much of the evidence is intangible and difficult to prove; therefore, input from many professionals is necessary to convince the court that a child is actually at risk for abuse or neglect. Evidence of risk might include the doctor's and nurse's notes on the child, the school nurse's report, and the social worker's impressions during a home visit regarding the child's physical appearance; interactions with parents, peers, and other adults; ability to respond to questions; and general development. Evidence of neglect might include developmental delays, substance abuse, poor medical care, poor school attendance, or lack of supervision. Careful documentation and recorded evidence is essential when presenting a case to the judicial system.

INVESTIGATIONS

An investigation is a fact-finding process undertaken to determine whether child abuse or neglect has occurred. Each state has a designated agency that provides services on a 24-hour basis. Services must be initiated within 72 hours (and in most instances within 48 hours). Agencies receiving abuse reports might include the children's protective services, law enforcement agencies, juvenile courts, county health departments, and state or central registries. The initial investigation focuses on the risks involved, the

family dynamics, the nature of the incident or injury, and the duration of dysfunctional parenting. The investigation entails data collection by gathering evidence and interviewing parents and children separately. Verification of abuse or neglect might occur through an admission by the parent or offender or through medical or other factual evidence. Supportive services might be provided to the family if abuse or neglect is verified, and court intervention might be necessary if the child has serious injuries, the parent refuses to allow an investigation, the child is in immediate danger, or the risks do not diminish over time (Munro 1984).

Under criminal codes, abusive parents might be charged with violating a criminal law. If a child recovers from the injury, the customary charge is assault and battery; if the child dies, prosecution is generally for manslaughter rather than intentional homicide. Although most experts agree that the parents are more in need of therapy than imprisonment, jail sentences are common. Most child abuse cases, however, are referred to juvenile court or family court rather than to criminal court. Juvenile and family courts have the power to declare abused or neglected children dependent on the court for proper care and protection. They also might, if necessary, remove children from their parents until the home problems can be resolved and the family safely reunited. In a few situations in which the parents disappear or cannot be located for long periods of time, the court terminates parental rights. This extreme measure is a last resort taken only after repeated instances of severe abuse or long-term abandonment and no response to rehabilitative efforts (Munro 1984).

Support Services

Various innovative programs have been developed specifically for the treatment of child abuse and neglect. One of the earliest of these programs is SCAN (Suspected Child Abuse and Neglect) Volunteer Service, Inc, which was organized in 1972. SCAN volunteers provide emergency intervention as well as long-term counseling and supportive services. Parents are offered the alternative of working with SCAN or facing law enforcement officials and possible foster placement of the child. Various other programs are modeled after SCAN and are intended to rehabilitate both the child and parent and to hold the family together.

Many communities use public health nurses in the treatment of abusive parents so that care focuses on all family members and not just the abused child. Once the nurse and family have established goals, the nurse listens carefully to the parents and children and looks for signs of further risks of abuse.

In planning interventions, the long-term goals are usually to rehabilitate the dysfunctional family and to support and encourage normal development. Short-term goals are best planned together with family members, but the developmental needs of children must be the nurse's prime consideration.

Interventions may be accomplished both in and out of the child's home. If the child remains at home and the primary nurturing figure remains the natural parent, that parent also receives support. Treatment at home might include play therapy, recreational activities, homemaker services, Big Sisters or Big Brothers, and services for special dental, medical, nutritional, or remedial education needs. Other services might be provided outside the home while the child continues to live at home. The responsibility for care is then shared with the natural parent by crisis nurseries, day-care centers, respite care providers, and schools.

Homemaker services can provide cooking, cleaning, bed making, and laundry as a step toward improving the child's standard of living. The homemaker might also be a role model, confidante, and "friend" of the parent. Other intermittent services include special education, health care, and "emergency parents" for short-term crises or stressors such as illness within the family.

If the child is removed from the care of the natural parent, nurturance becomes the sole responsibility of a substitute care giver. Additional social services are then necessary, particularly if the child has special needs. These services might include shelters with temporary removal to a foster home or institution on a short-term basis, foster care, longer-term care oriented toward an ultimate return of the child to the original family, special care for physical disabilities or emotional disturbances, and guardianship or adoption, in which the child is permanently removed from the original home and custody is given to another care giver.

Multidisciplinary Management

Because many complex factors must be assessed in evaluating suspected or known cases of child abuse or neglect, no single professional group can render all necessary services to a child or family. A multidisciplinary team approach to diagnosis, planning, and intervention is best. Teams can pool expertise from various fields and provide integrated planning and delivery of services. A multidisciplinary team might be composed of a mental health worker, lawyer, nurse, social worker, police officer, physician, teacher, juvenile division worker, and hospital or ancillary personnel. Ancillary personnel might include receptionists, drivers, custodians, secretaries, nutritionists, homemakers, or child-care workers. Some are volunteers who may or may not have expertise and training. Most personnel working with abusive or neglectful families need orientation concerning typical behaviors that suggest mistrust of the system, lack of self-esteem, or hostility and anger.

Ancillary personnel can help professionals convince dysfunctional families that change is worthwhile and that they are worth the team's efforts. Ancillary personnel can also provide additional insight and collaboration in a decision-making process. Because each team member brings a different range of experiences and knowledge of dysfunctional families and successful treatment, each is called on to define needs and, if necessary, find legal grounds for intervention. Team involvement offers planning coordination and a way to offset the frustration that professionals feel when nothing helpful can be done.

Child Abuse and the Role of the Nurse

By the nature of their work, nurses in a variety of settings are involved in the identification, treatment, and prevention of child abuse and neglect. Nurses who see medical problems that suggest abuse or neglect or who see children and parents whose behavior indicates the potential for abuse or neglect are called on to collaborate with members of other disciplines in protecting children at risk and advocating care for both children and families. Because each family is part of a community system, nurses also need to be aware of community resources. Early detection of child abuse and neglect is essential to intervene and provide services to the child and family.

NURSING ASSESSMENT

Childhood accidents are a common source of injuries; thus every parent who brings a child in for treatment of an injury should not automatically be suspected of abuse. Certain physical and behavioral findings are indicative of abuse, however, and the nurse should be aware of these clues. Tables 5–2 and 5–3 list the findings indicative of physical and sexual abuse.

In all cases of suspected abuse or neglect, the nurse needs to ask the child and family members present the following questions:

1. How did the accident (or incident) happen?

2. When did the accident happen?

3. Where were the child and other family members at the time?

4. Who was caring for the child at the time?

5. Who saw the accident?

6. What did the child do after the accident?

7. What measures were taken by the parent?

After recording answers to these questions, the nurse proceeds with the physical assessment, noting the location, color, and characteristics of all cutaneous lesions. Photographs might be needed as legal evidence, and orthopedic,

Table 5–2 Signs and Symptoms of Physical Abuse

Indication of Abuse	Assessment Findings
Bruises or welts on eyes, mouth, lips, torso, buttocks, genital areas, calves	Injuries in shape of object used to produce them (eg, sticks, belts, hairbrushes, buckles) Injuries located on parts of body not usually injured (normal bruises commonly appear on forehead, shins, knees, elbows) Injuries often in various stages of healing
Burns	Shape suggesting type of burn
Immersion burns	Immersion burns have "socklike" or "glovelike" appearance
Pattern burns	Pattern suggesting object used (eg, iron, stove grate, electric burner, heater); small, circular burns on feet, face, hands, chest, or buttocks suggest cigar or cigarette
Friction burns	Burns possibly caused by rope used to tie child's legs, arms, neck, or torso
Fractures of skull, face, nose, long bones	Multiple or spiral fractures caused by twisting motion Evidence of epiphyseal separations and periosteal shearing Shaft fractures from direct blows Fractures in various stages of healing if earlier fractures went untreated
Lacerations or abrasions on mouth, lips, gums, eyes, genitals	Possible human bite marks, especially those of adult size
Child's behaviors that indicate fear or apprehension	Extreme aggressiveness or withdrawal: wariness of adults; fear of going home; apprehension when other children cry Apparent fear of parents Vacant stare; no eye contact Wary, motionless surveying of environment Stiffening when approached as if in expectation of punishment of a physical nature

Source: Adapted from Mott SR, Fazekas NF, and James SR, *Nursing Care of Children and Families,* Menlo Park, Calif, Addison-Wesley, 1985, p 717.

Table 5–3 Signs of Sexual Abuse

Physical Signs	Behavior Signs
Laceration of labia, vagina, or perineum	Discussion of or implied involvement in sexual activity
Irritation, pain, or injury to genital area	Expression of severe emotional conflict at home with fear of intervention
Hematomas in genital area	Reluctance to participate in sports, showers, changing of clothes
Vaginal or penile discharge	Care in sitting because of injuries
Dysuria	Unusual interest in genital area (eg, "French kissing" or fondling of genitals)
Sexually transmitted disease in young child (on eyes, mouth, anus, or genitals)	Sleep disturbances (eg, nightmares, enuresis, fear of sleeping alone)
Pregnancy	Reluctance to participate in activities with a particular person or at a particular place
Itching, bruises, or bleeding in genital area	Increased number of new fears
Unexplained vaginal or rectal bleeding	Fear of being alone
	Poor peer relations
	Change in performance at school
	Vague somatic complaints

Source: Adapted from Mott SR, Fazekas NF, and James SR, *Nursing Care of Children and Families,* Menlo Park, Calif, Addison-Wesley, 1985, p 720.

surgical, ophthalmologic, and gynecologic examinations also might be needed depending on the type of injuries.

Skeletal radiographs should be obtained for all children under 5 years of age who are suspected of having been abused or neglected to identify any treated or untreated fractures. If the child has unexplained bruising, tests for blood dyscrasias are needed. In cases of sexual abuse, evidence must be gathered for legal proceedings.

This includes cultures for gonorrhea and other sexually transmitted diseases, microscopic examination for blood and sperm, pregnancy testing, and clothing examination for semen, blood, or pubic hairs. Strict procedures must be followed in collecting evidence and specimens to have data the courts will accept.

The most important determination to make is the risk of reinjury to the victim or injury to other children in the household. Assessment of family functioning, coping strategies, and current state of crisis provides valuable data for such determination. Sometimes, even when the injuries are not severe, hospitalization or foster home placement is necessary. Protection of the child (or children) is always the priority.

An interview is needed with parents or extended family members. Interviewing adult family members separately allows the interviewer to compare the facts and check the validity of the data.

In assessing neglected or abused children and their families, the nurse considers the long-term ramifications of neglect and their possible effects on family cooperation in meeting goals. Some considerations in planning interventions are:

- The parents' emotional ability to accept services

- Communication patterns within the family

- The range and availability of services

- The family's use of services

- Supportive counseling for all family members

- The children's growth and developmental patterns

- The parents' attempts to diminish isolation

- The parents' responses to expectations to change behaviors

- The quality of nurturance within the family

- Family dynamics and other risk factors such as substance abuse or violence

- Environmental stressors such as inadequate housing, hygiene, or nutrition

NURSING DIAGNOSIS

Once it has been determined that a child has been abused by a parent, the nurse should formulate nursing diagnoses based on the assessment findings. Examples of nursing diagnoses related to dysfunctional parenting are:

- Ineffective parental coping related to stress

- Knowledge deficit regarding the normal process of growth and development of children

- Disturbance in self-concept related to parent's low self-esteem

Examples of nursing diagnoses related to the abused child are:

- Developmental vulnerability related to dysfunctional parent-child interaction

- Potential for disturbance in self-concept related to parental abuse

NURSING GOAL: TO PROVIDE SUPPORT TO DYSFUNCTIONAL PARENTS

Providing parental supports to marginally functioning parents is preferable to removing the child from the home. Removing children is traumatic, and most communities lack adequate foster care homes. Foster care is more expensive than maintaining the family system. Dysfunctional parents also tend to continue the cycle of dysfunctional parenting with other children in the family.

Although both professionals and nonprofessionals acknowledge intense feelings concerning child abuse and neglect, they have little concern for the abusive parents. Jolly K, a former abusive parent (and the founder of Parents Anonymous), described the needs of abusive parents in this way:

> Child abusers are going through hell. We have a vision of how powerful our anger can be, a concept of where this anger will take us if we are pushed too far, and the constant dread that we will be pushed too far . . . We don't like being child abusers any more than society likes the problem of abuse. If a positive approach is offered to abusers, they will usually respond. We don't know how to listen— too many of us are afraid to go to agencies because of the fear that our children will be taken away (Reed 1975).

Abusive parents are afraid. They are afraid of what they are doing, what will happen if they go for help, and what might happen if they do not go for help.

Working with neglectful and abusive parents is emotionally draining and disturbing for all people involved. Seeing a child victimized calls forth strong emotions, particularly among nurses, who might be required to provide nursing care during the time of the acute injury. The tendency is to protect the victim, the innocent child, and to punish the parent, who after all is the offender, but the nurse who perceives the family as a system understands that both child and parent are victims (Smith 1981). The etiology of abuse is complex and multifaceted. Parents

bring to the family and to their roles as parents developmental histories that may predispose them to treat their offspring in an abusive/neglectful manner. Stress-promoting social forces both within the family (eg, handicapped child, marital conflict) and beyond (eg, social isolation, unemployment) increase the likelihood that parent-child conflict will occur (Belsky et al 1984, p 175).

Nurses need to avoid "rescuer fantasies," which can stem from caring for a child and wanting to save that child from harm. Unless recognized, these fantasies can blind the nurse to the real needs of the child and family. If the focus is the child's injuries, negative feelings toward the parent can multiply and ultimately affect interventions. Some nurses employ both overt (deliberately ignoring the parent or making accusatory remarks) and covert (supplying information in an offhand manner) behaviors toward abusive parents, thereby inhibiting rapport and parent teaching. One approach to this problem might be to have two nursing teams, one to care for the child and one to interact with the parent. This might help channel some negative feelings and maintain communication. Periodic discussions can help nurses focus on the identified needs of both the parent and child and allow for the appropriate release of tension. Nurses need to recognize and affirm that child abuse is not simply the problem of a disturbed parent but is a social problem of vast dimensions.

Nurses can avoid judgmental attitudes by first examining their own thoughts, feelings, and beliefs about poverty, neglect, alternative life-styles, and different ethnic and cultural groups. Nurses need to understand the complex relationships among poverty, alienation, and neglect, not only to identify risk factors but also to recognize the social forces that keep some families locked in a cycle of dysfunction.

Approximately 10 percent of all parents who abuse or neglect their children cannot be treated or helped (Medical News 1984). These parents are usually seriously mentally ill, and for them there is only one alternative—to sever the parent-child relationship. The child may be placed with relatives or in permanent foster care or may be placed for adoption after the formal termination of parental rights. The remaining 90 percent of parents might be helped, but of these, approximately 10 percent fail. The result is an overall rehabilitation rate of 80 percent (Kempe & Kempe 1978).

NURSING GOAL: TO HELP PARENTS COPE WITH STRESS

A major task is helping dysfunctional parents understand the impact of stress and crises in their lives and the appropriate responses to these crises.

In a family that is providing only marginal child care, any stress, however small, might create a crisis. Illness; separation of a family member; or problems with housing, heating, cooking, or laundry might trigger further neglect or apathy in an already fragile parent. The nurse who identifies stress in dysfunctional families therefore needs to assess coping strategies. Successful coping patterns sug-

gest growth and motivation. The nurse might be able to praise parents for positive coping behaviors or may need to teach appropriate ways to cope with stress. A family's reaction to stress is often a measure of the family's strength as a system.

Most parents need support services as they learn to develop new coping techniques. Group therapy might assist abusive parents through peer support because finding others with similar problems minimizes isolation. Nurse therapists can address and help parents verbalize common fears and misconceptions about parenting. The first signs of dysfunctional parenting, however, must be discussed with the family because the nurse needs to guard against becoming so involved with the family that early indicators of serious parenting problems go unrecognized. Progress might be slight at times but must always be identified, especially to the parent with low self-esteem.

Nurses and other professionals often need to make contracts and establish realistic deadlines in working with families. This in turn is good role modeling. Dysfunctional families need to be informed that the pattern of child care is inadequate and not acceptable to the community or school system. Facts of legal consequence, including removal of the children, need to be both verbalized and written out. These measures might seem drastic, but if they are handled in too gentle a manner and the family misinterprets the message, valuable time may be lost in mixed messages and conflicts.

Some parents appear to be docile, cooperative, and open but have merely learned responses that please. The nurse therefore is careful to identify concrete changes that indicate progress. Otherwise the therapeutic contact might end too early for a family that appears to have changed. Periodic evaluation of family dynamics and interagency accomplishments and conflicts should ensure that the family does not manipulate workers or agencies and decrease the effectiveness of the plan. In some instances a child protective worker is needed to function as coordinator.

NURSING GOAL: TO PROVIDE INFORMATION ABOUT COMMUNITY RESOURCES

Intervention at all levels is more effective when multiple resources are available and the family can help choose which resources to use. Most families need to draw on a variety of resources to break the cycle of a dysfunctional life-style (Broome & Daniels 1987). Nurses and other health professionals therefore need to be cognizant of the services available within their communities (Box 5–1). They need to help clients avail themselves of those programs most geared to their needs and then coordinate the program goals and the client's progress. The goals and philosophy of community outreach programs must be clearly defined for all concerned. Presenting prevention services positively increases the likelihood that they will be used.

For example, "positive parenting" is a better term than "prevention of child abuse and neglect," which tends to stigmatize the client. Some parents are reluctant to participate in any program, no matter how appropriate for them, that uses the word "abuse."

○   *CHILD-CARE CENTERS*   Child-care centers have been established by many communities in an effort to assist families. These centers provide child care for parents who need support services and time-out periods from their children. The philosophy of each center varies, but most centers encourage parents to use their respite time to attend to some of their own needs, thereby improving the quality of their relationships with their children. Some centers encourage or require parents to spend some portion of their time at the center learning child-care skills and seeing positive interaction with children. Participation is usually voluntary, although courts occasionally direct a parent to use these services. Most centers charge a minimal fee based on a sliding scale. Some centers even provide transportation to and from the center.

Box 5–1   Community Services Commonly Needed by Families Demonstrating Health-Threatening Parenting

Public housing
Welfare
Mental health centers
Emergency shelters
Subsidized child care
Homemaker services
WIC program
Food stamps
Free medical or dental care
Family or marital counseling
Vocational rehabilitation, employment services
Foster care
Parents Anonymous
Fuel assistance agencies
Child guidance centers
Child development clinics
Housing authorities
Alcoholics Anonymous, Al-Anon, Ala-Teen, Ala-Tot
Visiting Nurse Association
Juvenile authorities
DCYS (Division of Child and Youth Services)
Ambulatory care settings
Occupational health settings
Religious-affiliated groups

Source: Adapted from Mott SR, Fazekas NF, and James SR, *Nursing Care of Children and Families,* Menlo Park, Calif, Addison-Wesley, 1985, p 728.

Many centers conduct weekly group meetings for parents to discuss common problems and concerns. The group fosters a parental identity and stresses the importance of adequate child care. The sharing and collaboration elevates self-esteem and identifies feelings that might have been denied or repressed. Helping another parent cope with a problem that has been successfully resolved is a growth-producing experience and, for some parents, a first step out of isolation.

○   *LIFELINE TO AVOID ISOLATION*   Isolation and withdrawal, which prevent access to role models for child care, also foster lack of trust. An intervention program for isolated families needs to provide frequent home visits to foster parental maturity and encourage socialization. For many parents, such visits are the first attempts to remove the barrier of isolation.

Some communities have established "friendly visitor" programs to improve the health and quality of family life. The visitor compiles data showing family strengths and weaknesses, identifies families with the potential for change and growth, and devises a care plan. The goals vary depending on the specific needs of each family, but the overall goal is to improve family dynamics so that all members move toward wellness. Some specific areas of focus are (1) maintaining a stable home environment; (2) fostering feelings of adequacy as parents; (3) developing parenting skills; (4) learning effective ways to manage stress; (5) identifying ways of increasing self-esteem and self-acceptance; and (6) reducing social isolation.

○   *FOSTER GRANDPARENTS*   Grandparents play a special role in families. They usually have had years of successful living and bring warmth, love, and a sense of continuity to a family. Foster grandparents aim to provide such a role to children and families who have been fragmented or troubled.

Some foster grandparents are volunteers, whereas others are paid a minimum wage to augment their Social Security income. All are retired and usually donate time far in excess of the required hours. Many report an improvement in their physical health when they feel needed and have a defined purpose in living. Some are isolated from their own families and welcome the chance to interact socially with a new family or child. Foster grandparent programs are connected to social service agencies, community mental health groups, and many pediatric institutions, especially those whose clients are far from home.

○   *PARENT AIDES*   Parent aides visit selected homes several times a week, providing transportation and social experiences for either parent of a dysfunctional family. As paraprofessionals, parent aides are supervised by the health team and primarily provide long-term nurturing to parents rather than children, although children ultimately benefit.

Parent aides are parents themselves who have highly successful relationships and current support systems in their own lives. Proper selection and training are crucial to any parent aide program, and past family life experiences and parenting successes are the criteria for selecting parent aides. Many have experienced personal difficulties themselves; their problem-solving abilities and coping strategies are useful in working with troubled families. Experience has shown that parent aides with school-age children are most effective because dysfunctional parents can view them as peers or friends and accept nurturing from them (Hollen et al 1980).

○ *CHILDREN'S PROTECTIVE SERVICES* The children's protective service has a vested interest in the effectiveness and accessibility of a wide range of resources in the community and usually takes the lead in working with the family and mobilizing resources. A children's protective service office is generally located in the department of social services and is administered by the county, city, or state. Its prime functions include receiving, investigating, and evaluating reports of child abuse and neglect and providing necessary services, either directly or through referral. Its goals are to prevent injury to children, promote the development of healthy children, preserve and enhance family life, strengthen and support parents and families, and maintain children in their own homes and communities whenever possible.

The children's protective service usually coordinates fiscal and technical support to community-based child protection teams. Coordinated services are thus designed to:

● Maintain and improve the availability of community resources for the prevention and treatment of child abuse and neglect

● Strengthen cooperative working relationships through interdisciplinary teams

● Integrate clinical knowledge with child welfare practice

● Educate the public and professionals about the prevention and treatment of child abuse and neglect

○ *CRISIS INTERVENTION HOTLINES* Many communities have established "helplines" to help parents cope with frustrations. These telephone hotlines for crisis intervention are available 24 hours a day, 7 days a week, and generally are staffed by trained volunteers, professionals, and paraprofessionals. The hotline reassures many parents who just need to know that someone is there if they are unable to cope and might lead others to seek help at an earlier stage of frustration.

○ *PARENTS ANONYMOUS* Parents Anonymous is a self-help group that is especially effective in both the prevention and treatment of child abuse. The organization was founded in 1972 in California by Jolly K, who was both an abusive parent and an abused child who had lived in 35 foster homes. Meetings of Parents Anonymous are led by a parent, and participants are invited to share their feelings, concerns, and problems, but meetings are neither therapy nor classes in parenting. Members are often able to confront one another about parenting behaviors, especially if they have experienced the same problems, and they can also share possible solutions to family dilemmas.

All members are parents who need a support group to meet family stresses. Most attendance is on a voluntary basis, but some members are ordered to attend by the court system. Meetings are usually held once a week for two hours in accessible locations in the community. Professional sponsors who are present during the meeting are there as consultants rather than authorities. Members often exchange phone numbers to contact each other between meetings because Parents Anonymous suggests, "Reach for your phone instead of your kid."

Ideas for Informing Children About Sexual Abuse and Preventive Measures

1. A "good touch" is nice, like a hug, whereas a "bad touch" makes a person uncomfortable. Children need to be told, "Your body belongs to you; you can decide who touches it. Private areas are those covered by a bathing suit. If you are touched by someone and you don't like it, tell the person to stop and tell someone else about it."

2. Secrets and surprises are not the same. Secrets sometimes are not fair to keep. Surprises are fun; secrets are not fun if they make you feel funny or uncomfortable.

3. Strangers can be dangerous. Never go with someone you don't know who says anything like, "Your mother is ill and sent me to get you," or "Will you help me look for my lost puppy in the woods?"

4. Do not let others undress you, even if they promise to give you something such as candy or new clothes.

5. Do not listen when an older person tells you that they are going to help you grow up by showing you what big people do.

6. If you feel uncomfortable with someone, do not allow yourself to be left alone with that person.

Source: Adapted from Mott SR, Fazekas NF, and James SR, *Nursing Care of Children and Families,* Menlo Park, Calif, Addison-Wesley, 1985, p 719.

Two studies of Parents Anonymous have found that physical abuse usually stops within one month of the parent's joining and that verbal and emotional abuse decline significantly and continue to decline as long as the parent participates (Nix 1980). Formerly abusive parents often report increased self-esteem as they assist other parents in distress. Some continue to attend meetings long after their initial needs are met, and many parents report pleasurable relationships with their children for the first time in their lives.

NURSING GOAL: TO PROVIDE SUPPORT TO THE CHILD

If significant changes in the family are unavoidable, the child needs assistance in working through feelings of having caused the changes. Siblings also need to be included in the treatment plan of an abused or neglected child. If the child is hospitalized, fears of pain or violence are intensified by the unfamiliar surroundings and people. If a parent does visit, the parent is often unsupportive and may be angry with the child. The child is often confused, hurt, and frightened. Nurses and other hospital staff can identify pain, fear, and confusion and help the child discuss those feelings. The child needs to be told what will happen in developmentally appropriate terms and be reassured, as much as possible, that the parent will be back. The fewer the number of care givers, the most likely it is that the child will establish trusting relationships.

Some children have never heard their names spoken in a gentle voice, and a slow, gentle approach is essential to build any degree of trust. Children who withdraw from human contact must be allowed a reasonable period of time in which to grieve and appraise new people. If the child regresses, the regressive behavior needs to be accepted until the child can ease into a more appropriate developmental stage.

Younger children are likely to need nurturing in the form of rocking, cuddling, and soothing. The child initially might appear to reject any comforting, however, or become aggressive in response to overwhelming anxiety. The aggressive behaviors are learned responses to chaotic living and can become a problem if the child manages to manipulate many people. Team members need to set consistent limits in a firm but kindly manner and help the child learn more acceptable behaviors. Aggressive children usually have feelings of deprivation, sadness, and loneliness and may believe themselves to be unworthy and bad. Such children have little faith in their ability to inspire approval and affection (Kempe & Kempe 1978).

Individual therapy may help aggressive children to discuss the expectations their parents have for them and family dynamics. The therapeutic approach is to face reality honestly and not to arouse expectations in the child that

the parent cannot or will not fulfill (Kempe & Kempe 1978). Children who have been severely abused or have witnessed severe abuse of a sibling also need support in developing future relationships that are free of fears, guilt, and anxieties. Children facing loss or separation from their parents need therapeutic assistance to handle the loss and time to mourn the loss.

Box 5–2   Goals for Parental Behavior

Identifies problems in the family system

Identifies factors that contribute to potential or actual abusive behaviors

Demonstrates ability to meet own needs

Finds positive alternatives to present coping strategies by first identifying external stressors

Describes feelings toward self and children

Demonstrates alternative coping strategies in stressful situations

Demonstrates realistic expectations of children by identifying age-appropriate behaviors

Identifies methods of discipline

Demonstrates some consistency and appropriate use of discipline

Identifies a person or agency to contact in a crisis

Provides a safe environment for children by identifying an adequate caregiver during parental absence, identifying and correcting environmental hazards, providing ongoing health care for children

Identifies family members and friends available for support

Indicates frequency of visits to family and friends

Identifies ways in which family, friends, community supports (church, school, etc) can be helpful

Identifies ways in which health care system can be helpful

Demonstrates appropriate use of health care system and other agencies by keeping appointments

Earns income above the poverty level or receives and manages public assistance optimally (eg, food stamps used to buy food that is then allocated appropriately among family members)

Manages budget to purchase appropriate low-cost clothing for family members

Provides adequate housing that meets minimal requirements (heat, electricity, cooking and refrigeration facilites, some furnishings)

Remains at same residence without frequent moves

Adapted from Christensen ML, Schommer BL, Velasquez J: An interdisciplinary approach to preventing child abuse. Copyright © 1984 American Journal of Nursing Company. Reproduced with permission from *Am J Mat/Child Nurs* (March/April; 84(2)).

Long-term follow-up of dysfunctional families has no set time frame for completion. In some instances services are required until the children reach adulthood. Periodic evaluation of parental progress and family growth includes monitoring the behaviors of the children, who might exhibit anger, anxiety, intense loneliness, or apathy. The children's progress in school must also be assessed, together with their response to authority figures. Dysfunctional behaviors suggest that the child needs individual attention. Communication and caring, although time-consuming for the team members, does assist both parents and children in coping with the normal stress of development.

EVALUATION

The nurse who is caring for dysfunctional families must evaluate care on an ongoing basis. The nurse needs to see the family at regular intervals to identify specific evidence of progress or failure. Informing the parents of the consequences of failure to meet expectations and deadlines is a delicate and crucial issue for the nurse because most nurses find it difficult to discuss removing children from the family. Parents must know, however, that children's safety and security are of primary importance. The parents' failure to meet goals indicates a need for more intervention.

With a parent who has a history of inflicting trauma in response to personal stress, the expected behaviors need to be defined immediately. Box 5–2 lists specific goals for parental behavior. These can be used to determine the success of nursing interventions.

KEY CONCEPTS

Family violence occurs, with women and children being the most frequent targets, in families of all socioeconomic levels, races, and structure.

Family violence may result in physical and psychologic trauma to family members, removal of children from the parents' care, and legal proceedings against the perpetrators of the violence.

Spouse abuse is physical violence directed by one spouse at the other spouse.

Wife battering is a common occurrence, but it is the least reported serious crime in the United States.

Numerous factors contribute to continued family violence, such as sex-role stereotyping of traditional male and female behaviors and passive-aggressive interaction patterns between married couples.

Nurses are in an excellent position to intervene and assist battered women by recognizing their cues, diagnosing their problems appropriately, and providing information, medical attention, and emotional support.

Nurses must fully comprehend the complex dynamics of the battering family, use appropriate interpersonal skills in assisting battered women, and have a broad knowledge of available community resources.

All members of a violence-prone family are affected by the violent behavior; interventions should be directed at both victims and abusers.

Child abuse is physical violence or verbal assaults directed against a child.

Parents who abuse their children often feel isolated, are unable to trust others, have few supports for coping with stress, or have unrealistic expectations for their children's behavior.

Indicators of physical abuse include a series of injuries in various stages of healing (especially a series of similar injuries), the family's delay in seeking treatment, use of multiple treatment facilities, and attempts to hide or minimize the abuse, sometimes with special clothing.

Emotional abuse usually consists of name-calling, ridicule, and statements that make the child feel unlovable or unwanted.

Sexual abuse is the exploitation of a child for the sexual gratification of an adult; incest is sexual abuse by a family member.

The nurse documents evidence of child abuse by noting and specifically describing parent and child behaviors.

When a case of child abuse has been discovered, certain legal procedures are set in motion to protect the child from further abuse; abused children may be placed in foster homes for their protection.

Nursing actions in cases of child abuse include providing support to the parents and child and providing information about and referrals to community resources.

REFERENCES

Belsky J, Learner RM, Spanier GB: *The Child in the Family.* Reading, Mass, Addison-Wesley, 1984.
Broome ME, Daniels D: Child abuse: A multidimensional phenomenon. *Holistic Nurs Pract* 1987;1(2)13.

Densen-Gerger J, **Hutchinson** SF: Medical-legal and societal problems involving children—child prostitution, child pornography and drug-related abuse: Recommended legislation, in **Smith** SM (ed): *The Maltreatment of Children.* Baltimore, University Park Press, 1978.

Finley B: Nursing process with the battered woman. *Nurs Pract* 1981;6(July/August):11, 29.

Gelles RJ: *The Violent Home.* Beverly Hills, Calif, Sage, 1974.

Gelles RJ: Abused wives: Why do they stay? *J Marriage Fam* 1976;38:659.

Gelles RJ: The myths of battered husbands. *Ms* 1979; 8(4):65–66, 71.

Gelles RJ, **Cornell** CP: *Intimate Violence in Families.* Beverly Hills, Calif, Sage, 1985.

Gorline LL, **Ray** NM: Examining and caring for the child who has been sexually assaulted. *Am J Mat Child Nurs* 1979;4(March/April):110.

Heins M: The "battered child" revisited. *JAMA* 1984; 251(24):3295.

Hollen P, **Carroll** JF, **Carpenter** C: The pediatric home liaison in a private practice. *Pediatr Nurs* 1980;6(May/June):25.

Kempe CH, **Helfer** RE: *Helping the Battered Child and His Family.* Philadelphia, Lippincott, 1972.

Kempe RS, **Kempe** CH: *Child Abuse.* Cambridge, Mass, Harvard University Press, 1978.

Ledray LE: *Recovering from Rape.* New York, Henry Holt, 1986.

Lichtenstein VR: The battered woman: Guidelines for effective nursing intervention. *Issues Ment Health Nurs* 1981;3(July–September):237.

MacLeod L: *Wife Battering in Canada: The Vicious Cycle.* Ottawa, Canadian Advisory Council on the Status of Women, 1980.

Mahon L: Common characteristics of abused women. *Issues Ment Health Nurs* 1981;3(January–June):137.

McKittrick CA: Child abuse: Recognition and reporting by health professionals. *Nurs Clin North Am* 1981; 16(March):103.

Medical news, editorial. *JAMA* 1984;251(24):3201–3207.

Meiselman KC: Incest, in *A Psychological Study of Causes and Effects with Treatment Recommendations.* San Francisco, Jossey-Bass, 1978.

Mott SR, **Fazekas** NF, **James** SR: *Nursing Care of Children and Families.* Menlo Park, Calif, Addison-Wesley, 1985.

Munro JU: The nurse and the legal system: Dealing with abused children, in **Campbell** J, **Humphreys** J (eds): *Nursing Care of Victims of Family Violence.* Reston, Va, 1984.

Nix H: Why Parents Anonymous? *J Psychiatr Nurs* 1980;18(October):23.

Reed J: Working with abusive parents: A parent's view. *Child Today* 1975;4(3):6.

Sgroi SM: *Handbook of Clinical Intervention in Child Sexual Abuse.* Lexington, Mass, Lexington Books, 1982.

Sherman KO: The battered woman. *Dimens Crit Care Nurs* 1983;2(January/February):30.

Smith JB: Care of the hospitalized abused child and family. *Nurs Clin North Am* 1981;16(March):127.

Snell JE, et al: The wifebeater's wife. *Arch Gen Psychiatry* 1964;11:107.

Stark E, et al: *Wife Abuse in the Medical Setting.* Rockville, Md, National Clearinghouse on Domestic Violence, 1981.

Steele BF: Psychodynamic factors in child abuse, in **Kempe** CH, **Helfer** RE (eds): *The Battered Child.* Chicago, University of Chicago Press, 1980.

Straus MA, **Gelles** RJ, **Steinmetz** SK: *Behind Closed Doors.* Garden City, NJ, Anchor Books, 1980.

Tilden UR, **Shepherd** P: Battered women: The shadow side of families. *Holistic Nurs Pract* 1987;1(2):25.

Walker LE: *The Battered Woman.* New York, Harper & Row, 1979.

ADDITIONAL READINGS

Baum E, et al: Child sexual abuse: Criminal justice and the pediatrician. *Pediatrics* 1987;79(March):437.

Benton DA: Battered women: Why do they stay? *Health Care Int* 1986;7(6):403.

Bishop B: A guide to assessing parenting capabilities. *Am J Nurs* 1976;76(November):1784.

Campbell L: Hopelessness: A concept analysis. *J Psychosoc Nurs* 1987;25(February):25.

Cherry BS, **Carty** RM: Changing concepts of childhood in society. *Pediatr Nurs* 1986;12(November/December):421.

Christensen ML, **Schommer** BL, **Velasquez** J: An interdisciplinary approach to preventing child abuse. *Am J Mat Child Nurs* 1984;9(March/April):108.

Drake VK: Battered women: A health care problem in disguise. *Image* 1982;14(2):40.

Elbow M: Children of violent marriages: The forgotten victims. *Soc Casework J Contemp Soc Work* 1982;63:465.

Elkind D: David Elkind discusses parental pressures. *Pediatr Nurs* 1986;12(November/December):417.

Gelles RJ: *Family Violence.* Beverly Hills, Calif, Sage, 1979.

Hurwitz A, **Casteles** S: Misdiagnosed child abuse and metabolic disease. *Pediatr Nurs* 1987;13(January/February):33.

Kallman H: Detecting abuse in the elderly. *Human Sexuality* 1987(March suppl):89.

Kelley SJ: Learned helplessness in the sexually abused child. *Issues Compr Pediatr Nurs* 1986;9(3):193.

Lav EMC, Donnan SPB: Maternal and child factors for reported child abuse among Chinese in Hong Kong. *Soc Sci Med* 1987;24(5):449.

Ledray L: Victims of incest. *Am J Nurs* 1984;84(8):1010.

Leventhal JM, Berg A, Egerter SA: Is intrauterine growth retardation a risk factor for child abuse? *Pediatrics* 1987;79(April):515.

Limandri BJ: The therapeutic relationship with abused women. *J Psychosoc Nurs* 1987;25(February):8.

Lowery M: Adult survivors of childhood incest. *J Psychosoc Nurs* 1987;25(January):27.

Perch KL: The economics of changing household composition and family roles. *Fam Commun Health* 1987;9(February):1.

Rew L, et al: AFFIRM: A nursing model to promote role mastery in family caregivers. *Fam Commun Health* 1987;9(February):52.

Sideleau BF: Irrational beliefs and intervention. *J Psychosoc Nurs* 1987;25(March):18.

Sturfbergen AK: The impact of chronic illness on families. *Fam Commun Health* 1987;9(February):43.

Velasquez J, Christensen ML, Schommer BL: Intensive services help prevent child abuse. *Am J Mat Child Nurs* 1984;9(March/April):113.

Zdanuk JM, Harris CC, Wisian NL: Adolescent pregnancy and incest: The nurse's role as counselor. *J Obstet Gynecol Neonat Nurs* 16;(March/April):99.

One time when he beat me I started to fight back . . . . He threw kerosene around me and threatened to put a match to it . . . . I never fought back again . . . just kept trying to figure out what I was doing wrong that he would beat me that way. There were some good times together, like when we talked about going to college, and somehow I just kept hoping and believing he would change.

Before I came to this shelter I had no idea so many other women were going through the same thing I was . . . . I used to think the only way out of my situation would be a tragic one—to kill either myself or him.

I'd go to my friends' and mother's house, but I just couldn't make ends meet. I didn't have a baby sitter, money, or the physical and mental strength . . . . I was depressed about everything. My mother stuck it out for 40 years. I didn't believe in divorce, I believed in marriage. Basically it was my religion and for financial support [that she didn't leave earlier]. (Hoff, People in Crisis)

Reproductive Organs and Related Health Issues

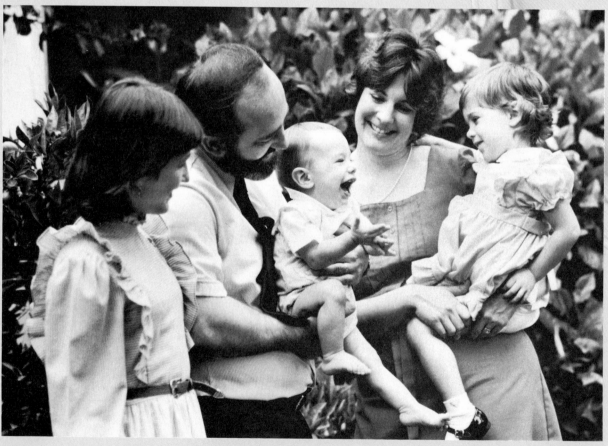

The physiology of reproduction always exists in a social context.

Part Three

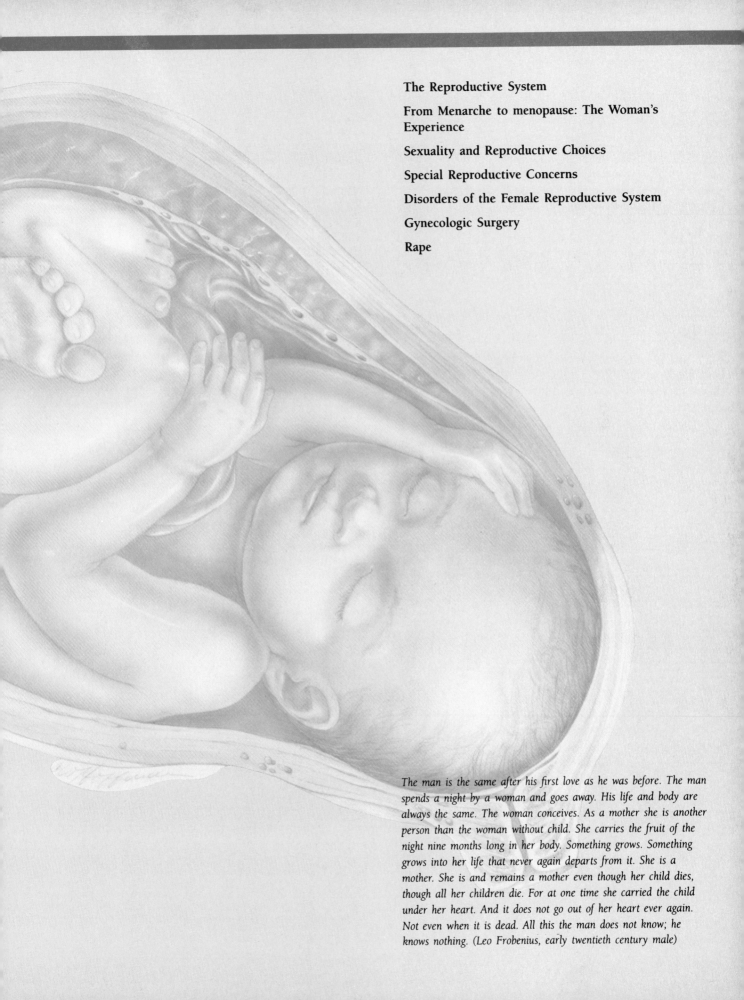

The man is the same after his first love as he was before. The man spends a night by a woman and goes away. His life and body are always the same. The woman conceives. As a mother she is another person than the woman without child. She carries the fruit of the night nine months long in her body. Something grows. Something grows into her life that never again departs from it. She is a mother. She is and remains a mother even though her child dies, though all her children die. For at one time she carried the child under her heart. And it does not go out of her heart ever again. Not even when it is dead. All this the man does not know; he knows nothing. (Leo Frobenius, early twentieth century male)

The Reproductive System

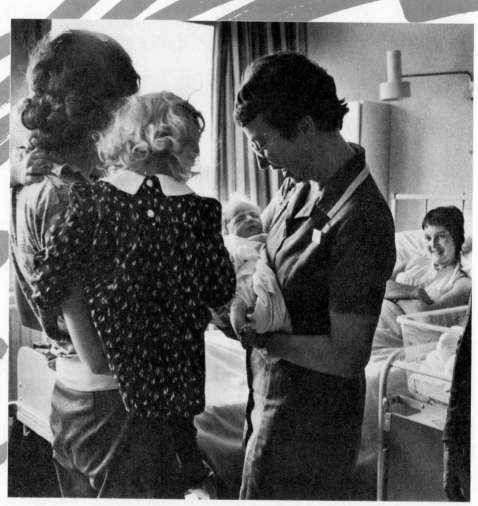

In England, where rooming-in is routine, the frequent visits of a nurse-midwife make life easier for the new mother.

Chapter Six

OBJECTIVES

- **Describe the prenatal development of the reproductive system.**
- **Summarize the major changes in the reproductive system that occur during puberty.**
- **Identify the structures and functions of the female and male reproductive systems.**
- **Describe the significance of specific female reproductive structures during childbirth.**

Understanding childbearing and life before birth requires more than understanding sexual intercourse or the process by which the female and male sex cells unite. One must become familiar with the structures and functions that make childbearing possible and the phenomena that initiate it. This chapter considers the anatomic, physiologic, and sexual aspects of the female and male reproductive systems. Information regarding embryologic development is also presented in order to increase understanding of anatomy, physiology, and function.

The female and male reproductive organs are homologous; that is, they are fundamentally similar in function and structure. The primary functions of both the female and male reproductive systems are to produce sex cells and to transport the sex cells to locations where their union can occur. The sex cells, called *gametes,* are produced by specialized organs called *gonads.* A series of ducts and glands within both the male and female reproductive systems contribute to the production and transport of the gametes.

● Early Development of Reproductive Structures and Processes

Although the genetic sex of an individual is determined at fertilization, for about the first eight weeks of gestation, the male and female reproductive systems are undifferentiated. This period, called the indifferent period, is followed by a period of rapid, dramatic changes as the reproductive organs differentiate and develop into recognizable structures.

Ovaries and Testes

During the fifth week of gestation, a primitive gonad arises from the medial aspect of the urogenital ridge. The gonad develops a medulla and cortex as primary sex cords appear in the underlying mesenchyme. In genetic males, during the seventh and eighth week the medulla develops into a testis, and the cortex regresses. In genetic females, by about the tenth week the cortex develops into an ovary and the medulla regresses.

The testis produces the male gametes, called *spermatozoa* or *sperm,* by a process called *spermatogenesis,* which is described in Chapter 13. Spermatogenesis of mature sperm does not occur until the onset of puberty.

Every egg available for maturation in a woman's reproductive life is present at her birth. During fetal life, the ovary produces *oogonia,* cells that become primitive eggs called *oocytes,* by the process of *oogenesis.* No oocytes are formed after fetal development. About 400,000 oocytes are contained in the ovary at birth. Each oocyte is contained in a small ovarian cavity called a *primordial* or *primitive follicle.*

During a female's reproductive years, every month one of the oocytes undergoes a process of cellular division and maturation that transforms it into a fertilizable egg, or *ovum.* At *ovulation,* the ovum is released from its follicle. Only about 400 ova are released during the reproductive years. The remaining follicles and oocytes degenerate over time.

Figure 6–1 illustrates the embryologic development of the gonads and other internal reproductive organs.

Other Internal Structures

During the indifferent period—the first seven weeks—two pairs of genital ducts develop: the *mesonephric* and *paramesonephric* ducts.

In genetic females, the fallopian tubes are formed from the unfused portions of the paramesonephric ducts, and the fused portions give rise to the epithelium and uterine glands. The endometrial stroma and the myometrium develop from the adjacent mesenchyme.

The vagina is derived from more than one embryologic structure. The vaginal epithelium develops from the endoderm of the urogenital sinus, and the musculature develops from the uterovaginal primordium.

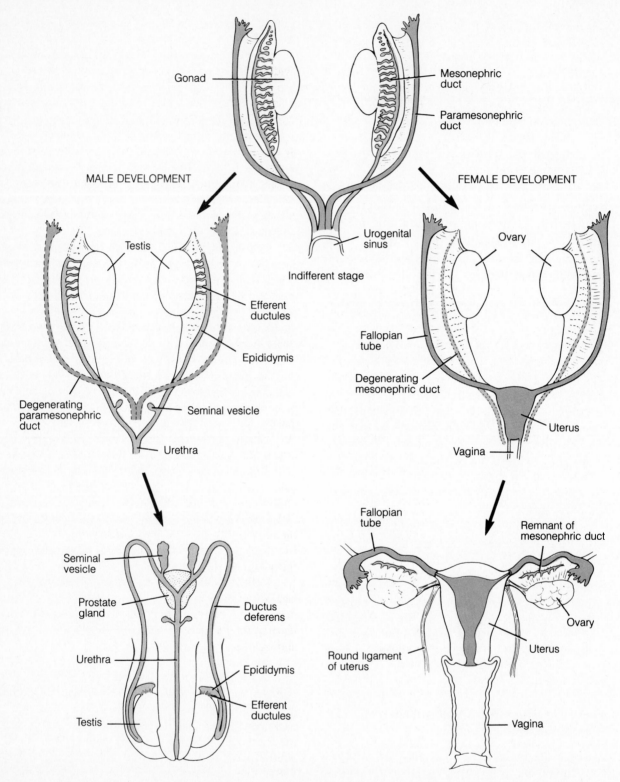

Figure 6–1   Embryonic differentiation of male and female internal reproductive organs (From Spence AP & Mason EB, *Human Anatomy and Physiology,* ed 3, Menlo Park, Calif, Benjamin/Cummings, 1987)

The urethral and paraurethral glands develop from outgrowths of the urethra into the surrounding mesenchyme. Bartholin's glands arise from similar structures.

In genetic males, the fetal testes secrete two hormones: Testosterone stimulates the mesonephric ducts to develop into the male genital tract, and the other hormone (müllerian regression factor) suppresses the development of the paramesonephric ducts, which would otherwise develop into the female genital tract.

From the mesonephric ducts comes development of the efferent ductules, vas deferens, epididymides, seminal vesicles, and ejaculatory ducts. Both the prostate and the bulbourethral glands develop from endodermal outgrowths of the urethra.

External Structures

Genetic males and females possess the same external genitals until the end of the ninth week. By the twelfth week, differentiation of the external genitals is complete.

The absence of fetal testosterone causes feminization of the indifferent external genitals. The phallus becomes the clitoris, and the urogenital folds remain open, forming the labia minora. The labioscrotal folds form the labia majora.

Because of the fetal testes' production of dihydrotestosterone, the indifferent external genitals become masculine. The phallus elongates, forming the penis. The fusion of the urogenital folds on the ventral surface of the penis forms the penile urethra, with the urethral meatus moving forward toward the glans penis.

● Puberty

The term *puberty* refers to the developmental period between childhood and attainment of adult sexual characteristics and functioning. Its onset is never sudden, although it may appear so to parents or to the young person who is not prepared for the physical and emotional changes of puberty. Boys generally mature physically about two years later than girls. In boys the age of onset of puberty ranges from 10 to 19 years; 14 years is the average age of onset. In girls the age of onset ranges from 9 to 17 years; 12 years is the average age of onset.

Puberty occurs over a period lasting 1½ to 5 years and involves profound physical, psychologic, and emotional changes. These changes result from the interaction of the central nervous system and the endocrine organs.

Major Physical Changes

In both boys and girls, puberty is preceded by an accelerated growth rate called *adolescent spurt*. Widespread body system changes occur at this time, including maturation of the reproductive organs.

The pattern of physical changes varies among individuals. Girls experience a broadening of the hips, then budding of the breasts, the appearance of pubic and axillary hair, and the onset of menstruation, called *menarche*.

The average time between breast development and menarche is 2.3 years (Stone 1981). A wide physiologic variation exists in the chronologic appearance and progression of the somatic puberty changes, and there is considerable overlapping of events. These variations are a result of different degrees of response of the gonads and adrenal gland to hypothalamic-pituitary stimulation and the target organ's sensitivity to sexual steroids.

Boys usually first note such changes as an increase in the size of the external genitals; the appearance of pubic, axillary, and facial hair; the deepening of the voice; and nocturnal seminal emissions without sexual stimulation (mature sperm are not usually contained in these earliest emissions).

Physiology of Onset

Puberty is initiated by the maturation of the hypothalamic-pituitary-gonad complex (the *gonadostat*) and input from the central nervous system. The process, which begins during fetal life, is sequential and complex.

The central nervous system releases a neurotransmitter that stimulates the hypothalamus to synthesize and release *gonadotropin*-releasing factor (GnRF) (Sloane 1985). GnRF is transmitted to the anterior pituitary, where it causes the synthesis and secretion of the gonadotropins, *follicle-stimulating hormone (FSH)* and *luteinizing hormone (LH)* (Figure 6–2).

Although the gonads do produce small amounts of *androgens* (male sex hormones) and *estrogens* (female sex hormones) before the onset of puberty, FSH and LH stimulate increased secretion of these hormones. Androgens and estrogens influence the development of secondary sex characteristics.

After puberty, more androgens and estrogens are required to inhibit the production of GnRF and the initiation of the negative feedback loop; therefore, the positive feedback loop predominates (Sloane 1985). One theory is that the brain becomes less sensitive to the inhibitory effects of gonadal steroids on the gonadotropin secretion (Ganong 1985). The gonadotropins FSH and LH stimulate the processes of spermatogenesis and maturation of ova.

Other hormones are involved in the onset of puberty. Although less direct, their action is essential. Abnormally high or low levels of adrenocorticotropic hormone (ACTH), thyroid hormone, or somatotropic (growth) hormone (STH) can disrupt the onset of normal puberty.

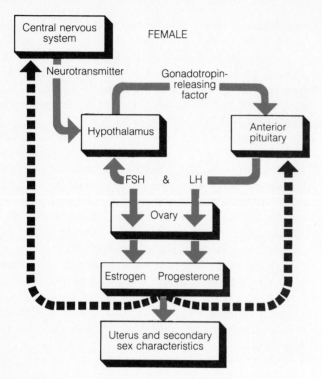

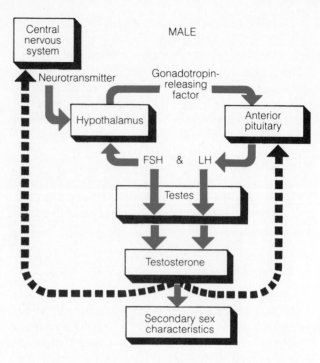

Figure 6–2   Positive feedback is illustrated with solid lines and negative feedback is illustrated with a broken line. Through a neurotransmitter, the CNS stimulates the hypothalamus, which in turn produces a gonadotropin-releasing factor that causes the anterior pituitary to produce gonadotropins (FSH or LH). These hormones stimulate specific structures in the gonads to secrete *steroid hormones (estrogen, progesterone, or testosterone). The rise in pituitary hormone production increases hypothalamus activity in a positive feedback relationship. Elevated steroid hormone levels stimulate the CNS and pituitary gland to inhibit hormone production in a negative feedback relationship.*

● Female Reproductive System

The female reproductive system consists of the external and internal genitals and the accessory organs of the breasts. The bony pelvis is also discussed in this section because of its importance in childbearing.

External Genitals

All the external reproductive organs, except the glandular structures, can be directly inspected. The size, color, and shape of these structures vary extensively among races and individuals.

The female external genitals, referred to as the *vulva* or *pudendum,* include the following structures (Figure 6–3):

- Mons pubis
- Labia majora
- Labia minora
- Clitoris
- Urethral meatus and opening of the paraurethral (Skene's) glands

- Vaginal vestibule (vaginal orifice, vulvovaginal glands, hymen, and fossa navicularis)
- Perineal body

Although not true parts of the female reproductive system, the urethral meatus and perineal body are considered here because of their proximity and relationship to the vulva.

The vulva has a generous supply of blood and nerves and is influenced by estrogenic hormones. As a woman ages, hormonal activity decreases, causing the vulvar organs to atrophy and become subject to a variety of lesions.

MONS PUBIS

The *mons pubis* is a softly rounded mound of subcutaneous fatty tissue beginning at the lowest portion of the anterior abdominal wall. Also known as the *mons veneris,* this structure covers the anterior portion of the symphysis pubis. The mons pubis is covered with pubic hair, typically with the hairline forming a transverse line across the lower abdomen (Figure 6–3). The hair is short and varies from sparse and fine in the Oriental woman to heavy, coarse, and curly in the Black woman.

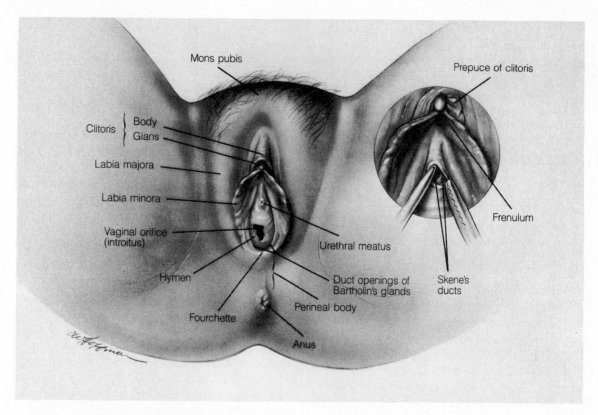

Figure 6–3   Female external genitals, longitudinal view

The mons pubis protects the pelvic bones, especially during coitus.

LABIA MAJORA

The *labia majora* are longitudinal, raised folds of pigmented skin, one on either side of the vulvar cleft (Figure 6–3). As the pair descend, they narrow, enclosing the vulvar cleft, and merge to form the *posterior commissure* of the perineal skin.

With each pregnancy, the labia majora become less prominent, so that in women who have had many children they may be obliterated as distinct structures. The labia majora are covered by stratified squamous epithelium containing hair follicles and sebaceous glands with underlying adipose and muscle tissue. Immediately under the skin is a sheet of dartos muscle called the *dartos muliebris*, which is responsible for the wrinkled appearance of the labia majora as well as for their sensitivity to heat and cold.

The inner surface of the labia majora in women who have not had children is moist and looks like a mucous membrane, whereas after many deliveries it is more skin-like (Pritchard et al 1985).

Arterial blood is supplied by the internal and external pudendal arteries. The venous drainage is composed of the area plexus connecting with the veins of the clitoris, labia minora, and perineum. Because of the extensive venous network in the labia majora, varicosities may occur during pregnancy and obstetric or sexual trauma may cause hematomas of these structures.

The labia majora share an extensive and diffuse lymphatic supply with the other structures of the vulva. Understanding this supply is important in understanding malignancies of the female reproductive organs.

The labia majora are supplied with an extensive network of nerve endings that make them extremely sensitive to touch, pressure, pain, and temperature. The nerves supplying the area are from the first lumbar and third sacral segment of the spinal cord. Because of the central nervous system innervation of this area, certain regional anesthesia blocks will affect it.

The chief function of the labia majora is protection of the structures lying between them.

LABIA MINORA

The *labia minora* are soft folds of skin within the labia majora that converge near the anus, forming the *fourchette* (Figure 6–3).

Each of the labia minora has the appearance of shiny mucous membrane, moist and devoid of hair follicles. Because the labia minora are rich in sebaceous glands that do not open into hair follicles but directly onto the surface of the skin, sebaceous cysts are common in this area. The labia minora are composed of erectile tissue containing loose connective tissue, blood vessels, numerous large venous spaces, and involuntary muscle tissue.

Vulvovaginitis in this area is very irritating because of the many tactile nerve endings.

The functions of the labia minora are to lubricate and waterproof the vulvar skin and to provide bactericidal secretions.

CLITORIS

The *clitoris* is the most erotically sensitive part of the female genital tract and is a common site of masturbation. The clitoris, located between the labia minora, is about 5 to 6 mm long and 6 to 8 mm across. Its tissue is essentially erectile.

The clitoris consists of the *glans,* the *corpus* or *body,* and two *crura* (Figure 6–3). The glans is partially covered by a fold of skin called the *prepuce.* This area often appears as an opening to an orifice, and may be confused with the urethral meatus. Attempts to insert a catheter here produce extreme discomfort.

The clitoris has very rich blood and nerve supplies. Overall, the clitoris has a richer nerve supply than the penis.

Clitoral innervation is through the terminal branch of the pudendal nerve. Its branches terminate in the glans and prepuce. Heightened clitoral sensation may depend on an abundance of Dogiel, Krause, and Ruffini corpuscles (specialized genital receptor nerve endings).

The clitoris exists primarily for female sexual enjoyment. In addition, it produces smegma. Along with other vulval secretions, smegma has a unique odor that may be erotically stimulating to the male.

URETHRAL MEATUS AND PARAURETHRAL GLANDS

The *urethral meatus* is 1 to 2.5 cm beneath the clitoris in the midline of the vestibule (Figure 6–3). At times the meatus is difficult to see because of the presence of blind dimples, small mucosal folds, or wide variance in location. Its appearance is often puckered and slitlike.

The *paraurethral,* or *Skene's, glands* open into the posterior wall of the female urethra close to its orifice (Figure 6–3). Their secretions help lubricate the vaginal vestibule, facilitating sexual intercourse.

VAGINAL VESTIBULE

The vaginal vestibule is a boat-shaped depression enclosed by the labia majora and visible when they are separated. It is bordered anteriorly by the clitoris and urethra, laterally by the labia minora, and posteriorly by the fourchette (Figure 6–3). The vestibule contains the vaginal opening, or *introitus,* which is the border between the external and internal genitals.

The *hymen* is a thin, stretchable membrane that partially closes the vaginal opening. Its strength, shape, and size vary greatly among women. The hymen is essentially avascular. The belief that the intact hymen is a sign of virginity and that it is broken at first sexual intercourse with resultant bleeding is not valid. The hymen can be broken through strenuous physical activity, masturbation, menstruation, or the use of tampons. Once it is broken, the irregular tags of tissue that remain are called the myrtiform or hymenal carbuncles.

External to the hymenal ring at the base of the vestibule are two small papular elevations containing the orifices of the ducts of the *vulvovaginal (Bartholin's) glands.* They lie under the constrictor muscle of the vagina. The vulvovaginal glands are not generally palpable upon examination, being placed deep in the perineal structures. Their ducts measure 1.5 to 2 cm in length and about 0.5 cm in diameter. The mucous secretion is clear and viscid, with an alkaline pH, all of which enhance the viability and motility of the sperm deposited in the vaginal vestibule.

These gland ducts can harbor gonococci and other bacteria, which can cause suppuration and Bartholin's gland abscesses (Pritchard et al 1985).

Innervation of the vestibular area is mainly by the perineal nerve from the sacral plexus. The area is not sensitive to touch generally, although the hymen contains numerous free nerve endings as receptors to pain.

PERINEAL BODY

The *perineal body* is a wedge-shaped mass of fibromuscular tissue, measuring about 4 × 4 × 4 cm, found between the lower part of the vagina and the anal canal (Figure 6–3). This area between the anus and the vagina is referred to as the *perineum.*

The muscles that meet at the perineal body are the external sphincter ani, both levator ani (the superficial and deep transverse perineal) and the bulbocavernosus. These muscles mingle with elastic fibers and connective tissue in an arrangement that allows a remarkable amount of stretching. The perineal body is much larger in the female than in the male and is subject to tearing during childbirth. It is the site of episiotomy during delivery (see Chapter 26).

Internal Genitals

The female internal reproductive organs—the vagina, uterus, fallopian tubes, and ovaries—are target organs for estrogenic hormones. These organs play a unique part in the reproductive cycle (Figure 6–4). The internal reproductive organs can be palpated during vaginal examination and assessed through use of a speculum, laparoscope, or

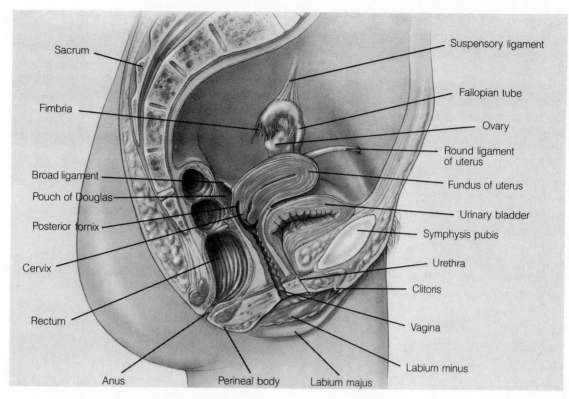

Figure 6–4   Female internal reproductive organs

culdoscope. Sonography has contributed greatly to the study of these reproductive organs and their functions.

VAGINA

The *vagina* is a muscular and membranous tube that connects the external genitals with the center of the pelvis (Figure 6–4). It passes from the vulva to the uterus in a position nearly parallel to the plane of the pelvic brim. This direction is optimal for coitus.

Because the cervix of the uterus projects into the upper part of the anterior wall of the vagina, the anterior wall is approximately 2.5 cm shorter than the posterior wall. Measurements range from 6 to 8 cm for the anterior wall and 7 to 10 cm for the posterior wall.

In the upper part of the vagina, which is called the vaginal *vault,* there is a recess or hollow around the cervix. This area is referred to as the vaginal *fornix.* Generally, the anterior and posterior vaginal walls meet; thus, on transverse sections, the vagina in repose is shaped like an **H.**

The walls of the vaginal vault are very thin. This structure facilitates pelvic examination. Various structures can be palpated through the walls and fornix of the vaginal vault, including the uterus, a distended bladder, the ovaries, the appendix, the cecum, the colon, and the ureters.

When a woman lies on her back, the space in the fornix permits the pooling of semen after intercourse. The

collection of a large number of sperm near the cervix in a favorable environment increases the chances of impregnation.

The walls of the vagina are covered with ridges, or *rugae,* crisscrossing each other. These rugae allow the vagina to stretch during the descent of the fetal head.

A rich blood supply is needed to maintain a high glycogen content in the epithelial cells as well as to nourish the underlying musculofascial layer, through which the vaginal vault has strong attachments to the cervix. The outer layer is composed of longitudinal muscle fibers, and the inner layer is composed of circular muscle fibers. These layers are continuous with the superficial muscle fibers of the uterus. A thin band of striated muscle, the sphincter vagina, is found at the lowest extremity of the vagina. However, the levator ani is the principal muscle that closes the vagina.

During a woman's reproductive life, an acidic vaginal environment is normal (pH 4–5). Secretion from the vaginal epithelium provides a moist environment. The acidic environment is maintained by a symbiotic relationship between lactic acid–producing bacilli (Döderlein bacillus or lactobacillus) and the vaginal epithelial cells. These cells contain glycogen, which is broken down by the bacilli into lactic acid. Figure 6–5 illustrates this process. The amount of glycogen is regulated by the ovarian hormones. Any interruption of this process can destroy the normal self-cleansing action of the vagina. Such interruption may be caused by antibiotic therapy, douching, or use of vaginal sprays or deodorants.

The acidic vaginal environment is normal only during the mature reproductive years and in the first days of life when maternal hormones are operating in the infant. A relatively neutral pH of 7.5 is normal from infancy until puberty and after menopause.

Each third of the vagina is supplied by a distinct vascular pattern. These include the cervicovaginal branches of uterine arteries (bladder arteries), the internal pudendal arteries, and the middle hemorrhoidal arteries (rectal arteries). Venous drainage is accomplished by the venous plexus, which is also anastomosed to the vertebral venous plexus. This anastomosis makes it possible for a pelvic embolism or carcinoma to bypass the heart and lungs and lodge in the brain, spine, or other remote part of the body.

Lymphatic drainage of the vagina follows a direct pattern. The upper third drains into the external and internal iliac nodes; the middle third, into the hypogastric nodes; and the lower third, into the inguinal glands. The posterior wall drains into nodes lying in the rectovaginal septum. Any vaginal infection follows these routes.

The vagina is a relatively insensitive organ, with meager somatic innervation to its lower third by the pudendal nerve and virtually no special nerve endings. Sensation during sexual excitement and coitus is minimal and pain during the second stage of labor is less than if somatic innervation were greater. Nervous supply to the vagina is predominantly autonomic. Sensation arises in the vagina and terminates at the S2-3-4 level.

The vagina is often called the birth canal because it forms the lower passageway through which the fetus moves during birth. It also permits the discharge of menstrual

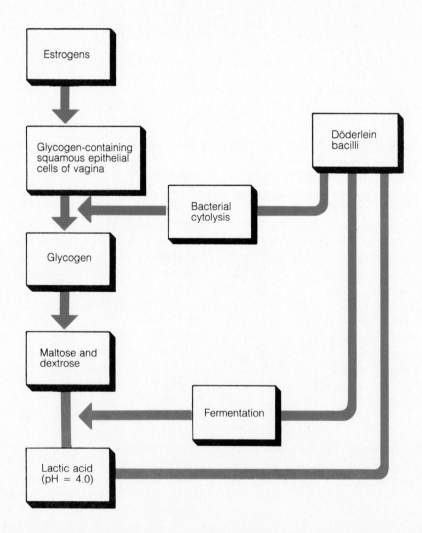

Figure 6–5   Scheme of biology of vagina: Reciprocal influence of the vaginal epithelium and Döderlein bacilli on maintenance of acidic vaginal milieu (From Beller FK, et al, *Gynecology: A Textbook for Students,* ed 3, New York, Springer-Verlag, 1980, p 220.)

products from the uterine endometrium to the outside of the body and protects against coital trauma and infection from pathogenic organisms.

UTERUS

Throughout the ages, the *uterus,* or womb, has been endowed with a mystical aura. As the core of reproduction and hence continuation of the human race, the uterus and its bearer have received particular attention and treatment. Numerous customs, taboos, mores, and values have evolved about women and their reproductive function. Although scientific knowledge has replaced much of this folklore, remnants of old ideas and superstitions persist. The nurse must be able to recognize and deal with such attitudes and beliefs so that nursing care can be effective.

The uterus is a hollow, muscular, thick-walled, pear-shaped organ lying centrally in the pelvic cavity between the base of the bladder and the rectum and above the vagina (Figure 6–6). It is level with or slightly below the brim of the pelvis, with the external os about the level of the ischial spines. Its anterior and posterior surfaces are in opposition, making its cavity potential rather than actual. The mature organ weighs about 60 g and is approximately 7.5 cm long, 5 cm wide, and 1 to 2.5 cm thick.

Many uterine anomalies are thought to be congenital and can be understood more easily by reviewing the embryologic development of the uterus. Between the sixth and ninth week of embryonic development, the two paramesonephric ducts, which are adjacent to the mesonephric ducts, grow caudally. Their ultimate fusion gives rise to the

fallopian tubes, uterine fundus, cervix, and upper vagina. A normal uterus therefore requires two symmetrical, parallel, equal-sized paramesonephric ducts to meet in the midline. Anomalies represent the absence of either one or both of the ducts, degrees of failure to fuse, or canalization defects. Figure 6–7 illustrates the normal uterus as contrasted with the common types of malformations. The bicornuate and didelphys uterine malformations are found most frequently and are associated with habitual abortion. Because both the urinary and reproductive systems develop from the common urogenital fold in the embryo, anomalies in one system are frequently accompanied by anomalies in the other. Problems of infertility and premature labor and delivery are common.

The uterus is kept in place by three sets of supports. The upper supports are the broad and round ligaments. The middle supports are the cardinal, pubocervical, and uterosacral ligaments. The lower supports are those structures considered to be the pelvic muscular floor.

The position of the uterus can vary, depending on a woman's posture, number of children borne, bladder and rectal fullness, and even normal respiratory patterns. Only the cervix is anchored laterally. The body of the uterus can move freely forward or backward. The axis also varies. The uterus generally bends forward, forming a sharp angle with the vagina. There is a bend in the area of the isthmus of the uterus; from there the cervix points downward. The uterus is said to be *anteverted* when it is in this position. The anteverted position is considered normal.

The isthmus, referred to earlier in this section, is a slight constriction in the uterus that divides it into two unequal parts. The upper two-thirds of the uterus is the *corpus,* or *body,* composed mainly of myometrium. The lower third is the *cervix,* or *neck.* The rounded uppermost portion of the corpus that extends above the points of attachment of the fallopian tubes is called the *fundus.* The elongated portion of the uterus where the fallopian tubes open is called the *cornua.*

The isthmus is about 6 mm above the internal os, and it is in this area that the uterine endometrium changes into the mucous membrane of the cervix. The isthmus takes on significance in pregnancy because it becomes the lower uterine segment. With the cervix, it is a passive segment and not part of the contractile uterus. At delivery, this thin lower segment, situated behind the bladder, is the site for lower-segment cesarean deliveries (see Chapter 26).

○   *THE CORPUS*   The *corpus* of the uterus is made up of three layers: outermost, or serosal (perimetrium); middle, or muscular (myometrium); and innermost, or mucosal (endometrium). Each layer is distinct in makeup and function.

The serosal layer of the uterus is made up of peritoneum, which runs directly onto the anterior surface of the uterus at the level of the internal os from the anterior

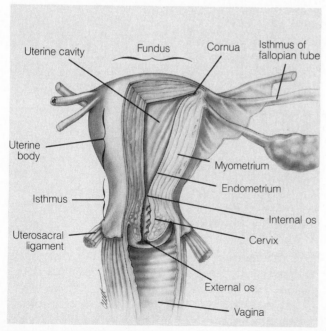

Figure 6–6   Structures of the uterus

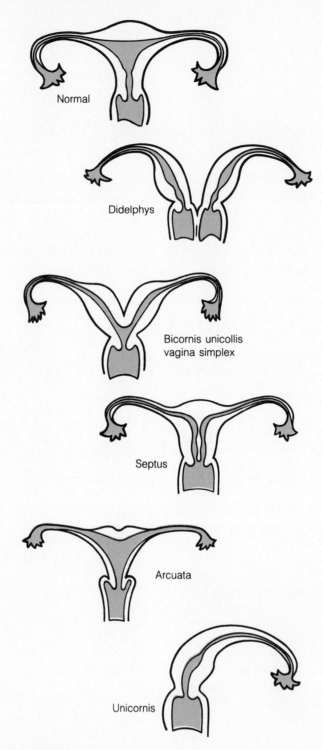

Figure 6–7   Congenital malformations of the uterus

abdominal wall, and continues over the fundus and down over the posterior surface of the corpus. It forms the anterior wall of the rectouterine pouch (pouch of Douglas). The two-layered folds of peritoneum, extending from the lateral uterine margins to the lateral pelvic walls, make up the broad ligament.

The muscular uterine layer has, in turn, three indistinct layers. It should be noted that myometrium is continuous with the muscle layer of the fallopian tubes as well as with that of the vagina. This helps these organs present a unified reaction to various stimuli—ovulation, orgasm, or the deposit of sperm in the vagina. These muscle fibers also extend into the ovarian, round, and cardinal ligaments and minimally into the uterosacral ligaments, which helps explain the vague but disturbing pelvic "aches and pains" reported by many pregnant women.

The myometrium has three distinct layers of uterine (smooth) involuntary mucles (Figure 6–8). The outer layer, found mainly over the fundus, is made up of longitudinal muscles especially suited to expel the fetus during birth. The middle layer is thick and made up of interlacing muscle fibers in figure eight patterns. These muscle fibers surround large blood vessels, and their contraction produces a hemostatic action. The inner muscle layer is made up of circular fibers, which form sphincters at the uterine tube attachment sites (tubia ostia) and at the internal os. The internal os sphincter inhibits the expulsion of the uterine contents during pregnancy. An incompetent cervical os can be caused by a torn, weak, or absent sphincter at the internal os. The sphincters at the fallopian tubes prevent menstrual blood from flowing backward into the fallopian tubal lumen from the uterus.

Although each layer of muscle has been discussed as having a unique function, it must be remembered that the uterine musculature works as a whole. The uterine contractions of labor are responsible for the dilation of the cervix and provide the major impetus for the passage of the fetus through the pelvic axis and vaginal canal at birth. The mucosal layer or endometrium of the uterine corpus is the innermost layer. This layer is composed of a single layer of columnar epithelium, glands, and stroma. From menarche to menopause, the endometrium undergoes monthly degeneration and renewal in the absence of pregnancy. As it responds to a governing hormonal cycle and prostaglandin influence as well, the endometrium varies in thickness from 0.5 to 5 mm.

The glands of the endometrium produce a thin, watery, alkaline secretion that keeps the uterine cavity moist. This "endometrial milk" not only assists the sperm on their journey to the fallopian tubes but also provides nourishment to the blastocyst prior to implantation (Chapter 13).

During the late luteal (secretory) phase of the menstrual cycle or in early pregnancy, the endometrium is composed of three layers. The *zona compacta* is in the region of the mouth of the glands. The *zona spongiosa* is the next deeper layer. Its glands are dilated and extremely tortuous. The deepest layer, next to the myometrium, is the *zona basalis*. The zona compacta and zona spongiosa, which are frequently combined to be called *zona functionalis,* are shed at menstruation.

The blood and lymphatic supplies to the uterus are extensive (Figure 6–9). The unique blood supply to the endometrium is important. In the myometrium, the radial arteries branch off from the arcuate arteries at right angles. Once inside the endometrium, they become the basal arteries supplying the zona basalis and ultimately become the coiled arteries supplying the zona functionalis. The

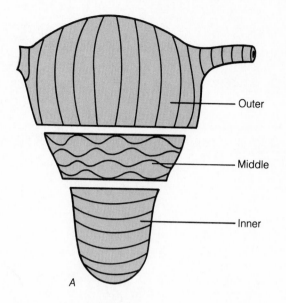

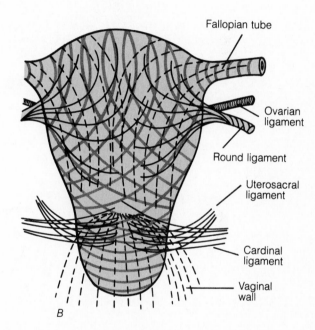

Figure 6–8   Uterine muscle layers: A Muscle fiber placement. B Interlacing of uterine muscle layers

straighter basal arteries are smaller than the coiled arteries; they are not sensitive to cyclic hormonal control. Hence the zona basalis remains intact and is the site of new endometrial tissue generation. The coiled arteries are extremely sensitive to cyclic hormonal control. Their response is alternate relaxation and constriction during the ischemic or terminal phase of the menstrual cycle.

When pregnancy occurs and the endometrium is not shed, the reticular stromal cells surrounding the endometrial glands become the decidual cells of pregnancy. The stromal cells are highly vascular, channeling a rich blood supply to the endometrial surface.

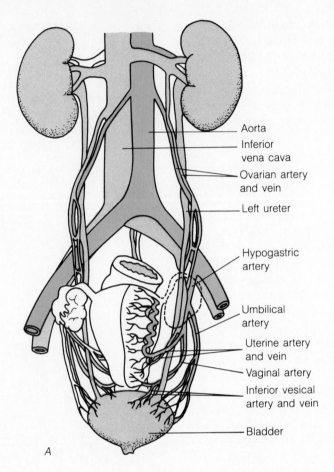

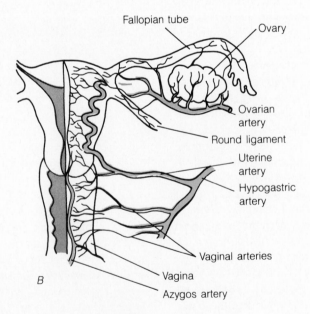

Figure 6–9   Blood supply to internal reproductive organs: A Pelvic blood supply. B Blood supply to vagina, ovary, uterus, and fallopian tubes

The uterus is innervated entirely by the autonomic nervous system, and innervation seems to more regulatory than primary in nature. It is helpful to recall that sympathetic fibers generally stimulate muscle contraction and vasoconstriction; parasympathetic fibers inhibit contractions and stimulate vasodilation. There is adequate contractility of the uterus without an intact nerve supply, as illustrated by the fact that hemiplegic patients have adequate uterine contractions (Beller et al 1980).

Uterine parasympathetic fibers arise from the second, third, and fourth sacral nerves to form the pelvic nerves. Sympathetic fibers enter the pelvis through the hypogastric plexus.

Both the sympathetic and parasympathetic nerves contain motor fibers and a few sensory fibers. Pain of uterine contractions is carried to the central nervous system by the eleventh and twelfth thoracic nerve roots. Pain from the cervix and upper vagina passes through the ilioinguinal and pudendal nerves. The motor fibers to the uterus arise from the seventh and eighth thoracic vertebrae. Because the sensory and motor levels are separated in this manner, caudal and spinal anesthesia can be used during labor and delivery.

The uterus is designed to provide a safe environment for fetal development. The uterine lining is cyclically prepared by steroid hormones for nidation (implantation of the embryo). Once the embryo is implanted, the developing fetus is protected until it is expelled.

Both the body of the uterus and the cervix are changed permanently by pregnancy. The body never returns to its prepregnant size, and the external os changes from a circular opening of about 3 mm to a transverse slit with irregular edges. Figure 6–10 illustrates the changes in size of the uterus and the external os during the life span of a parous woman.

○ *THE CERVIX* The cervix is about 2.5 cm in both length and diameter. It is canal-like; its exit into the vagina is called the *external os,* and its entrance into the corpus is called the *internal os* (Figure 6–6).

The cervix is a protective portal for the body of the uterus as well as the connection between the vagina and the uterus. The cervix is divided by its line of attachment into the vaginal and supravaginal areas. The *vaginal cervix* projects into the vagina at an angle of from 45° to 90°. The *supravaginal cervix* is surrounded by the attachments that give the uterus its main support: the uterosacral ligaments, the transverse ligaments of the cervix (Mackenrodt's ligaments), and the pubocervical ligaments.

The vaginal cervix appears pink and is covered by pale squamous stratified epithelium, which is continuous with the vaginal lining. The vaginal cervix ends at the external os. The cervical canal appears rosy red and is lined with columnar ciliated epithelium, which contain mucus-secreting glands. Most cervical cancer begins at this squamocolumnar junction. Its exact location varies with age and parity. Figure 6–11 shows this junction at various stages of a woman's life.

Elasticity is a chief characteristic of the cervix. Its ability to stretch is a result of the high fibrous and collagenous content of the supportive tissues and the vast number of folds in the cervical lining, which increases its actual area tremendously. About 10 percent of the cervix is composed of muscle cells.

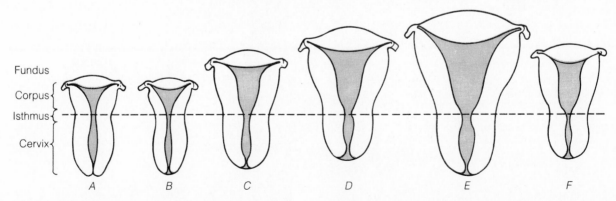

Fundus
Corpus
Isthmus
Cervix

A   B   C   D   E   F

Figure 6–10   Changes in size of uterus and external os during a woman's life. A Neonate: corpus ⅓ and cervix ⅔; length varies from 2.5 to 3.5 cm. B Childhood (preschool): same proportion; has elongated slightly. C Puberty: corpus ½ and cervix ½; length varies from 5 to 6 cm. D Adulthood (nulliparous): corpus ⅔ and cervix ⅓; *length varies from 6 to 8 cm. Weight varies from 50 to 70 g. E Adulthood (multiparous): corpus ⅔ and cervix ⅓; length varies from 9 to 10 cm. Weight 80 g or more. F Postmenopause: corpus* ⅔, *cervix ⅓; decrease in size and weight.*

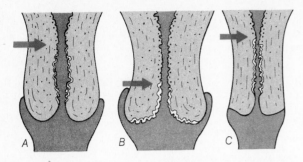

Figure 6–11 Changes in squamocolumnar junction (arrows) at various stages of life. A Childhood. B Reproductive years. C Old age (Modified from Beller FK, et al, *Gynecology: A Textbook for Students,* ed 3, New York, Springer-Verlag, 1980, p 34)

The cervical mucosa has three functions: (1) to provide lubrication for the vaginal canal, (2) to act as a bacteriostatic agent, and (3) to provide an alkaline environment to shelter deposited sperm from the acidic vagina. At ovulation, cervical mucus is clearer, thinner, and more alkaline than at other times.

○ **UTERINE LIGAMENTS** The uterine ligaments support and stabilize the various reproductive organs. The ligaments shown in Figures 6–8 and 6–12 are described in this section.

The *broad ligament* keeps the uterus centrally placed and provides stability within the pelvic cavity. It is a double mesenteric layer that is continuous with the abdominal peritoneum. The broad ligament covers the uterus anteriorly and posteriorly and extends outward from the uterus to enfold and stabilize the fallopian tubes. The round and ovarian ligaments are at the upper border of the broad ligament. At its lower border, it forms the cardinal ligaments. Between the folds of the broad ligament are connective tissue, involuntary muscle, blood and lymph vessels, and nerves.

The *round ligaments* help the broad ligament keep the uterus in place. Each of the round ligaments arises from the sides of the uterus near the fallopian tube insertion. They course outward between the folds of the broad ligament, passing through the inguinal ring and canals and eventually fusing with the connective tissue of the labia majora. Made up of longitudinal muscle, the round ligaments enlarge during pregnancy. During labor the round ligaments steady the uterus, pulling downward and forward so that the presenting part is forced into the cervix.

The *ovarian ligaments* are short, round, fibromuscular cords that anchor the lower pole of the ovary to the cornua of the uterus. They are composed of muscle fibers that allow the ligaments to contract. This contractile ability influences the position of the ovary to some extent, thus helping the fimbriae of the fallo-

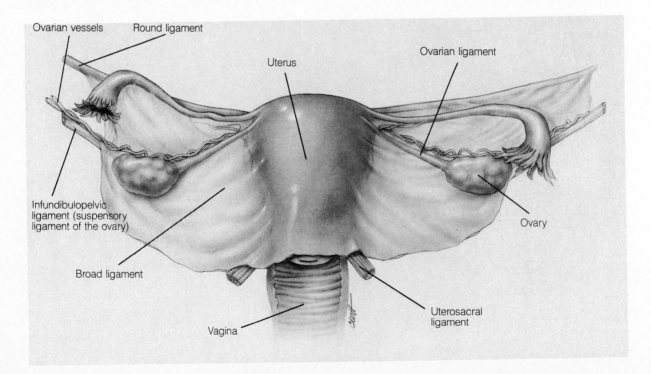

Figure 6–12 Uterine ligaments (cardinal ligaments not shown)

pian tubes to "catch" the ovum as it is released each month.

The *cardinal ligaments* are the chief uterine supports, suspending the uterus from the side walls of the true pelvis (Figure 6–8). These ligaments, also known as *Mackenrodt's,* or *transverse cervical, ligaments,* arise from the sides of the pelvic walls and attach to the cervix in the upper vagina. These ligaments prevent uterine prolapse and also support the upper vagina.

The *infundibulopelvic ligament* suspends and supports the ovaries (Figure 6–12). Arising from the outer third of the broad ligament, the infundibulopelvic ligament contains the ovarian vessels and nerves.

The *uterosacral ligaments* provide support for the uterus and cervix at the level of the ischial spines (Figure 6–12). Arising on each side of the pelvis from the posterior wall of the uterus, the uterosacral ligaments sweep back around the rectum and insert on the sides of the first and second sacral vertebrae. With the cardinal and pubovesical ligaments, the uterosacral ligaments make up a fibromuscular tissue support system extending from the pelvic wall to the uterus near the internal os.

The uterosacral ligaments contain smooth muscle fibers, connective tissue, blood and lymph vessels, and nerves. Providing support for the uterus and cer-

vix at the level of the ischial spines, they also contain sensory nerve fibers that contribute to dysmenorrhea.

FALLOPIAN TUBES

The fallopian tubes, also known as oviducts, arise laterally from the cornua of the uterus and reach almost to the side of the pelvis, where they turn posteriorly and medially toward the ovaries (Figure 6–13). Each tube is 8 to 13.5 cm long, lying in the superior border of the broad ligament (mesosalpinx). These tubes are not inert, rigid structures; they are dynamic and restless, constantly seeking the ovum to be released from the ovary. The fallopian tubes link the peritoneal cavity with the external environment by way of the uterus and vagina. This linkage increases a woman's biologic vulnerability to disease processes.

A short section of each fallopian tube is inside the uterus with its opening into the uterus (uterine ostium) only 1 mm in diameter.

Each tube may be divided into three parts: the isthmus, the ampulla, and the infundibulum (fimbria). The isthmus is straight and narrow, with a thick muscular wall and a lumen 2 to 3 mm in diameter. It is the site of tubal ligation (a surgical procedure to prevent pregnancy; see Chapter 8). Next to the isthmus is the curved ampulla, which comprises the outer two-thirds of the tube. Fertilization of the primary oocyte by a spermatozoon usually occurs here. The ampulla has the widest lumen, and its

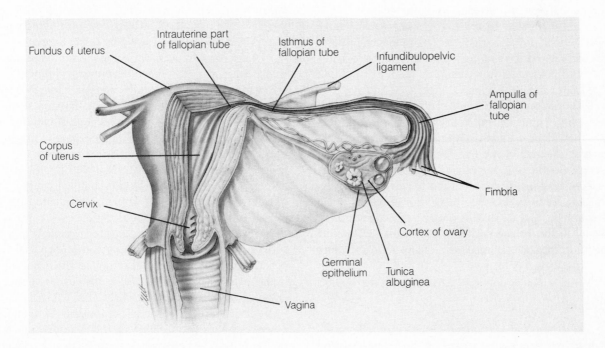

Figure 6–13   Fallopian tube and ovary

muscular wall is thin and distensible. It terminates in the infundibulum, which is a funnellike enlargement with many moving fingerlike projections (fimbriae) reaching out to the ovary. The longest of these, the fimbria ovarica, is attached to the ovary to increase the chances of intercepting the ovum as it is released.

The wall of the fallopian tube is made up of four layers: peritoneal (serous), subserous (adventitial), muscular, and mucous tissues. The peritoneum covers the tubes. The subserous layer contains the blood and nerve supply, and the muscular layer is responsible for the peristaltic movement of the tube created by smooth involuntary muscle fibers. The mucosal layer, immediately next to the muscular layer, is continuous with the uterine endometrium, although it is less sensitive to hormonal changes. This layer is arranged in longitudinal folds, or plicae, and is composed of ciliated and nonciliated cells with the number of ciliated cells more abundant at the fimbria. Nonciliated cells are goblet cells that secrete a protein-rich, serous fluid that nourishes the ovum. The constantly roving tubal cilia propel the ovum toward the uterus. Because the ovum is a large cell, this ciliary action is needed to assist the peristalsis of the tube's muscular layer. Any malformation or malfunction of the tubes could result in infertility or even sterility.

A well-functioning tubal transport system involves active fimbriae in close proximation to the ovary; peristalsis of the tube created by the muscular layer; ciliated currents beating toward the uterus; and the proximal contraction and distal relaxation of the tube caused by different types of prostaglandins (Marshall & Ross 1982).

Each fallopian tube is richly supplied with blood by the uterine and ovarian arteries. Thus the fallopian tubes have an unusual ability to recover from any inflammatory process. Venous drainage occurs through the pampiniform plexus and the ovarian and uterine veins. Lymphatic drainage occurs through the vessels close to the ureter into the lumbar nodes along the aorta.

Both parasympathetic and sympathetic motor and sensory nerves from the pelvic plexus and ovarian plexus supply the fallopian tubes. Pain arising from the tubes is referred to the area of the iliac fossa, because both areas are served by the same segment of skin innervation.

The functions of the tubes are to provide transport for the egg from the ovary to the uterus; to act as a site for fertilization; and to serve as a warm, moist, nourishing environment for the egg or zygote (Chapter 13). The time needed for transport through the fallopian tubes varies from 3 to 4 days.

OVARIES

The *ovaries* are two almond-shaped glandular structures lying on the posterior surface of the broad ligament, just below the pelvic brim and near the infundibulum

(Figure 6–13). Their size varies among women and with the stage of the menstrual cycle. Each ovary weighs 6 to 10 g and is 1.5 to 3 cm wide, 2 to 5 cm long, and 1 to 1.5 cm thick. The ovaries are small in girls but increase in size after puberty. They also change in appearance from a dull white, smooth-surfaced organ to a pitted gray organ because of scarring due to ovulation.

The typical position of each ovary is in the upper part of the pelvic cavity at the lateral wall in a depression created at the external iliac vein and ureteral junction. It is rare that both ovaries are at the same level. The ovary is held in place by the ovarian and infundibulopelvic ligaments (Figure 6–12). Blood vessels, nerves, and lymphatics enter the ovary through the hilum.

There is no peritoneal covering for the ovaries. Although this lack of covering assists the mature ovum to erupt, it also allows easier spread of malignant cells from cancer of the ovaries. A single layer of cuboidal epithelial cells, called the germinal epithelium, covers the ovaries. The ovaries are composed of three layers: the tunica albuginea, the cortex, and the medulla. The tunica albuginea is dense and dull white and serves as a protective layer. The cortex is the main functional part because it contains ova, graafian follicles, corpora lutea, degenerated corpora lutea (corpora albicantia), and degenerated follicles held together by the ovarian stroma. The medulla is completely surrounded by the cortex and contains the nerves and the blood and lymphatic vessels.

The motor and sensory parasympathetic and sympathetic nerves follow the ovarian artery across the infundibulopelvic ligament to reach the ovary. The ovaries are relatively insensitive unless they are squeezed or distended. *Mittelschmerz,* or midcycle pain, is caused by irritation of the peritoneum by fluid or blood escaping along with the ovum. Pain can also be caused by follicular cysts.

The ovary is a crucial component of reproduction. Even a small part of a functioning ovary will ovulate, providing an ovum for fertilization monthly. Close to a million oocytes are locked in the first meiotic division at birth.

The ovaries are the primary source of two important hormones: the estrogens and progesterone. *Estrogens* are associated with those characteristics contributing to femaleness including breast alveolar lobule growth and duct development. The ovaries secrete large amounts of estrogen, while the adrenal cortex (extraglandular sites) produces minute amounts of estrogen.

Progesterone is often called the *hormone of pregnancy* because its effects on the uterus allow pregnancy to be maintained. This hormone also inhibits the action of prolactin in α-lactalbumin synthesis, thereby preventing lactation during pregnancy (Pritchard et al 1985).

The interplay between the ovarian hormones and other hormones such as FSH and LH is responsible for the cyclic changes that allow pregnancy. Chapter 7 contains an in-depth discussion of the hormonal and physical changes that occur during the female reproductive cycle. When a woman reaches the age of 45 to 55 years, the ovaries no longer secrete estrogen. Ovulatory activity ceases and menopause occurs.

Bony Pelvis

The female *bony pelvis* has the unique functions of supporting and protecting the pelvic contents as well as forming the relatively fixed axis of the birth passage. For these reasons, structural aspects of the pelvis important to childbearing must be understood clearly.

BONY STRUCTURE

The pelvis is made up of two innominate bones, the sacrum, and the coccyx. The pelvis resembles a bowl or basin; its sides are the innominate bones, and its back is composed of the sacrum and coccyx. Lined with fibrocartilage and held tightly together by ligaments, the four bones join at the symphysis pubis, the two sacroiliac joints, and the sacrococcygeal joints (Figure 6–14).

The *innominate bones,* also known as the *hip bones* or *os coxae,* are actually made up of three separate bones: the ilium, the ischium, and the pubis. These bones fuse to form a circular cavity, the *acetabulum,* which articulates with the femur.

The *ilium* is the broad, upper prominence of the hip. The *iliac crest* is the margin of the ilium. The *iliac spine,* the foremost projection nearest the groin, is the site of attachment for ligaments and muscles.

The *ischium,* the stongest bone, is under the ilium and below the acetabulum. The L-shaped ischium ends in a marked protuberance, the *ischial tuberosity,* on which the weight of a seated body rests. The *ischial spines* arise near the junction of the ilium and ischium and jut into the pelvic cavity. The shortest diameter of the pelvic cavity is between the ischial spines. The ischial spines can serve as a reference point during labor to evaluate the descent of the fetal head into the birth canal.

The *pubis* forms the slightly bowed front portion of the innominate bone. Extending medially from the acetabulum to the midpoint of the bony pelvis, the two pubic bones meet to form a joint, the *symphysis pubis.* The triangular space below this junction is known as the *pubic arch.* The fetal head passes under this arch during birth. The symphysis pubis is formed by heavy fibrocartilage and the superior and inferior pubic ligaments. The mobility of the inferior ligament, also known as the *arcuate pubic ligament,* increases during pregnancy and to a greater extent in subsequent pregnancies than in first pregnancies.

The sacroiliac joints also have a degree of mobility that increases near the end of pregnancy as the result of an upward gliding movement. The pelvic outlet may be increased by 1.5 to 2 cm in the squatting, sitting, and dorsal lithotomy positions. These relaxations of the joints are induced by the hormones of pregnancy.

The *sacrum* is a wedge-shaped bone formed by the fusion of five vertebrae. On the anterior upper portion of the sacrum is a projection into the pelvic cavity known as the *sacral promontory.* This projection is another obstetric guide in determining pelvic measurements.

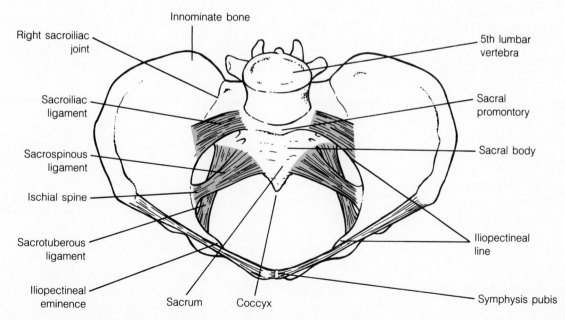

Figure 6–14   Pelvic bones with supporting ligaments

Table 6–1   Muscles of the Pelvic Floor

Muscle	Origin	Insertion	Innervation	Action
Levator ani	Pubis, lateral pelvic wall, and ischial spine	Blends with organs in pelvic cavity	Inferior rectal, second and third sacral nerves, plus anterior rami of third and fourth sacral nerves	Supports pelvic viscera; helps form pelvic diaphragm
Iliococcygeus	Pelvic surface of ischial spine and pelvic fascia	Central point of perineum, coccygeal raphe, and coccyx		Assists in supporting abdominal and pelvic viscera
Pubococcygeus	Pubis and pelvic fascia	Coccyx		
Puborectalis	Pubis	Blends with rectum; meets similar fibers from opposite side		Forms sling for rectum, just posterior to it; raises anus
Pubovaginalis	Pubis	Blends into vagina		Supports vagina
Coccygeus	Ischial spine and sacrospinous ligament	Lateral border of lower sacrum and upper coccyx	Third and fourth sacral nerves	Supports pelvic viscera; helps form pelvic diaphragm; flexes and abducts coccyx

The small triangular bone last on the vertebral column is the *coccyx*. It articulates with the sacrum at the sacrococcygeal joint. The coccyx usually moves backward during labor to provide more room for the fetus.

PELVIC FLOOR

A complementary structure of the bony pelvis is its muscular *pelvic floor,* which is designed to overcome the force of gravity exerted on the pelvic viscera and, to a lesser extent, on the abdominal viscera. It acts as a buttress to the irregularly shaped pelvic outlet, thereby providing stability and support for surrounding structures and organs.

Deep fascia and the levator ani and coccygeal muscles form the part of the pelvic floor known as the *pelvic diaphragm.* Superior to it is the pelvic cavity; inferior and posterior to it is the *perineum.* Laterally, the walls of the pelvis are composed of the obturator internus muscles and fascia, which form a band called the arcus tendineus. The sacrum is located posteriorly. Lateral and anterior to the sacrum are the many nerves of the sacral plexus, also covered with parietal pelvic fascia.

The sheetlike *levator ani muscle* makes up the major portion of the pelvic diaphragm and consists of four muscles: ileococcygeus, pubococcygeus, puborectalis, and pubovaginalis. Forming a sling for the pelvic structures, the levator ani is interrupted by the urethra, vagina, and rectum. The ileococcygeal muscle is a thin muscular sheet overlying the sacrospinous ligament and assists the levator ani in supporting the abdominal and pelvic viscera (Figure 6–15). The origins, insertions, innervations, and actions of these muscles are presented in Table 6–1.

Endopelvic fascia covers the pelvic diaphragm. The component parts function as a whole, yet are able to move over one another. This provides an exceptional capacity for dilation during birth and return to prepregnant condition following birth (Figure 6–15).

The *urogenital triangle* (diaphragm) is external to the pelvic diaphragm, in the triangular area between the ischial tuberosities and the hollow of the pubic arch. It is made up of superficial and deep perineal membranes extending from the rami of the ischial and pubic bones. Most important in this region are the deep transverse perineal muscles, which are flat bands of muscle arising from the ischiopubic rami and intertwining in the midline to form a seam, or raphe. These muscles are modified to encircle both the urinary meatus and the vaginal orifice, forming the urethral and vaginal sphincters.

PELVIC DIVISION

The pelvic cavity is divided into the false pelvis and the true pelvis (Figure 6–16A).

False pelvis. The false pelvis is the portion above the pelvic brim, or linea terminalis, bounded by the lumbar vertebrae posteriorly, the iliac fossae laterally, and the lower abdominal wall anteriorly. It supports the weight of the enlarged pregnant uterus and directs the presenting fetal part into the true pelvis below.

True pelvis. The true pelvis lies below the pelvic brim and is bounded superiorly by the promontory and alae of the sacrum and the upper margins of the pubic bones and inferiorly by the pelvic outlet. The true pelvis represents the bony limits of the birth canal. It measures about 5 cm at its anterior wall at the symphysis pubis and about 10 cm at its posterior wall. When a woman is standing upright, the upper portion of the pelvic cavity or canal is directed downward and backward and its lower portion,

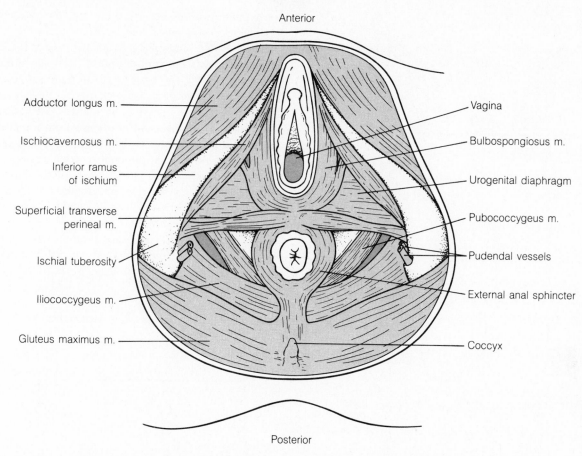

Anterior

Adductor longus m.

Ischiocavernosus m.

Inferior ramus
of ischium

Superficial transverse
perineal m.

Ischial tuberosity

Iliococcygeus m.

Gluteus maximus m.

Vagina

Bulbospongiosus m.

Urogenital diaphragm

Pubococcygeus m.

Pudendal vessels

External anal sphincter

Coccyx

Posterior

Figure 6–15 Muscles of the pelvic floor. The puborectalis, pubovaginalis, and coccygeal muscles cannot be seen from this view.

downward and forward. This forms an axis or curved canal through which the presenting part of the baby must pass during birth (Figure 6–16B). The inclination of the pelvis is the angle formed by two planes, a horizontal one through the tip of the coccyx and the superior border of the symphysis pubis and an inclined one through the sacral promontory and the superior border of the symphysis pubis. This pelvic angle of inclination usually measures 50° to 60° (Figure 6–17).

The bony circumference of the true pelvis is made up of the sacrum, coccyx, and innominate bones below the linea terminalis. This area is of paramount importance in obstetrics because its size and shape must be adequate for normal fetal passage during labor and at delivery. The relationship of the fetal head to this cavity is of critical importance.

The true pelvis is considered to have three parts: the inlet, the pelvic cavity, and the outlet. The pelvic planes are imaginary flat surfaces drawn across the three parts of the true pelvis at strategic levels (Figure 6–18). Associated with each part are distinct obstetric measurements that aid in evaluating the adequacy of the pelvis for childbearing.

The dimensions of the true pelvis and their obstetric implications are described here. Measurement techniques are discussed in Chapter 15. The effects of inadequate or abnormal pelvic diameters on labor and delivery are further considered in Chapter 25.

The *pelvic inlet* is the upper border of the true pelvis and typically is round in the female. The size and shape of the pelvic inlet are determined by assessing three anteroposterior diameters: the diagonal conjugate, obstetric conjugate, and conjugate vera (Figure 6–19). The *diagonal conjugate* extends from the subpubic angle to the middle of the sacral promontory and is 12.5 cm. The diagonal conjugate can be measured manually during a pelvic examination. The *obstetric conjugate* extends from the middle of the sacral promontory to an area approximately 1 cm below the pubic crest. Its length is estimated by subtracting 1.5 cm from the diagonal conjugate. The fetus passes through the obstetric conjugate, and the size of this diameter determines whether the fetus can move down into the birth canal and engagement will occur. The true (anatomic) conjugate, or *conjugate vera,* extends from the middle of the sacral promontory to the middle of the pubic crest (superior surface of the symphysis). One additional

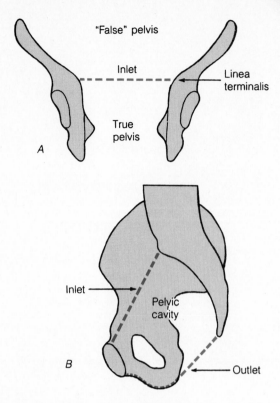

Figure 6–16 *Female pelvis: A False and true pelves. B Pelvic cavity*

measurement, the *transverse diameter,* helps determine the shape of the inlet. The transverse diameter is the largest diameter of the inlet and is measured using the linea terminales as the points of reference. This diameter assists in determining the shape of the inlet. It and the true conjugate lie at right angles to each other.

The *pelvic cavity* (canal) has varying diameters. The largest part of the pelvis is called the *plane of the greatest dimensions* (Figure 6–18). It is bounded by the junction of the second and third sacral vertebras posteriorly, the upper and middle thirds of the obturator foramen laterally, and the midpoint of the posterior surface of the pubis anteriorly. It is a curved canal with a longer posterior than anterior wall. A change in the lumbar curve can increase or decrease the pelvic inclination and can influence the progress of labor since the fetus has to adjust itself to a curved path as well as to the different diameters of the true pelvis (Figure 6–16).

The smallest part of the pelvis is called the *plane of the least dimensions,* or the midpelvic plane (Figure 6–18). Arrest of labor occurs most frequently because of contracture (narrowing) in this plane, so its diameters are of great importance. The plane extends from the lower margin of the symphysis pubis, through the ischial spines, to the junction of the fourth and fifth sacral vertebras. Its anterior and posterior borders are bounded by the lower margin of

the symphysis pubis, and fascia covering the obturator foramen, the ischial spines, the sacrospinous ligaments, and the sacrum. The anteroposterior diameter extends from the lower margin of the symphysis pubis to the junction of the fourth and fifth sacral vertebras. The transverse (interspinous) diameter extends between the ischial spines and measures about 10.5 cm; it is the shortest pelvic diameter. The posterior sagittal diameter extends from the bispinous diameter to the junction of the fourth and fifth sacral vertebras (Figure 6–19). At the midpelvic plane, the curve of the pelvic canal begins, and the axis of the birth canal changes. Until it reaches the ischial spines, the fetal head descends in a straight line. Then it curves forward toward the pelvic outlet (Figure 6–18).

The *pelvic outlet,* also called the *inferior strait,* is at the lower border of the true pelvis. It can be thought of as being composed of two triangles with a common base but in different planes. The common base as well as the most inferior part is the transverse diameter between the ischial tuberosities. The anterior triangle has as its apex the

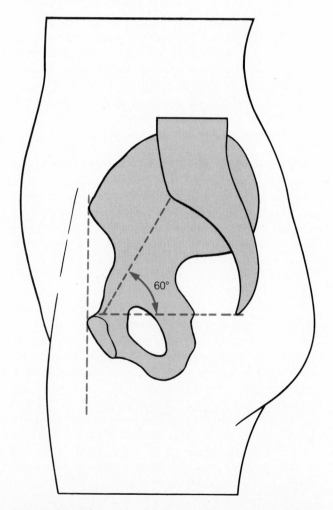

Figure 6–17 *Pelvic angle of inclination while woman is standing*

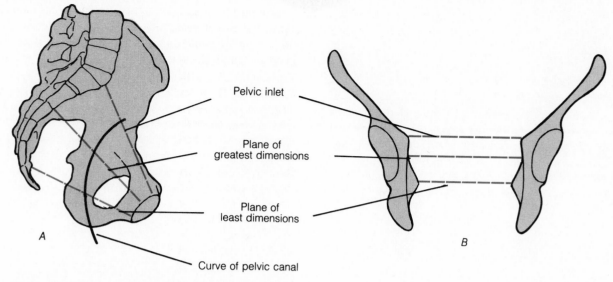

Pelvic inlet

Plane of
greatest dimensions

Plane of
least dimensions

Curve of pelvic canal

A

B

Figure 6–18   Pelvic planes: A Sagittal section. B Coronal section

lower margin of the symphysis pubis, and the posterior triangle, the tip of the sacrum (Figure 6–18).

The anteroposterior diameter of the pelvic outlet extends from the inferior margin of the symphysis to the tip of the coccyx. This is the anatomic diameter. The obstetric anteroposterior diameter extends to the sacrococcygeal joint (see Chapter 15). The anteroposterior diameter increases during delivery as the presenting part pushes the coccyx posteriorly at the mobile sacrococcygeal joint. Decreased mobility, a large fetal head, and/or a forceful delivery can cause the coccyx to snap. As the infant's head emerges, the long diameter of the head (occipital frontal) parallels the long diameter of the outlet (anteroposterior).

The transverse diameter (bi-ischial or intertuberous) extends from the inner surface of one ischial tuberosity to the other. It is the shortest diameter of the pelvic outlet

and becomes shorter as the pubic arch narrows. The anterior sagittal diameter extends from the middle of the transverse diameter to the suprapubic angle. The posterior sagittal diameter extends from the middle of the transverse diameter to the sacrococcygeal junction. This is the most significant diameter of the outlet because it is the smallest diameter through which the infant must pass as it descends through the pelvic canal. The pubic arch has great importance, because the baby must pass under it. If it is narrow, the baby's head may be pushed backward toward the coccyx, making the extension of the head difficult. This situation is known as *outlet dystocia,* and forceps (outlet) delivery is required.

TYPES OF PELVES

The Caldwell-Moloy classification of pelves is widely used to differentiate types of bony pelves (Caldwell & Moloy 1933). Gynecoid, android, anthropoid, and platypelloid are the four basic types. However, variations in the female pelvis from plane to plane are so great that classic types are not usual.

An imaginary line drawn through the greatest transverse diameter of the inlet divides it into anterior and posterior segments, and the pelvis type is always determined on the basis of the posterior segment of the inlet. With the posterior segment determining the type, the anterior segment of the inlet names variations. For example, an android pelvis with an anthropoid variation means that the posterior segment of the inlet is android and the anterior segment is anthropoid. Consideration is given to the size of the sacrosciatic notch, flaring of the pelvic brim, the shape of the inlet, and the relationship of the greatest anteroposterior diameter to the greatest transverse diameter.

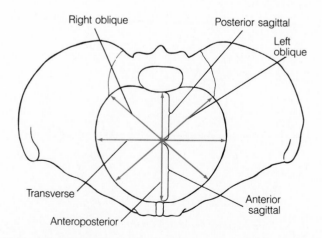

Right oblique

Posterior sagittal

Left oblique

Transverse

Anterior sagittal

Anteroposterior

Figure 6–19   Diameters of pelvic inlet

Each type of pelvis has implications for labor and delivery. These are described briefly here and in depth in Chapter 25.

○   *GYNECOID PELVIS*   The most common female pelvis is the gynecoid type (Figure 6–20). The inlet is rounded, with the anteroposterior diameter a little shorter than the transverse diameter. All the inlet diameters are at least adequate. The posterior segment is broad, deep, and roomy, and the anterior segment is well rounded. The gynecoid midpelvis has nonprominent ischial spines, straight and parallel side walls, and a wide, deep sacral curve. The sac-

rum is short and slopes backward. All of the midpelvic diameters are at least adequate. The gynecoid pelvic outlet has a wide and round pubic arch; the inferior pubic rami are short and concave. The anteroposterior diameter is long and the transverse diameter adequate. The capacity of the outlet is adequate. The bones are of medium structure and weight. Approximately 50 percent of female pelves are classified as gynecoid (Oxhorn 1986).

○   *ANDROID PELVIS*   The normal male pelvis is the android type (Figure 6–20). The inlet is heart-shaped. The anteroposterior and transverse diameters are adequate for

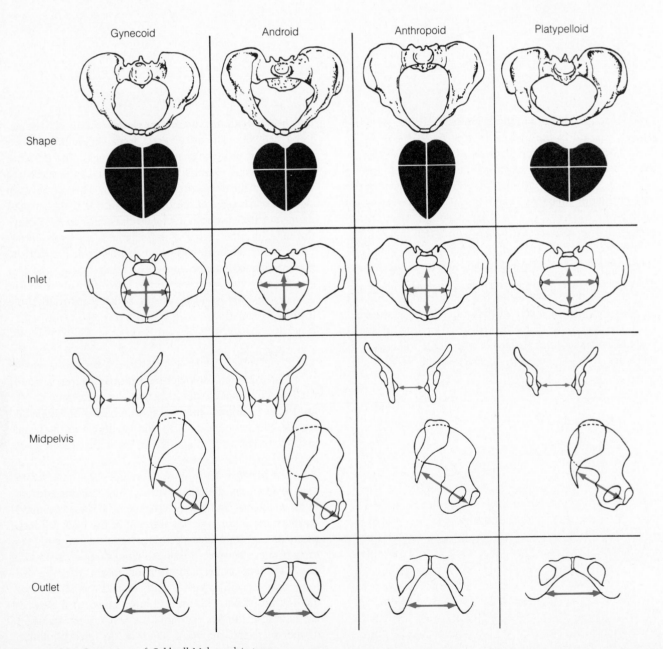

Figure 6–20   Comparison of Caldwell-Moloy pelvic types

delivery, but the posterior sagittal diameter is too short and the anterior sagittal diameter is long. The posterior segment is shallow because the sacral promontory is indented, resulting in a reduced capacity. The anterior segment is narrow, and the forepelvis is sharply angled. The android midpelvis has prominent ischial spines, convergent side walls, and a long, heavy sacrum inclining forward. All the midpelvic diameters are reduced. The distance from the linea terminalis to the ischial tuberosities is long, yet the overall capacity of the midpelvis is reduced. The android outlet has a narrow, sharp, and deep pubic arch; the inferior pubic rami are straight and long. The anteroposterior diameter is short and the transverse diameter is narrow. The capacity of the outlet is reduced. The bones are of medium to heavy structure and weight.

Approximately 20 percent of female pelves are classified as android.

The influence of an android pelvis on labor is not favorable. Descent into the pelvis is slow. The fetal head usually engages in the transverse or occipital posterior diameter in asynclitism with extreme molding. Arrest of labor is frequent, requiring difficult forceps manipulation (rotation and extraction), and the deep, narrow pubic arch may lead to extensive perineal lacerations. Cesarean delivery may be required.

○   *ANTHROPOID PELVIS*   The anthropoid pelvis (Figure 6–20) inlet is oval, with a long anteroposterior diameter and an adequate but rather short transverse diameter. Both the posterior and anterior segments are deep; the posterior sagittal diameter is extremely long, as is the anterior sagittal diameter. The anthropoid midpelvis has variable ischial spines, straight side walls, and a narrow and long sacrum that inclines backward. The midpelvic diameters are at least adequate, making its capacity adequate. The anthropoid outlet has a normal or moderately narrow pubic arch; the inferior pubic rami are long and narrow. The outlet capacity is adequate, and the bones are of medium weight and structure.

Approximately 25 percent of female pelves are classified as anthropoid.

○   *PLATYPELLOID PELVIS*   The platypelloid type refers to the flat female pelvis (Figure 6–20). The inlet is distinctly transverse oval, with a short anteroposterior and extremely short transverse diameter. The posterior sagittal and anterior sagittal diameters are short. Both the anterior and posterior segments are shallow. The platypelloid midpelvis has variable ischial spines, parallel side walls, and a wide sacrum with a deep curve inward. Only the transverse diameter is adequate; thus the midpelvic capacity is reduced. The platypelloid outlet has an extremely wide pubic arch; the inferior pubic rami are straight and short. The transverse diameter is wide but the anteroposterior diameter is

short. The outlet capacity may be inadequate. The platypelloid bones are similar to the gynecoid type.

Only 5 percent of female pelves are classified as platypelloid.

Breasts

The *breasts,* or *mammary glands,* considered accessories of the reproductive system, are specialized sebaceous glands. They are conical and symmetrically placed on the sides of the chest. The greater pectoral and anterior serratus muscles underlie each breast. Suspending the breasts are fibrous tissues, called *Cooper's ligaments,* that extend from the deep fascia in the chest outward to just under the skin covering the breast. The left breast is frequently larger than the right.

In the center of each mature breast is the *nipple,* a protrusion about 0.5 to 1.3 cm in diameter. The nipple is composed mainly of erectile tissue, which becomes more rigid and prominent during the menstrual cycle, sexual excitement, pregnancy, and lactation. The nipple is surrounded by the heavily pigmented *areola,* 2.5 to 10 cm in diameter. Both the nipple and areola are roughened by small papillae called *Montgomery's tubercles.* As an infant suckles, these tubercles secrete a fatty substance that helps lubricate and protect the breasts.

The breasts are composed of glandular, fibrous, and adipose tissue. The glandular tissue consists of acini or alveoli (Figure 6–21), which are arranged in a series of 15 to 24 lobes. These lobes are in a radial pattern and are separated from one another by varying amounts of adipose and fibrous tissue.

Each lobe of the breast is made up of several lobules, which in turn are made up of large numbers of alveoli in grapelike clusters around minute ducts. They are lined with a single layer of cuboidal epithelium, which secretes the various components of milk. The ducts from several lobules combine to form the larger lactiferous ducts or sinuses. Each lactiferous duct opens separately on the surface of the nipple and may be seen as a tiny isolated orifice. The smooth muscle of the nipple causes erection of the nipple on contraction.

Cyclic hormonal control of the mature breast is complex. Essentially, estrogenic hormones stimulate the growth and development of the ductal epithelium. Progesterone, in association with estrogen, is responsible for the acinar and lobular development during the luteal phase of menstruation. In addition, adrenal corticosteroids, prolactin, somatotropin (growth hormone), and thyroxine are necessary for estrogen and progesterone to act.

The arterial, venous, and lymphatic systems communicate medially with the internal mammary vessels and laterally with the axillary vessels. Therefore, in cancer of the breast, metastasis follows the vascular supply both medially and laterally (Figure 6–22).

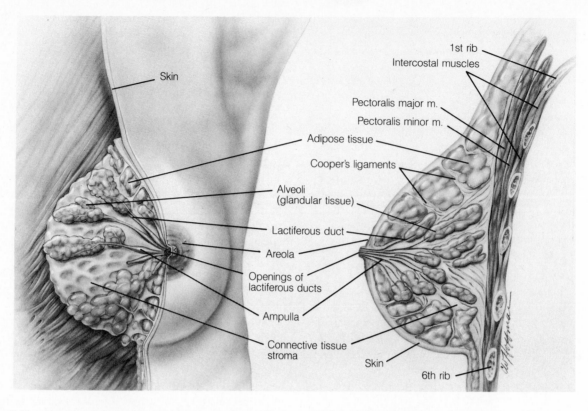

Figure 6–21 *Anatomy of the breast:* A *Anterior view of partially dissected left breast,* B *Sagittal view* (Adapted from Spence AP & Mason EB, *Human Anatomy and Physiology,* ed 3, Menlo Park, Calif, Benjamin/Cummings, 1987, p 830)

The cutaneous nerve supply to the upper breast is from the third and fourth branches of the cervical plexus, whereas the supply to the lower breast is from the thoracic intercostal nerve.

The biologic function of the breasts is to provide nourishment and protective maternal antibodies to infants through the lactation process. They are also a source of much pleasurable sexual sensation. In Western culture the breasts have become a sexual symbol; their size and sexual qualities receive more attention than their lactogenic functions.

● Male Reproductive System

Andrology is the study of the male reproductive organs. To date, the male organs have not been studied in the same depth as their female counterparts. New techniques are being applied to the study of male factors in such areas as infertility, contraception, congenital anomalies, and reproduction in general.

The primary reproductive functions of the male genitals are to produce and transport sperm through and eventually out of the genital tract into the female genital tract.

The male reproductive system consists of the external and internal genitals (Figure 6–23).

External Genitals

The two external reproductive organs are the penis and scrotum.

PENIS

The *penis* is an elongated, cylindrical structure consisting of a body, termed the *shaft,* and a cone-shaped end called the *glans.* The penis lies in front of the scrotum.

The shaft of the penis is made up of three longitudinal columns of erectile tissue: the paired *corpora cavernosa penis* and a third, the *corpus spongiosum penis.* These columns are covered by a dense fibrous connective tissue called the *tunica albuginea* and then enclosed by an elastic areolar tissue, the (Buck's) *fascia penis.* The penis is covered by a thin outer layer of skin (Figure 6–24).

The corpus spongiosum of the penis (also known as the corpus cavernosum urethra), contains the urethra, and extends beyond the corpora cavernosa to become the glans at the distal end of the penis. The urethra widens within

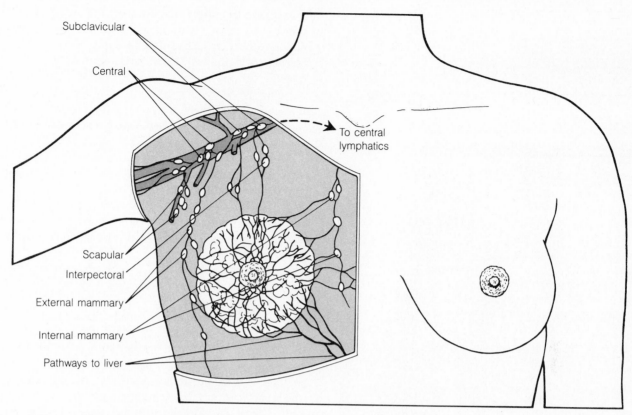

Subclavicular

Central

To central
lymphatics

Scapular

Interpectoral

External mammary

Internal mammary

Pathways to liver

Figure 6–22   Lymphatic drainage of the breast

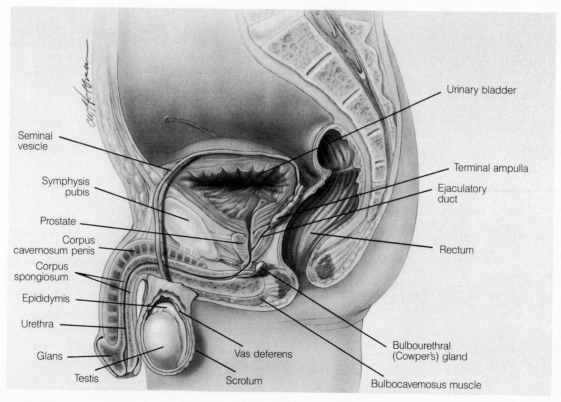

Seminal
vesicle

Symphysis
pubis

Prostate

Corpus
cavernosum penis

Corpus
spongiosum

Epididymis

Urethra

Glans

Testis

Vas deferens

Scrotum

Urinary bladder

Terminal ampulla

Ejaculatory
duct

Rectum

Bulbourethral
(Cowper's) gland

Bulbocavemosus muscle

Figure 6–23   Male reproductive system

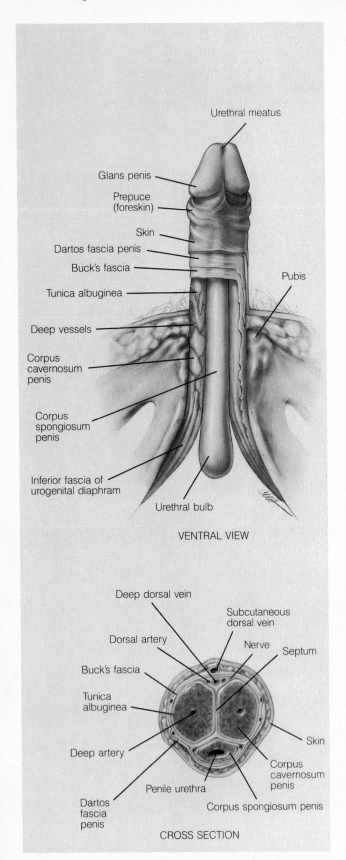

Urethral meatus

Glans penis

Prepuce
(foreskin)

Skin

Dartos fascia penis

Buck's fascia

Tunica albuginea

Deep vessels

Corpus
cavernosum
penis

Corpus
spongiosum
penis

Inferior fascia of
urogenital diaphram

Pubis

Urethral bulb

VENTRAL VIEW

Deep dorsal vein

Subcutaneous
dorsal vein

Dorsal artery

Nerve   Septum

Buck's fascia

Tunica
albuginea

Deep artery

Penile urethra

Dartos
fascia
penis

Skin

Corpus
cavernosum
penis

Corpus spongiosum penis

CROSS SECTION

Figure 6–24   Anatomy of the penis

the glans to form the *fossa navicularis* and ends in a slitlike orifice, located in the tip of the glans, called the *urethral meatus.* A circular fold of skin arises just behind the glans and covers it. Known as the *prepuce,* or foreskin, it is frequently removed by the surgical procedure of circumcision (Chapter 29). If the corpus spongiosum does not surround the urethra completely, the urethral meatus may occur on the ventral aspect of the penile shaft (hypospadias) or on the dorsal aspect (epispadias).

The suspensory ligament is the main attachment and support for the penis. It extends from the symphysis pubis and merges with the deep fascia of the penis.

The blood supply to the penis is a parallel system of internal and external pudendal arteries and veins. Blood to the cavernous sinuses is provided by two branches of the penile artery.

The penis is innervated by the pudendal nerve. Sympathetic fibers come from the hypogastric and pelvic plexuses, while parasympathetic fibers from the third and fourth sacral nerves form the splanchnic nerves. When the parasympathetic fibers are stimulated, the ischiocavernous muscle contracts, preventing the return of venous blood from the cavernous sinuses. The blood vessels of the penis engorge, causing the penis to become erect. During *erection,* the penis elongates, thickens, and stiffens.

Sexual stimulation causes the penis to become erect. If stimulation is intense enough, the forceful and sudden expulsion of semen occurs through the rhythmic contractions of the penile muscles. This phenomenon is called *ejaculation.*

The penis serves both the urinary and reproductive systems. Urine is expelled through the urethral meatus. However, the primary function of the penis is to deposit sperm in the female vagina during sexual intercourse to provide for fertilization of the ovum.

As the procreative functions of men and women have become minimized, the penis has assumed increasing importance as a provider of sexual pleasure. To many men, the penis is a symbol of virility and masculinity, and its loss or altered function results in a lessening of their self-esteem.

SCROTUM

The *scrotum* is a pouchlike structure suspended from the perineal region. It hangs anterior to the anus and posterior to the penis and may extend below it. Composed of skin and the *dartos* muscle, the scrotum shows increased pigmentation and scattered hairs. The sebaceous glands open directly onto the scrotal surface; their secretion has a distinctive odor. Contraction of the dartos and cremasteric muscles shortens the scrotum and draws it closer to the body, thus wrinkling its outer surface. The degree of wrinkling is greatest in young men and at cold temperatures and is least in older men and at warm temperatures.

Inside the scrotum are two lateral compartments separated by a medial septum derived from the dartos muscle. In each compartment is a testis with its related structures. Because the left spermatic cord grows longer during embryologic development, the left testis and its scrotal sac hang lower than the right. A ridge (raphe) on the external scrotal surface marks the position of the medial septum and continues anteriorly on the urethral surface of the penis but disappears in the perineal area.

The function of the scrotum is to protect the testes and the sperm by maintaining a temperature lower than that of the body. Spermatogenesis will not occur if the testes fail to descend and thus remain at body temperature. Because it is sensitive to touch, pressure, temperature, and pain, the scrotum defends against potential harm to the testes.

Internal Genitals

The male internal reproductive organs include the gonads (testes or testicles), a system of ducts (epididymis, vas deferens, ejaculatory duct, and urethra), and accessory glands (seminal vesicles, prostate gland, bulbourethral glands, and urethral glands).

TESTES

The *testes* are a pair of oval, compound glandular organs contained in the scrotum (Figure 6–25). In the sexually mature male, they are the site of spermatozoa production and the secretion of several male sex hormones (androgens).

Each testis is 4 to 6 cm long, 2 to 3 cm wide, and 3 to 4 cm deep and weighs 10 to 15 g. It is covered by a serous membrane known as the *tunica vaginalis.* Under this membrane is the *tunica albuginea,* which is a tough, white, fibrous capsule covering each testis. The tunica albuginea sends projections inward to form septa, thereby dividing the testis into 250 to 400 lobules. Each lobule contains one to three tightly packed, convoluted seminiferous tubules containing sperm cells in all stages of development.

The seminiferous tubules are surrounded by loose connective tissue, which houses abundant blood and lymph vessels and the Leydig's (interstitial) cells. The Leydig's cells produce testosterone, the primary male sex hormone. The seminiferous tubules come together to form the 20 or 30 straight tubules, or tubuli recti, which in turn form an anastomosing network of thin-walled spaces, the *rete testis.* At the upper border of the mediastinum, the rete testis forms 10 to 15 efferent ducts that perforate the tunica albuginea and empty into the duct of the epididymis. Prior to this, the efferent ducts enlarge and become convoluted.

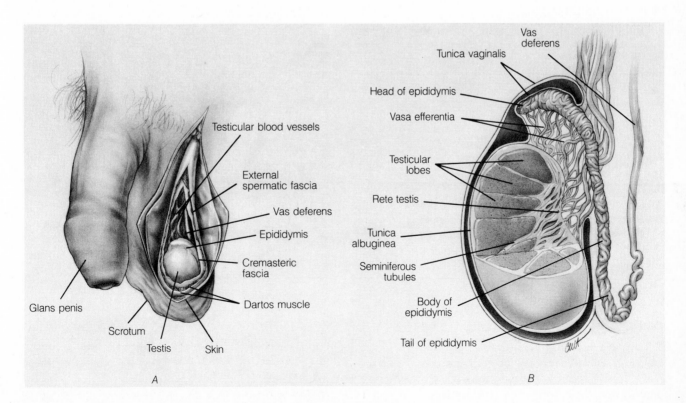

Figure 6–25   The testes: A External view. B Sagittal view showing interior anatomy

Most of the cells lining the seminiferous tubules undergo a process of maturation called *spermatogenesis*. (See Chapter 13 for further discussion of spermatogenesis.) Sperm production varies among and within the tubules, with cells in different areas of the same tubule undergoing different stages of spermatogenesis. The seminiferous tubules also contain Sertoli's cells, which nourish and protect the spermatocytes. Sertoli's cells undergo specific cyclic changes with each generation of spermatozoa. The sperm are eventually released from the tubules into the epididymis, where they mature further.

Like the female reproductive cycle, the process of spermatogenesis and other functions of the testes are the result of complex neural and hormonal controls. The hypothalamus secretes releasing factors, which stimulate the anterior pituitary to release the gonadotropins FSH and LH. The release of FSH is thought to be controlled by the hormone inhibin, which is released by the Sertoli's cells (Ganong 1985).

Along with testosterone and the other androgens, FSH maintains the spermatogenic function of the testes. LH is called *interstitial cell-stimulating hormone* (ICSH) in males because it stimulates the interstitial cells of the testes (Leydig's cells) to synthesize testosterone from cholesterol. Testosterone in turn inhibits the secretion of ICSH by the anterior pituitary. Most of the circulating testosterone is converted in the liver to 17-ketosteroids, which are secreted in the urine. About one-third of these ketosteroids are metabolized from testicular testosterone; the rest are adrenal in origin (Figure 6–2).

Testosterone is the most prevalent and potent of the testicular hormones. Its target organs are the testes, prostate, and seminal vesicles. In addition to being essential for spermatogenesis, it increases sperm production by the seminiferous tubules, stimulates production of seminal fluid, and is responsible for the development of secondary male characteristics and certain behavioral patterns. The effects of testosterone include structural and functional development of the male genital tract, emission and ejaculation of seminal fluid, distribution of body hair, promotion of growth and strength of long bones, increased muscle mass, and enlargement of the vocal cords. The action of testosterone on the central nervous system is thought to produce aggressiveness and sexual drive. The action of testosterone is constant, not cyclic like that of the female hormones, and is not limited to a certain number of years.

EPIDIDYMIDES

The *epididymis* is a duct about 5.6 m long, although it is convoluted into a compact structure about 3.75 cm long. An epididymis lies behind each testis. It arises from the top of the testis, courses downward, and then passes upward, where it becomes the vas deferens.

The epididymis provides a reservoir where spermatozoa can survive for a long period. When discharged from the seminiferous tubules into the epididymis, the sperm are immotile and incapable of fertilizing an ovum. The

Box 6–1 Male Reproductive Organ Functions

Testes:	House seminiferous tubules and gonads.
Seminiferous tubules:	Contain sperm cells in various stages of development and undergoing meiosis.
Sertoli's cells:	Nourish and protect spermatocytes (phase between spermatids and spermatozoa)
Leydig's cells:	Main source of testosterone.
Epididymides:	Provide an area for maturation of sperm and a reservoir for mature spermatozoa.
Vas deferens:	Connect epididymis with prostate gland, then connects with ducts from seminal vesicle to become ejaculatory duct.
Ejaculatory ducts:	Provide passageway for semen and seminal fluid into urethra.
Seminal vesicles:	Secrete yellowish fluid rich in fructose, prostaglandins, and fibrinogen. Provide nutrition that increases motility and fertilizing ability of sperm. Prostaglandins also aid fertilization by making the cervical mucus more receptive to sperm.
Prostate gland:	Secretes thin, alkaline fluid containing calcium, citric acid, and other substances. Alkalinity counteracts acidity of ductus and seminal vesicle secretions.
Bulbourethral (Cowper's) glands:	Secrete alkaline, viscous fluid into semen aiding in neutralization of acidic vaginal secretions.

spermatozoa remain in the epididymis for 2 to 10 days, until maturation is complete.

VAS DEFERENS AND EJACULATORY DUCTS

The *vas deferens,* also known as the *ductus deferens,* is about 40 cm long and connects the epididymis with the prostate. One vas deferens arises from the posterior border of each testis. It joins the spermatic cord and weaves over and between several pelvic structures until it meets the vas deferens from the opposite side. Each vas deferens then unites with a seminal vesicle duct to form the *ejaculatory ducts,* which enter the prostate gland, terminating in the prostatic urethra. These ducts form a passageway for semen and for fluid secreted by the seminal vesicles. The vas deferens can be divided into five parts. The scrotal portion is usually the surgical site of a vasectomy, the male sterilization procedure.

Prior to its entrance into the prostate, the vas deferens enlarges. This enlargement is called the *terminal ampulla* and serves as the primary storehouse for spermatozoa, which are still relatively immotile, and tubule secretions. The sperm are immobile because the metabolic production of carbon dioxide by the sperm creates an acidic environment that inhibits motility, and because the vas deferens secretions do not provide high-energy nutrients that can be metabolized into lactic acid as do the seminal fluids.

URETHRA

The male urethra is a common passageway for urine and semen. The urethra begins in the bladder and passes through the prostate gland, where it is called the *prostatic urethra.* The surrounding connective tissue is highly vascular and contains glands, elastic fibers, and smooth muscles arranged in an inner longitudinal layer and an outer circular layer. These circular fibers form the internal urethral sphincter.

The urethra emerges from the prostate gland to become the *membranous urethra.* As it passes through the urogenital diaphragm, skeletal muscle fibers form the external urethral sphincter. It terminates in the penis, where it is called the penile urethra. In the penile urethra, goblet secretory cells are present, and smooth muscle is replaced by erectile tissue.

Accessory Glands

The male accessory glands are specialized structures under endocrine and neural control (see Box 6–1). Each secretes a unique and essential component of the total seminal fluid in an ordered sequence.

The *seminal vesicles* are two glands composed of many lobes. Each vesicle is about 7.5 cm long. They are situated between the bladder and rectum and immediately above the base of the prostate. The epithelium lining the seminal vesicles secretes an alkaline, viscid, clear fluid rich in high-energy fructose, prostaglandins, fibrinogen, and proteins. During ejaculation, this fluid empties into the ejaculatory ducts and mixes with the sperm. An activating principle is present in the secretions that acts on the sperm to increase their motility. This fluid helps provide an environment favorable to sperm motility and metabolism. It is believed that prostaglandins aid fertilization by causing uterine contractions that move the sperm toward the fallopian tubes (Vick 1984), while the fibrinogen increases the viscosity of the semen.

The *prostate gland* surrounds the upper part of the urethra and lies below the neck of the urinary bladder. Made up of several lobes, it measures about 4 cm in diameter and weighs 20 to 30 g. The prostate is made up of both glandular and muscular tissue. It secretes a thin, milky, slightly acidic fluid (pH 6.5) containing high levels of zinc, calcium, citric acid, and acid phosphatase. This fluid protects the sperm from the acidic environment of the vagina and the male urethra, which could be spermicidal (Vick 1984).

The *bulbourethral* or *Cowper's glands* are a pair of small round structures on either side of the membranous urethra. The glands secrete a clear, viscous, alkaline fluid rich in mucoproteins that becomes part of the semen. This secretion also lubricates the penile urethra during sexual excitement and neutralizes the acid in the male urethra and the vagina, thereby enhancing sperm mobility.

The *urethral* or *Littre's glands* are tiny mucous-secreting glands found throughout the membranous lining of the penile urethra. Their secretions add to those of the bulbourethral glands.

SEMEN

The male ejaculate, *semen* or *seminal fluid,* is made up of spermatozoa and the secretions of the bulbourethral glands, urethral glands, prostate, epididymides, and seminal vesicles. The seminal fluid transports viable and motile sperm to the female reproductive tract. Effective transportation of sperm requires adequate nutrients, an adequate pH (about 7.5), a specific concentration of sperm to fluid, and an optimal osmolarity.

A spermatozoon is made up of a *head* and a *tail* (Figure 6–26). The tail is divided into the middle piece and end piece. The head's main components are the *acrosome, nucleus,* and *nuclear vacuoles.* The head carries the haploid number of chromosomes (23), and it is the part that enters the ovum at fertilization (Chapter 13). The tail, or *flagellum,* is specialized for motility. Figure 6–27 shows a scanning electron micrograph of human spermatozoa.

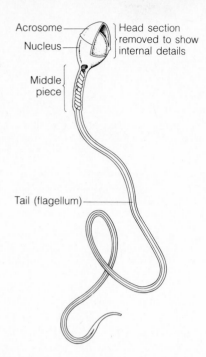

Acrosome — Head section removed to show internal details

Nucleus —

Middle piece

Tail (flagellum) —

Figure 6–26 Schematic representation of a mature spermatozoon

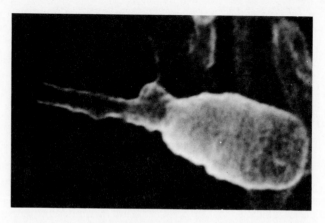

Figure 6–27 Scanning electron micrograph of human spermatozoa (Courtesy Dr Landrum B. Shettles)

Sperm may be stored in the male genital system for up to 42 days, depending primarily on the frequency of ejaculations. The average volume of ejaculate following abstinence for several days is 2 to 5 mL but may vary from 1 to 10 mL. Repeated ejaculation results in decreased volume. Once ejaculated, sperm can live only two or three days in the female genital tract.

KEY CONCEPTS

Reproductive system activities include developmental changes that lead to puberty, gametogenesis (spermatogenesis and oogenesis), sexual intercourse, development of sense of sexuality, pregnancy, embryo development, parturition, and lactation.

Reproductive activities require a complex interaction between the reproductive structures, the central nervous system, and such endocrine glands as the pituitary, hypothalamus, testes, and ovaries.

At puberty, an alteration in brain sensitivity leads to an increased release of GnRH, which stimulates LH and FSH leading in the male to an increase in testosterone; and in the female, to an increase in estrogen and progesterone.

Estrogen is the principal cause of the events of puberty (maturation of ova, enlargement of the uterus and fallopian tubes, deposition of fat in the breasts and hips, and characteristic hair growth) in females.

Puberty changes for the male (onset of spermatogenesis; enlargement of the penis, scrotum, and testes; voice changes; and characteristic hair growth) occur as a result of increased testosterone production by the testes.

The female reproductive system consists of: the ovaries, where female germ cells and female sex hormones are formed; the fallopian tubes, which capture the ovum and allow transport to the uterus; the uterus, whose lining is shed during menstruation or is the implantation site for the fertilized ovum (blastocyst); the cervix, which is a protective portal for the body of the uterus and the connection between the vagina and the uterus (it must thin and dilate to allow passage of a baby); and the vagina, which is the passageway from the external genitals to the uterus and provides for discharge of menstrual products to the outside of the body.

The male reproductive system consists of: the testes, where male germ cells and male sex hormones are formed; a series of continuous ducts through which spermatozoa are transported outside the body; accessory glands that produce secretions important to sperm nutrition, survival, and transport; and the penis, which serves as the organ of copulation.

REFERENCES

Beller FK, et al: *Gynecology: A Textbook for Students,* ed 3. New York, Springer-Verlag, 1980.

Caldwell WE, **Moloy** HC: Anatomical variations in the female pelvis and their effect on labor with a suggested classification. *Am J Obstet Gynecol* 1933;26:479.

Ganong WF: *Review of Medical Physiology,* ed 12. Los Altos, Calif, Lange Medical Publishing, 1985.

Oxhorn H: *Human Labor and Birth,* ed 5. East Norwalk, Conn, Appleton-Century-Crofts, 1986.

Marshall JR, **Ross** J: Other aspects of the endocrine physiology of reproduction, in **Danforth** DN (ed): *Obstetrics and Gynecology* ed 4. Philadelphia, Pa, Harper & Row, 1982.

Pritchard JA, **MacDonald** PC, **Gant** NF: *Williams Obstetrics,* ed 17. East Norwalk, Conn, Appleton-Century-Crofts, 1985.

Sloane E: *Biology of Women,* ed 2. New York, John Wiley, 1985.

Spence AP, **Mason** EB: *Human Anatomy and Physiology,* ed 3. Menlo Park, Calif, Benjamin/Cummings, 1987.

Stone SC: Physiology of puberty, in **Sciarra** JJ, et al (eds): *Gynecology and Obstetrics.* Hagerstown, Md, Harper & Row, 1981, vol 5.

Vick RL: *Contemporary Medical Physiology.* Menlo Park, Calif, Addison-Wesley, 1984.

ADDITIONAL READINGS

Catanzarite VA, et al: Successful pregnancy after hysterectomy in a patient with uterus didelphys: Case report. *J Reprod Med* 1986;31(February):133–135.

Cooper TG: *The Epididymis, Sperm Maturation and Fertilization.* New York, Springer-Verlag, 1986.

Embrey MP: Prostaglandins in human reproduction. *Br Med J* 1981;238:1563.

Goss CM (ed): *Gray's Anatomy of the Human Body,* ed 30. Philadelphia, Lea & Febiger, 1984.

Hafez ESE, **Ludwig** H: Scanning electron microscopy of human reproduction, in **Danforth** DN, **Scott** JR (eds): *Obstetrics and Gynecology,* ed 5. Philadelphia, Harper & Row, 1986.

Lierse W: *Applied Anatomy of the Pelvis.* New York, Springer-Verlag, 1987.

Mauras N, et al: Augmentation of growth hormone secretion during puberty: Evidence for a pulse amplitude–modulated phenomenon. *J Clin Endocrinol Metabol* 1987;64(3):596.

Page EW, et al: *Human Reproduction: Essentials of Reproduction and Perinatal Medicine,* ed 3. Philadelphia, WB Saunders, 1981.

Speroff L, **Glass** RH, **Kase** NG: *Clinical Gynecologic Endocrinology and Infertility,* ed 3. Baltimore, Williams & Wilkins, 1984.

Tyler SL, **Woodall** GM: *Female Health and Gynecology: Across the Life Span.* Bowie, Md, Brady, 1982.

Urban DJ, et al: Nurse specialization in reproductive endocrinology. *J Obstet Gynecol Neonat Nurs* 1982;11(May/June):167.

Yen SS, **Jaffe** RB: *Reproductive Endrocrinology: Physiology, Pathophysiology and Clinical Management,* ed 2. Philadelphia, Saunders, 1985.

I always thought it was so boring to study anatomy and physiology. Who cares how many bones there are in the pelvis, or the muscles involved. But now I'm with mothers having babies and now it all makes sense. (A nursing student)

From Menarche to Menopause: The Woman's Experience

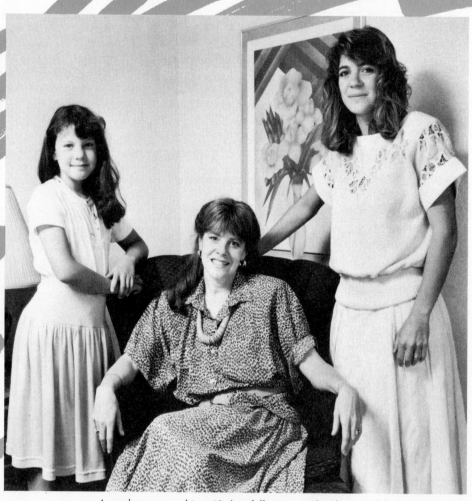

A mother approaching 40, her fully mature daughter, and her preadolescent daughter represent three of the stages of womanhood.

Chapter Seven

OBJECTIVES

- Summarize the action of the hormones that affect reproductive functioning.
- Describe the menstrual cycle, correlating the phases of the cycle with their dominant hormones and the changes that occur in each phase.
- Explain the physiologic and psychologic aspects of the female reproductive cycle.
- Review the origin of the myths surrounding menstruation and the impact of these beliefs on women today.
- Describe the information women may need to develop healthy, positive perceptions of this area of their lives and the self-care comfort measures they can use.
- Summarize the theories about premenstrual tension syndrome and dysmenorrhea, their medical management, and self-care measures.
- Explain the physiologic and psychologic aspects of menopause.

Menstruation and menopause are physiologic events shared by all women, yet each woman's experience is unique. How a woman experiences menstruation and menopause depends on sociocultural factors and her attitudes about her body, sexuality, and reproductive function.

Menstruation can be defined as cyclic uterine bleeding in response to hormonal changes. Menarche is the onset of menstruation. Menopause is the cessation of menstruation, and it occurs during the climacteric, a transitional period of major physiologic and resultant psychologic changes.

Menstruation in the sexually mature female occurs as the result of a series of monthly rhythmic changes, including ovulation. These changes are collectively referred to as the *female reproductive cycle (FRC)* (Figure 7–1). The FRC is composed of the *ovarian cycle,* during which ovulation occurs, and the *menstrual (uterine) cycle,* during which menstruation occurs. These two cycles take place simultaneously.

● Characteristics of Menstruation

Menarche occurs at approximately 12 to 13 years of age. Early cycles are often anovulatory and irregular in frequency, amount of flow, and duration. Within several months to 2 or 3 years, a regular cycle becomes established.

Menstrual parameters vary greatly among individuals. Menses generally occur every 28 days, plus or minus 5 to 10 days. Approximately 60 percent of women experience menses every 25 to 30 days, but 1 percent menstruate as frequently as every 20 days or less and another 1 percent have periods 36 to 40 days apart. Emotional and physical factors such as illness, excessive fatigue, high levels of stress or anxiety, and rigorous exercise programs can alter the cycle interval. In addition, environmental factors such as temperature and altitude may influence the cycle.

The duration of menses is from 2 to 8 days, with the blood loss averaging 30 to 100 mL and the loss of iron averaging 0.5 to 1 mg daily.

The menstrual discharge or flow is composed of blood mixed with fluid, cervical and vaginal secretions, bacteria, mucus, leukocytes, and partially autolyzed cellular debris. The menstrual discharge is dark red and has a distinctive odor. It results from physiologic tissue necrosis caused by ischemia and anoxia of the endometrium. Menstruation occurs when the ovum is not fertilized.

A review of the endometrium and its arterial blood supply will provide further understanding of this process. Blood flow from the spiral arterioles in the superficial endometrium is reduced, with resultant ischemia and anoxia, which in turn produce necrosis and discharge of the superficial endometrium (menses). Concurrently, the straight arterioles provide the basal endometrium with sufficient blood flow to maintain it and the endometrial glands or seeds that are responsible for the regeneration of the en-

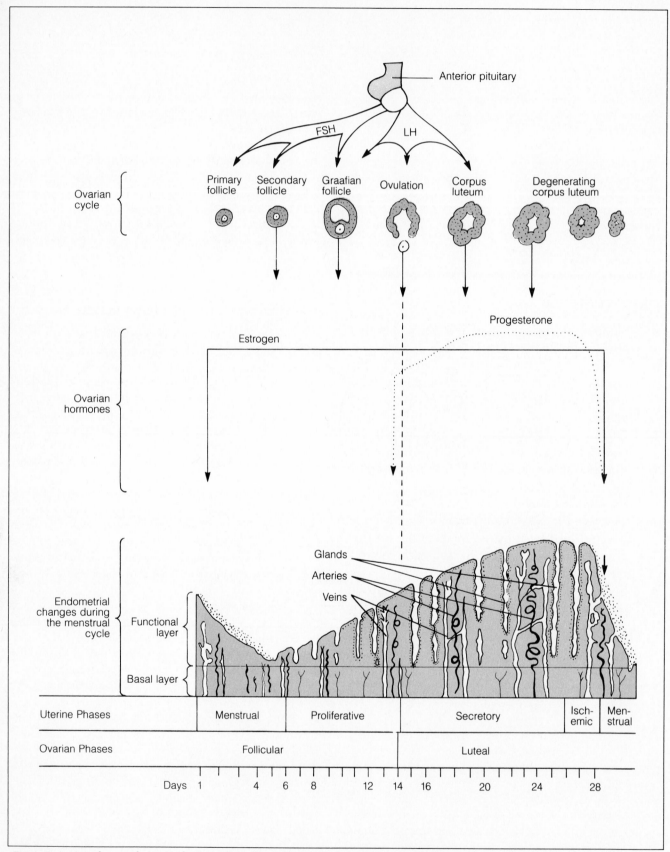

Figure 7–1   Female reproductive cycle: Interrelationships of hormones and the four phases of the uterine cycle and the two phases of the ovarian cycle

dometrium in the next female reproductive or menstrual cycle (Figure 7–2). Bleeding is controlled by vasospasm of the straight basal arterioles, resulting in coagulative necrosis at the vessel tips.

● Physiologic Aspects of the Female Reproductive Cycle (FRC)

Effects of Female Hormones

After menarche, a female undergoes a cyclic pattern of ovulation and menstruation (if pregnancy does not occur) for a period of 30 to 40 years. This cycle is an orderly process under neurohormonal control: Each month one oocyte matures, ruptures from the ovary, and enters the

fallopian tube. The ovary, vagina, uterus, and fallopian tubes are major target organs for female hormones. Each organ undergoes changes indicative of the exact point in time of any menstrual cycle.

The ovaries produce mature gametes and secrete hormones. Ovarian hormones include the estrogens, progesterone, and testosterone. The ovary is sensitive to FSH and LH. The uterus is sensitive to estrogen and progesterone. The relative proportion of these hormones to each other controls the events of both ovarian and uterine cycles.

ESTROGENS

Estrogens are associated with those characteristics contributing to "femaleness." The major estrogenic effects

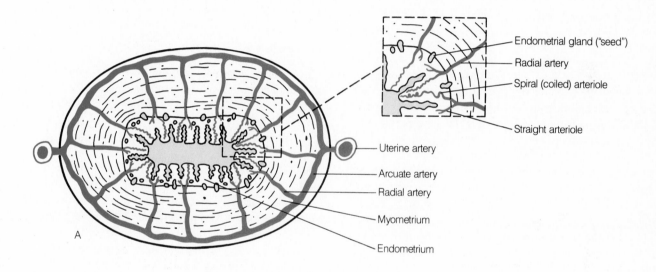

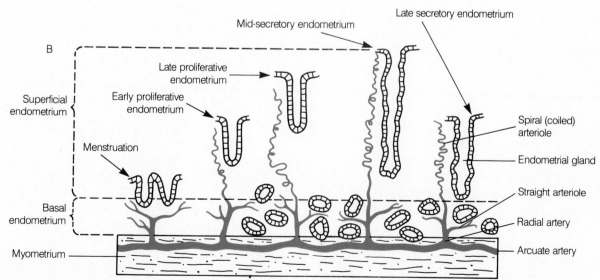

Figure 7–2   A blood supply to the endometrium (cross-section view of the uterus); B Schematic representation of blood supply during complete menstrual cycle (Modified from Bloom ML and Van   Doungen L. *Clinical Gynaecology: Integration of Structure and Function.* London: Williams Heinemann, 1972, p 144.)

are due primarily to three classical estrogens: estrone, β-estradiol, and estriol. β-Estradiol is the major estrogen. Estrogens are secreted in large amounts by the ovaries in nonpregnant women; minute amounts are secreted by the adrenal cortex.

Estrogens control the development of the female secondary sex characteristics: breast development, widening of the hips, and adipose deposits in the buttocks and mons pubis. Certain characteristics, such as a high-pitched voice, occur because of low androgen levels, although the adrenal cortex supplies sufficient androgens to cause hair growth. The female pattern of hair growth is influenced by estrogens. Estrogens assist in the maturation of the ovarian follicles and cause the endometrial mucosa to proliferate following menstruation. The amount of estrogens is greatest during the proliferative (follicular or estrogenic) phase of the menstrual cycle (p 00). Estrogen also causes the uterus to increase in size and weight because of increased glycogen, amino acids, electrolytes, and water. Blood supply is augmented as well. Under the influence of estrogens, myometrial contractility increases in both the uterus and the fallopian tubes, and there is increased uterine sensitivity to oxytocin. The vaginal epithelium becomes thicker. More sodium and chloride are retained by the kidneys, causing mild edema and body weight increase. Estrogens inhibit FSH production and stimulate LH production.

Estrogens have effects on many hormones and other carrier proteins. This explains, for example, the increased amount of protein-bound iodine in pregnant women and in women who use oral contraceptives containing estrogen (Little & Billiar 1981).

Estrogens may increase libidinal feelings in humans. They decrease the excitability of the hypothalamus, which may cause an increase in sexual desire.

For many years estrogens have been considered a preventive factor for coronary artery disease in women up to menopause, in the absence of diabetes or hypertension. Both lipoprotein and triglyceride metabolism are altered by estrogens. Although low estrogen levels do decrease serum cholesterol and β-lipoprotein levels and increase phospholipids and α-lipoprotein levels, numerous other factors must be considered in the development of coronary artery disease. Recent studies indicate that persistent high stress, coupled with specific types of personality patterns, diet (excessive calories, sodium, and saturated fats), smoking (especially in women taking oral contraceptives), obesity, and lack of exercise are influencing today's rise in incidence of coronary artery disease in women (Griffith-Kenney 1986).

PROGESTERONE

Progesterone is secreted by the corpus luteum and is found in greatest amounts during the secretory (luteal or progestational) phase of the menstrual cycle. It decreases the motility and contractility of the uterus caused by estrogens, thereby preparing the uterus for implantation after fertilization of the ovum. The endometrial mucosa is in a ready state as a result of estrogenic influence. Progesterone causes the uterine endometrium to further increase its supply of glycogen, arterial blood, secretory glands, amino acids, and water. This hormone is often called the *hormone of pregnancy* because its effects on the uterus allow pregnancy to be maintained.

Under the influence of progesterone, the vaginal epithelium proliferates and the cervix secretes thick, viscous mucus. Breast glandular tissue increases in size and complexity. Progesterone also prepares the breasts for lactation.

The temperature rise of about 0.35C (0.5F) that accompanies ovulation and persists throughout the secretory phase of the menstrual cycle is probably due to progesterone.

PROSTAGLANDINS

Prolific research continues to determine the definite and complete role of *prostaglandins* (PGs) in human reproduction (Caldwell & Behrman 1981; Wilhelmson et al 1981).

Prostaglandins are complex lipid compounds that are rapidly synthesized throughout the body from arachidonic acid. Three classes of PGs have been identified and categorized according to their molecular structure (Aten et al 1986). Because PGs are tissue hormones, not humoral, only small amounts circulate in the bloodstream (Lackritz 1981). Prostaglandins have a very short half life.

The actions of PGs are more varied than any other compound occurring naturally in the body. Certain PGs are known to have a major role in the regulation of reproductive processes. For example, PGE_1 and PGE_2 appear to affect gonadotropin secretion by acting on the hypothalamus (Aten et al 1986). In the female, PGE_2 and $PGE_{2\alpha}$ are the most important. Generally PGEs relax smooth muscles and are potent vasodilators; PGFs are potent vasoconstrictors and increase the contractility of muscles and arteries. While their primary actions seem antagonistic, their basic regulatory functions in cells are achieved through an intricate pattern of reciprocal events. The discussion here will summarize their role in ovulation and menstruation.

Authorities differ about the precise mechanisms by which PGs control or mediate ovulation. Prostaglandin formation increases during follicular maturation, is dependent on gonadotropins, and is essential to ovulation. Extrusion of the ovum, resulting from the increased contractility of the smooth muscle in the theca layer of the mature follicle, is thought to be caused by $PGF_{2\alpha}$. Significant amounts of PGs are found in and around the follicle at the time of ovulation. Prostaglandins may act as intracellular regulators in hormone action. For example, $PGF_{2\alpha}$ receptors have been demonstrated in the human corpus luteum (Aten et al 1986), and $PGF_{2\alpha}$ is known to cause luteolysis. While the exact mechanism by which the corpus luteum regresses remains obscure, $PGF_{2\alpha}$ is postulated to induce progesterone withdrawal, the lowest point of which coincides with the onset of early menses.

Endometrium and menstrual fluid are known to be rich sources of PGs. It is thought that estrogen acts on the uterus primed by progesterone to produce PGs. One study (Vijayakumar et al 1981) suggests that the ratio of PGF to PGE is a critical factor in the endometrial cycle. Both PGE and PGF peak during the proliferative phase, but PGE peaks at a higher level, which increases through vasodilation of the blood supply for the regenerating endometrium. The level of PGE then steadily falls during the secretory phase while the $PGF_{2\alpha}$ level rises. Only during the late secretory phase is the level of $PGF_{2\alpha}$ higher than that of PGE. This event increases vasoconstriction and contractility of the myometrium, which contributes to the ischemia preceding menstruation. High concentration of PGs may also account for the vasoconstriction of the endometrium venous lacunae allowing for platelet aggregation at vascular rupture points, thereby preventing a rapid blood loss during menstruation. The menstrual flow's high concentration of PGs may also facilitate the process of tissue digestion, which allows for an orderly desquamation of the endometrium during menstruation.

Neurohumoral Basis of the FRC

The FRC is controlled by complex interactions between the nervous and endocrine systems and their target tissues. These interactions involve the hypothalamus, anterior pituitary, and ovaries; their functions are reciprocal.

The hypothalamus controls anterior pituitary hormone production by secretion of gonadotropin-releasing hormone (GnRH). This releasing hormone is often called both luteinizing hormone–releasing hormone (LHRH) and follicle-stimulating hormone–releasing hormone (FSHRH).

In response to the hypothalamic-releasing hormone GnRH, the anterior pituitary secretes gonadotropic hormones: follicle-stimulating hormone (FSH) and luteinizing hormone (LH). The ovaries contain specialized FSH and LH receptor cells. These receptor cells activate the production of adenylcyclase, causing increased cell growth and hormone secretion through the cyclic adenosine monophosphate (cAMP) mechanism.

The FSH is primarily responsible for the maturation of the follicle. During this process, the maturing follicle secretes increasing amounts of estrogen, which enhance the growth and maturation of the follicle. (The excessive amounts of estrogen are also responsible for the rebuilding/proliferation phase of the endometrium following its desquamation during menses.) In spite of the rich supply of FSH, final maturation of the follicle will not come about without the synergistic action of LH. The anterior pituitary's production of LH increases sixfold to tenfold. About 18 hours after the peak production, ovulation occurs. The LH is also responsible for the "luteinizing" of the theca and granulosa cells of the ruptured follicle (described in the next section). As a result, estrogen production is reduced and progesterone secretion continues. Thus estrogen levels fall a day before ovulation; tiny amounts of progesterone are in evidence. Ovulation takes place following the very rapid growth of the follicle, as the sustained high level of estrogen diminishes, and progesterone secretion begins.

The ruptured follicle undergoes rapid change; luteinization is accomplished and the mass of cells becomes the corpus luteum. The lutein cells secrete large amounts of progesterone with smaller amounts of estrogen. (Concurrently, the excessive amounts of progesterone are responsible for the secretory phase of the uterine cycle.) Seven or eight days following ovulation, the corpus luteum begins to involute, losing its secretory function. The production of both progesterone and estrogen is severely diminished. The anterior pituitary responds with increasingly large amounts of FSH; a few days later LH production begins. As a result, new follicles become responsive to another ovarian cycle and begin maturing.

As has been described, hypothalamic-releasing hormones, anterior pituitary gonadotropic hormones (FSH and LH), and ovarian estrogen and progesterone comprise the neurohormonal hypothalamic-pituitary-ovarian axis system controlling the FRC. The hormones are secreted in continuously fluctuating amounts throughout the female reproductive cycle in precarious and miraculous interrelationships, which are still incompletely understood.

Ovarian Cycle

The ovarian cycle has two phases: the follicular phase (days 1 through 14) and the luteal phase (days 15 through 28). During the *follicular phase,* the primordial follicle matures as a result of FSH. The oocyte grows within the primordial follicle. Follicular cells increase in number, and a fluid space (antrum) appears and increases in size. Under the dual control of FSH and LH, as previously described, a mature *graafian follicle* appears about day 14. Figure 7–3 shows a mature graafian follicle in diagrammatic form.

In the mature graafian follicle, the cells surrounding the antral cavity are granulosa cells. The oocyte and follicular fluid are enclosed in the cumulus oophorus. The stromal elements of the ovary are condensed around the follicle in two layers: the *theca interna,* a vascular, hypertrophied layer; and the *theca externa,* an avascular layer of connective tissue. The theca interna cells resemble the luteal cells of the corpus luteum. The zona pellucida

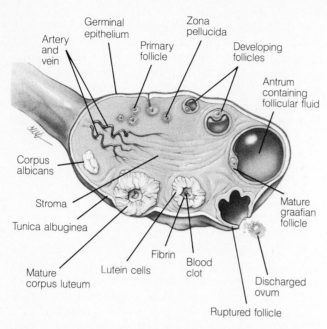

Figure 7–3   Various stages of development of the ovarian follicles

(oolemma), a thick elastic capsule, develops around the oocyte. The fully mature graafian follicle is a large structure, measuring 5 to 10 mm. The mature follicle produces increasing amounts of estrogen.

Just before ovulation the mature oocyte completes its first meiotic division, in which the diploid number of 46 chromosomes found in somatic cells is reduced to the haploid number of 23. As another result of this division, the first polar body and the secondary oocyte are formed (see Chapter 13). The secondary oocyte matures into the ovum. As the graafian follicle matures and enlarges, it comes close to the surface of the ovary. The ovary surface has a blisterlike protrusion 10 to 15 mm in diameter, and the follicle's walls become thin. Extrusion of the ovum is aided by proteolytic enzyme formation by the theca externa and prostaglandin secretion into the follicular tissues. Thus the secondary oocyte, the polar bodies, and the follicular fluid are pushed out. The egg (ovum) carries with it the cumulus oophorus. Discharged near the fimbriated end of the fallopian tube, the ovum is pulled into the tube and begins its journey through it.

Occasionally ovulation is accompanied by midcycle pain, known as *mittelschmerz,* which may be caused by a thick ovarian tunica albuginea or by a local peritoneal reaction to the expelling of the follicular contents. Vaginal secretion may increase during ovulation, and a small amount of blood (midcycle spotting) may be discharged as well.

The body temperature increases 0.3 to 0.6C (0.5 to 1.0F) at the time of ovulation or shortly thereafter and remains elevated until the second or third day after ovu-

lation. There may be an accompanying sharp temperature drop just before the increase. These temperature changes are clinically useful in determining the approximate time of ovulation (see Chapter 9).

The ovum generally takes several minutes to travel from the ruptured follicle to the fallopian tube opening. The contractions of the fallopian tube smooth muscle and ciliary action propel the ovum through the tube. The ovum is thought to be fertile for only 6 to 24 hours. The ovum remains in the ampulla, where it may be fertilized and cleavage can begin. It reaches the uterus 72 to 96 hours after it is released from the ovary.

The *luteal phase* begins when the ovum leaves its follicle. Under the influence of LH, the *corpus luteum* develops from the ruptured follicle. Within two or three days, the corpus luteum becomes yellowish and spherical and increases in vascularity. If the ovum is fertilized and implants in the endometrium, the fertilized egg begins to secrete human chorionic gonadotropin (hCG), which is needed to maintain the corpus luteum. If fertilization does not occur, within about a week after ovulation the corpus luteum begins to degenerate, eventually becoming a connective tissue scar called the *corpus albicans.* Approximately 14 days after ovulation (in a 28-day cycle), in the absence of pregnancy, menstruation begins. Figure 7–3 depicts the changes that the follicle undergoes during the ovarian cycle.

Menstrual Cycle

The menstrual cycle has four phases: the menstrual phase, proliferative phase, secretory phase, and ischemic phase (see Box 7–1). Menstruation occurs during the *menstrual phase.* Some endometrial areas are shed, while others remain. Some of the remaining tips of the endometrial glands begin to regenerate. The endometrium is in a resting state following menstruation. Estrogen levels are low, and the endometrium is 1 to 2 mm deep. During this part of the cycle, the cervical mucosa is scanty, viscous, and opaque.

The *proliferative phase* begins when the endometrial glands enlarge, becoming tortuous and longer, in response to increasing amounts of estrogen. The blood vessels become prominent and dilated, and the endometrium increases in thickness sixfold to eightfold. This gradual process reaches its peak just before ovulation. The cervical mucosa becomes thin, clear, watery, and more alkaline, making the mucosa more favorable to spermatozoa. As ovulation nears, the cervical mucosa shows increased elasticity, called *spinnbarkheit.* At ovulation, the mucus will stretch more than 5 cm. The cervical mucosa pH increases from below 7.0 to 7.5 at the time of ovulation. On microscopic examination, the mucosa shows a characteristic ferning pattern (see Figure 9–4B). This fern pattern is a useful aid in assessment of ovulation time. For in-depth discussion, see Chapter 9.

Box 7–1 Characteristics of Menstrual Cycle and Ovulation

Menstrual phase (Days 1–5)	Estrogen levels are low. Cervical mucus is scanty, viscous and opaque. Endometrium is shed.
Proliferative phase (Days 6–14)	Endometrium and myometrium thickness increases. Estrogen peaks just before ovulation. Cervical mucosa at ovulation: Is clear, thin, watery, and alkaline. Is more favorable to sperm. Has *Spinnbarkheit* greater than 5 cm. Shows ferning pattern on microscopic exam. At ovulation body temperature increases 0.3 to 0.6C, and *mittelschmerz* and/or midcycle spotting may occur.
Secretory phase (Days 15–26)	Estrogen drops sharply, and progesterone dominates. Vascularity of entire uterus increases. Tissue glycogen increases, and the uterus is made ready for implantation.
Ischemic phase (Days 27–28)	Both estrogen and progesterone levels fall. Spiral arteries undergo vasoconstriction. Endometrium becomes pale. Blood vessels rupture. Blood escapes into uterine stromal cells.

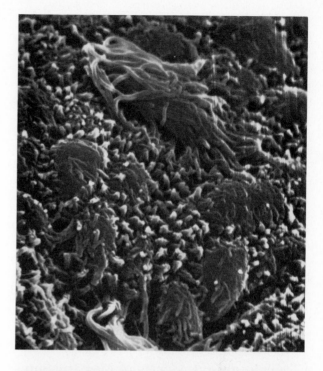

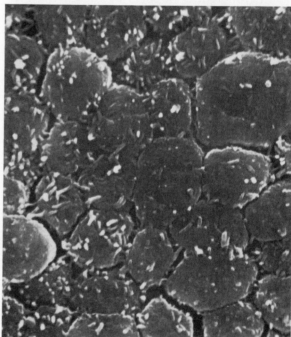

Figure 7–4 Scanning electron micrographs of the uterine lining during different phases of the uterine cycle. During the luteal phase (A) some of the cells have cilia and some are secreting droplets. The secreting cells are covered with microvilli. In the secretory phase (B), microvilli are still present on the surface of the secreting cells, but the general surface of the lining has a lumpier appearance than during the proliferative phase, and the cilia appear shorter and less numerous. The named phases refer to the uterine condition at the time the photographs were taken. (Courtesy Dr E S E Hafez, Wayne State University, Detroit, Michigan)

The *secretory phase* follows ovulation. The endometrium, under estrogenic influence, undergoes slight cellular growth. Progesterone, however, causes such marked swelling and growth that the epithelium is warped into folds (Figure 7–4). The amount of tissue glycogen increases. The glandular epithelial cells begin to fill with cellular debris, become tortuous, and dilate. The glands secrete small quantities of endometrial fluid in preparation for a fertilized ovum. The vascularity of the entire uterus increases greatly, providing a nourishing bed for implantation. If implantation occurs, the endometrium, under the influence of progesterone, continues to develop and become even thicker (Figure 7–5; see Chapter 13 for an in-depth discussion of implantation).

If fertilization does not occur, the *ischemic phase* begins. The corpus luteum begins to degenerate, and as a result both estrogen and progesterone levels fall. Areas of necrosis appear under the epithelial lining. Extensive vascular changes also occur. Small blood vessels rupture, and the spiral arteries constrict and retract, causing a deficiency of blood in the endometrium, which becomes pale. This ischemic phase is characterized by the escape of blood into the stromal cells of the uterus. The menstrual flow begins, thus beginning the menstrual cycle again. After menstruation the basal layer remains, so that the tips of the glands can regenerate the new functional endometrial layer.

● Sociocultural Aspects of Menstruation

Cultural Myths and Themes Related to Menstruation

The consistent and somewhat mysterious recurrence of menstruation over the millennia has engendered menstrual belief systems that remain with us and become the social reality. Cultural, religious, and personal attitudes about menstruation are part of the menstrual experience and, unfortunately, often reflect negative attitudes toward

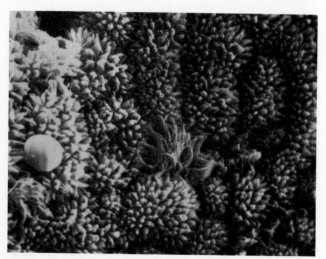

Figure 7–5   Scanning micrograph of the inner lining of the uterus at the time of implantation of the blastocyst. The blastocyst is an embryo at an early stage of development. (Courtesy Dr E S E Hafez, Wayne State University, Detroit, Michigan)

women. Consider how you have been influenced by attitudes and customs about menstruation. How did you first hear about it: family, friends, advertising, books, films, teachers, nurses, doctors, taboos, slang, names, jokes? What particular experiences stand out in your mind? How did they make you feel? Are your current experiences different? How is menstruation a part of your life now?

Some cultures have isolated women entirely (in menstrual huts, for example), or restricted them to the company of other women, during menstruation because they believed that menstrual blood was "unclean" and dangerous. Some beliefs emanating from this myth are that menstruating women have the ability to harm growing crops, wither flowers, and cause bread not to rise. Paramount is the belief that menstruating women are able to contaminate their husbands, so sexual intercourse is contraindicated (see Leviticus 15 and the Talmud). Menstruating women have been accused of having supernatural powers (since bleeding was usually associated with death)—sometimes good but more often destructive (Delaney et al 1976).

Although many of these myths have disappeared, there is a tendency to regard the menstruating woman as vulnerable or less capable. Current customs include refraining from exercise, showers, and sexual intercourse and hiding the fact of menstruation entirely. Note the wording in ads for menstrual products to see how this is reinforced in our country.

Some people have used these myths to deny jobs to women and treat them as inferior. The belief that women lose a lot of time from work is largely unsupported. Women still work where they are needed at home, in factories, or in offices with no concessions in schedules or routines to take account of individual differences in cycles. It is interesting to note that men, who are more prone to incapacitating and unpredictable diseases such as heart problems, are encouraged to continue in highly responsible positions. The theme that women are less capable and vulnerable is constantly evolving into new applications. For example, lawyers in Britain and the United States recently used the premenstrual syndrome for a mental incompetence alibi (Tybor 1982). In post–World War II Japan, the legislative body passed laws allowing for a "menstrual leave" for the supposed incapacity of women at this time (Dan 1983). Orthodox Judaism still prescribes the ritual bath (mikvah) following menstruation (Siegel 1983), and fear of contamination occurs in other societies as well. These beliefs relate not only to the menstruating woman but also to the menopausal woman, who is expected to be asexual or depressed at this time.

Many if not all the applications of this theme can be regarded as "put-downs" of women; most are not supported by scholarly research. These general belief systems influence our personal subjective beliefs and experiences. They persist and are continually recreated as part of the shared experience of women.

Male Attitudes and Sexual Activity

Most women have been socialized to refrain from discussing menstruation with men. In a survey of midwestern preteen girls, 85 percent expressed the belief that menstruation should not be discussed with boys, although 59 percent felt it was all right to discuss it with their fathers (Williams 1983). This cultural taboo is usually supported by the tendency to separate into gender groups for school discussions of growth and development.

Golub (1981) asked male and female college students for their attitudes and beliefs about menstruation. Although men lacked knowledge, they did not report any differences in their feelings toward women who were menstruating. Women reported that they felt less affectionate and less interested in sex at this time. In a study of marital sex by Morris (1983), a sample of American college-educated women reported that they were less easily aroused sexually during menstruation, although they reported a high incidence of noncoital orgasm at this time. There were few differences in their husbands during this time. These writers suggested that decreased arousal in females may be related to a biologic, hormonal influence.

Cultural taboos against coitus during menses are of long duration, but the health reasons for such taboos have been found to be invalid. Nurses discussing this area with clients may want to confirm that sexual activity during menses is common practice (Morris 1983) and is not contraindicated; however, not all couples desire it.

Alpern (1983) found that men, even male physicians, lacked information about menstruation. The showing of a modern, graphic film on menstruation to a sample of 13 men increased their understanding of the female experience. It is important to be open and tell both daughters and sons about the many changes of the life cycle so that they can be comfortable and open about these changes and maturational processes.

● Nursing Role

The nurse's primary role is to provide accurate information and assist in clearing up misconceptions so that girls and women will develop positive self-images and progress smoothly through this maturational phase.

The biophysical aspects of the menstrual cycle have been discussed already. It is important to remember, however, that the cyclic changes in body structures triggered by hormonal feedback mechanisms are influenced by social and environmental factors. McClintock (1981) described some of these interrelationships and suggested research in this area. For example, researchers have confirmed that women living in close proximity to each other tend to have concurrent menstrual cycles (McClintock 1981). Gardner (1983) noted that adolescents who have painful and irregular menstrual cycles tend to have gynecologic difficulties

in later life. In both of these instances, it is virtually impossible to distinguish psychosocial effects from physiologic effects, but the findings imply a complex relationship of both types of factors.

Nursing Goal: Assisting the Woman to Understand Her Menstrual Experience

The nurse provides information about what is normal and expected. Some of the objective data that nurses need to assess with the woman and use to resolve the question of normality include:

● *Length of the average cycle.* Early in a female's menstrual life, the median cycle length is 29 days; this will decrease slightly to a median of 25+ days prior to menopause. There is a wide variation among women.

● *Individual variability.* The typical month-to-month variation in an individual's cycle is plus or minus two days, although greater normal variations are frequently noted. No woman's cycle is exactly the same length every month.

● *Amount of flow.* The average flow is approximately 30 mL in a period; users of IUDs will usually have double this amount. The average woman will report amounts of flow in the number of pads or tampons used. Increase or decrease in the number of pads or tampons used is a good subjective indicator of changes in menstrual flow.

● *Length of menses.* The length of the menses is usually from two to eight days. Here again, there is wide variability. The number of days is another indicator of amount of flow.

Information of a more subjective nature may be elicited by more general questions such as, "How do you feel?" "Has there been any change?" "Do you have any problems with your menstrual period?" Skilled interviewing will reveal the social, environmental, and biophysiology of the individual menstrual cycle.

Nursing guidance is frequently concerned with the subjective reality of the woman, which is based on a variety of beliefs, feelings, and symptoms. In some cases a nurse may find it advisable to support a strong cultural tradition, such as the ritual bath, if taking part in a traditional act promotes a sense of belonging.

Nursing Goal: Promotion of Successful Adaptation to Menarche

Many young women find it embarrassing or stressful to discuss the menstrual experience, both because of the many taboos associated with the subject and because of their immaturity. The young woman who matures earlier than her peers is especially likely to be at a disadvantage; because the event has not been expected to occur so soon, she is less likely to have an adequate knowledge base for coping with her experience. A girl 10 or 11 years of age is also limited by her cognitive immaturity; the "magical thinking" typical of her developmental stage may lead to such thoughts as "everyone will know I have my period."

The most critical factor in successful adaptation to menarche is the adolescent's level of preparedness. A recent study revealed that one third of American women had not been prepared for their first "period," although women under 35 years of age were more likely than older women to have received preparation. Two-fifths of the women studied reported that their initial menstrual experience was negative.

Rierdan (1983) reported a direct relationship between adequacy of preparation and the degree to which the menarcheal experience is positive. Rierdan noted three areas in which girls require information:

- *Physiology of the experience.* Why does menstruation occur? How is it related to conception and childbirth? What anatomic and physiologic changes occur?

- *Menstrual hygiene.* What equipment is needed? How is it worn or used? Is it safe to take a bath or shower? What are the advantages and disadvantages of pads? Of tampons?

- *Concrete facts about the experience.* What color is the normal flow? What consistency? How does it smell?

The nurse should make it clear that variations in age at menarche, length of cycle, and duration of menses are normal because girls are likely to become concerned if they are not "on time" as compared with their peers. Rierdan (1983) also reported that it is helpful to acknowledge the negative aspects of menstruation (messiness, embarrassment), as well as its positive role as a symbol of maturity and womanhood.

Information should be given to premenstrual girls over time rather than all at once. In a study conducted by a student nurse (Wilke 1983), sixth-grade girls anonymously submitted questions after the school nurse had presented two classes on human development and sexuality. Even after these informative sessions, the girls asked many questions (Box 7–2).

The menarcheal client encountered by a nurse may be his or her own daughter, a hospitalized adolescent, a camper or student, or the client of a community health program. School nurses, especially, relate both to young women and their parents as part of planning for health and sex education curricula. Nursing assessment should address the stage of physical development, the client's need

for information, and the needs of parents for support in their role.

Nursing Goal: Education About Comfort Measures and Issues During Menstruation

Menstrual fluid contains blood; cervical mucus; vaginal secretions, mucus, and cells; and degenerated endometrial particles. It is important to remember that this fluid usually does not smell until it makes contact with bacteria on the skin or in the air.

TAMPONS AND PADS

Women in different cultures have handled their menstrual flow in many ways, including using nothing at all. Since early times, women have made tampons and pads from cloths or rags, which required washing but were reusable. Some women made them from gauze or cotton balls. Commercial tampons were introduced in the 1930s.

Today's adhesive stripped mini- and maxipads and flushable tampons have made life easier. Unfortunately, in their zeal to perfect a comfortable, convenient, leak- and odorproof product, manufacturers have added deodorants to both sanitary napkins and tampons and have increased their absorbency. (Consider why women need to deodorize internally if odor occurs only when the flow comes in contact with the air.)

Both these "improvements" may prove harmful. The chemical used to deodorize can create a rash on the vulva, or outer vaginal lips and can do worse damage to the tender mucous lining of the vagina itself. Excessive or inappropriate use of superabsorbent tampons can produce dryness and even small sores or ulcers in the vagina.

Superabsorbent tampons are to be used only for exceptionally heavy menstrual flow (during the first two or three days of the period), not during the whole period. In the absence of a heavy menstrual flow, these tampons will absorb all moisture, leaving the vaginal walls dry and subject to injury. The absorbency of even regular tampons can vary. If the tampon is hard to pull out or shreds when removed or if the vagina becomes dry, the tampon is probably too absorbent. If a woman is worried about accidental spotting, she should check the diagrams on the packages of regular tampons. Those that expand in width are better able to prevent leakage without being too absorbent.

A woman may want to use tampons only during the day and switch to napkins at night to avoid vaginal irritation. Tampons should be avoided on the last spotty days of the period. If a woman experiences vaginal irritation, itching, soreness, unusual odor, or bleeding while using tampons, she should stop using them or change brands or absorbencies to see if that helps. Some suggested guidelines for tampon use appear in Box 7–3.

Box 7–2 Questions Related to Sexuality Submitted by Sixth-Grade Girls Surveyed by Wilke (1983)

Subject Area	Number of Questions
Menstruation	21
Pregnancy	21
Sexual intercourse	18
Female growth and development	12
Breast-feeding	10
Masturbation	8
Multiple births	7
Abortion	7
Herpes	7
Ovulation	7
Male growth and development	4
Nocturnal emissions	4
Sexually transmitted disease	4
Ejaculation	3
Fertilization	3
Tampons	2
Vaginal discharge	2
Cesarean section	1
Uterine cancer	1
Other questions unrelated to growth and development	12

Wilke L: Presenting sex education in elementary schools; unpublished paper. University of Alaska, Anchorage, 1983.

There has been a question about the link between toxic shock syndrome (TSS) and tampon use. It is postulated that small vaginal ulcers or sores may allow or be the route by which the bacteria enters the bloodstream, causing TSS.

The choice of sanitary protection must meet the individual's needs, and she should feel comfortable using it whether it be napkins or tampons.

VAGINAL SPRAYS AND DOUCHING

Another comfort issue is the use of douching and vaginal sprays. Women have been led to believe that regular douching is as fundamental as a morning shower and use of hygiene spray deodorant as essential as underarm deodorant. In fact these douches and deodorants are not only unnecessary but also can be harmful. Vaginal sprays can cause infections, itching, burning, irritation, vaginal discharge, rashes, and other problems.

Women should carefully follow the directions for proper use of deodorant sprays. It is recommended that these sprays be used externally only and not be used with sanitary napkins or applied to broken, irritated, or itching skin. The two circumstances in which women may be most concerned with vaginal odor are during menstruation and during intercourse, and these are times when use of feminine deodorant sprays is clearly contraindicated.

Douching is unnecessary since the vagina cleanses itself; simply wiping the vaginal lips is sufficient for cleanliness. Douching washes away the natural mucus and upsets the vaginal ecology, which can make the vagina more susceptible to infection. Douching with one of the perfumed or flavored douches can cause allergic reactions, and too frequent use of an undiluted or strong douche solution can induce severe irritation and even tissue damage. Propelling water up the vagina may also erode the antibacterial cervical plug and force bacteria and germs from the vagina into the uterus. Women should not douche during menstruation because the cervix is dilated to permit the downward flow of menstrual flow from the uterine lining. Douching may force tissue back up into the uterine cavity, which could create endometriosis.

Women need to remember that there is nothing offensive about a healthy vagina. The mucous secretions that continually bathe the vagina are completely odor free while they are in the vagina; only when they mingle with per-

Box 7–3 Guidelines for Tampon Use

- Eliminate the use of tampons, or reduce use by substituting sanitary pads part of the time, especially at night.
- Avoid tampons at the end of the period when vaginal walls are drier.
- Avoid superabsorbent tampons. Do not use more than one tampon at a time.
- Avoid deodorant tampons and feminine deodorants.
- If toxic shock syndrome occurs, eliminate all use of tampons, until *Staphylococcus aureus* is eliminated from the vagina.
- If high fever, vomiting, diarrhea, vaginitis, or any sign of vaginal ulceration, occur while using tampons, consult a health care professional.
- If milder forms of illness, such as weakness, skin rash, and sore throat, occur while using tampons, discontinue tampon use and consult a health care provider.

Adapted from Cibulka NJ: Toxic shock syndrome and other tampon-related risks. *J Obstet Gynecol Nurs* 1983;(March/April)12(2):94.

spiration and hit the air does odor develop. Keeping one's skin clean and free of bacteria with plain soap and water is the most effective method of controlling odor. A soapy finger should be used to wash gently between the vulvar folds. Bathing is as important (if not more so) during your period as at any other time. There is no evidence that bathing will bring on cramps or interrupt blood flow. On the contrary, a long leisurely soak in a warm tub will promote menstrual blood flow and relieve cramps by relaxing the muscles.

Keeping the vaginal area fresh throughout the day means keeping it dry and clean. After bathing or showering and patting herself dry a woman should powder her bottom with cornstarch or powdered natural clay (available at many health food stores) and wear cotton panties. She should make sure that her clothes are loose enough to permit the vaginal area to breathe. After using the toilet, a woman should always wipe herself from front to back and if necessary, follow up with a moistened paper towel or toilet paper.

The most important thing to remember is that if an unusual odor persists despite these efforts, it may be a sign that something is awry. Certain conditions such as vaginitis produce a foul-smelling discharge.

DISCOMFORT

Cramping and general discomfort may be alleviated by instituting certain nutritional practices, exercise, and use of heat and massage.

○ *NUTRITIONAL SELF-CARE* Vitamins such as B and E have been found helpful in relieving the discomforts associated with menstruation. The B complex vitamins play a key role in neutralizing the excessive amounts of estrogen produced by the ovaries during the course of normal menstrual cycles and therefore may protect against the bloating and bristling nervousness that sometimes occur premenstrually. Vitamin B_6 in particular can relieve the heavy, bloated puffy feeling that is often experienced a week or so before the period starts. Vitamin E is also an excellent weapon against menstrual pain and swelling. Vitamin E is a mild prostaglandin inhibitor similar to aspirin but without the side effects. Vitamin E is also able to improve circulation, which will reduce muscular spasms and pain by reducing the uterus's need for oxygen. Calcium may also provide relief from menstrual symptoms.

Supplements are probably the best way to get concentrated nutrients when you need them, but all these vitamins and minerals are readily available in well-balanced diets. Foods high in vitamin B complex are lean meats, whole grains, dark green leafy vegetables, and brewer's yeast; wheat germ is high in vitamin E; and low-fat milk, yogurt, and cottage cheese are good sources of calcium.

Women should avoid salt as it is a potential contributor to menstrual problems.

○ *EXERCISE* Exercise can not only ease existing menstrual discomfort but if performed daily can also help prevent cramps and other common menstrual complaints before they start. It relieves constipation by increasing intestinal contractions and curbs bloating by increasing perspiration. The deep breathing required by exercise brings more oxygen to the blood, which relaxes the uterus and can ease even the painful contractions of childbirth. It has been known to alleviate irritability and tension. Helpful exercises include jogging, swimming, cycling, or fast-paced walking. Menstrual relaxation exercises have also been found helpful.

○ *HEAT AND MASSAGE* Heat is a wonderful soother and promoter of blood flow. Any type of warmth, from sipping herbal tea to soaking in a hot tub or using a heating pad, may be beneficial during painful periods. Massage can also soothe aching back muscles and promote relaxation and blood flow.

Research Note

Patterson and Hale used grounded theory methodology to investigate how women integrate menstrual care practices into their daily activities. The theory that emerged (primarily through interviews and observations) was that women have developed the self-care process of "making sure" in order to meet continuous menstrual demands in a way that does not excessively interfere with other activities. The study revealed several subprocesses of "making sure": attending (assessing the demand), calculating (deciding appropriate action to meet the demand), and juggling (finding time, space, supplies).

The study speaks to the changing attitudes toward menstruation. With increased knowledge about female physiology and the development of menstrual absorbents women are no longer confined to their homes during their menses as they were in the 19th century. Despite these advances menstruation is not a topic for open discussion. Women are encouraged to continue usual activities during their menses, as long as they "make sure" to conceal the reality of their menstruation.

This study will help nurses become sensitive and provide support to teens approaching menarche.

Patterson ET, Hale ES: Making sure: Integrating menstrual care practices into activities of daily living. Adv Nurs Sci 1985;7 (April): 18.

● **Associated Menstrual Conditions**

Premenstrual Syndrome

Progesterone withdrawal and a decreased progesterone-to-estrogen ratio with its resultant physiologic and metabolic changes in the late luteal/secretory phase may produce a cluster of symptoms known as premenstrual syndrome (PMS).

Premenstrual syndrome is a term that refers to a variety of luteal phase target organ symptoms. The syndrome has not yet been clearly defined as an entity by carefully designed studies, but it is real and has become part of the "menstrual mystique" for some women because of the recent publicity.

Women over 30 years of age are most likely to have PMS. It has been estimated that from 30 percent to 50 percent of ovulating women have mild or severe episodes of some or all of the following types of symptoms (Chihal 1982, Pariser et al 1985):

- *Psychologic*—irritability, lethargy, depression, low morale, anxiety, sleep disorders, crying spells, and hostility

- *Neurologic*—classic migraine, vertigo, syncope

- *Respiratory*—coryza, hoarseness, asthma

- *Gastrointestinal*—nausea, vomiting, constipation, abdominal bloating, craving for sweets

- *Urinary*—retention and oliguria

- *Dermatologic*—acne

- *Mammary*—swelling and tenderness

Most women do not experience all of these symptoms. The symptoms are most pronounced two or three days before the onset of menstruation (although they may be present for up to two weeks before the onset of menstruation) and subside as menstrual flow begins, with or without treatment. It is less well known that some women experience feelings of heightened creativity, increased powers of concentration, and more productive mental and physical activity (Fogel & Woods 1981).

NURSING ROLE

The nurse uses a self-care model to assist the woman in identifying specific symptoms and to support healthy behavior. After assessment, counseling for PMS may include restriction of foods containing methylxanthines (eg, chocolate and coffee), salt, and sugar; increased intake of complex carbohydrates and protein; and increased frequency of meals. Supplementation with B complex vitamins, especially B_6, and magnesium and zinc are also effective in some cases (Abraham 1982, Schaumburg 1984). Vitamin

Research Note

Premenstrual syndrome (PMS) is experienced, with a wide variety of symptoms, by 70% to 90% of women in the United States. Brown and Zimmer explored the impact of PMS symptoms on a woman's personal life and on family functioning. The 83 women and 32 men who attended a lecture on PMS were given a short questionnaire to complete prior to the lecture, including questions about their motivation for attending, coping strategies, symptoms, and personal and family distress.

Responses to the questionnaire indicated that women came to the lecture because they were concerned about their male partner's interpretation and response to PMS and wanted to learn self-care. Men came in an effort to handle their responses and learn ways in which to help their partners. The women reported 74 different regularly recurring symptoms, mostly related to "tension states" (eg, irritability, anxiety, frustration, argumentativeness). Moderate to severe life disruption from PMS was reported by 76% of the men and 89% of the women. Men reported that PMS increased conflict; disrupted family communication; and decreased participation in enjoyable activities, participation in housework by the woman, contact among family members, and family cohesion. Men said that they coped with their partners' PMS by offering support, expressing anger, seeking outside help, ignoring symptoms, participating more in childrearing, involving themselves more in work, and seeking marital counseling.

Women with PMS are often seen in settings where nurses offer primary care. Nurses can use this opportunity to validate womens' symptoms as PMS, facilitate positive coping, coordinate referral, and provide general support and counseling.

Brown MA, Zimmer PA: Personal and family impact of premenstrual symptoms. J Obstet Gynecol Neonatal Nurs, 1986;15 (January/February):31.

E supplementation to decrease food cravings has also been suggested. A balance between rest periods and a program of aerobic exercises such as fast walking, jogging, and aerobic dancing is suggested.

Two widely prescribed pharmaceutical treatments for PMS are progesterone supplementation by means of vaginal or rectal suppositories and spironolactone orally; but these treatments are under dispute (Griffith-Kenney 1986). Other drugs that may be advocated depending on symptomatology include prostaglandin inhibitors, psychoactive drugs, diuretics, and bromocriptine for treatment of mastodynia (Pariser et al 1985).

An emphathetic relationship with a health care professional to whom the woman feels free to voice her concerns is highly beneficial. Encouragement to keep a diary may help the woman identify life events associated with PMS. Self-care groups and self-help literature both help women gain control over their bodies. Group members share helpful therapies including nutrition information and exercise and relaxation techniques. Biofeedback techniques can be learned and used to treat specific symptoms such as headache. Nurses can assist women who feel the negative aspects of the PMS publicity that focuses on labeling women as ill and not having control over their bodies. Support groups also assist in reducing the stress women may feel.

Dysmenorrhea

Dysmenorrhea, or painful menstruation, occurs at or a day before the onset of menstruation and disappears by the end of menses. Sloane (1985) reports that 90 percent of women experience some pain with menses, and 50 percent to 60 percent require analgesia some of the time. Dysmenorrhea is classified as primary or secondary. Primary or essential dysmenorrhea usually appears within 12 months after menarche, and occurs for the first one or two days of the menstrual flow. It presents as waves of lower abdominal cramps radiating to the lower back or upper thighs and often both areas. These cramps may be accompanied by headache, nausea, vomiting, and diarrhea. Dysmenorrhea is absent when ovulation does not occur. Nulliparous teens and women under 25 years of age experience it more often, and it usually disappears after the first pregnancy (Ganong 1985).

The causes of dysmenorrhea seem to be intrinsic to the uterus itself. Hypercontractibility of the uterus (as well as the gastrointestinal tract) may result from excessive production of prostaglandins F_2 and $F_{2\alpha}$, which occurs following ovulation and peaks at menstruation. An increase in prostaglandins is thought to result in an increase in uterine contractions, ischemia from the decrease in uterine arterial blood flow, and a lowering of the pain threshold of the nerves of the uterus. Dysmenorrhea usually corresponds to the secretory phase of the endometrium and indicates that ovulation has occurred.

Secondary dysmenorrhea is associated with pathology of the reproductive tract and usually appears after menstruation has been established. Conditions that most frequently cause secondary dysmenorrhea include endometriosis, residual pelvic inflammatory disease, and anatomic anomalies such as cervical stenosis, imperforate hymen, or uterine displacement (Fogel & Woods 1981). Because primary and secondary dysmenorrhea may coexist, accurate differential diagnosis is essential for appropriate treatment.

Treatment of physiologic primary dysmenorrhea includes hormonal therapy, such as oral contraceptives; nonsteriodal anti-inflammatory drugs or prostaglandin inhibitors, such as ibuprofen; or cervical dilatation (Fraser et al 1983). Cervical dilatation produces relief in 25 percent of cases, but even for these women dysmenorrhea can recur after the procedure (Sloane 1985). Women need to be informed that there may be side effects of these drug therapies and procedures and that they should be undertaken only under medical supervision.

NURSING ROLE

The nurse can assist women by becoming informed about self-care measures for dysmenorrhea. Self-care measures include starting an exercise program; using the pelvic rock exercise, which can decrease the pain; using heat in the form of baths, showers, or heating pads to relieve discomfort by increasing blood flow and decreasing muscle spasm; and getting more rest during menstruation. Hot drinks like soups or spiced or herbal teas are soothing and relaxing and can help break the pain-tension cycle. Good nutrition can also promote a sense of well-being.

Biofeedback has been used against dysmenorrhea with some success (Heczy 1980, Balick et al 1982). Clients using biofeedback techniques perceived some control over their bodies and also appeared more relaxed.

Menstrual Cycle Variations

Amenorrhea, the absence of menses, is classified as primary or secondary. Primary amenorrhea is said to occur if menstruation has not been established by age 18 years. Secondary amenorrhea is said to occur when an established menses (of longer than three months) ceases. Any of the functional causes of delayed menarche may also cause secondary amenorrhea.

Primary amenorrhea necessitates a thorough assessment of the young woman to determine its cause. Identified causes include congenital obstructions, congenital absence of the uterus, testicular feminization, or absence or imbalance of hormones. Successful treatment is limited by causative factors. Many causes are not correctable, and infertility will persist (Fogel & Woods 1981).

Secondary amenorrhea is caused most frequently by pregnancy. Additional causes include lactation, hormonal imbalances, poor nutrition (anorexia nervosa, obesity, fad dieting), ovarian lesions, strenuous exercise (associated with long-distance runners with low body fat ratios), debilitating systemic diseases, stress of high intensity and/or long duration, stressful life events, a change in season or climate, use of oral contraceptives, the phenothiazine and chlorpromazine group of tranquilizers, and syndromes such as Cushing and Sheehan. Treatment is dictated by causative factors (Gaines 1981, Griffith-Kenney 1986). If the cause is related to such conditions the nurse can explain that once the underlying condition has been corrected—for example, when sufficient body weight is gained—menses will resume. Female athletes and women who participate in strenuous exercise routines may be advised to increase their caloric intake or reduce their exercise levels for a month or two to see whether a normal cycle ensues. If it does not, medical referral is indicated.

An abnormally short menstrual cycle is termed *hypomenorrhea*; an abnormally long one is called *hypermenorrhea*. Excessive, profuse flow is called *menorrhagia*, and bleeding between periods is known as *metrorrhagia*. Infrequent and too frequent menses are termed *oligomenorrhea* and *polymenorrhea*, respectively. Such irregularities should be investigated to rule out any disease process.

Anovulatory Cycle

An anovulatory cycle is a cycle in which ovulation does not occur, even though the woman is not taking oral contraceptives. These cycles are noted for their irregularity, the absence of any symptoms of menstrual distress, and (often) heavy bleeding (Charpentier 1983). In cases of this kind, hormonal disturbances result in the proliferation of endometrial growth because the secretory changes stimulated by progesterone fail to occur.

In women taking oral contraceptives, however, an ovulation-suppressed cycle occurs. Although administration of the birth control pill is interrupted each month so that cyclic bleeding can occur, these episodes of bleeding are unlike normal menses in some respects. The hygienic requirements of these "artificial periods" are the same as those for normal menses, but research regarding their emotional and behavioral aspects has so far been inconclusive. "Breakthrough bleeding," or spotting, also occurs in some women between "periods." Controversy still exists over the potential risks involved in pharmacologic suppression of ovulation.

● Menopause

The climacteric occurs near the end of middle age. This period is commonly called the change of life. It is a transitional phase for women, marking the end of their reproductive abilities. A variety of physiologic and hormonal changes occur during this period, including menopause or cessation of menses.

Psychologic Aspects

Menopause is to the climacteric as menarche is to puberty—one indication of a larger, complex process. In addition to the normal physiologic cessation of ovarian function in women at about the age of 50, menopause can appear prematurely or can be surgically induced.

A woman's approach to the climacteric is influenced by social forces in her culture. It is important to determine if she has internalized Victorian beliefs about reproductive and sexual behaviors. Does she believe that sex should be limited to procreative purposes only? Is she intimidated by stereotypes of "older women" portrayed in the media? Is she bound by the traditional double standard? Is she ashamed or bewildered by an increased libido? These and other questions may help nurses understand a particular woman's response to this stage in her life. Spurred by the feminist movement, research is increasing in the area of adjustment and behaviors before, during, and after menopause. Fogel and Woods (1981) present an excellent summary of numerous studies. Of particular interest is a study by Uphold and Susman (1981). The results stress the importance of the quality of marital relationships as correlated with the reporting of climacteric symptoms. The most frequent and severe symptoms were reported by women whose marital adjustment was low. Symptoms were not related to the "empty nest" stage of childrearing as has often been assumed. Further research should consider the presence of and satisfaction with the support systems in women's lives.

Physical Aspects

The physical characteristics of menopause are linked to the shift from a cyclic to a noncyclic hormone pattern. Menopause usually occurs between 45 and 52 years of age. The age of onset may be influenced by nutritional, cultural, or genetic factors. The physiologic mechanisms initiating its onset are not exactly known. The onset of menopause occurs when estrogen levels become so low that menstruation ceases.

Generally, ovulation ceases 1 or 2 years prior to menopause. However, individual variation does exist; as much as 6 to 8 years of transition prior to menopause has been noted. The change is usually gradual, and normal menstrual irregularities do not include menorrhagia or metrorrhagia. Atrophy of the ovaries occurs gradually; FSH levels rise permanently and less estrogen is produced. The endometrium remains in a persistent state of proliferation, increasing a tendency toward uterine fibroids and endometriosis. Menopausal symptoms include atrophic changes in the vagina, vulva, and urethra and in the trigonal area of the bladder.

Most menopausal women experience certain vasomotor disturbances that are clearly related to hormonal changes and the cessation of menstruation. Fifty percent of women report symptoms of heat arising on the chest and spreading to the neck and face (caused by vasodilation), sweating (mild to drenching), sleep disturbances, and occasional chills. This cluster of symptoms is often called hot flashes. There may be 20 to 30 of these a day, lasting 3 to 5 minutes. Dizzy spells, palpitations, and weakness are also reported by some women. Increased perspiration may occur at night as well as during the hot flash.

Most women deal with hot flashes without much difficulty or behavior change. Some report that using a fan or drinking cool liquids is helpful.

Long-range physical changes may include osteoporosis, a decrease in the bony skeletal mass. The bones become more brittle and can more easily be broken. This change is thought to occur in association with lowered estrogen and androgen levels, lack of physical exercise, and a chronic low intake of calcium. The occurrence of diabetes mellitus increases at this age. Loss of protein from the skin and supportive tissues causes wrinkling. Postmenopausal women frequently gain weight, which may be due to excessive caloric intake rather than to a change in adipose deposits.

Vulvar atrophy occurs late, and the pubic hair thins, turns gray or white, and may ultimately disappear. The labia shrivel and lose their heightened pigmentation. Pelvic fascia and muscles atrophy, resulting in decreased pelvic support. The breasts become pendulous and decrease in size and firmness.

The uterine endometrium and myometrium atrophy, as do the cervical glands. The uterine cavity becomes stenosed. The fallopian tubes atrophy extensively. The vaginal mucosa becomes smooth and thin and the rugae disappear, leading to loss of elasticity. As a result, intercourse may be painful. Dryness of the mucous membrane can lead to burning and itching. The vaginal pH level increases as the number of Döderlein's bacilli decreases.

Atrophy of the vagina may also cause discomfort during intercourse, but this may be overcome with the use of lubricating gel or saliva. Women are still multiorgasmic and sexual interest and activity may even improve as the need for contraception disappears and personal growth and awareness increase.

Until recently, menopausal symptoms were primarily treated with supplementary estrogen. However, estrogen therapy has been challenged in recent years. It has been determined that only vasomotor symptoms and vaginal atrophy are related to low estrogen levels. Also, sustained high-dosage estrogen therapy has been reported to predispose women to malignancy of the reproductive tract. Currently, the prescription of short-term, low-dose estrogenic therapy for extensive troublesome vasomotor disruptions and of intravaginal estrogenic creams for vaginal atrophy are preferred treatment measures.

To complicate the estrogen use issue, there is evidence that the use of estrogen delays bone loss in age-related osteoporosis in older women (Riis et al 1987). There are also some reports that administration of estrogens reduces the incidence of cardiovascular disease (Friederich 1982). Henderson (1983) also reported this effect of estrogens. This is a comparatively new area of research, and nurses should use discretion in advising women until more information is available.

Another controversial treatment method is the use of calcium supplements to reduce bone disease in women. It is currently felt that calcium supplementation will not prevent bone disease. Women are advised, however, to include more calcium in their diets beginning when they are young so that their bones are as thick as possible. They may thus be able to avoid the onset of osteoporosis (Waldholz 1986).

Nursing Role

Menopausal women may need assistance, in the form of counseling, to adjust successfully to this developmental phase of life. Reaction to menopause is determined to a large extent by the kind of life the woman has lived, by the security she has in her feminine identity, and by her feelings of self-worth and self-esteem.

Nurses or other health professionals can help the menopausal client achieve high-level functioning at this time in her life. Of paramount importance is the nurse's ability to understand and provide support for the client's views and feelings. Whether the woman expresses "relief and delight" or "tearfulness and fear," the nurse needs an empathetic approach in counseling, health teaching, or providing physical care. Touch and caring as nursing measures may enhance the self-actualization of both nurse and client.

Nurses should explore the question of comfort during sexual intercourse. Dryness and shrinking of the vagina can cause discomfort and difficulty during intercourse. Lubrication with a water-soluble jelly will help provide relief. Use of estrogen, orally or in vaginal creams, may also be indicated. Increased frequency of intercourse will maintain some elasticity in the vagina.

When assessing the menopausal client, the nurse should address the question of sexual activity openly but tactfully because many clients in this age group may have been socialized to be reticent in discussing sex.

The nurse can offer counsel and support to women experiencing psychosocial and emotional stresses associated with menopause. MacPherson (1981) suggested an alliance of nurses and feminist health workers to encourage women to develop a more positive attitude toward the menopausal experience. The client can be referred to self-help groups that focus on understanding, ownership, and control of one's body. These groups are composed of both premenopausal and postmenopausal women and are usually small enough to facilitate easy interaction among members. They are led by lay health care workers or health professionals whose goals are in accordance with those of the group. Women may find that attending such a group for several months helps satisfy their personal needs.

The crucial need of women in the perimenopausal phase of life is adequate information about the changes taking place in their bodies and their lives. Supplying that information provides both a challenge and an opportunity for employing the advocacy approach to nursing for the benefit of both client and nurse.

A woman at menopause looks forward to about 30 more years of life. As she accomplishes the developmental tasks of the climacteric period and adjusts to changes through incorporation of role transitions, she can affirm her worth and go on to an exciting and challenging time of her life.

KEY CONCEPTS

The female reproductive cycle is composed of the ovarian cycle, during which ovulation occurs, and the menstrual cycle, during which menstruation occurs. These two cycles take place simultaneously and are under neurohormonal control.

The ovarian cycle has two phases: the follicular phase and the luteal phase. During the follicular phase the primordial follicle matures under the influence of FSH and LH until ovulation occurs. The luteal phase begins when the ovum leaves the follicle and the corpus luteum develops under the influence of LH. The corpus luteum produces high levels of progesterone and low levels of estrogen.

The menstrual cycle has four phases: menstrual, proliferative, secretory, and ischemic. Menstruation is the actual shedding of the endometrial lining, when estrogen levels are low. The proliferative phase begins when the endometrial glands begin to enlarge under the influence of estrogen and cervical mucosa changes occur; the changes peak at ovulation. The secretory phase follows ovulation and under the influence primarily of progesterone the uterus increases its vascularity to make it ready for possible implantation. The ischemic phase is characterized by degeneration of the corpus luteum, fall in both estrogen and progesterone levels, constriction of the spiral arteries, and escape of blood into the stromal cells of the endometrium.

Menstruation is steeped in myths and the resulting taboos place restraints on women. These come from the beliefs that menstruation causes the woman to be less capable and vulnerable, unclean while menstruating or possessing supernatural powers. These beliefs have no logical documentable basis.

Girls and women should be provided with clear information about comfort issues, such as tampons (deodorant and absorbency); vaginal spray and douching practices; and self-care comfort measures, such as nutrition, exercise, and use of heat and massage during menstruation.

Premenstrual syndrome occurs most often in women over 30, and symptoms occur 2 to 3 days before onset of menstruation and subside as menstruation starts with or without treatment. Medical management usually includes progesterone agonists and prostaglandin inhibitors. Self-care measures include improved nutrition (vitamin B complex and E supplementation and avoidance of methylxanthines, such as in chocolate and caffeine), a program of aerobic exercise, and participation in self-care support groups.

Dysmenorrhea usually begins at, or a day before, onset of menses and disappears by the end of menstruation. Therapy with hormones such as oral contraceptives or the use of nonsteroidal anti-inflammatory drugs or prostaglandin inhibitors is useful. Self-care measures include improved nutrition, exercise, applications of heat, and extra rest.

Menopause is a physiologic maturational change in a woman's life that may be associated with emotional attributes. It is a time of reflection on a woman's life up to this point and gives impetus to evaluate desired future directions. Physiologic changes include the cessation of menses and decrease in circulating hormones. The more common physiologic symptoms are "hot flashes," palpitations, dizziness, and increased perspiration at night. The woman's anatomy also undergoes changes such as atrophy of the vagina, reduction in size and pigmentation of the labia, and myometrial atrophy. Osteoporosis becomes an increasing concern.

Current management of menopause still centers around estrogen replacement and calcium supplementation therapy.

REFERENCES

Abraham G: The nutritionist approach, in **Debrovener** CH (ed): *Premenstrual Tension: A Multidisciplinary Approach.* New York, Human Sciences Press, 1982.
Alpern N: Men and menstruation: A phenomenological investigation of men's experiences of menstruation. Presented at Socio-Cultural Issues in Menstrual Cycle Research, an Inter-Disciplinary Conference/Workshop, University of California, San Francisco, May 20–21, 1983.

Aten RF, **Luborsky** JL, **Behrman** HR: Prostaglandins: Basic chemistry and action, in **Sciarra** JJ et al (eds): *Gynecology and Obstetrics*. Hagerstown, Md, Harper & Row, 1986, vol 5.

Balick L, et al: Biofeedback treatment and dysmenorrhea. *Biofeedback Self-Regulation* 1982;7:499.

Bloom ML, **Van Dongen** L: *Clinical Gynaecology: Integration of Structure and Function*. London, Williams Heinemann, 1972.

Boston Women's Health Book Collective: *The New Our Bodies, Ourselves*. New York, Simon & Schuster, 1984.

Caldwell BV, **Behrman** HR: Prostaglandins in reproductive processes. *Med Clin North Am* 1981;65:927.

Charpentier LA: When anovulation is the cause. *Consultant* 1983;23:273.

Chihal HJ: Painful periods and preludes. *Emergency Med* 1982;14(17):33.

Cibulka NJ: Toxic shock syndrome and other tampon related risks. *J Obstet Gynecol Neonat Nurs* 1983;(March/April)12(2):94.

Dan A: The law and women's bodies: Menstruation leave in Japan. Presented at Socio-Cultural Issues in Menstrual Cycle Research, an Inter-Disciplinary Conference/Workshop, University of California, San Francisco, May 20–21, 1983.

Delaney J, **Lupton** MJ, **Toth** E: *The Curse: A Cultural History of Menstruation*. New York, New American Library, 1976.

Fogel CI, **Woods** NF: *Health Care of Women: A Nursing Perspective*. St. Louis, Mosby, 1981.

Fraser IS, et al: Long term treatment of menorrhagia with mefenamic acid *Obstet Gynecol* 1983;61(1):109.

Friederich MA: Aging, menopause, and estrogens: The clinician's dilemma, in **Voda** A, **Dinnerstein** M, **O'Donnell** S (eds): *Changing Perspectives on the Menopause*. Austin, University of Texas Press, 1982.

Gaines F: Secondary amenorrhea: Assessment and plans. *Nurs Pract* 1981;6(September/October):14.

Ganong WF: *Review of Medical Physiology*, ed 12. Los Altos, Calif, Lange Medical Publishing, 1985.

Gardner J: Adolescent menstrual characteristics and predictors of gynaecological health. *Ann Hum Biol* 1983; 10:31.

Golub S: Sex differences in attitudes and beliefs regarding menstruation, in **Komnenich** P, et al (eds): *The Menstrual Cycle*. New York, Springer, 1981, vol 2.

Griffith-Kenney J: *Contemporary Women's Health: A Nursing Advocacy Approach*. Menlo Park, Calif, Addison-Wesley, 1986.

Heczy MD: Effects of biofeedback and autogenic training on dysmenorrhea, in **Dan** A, **Graham** E, **Beecher** C (eds): *The Menstrual Cycle*. New York, Springer, 1980, vol 1.

Henderson BE: Arteriosclerotic heart disease and endometrial cancer. *Ann Intern Med* 1983;98:195.

Lackritz RM: Prostaglandins in pregnancy, in **Sciarra** JJ, et al (eds): *Gynecology and Obstetrics*. Hagerstown, Md, Harper & Row, 1981, vol 5.

Little AB, **Billiar** RB: Endocrinology, in **Romney** SL, et al (eds): *The Health Care of Women*, ed 2. New York, McGraw-Hill, 1981.

MacPherson K: Menopause as a disease: The social construction of a metaphor. *Adv Nurs Sci* 1981;3(January):95.

McClintock MK: Major gaps in menstrual cycle research: Behavioral and physiological controls in a biological context, in **Komnenich** P, et al (eds): *The Menstrual Cycle*. New York, Springer, 1981, vol 2.

Morris NM: Menstruation and marital sex. *J Biosoc Sci* 1983;15:173.

Pariser SF, et al: Premenstrual syndrome: Concerns, controversies, and treatment. *Am J Obstet Gynecol* 1985; 153(6):599.

Rierdan J: Variations in the experience of menarche as a function of preparedness, in **Golub** S (ed): *Menarche*. Lexington, Mass, Lexington Books, 1983.

Riis B, **Thomsen** K, **Christiansen** C: Does calcium supplementation prevent postmenopausal bone loss? *N Engl J Med* 1987;316(January):173.

Schaumburg H, et al: Sensory neuropathy from pyridoxine abuse. *N Engl J Med* 1984;309:445.

Siegel SJ: The effect of culture on the way women experience menstruation: Jewish women and mikvah. Presented at Socio-Cultural Issues in Menstrual Cycle Research, an Inter-Disciplinary Conference/Workshop, University of California, San Francisco, May 20–21, 1983.

Sloane E: *Biology of Women*, ed 2. New York, John Wiley, 1985.

Tybor JR: Premenstrual tension tested as legal defense. *Chicago Tribune*, May 23, 1982.

Uphold CR, **Susman** EJ: Self-reported climacteric symptoms as a function of the relationship between marital adjustment and childrearing stage. *Nurs Res* 1981;30(March/April):84.

Vijayakumar R, et al: Myometrial prostaglandins during human menstrual cycle. *Am J Obstet Gynecol* 1981; 141(3):313.

Waldholz M: Research suggest calcium supplements fail to prevent a bone disease in women. *The Wall Street Journal*, July 29, 1986, p 6.

Wilhelmson L, et al: Effects of prostaglandins on the isolated uterine artery of the nonpregnant woman. *Prostaglandins* 1981;22(2):223.

Williams LR: Beliefs and attitudes of young girls regarding menstruation, in **Golub** S (ed): *Menarche*. Lexington, Mass, Lexington Books, 1983.

Wilke L: *Presenting Sex Education in Elementary Schools*, unpublished paper. University of Alaska, Anchorage, 1983.

ADDITIONAL READINGS

Beach RK: Help for the dysmenorrheic adolescent. *Patient Care* 1986;20(December 15):100.

Bell SE: Changing ideas: The medicalization of menopause. *Soc Sci Med* 1987;24(6):535.

Calesnick B, **Dinan** A: Prostaglandins and NSIADs in primary dysmenorrhea. *AFP* 1987;35(January):223.

Chard T, **Liford** R: *Basic Sciences for Obstetrics and Gynaecology,* ed 2. New York, Springer-Verlag, 1986.

Coyne CM, **Woods** NF, **Mitchell** ES: Premenstrual tension syndrome. *J Obstet Gynecol Neonatal Nurs* 1985;14(6):446.

Gardner J: Adolescent menstrual characteristics and predictors of gynaecological health. *Ann Hum Biol* 1983; 10:31.

Harlow SD: Function and dysfunction: A historical critique of the literature on menstruation and work. *J Health Care for Women Int'l* 1986;7:39.

Heinz SA: Premenstrual syndrome: An assessment, education, and treatment model. *J Health Care for Women Int'l* 1986;7:153.

McKeever P, **Galloway** S: Effects of nongynecological surgery on the menstrual cycle. *Nurs Res* 1984;33(January–February):42.

Nagamani M, **Kelvin** ME, **Smith** ER: Treatment of menopausal hot flashes with transdermal administrations of clonidine. *Am J Obstet Gynecol* 1987;156(March):561.

Ouellette MD, et al: Relationship between percent body fat and menstrual patterns in athletes and nonathletes. *Nurs Res* 1986;35(6):330.

Posthuma BW, et al: Detecting changes in functional ability in women with premenstrual syndrome. *Am J Obstet Gynecol* 1987;156(February):275.

Reame NE: Women in wheelchairs: Menstrual health and hygiene practices. Presented at Socio-Cultural Issues in Menstrual Cycle Research, an Inter-Disciplinary Conference/Workshop, University of California, San Francisco, May 20–21, 1983.

Simon JA, et al: Variability of midcycle estradiol: Positive feedback evidence for unique pituitary responses in individual women. *J Clin Endocrinol Metab* 1987;64(4):789.

Sloss EM, **Frerichs** RR: Smoking and menstrual disorders. *Int J Epidemiol* 1983;12(1):107.

Speroff L, et al: ERT-Whom to treat and how. *Contemp OB/GYN* 1987;29(April):179.

Urban DJ, et al: Nurse specialization in reproductive endocrinology. *J Obstet Gynecol Neonatol Nurs* 1982;11(May/June):167.

Voda M: The menopausal hot flash, in **Voda** A, **Dinnerstein** M, **O'Donnell** S (eds): *Changing Perspectives on the Menopause.* Austin, University of Texas Press, 1982.

Wager GP: Toxic shock syndrome: A review. *Am Obstet Gynecol* 1983;146:93.

Woods NF: Socialization and social context: Influence on perimenstrual symptoms, disability and menstrual attitudes. *J Health Care for Women Int'l* 1986;7:115.

I think that one of the most difficult things for me as a woman is trying to put myself into all these different places, be a wife, and be a mother, and also have a job, and trying to look where that goes and what's important to me in my life, and to form a kind of balance so I am not all mother and not all wife, and I am not all worker. Somehow all of that is important to make me see myself as a whole person. (Ourselves and Our Children)

Sexuality and Reproductive Choices

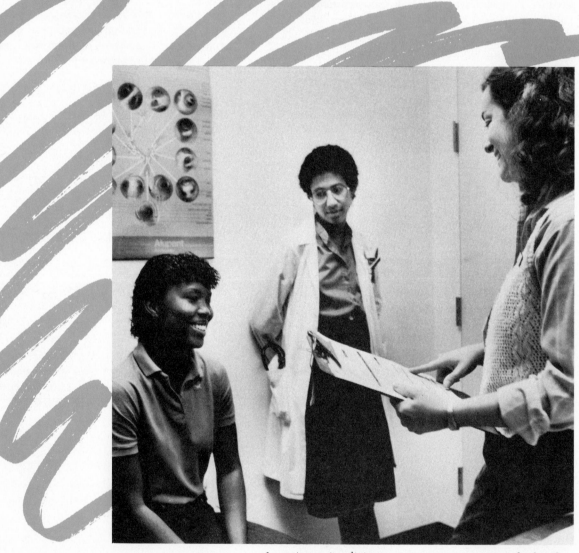

In an inner-city clinic, a nurse prepares a teenager for her first contraceptive consultation.

Chapter Eight

OBJECTIVES

- Summarize the factors that influence the development of attitudes about sexuality.
- Compare the sexual responses of males and females as identified by Masters and Johnson.
- Identify three factors that are necessary for the nurse to be an effective sexual counselor.
- Describe techniques a nurse can use to be more effective when taking a sexual history.
- Relate the basic content of preconception counseling to its rationale.
- Compare the various methods of fertility control with regard to advantages, disadvantages, and effectiveness.
- Develop a teaching plan that could be used to instruct a woman about a specific method of contraception.

People are sexual beings. Men and women develop sexual identities, make sexual choices, and establish personal standards of appropriate sexual behavior. Human sexuality begins developing at conception and evolves throughout an individual's life. The sexual experimentation and exploration of children gives way to the more urgent activities of the adolescent. With maturity, sexual contact becomes part of a broader and usually more meaningful relationship.

People make many choices related to their sexual activity. They can choose to be sexually active or celibate. They can choose a monogamous relationship or relationships with many partners. They can choose heterosexual or homosexual activity. They can choose to be parents or to remain childless. They can choose unprotected intercourse, or they can use contraceptives. They can continue in a sexual relationship, or they can end it.

This chapter focuses on the concept of sexuality particularly as it relates to people of childbearing age. The initial discussion relates to human sexuality and human sexual response. Information designed to help nurses take effective sexual histories and do basic counseling is included.

This chapter also provides information on preconception planning for women or couples who choose to become parents. What can couples do to ensure that they are in optimum health when they choose to have a child? The remainder of the chapter focuses on available methods of contraception.

Development of Sexuality

Sexual development begins at conception, when biologic sex is determined: XX, a female, XY, a male. As the embryo becomes a fetus and development continues, sexual differentiation takes place (See Figure 6–1), and the sex organs begin functioning. For example, on sonography male fetuses have been noted to have cyclical erections (Calderone 1983). Even as the sex organs are developing, other senses and systems are developing that enable the infant to react to sexual stimuli at birth. The sense of touch, for example, which is fundamental in the development of sexuality, is highly developed by eight weeks' gestation.

The stimuli, experiences, and relationships that are essential to the development of sexuality come into play at birth. The infant learns to find satisfaction through oral stimuli, through contact with another, and through cuddling and holding. Young infants learn to touch and stroke their genitals and seem to be capable of sexual arousal.

Toddlers facing toilet training become even more aware of their bodies and may more consciously practice masturbation although their parents often discourage it. By age 3 most children are aware of their sexual identity as a result of consistent parental and social reinforcement. During the childhood years, from 5 through 12, sexual activity and interest may be less apparent but it has not disappeared. Games such as "playing house" or "playing doctor" help children learn sex roles and more about the differences between the sexes. Children show a preference for playmates of the same sex, although they may also show some romantic interest in members of the opposite sex.

Puberty and adolescence are a time of transition from childhood to adulthood. Adolescence finds sexually mature young people trying to cope with new situations and sensations while they are still psychologically immature. Sexual experimentation begins, and masturbation accompanied by fantasy is common. Homosexual experiences may occur, and mutual masturbation for boys is not uncommon. Heterosexual contacts progress over four or five years from initial kissing and fondling, to mutual body exploration and masturbation, to sexual intercourse.

With adulthood comes responsibility and choice. Because sexual expression in marriage has the most legitimacy in our society, many adults choose to marry. However, new life-styles, changing morality, and contraceptive choices have made available other situations in which sexuality can be expressed.

Sexual Attitudes

Attitudes about sex are influenced by a variety of factors. The home environment is one of the greatest influences. Children raised by parents who are comfortable with and open about sexuality will probably be more comfortable with their sexuality than children raised in more restrictive environments. The following anecdote from a young mother provides an example.

When I was growing up, my parents always showed affection for each other and for us. Hugs, kisses, and pats on the shoulder were common. In discussing sexual issues with me, my mother was very direct and always used correct terminology. She never seemed embarrassed to answer questions. My closest girlfriend couldn't talk to her mother about anything. She told me once that she had never seen her parents show any physical affection for each other. They never kissed or hugged her either. She had an older sister, but they weren't close, so I ended up telling her what my mother told me. When we started high school and had so many questions, it was harder. One day a neat thing happened. My mom made some cocoa, and the three of us sat and talked all afternoon. Mom answered our questions about sex and got us thinking about more abstract aspects of sexuality like ethics and choices. It was one of the most special times I ever shared with my mother. I hope I can do the same for my children.

Even if parents are not openly demonstrative, they can convey to children that sexuality is a natural, acceptable, and satisfying part of life by creating a positive home atmosphere.

Cultural background can profoundly influence the home and environment and thereby have a major impact on the child's socialization. Individuals raised in a male dominated or strongly moralistic culture will usually have very different attitudes from those of individuals raised in a culture that views sexual expression as a shared experience between equals. People can reject cultural norms as adults, but it is often difficult and may cause stress. Thiederman (1986) describes the difficulties experienced by Indian and Pakistani women who have emigrated to Great Britain. These women have been exposed to pressure from those trying to "educate" them about the value of self-reliance and independence. The effort to "raise their consciousness" has caused stress, anxiety, and emotional problems for these women.

Attitudes about sex are also influenced by education and socioeconomic level. People with more income and education tend to be more comfortable with a wider variety of sexual activities. Sexual attitudes can be profoundly affected by previous sexual experiences, especially very intense experiences such as incest, rape, or severe punishment for sexual experimentation.

The personal characteristics of the individual are also influential in the development of sexual attitudes. Although it is difficult to negate the influence of environment, people are born with different personality characteristics: Some are shy, others more adventuresome, and so forth. There are also variations in sex drive or libido that significantly influence an individual's view of sexuality.

Ethics and Sexuality

Sexuality must be considered within the context of a person's life and life choices. Sex is a major focus to some and a minor consideration to others. Some feel sex is only appropriate in a close and loving relationship; others feel that love and sex are separate and do not necessarily have to occur together.

Opinions also vary about the purpose of sex. More traditional views hold that the sole purpose of sex is procreation. Pleasure may be experienced, but it is not essential. While it is obviously necessary for the man to experience an orgasm, a woman may or may not achieve one. Any sexual activities engaged in for pleasure only are selfish and immoral. Others believe that the purpose of sex is pleasure: If an action brings pleasure it is good. Nothing is unacceptable as long as it provides pleasure and release. Sex is only "bad" if it does not bring satisfaction to either or both parties. Sexual expression can also be viewed as a means of expression, a sharing of feelings, a union of two individuals seeking to communicate. This communication may involve demonstration of a variety of messages: tenderness, domination, passion, or even anger (Fromer 1983).

Although the basic patterns of psychosexual development are established by the end of adolescence, a person continues to develop and modify beliefs and attitudes throughout life. Many adults broaden their attitudes about sexual activities and experiment with different sexual life-styles. During adulthood an individual resolves any psychosexual conflicts and develops a set of sexual values. Fromer suggests that these values must be in accord with the moral values that influence other aspects of a person's life. If they are not, conflict may result. Because sexual activity (except for masturbation) usually involves another person, it also requires respect for other people. "Any form of sexuality that involves depersonalization, that is, treating the sex partner as anything less than a freely autonomous person, signifies a failure of both sexual and moral development" (Fromer 1983, p 41).

● Sexual Response Cycle

People obtain sexual satisfaction in a variety of ways. A person alone may find sexual pleasure in a book, a film, or a stirring musical piece; he or she may also derive pleasure from fantasy or masturbation. Couples may experience sexual pleasure through a shared experience, through physical closeness such as holding each other or cuddling together; through touching, kissing, and stroking each other; through mutual masturbation; or through sexual intercourse.

Many terms are used to describe the sexual mating of a sexually mature male and female. These include *coitus, sexual intercourse, copulation, making love,* and *the sex act.* Coitus is defined as the insertion of the erect penis into the vagina. After repeated thrusting movements of the penis, the man experiences ejaculation of semen concurrent with orgasm. *Orgasm* is the involuntary climax of the sexual experience, involving a series of muscular contractions, profound physiologic bodily response, and intense sensual pleasure. Orgasm may be achieved by other methods of sexual stimulation besides sexual intercourse, such as masturbation and oral stimulation. Although the basic events of coitus are the same for all couples, wide variation exists in sexual positions, technique, duration, intent, meaning, and reactions among individuals.

Coitus is a personal act between two consenting adults. It can signify a variety of feelings, beliefs, and attitudes.

The traditional purpose of coitus is procreation. However, with the availability of contraceptive methods and changing social mores, sexual intercourse has become accepted as a pleasurable and personally gratifying experience in itself. The sexual union of two individuals may reflect their mutual commitment and caring, or it may be a more immediate interaction for the purpose of personal pleasure or merely temporary companionship. In our society, sexual intercourse ideally is the sharing by two persons of their emotions and bodies in the context of the larger sharing of their lives. Such sexual interactions are the result of mutual caring and love.

Physiology of Sexual Response

Masters and Johnson (1966) have identified and described the physiology of the sexual response in both males and females. All the responses can be classified as either vasocongestive or myotonic. *Vasocongestion* involves the congestion or engorgement of blood vessels and is the most common physiologic response to sexual arousal. *Myotonia,* a secondary physiologic response, is increased muscular tonus, which produces tension.

Sexual response occurs in four phases: excitement, plateau, orgasm, and resolution. Essentially, the sexual response of males (Table 8–1) and females (Table 8–2) is similar, involves the total body, and is continuous. Individual variations do occur.

Female sexual response varies considerably. Not all women experience orgasm consistently; they are influenced by their psychologic state, health, current sexual motivation, and environmental distractions. A woman may not experience orgasm during a particular act of coitus, or she may experience one or multiple orgasms of varying intensity (Figure 8–1A). Such variation is usual in a woman of "normal" sexual activity, interest, and response.

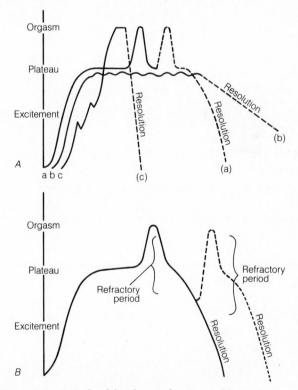

Figure 8–1 A Cycle of female sexual response: (a) reaction pattern with single or multiple orgasms; (b) reaction pattern without orgasm; (c) reaction pattern without distinct plateau. B Cycle of male sexual response. (From Masters WH and Johnson VE: Human Sexual Response. Boston, Little, Brown, 1966, p 55)

Table 8–1   Summary of Male Sexual Response

Organ	Excitement (foreplay)	Plateau (entry and coital movements)	Orgasm (climax)	Resolution (relaxation)
Scrotum	Skin thickens; scrotal sac elevates and flattens against body (spermatic cord contracts)	Remains tense and close to body		
Testes	Elevate with scrotum	May increase in size by 50%; remain elevated		
Penis	Engorgement and erection is rapid; size increases; position changes; angle of protrusion created	Coronal ridge size increases; glans becomes purplish	Contracts	Becomes flaccid; refractory period: erection may not be experienced
Urethra	Moistened with mucus	Mucus increases; becomes distended with semen just before orgasm	Semen ejected with force as bulb contracts	Minor contractions persist even after semen is ejected
Seminal vesicles			Semen is discharged into urethral bulb	
Prostate			Contracts, expelling fluid into urethral bulb	
Bulbourethral glands		Few drops of fluid may be discharged (contain sperm)		
Breasts	Nipple erections; sex flush may appear		Sex flush most pronounced	Slow return to normal; sex flush fades slowly

The male physical response is relatively constant, resulting in orgasm if erection and sexual stimulation are maintained (Figure 8–1B).

Men and women exhibit several identical responses. The *sex flush* is a maculopapular rash that usually begins in the epigastric area and spreads quickly to the breasts. Less than half of men exhibit the sex flush, whereas more than half of women do. Heart rate and blood pressure increase in proportion to the degree of sexual excitement. Muscles tense beginning in the excitement phase. This tension increases during the plateau phase. Hyperventilation occurs just before and during orgasm. At orgasm, muscle tension is extreme. The face may contort, while muscles of the neck, extremities, abdomen, and buttocks contract tightly. Individuals may moan, murmur, or cry out and will experience a total surrender to bodily responses, accompanied by acute pleasure and relief.

During resolution the body returns to the unaroused state. Muscular tension is dramatically reduced, and blood is released from the engorged tissues. If orgasm did not occur, the lingering vasocongestion may cause feelings of pelvic fullness and pressure that take a longer time to resolve.

Although women are capable of achieving multiple orgasms, men are more limited in that respect. Practically all men experience a refractory period as part of their resolution phase. During this period, which may last from a few minutes in young men to several hours in older men, a man is physiologically unable to achieve another erection. Some men, however, can achieve two or more ejaculations with such a short refractory time between that it may be compared to multiple orgasm.

● The Nurse as Counselor on Sexuality and Reproduction

On occasion most people experience concern and even anxiety about some aspect of sexuality. Societal standards and pressures can cause people to evaluate and compare with others their sexual attractiveness, technical abilities, the frequency of sexual interaction, and so on. Appearance and sexual behavior are not the only causes for concern; the reproductive implications of sexual intercourse must also be considered. Some people desire conception; others wish to avoid it at all costs. Health factors are another consideration. The increase in the incidence of sexually transmitted diseases, especially AIDS and herpes, have caused many people to modify their sexual practices and activities.

Because sexuality and its reproductive implications are such an intrinsic and emotion-laden part of life, people have many concerns, problems, and questions about sex roles, sexual behaviors, sex education, family planning, sex-

Table 8–2 Summary of Female Sexual Response

Organ	Excitement (foreplay)	Plateau (entry and coital movements)	Orgasm (climax)	Resolution (relaxation)
Clitoris	Size of glans increases; engorgement of dorsal vein occurs; shaft elongates	Glans retracts under hood after erection	Rhythmic muscular contractions occur, ranging from mild to intense	Returns to normal; no refractory period; multiple orgasms possible
Labia majora	Vasocongestion and swelling occurs; nulliparous: flatten and widen; multiparous: widen by movement from vaginal introitus	Increases		Return to normal size and color
Labia minora	Vasocongestion of erectile tissue occurs; color darkens; extension of tissue	Increases		Return to normal size and color
Vagina	Vaginal lubrication appears; in 10–30 seconds, widens and lengthens 1 cm; walls become purplish; progressive distention occurs; upper portion "tents"; rugae become smooth	Engorgement occurs; outer third of vagina swells; "orgasmic platform" develops; interior lumen decreases to "grasp" penis	Outer third has spasm, then rhythmic contractions; perivaginal muscles contract	Outer third relaxes after clitoris returns to normal; remaining portion returns to normal
Cervix	Moves upward and backward posteriorly	Cervical os opens slightly		Returns to normal position; os closes in 20–30 minutes
Uterus	Moves upward and backward	Increases in size	Rhythmic contractions from fundus to cervix occur	Returns to precoital size slowly
Breasts	Areolae increase in size; nipples become erect and size increases; sex flush may appear		Sex flush most pronounced	Slow return to normal; sex flush disappears

ual inhibitions, sexual morality, and related areas. Child-bearing women frequently voice these concerns to the nurse, who may need to assume the role of counselor on sexual and reproductive matters.

To be effective in providing sexual health care, nurses must develop an awareness of their own feelings, values, and attitudes about sexuality. Often people believe that their own sexual values and patterns of sexual behavior are the best ones, the "right" ones. This of course implies that all other attitudes and practices are not as good or are "wrong." Nurses must recognize their own beliefs and attitudes so that they can be more sensitive when confronted with the beliefs of others. As Hogan (1980) points out, "Nurses are entitled to their individual feelings, attitudes, beliefs, and standards in relation to sexuality, but they must remain objective when caring for people and when dealing with their sexuality" (p 24). The nurse may develop more personal insight by reading, undertaking thoughtful self-evaluation, and participating in programs or workshops on the subject. The nurse who recognizes that he or she is not comfortable dealing with issues related to sexuality

should avoid situations that require sexual counseling or should refer the client to a nurse who is more skilled in this area.

Many nurses who care for childbearing families will be faced with questions about sexuality, sexual practices, and so forth. These nurses have a responsibility to have accurate, up-to-date knowledge about these topics. They should also know about the structure and functions of the male and female reproductive systems.

Continuing education for the practicing nurse and appropriate courses in undergraduate and graduate nursing education programs can help nurses achieve this knowledge about aspects of sexuality. These courses can teach nurses about sexual values, attitudes, alternative life-styles, cultural factors, and misconceptions and myths about sex and reproduction. The nurse can then maintain this knowledge by regular reading so that he or she is familiar with current literature on the subject.

Self-awareness and a sound knowledge base are not, by themselves, sufficient to make the nurse an effective counselor. The nurse also needs to develop skills in listen-

CONTEMPORARY DILEMMA

Sex Selection: Possible? Yes. But Ethical?

For couples who strongly desire a child of a certain sex, the possibility of sex selection holds tremendous appeal. Earlier theories, such as Dr. Landrum B Shettles's belief that sex could be determined by controlling the time within a woman's cycle when conception occurred, were controversial and not always successful.

Recently Ronald Ericsson developed a procedure for sperm separation, which is marketed by Gametrics. The technique uses a filtering process based on the superior swimming ability of sperm bearing the Y chromosome. The filtration process eliminates the slower-swimming X sperm, leaving a solution that is composed of about 80 percent Y sperm. If a couple strongly desires a boy, the man obtains a specimen of his semen near the time when the woman ovulates. The specimen undergoes the filtration process and is artificially inseminated into the woman at the time of ovulation. Another process is being developed for isolating X sperm.

For couples unable to afford the Gametrics procedure, a home fertility lab kit is now available for determining sex. The kit is based on the Billings method of timing ovulation and the work of Dr. Shettles; its success rate is not yet clear.

Proponents suggest that the process offers choice for couples and will improve family relationships because a child of the desired sex will be especially cherished.

Opponents believe that the process is unnatural and demeaning to babies. They suggest that in a male-dominated world with its recognized preference for boy children, the process is another indication of a deep-seated, if unconscious, prejudice against women.

The availability of this technique raises several difficult questions:

- If the process becomes widespread, will the balance of world population shift to males?
- Will the availability of the process strengthen and foster negative attitudes about women?
- Will religious groups view the technique as another form of unnatural technology and speak out against it? (The Catholic Church has already spoken out against the process of artificial insemination, which forms part of this procedure.)
- What will be the impact on a child born following the procedure if he or she is not the desired sex?
- Is the next step amniocentesis or chorionic villus sampling (CVS) to confirm the sex, followed by abortion if the fetus is not the desired sex? (Currently most medical facilities refuse to do amniocentesis or CVS solely for sex selection, except in cases of serious sex-linked disorders such as hemophilia.)

---

ing, communicating, interviewing, assessing, and intervening. Communication skills are essential. Discussions about sexual concerns are difficult for many people. For a young woman seeking contraception or prenatal care, this may be the first time she has been asked questions related to her sexuality. The nurse must be able to put the woman at ease and gain necessary information. Opening the discussion with a brief explanation of the purpose of such questions is often helpful. For example the nurse might say,

> As your nurse I'm interested in all aspects of your well-being. Often women have concerns or questions about sexual matters, especially when they are pregnant (starting to be sexually active). I will be asking you some questions about your sexual history as part of your general health history.

The nurse may find the following additional suggestions useful when taking a sexual history:

- Provide a quiet, private place, free of distractions.

- Approach the situation in a relaxed unhurried way and with an attitude of honesty and acceptance.

- Use direct eye contact as much as possible unless you know that this is culturally unacceptable to the woman.

- Fit the taking of the sexual history into the gynecologic and obstetric history rather than isolating it.

- Do little if any writing during the discussion, especially if the woman seems ill at ease or is discussing very personal issues.

- Avoid sitting across a desk. Sit as close to the woman as seems comfortable to you both.

- Pay attention to nonverbal cues and body language.

- Ask open-ended questions. Often nurses develop the habit of asking questions that require a "yes" or "no" response. Open-ended questions often elicit far more information. For example, "What, if anything, would you change about your current sex life?" will produce more information than "Are you happy with your sex life now?"

- If the woman has no questions or concerns, it is not necessary to press for a lengthy discussion. It may be that she is satisfied, or that your relationship has not reached the point where she is comfortable with such a discussion.

- Clarify terminology. If the woman uses a slang term find out what she means by it. If the word she uses is not comfortable for you, use one that is comfortable without being too clinical.

- Proceed from easier topics to those that are more difficult to discuss. Often it is easier to discuss the menstrual history, for example, before considering sexually transmitted diseases or unusual sexual practices.

- Before asking direct questions it is often useful to make a generality or normalcy statement such as "Many women worry about . . ." or "Often women have questions about . . ."

- Try to determine whether the woman has already identified specific concerns or if she attributes problems to something specific. For example, you might ask, "Do you feel that anything is affecting your sexual health or happiness in any way?"

- The phrase "How do you feel about that?" is used so often that it has become trite. Instead try "What would you like to change about that situation?" or "You seem uncomfortable. What are you thinking about now?"

- Self-disclosure can occasionally help the woman be more at ease. Before any self-disclosure statement, however, the nurse should internally question whose needs will be met by the disclosure and whether there is any sense of being in competition with the client.

Applying the Nursing Process

After completing the sexual history, the nurse assesses the information obtained. If the nurse identifies a problem that requires further medical tests and assessments, he or she will refer the woman to a nurse practitioner, nurse-midwife, physician, or counselor as necessary. In many instances the nurse alone will be able to develop a nursing diagnosis and then plan and implement therapy. For example, if the nurse determines that a woman who is interested in conceiving a child does not have a clear understanding of when she ovulates, the nurse may formulate the nursing diagnosis: Knowledge deficit related to the timing of ovulation. The nurse could then evaluate the woman's knowledge through discussion and review and work with the woman to provide necessary knowledge. The

nurse might also suggest that the woman keep a menstrual calendar and monitor basal body temperatures to identify the time of ovulation.

The nurse must be realistic in making assessments and planning interventions. It requires insight and skill to recognize when a woman's problem requires interventions that are beyond a nurse's preparation and ability. In such situations, appropriate referrals should be made.

●   Preconception Counseling

Pregnancy is often unplanned and unexpected. It may be the result of a contraceptive failure or a decision by the woman and her partner not to use any method of fertility control. For many women this decision is made for religious or philosophical reasons; some women have no strong feelings about avoiding pregnancy and decide to "let nature take its course"; some women get caught up in a romantic sexual encounter that they failed to anticipate and have no method of contraception available; and some women have unprotected intercourse because they are the victims of sexual assault.

Not all people wish to become parents. Society still puts pressure on couples to have children. Couples who choose to remain childless are often labeled "selfish" and "short-sighted." They are told that they are "missing out" on a unique experience. Despite the pressure, more couples are beginning to speak up for the right of choice.

Thus one of the first questions a couple should ask prior to conception is whether they wish to have children. This involves consideration of each person's personal goals, expectations of their relationship, and desire to be a parent. Often one individual wishes to have a child while the other does not. In such situations open discussion is essential to reach a mutually acceptable decision. In some cases this may require marital counseling.

Couples who wish to have children face a decision about the timing of pregnancy. At what point in their lives do they believe it would be best to become parents: when they are young or when they are older? After two years in their relationship? Or five? Or eight? Do they want to be well-established in careers first? Pregnancy comes as a surprise even when the decision about timing is made, but at least the couple has some control over it.

For couples who believe children are a gift and a responsibility from God or for couples who feel that fertility planning is unnatural and wrong, issues of timing of pregnancy are unacceptable and irrelevant. These couples can still take steps to ensure that they are in the best possible physical and mental health when pregnancy occurs.

Only one person gave me any idea of what having a baby would be like. She said the nearest thing to it was a passionate love affair. (Sally Emerson, A Celebration of Babies)

Preconception Health Measures

If a couple has decided to have a child or if the couple does not find planning acceptable, the couple may make an effort to maximize the quality of their health. This effort should include making life-style changes to avoid known or potential health risks such as alcohol use.

Because there is no definite safe level for alcohol consumption during pregnancy, and because the woman is often pregnant before she realizes it, a woman planning to become pregnant should be advised to stop drinking totally if possible. Because the effects on the embryo of heavy drinking by the father are not as well understood, less emphasis has been placed on male drinking. However, studies suggest that heavy alcohol consumption may decrease a man's fertility. Furthermore, his partner may find it more difficult to avoid alcohol if the man continues to drink. Thus it is helpful if the man, too, restricts his alcohol intake.

Smoking has been linked to preterm labor and intrauterine growth retardation in the fetus. The woman is advised to cease smoking if possible or at least limit her intake to less than half a pack a day. Because exposure to cigarette smoke from another smoker also poses a risk and because of the difficulty most people have in stopping smoking, it is especially helpful if the man doesn't smoke either.

The effects of caffeine are less clearly understood. Because it poses a potential risk, women are advised to stop drinking beverages containing caffeine completely if possible, or at least limit them to two drinks per day.

Many of the social (cocaine, marijuana, LSD) and street (heroin, crack, etc) drugs pose a real threat to a fetus. Prescription drugs can also be hazardous. A woman who uses any drugs or medications should discuss the implications of their use with her health care provider. In most cases it is best to avoid the use of medication whenever possible.

Certain jobs result in exposure to agents that can reduce a man's or woman's fertility or that might cause harm to the fetus if the woman becomes pregnant. This is especially true of exposure to radiation, photographic chemicals, and anesthetic agents. When a couple is contemplating pregnancy, they should carefully consider whether they are exposed to any environmental hazards at work or in their community.

Physical Examination

It is advisable for both partners to have a physical examination to identify any health problems so that they can be corrected if possible. These might include medical conditions such as high blood pressure or obesity; problems that pose a threat to fertility, such as certain sexually transmitted diseases; or conditions that keep the individual from achieving optimal health, such as anemia or colitis. If the family history indicates previous genetic disorders or if the couple is planning pregnancy when the woman is over age 35, the health care provider may suggest that the couple consider genetic counseling (see Chapter 9 for further discussion).

Prior to conception the woman is also advised to have a dental examination and any necessary dental work.

Nutrition

Prior to conception it is advisable for the woman to be at a suitable weight for her body build and height. She should follow a nutritious diet that contains ample quantities of all the essential nutrients. Some nutritionists advocate emphasizing the following nutrients: calcium, protein, iron, B complex vitamins, vitamin C, folic acid, and magnesium.

Exercise

A woman is advised to establish a regular exercise plan beginning at least three months before she plans to attempt to become pregnant. The exercise chosen should be one she enjoys and will continue. It should provide some aerobic conditioning and some general toning. Exercise improves the woman's circulation and general health and tones her muscles. Once an exercise program is well-established, the woman is generally encouraged to continue it during pregnancy. For a discussion of exercise during pregnancy see p 388.

Contraception

Women who wish to conceive and who take birth control pills are advised to stop the pill two to three months before attempting to get pregnant. Women with IUDs are advised to have them removed three months before attempting to conceive. During the three months, barrier methods of contraception (condom or diaphragm) are acceptable. Currently some clinicians are questioning the necessity of delaying pregnancy. They suggest that if pregnancy occurs before the woman has a menstrual period, the gestation of the pregnancy can be determined with ultrasound.

Conception

Most preconception recommendations focus on helping the couple attain their best possible health state so that they do not enter pregnancy with unnecessary risks. Conception is a personal and emotional experience, and even if a couple is prepared they may feel some ambivalence. This is a normal response, but they may require reassurance that the ambivalence will pass. A couple may get so caught up in preparation and in their efforts to "do things right" that they lose sight of the pleasure they derive from each other and their lives together, and cease to value the joy of spontaneity in their relationship. It is often helpful for the health care provider to remind an overly zealous couple that moderation is always appropriate and that there is value in taking "time to smell the roses."

● Reproductive Choices (Contraception)

A couple's decision to use a method of contraception is often motivated by a desire to gain control over the number of children they will conceive and/or to determine the spacing of future children. In choosing a specific method, consistency of use outweighs the absolute reliability of a given method. Other factors to be considered are the side effects and contraindications for use of a particular contraceptive method.

The nurse often assists the couple in selecting a contraceptive method. To be able to suggest a method that has practical application and is compatible with the couple's health and physical needs, the nurse must assess the couple to gather relevant data. The woman's past medical, surgical, menstrual, and obstetrical history, including former contraceptive use, should be reviewed. The history should include immediate family incidences of diabetes, bleeding or clotting problems, heart problems or high blood pressure, migraine headaches or seizure disorders, kidney or liver disease, anemia, tuberculosis, stroke, cancer, or mental problems. This information provides a baseline of risk factors that could influence or contraindicate the prescription of oral contraceptives.

A precontraception physical examination should include, at a minimum, breast and pelvic examinations. Weight, age, and blood pressure can indicate risk factors that may preclude prescribing certain forms of birth control. Minimal laboratory testing is necessary. This includes a hemoglobin/hematocrit analysis; urinalysis for sugar and protein; Pap smear; endocervical culture for *Neisseria gonorrhoeae;* serologic test for syphilis; and any other test identified during the history or physical as being appropriate. For women who are resuming contraception postpartally, the laboratory data obtained during pregnancy may be used.

The couple's decisions about contraception should be made voluntarily, with full knowledge of options, advantages, disadvantages, effectiveness, side effects, and long-range effects; with access to alternatives; without pressure by health professionals; and with the strictest confidentiality. Many outside factors influence a couple's choice, including cultural influences, religious beliefs, personality, cost, effectiveness, misinformation, practicability of method, and self-esteem. Different methods of contraception may be appropriate at different times in a couple's life.

Following is a review of the major contraceptive methods available, with an examination of their advantages and disadvantages. Table 8–3 identifies first-year failure rates for the various birth control methods.

Fertility Awareness Methods

Increasing numbers of couples are becoming interested in methods of contraception that do not use artificial devices or substances. These methods have been called "natural family-planning" or fertility awareness methods. Periodic abstinence from sexual intercourse is a requirement of all methods, as is the recording of certain events during the menstrual cycle; hence cooperation of the partner is important. Advantages of the natural methods include an increased awareness of one's body and avoidance of artificial substances. These methods are not as predictable to use during lactation, however, since menses may be suppressed and ovulation erratic.

The *basal body temperature (BBT) method* to detect ovulation requires that the woman take her BBT every morning and record the readings on a temperature graph. The completed graph then provides data to identify the safe and unsafe periods of the menstrual cycle. Intercourse is avoided on the day of temperature rise and for the following three days. Not all temperature curves are interpretable, however, so many abstain from intercourse for an extended period of time, between days 12 and 18 in a cycle, to ensure safety.

The *calendar rhythm method* first requires the recording of each menstrual cycle for at least six months so that the shortest and longest cycles can be identified. The first day of menstruation is the first day of the cycle. The fertile phase is calculated from 18 days before the end of the shortest recorded cycle through 11 days from the end of the longest recorded cycle (Hatcher et al 1986). For example, if a woman's cycle lasts from 24 to 28 days, the fertile phase would be calculated as days 6 through 17. Once this information is obtained, the woman can identify the fertile and infertile phases of her cycle. For effective use of the method, she must abstain from intercourse during the fertile phase.

Rhythm is a variation of the calendar rhythm method previously discussed. It is based on identification of the "unsafe period" of a menstrual cycle, which is a period of time immediately before and after ovulation. Theoretically, conception may occur on only three days in each cycle, but women who have irregular cycles find it difficult to pinpoint the time of ovulation. The irregularity of menses during the postpartum period and lactation obviously limits the effectiveness of this method of contraception.

The *ovulation method,* sometimes called the *Billings method,* involves the assessment of cervical mucus changes that occur during the menstrual cycle. The amount and character of cervical mucus change as a result of the in-

Table 8–3 First-Year Failure Rates of Birth Control Methods

Method	Lowest observed failure rate* (%)	Failure rate in typical users† (%)
Tubal sterilization	0.4	0.4
Vasectomy	0.4	0.4
Injectable progestin	0.25	0.25
Combined birth control pills	0.5	2
Progestin-only pill	1	2.5
IUD	1.5	5
Condom	2	10
Diaphragm (with spermicide)	2	19
Sponge (with spermicide)	9–11	10–20
Cervical cap	2	13
Foams, creams, jellies, and vaginal suppositories	3–5	18
Coitus interruptus	16	23
Fertility awareness techniques (basal body temperature, mucus method, calendar, and "rhythm")	2–20	24
Douche	—	40
Chance (no method of birth control)	90	90

*Designed to complete the sentence: "In 100 users who start out the year using a given method and who use it correctly and consistently, the lowest observed failure rate has been _____."
†Designed to complete the sentence: "In 100 typical users who start out the year using a given method, the number of pregnancies by the end of the year will be _____."

Source: Hatcher RA, et al: *Contraceptive Technology 1986–1987,* ed 13. New York, Irvington Publishers, 1986, p 102.

fluence of estrogen (type E mucus) and progesterone (type G mucus) on the mucous secretory units present in the cervix.

At ovulation, type E mucus is greatest in amount and stretchability. The woman notices a feeling of wetness around the vagina. This mucus shows a fern pattern that becomes apparent when the mucus is placed on a glass slide and allowed to dry (see Figure 9–4). The stretchability (spinnbarkheit) of the cervical mucus is greatest at the time of ovulation and may vary from 5 to 20 cm. Type E mucus allows increased permeability to sperm.

During the luteal phase, the characteristics of the cervical mucus change. This type G mucus becomes thick and sticky and forms a network in the cervical canal that traps the sperm and makes their passage more difficult.

To use the ovulation method, the woman should abstain from intercourse for the first menstrual cycle. Cervical mucus should be assessed on a daily basis for the woman to become more familiar with varying characteristics. After a pattern has been established, abstinence from intercourse is necessary when type E mucus predominates and for four days following ovulation.

The *symptothermal method* consists of various assessments that are made and recorded by the couple. They use a chart to record information regarding cycle days, coitus, cervical mucus changes, and secondary signs such as increased libido, abdominal bloating, mittelschmerz, and

basal body temperature. Through the various assessments, the couple learns to recognize signs that indicate ovulation. This combined approach tends to improve the effectiveness of fertility awareness contraception methods.

Situational contraceptives also fall under the heading of natural family planning. These methods involve no prior preparation of the couple but involve motivation to abstain from intercourse or to interrupt the sexual act prior to the ejaculation of the sperm into the vagina. *Coitus interruptus,* or withdrawal, is the oldest method of contraception but has limited effectiveness as a birth preventive.

Douching after intercourse is an ineffective method of contraception. It may actually facilitate conception by pushing the sperm farther up the birth canal. Furthermore, sperm have been identified in the fallopian tubes as soon as 90 seconds after ejaculation.

Mechanical Contraceptives

Mechanical contraceptive methods act either as barriers preventing the transport of sperm to the ovum or by preventing implantation of the ovum/zygote.

CONDOM

Condoms offer a viable means of contraception when used consistently and properly (Figure 8–2). Acceptance has been increasing as a growing number of men are assuming responsibility for regulation of fertility. Another reason for the increased use of condoms is the protection they afford against sexually transmitted diseases, especially AIDS. Condoms are applied to the erect penis, rolled from the tip to the end of the shaft, before vulvar or vaginal contact is made. A small space must be left at the end of the condom to allow for collection of the ejaculate so that the condom will not break at the time of ejaculation. Vaginal jelly should be used if the condom and/or vagina are dry to prevent irritation and possible condom breakage. For optimum effectiveness, the penis should be withdrawn from the vagina while still erect and the condom rim held to prevent spillage. If after ejaculation the penis becomes flaccid while still in the vagina, the male should hold onto the edge of the condom while withdrawing from the vagina to avoid spilling the semen and to prevent the condom from slipping off. The effectiveness of condoms is largely determined by their use. The condom is small, lightweight, disposable, and inexpensive; has no side effects; requires no medical examination or supervision; offers visual evidence of effectiveness; and protects against sexually transmitted diseases. Breakage, displacement, possible perineal or vaginal irritation, and dulled sensation are cited as disadvantages.

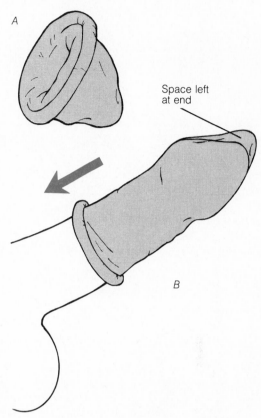

Space left at end

Figure 8–2   A Condom, B Condom applied to penis. Note space left at end to allow collection of ejaculate.

Research Note

Ewald and Roberts used Fishbein's belief-attitude-intention-behavior model to investigate the contraceptive behavior of 54 sexually active college men. The model argues that behavior is based on intention, that intention is based on attitudes, and that attitudes are based on beliefs.

Responses to the 51-item questionnaire confirmed that for these men beliefs about condoms were associated with attitudes about condom use, attitudes were associated with the intention of these men to use condoms in the coming month, and that intention to use in the coming month was associated with actual use in the past month. The results suggest that recent past behavior and immediate future behavior are highly correlated with condom use.

Nursing interventions are usually directed at altering health-related behaviors. This study indicates that the logical point of intervention to alter contraceptive use in college-aged men is at the level of belief rather than behavior. The nurse could expect that a change in beliefs about condom use would change attitudes, intentions, and behaviors in the same direction.

Ewald, BM, Roberts CS: Contraceptive behavior in college-age males related to Fishbein model. Adv Nurs Sci 1985:7(April):63.

DIAPHRAGM

The *diaphragm* (Figure 8–3) offers a good level of protection from conception when used with spermicidal creams or jellies. The woman must be fitted with a diaphragm and instructions given by trained personnel. The diaphragm should be rechecked for correct size after each childbirth and if a woman has gained or lost 15 pounds or more.

The diaphragm must be inserted before intercourse, with approximately 1 teaspoonful (or 1½ inches from the tube) of spermicidal jelly placed around its rim and in the cup. This serves as a chemical barrier to supplement the mechanical barrier of the diaphragm. The diaphragm is inserted through the vagina and covers the cervix. The last step in insertion is to push the edge of the diaphragm under the symphysis pubis, which may result in a "popping" sensation. When fitted properly and correctly in place, the diaphragm should not cause discomfort to the wearer or her partner. Correct placement of the diaphragm can be checked by touching the cervix with a fingertip through the cup. The cervix feels like a small rounded structure and has a consistency similar to that of the tip of the nose. The center of the diaphragm should be over the cervix. Women who have chronic urinary tract infec-

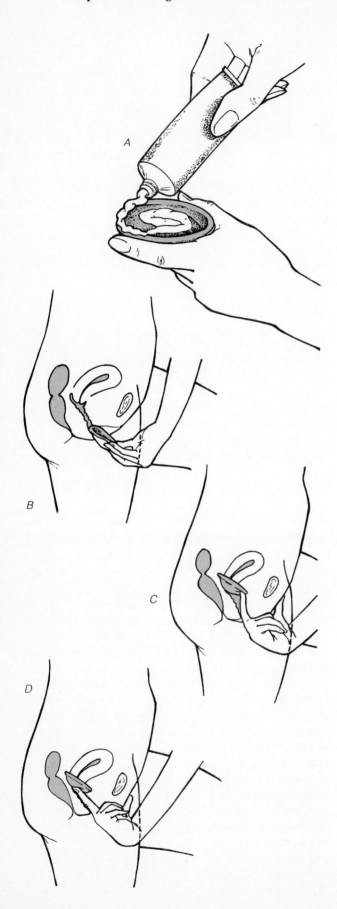

tions should not use the diaphragm. Those who object to manipulation of the genitals for insertion, determination of correct placement, and removal may find this method offensive. If more than four hours elapse between insertion of the diaphragm and intercourse, additional spermicidal cream should be used. It is necessary to leave the diaphragm in for six hours after coitus. Some couples feel that the use of a diaphragm interferes with the spontaneity of intercourse. To overcome this idea, it can be suggested that the partner insert the diaphragm as part of foreplay. If intercourse is again desired within the next six hours, another type of contraception must be used or additional spermicidal jelly placed in the vagina with an applicator, taking care not to disturb the placement of the diaphragm. The diaphragm should be periodically held up to a light and inspected for tears or holes.

Diaphragms are an excellent contraceptive means for women who are lactating, who cannot or do not wish to use the pill (hormonal contraceptives), or who wish to avoid exposure to the increased risk of pelvic inflammatory disease associated with intrauterine devices.

CERVICAL CAP

The *cervical cap* is a cup-shaped "diaphragm" that stays in place over the cervix by suction. The degree of suction depends on the tightness of the fit between the cap and the cervix. Since pregnancies have occurred without cap displacement, spermicidal jelly should be used in the cap. It can remain in place for one or more days. In March 1988, the FDA approved the use of cervical caps.

Intracervical devices made of either plastic or metal are under current investigation. Expulsion rates are unacceptable, but new models offer promise.

CONTRACEPTIVE SPONGE

Contraceptive sponges were approved by the FDA for use in 1983. The contraceptive sponge, available without prescription, is a small pillow-shaped polyurethane sponge with a concave cupped area on one side designed to fit over the cervix (Figure 8–4). The sponge currently available, Today® Vaginal Contraceptive Sponge, contains spermicide. Although the sponge is slightly less effective than the diaphragm, it is easier to use (Rosenfield 1985). It has been shown to be slightly less effective with multiparas, presumably due to the relaxation of vaginal walls. The sponge is moistened with water prior to use and inserted into the vagina so that the cupped area fits snugly over the cervical os. This decreases the chance of the sponge dis-

Figure 8–3 A Applying jelly to the rim and center of the diaphragm. B Inserting the diaphragm. C Pushing the rim of the diaphragm under the symphysis pubis. D Checking placement of the diaphragm. Cervix should be felt through the diaphragm.

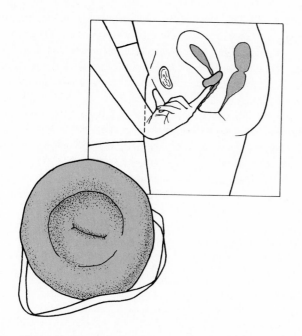

Figure 8–4   Contraceptive sponge is moistened with water and inserted into the vagina with concave portion over the cervix

lodging during intercourse. It should be left in place for six hours after coitus.

Advantages of the sponge are: Professional fitting is not required as for the diaphragm; it may be used for multiple coitus up to 24 hours unlike the single-use condom; one size fits all; and it is both barrier and spermicide. Problems associated with sponge use include difficulty in removing the sponge, cost (approximately one dollar per sponge), and irritation or allergic reactions. Some women also report that vaginal dryness is sometimes a problem because the sponge absorbs vaginal secretions. Research suggests that women who use the sponge on nonmenstrual days have a slightly increased risk of developing toxic shock syndrome (Faich et al 1986). Women with a history of toxic shock syndrome should not use vaginal sponges (Hatcher et al 1986).

INTRAUTERINE DEVICE

Intrauterine devices (IUDs) come in many types and shapes, but primarily work by producing a local reaction in the endometrium. It is generally accepted that the IUD produces a local, sterile inflammatory reaction. The inflammatory reaction increases the number of uterine leukocytes whose tissue breakdown products are toxic to the sperm and the blastocyst. Implantation is inhibited if fertilization occurs.

Possible adverse reactions to the IUD include discomfort to the wearer, increased bleeding during menses, pelvic inflammatory disease, perforation of the uterus, intermenstrual bleeding, dysmenorrhea, expulsion of the de-

vice, and ectopic pregnancy. Advantages include convenience, no coitus-related activity, and duration of effectiveness.

The Progestasert was the only IUD on the market in 1987, but the Copper T 380A is due out in late 1988.

Oral Contraceptives

The use of hormones, specifically the combination of estrogen and progesterone, succeeds as a birth control method by inhibiting the release of an ovum and by maintaining type G mucus, which interferes with the passage of sperm through the cervix.

Numerous oral contraceptives are available. The dosage regime consists of taking one pill daily for 21 days beginning on the Sunday after the first day of the menstrual cycle. In most cases menstrual bleeding will occur one to four days after the last tablet. Some pharmaceutical companies have added seven "blank" tablets so the woman can continue to take one tablet daily. With the 21-day package, the woman goes off the pill for 7 days and restarts the pill on the following Sunday. The pill should be taken at the same time each day for optimum effectiveness. The oral contraceptives recommended for general use are low-dose (35 mcg or less) estrogen preparations. Progesterone preparation and dosage varies according to the specific pill used.

Although they are highly effective, oral contraceptives may produce side effects ranging from breakthrough bleeding to thrombus formation. Side effects from oral contraceptives may be either progesterone- or estrogen-related (Table 8–4). Regulation of dosages has reduced many of the side effects, but the threat of potential risk is sufficient to deter some women from using oral contraceptives.

Another oral contraceptive is the seldom-used progesterone-only pill, also called the *minipill*. It is used primarily with women who have a contraindication to the estrogen component of the combination preparation, such as history of thrombophlebitis, but are strongly motivated toward this form of contraception. The major problems with this preparation are amenorrhea or irregular spotting and bleeding patterns.

Contraindications to the use of oral contraceptives include pregnancy, previous history of thrombophlebitis or thrombolic disease, acute or chronic liver disease of cholestatic type with abnormal function, presence of estrogen-dependent carcinomas, undiagnosed uterine bleeding, heavy smoking, hypertension, diabetes, toxemia, age over 40, lack of regular menstrual cycles for at least one to two years in adolescents, and hyperlipoproteinemia. In addition, women with the following conditions who use oral contraceptives should be examined every three months: migraine headaches, epilepsy, depression, oligomenorrhea, and amenorrhea. Women who choose this method of contraception should be fully advised of potential side effects. See Table 8–4 for side effects of oral contraceptives.

A once-a-month oral contraceptive (RU 486) is in early clinical trials. It is an antiprogestin that binds to the progesterone receptors in the endometrium and blocks the action of progesterone. This drug represents a prototype of a new class of compounds for fertility control (Spitz & Bardin 1985). Many issues need to be resolved and large randomized trials conducted before this drug can be made available for general use.

Injectable and Sustained-Release Contraceptives

Two injectable steroid contraceptives are available and marketed in other areas of the world at present. Depomedroxyprogesterone acetate (Depo-Provera) is a microcrystalline suspension of progestins, and Norethindrone enanthate (Noristat) is an oily suspension with a shorter duration than Depo-Provera. Depo-Provera is a controversial contraceptive in the United States. The FDA had recommended its approval for women who could not use other forms of contraception, but withdrew the approval, pending further review, in response to consumer group pressures. It has been approved in more than 80 countries around the world. It is the most effective reversible form of contraception currently available (Rosenfield 1985). Since it is given as an injection once every three months, the practical and theoretical effectiveness are equal. The most pressing concerns are reversibility and safety. It may take the woman longer to conceive after use, and breast cancer has been found in laboratory animals given the drug.

Steroid implants are biodegradable rods or microcapsules containing a sustained-release, low-dose progesterone. If they are approved for use, the safety of the currently available injectable forms of contraception will be a moot question. The drugs inhibit secretion of gonadotropins, including midcycle LH release.

Vaginal and cervical devices are being considered for the sustained release of combined steroids or progesterone. Vaginal rings containing contraceptive substances are as effective as oral contraceptives but retention, comfort, bleeding, and irritation present problems. Prolonged amenorrhea or increased uterine bleeding or both have occurred during and after steroid contraceptive use, and thromboembolism has also been noted (Schwallie 1974). Clinical trials with several different agents are currently underway (Darney 1984). The effectiveness will not change remarkably, but they could be less irritating to the tissues.

Spermicides

A variety of creams, jellies, foams, and suppositories, inserted into the vagina prior to intercourse, destroy sperm or neutralize vaginal secretions and thereby immobilize sperm. Spermicides that effervesce in a moist environment

offer more rapid protection and coitus may take place immediately after they are inserted. Suppositories may require up to 30 minutes to dissolve and will *not* offer protection until they do so. The woman should be instructed to insert these spermicide preparations high in the vagina and maintain a supine position.

Spermicides are minimally effective when used alone, but their effectiveness increases in conjunction with a diaphragm or condom. They provide a high degree of protection from exposure to gonorrhea, and are also useful against chlamydia, trichomonas, and herpes organisms (Hatcher et al 1986). Recently a civil suit was decided in favor of a woman who contended that spermicide use around the time of conception contributed to the development of the congenital anomalies with which her infant was born. It is not yet apparent what this finding will mean with regard to the availability of spermicides.

Male Contraception

The vasectomy and condom are currently the only forms of male contraception available in the United States. Hormonal contraception for men remains a perplexing problem. Numerous investigations are underway. Antagonists to gonadotropin-releasing hormone (GnRH), which stimulates the pituitary release of LH and FSH, work by preventing the LH and FSH surges necessary for spermatogenesis. These substances have been shown to cause a 50 percent drop in hormone levels but not completely stop sperm production (Darney 1984).

Long-acting androgen-progestin combinations may stop sperm production but none have proved reliable to date. The most promising, inhibin, is a hormone found naturally in the semen. It inhibits FSH release.

Gossypol, a cottonseed derivative first developed in China, is being evaluated in the United States. Its effectiveness, side effects, reversibility, method of action, and carcinogenicity are being assessed.

Operative Sterilization

Before sterilization is performed on either partner, a thorough explanation of the procedure should be given to both. Each should understand that sterilization is not a decision to be taken lightly or entered into when psychologic stresses, such as separation or divorce, exist. Even though male and female procedures are theoretically reversible, the permanency of the procedure should be stressed and understood. All forms of reversible contraception should be explained and discussed in detail to assist the client in making an informed decision.

Male sterilization is achieved by a relatively minor procedure called a *vasectomy*. Under local anesthesia, a 2 to 3 cm incision is made over the vas deferens on each side of the scrotum. The ducts are isolated; severed; and

Table 8–4 Side Effects of Oral Contraceptives

Estrogen Component	Progestin Component
Altered carbohydrate metabolism	Acne
Altered clotting factors—thrombophlebitis	Amenorrhea
Altered convulsive threshold	Anabolic weight gain
Altered lipid metabolism	Breast regression
Breast tenderness or engorgement	Depression and altered libido
Chloasma	Fatigue
Edema and cyclic weight gain	Hirsutism
Excessive menstrual flow	Increased appetite
Headache	Loss of hair
Hypertension	Moniliasis
Irritability, nervousness	Oligomenorrhea
Leukorrhea, cervical erosion, or polyposis	
Nausea, bloating	
Venous or capillary engorgement (spider nevi)	

occluded by ligation of the ends, by coagulation of the lumen, by burial of the cut ends, or by use of clips or polyethylene tubing with a stopcock for potentially reversible procedures. Absorbable sutures are used to close the skin. The man is instructed to apply ice when pain or swelling occurs and to use a scrotal support for a week. It takes about 4 to 6 weeks and 6 to 36 ejaculations to clear remaining sperm from the vas deferens. During that period, the couple is advised to use another method of birth control and to bring in two or three sperm samples for a sperm count. The man is rechecked at 6 and 12 months to ensure that fertility has not been restored by recanalization. Side effects of a vasectomy include hematoma, sperm granulomas, and spontaneous reanastomosis.

Vasectomies can be reversed with the use of microsurgery techniques, but fertility is restored in only about 18 percent to 60 percent of cases (Hatcher et al 1986).

Female sterilization (tubal ligation) can be accomplished by several abdominal and vaginal procedures. The fallopian tubes are transected or occluded by electrocautery. The postpartal laparotomy is done 1 to 3 days after delivery, under general anesthesia and usually with a small subumbilical incision. The tubes are isolated and may then be crushed, ligated, electrocoagulated, banded, or plugged (in the newer reversible procedures). The interval minilaparotomy uses a suprapubic incision with similar techniques for interrupting tubal patency.

Laparoscopic sterilization may be done at any time. One or two incisions are made in the subumbilical area. The abdomen is distended with carbon dioxide gas, the laparoscope is introduced through a trocar, and the fallopian tube is visualized. The isthmic portion of the tube is grasped and coagulated and may be transected. The procedure is repeated on the other tube.

Complications of female sterilization procedures include coagulation burns on the bowels, bowel perforation, infection, hemorrhage, and adverse anesthesia effects. Reversal of a tubal ligation depends on many factors, including the portion of the tube excised, the presence or absence of the fimbriae, and the length of the tube remaining. With microsurgical techniques, a pregnancy rate of approximately 70 percent is possible (Siber & Cohen 1980).

No reversible form of sterilization holds promise of widespread use at the present time. However, a reversible form of sterilization is currently being investigated. It incorporates the use of a hysteroscope for direct visualization of the tubal openings into the uterus. The openings are injected with a silicone substance that hardens and occludes the cornual section of the fallopian tube. Hysterosalpingography confirms the success of the procedure and a thread is left in the uterine cavity for future removal.

I think I'm like a lot of women. During my life I've used a variety of contraceptive methods. I took the pill back when the doses were higher, I used foam alone and had a baby, then used spermicidal cream and condoms more successfully. I never wanted a tubal and my husband refuses to consider vasectomy, so the IUD was a perfect alternative. I'm 41 and I like something I don't have to think about every time we want to make love. This is my second Copper 7, but it's been in three years and now it's no longer available. I hear that a new copper IUD is coming out. I hope so. Women my age need choices, too. Why, with all the technological advances around, can't someone come up with safe, convenient, and effective methods for women like me? I feel frustrated and angry every time I think about it.

The Role of the Nurse

In most cases the nurse who provides information and guidance about contraceptive methods works with a woman because most contraceptive methods are female oriented. Since a man can purchase condoms without seeing a health care provider, only in the case of vasectomy does a man require counseling and interaction with a nurse. The nurse can play an important role in helping a woman choose a method of contraception that is acceptable to her and to her partner.

In addition to the assessments described on page 161, the nurse can spend time with the woman learning about her life-style, personal attitudes about particular contraceptive methods, and plans for future childbearing. If a woman has multiple sexual partners and a high rate of sexual activity, for example, a spermicide alone offers only limited protection against pregnancy, while an IUD greatly increases her chances of developing pelvic inflammatory disease. Birth control pills may provide the greatest protection for this woman if future childbearing ability is important to her. The woman who has just stopped taking oral contraceptives in order to become pregnant can use spermicides and condoms effectively for a few months to allow her body to return to its prepill state.

Religious beliefs are an important issue in selecting a method of fertility control, and the nurse counseling women about contraception should be sensitive to its importance. Some women accept only fertility awareness methods of contraception. The nurse working with these women can help by providing them with the information and support they need to follow this method effectively.

Personal bias also plays a role in selection of method. Some women are reluctant to take birth control pills because they fear the associated risk factors. If the woman remains fearful even after careful explanation and reassurance that the risks of the pill are limited in women who are good candidates for the pill, the nurse should recommend another method. By the same token, if a woman is uncomfortable with touching her genitals and thus finds the diaphragm distasteful, she should choose another method.

Personal bias can also influence the nurse unless care is taken. Nurses tend to recommend the methods they prefer and have confidence in. While this is understandable, it could also interfere with the effectiveness of the counseling the nurse provides. It is important for nurses to examine their own feelings, attitudes, and biases about contraceptive choices.

Once a method is chosen, the nurse can help the woman learn to use it effectively. Often it is the nurse who is available to answer questions about a particular method. For example a woman might ask:

What do I do if I get sick and have problems with diarrhea for several days when taking the pill?

What if I am using a diaphragm, and we want to make love a second time?

In the first case the nurse would advise the woman to continue taking the pills but use a backup method of contraception for the remainder of the cycle. In the second situation the nurse would advise the woman to leave the diaphragm in place but insert an applicatorfull of spermicide cream or jelly prior to a second episode of intercourse.

If a woman is considering a tubal ligation or her partner is considering a vasectomy, careful preoperative preparation and explanation is essential. The couple should clearly understand the risks and the surgical techniques used and should accept the idea that the method is essentially irreversible. Although the physician does much of the counseling for these procedures, nurses are often responsible for reinforcing the information and for answering questions.

The nurse also reviews any possible side effects and warning signs of the method chosen and counsels the woman about what action to take if she suspects she is pregnant. In many cases the nurse may become involved in telephone counseling for women who call with questions and concerns. Thus, it is vital that the nurse be knowledgeable about this topic and have resources available to find answers to less-common questions.

KEY CONCEPTS

Sexual development begins at conception. The development of sexuality continues throughout an individual's lifetime.

Attitudes about sex are influenced by a variety of factors including: family and home environment, culture, education, socioeconomic level, previous sexual experiences, and individual personality characteristics.

People obtain sexual satisfaction in a variety of ways, not only through sexual intercourse.

Masters and Johnson (1966) have identified four phases to the human sexual response cycle: excitement, plateau, orgasm, and resolution.

Nurses in maternity and women's health settings may become involved in counseling about sexual issues.

To be effective as a counselor on sexual matters nurses must be aware of and comfortable with their feelings and attitudes; have accurate, up-to-date knowledge; and be skilled in communicating.

The nursing process can be used effectively when working with women concerned about sexual issues. The nurse must be insightful enough to recognize those occasions when a woman's problem requires more specialized intervention so that appropriate referral can be made.

Preconception counseling focuses on the decision to have children (if this decision is morally acceptable to the couple). It also includes counseling about health measures, physical examination, nutrition, exercise, and contraception.

Contraception is used by couples to decide when to have children and to help with the spacing of children.

Fertility awareness methods are "natural," noninvasive methods often used by people whose religious beliefs keep them from using other methods of contraception.

Mechanical contraceptives such as the diaphragm, cervical cap, contraceptive sponge, and condom act as barriers to prevent the transport of sperm. These methods are used in conjunction with a spermicide.

The IUD is another mechanical contraceptive that works primarily by preventing the implantation of a fertilized ovum.

Oral contraceptives (the "pill") are combinations of estrogen and progesterone. When taken correctly they are the most effective of the reversible methods of fertility control.

Spermicides are far less effective in preventing pregnancy when they are not used with a barrier method.

A variety of experimental approaches to contraception are currently being tested.

Permanent sterilization is accomplished by tubal ligation for women and vasectomy for men. Clients are advised that the method should be considered irreversible.

REFERENCES

Calderone MS: Fetal erection and its message to us. *SIECUS Rep,* May–July, 1983.

Darney PD: What's new in contraception? *Contemp OB/GYN* 1984;23(6):117.

Faich G, et al: Toxic shock syndrome and the vaginal contraceptive sponge. *JAMA* 1986;225:216.

Fromer MJ: *Ethical Issues in Sexuality and Reproduction.* St. Louis: Mosby, 1983.

Hatcher RA, et al: *Contraceptive Technology 1986–1987,* ed 13. New York, Irvington Publishers, 1986.

Hogan RM: *Human Sexuality.* New York, Appleton-Century-Crofts, 1980.

Masters WH, **Johnson** VE: *Human Sexual Response.* Boston, Little, Brown, 1966.

Rosenfield AG: Contraception: Where are we in 1985? *Contemp OB/GYN* 1985;25(2):79.

Schwallie PC: Experience with Depo-Provera as an injectable contraceptive. *J Reprod Med* 1974;13:113.

Siber SJ, **Cohen** R: Microsurgical reversal of female sterilization: Role of tubal length. *Fertil Steril* 1980;33(6):598.

Spitz IM, **Bardin** CW: Antiprogestins: Prospects for a once-a-month pill. *Fam Plan Perspect* 1985;17(6):260.

Thiederman SB: Ethnocentrism: A barrier to effective health care. *Nurse Prac* 1986;11(August):52.

ADDITIONAL READINGS

Alzate H, **Hoch** Z: The "G spot" and "female ejaculation": A current appraisal. *J Sex Marital Ther* 1986;12(Fall):211.

Combination oral contraceptive use and the risk of endometrial cancer. *JAMA* 1987;257(6):796.

Crooks R, **Baur** K: *Our Sexuality.* Menlo Park, Calif, Benjamin/Cummings, 1987.

Eisen M, et al: The role of health belief attitudes, sex education, and demographics in predicting adolescents' sexuality knowledge. *Health Educ Q* 1986;13(Spring):9.

Ford K, et al: Contraceptive usage during lactation in the United States: An update. *Am J Pub Health* 1987;77(1):79.

Greener D, et al: Sexuality: Knowledge and attitudes of student nurse-midwives. *J Nurse Midwife* 1986;31(January/February):30.

Howe CL: Developmental theory and adolescent sexual behavior. *Nurse Pract* 1986;11(February):65.

Kurtzman C, **Block** DE: Family planning: Beyond contraception. *MCN* 1986;11(September/October):340.

Rosenbaum J, et al: A sexuality workshop: Increasing sexual self-awareness. *Can J Psychiatr Nurs* 1986;27(April):8.

Schaninger MC, **Buss** WC: The relationship of sex-role norms to couple and parental demographics. *Sex Roles* 1986;15(July):77.

Schinfeld JS: Does exercise affect sexuality? *Contemp OB/GYN* 1986;28(August):63.

Speroff L: Which birth control pill should be prescribed? *Contemp OB/GYN* 1987;29(3):102.

The aftermath of love . . . injuries associated with sexual behavior. *Emerg Med* 1987;19(1):24.

White JH, et al: Femininity, image, feminism and a decision to seek treatment in obese women. *Health Care Women Int* 1986;7(6):455.

Youngkin EQ, et al: The triphasics: Insights for effective clinical use. *Nurse Pract* 1987;12(2):17.

Zimmet JA, et al: An historical look at a contemporary question: The cervical cap. *Health Educ* 1986;17(5):53.

I've never thought about a baby before. In fact, now I find myself thinking of nursing a child or holding one, or even looking at them. I hated babysitting. I . . . never took that much notice. I'm real excited. But its taken me months to really feel good about it, really positive about it. (Lederman, Psychosocial Adaptation to Pregnancy)

Special Reproductive Concerns

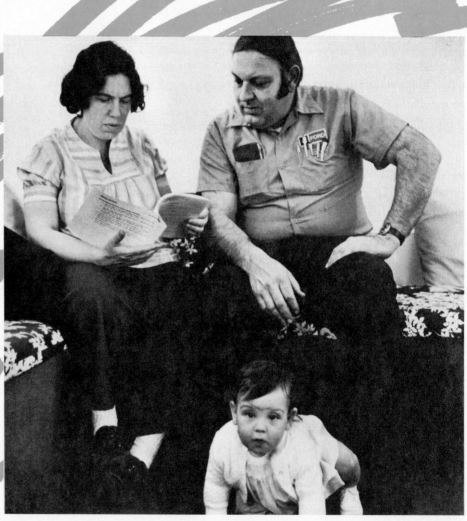

A nurse must be sensitive to the unspoken fears of parents asked to
assimilate complex information.

Chapter Nine

OBJECTIVES

- Summarize the physiologic and psychologic effects of infertility on a couple.
- Identify the various tests done in an infertility workup.
- Discuss the indications for chromosomal analysis and genetic amniocentesis.
- Relate the significance of the Barr chromatin body to identifying sex chromosome abnormalities.
- Identify the general characteristics of an autosomal dominant disorder.
- Compare autosomal recessive disorders with X-linked (sex-linked) recessive disorders.
- Compare prenatal and postnatal diagnostic procedures that may be used to determine the presence of genetic disease.
- Explore the emotional impact on a couple undergoing genetic testing and/or the birth of a baby with a genetic disorder.
- Explain the nurse's responsibility in genetic counseling.

Most couples who want children are able to have them with little trouble. Pregnancy and childbirth usually take their normal course, and a healthy baby is born. But some couples are not so fortunate and are unable to fulfill their dream of having a healthy baby because of special reproductive problems.

This chapter explores two particularly troubling reproductive problems facing some couples: the inability to conceive and the risk of bearing babies with genetic abnormalities.

Infertility

Infertility can be defined as the inability of a couple to produce a living child as a result of failure to conceive or of failure to carry the conceived baby to a viable state. It has been estimated that in the United States there are at least 2.8 million infertile couples who want to have children (Mosher 1983).

Primary infertility indicates those women who have never conceived, whereas secondary infertility identifies the woman who has formerly been pregnant but has not conceived during one or more years of unprotected intercourse (Coulam 1982). *Sterility* is a term applied when there is an absolute factor preventing reproduction. The incidence of infertility appears to be increasing, which may be related to the trend toward delaying marriage and postponing childbearing until the couple has passed the age of optimal fertility. Other factors in infertility include increased risk of prolonged anovulation following the use of birth control pills, infections associated with abortions or use of intrauterine devices, and obstructive diseases of the female and male reproductive systems caused by the current epidemic of sexually transmitted diseases.

Essential Components of Fertility

Understanding the elements essential for normal fertility can help the nurse identify the many factors that may cause infertility. The following essential components must be present for normal fertility:

Female partner:

1. The vaginal secretions and cervical mucus must be favorable for survival of spermatozoa.

2. There must be clear passage between the cervix and the fallopian tubes.

3. Fallopian tubes must be patent and have normal peristaltic movement to allow ascent of spermatozoa and descent of ovum.

4. Ovaries must produce and release normal ova.

5. There must be no obstruction between the ovaries and the uterus.

6. The endometrium must be in a normal physiologic state to allow implantation of the blastocyst and to sustain normal growth.

Male partner:

1. The testes must produce spermatozoa of normal quality and quantity.

2. The male genital tract must not be obstructed.

3. The male genital tract secretions must be normal.

171

4. Ejaculated spermatozoa must be deposited in the female genital tract in such a manner that they reach the cervix.

These normal findings are correlated with possible causes of deviation in Table 9–1. In addition to these necessary elements, certain general physiologic and psychologic conditions must be present to support conception.

With intricacies of timing and environment playing such a crucial role, it is an impressive natural phenomenon that approximately 85 percent of couples in the United States are able to conceive (Templeton & Penney 1982, Andrew 1984). Of the remaining 15 percent, for every 100 couples about 40 will show a male deficiency, 10 to 15 a female hormonal defect, 20 to 30 a female tubal disorder, 5 a cervical defect, and 10 to 20 couples have no discernible cause of their infertility (Coulam 1982). In 35 of the couples there are multiple etiologies. Professional intervention can help 30 percent to 50 percent of infertile couples achieve pregnancy.

Couples are usually concerned about infertility following their inability to conceive after at least one year of attempting to achieve pregnancy. At the age of 25 years, which is identified as the couple's most fertile time, the average length of time needed to achieve conception is 5.3 months. The average 20- to 30-year-old American couple has intercourse one to three times a week, a frequency that should be sufficient to achieve pregnancy if all other factors are satisfactory. In about 20 percent of cases, conception occurs within the first month of unprotected intercourse (Zacur & Rock 1983). Between 1975 and 1980 there was a 94 percent increase in the number of women who gave birth to their first child after the age of 30, and this trend is predicted to increase. Delaying parenthood appears to increase the risk to the success of each of the physiologic processes necessary for conception (Berg 1984).

Preliminary Investigation

Evaluation and preliminary investigation should be available for couples seeking help for infertility. The easiest and least intrusive approach is used first. Extensive testing is avoided until data confirm that the timing of intercourse and the length of coital exposure have been adequate. The couple should be informed of the appropriate times to have intercourse during the menstrual cycle. Teaching the couple the signs of and timing of ovulation within the cycle and effective sexual techniques may solve the problem before extensive testing needs to be initiated (see Box 9–1). Primary assessment, including a comprehensive history and physical examination for any obvious causes of infertility, is done before a costly, time-consuming, and emotionally trying investigation is initiated. During the first visit for the preliminary investigation, the basic infertility workup is explained. The basic investigation usually includes assessment of ovarian function, cervical mucosal adequacy and receptivity to sperm, sperm adequacy, tubal patency, and the general condition of the pelvic organs.

Table 9–1   Possible Causes of Infertility

Necessary norms	Deviations from normal
FEMALE	
Favorable cervical mucus	Cervicitis, immunologic response ("hostile" mucus), use of coital lubricants, antisperm antibodies
Clear passage between cervix and tubes	Myomas, adhesions, adenomyosis, polyps, endometritis, cervical stenosis, endometriosis, congenital anomalies (for example, septate uterus)
Patent tubes with normal motility	Pelvic inflammatory disease, peritubal adhesions, endometriosis, IUD, salpingitis (for example, tuberculosis), neoplasm, ectopic pregnancy, tubal ligation
Ovulation and release of ova	Primary ovarian failure, polycystic ovarian disease, hypothyroidism, pituitary tumor, lactation, periovarian adhesions, endometriosis, medications (for example, oral contraceptives), premature ovarian failure, hyperprolactinemia
No obstruction between ovary and fimbria	Adhesions, endometriosis, pelvic inflammatory disease
Endometrial preparation	Anovulation, luteal phase defect, IUD
MALE	
Normal semen analysis	Abnormalities of sperm or semen, polyspermia, congenital defect in testicular development, mumps after adolescence, cryptorchidism, infections, gonadal exposure to x rays, chemotherapy, smoking, alcohol abuse, malnutrition, chronic or acute metabolic disease, medications (for example, morphine and cocaine), marijuana use, constrictive underclothing
Unobstructed genital tract	Infections, tumors, congenital anomalies, vasectomy, strictures, trauma, varicocele
Normal genital tract secretions	Infections, autoimmunity to semen, tumors
Ejaculate deposited at the cervix	Premature ejaculation, hypospadias, retrograde ejaculation (for example, diabetic), neurologic cord lesions, obesity (inhibiting adequate penetration)

Box 9–1 Fertility Awareness

Avoid douching and artificial lubricants. Prevent alteration of pH of vagina and introduction of spermicidal agents.

Promote retention of sperm. The male superior position with female remaining recumbent for at least one hour after intercourse maximizes the number of sperm reaching the cervix.

Avoid leakage of sperm. Elevate the woman's hips with a pillow after intercourse. Avoid getting up to urinate for one hour after intercourse.

Maximize the potential for fertilization. Have intercourse one to three times per week and at intervals of no less than 48 hours.

Avoid emphasizing conception during sexual encounters to decrease anxiety and potential sexual dysfunction.

Maintain adequate nutrition and reduce stress. Using stress reduction techniques and good nutrition habits increases sperm production.

Explore other methods to increase fertility awareness, such as home assessment of cervical mucus and basal body temperature recordings.

It is never easy to discuss one's sexual activity, especially when potentially irreversible problems with fertility may exist. The mutual desire to have children is the basis of many marriages. A fertility problem is a deeply personal, emotion-laden area in a couple's life. The self-esteem of one or both partners may be threatened if the inability to conceive is perceived as a lack of virility or femininity. The nurse can provide comfort to the client by offering a sympathetic ear, a nonjudgmental atmosphere, and appropriate information and instructions. Since counseling includes discussion of very personal matters, nurses who are comfortable with their own sexuality are more capable of establishing rapport and eliciting relevant information.

Health care interventions in cases of infertility are illustrated in Figure 9–1. Following the initial interview with the infertile couple, a comprehensive history (including a detailed sexual history) is taken and a physical examination is performed. The historical data base for the couple should include the following information.

A. Female

1. Menstrual history

   a. Age of menarche; interval, duration, and quantity of menses; dysmenorrhea

   b. Ovulation: symptoms, including PMS (premenstrual symptoms such as mood changes, breast tenderness, acne), mittelschmerz (midcycle ovulatory pain), intermenstrual spotting, increased midcycle discharge

   c. Date of last menstrual period

   d. Current lactation (amenorrhea)

2. Medical history

   a. Diabetes

   b. Genital tuberculosis

   c. Use of intrauterine device (IUD), which may cause increased bacterial growth on endometrial surfaces or tube damage

   d. Pelvic inflammatory disease

   e. Sexually transmitted disease (gonorrhea, syphilis, chlamydia, herpes)

   f. Polycystic ovarian disease (Stein-Leventhal syndrome)

   g. Hyperprolactinemia

3. Surgical history

   a. Appendectomy (appendicitis may cause tubal obstruction or adhesions)

   b. Reproductive surgery

   c. Endometriosis

   d. Cone biopsy

   e. Intra-abdominal surgery that resulted in inflammatory complications

   f. Abortions

4. Fertility history

   a. Length of time without contraception

   b. Duration of infertility

   c. Fertility testing in the past

   d. Previous pregnancy: number and age at time of conception

   e. Family reproductive history

   f. Contraception use (type, duration, complications)

   g. Previous labor or postpartum circumstances surrounding pregnancy loss

5. Sexual history: practices and knowledge

   a. Frequency of intercourse

   b. Timing of intercourse (ie, ovulatory cycle)

   c. Sexual positions used

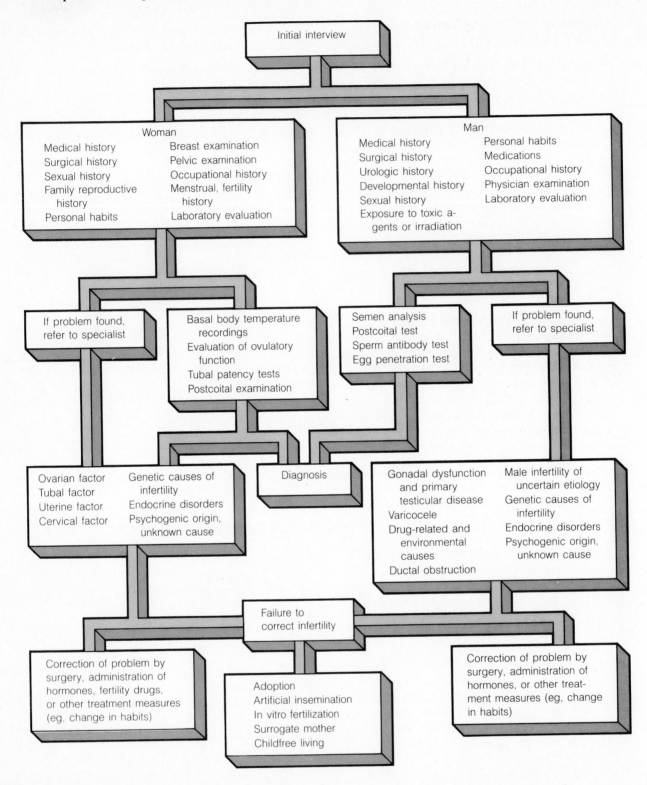

Figure 9–1　Flow chart for management of the infertile couple

d. Fertility with the other partners

e. Number of partners (over time multiple partners can create cervical antibody reactions against different men's semen)

f. Use of coital lubricants

g. Influence of religious, educational, and social factors

6. Occupation

　a. Exposure to toxic substances (x rays, lead, chemicals, anesthetic gases)

　b. Irradiation may cause ovarian failure

7. Medications

　a. Oral contraceptives or other medications affecting fertility

　b. In utero exposure to DES

8. Personal habits

　a. Alcohol consumption

　b. Smoking

　c. Strenuous exercise (long-distance running or professional dancing may cause reversible amenorrhea)

　d. Douching, vaginal deodorants, and timing of douching

　e. Weight history, especially if amenorrhea has resulted from weight loss or gain

　f. Use of recreational drugs (such as marijuana)

B. Male

1. Age (sperm count decreases with age)

2. Occupation (some occupations expose the scrotum to excessive heat, which is harmful to spermatogenesis, for example, cross-country truck driving)

3. Medical history

　a. Mumps after adolescence

　b. Diabetes

　c. Tuberculosis

　d. Sexually transmitted disease, epididymitis, orchitis, hypospadias, prostatitis, or other medical conditions

　e. Renal disease

　f. Acute viral or febrile illness in past three months (the complete cycle of spermatogenesis is approximately three months)

4. Surgical history

　a. Accidental damage to testes

　b. Previous hernia repairs, vasectomy, cryptorchidism, circumcision, hypospadias, or other conditions requiring surgical intervention

　c. Retroperitoneal surgery

5. Developmental history

　a. Endocrine diseases: thyroid or hypoprolactinemia

　b. Age when growth spurt occurred; acne; appearance of facial hair

6. Sexual history

　a. Sexual technique

　b. Frequency of intercourse

　c. Adequacy of erection

　d. Presence of orgasm during coitus and ejaculation with orgasm

　e. Previous fathering of other children with different sexual partner

　f. Family reproductive history

　g. Use of coital lubricants

7. Exposure to toxic substances or irradiation

　a. Toxic substance exposure (such as x rays, lead, chemicals: can produce low sperm counts and defective sperm cells)

　b. Irradiation in work place or for genital cancer

　c. Chemotherapy (reduces sperm count and increases abnormal sperm cells) (Smith 1982a)

8. Medications

　a. Drugs affecting potency (such as narcotics; alcohol; tranquilizers; antihypertensives [erectile dysfunction]; monoamine oxidase inhibitors; and guanethidine and methyldopa, which interfere with the autonomic nervous system and cause retrograde ejaculations)

　b. Drugs affecting spermatogenesis (including amebicides, antimalarial drugs, nitrofurantoin, and methotrexate)

9. Personal habits

　a. Smoking and alcohol consumption

b. Type of underwear worn (tight underwear may raise scrotal temperature)

c. Bathing habits (hot baths and saunas may harm sperm)

d. Use of recreational drugs (marijuana may depress androgen levels) (La Nasa 1980); PCP or angel dust and heroin addiction may cause low testosterone levels and loss of libido (Smith 1982a)

Following completion of the couple's histories, a complete physical examination of each partner is performed. See Table 9–2.

Tests for Infertility

After a thorough history and physical examination of both partners, tests may be initiated to identify other causes of infertility. More assessment tests have been developed for women than for men. At present, unless obvious pa-thology is identified in the male partner, male infertility assessments are usually limited to evaluating sperm production and viability and determining whether any obstruction interferes with ejaculation.

Four general areas are investigated to evaluate the anatomy, physiology, and sexual compatibility of the couple. The female's fertility assessments are discussed first. For review of female reproductive cycle characteristics see Box 9–2.

OVULATORY FUNCTION

Ovulation problems account for approximately 15 percent to 20 percent of female infertility (Moghissi & Wallach 1983). The most accurate ways of monitoring ovulation are recording BBT, observing cervical mucus changes, and obtaining endometrial biopsies.

One basic test of ovulatory function is the basal body temperature recording (BBT), which aids in identification of follicular and luteal phase abnormalities. At the initial visit, the woman is instructed in the technique of recording

Table 9–2 Infertility Physical Workup

Female	Male

1. Physical examination
  a. Assessment of height, weight, blood pressure, temperature, and general health status
  b. Endocrine evaluation of thyroid for exophthalmos, lid lag, tremor, or palpable gland
  c. Optic fundi evaluation for presence of increased intracranial pressure especially in oligomenorrheal or amenorrheal women (possible pituitary tumor)
  d. Reproductive features (including breast and external genital area)
  e. Physical ability to tolerate pregnancy
2. Pelvic examination
  a. Papanicolaou smear
  b. Culture for gonorrhea
  c. Signs of vaginal infections (see Chapter 10)
  d. Shape of escutcheon (for example, does pubic hair distribution resemble that of a male?)
  e. Size of clitoris (enlargement caused by endocrine disorders)
  f. Evaluation of cervix: old lacerations, tears, erosion, polyps, condition and shape of os, signs of infections, cervical mucus (evaluate for estrogen effect of spinnbarkheit and cervical ferning)
3. Bimanual examination
  a. Size, shape, position, and mobility of uterus
  b. Presence of congenital anomalies
  c. Presence of endometriosis
  d. Evaluation of adnexa: ovarian size, cysts, fixations, or tumors
4. Rectovaginal examination
  a. Presence of retroflexed or retroverted uterus
  b. Presence of rectouterine pouch masses
  c. Presence of possible endometriosis
5. Laboratory examination
  a. Complete blood count
  b. Sedimentation rate if indicated
  c. Serology
  d. Urinalysis
  e. Rh factor and blood grouping
  f. If indicated, thyroid function tests, glucose tolerance test, 17-ketosteroid assay, 17-hydrocorticoid assay, urine pregnanediol level
	1. Physical examination
	  a. General health (assessment of height, weight, blood pressure)
	  b. Endocrine evaluation (for example, presence of gynecomastia)
	  c. Visual fields evaluation for bitemporal hemianopia
	  d. Abnormal hair patterns
	2. Urologic examination (includes presence or absence of phimosis; location of urethral meatus; size and consistency of each testis, vas deferens, and epididymis; presence of varicocele)
	3. Rectal examination
	  a. Size and consistency of the prostate, with microscopic evaluation of prostate fluid for signs of infection
	  b. Size and consistency of the seminal vesicles
	4. Laboratory examination
	  a. Complete blood count
	  b. Sedimentation rate if indicated
	  c. Serology
	  d. Urinalysis
	  e. Rh factor and blood grouping
	  f. Semen analysis
	  g. If indicated, testicular biopsy, buccal smear

Box 9–2   Female Reproductive Cycle

FRC includes the ovarian cycle and the menstrual cycle

Ovarian Cycle

Follicular phase (days 1–14): Primordial follicle matures under influence of FSH and LH up to the time of ovulation.

Luteal phase (days 15–28): Ovum leaves follicle; corpus luteum develops under LH influence and produces high levels of progesterone and low levels of estrogen.

Menstrual Cycle

Menstrual phase (days 1–5)

Proliferative phase (days 6–14): Estrogen peaks just prior to ovulation. Cervical mucus at ovulation is clear, thin, watery, alkaline, and more favorable to sperm; shows ferning pattern; and has spinnbarkheit greater than 5 cm. At ovulation body temperature drops, then rises sharply and remains elevated.

Secretory phase (days 15–26): Estrogen drops sharply and progesterone dominates.

Ischemic phase (days 27–28): Both estrogen and progesterone levels drop.

---

basal body temperature, which may be taken with a BBT thermometer. This special kind of thermometer measures temperature between 96F and 100F and is calibrated by tenths of a degree, thereby facilitating identification of slight temperature changes. The woman may choose the site to obtain the temperature. Possible sites include oral, axillary, rectal, or vaginal, and the same site should be used each time. For best results the thermometer should be kept beside the bed, and the woman should take her temperature upon awakening, before any activity. After obtaining her temperature, she shakes the thermometer down to prepare it for use the next day. This step is important, as even the activity of shaking the thermometer immediately before use can cause a small increase in the basal temperature. Other factors that may produce temperature variation are sleeplessness, digestive disturbances, illness, fever, and emotional upset. Daily variations should be recorded on the temperature graph. The temperature graph and the readings are used for detecting ovulation and timing intercourse (Figure 9–2).

Basal temperature for females in the preovulatory phase is usually below 98F (36.7C). An ovulatory menstrual cycle is characterized by a biphasic basal body temperature pattern. As ovulation approaches, production of

estrogen increases and at its peak may cause a drop in the basal temperature. When ovulation occurs, there is a surge of LH, and progesterone is produced by the corpus luteum, causing a 0.5 to 1.0F (0.3 to 0.6C) rise in basal temperature. Figure 9–2B shows a biphasic ovulatory BBT chart. Progesterone is thermogenic, thereby maintaining the temperature increase during the second half of the menstrual cycle. Temperature elevation does not predict the day of ovulation but provides supportive evidence of ovulation about a day after it has occurred. Actual release of the ovum probably occurs 24 to 36 hours prior to the first temperature elevation (Coulam 1982).

With the additional documentation of coitus, serial BBT charts can be used to indicate if, and approximately when, the woman is ovulating and if intercourse is occurring at the proper time to achieve conception. A proposed schedule for intercourse based on serial BBT charts might be to recommend sexual intercourse *every other day* in the period of time beginning 3 to 4 days prior to and continuing for 2 to 3 days following the expected time of ovulation.

Hormonal assessments of ovulatory function fall into two categories:

1. *LH assays.* Daily samplings of serum LH at midcycle can detect the LH surge. The day of the LH surge is believed to be the day of maximum fertility. LH assay testing can be done using a home urine test or a laboratory serum test. Normal serum values vary depending on the phase of the menstrual cycle: proliferative phase: 5 to 15 mIU/ml; midcycle peak: 30 to 60 mIU/ml; and secretory phase: 5 to 15 mIU/ml.

2. *Progesterone assays.* Progesterone levels furnish the best evidence of ovulation and corpus luteum functioning. Plasma progesterone levels begin to rise with the LH surge and peak about eight days after the LH surge. Two blood samples, on days 8 and 21, showing an increase of from less than 1 ng/mL to greater than 5 ng/mL indicates ovulation. A normal serum progesterone level is 10 ng/mL or higher on day 21. Urinary pregnanediol reaches levels of 4 to 6 mg at 24 hours after ovulation; a level of 2 mg at 24 hours or greater indicates ovulation. Serum progesterone levels may be done instead of endometrial biopsy.

Further evaluation of ovulatory function is made by performing a biopsy of the endometrium. This procedure can determine the presence and adequacy of secretory tissue as a result of progesterone produced by the corpus luteum after ovulation.

The biopsy is usually performed in a physician's office 2 to 6 days before menstruation as this is the time of the greatest luteal function. A sample of endometrium from the fundal area of the uterus is obtained by use of a special

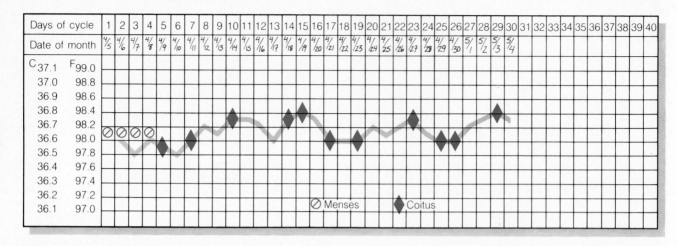

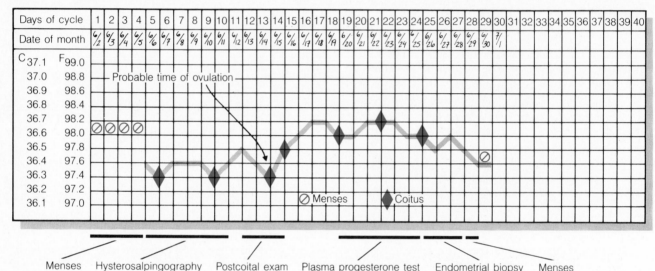

Figure 9–2 A *A monophasic, anovulatory basal body temperature chart.* B *A biphasic basal body temperature chart illustrating ovulation, the different types of testing, and the time in the cycle that each would be performed*

small tubular curet, which is attached to either electric, water, or syringe suction. The woman should be informed that she will experience cramping similar to menstrual cramps at the time the actual specimen is taken.

A dysfunction may exist if the endometrial lining does not show the expected amount of secretory tissue for that day of the women's menstrual cycle. Endometrial biopsies and serum progesterone assay may both be necessary to confirm luteal phase dysfunction.

Ultrasound is now also being used to detect ovulation and changes in follicular development to determine the best time for artificial insemination or in vitro fertilization.

CERVICAL MUCOSAL TESTS

The cervical mucous cells of the endocervix consist predominantly of water. As ovulation approaches, the ovary increases its secretion of estrogen and produces changes in the cervical mucus. The amount of mucus increases tenfold

and the water content rises significantly. To be receptive to sperm, cervical mucus must be thin, clear, watery, profuse, alkaline, and acellular. As shown in Figure 9–3, the maze-like microscopic mucoid strands align in a parallel manner to allow for easy sperm passage (Poon & McCoshen 1985). The mucus is termed *hostile* if these changes do not occur.

Cervical mucus hostile to sperm survival can have several causes, some of which are treatable. For example, estrogen secretion may be inadequate for the development of receptive mucus. Therapy with supplemental estrogen for approximately six days before expected ovulation permits the formation of suitable spinnbarkheit. Cervical infection, another cause of mucosal hostility to sperm, can be treated, depending on the type of infection. Cone biopsy, electrocautery, or cryosurgery to the cervix may remove large numbers of mucus-producing glands and cervical crypts, creating a "dry cervix" inhospitable to sperm survival (Hammond & Talbert 1985).

The cervix can also be the site of secretory immunologic reactions in which antisperm antibodies are

- Corticosteroid therapy for immunosuppression to reduce IgG antibody concentration (Sogor 1986)

- When only the woman has a positive antibody titer condom use for six months, to reduce the titer by decreasing the exposure to the antigen (McShane et al 1985).

Elasticity or *spinnbarkheit* increases and the viscosity decreases at ovulation. Excellent *spinnbarkheit* exists when the mucus can be stretched 5 to 6 cm or longer (Zacur & Rock 1983). This is accomplished by using two glass slides (Figure 9–4A) or by grasping some mucus at the external os and stretching it in the vagina toward the introitus. Studies are exploring the possibility of cervical mucus strand size and spacing as causes of infertility (Poon & McCoshen 1985).

The *ferning capacity* (Figure 9–4B) of the cervical mucus also increases as ovulation approaches. Ferning, or

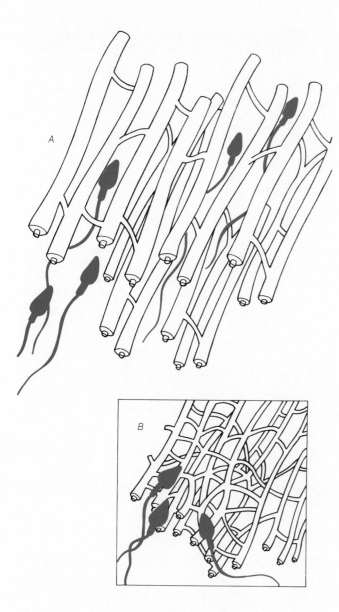

Figure 9–3 Sperm passage through cervical mucus. A Receptive mucus under estrogen influence coincides with ovulation. B Nonreceptive mucus under influence of progesterone, endogenous or exogenous (From Fogel CL, Woods NP. Health Care of Women. St. Louis, Mosby, 1981.)

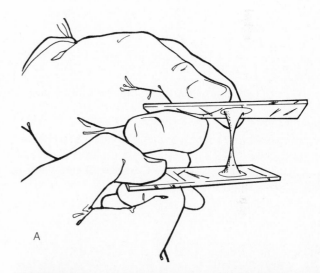

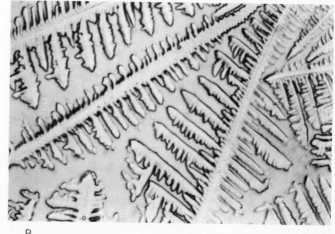

Figure 9–4 A Spinnbarkheit (elasticity) B Ferning (Courtesy Lovena L Porter)

produced, causing agglutination or immobilization of sperm. A mucus-sperm contact or sperm penetration test has been developed in which initial interaction is observed microscopically (Bronson 1984). The most widely used serum-sperm bioassays are the gelatin agglutination test and the sperm immobilization test. Radioimmunoassays have been developed to detect specific classes of antibodies in serum and seminal fluid. Measures used to decrease antibody concentrations are:

crystallization, is caused by increased levels of salt and water interacting with the glycoproteins in the mucus during the ovulatory period and is thus an indirect indication of estrogen production. To test for ferning, mucus is obtained from the cervical os, spread on a glass slide, allowed to air dry, and examined under the microscope.

POSTCOITAL TEST

The postcoital examination (Huhner test) is performed one or two days prior to the expected date of ovulation. This examination evaluates the cervical mucus and the number and motility of the sperm at the endocervix. The procedure assesses the sperm's ability to negotiate the cervical barrier and the interaction of sperm and mucus.

The couple is asked to have intercourse four to six hours before the examination. A small plastic catheter, attached to a 10-mL syringe, is placed in the cervix. Mucus is aspirated from the internal and external os, measured, and examined microscopically for signs of infection, number of active spermatozoa per high-powered field, and number of spermatozoa with poor or no motility.

SPERM ADEQUACY TESTS

A semen analysis is the most important initial diagnostic study of the male. It is one of the first steps in infertility testing because it is relatively simple and precludes unnecessary exposure of the female partner to high-risk painful procedures. Optimum results are obtained when a specimen is collected after two days of abstinence. If the male has difficulty producing sperm other than with intercourse, special sheaths are available to collect the sperm. Regular condoms should not be used because they contain spermicidal agents and sperm can be lost on the condom. The specimen should be placed in a glass container and brought to the laboratory within an hour of collection if possible (2 to 3 hours maximum). It should be marked with the time of collection and date of previous ejaculation and maintained at body temperature. Repeated semen analysis may be required to identify the male's fertility potential adequately. Semen collections should be repeated at least 74 days apart to allow for new germ cell maturation (Speroff et al 1983).

Sperm analysis provides information about sperm motility and morphology as well as a determination of the absolute number of spermatozoa present (Table 9–3). Debate exists over the absolute number of sperm required for fertility. It has been reported that men with counts of 20 million per milliliter are able to impregnate their partners (Glass 1981). The chance for conception is remote if the semen analysis reveals fewer than 10 million sperm per milliliter, less than 50 percent to 60 percent active sperm, or less than 70 percent normal sperm forms.

Table 9–3　Normal Semen Analysis

Factor	Value
Volume	2–5 mL (range 1–7 mL)
pH	7.2–8.9
Total sperm count	≥50 million/mL preferably
Liquification time	5–20 minutes after collection
Motility	
Immediate	>60%
4 hours	>50%
Forward movement	>30%
Normal forms	>60%
No agglutination of sperm	

Source: Ansbacher R: Male Infertility. Clin Obstet Gynecol *1982;25(3):461.*

Spermatozoa have been shown to possess intrinsic antigens that can provoke male immunologic infertility. This is especially apparent following vasectomy reversals where an autoimmunity (male produces antibodies to his sperm) to sperm develops (Bronson 1984). Research now indicates that it is the actual presence of antibodies on the spermatozoal surface (not just the presence of antibodies in the serum) that affects sperm function and thus leads to subfertility (Sogor 1986). Treatment for the presence of antibodies in the male ejaculate may include immunosuppression, and sperm washing–dilution insemination techniques. The prostaglandin inhibitor effect of anti-inflammatory drugs has been shown to increase the sperm count, sperm motility, and fertilizing capacity (Barkay 1984).

TUBAL PATENCY TESTS

Tubal patency tests are usually done after BBT evaluation, semen analysis, and the other less invasive tests have been done and results evaluated. Tubal patency is confirmed usually by hysterosalpingography. Other invasive tests of tubular function are laparoscopy and culdoscopy.

Hysterosalpingography, or *hysterogram,* involves an instillation of a radiopaque substance into the uterine cavity. As the substance fills the uterus and fallopian tubes and spills into the peritoneal cavity, it is viewed with x-ray techniques. This procedure can reveal tubal patency and any distortions of the endometrial cavity. Hysterosalpingography has also been known to have a therapeutic effect. Pregnancy is frequently achieved within the first three cycles following the test. This effect may be caused by the flushing of debris, breaking of adhesions, or induction of peristalsis by the instillation.

The hysterosalpingogram should be performed in the proliferative phase of the cycle to avoid interrupting an early pregnancy. This timing also avoids the lush secretory changes in the endometrium that occur after ovulation, which may prevent the passage of the dye and present a false picture of cornual obstruction.

Hysterosalpingography causes moderate discomfort. The pain is referred from the peritoneum, which is irritated by the subdiaphragmatic collection of gas, to the shoulder. Some are now advocating hysteroscopy to detect peritubal disease, for which hysterosalpingography has limited value (Daly 1986).

Laparoscopy enables direct visualization of the pelvic organs and is usually done six to eight months after the hysterogram. The woman usually is given a general anesthetic for this procedure. Entry is generally made through an incision in the umbilical area, although it is occasionally done suprapubically. The peritoneal cavity is distended with carbon dioxide gas, and the pelvic organs can be directly visualized. Tubular function can be assessed by instillation of dye into the uterine cavity from below. The pelvis is evaluated for endometriosis, adhesions, organ fixations, pelvic inflammatory disease, tumors, and cysts. Visualization is best when the procedure is performed in the early follicular stage of the cycle (Valle 1984). The intraperitoneal gas is usually manually expressed at the end of the procedure. Routine preanesthesia instructions should be given. The woman is told she may have some discomfort from organ displacement and shoulder and chest pain caused by gas in the abdomen lasting 24 to 48 hours after the procedure. She should be informed that she can resume normal activities after resting for about two days.

Culdoscopy is sometimes used to assess tubular function. The posterior cul-de-sac is infiltrated with local anesthetic and entered with a metallic trocar. Culdoscopic examination of pelvic structures is accomplished by injecting indigo, carmine, or similar dyes through a cannula inserted into the cervix.

Methods of Infertility Management

PHARMACOLOGIC METHODS

If a defect in ovulation has been detected during the fertility testing, the treatment depends on the specific cause of the problem. In the presence of normal ovaries and an intact pituitary gland, *clomiphene citrate* (Clomid) is often used. This medication induces ovulation in 80 percent of women by actions at both the hypothalamic and ovarian levels, and 40 percent of these women will become pregnant (Speroff et al 1983). Clomiphene works by increasing the secretion of FSH and LH, which stimulates follicle growth. The woman is instructed to take the medication daily for five days beginning on day 5 of the menstrual cycle. She is informed that if ovulation occurs, it will be on cycle day 14 to 16. The presence of ovulation and evaluation of response to therapy should be assessed by BBT, plasma progesterone, or cervical mucus and vaginal cytology studies.

A pelvic exam should be done to rule out ovarian enlargement, hyperstimulation syndrome, or the presence of pregnancy before another cycle is begun. Ovarian enlargement and abdominal discomfort may result from follicular growth and development and multiple corpus luteum formation. Persistence of ovarian cysts is a contraindication for further clomiphene administration. Other side effects include vasomotor flushes, abdominal distention, bloating, breast discomfort, nausea and vomiting, vision problems (such as visual spots), headache, and dryness or loss of hair. Supplemental low-dose estrogen may be given to ensure appropriate quality and quantity of cervical mucus, since clomiphene has been shown to inhibit mucus production.

Human menopausal gonadotropin (hMG), a potent hormone, is capable of causing mild to severe reactions. It is a combination FSH and LH obtained from postmenopausal women's urine and administered intramuscularly every day for varying periods of time during the first half of the cycle to stimulate follicular development (Smith 1985). To effect ovulation, hMG must be given intramuscularly. Ovarian hyperstimulation syndrome may develop with this form of therapy. Follicle size and number should be monitored by real time ultrasound, and the hMG can be administered accordingly to match the LH surge and follicle development. The couple is advised to have intercourse on the day of hMG administration and for the next two days. Multiple birth rate is reported to be about 20 percent, with 15 percent twins. Women who elect to have hMG medication usually have passed through all other forms of management without conceiving. Strong emotional support is needed because of the numerous office visits, injections, monthly ultrasounds, and stress in the woman's relationship.

Regimens combining clomiphene and hMG have been recommended for some women who respond poorly to clomiphene. This reduces the amount of hMG required per cycle.

When hyperprolactinemia accompanies anovulation, the infertility may be treated with *bromocriptine*. This medication acts directly on the prolactin-secreting cells in the anterior pituitary. It inhibits the pituitary's secretion of prolactin—thus preventing suppression of the pulsatile secretion of FSH and LH. This restores normal menstrual cycles—and induces ovulation by allowing FSH and LH production. High prolactin levels may impair the glandular production of FSH and LH and/or block their action on the ovaries. If treatment is successful, the BBT record will show a normal biphasic pattern. The drug should be discontinued if pregnancy is suspected or at the anticipated time of ovulation because of its possible teratogenic effects. Other side effects include nausea, diarrhea, dizziness, headache, and fatigue.

When endometriosis is determined to be the cause of the infertility, *danazol* (Danocrine) may be given to suppress ovulation and menstruation, and effect atrophy of the ectopic endometrial tissue. It has an antigonadotropin effect and suppresses both FSH and LH. Temporary suppression has been shown to result in healing of the endometriosis. The treatment regimen may last for 6 to 12 months or longer, depending on the severity of the disease (Bultram et al 1982). The return of menstrual function and fertility is prompt after discontinuation of danazol, with the first menstrual period occurring within four to six weeks. (This same suppression can be achieved with the continuous use of oral contraceptives. However, troublesome side effects are much more frequent and symptomatic relief is less.) The woman is instructed to take danazol four times a day for 6 to 12 months. The nurse should inform the woman about measures to minimize the side effects of the drug. Women should avoid foods containing excessive sodium that may increase fluid retention and add potassium foods to reduce muscle cramps. If mild hirsutism occurs she can use tweezers or a depilatory agent to remove the temporary hair. Conscientious skin care will minimize skin oiliness and acne. Another side effect, atropic vaginitis, can be dealt with by using an iodine douche if it occurs and using additional lubricants during intercourse.

Gonadotropin-releasing hormone is a new therapeutic tool being tested in the United States for ovulation stimulation. It is used for women who have insufficient endogenous release of GnRH. Administration is either by subcutaneous injection or intravenous infusion. Subcutaneous injection is accomplished by a portable infusion pump with a pulsatile mechanism worn on a belt around the waist (Loucopoulos et al 1984). The length of treatment varies from two to four weeks and hCG is also given to stimulate ovulation. Reports state that side effects such as multiple births and hyperstimulation syndrome are less than with combination hMG-hCG therapy (Hammond & Talbert 1985).

Progesterone therapy for luteal phase defects is also being done. Most authorities recommend the use of natural progesterone in conjunction with clomiphene or clomiphene and hCG for these problems (Wentz 1982).

ARTIFICIAL INSEMINATION

Artificial insemination, with either the husband's semen (AIH) or that of a donor (AID), is the depositing of semen at the cervical os or in the uterus by mechanical means. The conception rates vary widely between centers. AIH is used in cases of insufficient semen, oligozoospermia or polyzoospermia, low levels of spermatozoal motility, anatomic defects accompanied by inadequate deposition or penetration of semen, or retrograde ejaculation.

AID is considered in cases of azoospermia, antisperm antibodies, total lack of sperm motility or combination of inadequate motility and viability of sperm, recurrent abortions resulting from male cytogenetic abnormality, or male homologous translocation carrier. AID is not appropriate therapy in cases of women with antibodies, since they have antibodies against antigens common to all human sperm cells, not just to their partner's sperm.

Numerous factors need to be evaluated before AID is performed. Has every possible effort been made to diagnose and treat the cause of the male infertility? Do tests indicate normal fertility and sperm/ovum transport in the woman? Is each member psychologically stable? Is this a voluntary decision on the part of the male partner? Are there any religious contraindications?

Artificial insemination is accomplished by collecting semen from the male in a glass container. The semen then is drawn into a syringe and placed in a small plastic cervical cup. The cup is put in place at the cervical os, and the woman remains in the supine position with the hips elevated for about 30 minutes. An alternate method is to instill the semen directly into the uterus using a small plastic catheter on a syringe. The semen must first be chemically cleansed and centrifuged. This method enables the semen to bypass possible cervical or immunologic factors.

IN VITRO FERTILIZATION

The first birth conceived by *in vitro fertilization* (IVF) was achieved in Great Britain in 1978. This procedure is selectively used in cases in which infertility has resulted from tubal factors, mucus abnormalities, and immunity to spermatozoa in either partner and when infertility is long-term and unexplained. IVF is felt to be the only hope for up to 25 percent of infertile couples (Phillips 1985).

Ovulation is induced using fertility drugs, and ovarian function is monitored daily with blood tests, cervical mucus tests, and ultrasound. Just before ovulation, the ripened ova are aspirated from the ovaries during a laparoscopy. The ova are fertilized with the prospective father's sperm and transferred to the mother's uterus when they reach the four- to eight-cell stage of development (Dodson et al 1986). A series of progesterone injections are given to assist the process of implantation. The procedure has had a success rate of up to 20 percent, with a spontaneous abortion rate of one in three.

In vitro fertilization is an invasive method of treating infertility. The risk to offspring can only be assessed with more experience. Controversy concerning IVF has elicited concern, criticism, opinions, and condemnation from a variety of church leaders and scientists. In spite of the ethical and legal issues, it has found fairly wide acceptance with childless couples. In the near future, it may be a routine treatment for many infertile couples (Creighton 1985).

ADOPTION

The adoption of an infant is not as satisfactory an alternative to infertility today as it was in the past. In fact there are 44 couples waiting to adopt each available white infant (Phillips 1985). A waiting period as long as seven years even to begin the adoption process is not uncommon. The decrease in number of available infants has occurred because many infants are reared by their single mothers instead of being relinquished for adoption as was customary in the past. In addition, many unwanted pregnancies are being terminated by elective abortion. Some couples seek international adoptions or consider adopting older children, children with handicaps, or children of mixed parentage. The adoption process is quicker and more children are available in these groups.

The Nurse's Role

Approximately 15 percent of the childbearing population in the United States (one out of six couples) is unable to conceive or carry a pregnancy to term (Darland 1985). The couple may incur tremendous emotional and physical stress, as well as financial expense for infertility testing. Treatment can cost an average of $20,000 a year. Years of effort and numerous evaluations and examinations may take place before a conception occurs, if one occurs at all. In a society that values children and considers them to be the natural result of marriage, infertile couples may face a myriad of tensions and discrimination.

The nurse must be constantly aware of the emotional needs and sometimes irrational thoughts and fears of the couple with a fertility problem. The emotional aspect of infertility is often more difficult for the couple than the testing and treatment. Constant attention to temperature charts and instructions about their sex life from a person outside the relationship naturally affects the spontaneity of a couple's interactions. Their relationship will be stressed by these and other intrusive but necessary measures. The tests may heighten feelings of frustration or anger between the partners. Correction of infertility may require surgery, administration of hormones, and other treatment measures. The need to share this intimate area of a relationship may cause feelings of guilt and shame. Throughout the evaluations and emotional-financial strains one or both partners may undergo at this time, the nurse plays a major role in teaching and offering emotional support. Extensive and repeated explanations may be necessary to help relieve anxiety.

Infertility may be perceived as a loss by one or both partners, and as in the loss of a loved one who dies, this

Research Note

Experts estimate that 20% of couples in the United States experience difficulty conceiving. Olshansky used an inductive method to clarify the human response to infertility. Qualitative data was collected through observations and open-ended interview questions of 15 married couples and two married women who were at various stages of an infertility workup.

This researcher found that infertile persons who are distressed by their infertility undergo a process of "taking on" an identity of themselves as infertile. As these couples attempt pregnancy and fail, they experience "reluctant acceptance" of an identity as infertile and begin informal fertility work using suggestions from friends or the media to achieve pregnancy. When these also fail, they seek medical diagnosis and treatment, taking on a "formal identity" of infertility, and begin formal fertility work by following a medical regimen.

The identity of infertility takes a central place in the person's self-concept, pushing other identities to the periphery. Finally, the individual either manages the identity by overcoming it (becoming pregnant), circumventing it (achieving pregnancy through artificial insemination or in vitro fertilization), or reconciling oneself to it (adopting or choosing to be child free) or remains in limbo.

Nurses can use an awareness of this process to provide sensitive support and anticipatory guidance to infertile clients.

Olshansky EF: Identity of self as infertile: An example of theory generating research. Adv Nurs Sci 1987;9(Jan):54.

situation is attended by feelings of grief and mourning. Each couple passes through several stages of feelings, not unlike those identified by Kübler-Ross: surprise, denial, anger, isolation, guilt, grief, and resolution (Menning 1980). Nonjudgmental acceptance and a professional caring attitude on the nurse's part can go far to dissipate the negative emotions the couple may experience while going through this process. This is also a time when the nurse may assess the quality of the couple's relationship: Are they able and willing to communicate verbally and share feelings? Are they mutually supportive? The answers to such questions may help the nurse identify areas of strength and weakness and construct an appropriate plan of care. At times, individual or group counseling with other infertile couples may facilitate the couple's resolution of feelings brought about by their own difficult situation. Sawatzky (1981) has identified the essential tasks of the infertile couple (Table 9–4).

Table 9–4 Tasks of the Infertile Couple

Tasks	Nursing interventions
1. Recognition of how infertility affects their lives and expression of feelings (may be negative toward self or mate)	1. Supportive: help to understand and facilitate free expression of feelings
2. Grieving the loss of potential offspring	2. Help to recognize feelings
3. Evaluation of reasons for wanting a child	3. Help to understand motives
4. Decision making about management	4. Identify alternatives; facilitate partner communication

Source: Sawatzky, M: Tasks of the Infertile Couple. J Obstet Gynecol Neonat Nurs 1981;10:132.

● Genetic Disorders

Even when conception has been achieved, families can have special reproductive concerns. The desired and expected outcome of any pregnancy is the birth of a healthy "perfect" baby. Unfortunately, a small but significant number of parents experience grief, fear, and anger when they discover that their baby has been born with a defect or a genetic disease. Such an abnormality may be evident at birth or may not appear for some time. The baby may have inherited a disease from one parent, creating guilt and strife within the family.

Regardless of the type or scope of the problem, parents will have many questions: "What did I do?" "What caused it?" "Will it happen again?" The nurse must anticipate the parents' questions and concerns and guide, direct, and support the family. To do so, the nurse must have a basic knowledge of genetics and genetic counseling. Many congenital anomalies and diseases are genetic or have a strong genetic component. Others are not genetic at all. The genetic counselor attempts to categorize the problem and answer the family's questions. Professional nurses can help expedite this process if they already have an understanding of the principles involved and are able to direct the family to the appropriate resources.

Chromosomes and Chromosomal Abnormalities

All hereditary material is carried on tightly coiled strands of DNA known as *chromosomes*. The chromosomes carry the genes, the smallest unit of inheritance, as discussed in greater detail in Chapter 13.

All somatic (body) cells contain 46 chromosomes, which is the *diploid* number, while the sperm and egg contain 23 chromosomes, or the *haploid* number (see Chapter 13). There are 23 pairs of *homologous* chromosomes (a matched pair of chromosomes, one inherited from each parent). Twenty-two of the pairs are known as *autosomes*

CONTEMPORARY DILEMMA

How Many Is Too Many?

In vitro fertilization has been an answer for many couples who are unable to conceive. The procedure involves retrieval of the woman's ovum at the time of ovulation. After conception occurs, using the husband's sperm, the fertilized ovum is replaced in the woman's uterus. The chance of success is increased when more than one ovum is removed and fertilized.

Although in vitro fertilization has been viewed as a tremendous new development by many childless couples, some groups have raised questions about the procedure. Some of the issues are the following:

● If more than one fertilized ovum is returned to the uterus, it may be possible for the woman to have a multiple pregnancy of two to eight fetuses. This multiple pregnancy creates problems when delivery occurs long before the estimated date of delivery. The financial and emotional costs are great when the parents have more than one baby in an intensive care setting.

● If more than one ovum is fertilized and they are not returned to the uterus, what should be done with them? If they are kept, are the embryos entitled to inheritance from their family? If the embryos are destroyed, is it murder?

● Should "extra" embryos be made available for implantation into another woman's uterus?

● Should research be allowed on the extra embryos? If so under what conditions and for what purposes? Who should approve the research that is done? Is approval needed?

● If extra embryos are frozen and kept, how long should the facility be required to keep them? Does prolonged freezing harm the embryo?

● If sperm other than the husband's is used to fertilize the ovum, does it create special problems? Who does the child belong to? Does the husband need to adopt the child?

● With a success rate of approximately 10 to 20 percent, does in vitro fertilization take advantage of childless couples rather than helping them?

● Does the procedure move conception out of the human range entirely?

(nonsex chromosomes), and one pair are the *sex chromosomes*, X and Y. A normal female has a 46,XX chromosome constitution; the normal male, 46,XY (Figures 9–5 and 9–6.).

The *karyotype*, or pictorial analysis of an individual's chromosomes, is usually obtained from specially treated and stained peripheral blood lymphocytes. Once obtained, the cells are stimulated to undergo mitosis. The mitotic process is stopped during a phase called metaphase, the preparation is then stained and the chromosomes become visible (Figure 9–7). Although the use of peripheral blood is an easy convenient method of obtaining chromosomes, almost any tissue can be examined to get this information. In the case of a stillbirth or perinatal death in which there are multiple congenital abnormalities and there is a question of diagnosis or cause, karyotypes of cells in the child's thymus can be examined if it has not been fixed in formalin.

Chromosome abnormalities can occur in either the autosomes or the sex chromosomes and can be divided into two categories: abnormalities of number and abnormalities of structure. With the advent of quinacrine mustard staining of chromosomes, begun by Caspersson in 1970, it is possible to identify not only those cases in which an entire chromosome has been added or deleted but also those in which the addition or deletion of chromosomal material has been very small. Many children who received chromosomal analysis prior to this test were said to have normal chromosomes. But when examined with the new banding techniques, many were found to have additions or deletions of chromosomal material.

Even small aberrations in chromosomes can cause problems, especially those associated with slow growth and development or with mental retardation. The child need not have obvious major malformations to be affected (Figure 9–8). Some of these abnormalities can also be passed on to other offspring. In some cases, chromosomal analysis is appropriate even if clinical manifestations are mild. Whatever the case, too much or too little genetic material usually produces adverse effects on normal growth and development.

Indications for chromosomal analysis include:

- Chromosome syndrome suspected (or clients with a clinical diagnosis of Down syndrome)

- Mental retardation and congenital malformations

- Abnormal sexual development (primary amenorrhea, lack of secondary sex characteristics)

- Ambiguous genitals

- Multiple miscarriages

- Possible balanced translocation carrier

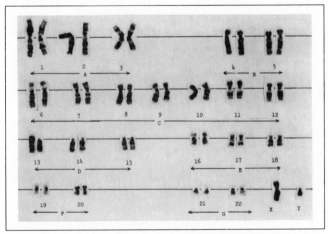

Figure 9–5   Normal male karyotype (Courtesy Dr Arthur Robinson, National Jewish Hospital and Research Center)

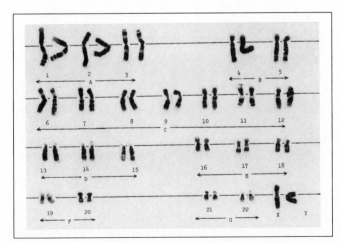

Figure 9–6   Normal female karyotype (Courtesy Dr Arthur Robinson, National Jewish Hospital and Research Center)

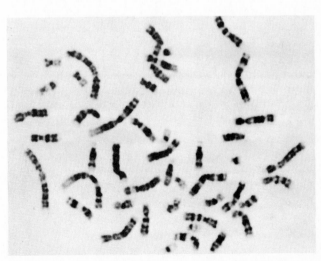

Figure 9–7   Chromosomes in metaphase spread (Courtesy Dr Arthur Robinson, National Jewish Hospital and Research Center)

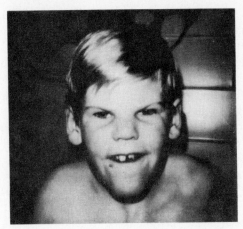

Figure 9–8   Ten-year-old boy who has a partial trisomy for short arm of chromosome number 4: He is mentally retarded and has minor abnormalities.

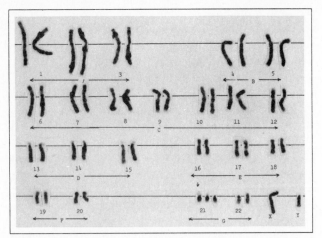

Figure 9–9   Karyotype of a male who has trisomy 21, Down syndrome: Note the extra 21 chromosome. (Courtesy Dr Arthur Robinson, National Jewish Hospital and Research Center)

AUTOSOME ABNORMALITIES

○   *ABNORMALITIES OF CHROMOSOME NUMBER*   Abnormalities of chromosome number are most commonly seen as trisomies, monosomies, and as mosaicism. In all three cases, the abnormality is most often caused by *nondisjunction*. Nondisjunction occurs when paired chromosomes fail to separate during cell division. If nondisjunction occurs in either the sperm or the egg before fertilization, the resulting zygote will have an abnormal chromosome makeup in all of the cells (trisomy or monosomy). If nondisjunction occurs after fertilization, the developing cell (zygote) will have cells with two or more different chromosome makeups, evolving into two or more different cell lines (mosaicism).

Trisomies are the product of the union of a normal gamete (egg or sperm) with a gamete that contains an extra chromosome. The individual will have 47 chromosomes and is trisomic (has three chromosomes the same) for whichever chromosome is extra. Down syndrome, or mongolism, is the most common trisomy abnormality seen in children (Figure 9–9). The presence of the extra chromosome 21 produces distinctive clinical features (see Table 9–5 and Figure 9–10). With the advent of modern surgical techniques and antibiotics, children with Down syndrome are now living into their fifth or sixth decade of life.

Trisomies can occur among other autosomes, the two most common being trisomy 18 and trisomy 13 (see Table 9–5 and Figures 9–11 and 9–12). The prognosis for children with trisomy 13 and 18 is extremely poor. Most children (70 percent) die within the first three months of life. The major cause of death is usually secondary complications related to cardiac and respiratory abnormalities.

Monosomies occur when a normal gamete unites with a gamete that is missing a chromosome. In this case, the individual will have only 45 chromosomes and is said to be monosomic. Monosomy of an entire autosomal chro-

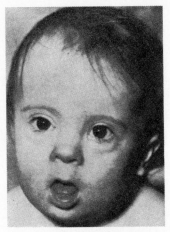

Figure 9–10   A child with Down syndrome (From Smith DW: *Recognizable Patterns of Human Malformations*. Philadelphia, Saunders, 1982b.)

mosome is incompatible with life. The only exception is in the sex chromosomes. A female can survive with only one X chromosome; this condition is known as *Turner syndrome* (Table 9–5 and Figure 9–13).

Mosaicism occurs after fertilization and results in an individual with two different cell lines, each with a different chromosomal number. Mosaicism tends to be more common in the sex chromosomes, but when it does occur in the autosomes, it is most common in Down syndrome.

Different body tissues may have different chromosome makeups, depending on when the nondisjunction occurs. Or the tissue may have a mixture of cells, and the ratio of normal to abnormal cells may vary from one tissue to the next. For instance, in Down syndrome, one cell line contains the normal 46 chromosomes while the other cell

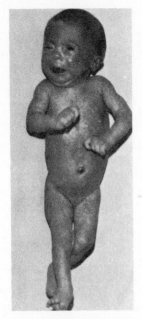

Figure 9–11   Infant with trisomy 18
(From Smith DW: Recognizable
Patterns of Human Malformations.
Philadelphia, Saunders, 1982b.)

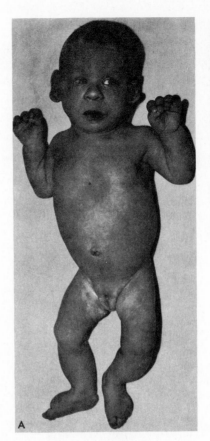

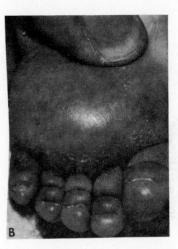

Figure 9–13   Infant with Turner
syndrome at one month of age. Note:
A Prominent ears. B Lymphedema.
(From Lemli L, Smith DW: The
XO syndrome: A study of the
differentiated phenotype in 25
patients. J Pediatr 1963;63:577.)

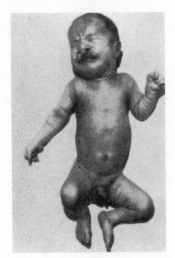

Figure 9–12   Infant with trisomy 13. (From Smith DW:
Recognizable Patterns of Human Malformations. Philadelphia,
Saunders, 1982b.)

line contains 47 chromosomes, that is, an extra number
21. Or within a single tissue, some of the cells may be
normal while others contain the extra chromosome 21.

Clinical signs and symptoms may vary if mosaicism
is present. In Down syndrome the clinical signs may be
classic, minimal, or not apparent, depending on the number and location of the abnormal cells. An individual with
many of the classic signs of Down syndrome but with normal intelligence should be investigated for the possibility

of mosaicism. In these cases, more than one tissue may
have to be examined to make the diagnosis. The peripheral
blood may contain 46 chromosomes while the skin fibro-
blasts contain 47, +21.

○   *ABNORMALITIES OF CHROMOSOME STRUCTURE* Abnormalities of chromosome structure involving only parts of
the chromosome generally occur in two forms: translocation and deletions and/or additions. Over 100 such abnormalities have been described in the literature. Again,
Down syndrome is one of the most common syndromes
described (see Table 9–6).

Not all children born with Down syndrome have trisomy 21. Instead, they may have an abnormal rearrangement of chromosomal material known as a *translocation*.
Clinically, the two types of Down syndrome are indistinguishable. What is of major importance to the family is
that the two different types have significantly different risks
of recurrence. The only way to distinguish the two is to
do a chromosome analysis.

The translocation occurs when the carrier parent has
45 chromosomes, usually with one of the number 21 chromosomes fused to one of the number 14 chromosomes.
The parent has one normal 14, one normal 21, and one

Table 9–5 Chromosomal Syndromes

Altered chromosome	Genetic defect and incidence	Characteristics

21	Trisomy 21 (Down's syndrome) (secondary to nondisjunction or 14/21 unbalanced translocation)
	1 in 700 live births
	(Figure 9–10)
		CNS: Mental retardation
		      Hypotonia at birth
		Head: Flattened occiput
		      Depressed nasal bridge
		      Mongoloid slant of eyes
		      Epicanthal folds
		      White speckling of the iris
		      (Brushfield's spots)
		      Protrusion of the tongue
		      High, arched palate
		      Low-set ears
		Hands: Broad, short fingers
		      Short fingers
		      Abnormalities of finger and foot
		      dermal ridge patterns
		      (dermatoglyphics)
		      Transverse palmar crease (simian line)
		Other: Congenital heart disease

21	2° mosaicism (Down syndrome) Incidence 1%	Classic symptoms as described in trisomy 21 except that the child has normal intelligence

18	Trisomy 18
	1 in 3000 live births
	(Figure 9–11)
		CNS: Mental retardation
		      Severe hypertonia
		Head: Prominent occiput
		      Low-set ears
		      Corneal opacities
		      Ptosis (drooping of eyelids)
		Hands: Third and fourth fingers overlapped by
		      second and fifth fingers
		      Abnormal dermatoglyphics
		      Syndactyly (webbing of fingers)
		Other: Congenital heart defects
		      Renal abnormalities
		      Single umbilical artery
		      Gastrointestinal tract abnormalities
		      Rocker-bottom feet
		      Cryptorchidism
		      Various malformations of other organs

18	Deletion of long arm of chromosome 18	CNS: Severe psychomotor retardation
		Head: Microcephaly
		      Stenotic ear canals with conductive
		      hearing loss
		Other: Various other organ malformations

14/21 chromosome. Since all the chromosomal material is present and functioning normally, the parent is clinically normal. This individual is known as a *balanced translocation carrier.*

When a balanced translocation carrier person has a child with a person who has a structurally normal chromosome constitution, there are several possible outcomes (Figure 9–14). The offspring can receive the carrier parent's normal number 21 and normal number 14 chromosomes in combination with the noncarrier parent's normal chromosomes 21 and 14. In this case the offspring is chromosomally normal. Or the child may receive one of the balanced translocations, thus becoming a carrier like the carrier parent—chromosomally abnormal but clinically normal. If, however, the offspring receives the carrier parent's normal number 21 chromosome and the 14/21 chromosome and the noncarrier parent's normal chromosomes, the offspring receives two functioning number 14 chromosomes and three functioning number 21 chromosomes. At first glance, the child seems to have 46 chromosomes but actually has an extra chromosome 21. Thus the child has an *unbalanced translocation* and has Down syndrome. Other types of translocations can occur. But regardless of the chromosome involved, any person having a balanced chromosome rearrangement (translocation) has the potential of having a child with an unbalanced chromosome constitution. This usually means a substantial negative effect on normal growth and development.

The other type of structure abnormality seen is caused by *additions and/or deletions* of chromosomal material. Any portion of a chromosome may be lost or added, generally leading to some adverse effect. Depending on

Table 9–5 Chromosomal Syndromes (continued)

Altered chromosome	Genetic defect and incidence	Characteristics	
13	Trisomy 13 1 in 5000 live births (Figure 9-12)	CNS:	Mental retardation Severe hypertonia Seizures
		Head:	Microcephaly Microphthalmia and/or coloboma Malformed ears Aplasia of external auditory canal Micrognathia Cleft lip and palate
		Hands:	Polydactyly (extra digits) Abnormal posturing of fingers Abnormal dermatoglyphics
		Other:	Congenital heart defects Hemangiomas Gastrointestinal tract defects Various malformations of other organs
5	Deletion of short arm of chromosome 5 (cri du chat—cat cry syndrome) 1 in 20,000 live births (Figure 9–15)	CNS:	Severe mental retardation A catlike cry in infancy
		Head:	Microcephaly Hypertelorism Epicanthal folds Low-set ears
		Other:	Failure to thrive Various organ malformations
X (sex chromosome)	Only one X chromosome in female (Turner syndrome) 1 in 300 to 7000 live female births (Figure 9–13)	CNS:	No intellectual impairment Some perceptual difficulties
		Head:	Low hairline Webbed neck
		Trunk:	Short stature Cubitus valgus (increased carrying angle of arm) Excessive nevi Broad shieldlike chest with widely spaced nipples Puffy feet No toe nails
		Other:	Fibrous streaks in ovaries Underdeveloped secondary sex characteristics Primary amenorrhea Usually infertile Renal anomalies Coarctation of the aorta
X	Extra X in male (Klinefelter syndrome) 1 in 1000 live male births, approx. 1%–2% of institutionalized males (Figure 9–18)	CNS: Trunk:	Mild mental retardation Occasional gynecomastia Eunuchoid body proportions
		Other:	Small, soft testes Underdeveloped secondary sex characteristics Usually sterile

how much chromosomal material is involved, the clinical effects may be mild or severe. Many types of additions and deletions have been described, such as the deletion of the short arm of chromosome 5 (cri du chat syndrome) or the deletion of the long arm of chromosome 18 (see Table 9–5 and Figure 9–15).

○ *SEX CHROMOSOME ABNORMALITIES* To better understand normal X chromosome function and thus abnormalities of the sex chromosomes, the nurse should know that in females, at an early embryonic stage, one of the two normal X chromosomes becomes inactive. The inactive X chromosome forms a dark staining area known as the *Barr body,* or *sex chromatin body* (Figure 9–16).

The Barr body may be seen by examining the cells scraped from the inside of a woman's mouth. This procedure, the *buccal smear,* will show the number of inactivated X chromosomes or Barr bodies present. The normal

Table 9–6 Risk of Down Syndrome in Fetuses at Amniocentesis and in Live Births

Maternal age*	Frequency of Down syndrome	
	FETUSES	LIVE BIRTHS
–19	—	1/1550
20–24	—	1/1550
25–29	—	1/1050
30–34		1/700
35	1/350	1/350
36	1/260	1/300
37	1/200	1/225
38	1/160	1/175
39	1/125	1/150
40	1/70	1/100
41	1/35	1/85
42	1/30	1/65
43	1/20	1/50
44	1/13	1/40
45+	1/25	1/25

*Approximate (rounded) estimates chiefly from data of: Hook EB, Cross PK, Schreimachers DM: Chromosomal abnormality rates at amniocentesis and in live-born infants. JAMA 1983;249:2034.

female has one Barr body, since one of her two X chromosomes has been inactivated. The normal male has no Barr bodies, since he has only one X chromosome to begin with. The number of Barr bodies seen on the buccal smear *is always* one less than the number of X chromosomes present in the client's cells.

When Y cells are stained and viewed, the Y chromosome appears as a bright body within the nucleus (Figure 9–17). The number of Y bodies present is equal to the number of Y chromosomes present. Males should have one Y body, and females should have none.

The most common sex chromosome abnormalities are *Turner syndrome* in females (45,X with no Barr bodies present) and *Klinefelter syndrome* in males (47,XXY with one Barr body present) (Figure 9–18). See Table 9–5 for clinical description of these abnormalities. During the newborn period, clinical signs and symptoms of Turner syndrome are lymphedema of the dorsum of the hands and feet and excessive skin in the neck.

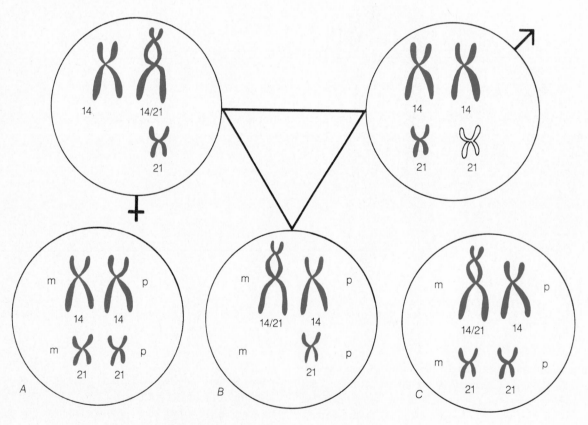

m = maternal origin
p = paternal origin

Figure 9–14 *Diagram of various types of offspring when mother has a balanced translocation between 14 and 21 and father has a normal arrangement of chromosomal material. A Normal offspring;*

B *Balanced translocation carrier; C Unbalanced translocation: Child has Down syndrome.*

Other sex chromosome abnormalities may occur. Whether it is an increased number of X chromosomes or Y chromosomes or both, the affected individual generally has an increased number of abnormalities and increased severity of mental retardation.

Patterns of Inheritance

Many inherited diseases are produced by an abnormality in a single gene or pair of genes. In such instances, the chromosomes are grossly normal. The defect is at the gene level and cannot be detected by present laboratory techniques. Therefore the pattern of inheritance for a particular disease or defect is determined by two methods: (a) close examination of the family in which the disease appears and (b) knowledge of how the disease has been previously inherited.

There are two major categories of inheritance: *Mendelian* or *single gene inheritance,* and *non-Mendelian,* or *multifactorial inheritance.* Each single-gene trait is determined by a pair of genes working together. These genes are re-

sponsible for the observable expression of the trait, referred to as the phenotype (eg, blue eyes, fair skin). The total genetic makeup of an individual is referred to as the genotype (ie, chromosomal structure). One of the genes for a trait is inherited from the mother; the other, from the father. An individual who has two identical genes at a given locus is considered to be *homozygous* for that trait. An individual is considered to be *heterozygous* for a particular trait when he or she has two different *alleles* (alternate forms of the same gene) at a given locus on a pair of homologous chromosomes.

The well-known modes of single-gene inheritance are autosomal dominant, autosomal recessive, and X-linked (sex-linked) recessive. There is also a less-common, X-linked dominant mode of inheritance.

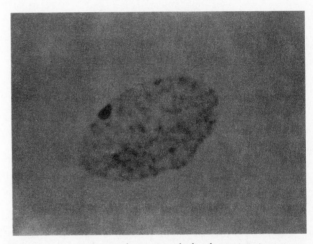

Figure 9–16   Nucleus with one Barr body; the patient is sex chromosome positive (Courtesy Dr Arthur Robinson, National Jewish Hospital and Research Center)

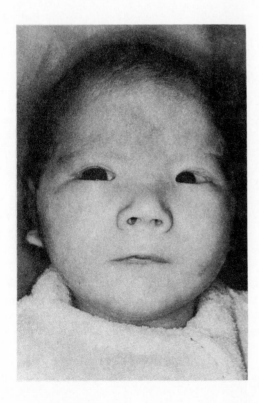

Figure 9–15   Infant with cri du chat syndrome resulting from deletion of part of the short arm of chromosome 5. Note characteristic facies with hypertelorism, epicanthus, and retrognathia. (From Thompson JS, Thompson MW: *Genetics in Medicine,* ed 4. Philadelphia, Saunders, 1986.)

Figure 9–17   Nucleus with a Y body present (Courtesy Dr Arthur Robinson, National Jewish Hospital and Research Center)

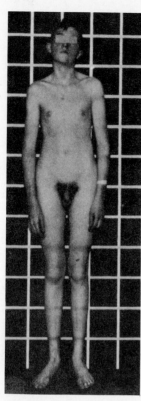

Figure 9-18 Boy with Klinefelter syndrome: 47, XXY karyotype. Note relatively small genitalia and long arms. Gynecomastia may or may not be present (From Smith DW: Recognizable Patterns of Human Malformations. Philadelphia, Saunders, 1982b.)

AUTOSOMAL DOMINANT INHERITANCE

An individual is said to have an autosomal dominantly inherited disorder if the disease trait is heterozygous. That is, the abnormal gene overshadows the normal gene of the pair to produce the trait. It is essential to remember that in autosomal dominant inheritance:

1. An affected individual generally has an affected parent. The family pedigree (graphic representation of a family tree) usually shows multiple generations having the disorder (Figure 9-19).

2. The affected individual has a 50 percent chance of passing on the abnormal gene to each of his or her offspring (Figure 9-19).

3. Both males and females are equally affected, and a father can pass the abnormal gene on to his son. This is an important principle when distinguishing autosomal dominant disorders from X-linked disorders.

4. An unaffected individual in most cases cannot transmit the disorder to his or her children.

5. A mutation or a change of a normal gene into a dominant abnormal gene is possible. In this case, this is the first time the disorder is seen in the family; an affected child is born to parents who are unaffected. In such instances, there is not an increased

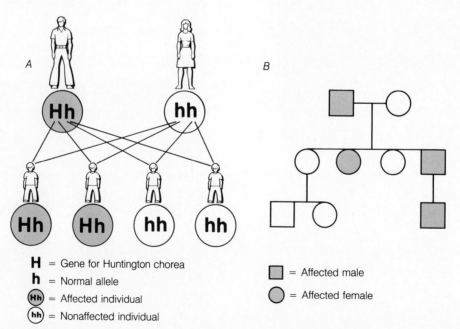

H = Gene for Huntington chorea
h = Normal allele
(Hh) = Affected individual
(hh) = Nonaffected individual

■ = Affected male
● = Affected female

Figure 9-19 A Autosomal dominant inheritance. One parent is affected. Statistically, 50 percent of offspring will be affected, regardless of sex. B Autosomal dominant pedigree

risk for future children of the same parents to be affected. The child, however, now has a 50 percent chance of passing the abnormal gene on to each of his or her offspring.

6. Autosomal dominant inherited disorders have varying degrees of presentation. This is an important factor when counseling families concerning autosomal dominant disorders. Although a parent may have a mild form of the disease, the child may have a more severe form. Unfortunately there is no method for predicting whether a child will be only mildly affected or more severely affected. The geneticist or health care provider must be thorough in the examination of family members to discern whether any of those individuals are indeed affected. They may express the disease in such a mild form that a cursory examination may miss clinical signs of the disease.

Some common autosomal dominantly inherited disorders are Huntington chorea, polycystic kidney disease, neurofibromatosis (von Recklinghausen disease), and achondroplastic dwarfism.

AUTOSOMAL RECESSIVE INHERITANCE

An individual has an autosomal recessively inherited disorder if the disease manifests itself only as a homozygous trait. That is, because the normal gene overshadows the abnormal one, the individual must have two abnormal genes to be affected. The notion of a *carrier state* is appropriate here. An individual who is heterozygous for the

abnormal gene is clinically normal. It is not until two individuals mate and pass on the same abnormal gene that affected offspring may appear. It is essential to remember that in autosomal recessive inheritance:

1. An affected individual has clinically normal parents, but they are both carriers of the abnormal gene (Figure 9–20).

2. Parents who are both carriers of the same abnormal gene have a 25 percent chance of both passing the abnormal gene on to any of their offspring (Figure 9–20).

3. If the offspring of two carrier parents is clinically normal, there is a 50 percent chance that he or she is a carrier of the gene (Figure 9–20).

4. Both males and females are equally affected.

5. The family pedigree usually shows siblings affected in a horizontal fashion (Figure 9–20). Future generations are not affected unless both parents carry the same abnormal gene.

6. There is often an increased incidence of consanguineous matings. Parents who are closely related are more likely to have the same genes in common than two parents who are unrelated.

7. Recessively inherited disorders tend to be more severe in their clinical manifestations. Clinically normal carrier parents pass on the disorder, and the affected offspring will often not reproduce. If an af-

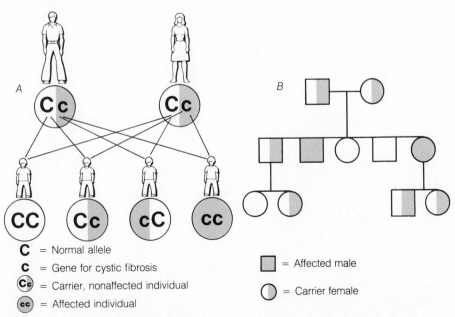

C = Normal allele
c = Gene for cystic fibrosis
Cc = Carrier, nonaffected individual
cc = Affected individual

= Affected male
= Carrier female

Figure 9–20   A Autosomal recessive inheritance. Both parents are carriers. Statistically, 25 percent of offspring are affected, regardless of sex. B Autosomal recessive pedigree

fected individual does reproduce, all the offspring will be carriers for the disorder.

8. The presence of the abnormal gene for some autosomal recessively inherited disorders can be detected in a normal carrier parent. For instance, Tay-Sachs disease is caused by an inborn error of metabolism—that is, a deficiency of the enzyme hexosaminidase A. An affected individual has little or no enzyme activity present, whereas a carrier parent usually has 50 percent normal enzyme activity present. Biochemically the carrier is abnormal, and the heterozygous state can be detected, even though it is asymptomatic.

Some common autosomal recessive inherited disorders are cystic fibrosis, phenylketonuria (PKU), galactosemia, sickle cell anemia, Tay-Sachs disease, and most metabolic disorders.

X-LINKED RECESSIVE INHERITANCE

X-linked or sex-linked disorders are those for which the abnormal gene is carried on the X chromosome. A female may be heterozygous or homozygous for a trait carried on the X chromosome, since she has two X chromosomes. A male, however, has only one X chromosome, and there are some traits for which no comparable genes are located on the Y chromosome. The male in this case is considered to be *hemizygous*, having only one alternate form of the gene instead of a pair for a given trait or disorder. Thus

an X-linked disorder is manifested in a male who carries the abnormal gene on his X chromosome. His mother is considered to be a carrier when the normal gene on one X chromosome overshadows the abnormal gene on the other X chromosome. It is essential to remember that in X-linked recessive inheritance:

1. There is no male-to-male transmission. Fathers pass only their Y chromosomes to their sons and their X chromosomes to their daughters. Daughters receive one X chromosome from the mother and one from the father.

2. Affected males are related through the female line (Figure 9–21B).

3. There is a 50 percent chance that a carrier mother will pass the abnormal gene to each of her sons, who will thus be affected. There is a 50 percent chance that a carrier mother will pass the normal gene to each of her sons, who will thus be unaffected. Finally, there is a 50 percent chance that a carrier mother will pass the abnormal gene to each of her daughters, who become carriers like their mother (Figure 9–21).

4. Fathers affected with an X-linked disorder cannot pass the disorder to their sons, but *all* their daughters become carriers of the disorder.

5. Occasionally, a female carrier may show some symptoms of an X-linked disorder. This situation is prob-

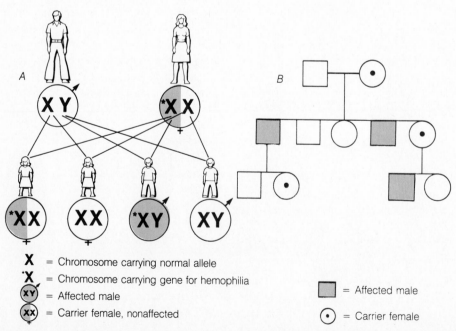

X = Chromosome carrying normal allele
˙X = Chromosome carrying gene for hemophilia
(XY) = Affected male
(XX) = Carrier female, nonaffected

☐ = Affected male
⊙ = Carrier female

Figure 9–21   A X-linked recessive inheritance. The mother is the carrier. Statistically, 50 percent of male offspring are affected, and 50 percent of female offspring are carriers. B X-linked pedigree

ably due to random inactivation of the X chromosome carrying the normal allele. Thus a heterozygous female may show some manifestation of an X-linked disorder.

Common X-linked recessive disorders are hemophilia, Duchenne muscular dystrophy, and color blindness.

X-LINKED DOMINANT INHERITANCE

X-linked dominant disorders are extremely rare, the most common being vitamin D-resistant rickets. When X-linked dominance does occur, the pattern is similar to X-linked recessive inheritance except that heterozygous females are affected. It is essential to remember that in X-linked dominant inheritance:

1. The abnormal gene is dominant and overshadows the normal gene on the female's other X chromosome.

2. There is no male-to-male transmission. An affected father will have affected daughters, but no affected sons.

A newly identified chromosomal disorder is the *fragile-X syndrome*. It is a central nervous system disorder linked to a "fragile site" on the X chromosome. This fragile site is seen when cells are grown in a folic acid–deficient media and detectable in both affected males and heterozygote carrier females (Shapiro 1982). Fragile-X syndrome is characterized by moderate mental retardation, large protuberant ears, and large testes after puberty (Thompson & Thompson 1986).

MULTIFACTORIAL (POLYGENIC) INHERITANCE

Many common congenital malformations, such as cleft palate, heart defects, spina bifida, dislocated hips, clubfoot, and pyloric stenosis are caused by an interaction of many genes and environmental factors. They are, therefore, multifactorial in origin. It is essential to remember that in multifactorial inheritance:

1. The malformations may vary from mild to severe. For example, spina bifida may range in severity from mild, as spina bifida occulta, to more severe, as a myelomeningocele. It is believed that the more severe the defect, the greater the number of genes present for that defect.

2. There is often a sex bias. Pyloric stenosis is more common in males, whereas cleft palate is more common among females. When a member of the less commonly affected sex shows the condition, a greater number of genes must usually be present to cause the defect.

3. In the presence of environmental influence (such as seasonal changes, altitude, irradiation, chemicals in the environment, or exposure to toxic substances), it may take fewer genes to manifest the disease in the offspring.

4. In contrast to single-gene disorders, there is an additive effect in multifactorial inheritance. The more family members who have the defect, the greater the risk that the next pregnancy will also be affected.

5. Risk factors are determined by the distribution of cases found in the general population. The risk of recurrence is usually 2 percent to 5 percent for all first-degree relatives (ie, parents, siblings, and offspring) if one family member is affected. The recurrence figure decreases with second-degree relatives (ie, grandparents, grandchildren, aunts, and uncles) and so forth.

Although most congenital malformations are polygenic traits, a careful family history should always be taken, since occasionally cleft lip and palate, certain congenital heart defects, and other malformations can be inherited as autosomal dominant or recessive traits. Other disorders thought to be within the multifactorial inheritance group are diabetes, hypertension, some heart diseases, and mental illness.

Nongenetic Conditions

Not all disorders or congenital malformations are inherited or have an inherited component. Malformations present at birth may represent an environmental insult during pregnancy, such as exposure to a drug or an infectious agent (see Chapter 16). Some malformations, however, cannot be explained by genetic mechanisms or teratogens. These disorders are considered to have a developmental cause. A couple who has a child with phocomelia (abnormality of the limbs), in the absence of any other problems or family history, may be reassured that the problem is developmental in etiology and the risk for future pregnancies is low. Such reassurance is also appropriate for families concerned about a child's seizures or developmental delays, if they can be attributed to an acquired problem.

Prenatal Diagnosis

Parent-child and family planning counseling have become a major responsibility of professional nurses. To be effective counselors, nurses must have the most current knowledge available concerning prenatal diagnosis.

It is essential that the couple be completely informed as to the known and potential risks of each of the genetic diagnostic procedures. The nurse must recognize the emotional impact on the family of a decision to have or not to have a genetic diagnostic procedure.

The ability to diagnose certain genetic diseases by various diagnostic tools has enormous implications for the practice of preventive health care. Several methods are available for prenatal diagnosis, although some are still being used on an experimental basis.

GENETIC ULTRASOUND

Ultrasound may be used to assess the fetus for genetic and/or congenital problems. With ultrasound, one can visualize the fetal head for abnormalities in size, shape, and structure. Craniospinal defects (anencephaly, microcephaly, hydrocephalus), gastrointestinal malformations (omphalocele, gastroschisis), renal malformations (dysplasias or obstruction), and skeletal malformations are only some of the disorders that have been diagnosed in utero by ultrasound. As ultrasound technology improves, the number of structural abnormalities being detected will increase. Screening for congenital anomalies is best done at 16 to 18 weeks when fetal structures have completed develop-

ment (Lange 1985). Information about possible harmful effects to either the mother or the fetus from exposure to ultrasound is still limited (Kremkau 1984). The ACOG recommends that ultrasound be used only in medically indicated situations.

GENETIC AMNIOCENTESIS

The major method of prenatal diagnosis is genetic amniocentesis (Figure 9–22). The procedure is described in Chapter 20. The indications for genetic amniocentesis include:

1. Advanced maternal age. Any woman 35 or older is at greater risk for having children with chromosome abnormalities. Approximately 85 percent of all amniocentesis is done because of advanced maternal age (Verp 1984). See Chapter 20 for further discussion. This maternal age effect is most pronounced for trisomy 21. For women over 35 the risk for having children with Down syndrome is 1 in 385; at age 39 the risk is 1 in 137, and at age 45 the risk is 1

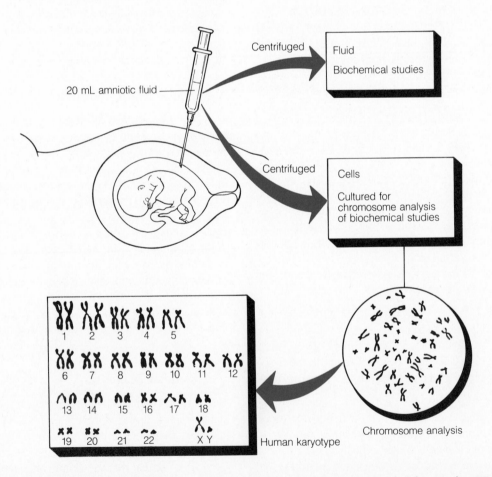

Figure 9–22   Genetic amniocentesis for prenatal diagnosis is done at 14 to 16 weeks' gestation. (Modified from Richie DD, Carola R: *Biology.* Reading, Mass, Addison-Wesley, 1979, p 302).

in 30 (Hook et al 1983). Table 9–6, on page 190, presents the risk of Down syndrome.

The occurrence of other autosomal trisomies (trisomy 13 and 18) also shows a correlation with increasing maternal age, although it is not as marked as in trisomy 21.

2. Previous child born with a chromosomal abnormality. Young couples who have had a child with trisomy 21 have approximately a 1 to 2 percent risk of a future child having a chromosome abnormality. Although no statistics of recurrence risks for other chromosome abnormalities have been established, genetic amniocentesis is made available to any couple who has already had a child with a chromosome abnormality.

3. Parent carrying a chromosomal abnormality (balanced translocation). Any couple in which one of the partners is a carrier of a balanced translocation should be considered for prenatal diagnosis. Although the person with the chromosome rearrangement is clinically normal, he or she has the potential for conceiving a child with an unbalanced chromosome constitution, which usually has substantial adverse effects on normal development. For example, a woman who carries a balanced 14/21 translocation has a risk of approximately 10 percent to 15 percent that her offspring will be affected with the unbalanced translocation of Down syndrome; if the father is the carrier, there is a 2 percent to 5 percent risk (Henry & Robinson 1978).

4. Mother carrying an X-linked disease. In families in which the woman is a known or possible carrier of an X-linked disorder, such as hemophilia or Duchenne muscular dystrophy, genetic amniocentesis may be an appropriate option for the family. These disorders are becoming increasingly diagnosable in utero. Since they usually affect only males, the sex of the fetus can be determined and termination of pregnancy considered when it is found to be male. For a known female carrier, the risk of an affected male fetus is 50 percent. The decision to abort a possibly normal male fetus must be discussed and made within each family. Similarly, couples in which the father is affected with an X-linked disorder may elect to have only male children so that the gene would not be continued in the family; all females (who would have to be carriers) could be aborted. Since many males with X-linked disorders, especially hemophilia, are surviving to reproduce as greater advances in medical treatment become available, genetic amniocentesis for these reasons may become more common.

5. Parents carrying an inborn error of metabolism that can be diagnosed in utero. The number of inherited metabolic disorders that can be diagnosed in utero is increasing at a rapid rate (Hogge & Golbus 1984)

Metabolic disorders detectable in utero include (partial list):
Argininosuccinicaciduria
Cystinosis
Fabry disease
Galactosemia
Gaucher disease
Homocystinuria
Hunter syndrome
Hurler disease
Krabbe disease
Lesch-Nyhan syndrome
Maple syrup urine disease
Metachromatic leukodystrophy
Methylmalonic aciduria
Niemann-Pick disease
Pompe disease
Sanfilippo syndrome
Tay-Sachs disease

6. Both parents carrying an autosomal recessive disease. When both parents are carriers of an autosomal recessive disease, there is a 25 percent risk for each pregnancy that the fetus will be affected. Diagnosis is made by testing the cultured amniotic fluid cells (either enzyme level, substrate level, or product level) or the fluid itself. Autosomal recessive diseases identified by amniocentesis are hemoglobinopathies such as sickle cell anemia and thalassemia. Most research to date has been in the prenatal diagnosis of hemoglobinopathies. Both sickle cell anemia and β-thalassemia once were diagnosed using fetal blood samples obtained by amnioscopy, which has 3 percent to 5 percent risk of fetal demise and spontaneous abortion. Now prenatal diagnosis of these conditions can be accomplished on uncultured amniotic fluid from an amniocentesis by a restriction endonuclease analysis of DNA test (Hogge & Golbus 1984).

Perhaps one of the most promising breakthroughs is the prenatal diagnosis of cystic fibrosis. Walsh and Nadler (1984) report reduced amounts of 4-methylumbelliferyl quanidinobenzoate (MUGB) reactive proteases in amniotic fluid samples from fetuses with cystic fibrosis. If these findings continue to be confirmed, the prenatal diagnosis of cystic fibrosis may become a reality (Brock et al 1985).

7. Family history of neural tube defects (anencephaly or spina bifida). Recently, genetic amniocentesis has been made available to those couples who have had

a child with neural tube defects or who have a family history of these conditions, which include anencephaly, spina bifida, and myelomeningocele. Neural tube defects are usually polygenic traits.

Regardless of the statistical risk for a given family, whether for an isolated neural tube defect or a disorder in which a neural tube defect is a constant feature, the risk of recurrence can be reduced (possibly by as much as 90 percent) through α-fetoprotein (AFP) determination of the amniotic fluid (Main & Mennuti 1986). Normally α-fetoprotein is a substance found in high levels in a developing fetus and in low levels in maternal serum and in amniotic fluid. In pregnancies in which the fetus has an open neural tube defect, α-fetoprotein leaks into the amniotic fluid and levels are elevated (Davis et al 1985). Thus, genetic amniocentesis allows those families for whom the risk of a neural tube defect is increased the opportunity to choose whether to have a child affected with such a disorder.

CHORIONIC VILLUS SAMPLING (CVS)

Chorionic villus sampling is a new technique that is used in selected regional centers. Its diagnostic capability is similar to amniocentesis. Its advantage is that diagnostic information is available before the completion of the first trimester of pregnancy. (For further discussion, see Chapter 20.)

AMNIOGRAPHY AND AMNIOSCOPY

Amniography (instillation of dye into the amniotic cavity to outline the fetus) and aminoscopy (direct visualization of the fetus through a scope) are two methods of prenatal diagnosis that are not yet available for general clinical use. These methods are used primarily to observe the fetus for major structural abnormalities or to obtain fetal blood and tissue.

IMPLICATIONS OF PRENATAL DIAGNOSTIC TESTING

With the advent of diagnostic techniques such as amniocentesis, couples at risk, who would not otherwise have additional children, can decide to conceive. The percentage of therapeutic abortions after amniocentesis is small; most couples find peace of mind throughout the remainder of the pregnancy after prenatal diagnosis.

After prenatal diagnosis, a couple can decide not to have a child with a genetic disease. For many couples, however, prenatal diagnosis is not a solution, since the only method of preventing a genetic disease is preventing the birth by aborting the affected fetus. This decision can only be made by the family.

Genetic counselors do, however, discuss with the family all available options if an abnormal fetus is discovered or suspected. A couple is at the same risk as the general population or at the risk calculated for their individual cases based on their family history for any other disorder. It becomes imperative, then, that preamniocentesis counseling precede any procedure for prenatal diagnosis. Many questions and points must be considered if the family is to reach a satisfactory decision.

Prenatal diagnosis cannot guarantee the birth of a normal child. It can only determine the presence or absence of specific disorders (within the limits of laboratory error). Nonspecific mental retardation, cleft lip and palate, and PKU are a few of the disorders that cannot be determined by intrauterine diagnosis.

In the future, cure or treatment of diagnosable disorders may be possible. Prenatal diagnosis may allow for treatment to begin during the pregnancy, thus possibly preventing irreversible damage. For other disorders, effective postnatal treatment may make prenatal diagnosis unnecessary. The ability to diagnose many diseases in utero is proved every day. In light of the philosophy of preventive health care, this information should be made available to all couples who are expecting a child or who are contemplating pregnancy.

Postnatal Diagnosis

Questions concerning genetic disorders, cause, treatment, and prognosis are most often first discussed in the newborn nursery or during the infant's first few months of life. When a child is born with anomalies, has a stormy neonatal period, or does not progress as expected, a genetic evaluation may well be warranted.

Accurate diagnosis and optimal treatment plan incorporates a complete and detailed history, pedigree, thorough physical examination, dermatoglyphic analysis, and laboratory analysis. To make an accurate diagnosis the geneticist consults with other specialists and reviews the current literature. This permits the geneticist to evaluate all the available information before arriving at a diagnosis and plan of action.

PHYSICAL EXAMINATION

The physical examination is paramount in helping to establish the diagnosis. The geneticist must attend to minute details and look for specific patterns of abnormalities. Two major questions should be kept in mind: Is just one organ system involved or are multiple systems involved? Does the abnormality have a prenatal or postnatal onset? If only a single malformation is present, such as cleft palate, or only one organ system is involved (the skin), the geneticist tends to think in terms of polygenic, single-gene disorders, or developmental causes. If multiple malformations are present, chromosomal and teratogenic causes are often the first possibilities to consider. Many chromosomal abnormalities and single-gene disorders are associated with a specific pattern of malformations. Thus one must have expertise in syndrome recognition to be able to arrive at an accurate diagnosis.

DERMATOGLYPHIC ANALYSIS

Dermatoglyphics (Figure 9–23) are the patterns of the ridged skin found on the fingers, palms, toes, and soles (Thompson & Thompson 1986). Although each individual has a unique ridge pattern, specific types of patterns exist that can be systematically classified. Since differentiation of dermal ridges is complete by the end of the fourth month of gestation, many genetic disorders that affect multiple systems also affect the dermatoglyphics. Thus, a child with a chromosomal abnormality often exhibits certain characteristic dermatoglyphics.

Pattern combinations and frequencies considered together are more significant than pattern types alone. In Down syndrome or any other abnormality, any one of the particular specific patterns seen can also be found in normal individuals. It is when these patterns are in *combination* that they are associated with a specific disorder, such as Down syndrome.

Children with Down syndrome often have a single flexion crease (simian line) on the palms, an increased number of ulnar loops on the fingertips (often on all ten fingers), and a characteristic pattern on the soles of the feet (the hallucal pattern), known as an arch tibial (Figure 9–23). Children with trisomy 13 are found to have an increase in the number of arch patterns on the fingertips and

also single flexion creases of the palms (Thompson & Thompson 1986). Chromosome abnormalities are only one area in which unusual dermatoglyphics have been described and can be associated with other single-gene or polygenic disorders.

LABORATORY ANALYSIS

Laboratory studies include chromosome analysis (discussed on p 196), enzyme assays, and serologic and microscopic studies. Enzyme assays are performed to diagnose inherited metabolic diseases. These usually are done if the result on newborn screening is abnormal or if the child has any combination of the following: nausea and vomiting, enlarged viscera, poor feeding, lethargy, and seizures. Metabolic abnormalities should also be considered in any child who does well during the neonatal period with normal developmental milestones, but then deteriorates, particularly in CNS functioning. The major assays done are of amino and organic acids. Other specific enzyme assays are performed only if the clinical picture warrants doing them.

As mentioned, some genetic disorders are identified on newborn screening. Many institutions now screen for six inborn errors of metabolism: PKU, galactosemia, hypothyroidism, sickle cell anemia, maple syrup urine disease, and homocystinuria. These tests all use the same dried blood spot. The major purpose of these screening programs is to identify affected newborns as soon as possible after birth so that corrective treatment can be instituted before irreversible damage is done. (See Chapter 32 for further discussion of these conditions.)

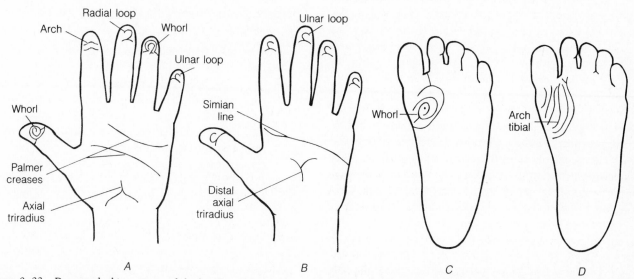

Figure 9–23 Dermatoglyphic patterns of the hands and feet in a normal individual (A and C) and those commonly found in a child with Down syndrome (B and D). Note the simian line, distally placed axial triradius, and increased number of ulnar loops on the hand and the arch tibial pattern on the hallucal area of the foot.

Other laboratory analyses that may be appropriate are serologic and microbiologic studies to identify infectious teratogens, such as a serum TORCH screen. The TORCH screen tests the child's serum for antibodies against toxoplasmosis, rubella, cytomegalovirus, and herpesvirus type 2 (see Chapter 19).

The Family, The Nurse, and The Genetic Counseling Process

Genetic counseling is a communication process in which the genetic counselor tries to provide a family with the most complete and accurate information on the occurrence or the risk of recurrence of a genetic disease in that family. The goals inherent in this definition are threefold. First, genetic counseling allows families to make informed decisions about reproduction. Second, it assists families in assessing the available treatments, examining appropriate alternatives to decrease the risk, learning about the usual course and outcome of the genetic disease or abnormality, and dealing with the psychologic and social implications that often accompany such problems. Finally, it is hoped that genetic counseling will help decrease the incidence and impact of genetic disease. The use of a team approach and appropriate timing are important considerations in genetic counseling.

TEAM APPROACH

Because genetic counseling is a complex and multidimensional process, it cannot be done efficiently or effectively in isolation. The genetics team consists of health professionals and scientists with a variety of backgrounds and expertise. The genetics unit itself usually includes a medical geneticist, a genetic associate, and/or a nurse-geneticist. Often a social worker is directly involved. This group works closely with cytogeneticists, biochemists, and other specialty groups to clarify the situation for families. Many genetics groups also work closely with clergy and family support groups to provide the family with additional resources.

The genetics team continually tries to inform and assist the primary health care provider before, during, and after counseling. Ideally, the primary physician or nurse clinician will feel free to consult the genetics team as a resource group for information, assistance, and support in the care of their clients.

TIMING

Timing is an important aspect of the counseling process. When should genetic counseling be initiated? Preferably, counseling should be *prospective*—before the birth of an affected child. Increasing numbers of young couples who are contemplating childbearing are seeking genetic counseling to discover their risk of having children with an abnormality or genetic disease. However, many genetic diseases do not present themselves until after an affected child is born. Genetic counseling in this case is *retrospective*.

In retrospective genetic counseling, time is a crucial factor. One cannot expect a family who has just learned that their child has a birth defect or has Down syndrome to assimilate any information concerning future risks. However, the couple should never be "put off" from counseling for too long a period, only to find that they have borne another affected child. Here the nurse can be instrumental in directing the parents into counseling at the appropriate time. At the birth of an affected child, the nurse can inform the parents that genetic counseling is available before they attempt having another child. Asking one or two members of a genetics team to introduce themselves to the family is often enough to bring up the subject of genetic counseling. When the parents have begun to recover from the initial shock of bearing a child with an abnormality, or when they begin to contemplate having more children, the nurse can encourage the couple to seek counseling.

THE NURSE'S ROLE

Nurses who are aware of families at an increased risk for having a child with a genetic disorder are in an ideal position to make referrals. Genetic counseling is an appropriate course of action for any family wondering, "Will it happen again?" The nursery nurse frequently has the first contact with the family and newborn with a congenital abnormality. The family nurse practitioner or family-planning nurse is in an excellent position to reach at-risk families before the birth of another baby with a congenital problem. Genetic counseling referral is advised for any of the following categories:

1. *Congenital abnormalities, including mental retardation.* Any couple who has a child or a relative with a congenital malformation may be at an increased risk and should be so informed. If mental retardation of unidentified cause has occurred in a family, there may be an increased risk of recurrence.

   In many cases, the genetic counselor will identify the cause of a malformation as a teratogen (see Chapter 16). The family should be aware of teratogenic substances so they can avoid exposure during any subsequent pregnancy.

2. *Familial disorders.* Families should be told that certain diseases may have a genetic component and that the risk of their occurrence in a particular family may be higher than that for the general population. Such disorders as diabetes, heart disease, cancer, and mental illness fall into this category.

3. *Known inherited diseases.* Families may know that a disease is inherited but not know the mechanism or the specific risk for them. An important point to remember is that family members who are not at risk for passing on a disorder should be as well informed as family members who are.

4. *Metabolic disorders.* Any families at risk for having a child with a metabolic disorder or biochemical defect should be referred. Because most inborn errors of metabolism are autosomal recessively inherited ones, a family may not be identified as at risk until the birth of an affected child.

Carriers of the sickle cell trait can be identified before pregnancy is begun, and the risk of having an affected child can be determined. Prenatal diagnosis of an affected fetus is available on an experimental basis only.

5. *Chromosomal abnormalities.* As discussed previously, any couple who has had a child with a chromosomal abnormality may be at an increased risk of having another child similarly affected. This group would include families in which there is concern for a possible translocation.

The process of genetic counseling usually begins after the birth of a child diagnosed as having a congenital abnormality or genetic disease. After the parents have been referred to the genetic clinic, they are sent a form requesting information on the health status of various family members. The nurse can help by discussing the form with the

family or clarifying the information needed to complete it. A pedigree and history facilitate identification of other family members who might also be at risk for the same disorder. The family being counseled may wish to notify those relatives at risk so that they, too, can be given genetic counseling. When done correctly, the family history and pedigree become one of the most powerful and useful tools for determining a family risk.

A screening pedigree generally includes the affected individual, siblings, parents, aunts and uncles, and grandparents (Figure 9–24). If the family does not have all the necessary information at hand, the nurse can urge them to obtain the information in time for their first genetic counseling session, when a more complete pedigree will be taken.

The pedigree is a fairly easy and productive method for screening families. The nurse can obtain the necessary information and draw a screening pedigree in approximately 15 minutes. Information that should be obtained when drawing the family pedigree includes names (maiden names if appropriate) and birth dates of members of the immediate family; names and ages of the remainder of the family (including deceased members), with a description of their health status; causes of death of family members; and any other information the family feels is significant. In discussing the affected individual, the nurse should obtain information on the pregnancy history of the mother (including miscarriages), medications and drugs taken during pregnancy, x-ray exposure, infections or illness during pregnancy, the type of birth control used prior to pregnancy, and the method used to diagnose the pregnancy. A

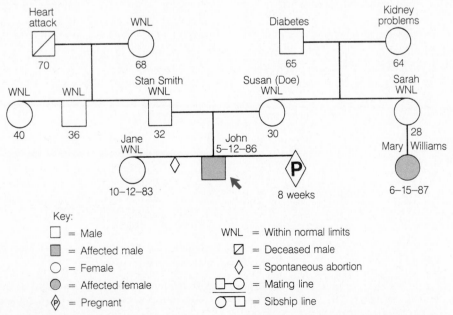

Figure 9–24 Screening pedigree. Arrow indicates the nearest family member affected with the disorder being investigated. Basic *data have been recorded. Numbers refer to the ages of the family members.*

complete delivery history should be taken, including a description of any complications. It is also appropriate for the nurse to ask the family when the problem was evident to them or was diagnosed.

The nurse should inquire about the affected child's growth and development. The information obtained should include developmental milestones, growth in comparison to siblings or other children the same age, symptoms of a problem, school records, and any previous testing.

Finally, information concerning ethnic background, family origin, and/or religion should be elicited. Many genetic disorders are more common among certain ethnic groups or more commonly found in particular geographic areas. For example, families from the British Isles are at higher risk of having children with neural tube defects; the Ashkenazi Jews are at higher risk for being carriers of Tay-Sachs disease; blacks have a high risk of sickle cell anemia; and people of Mediterranean heritage have a higher risk of thalassemias.

○ *FOLLOW-UP COUNSELING* When all the data have been carefully examined and analyzed, the family returns for a follow-up visit. At this time, the parents are given all the information available, including the medical facts, diagnosis, probable course of the disorder, and any available management; the inheritance pattern for this particular family and their risk of recurrence; and the options or alternatives for dealing with the risk of recurrence. The remainder of the counseling session is spent discussing the course of action that seems appropriate to the family in view of their risk and family goals.

Among those options or alternatives are prenatal diagnosis and early detection and treatment, and in some cases, adoption, artificial insemination, or delayed childbearing.

The family may consider *artificial insemination by donor* (AID), discussed earlier in this chapter. This alternative is appropriate in several instances; for example, if the male partner is affected with an autosomal dominant disease, AID would decrease the risk of having an affected child to zero, since the child would not inherit any genes from the affected parent. If the man is affected with an X-linked disorder and does not wish to continue the gene in the family (all his daughters will be carriers), AID would be an alternative to terminating all pregnancies with a female fetus. If the man is a carrier for a balanced translocation and if termination of pregnancy is against family ethics, AID is the most appropriate alternative. AID is also appropriate if both parents are carriers of an autosomal recessive disease. AID lowers the risk to a very low level or to zero if a carrier test is available. Finally, AID may be appropriate if the family is at high risk for a polygenic disorder.

Couples who are young and at risk may decide to delay childbearing for a few years. Medical science and medical genetics are continually making breakthroughs in early detection and treatment. These couples may find in a few years that prenatal diagnosis will be available or that a disease can be detected and treated early to prevent irreversible damage.

When the parents have completed the counseling sessions, the counselor sends them a letter detailing the contents of the sessions. The family keeps this document for reference.

The family may return a number of times to air their questions and concerns. It is most desirable for the nurse working with the family to attend many or all of these counseling sessions. Since the nurse has already established a rapport with the family, the nurse can act as a liaison between the family and the genetic counselor. Hearing directly what the genetic counselor says helps the nurse clarify issues for the family, which in turn helps them formulate questions.

Perhaps one of the most important and crucial aspects of genetic counseling in which the nurse is involved is follow-up counseling. The nurse with the appropriate knowledge of genetics is in an ideal position to help families review what has been discussed during the counseling sessions and to answer any additional questions they might have. As the family returns to the daily aspects of living, the nurse can provide helpful information on the day-to-day aspects of caring for the child, answer questions as they arise, support parents in their decisions, and refer the family to other health and community agencies.

If the couple is considering having more children or if siblings want information concerning their affected brother or sister, the nurse should recommend that the family return for another follow-up visit with the genetic counselor. Appropriate options can again be defined and discussed, and any new information available can be given to the family. Many genetic centers have found the public health nurse to be the ideal health professional to provide such follow-up care.

KEY CONCEPTS

A couple is considered infertile after one year of unprotected coitus.

At least 2.8 million couples in the United States have undesired infertility.

A thorough history and physical of both partners is essential as a basis for infertility investigation.

General areas of fertility investigation are evaluation of ovarian function, cervical mucus adequacy and recep-

tivity to sperm, sperm adequacy, tubal patency, general condition of the pelvic organs, and certain laboratory tests.

Among cases of infertility, 40 percent involve male factors, 10 percent to 15 percent involve female hormonal defects, 20 percent to 30 percent involve female tubal disorders, 5 percent involve cervical factors, 10 percent to 20 percent have no identifiable cause, and 35 percent have multifactorial etiologies.

Medications may be prescribed to induce ovulation, facilitate cervical mucus formation, reduce antibody concentration, increase sperm count and motility, and suppress endometriosis.

The emotional aspect of infertility may be more difficult for the couple than the testing and therapy.

Based on a sound knowledge base regarding common genetic problems, the nurse should initiate referrals, prepare the family for counseling, and act as a resource person during and after the counseling sessions.

Those genetic conditions that can currently be diagnosed prenatally are craniospinal defects; renal malformations; hemophilia; fragile-X syndrome; thalassemia; cystic fibrosis; many inborn errors of metabolism, such as Tay-Sachs disease or maple syrup urine disease; and neural tube defects.

Autosomal dominant disorders are characterized by an affected parent who has a 50 percent chance of having an affected child and equally affects both males and females. The characteristic presentation will vary in each individual with the gene. Some of the common autosomal dominant inherited disorders are Huntington chorea, polycystic kidney, and neurofibromatosis (von Recklinghausen disease).

Autosomal recessive disorders are characterized by both parents being carriers; each offspring having a 25 percent chance of having the disease, a 25 percent chance of not being affected, and a 50 percent chance of being a carrier; and males and females being equally affected. Some common autosomal recessive inheritance disorders are cystic fibrosis, PKU, galactosemia, sickle cell anemia, Tay-Sachs disease, and most metabolic disorders.

X-linked recessive disorders are characterized by no male-to-male transmission; effects limited to males, a 50 percent chance that a carrier mother will pass the abnormal gene to her son, a 50 percent chance that she will not transmit the abnormal gene to her son, a 50 percent chance that a daughter will be a carrier, and a 100 percent chance that daughters of affected fathers will be carriers. Common X-linked recessive disorders are hemophilia, color blindness, and Duchenne disease.

Multifactorial inheritance disorders include cleft lip and palate, spina bifida, dislocated hips, clubfoot, and pyloric stenosis.

The chief tools of prenatal diagnosis are ultrasound, amniocentesis, and chorionic villus sampling.

REFERENCES

Andrew LB: *New Conceptions: A Consumers Guide to the Newest Infertility Treatments.* New York, St. Martin's Press, 1984.

Ansbacher R: Male infertility. *Clin Obstet Gynecol* 1982;25(3):461.

Attending OB/GYN Patients, Nursing 86 Books. Springhouse, Pa, Springhouse Corp, 1986.

Barkay J, et al: The prostaglandin inhibitory effect of anti-inflammatory drugs in the therapy of male infertility. *Fertil Steril* 1984;42(3):406.

Berg B: Early signs of infertility. *Ms* 1984;6(8):72.

Brock DJH, et al: Prospective prenatal diagnosis of cystic fibrosis. *Lancet* 1985;1:1175.

Bronson R, et al: Sperm antibodies: Their role in infertility. *Fertil Steril* 1984;42:(2):171.

Bultram VC, **Belne** JB, **Reiter** R: Interim report of a study of danazol for the treatment of endometriosis. *Fertil Steril* 1982;37:478.

Coulam CB: The diagnosis and management of infertility, in **Sciarra** JJ, et al (eds): *Gynecology and Obstetrics.* Hagerstown, Md, Harper & Row, 1982, vol 5.

Creighton H: In vitro fertilization. *Nurs Manage* 1985;16(April):12.

Daly DC: Hysteroscopy and infertility, in **Sciarra** JJ, et al (eds): *Gynecology and Obstetrics.* Hagerstown, Md, Harper & Row, 1986, vol 5.

Darland NW: Infertility associated with luteal phase defect. *J Obstet Gynecol Neonat Nurs* 1985;14(May/June):212.

Davis RO, et al: Decreased levels of amniotic fluid alpha-fetoprotein associated with Down syndrome. *Am J Obstet Gynecol:* (November) 1985, 185:541.

Dodson MG: A detailed program review of in vitro fertilization with a discussion and comparison of alternative approaches. *Surg Gynecol & Obstet* 1986;162(January):89.

Fogel CL, **Woods** NP: *Health Care of Women.* St. Louis, Mosby, 1981.

Glass RH: Infertility, in **Glass** RH (ed): *Office Gynecology,* ed 2. Baltimore, Williams & Wilkins, 1981.

Hammond M, **Talbert** L: *Infertility.* Oradell, NJ, Medical Economics Books, 1985.

Henry GP, **Robinson** A: Prenatal diagnosis. *Clin Obstet Gynecol* 1978;21:329.

Hogge WA, **Golbus** MS: Antenatal diagnosis of mendelian disorders, in **Sciarra** JJ, et al (eds): *Gynecology and Obstetrics.* Hagerstown, Md, Harper & Row, 1984, vol 3.

Hook EB: Rates of chromosome abnormalities of different maternal ages. *Obstet Gynecol* 1981;58:282.

Hook EB, **Cross** PK, **Schreimachers** DM: Chromosomal abnormality rates at amniocentesis and in live-born infants. *JAMA* 1983;249:2034.

Jackson L: Prenatal genetic diagnosis by chorionic villus sampling (CVS). *Semin Perinatol* 1985;9(April):209.

Kremkau F: Safety and long term effects of ultrasound. *Clin Obstet Gynecol* 1984;27(2):269.

Lange IR: Congenital anomalies: Detection and strategies for management. *Semin Perinatol* 1985;9(October):151.

La Nasa J: Office evaluation of the infertile couple. *Urol Clin North Am* 1980;7:121.

Lemli L, **Smith** DW: The XO syndrome: A study of the differentiated phenotype in 25 patients. *J Pediatr* 1963;63:577.

Loucopoulos A, et al: Pulsatile administrations of gonadotropin-releasing hormone for induction of ovulation. *Am J Obstet Gynecol* 1984;148:895.

Main DM, **Mennuti** MT: Neural tube defects: Issues in prenatal diagnosis and counseling. *Obstet Gynecol* 1986;67(January):1.

McShane PM, **Schiff** I, and **Trentham** DE: Cellular immunity to sperm in infertile women. *JAMA* 1985; 253(24):3555.

Menning BE: The emotional needs of the infertile couple. *Fertil Steril* 1980;34(4):313.

Moghissi K, **Wallach** E: Unexplained infertility. *Fertil Steril* 1983;39:5.

Mosher WF: Reproductive impairment among married couples in the U.S. *Natl Fam Growth Ser* 1983;23:11.

Phillips M: One woman's courage. *Am Health,* November 1985, p 76.

Poon WW, **McCoshen** JA: Variances in mucus architecture as a cause of cervical factor infertility. *Fertil Steril* 1985;44(3):361.

Richie DD, **Carola** R: *Biology.* Reading, Mass, Addison-Wesley, 1979.

Sawatzky M: Tasks of the infertile couple. *J Obstet Gynecol Neonat Nurs* 1981;10:132.

Schmickel RD: Chromosomal deletions and enzyme deficiencies. *J Pediatr* 1986;108(2):244.

Shane JM, **Schiff** I, **Wilson** EA: The infertile couple. *Clin Symp* 1976;28(5):2.

Shapiro LR, et al: Prenatal diagnosis of fragile X chromosome. *Lancet* 1982;1:99.

Smith C: Drug effects on male sexual function. *Clin Obstet Gynecol* 1982a;25:525.

Smith DW: *Recognizable Patterns of Human Malformations.* Philadelphia, Saunders, 1982b.

Smith P: Ovulation induction. *J Obstet Gynecol Neonat Nurs* 1985;14(November/December):37s.

Speroff L, **Glass** RH, **Kase** NG: *Clinical Gynecologic Endocrinology and Infertility,* ed 3. Baltimore, Williams & Wilkins, 1983.

Sogor L: Immune aspects of infertility, in **Sciarra** JJ, et al (eds): *Gynecology and Obstetrics.* Hagerstown, Md, Harper & Row, 1986, vol 5.

Templeton A, **Penney** G: The incidence, characteristics, and prognosis of patients whose infertility is unexplained. *Fertil Steril* 1982;37:175.

Thompson JS, **Thompson** MW: *Genetics in Medicine,* ed 4. Philadelphia, Saunders, 1986.

Valle RF: How endoscopy aids the infertility workup. *Contemp OB/GYN* 1984;23:191.

Verp MS: Antenatal diagnosis of chromosome abnormalities, in **Sciarra** JJ, et al (eds): *Gynecology and Obstetrics.* Hagerstown, Md, Harper & Row, 1984, vol 3.

Walsh MMJ, **Nadler** HL: Methylumbelliferyl quanidinobenzoate-reactive proteases in human amniotic fluid: Promising market for the intrauterine detection in cystic fibrosis. *Am J Obstet Gynecol* 1984;137:978.

Wentz AC: Progesterone therapy of the inadequacy luteal phase. *Cur Prob Obstet Gynecol* 1982;6:1.

Zacur H, **Rock** J: Diagnosis and treatment of infertility. *Female Patient* 1983;8:52.

ADDITIONAL READINGS

Carothers GP: Down syndrome and maternal age: The effect of erroneous assignment of parental origin. *Am J Human Genetics* 1987;40(February):147.

Clapp D: Emotional responses to infertility: Nursing interventions. *J Obstet Gynecol Neonat Nurs* 1985; 14(November/December):32.

Cohen FL: *Clinical Genetics in Nursing Practice.* Philadelphia, Lippincott, 1984.

Christianson C: Support groups for infertile patients. *J Obstet Gynecol Neonat Nurs* 1986;15(July/August):293.

Embury SH, et al: Rapid prenatal diagnosis of sickle cell anemia by a new method of DNA analysis. *N Engl J Med* 1987;316(March 12):656.

Fayez JA, et al: The diagnostic value of hysterosalpingography and hysteroscopy in infertility investigation. *Am J Obstet Gynecol* 1987;156(March):558.

Feichtinger W, **Kemeter** P (eds): *Future Aspects in Human In Vitro Fertilization.* New York, Springer-Verlag, 1987.

Hearn MT, et al: Psychological characteristics of in vitro fertilization participants. *Am J Obstet Gynecol* 1987; 156(February):269.

Keating C: The impact of sexually transmitted diseases on human fertility. *Health Care Women Inter* 1987;8(1):33.

Kogan BA, et al: Fertility in cryptorchism: Further development of an experimental model. *J Urol* 1987; 137(January):128.

Olshansky EF: Identity of self as infertile: An example of theory-generating research. *ANS* 1987;9(January):54.

Pace-Owens S: In vitro fertilization and embryo transfer. *J Obstet Gynecol Neonat Nurs* 1985;14(November/December):44.

Policy Statement for maternal serum alpha-fetoprotein screening program. *Am J Human Genetics* 1987; 40(February):75.

Sandelowski M, et al: Women's experiences of infertility. *Image* 1986;18(Winter):140.

Schlaff WD: New ways to prepare semen for IUI. *Contemp OB/GYN* 1987;29(April):79.

Schulman JD, et al: Outpatient in vitro fertilization using transvaginal ultrasound guided oocyte retrieval. *Obstet Gynecol* 1987;69(April):665.

Schuwager EJ, **Weiss** BD: Prenatal testing for maternal serum alpha-fetoprotein. *Am Fam Physician* 1987; 35(April):169.

Sermer M, et al: Prenatal diagnosis and management of congenital defects of the anterior abdominal wall. *Am J Obstet Gynecol* 1987;156(February):308.

Simpson JL, **Nadler** HL: Maternal serum alpha-fetoprotein screening in 1987. *Obstet Gynecol* 1987;69(January):134.

Sokoloff BZ: Alternative methods of reproduction: Effects on the child. *Clin Pediatr* 1987;26(January):11.

Syrop CH, **Halme** J: Cyclic changes of peritoneal fluid parameters in normal and infertile patients. *Obstet Gynecol* 1987;69(March pt 1):416.

Wallach EE, et al: Ethical dilemmas of infertility. *Contemp OB/GYN* 1987;29(March):170.

Williamson RA, et al: Abnormal pregnancy sonogram: Selective indications for fetal karyotype. *Obstet Gynecol* 1987;69(January):15.

Ying YK, et al: Luteal phase defect and premenstrual syndrome in an infertile population. *Obstet Gynecol* 1987;69(January):96.

I was sure John must hate me for not being able to have a child like other women. No matter what he said, I was convinced he would want a divorce. I pounced on every ambiguous comment. Every time he turned his head the wrong way or came home five minutes late—everything was proof that our marriage was over. And I guess I started acting cold toward him, withdrawing into myself as protection. We finally had it out one night. When I told him what I felt, he was shocked. He said he was distant because he was feeling bad about the baby and didn't know how to talk to me about it. Once we started to talk, I realized my worry about divorce had been only in my own mind. (When Pregnancy Fails)

Disorders of the Female Reproductive System

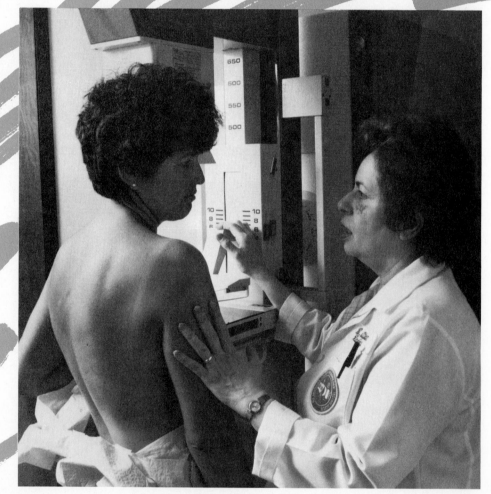

It is especially important for the nurse to provide emotional support during a mammogram and other procedures that aid in the diagnosis of breast disorders.

Chapter Ten

OBJECTIVES

- **Compare the common benign breast disorders.**
- **Describe the tests available to diagnose carcinoma of the breast.**
- **Develop a plan of care to meet the nursing needs of a woman with cancer of the breast.**
- **Discuss the signs, symptoms, and treatment of endometriosis.**
- **Describe toxic shock syndrome.**
- **Compare the common sexually transmitted diseases with regard to causative organism, signs and symptoms, treatment, and long-term implications.**

- **Summarize health teaching the nurse should provide to a woman with a sexually transmitted disease.**
- **Relate the development and progress of pelvic inflammatory disease to the possible development of infertility.**
- **Identify diagnostic measures that should be employed to establish a diagnosis when a woman has an abnormal finding during a pelvic examination.**
- **Compare lower urinary tract infections with upper urinary tract infections.**

Throughout her life span the contemporary woman is likely to encounter various major or minor gynecologic and urinary problems, and some women will face disorders of the breast. These problems may provoke a variety of psychologic responses and physical concerns. A woman's encounters with health care providers may be satisfying or complex, frustrating, and disappointing. Traditional health care professionals have tended to view women as passive and indecisive and have, therefore, often treated them in an insensitive or patronizing manner. As women become better able to speak up for their right to effective and respectful care, this traditional approach is becoming less prevalent.

A woman expects a health care provider to provide information about such concerns as: Is my condition contagious? Is it my fault? What did I do wrong? Will it recur? Will the medication work? Does it have side effects? Is the problem serious?

Nurses can assist women by providing them with accurate, sensitive, and supportive health education and counseling. The nurse's role is to assess the woman's needs, determine nursing diagnoses, plan interventions and follow-up, and evaluate the effectiveness of the care provided. As part of this process the nurse can clarify misconceptions and handle psychosocial aspects of specific health problems that concern the woman.

To meet the woman's needs the nurse needs up-to-date information about the various diagnostic and treatment options available. This chapter provides general information about breast disorders, followed by information about gynecologic and urinary problems.

- ## The Female Breast

Psychosocial Considerations

In the United States today, the female breast is the primary symbol of female sexuality. Idealized images of "perfect" breasts are used by the media to sell all manner of products and services. Yet there is a strong cultural taboo against exposing the breasts in the everyday environment. The breasts revealed in popular periodicals and in advertisements are the breasts of women with very restricted, glamorous physical qualifications, and the focus of these glorified images has been on the erotic function of the breast. The primary function of the female breast, nourishment of the infant, has been virtually ignored. These cultural attitudes have had profound effects on the body image of the contemporary woman.

According to developmental theory, secondary sexual characteristics, especially the breasts, are vital to the adolescent female's concept of her body image. Her breasts are visible both to herself and to others; she can observe their development. Her primary sexual organs cannot be observed. Breast development provides visual confirmation that the adolescent is becoming a woman.

Earlier studies corroborated an association between physical attractiveness and feelings of self-worth and self-acceptance. Various investigators have observed that women have positive feelings when their bodies correspond to the "ideal." From this observation, some authors concluded that women might base their status and security on their attractiveness to men (Bard & Sutherland 1955, Jourand & Secord 1955). More recent observers have suggested that the breasts are a prized physical attribute and a means of attracting men and therefore are a part of a women's overall feminine identity (Hyde 1979).

Others have proposed a slightly different analysis, observing that the actual physical appearance of a female's breasts is less important than her individualized interpretation of what her breasts mean to her as a woman and as a sexual being (Wabrek and Wabrek 1979). These authors believe that there is a complex interaction among the cultural psychologic factors that determine the individual meaning of the breasts for each woman. Consequently, each woman translates the idealized media images and her own degree of acceptance of her real breasts into something uniquely meaningful to her.

Normal Cyclic Changes in the Nonlactating Breast

Like the uterus, the breast functions dynamically in a cyclic process that is regulated by the nervous and hormonal systems. Each month, in rhythm with the cycle of ovulation, the breasts become engorged with fluid in anticipation of pregnancy. The contours of the breasts' lobular structure become apparent, producing the sensations of lumpiness, tenderness, and perhaps pain. If conception does not occur, the accumulated fluid drains away via the lymphatic network. *Mastodynia* (premenstrual swelling and tenderness of the breasts) is common. It usually lasts for

3 to 4 days prior to the onset of menses, but the symptoms may persist throughout the month. Such symptoms may be diagnosed erroneously as fibrocystic breast disease but are more properly identified as increased physiologic nodularity, an exaggerated response to normal cyclic changes (Mann 1983).

In women who never become pregnant, a degree of breast swelling may become chronic, with breast tissue assuming a lumpy texture, which may remain even after menopause. This lumpiness may take the form of multiple tiny nodules (fibroadenosis) or cystic masses (often identified as fibrocystic breast disease).

After menopause, adipose breast tissue atrophies and is replaced by connective tissue. Elasticity is lost, and the breasts may droop and become pendulous. The skin of the breasts in the older woman tends to wrinkle, appearing loose and flabby. There is continuous involution of the breasts, accompanied by loss of the glandular elements and atrophy. Recurring breast engorgement, which can be increasingly troublesome to women in middle age, is relieved by menopause. If estrogen replacement therapy is used to counteract other symptoms of menopause, however, breast engorgement will resume.

● Care of the Woman With Fibrocystic Breast Disease

Fibrocystic breast disease is the most common of the benign breast disorders. *Mammary dysplasia* or *chronic cystic mastitis* are also terms used to describe this benign condition. It is estimated that 1 woman in 20 will have palpable evidence of cystic disease sometime during her reproductive years (Parsons & Sommers 1978). Kister (1984) observed that fibrocystic breast disease has become an all-purpose term denoting a variety of breast conditions ranging from painful, lumpy breasts to true cystic disease. Kister further stated that the use of one term to encompass such a range of conditions is unfortunate because other benign conditions do not present a risk, whereas true cystic disease is seen as an increased risk factor in breast cancer. Wynn (1983) stated that there is an increased risk for subsequent breast cancer in women with dysplastic fibrocystic changes. *Dysplasia* is determined by histologic examination and is seen as irregular cell growth. Multiple or solitary cysts occurring in fibrocystic disease that are not found to be dysplastic are not a risk factor for breast cancer.

Fibrocystic breast disease appears to be a problem for some women during the childbearing years, improving during pregnancy and lactation and resolving with menopause. Early cystic changes have been found in teenagers and women in their twenties; however, the occurrence of breast cysts is most prevalent in women 30 to 50 years of age (Wynn 1983).

Fibrosis is a thickening of normal breast tissue. In later stages the breast may become multinodular with a periodic mass. Cyst formation that may accompany fibrosis is considered a later change in fibrocystic disease. Cyst formation may result when normal secretions within the ductal network are unable to drain away. Their accumulation can then create a fluid-filled sac or cyst.

Fibrocystic breast disease is probably caused by an imbalance in estrogen and progesterone, which distorts the normal changes of the menstrual cycle. Because the condition responds to the changes of the menstrual cycle, a woman may actually observe a lessening in the size of a lump with the onset of her menstrual cycle. The symptoms often increase as the woman approaches menopause, while the condition generally improves following menopause.

Medical Therapy

The woman often complains of pain, tenderness, and swelling that occurs cyclically and is most pronounced just before her menses begins. Physical examination may reveal only mild signs of irregularity, or the breasts may feel dense, with areas of irregularity and nodularity. Women often refer to this as "lumpiness." Some women may also have expressible nipple discharge.

If the woman has a large, fluid-filled cyst she may experience a localized painful area as the capsule containing the accumulated fluid distends coincident with her cycle. However, if small cyst formation occurs, the woman may experience not a solitary tender lump but a diffuse tenderness.

Mammography, palpation, and fine-needle aspiration are used to confirm fibrocystic breast disease. Often, fine-needle aspiration is the treatment as well, affording relief from the tenderness or pain. Kister (1984) identified candidates for gross cystic disease to be primarily premenopausal women or postmenopausal women receiving exogenous estrogens. He defined gross cystic disease for this group of women according to following criteria (Kister 1984):

● A palpable, fluid-filled mass is felt.

● The mass can be aspirated.

● Histologic examination confirms cystic disease.

● Mammography indicates cystic formation.

Physical examination reveals that cysts are round, movable, and well delineated in appearance. Specific characteristics that differentiate a cyst from a malignant neoplasm are mobility, tenderness, and the absence of skin retraction (or pulling) in surrounding tissue (Parsons & Sommers 1978). Although fibrocystic disease is nonmalignant, a coexisting, hidden malignancy can be present, making it essential that the diagnosis be thorough (Vaughn 1983).

Fine-needle aspiration, an office procedure, is used in conjunction with physical examination. Fluid withdrawal confirms the presence of a cyst. The fluid aspirated is sent for cytologic examination. If aspiration is incomplete, yielding no fluid, or yields bloody fluid, a biopsy is necessary (Wynn 1983). If the physical findings remain unclear, a mammogram is ordered to clarify the diagnosis. A mammogram revealing an unexplained or suspicious area warrants surgical exploration or biopsy.

Treatment of palpable cysts is conservative; invasive procedures such as biopsy are used only if the diagnosis is questionable. If a question persists, surgical exploration of the tissue and removal of the affected area are scheduled as an outpatient procedure. Fine-needle aspiration of the mass commonly confirms cystic disease and relieves pain. The mass or affected area is reexamined after four weeks to determine if the cyst has refilled.

Women with mild symptoms may benefit from restricting sodium intake and taking a mild diuretic during the week before the onset of menses. This counteracts fluid retention, relieves pressure in the breast, and helps decrease the pain. In other cases a mild analgesic is necessary.

Controversy surrounds the practice of limiting caffeine to relieve symptoms. One source (Minton et al 1981) proposed that methylxanthines (eg, coffee, tea, colas, chocolate, and some medications) may predispose to fibrocystic breast changes and suggested that limiting caffeine intake would help decrease fibrocystic changes. However, a recent review of research studies on the effect of limiting methylxanthines failed to demonstrate a clear association between caffeine and fibrocystic breast changes (Levinson & Dunn 1986).

Other approaches that are occasionally advocated include daily intake of 50 to 100 mg of thiamine daily. Thiamine plays a role in the detoxification of estrogen and might decrease levels of available estrogen. This method is not yet supported by good clinical trials (Havens et al 1986). Vitamin E is sometimes advocated, but its value is questionable.

In severe cases of fibrocystic disease, the hormone inhibitor danazol (Danocrine) is the drug of choice. The drug produces marked relief within four to six months. In most cases the medication is discontinued after six to eight months, and the improvement lasts for years. Danazol does have some troublesome side effects, especially weight gain, amenorrhea, and masculinization.

In rare instances the condition can become so severe that the woman is incapacitated by pain and must undergo multiple biopsies for questionable masses. After careful evaluation and counseling the woman may elect to undergo simple mastectomy with or without implants. This is a drastic intervention and should never be undertaken without a second medical opinion.

Nursing Assessment

The nurse assesses the woman's understanding of fibrocystic breast disease and the importance of regular breast self-examination. Some specially trained nurses perform breast examinations of healthy women. The nurse also reviews the woman's history for close relatives with fibrocystic breast disease or cancer of the breast. The nurse also obtains information on relief measures that have been effective for the woman.

Nursing Diagnosis

Nursing diagnoses that may apply to a woman with fibrocystic breast disease include:

- Noncompliance with the recommendation to do monthly breast self-examination related to a lack of understanding of its importance in detecting abnormalities

- Alteration in comfort: acute pain related to the breast changes that occur premenstrually

- Fear related to the increased incidence of breast cancer in women with fibrocystic breast disease

Nursing Goal: Education for Self-Care

The nurse suggests measures the woman can employ to help alleviate her discomfort. These include:

- Wearing a well-fitting, supportive bra, at night as well as during the day when symptoms are severe

- Applying ice packs to tender areas of the breasts

- Using nonprescription salicylates or anti-inflammatory medication

The nurse also plays a significant role in helping the woman understand the importance of performing careful, monthly breast self-examination (BSE). When a woman knows the feel and texture of her own breasts, she is far more likely to detect any changes that develop.

Nursing Goal: Provision of Psychologic Support

Women with fibrocystic breast disease have an increased risk of developing cancer and many feel a great deal of fear about the possibility. By carefully explaining fibrocystic disease and its relationship to the monthly cycle, the nurse can alleviate the woman's anxiety while reinforcing the importance of having any suspected abnormality evaluated thoroughly.

The nurse can also point out that frequent professional breast examination and regular mammograms are tools that help detect any abnormalities and that the woman who practices monthly BSE, follows her care giver's advice, and is examined regularly has taken positive action to protect her health.

Evaluative Outcome Criteria

Anticipated outcomes of nursing care include the following:

- The woman incorporates monthly BSE into her personal routine.

- The woman implements measures to help alleviate her discomfort.

- The woman understands fibrocystic breast disease, deals with her anxiety over the potential complications, and takes positive action to protect her health.

• Care of the Woman With a Disorder of the Breast

Table 10–1 summarizes common breast disorders. Mastitis is discussed in Chapter 36.

Fibroadenoma

The fibroadenoma is a common tumor seen in women in their teens and early twenties. It is the third most common tumor of the breast; its incidence is exceeded only by carcinoma and fibrocystic disease. The cause of fibroadenomas found in adolescent breasts appears closely linked to that of breast hypertrophy, which may occur during the pubertal growth spurt. Fibroadenomas will respond to hormonal influence and are known to increase in size and secrete milk during pregnancy. Unlike cystic disease, fibroadenoma has not been significantly associated with malignant neoplasms.

Fibroadenomas are solid tumors that are well defined, sharply delineated, and rounded, with a rubbery firmness. These tumors can be moved freely within the breast tissue and are not associated with any fibroblastic response in surrounding tissue. A solitary nodule is common, but multiple tumors have been observed in about 15 percent of cases (Parsons & Sommers 1978). The size of a fibroadenoma ranges from 1 to 5 cm, with the nodule commonly occurring around the nipple or in the upper quadrant of the breast along the lateral side. Fibroadenomas are asymptomatic and nontender. They are usually discovered by accident.

MEDICAL THERAPY

Fibroadenomas are characterized by their appearance on physical examination. They are:

- Well outlined

Table 10–1   Summary of Common Breast Disorders

Condition	Age	Pain	Nipple Discharge	Location	Consistency and Mobility	Diagnosis and Treatment
Duct ectasia	35–55 years; median age 40	Burning around nipple	Sticky, multicolored; usually bilateral	No specific location	Retroareolar mass with advanced disease	Open biopsy; local excision of diseased portion of breast
Fibroadenoma	15–39 years; median age 20	No	No	No specific location	Mobile, firm, smooth, well delineated	Mammography, xeromammography; surgical or needle biopsy; excision of the tumor
Fibrocystic breast disease	20–49 years; median age 30 (may subside with menopause)	Yes	No	Upper outer quadrant	Bilateral multiple lumps influenced by the menstrual cycle	Needle aspiration; observation; biopsy if there is an unresolved mass or mammographic changes
Intraductal papilloma	35–55 years; median age 40	Yes	Serous or serosanguineous; usually unilateral from one duct	No specific location	Usually soft, poorly delineated	Pap smear of nipple discharge; biopsy; wedge resection
Mastitis	Childbearing years	Tenderness, pain	No	No specific location	Generalized redness of overlying skin	Antibiotic therapy; incision and drainage if mastitis progresses to an abscess

Source: Modified from Fogel CI, Woods NF (eds): *Health Care of Women: A Nursing Perspective.* St. Louis, Mosby, 1981, p 337.

- Rounded

- Lobulated in appearance

- Often rubbery in firmness

- Relatively movable

If there are any disquieting features to the appearance of the lump, fine-needle biopsy and/or excision of the mass may be indicated. Caution is exercised when deciding upon biopsy because excision of the mass in a young girl may interfere with normal breast development. Watchful observation and possible surgical excision are the only treatments for fibroadenomas. Surgery is often deferred. When advisable, surgical removal of the fibroadenoma concludes its treatment.

Intraductal Papilloma

Papillomas do not appear as often as carcinomas and have no particular predilection for any age group. Papillomas are tumors growing in the terminal portion of a duct or sometimes throughout the duct system within a section of the breast. Papillomas are typically benign, but have the potential to become malignant (Havens et al 1986).

MEDICAL THERAPY

The majority of papillomas present as solitary nodules or, more frequently, as multiple lesions. These small ball-like lesions may be detected on mammography. The presence of a papilloma is often frightening to the woman because her primary symptom is a discharge from the nipple that may be serosanguineous or brownish-green due to old blood. The location of the papilloma within the duct system and its pattern of growth determine whether nipple discharge will be present. The tumor frequently is not palpable, although a small soft tumor in a central or peri-areolar portion of the breast can sometimes be palpated.

If the woman reports a nipple discharge, the breast should be milked to obtain fluid. The fluid obtained is sent for a Papanicolaou (Pap) smear. The diagnosis is confirmed if papilloma cells are present (Havens et al 1986). The lesion must be excised and histologically examined because of the difficulty in differentiating between a benign papilloma and a papillary carcinoma. A permanent paraffin section is indicated because a frozen section may not differentiate the two conditions conclusively. A permanent paraffin section requires several days, lengthening the time of diagnosis, whereas a frozen section provides immediate findings. The woman may need emotional support while awaiting the diagnosis. Treatment for benign papilloma is excision. Medical follow-up visits may be more frequent

because of the possibility of recurrence and the similarity of papillary carcinoma to the benign condition.

Duct Ectasis (Comedomastitis)

Ectasis of the duct, a disease of the aging breast, occurs commonly during or near the onset of menopause. Comedomastitis is not associated with carcinoma. The condition typically occurs in women who have borne and nursed children.

MEDICAL THERAPY

The woman will report a thick, sticky nipple discharge with burning pain, pruritus, and inflammation. Treatment is conservative, with drug therapy aimed at symptomatic relief. The major central ducts of the breast occasionally have to be excised. The symptoms may be frightening, and the woman may need emotional support in addition to reassurance that this disorder is not associated with cancer.

Nursing Assessment

During the period of diagnosis, the woman may be anxious about a possible change in body image or a diagnosis of cancer. The nurse can use therapeutic communication to assess the significance the woman places on her breasts; her current emotional status, coping mechanisms used during periods of stress, and knowledge and beliefs about cancer; and other variables that may influence her coping and adjustment.

Nursing Diagnosis

Nursing diagnoses that may apply to a woman with a benign disorder of the breast include:

- Knowledge deficit related to a lack of understanding of diagnostic procedures

- Anxiety related to possible diagnosis of breast cancer

Nursing Goal: Provision of Emotional Support During the Period of Diagnosis

During the prediagnosis period the woman should be encouraged to express her anxiety. Misconceptions need to be clarified, and the woman should be allowed to express her fears. The woman may find herself considering the implications for her personal life, her family, and the future if the diagnosis is cancer. This "what if" concern helps the woman consider the implications of cancer and enables her to begin planning. It is tempting to disregard these concerns by simply responding, "Oh, don't think like that. Everything will be fine." Such an approach, however, invalidates the woman's concerns and denies her the opportunity to begin considering the future. The sensitive nurse will avoid unnecessary pessimism, while recognizing that the woman's concerns are valid.

Nursing Goal: Teaching Breast Self-Examination (BSE)

The knowledge that a breast lump is benign fills a worried woman with relief and the desire to put the incident behind her. Yet this relief must not minimize the woman's personal accountability and commitment to practice monthly breast self-examination (BSE).

Common breast disorders may be medically treated as an acute episode or, as in the case of fibrocystic breast disease, as a condition that necessitates vigilant follow-up. For the teenager with a fibroadenoma or the older woman with chronic cystic disease, BSE should be a routine part of life. Women at high risk for breast cancer (see Table 10–2) must become especially attentive to the importance of early detection through routine BSE. Despite recent advances in mechanical screening procedures, manual BSE remains the primary diagnostic tool for early detection of cancer.

In the course of a routine physical examination or during an initial visit to the care giver, the BSE technique should be taught and its importance as a monthly practice emphasized by the nurse. The effectiveness of BSE is determined by the woman's skill. Traditional methods of instruction in BSE have been cognitive in orientation and have not allowed the woman sufficient training or manual practice under supervision. Offering a woman a brochure or having her view a film without actually performing BSE is inadequate. Women who receive personal training and instruction report greater frequency of examination than those who read pamphlets or see films (Hall et al 1977). The woman must use her own hands to become familiar with the contours of her breasts. She needs to be reassured and emotionally supported if she becomes alarmed at nodularity or lumpiness of her breasts. With familiarity and practice the woman will learn not to be afraid that every thickening is a potential cancer.

Breast self-examination should be performed on a regular, monthly basis about one week after each menstrual period when the breasts are typically not tender or swollen. After menopause, BSE should be performed on the same day each month (the woman can choose the particular day).

The nurse is the woman's advocate in the community, industrial setting, hospital, or physician's office. Through routine health screening and assessment, the nurse has an opportunity to provide emotional support, evaluate the woman's risk of developing breast cancer, and teach BSE. A return demonstration of BSE by the woman during a routine health examination facilitates understanding of the procedure and encourages the woman's commitment to her own health care. A method of record keeping also should be mutually determined by the nurse and the woman. Ongoing spoken feedback about the woman's performance of BSE should be part of the visit in which the technique is taught, as well as subsequent visits. Nurse and client should review the woman's record of breast examination during follow-up visits to ensure that a monthly pattern has been established.

Nurses involved in breast inspection should also develop a systematic approach. Procedure 10–1 describes a logical approach to breast inspection.

Evaluative Outcome Criteria

Anticipated outcomes of nursing care include the following:

- The woman feels comfortable discussing her fears, concerns, and questions during the period of diagnosis.

- The diagnosis is made quickly and accurately.

- The woman incorporates monthly BSE into her personal routine.

● Care of the Woman With Carcinoma of the Breast

Approximately 38,400 deaths were estimated to have occurred as a result of breast cancer during 1985. During that same year 119,000 American women were diagnosed as having breast cancer. More specifically, 1 woman out of 11 will develop breast cancer during her lifetime (American Cancer Society 1984). Most women are likely to know a family member or friend who has had a mastectomy. Myths concerning the causes and treatment of breast cancer are commonplace and can be heard around coffee tables and in boardrooms. Concerted efforts on the part of health organizations and the media have begun to dispel myths, supplanting misinformation with health education.

The mastectomies of Betty Ford and "Happy" Rockefeller in September and October 1974 brought the importance of breast cancer, its detection, and its treatment to the attention of the American public. The feminist and consumer rights movements have also been instrumental in raising the women's consciousness about their accountability for personal health care. As a result of this awareness, many women today expect a voice in any decisions made about their health and proposed treatments.

Procedure 10–1　Inspection of the Breasts

Look at the breasts individually and in comparison with one another. Note and record the following characteristics:

Size and Symmetry of the Breasts

1. Breasts may vary, but the variations should remain constant during rest or movement—note abnormal contours.
2. Some size difference between the breasts is normal.

Shape and Direction of the Breasts

1. The shape of the breasts can be rounded or pendulous with some variation between breasts.
2. The breasts should be pointing slightly laterally.

Color, Thickening, Edema, and Venous Patterns

1. Check for redness or inflammation.
2. A blue hue with a marked venous pattern that is focal or unilateral may indicate an area of increased blood supply due to tumor. Symmetric venous patterns are normal.
3. Skin edema observed as thickened skin with enlarged pores ("orange peel") may indicate blocked lymphatic drainage due to tumor.

Surface of the Breasts

1. Skin dimpling, puckering, or retraction (pulling) when the woman presses her hands together or against her hips suggests malignancy.
2. Striae (stretch marks) red at onset and whitish with age are normal.

Nipple Size and Shape, Direction, Rashes, Ulcerations, and Discharge

1. Long-standing nipple inversion is normal, but an inverted nipple previously capable of erection is suspicious. Note any deviation, flattening, or broadening of the nipples.
2. Check for rashes, ulcerations, or discharge.

Within the medical profession, controversy persists regarding the treatment alternatives for breast cancer. What the physician decides is the best treatment for a woman with a newly diagnosed breast cancer may not be what the woman wishes. The physician's major concern may be the attainment of cure, necessitating a more radical surgical treatment, whereas the woman may feel that the threatened loss of a valued body part is equally important.

Theories of causation include hormonal mechanisms, viral agents, and immunological processes. The fact that breast cancer does not occur in the prepubertal female suggests that prior conditioning of the breast tissue by endogenous steroids may be essential for neoplastic development (Rickel et al 1982). The incidence of carcinoma of the breast increases in women after the age of 35. Most lumps (95 percent) are discovered by women themselves.

Factors placing women at risk for breast cancer have been studied extensively by epidemiologists and other clinical researchers. The risk factors associated with carcinoma of the breast in women are summarized in Table 10–2.

Screening and Detection

The purpose of breast screening programs is to identify women who have no clinical signs of breast cancer but have covert signs suggesting the presence of the disease. The chances of cure improve dramatically when breast cancer is detected when the tumor is small and located in only one breast. In fact, the cure rate for noninvasive or minimally invasive cancers is greater than 95 percent (Donegan 1986).

The primary screening tools currently available include regular breast self-examination, examination by a health professional, and mammogram. Other screening methods include thermography and ultrasonography.

BREAST SELF-EXAMINATION (BSE)

Monthly breast self-examination is the best method for detecting masses early. All health professionals need to include breast examination and the teaching of routine BSE in routine checkups.

It is difficult to convince women of the need to perform regular BSE. One study (Foster et al 1978) revealed that only 24 percent of the breast cancer patients interviewed had performed regular BSE, and 47 percent had never performed the examination all. Schlueter (1982) concluded in her study of 204 women of high socioeconomic backgrounds, primarily college graduates, that knowledge of breast cancer, beliefs about perceived susceptibility to breast cancer, and beliefs about the perceived benefits of BSE do not affect the practice of BSE. She also observed that women who engage in the preventive health practice of regular exercise do not practice BSE more regularly than those who do not exercise. Explanations offered by women for not regularly examining their breasts include being too busy, being unfamiliar with the technique, not wanting to think about it, forgetting it, lacking motivation, lacking confidence in performing self-examination correctly, fear, and anxiety.

The American Cancer Society (1973) recommends a three-step procedure for self-examination of the breasts. The pamphlet "How to Examine Your Breasts" can easily

Table 10-2 Risk Factors Associated With Increased Incidence of Breast Cancer

Variable	High Risk	Low Risk
Age	Over 50 years of age	Under 50 years of age
Family history	Breast cancer in grandmother, mother, aunt, or sister	No family history of breast cancer
Marital status	Unmarried	Married
Medical history	Cancer in the other breast Fibrocystic breast disease with dysplasia Endometrial cancer Other organ cancers Lowered immunologic competence	No breast cancer No fibrocystic breast disease No endometrial cancer No other organ cancers No other systemic disorders
Menstrual history	Early menarche (before 12 years of age) Late menopause (after 50 years of age) More than 30 years of menstrual activity	Menarche after 12 years of age Menopause before 50 years of age Less than 30 years of menstrual activity
Nutrition	High fat intake High protein intake Low selenium intake	Low fat intake Moderate protein intake High selenium intake
Race	Caucasian	Noncaucasian
Socioeconomic status	Upper middle class	Lower class

Source: Scholtenfeld D, Fraumeni J (eds): *Cancer Epidemiology and Prevention.* Philadelphia: Saunders, 1982. Dunphy J, Way L: *Current Surgical Diagnosis and Treatment.* Los Altos, Calif: Lange, 1980.

be obtained free of charge from the American Cancer Society. Procedure 10-2 describes the recommended technique.

The physician also felt the lump and thickening, and now I'm waiting for my mammogram. In these few days my thoughts and feelings have been a roller coaster. I'm 46, and I'm wondering if this is it. Am I dying? Now? I'm afraid as I have not been afraid since one of our children was very ill. Try as I may to fill my head with other thoughts, it keeps slipping back to this.

MAMMOGRAPHY

A mammogram is a soft tissue radiograph of the breast without the injection of a contrast medium. Mammography can detect lesions in the breast before they can be palpated. A mammogram also functions as a diagnostic tool in facilitating a differential diagnosis.

The ionizing radiation in mammography has been implicated as a risk factor associated with breast cancer, although newer equipment has significantly decreased the radiation levels required for the procedure. In fact, now that two-view studies can be obtained using only 0.2 rad (cancer has been linked to doses above 100 rads), the risk is approximately one in a million. When this information is considered with the data that demonstrates a 25 percent to 35 percent reduction in mortality from breast cancer when mammography is used (Kopans 1985), the fear of exposure to the radiation should not deter women from taking advantage of this valuable screening tool.

Currently the American Cancer Society and the American College of Radiology suggest the following mammogram screening guidelines (Kopans 1985):

● Baseline mammogram between ages 35 and 40

● Mammogram every 1 to 2 years between ages 40 and 49

● Mammogram annually for all women over age 50

Mammograms are a useful tool, but they cannot replace BSE or physical examination. Up to 15 percent of early breast cancers are detected by physical examination and are not detected by mammogram (Donegan 1986). In addition, while mammograms can detect a suspicious lesion, they are not always precise enough to identify the specific type of lesion.

Kopans and Meyer observed that physicians may view physical examination and mammography as competing techniques when in fact they are complementary. "It is necessary for the medical community and the public to realize that high quality mammography will reveal a vast majority of breast cancers but this fact does not obviate the need for a thorough routine physical examination and breast self-examination" (Kopans & Meyer 1980, p 60).

THERMOGRAPHY

The thermographic photograph is a pictorial representation of heat patterns on the surface of the breast. This diagnostic technique can sometimes indicate breast cancer or inflammation because these processes have a higher rate of metabolic activity and will generate a higher than normal temperature, or "hot spot," on the photograph. The advantage of thermography over mammography is that thermography does not expose the woman to radiation. However, because up to 67 percent of cancers are missed, while 12 percent of examinations are falsely positive, the technique has gained very little acceptance in clinical practice (Donegan 1986).

ULTRASONOGRAPHY

Ultrasonography is not sufficiently accurate to differentiate various breast disorders. The technique produces an image created by inaudible sound waves that reflect from tissue. It is quite accurate in distinguishing cysts from solid masses but cannot differentiate between malignant cells and nonmalignant cells. It is used as an adjunct screening procedure. It is primarily used to identify the location of a cyst for needle aspiration.

PATHOPHYSIOLOGY OF BREAST CANCER

The most common malignancy in women is breast cancer, which has its peak incidence prior to menopause (Parsons & Sommers 1978). No method for preventing breast cancer is known. Cancer of the breast has an unpredictable course, with a long-term risk—20 years or more—of metastasis (Keyes et al 1983). A secondary rise in the incidence of breast cancer is observed following menopause. Practitioners tend to follow the informal rule that the older the woman, the greater the chance that malignant disease will appear.

A malignant breast neoplasm may originate either in a duct or in the lobular epithelium. It may be infiltrating (penetrating the limiting basement membranes) or noninfiltrating (nonpenetrating). All forms of breast cancer can spread locally by invasion. A breast tumor tends to adhere to the pectoral muscles or deep fascia of the chest wall beneath the breast and the skin overlying the breast. This adherence of the tumor can cause an appearance of skin dimpling and retraction in the later stages of the disease ("orange peel sign"). About 50 percent of all breast cancers originate in the upper outside quadrant and metastasize to the axillary lymph nodes. Approximately 25 percent of all breast cancers arise in the central portion of the breast and metastasize to the mammary lymph node chain (Rickel et al 1982).

In more than half of all women with breast cancer, systemic metastasis either has occurred by the time the woman seeks professional assistance or develops later. Malignant breast neoplasms spread from the breast to the axillary nodes, to the internal mammary nodes, and to the supraclavicular nodes. Of the women seeking medical care for a breast mass, 50 percent with a palpable lump of one month's duration have positive axillary nodes and 68 percent with a palpable lump of six months' duration have positive axillary nodes (Rubin 1978). Wider dissemination of the breast neoplasm is primarily hematogenous, with the common sites of distant metastasis being the lymph nodes, lungs, bone marrow, liver, brain, and bone.

Cancer of the breast is often discovered accidentally by the woman or her sexual partner. During the early stages of development, the lump is usually isolated, movable, and painless. A hard, circumscribed mass that is not freely movable also suggests malignancy. More advanced signs, such as fixation to the skin, skin edema, nipple retraction, or deep fixation, are further evidence of cancer.

Diagnosis

In diagnosing breast lesions, physical examination, radiographic or other diagnostic techniques, and biopsy are the most common procedures.

PHYSICAL EXAMINATION

During a physical examination of the breast, inspection and palpation are the primary methods of assessment. A health history focusing on breast problems is also necessary. Table 10–3 describes the areas relevant to history taking.

For breast examination, the woman is asked to disrobe to the waist. She sits in four different positions while the breasts are examined individually and in comparison to each other. Positions include:

1. Sitting upright with arms at the side.

2. Sitting upright with arms abducted over the head.

3. Sitting upright with hands pressed against the hips (to contract the pectoral muscles).

4. Leaning forward from a sitting position to allow the breasts to hang freely.

In each position the breasts are carefully observed for symmetry, bulging, retraction, and fixation. A mass not apparent while the breast is at rest may be detected. A tumor can fix tissue to the chest wall, preventing forward or upward movement of the breast in various positions. Dimpling is most likely to be seen in position 3, which calls for contraction of the pectoral muscles.

The purpose of palpation is to discover any masses in the breasts. Both breasts should be palpated with equal care. If the woman suspects a lump in one breast, the other should be examined first for a basis of comparison (King 1982). The breasts should be palpated first while the woman is sitting and then when she is supine. When the woman is supine, she should be asked to raise her arm

Procedure 10–2   Breast Self-Examination

Objective	Nursing action	Rationale

Provide instruction

Figure 10–1A

Instruct woman as follows:
1. Lie down. Put one hand behind your head. With the other hand, fingers flattened, gently feel your breast. Press lightly (Figure 10–1A). Now examine the breast.

Over 74,000 American women develop breast cancer every year. About half die within 5 years. Experience shows that 95 percent of breast cancers are found by women themselves. When women discover lumps in their breasts at a very early stage, surgery can save 70 percent–80 percent of proven cancer cases.

Figure 10–1B

2. Figure 10–1B shows you how to check each breast. Begin as you see in C and follow the arrows, feeling gently for a lump or thickening. Remember to feel all parts of each breast.

Figure 10–1C

3. Now repeat the same procedure sitting up, with the hand still behind your head (Figure 10–1C).

Instruct woman to perform breast self-examination on a monthly basis.

Monthly assessment will increase opportunity to identify breast changes. Nonpregnant women should check breasts at end of menstrual period.

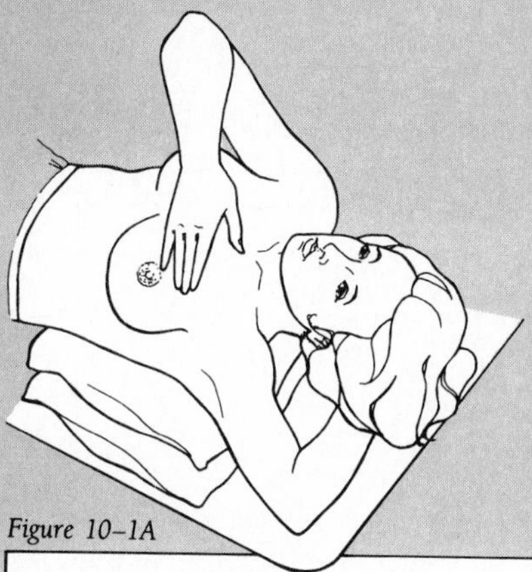

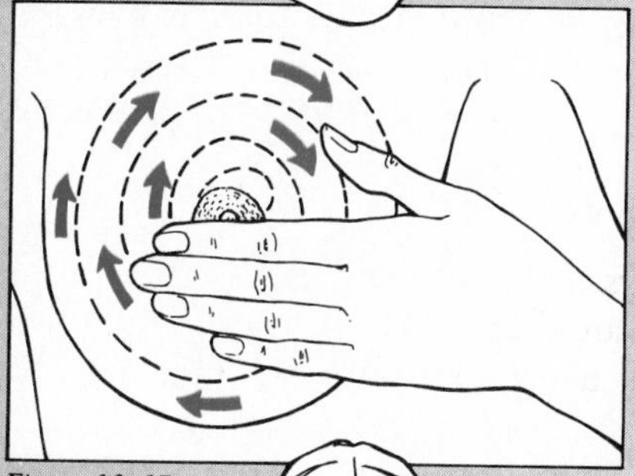

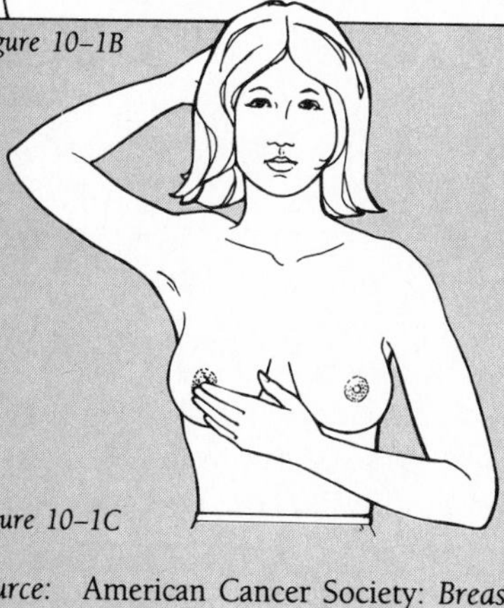

Source: American Cancer Society: *Breast Self-Examination and the Nurse,* No. 3408 PE. New York, 1973.

above her head or place it underneath her neck, which causes the breast to spread over the chest and makes any nodules more apparent. The nurse should develop a system of palpation starting and ending at an arbitrary fixed point on the breasts. Areolar areas are also carefully palpated to determine whether underlying masses are present. Each nipple should be compressed to check for discharge. The lymph nodes are palpated with the woman in a sitting position. When examining the axillas for nodes, tissues are best felt if the muscles are relaxed because contracted muscles can obscure slightly enlarged nodes. Relaxation of the

muscles can be accomplished by having the woman relax her arm while the examiner supports it from underneath during the palpation of the axilla. The characteristics of masses that should be noted and recorded following palpation of the breast are:

● Location—where found (provide diagram)

● Size—in centimeters

● Shape—type of shape (round, oval, oblong, tubular, or irregular)

Table 10–3　Brief Health History for Women With Breast Disorders

Area	Assessment Guidelines	Area	Assessment Guidelines
Description of presenting symptoms	Symptoms: How discovered: Date of onset: Date of visit:	Related medical history	Fibrocystic breast disease: Breast cancer: Reproductive cancer: Other cancers: Pertinent medical history not mentioned above:
Demographic information	Age: Race: Marital status:		
Family history of breast problems	Family member(s) problem 　Grandmother: 　Mother: 　Aunt: 　Sister:	Life-style patterns	Caffeine ingestion: Dietary habits:
Menstrual patterns	Age of menarche: Age of menopause: Regularity of menses: Difficulty/discomfort:	Psychosocial information	What does the woman perceive to be the problem? What significance does she attach to her breasts? Does she identify any specific fears?
Pregnancies and lactation	Age of first pregnancy: Number of pregnancies: Number of children: Breast-feeding: 　How long: 　Problems:		What are her support systems?
Use of estrogen	Type(s): How long:	Other risk factors	Identify:

- Consistency—soft, hard, indurated, or cystic
- Mobility—movable or fixed (attachment and/or fixation)
- Borders—well defined or poorly demarcated
- Tenderness—pain or tenderness on palpation

MAMMOGRAPHY

Mammography is used as a diagnostic tool for women with a palpable lump or for women who have noticed breast changes, such as abnormalities in the skin (dimpling, discoloration, or puckering) or a change in the size or shape of the breast. On mammography, the malignant lesion may have a poorly circumscribed, irregular appearance. Lesions are often nonhomogeneous in density and may exhibit tentaclelike infiltrations into tissue. In contrast, benign lesions tend to have sharp margins, are homogeneous in density, and are frequently surrounded by a radiolucent halo of fat. Benign masses push tissue aside as they expand rather than invading it (Rickel et al 1982). Mammography helps the physician determine whether a biopsy should be performed by fine-needle aspiration or excision. The mammogram can also be a definitive tool in choosing a medical treatment course of careful observation.

NEEDLE BIOPSY

Definitive diagnosis of a suspicious mass beyond the noninvasive preliminary screening and diagnostic techniques already mentioned always involves biopsy of some kind, either by aspiration or incision.

An aspiration (needle) biopsy is accomplished by inserting a needle into the mass to withdraw cells or cystic fluid for microscopic examination. A fine needle on a hypodermic syringe is typically used by physicians to aspirate cystic fluid. Aspiration biopsy may be done in the physician's office or as an outpatient procedure. A wider needle may be used when removing a biopsy sample of cells from a solid mass. Needle biopsy is not always a definitive diagnostic procedure, and surgical (incisional) biopsy may still be necessary. Needle biopsies cannot conclusively rule out the presence of cancerous cells. Hence aspiration biopsy has been viewed by practitioners as only a supplemental diagnostic technique.

SURGICAL (INCISIONAL) BIOPSY

Incisional biopsy is the primary diagnostic technique for confirming the presence of cancer in a solid breast mass. Incisional biopsy involves direct examination of a portion of the tumor for microscopic evaluation by either frozen section or permanent section. Staging the cancer to determine its extent may follow the biopsy.

Incisional biopsy requires the woman to undergo surgery. Historically, incisional biopsy of the breast mass was done under general anesthesia while the surgeon awaited the pathologist's report on the tissue obtained. If the frozen section was determined to be malignant, a radical mastectomy was performed at that time. Prior to surgery, the woman was informed of the possibility of mastectomy as a result of her biopsy. The fear of not knowing whether her breast would be removed became a real issue of concern for most women undergoing biopsy. Health professionals, particularly nurses, were often faced with assisting the woman to cope with this fear both preoperatively and postoperatively.

As hospital costs have increased and more treatment alternatives have become available to the woman diagnosed with breast cancer, the treatment approach to incisional biopsy has changed. Outpatient surgery for breast biopsy has become the approved method of treatment for third-party reimbursement. Surgical biopsy is performed on an outpatient basis with the woman under local anesthesia. Using local anesthesia also has eliminated the postoperative complications common with general anesthesia. The tissue sample obtained during biopsy is sent out as a permanent section, and a pathologist's report is sent to the surgeon within a few days. During a follow-up office visit to the surgeon, the woman is given the results and the opportunity to discuss the best breast cancer treatment alternative for her. This two-step approach to breast cancer treatment

has gained a great deal of support from women and health care professionals alike. Participation in choosing treatment incorporates the woman, and possibly her family, as active partners. A decision made in this fashion is not as likely to be regretted later.

STAGING OF BREAST CANCER

Breast cancer staging is usually done through surgical dissection of the axillary lymph nodes to determine the type and extent of the carcinoma. Staging is based on three criteria (Pattison & Sorensen 1980):

1. The size of the primary tumor

2. The extent of the spread to the regional lymph nodes

3. The presence or absence of metastasis

A frequently used method of staging involves the TNM staging system, which determines the classifications according to the characteristics of the primary tumor (T), regional lymph nodes (N), and distant metastases (M). Subgroups within the TNM classification are based on tumor size, tumor attachment to underlying structures, and other demonstrable characteristsics (eg, nipple discharge, edema). Other systems of classification for breast cancer are also used, although all staging systems are similar. Table 10–4 describes the TNM staging system for breast carcinoma.

Table 10–4 Staging of Breast Carcinoma and Its Relation to Survival

Clinical staging (American Joint Committee)	Crude 5-year survival (%)	Histologic staging	Crude survival (%)	
			5 YEARS	10 YEARS
Stage I	85	Negative axillary nodes	78	65
(T) Tumor less than 2 cm in diameter		Positive axillary nodes		
(N) Nodes, if present, not felt to contain		One to three positive nodes	62	38
metastasis		More than four positive nodes	32	13
(M) Without distant metastases				
Stage II	66			
(T) Tumor less than 5 cm in diameter				
(N) Nodes, if palpable, not fixed				
(M) Without distant metastases				
Stage III	41			
(T) Tumor greater than 5 cm or tumor of any size with skin invasion or attachment				
(N) Nodes in supraclavicular area				
(M) Without distant metastases				
Stage IV	10			
(T) Tumor of any size with extension to chest wall and skin				
(N) Any amount of nodal involvement				
(M) Distant metastases				

Source: Dunphy J, Way L: *Current Surgical Diagnosis and Treatment.* Los Altos, Calif: Lange, 1980.

Surgical Treatment Alternatives

As early as 1650, treatment of breast cancer involved removal of the affected breast (Weber 1983). The standard American surgical treatment was established in the 1890s when Halsted described the procedure now known as the Halsted radical mastectomy. This procedure entailed the removal of the entire breast, skin, pectoralis major and minor muscles, lymph nodes of the axilla, and surrounding fat tissue. For over 50 years, the radical mastectomy was the treatment of choice for many surgeons despite advances in breast cancer screening and treatment that have facilitated discovery of earlier, more localized, and treatable breast tumors.

The unfortunate aspect of radical breast surgery is its mutilation. Breast cancer treatment has a significant emotional impact on the woman's integrity, body image, self-concept, and sexual identity. O'Brien observed that breast cancer treatment has even become "a feminist issue with some women blaming the predominantly male medical establishment for introducing mutilating therapy and resisting the development of therapies that are less disfiguring" (O'Brien 1983, p 125).

The most effective treatment for breast cancer tends to divide along the lines of each medical discipline's professional views: surgery, medical oncology, or radiotherapy (O'Brien 1983). Clinical stages I (tumor less than 2 cm with negative axillary nodes) and II (tumor less than 5 cm with movable homolateral axillary nodes) breast disease offer the greatest possibility for breast preservation and hence have become the two diagnoses about which the greatest treatment controversy exists (Rickel et al 1982). Many oncologists and radiotherapists feel that the lack of definitive proof that one surgical technique is more effective than another indicates that surgery alone cannot determine efficacy and that other therapies need to be investigated more fully.

Historically, surgical treatment has been the primary method of intervention for breast cancer. The principal issues regarding the choice of one surgical method over the other are the possibility that cancer cells may be present after surgery and clinical evidence verifying lengthened rates of survival. Because of the possibility of residual cancer cells after surgical intervention, many surgeons believe it is logical to remove the greatest amount of tissue in the hope of curative treatment. The second concern is that no single type of surgery can be considered preferable to another until sufficient clinical study yields proof of lengthened survival. However, recent studies (Fisher et al 1985) have offered proof, in their study of 1843 women at five-year follow-up, that conservative breast surgery in early disease, combined with radiotherapy, gives survival results that are as satisfactory as the modified radical mastectomy. It is important for the nurse to realize that the aim of surgical breast cancer treatment is threefold:

1. To preserve the woman's life
2. To minimize recurrence
3. To provide the best cosmetic results possible

From a surgical perspective, the goal of disease control (preserving the woman's life and minimizing recurrence) takes precedence over the woman's psychosocial concerns that may center on body image and cosmetic results.

A woman with a breast lump may have some definite ideas, gleaned from family, friends, or the media, about what surgical treatment she favors. However, the stage of her disease and her surgeon's treatment goals may indicate a more radical procedure than she anticipated. The following discussions of treatment methods are based on current practice in the United States.

RADICAL MASTECTOMY

Halsted believed that cancer spread directly from the tumor into adjoining tissue and that radical removal of the breast, skin, chest muscles, axillary lymph nodes, and surrounding fat tissue would therefore be the best method of arresting the disease. This "permeation theory" of cancer metastasis persisted until Halsted's rationale was refuted (Fisher et al 1975). Researchers observed that cancer cells circulated in the lymphatic and circulatory systems, confirming that cancer is present as a systemic disease before a clinical diagnosis is established. Given this knowledge, how effective can the most extensive of radical surgical procedures be against a systemic disease?

EXTENDED RADICAL MASTECTOMY

As early as the first decade of the twentieth century, it was apparent that the Halsted radical procedure did not always arrest the disease. Radiation therapy began to supplement the surgery, particularly if axillary nodes were found to be involved. Surgeons also believed that Halsted's approach ignored the internal mammary lymph nodes, a primary site for spread, and thus the extended radical mastectomy was developed. The extended radical mastectomy encompassed the Halsted procedure plus resection of the internal mammary lymph nodes. To gain access to these nodes, a portion of the rib cage was removed. This operation became quite popular with surgeons in the 1950s and 1960s, who nicknamed it, with black humor, "upper-body amputation" (Weber 1983). These radical procedures left the woman with a flattened or sunken chest wall, lymphedema of the affected arm, and shoulder stiffness.

MODIFIED RADICAL MASTECTOMY

The modified radical mastectomy involves removing the entire breast and axillary contents; however, the pectoralis major muscle is preserved. Pilch (1983, p 127) stated that "while benefits of preserving this muscle are entirely cosmetic, they are significant." The normal contours of the shoulder and chest wall are maintained, hollowness under the clavicle is eliminated, the arm retains its strength, and lymphedema is lessened. The placement of the incisions avoids shoulder scarring, and breast reconstruction may be possible. In fact some major medical centers report great success when reconstruction is done at the same time as the modified radical mastectomy. This approach helps alleviate the depression that generally occurs following mastectomy (Feller et al 1986).

The stated benefits of modified radical mastectomy appear to go beyond purely cosmetic effects because function of the shoulder and arm is preserved. Two versions of the modified radical mastectomy have been developed: One technique leaves the pectoralis minor muscle intact, while the other resects it. Today, the modified radical mastectomy has become the surgical procedure of choice, replacing the radical mastectomy as the standard treatment for stage I and II breast cancer and occasionally for stage III disease (Pilch 1983).

TOTAL (SIMPLE) MASTECTOMY

Simple mastectomy, followed by postoperative radiation of regional lymph nodes, has been used for early stage breast cancer. The results of this method are similar to those of modified radical mastectomy. The issue in choosing the total over the modified radical mastectomy is one of whether nodal radiation is as effective as surgical removal. Total mastectomy avoids a sunken chest. Lymphedema of the arm is reduced or nonexistent because the chest muscles are left intact and only the axillary nodes closest to the breast are dissected for staging purposes. Radiation of the regional lymph nodes commonly follows the surgical treatment. Breast reconstruction can be combined with the resection; the surgeon inserts a suitable prosthesis under the skin to produce a breast shape. When skin grafting is involved, a more elaborate reconstruction occurs during two or more procedures following simple mastectomy.

Simple mastectomy is rarely done as the sole treatment. Radiation of the lymph nodes or surgical removal is usually necessary. If staging for axillary lymph node involvement is done during the biopsy phase of the two-step procedure and the nodes are found to be negative, the simple mastectomy may be the only treatment. However, if the physician believes that prophylactic treatment of negative axillary lymph nodes is necessary despite the negative findings, radiation of the nodes follows.

SUBCUTANEOUS MASTECTOMY

Subcutaneous mastectomy evolved as a procedure to complement breast reconstruction. The internal breast tissue is removed and the skin of the breast remains. The excised breast tissue is examined histologically to determine if any invasive cancer is present. If invasive carcinoma is found, more radical surgery will need to be done. If staging took place earlier during biopsy, subcutaneous mastectomy and augmentation may be done in one surgical procedure.

An implant is inserted in the chest cavity to restore the contour of the breast after breast tissue has been removed. Subcutaneous mastectomy is particularly beneficial in breast cancers that are noninvasive and located away from the nipple (US Department of Health, Education, and Welfare 1979). In this procedure, all underlying tissue cannot be removed from the nipple area, and the problem of recurrence with invasive disease is not eradicated. Occasionally this procedure is recommended for women at high risk for breast cancer or those with serious chronic fibrocystic disease. It may also be performed on the unaffected breast when a woman with fibrocystic disease has breast cancer.

PARTIAL (SEGMENTAL) MASTECTOMY

Partial mastectomy removes the tumor and 2 to 3 cm of surrounding tissue. Some of the breast remains. Initially the procedure of segmented mastectomy was performed on individuals with serious coexisting systemic disease, on women of advanced age, and occasionally on women who refused mastectomy (Pilch 1983). A partial mastectomy may be attractive to women because it does not mean complete breast loss. The procedure may offer survival rates comparable to other more extensive procedures.

In 1976 the National Surgical Adjuvant Breast Project (NSABP) began a protocol (B-06) that prospectively randomized a clinical trial of 1843 women at five-year follow-up. Segmental mastectomy with and without radiation was compared with the modified radical mastectomy. Researchers stated that the results of the NSABP protocol of segmental mastectomy with axillary dissection and with or without postoperative radiation have achieved survival results as satisfactory as the modified radical mastectomy (Fisher et al 1985). Current trends support the use of both radiation and chemotherapy in women who have positive lymph nodes when segmental mastectomy is done (Margolese 1986). The cosmetic results were reported earlier as good to excellent (Fisher and Gebhardt 1978). In addition, results on 1593 women undergoing various conservative treatment protocols for breast cancer at the Cleveland Clinic between 1957 and 1975 have been reported for 5-, 10-, and 15-year survival rates. Segmental mastectomy without radiation was performed on 291 patients who qualified for that procedure. The 5- to 15-year survival rates for segmental mastectomy were equal to the survival rates for modified radical and simple (total) mastectomies (Hermann et al 1985).

The major argument against this procedure is that the tendency for breast cancer to appear in another part of the breast or in the opposite breast remains if all breast tissue is not removed. Radiation of breast tissue is often done to kill any cancer cells remaining in the breast. Axillary node dissection and removal of at least a portion of the nodes are also recommended. Despite recent findings, some physicians still view segmental mastectomy as experimental.

LOCAL WIDE EXCISION (TYLECTOMY OR LUMPECTOMY)

Local wide excision removes only the tumor mass and a narrow margin of normal tissue surrounding the mass. Local excision is less traumatic and less disfiguring than mastectomy. In early breast cancer, stages I and II, simple excision followed by definitive radiation yields local tumor control and survival rates that compare favorably with those of other treatments (Wilson 1983). Local wide excision with radiation is suitable for women with early operable breast cancer (tumor less than 5 cm with negative axillary nodes or palpable, nonfixed nodes). Aggressive radiation following excision is indicated for invasive breast carcinoma, particularly those originating in the ducts. Limited dissection of the axillary nodes is done for staging and to determine whether a regimen of adjuvant chemotherapy is necessary. Few surgeons would perform wide excision of the mass without follow-up radiotherapy. Radiation is delivered to the entire breast and the associated regional lymph nodes in a series of outpatient treatments over five weeks. After the last treatment, a supplementary dose is usually administered through radioactive implants in the breast.

Conservative breast cancer surgery presents other considerations because cosmetic effect is of primary importance when preserving the breast (Eich 1985). The size of the tumor in relation to the breast's total volume is important; even the most limited surgical procedure can deform or significantly alter a small breast. Lumpectomy with radiation also may be contraindicated in women with large breasts because radiation can cause fibrosis and skin retraction.

Therapy for breast cancer that offers breast preservation has received a great deal of media attention. These procedures have been presented as suitable for every woman, leading some to believe that radical treatment is unnecessary. Many women are not suitable candidates for excision and radiation because of the stage or type of cancer they have. Other women may not feel breast loss is that significant and believe that a more radical treatment may offer them a better chance of cure. The woman who is a suitable candidate for excision and radiation must be highly motivated, possessing patience and desiring breast preservation strongly. Treatment may be 10 to 12 weeks in duration and is very time-consuming. The desire of women of all ages to preserve the breasts and protect their femininity should not be underestimated (Wilson 1983). The woman needs to feel secure in her treatment choice and realize that conservative treatment is often viewed by the medical community as experimental and possibly not curative.

BREAST RECONSTRUCTION

As less-extensive surgical procedures for breast cancer become increasingly viable, more women have become candidates for reconstruction. The American Society of Plastic and Reconstructive Surgeons (1982) estimates that 20,000 women annually will undergo breast reconstruction in conjunction with or following mastectomy.

Reconstruction may not be presented as an option if the surgeon fears that implants may cause sarcomas of the chest wall, that the less radical resections used in successful reconstruction (eg, subcutaneous mastectomy) will not remove all cancerous tissue, or, perhaps most important, that the woman will not be pleased with the results. Evidence of cancer developing in reconstructed breasts has been reported, leading some plastic surgeons to postpone breast reconstruction until the woman has remained free of cancer for two years after the initial surgery.

Candidates for breast reconstruction are women with a mass less than 2 cm and fewer than three positive nodes. Women who have received a Halsted radical mastectomy or the extended mastectomy are not good candidates because they lack sufficient amounts of skin and muscle. Table 10–5 summarizes breast reconstruction procedures.

Medical Therapy

RADIATION THERAPY

Radiation therapy has played an increasingly significant role in breast cancer treatment. There is considerable controversy about the effectiveness of radiation as sole treatment. Four specific purposes of radiation therapy are:

1. As primary treatment for inflammatory breast cancer or for local control of inoperable breast cancer.

2. As an adjunct to mastectomy or local excision.

3. As a method of shrinking a large tumor to operable dimensions.

4. As palliation to relieve the pain caused by metastasis.

Although radiation is beneficial in achieving local control of breast carcinoma, cancer is now thought to be a systemic disease even in its early stages (Fisher et al 1975). Therefore radiation is considered inadequate without adjuvant chemotherapy (Pattison & Sorensen 1980).

Table 10–5 Breast Reconstruction Procedures

Type	Procedure	Surgical Treatment Amenable to Reconstruction	Treatment Considerations
Implant methods Silicone gel implants	Internal prosthesis is inserted through a small incision at the base of the fold area of the affected breast. The implant is positioned underneath the breast skin	Used with modified radical mastectomy, simple mastectomy, partial mastectomy, subcutaneous mastectomy, or lumpectomy	1. General side effects of surgery, including hemorrhage, infection, and edema. 2. Necrosis of the covering skin or discoloration of the skin over the implant. 3. The breast may harden into a baseball shape as a result of a fibrous capsule of scar tissue. 4. Improper placement may lead to an undesirable shape. 5. Inflatable implants can leak and deflate, necessitating their removal. 6. The size and shape of the remaining breast may need alteration, requiring a subsequent procedure to reduce/increase the unaffected breast. 7. Several basic surgical procedures allow the implant to be inserted at the time of the cancer surgery. 8. This is the least expensive and complicated of breast reconstruction surgeries.
Inflatable implants	After the implant is inserted in the above fashion, a saline solution is injected into the saucer-shaped form, and the wound is closed		
Flaps	Series of procedures: 1. A flap is created from upper/lower abdomen, thigh, buttocks, or back into a tube of skin (pedicle) 2. Pedicle is attached to the chest 3. Lower end of the pedicle is severed, and the tube of tissue is twisted and sutured over the missing breast area 4. After the skin covering is sufficiently thick, an incision is made at the base of the skin mound, and an implant is inserted	Used with Halsted radical mastecomy or extended radical mastectomy	1. General side effects of surgery, including hemorrhage, infection, and edema. 2. Flap methods can result in infection and tissue rejection. 3. More scarring occurs due to the numerous surgeries. 4. Symmetry between the breasts is difficult to achieve, and augmentation or reduction of the unaffected breast is usually necessary. 5. Flap method involves four to five hospitalizations and is very expensive.
Areola-nipple reconstruction	Nipple may be removed at the time of cancer surgery and checked by pathology. If it is free of carcinoma, it may then be sewn on the thigh or abdomen for transplantation later. Nipples also have been removed and put in a nipple bank until reconstruction is done. The nipple is grafted onto the reconstructed breast as a separate procedure.	Used with any of the breast cancer surgeries following other reconstruction	1. General side effects of surgery, including hemorrhage, infection, and edema. 2. Nipple may become discolored. 3. Nipple graft may not take. 4. A new nipple may need to be created using skin from the labia or earlobe, and tatooing can be necessary to achieve pigmentation. 5. Many women are content with a created breast form and don't choose to have the additional procedure of nipple grafting. 6. Because of the potential problems and the risk that the woman's nipple may contain malignant cells, there is a trend toward constructing a new nipple rather than using the woman's nipple.

Radiation therapy produces side effects that may be very uncomfortable. Loss of appetite, occasional nausea, and skin reactions commonly occur. Erythema is often followed by sloughing of skin tissues, although the tissue will gradually regain its normal color. If advanced radiation therapy is used as a primary treatment, skin reactions may range from mild erythema to blistering, pain, and weeping. The woman may report lethargy, fatigue, nausea, and digestive disorders. Radiation may irritate the trachea or esophagus, leading to coughing or dysphagia. The woman needs reassurance that these symptoms will subside once the treatment is stopped.

CHEMOTHERAPY

The purpose of chemotherapy is to kill circulating cancer cells that are shed from the primary tumor and circulated in the blood and lymph. The antineoplastic drugs are effective against cancer cells that are undergoing rapid cellular division. For this reason, drug therapy regimens often consist of three or more drugs given at different intervals to kill a maximum number of dividing cells at any one time. High therapeutic levels of each neoplastic drug may be used because each drug has a different mechanism of action and the side effects are not additive. Chemotherapy has substantial side effects, and discomfort related to drug side effects is a major nursing concern. Side effects from chemotherapy protocols are clustered in five groups (Rickel et al 1982):

1. Bone marrow depression

2. Gastrointestinal disturbances

3. Fluid retention

4. Neuropathy

5. Alopecia

For information on specific chemotherapeutic agents and their associated side effects, the reader is referred to current oncology literature.

Chemotherapy is not used alone in breast cancer; adjuvant chemotherapy following intervention is the currently preferred protocol when positive axillary nodes are found. The aim of adjuvant therapy is to cure microscopic metastatic disease and lengthen the period before relapse. The cancer-free period ranges from 1½ to 5 years, depending on the extent of lymphatic metastasis. Most studies indicate that in premenopausal women with early breast cancer, the use of adjuvant chemotherapy improves the survival rate, especially when combination drug therapy is used (Mitchell 1983). Adjuvant chemotherapy for advanced breast cancer has been less successful; it is used primarily as a palliative measure. In summary, the three uses of chemotherapy are:

1. As adjuvant therapy (in early disease as part of a combined treatment approach)

2. At the time of disease recurrence

3. When metastasis is present at the time of diagnosis

ENDOCRINE THERAPY

The endocrine glands secrete hormones that affect breast growth and function (see the section entitled "Normal Cyclic Changes in the Nonlactating Breast" earlier in this chapter), and the presence of these hormones can also affect the growth of breast cancer. Women with breast cancer whose tumors are influenced by hormones may respond to treatment involving endocrine manipulation. Three endocrine glands affect breast cancer growth: the ovaries, the adrenals, and the pituitary. An estrogen-receptor assay (determined by tissue biopsy) will identify a tumor as estrogen-dependent or estrogen-receptor positive. If endocrine manipulation is indicated, treatment may be surgical or chemical. Ablative surgery involves removing one or more of the glands that secrete hormones. An oophorectomy, adrenalectomy, or hypophysectomy (removal of the pituitary) may be indicated. In premenopausal women with estrogen-receptor positive tumors, oophorectomy can provide about a 65 percent chance of tumor remission (US Department of Health, Education, and Welfare 1979). The nurse should consult the surgical literature because each of these procedures requires different nursing management.

Additive hormonal therapy involves administering large doses of estrogen, androgen, or progestin in postmenopausal women. High doses of these hormones have been observed to cause tumor regression, although the exact mechanism of interaction is unknown. Some physicians consider chemical endocrine manipulation to be as effective as surgical intervention. In addition, certain drugs that can inhibit estrogen-dependent tumors (antiestrogens) may be tried before surgery is considered. Antiestrogen therapy has produced responses in about 70 percent of women who had estrogen-receptor positive tumors or had previously responded to hormone therapy (Legha et al 1976). Tamoxifen, an antiestrogen, is now commonly used in adjuvant therapy of postmenopausal women with receptor-positive neoplasms (Donegan 1986). Data from the NSABP and other studies examining the use of hormone therapy alone or as an adjuvant treatment are preliminary because long-term follow-up has so far been limited. More definitive studies are needed.

A major problem associated with hormone therapy is discomfort related to side effects. Symptoms may include the discomforts that accompany menopause, such as hot flashes. Estrogen taken in large doses may cause fluid retention, breast tenderness, and urinary incontinence. Hypercalcemia also may become a problem for approximately 10 percent of the women taking large doses of estrogen. Androgens may cause masculinizing side effects such as deepening of the voice, facial hair, and emotional and libidinal changes. These symptoms may cause body image disturbance for some women. Antiestrogens are accompanied by side effects of nausea, vomiting, hot flashes, lightheadedness, headaches, vaginal bleeding, and itching of the vulva.

Metastatic Disease

Metastatic breast cancer is characterized by the presence of cancer cells in distant parts of the body. Four sites of metastasis are the lungs, the viscera (liver), the brain, and bone. The woman with breast cancer metastasis has a shortened life expectancy, and her survival is frequently contingent on the organ systems involved in the metastasis and her response to therapy. In metastatic disease endocrine manipulation and chemotherapy are used to interrupt the cellular growth and spread of the cancer cells. Radiation therapy to a specific area and surgery are used palliatively to relieve the pain or obstruction associated with metastatic tumor spread. Metastatic disease is considered to be advanced or terminal when the cancer spread cannot be controlled by any of the therapeutic interventions previously discussed.

Metastatic breast cancer can cause various symptoms, depending in part on the organ affected. Metastasis to bone can cause a great deal of pain that is exacerbated by movement. Analgesics must be taken on a regular schedule to maintain a constant serum level of analgesia. Radiation therapy to the affected areas may alleviate skeletal pain. Visceral metastasis can involve ascites, which require diuretic therapy and possibly paracentesis. Lung metastasis often results in pleural effusions and difficulty in breathing. Brain metastasis can produce an alteration in sensorium, particularly memory loss, headaches, visual disturbances, seizures, and ataxic gait.

Women become aware of their increasing dependence and often feel that they can adjust to it, but the pain becomes an almost continual reminder of the disease and the inevitability of death (McCorkle 1973).

Psychosocial Concerns of the Woman With Breast Cancer

DELAY IN SEEKING DIAGNOSIS

Much of the literature written about women who discover lumps in their breasts centers on the problem of delay. A woman not seeking medical attention following discovery of a lump is considered to be delaying. Studies usually focus on women who have delayed more than one month after discovery of a mass. Factors observed to be significant in delay are:

- Attempts to deny the presence of a lump

- Lack of education about breast disorders

- Fear of mutilating surgery

- Fear of body image change resulting from treatment

- Fear of changes in relationships because of the disease

- Reluctance to submit to diagnostic and therapeutic procedures

Upon discovery of a lump, the woman will interpret the symptom in an effort to assign it meaning or put it into perspective; it is not the lump per se that influences action but the woman's interpretation of it (Green & Roberts 1974). Earlier studies of symptom interpretation in general found that women who delayed seeking treatment were often (a) unconcerned about their symptoms, viewing them as a recurrence of an old illness (eg, fibrocystic breast disease); (b) hesitant to know what the illness was; or (c) fearful of the effects of the suspected disease.

Women who delay seeking treatment have been observed to employ some common defense mechanisms such as denial. Compared with women who seek treatment promptly, women who delay tend to believe more strongly that the condition is not serious, experience a greater sense of powerlessness, and use more avoidance defenses in coping. They are also more likely to be depressed. Related psychosocial problems of delaying women have included marital problems, rejection by family members, and a general sense of isolation related to living alone.

DILEMMAS IN CHOOSING TREATMENT

When a woman is confronted with a breast mass, she initiates a formal or informal decision-making process that may involve a variety of factors and individuals other than herself. The decision-making process entails:

- Clarification of personal values and the formation of behavioral outcomes based on these values

- Recognition of an actual or potential threat to these values or beliefs

- Identification of alternatives

- Selection of alternatives

- Evaluation of alternatives

The optimal solution is more likely to be achieved if the decision maker uses reason and acts systematically. The best decision is consistent with the person's preferences and beliefs.

A study in which 138 healthy women were asked to choose breast cancer therapy under various conditions found that women may be willing to trade some physical safety for psychologic comfort (Valanis & Rumpler 1982). For treatment of a localized tumor, the majority chose a lumpectomy. For a metastatic tumor, 51.2 percent chose simple mastectomy; only 20.3 percent chose the radical mastectomy, which until very recently was preferred by most surgeons.

The most consistent influence on a woman's decision making is her physician. The traditional doctor-patient relationship places women in a passive, dependent role and limits their responsibility to seeking competent help and cooperating with the physician to get well.

Client involvement in treatment decisions has often been limited rather than encouraged. Not all women want to take full responsibility for their health care decisions, and some physicians wish to retain the traditional doctor-patient relationship, maintaining the woman's dependence on the physician's expertise and limiting her role in the decision making. Nevertheless, the woman is the only person who can decide what benefits of surgery are worth what personal risks. Despite the seriousness of the diagnosis, the time constraints, and expense involved, the woman should be encouraged to seek a second opinion. Many third-party payment plans now pay for this.

DILEMMAS IN COPING: BREAST CANCER VERSUS BREAST LOSS

Breast cancer is a health problem that engenders several psychosocial issues. In the early phases of treatment, an emotional dichotomy often prevails: The woman experiencing a mastectomy deals with either the cancer or the breast loss. Many authors and investigators claim that the emotional impact on body image is more devastating than the cancer itself; others believe that the diagnosis of cancer is more emotionally destructive than loss of a breast.

Unfortunately, health professionals, family, and friends may fall prey to this dichotomy. In an effort to comfort the woman, they complicate her feelings by commenting: "How awful to lose your breast, but you must feel grateful (happy, relieved) that the cancer is gone." In an earlier work, Quint (1963) and associates were impressed by the loneliness of women who had sustained mastectomy. The loneliness stemmed from two sources: body disfigurement and the possibility of dying from cancer. These issues assume equal importance in the woman's mind. To emphasize either issue only postpones resolution of the other. Yet in in the period immediately preceding and following mastectomy, health professionals tend to emphasize treatment of the cancer so that the woman will comply with her therapeutic regimen. The issue of breast loss is postponed. In the early postoperative phase, the woman may experience strong pressure from her husband, family, friends, and health care team to "do well" by adjusting quickly and easily to the surgery. Most American women have been socialized to be "good" by pleasing others. To please her mate or her physician, a woman may begin to deny some of her feelings, particularly about the loss of the breast. She may hold back her questions and refrain from talking about her feelings to impart a good impression. Yet it is known that gynecologic and breast cancers and the surgical procedures employed to treat them possess a unique potential for emotional devastation. The woman's self-concept and psychologic integration are severely threatened. The issue of sexuality is not secondary to the issue of physical survival; it is central to the woman's well-being (Derogatis 1980).

PERSONAL RESOURCES FOR COPING

Information about coping related specifically to breast cancer is limited. There is some evidence that coping

patterns displayed before the diagnosis of cancer are good predictors of postsurgery coping and eventual adjustment. A study of 60 terminally ill cancer patients indicated that women who had been "good copers" revealed less depression, anxiety, and social withdrawal. These women had a capacity for facing problems, a sense of life fulfillment, and a positive marital relationship (Hinton 1975). Some evidence suggests that religious affiliation promotes good coping.

Various studies suggest that age also influences women's ability to cope with breast cancer and/or mastectomy. In one study of 41 women with mastectomies, women under 45 years of age gave significantly poorer ratings of their postmastectomy adjustment than older women did. Women under 45 years of age were also more likely to seek psychologic counseling and to perceive mastectomy as having a negative influence on their sexual relationships. Derogatis (1980) suggested that the difference in perceptions may be related to the life events (eg, marriage and childbearing) anticipated by younger women in contrast to the perceptions of postmenopausal women. An older woman might not associate the illness with loss of sexual and reproductive functioning.

Gender role identification also affects a woman's adjustment to her breast loss and her disease. A woman who derives her sense of being "feminine" from her appearance may be at greater emotional risk than a woman whose self-concept is more expansive. Woods (1975) hypothesized that women whose breasts were smaller or larger than the norm would have strong positive or negative feelings about their breasts and therefore would experience the greatest psychologic trauma.

FAMILY AND FRIENDS

A woman's family and friends significantly influence her decision regarding surgery and her convalescence. A study of 41 mastectomy patients and 31 husbands concluded that women tended to perceive their husbands as their primary source of emotional support; health care professionals (surgeons and nurses) were evaluated as least supportive. The ability of a couple to adjust to breast cancer is related to (Jamison et al 1978):

● The partner's involvement in the decision-making process leading to the mastectomy

● The number of hospital visits the partner makes

● The resumption of the sexual relationship

● The husband looking at his wife's body after surgery

In addition to an alteration in sexual intimacy, the outside interests and social activities of the woman may decline despite physical recovery. Maguire (1975) reported that all the women in her sample of 450 experienced a decline in social and leisure activities. This decline may be related to reluctance of friends and family to initiate interactions with the ill woman (Lewis & Bloom 1978–1979). The woman's own uncertainty about resuming previous activities coupled with friends' reticence about "pushing" her may result in self-fulfilling behavior—a more withdrawn life-style.

Treatment of the woman as an isolated individual remains prevalent despite medicine's emphasis on family-centered health care. Significant others are not overlooked in health care team conferences, yet few planned interventions involve the woman's partner or significant other. This noninvolvement with significant others occurs despite professionals' awareness that the family is the primary source of social intervention and emotional support during adjustment to a stressful situation. Perhaps intervention with significant others is sporadic because family and friends are not easily accessible to the physician and other health team members. The professional nurse who is responsible for 24-hour primary care can often be instrumental in determining a multidisciplinary treatment focus that involves the woman and her partner.

LONG-TERM ADJUSTMENT: LIFE AFTER BREAST CANCER

The course of adjustment confronting the woman with breast cancer has been identified as a series of phases. Gyllenskold's (1982) in-depth interviews of 21 women with breast cancer reveal four phases of adjustment: shock, reaction, recovery, and reorientation.

In the shock phase, women made statements like "Everything is unreal" or "I can't understand what is happening to me." Shock extends from the discovery of the lump and throughout the process of diagnosis.

Reaction occurs in conjunction with the initiation of treatment. As treatment begins, the woman is compelled to face what has occurred and begins to take in what has happened. Coping mechanisms become evident during this phase. Reaction coincides with the length of treatment, and for many women radiation treatment or chemotherapy prolongs this period to months. During the phases of shock and reaction, the woman is completely absorbed with what has caused the problem (Gyllenskold 1982). Treatment reinforces the diagnosis of cancer and the immediate consequences of the disease. Physicians, intent on cure, emphasize survival and the importance of follow-up therapy. The woman wishes to "do well" and complies with the proposed adjuvant treatment. Denial of breast loss and the reality of her illness is common during the periods of diagnosis and treatment. Denial protects the woman, making therapy tolerable and enhancing her compliance.

Recovery begins during convalescence following the completion of medical treatment. Anxiety about her illness diminishes and the woman looks to the future once more

(Gyllenskold 1982). She turns outward and gradually resumes her former activities. Conversely, depression and social isolation occur if the woman is unable to negotiate this recovery phase successfully, and a chronic state of emotional and physical disability may result (Schmale 1979). Polivy (1977) indicated recovery to be a particularly vulnerable time. In her study of 40 women with mastectomies, denial remained strong well after discharge until the period of convalescence, when feelings of loss, devastation, and isolation would begin to emerge.

Reorientation follows recovery and is unending. It is accomplished when the woman can acknowledge that breast cancer is a part of her life, yet living, for her, has returned to or perhaps exceeded its former fullness and meaning.

Nursing Care During the Diagnostic Period

Nursing care begins before a woman faces a diagnosis of breast cancer. Indeed, the nurse can significantly affect the woman's prognosis by encouraging early detection of malignant tumors. Health teaching can assist the woman in understanding breast cancer treatment alternatives before disease occurs. Awareness of possible choices enables a woman to select the treatment regimen she perceives is best for her individual needs. Women are frequently overwhelmed by the amount of new information they must absorb while coping with the possibility of a frightening diagnosis. Anxiety can confuse and distort the decision-making process.

An effective nursing strategy involves systematically identifying women at risk for breast cancer and women at risk for ineffective coping after mastectomy. In the course of routine health checkups, nurses can identify risk factors and explore the woman's feelings about possible breast loss. During routine visits, the nurse can teach breast self-examination (BSE), and provide opportunities for return demonstration, and plan with the woman for monthly BSE and follow-up evaluations. The nurse also can assess and record the woman's knowledge about breast cancer and its treatment alternatives. The nurse should present information in a straightforward fashion in terms appropriate to the woman's education and cognitive level. Throughout interactions with the woman, the nurse should emphasize the value of BSE in early detection.

NURSING ASSESSMENT

The woman seeking health care following discovery of a lump is likely to be apprehensive. She may hold unfounded beliefs about breast cancer. Holistic health assessment should be conducted in an understanding, unhurried, emotionally supportive atmosphere. Such an assessment has therapeutic value in itself. It should include:

- A systems review emphasizing the reproductive system, particularly the breast

- The significance the woman attributes to her breasts

- The woman's knowledge and beliefs about breast cancer

- Identification of social support

- The woman's emotional status and coping mechanisms she has used during periods of stress

- Environmental factors that may influence coping and adjustment

Assessment of the woman facing a diagnosis of breast cancer must be an ongoing process. Sufficient data must be obtained to provide the nurse and other health team members with increasing insight into the client's biophysical, mental, emotional, and social situation.

NURSING DIAGNOSIS

Nursing diagnoses that may apply during the diagnostic period include:

- Knowledge deficit related to the diagnostic procedures

- Fear related to the possibility of a diagnosis of cancer

NURSING GOAL: PROVISION OF ADEQUATE INFORMATION AND EMOTIONAL SUPPORT

The nurse should explain the two-step procedure to assure the woman that she will be able to participate in deciding about her treatment once the biopsy results are known. If the woman has reservations or doubts about the proposed course of treatment or her relationship with her physician, the nurse can encourage her to discuss her desire for a second medical opinion with her physician. In fact many third-party payment plans now encourage and pay for a second opinion. Nursing advocacy involves supporting the woman's right to make the best decision for her. The woman who has discovered a breast lump is often so upset and fearful that she finds it difficult to voice her concern or even ask questions. She may be afraid that seeking another medical opinion will waste precious time and compromise her prognosis. With the assistance of the nurse she can explore her fears, clarify her values, and identify what treatment alternatives would be personally acceptable. Once the woman has made an informed decision, the nurse's function becomes one of support.

Once the results of the biopsy are known, the woman and her partner should hear the treatment alternatives together. They need adequate time to make a decision that is best for her as a woman and them as a couple. Illness is a family affair; failure to include family or friends in the

decision-making process limits the woman's resources and hampers decision making.

Nursing Care During the Preoperative Period

If a diagnosis of cancer is made and the woman elects to have a surgical intervention, nursing care is directed to the assessments and care typically indicated prior to any surgery, as well as the assessments indicated by the woman's diagnosis.

NURSING ASSESSMENT

The nurse assesses the woman's health status with regard to any evidence of infection, especially respiratory infection, which would increase her risk of complications. The nurse inquires about medication allergies, previous experience with surgery, and any factors in the woman's history (for example, previous episodes of thrombophlebitis or routine use of steroid medication) that increase her risk.

The nurse also assesses the woman's knowledge of her condition, what to expect from surgery, and what postoperative care involves. Finally the nurse assesses the woman's and her family's emotional state and attitude toward surgery.

NURSING DIAGNOSIS

Nursing diagnoses that might apply preoperatively include:

- Knowledge deficit related to the surgical procedure

- Anxiety related to possible change in body image following surgery

- Ineffective individual coping related to inability to accept the reality of the cancer diagnosis

NURSING GOAL: PROVISION OF EFFECTIVE PREOPERATIVE TEACHING

The nurse explains routines and procedures of surgery that are pertinent to the woman's hospital stay. This includes, but is not limited to, information about preoperative skin preparation, having nothing to eat or drink for several hours before surgery, any preoperative medication, the series of events that will occur on the day of surgery, and the assessments that will be made in the recovery room. The nurse also discusses with the family the care and assessments that will be made postoperatively. The nurse includes information on the dressing, wound suction device (if indicated), availability of pain medication, rationale for early ambulation, and respiratory and arm exercises. The nurse may also have the woman practice deep breathing and coughing as well as leg exercises.

NURSING GOAL: PROVISION OF EMOTIONAL SUPPORT

The nurse provides the woman with opportunities to ask questions and clarifies any misconceptions. The nurse also helps the woman verbalize her fears or concerns about the treatment and the implications of her diagnosis. The nurse is also alert to the coping abilities and needs of the woman's family. It is very important for the woman to feel that she is receiving nursing care from individuals who are skilled technically but also recognize the impact of a diagnosis of breast cancer and are committed to helping the woman in a holistic way.

Nursing Care During the Postoperative Period

Nursing care during the postoperative period changes as the woman progresses and adapts following surgery. The woman's needs in the immediate postoperative period, for example, are somewhat different from those on the third postoperative day.

NURSING ASSESSMENT

The nurse assesses the woman's condition postoperatively to detect any potential complications. Vital signs are assessed regularly for evidence of change, and the nurse is alert to other signs that might indicate shock. The dressing is inspected and reinforced as necessary, and the quantity of drainage in the wound suction device (Hemovac) is monitored.

In addition, other routine postoperative assessments are made: The nurse auscultates the woman's lungs, assesses the abdomen for distention, evaluates urinary output, monitors the intensity of the woman's discomfort, and regulates the intravenous fluids.

After the immediate postoperative period, the nurse continues to assess the woman for evidence of infection, discomfort, and emotional problems. Throughout the postoperative period the nurse evaluates the woman's teaching needs and plans appropriate interventions.

NURSING DIAGNOSIS

Nursing diagnoses that may apply during the postoperative period include:

- Potential alteration in respiratory function related to the effects of anesthesia and immobility
- Potential for infection related to surgical intervention
- Alteration in comfort: acute pain related to surgery

- Potential sexual dysfunction related to loss of a body part
- Knowledge deficit related to a lack of understanding of the importance of follow-up care

NURSING GOAL: PREVENTION OF RESPIRATORY COMPLICATIONS

Following surgery the woman is at increased risk for respiratory complications. The nurse monitors the respiratory rate and breath sounds regularly to prevent respiratory complications. The woman is encouraged to turn, cough, and deep breathe every two hours. This is especially important for the woman who had a mastectomy because the pressure dressing may constrict chest expansion. In addition pain and pain medication also decrease the depth of respirations. Deep breathing may be facilitated by the use of an incentive spirometer or blow bottles. Early ambulation also helps prevent respiratory complications.

NURSING GOAL: PREVENTION OF INFECTION

Because fever is generally indicative of infection, the woman's temperature is assessed regularly. The wound is also evaluated for signs of infection (redness, edema, ecchymosis, drainage, and poor approximation) at least three times daily once the initial pressure dressing has been changed. Sterile technique is essential during regular dressing changes. The type of drainage in the Hemovac is also useful in monitoring for infection. Purulent drainage is always suspect. The nurse also administers antibiotics as ordered.

The woman is instructed not to permit blood pressure assessment, venipunctures, or injections to be done on the infected side, especially if lymph nodes have been removed.

NURSING GOAL: PROVISION OF COMFORT AND PAIN RELIEF

The nurse is alert to verbal and nonverbal clues that the woman is experiencing pain. The nurse assists the woman in achieving a position of comfort, and provides alternative methods to promote comfort. These include oral care, back rubs, use of imagery, and a restful environment. The nurse also provides pain medication as needed. The astute nurse provides pain medication prior to morning care, ambulation, or turning and coughing so that the woman can accomplish these tasks more effectively.

NURSING GOAL: PREVENTION OF LYMPHEDEMA

The woman who has lymph nodes removed as part of her surgical treatment is at risk of swelling and pain in the arm on her affected side. This is especially true if a radical or modified radical mastectomy is done. Postoperatively the nurse maintains the woman's arm in an elevated position to facilitate drainage. This can be done by propping it on pillows so that the hand is higher than the elbow and the elbow is higher than the shoulder. The circumference of the forearm and upper arm are measured regularly to monitor the amount of edema. Forearm exercises are generally ordered to begin as early as the first postoperative day. The nurse can also encourage the woman to use her affected arm for feeding, washing, and hair combing. The nurse should also give the following information on arm care:

- Do not have blood drawn, injections given, or blood pressures taken from the affected arm without the physician's permission.

- Wear a mitt when cooking to avoid burns.

- Use a lanolin-based cream to keep cuticles soft rather than cutting them.

- Protect the affected arm and hand during other activities such as gardening, sewing, or washing dishes.

- Wear a Medic Alert tag that indicates lymphedema arm—no blood tests or needle injections.

- See a physician if there is swelling, hardness, or redness in the arm.

The nurse teaches arm exercises, such as wall climbing, forward and lateral arm lifting, and pendulum swinging (across the body, in circles, and forward and backward); exaggerated deep breathing; and pulley exercises. The nurse advises the woman to avoid lifting heavy objects with the affected arm and to maintain an upright posture with her back straight, shoulders back, and arms hanging loosely at her sides when ambulating.

NURSING GOAL: PROVISION OF PSYCHOLOGIC SUPPORT

Breast cancer is a situational crisis that affects the woman's ability not only to cope but also to make the best treatment decision. If the woman is displaying a great deal of anxiety about treatment, she may need counseling both preoperatively and postoperatively. Arrangements for psychotherapy may need to be made if the woman appears to be at high risk for postmastectomy depression. Sexual counseling should also be made available for those who believe their sexual relationships will suffer. A psychiatric clinical nurse specialist who is a liaison to the medical-surgical units may be a valuable resource. The clinical nurse specialist also can provide continuity of emotional support for the woman throughout the treatment process.

The emotional dilemma of breast cancer versus breast loss that often confronts the woman who is newly recovering from mastectomy has already been discussed. The nurse providing emotional support must allow the woman to express her feelings of both death and disfigurement. The health care team must avoid exerting subtle pressure on the woman to "do well" by discouraging her from talking about her fears or providing only superficial information about her recovery. The nurse must be skillful in crisis theory and intervention. The nurse who is intimately involved with the woman's care should watch for signs that the woman is shifting her focus from the cancer itself to the loss of the breast. Is she coping with both issues simultaneously, or is she remaining preoccupied with one or the other? How a woman integrates her disease and her breast loss into her psychologic and physical rehabilitation is of cardinal concern to the professional nurse.

A client-centered conference dealing with the woman's psychosocial response to her mastectomy is beneficial. The nurse with primary care responsibility may be in a position to teach the health care team about the woman's coping behaviors and her need to verbalize her distress. A consistent, individualized approach to the woman's psychosocial needs should be noted in the nursing care plan. Ideally, one nurse would assume the primary therapeutic role. Psychosocial support for the woman's sexual partner is also vital, and the sexual partner should be included in teaching and counseling sessions.

The nurse who assumes primary responsibility for helping the woman deal with the psychosocial aspects of her breast loss should provide the woman with opportunities to express her feelings about her breast and its loss. The nurse must be sensitive to the woman's cues as to when it is acceptable to involve the sexual partner in the observation of the woman's incision and in counseling about the woman's altered appearance. The nurse can also discuss the types of prostheses available if reconstruction is not possible or if the woman has decided against it. Even if the woman will be having reconstruction at a later time, she will probably be interested in using a prosthesis temporarily.

The nurse can help the woman plan the resumption of her normal daily activities and interests. Sexual activity can be resumed when the woman's energy level permits. The nurse can help the couple explore alternative methods of sexual expression if sexual intercourse is too difficult initially. The nurse can tactfully assess the woman's prior sexual activity and discuss modifications in sexual activity that may make sexual expression easier. These modifications may be as simple as changing the sides of the bed so that the partner can more easily caress the remaining breast or having the woman wear her prosthesis and an attractive nightgown to bed. Sexual or marital counseling is valuable for some couples and should be initiated if requested.

NURSING GOAL: EFFECTIVE DISCHARGE
PLANNING

The woman should have a clear understanding of follow-up treatment and care prior to discharge. The nurse can collaborate with the physician regarding planned post-operative therapy. The woman should clearly understand her prescribed chemotherapeutic drugs and their side effects. She should have a clear understanding of other possible therapies as well. Furthermore the woman should thoroughly understand the importance of preventive health care such as BSE and the need to comply with scheduled routine physical examinations and medical evaluations.

Referrals to either a community health nurse or a "Reach to Recovery" volunteer should be initiated and the date of the visit confirmed with the woman. A "Reach to Recovery" volunteer from the American Cancer Society is invaluable in helping the woman adjust to her mastectomy. Each volunteer has had a mastectomy herself and often serves as a role model for the woman with a new mastectomy. The American Cancer Society volunteer can provide the woman with information about breast prostheses and guidelines for arm exercises and self-care.

The woman who has had a mastectomy must continually monitor the information she divulges to society about her self-identity. Her altered self-identity will influence her pattern of interactions with others. She may choose to deal with her "difference" and resolve it, or she may choose not to adjust but to withdraw socially and emotionally. The woman needs to experience sorrow that accompanies her breast loss. She must then integrate her changed image of her feminine self into an overall self-concept that affirms her as a vital, sexual woman. When a woman can discuss her breast cancer as part of her history while affirming her life as full and sexually satisfying, her adjustment to her illness is complete.

Nursing Care of the Woman Choosing Reconstructive Surgery

Reconstructive surgery is becoming increasingly common following mastectomy. In some cases it is done at the same time as the mastectomy; in other instances the woman returns for reconstruction at a later time. The nurse who works with a woman considering reconstruction plays a vital role in providing information to help the woman make an informed decision.

The nurse and the woman should discuss the advantages and disadvantages of breast reconstructive surgery. Women are learning about the variety of surgical treatments, and many women are now asking about reconstruction. The nurse, as the woman's advocate, is responsible for making sure that the woman has been fully informed about the advantages and disadvantages of this procedure. Advantages of breast reconstruction include:

- Improved physical appearance

- An invaluable psychologic lift and improvement of body image

- The ability to wear normal clothing without worrying about exposing a prosthesis

- The opportunity to resume more strenuous activities (eg, sports) without being concerned about exposing a prosthesis

Disadvantages include:

- The reality that the reconstructed breast is never identical to the unaffected breast

- The expense and risk of further surgical procedures

- The possibility of an unsatisfactory result or surgical complications

- The fact that the reconstructed breast will never replace the lost one

Nursing responsibilities include health education and emotional support. Following discharge, the woman is often instructed to keep the elbow on the affected side close to her body for several days to a week. Within a month, full use of her arm should be possible. Her physician may provide her with specific recommendations about strenuous exercise (eg, golf or swimming). The nurse should stress the need for full compliance with any restrictions. Often a specifically designed bra is to be worn day and night to assist the reconstructed breast to take on the appropriate shape. The psychologic victory that a woman may experience as a result of breast reconstruction should not be underestimated. The nurse working with a woman considering breast reconstruction should be experienced in psychosocial assessment and counseling.

Nursing Care of the Woman With Metastatic Breast Cancer

A woman with metastatic breast cancer simultaneously faces the difficulty of dealing with the pain she is experiencing and the reality that she is going to die. Nursing interventions must be directed toward alleviating pain and enhancing comfort. The nurse should support and encourage the woman's independence and efforts at self-care and provide time for recreation and ambulation within the hospital routine. The potential for pathologic fractures in bones with metastasis must be carefully monitored; teaching the woman good body mechanics helps prevent fractures.

Psychosocial support becomes paramount for the woman who is terminally ill. The nurse plays a significant role in assisting the woman to grieve and eventually to come to terms with her impending death. Family members also need emotional support and the opportunity to begin their grief work. As the woman attempts to confront her death, she may wish to return home. Community resources, home health care services, or hospice care are often instrumental in providing the necessary support for a comfortable, dignified death. The nurse should review the nursing literature that deals with care of the terminally ill. The nurse must be comfortable in establishing a therapeutic, helping relationship with the woman and her family. Perhaps at no other point in nursing practice is the therapeutic use of self more important.

Evaluative Outcome Criteria

Anticipated outcomes of nursing care include the following:

- The woman copes successfully with the diagnosis of breast cancer and the therapy she chooses.

- The woman clearly understands her diagnosis and treatment, her therapy, and her long-term prognosis.

- If she receives surgery, the woman has a successful recovery period. If complications do occur they are quickly recognized and treatment is begun.

- The woman participates in planning her recovery program.

- The woman completes planned exercises, activities, follow-up, and additional therapy.

● Care of the Woman With Endometriosis

Endometriosis is a condition characterized by the presence of endometrial tissue outside the endometrial cavity. This tissue responds to the hormonal changes of the menstrual cycle and bleeds in a cyclic fashion. This bleeding results in inflammation, scarring of the peritoneum, and formation of adhesions. The most common symptoms include progressive dysmenorrhea, dyspareunia, and infertility.

Endometriosis may occur at any age after puberty, although it is most common in women between 30 and 40 and is rare in postmenopausal women. A familial tendency does seem to exist.

The exact cause of endometriosis is not known. One of the oldest theories suggests that endometriosis is caused by a reflux of endometrial cells through the fallopian tubes during menstruation and their implantation in the abdominal cavity. Another theory suggests that endometrial cells are carried to distant sites through the venous and lymphatic systems. Hormonal causes have also been suggested. To date, however, no single theory provides an adequate explanation (Garner & Webster 1985).

Medical Therapy

Somewhat paradoxically, the extent of a woman's symptoms does not necessarily indicate the extent of her endometriosis. A woman may have extensive involvement with few symptoms or only a few lesions with severe incapacitation. The most common symptom is pelvic pain, which is often a dull ache or cramping sensation. It is often related to menstruation and generally ceases following the completion of the woman's menses. Dyspareunia, another common symptom, occurs most frequently if the uterus is retroverted and lesions are present in the area of the posterior vaginal fornix or the uterosacral ligaments.

Another frequently cited symptom is abnormal uterine bleeding. No specific pattern exists, although it may be frequent, prolonged, and excessive (Merrill 1986).

Endometriosis is often diagnosed when a woman seeks treatment or evaluation for infertility. Bimanual examination may reveal a fixed, tender, retroverted uterus and palpable nodules in the cul-de-sac. The diagnosis can be confirmed by laparoscopy.

Treatment may be medical, surgical, or a combination of the two. During the laparoscopic examination, the physician may surgically resect any visible implants of endometrial tissue, taking care to avoid damaging any organs. If the woman does not desire pregnancy at the present time, she may be started on oral contraceptives. The woman who desires pregnancy and has been unsuccessful in her attempts to conceive is treated with a six-month course of danazol (Wedell et al 1985). Danazol alters estrogen production, which results in endometrial suppression by blocking pituitary secretion of gonadotropins. Because it has some androgenic effects, side effects may include fluid retention, mild weight gain, acne, hirsutism, depression, decreased breast size, rash, and deepening of the voice (Malinak & Wheeler 1985).

In more advanced cases surgery may be done to remove implants and break up adhesions. If severe dyspareunia or dysmenorrhea are symptoms, the surgeon may perform a presacral neurectomy. In advanced cases in which childbearing is not an issue, a hysterectomy with bilateral salpingo-oophorectomy may be done.

Nursing Assessment

The nurse should be aware of the common symptoms of endometriosis and elicit an accurate history if a woman mentions these symptoms. If a woman is being treated for endometriosis, the nurse should assess the woman's understanding of the condition, its implications, and the treatment alternatives.

Nursing Diagnosis

Nursing diagnoses that may apply to a woman with endometriosis include:

- Alteration in comfort: acute pain related to dysmenorrhea

- Knowledge deficit related to a lack of understanding of the disease process

- Ineffective individual coping related to depression secondary to infertility

Nursing Goal: Provision of Effective Education

The nurse can be available to explain the condition, its symptoms, treatment alternatives, and prognosis. The nurse can help the woman evaluate treatment options and make choices that are appropriate for her. If medication is begun, the nurse can review the dosage, schedule, possible side effects, and any warning signs. Women are often advised to avoid delaying pregnancy because of the risk of infertility. The woman may wish to discuss the implications of this on her life choices, relationship with her partner, and personal preferences. The nurse can be a nonjudgmental listener and help the woman consider her options.

Nursing care for a woman with infertility are discussed in Chapter 9.

Evaluative Outcome Criteria

Anticipated outcomes of nursing care include the following:

- The woman clearly understands her condition, its implications for fertility, and her treatment options.

- The woman successfully copes with the discomfort and long-term implications of her diagnosis.

● Care of the Woman With Toxic Shock Syndrome

Toxic shock syndrome (TSS) was first described in children (Todd et al 1978). Two years later the association between TSS and menstruation was identified (Johnson 1985). Although TSS has been reported in children, postmenopausal women, and men, it is primarily a disease of reproductive age women, especially women at or near menses or during the postpartum period. The causative organism is a strain of *Staphylococcus aureus* that produces a specific toxin called TSST-1. Although the vast majority of women have antibodies to *S. aureus*, only a few ever develop signs of the disease. Research indicates a possible link between high levels of estradiol and inhibition of toxin production. If this is the case, it would explain the higher incidence of TSS during menstruation and the postpartal period when estradiol levels are low (Connell 1985).

The use of high absorbency tampons has been widely related to an increased incidence of TSS. However, occluding the cervical os with a contraceptive device such as a diaphragm or contraceptive sponge, especially if they are left in place for more than 24 hours, may also increase the risk of TSS (Connell 1985).

Medical Therapy

Early diagnosis and treatment are important in preventing a fatal outcome. The case-to-fatality ratio has decreased from 15 percent to 3 percent (Eschenbach 1986).

The most common signs of TSS include fever (often greater than 38.9C [102F]); desquamation of the skin, especially the palms and soles, which usually occurs one to two weeks after the onset of symptoms; rash; hypotension; and dizziness. Systemic symptoms often include vomiting, diarrhea, severe myalgia, and inflamed mucous membranes (oropharyngeal, conjunctival, or vaginal). In addition, disorders of the central nervous system, including alterations in consciousness, disorientation, and coma, may occur.

Laboratory findings reveal elevated BUN, creatinine, SGOT, SGPT, and total bilirubin, while platelets are often less than $100,000/mm^3$. Blood, throat, and CSF cultures are negative, as are tests for Rocky Mountain spotted fever (Connell 1985).

Women with TSS are generally hospitalized and given supportive therapy, including intravenous fluids to maintain blood pressure. Severe cases may require renal dialysis, administration of vasopressors, and intubation. Penicillinase-resistant antibiotics, while of limited value during the acute phase, do help reduce the risk of recurrence (Eschenbach 1986).

Nursing Assessment

Nurses caring for women should ask about their clients' tampon use practices. The nurse should pay special attention to women who customarily wear their tampons for extended periods of time or who leave a diaphragm or contraceptive sponge in place longer than six hours after intercourse. The nurse should also be alert for early signs of TSS and refer women with them to a physician for further evaluaton.

Nursing Diagnosis

Nursing diagnoses that may apply to a woman with TSS include:

- Knowledge deficit related to ways of preventing the development of TSS

- Alteration in comfort: acute pain related to severe myalgia secondary to TSS

Nursing Goal: Education for Self-Care

Nurses play a major role in helping educate women about ways of preventing the development of TSS. Women should understand the importance of avoiding prolonged use of tampons. Some women may choose to use other products, such as sanitary napkins or minipads. The woman who chooses to continue using tampons may reduce her risk by alternating them with napkins and by avoiding overnight use of tampons.

Postpartal women are advised to avoid the use of tampons for six to eight weeks after delivery. Women with a history of TSS should totally refrain from using tampons (Eschenbach 1986).

Women who use barrier contraceptives such as diaphragms or contraceptive sponges should avoid leaving them in place for prolonged periods.

Nurses can also help make women aware of the signs and symptoms of TSS so that women will seek treatment promptly if signs occur.

Evaluative Outcome Criteria

Anticipated outcomes of nursing care include the following:

- The woman understands the cause of toxic shock syndrome and modifies any personal practices that might increase her risk of developing TSS.

- If a woman develops TSS, treatment is effective and any potential problems are quickly identified and corrected.

● Infectious Disorders of the Genital Tract

The occurrence of sexually transmitted diseases (STDs) has increased over the past few decades. The terms *venereal disease* and *VD* are being used less frequently; they appear outdated and carry value-laden, negative connotations. Moreover, not all sexually transmitted infections are included among those that have been classified as venereal disease. Many health professionals do not acknowledge the distinction between sexually transmitted infections and vaginitis, yet it is important to differentiate minor or recurring infections from those that can cause serious health problems. No matter how these infections are classified, women often feel anxious, guilty, embarrassed, or fearful when they have or suspect they have vaginitis or a sexually transmitted infection.

Vaginitis is an inflammation of the vulva and/or vagina. Symptoms of vaginitis and STDs include pain, discharge, foul odor, and/or pruritus. Vaginitis is sometimes but not always sexually related, whereas STDs include infections that are either definitely or potentially sexually related. Transmission of STDs can occur during various types of heterosexual or homosexual contact, including nongenital (eg, oral-genital) as well as genital contact.

Vaginitis and sexually transmitted infections are the most common reasons for outpatient treatment of women. Because vaginitis is a common, supposedly simple disorder, diagnosis and prescription of therapy are frequently done over the phone. Often clinicians fail to appreciate all aspects of these infections as they relate to discomfort and concerns of their clients.

Basic information applicable to all infections that may be sexually transmitted is listed in Table 10–6. Precautions specific to a particular sexually transmitted infection are noted with discussion of that infection.

● Care of the Woman With a Vaginal Infection

Candida albicans (Moniliasis)

Moniliasis (often called "yeast infection") is the most common form of vaginitis affecting the vagina and vulva. Recurrences are frequent for some women. Factors that contribute to occurrence of this infection are use of oral contraceptives, use of antibiotics, pregnancy, diagnosed diabetes mellitus, and other premenstrual factors that are un-

Table 10–6 Ten Basic Points About Sexually Transmitted Infections

1. Use of condoms and spermicidal contraceptives can reduce the possibility of infection.
2. Women with a new sexual partner or more than one sexual partner may be more likely to develop an infection.
3. If symptoms of infections are suspected, the client should avoid intercourse or instruct her male partner or partners to use condoms.
4. Clients should *complete* the prescribed medication regimen. Disappearance of symptoms is not evidence that the infection has been cured.
5. Nurses should encourage women to have an examination and specific testing. Second guessing or phone diagnosing (eg, "I think it's what I had last year") should be avoided.
6. Women in poor general health and those with certain chronic health problems are more susceptible to infection.
7. If one sexually transmitted infection is present, it is common to have another infection.
8. The presence of infection can contribute to an abnormal Pap smear report.
9. Informing a sexual partner of the possible need for treatment is essential.
10. Cleansing genitals before and after intercourse and postcoital urination may prevent sexually transmitted infections.

Source: Keith L, Brittain J: *Sexually Transmitted Diseases.* Aspen, Colo., Creative Informatics, 1978.

clear. A gram-positive fungus (*Candida albicans*) is the causative organism. *Candida* is a resident of the mouth, intestines, and vagina in 25 percent to 50 percent of healthy women (Sonstegard et al 1982). Infection seems to occur when there is overgrowth of this organism.

MEDICAL THERAPY

The goal of medical therapy is to diagnose the infection and treat it effectively. The woman will often complain of thick, curdy vaginal discharge; severe itching; dysuria; and dyspareunia. A male sexual partner may experience a rash or excoriation of the skin of the penis, and possibly pruritus. The male may be symptomatic and the female asymptomatic.

On physical examination the woman's labia may be swollen and excoriated if the pruritus has been severe. A speculum examination reveals thick, white, tenacious cheeselike patches adhering to the vaginal mucosa. Diagnosis is confirmed by microscopic examination of the vaginal discharge; hyphae and spores will usually be seen on a wet mount preparation (Figure 10–2).

Medical treatment of monilial vaginitis includes intravaginal insertion of miconazole or clotrimazole suppositories or cream at bedtime for one week. If the vulva is also infected, the cream is prescribed and may be applied topically.

Because *Candida* may be harbored in the folds of skin of the penis, it is important to treat the sexual partner to

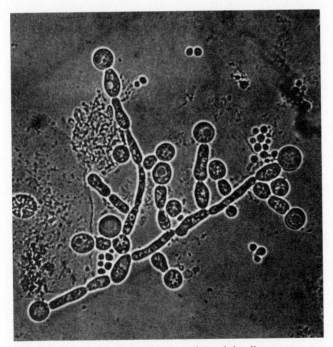

Figure 10–2   The hyphae and spores of Candida albicans (Courtesy of Tortora G, et al: *Microbiology.* Menlo Park, Calif, Benjamin/Cummings, 1982)

prevent recurrence of the vaginitis in the woman. Topical miconazole usually eliminates the yeast infection from the male.

If miconazole cream is being used by both partners, sexual intercourse is permitted and may assure the spread of the cream throughout the vagina. With other methods of treatment, abstinence is recommended until both partners are cured.

Systemic nystatin therapy may be prescribed for recurrences when intestinal colonization is suspected (Keith & Brittain 1978). If a woman experiences frequent recurrences of monilial vaginitis, she should be tested for an elevated blood glucose level to determine whether a diabetic or prediabetic condition is present. A pregnant woman should be aware that infection at the time of delivery could cause thrush in the neonate.

NURSING ASSESSMENT

The nurse caring for the woman should suspect monilial vaginitis if the woman complains of intense vulvar itching and a curdy, white discharge. Because the woman with diabetes mellitus during pregnancy is especially susceptible to this infection, the nurse should be alert for symptoms in these women. In some areas, nurses are trained to do speculum examinations and wet mount preparations and can, therefore, confirm the diagnosis themselves. In most cases, however, the nurse who suspects a vaginal infection reports this to the woman's physician, nurse practitioner, or certified nurse-midwife.

NURSING DIAGNOSIS

Nursing diagnoses that might apply to the woman with monilial vaginitis include:

- Alteration in comfort: acute itching related to the effects of the monilial infection

- Knowledge deficit related to ways of preventing the development of monilial vaginitis

NURSING GOAL: EDUCATION FOR SELF-CARE

If the woman is experiencing discomfort due to the pruritus, the nurse can recommend gentle bathing of the vulva with a weak sodium bicarbonate solution. If a topical treatment is being used, the woman should bathe the area before applying the medication.

The nurse will also discuss with the woman the factors that contribute to the development of monilial vaginitis and can suggest ways to prevent recurrences, such as wearing cotton underwear, careful wiping front to back following elimination, and avoiding vaginal powders or sprays that may irritate. Some women report that the addition of yogurt to the diet or the use of activated culture of plain yogurt as a vaginal douche helps prevent recurrence by maintaining high levels of lactobacillus.

EVALUATIVE OUTCOME CRITERIA

Anticipated outcomes of nursing care include the following:

- The woman's symptoms are relieved and the infection is cured.

- The woman is able to identify self-care measures to prevent further episodes of monilial vaginitis.

Bacterial Vaginosis (*Gardnerella vaginalis* Vaginitis)

Many flora normally inhabit the vagina of the healthy woman. Some of these organisms are potentially pathogenic. In some women these bacteria begin to "overgrow," causing a vaginitis. The cause of this overgrowth is not clear, although tissue trauma and sexual intercourse are sometimes identified as contributing factors. The *Gardnerella vaginalis* organism (formerly referred to as *Hemophilus vaginalis*) has been found in the vast majority of cases, along with an increased concentration of anaerobic bacteria. The infected woman often notices an excessive amount of thin, watery, yellow-gray vaginal discharge with a foul odor described as "fishy." The characteristic "clue" cell is seen on vaginal smear (Figure 10–3).

The nonpregnant woman is generally treated with metronidazole (Flagyl). Because of its potential teratogenic effects, metronidazole is avoided during pregnancy; 500 mg ampicillin every six hours for seven days is used instead.

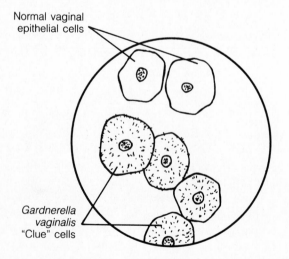

Normal vaginal
epithelial cells

Gardnerella vaginalis "Clue" cells

Figure 10–3   Depiction of the "clue cells" characteristically seen in bacterial vaginosis (Gardnerella vaginalis)

Care of the Woman With a Sexually Transmitted Disease

Trichomoniasis

Between 15 percent and 20 percent of all women are infected with trichomoniasis at some time. This infection is most frequently seen in females 16 to 35 years of age (Sonstegard et al 1982). Women are usually symptomatic. Between 60 percent and 70 percent of male partners may be asymptomatic carriers (Mims & Swenson 1980).

Trichomonas is a microscopic motile protozoan that thrives in an alkaline environment. Most infections are acquired through sexual intimacy. Transmission by shared bath facilities, wet towels, or wet swimsuits may be possible (Sonstegard et al 1982).

MEDICAL THERAPY

Symptoms of trichomoniasis include a yellow-green, frothy, odorous discharge frequently accompanied by inflammation of the vagina and cervix, dysuria, and dyspareunia. There is a wide variation of symptoms from woman to woman, including the symptomatic presence of *Trichomonas*. Visualization of *Trichomonas* under the microscope on a wet-mount preparation of vaginal discharge will confirm the diagnosis (Figure 10–4).

Prescriptive treatment for trichomoniasis is metronidazole administered over 7 days or in a single 2 g dose for both male and female sexual partners. Intercourse should be avoided until both partners are cured.

The woman should be informed that metronidazole is contraindicated in the first trimester of pregnancy because of possible teratogenic effects on the fetus. The woman and her partner should be cautioned to avoid alcohol while taking metronidazole; the combination has an effect similar to that of alcohol and Antabuse—abdominal pain, flushing, or tremors (Sciarra et al 1984).

Various vaginal creams, suppositories, or douches may decrease symptoms without clearing up the infection. The woman should be tested for other sexually transmitted infections such as gonorrhea and chlamydia.

Chlamydial Infection

Chlamydial infection, caused by *Chlamydia trachomatis,* is the most common STD in the United States. The organism is an intracellular bacterium with several different immunotypes. Immunotypes of *Chlamydia* are responsible for lymphogranuloma venereum and trachoma, which is the world's leading cause of preventable blindness.

Chlamydia is a major cause of nongonococcal urethritis (NGU) in men. In women it can cause infections similar to those that occur with gonorrhea. It can infect the fallopian tubes, cervix, urethra, and Bartholin's glands.

Pelvic inflammatory disease, infertility, and ectopic pregnancy are associated with chlamydia.

The infant of a woman with untreated chlamydia is at risk to develop ophthalmia neonatorum, which, although responsive to erythromycin ophthalmic ointment, does not respond to silver nitrate eye prophylaxis. The newborn may also develop chlamydial pneumonia. In fact, approximately 30,000 cases of pneumonia in infants 6 months old or less are traceable to chlamydial infections (Sweet et al 1983). Pregnant women with asymptomatic cases of chlamydia have a 40 percent to 70 percent incidence of neonatal chlamydial infection. Chlamydia may also be responsible for premature labor and fetal death.

Symptoms of chlamydia include a thin or purulent discharge, burning and frequency of urination, and lower abdominal pain. Women, however, are often asymptomatic. Diagnosis is frequently made after treatment of a male partner for NGU or in a symptomatic woman with a negative gonorrhea culture. Laboratory detection is now simpler due to the availability of a test to detect monoclonal antibodies specific for *Chlamydia*.

The usual prescribed treatment is tetracycline or doxycycline. Pregnant women should be treated with erythromycin ethyl succinate (Schachter 1986). Many authorities are recommending routine treatment of newborns with tetracycline or erythromycin eye ointment to avoid the possibility of conjunctivitis.

Herpes Genitalis (Herpes Simplex Virus)

Herpes infections are seen in private offices more often than gonorrhea. Accurate incidence statistics are not available because herpes is not a reportable infection. The herpes simplex virus is the causative organism. There are two types of herpes:

- Type 1—usually noted to be present above the waist and not usually sexually transmitted (the "cold sore" is the most common herpes type 1 lesion). This type may occur in the genital area, usually as a result of oral-genital sexual contact.

- Type 2—usually associated with genital infections. This type can occur as oral lesions after oral-genital sexual contact if genital lesions are present.

The clinical symptoms and treatment of type 1 and type 2 herpes are the same when they occur in the genital area.

PRIMARY EPISODE

Single or multiple blisterlike vesicles appear, usually in the genital area and sometimes affecting the vaginal walls, cervix, urethra, and anus. The vesicles may appear within a few hours to 20 days after exposure and rupture spontaneously to form extremely painful, open, ulcerated

lesions. Inflammation and pain secondary to the presence of herpes lesions can cause difficult urination and urinary retention. Inguinal lymph node enlargement may be present. Flulike symptoms and genital pruritus or tingling also may be noticed. A severe primary episode does not necessarily indicate that a woman will be predisposed to frequent or severe recurrences. Primary episodes usually last the longest and are the most severe. Lesions heal spontaneously in 2 to 4 weeks.

RECURRENT EPISODES

After the lesions heal, the virus enters a dormant phase, residing in the nerve ganglia of the affected area. Some individuals never have a recurrence, whereas others have regular recurrences. Recurrent lesions usually occur at the site of the primary episode. Recurrences are usually less severe than the initial episode and seem to be triggered by emotional stress, menstruation, ovulation, pregnancy, frequent or vigorous intercourse, poor health status or a generally rundown physical condition, tight clothing, or overheating. Diagnosis is made on the basis of the clinical

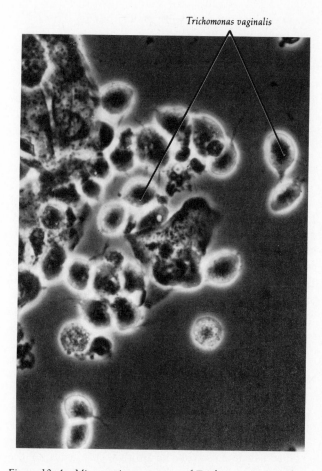

Figure 10–4 Microscopic appearance of Trichomonas vaginalis (Courtesy of Tortora G, et al: *Microbiology*. Menlo Park, Calif: Benjamin/Cummings, 1982)

appearance of the lesions, Pap smear or culture of the lesions, and sometimes blood testing for antibodies.

Recent studies suggest a possible link between genital herpes and dysplasia (abnormal cells) of the cervix or cervical cancer. This connection is still unclear. Women with a diagnosis of herpes should have yearly Pap smears.

MEDICAL THERAPY

There is no known cure for herpes. Prescriptive treatment is available to provide relief from pain and prevent complications from secondary infection. Women may apply acyclovir (Zovirax) ointment to reduce viral shedding and healing time of the lesions. Oral acyclovir can be considered for women with primary episodes and for recurrences.

Self-help suggestions include cleansing with povidone-iodine (Betadine) solution to prevent secondary infection and Burow's solution to relieve discomfort. Use of vitamin C or lysine is frequently suggested to prevent recurrence, although studies have not documented the effectiveness of these supplements. Keeping the genital area clean and dry, wearing loose clothing, and wearing cotton underwear or none at all will promote healing. Primary or recurrent lesions will heal without prescriptive therapies.

If herpes is present in the genital tract of a woman during childbirth, it can have a devastating, even fatal, effect on the newborn. In fact, herpes is one of a group of infections referred to as TORCH (TOxoplasmosis, Rubella, Cytomegalovirus, Herpes) that can have serious implications for pregnancy. For further discussion, see Chapter 19.

Syphilis

Syphilis is a chronic infection caused by a spirochete, *Treponema pallidum*. Syphilis can be acquired congenitally through transplacental inoculation, and can result from maternal exposure to infected exudate during sexual contact, or from contact with open wounds or infected blood. The incubation period varies from 10 to 90 days, and even though no symptoms or lesions are noted during this time, the woman's blood contains spirochetes and is infectious.

Syphilis is divided into early and late stages. During the early stage (primary), a chancre appears at the site where the *Treponema pallidum* organism entered the body. Symptoms include slight fever, loss of weight, and malaise. The chancre persists for about four weeks and then disappears. In six weeks to six months, secondary symptoms appear. Skin eruptions called condylomata lata, which resemble wartlike plaques, may appear on the vulva. Other secondary symptoms are acute arthritis, enlargement of the liver and spleen, iritis, and a chronic sore throat with hoarseness. When infected in utero, the newborn will exhibit secondary stage symptoms of syphilis.

The incidence of syphilis declined after the discovery of penicillin, but since 1958 the incidence has been increasing. As a result of the increased incidence and the disease's impact on the fetus in utero, serologic testing of every pregnant woman is recommended, and required by some state laws. Testing is done at the initial prenatal screening and repeated in the third trimester.

With adequate early treatment congenital syphilis is preventable. However, one of the following outcomes can occur in the presence of untreated maternal syphilis: (a) second trimester abortion, (b) a stillborn infant at term, (c) a congenitally infected infant born prematurely or at term, or (d) an uninfected live infant. The clinical manifestations and treatment of the syphilitic newborn are discussed in Chapter 32.

MEDICAL THERAPY

The goal of medical therapy is to identify women with syphilis and begin antibiotic treatment.

Diagnosis is made by dark-field examination for spirochetes. Blood tests such as VDRL (Venereal Disease Research Laboratories), RPR (Rapid Plasma Reagin), or the more specific FTA-ABS (fluorescent treponemal antibody absorption test) are commonly done. Blood studies may be negative if blood is drawn too early.

For women with syphilis of less than a year's duration, the Centers for Disease Control (CDC) recommend 2.4 million units of benzathine penicillin G intramuscularly. If syphilis is of long (more than a year) duration, 2.4 million units of benzathine penicillin G is given intramuscularly once a week for three weeks. If a woman is allergic to penicillin, erythromycin can be given. Maternal serologic testing may remain positive for eight months, and the newborn may have a positive test for three months.

In the pregnant woman, treatment with penicillin should begin after the first positive test rather than waiting for further testing.

Gonorrhea

Gonorrhea (popularly called "clap," "GC," "drip," or "dose") is an infection caused by the bacteria *Neisseria gonorrhoeae*. If a nonpregnant woman contracts the disease, she is at risk to develop pelvic inflammatory disease. If a woman becomes infected after the third month of pregnancy, the mucous plug in the cervix will prevent the infection from ascending, and it will remain localized in the urethra, cervix, and Bartholin's glands until the membranes rupture. Then it can spread upward.

MEDICAL THERAPY

The majority of women with gonorrhea are asymptomatic. Thus it is accepted practice to screen for this infection by doing a cervical culture during the initial prenatal examination. Cultures of the urethra, throat, and rectum may also be required for diagnosis, depending on the body orifices used for intercourse.

The most common symptoms of gonorrheal infection include a purulent, greenish-yellow vaginal discharge; dysuria; and urinary frequency. Some women also develop inflammation and swelling of the vulva. The cervix may appear swollen and eroded and may secrete a foul-smelling discharge in which gonococci are present.

Treatment consists of antibiotic treatment with aqueous procaine penicillin G given intramuscularly to the infected woman. A total dosage of 4.8 million units is administered, with 2.4 million units injected into each buttock with 1.0 gm probenecid by mouth. If the woman is allergic to penicillin, spectinomycin is given. Additional treatment may be required if the cultures remain positive 7 to 14 days after completion of treatment. All sexual partners must also be treated or the woman may become reinfected.

Women should be informed of the need for reculture to verify cure and the need for abstinence or condom use until cure is confirmed. Both sexual partners should be treated if either has a positive test for gonorrhea. It is important to explain why treatment is necessary even if the client has a negative culture or is asymptomatic. For example, false negative reports are possible. Gonorrhea may be asymptomatic. Untreated infections are associated with the following risks:

- The possibility of pelvic inflammatory disease and secondary infertility.

- Disseminated gonorrhea can involve joints or cause septicemia.

- Infection present at the time of delivery causes opthalmia neonatorum in the infant.

Acquired Immunodeficiency Syndrome (AIDS)

Acquired immunodeficiency syndrome (AIDS) is a fatal disorder caused by a virus and occurs most commonly in homosexual or bisexual men, heterosexual partners of persons with AIDS, drug users, recipients of blood transfusions, Haitians, and Africans in Zaire. It can also be transmitted to a fetus in utero from an infected mother.

The care of a person with AIDS is primarily supportive, although some medications are being developed that seem to prolong life. The reader is referred to a medical-surgical text for a description of this care.

However, because the diagnosis of AIDS or the presence of the AIDS antibody has profound implications for a fetus if the woman is pregnant, AIDS is discussed in greater detail in Chapter 19.

Condyloma Accuminata (Venereal Warts)

Venereal warts occur in all age groups and develop in more than 50 percent of sexual partners of infected individuals (Sonstegard et al 1982). The causative organism is a papovavirus. A woman often seeks medical care after noting "bumps" in the genital area. Single or multiple soft, grayish-pink, cauliflowerlike lesions may be observed.

The moist warmth of the genital area is conducive to the growth of the warts, which may be present on the vulva, vagina, cervix, and anus. The virus is transmitted through sexual contact. The incubation period following exposure is one to three months.

MEDICAL THERAPY

Because condyloma sometimes resembles other lesions and malignant transformation is possible, all large areas of genital warts should be biopsied and treatment should be instituted promptly (Ferenczy 1986). Small lesions can be treated with topically applied podophyllin, which the woman is instructed to wash off four hours after application. The drug is not used during pregnancy because it is thought to be teratogenic and in large doses has been associated with fetal death. If the woman is pregnant or if the lesions do not respond to podophyllin, trichloroacetic acid, liquid nitrogen, or cryocautery may be used (Eschenbach 1986). Carbon dioxide laser therapy, performed under colposcopy, has a good success rate. This is probably due to the fact that use of the colposcope aids in detecting tiny "satellite" lesions (Ferenczy 1986).

Medical literature has indicated a link between the occurrence of condylomas and abnormal cell changes of the cervix or possibly cervical cancer (Contemporary OB/GYN 1982). Women with a history of this lesion should have yearly Pap smears.

Pediculosis Pubis (Pubic or Crab Louse)

Pubic lice occur more commonly in adults than in children. Pediculosis pubis is caused by Phthirus, a grayish parasitic "crab" louse that lays eggs that attach to the hair shaft. Transmission is primarily by sexual contact, but transmission through shared towels and bed linens is possible.

MEDICAL THERAPY

Symptoms include intense pruritus in areas covered by pubic hair. Occasionally lice are present in chest hair, armpits, eyelashes, and eyebrows. "Crabs" or brown-red spots may be noted in the underwear. Diagnosis is made by clinical and microscopic identification of adult lice or nits (eggs). Pediculosis is treated with 1 percent gamma benzene (Kwell) shampoo to the affected area, plus combing of the pubic hair with a fine-tooth comb. This is repeated in 24 hours. Over-the-counter medications are safe but less effective. Women should be instructed to launder, dry clean, or expose to sunlight all contaminated linens or clothing. All sexual partners or members of the household should be treated. The woman should be warned of possible toxicity with overuse of the medication. Women should be cautioned not to use medication in or around their eyes.

Scabies

Sarcoptes scabiei is an ectoparasitic itch mite. The female mite burrows under the skin to deposit her eggs. Transmission is by intimate sexual contact and contact with household members.

MEDICAL THERAPY

Symptoms include pruritus that worsens at night or when the individual is warm. Noticeable erythematous, papular lesions or furrows may be present. Diagnosis is made by confirmation of the symptoms or scraping of the furrows to obtain mites. Prescriptive therapy is 1 percent gamma benzene lotion applied from the neck down after taking a bath.

The woman should be advised that sexual partners and other household members should also be treated. Clothing and household linens should be laundered and air dried or dry cleaned. Persistent pruritus often occurs after treatment; the woman should be aware that pruritus does not signify that the treatment is ineffective. She should be cautioned that overuse of lotion can cause toxicity.

General Principles of Nursing Intervention

NURSING ASSESSMENT

The nurse working with women must become adept at taking a thorough history and identifying women at risk for sexually transmitted diseases. The nurse should be alert for signs and symptoms of sexually transmitted diseases and familiar with diagnostic procedures if STD is suspected.

While each STD has certain distinctive characteristics, the following complaints suggest the possibility of infection and warrant further investigation:

● Presence of a "sore" or lesion on the vulva

● Increased vaginal discharge or malodorous vaginal discharge

● Burning with urination

In many instances the woman is asymptomatic, but may report symptoms in her partner, especially painful urination or urethral discharge. It is often helpful to ask the woman whether her partner is experiencing any symptoms.

NURSING DIAGNOSIS

Nursing diagnoses that may apply when a woman has a sexually transmitted disease include:

● Alterations in family processes related to the effects of a diagnosis of STD on the couple's relationship

● Knowledge deficit related to the long-term effects of the diagnosis on childbearing status

● Disturbance in self-concept related to difficulty in accepting the knowledge that the condition is sexually transmitted

NURSING GOAL: EDUCATION FOR SELF-CARE

In a supportive and nonjudgmental way the nurse provides the woman who has a sexually transmitted disease with information about the disease, methods of transmission, implications for pregnancy or future fertility, and importance of thorough treatment. If treatment of her partner is indicated, the woman must understand that it is important to prevent a continuous cycle of reinfection. She should also understand the need to abstain from sexual activity, if necessary, during treatment.

The woman should be instructed about the correct procedure for taking her medication and should clearly understand the importance of any follow-up assessments.

NURSING GOAL: PROVISION OF PSYCHOLOGIC SUPPORT

Some sexually transmitted diseases such as trichomoniasis or chlamydia may cause a woman concern but once diagnosed are rather simply treated. Other STDs may also be fairly simple to treat medically but may carry a stigma and be emotionally devastating for the woman. Diseases such as pediculosis pubis may cause a woman to feel "unclean," while syphilis, since it is reportable, may leave the woman feeling exposed and vulnerable. Herpes can be especially difficult to deal with emotionally because it causes discomfort and is not presently curable.

The sensitive nurse can be especially helpful in encouraging the woman to explore her feelings about the diagnosis. She may experience anger or feel "betrayed" by a partner; she may feel guilt or see her diagnosis as a form of "punishment"; or she may feel concern about the long-term implications for future childbearing or ongoing intimate relationships. She may experience a myriad of differing emotions that she never expected. Opportunities to discuss her feelings in a nonjudgmental environment can be especially helpful. The nurse can offer suggestions about support groups if indicated and assist the woman in planning for her future with regard to sexual activity.

More subtly, the nurse's attitude of acceptance and matter-of-factness conveys to the woman that she is still an acceptable person who happens to have an infection.

EVALUATIVE OUTCOME CRITERIA

Anticipated outcomes of nursing care include the following:

- The STD is identified and cured if possible. If not, supportive therapy is provided.

- The woman and her partner understand the infection, its method of transmission, its implications, and the therapy.

- The woman copes successfully with the impact of the diagnosis on her self-concept.

● Care of the Woman With Pelvic Inflammatory Disease

Pelvic inflammatory disease (PID) occurs in approximately 1 percent of women between 15 and 39, although sexually active young women between 15 and 24 have the highest infection rate (Eschenbach 1986). The disease is more common in women who have had multiple sexual partners, a history of PID, or an intrauterine device. It usually produces a tubal infection (salpingitis) that may or may not be accompanied by a pelvic abscess. However, perhaps the greatest problem of PID is that postinfection tubal damage is associated with a high incidence of infertility.

The organisms most frequently identified with PID include *Chlamydia trachomatis, Neisseria gonorrhoeae,* and *Mycoplasma hominis,* although other aerobic and anaerobic organisms that are often part of the normal vaginal flora have also been found in women with PID (Torrington 1985).

Medical Therapy

Symptoms of PID include bilateral sharp, cramping pain in the lower quadrants, fever, chills, purulent vaginal discharge, irregular bleeding, malaise, nausea, and vomiting. However, it is possible to be asymptomatic and have normal laboratory values.

Diagnosis consists of a clinical examination to define symptoms plus blood tests and a gonorrhea culture and test for chlamydia. Other diagnostic procedures that may

be helpful in confirming the diagnosis include the following:

- Elevated white blood count and sedimentation rate

- Wet prep of vaginal secretions that reveals the presence of numerous inflammatory cells and coccoid bacteria

- Culdocentesis that provides fluid containing an elevated white blood count

- Ultrasound to detect the presence of a pelvic abscess

- Laparoscopy to confirm the diagnosis and enable the examiner to obtain cultures from the fimbriated ends of the fallopian tubes

In stressing the accuracy of confirming a diagnosis of PID by the use of laparoscopy, Eschenbach (1986) states:

> It is estimated that for every 100 times a clinical diagnosis of pelvic inflammatory disease is made without visual confirmation, four patients with ectopic pregnancy and three patients with appendicitis are treated for pelvic inflammatory disease, resulting in a critical delay in the correct diagnosis (p 992).

Except in very mild cases, the woman is hospitalized and treated with intravenous antibiotics. Antibiotics such as doxycycline and cefoxitin are used if the causative organism is either *Chlamydia trachomatis* or *Neisseria gonorrhoeae,* while an abscess or the presence of anaerobes or gram-negative rods indicates treatment with clindamycin and an aminoglycoside (Mead 1985). In addition, supportive therapy is often indicated for severe symptoms. The sexual partner should also be treated. If the woman has an IUD, it is generally removed 24 to 48 hours after antibiotic therapy is started (Eschenbach 1986).

After the infection is treated, microsurgical techniques are sometimes used to release any adhesions and repair tubal damage.

Nursing Assessment

The nurse is alert to factors in a woman's history that put her at risk for PID. Even though fewer IUDs are available, many women still have them, and the nurse should question the woman about possible symptoms, such as aching pain in the lower abdomen, foul-smelling discharge, malaise, and the like. The woman who is acutely ill will have obvious symptoms, but a low-grade infection is more difficult to detect.

Nursing Diagnosis

Nursing diagnoses that may apply to a woman with PID include:

- Alteration in comfort: acute pain related to peritoneal irritation

- Knowledge deficit related to a lack of understanding of the possible effects of PID on fertility

Nursing Goal: Provision of Information

The nurse plays a vital role in helping to prevent or detect PID. The nurse should spend time discussing risk factors related to this infection. The woman who uses an IUD for contraception and has multiple sexual partners should clearly understand the risk she faces. The nurse should discuss signs and symptoms of PID and stress the importance of early detection should the woman develop symptoms.

The woman who develops PID should understand the importance of completing her antibiotic treatment and of returning for follow-up evaluation. She should also understand the possibility of decreased fertility following the infection. If appropriate, the nurse can also answer the woman's questions about microsurgical techniques.

The care of the woman who is acutely ill with pelvic abscess is discussed in Chapter 36.

Evaluative Outcome Criteria

Anticipated outcomes of nursing care include the following:

- The woman clearly understands her condition, her therapy, and the possible long-term implications of PID on her fertility.

- The woman completes her course of therapy, and the PID is cured.

● Care of the Woman With Vulvitis

Genital pruritus and soreness may be secondary to a nonpathogenic process. Common causes are:

- Frequent douching or use of over-the-counter douches

- Feminine deodorant spray

- Detergents or harsh soaps

- Colored or perfumed toilet paper

- Contraceptive creams, foams, or suppositories

- Dye as in new clothing

- Synthetic clothing that traps moisture, such as nylon underwear, polyester slacks

Nursing Goal: Education for Self-Care

Although women are often told that the practices listed above contribute to vaginitis, this is not necessarily so. In many cases the woman may be experiencing vulvitis without vaginitis (Ervin et al 1982).

The nurse can inform women of the possible factors contributing to local irritation and encourage them to avoid practices that contribute to symptoms. Suggestions for good genital hygiene are advisable. The nurse should encourage medical evaluation if symptoms persist.

● Care of the Woman With Cervicitis

Cervicitis is an inflammation of the cervix. It may be caused by an infective process such as gonorrhea, herpes, *Trichomonas*, *Candida*, or *Gardnerella*. Chemical or hygienic products used in the vagina or the presence of foreign bodies may cause cervicitis.

Medical Therapy

Symptoms of cervicitis include yellow discharge with odor, dyspareunia, and irregular bleeding. A woman may be asymptomatic. Diagnosis consists of a clinical examination and appropriate wet smear, cultures, or Pap smear. Appropriate treatment is antibiotic therapy, cryotherapy, or removal of any foreign object (IUD or tampon).

Nursing Goal: Education for Self-Care

The woman should be advised to avoid possible vaginal irritants such as douches or tampons. Medical care should be sought if the woman is symptomatic. If an abnormal reading occurs on a Pap smear report, the nurse should clarify the report for the woman. It is reassuring to inform women that an infectious process and cervical irritants can result in an abnormal Pap smear reading. The Pap smear should be repeated after these problems are eliminated.

● Care of the Woman With an Abnormal Finding During Pelvic Examination

Abnormal Pap Smear Results

Women tend to expect a report of negative or normal when having a Pap smear done, but various abnormal findings are common. The original purpose of the Pap smear was to detect the presence of cellular abnormalities by obtaining a smear containing cells from the cervix and the endocervical canal. Precancerous or potentially cancerous conditions, as well as cervical cancer, can be identified by microscopic identification.

Early detection of abnormalities allows early changes to be treated before cells reach a precancerous or cancerous stage. For this reason, women should be encouraged to have regular physical examinations, including Pap smears. Noncancerous changes in cervical cells may be found, or a false negative report may occur. Some findings that are classified as abnormal, such as inflammatory or "atypical" cells, are not indicative of cancer.

MEDICAL THERAPY

Diagnostic or therapeutic procedures employed in cases of cellular abnormalities include repetition of Pap smears at shorter intervals, colposcopy and endocervical biopsy, cryotherapy, or laser conization. Decisions for management are based on the specific report.

Women who have multiple sexual partners or a history of herpes, condyloma accuminata, or other STDs have an increased risk of abnormal cell changes and cervical cancer. Some researchers believe that precancerous cervical cell changes are more common in women who have been exposed to diethylstilbestrol (DES), but other researchers disagree.

Ovarian Masses

Between 70 percent and 80 percent of ovarian masses are benign (Martin 1978). More than 50 percent are functional cysts occurring most commonly in women 20 to 40 years of age (Martin 1978). Functional cysts are rare in women who take oral contraceptives.

Ovarian cysts usually represent physiologic variations in the menstrual cycle (Sciarra et al 1984). Dermoid cysts (cystic teratomas) comprise 10 percent of all benign ovarian masses. Cartilage, bone, teeth, skin, or hair can be observed in these cysts. Endometriomas, or "chocolate cysts," are another common type of ovarian mass.

MEDICAL THERAPY

A woman with an ovarian mass may be asymptomatic; the mass may be noted on a routine pelvic examination. She may experience a sensation of fullness or cramping in the lower abdomen (often unilateral), dyspareunia, irregular bleeding, or delayed menstruation.

Diagnosis is made on the basis of a palpable mass with or without tenderness and other related symptoms. Radiography or ultrasonography may be used to assist or confirm the diagnosis.

The woman is frequently kept under observation for a month or two because most cysts will resolve on their own and are harmless. Alternatively, oral contraceptives may be prescribed for one to two months to suppress ovarian function. If this regimen has been effective, a repeat

pelvic examination should be normal. If the mass is still present after 60 days of observation and oral contraceptive therapy, a diagnostic laparoscopy or laparotomy may be considered (Merrill 1986). Tubal or ovarian lesions, ectopic pregnancy, cancer, infection, or appendicitis also must be ruled out before a diagnosis can be confirmed.

Surgery is not always necessary but will be considered if the mass is larger than 6 to 7 cm in circumference; if the woman is over 40 years of age with an adnexal mass, a persistent mass, or continuous pain; and if the woman is taking oral contraceptives. Surgical exploration is also indicated when a palpable mass is found in an infant or young girl or in a postmenopausal woman (Merrill 1986).

Women who are taking oral contraceptives should be informed of their preventive effect against ovarian masses (Dickey 1983). Women may need clear explanations about why the initial therapy is observation. A discussion of the origin and resolution of ovarian cysts may clarify this treatment plan. If surgery should involve removal or impaired function of one ovary, the woman should be assured that the remaining ovary should take over ovarian functioning and that pregnancy is still possible.

Uterine Masses

Fibroid tumors or leiomyomas are among the most common benign disease entities in women and are the most common reason for gynecologic surgery. Between 20 percent and 50 percent of women develop leiomyomas by 40 years of age (Sciarra et al 1984). The potential for cancer is minimal. Leiomyomas are more common in black women.

MEDICAL THERAPY

Smooth muscle cells are present in whorls and arise from uterine muscles and connective tissue. The size varies from 1 to 2 cm to the size of a 10-week fetus. Frequently the woman is asymptomatic. Lower abdominal pain, fullness or pressure, menorrhagia, metrorrhagia, or increased dysmenorrhea may occur, particularly with large leiomyomas. Ultrasonography revealing masses or nodules can assist in and confirm the diagnosis. Leiomyoma is also considered a possible diagnosis when masses or nodules involving the uterus are palpated on a pelvic examination.

The majority of these masses require no treatment and will shrink after menopause. Close observation for symptoms or an increase in size of the uterus or the masses may be the only management most women will require. Routine repeat pelvic examinations every three to six months are commonly recommended unless there are other symptoms.

If a woman notices symptoms, or pelvic examination reveals that the mass is increasing in size, surgery (myomectomy, dilation and curettage, or hysterectomy) will be recommended. The choice of surgery depends on the age and reproductive status of the woman and/or the significance of the noted changes. There are no medications or therapies to prevent fibroids.

General Principles of Nursing Intervention

NURSING ASSESSMENT

Except for those nurses specially trained to do pelvic examinations and Pap smears, these procedures are not routinely done by nurses. In most cases, nursing assessment is directed toward an evaluation of the woman's understanding of the findings, their implications, and her psychosocial response.

NURSING DIAGNOSIS

Nursing diagnoses that might apply to a woman with an abnormal finding from a pelvic examination include:

- Anxiety related to the significance of the finding
- Fear related to the possibility of cancer
- Knowledge deficit related to the meaning of the diagnosis

NURSING GOAL: PROVISION OF INFORMATION AND EMOTIONAL SUPPORT

The woman needs accurate information on etiology, symptomatology, and treatment options. She should be encouraged to report symptoms and keep appointments for follow-up examination and evaluation. The woman needs realistic reassurance if her condition is benign; she may require counseling and effective emotional support if a malignancy is likely. If the management plan includes surgery, she may need the nurse's support in obtaining a second opinion and making her decision.

EVALUATIVE OUTCOME CRITERIA

Anticipated outcomes of nursing care include the following:

- The woman understands the abnormal finding, the diagnostic procedures that are indicated, and the possible causes of the abnormal finding.
- The woman copes successfully with the stress associated with waiting for a definite diagnosis.

● Care of the Woman With a Urinary Tract Infection

A urinary tract infection (UTI) may be a mere inconvenience or may reach life-threatening severity. Bacteria usually enter the urinary tract at its distal end; that is, by way of the urethra. The organisms are capable of migrating against the downward flow of urine. The shortness of the female urethra facilitates the passage of bacteria into the bladder. Other conditions that facilitate bacterial entry are relative incompetence of the urinary sphincter, frequent enuresis (bedwetting) prior to adolescence, and urinary catheterization (Sciarra et al 1984). A habit of wiping from back to front after urination may transfer bacteria from the anorectal area to the urethra.

About 5 percent of women have at least one UTI before becoming sexually active. The prevalence increases 1 percent per decade of life (Sciarra et al 1984). Voluntarily suppressing the desire to urinate is a predisposing factor. Retention overdistends the bladder and can lead to an infection. For reasons that are unclear, there seems to be a relationship between recurring UTI and sexual intercourse. General poor health or lowered resistance to infection can also increase a woman's susceptibility to UTI. Stasis of urine, compression of ureters (especially the right ureter), decreased bactericidal capabilities of leukocytes in the urine, and vesicoureteral reflux (backward urine flow) make the pregnant woman even more susceptible to UTI.

The highest prevalence of UTI is among women of high parity in the low socioeconomic level, women with a history of UTI, and women with sickle cell disease or sickle cell trait (Pritchard et al 1985).

Asymptomatic bacteriuria (ASB) (bacteria in the urine actively multiplying without accompanying clinical symptoms) constitutes about 6 percent to 8 percent of UTI. This becomes especially significant if the woman is pregnant (Fantl 1986). Between 20 percent and 30 percent of pregnant women with untreated ASB will go on to develop cystitis or acute pyelonephritis by the third trimester (Whalley 1986). Asymptomatic bacteriuria is almost always caused by a single organism. If more than one type of bacteria is cultured, the possibility of urine culture contamination must be considered.

The most common cause of ASB is *Escherichia coli.* Other commonly found causative organisms include *Klebsiella* and *Proteus.*

A woman who has had a UTI is more susceptible to a recurrent infection. If a pregnant woman develops an acute UTI, especially with high temperature, amniotic fluid infection may develop and retard the growth of the placenta. Increased risk of premature labor exists if the infection occurs near term.

Lower Urinary Tract Infection (Cystitis)

Because urinary tract infections are ascending, it is important to recognize and diagnose a lower UTI early to avoid the sequelae associated with upper UTI.

MEDICAL THERAPY

Symptoms of frequency, pyuria, and dysuria without bacteriuria may indicate urethritis caused by *Chlamydia trachomatis*. It has become a common pathogen in the genitourinary system.

When cystitis develops, the initial symptom is often dysuria, specifically at the end of urination. Urgency and frequency also occur. Cystitis is usually accompanied by a low-grade fever (101F or lower), and hematuria is seen occasionally. Urine specimens usually contain an abnormal number of leukocytes and bacteria.

Oral sulfonamides, particularly sulfisoxazole, are generally effective against lower UTI. If the woman is pregnant these should only be used in early pregnancy since they interfere with protein binding of bilirubin in the fetus. Use in the last few weeks of pregnancy can lead to neonatal hyperbilirubinemia and kernicterus. Other drugs that are usually effective (and apparently safe for a fetus) are ampicillin and nitrofurantoin (Furadantin). Nitrofurantoin crosses the placenta, but no harm to the fetus has been demonstrated.

NURSING ASSESSMENT

During each visit the nurse notes any complaints from the woman of pain on urination or other urinary difficulties. If any concerns arise, the nurse obtains a clean-catch urine specimen from the woman.

NURSING DIAGNOSIS

Nursing diagnoses that may apply to a woman with a lower UTI include:

- Alteration in comfort: acute pain related to dysuria secondary to the urinary tract infection

- Knowledge deficit related to a lack of understanding of self-care measures to help prevent recurrence of UTI

NURSING GOAL: EDUCATION FOR SELF-CARE

The nurse should make sure the woman is aware of good hygiene practices, since most bacteria enter through the urethra after having spread from the anal area. Table 10–7 identifies measures for preventing cystitis. The nurse should also reinforce instructions or answer questions regarding the prescribed antibiotic, the amount of liquids to take, and the reasons for these treatments. Cystitis usually responds rapidly to treatment, but follow-up urinary cultures are important.

EVALUATIVE OUTCOME CRITERIA

Anticipated outcomes of nursing care include the following:

- The woman implements self-care measures to help prevent cystitis as part of her personal routine.

- The woman can identify the signs, symptoms, therapy, and possible complications of cystitis.

- The woman's infection is cured.

Upper Urinary Tract Infection (Pyelonephritis)

Pyelonephritis (inflammatory disease of the kidneys) is less common but more serious than cystitis and is often preceded by lower UTI. It is more common during the latter part of pregnancy or early postpartum and poses a serious threat to maternal and fetal well-being. Women with symptomatic pyelonephritis during pregnancy have an increased risk of premature deliveries as well as intrauterine growth retardation (Hawkins & Whalley 1985).

MEDICAL THERAPY

The goal of medical intervention is to diagnose acute pyelonephritis and begin treatment as soon as possible.

Table 10–7 Measures for Preventing Cystitis

○ If you use a diaphragm for contraception try changing methods or using another size of diaphragm. ○ Avoid bladder irritants such as alcohol, caffeine products, and carbonated beverages. ○ Increase fluid intake, especially water, to a minimum of six to eight glasses per day. ○ Make regular urination a habit; avoid long waits. ○ Practice good genital hygiene including wiping from front to back after urination and bowel movements.	○ Be aware that vigorous or frequent sexual activity may contribute to urinary tract infection. ○ Urinate before and after intercourse to empty the bladder and cleanse the urethra. ○ Complete medication regimens even if symptoms decrease. ○ Do not use medication left over from previous infections. ○ Drink cranberry juice to acidify the urine. This has been found to relieve symptoms in some cases.

Acute pyelonephritis has a sudden onset with chills, high temperature of 39.6–40.6C (103–105F), and flank pain (either unilateral or bilateral). The right side is almost always involved if the woman is pregnant because the large bulk of intestines to the left pushes the uterus to the right, putting pressure on the right ureter and kidney. Nausea, vomiting, and general malaise may ensue. With accompanying cystitis, frequency, urgency, and burning with urination may be experienced.

Edema of the renal parenchyma or ureteritis with blockage and swelling of the ureter may lead to temporary suppression of urinary output. This is accompanied by severe colicky pain, vomiting, dehydration, and ileus of the large bowel. The woman with acute pyelonephritis will generally have increased diastolic blood pressure, positive fluorescent antibody titer (FA-test), low creatinine clearance, significant bacteremia in urine culture, pyuria, and presence of white blood cell casts.

During pregnancy, acute pyelonephritis can lead to maternal sepsis, and is life threatening to both the woman and her unborn child. Consequently the woman is hospitalized and started on intravenous antibiotic therapy as soon as an acute upper UTI is diagnosed by symptoms and urine culture. In the case of obstructed pyelonephritis, a blood culture is necessary. The woman is kept in bed. After a sensitivity report, the antibiotic may be changed to one more specific for the infecting organism. Ampicillin, or nitrofurantoin, or one of these in combination with a sulfonamide, is commonly prescribed. Other antibiotics considered safe during pregnancy include cephalexin, sulfisoxazole, and methenamine (Harris 1986).

If signs of urinary obstruction occur or continue, the ureter may be catheterized to establish adequate drainage.

With appropriate drug therapy, the woman's temperature should return to normal. The pain subsides and the urine shows no bacteria within two to three days. Follow-up urinary cultures are needed to assure that the infection has been eliminated completely.

NURSING ASSESSMENT

During the woman's visit the nurse obtains a sexual and medical history to identify the woman at risk for UTI. A clean-catch urine specimen is evaluated for evidence of ASB.

NURSING GOAL: EDUCATION FOR SELF-CARE

The nurse provides the woman with information to help her recognize the signs of UTI, so she can contact her care giver as soon as possible. The nurse also discusses hygiene practices, the advantages of wearing cotton underwear, and the need to void frequently to prevent urinary stasis.

The nurse stresses the importance of maintaining a good fluid intake. Drinking cranberry juice daily and taking 500 mg Vitamin C both help acidify the urine and may help prevent recurrence of infection. Women with a history of UTI find it helpful to drink a glass of fluid prior to sexual intercourse and void afterward.

Cystocele and Pelvic Relaxation

A cystocele is the downward displacement of the bladder, which appears as a bulge in the anterior vaginal wall. Arbitrary classifications of mild to severe are frequently given. Genetic predisposition, childbearing, obesity, and increased age are factors that may contribute to cystocele.

MEDICAL THERAPY

Symptoms of stress incontinence are most common, including loss of urine with coughing, sneezing, laughing, or sudden exertion. Vaginal fullness, a bulging out of the vaginal wall, or a dragging sensation may also be noticeable.

If pelvic relaxation is mild, Kegel exercises are helpful in restoring tone. The exercises involve contraction and relaxation of the pubococcygeal muscle. Women have found these exercises helpful before and after childbirth in maintaining vaginal muscle tone. Estrogen may improve the condition of vaginal mucous membranes—especially in menopausal women (see Chapter 7). Vaginal pessaries or rings may be used if surgery is undesirable or impossible or until surgery can be scheduled. Surgery may be considered for cystoceles considered moderate to severe.

NURSING GOAL: EDUCATION FOR SELF-CARE

The nurse may instruct the woman in the use of Kegel exercises. Information on causes and contributing factors and discussion of possible alternative therapies will greatly assist the woman.

KEY CONCEPTS

The breasts function in a cyclic process that is regulated by nervous and hormonal systems. Thus many women experience breast tenderness and swelling premenstrually.

In fibrocystic breast disease the cysts tend to be round, mobile, and well delineated. The woman generally ex-

periences increased discomfort premenstrually. Because of the increased risk of developing breast cancer, women with FBD should understand the importance of monthly BSE.

Factors that increase a woman's risk of developing breast cancer include: advancing age (most occur after age 40), family history (especially mother or sister) of breast cancer, early menarche, late menopause, personal history of cancer in one breast, high levels of dietary fat, and high protein and low selenium diet.

Mammography is a valuable tool because breast lesions can be detected before they are palpable.

Recommendations for frequency of screening mammograms are:
- Baseline mammogram between ages 35 and 40
- Mammogram every one to two years between ages 40 and 50
- Mammogram annually for all women after age 50

Diagnosis of a suspicious breast mass is made by fine-needle biopsy.

A variety of surgical treatment alternatives now exist for women with breast cancer, including radical mastectomy, modified radical mastectomy, simple mastectomy, subcutaneous mastectomy, partial mastectomy, and lumpectomy. Breast reconstruction following surgery is becoming a more common alternative. Other treatment modalities for breast cancer include radiation therapy, chemotherapy, and endocrine therapy.

A woman with breast cancer faces many psychologic concerns including fear of the diagnosis, altered body image, and the response of family and friends. She must also deal with the long-term prognosis, and her physical response to the treatment she receives. Nurses play a vital role in providing information and psychologic support.

Endometriosis is a condition in which endometrial tissue occurs outside the endometrial cavity. This tissue bleeds in a cyclic fashion in response to the menstrual cycle. The bleeding leads to inflammation, scarring, and adhesions. The prime symptoms include dysmenorrhea, dyspareunia, and infertility.

Treatment of endometriosis may be medical, surgical, or a combination. For the woman not desiring pregnancy at present, oral contraceptives are used. Women desiring pregnancy are treated with a course of danazol.

Toxic shock syndrome, caused by a toxin of *Streptococcus aureus*, is most common in women of childbearing age. There is an increased incidence in women who use tampons or barrier methods of contraception such as the diaphragm and sponge.

Moniliasis, a vaginal infection caused by *Candida albicans,* is most common in women who use oral contraceptives, are on antibiotics, are currently pregnant, or have diabetes mellitus. It is generally treated with intravaginal miconazole or clotrimazole suppositories.

Bacterial vaginosis (*Gardnerella vaginalis* vaginitis), a common vaginal infection, is diagnosed by its characteristic "fishy" odor and by the presence of clue cells on a vaginal smear. It is treated with metronidazole unless the woman is pregnant.

Chlamydial infection is difficult to detect in a woman, but may result in PID and infertility. It is treated with antibiotic therapy.

Herpes genitalis, caused by the herpes simplex virus, is a recurrent infection with no known cure. Acyclovir (Zovirax) may provide a reduction in symptoms.

Syphilis, caused by *Treponema pallidum,* is a sexually transmitted disease that is treatable if diagnosed. The characteristic lesion is the chancre. Syphilis can also be transmitted in utero to the fetus of an infected woman. The treatment of choice is penicillin.

Gonorrhea, a common sexually transmitted disease, may be asymptomatic in women initially but may cause PID if not diagnosed early. The treatment of choice is penicillin.

Condyloma accuminata (venereal warts) is transmitted by a virus. Treatment is indicated because research suggests a possible link with abnormal cervical changes. The treatment chosen depends on the size and location of the warts.

Nurses caring for women with a STD should discuss methods of prevention, signs and symptoms, and treatment alternatives in a supportive, nonjudgmental way.

Pelvic inflammatory disease may be life threatening and may lead to infertility.

Women with an abnormal finding on a pelvic examination will need careful explanation of the finding and techniques of diagnosis and emotional support during the diagnostic period.

The classic symptoms of a lower UTI are dysuria, urgency, frequency, and sometimes hematuria. Oral sulfonamides are the treatment of choice.

An upper UTI is a serious infection that can permanently damage the kidneys if untreated. Generally the woman is acutely ill and may require supportive therapy as well as antibiotics.

A cystocele is a downward displacement of the bladder into the vagina. Often it is accompanied by stress incontinence. Kegel exercises may help restore tone in mild cases.

REFERENCES

American Cancer Society: *Breast Self-Examination and the Nurse*, No. 3408 PE. New York, 1973.

American Cancer Society: *Cancer Facts and Figures*. New York, 1984.

American Cancer Society: *A Cancer Source Book for Nurses*. New York, 1981.

American Society of Plastic and Reconstructive Surgeons: *Breast Reconstruction Following Mastectomy* (pamphlet). 1982.

Bard M, **Sutherland** A: The psychological impact of cancer and its treatment. IV. Adaptation to radical mastectomy. *Cancer* 1955;8:656.

Connell EB: Which contraceptives *don't* cause TSS? *Contemp OB/GYN* 1985;26(October):127.

Contemporary OB/GYN, Symposium on Advances in Managing Condylomas. 1982;20(September):92.

Derogatis LR: Breast and gynecologic cancers: Their unique impact on body image and sexual identity in women. *Front Radiat Ther Oncol* 1980;14:1.

Dickey RP: *Managing Contraceptive Pill Patients*. Durant, Okla, Creative Informatics, 1983.

Donegan WL: Diseases of the breast, in **Danforth** DN, **Scott** JR (eds): *Obstetrics and Gynecology*, ed 5. Philadelphia, Lippincott, 1986.

Dunphy J, **Way** L: *Current Surgical Diagnosis and Treatment*. Los Altos, Calif, Lange, 1980.

Eich SJ: Promising early breast cancer treatment—without mastectomy. *Cancer Nurs*, February 1985;51.

Ervin CT, et al: Behavioral factors and vaginitis, in *The Nurse Practitioner*. Seattle, Wash, Vernon Publications, 1982.

Eschenbach DA: Pelvic infections, in **Danforth** DN, **Scott** JR (eds): *Obstetrics and Gynecology*, ed 5. Philadelphia, Lippincott, 1986.

Fantl JA: The urinary tract as it is related to gynecology, in **Danforth** DN, **Scott** JR (eds): *Obstetrics and Gynecology*, ed 5. Philadelphia, Lippincott, 1986.

Feller WF, et al: Modified radical mastectomy with immediate breast reconstruction. *Amer Surg* 1986;52(March):129.

Ferenczy A: To contain spread of condyloma: Treat your patient's partner. *Contemp OB/GYN* 1986;27(June):51.

Fisher B, **Gebhardt** M: The evolution of breast cancer surgery: Past, present and future. *Sem Oncol* 1978;5(4):385.

Fisher B, et al: Five-year results of a random clinical trial comparing total mastectomy and segmental mastectomy with or without radiation in the treatment of breast cancer. *N Engl J Med* 1985;312(11):665.

Fisher B, et al: L-Phenylalanine mustard (L-PAM) in the management of primary breast cancer. *N Engl J Med* 1975;292:11.

Fogel CI, **Woods** NF (eds): *Health Care of Women: A Nursing Perspective*. St. Louis, Mosby, 1981.

Foster RS, et al: Breast self-examination practices and breast cancer stage. *N Engl J Med* 1978;299:265.

Garner CH, **Webster** BW: Endometriosis. *J Obstet Gynecol Neonat Nurs* 1985;14(6)S:10S.

Green LW, **Roberts** BJ: The research literature on why women delay in seeking medical care for breast symptoms. *Health Educ Monogr* 1974;2(2):129.

Gyllenskold K: *Breast Cancer: The Psychological Effects of the Disease and Its Treatment*. London, Tavistock, 1982.

Hall D, **Goldstein** M, **Stein** G: Progress in manual breast exam. *Cancer* 1977;40(1):364.

Harris RE: Urinary tract infections during pregnancy, in **Sciarra** JJ (ed): *Gynecology and Obstetrics*. Philadelphia, Harper & Row, 1986.

Havens C, **Sullivan** ND, **Tilton** P: *Manual of Outpatient Gynecology*. Boston, Little, Brown, 1986.

Hawkins G, **Whalley** PJ: Acute urinary tract infections in pregnancy. *Clin Obstet Gynecol* 1985;28(2):266.

Hermann RE, et al: Results of conservative operations for breast cancer. *Arch Surg* 1985;120(6):746.

Hinton J: The influence of previous personality on reactions to having terminal cancer. *Omega* 1975;6:95.

Hyde JS: *Understanding Human Sexuality*. New York, McGraw-Hill, 1979.

Jamison K, **Welisch** D, **Pasnau** R: Psychosocial aspects of mastectomy: I. The woman's perspective. *Am J Psychiatry* 1978;135(4):432.

Johnson SR: TSS: Don't overlook less obvious cases. *Contemp OB/GYN* 1985;25(June):131.

Jourand S, **Secord** P: Body cathexis and the ideal female figure. *J Abnorm Soc Psychol* 1955;50:243.

Keith L, **Brittain** J: *Sexually Transmitted Diseases*. Aspen, Colo, Creative Infomatics, 1978.

Keyes HM, **Bakemeier** RF, **Savlov** ED: Breast cancer, in **Rubin** P (ed): *Clinical Oncology for Medical Students and Physicians*. New York, American Cancer Society, 1983.

King C: Detailed guidelines for a thorough examination of the breast. *RN*, July, 1982, p 57.

Kister SJ: Diseases of the breast, in **Rokel** RF (ed): *Conn's Current Therapy*. Philadelphia, Saunders, 1984.

Kopans DB: Use mammography to detect cancer earlier. *Contemp OB/GYN* 1985;26(September):170.

Kopans D, **Meyer** J: Screening for breast cancer. *N Engl J Med* 1980;302(1):59.

Legha S, **Slavik** M, **Carter** S: Nafoxidine: An anti-estrogen for the treatment of breast cancer. *Cancer* 1976; 38:1535.

Levinson W, **Dunn** PM: Nonassociation of caffeine and fibrocystic breast disease. *Arch Intern Med* 1986; 146(September):1773.

Lewis F, **Bloom** F: Psychological adjustment to breast cancer: A review of selected literature. *Int J Psychiatry Med* 1978–1979;9(1):1.

Lubin R, et al: A case control study of caffeine and methylxanthines in benign breast disease. *JAMA* 1985; 253(16):2388.

Maguire P: The psychological and social consequences of breast cancer. *Nurs Mirror* 1975;140:54.

Malinak LR, **Wheeler** JM: A practical approach to endometriosis: II. Treatment. *Female Patient* 1985;10(June):15.

Mann C: Cystic breasts: A condition, not a disease. *Ms,* April, 1983, p 84.

Margolese RG: Breast Ca treatment: Where do we stand? *Contemp OB/GYN* 1986;28(July):39.

Martin I: *Health Care of Women.* Philadelphia, Lippincott, 1978.

McCorkle M: Coping with physical symptoms in metastatic breast cancer. *Am J Nurs* 1973;73(June):1034.

Mead PB: PID: A critique of current therapies. *Contemp OB/GYN* 1985;26(2):111.

Merrill JA: Endometriosis, in **Danforth** DN, **Scott** JR (eds): *Obstetrics and Gynecology,* ed 5. Philadelphia, Lippincott, 1986.

Mims FH, **Swenson** M: *Sexuality: A Nursing Perspective.* New York, McGraw-Hill, 1980.

Minton JP, et al: Clinical and biochemical studies on methylxanthine-related fibrocystic breast disease. *Surgery* 1981; 90:299.

Mitchell M: Breast cancer treatment—current status: 4. Adjuvant therapy. *Postgrad Med* 1983;74(3):161.

O'Brien R: Breast cancer treatment—current status. *Postgrad Med* 1983;74(3):125.

Parsons L, **Sommers** S: *Gynecology.* Philadelphia, Saunders, 1978.

Pattison J, **Sorensen** K: Neoplasms, in **Luckman** J, **Sorensen** K (eds): *Medical-Surgical Nursing: A Psychophysiologic Approach.* Philadelphia, Saunders, 1980.

Pilch Y: Breast cancer treatment—current status: Standard surgical approach. 2. Segmental mastectomy, alternative to total breast excision? *Postgrad Med* 1983;74(3):126.

Polivy J: Psychological effects of mastectomy on a woman's feminine self-concept. *J Nerv Ment Dis* 1977;164(2):77.

Pritchard JA, **MacDonald** P, **Gant** NF: *Williams Obstetrics,* ed 17. New York, Appleton-Century-Crofts, 1985.

Quint JC: The impact of mastectomy. *Am J Nurs* 1963; 63:88.

Rickel L, **Davis** A, **Sigler** B: Solid neoplasms, in **Jones** D, **Dunbar** C, **Jirovec** M (eds): *Medical-Surgical Nursing—A Conceptual Approach.* New York, McGraw-Hill, 1982.

Rubin P: *Clinical Oncology for Medical Students and Physicians.* New York: American Cancer Society, 1978.

Schachter J, et al: Experience with routine use of erythromycin for chlamydial infections in pregnancy. *N Engl J Med* 1986;314:276.

Schlueter LA: Knowledge and beliefs about breast cancer and breast self-examination among athletic and nonathletic women. *Nurs Res* 1982;31(November/December):348.

Schmale A: Reactions to illness: Convalescence and grieving. *Psychiatr Clin North Am* 1979;2(2):321.

Scholtenfeld D, **Fraumeni** J (eds): *Cancer Epidemiology and Prevention.* Philadelphia, Saunders, 1982.

Sciarra JJ, et al: *Gynecology and Obstetrics.* New York, Harper & Row, 1984, vol 1.

Sonstegard L, et al: *Women's Health.* New York, Grune & Stratton, 1982, vol 1.

Sweet RL, et al: Chlamydial infections in obstetrics and gynecology. *Clin Obstet Gynecol* 1983;26(1):143.

Todd J, et al: Toxic-shock syndrome associated with phage-group-1 staphylococci. *Lancet* 1978;2:1116.

Torrington J: Pelvic inflammatory disease. *J Obstet Gynecol Neonat Nurs* 1985;14(6)S:21S.

Tortora G, et al: *Microbiology.* Menlo Park, Calif: Benjamin/ Cummings, 1982.

US Department of Health, Education, and Welfare: *The Breast Cancer Digest.* Bethesda, Md, National Cancer Institute, 1979.

Valanis B, **Rumpler** C: Factors affecting healthy women's expressed preferences for breast cancer treatment. *J Am Med Wom Assoc* 1982;37(12):311.

Vaughn TC: Axioms on managing the lumpy breast. *Consultation* 1983;23(6):137.

Wabrek AJ, **Wabrek** CJ: Mastectomy: Sexual implications. *Primary Care* 1979;3(4):803.

Weber M: Breast cancer: Odds, options, arguments. *Vogue,* August 1983, p 334.

Wedell MA, et al: Endometriosis and the infertile patient. *J Obstet Gynecol Neonat Nurs* 1985;14(4):280.

Whalley PJ: Value of treating UTI during pregnancy. *Contemp OB/GYN* 1986;27(5):134.

Wilson JF: Breast cancer treatment—current status: 3. Simple excision with irradiation. *Postgrad Med* 1983; 74(3):151.

Woods NF: Influences on sexual adaptation to mastectomy. *J Obstet Gynecol Nurs* 1975;4:33.

Wynder EL, **Rose** DP: Diet and breast cancer. *Hosp Pract* 1984:73.

Wynn RM: *Obstetrics and Gynecology: The Clinical Case.* Philadelphia, Lea & Febiger, 1983.

ADDITIONAL READINGS

Bourcier KM, **Seidler** AJ: Chlamydia and condylomata accuminata: an update for the nurse practitioner. *J Obstet Gynecol Neonat Nurs* 1987;16(January/February):17.

Chagares R: Intrathoracic endometriosis: a women's health issue. . .perimenstrual spontaneous pneumothorax. *Heart Lung* 1987;16(March):183.

Conti MT et al: Preventing UTIs: what works? *Am J Nurs* 1987;87(March):307.

Deckers PJ: Current strategies in operable breast cancer. *Hosp Pract* 1987;22(January 30):41.

Edlund BJ et al: Herpes: a dilemma for client and clinician. *Health Care Women Int* 1987;8(1):43.

Evans KM: The female AIDS patient. *Health Care Women Int* 1987;8(1):1.

Fisher S et al: Women and preventive health care: an exploratory study of the use of Pap smears in a potentially high-risk Appalachian population. *Women Health* 1986;11(Fall/Winter):83.

Fogel CI et al: Gonorrhea in women: a serious health problem. *Health Care Women Int* 1987;8(1):75.

Foley SF: Preventive gynecologic nursing in an inpatient setting. *J Obstet Gynecol Neonat Nurs* 1987:16 (May/June):160.

Funch DP: Socioeconomic status and survival for breast and cervical cancer. *Women Health* 1986;11(Fall/Winter):37.

Larson E: Chlamydia: the most prevalent cause of sexually transmitted disease. *Health Care Women Int* 1987;8(1):19 Leads from the MMWR. Progress toward achieving the national 1990 objectives for sexually transmitted diseases. *JAMA* 1987;257(April 24):2141.

Lee GF: Fine-needle aspiration of the breast: the outpatient management of breast lesions. *Am J Obstet Gynecol* 1987;156(June):1532.

Lindsey AM et al: Endocrine mechanisms and obesity; influences in breast cancer. *Oncol Nurs Forum* 1987;14(March/April):47.

Matsunaga J et al: Genital condylomata accuminata in pregnancy: effectiveness, safety and pregnancy outcome following cryotherapy. *Br J Obstet Gynaecol* 1987;94 (February):168.

McGee JE: Management of cervical dysplasia in pregnancy. *Nurse Pract* 1987;12(March):34.

Mechcatie E: Fibrocystic breasts: long-term care. *Patient Care* 1987;21(March):41.

Rutledge DN: Factors related to women's practice of breast self-examination. *Nurs Res* 1987;36(March/April):117.

Shull BL: Female urinary incontinence: tips on office diagnosis and treatment. *Consultant* 1987;27(March):147.

I was 35 when my husband divorced me for another woman. During the following year I had sex with only two men, but one of them gave me herpes. I was devastated when my nurse practitioner diagnosed it. I felt embarrassed, ashamed, dirty. My self-esteem had never been lower. My nurse practitioner was wonderful. She explained the disease and how it was spread and helped me find ways to relieve the symptoms. More than that, though, I always knew she cared about me personally. She helped me realize I was still a worthwhile person. Knowing she still liked and respected me helped me start feeling good about myself again. When I met a man I really cared about, she helped me figure a way to tell him about my herpes. He was able to accept it and still love me. We are married now and I've never been happier. We've followed my practitioner's advice about ways to avoid infecting my husband and he hasn't had any sign of infection. When I think about all the changes and stress in my life I can't imagine how I would have coped without my practitioner. She gave me support when I needed it and encouraged me to stand alone when I was ready. She's a special woman.

Gynecologic Surgery

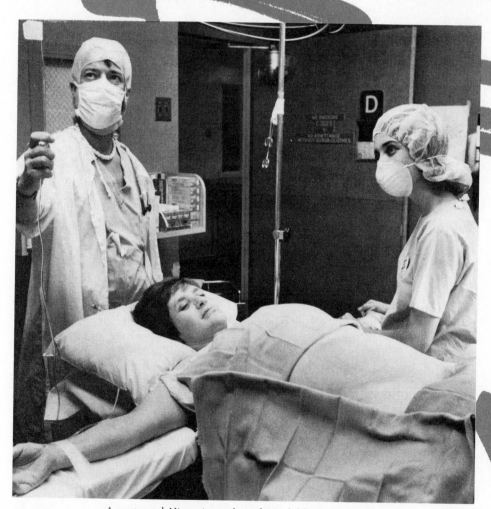

A postpartal Hispanic mother of 11 children is being prepared for the tubal ligation she has chosen.

Chapter Eleven

OBJECTIVES

- **Discuss the issues and concerns surrounding gynecologic surgery.**
- **Describe the most common gynecologic surgical rocedures.**
- **Discuss the nursing care of women during gynecologic surgery.**

The women's health movement has increased public and professional awareness of issues related to gynecologic problems and treatments. Information on new, improved diagnostic and surgical techniques that may be used as alternatives to major surgery is being disseminated to consumers and nurses by various groups. The field of reproductive surgery has changed considerably since the late nineteenth century when an oophorectomy was performed to treat "female unruliness" and hysterectomies were used to treat backaches and "prevent" cancer (Holt & Weber 1982).

Continuing increases in the number of reproductive surgical procedures being performed, particularly hysterectomies, are still cause for concern, however. This chapter identifies gynecologic surgery issues of interest to nurses and women facing the prospect of surgery. It provides an overview of the most common reproductive surgical procedures, including dilation and curettage, hysterectomy, tubal surgery, and termination of pregnancy. It describes indications for surgery, techniques, risks and complications, pre- and postoperative nursing interventions, and psychosexual responses to surgery. It also explains evaluation and treatment of women having surgery because of abnormal cytologic findings and presents an overview of surgical management for gynecologic cancer.

● Issues and Concerns for Women Facing Surgery

There are many components to an informed decision to undergo reproductive surgery. The first question that should be addressed is: What are the indications for having the surgery? An explanation of the surgical procedure and the reasons it was selected over other available alternative procedures should be given to the woman. Effects on childbearing ability and/or sexual performance should be explained, as well as effects on the general functioning of the body. An explanation of the risks of the surgery should include the common risks, the nonserious ones, the rare or unusual complications, and the risk of not surviving (Holt & Weber 1982).

The question whether a second opinion on the necessity for surgery should be sought is somewhat controversial. In the case of elective surgery, different physicians may have different opinions. A woman should be encouraged to consult other physicians when there is controversy about a treatment (such as, for example, treatment of early cervical cancers) or when the surgeon is unknown to the woman. A specialist in gynecology is the preferred source for a second opinion (Holt & Weber 1982). Some third-party payment plans encourage second opinions. The woman can analyze the information and discuss her concerns with the nurse or physician before she legally authorizes the surgery. Usually she is asked to sign a written consent that acknowledges the information given and the authorization for the surgery.

Other concerns that may influence the decision to have reproductive surgery may be categorized as general concerns about surgery and specific concerns related to gynecologic surgery. General concerns include:

- Anesthesia: fear of general anesthesia because of loss of control; fear of regional anesthesia because of possible postoperative problems and concern about being awake during surgery

- Anticipation of postoperative pain

- Fear of death or disability

- Concerns about limitation of normal functioning and dependency during recovery

- Financial coverage

- Family members: welfare of family members while the woman is undergoing surgery (eg, child care, loss of wages, help for household chores) (Webb 1986, Tyler & Woodall 1982)

Specific concerns related to gynecologic surgery are related to the significance of the reproductive organs for the woman. Surgery to alter or remove a reproductive organ may be perceived as a threat to self-concept.

Body image is affected whenever a body part is lost. The degree of mourning for that loss is related to the significance attached to it. Even though there is no outwardly apparent change with a hysterectomy, the loss may be felt strongly. Many women fear postoperative changes such as masculinization, weight gain, and loss of sexuality. Reproductive surgery may also be seen as a threat to femininity in our society, which emphasizes childbearing and motherhood. A woman whose self-esteem comes from sources other than attractiveness and the ability to bear children will usually adjust bettter to reproductive surgery.

● Issues and Concerns for Nurses

Two major areas of concern to the nurse advocate are:

What information does the woman need to make an informed decision about surgery?

What assessment data about the woman are needed to implement a plan of care?

The nurse needs a broad knowledge of gynecology to assist women in making informed decisions. The practitioner must be able to explain a planned surgical intervention at the woman's level of understanding. Before providing explanations, the nurse may have to assess what the woman has already been told by the physician and whether she has any misconceptions about the procedure or its effects.

The nurse needs physical and psychosexual assessment data to plan comprehensive care of the woman. The nurse considers the woman as a total person from the woman's point of view. This self-concept is assessed in terms of body image and feelings of self-worth as influenced by family, society, and culture. For example, religion may be an important factor in decision making. A woman who is a Jehovah's Witness may decline surgery because according to her beliefs she must refuse to accept blood transfusions. However, major gynecologic surgery can be performed with minimum morbidity and mortality, and the woman should have this information (Bonakdar et al 1982). The nurse needs to assess the woman's feelings about the surgery or its effects and encourage her to express her concerns.

● Care of the Woman During Gynecologic Surgery

Hysterectomy

A hysterectomy involves the removal of the uterus through an abdominal incision or through the vagina. When the fallopian tubes and both ovaries are also removed, the procedure is called a total abdominal hysterectomy with bilateral salpingo-oophorectomy (TAH-BSO) or panhysterectomy. At this time, approximately 600,000 to 700,000 total abdominal hysterectomies are performed every year (Wells & Villano 1986).

The necessity of the large number of hysterectomies has recently been questioned. When a hysterectomy is recommended, the woman needs to be aware of her right to a second opinion before making her final decision. The nurse has an important role in providing information to women about issues such as hysterectomy and other reproductive surgery.

INDICATIONS

Hysterectomy is the usual treatment for several conditions, although there is no medical consensus about absolute indications. Abdominal hysterectomies are generally performed for cancer of the cervix, endometrium, and ovary; fibroids; endometriosis; chronic pelvic inflammatory disease; and adenomyosis.

SURGICAL PROCEDURE

The types of hysterectomy include those already described and total vaginal hysterectomy (TVH), the removal of the uterus through the vagina. An anterior and/or posterior repair of the vaginal walls may also be performed with vaginal hysterectomy. This surgical repair is done when weakened pelvic supports have displaced one or more of the pelvic organs (urethra, bladder, rectum), causing urinary incontinence, constipation, or defecation problems.

Abdominal procedures are usually performed if the woman has had previous pelvic surgery or if the fallopian tubes and ovaries are also to be removed. Abdominal hysterectomy is also preferred when malignancy is suspected or confirmed because the procedure allows exploration of the abdomen and pelvis to locate tumor extension. Disadvantages of the abdominal procedure over the vaginal procedure include scarring, more postoperative pain, slower recovery, and more problems with bowel functions.

Vaginal hysterectomy is usually the treatment of choice for uterine prolapse and pelvic relaxation. The advantages of vaginal hysterectomy include earlier ambulation, less postoperative pain, less anesthesia and operative time, less blood loss, no visible scar, and a shorter hospital stay. The vaginal route is preferred for the elderly, obese, or debilitated woman who is a poor risk for abdominal surgery. The major disadvantage of a vaginal hysterectomy is the increased risk of postoperative infection.

Removal of the ovaries with the uterus remains controversial. Some surgeons recommend that the ovaries never be removed in premenopausal women because bilateral oophorectomy results in surgical castration and menopause. Other physicians recommend removal of the ovaries in all hysterectomy patients over 40 years of age because of the risk of ovarian cancer. In any case, oophorectomy should not be considered routine with hysterectomy. The woman should be informed about the alternatives so that she can decide which alternative she prefers. If the ovaries are removed in a premenopausal woman, estrogen replacement therapy is considered. Further discussion of this treatment appears in the following section on oophorectomy.

Preoperative preparation for the hysterectomy generally includes:

- Laboratory work (complete blood count, hemoglobin, hematocrit, type and cross-match of blood, urinalysis, chest radiographs, electrocardiogram)

- Vaginal examination and/or complete physical examination

- Surgical preparation (enema, douche, abdominal-pubic or perineal shave)

- Emptying of the stomach and bladder prior to surgery

- Preoperative medication and intravenous fluids

NURSING ASSESSMENT

Nursing assessment of the woman undergoing a hysterectomy will include psychosocial aspects and determination of the learning needs of the woman.

The initial reaction to the need for hysterectomy has been related to the grief responses identified by Kübler-Ross and described by Stanfill (1982). The first response may be shock, disbelief, or denial, especially if the surgery is an emergency procedure. The woman may not realize the impact of the surgery. Anger may result when there is a waiting period between diagnosis and surgery. This anger often results from the loss of reproductive function or conceptual loss of femininity. Bargaining may be noted in childless women who express the desire to have a child before having the surgery. Depression can occur preoperatively if the woman is very sensitive about her impending loss and is upset by the sight of a pregnant woman or comments about attractiveness.

The nurse must thoroughly assess the physiologic, psychosocial, and sexual needs of the woman. Factors known to affect psychologic adjustment after surgery include the age of the woman, her cultural background and educational level, the attitude of her husband or sexual partner, her family situation, her preoperative preparation, and whether or not cancer is involved. The significance of the uterus in the woman's self-image will be reflected in her attitudes about menstruation, childbearing, body image, and sexuality. If the woman equates her uterus with femininity, she may feel an acute loss. She may feel that she will become an "empty shell." If she sees childbearing as a major role in life, loss of reproductive ability can cause problems. The loss of menses is viewed with relief if there has been dysmenorrhea or other menstrual problems, but with sadness if menses is seen as a cleansing process or a sign of youth. The woman may feel that sexual ability and desire depend on the presence of the uterus and that hysterectomy will affect satisfaction and ability (Christiano 1981).

Misconceptions and fears about the effects of hysterectomy need to be identified preoperatively so that correct information is provided to the woman and reassurances are given that assist her in making a positive emotional adjustment to surgery.

NURSING DIAGNOSIS

Examples of nursing diagnoses that may apply include:

- Knowledge deficit related to lack of information regarding the indications, procedure, advantages and disadvantages, risks, and future implications of hysterectomy

- Fear related to unknown outcome of surgery

NURSING GOAL: PROVISION OF PREOPERATIVE TEACHING

During teaching sessions, the nurse can be a counselor, support person, listener, and teacher. Involvement of the husband or significant others in the discussions can help them accept the surgery and support the woman. Techniques that will encourage the woman to express her feelings and concerns include active listening, sitting down with the woman, eye contact, use of open-ended questions, nonverbal communication, and touch.

Preoperative information and teaching can be done individually or in groups. Being informed about hysterectomy prior to surgery can decrease anxiety and prepare the woman for the procedure and the postoperative period. The preoperative information given should include the consequences of the surgery (what is removed, effect on reproductive ability, and so on), the type of anesthesia used, possible risks and complications, postoperative care routines, convalescence, and resumption of activities.

NURSING GOAL: PROMOTION OF PHYSICAL WELL-BEING IN THE POSTOPERATIVE PERIOD

Routine postoperative care includes monitoring vital signs, temperature, and fluid intake and output; checking the amount of bleeding by assessing the abdominal dressing and/or perineal pads; assessing the need for pain relief; and encouraging early ambulation, leg exercises, and turning, coughing, and deep breathing. In addition to these routine interventions, the diet will be advanced from clear liquids to a regular diet when bowel sounds are present. Sitz baths, heat lamps, and ice packs may be used to relieve perineal discomfort (for vaginal hysterectomy). Foley catheters are usually discontinued 24 to 48 hours after surgery unless anterior repairs were done with vaginal hysterectomy, in which case the Foley or suprapubic catheter may remain in place for up to seven days.

Postoperative complications can occur with both abdominal and vaginal hysterectomies. Hemorrhage, urinary tract complications, and wound infections occur more frequently with the vaginal procedure. Complications associated more frequently with abdominal procedures include intestinal obstruction (paralytic ileus), thromboembolism, pulmonary embolism, atelectasis, pneumonia, and wound dehiscence. Emotional complications can occur with both procedures (see the following section on psychosexual reactions).

Discharge planning begins early in the postoperative period. The nurse and other members of the health care team should discuss and reinforce information concerning physical and emotional recovery. Topics to be covered include physical changes the woman can expect, physical limitations or restrictions during convalescence, anticipatory guidance, and emotional reactions that can occur.

Anticipated physical changes include weakness and fatigue, cessation of menses, inability to become pregnant, possibility of painful intercourse after vaginal hysterectomy with repair (until vaginal walls are stretched), possible bowel irregularity, possible lack of appetite, possible phantom pain (uterine cramps), and possible temporary loss of vaginal sensation after vaginal hysterectomy. Restrictions after surgery may include avoidance of heavy lifting, strenuous housework, or active sports for at least one month; avoidance of tub baths, douches, and sexual intercourse for three to six weeks; and avoidance of sitting for long periods of time to prevent pelvic congestion. Anticipatory guidance is given to stress the need for the postoperative checkup in four to six weeks. The woman also should be taught the signs of infection, hemorrhage, and bladder problems because these complications can occur after discharge. Discussions about possible emotional responses should clear up any misconceptions about hysterectomy causing masculinization, detrimental effects on sexual responses, or mental illness (Tyler & Woodall 1982).

NURSING GOAL: ADDRESSING PSYCHOSEXUAL CONCERNS

Depression is the most frequently reported psychologic reaction after pelvic surgery, especially hysterectomy. Other reactions reported are feelings of loss of femininity and decreased desire for sex. The most common factors in poor adjustment after surgery are the woman's feminine self-concept, previous adverse reactions to stress, previous depression, multiple physical complaints, numerous surgical experiences prior to the hysterectomy, age (under 35 years of age), the wish for more children, fear of loss of interest in or satisfaction with sex, a negative attitude to the surgery on the part of the husband or significant other, marital instability, religious or cultural disapproval of hysterectomy, lack of vocational or avocational involvement, presence of misconceptions, and lack of preoperative anx-

iety (Humphries 1980). Severe depression may occur if the hysterectomy is performed for malignancy because the woman may be faced with the possibility of death.

Emotional responses to vaginal hysterectomy may be different from those to abdominal hysterectomy because there is no external focus for feelings (no obvious physical change to mourn). The woman may need to be encouraged to recognize and express her feelings about having the surgery.

These reactions can occur from three months to three years after the surgery. The woman who has any of the above risk factors should be closely observed during the postoperative period for signs that follow-up or referral is needed after discharge.

There are wide variations in sexual adjustment after hysterectomy. Drellich (1967) reported reactions ranging from increased satisfaction to no change to loss of desire and concluded that these reactions were related to psychologic consequences of reproductive surgery. Another study (Zussman et al 1981), however, suggested that sexual responses after surgery could have physiologic as well as psychogenic causes and suggested sexual counseling, as well as possible hormonal therapy.

Humphries (1980) suggested that the nurse could develop a profile of the woman's sexual behavior prior to surgery to determine her postoperative needs. Specific information that may assist with sexual adjustment after surgery includes the following (Zussman et al 1981):

- Coitus will help stretch the vagina after the temporary shrinking postoperatively.

- Clitoral orgasm can be encouraged.

- Overall sensual enjoyment should be emphasized.

Nurses who are not comfortable or knowledgeable about sexual counseling should be encouraged to seek more education in human sexuality.

EVALUATIVE OUTCOME CRITERIA

Anticipated outcomes of nursing care include the following:

- The woman understands the reason for the hysterectomy, the alternatives, the expected outcome of surgery, the risks, and aspects of self-care after surgery.

- The woman has an uneventful recovery without complications.

- The woman feels she is able to ask questions and obtain support.

- The woman is able to participate in decision making as she desires.

Dilation and Curettage

Dilation and curettage (D & C) is the most frequently performed minor gynecologic surgical procedure. Indications for D & C can be diagnostic or therapeutic. Diagnostic indications include checking for uterine malignancy, evaluating infertility causes, and investigating dysfunctional uterine bleeding. Therapeutic indications include treatment of heavy bleeding, incomplete abortion, therapeutic abortion, dysmenorrhea, and removal of polyps.

A D & C may be performed as inpatient or outpatient surgery. Anesthesia may be regional or local but frequently is general. With the woman in a lithotomy position, a speculum is inserted in the vagina to visualize the cervix. The cervical os is dilated and a curette is used to scrape out the endometrium. Complications associated with a D & C are infection, cervical lacerations, uterine perforation, and secondary hemorrhage (7 to 14 days postoperatively).

Salpingectomy

Salpingectomy is the unilateral or bilateral removal of the fallopian tubes. Indications include diseases of the tubes, sepsis, malignancy, and tubal pregnancy. Salpingectomy for tubal pregnancy is generally an emergency procedure because of the danger of hemorrhage from the placenta, which erodes the tube.

Tubal Reconstruction

Microsurgery has significantly affected gynecologic surgery primarily in the treatment of infertility and reversal of sterilization. The procedure involves "unblocking" the tubes and reconnecting the remaining portions (tubal reanastomosis), using magnification and microsurgical techniques to obtain proper alignment and accurate approximation of the tubes.

Oophorectomy

Oophorectomy is unilateral or bilateral removal of the entire ovary. Indications may include severe pelvic inflammatory disease, malignancy, ectopic pregnancy, and ovarian cysts. Ovaries may be removed when a hysterectomy is performed if the woman is menopausal but may not be removed in premenopausal women, depending on the indication for the hysterectomy. Reasons for oophorectomy with hysterectomy are related to the risk of ovarian cancer, whereas the reasons for not performing oophorectomy are related to the superiority of hormones produced by the body over hormone replacement therapy in younger women.

When both ovaries are removed, abrupt surgical menopause occurs in premenopausal women. This may cause decreased libido, decreased vaginal lubrication, and decreased sensations in the lower vaginal tract. Symptoms of menopause—such as hot flashes and atrophy of the vaginal epithelium—may be treated with estrogen replacement therapy. Estrogen is usually given orally on a cyclic basis, in the lowest doses compatible with effective treatment of symptoms (0.3 to 0.625 mg) to reduce severe menopausal symptoms and the risk of osteoporosis. Women on estrogen replacement therapy are at risk for hypertension, gallbladder disease, angina pectoris, breast cancer, and endometrial cancer (if they have not had a hysterectomy). Topical application of estrogen may relieve vaginal atrophy and dyspareunia, although water-soluble lubricants may work as well (Judd et al 1981). There is no consensus on the risk factors, benefits, or side effects of the use of estrogen replacement therapy in women who have had hysterectomies. Some clinicians advocate administration of progesterone for a portion of each cycle to oppose the estrogen effects. There is a need for further research on this controversial issue.

NURSING ASSESSMENT

The nurse assesses the woman's knowledge of the surgery, the indications for it, the risks, and self-care information. The nurse also assesses the woman's knowledge of the need for estrogen replacement and the associated problems of this therapy.

NURSING DIAGNOSIS

Examples of possible nursing diagnoses include:

- Knowledge deficit related to inadequate knowledge about the proposed surgery, indications, risks, expected outcome, and associated self-care measures

- Potential sexual dysfunction related to distress over surgery

NURSING GOAL: PROVISION OF CLIENT TEACHING

The nurse provides information regarding the expected surgery, the expected benefit, the risks, and associated complications. The woman will need to know the expected activities during hospitalization and self-care after discharge. The woman will also require information about estrogen replacement therapy in order to make an informed decision about whether she wants to receive it.

EVALUATIVE OUTCOME CRITERIA

Anticipated outcomes of nursing care include the following:

- The woman understands the surgery, and is able to participate in decision making at the level she wishes.

- The woman's recovery is uneventful without complications.

Surgical Interruption of Pregnancy

Although for centuries abortion was banned by both church and public law, many women still sought to terminate their pregnancies. Because of the illegal status of abortion, however, the procedure was always dangerous. Illegal abortions became the single highest cause of maternal death in this country. Since 1973, when induced abortion became a legal option, the maternal mortality rate has steadily declined.

Although legalized abortion has been in effect for several years, the controversy over the moral and legal issues continues. This controversy is as readily apparent in the medical and nursing professions as among other groups. See Chapter 4 for further discussion of the belief system and social issues surrounding abortion.

FACTORS INFLUENCING THE DECISION TO SEEK ABORTION

A number of physical and psychosocial factors influence a woman's decision to seek an abortion. The presence of a disease or health state that jeopardizes the mother's life and serious, life-threatening fetal problems are frequently suggested as indications for abortion. In other instances, the timing or circumstance of the pregnancy creates an inordinate stress on the woman and she chooses an abortion. Some of these situations may involve contraceptive failure, rape, or incest. In all cases, the decision is best made by the woman or couple involved. A mother whose life is threatened by the pregnancy may choose to continue the pregnancy while one with no obvious threat may choose abortion. Many feel this is as it should be because the decision must rest with the individuals who bear the impact of the continuance or termination of the pregnancy.

METHODS

The method of abortion differs depending on the length of gestation. See Table 11–1 for various techniques.

NURSING ASSESSMENT

The nurse must assess the woman's knowledge base regarding the abortion and her emotional status in order to devise a teaching plan and provide emotional support.

NURSING DIAGNOSIS

Examples of possible nursing diagnoses include:

- Knowledge deficit related to the abortion procedure, alternatives, risks, and associated self-care

- Alteration in comfort related to pain during the procedure

NURSING GOAL: PROVISION OF CLIENT TEACHING

As the woman makes her decision regarding an abortion she will need information regarding the types of abortion and the associated risks. The woman needs to understand the available alternatives and the possible problems. The debate about abortion is frequently empassioned, which makes it very difficult to obtain accurate, unbiased facts on which to base a decision. The nurse helps provide valuable information so that the woman can make an informed choice.

The need for teaching continues during the procedure and afterward for self-care measures.

NURSING GOAL: PROVISION OF SUPPORT

Important aspects of care include allowance for verbalization by the woman; support before, during, and after the procedure; monitoring of vital signs, intake, and output; providing for physical comfort and privacy throughout the procedure; and health teaching regarding self-care, the importance of the postabortion checkup, and contraception review.

EVALUATION OUTCOME CRITERIA

Anticipated outcomes of nursing care may include the following:

- The woman understands the procedure, the alternatives, and the associated risks.

- The woman has been able to participate in informed decision making.

- The woman has not suffered any complications of the procedure.

Table 11–1 Methods Used in Termination of Pregnancy

First-trimester abortion	Complications
DILATION AND CURETTAGE Dilation and curettage is the oldest method. It involves the use of a metal curette to scrape out the inside of the uterus. It is not done frequently now because other methods are deemed safer and less traumatic.	Perforation of the uterus, laceration of the cervix, systemic reaction to the anesthetic agent, hemorrhage
MINISUCTION A minisuction is accomplished with a small-bore cannula and a 50 mL syringe as a vacuum source. This technique is also called menstrual regulation or menstrual extraction.	Perforation of the uterus, laceration of the cervix, systemic reaction to the anesthetic agent, hemorrhage
VACUUM CURETTAGE After a paracervical block, the cervix is dilated and a vacuum suction cannula is inserted to remove the contents of the uterus. A laminaria may be inserted into the cervix the day before to dilate the cervix.	Perforation of the uterus, laceration of the cervix, systemic reaction to the anesthetic agent, hemorrhage (Gabbe et al 1986)

Second trimester (mid-trimester)	Complications
HYPERTONIC SALINE Hypertonic saline is still a common method after 20 weeks. A laminaria is inserted the day before. Hypertonic saline is injected or infused into the amniotic cavity. The procedure takes an average of 33 to 35 hours to completion. Some clinicians begin intravenous oxytocin a few hours after the instillation of hypertonic saline. In this case the procedure takes an average of 25 hours (Gabbe et al 1986). The addition of oxytocin increases the risk to the woman.	Cervical laceration, uterine rupture, cardiovascular collapse, pulmonary and/or cerebral edema, renal failure, failed abortion, hemorrhage, infection, embolism
DILATION AND EXTRACTION (D & E) Laminaria are inserted one or two days before the procedure. During the D & E an IV is started, local anesthesia is administered, and the pregnancy is removed with a combination of suction and forceps. The procedure usually take 10 to 20 minutes.	Perforation of the uterus with bladder or intestinal injury, amniotic fluid embolism, disseminated intravascular coagulation (Gabbe et al 1986)
SYSTEMIC PROSTAGLANDINS Prostaglandin E_2 vaginal suppositories or 15-methyl $PGF_{2\alpha}$ (Prostin 15M) may be used. The average time for either of these procedures is 13 to 15 hours.	Nausea, vomiting, fever (Gabbe et al 1986)
INTRAUTERINE PROSTAGLANDINS Insertion of laminaria is done the night before. Prostaglandin $F_{2\alpha}$ is injected into the amniotic sac. The abortion procedure usually averages about 14 hours after the $PGF_{2\alpha}$ is instilled. In some instances, urea is also instilled.	Vomiting, diarrhea, fever, cervical rupture, hemorrhage, infection (Gabbe et al 1986)

● The woman has a support base and knows community resources to use if needed.

Surgical Interventions for Abnormal Cytology

Whenever a Pap smear report for a woman is abnormal, the cytologic study should be repeated. If an abnormal smear is reported again, a colposcopy can be performed to examine the cervix more closely. If the initial Pap report reveals mild dysplasia or a more serious finding, colposcopy should be done immediately. If abnormal tissue is detected, punch biopsies and endocervical curettage

(ECC) are carried out. If cervical intraepithelial neoplasia (CIN) is detected, five possible treatments are suggested based on whether the ECC was negative or positive and whether invasive cancer was found. Treatment alternatives are conization, cryosurgery, electrocautery, carbon dioxide laser, and hysterectomy.

COLPOSCOPY

Colposcopy is used to rule out invasive cancer of the cervix and is a diagnostic tool for women exposed to diethylstilbestrol (DES). A stereoscopic viewing instrument can magnify the tissues observed from 6 to 40 power. The area viewed is the transformation zone, the area of the cervix where columnal epithelium has been changed by the process of metaplasia to squamous epithelium. Dysplasia, CIN, and carcinoma in situ (CIS) usually originate in this area.

The woman assumes a lithotomy position after she has emptied her bladder. A speculum is inserted in the vagina and the cervix is cleansed with a solution of 3% acetic acid. This softens the mucosa and causes the tissues to swell which aids in visualizing the epithelium. The examiner looks through the scope (which is not inserted in the vagina) for areas of irregular punctuation or mosaic white epithelium. If abnormal tissue is detected and a punch biopsy of the tissue is performed, the woman may experience a pinching or stinging sensation. She also may become tired in the lithotomy position.

Colposcopy is performed as an outpatient procedure. Although it is expensive, the costs are usually covered by insurance; women without medical insurance may be referred to special colposcopy clinics at large teaching hospitals (Benedet et al 1982). The nurse should tell the woman what to expect and remain with her to assist and encourage slow breathing or other relaxation techniques during the procedure.

BIOPSY

A cervical biopsy is performed to investigate suspicious cervical tissue to diagnose or rule out cancer of the cervix at its earliest stages. An endometrial biopsy is used to diagnose functional menstrual disorders, infertility problems related to ovulation, and benign or malignant lesions.

The woman may experience moderate to severe cramplike pains. A small amount of bleeding also may be experienced after the biopsy, and this may continue for up to two weeks. Bleeding as heavy as a menstrual period should be reported to the physician or clinic. The woman should be advised to avoid douches and sexual intercourse for five days (Winer 1982, Tyler & Woodall 1982).

An endocervical curettage is performed prior to biopsies to confirm the presence or absence of disease in the endocervix. The endocervical canal is scraped from the internal to external os. The woman needs to be prepared for some cramping and pain during the procedure.

CONIZATION

A conization is generally performed when the entire lesion cannot be visualized by colposcopic examination. In this procedure a cone of tissue, the size and length of which are determined by the extent of the lesion, is surgically removed. A large amount of normal tissue is removed along with the abnormal tissue. Conization can be performed as an inpatient or outpatient procedure and under local or general anesthesia. There is a risk of postop-

erative infection and hemorrhage, and premature labor and abortion may be experienced in future pregnancies. A prolonged or profuse menstrual period can occur with the next two or three cycles (Winer 1982).

CRYOSURGERY

Cervical dysplasia, endocervicitis, and nabothian cysts may be treated by cryosurgery. The procedure causes tissue necrosis by freezing. A double freeze method is advocated, with nitrous oxide or carbon dioxide as the refrigerant. The freezing also can destroy normal tissue. The failure rate for treatment of stage II and III CIN is as high as 30 percent.

The procedure is usually performed a week after the menstrual period to avoid disturbing a pregnancy and to allow new tissue to generate before the next period. Cryosurgery can be performed in the physician's office or clinic without anesthesia. It is not a painful procedure, although the woman may experience some cramping.

The woman should be told to expect a heavy, persistent watery discharge for several weeks. She should not use tampons and should avoid sexual intercourse while the discharge is present, because the cervix is friable.

LASER THERAPY

The laser is used to treat both CIN and vaginal and vulvar intraepithelial neoplasia. It is reported to be safer, less mutilating, and less costly than conization and hysterectomy. The laser is used when all boundaries of the lesion are visible on colposcopy and the endocervical curettage is negative. The invisible, highly concentrated beam is absorbed by water in the tissues, and the energy is converted to heat, causing evaporation of the cellular water and cellular death.

The laser can be used in outpatient settings. No anesthesia is necessary for cervical lesions, and there is minimal bleeding. The woman may experience minor cramping and a slight discharge for 5 to 7 days. She should avoid the use of tampons, douching, and sexual intercourse for two weeks. Healing may take 6 to 12 weeks. Fertility remains intact (Winer 1982).

Surgical Management of Gynecologic Cancer

Reproductive malignancies can be treated with surgery, radiation, chemotherapy, or a combination of the three methods depending on the type of cancer and the extent of disease. A discussion of reproductive oncology and all the treatment modalities is beyond the scope of this chapter; this discussion focuses on surgical management, emphasizing radical surgery and its physiologic, psychosocial, and sexual implications.

TYPES OF CANCER

○ *CERVICAL CANCER* Microinvasive cancer of the cervix (depth of penetration of the tumor into submucosal tissues up to 3 mm) is treated with hysterectomy. Invasive cancer of the cervix is treated according to the extent of the cancer, the woman's health, and her age. Staging of the cancer is an evaluation process that identifies the extent of spread of the tumor based on routine studies such as intravenous pyelography, complete blood count, barium enema, cystoscopy, lymphangiography, bone scan, and proctoscopy (see Table 11–2). TAH and bilateral lymphadenectomy are recommended for stage Ib and IIa. Stage Ia cancer of the cervix is treated with hysterectomy or radiotherapy. In this stage the cancer is confined to the cervix. Stages IIb through IV involve tumor growth beyond the cervix (ie, vagina, pelvis, ureters, and outside the reproductive organs), and the treatment of choice is radiotherapy (Kneisl & Ames 1986).

○ *OVARIAN CANCER* Ovarian cancer is very difficult to diagnose and frequently it has spread before it has been detected. All stages of ovarian cancer are treated with a total abdominal hysterectomy and bilateral salpingo-oophorectomy. Radiation and chemotherapy are often used following surgery. Chemotherapy is frequently begun the day of surgery (Danforth & Scott 1986) and radiation may also be used.

Table 11–2 Staging of Cervical Cancer

Stage 0: Carcinoma in situ, intraepithelial carcinoma.

Stage I: Carcinoma strictly confined to the cervix (extension to the corpus should be disregarded).
Ia: Microinvasive carcinoma (early stromal invasion)
Ib: All other cases of stage I; occult cancer should be marked "occ"

Stage II: Carcinoma extends beyond the cervix, but not to the pelvic wall; the carcinoma involves the vagina, but not as far as the lower third.
IIa: No obvious parametrial involvement
IIb: Obvious parametrial involvement

Stage III: Carcinoma extends to the pelvic wall; on rectal examination, there is no cancer-free space between the tumor and the pelvic wall; the tumor involves the lower third of the vagina; all cases with a hydronephrosis or nonfunctioning kidney are included.
IIIa: No extension to the pelvic wall
IIIb: Extension to the pelvic wall and/or hydronephrosis or nonfunctioning kidney

Stage IV: Carcinoma extends beyond true pelvis or has clinically involved the mucosa of the bladder or rectum; a bullous edema as such does not permit a case to be allotted to stage IV.
IVa: Spread of the growth to adjacent organs
IVb: Spread to distant organs

From Kneisl C, Ames S: *Adult Health Nursing*. Menlo Park, Calif, Addison-Wesley, 1986.

Table 11–3 Staging of Endometrial Cancer

Stage I: Carcinoma is confined to the corpus.

Subdivision according to size of uterus:
Ia: Uterine cavity sounds to 8 cm or less
Ib: Uterine cavity sounds to more than 8 cm

Subdivision according to histology:
G1: Highly differentiated adenomatous carcinomas
G2: Differentiated adenomatous carcinomas with partly solid areas
G3: Predominantly solid or entirely undifferentiated carcinomas

Stage II: Carcinoma has involved corpus and cervix.

Stage III: Carcinoma has extended outside uterus but not outside true pelvis.

Stage IV: Carcinoma has extended outside true pelvis or has obviously involved mucosa of bladder or rectum. Bullous edema as such does not permit allotment of a case to stage IV.

Source: Kneisl C, Ames S: *Adult Health Nursing*. Menlo Park, Calif, Addison-Wesley, 1986.

○ *ENDOMETRIAL CANCER* Stage I tumors, which involve only the corpus, are treated with TAH-BSO (Table 11–3). Stage II tumors, which involve the corpus and cervix, require TAH-BSO with lymph node dissection and radiation therapy. Stages III and IV are usually treated with external and/or intracavitary irradiation (Kneisl & Ames 1986).

○ *VULVAR CANCER* Cancer of the vulva is more common in women between 70 and 80 years of age who have had chronic vulvitis. Treatment usually includes vulvectomy and removal of superficial inguinal lymph nodes.

Before I was faced with cancer, I thought that doctors were the people with all the information. But it was the nurse who explained the test results and the diagnosis the doctor had given me. Because of my nurse, I know just what to expect and how to take care of myself. I think nurses should speak up more, so people know all the wonderful things they do.

VULVECTOMY

A simple vulvectomy is performed for leukoplakia and intractible pruritus, whereas a radical procedure is done for malignant disease. A simple vulvectomy is the removal of the labia majora and minora and the clitoris. Radical vulvectomy is the removal of the whole vulva, the skin and fat of the femoral triangle, and the pelvic lymph nodes. Skin grafts may be necessary.

This disfiguring procedure is associated with marked psychosexual disturbances. Most women report greatly decreased sexual arousal levels and low self-image (Hacker et al 1984). The woman may express grief over her loss by crying, withdrawing, or becoming depressed or angry.

Sexual activity can be resumed within three months but adjustments are necessary owing to the loss of sensory perception for foreplay. Stimulation of the breast, thighs, buttocks, or anterior abdominal wall can be suggested (Jusenius 1981).

PELVIC EXENTERATION

A pelvic exenteration is performed for recurrence of cervical cancer. Only about 5 percent of women with recurrence are candidates for the procedure, which will not be performed if there is any evidence of tumor outside of the pelvis, if the lymph nodes have metastatic tumor, or if all of the tumor cannot be removed.

Exenteration can be of the anterior or posterior pelvis or the total pelvis. Anterior exenteration is the removal of the uterus, ovaries, fallopian tubes, vagina, bladder, urethra, and pelvic lymph nodes. Urine is diverted through an ileal conduit. Posterior exenteration is the removal of the uterus, tubes, ovaries, descending colon, rectum, and anal canal. A colostomy is created. A total exenteration is a combination of the anterior and posterior procedures. A vagina can be reconstructed from split-thickness skin grafts or a segment of small bowel.

Complications associated with exenteration include intestinal and urinary obstruction, thrombophlebitis, pulmonary embolism, pyelonephritis, hypovolemia, peritonitis, pneumonia, and wound infection.

NURSING ASSESSMENT

The nurse frequently has contact with the woman shortly after she has been told of the possible diagnosis. The woman may be confused and stunned by the diagnosis or unclear about what is happening. The nurse can provide support as she begins to establish a relationship with the woman. Initial assessments may focus on the information the woman has and desires, on clarifying information, and on assessing the coping style and strengths of the woman. It may be helpful to ask the woman to explain her diagnosis and anticipated treatment in order to determine her understanding and the need for further information. After these beginning assessments the nurse extensively assesses preoperative physical and emotional states and potential problems with adjustment related to the woman's body image. The main question is whether the woman's self-concept and feelings of self-worth are based on her appearance or ability to have normal body functions. The sociocultural (religious, racial) influences on the woman also need to be assessed. Another major assessment area is the impact of the surgery on sexual functioning due to the alteration of excretory function and obliteration of the vagina with pelvic exenteration. The feelings and reactions of the sexual partner are crucial to the woman's adjustment. The nurse or counselor should explore with the woman and her partner new ways of physical contact. Often the woman is so anxious about the recurrence of her cancer that she is willing to accept the body changes preoperatively because she is hopeful for a cure.

NURSING DIAGNOSIS

Examples of nursing diagnoses that may apply include:

- Knowledge deficit related to lack of information regarding the diagnosis, suggested therapy and alternatives available, risks, and associated complications

- Ineffective coping, related to stress associated with the diagnosis and anticipated treatment

- Grieving related to loss of body part and/or life-style changes

NURSING GOAL: PROVISION OF PREOPERATIVE TEACHING

Many times the initial contact with the woman occurs in the hospital setting as the woman is admitted for diagnostic testing or a surgical procedure. It is important to provide information related to the procedures and to be available to validate any information that the woman has. Prior to a surgical procedure the nurse provides information specific to the procedure, the associated nursing care, and the expected postsurgical course.

NURSING GOAL: PROMOTION OF EMOTIONAL SUPPORT

The woman must deal not only with the diagnosis of cancer but also with a surgical procedure that will make many changes in her body. The nurse has the vital role of providing emotional support, information, and counseling.

NURSING GOAL: PROVISION OF POSTOPERATIVE CARE

Postoperative care for vulvectomy includes urinary drainage via an indwelling catheter to prevent wound contamination and meticulous wound care to debride and provide healing. Wound care usually consists of debriding with a solution of half-strength peroxide followed by normal saline. The wound is then dried with either a heat lamp or a hair dryer (cold air) (Lowdermilk 1981).

Postoperative care for the woman with pelvic exenteration usually begins with three or four days in the intensive care unit because of the risk of shock, cardiac changes, and kidney failure. Once the woman returns to the regular postoperative unit, care includes the usual postoperative interventions, as well as care for the ileal conduit and/or colostomy. The nurse needs to continue to assess the woman for a grief reaction to the drastic changes in her body and should expect emotional fluctuations.

EVALUATIVE OUTCOME CRITERIA

Anticipated outcomes of nursing care may include the following:

- The woman understands the diagnosis, the recommended and alternative procedures, and the associated risks and complications.

- The woman is able to participate in the decision-making process as much as she desires.

- The woman recovers without complications.

- The woman knows resources in her community that she may use if desired.

KEY CONCEPTS

Components of an informed decision regarding reproductive surgery include an explanation of the indications for the surgery, the surgical procedure, the treatment and alternatives, the risks and the effects on the woman.

The nurse focuses on the information the woman needs to make an informed decision and on the assessment of data and implementation of nursing care.

A hysterectomy involves the removal of the uterus. It may be done abdominally or vaginally.

Dilation and curettage is the most frequently performed minor gynecologic surgical procedure. It is done for heavy bleeding, incomplete abortion, therapeutic abortion, dysmenorrhea, or removal of a polyp.

A number of physical and psychosocial factors influence a woman's decision to seek an abortion.

When abnormal Pap smear results are discovered, associated procedures may include colposcopy, biopsy, conization, cryosurgery, or laser surgery.

Gynecologic cancer involves carcinoma of the cervix, ovaries, uterus, endometrium, and/or vulva.

REFERENCES

Averette HE (mod): Symposium: Ovarian Cancer: Optimal chemotherapy regimens. *Contemp OB/GYN* 1986; 28(December):108.

Benedet IL, et al: Colposcopy, conization and hysterectomy practices: A current perspective. *Obstet Gynecol* 1982; 60(5):539.

Bonakdar MI, et al: Major gynecologic and obstetric surgery in Jehovah's Witnesses. *Obstet Gynecol* 1982; 60(5):587.

Christiano MY: Hysterectomy, in **Smith** ED (ed): *Women's Health Care: A Guide for Patient Education.* New York, Appleton-Century-Crofts, 1981.

Danforth DN, **Scott** JR: *Obstetrics and Gynecology.* Philadelphia, J.B. Lippincott, 1986.

Drellich MG: Sex after hysterectomy. *Med Aspects Hum Sex* 1967;(3):62.

Gabbe SG, **Niebyl** JR. **Simpson** JL: *Obstetrics.* New York: Churchill Livingstone, 1986.

Hacker NF, et al: Guide to conservative management of stage 1 vulvar cancer. *Contemp OB/GYN* 1984; 24(December):105.

Holt LH, **Weber** M: *The American Medical Association Book of Woman Care.* New York, Random House, 1982.

Humphries PT: Sexual adjustment after hysterectomy. *Health Care Wom* 1980;2(2):1.

Judd HL, et al: Estrogen replacement therapy. *Obstet Gynecol* 1981;58(3):267.

Jusenius K: Sexuality and gynecologic cancer. *Cancer Nurs* 1981;4(December):479.

Kneisl CR, **Ames** SA: *Adult Health Nursing.* Menlo Park, Calif, Addison-Wesley, 1986.

Lowdermilk DL: Reproductive malignancies, in **Fogel** CI, **Woods** NF (eds): *Health Care of Women: A Nursing Perspective.* St. Louis, Mosby, 1981.

National Center for Health Statistics: *Utilization of Short-Stay Hospitalization—United States 1982.* Department of Health and Human Services. Publication No. (PHS) 84-1739. Government Printing Office, 1984.

Stanfill PH: The psychosocial implications of hysterectomy. *J Obstet Gynecol Neonat Nurs* 1982;11(5):318.

Tyler SL, **Woodall** GM: *Female Health and Gynecology Across the Lifespan.* Bowie, Md, Brady, 1982.

Webb C: Professional and lay social support for hysterectomy patients. *J Admin Nurs* 1986;11:167.

Wells MP, **Villano** K: Total abdominal hysterectomy. *AORN J* 1986;42:368.

Winer WK: Laser treatment of cervical neoplasia. *Am J Nurs* 1982;82(September):1384.

Zussman L, et al: Sexual responses after hysterectomy oophorectomy: Recent studies and consideration of psychogenesis. *Am J Obstet Gynecol* 1981;140(7):725.

ADDITIONAL READINGS

Arneson AN, **Kao** MS: Long term observation of cervical cancer. *Am J Obstet Gynecol* 1987;156(March):614.

Bates MS: Ethnicity and pain: A biocultural model. *Soc Sci Med* 1987;24(1):47.

Benotti PN, et al: Management of recurrent pelvic tumors. *Arch Surg* 1987;122(April):457.

Buehler JW, et al: The risk of serious complications from induced abortion: Do personal characteristics make a difference? *Am J Obstet Gynecol* 1985;153(September):14.

Collison C, **Miller** S: Using images of the future in grief work. *Image* 1987;19(Spring):9.

DiSaia PJ: Diagnosis and management of ovarian cancer. *Hosp Pract* 1987;22(April):235.

Elder JP, **Neef** NA: Behavior modification and the primary and secondary prevention of cancer. *Fam Commun Health* 1987;9(November):14.

Geach B: Pain and coping. *Image* 1987;19(Spring):12.

Gilman CJ: Management of early-stage endometrial carcinoma. *Am Fam Physician* 1987;35(April):103.

Green CP: Changes in responsibility in women's families after the diagnosis of cancer. *Health Care Women Int* 1986;7(3):221.

Griggin D, **Said** HM: The enterohepatic circulation of methotrexate in vivo: Inhibition by bile salt. *Ca Chemother Pharm* 1987;19(1):40.

Hassey KM: Principles of radiation safety and protection. *Semin Oncol Nurs* 1987;3(February):23.

Herbath L, **Gosnell** DJ: Nursing diagnosis for oncology nursing practice. *Cancer Nurs* 1987;10(February):41.

Howard J: 'Avoidable mortality' from cervical cancer: Exploring the concept. *Soc Sci Med* 1987;24(6):507.

Irwin M, et al: Life events, depressive symptoms and immune function. *A J Psychiatr* 1987;144(April):437.

Ladermen C: The ambiguity of symbols in the structure of healing. *Soc Sci Med* 1987;24(4):293.

Littlefield VM: *Health Education for Women.* Norwalk, Conn, Appleton-Century-Crofts, 1986.

Macinick CG, **Macinick** JW: Toxic new world: What nurses can do to cope with a polluted environment. *Int Nurs Rev* 1987;34(March):40.

Tiffany R: The development of cancer nursing as a specialty. *Int Nurs Rev* 1987;34(March):35.

Wang JF: Induced abortion: Reported and observed practice in Taiwan. *Health Care Women Int* 1985;6(5–6):383.

When I went in for surgery, I was very frightened. The hospital seemed so cold and crisp. The nurse who admitted me knew I was afraid. She talked with me and explained what was planned and said she would be with me. She made all the difference.

Rape

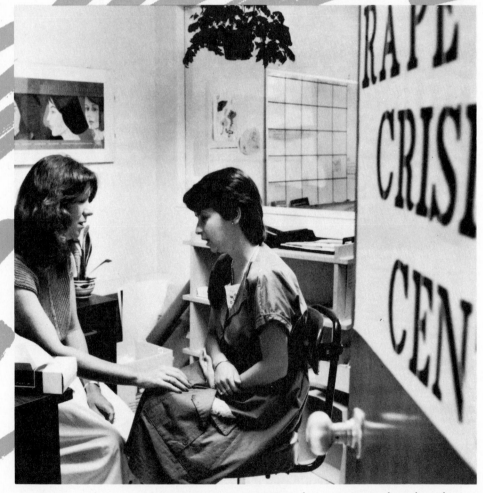

A nurse's greatest sensitivity and compassion are brought to bear in counseling a rape survivor.

Chapter Twelve

Rape as a Community Responsibility
Preventive Education
Rape Crisis Counseling
Prosecution of the Rapist

OBJECTIVES

- **Contrast the nonsexual and sexual aspects of rape.**
- **Compare the types of rape.**
- **Identify the phases of the rape trauma syndrome.**
- **Discuss the importance of values clarification for nurses caring for rape survivors.**
- **Discuss the nurse's role as client advocate and counselor with rape survivors.**
- **Summarize the procedures for collecting and preserving physical evidence of sexual assault.**
- **Discuss the preventive and legal responsibilities of the community.**

Rape can happen to women of all ages, ethnic backgrounds, and walks of life. No woman is immune. As rape is being recognized as one of today's most serious violent crimes, rape crisis counseling centers are emerging to meet the needs of rape survivors. Nevertheless, society continues to harbor many myths and misconceptions about rape and rape survivors. Fear related to these myths may discourage the rape survivor from reporting the assault and may deprive her of the care she needs.

To assist the rape survivor in overcoming this horrifying trauma, the nurse must be able to refute societal myths and must understand the legal definitions of rape, the personality patterns of rapists, and the ways in which survivors are likely to respond. With this information, the nurse can apply specific nursing strategies to benefit the rape survivor and her loved ones.

● Definitions and Perspectives

Defining Rape

According to Ledray (1986, p 10), "rape occurs anytime a person is forced or coerced, physically or verbally, into any type of sexual contact with another person." The person who rapes may be a stranger, acquaintance, husband, or employer. The sexual component usually involves penetration of the genitals by a penis, hand, or other object, but any type of coerced sexual contact can be considered rape. The term *sexual assault* is also used to label such acts.

Legally, there are three preconditions for a valid charge of rape:

- The use of threat, physical force, intimidation, or deception.
- Nonconsent of the victim.
- Coitus or vaginal penetration, however slight.

However one chooses to define it, rape is an act of savagery and terror. It is not an act of sex but an act of violence expressed sexually—a man's aggression and rage acted out against a female. The woman who survives such an act may bear its scars for life.

The Incidence of Rape

Between 1971 and 1981, the incidence of forcible rape rose more sharply than that of any other Crime Index offense (Uniform Crime Reports 1982). In the United States, an estimated 330,000 to 810,000 women are raped every year (Ledray 1986). Of these, only 82,000 women report their rapes. At one time, the estimated ratio of unreported rapes to reported rapes ranged as high as 20 to 1. This ratio is probably declining as states change their laws to allow women to prosecute their assailants without being victimized a second time by the judicial system. Nevertheless, the National Center for the Prevention and Control of Rape estimates that one out of every three women will be raped at some time in her life.

Societal Views of Rape

RAPE AS CONQUEST

The act of rape is ages old. Traditionally, it was viewed, not as an act of a man against a woman, but as an act of aggression against another man—the woman's husband or father; that is, her "owner." To rape a man's daughter or wife was the ultimate insult, an act of power. On conclusion of a battle, rape of the wives and daughters of the losers symbolized the triumph of the conquerors and the humiliation of the vanquished.

THE VICTIM AS TEMPTRESS

Recently, rape survivors have been accused of provoking the assault by their appearance or behavior or merely by being present in a secluded area. This neomedieval concept of rape portrays woman as a temptress preying on men's susceptibility to passion, destroying their always tenuous control, until she "gets what she is asking for."

Various studies have refuted the myth that rape is passion out of control. Groth and Burgess (1977), for example, interviewed 170 convicted rapists. Virtually none of these men reported sexual dysfunction in consenting sexual relations, but 59 percent reported sexual dysfunction during the rape. Moreover, 9 percent of these men admitted that coitus was not their intent.

Rape has also been portrayed as a universal female fantasy—the secret dream of every American girl. Sudden attack, physical abuse, and the threat to her life were believed to "turn her on." Actually, rape appears to be the fantasy of some men. Malamuth (1981) asked male students at the University of California whether they would rape a woman if they knew they would not be caught and punished. Approximately 35 percent said they might.

● Who Commits Rape—and Why?

Characteristics of Rapists

Like their victims, rapists come from all ethnic backgrounds and walks of life. More than half are under 25 years of age, and three out of five are married and leading "normal" sex lives. Why do these men rape? Of the many theories proposed in answer to this question, none provides a concrete explanation.

Freud viewed rape as an instinctual expression of male aggression usually blocked by civilization. Groth and Burgess (1977) found that 33 percent of the rapists they interviewed had been sexually abused as children. Their assaults appeared to replicate their childhood experiences. Groth and Burgess's study has been criticized as being biased because all their subjects were incarcerated and therefore not representative of male sexual offenders, the vast majority of whom are not imprisoned.

Rapists also have been examined for biologic abnormalities; for example, the extra Y chromosome (XYY) phenomenon. The extra Y chromosome is thought to cause elevated levels of testosterone, leading to increased aggression. The finding that few incarcerated rapists had ex-

tremely high levels of testosterone appears to invalidate this theory (Rada et al 1976).

Feminist theorists link rape with sociocultural conditions. Brownmiller (1975) proposed that rape helps maintain patriarchy by keeping females dependent on males for protection. Sanday studied reports of primitive tribal societies and concluded that rape is not integral to male nature; rather, it is "the means by which men programmed for violence express their sexual selves" (Garrison 1983, p 6).

Types of Rape

Rape assaults are categorized statistically according to the style of the rape and its suspected motivation. Five categories have been identified: blitz rape, acquaintance or date rape, power rape, anger rape, and sadistic rape.

BLITZ RAPE

In the blitz rape, victim and assailant are strangers. The assault occurs suddenly and by surprise. An attack on a nurse who is walking to her car after working an evening shift is an example of a blitz rape.

ACQUAINTANCE OR DATE RAPE

In acquaintance rape, the assailant obtains sex from a reluctant, unconsenting victim by betrayal or coercion, for example, after a date. This kind of rape is commonly found on college campuses. Koss and Oros (1982) questioned 1846 male students at Kent State University about using coercion to obtain sexual relations. Over 9 percent had attempted or committed rape in this manner without being reported. Women in such situations may not report the rapist for fear of being blamed for the rape.

POWER RAPE

Power rape accounts for 55 percent to 65 percent of all reported rapes. The power rapist is dominated by conflicts about power and mastery. His self-esteem is low; he feels worthless. In capturing a woman, he places her in the powerless position he has frequently experienced and despised. By raping her, he proves to himself that he is desirable, potent, and strong. He fantasizes about sexual conquest of women and often believes that the victim enjoys the assault. His victims are usually strangers whom he captures by a blitz attack. He exerts only the amount of force needed to subdue his victim. Usually a power rape is planned (Foley & Davies 1983).

ANGER RAPE

In 35 percent to 40 percent of cases, the rapist uses the act to release pent-up anger. This type of rapist feels mistreated and mentally abused by significant women in his life; the rape becomes a symbolic expression of his anger toward them, an act of revenge. The man's feelings may or may not be based on reality, but he perceives them as real. Anger rape usually occurs on impulse and is characterized by considerable brutality and trauma. The rapist derives sexual satisfaction from his ability to hurt the victim (Foley & Davies 1983).

SADISTIC RAPE

Some 5 percent of rapes are sadistic. The sadistic rapist has an antisocial personality, and sadism usually characterizes all his relationships. Theorists propose that during their childhoods, such men develop a view of the world as a hostile environment from which they must aggressively defend themselves. During puberty, such men learn to eroticize their aggression, eventually requiring violence to experience sexual excitation. The sadistic rapist delights in his victim's struggle and pain. Often he abuses and tortures the woman until he is completely out of control. "A self-perpetuating cycle of increasing intensity results: the more aggression aroused, the more powerful he feels, the more excited he becomes—to the extent that he may, in a frenzy, commit a lust murder" (Foley & Davies 1983, p 34). In this type of rape, victim and assailant are usually strangers, and the assault is planned. This type of rape usually receives media attention.

The foregoing classifications are not mutually exclusive; they categorize the dominant motive in a given rape. Regardless of the style of attack, anger, power, and sadism are components of any rape, which is essentially the use of sexual behavior to meet nonsexual needs.

● How Do Rape Survivors Respond?

Rape is viewed as a situational crisis; that is, an unanticipated traumatic event that the victim is generally unprepared to handle because it is unforeseen. The victim experiences disequilibrium and loss of control. According

CONTEMPORARY DILEMMA

Does No Mean "No?"

Date rape is a significant, underreported problem on many college campuses. A recent study indicates that one in eight women on college campuses are the victims of rape. Of these, 47 percent involved rape by a date or acquaintance (Sweet 1985). Since date rape occurs within the context of a shared social experience, the woman who reports this type of rape is often labeled a liar. Consequently she suffers in three ways:

1. She is the victim of a forceful act of aggression.

2. Her honesty and integrity are questioned.

3. Her confidence in her ability to judge people is shaken because a man she trusted betrayed that trust.

Often the woman herself fails to identify the act as rape. She assumes that in some way she is responsible for the act. Furthermore, if she believes that only "bad" girls get raped, then to view the act as rape means that she must see herself as "bad."

Why do certain men rape? Some men have strongly traditional "macho" male attitudes. They subscribe to the notion that a woman who says "no" really means "yes." They consider aggression and force normal male patterns of behavior and do not view their actions as rape.

Researchers also suggest that some men are very insensitive to negative cues from women. Consequently it is difficult for them to realize when a woman is not interested in a sexual relationship.

A man may deny the possibility that his action was rape because it contradicts his self-image as a nice person. Moreover, he must not be sexually desirable if he can only obtain sex by force.

Colleges have failed to recognize and take action to counteract the problem of date rape for pragmatic reasons: The topic is inflammatory and alarming and might result in decreased student enrollment.

Many questions arise about this subject. For instance:

● What can be done to help women realize that accepting a date does not automatically mean consenting to sexual intercourse?

● How can men learn to recognize when a woman means "no?"

● Are there behavioral cues that can help women recognize men who are potential rapists?

● How can we help women overcome the emotional turmoil resulting from date rape?

● What role should colleges and universities play in preventing date rape?

● How should date rape situations be handled?

to Foley and Davies (1983, p 238), the survivor's crisis response after a rape develops in four stages:

1. Tension rises as the survivor tries her habitual problem-solving techniques.

2. She does not succeed in coping and cannot restore homeostasis with her usual coping mechanisms; her stress and discomfort increase.

3. Additional increase in stress acts as a powerful internal stimulus; the woman mobilizes her internal and external resources to solve her problem and reduce her powerful anxiety.

4. If the disequilibrium continues and can neither be resolved nor avoided, tension increases and a major disorganization and/or disintegration of personality occurs.

A crisis state does not necessarily follow rape; some survivors possess the resources necessary to avoid it. Many rape survivors are able to cope constructively with their anxiety. Nevertheless, the rape survivor's response usually parallels the four phases of crisis development.

Rape Trauma Syndrome

Following rape, the survivor may experience a cluster of symptoms described by Burgess and Holmstrom (1979) as "rape trauma syndrome." Burgess and Holmstrom originally described this syndrome as having two phases: the acute phase and adjustment or reorganization phase. Sutherland and Scherl proposed an intermediate "outward adjustment" phase (Golan 1978). These phases are summarized in Table 12–1. Other authors have described an alternative "silent reaction." Survivors also suffer long-term effects.

Although the phases of response are discussed individually in the following sections, they often overlap. Individual responses and their duration vary greatly.

ACUTE PHASE

The acute phase of rape trauma syndrome begins during the rape and may last up to a week. The woman's primary reaction is intense fear; during the rape she is likely to fear being killed (Ferris 1983). Other early reactions may include shock and disbelief and sometimes denial. The woman may feel embarrassed, humiliated, and unclean; her wish to cleanse herself by bathing or douching may be overpowering, even if she knows that by doing so she is destroying evidence. She may feel angry or anxious, powerless or helpless. Some women blame themselves and feel guilty or feel compelled to "play the scene over and over in their minds."

The rape survivor may suppress her emotions or may reveal them by crying, sobbing, or acting tense and restless. Survivors who control or mask their emotions may appear calm, composed, or subdued. Physical manifestations of rape trauma syndrome include (Burgess & Holmstrom 1979, p 234):

- *Circulatory*—flushing, perspiration, feeling hot or cold.
- *Respiratory*—sighing respirations, hyperventilation, dizziness.
- *Gastrointestinal*—abdominal pain, nausea, anorexia, diarrhea, constipation.
- *Genitourinary*—urinary frequency; interference with sexual function.
- *Mental*—impaired attention, poor concentration, poor memory, changes in outlook and planning.

Many rape survivors also experience alterations in sleep patterns such as insomnia, nightmares, or crying out at night.

OUTWARD ADJUSTMENT PHASE

Once the acute stage has passed, the survivor may appear adjusted. She returns to work or school and resumes her usual roles. But although she appears composed she is actually coping by denial and suppression (Fogel & Woods 1981). Sutherland and Scherl suggested that the survivor needs the outward adjustment phase to cope with the experience of rape; it is a means of regaining control of her life (Golan 1978). During this time, she may move to a different house or apartment or may institute security measures such as installing extra locks or requesting an unlisted telephone number. She may buy a weapon or take a course in self-defense. These activities do not resolve her emotional trauma; they simply push it further into her subconscious.

Table 12–1 Phases of the Rape Trauma Syndrome

Phase	Response
Acute phase	Fear, shock, disbelief, desire for revenge, anger, denial, anxiety, guilt, embarrassment, humiliation, helplessness, dependency; survivor may seek help or may remain silent.
Outward adjustment phase	Survivor appears outwardly composed, denying and repressing feelings; for example, she returns to work, buys a weapon, adds security measures to her residence, and denies need for counseling.
Reorganizational phase	Survivor experiences sexual dysfunction, phobias, sleep disorders, anxiety, and a strong urge to talk about or resolve feelings; victim may seek counseling or may remain silent.

REORGANIZATIONAL PHASE

Because the rape experience had not been resolved, denial and suppression cannot sustain the survivor for long. These coping mechanisms deteriorate; she becomes depressed and anxious and feels a strong urge to talk about the rape. At this point, the woman enters the reorganizational phase of the rape trauma syndrome. She must alter her self-concept and resolve her feelings about the rape.

During this phase, the rape survivor experiences numerous difficulties. Survivors frequently report prolonged menstrual and/or gynecologic disorders. The woman may develop phobias about being in crowds or alone or about sensory impressions related to her assailant. For example, a distinctive odor the assailant possessed, such as alcohol or gasoline, may precipitate a painful memory or an emotional crisis. Fears of being indoors or outdoors or of being attacked from behind—depending on how the attack took place—are common. Because of these fears, the woman may alter her life-style. If she is afraid of crowds, of being out after dark, or of returning to an empty house, she may become a virtual recluse.

Rape survivors frequently report sexual dysfunction. Some women become totally averse to sexual activity. Those who do try to engage in sex often report a decrease in vaginal lubrication, inability to be aroused, unusual sensations in the genital area, and inability to achieve orgasm (Foley & Davies 1983).

Sleep disorders persist. Survivors report repeated nightmares in which they either relive the rape or thwart the rapist's attempt. In either case the dream contains disturbing violence. The woman repeatedly replays the role of victim until she comes to terms with the experience.

The Silent Reaction

Women who do not report the rape go through the phases of the rape trauma syndrome without using available support systems. Their reasons for keeping silent vary; a woman may be embarrassed, she may accept society's "temptress view" and blame herself, or she may fear retaliation. Her experience may be discovered much later, perhaps when she seeks professional help in resolving a different crisis. Some women seek medical help for their physical injuries without disclosing that a rape was the cause. The nurse who suspects that a woman has been raped should seek validation through sympathetic questioning. Public health nurses are often able to identify silent victims by their observations of violent family interactions.

LONG-TERM EFFECTS

Although not enough research has been devoted to determining the long-term effects of rape, the most prevalent sequelae appear to be sexual problems, fear, and anxiety. In summing up the few studies conducted to date, Ferris (1983) compared the long-term reactions of survivors with those related to war, hurricanes, floods, or similar major disasters.

● The Rape Survivor and the Role of the Nurse

Rape survivors often enter the health care system by way of the emergency room; nurses are often the first to counsel them. It is essential to remember that the rape survivor is not sick; she is in a crisis state. Counseling should follow the crisis intervention pattern outlined in Box 12–1.

Clarifying the Nurse's Reaction

The values, attitudes, and beliefs of a care giver will necessarily affect the competency and focus of the care that that person gives. Because rape arouses such strong reactions, it is especially important that the nurse's values be clarified. Interaction with a rape survivor may provoke anxiety, ambivalence, or feelings of personal vulnerability to rape. The nurse may feel overwhelmed by sympathetic feelings or by a sense of inadequacy. Conversely, the nurse may consciously or subconsciously accept the view that a

---

Box 12–1 Nursing Strategies to Assist the Client in Crisis

The nurse:

Listens actively and with concern

Encourages the open expression of feelings

Assists the woman in gaining an understanding of the crisis

Assists the woman to accept reality gradually

Assists the woman to explore new ways of coping with her problems

Links the woman to a social network

Assists the woman to make decisions about:
What problem needs to be solved
How it is to be solved
When and where it should be solved
Who should be solving it

Reinforces newly learned coping strategies

Encourages follow-up contact

Source: Adapted from Kozier B, Erb G: *Fundamentals of Nursing,* ed 3. Menlo Park, Calif, Addison-Wesley, 1987.

woman was "asking for it." Such feelings interfere with the nurse's ability to give empathic, advocative assistance. Moreover, the nurse may silently convey these feelings to the woman, thus increasing her distress.

By using value clarification to discover their own beliefs, nurses can improve their effectiveness in assisting rape survivors. Clarification may be enhanced in a group setting. With the aid of a skilled facilitator, nurses can discuss their feelings about rape and rape survivors and resolve any conflicts.

Acute Phase

Policies for admitting and examining rape survivors vary among institutions. A woman who has been raped is under great stress and needs the sensitive care of professionals who are aware of her special needs. The manner in which she is treated at this crucial time will strongly affect her ability to function in the future. Table 12–2 outlines the general principles of nursing actions during the various phases of the rape trauma syndrome.

The first priority is creating a safe, secure milieu. Admission information should be gathered in a quiet, private room. The woman should be reassured that she is not alone and will not be abandoned and that she is safe from a second attack. During this time, the nurse can develop a primary nurse relationship so that the rape survivor has one person to whom she can relate consistently throughout her hospital experience.

The survivor's level of emotional distress must be assessed, both for the purpose of planning care and as possible courtroom evidence. Scrupulous documentation is essential because the survivor's medical record is often used

Table 12–2 Nursing Actions Appropriate to Phases of the Rape Trauma Syndrome

Phase	Nursing action
Acute phase	Creating a safe milieu
	Explaining the sequence of events in the health care facility
	Allowing the woman to grieve and express her feelings
	Providing care for significant others
Outward adjustment phase	Providing advocacy and support at the level requested by the woman
	Providing assistance to significant others
Reorganizational phase	Establishing a trusting relationship
	Assisting the woman to understand her role in the assault
	Clarifying and enhancing the woman's feelings
	Assisting the woman in planning for her future

in the courtroom to verify her testimony. The mental status examination includes:

- *General appearance and behavior.* What is the woman's attitude? Her posture? What mannerisms does she display?

- *Consciousness/awareness.* Is the woman oriented to time, place, and identity? Is she able to focus on a subject, theme, or event?

- *Affectivity and mood.* Is the woman depressed? Anxious? Displaying elation anxiety? Is she fearful or apathetic? Is she expressing her feelings or controlling them?

- *Motor behavior.* Is the woman inactive, hyperactive, or underactive?

- *Thought control.* How logical is the woman's flow of ideas and associations?

- *Intellectual functioning.* How intelligent does the woman appear? What is her level of general knowledge? How well does she remember events? How sound is her judgment?

It is imperative that control be returned to the woman as quickly as possible. She has suffered trauma in which all control was taken from her. The nurse can return control by encouraging the woman to make contact. When feasible, the woman should decide on the sequence of hospital events. In this way the nurse helps her deal with her crisis in small, manageable increments.

The woman should be encouraged to express her feelings and reassured that anger and fear are normal, appropriate responses. The nurse can also address expressed or unexpressed guilt by assuring the woman that the rape was not her fault.

By explaining the medical examination and the sequence of events in the emergency department, the nurse alleviates anxiety related to fear of the unknown. The woman should know what is going to happen and why, and how she can assist in each phase of the examination. (Examination of the rape survivor and collection of evidence are discussed later in this chapter.)

Throughout the experience, the nurse acts as the survivor's advocate, providing support without usurping decision making (see Chapter 1). The nurse need not agree with all the survivor's decisions but should respect and defend the survivor's right to make them.

The family members or friends on whom the survivor calls also need nursing care. Like the survivor, the reactions of the family will depend on the values to which they ascribe. Sonstegard et al (1982) reported that the most common reaction is to regard rape as a sexual act rather than an act of violence. Many families or mates blame the survivor for the rape and feel angry with her for not being more careful. They may feel personally wronged or attacked and see the survivor as being devalued or unclean. These reactions compound the survivor's crisis.

By spending some time with family members before their first interaction with the survivor, the nurse can reduce their anxiety and absorb their frustrations, sparing the woman further trauma.

Outward Adjustment Phase

A survivor who is in the outward adjustment phase may deny any need for counseling. The nurse, respecting the woman's wishes, does not force counseling on her. The family, however, may still be in need of assistance in coping with anger or guilt. The survivor's behavior may confuse them. By providing information and support, the nurse can assist them in examining and reconciling their feelings.

Reorganizational Phase

As the woman enters the reorganizational phase, she usually feels a strong urge to discuss and resolve her feelings about herself and her assailant. "This means that she must come to terms intellectually and viscerally (her head and heart) by acknowledging the impact of the rape on her life and incorporating it as a stressful memory in her total life experience" (Burgess & Holmstrom 1979, p 330). During this phase, the survivor may benefit from counseling.

Rape Counseling

Foley and Davies (1983) identified three phases of rape counseling: self-exploration, self-understanding, and action.

SELF-EXPLORATION

Counselor and survivor explore the survivor's feelings and establish rapport. Feelings that have been denied and suppressed are brought into the woman's awareness. She should be encouraged to express those feelings openly, identify their source, and understand that they belong to her. The nurse employs a nondirective therapeutic use of self, responding empathically to the survivor's feelings and demonstrating perception of and sensitivity to the woman's feelings, thoughts, and experiences. Acceptance of the woman and respect for her are essential. The woman must feel that she can come to the nurse in a safe, stable, non-judgmental environment to express her feelings fully and get in touch with them.

During this time, the nurse also uses reflective and enhancing responses with the woman. Reflective responses demonstrate that the nurse comprehends the woman's feelings; enhancing responses promote fuller awareness. An example of a reflective response is:

Survivor: I feel so ashamed and dirty. I feel like everyone is looking at me.

Nurse: It sounds as if you feel humiliated.

An example of an enhancing response is:

Survivor: My parents keep telling me that if I had been more careful this would not have happened. They don't understand.

Nurse: You are feeling hurt and rejected by your parents.

These techniques assist the woman gradually to go beyond superficial feelings and enter the self-understanding phase.

SELF-UNDERSTANDING

Having identified the woman's feelings, she and the nurse go on to clarify them and understand their source. Understanding the reasons for her feelings enables the woman to decide on actions that will resolve her problems. The nurse can assist her in understanding the larger context of the rape. It is important for the nurse to avoid reinforcing the prevalent myth that rape is the survivor's "fault." Rather, the nurse can use questions and discussion to encourage the woman to conclude that the blame lies with the rapist. Similarly, the nurse assists the individual in formulating strategies for returning to her prerape level of functioning.

ACTION

In this phase the survivor makes specific plans for overcoming her problems and tests them with the nurse's support. With the nurse, the woman explores her thoughts and feelings about self-care, celebrates her victories, and evaluates her defeats. It is important to emphasize that the loss of control that occurred during the rape was temporary and that the woman does have control over other aspects of her life. "The counselor can conclude that the victim has come to terms with the rape when the victim can honestly say that the memory is not as frequent, the physical distress is not as great, and the intensity of the memory has decreased" (Burgess & Holmstrom 1979, p 331).

● Physical Care of the Rape Survivor

Traditionally, the health care system has met the physical needs of the rape survivor (often to the detriment of emotional needs). Repair of tissue damage and prevention of complications are primary concerns. Because rape is a crime as well as a traumatic emergency, however, some aspects of medical care are governed by the need to collect and preserve legal evidence for use in prosecuting the assailant. In so doing, health care providers must respect the rights of the rape victim, which are summarized in Box 12–2. The nurse as client advocate is responsible for defending those rights.

Collection of Evidence

For the rape survivor, who has already been violated and deprived of control, further invasion of her body for the collection of evidence can be traumatic. The nurse can assist her in coping with this procedure by carefully explaining what will be done and why it is necessary.

Specimens to be collected include:

The survivor's clothing

- Swabs of body stains
- Oral swabs
- Vaginal and rectal swabs
- Fingernails or scrapings
- Combings of pubic hair
- Blood samples
- Photographs (sometimes)

Vaginal and rectal examinations are also performed, along with a complete physical examination for trauma. Any lacerations of the vaginal wall are repaired and noted.

Box 12–2   The Rights of the Rape Victim

The rape victim has the right:

1. To transportation to a hospital when incapacitated.
2. To emergency room care with privacy and confidentiality.
3. To be listened to carefully and treated as a human being, with respect, courtesy, and dignity.
4. To have an advocate of choice accompany her through the treatment process.
5. To be given as much credibility as a victim of any other crime.
6. To have her name kept from the news media.
7. To be considered a victim of rape regardless of the assailant's relationship to her.
8. Not to be exposed to prejudice against race, age, class, life-style, or occupation.
9. Not to be asked questions about prior sexual experience.
10. To be treated in a manner that does not usurp her control but enables her to determine her own needs and how to meet them.
11. To be asked only those questions that are relevant to a court case or to medical treatment.
12. To receive prompt, free medical and mental health services, regardless of whether the rape is reported to the police.
13. To be protected from future assault.
14. To accurate collection and preservation of evidence for court in an objective record that includes the signs and symptoms of physical and emotional trauma.

15. To receive clear explanations of procedures and medication in language she can understand.
16. To know what treatment is recommended, for what reasons, and who will administer the treatment.
17. To know any possible risks, side effects, or alternatives to proposed treatments, including all drugs prescribed.
18. To ask for another physician, nurse practitioner, or nurse.
19. To consent to or refuse any treatment, even when her life is in serious danger.
20. To refuse to be part of any research or experiment.
21. To make reasonable complaints and to leave a care facility against the physician's advice.
22. To receive an explanation of and understand any papers she agrees to sign.
23. To be informed of continuing health care needs after discharge from the emergency room, hospital, physician's office, or care facility.
24. To receive a clear explanation of the bill and review of charges and to be informed of available compensation.
25. To have legal representation and be advised of her legal rights, including the possibility of filing a civil suit.

Source: Adapted from Foley TS, Davies MA: *Rape: Nursing Care of Victims.* St. Louis, Mosby, 1983.

CLOTHING

Clothing will be inspected for the presence of semen, because a rapist will frequently ejaculate outside the vagina. Clothing should be placed in a paper bag, sealed, and labeled appropriately.

SWABS OF STAINS AND SECRETIONS

Swabs of body stains are analyzed for semen or sperm. Because victims are often forced to commit fellatio, oral swabs are examined for semen. Gonorrhea cultures also are taken from oral swabs. Specimens of the woman's saliva will be examined to determine whether she is a secretor or nonsecretor of certain blood-group antigens. If she is a nonsecretor—that is, if these antigens are not present in her saliva—the presence of antigens in her mouth and/or vagina may be evidence of semen from the assailant (Foley & Davies 1983).

Vaginal and rectal swabs are necessary to document the presence of sperm. Because sperm are sensitive to air and do not survive for long periods, a screen for vaginal sperm is performed as soon as possible. A vaginal smear is placed on a wet mount and stained; any sperm that are present will appear light blue. The absence of sperm, however, does not signify that no rape has occurred. As discussed earlier, many rapists suffer sexual dysfunction during the rape and do not ejaculate.

HAIR AND SCRAPINGS

Clippings or scrapings of the woman's fingernails are examined for blood or tissue from the assailant. Her pubic hair is combed to check for loose pubic hair that may have been transferred from the rapist.

BLOOD SAMPLES

Blood is drawn to be tested for gonorrhea and syphilis and to determine whether the woman is pregnant.

PHOTOGRAPHS

The procedure for taking photographs, if any, is determined by institutional policy.

Prevention of Sexually Transmitted Disease

The survivor is offered prophylactic treatment for syphilis and gonorrhea. If she is not allergic to penicillin, she is usually given 4.8 million units of procaine penicillin intramuscularly and 1 g of probenecid orally. A woman who is allergic to penicillin may be given 500 mg of tetracycline orally four times a day for 10 days. Tetracycline should not be given to a woman who is pregnant. If the survivor chooses not to receive prophylactic treatment, the nurse should instruct her to return in two weeks to be tested for gonorrhea and again in four to six weeks to be tested for syphilis.

Prevention of Pregnancy

The woman is questioned about her menstrual cycle and contraceptive practices. If she could become pregnant as a result of the rape, postcoital therapy is offered. Synthetic estrogens are most often used for this purpose. Although diethylstilbestrol (DES) was frequently used in the past, it has been linked to cervical cancer in female offspring. Equally effective in preventing pregnancy are:

Premarin: 50 mg intravenously or 2.5 mg orally four times per day for five days

Estinyl: 0.5 mg orally four times per day for five days

The initial dose of estrogen must be taken within 72 hours of intercourse to be effective.

Estrogen therapy causes such side effects as nausea, vomiting, headaches, breast tenderness, and menstrual irregularities. The woman should be advised that these effects may occur and should be given antiemetics to assist her in completing the prescribed regimen.

If the woman chooses not to be treated for the prevention of pregnancy, she may need information in the future about abortion or adoption agencies. She has the right to be informed of all alternatives.

● Rape as a Community Responsibility

Preventive education, funding of rape crisis counseling centers, and prosecution of the rapist are community responsibilities.

Preventive Education

Community colleges or local rape awareness groups may offer courses in preventive strategies. Some classes focus on increasing women's awareness of situations in which they are at risk. Others are concerned with changing societal attitudes about rape and rape survivors. Because rape is a considerable risk for any woman, courses in what to do during and after a rape may also be helpful. Nurses are well qualified to initiate or participate in preventive instruction. Some do's and don'ts for rape victims are listed in Box 12–3.

Rape Crisis Counseling

Most rape crisis counseling centers operate 24 hours a day, seven days a week. Their services are invaluable. Properly trained telephone counselors can help the woman regain control early in the crisis. Early crisis intervention

---

Box 12–3   Do's and Don'ts for the Rape Victim

1. Try to remain calm and use your head. Escape from the situation with the least amount of harm to yourself.

2. Be able to identify your assailant.

3. Call the police immediately.

4. Avoid cleaning yourself or the area where the assault occurred. Physical evidence is essential for the apprehension and prosecution of your assailant.

5. Call a rape crisis center. A volunteer will counsel you, tell you what to expect, and how they can help you. They understand! Don't be afraid to call!

Source: National Center for the Prevention and Control of Rape: *Rape and Older Women: A Guide to Prevention.* Rockville, Md, NIMH, 1979.

---

often encourages the woman to seek professional treatment and assistance. Many rape crisis centers offer free counseling to rape survivors or can refer them to qualified counselors. Information on sexually transmitted disease and pregnancy alternatives may also be obtained from these centers.

Prosecution of the Rapist

Legally, rape, like any criminal action, is considered a crime against the state rather than against the victim. Therefore, prosecution of the assailant is a community responsibility in which the district attorney will act on the victim's behalf. The victim, however, must initiate the process by reporting the crime and pressing charges against her assailant. Once authorities have apprehended the alleged rapist, the judicial system is set into motion.

Procedures vary from state to state. A judge or magistrate generally conducts a hearing to determine whether there is sufficient evidence that a crime has in fact been committed and that the accused has committed it. If so, the alleged assailant will be bound over for the grand jury. The grand jury will hear the state's evidence (not the defense), again to determine whether the evidence is sufficient for trial. If so, the defendant is indicted; if not, he is acquitted. Once indicted, a defendant must stand trial unless he waives this right. He may elect to have his case heard by a judge rather than a jury. Either a judge or a jury will find the defendant guilty or not guilty, and he will be retained or set free accordingly.

Many rape survivors who have gone through the judicial process refer to it as a second rape—and sometimes a more damaging one. The survivor will be repeatedly asked to identify the assailant and describe the rape in intimate detail. Throughout the pretrial period, the defense attorney may use delaying tactics, obtaining continuances or postponements, further frustrating the survivor and her support system. Publicity may intensify her feelings of humiliation, and if the assailant is released on bail, she may fear retaliation.

During the trial itself, cross-examination by the defense attorney can be a severely degrading experience in which the "victim as temptress" myth is continually evoked. Although some states have altered their laws so that the survivor's sexual history may not be made public, others have not. The defense attorney will try to discredit her testimony, causing her to feel victimized a second time.

The nurse acting as a counselor needs to be aware of the judicial sequence to anticipate rising tension and frustration in the survivor and her support system. They will need consistent, effective support at this crucial time.

KEY CONCEPTS

A rape occurs every ten minutes in the United States, yet a majority of rapes are unreported.

Why men rape remains a mystery, although it has been established that rape is an act of eroticized aggression.

Following rape, the survivor will usually experience an assortment of symptoms known as the rape trauma syndrome.

The responses demonstrated by the survivor and the duration of each phase of the syndrome are highly individual.

The nursing actions to assist rape survivors are encompassed in the roles of advocate, educator, and counselor.

Nurses inform the woman of the sequence of events and her options and support the survivor's decisions.

The counseling process used by the nurse follows the crisis intervention model because the survivor is in a situational crisis rather than being ill.

Nursing research is needed on the long-term effects of rape on survivors and their families, positive coping mechanisms used by past survivors, and effective counseling strategies.

Widespread education is also needed to abolish societal myths surrounding rape.

REFERENCES

Brownmiller S: *Against Our Will: Men, Women, and Rape.* New York, Simon & Schuster, 1975.

Burgess AW, **Holmstrom** LL: *Rape: Crisis and Recovery.* Englewood Cliffs, NJ, Prentice-Hall, 1979.

Ferris E: *Long-Term Consequences of Adult Rape.* Response to Violence in the Family and Sexual Assault. Vol 6, No 1. Rockville, Md, National Center for the Prevention and Control of Rape, January/February, 1983.

Fogel CI, **Woods** NF (eds): *Health Care of Women: A Nursing Perspective.* St. Louis, Mosby, 1981.

Foley TS, **Davies** MA: *Rape: Nursing Care of Victims.* St. Louis, Mosby, 1983.

Garrison J: *Research on Rapists.* Response to Violence in the Family and Sexual Assault. Vol 6, No 2. Rockville, Md, National Center for the Prevention and Control of Rape, March/April, 1983.

Golan N: *Treatment in Crisis Situations.* New York, Free Press, 1978.

Groth AN, **Burgess** AW: Sexual dysfunction during rape. *N Engl J Med* 1977;297(14):764.

Koss MP, **Oros** CJ: The sexual experience survey: An empirical instrument for investigating sexual aggression and victimization. *J Consult Clin Psychol* 1982;50:455.

Kozier B, **Erb** G: *Fundamentals of Nursing,* ed 3. Menlo Park, Calif, Addison-Wesley, 1987.

Ledray LE: *Recovering from Rape.* New York, Henry Holt, 1986.

Malamuth N: Rape proclivity among males. *J Soc Issues* 1981;37:138.

National Center for the Prevention and Control of Rape: *Rape and Older Women: A Guide to Prevention.* Rockville, Md, NIMH, 1979.

Rada RT, **Laws** DR, **Kellner** R: Plasma testosterone levels in the rapist. *Psychosom Med* 1976;38(4):257.

Sonstegard LJ, **Kowalski** KM, **Jennings** B: *Women's Health: Ambulatory Care.* New York, Grune & Stratton, 1982, vol 1.

Sweet R: Date rape: The story of an epidemic and those who deny it. *Ms.* 1985;14(October):56.

Uniform Crime Reports: *Crime in the United States.* National Center for the Prevention and Control of Rape. National Institute of Mental Health. Government Printing Office, 1982.

Becker JV, et al: Level of postassault sexual functioning in rape and incest victims. *Arch Sex Behav* 1986; 15(February):37.

Costin F: Beliefs about rape and women's social roles. *Arch Sex Behav* 1985;14(August):319

DeNitto D, et al: After rape: Who should examine rape survivors? . . . Nurse rape examiners? *Am J Nurs* 1986;86(May):538.

D'Epiro P: Examining the rape victim. *Pt Care* 1986;20(April 20):98.

Ellison ES: Social support and the constructive development model. *West J Nurs Res* 1987;9(1):19.

Freund K, et al: Males disposed to commit rape. *Arch Sex Behav* 1986;15(February 15):23.

Goldenring JM: Inadequate care of rape cases in emergency rooms of hospitals with religious affiliation. *J Adolesc Health Care* 1986;7(March):141.

Heinrich KT: Effective responses to sexual harrassment. *Nurs Out* 1987;35(March/April):70.

Hibbard RA, et al: Genitalia in children's drawing. *Pediatr* 1987;79(January):129.

Kohnke M: *Advocacy: Risk and Reality.* St. Louis, Mosby, 1982.

Limandri BJ: The therapeutic relationship with abused women. *J Psychosoc Nurs* 1987;25(February):8.

Lowery M: Adult survivors of childhood incest. *J Psychosoc Nurs* 1987;25(January):27.

Martin CA, et al: Psychotherapy of rape. *Curr Psychiatr Ther* 1986;23(May):65.

Meyer CB, et al: Adjustment to rape. *J Pers Soc Psychol* 1986;50(June):1226.

Mishel MH, **Braden** CJ: Uncertainty: A mediator between support and adjustment. *West J Nurs Res* 1987;9(1):43.

Sanday PR: The socio-cultural context of rape: A cross-cultural study. *J Soc Issues* 1981;37(4):5.

Zdanuk JM, **Harris** CC, **Wisian** NL: Adolescent pregnancy and incest: The nurse's role as counselor. *J Obstet Gynecol Neonat Nurs* 1987;16(March/April):99.

ADDITIONAL READINGS

Bateman AW: Rape: The forgotten victim. *Br Med J* 1986;292(May 17):1306.

Barnell MA: Similarity and empathy: The experience of rape. *J Soc Psychol* 1986:126(February):47.

If you really want to help her, the first thing you must do is believe her—even if no weapons were used, she knew the single assailant, she didn't make a police report, and/or there is no evidence of harm. It's not necessary for you to decide if she was "really raped." She says she was raped and that's enough. She feels raped, and she needs your support. (Linda E. Ledray, Recovering from Rape)

Pregnancy

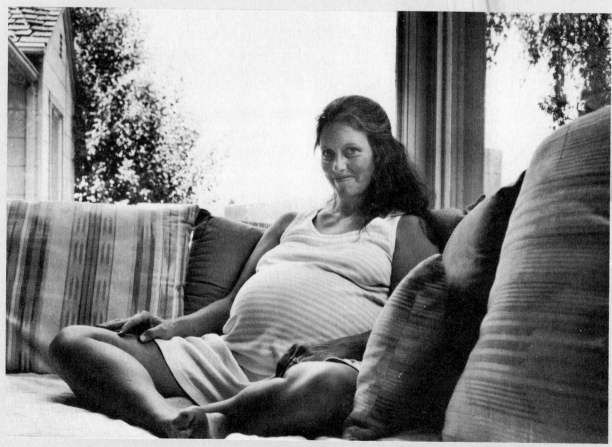

Pregnancy for a woman in the middle of a successful career demands a shift in focus from the outer to the inner world.

Part Four

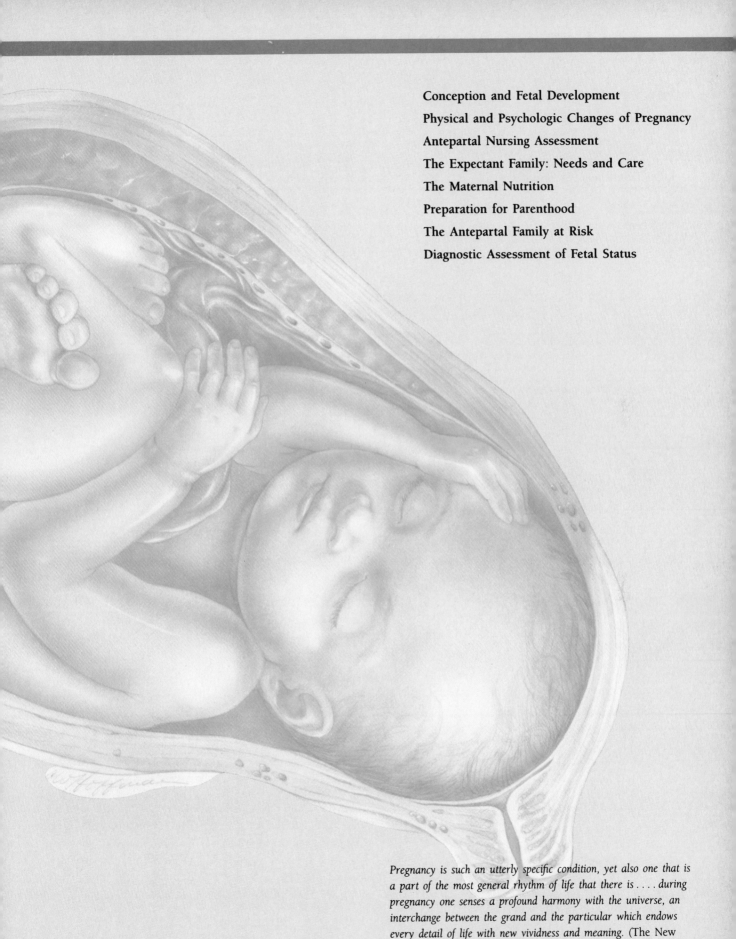

Pregnancy is such an utterly specific condition, yet also one that is a part of the most general rhythm of life that there is . . . . during pregnancy one senses a profound harmony with the universe, an interchange between the grand and the particular which endows every detail of life with new vividness and meaning. (The New Yorker, "Talk of the Town")

Conception and Fetal Development

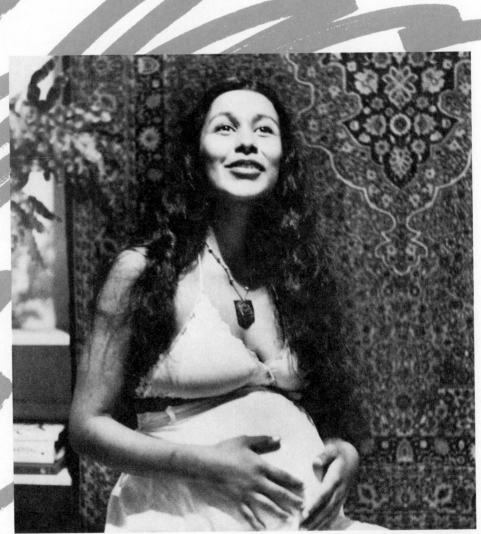

In the best of circumstances, pregnancy is a time of radiant health and optimism.

Chapter Thirteen

Embryo and Fetal Development and Organ Formation
Preembryonic Stage
Embryonic Stage
Fetal Stage
Factors Influencing Embryonic and Fetal Development
Twins

OBJECTIVES

- **Explain the difference between meiotic cellular division and mitotic cellular division.**
- **Describe the development, structure, and functions of the placenta and umbilical cord during intrauterine life.**
- **Summarize the significant changes in growth and development of the fetus in utero at 4, 6, 12, 16, 20, 24, 28, 36, and 40 weeks' gestation.**
- **Identify the vulnerable periods during which malformations of the various organ systems may occur, and describe the resulting congenital malformations.**

Every person is unique. What is interesting about this uniqueness is that all of us have most if not all the same "parts," and these parts usually function similarly. Even our chromosomes, those determiners of the structure and function of our organ systems and traits, are made of the same biochemical substances. How do we become unique, then? The answer lies in the physiologic mechanisms of heredity, the processes of cellular division, and the environmental factors that influence our development from the moment we are conceived. This chapter explores the processes involved in conception and fetal development—the basis of our uniqueness.

● Chromosomes

The body (somatic) cells of each individual contain within their nuclei threadlike bodies known as chromosomes, which are composed of strands of deoxyribonucleic acid (DNA) and protein. Genes are regions in the DNA strands that contain coded information used to determine the unique characteristics of the individual; they are arranged in linear order on the chromosomes.

As the storage place for genetic information, DNA does not leave the cell nucleus. The DNA strand splits and forms the basis for a ribonucleic acid (RNA) molecule. The RNA passes out of the nucleus and carries coded information to the cytoplasm of the cell. A single error in the "reading" of the code can cause a change that may have serious effects on the functioning of the organism.

Each chromosome contains two longitudinal halves called chromatids, which are joined together at a point called the centromere. Each animal species tends to have a constant number of chromosomes. Human beings have 46 chromosomes divided into 23 pairs: 22 pairs of autosomes and one pair of sex chromosomes. Each member of a pair carries either similar genes referred to as homologous, or dissimilar, allelic, genes referred to as heterozygous (Figure 13–1A).

The chromosomes are classified according to their length and to the position of their centromere. When the centromere is centrally located, the longitudinal halves are divided into arms of approximately equal length, and the chromosome resembles an X (Figure 13–1B).

● Cellular Division

All humans begin life as a single cell (zygote). This single cell reproduces itself, and in turn each new cell also reproduces itself in a continuing process. The new cells must be similar to the cells from which they came.

Cells are reproduced either by mitosis or meiosis, two different but related processes. *Mitosis* results in the production of additional somatic cells. Mitosis makes growth and development possible, and in mature individuals it is the process by which our body cells continue to divide and replace themselves. *Meiosis,* by contrast, leads to the development of a new organism.

Mitosis

During mitosis the cell undergoes several changes, ending in cell division. Although mitosis is a continuous process, it is generally divided into five stages: interphase, prophase, metaphase, anaphase, and telophase (Figure 13–2).

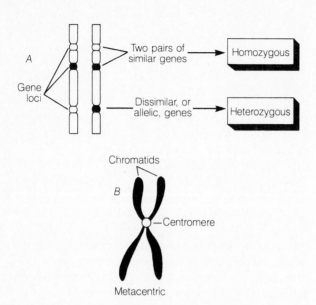

Figure 13–1   A *Pair of chromosomes with similar (homozygous) and dissimilar (heterozygous) genes. B Classification of chromosomal joining* (From Whaley LE: *Understanding Inherited Disorders.* St Louis, Mosby, 1974, p 6)

During interphase, before cell division takes place, the DNA within the chromosomes replicates so that the genes will be doubled. Mitosis begins when the cell enters prophase. The strands of chromatin shorten and thicken, and the chromosomes reproduce themselves by doubling the strands of chromatin. Next comes the appearance of a mitotic apparatus known as a spindle, in which fine threads extend from the top and bottom poles of the nucleus. At each pole of the spindle, a body known as the centriole is formed, so that the threads of the spindle extend from one centriole to the other. Next the nuclear membrane, which separates the nucleus from the cytoplasm, disappears; the nucleus as a separate entity disappears, and the cell enters metaphase.

During metaphase, the chromosomes line up at the equator (midway between the poles) of the spindle. Metaphase is followed by anaphase, in which the two chromatids of each chromosome separate and move to opposite ends of the spindle, where they cluster in masses near the two poles of the cell.

Telophase is essentially the reverse of prophase. A new nuclear membrane forms, separating each newly formed nucleus from the cytoplasm. The spindle disappears and the centrioles relocate outside of each new nucleus. Within the nucleus the nucleolus again becomes visible, and the chromosomes lengthen and become thread-like. As telophase nears completion, a furrow develops in the cytoplasm at the midline of the cell and divides it into two daughter cells, each with its own nucleus. Daughter

cells have the same diploid number of chromosomes and the same genetic makeup as the cell from which they came.

In other words, after a cell with 46 chromosomes goes through mitosis, the result is two identical cells, each of them having 46 chromosomes.

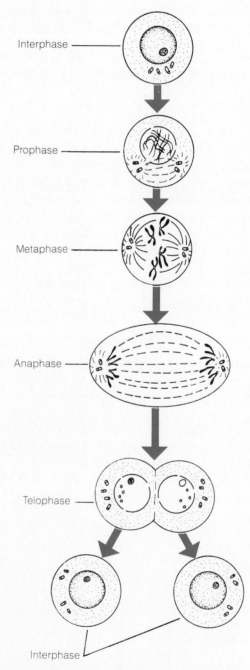

Figure 13–2   Somatic cell undergoing mitosis. Only four chromosomes are illustrated. (From Whaley LE: *Understanding Inherited Disorders.* St Louis, Mosby, 1974, p 11)

Meiosis

Meiosis consists of two successive cell divisions, each of which includes the stages of interphase, prophase, metaphase, anaphase, and telophase (Figure 13–3).

In the first division the chromosomes replicate. Instead of separating immediately as in mitosis, the similar chromosomes become closely intertwined. An exchange of parts between chromatids (the arms of the chromosomes) often takes place. At each point of contact, there is also a physical exchange of genetic material between the chromatids. New combinations are provided by the newly formed chromosomes; these combinations account for the wide variation of traits in people. The chromosome pairs then separate, each member of a pair moving to opposite sides of the cell. (In contrast, during mitosis the chromatids of each chromosome move together toward the poles.) The cell divides, forming two daughter cells, each with half (23) of the usual number of chromosomes. In the second division, the chromatids of each chromosome separate and move to opposite poles of each of the daughter cells. Cell division occurs, resulting in the formation of four cells, each containing 23 chromosomes (*the haploid number of chromosomes*).

Occasionally during the second meiotic division, two of the chromatids may not move apart rapidly enough when the cell divides. The still-paired chromatids are carried into one of the daughter cells and eventually form an extra chromosome. This condition is referred to as an autosomal nondisjunction (chromosomal mutation) and is harmful to the offspring that may result should fertilization occur. The implications of nondisjunction are discussed in Chapter 9.

Another type of chromosomal mutation can occur if chromosomes break during meiosis. If the broken segment is lost, the result is a shorter chromosome; this situation is known as deletion. If the broken segment becomes attached to another chromosome, it is called translocation, which often results in harmful structural mutations (Thompson & Thompson 1986). The effects of translocation are described in Chapter 9.

● Gametogenesis

Meiosis occurs during *gametogenesis,* the process by which germ cells, or gametes, are produced. The gametes must have a haploid number (23) of chromosomes so that when the female gamete (ovum) and the male gamete (spermatozoon) unite to form the zygote, the normal human diploid number of chromosomes (46) is reestablished.

Ovum

As discussed in Chapter 6 the ovaries begin to develop early in the fetal life of the female. All the ova that the female will produce are formed by the sixth month of fetal life. The ovary gives rise to oogonial cells, which develop into oocytes. Meiosis begins in all oocytes before the female infant is born but stops before the first meiotic di-

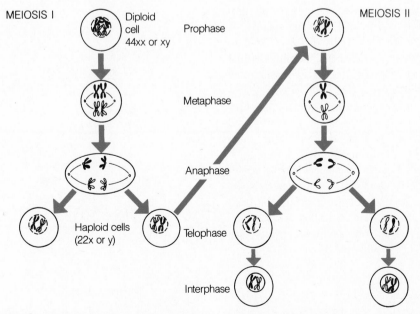

Figure 13–3 Meiosis in a germ cell. This illustration indicates the behavior of two pairs of homologous chromosomes. (From Whaley LE: Understanding Inherited Disorders. St Louis, Mosby, 1974, p 13)

vision is complete and remains in this arrested phase until puberty. During puberty the mature primary oocyte continues (by oogenesis) through the first meiotic division in the graafian follicle of the ovary.

At the time of ovulation, the first meiotic stage is completed (Thompson & Thompson 1986). As shown in Figure 13–4 the first meiotic division produces two cells of unequal sizes with unequal amounts of cytoplasm but the same number of chromosomes. These two cells are the secondary oocyte and a minute polar body (half of the chromosomes are actually extruded outside the secondary oocyte's cell membrane). Both the secondary oocyte and the first polar body contain 22 autosomal chromosomes and one sex chromosome (X). At the time of ovulation second meiotic division begins immediately and proceeds as the oocyte moves down the fallopian tube. Division is again not equal and the secondary oocyte proceeds to metaphase where its meiotic division is arrested.

Only when fertilized by the sperm does the secondary oocyte complete the second meiotic division, becoming a mature ovum with the haploid number of chromosomes and having virtually all the cytoplasm. The second polar body is also formed at this time (Figure 13–4). The first polar body has now also divided, producing two additional polar bodies. Thus, when meiosis is completed, four haploid cells have been produced: three small polar bodies, which eventually disintegrate, and one ovum (Figure 13–5).

Sperm

During puberty the germinal epithelium in the seminiferous tubules of the testes begins the process of spermatogenesis, which produces the male gamete (sperm). As the diploid spermatogonium enters the first meiotic division, it is called the primary spermatocyte. During this first meiotic division, the spermatogonium forms two haploid cells termed secondary spermatocytes, each of which contains 22 autosomal chromosomes and either an X sex chromosome or a Y sex chromosome. During the second meiotic division they divide to form four spermatids, each with the haploid number of chromosomes (Figure 13–5). The spermatids undergo a series of changes during which they lose most of their cytoplasm and become sperm (spermatozoa). The nucleus becomes compacted into the head of the sperm, which is covered by a cap called an acrosome. A long tail is produced from one of the centrioles (see Figure 6–26).

● Sex Determination

The two chromosomes of the twenty-third pair (either XX or XY) are called *sex chromosomes*. The larger of the sex chromosomes is designated X, and the smaller sex

chromosome is called Y. Females have two X chromosomes, and males have an X and a Y chromosome. Because male cells contain both an X and a Y chromosome, meiosis in the male produces two gametes with an X chromosome and two gametes with a Y chromosome from each primary spermatocyte. The sex chromosomes in oocytes are both X, and thus the mature ovum can have only one type of sex chromosome. To produce a female child each parent must contribute an X chromosome. To produce a male, the mother must contribute an X chromosome and the father a Y chromosome.

The Y chromosomes contain mainly genes for maleness. The X chromosomes carry several genes other than those for sexual traits. As discussed in Chapter 9, these other traits are termed *sex linked* because they are controlled by the genes of the X chromosome. Two examples of sex-linked traits are color blindness and hemophilia.

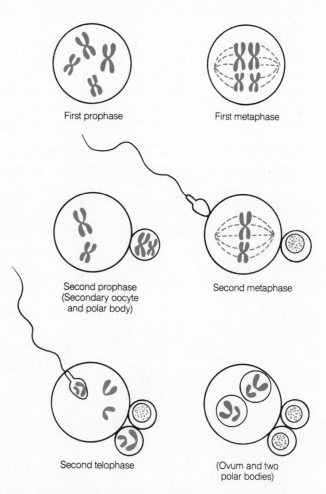

First prophase   First metaphase

Second prophase
(Secondary oocyte
and polar body)   Second metaphase

Second telophase   (Ovum and two
polar bodies)

Figure 13–4 Human oogenesis and fertilization (From Thompson JS, Thompson MW: *Genetics in Medicine,* ed 4. Philadelphia, Saunders, 1986, p 23)

It seems that I knew the moment you began. We had been planning and wanting the pregnancy for months. We carefully kept track of my menstrual periods and calculated the time of ovulation, and yet pregnancy kept eluding us. Then suddenly one night, I knew that you were there. This had been the moment, and even as I lay quietly I somehow could sense your presence. That feeling never changed, it just grew stronger as you grew inside me.

I haven't told many people about this. People look at me like I'm crazy. But I think if we would ask mothers, we would be surprised to find out just how many know exactly the moment that conception occurs.

● Fertilization

The process of *fertilization* takes place in the ampulla (or outer third) of the fallopian tube. High estrogen levels during ovulation increase the ability of the fallopian tubes to contract, which helps move the ovum down the tube. The high estrogen levels also cause a thinning of the cervical mucus, facilitating penetration by the sperm.

The ovum's cell membrane is surrounded by two layers of tissue. The layer closest to the cell membrane is called the *zona pellucida*. It is a clear, noncellular layer whose function is not known. Surrounding the zona pel-

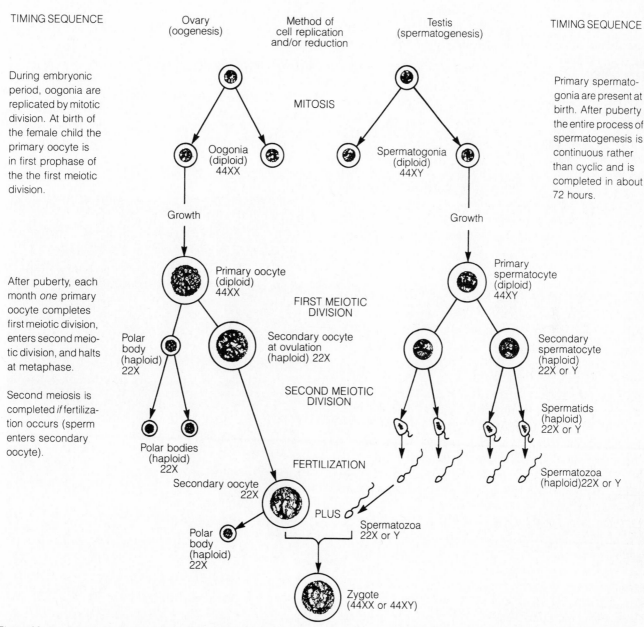

Figure 13–5 Gametogenesis involves meiosis within the ovary and testis. Note that during meiosis, each oogonium produces a single haploid ovum, whereas each spermatogonium produces four haploid spermatozoa. (Modified from Spence AP, Mason EB: Human Anatomy and Physiology, ed 3. Menlo Park, Calif, Benjamin/ Cummings, 1987, pp 822, 832)

lucida is a ring of elongated cells, called the *corona radiata* because they radiate from the ovum like the gaseous corona around the sun. These cells are held together by hyaluronic acid.

The mature ovum and spermatozoa have only a brief time to unite. Ova are considered fertile for about a 24-hour period after ovulation. Sperm can survive in the female reproductive tract for up to 72 hours but are believed to be healthy and highly fertile for only about 24 hours (Silverstein 1980).

In a single ejaculation the male deposits approximately 200 to 400 million spermatozoa in the vagina, of which fewer than 200 actually reach the ampulla (Eddy & Pauerstein 1980). The spermatozoa move up the female tract by the flagellar movement of their tails. Transit time from the cervix into the fallopian tube can be as short as five minutes but usually takes an average of four to six hours after ejaculation (Pritchard et al 1985). Prostaglandins in the semen may increase uterine smooth muscle contractions, which help transport the sperm (Spence 1982). The fallopian tubes have a dual ciliary action that facilitates movement of the ovum toward the uterus and movement of the sperm from the uterus toward the ovary. The ovum has no inherent power of movement.

The sperm must undergo two processes before fertilization can happen: capacitation and the acrosomal reaction. *Capacitation* is the removal of the plasma membrane overlying the spermatozoa's acrosomal area and loss of seminal plasma proteins and glycoprotein coat. Capacitation must occur in the female reproductive tract and is thought to last up to seven hours.

The acrosomal reaction follows capacitation. The acrosomal covering of the head of the sperm contains the enzyme hyaluronidase. As millions of sperm surround the ovum, they deposit minute amounts of hyaluronidase in the corona radiata, the outer layer of the ovum. This activity is the *acrosomal reaction*. The hyaluronidase breaks down enough hyaluronic acid in the corona radiata layer of the ovum for one spermatozoon to penetrate the zona pellucida of the ovum (Figure 13–6). At the moment the sperm penetrates the zona pellucida and makes contact with the vitelline membrane, a cellular change occurs in the ovum that renders it impenetrable by other spermatozoa; thus only one spermatozoon enters a single ovum. The cellular change that blocks other sperm from entering the ovum is mediated by release of materials from the cortical granules, organelles found just below the egg surface (Glass 1984).

At the moment of penetration the second meiotic division is completed in the nucleus of the oocyte, and the second polar body is produced. At the union of the gametes, each containing a haploid number of chromosomes (23), the diploid number (46) is restored. Also at this time, the sex of the new individual is established. Within the cell the nuclei of the spermatozoon and oocyte unite, and

their individual nuclear membranes disappear. Their chromosomes pair up, and a new cell, the *zygote*, is created. The zygote contains a new combination of genetic material, which creates an individual different from either parent and from anyone else.

● Intrauterine Development

Intrauterine development after fertilization can be divided into three phases: cellular multiplication, cellular (embryonic membrane) differentiation, and development of organ systems. These phases and the process of implantation will be discussed next.

Cellular Multiplication

Cellular multiplication begins as the zygote moves through the fallopian tube into the cavity of the uterus. This transport takes three days or more and is effected mainly by a very weak fluid current in the fallopian tube

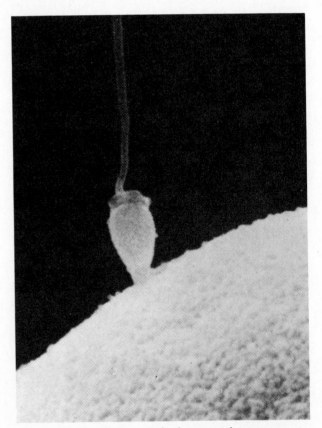

Figure 13–6 Electron micrograph of a sperm about to penetrate the surface of an ovum (From Bloom W, Fawcett DW: A Textbook of Histology, ed 10. Philadelphia, Saunders, 1975, p 807)

resulting from the beating action of the ciliated epithelium that lines the tube.

The zygote now enters a period of rapid mitotic divisions called *cleavage,* in which it divides into two cells, four cells, eight cells, and so on. These cells, called *blastomeres,* are so small that the developing cell mass is only slightly larger than the original zygote. The blastomeres are held together by the zona pellucida, a layer of cells under the corona radiata. The blastomeres will eventually form a solid ball of cells called the *morula.* Upon reaching the uterus, the morula floats freely for a few days, and then a cavity forms within the cell mass. The inner solid mass of cells is called the *blastocyst.* The outer layer of cells that surround the cavity and have replaced the zona pellucida is the *trophoblast.* Eventually, the trophoblast develops into one of the embryonic membranes, the chorion. The blastocyst develops into the embryo and the other embryonic membrane (the amnion). The journey of the fertilized ovum to its destination in the uterus is illustrated in Figure 13–7.

Implantation

While floating in the uterine cavity, the blastocyst is nourished by the uterine glands, which secrete a mixture of lipids, mucopolysaccharides, and glycogen. The trophoblast attaches itself to the surface of the endometrium for further nourishment. The most frequent site of attachment is the upper part of the posterior uterine wall (Figure 13–7). Between days 7 and 9 after fertilization the blastocyst implants itself by burrowing into the uterine lining and penetrating down toward the maternal capillaries until it is

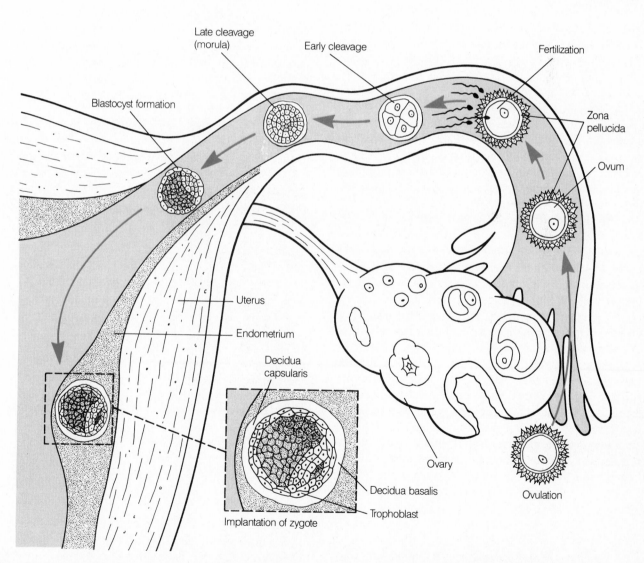

Figure 13–7   During ovulation the ovum leaves the ovary and enters the fallopian tube. Fertilization generally occurs in the outer third of the fallopian tube. Subsequent changes in the fertilized ovum from conception to implantation are depicted.

completely covered. In order for implantation to occur, the zona pellucida must disappear (Glass 1984). The lining of the uterus thickens below the implanted blastocyst, and the cells of the trophoblast grow down into the thickened lining, forming processes called *villi*.

Under the influence of progesterone, the endometrium increases in thickness and vascularity in preparation for implantation and nutrition of the ovum. After implantation the endometrium is called the *decidua*. The portion of the decidua that covers the blastocyst is called the decidua capsularis; the portion directly under the implanted blastocyst is the decidua basalis; and the portion that lines the rest of the uterine cavity is the decidua vera (parietalis). The decidua basalis forms the area where the chorionic villi (the chorion frondosum) will form the fetal component of the placenta. The maternal part of the placenta develops from the decidua basalis, which contains large numbers of blood vessels.

Cellular Differentiation

EMBRYONIC MEMBRANES

The embryonic membranes begin to form at the time of implantation (Figure 13–8). These membranes protect and support the embryo as it grows and develops inside the uterus. The first membrane to form is the *chorion,* the outermost embryonic membrane that encloses the amnion, embryo, and yolk sac. The chorion is a thick membrane that develops from the trophoblast and has many fingerlike projections, called chorionic villi, on its surface. The villi begin to degenerate, except for those just under the embryo, which grow and branch into depressions in the uterine wall, forming the embryonic portion of the placenta. By the fourth month of pregnancy, the surface of the chorion is smooth except at the place of attachment to the uterine wall.

The second membrane, the *amnion*, originates from the ectoderm, a primary germ layer, during the early stages of embryonic development. The amnion is a thin protective membrane that contains amniotic fluid. The space between the amniotic membrane and the embryo is the *amniotic cavity*. This cavity surrounds the embryo and yolk sac, except where the developing embryo (germ layer disk) attaches to the trophoblast via the umbilical cord. As the embryo grows, the amnion expands until it comes in contact with the chorion. These two slightly adherent membranes form the fluid-filled sac that protects the floating embryo.

AMNIOTIC FLUID

Amniotic fluid functions as a cushion to protect against mechanical injury. It also helps control the embryo's temperature, permits symmetrical external growth of the embryo, prevents adherence to the amnion, and allows freedom of movement so that the embryo-fetus can change position freely, thus aiding in musculoskeletal development.

The amount of amniotic fluid is about 30 mL at 10 weeks and increases to 350 mL at 20 weeks. After 20 weeks, the volume ranges from 500 to 1000 mL (Moore 1982). The amniotic fluid volume is constantly changing as the fluid moves back and forth across the placental membrane. As the pregnancy continues, the fetus contributes to the volume of amniotic fluid by excreting urine. The fetus also swallows up to 400 mL of the fluid every 24 hours. Between 600 and 800 mL of amniotic fluid flows in and out of the fetal lung each day (Creasy & Resnik 1984). Amniotic fluid is slightly alkaline and contains albumin, urea, uric acid, creatinine, lecithin, sphingomyelin, bilirubin, fat, fructose, leukocytes, proteins, epithelial cells, enzymes, and lanugo hair.

Moore (1982) postulates that some amniotic fluid is formed by the amniotic membrane cells. Other sources suggest that amniotic fluid may be a transudate of maternal plasma. More probably, it is a transudate of fetal plasma, since a close relationship exists between fetal size and amount of amniotic fluid up to 20 weeks' gestation.

Water and solutes must pass between the amniotic fluid and fetus; Figure 13–9 summarizes the major pathways of exchange. During the first half of pregnancy water is transported across the highly permeable skin of the fetus, since the amniotic fluid composition resembles fetal extracellular fluid. After 24 weeks cornification of the fetal skin inhibits the diffusion. The major pathway for intrauterine water accumulation in pregnancy appears to be across the chorionic villi between the maternal and fetal compartments (Creasy & Resnik 1984).

YOLK SAC

In humans the yolk sac is small and functions only in early embryonic life. It develops as a second cavity in the blastocyst about day 8 or 9 after conception, and it forms primitive red blood cells during the first six weeks of development until the embryo's liver takes over the process. As the embryo develops, the yolk sac is incorporated in the umbilical cord, where it can be identified as a degenerate structure.

PRIMARY GERM LAYERS

About day 10 to 14 after conception the homogenous mass of blastocyst cells differentiate into the primary germ layers. These layers, the ectoderm, mesoderm, and endoderm (Figure 13–10), are formed at the same time as the embryonic membranes. All tissues, organs, and organ systems will develop from these primary germ cell layers (Table 13–1).

How and why differentiation occurs are not clearly understood. Differentiation is believed to be a gene-directed phenomenon that originates in the DNA of the zygote and is carried out in the cytoplasm by an elaborate set of chemical reactions caused by the RNA-controlled synthesis of specific enzymes.

Intrauterine Organ Systems

PLACENTA

The placenta is the means of metabolic and nutrient exchange between the embryonic and maternal circulations. Placental development and circulation does not begin until the third week of development. The placenta develops at the site where the developing embryo attaches to the

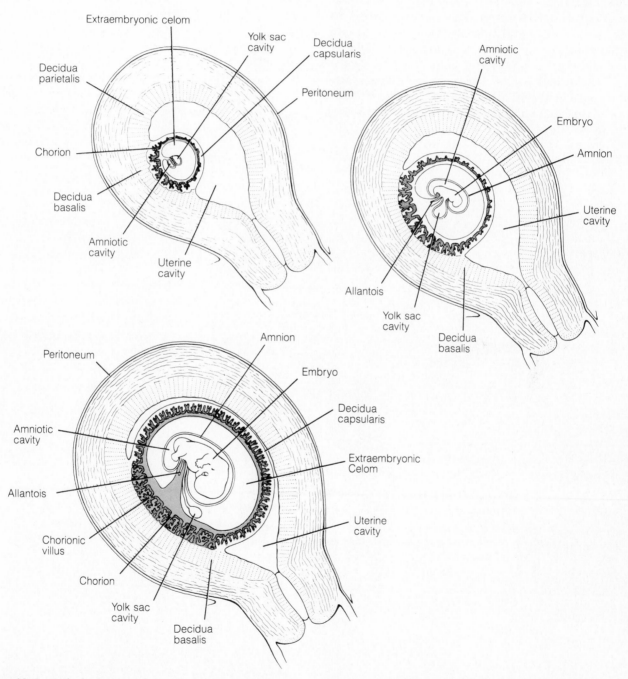

Figure 13–8 Early development of the embryonic membranes. The early development of selected structures is depicted starting at the top left and moving clockwise. The time sequence is from day 10 to day 14 after conception to approximately eight weeks. (From Spence AP, Mason EB: Human Anatomy and Physiology, ed 3. Menlo Park, Calif, Benjamin/Cummings, 1987, p 851)

uterine wall. Expansion of the placenta continues until about 20 weeks, when it covers about one-half the internal surface of the uterus. After 20 weeks' gestation, the placenta becomes thicker but not wider. At 40 weeks' gestation, the placenta is about 15 to 20 cm (5.9 to 7.9 in) in diameter and 2.5 to 3.0 cm (1.0 to 1.2 in) in thickness. At that time, it weighs about 400 to 600 g (14 to 21 oz).

The placenta has two parts: the maternal portion and the fetal portion. The maternal portion consists of the decidua basalis and its circulation. Its surface is red and flesh-like. The fetal portion consists of the chorionic villi and their circulation. The fetal surface of the placenta is covered by the amnion, which gives it a shiny, gray appearance. (See Color Plates III and IV.)

Development of the placenta begins with the chorionic villi. The trophoblast cells of the chorionic villi form spaces in the tissue of the decidua basalis. These spaces fill with maternal blood, and the chorionic villi grow into these spaces. As the chorionic villi differentiate, two trophoblastic layers appear: an outer layer called the syncy-

tium (consisting of syncytiotrophoblasts) and an inner layer known as the cytotrophoblast (Figure 13–11). The cytotrophoblast thins out and disappears about the fifth month, leaving only a single layer of syncytium covering the chorionic villi. The syncytium is in direct contact with the maternal blood in the intervillous spaces. It is the functional layer of the placenta and secretes the placental hormones of pregnancy.

A third, inner layer of connective mesoderm develops in the chorionic villi, forming anchoring villi. These anchoring villi eventually form the septa (partitions) of the placenta. These septa divide the mature placenta into 15 to 20 segments called *cotyledons*. In each cotyledon, the branching villi form a highly complex vascular system that allows compartmentalization of the uteroplacental circulation. The exchange of gases and nutrients takes place across these vascular systems.

Exchange of substances across the placenta is minimal during the early months of development because of limited permeability. The villous membrane is too thick.

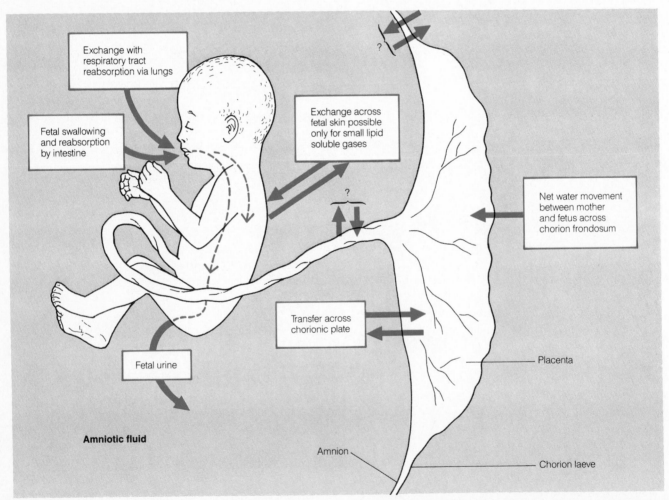

Figure 13–9   Summary of the significant pathways of water and solute exchange between the amniotic fluid and fetus (From Seeds AE: Current concepts of amniotic fluid dynamics. Am J Obstet Gynecol 1980;138(November):575)

Placental permeability increases (as the villous membrane thins) until about the last month of pregnancy, when it begins to decrease as the placenta ages.

As the placenta is developing, the *umbilical cord* is also being formed from the amnion. The body stalk, which attaches the embryo to the yolk sac, contains blood vessels that extend into the chorionic villi. The body stalk fuses with the embryonic portion of the placenta to provide a circulatory pathway from the chorionic villi to the embryo. As the body stalk elongates to become the umbilical cord or funis, the vessels in the cord decrease to one large vein and two smaller arteries. About 1 percent of umbilical cords have only two vessels, an artery and a vein; this condition is associated with congenital malformations. A

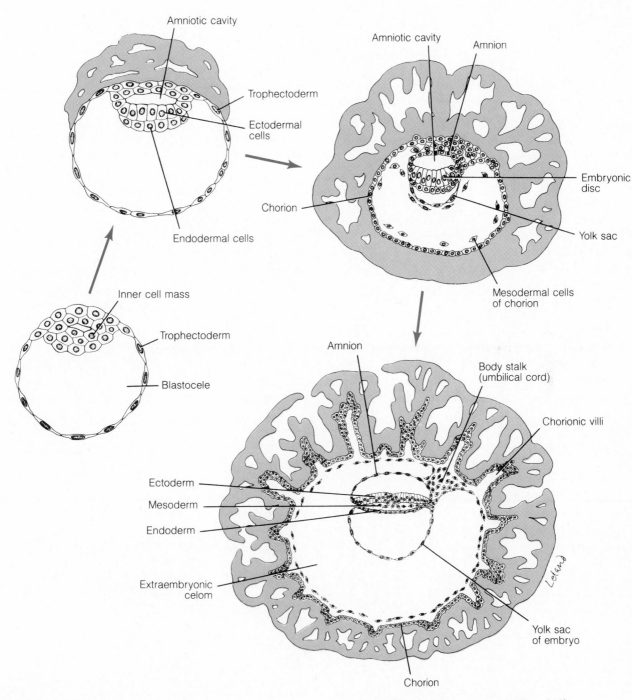

Figure 13–10 Formation of primary germ layers (From Spence AP, Mason EB: *Human Anatomy and Physiology,* ed 3. Menlo Park, Calif, Benjamin/Cummings, 1987, p 849)

Table 13–1 Derivation of Body Structures from Primary Cell Layers

Ectoderm	Mesoderm	Endoderm
Epidermis	Dermis	Respiratory tract epithelium
Sweat glands	Wall of digestive tract	Epithelium (except nasal), including
Sebaceous glands	Kidneys and ureter (suprarenal cortex)	pharynx, tongue, tonsils, thyroid,
Nails	Reproductive organs (gonads, genital	parathyroid, thymus, tympanic cavity
Hair follicles	ducts)	Lining of digestive tract
Lens of eye	Connective tissue (cartilage, bone, joint	Primary tissue of liver and pancreas
Sensory epithelium of internal and	cavities)	Urethra and associated glands
external ear, nasal cavity, sinuses,	Skeleton	Urinary bladder (except trigone)
mouth, anal canal	Muscles (all types)	Vagina (parts)
Central and peripheral nervous systems	Cardiovascular system (heart, arteries,	
Nasal cavity	veins, blood, bone marrow)	
Oral glands and tooth enamel	Pleura	
Pituitary glands	Lymphatic tissue and cells	
Mammary glands	Spleen	

specialized connective tissue known as *Wharton's jelly* surrounds the blood vessels. This tissue, plus the high blood volume pulsating through the vessels, prevents compression of the umbilical cord in utero. At term the average cord is 2 cm (0.8 in) across and about 55 cm (22 in) long.

The cord can attach itself to the placenta in various sites. Central insertion into the placenta is considered normal. A peripheral insertion is called *battledore* insertion. In rare circumstances the cord inserts away from the placenta so that vessels run along the membranes from the site of cord insertion to the surface of the placenta. This configuration is called a *velamentous* placenta. See Chapter 19 for a discussion of the various attachment sites.

Umbilical cords appear twisted or spiraled. This is most likely caused by fetal movement (Benirschke 1981). A true knot in the umbilical cord rarely occurs and, if it does, the cord is usually long. More common are so-called false knots. False knots are caused by the folding of cord

vessels. A *nuchal cord* is said to exist when the umbilical cord is around the back of the neck.

○   *CIRCULATION*   After implantation of the blastocyst, the cells distinguish themselves into fetal cells and trophoblastic cells. The proliferating trophoblast successfully invades the decidua basalis of the endometrium, first opening the uterine capillaries and later opening the larger uterine vessels. The chorionic villi are an outgrowth of the blastocystic tissue. As these villi continue to grow and divide, the fetal vessels begin to form. The intervillous spaces in the decidua basalis develop as the endometrial spiral arteries are opened.

By the fourth week the placenta has begun to function as a means of metabolic exchange between embryo and mother. The completion of the maternal–placental–fetal circulation occurs about 17 days after conception when the embryonic heart begins functioning (Ahokas

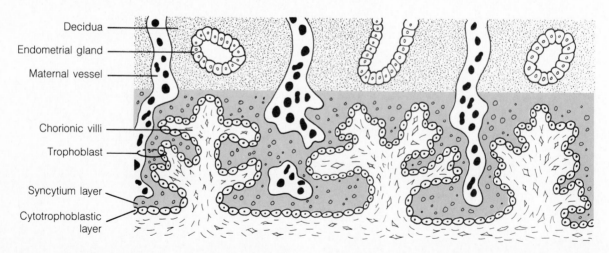

Figure 13–11   Longitudinal section of placental villus. Spaces formed in the maternal decidua are filled with maternal blood;   *chorionic villi proliferate into these maternal-blood-filled spaces and differentiate into a syncytium layer and a cytotrophoblast layer.*

1985). By 14 weeks, it is a discrete organ. The placenta has grown in thickness as a result of growth in the length and size of the chorionic villi and accompanying expansion of the intervillous space.

The cotyledons of the maternal surface contain branches of a single placental mainstem villus, allowing for some compartmentalization of the uteroplacental circulation. Each cotyledon is a natural vascular unit containing branching vessels distributed throughout that particular lobule and partially separated from other lobules by the cotyledon's thin septal partitions.

In the fully developed placenta, fetal blood in the villi and maternal blood in the intervillous spaces are separated by three to four thin layers of tissue. The capillaries of the villi are lined with an extremely thin endothelium and are surrounded by a layer of mesenchymal (connective) tissue that is covered by chorionic epithelium consisting of cytotrophoblast and syncytiotrophoblast (see Figure 13–11). As previously discussed, the cytotrophoblast thins out and disappears after the fifth month.

Fetal blood flows through the two umbilical arteries to the capillaries of the villi and back through the umbilical vein into the fetus (Figure 13–12). During late pregnancy a soft blowing sound (funic souffle) can be heard over the location of the umbilical cord of the fetus. The rate of the sound is synchronous with the fetal heartbeat and the flow of fetal blood through the umbilical arteries.

Maternal blood, rich in oxygen and nutrients, spurts from the spiral uterine arteries into the intervillous spaces. These spurts are produced by the maternal blood pressure. The spurt of blood is directed toward the chorionic plate, and as the blood flow loses pressure, it becomes lateral (spreads out). Fresh blood continually enters and exerts pressure on the contents of the intervillous spaces, pushing blood toward the exits in the basal plate. Blood is then drained through the uterine and other pelvic veins. A uterine souffle is also heard during the last months of pregnancy. It is identified as a loud blowing murmur or swishing sound heard just above the symphysis pubis and timed precisely with the mother's pulse. This sound is caused by the augmented blood flow entering the dilated uterine arteries.

Circulation within the intervillous spaces depends on maternal blood pressure producing a gradient between ar-

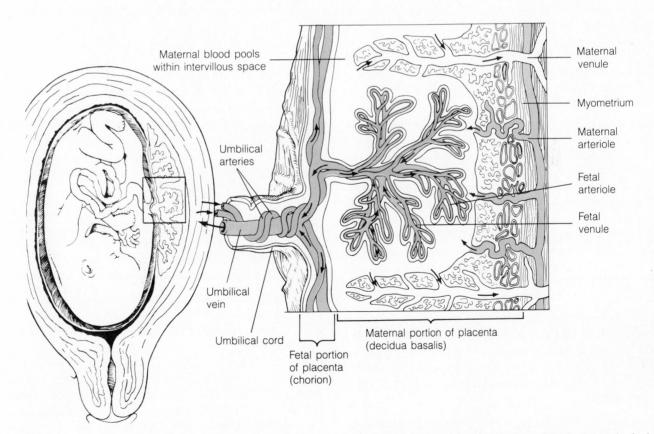

Figure 13–12 Vascular arrangement of the placenta. Arrows indicate the direction of blood flow. Maternal blood flows through the uterine arteries to the intervillous spaces of the placenta and returns through the uterine veins to maternal circulation. Fetal blood flows through the umbilical arteries into the villous capillaries of the placenta and returns through the umbilical veins to the fetal circulation. (From Spence AP, Mason EB: Human Anatomy and Physiology, ed 3. Menlo Park, Calif, Benjamin/Cummings, 1987, p 850)

terial and venous channels. The lumen of the spiral uterine artery is narrow when it pierces the chorionic plate and enters the intervillous space, resulting in an increased blood pressure. The pressure in the arteries forces the blood into the intervillous spaces and bathes the numerous small villi in oxygenated blood. As the pressure decreases, the blood flows back from the chorionic plate toward the decidua where it enters the endometrial veins. Naeye (1981) found that in women whose blood pressure did not exceed 110/65 during pregnancy, the uteroplacental blood flow was low and the resulting term newborns were underweight. Ahokas (1985) postulated that prostaglandins are implicated in the regulation of uterine and placental blood flow because of their vasoconstrictive and vasodilative effects.

Braxton Hicks contractions (Chapter 14) are believed to facilitate placental circulation by enhancing the movement of blood from the center of the cotyledon through the intervillous space.

○ *FUNCTIONS* Placental exchange functions occur only in those fetal vessels in intimate contact with the covering syncytial membrane. The syncytium villi have brush borders containing many microvilli, which greatly increase the exchange rate between maternal and fetal circulation (Sadler 1985).

The placental functions, many of which begin soon after implantation, include fetal respiration, nutrition, and excretion. To carry out these functions, the placenta is involved in metabolic and transfer activities. It also has endocrine functions and special immunologic properties.

Metabolic Activities The placenta has a metabolic rate comparable to that of an adult liver or kidney. Glycogen, cholesterol, and fatty acids are continuously synthesized by the placenta for fetal use and hormone production. The placenta also produces the numerous enzymes necessary for fetoplacental transfer, and it breaks down such substances as epinephrine and histamine by enzymatic deamination. It also functions as a storage unit for glycogen and iron.

Transport Mechanisms The placenta is no longer considered to be an inert barrier with pores that prevent the transfer of large molecules and permit the transfer of small molecules. It is a functional membrane that controls the transfer of a wide range of substances by five major mechanisms:

1. *Simple diffusion.* This type of transport requires no energy output. Molecules move from an area of higher concentration to an area of lower concentration until equilibrium is established. Substances that transfer across the placental membrane by simple diffusion have a molecular weight of less than 500 and include water, electrolytes such as sodium and chloride, carbon dioxide, anesthetic gases, and drugs. Insulin and steroid hormones originating from the adrenals and thyroid hormones also cross the placenta but at a very slow rate. The rate of oxygen transfer across the placental membrane is greater than that allowed by simple diffusion, indicating that oxygen is also transferred by facilitated diffusion of some type.

2. *Facilitated transport.* This type of transport involves a carrier system to move molecules from an area of greater concentration to an area of lower concentration, thereby speeding up the transfer of certain substances through the placental membrane. Among the molecules carried by facilitated placental transport are glucose, galactose, and some oxygen. The glucose level in the fetal blood ordinarily is approximately 20 percent to 30 percent lower than the glucose level in the maternal blood because glucose is being metabolized rapidly by the fetus (Vorherr 1982). This in turn causes rapid transport of additional glucose from the maternal blood into the fetal blood.

3. *Active transport.* This type of transport requires energy, involves an enzymatic pathway, and can work against a concentration gradient, with molecules moving from an area of lower concentration to an area of higher concentration. Amino acids, calcium, iron, iodine, water-soluble vitamins, and glucose transfer across the placental membrane by active transport. The measured amino acid content of fetal blood is greater than that of maternal blood, and calcium and inorganic phosphate occur in greater concentration in fetal blood than in maternal blood (Aladjem & Lueck 1982).

4. *Pinocytosis.* In this type of transport, materials are engulfed by amebalike cells forming plasma droplets. This mechanism is important for transferring large molecules, such as albumin and gamma globulins, across the placental membrane.

5. *Bulk flow.* Water and some solutes are transported across the placental membrane by hydrostatic and osmotic pressures. Most fetal water comes from the mother.

Other modes of transfer exist. For example, fetal red blood cells pass into the maternal circulation through breaks in the placental membrane, particularly during labor and delivery. Certain cells, such as maternal leukocytes, and microorganisms, such as viruses and *Treponema pallidum* (which causes syphilis), can also cross the placental membrane, but the exact mechanism is not known. Some bacteria and protozoa infect the placenta by causing lesions and then entering the fetal blood system.

Several factors affect transfer rate: (a) molecular size, (b) electrical charge, (c) lipid solubility, (d) placental area, (e) diffusion distance, (f) maternal–fetal–placental blood flow, (g) blood saturation with gases and nutrients, (h) pka of the substance, and (i) maternal–placental–fetal metabolism of the substance. Substances that have a molecular weight of 1000 daltons or more have difficulty crossing the placenta by simple diffusion. Therefore heparin, with a molecular weight above 6000, does not cross the placenta, while warfarin sodium (Coumadin), which has a molecular weight in the 300 to 400 range, crosses easily (Dilts 1981).

Electrically charged molecules pass across the placenta more slowly. An example is the muscle relaxant, succinylcholine. A lipid-soluble substance moves quickly across the placenta into the fetal circulation. Reduction of the placental surface area, as with abruptio placentae, will lessen the area that is functional for exchange. Placental diffusion distance also affects exchange; in conditions such as diabetes and placental infection, edema of the villi increases the diffusion distance, thus increasing the distance the substance has to be transferred.

The placental concentration gradient is altered by the concentration of substances in the maternal and fetal blood, by the placental blood flow from the fetus and the intervillous space blood flow from the mother, by the ratio of blood on each side of the placenta, and by the functioning of the carrier molecules in binding and dissociating. Decreased intervillous space blood flow is seen in labor and with certain maternal disease conditions such as hypertension. Mild hypoxia in the fetus increases the umbilical blood flow, but severe hypoxia results in decreased blood flow.

As the maternal blood picks up fetal waste products and carbon dioxide, it drains back into the maternal circulation through the veins in the basal plate. Fetal blood is hypoxic; it therefore attracts oxygen from the mother's blood. In addition, affinity for oxygen increases as the fetal blood gives up its carbon dioxide, which also decreases its acidity.

Endocrine Functions The placenta produces hormones that are vital to the survival of the fetus. The syncytium is believed to be the site of hormone production. Four hormones are known to be produced by the placenta: two protein hormones—human chorionic gonadotropin (hCG) and human placental lactogen (hPL)—and two steroid hormones, estrogen and progesterone.

Biochemically, hCG is similar to pituitary luteinizing hormone (LH), and its most important function is to prevent the normal involution of the corpus luteum at the end of the menstrual cycle. The hCG causes the corpus luteum to secrete increased quantities of estrogen and progesterone. Spontaneous abortion occurs if the corpus luteum ceases functioning before 11 weeks of pregnancy. After the eleventh week the placenta produces enough progesterone

and estrogen to maintain pregnancy. In the male fetus hCG also exerts an interstitial cell-stimulating effect on the testes, resulting in the production of testosterone. This small secretion of testosterone during embryonic development is the factor that causes male sex organs to grow. hCG may play a role in the trophoblasts' immunologic capabilities (ability to mask pregnancy) (Pritchard et al 1985). hCG is present in maternal blood serum eight to ten days after fertilization, just as soon as implantation has occurred, and is detectable in maternal urine a few days after the missed menses. Chorionic gonadotropin reaches its maximum level at 50 to 70 days' gestation and then begins to decrease as placental hormone production increases.

Progesterone is a hormone essential for pregnancy. It increases the secretions of the fallopian tubes and uterus to provide appropriate nutritive matter for the developing morula and blastocyst. It also appears to aid in ovum transport through the fallopian tube (Ahokas 1985). Progesterone causes decidual cells to develop in the uterine endometrium, and it must be present in high levels for implantation to occur. It also decreases the contractility of the uterus, thus preventing uterine contractions from causing spontaneous abortion.

Prior to stimulation by hCG, the production of progesterone by the corpus luteum reaches a peak about seven to ten days after ovulation. Implantation occurs at about the same time as this peak. At 16 days after ovulation, progesterone reaches a level between 25 and 50 mg per day and continues to rise slowly in subsequent weeks (Pritchard et al 1985). After ten weeks the placenta (syncytiotrophoblast) takes over the production of progesterone and secretes it in tremendous quantities, reaching levels late in pregnancy of more than 250 mg per day.

By seven weeks the placenta produces more than 50 percent of the estrogens in the maternal circulation. Estrogens serve mainly a proliferative function, causing enlargement of the uterus, breasts, and breast glandular tissue. Estrogens also have a significant role in increasing vascularity and vasodilation, particularly in the villous capillaries near the end of pregnancy. Placental estrogens increase markedly toward the end of pregnancy, to as much as 30 times the daily production in the middle of a normal monthly menstrual cycle. The primary estrogen secreted by the placenta is different from that secreted by the ovaries: The placenta secretes mainly estriol, whereas the ovaries secrete primarily estradiol. The placenta by itself cannot synthesize estriol. Essential precursors are provided by the adrenal glands of the fetus and are transported to the placenta for the final conversion to estriol. Measurement of the presence of estriol is a clinical test for both fetal well-being and placental functioning.

The hormone hPL (sometimes referred to as human chorionic somatomammotropin or hCS) is biochemically similar to human pituitary growth hormone. Secretion of this protein hormone can be detected by about four weeks (Batzer 1980). Placental lactogen stimulates key maternal metabolic adjustments, which ensure that more protein, glucose, and minerals are available for the fetus.

Immunologic Properties The placenta is a transplant of living tissue within the same species and is therefore considered a homograft. Ordinarily, homografts are destroyed by the host within a week or two. The placenta and embryo, however, seem to be exempt from their host's immunologic reactivity. In fact a totally unrelated embryo will grow after being transferred to a second uterus. One theory used to explain this phenomenon postulates that trophoblastic tissue is immunologically inert. It may contain a cell coating that masks transplantation antigens and that repels sensitized lymphocytes (Pritchard et al 1985). Data suggest that cellular immunity is suppressed during pregnancy by the placental hormones, specifically progesterone and hCG (Gudson & Sain 1981).

FETAL CIRCULATORY SYSTEM

The fetus must maintain the blood flow to the placenta to obtain oxygen and nutrients and to remove carbon dioxide and other waste products. Thus the fetal circulatory system has several unique features.

The lungs of the fetus do not carry out respiratory gas exchange in utero. Therefore a special circulatory system is required to bypass the blood supply to the lungs:

1. The placenta assumes the function of the fetal lungs by supplying oxygen and allowing the fetus to excrete carbon dioxide into the maternal bloodstream.

2. The blood from the placenta is carried through the umbilical vein, which penetrates the abdominal wall of the fetus. It divides into two branches, one of which circulates a small amount of blood through the liver and empties into the inferior vena cava through the hepatic vein. The second and larger branch, called the ductus venosus, empties directly into the vena cava. This blood then enters the right atrium, passes through the foramen ovale into the left atrium, and pours into the left ventricle, which pumps it into the aorta. Some blood returning from the head and upper extremities by way of the superior vena cava is emptied into the right atrium and passes through the tricuspid valve into the right ventricle. This blood is pumped into the pulmonary artery, and a small amount passes to the lungs, to provide nourishment only. The larger portion of blood passes through the ductus arteriosus into the descending aorta, thus bypassing the lungs. Finally the blood returns to the placenta through the two umbilical arteries, and the process is repeated (Figure 13–13).

The fetus receives oxygen via diffusion from the maternal circulation across a gradient of a mean PO_2 of 50 mm Hg in maternal blood in the placenta to a 30 mm Hg mean PO_2 in the fetus. At term the fetus receives oxygen from maternal circulation at the rate of 20 to 30 mL/min (Sadler 1985). The fetus is able to obtain sufficient oxygen due to:

- Special fetal hemoglobin, which carries as much as 20 percent to 30 percent more oxygen than adult (mature) hemoglobin.

- The hemoglobin concentration in the fetus, which is about 50 percent greater than that of the mother.

- The higher cardiac output per unit of body weight in the fetus than in adults.

For further discussion see Chapter 27. The fetal circulatory pathway provides the highest available oxygen concentration to the head, neck, brain, and heart (coronary circulation), while a lesser degree of oxygenation and blood goes to the abdominal organs and the lower body (Koffler 1981). This circulatory pattern leads to cephalocaudal (head-to-toe) development.

FETAL HEART

The heart of the fetus, as of the adult, is under the control of its own pacemaker. The sinoatrial (S-A) node sets the rate and is supplied by the vagus nerve. Bridging the atrium and the ventricle is the atrioventricular (A-V) node. It is also supplied by the vagus nerve. Baseline variability of the fetal heartbeat has been shown to be under the influence of this nerve. Atropine will block this effect.

Under the influence of the sympathetic nervous system, norepinephrine is released when the fetus is stressed, causing an increase in the fetal heart rate. To counteract the increase in blood pressure, baroreceptors, which respond to stretch, are present in the vessel walls at the junction of the internal and external carotid arteries. When stimulated, these receptors, under the influence of the vagus and glossopharyngeal nerves, cause the fetal heart rate to slow.

Chemoreceptors in the fetal peripheral and central nervous systems respond to decreased oxygen tensions and to increased carbon dioxide tensions, leading to fetal tachycardia and an increase in blood pressure. The central nervous system (CNS) also has control over heart rate. Increased activity of the fetus in a wakeful period was exhibited in an increase in the beat-to-beat variability of the fetal heart baseline. Sleep patterns demonstrated a decrease in the beat-to-beat baseline variability. In cases of severe hypoxia, increased levels of epinephrine and norepinephrine act on the fetal heart to produce a faster and stronger rate.

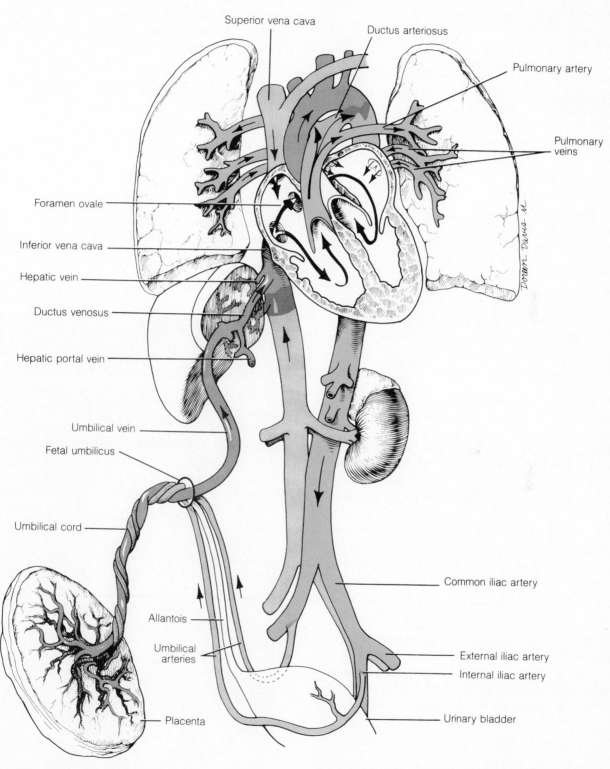

Figure 13–13 Fetal circulation. Blood leaves the placenta and enters the fetus through the umbilical vein. After circulating through the fetus the blood returns to the placenta through the umbilical arteries. The ductus venosus, the foramen ovale, and the ductus arteriosus allow the blood to bypass the fetal liver and lungs. (From Spence AP, Mason EB: Human Anatomy and Physiology, ed 3. Menlo Park, Calif, Benjamin/Cummings, 1987, p 862)

Embryo and Fetal Development and Organ Formation

Pregnancy is calculated to have an average of ten lunar months, 40 weeks, or 280 days. This period of 280 days is calculated from the beginning of the last menstrual period to the time of delivery. The fertilization age or post-conception age of the fetus is calculated to be about 2 weeks less, or 266 days (38 weeks). The latter measurement is more accurate because it measures time from the fertilization of the ovum, or conception. The basic events of organ development in the embryo and fetus are outlined in Table 13–2. The time periods in the table are postconception age periods.

Preembryonic Stage

The first 14 days of human development, starting on the day the ovum was fertilized (conception), are referred to as the preembryonic stage, or the stage of the ovum. This period is characterized by extremely rapid cellular multiplication and differentiation and the establishment of the embryonic membranes and germ layers described earlier in this chapter.

Embryonic Stage

The stage of the embryo starts on day 15 (begins the third week after conception or fertilization) and continues until approximately eight weeks or until the embryo reaches a crown-to-rump length of 3 cm or 1.2 in. This length is usually attained about 49 days after fertilization. The embryonic stage is a period of differentiation of tissues into essential organs and development of the main external features.

THREE WEEKS

In the third week the embryonic disk becomes elongated and pear-shaped, with a broad cephalic end and a narrow caudal end (Figure 13–14). The ectoderm has formed a long cylindrical tube for brain and spinal cord development. The gastrointestinal tract, created from the endoderm, appears as another tubelike structure communicating with the yolk sac. The most advanced organ is the heart. At three weeks a single tubular heart forms just outside the body cavity of the embryo.

FOUR TO FIVE WEEKS

During days 21 to 32, somites, a series of mesodermal blocks, form on either side of the embryo's midline. The vertebrae that form the spinal column will develop from these somites. Prior to 28 days, arm and leg buds are not visible, but the tail bud is present. The pharyngeal arches—which will form the lower jaw (mandibular arch), hyoid bone, and cartilage of the larynx—develop at this time. The pharyngeal pouches appear now; these pouches will form the eustachian tube and cavity of the middle ear, the tonsils, and the parathyroid and thymus glands. The primordia of the ear and eye are also present. By the end of 28 days, the tubular heart is beating at a regular rhythm and pushing its own primitive blood cells through the main blood vessels.

During the fifth week, the optic cups and lens vesicles of the eye form and the nasal pits develop. Partitioning in the heart occurs with the dividing of the atrium. The embryo has a marked C-shaped body, accentuated by the rudimentary tail and the large head folded over a protuberant trunk (Figure 13–15). By day 35, the arm and leg buds are well developed, with paddle-shaped hand and foot plates. The heart, circulatory system, and brain show the most advanced development. The brain has differentiated into five areas, and ten pairs of cranial nerves are recognizable.

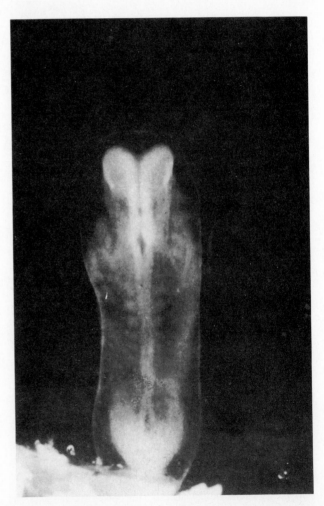

Figure 13–14 The embryo at three weeks (Courtesy Drs Roberts Rugh and Landrum B Shettles)

SIX WEEKS

At six weeks the head structures are more highly developed and the trunk is straighter than in earlier stages (Figure 13–16). The upper and lower jaws are recognizable, and the external nares are well formed. The trachea has developed, and its caudal end is bifurcated for beginning lung formation. The upper lip has formed, and the palate is developing. The ears are developing rapidly, as are the other postbranchial body parts. The arms have begun to extend ventrally across the chest, and both arms and legs have digits, although they may still be webbed. There is a slight elbow bend in the arm, and the arm is more advanced in development than the leg. Beginning at this stage the prominent tail will recede. The heart now has most of its definitive characteristics, and fetal circulation begins to be established. The liver begins to produce blood cells.

SEVEN WEEKS

At seven weeks the head of the embryo is rounded and nearly erect (Figure 13–17). The eyes have shifted from their original lateral position to a forward location, where they are closer together, and the eyelids are beginning to form. The palate is nearing completion, and the tongue is developing in the formed mouth. The gastrointestinal and genitourinary tracts undergo significant changes during the seventh week. Prior to this time the rectal and urogenital passages formed one tube that ended in a blind pouch; they now separate into two tubular structures. The intestines enter the extraembryonic celom in the area of the umbilical cord (called umbilical herniation) (Moore 1982). At this point the beginnings of all essential external and internal structures are present.

EIGHT WEEKS

At eight weeks the embryo is approximately 3 cm (1.2 in) long crown to rump (C–R) and clearly resembles a human being (Figure 13–18). Facial features continue to develop. The eyelids begin to fuse. Auricles of the external ears begin to assume their final shape, but they are still set low (Moore 1982). External genitals appear but are not discernible, and the rectal passage opens with the perforation of the anal membrane. The circulatory system through the umbilical cord is well established. Long bones are beginning to form, and the large muscles are now capable of contracting.

Fetal Stage

By the end of eight weeks, the embryo is sufficiently developed to be called a *fetus*. Every organ system and

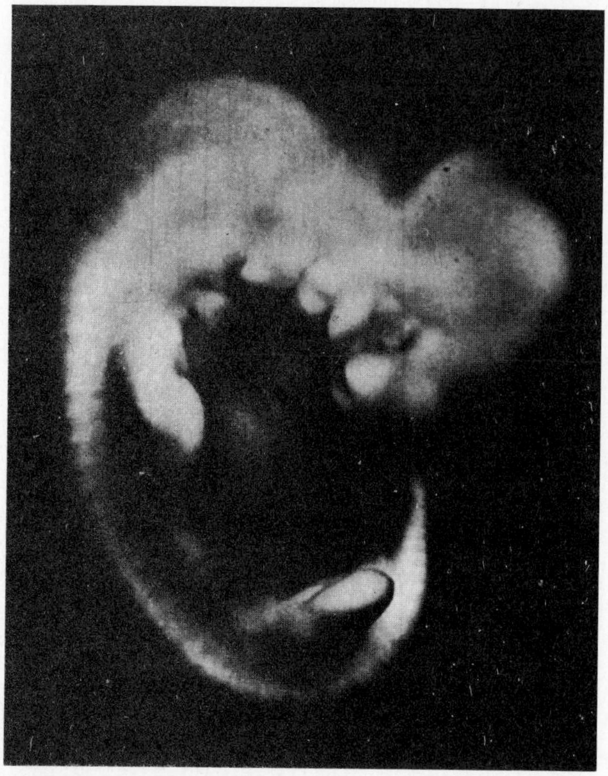

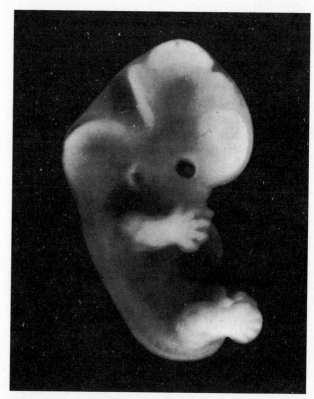

Figure 13–15 The embryo at five weeks (Courtesy Drs Roberts Rugh and Landrum B Shettles)

Figure 13–16 The embryo at six weeks (Courtesy Drs Roberts Rugh and Landrum B Shettles)

Table 13-2   Classification of Organ System Development

Postconception age*	Length†	Weight	Nervous system	Musculoskeletal system	Cardiovascular system	Gastointestinal system
CONCEPTION						
2–3 weeks	2mm C–R		Groove is formed along middle of back as cells thicken; neural tube formed from closure of neural groove		Beginning of blood circulation; tubular heart begins to form during third week	
4 weeks	4–6 mm C–R	0.4 g	Anterior portion of neural tube closes to form brain; closure of posterior end forms spinal cord	Noticeable limb buds	Tubular heart is beating at 28 days and primitive red blood cells are circulating through fetus and chorionic villi	Mouth: formation of oral cavity; primitive jaws present; esophagotracheal septum begins division of esophagus and trachea. Digestive tract: stomach forms; esophagus and intestine become tubular; ducts of pancreas and liver forming
5 weeks	8 mm C–R	Only 0.5% of total body weight is fat (to 20 weeks)	Brain has differentiated and cranial nerves are present	Developing muscles have innervation	Atrial division has occurred	
6 weeks	12 mm C–R			Bone rudiments present; primitive skeletal shape forming; muscle mass begins to develop; ossification of skull and jaws begins	Chambers present in heart; groups of blood cells can be identified	Oral and nasal cavities and upper lip formed
7 weeks	18 mm C–R				Fetal heartbeats can be detected	Mouth: tongue separates; palate folds. Digestive tract: stomach attains final form
8 weeks	2.5–3 cm C–R	2 g		Digits formed; further differentiation of cells in primitive skeleton; cartilaginous bones show first signs of ossification; development of muscles in trunk, limbs, and head; some movement of fetus is now possible	Development of heart is essentially complete; fetal circulation follows two circuits—four extraembryonic and two intraembryonic	Mouth: completion of lip fusion. Digestive tract: rotation in midgut; anal membrane has perforated

*Refers to gestational age of fetus/conceptus; fertilization age.
†C–R = crown–rump; C–H = crown–heel

Sources: Langman J: *Medical Embryology,* ed 5. Baltimore, Williams & Wilkins, 1985; and Moore KL: *The Developing Human: Clinically Oriented Embryology,* ed 3. Philadelphia, Saunders, 1982.

Table 13–2   Classification of Organ System Development (continued)

Genitourinary system	Respiratory system	Skin	Specific organ systems	Sexual development
Formation of kidneys beginning	Nasal pits forming		Endocrine system: thyroid tissue appears Eyes: optic cup and lens pit have formed; pigment in eyes Ear: auditory pit is now enclosed structure Liver function begins	
	Trachea, bronchi, and lungs buds present		Ear: formation of external, middle, and inner ear continues Liver begins to form red blood cells	Embryonic sex glands appear
Separation of bladder and urethra from rectum	Diaphragm separates abdominal and thoracic cavities		Eyes: optic nerve formed; eyelids appear; thickening of lens	Differentiation of sex glands into ovaries and testes begins
			Ear: external, middle, and inner ear assuming final structure forms	Male and female external genitals appear similar until end of ninth week

Table 13–2   Classification of Organ System Development (continued)

Postconception age*	Length†	Weight	Nervous system	Musculoskeletal system	Cardiovascular system	Gastrointestinal system
10 weeks	5–6 cm C–H	14 g	Neurons appear at caudal end of spinal cord; basic divisions of the brain present	Fingers and toes begin nail growth		Mouth: separation of lips from jaw; fusion of palate folds. Digestive tract: developing intestines enclosed in abdomen
12 weeks	8 cm C–R, 11.5 cm C–H	45g		Clear outlining of miniature bones (12–20 weeks); process of ossification is established throughout fetal body; appearance of involuntary muscles in viscera		Mouth: completion of palate. Digestive tract: appearance of muscles in gut; bile secretion begins; liver is major producer of red blood cells
16 weeks	13.5 cm C–R, 15 cm C–H	200 g		Teeth: beginning formation of hard tissue that will become central incisors		Mouth: differentiation of hard and soft palate. Digestive tract: development of gastric and intestinal glands; intestines begin to collect meconium
18 weeks				Teeth: beginning formation of hard tissue (enamel and dentine) that will become lateral incisors	Fetal heart tones audible with fetoscope at 16–20 weeks	
20 weeks	19 cm C–R, 25 cm C–H	435 g (6% of total body weight is fat)	Myelination of spinal cord begins	Teeth: beginning formation of hard tissue that will become canine and first molar. Lower limbs are of final relative proportions		Fetus actively sucks and swallows amniotic fluid; peristaltic movements begin
24 weeks	23 cm C–R, 28 cm C–H	780 g	Structure of brain: looks like mature brain	Teeth: beginning formation of hard tissue that will become second molar		
28 weeks	27 cm C–R, 35 cm C–H	1200–1250 g	Nervous system begins regulation of some body functions			
32 weeks	31 cm C–R, 38–43 cm C–H	2000 g	More reflexes present			

Table 13–2 Classification of Organ System Development (continued)

Genitourinary system	Respiratory system	Skin	Specific organ systems	Sexual development
Bladder sac formed Urine formed			Eyelids fused closed Endocrine system: islets of Langerhans differentiated Eyes: development of lacrimal duct	
	Lungs acquire definitive shape	Skin pink, delicate	Endocrine system: hormonal secretion from thyroid Immunologic system: appearance of lymphoid tissue in fetal thymus gland	
Kidneys assume typical shape and organization		Appearance of scalp hair; lanugo present on body; transparent skin with visible blood vessels	Eye, ear, and nose formed Sweat glands developing	Sex determination possible
		Lanugo covers entire body; brown fat begins to form; vernix caseosa begins to form	Immunologic system: detectable levels of fetal antibodies (IgG type) Blood formation: iron is stored and bone marrow is increasingly important	
	Respiratory movements may occur (24–40) weeks) Nostrils reopen Alveoli appear in lungs and begin production of surfactant; gas exchange possible	Skin reddish and wrinkled, vernix caseosa present	Immunologic system: IgG levels reach maternal levels Eyes structurally complete	
		Adipose tissue accumulates rapidly; nails appear; eyebrows and eyelashes present	Eyes: eyelids open (28–32 weeks)	Testes descend into inguinal canal and upper scrotum

Table 13–2 Classification of Organ System Development (continued)

Postconception age*	Length†	Weight	Nervous system	Musculoskeletal system	Cardiovascular system	Gastrointestinal system
36 weeks	35 cm C–R, 42–48 cm C–H	2500–2750 g		Distal femoral ossification centers present		
40 weeks	40 cm C–R, 48–52 cm C–H	3200+ g (16% of total body weight is fat)				

external structure that will be found in the full-term newborn is present. The remainder of gestation is devoted to refining structures and perfecting function.

9 TO 12 WEEKS

By ten weeks the fetus reaches a C–R length of 5 cm (2 in) and weighs about 14 g. The head is large and comprises almost half of the fetus's entire size (Figure 13–19). The neck is distinct from the head and body, and both the head and neck are straighter than in previous stages of development.

By 12 weeks, the fetus reaches an 8 cm (3.2 in) C–R length and weighs about 45 g (1.6 oz). The face is well formed, with the nose protruding, the chin small and receding, and the ear acquiring a more adult shape. The eyelids close at about the tenth week and will not reopen until about 28 weeks. Some reflex movements of the lips suggestive of the sucking reflex have been observed at three months. Tooth buds now appear for all 20 of the child's first teeth (baby teeth). The limbs are long and slender, with well-formed digits. The fetus can curl the fingers toward the palm and make a tiny fist. The legs are still shorter and less developed than the arms. The urogenital tract completes its development, well-differentiated genitals appear, and the kidneys begin to produce urine. Red blood cells are produced primarily by the liver. Spontaneous movements of the fetus now occur.

13 TO 16 WEEKS

This is a period of rapid growth. At 13 weeks the fetus weighs 55 to 60 g and is about 9 cm (3.6 in) in C–

R length. Downy lanugo hair begins to develop, especially on the head. The fetal skin is so transparent that blood vessels are clearly visible beneath it. More muscle tissue and body skeleton have developed, which tend to hold the fetus more erect. Active movements are present—the fetus

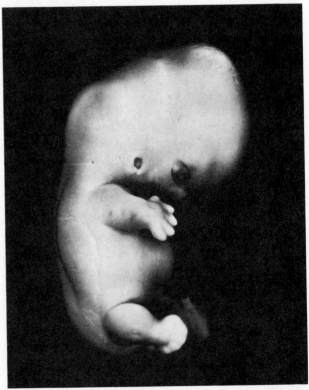

Figure 13–17 The embryo at seven weeks (Courtesy Drs Roberts Rugh and Landrum B Shettles)

Table 13-2 Classification of Organ System Development (continued)

Genitourinary system	Respiratory system	Skin	Specific organ systems	Sexual development
		Skin pale; body rounded; lanugo disappearing; hair fuzzy or woolly; few sole creases; sebaceous glands active and helping to produce vernix caseosa (36–40 weeks)	Ear lobes soft with little cartilage	Scrotum small and few rugae present; descent of testes into upper scrotum to stay (36–40 weeks)
At 38 weeks, lecithin-sphingomyelin (L/S) ratio approaches 2:1		Skin smooth and pink; vernix present in skin-folds; moderate to profuse silky hair; lanugo hair on shoulders and upper back; nails extend over tips of digits; creases cover sole	Ear lobes stiffened by thick cartilage	Males: rugous scrotum Females: labia majora well developed

stretches and exercises its arms and legs. It makes sucking motions, swallows amniotic fluid, and produces meconium in the intestinal tract. Bronchial tubes are branching out in the primitive lungs, and sweat glands are developing. The liver and pancreas now begin production of their appropriate secretions. By the beginning of week 16, skeletal ossification is clearly identifiable.

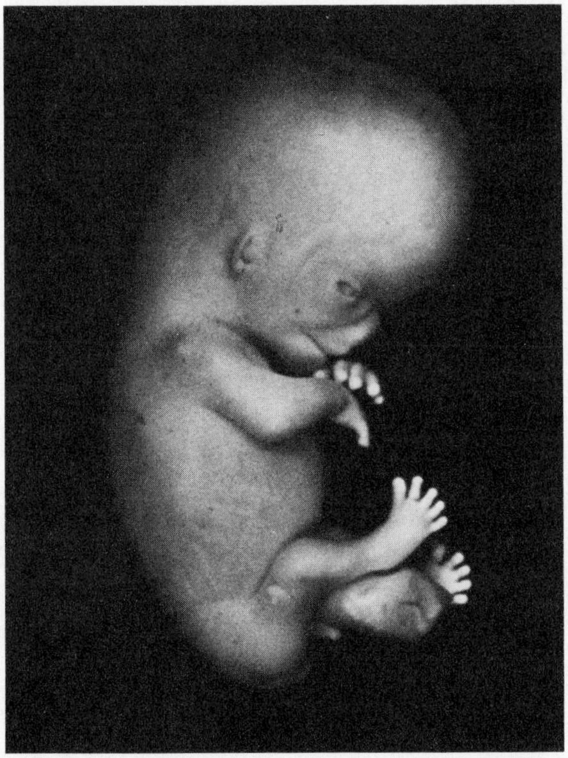

17 TO 20 WEEKS

The fetus almost doubles its length and at 20 weeks now measures about 19 cm (8 in) and fetal weight increases to between 435 and 465 g. Lanugo covers the entire body and is especially prominent on the shoulders. Subcutaneous deposits of brown fat have made the skin a little less transparent. Nipples now appear over the mammary glands. The head sports fine, "wooly" hair, and the eyebrows and eyelashes are beginning to form. The fetus has nails on both fingers and toes. Muscles are well developed, and the fetus is active. Fetal movement, known as quickening, is felt by the mother. The heartbeat is audible with the use of a stethoscope. Quickening and fetal heartbeat can assist in reaffirming maternal estimated delivery date.

24 WEEKS

The fetus at 24 weeks reaches a crown-to-heel (C–H) length of 28 cm (11.2 in). It weighs about 780 g (1 lb, 10 oz). The hair on the head is growing long, and eyebrows and eyelashes have formed. The eye is structurally complete and will soon open. The fetus has a reflex hand grip (grasp reflex), and by the end of six months will have a startle reflex. Skin covering the body is reddish and wrinkled, with little subcutaneous fat. Skin on the hands and feet has thickened, with skin ridges on palms and soles forming distinct footprints and fingerprints. The skin over the entire body is covered with a protective cheeselike fatty substance secreted by the sebaceous glands called *vernix caseosa*. The alveoli in the lungs are just beginning to form.

Figure 13-18 The fetus at eight weeks (Courtesy Drs Roberts Rugh and Landrum B Shettles)

25 TO 28 WEEKS

At six calendar months the fetal skin is still red, wrinkled, and covered with vernix caseosa. During this time the brain is developing rapidly, and the nervous system is complete enough to provide some regulation of body functions. The eyelids open and close under neural control. If the fetus is a male, the testes begin to descend into the scrotal sac. Respiratory and circulatory systems have developed sufficiently. Even though the lungs are still physiologically immature, they are sufficiently developed to provide gas exchange. A fetus born at this time will require intensive care in order to survive and to decrease the risk of major handicap. The fetus at 28 weeks (Figure 13–20) is about 35 to 38 cm (14–15 in) long C–H and weighs about 1200 to 1250 g (2 lbs, 10.5 oz to 2 lbs, 12 oz).

29 TO 32 WEEKS

At 30 weeks the pupillary light reflex is present (Moore 1982). The fetus is gaining weight from an increase in body muscle and fat and weighs about 2000 g (4 lbs,

6.5 oz) with a length of about 38 to 43 cm (15 to 17 in) by 32 weeks of age. The CNS has matured enough to direct rhythmic breathing movements and partially control body temperature. However, the lungs are not yet fully mature. Bones are now fully developed but are soft and flexible. The fetus begins storing iron, calcium, and phosphorus. In males the testicles may be located in the scrotal sac but are often still high in the inguinal canal.

33 TO 36 WEEKS

The body and extremities of the fetus are "filling out" by 33 to 36 weeks. The fetus is beginning to get plump, with less-wrinkled skin covering the deposits of subcutaneous fat. Lanugo hair is beginning to disappear, and the nails reach the edge of the fingertips. By 35 weeks the fetus has a firm grasp and exhibits spontaneous orientation to light (Page et al 1981). By 36 weeks of age the weight is usually 2500 to 2750 g (5 lb, 12 oz to 6 lb, 11.5 oz), and the C–H length of the fetus is about 42 to 48 cm (16 to 19 in). An infant born at this time has a good chance of surviving but may require some special care.

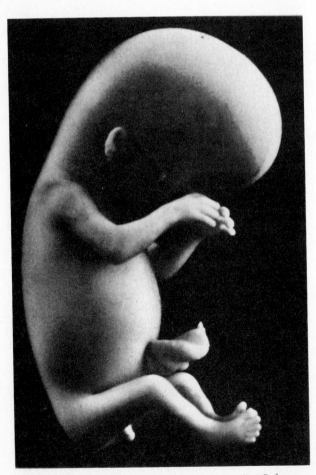

Figure 13–19   The fetus at nine weeks (Courtesy Drs Roberts Rugh and Landrum B Shettles)

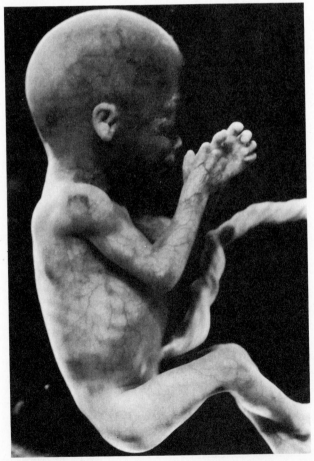

Figure 13–20   The fetus at 28 weeks (Courtesy Drs Roberts Rugh and Landrum B Shettles)

37 TO 40 WEEKS

The fetus is considered full term at 38 weeks after conception. The C–H length varies from 48 to 52 cm (19 to 21 in) with males usually longer than females. Males also usually weigh more than females. The weight at term is about 3000 to 3600 g (6 lb, 10 oz to 7 lb, 15 oz). The skin is pink and smooth with a polished look. The only lanugo hair remaining is on the upper arms and shoulders. The hair on the head is no longer woolly but coarse and about an inch long. Vernix caseosa is still present but varies in amount, with heavier deposits remaining in creases and folds of the skin. The body and extremities are plump, with good skin turgor, and the fingernails extend beyond the fingertips. The chest is prominent but still a little smaller than the head, and mammary glands protrude in both sexes. The testes are in the scrotum or are palpable in the inguinal canals. As the fetus enlarges, amniotic fluid diminishes to about 500 mL or less, and the fetal body mass fills the uterine cavity. The fetus assumes what is referred to as its position of comfort, or lie. The head is generally pointed downward because of the shape of the uterus and also possibly because the head is heavier than the feet. The extremities and often the head are well flexed. After five months, feeding patterns, sleeping patterns, and activity patterns become established, so that at term the fetus has its own body rhythms and individual style of response.

Factors Influencing Embryonic and Fetal Development

Among factors that may affect embryonic development are the quality of the sperm or ovum from which the zygote was formed and the genetic code established at fertilization. In addition, the adequacy of the intrauterine environment is important for optimal growth. If the environment is unsuitable before cellular differentiation occurs, all the cells of the zygote are affected. The cells may die, which causes spontaneous abortion, or growth may be slowed, depending on the severity of the situation. When differentiation is complete and the fetal membranes have formed, an injurious agent has the greatest effect on those cells undergoing the most rapid growth. Thus the time of injury is critical in the development of anomalies.

Because organs are formed primarily during embryonic development, the growing organism is considered most vulnerable to noxious agents during the first months of pregnancy. Table 13–3 lists potential malformations related to the time of insult. Any agent, such as a drug, virus, or radiation, that can cause development of abnormal structures in an embryo is referred to as a teratogen. Chapter 14 discusses the effects of specific teratogenic agents on the developing fetus.

The adequacy of the maternal environment is also extremely important to embryonic and fetal development.

The substances required for growth of a particular structure must be readily available at its time of development. In general the raw materials for development come from the mother's diet and not from her bodily reserves. Thus temporary deficiencies in the mother's diet, which may cause no manifest symptoms in her, may damage the developing embryo or fetus. Data concerning infants born to mothers with reportedly deficient diets during pregnancy indicate smaller intrauterine growth and more susceptibility to infections, particularly respiratory infections, during the first year of life. Barely adequate maternal nutritional intake may sustain growth and development during early pregnancy but may not meet the needs of the rapidly growing fetus during late pregnancy and thus produce underweight newborns (Page et al 1981).

Maternal nutrition can also affect brain development. The period of maximum brain growth and myelination begins with the fifth lunar month before birth and continues during the first six months after birth. During the first six months after birth there is a twofold increase in myelination, in the second six months to two years of age there is about a 50 percent further increase (Volpe 1987). Amino acids, glucose, and fatty acids are considered to be the

Table 13–3 Developmental Vulnerability Timetable

Weeks since conception	Potential teratogen-induced malformation
3	Ectromelia (congenital absence of one or more limbs) Ectopedia cordis (heart lies outside thoracic cavity)
4	Omphalocele Tracheoesophageal fistula (4–5* weeks) Hemivertebra (4–5* weeks)
5	Nuclear cataract Microphthalmia (abnormally small eyeballs; 5–6* weeks) Facial clefts Carpal or pedal ablation (5–6* weeks)
6	Gross septal or aortic abnormalities Cleft lip, agnathia (absence of the lower jaw)
7	Interventricular septal defects Pulmonary stenosis Cleft palate, micrognathia (smallness of the jaw) Epicanthus Brachycephalism (shortness of the head; 7–8* weeks) Mixed sexual characteristics
8	Persistent ostium primum (persistent opening in atrial septum) Digital stunting (shortening of fingers and toes)

May occur in several different time periods after conception.

Modified from Danforth DN, Scott JR: *Obstetrics and Gynecology,* ed 5. Philadelphia, Lippincott, 1986, p 319.

primary dietary factors in brain growth. A subtle type of damage that affects the associative capacity of the brain, possibly leading to learning disabilities, may be caused by nutritional deficiency at this stage. (Maternal nutrition is discussed in depth in Chapter 17.)

Another prenatal influence on the intrauterine environment is maternal hyperthermia associated with sauna baths or hot tub use (Jones & Chernoff 1984). Studies of the effects of maternal hyperthermia during the first trimester have raised concern about possible central nervous sys-

tem defects and failure of neural tube closure (Pleet et al 1980).

Twins

Twins have been reported to occur more often among black than among white women and more often among white individuals than among Orientals. Among all groups, as parity increases so does the chance for multiple births.

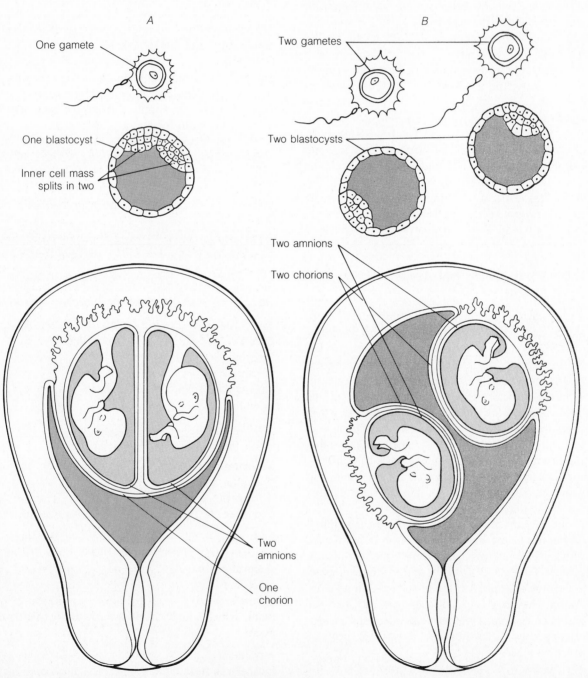

Figure 13–21   A *Formation of identical twins.* B *Formation of fraternal twins*

Twins may be either fraternal or identical. If they are fraternal, they are dizygotic, which means they arise from two separate ova fertilized by two separate spermatozoa (Figure 13–21). There are two placentas, two chorions, and two amnions; however, the placentas sometimes fuse together and look as if they are one. Despite their birth relationship, fraternal twins are no more similar to each other than they would be to siblings born singly. They may be the same or different sex.

Dizygotic twinning increases with maternal age up to about 35 years of age and then decreases abruptly. The chance of dizygotic twins increases with parity, decreases in periods of malnutrition, increases in conceptions that occur in the first three months of marriage, and increases with coital frequency (James 1981). Studies indicate dizygotic twins occur in certain families, perhaps because of genetic factors leading to double ovulation (Creasy & Resnik 1984).

Identical, or monozygotic, twins develop from a single fertilized ovum. Consequently, they are of the same sex and have the same genotype (appearance). Identical twins usually have a common placenta (Figure 13–21).

Monozygotic twins originate from division of the fertilized ovum at different stages of early development (Pritchard et al 1985). The division of the single fertilized ovum occurs only after the embryo consists of thousands of cells; complete separation of the cellular mass into two parts is necessary for twin formation. The number of amnions and chorions present depends on the timing of the division:

1. If division occurs within the first 72 hours after fertilization (before the inner cell mass and chorion is formed), two embryos, two amnions, and two chorions will develop. This occurs about 20 percent to 30 percent of the time, and there may be distinct placentas or a single fused placenta.

2. If division occurs between four and eight days after fertilization (when the inner cell mass is formed and the chorion cells have differentiated but those of the amnion have not), two embryos develop with separate amnionic sacs. These sacs will eventually be covered by a common chorion.

3. If the amnion has already developed approximately eight days after fertilization, division results in two embryos with a common amnionic sac and a common chorion. This type occurs about 1 percent of the time (Creasy & Resnik 1984).

Monozygotic twinning is considered a random event and occurs in approximately 1 of 250 births. The survival rate of monozygotic twins is 10 percent lower than that of dizygotic twins, and congenital anomalies are more prevalent. Both twins may have the same malformation (Oxorn 1986).

KEY CONCEPTS

Chromosomes are threadlike bodies composed of strands of deoxyribonucleic acid (DNA) and protein. Each chromosome contains two longitudinal halves called chromatids, which are joined together at a point called the centromere.

Humans have 46 chromosomes, which are divided into 23 pairs—22 pairs of autosomes and one pair of sex chromosomes.

Each member of a chromosome pair carries either similar (homologous) genes or dissimilar (heterozygous) genes.

Mitosis is the process by which additional somatic (body) cells are formed. It provides growth and development of the organisms and replacement of body cells.

Meiosis is the process by which new organisms are formed. It occurs during gametogenesis and consists of two successive cell divisions (reduction division), which produce a gamete with 23 chromosomes (22 chromosomes and 1 sex chromosome)—the haploid number of chromosomes.

Gametes must have a haploid number (23) of chromosomes so that when the female gamete (ovum) and the male gamete (spermatozoon) unite (fertilization) to form the zygote, the normal human diploid number of chromosomes (46) is reestablished.

Sex chromosomes are referred to as X and Y. Females have two X chromosomes and males have an X and a Y chromosome. Y chromosomes are carried only by the sperm. To produce a male child the mother contributes an X chromosome and the father contributes a Y chromosome.

Fertilization usually takes place in the ampulla (outer third) of the fallopian tube.

An ovum is considered fertile for about a 24-hour period after ovulation, and the sperm is capable of fertilizing the ovum for only about 24 hours after it is deposited in the female reproductive system.

Both capacitation and acrosomal reaction must occur for the sperm to fertilize the ovum. Capacitation is the removal of the plasma membrane, which exposes the acrosomal covering of the sperm head. Acrosomal reaction is the deposit of hyaluronidase in the corona radiata, which allows the sperm head to penetrate the ovum.

Intrauterine development first proceeds via cellular multiplication in which the zygote undergoes rapid mitotic division called cleavage. As a result of cleavage the zygote divides and multiplies into cell groupings called blastomeres, which are held together by the zona pellucida. The blastomeres will eventually become a solid ball of cells called the morula. When the cavity forms in the morula cell mass, the inner solid cell mass is called the blastocyst.

Implantation usually occurs in the upper part of the posterior uterine wall when the blastocyst burrows into the uterine lining.

After implantation the endometrium is called the decidua. Decidua capsularis is the portion that covers the blastocyst. Decidua basalis is the portion that is directly under the blastocyst. Decidua vera is the portion that lines the rest of the uterine cavity.

Embryonic membranes are called the amnion and the chorion. The amnion is formed from the ectoderm and is a thin protective membrane that contains the amniotic fluid and the embryo. The chorion is a thick membrane that develops from the trophoblast and encloses the amnion, embryo, and yolk sac.

Amniotic fluid cushions the fetus against mechanical injury, controls the embryo's temperature, allows symmetrical external growth, prevents adherence to the amnion, and permits freedom of movement.

Amniotic fluid is made up of albumin, creatinine, lecithin, sphingomyelin, fat, bilirubin, proteins, epithelial cells, and lanugo. Normal volume is 500 to 1000 cc/day after about 20 weeks. The fetus contributes to the amniotic fluid via urination.

Primary germ layers will give rise to all tissues, organs, and organ systems. The three primary germ cell layers are ectoderm, endoderm, and mesoderm.

The placenta develops from the chorionic villi and has two parts: The maternal portion, consisting of the decidua basalis, is red and freshlooking. The fetal portion, consisting of chorionic villi, is covered by the amnion and appears shiny and gray. The placenta is made up of 15 to 20 segments called cotyledons.

The placenta serves endrocrine (production of hPL, hCG, estrogen, and progesterone), metabolic, and immunologic functions; it acts as the fetus's respiratory organ, is an organ of excretion, and aids in the exchange of nutrients.

The umbilical cord contains two umbilical arteries, which carry deoxygenated blood from the fetus to the placenta, and one umbilical vein, which carries oxygenated blood from the placenta to the fetus. The umbilical cord has a central insertion into the placenta. Wharton's jelly, a specialized connective tissue, prevents compression of the umbilical cord in utero.

Fetal circulation is a specially designed circulatory system that provides for oxygenation of the fetus while bypassing the fetal lungs.

Stages of fetal development include the preembryonic stage (the first 14 days of human development starting at the time of fertilization), the embryonic stage (from day 15 after fertilization, or the beginning of the third week, until approximately eight weeks after conception), and the fetal stage (from 8 weeks until delivery at approximately 40 weeks postconception).

Some significant events that occur during the embryonic stage are: at four weeks, the fetal heart begins to beat and at six weeks, fetal circulation is established.

The fetal stage is devoted to refining structures and perfecting function. Some significant developments during the fetal stage are:

At 16 weeks sex can be determined visually.

At 20 weeks fetal heartbeat can be auscultated by a fetoscope, and the mother can feel movement (quickening).

At 24 weeks vernix caseosa covers the entire body.

At 26 to 28 weeks the eyes reopen.

At 36 weeks fingernails reach the ends of fingers.

At 40 weeks fingernails extend beyond fingertips, vernix is apparent only in creases and folds of skin, and lanugo remains on upper arms and shoulders only.

Twins are either monozygotic (identical) or dizygotic (fraternal). Dizygotic twins arise from two separate ova fertilized by two separate spermatozoa. Monozygotic twins develop from a single fertilized ovum.

REFERENCES

Ahokas RA: Development and physiology of the placenta and membranes, in Sciarra JJ, et al (eds): Gynecology and Obstetrics. Hagerstown, Md, Harper & Row, 1985;2(11):1.
Aladjem S, Lueck J: Placental physiology, in Sciarra JJ, et al (eds): Gynecology and Obstetrics. Hagerstown, Md, Harper & Row, 1982;3(8):1.
Batzer FR: Hormonal evaluation of early pregnancy. Fertil Steril 1980;34(July):1.
Benirschke K: Anatomy, in Berger GS, Brenner WE, Keith LG (eds): Second Trimester Abortion. Boston, John Wright, 1981.

Bloom W, Fawcett DW: *A Textbook of Histology,* ed 10. Philadelphia, Saunders, 1975.

Creasy RK, Resnik JR: *Maternal Fetal Medicine Principles and Practice.* Philadelphia, Saunders, 1984.

Danforth DN, Scott JR: *Obstetrics and Gynecology,* ed 5. Philadelphia, Lippincott, 1986.

Dilts PV: Placental transfer. *Clin Obstet Gynecol* 1981; 24(June):555.

Eddy CA, Pauerstein CJ: Anatomy and physiology of the fallopian tube. *Clin Obstet Gynecol* 1980;23:1177.

Glass RH: The placenta-sperm and egg transport, fertilization and implantation, in Creasy RK, Resnik JR (eds): *Maternal-Fetal Medicine Principles and Practice.* Philadelphia, Saunders, 1984, p 115.

Gudson JP, Sain LE: Uterine and peripheral blood concentrations and human chorionic gonadotropin and human placental lactogen. *Am J Obstet Gynecol* 1981;39 (March):705.

James WH: Dizygotic twinning, marital stage and status and coital rates. *Ann Hum Biol* 1981;8:371.

Jones KL, Chernoff GF: Effects of chemical and environmental agents, in Creasy RK, Resnik JR (eds): *Maternal-Fetal Medicine Principles and Practice.* Philadelphia, Saunders, 1984, p 190.

Koffler H: Fetal and neonatal physiology. *Clin Obstet Gynecol* 1981;24(June):545.

Langman J: *Medical Embryology.* ed 5. Baltimore, Williams & Wilkins, 1985.

Moore KL: *The Developing Human: Clinically Oriented Embryology,* ed 3. Philadelphia, Saunders, 1982.

Naeye RL: Maternal blood pressure and fetal growth. *Am J Obstet Gynecol* 1981;141(December):780.

Oxorn H: *Oxorn-Foote Human Labor and Birth,* ed 5. Norwalk, Conn, Appleton-Century-Crofts, 1986.

Page EW, Villee CA, Villee DB: *Human Reproduction: Essentials of Reproductive and Perinatal Medicine,* ed 3. Philadelphia, Saunders, 1981.

Pleet HB, et al: Patterns of malformations resulting from the teratogenic effects of first trimester hyperthermia. *Pediatr Res* 1980;14:587.

Pritchard JA, MacDonald PC, Gant NF: *Williams Obstetrics,* ed 17. New York, Appleton-Century-Crofts, 1985.

Sadler TW: *Langman's Medical Embryology,* ed 5. Baltimore, Williams & Wilkins, 1985.

Seeds AE: Current concepts of amniotic fluid dynamics. *Am J Obstet Gynecol* 1980;138(November):575.

Silverstein A: *Human Anatomy and Physiology.* New York, John Wiley, 1980.

Spence AP: *Basic Human Anatomy,* Menlo Park, Calif, Benjamin/Cummings, 1982.

Spence AP, Mason EB: *Human Anatomy and Physiology,* ed 3. Menlo Park, Benjamin/Cummings, 1987.

Thompson JS, Thompson MW: *Genetics in Medicine,* ed 4. Philadelphia, Saunders, 1986.

Volpe JJ: *Neurology of the Newborn,* ed 2. Philadelphia, Saunders, 1987.

Vorherr H: Factors influencing fetal growth. *Am J Obstet Gynecol* 1982;142(March):577.

Whaley LE: *Understanding Inherited Disorders.* St Louis, Mosby, 1974.

ADDITIONAL READINGS

Bernhardt J: Sensory capabilities of the fetus. *Am J Mat Child Nurs* 1987;12(January/February):44.

Bingol N, et al: Teratogenicity of cocaine in humans. *J Pediatr* 1987;110(January):93.

Boylan P, Parisi V: An overview of hydramnios. *Semin Perinatol* 1986;10(April):136.

Cohen-Overbeek T, et al: The antenatal assessment of utero-placental and feto-placental blood flow using doppler ultrasound. *Ultrasound in Med & Biol* 1985;11(2):329.

Frank L, et al: Development of lung antioxidant enzyme system in late gestation: Possible implications for the prematurely born infant. *J Pediatr* 1987;110(January):9.

Fritz MA, et al: Maternal estradiol response to alterations in uteroplacental blood flow. *Am J Obstet Gynecol* 1986;155(December):1317.

Hill LM, et al: Polyhydramnios: Ultrasonically detected prevalence and neonatal outcome. *Obstet Gynecol* 1987; 69(January):21.

Hertzberg BS, et al: Significance of membrane thickness in the sonographic evaluation of twin gestation. *AJR* 1987;148(January):151.

Levine J, et al: Help from the unborn: Fetal-cell surgery raises hopes—and issues. *Time,* January 12, 1987, p 62.

Lee ML, Yeh Ming-neng: Fetal microcirculation of abnormal human placenta. I. Scanning electron microscopy of placental vascular casts from small for gestational fetus. *Am J Obstet Gynecol* 1986;154(May):1133.

Nazir MA, et al: Antibacterial activity of amniotic fluid in the early third trimester: Its association with preterm labor and delivery. *Am J Perinatol* 1987;4(January):59.

Niesert S, et al: The effect of fetal urine on arachidonic acid metabolism in human amnion cells in monolayer culture. *Am J Obstet Gynecol* 1986;155(December):1310.

O'Grady JP: Clinical management of twins. *Contemp OB/GYN,* April 1987, p 126.

Ramsay J: Prenatal influences on fetal development. *Nursing* 1986;3(December):432.

Roger JC, Drake BL: The enigma of the fetal graft. *Am Sci* 1987;75(January/February):51.

Winick M: Maternal nutrition and fetal growth. *Perinat Neonat* 1986;10(September/October):28.

Physical and Psychologic
Changes of Pregnancy

Anatomy and Physiology of Pregnancy
Reproductive System
Respiratory System
Cardiovascular System
Gastrointestinal System
Urinary Tract
Skin
Skeletal System
Metabolism
Endocrine System

Subjective (Presumptive) Changes
Objective (Probable) Changes
Pregnancy Tests
Immunoassay
Radioreceptor Assay (RRA)
Over-the-Counter Pregnancy Tests

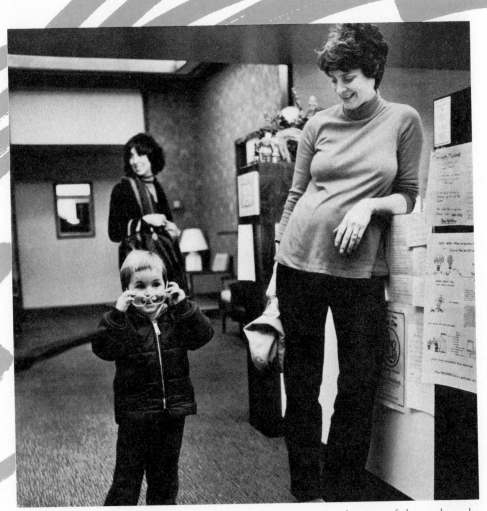

There are many extra demands on the time and energy of the mother who already has children.

Chapter Fourteen

OBJECTIVES

- **Compare subjective (presumptive), objective (probable), and diagnostic (positive) changes of pregnancy.**
- **Describe the various types of pregnancy tests.**
- **Relate the physiologic changes that occur in the body systems as a result of pregnancy to the signs and symptoms that develop.**
- **Discuss the emotional and psychologic changes that commonly occur in a woman during pregnancy.**
- **Summarize cultural factors that may influence a family's response to pregnancy.**

Through modern technology and highly evolved research methods, we know a great deal about how pregnancy occurs and what happens to the fetus and the woman's body during gestation. Yet no matter how much we learn about this event, it never ceases to amaze us. First, it is nothing short of a miracle that the union of two microscopic entities—an ovum and a sperm—can produce a living being. Second, the woman's body must undergo extraordinary physical changes to sustain a pregnancy. A pregnant woman's body changes in size and shape, and all her organ systems modify their functions to create an environment that protects and nurtures the growing fetus.

The duration of human pregnancy is nine calendar months, ten lunar months, 40 weeks, or 280 days. The date of delivery is calculated from the first day of the last menstrual period (LMP). However, ovulation actually occurs about two weeks before the next menstrual period begins. Thus the real length of gestation is about 266 days, although considerable variation is possible. The LMP is used because it provides the most specific time for dating a pregnancy since the actual time of fertilization is usually not known.

Pregnancy is divided into three trimesters, each a three-month period. Each trimester has its own predictable developments, both fetally and maternally.

The diagnosis of pregnancy is generally not difficult for the clinician. In most cases the woman is fairly certain of the diagnosis when she presents herself for the initial office visit. For a woman with regular menstrual periods, the absence of one or more menses usually confirms the diagnosis. The objective diagnosis is based on the subjective symptoms of the pregnant woman and on certain clinical signs, which can be noted on physical examination and through laboratory procedures.

This chapter describes both obvious and subtle physical and psychologic changes caused by pregnancy. It also discusses the various cultural factors that can affect a woman's well-being during pregnancy.

Anatomy and Physiology of Pregnancy

The changes that occur in the pregnant woman's body are caused by several factors. Many changes are the results of hormonal influences, some are caused by the growth of the fetus inside the uterus, and some are a result of the mother's physical adaptation to the changes that are occurring.

Reproductive System

The changes in the body during pregnancy are most obvious in the organs of the reproductive system.

UTERUS

The changes in the uterus during pregnancy are phenomenal. Before pregnancy the uterus is a small, semisolid, pear-shaped organ measuring approximately 7.5 × 5 × 2.5 cm and weighing about 60 g (2 oz). At the end of pregnancy the dimensions are approximately 28 × 24 ×

311

21 cm, with an organ weight of approximately 1000 g (2.2 lb). Its capacity increases from 10 mL to 5 L or more.

The enlargement of the uterus is primarily a result of an increase in size (hypertrophy) of the preexisting myometrial cells. There is only a limited increase in cell number (hyperplasia). Individual cells have been shown to increase 17 to 40 times their prepregnancy size as a result of the stimulating influence of estrogen and the distention caused by the growing fetus. The amount of fibrous tissue between the muscle bands increases markedly, which adds to the strength and elasticity of the muscle wall.

The uterine walls are considerably thicker during the first few months of pregnancy than during the nonpregnant state. The initial changes are stimulated by increased estrogen and progesterone levels and not by mechanical distention by the products of conception. After approximately the third month, intrauterine pressure begins to be exerted by the uterine contents. The myometrial hypertrophy ceases at about the fifth lunar month and the musculature begins to distend, resulting in a thinning of the muscle wall to a thickness of about 5 mm or less at term. The ease of palpating the fetus through the abdominal wall attests to this thinning.

The circulatory requirements of the uterus increase as the uterus enlarges and the fetus and placenta develop. The size and number of the blood vessels and lymphatics increase greatly. By the end of pregnancy, one-sixth the total maternal blood volume is contained within the vascular system of the uterus.

Braxton Hicks contractions—irregular, generally painless contractions of the uterus—occur intermittently throughout pregnancy. They may be felt by careful palpation beginning about the fourth month of pregnancy. During a contraction, the previously relaxed uterus becomes firm or hard and then returns to the relaxed state. These contractions help stimulate the movement of blood through the intervillous spaces of the placenta (Danforth & Ueland 1986). Some mothers report that Braxton Hicks contractions late in pregnancy are more uncomfortable than early labor contractions. Multigravidas tend to report greater incidence of Braxton Hicks contractions than do primigravidas.

CERVIX

Estrogen stimulates the glandular tissue of the cervix, which increases in cell number and becomes hyperactive. The endocervical glands occupy about half the mass of the cervix at term, as compared to a small fraction in the nonpregnant state. They secrete a thick, tenacious mucus, which accumulates and thickens to form the mucous plug that seals the endocervical canal and prevents the ascent of bacteria or other substances into the uterus. This plug is expelled when cervical dilatation begins. The hyperactive glandular tissue also causes an increase in the normal phys-

iologic mucorrhea, at times resulting in a profuse discharge. Increased vascularization causes both softening and a blue-purple discoloration of the cervix (Chadwick's sign). Increased vascularization is a result of hypertrophy and engorgement of the vessels below the growing uterus.

OVARIES

The ovaries cease ovum production during pregnancy. Many follicles develop temporarily but never to the point of maturity. The cells lining these follicles, the thecal cells, become active in hormone production and have been called the *interstitial glands of pregnancy.*

The corpus luteum persists and produces hormones until about week 10 to 12 of pregnancy. It engulfs approximately a third of the ovary at its peak of hypertrophy. By the middle of pregnancy, it has regressed to almost complete obliteration. The progesterone it secretes maintains the endometrium until adequate progesterone is produced by the placenta to maintain the pregnancy.

VAGINA

The vaginal epithelium undergoes hypertrophy, increased vascularization, and hyperplasia during pregnancy. As with the cervical changes, these changes are estrogen-induced and result in a thickening of mucosa, a loosening of connective tissue, and an increase in vaginal secretions. The secretions are thick, white, and acidic (pH 3.5–6.0). The acid pH plays a significant role in preventing infections. However, it also favors the growth of yeast organisms, resulting in moniliasis, a common vaginal infection during pregnancy.

As in the uterus, the smooth muscle cells of the vagina become hypertrophied, with an accompanying loosening of the supportive connective tissue. By the end of pregnancy, the vaginal wall and perineal body have become sufficiently relaxed to permit distention of the tissues and passage of the infant.

Because the blood flow to the vagina is increased, it may show the same blue-purple color (Chadwick's sign) seen in the cervix.

BREASTS

Soon after the first menstrual period is missed, estrogen- and progesterone-induced changes are noted in the mammary glands. Increases in breast size and nodularity are the result of glandular hyperplasia and hypertrophy in preparation for lactation. By the end of the second month superficial veins are prominent, nipples are more erectile, and pigmentation of the areola is obvious. Hypertrophy of Montgomery's follicles is noted within the primary areola. Striae may develop as the pregnancy progresses. Breast changes are often most noticeable in the primigravida.

Colostrum, a yellow secretion, may be expressed or may leak from the breasts during the last trimester of pregnancy. This substance has more protein and minerals but less sugar and fat than mature milk. The antibody-rich colostrum persists for 2 to 4 days after delivery, gradually undergoing conversion to milk.

Respiratory System

Pulmonary function is modified throughout pregnancy (Table 14–1). Pregnancy induces a small degree of hyperventilation as the tidal volume (amount of air breathed with ordinary respiration) increases steadily throughout pregnancy. There is a 30 to 40 percent rise from nonpregnant values in the volume of air breathed each minute. Between weeks 16 and 40, oxygen consumption increases approximately 15 to 20 percent to meet the increased needs of the mother as well as those of the fetus and placenta. The vital capacity (maximum amount of air that can be moved in and out of the lungs with forced respiration) increases slightly, while lung compliance and pulmonary diffusion remain constant. Measurements of airway resistance show a marked decrease in pregnancy in response to elevated progesterone levels. This permits increases in oxygen consumption, carbon dioxide production, and in the respiratory functional reserve.

Table 14–1 Measurable Pregnancy Changes*

Parameter	Increase (%)	Decrease (%)	Unchanged
Respiratory system			
Tidal volume	30–40		
Respiratory rate			X
Resistance in tracheobronchial tree		36	
Expiratory reserve		40	
Residual volume		40	
Functional residual capacity		25	
Vital capacity			X
Respiratory minute volume	40		
Cardiovascular system			
Heart			
Rate	0–20		
Stroke volume	X		
Cardiac output	20–30		
Blood pressure			X
Peripheral blood flow	600		
Blood volume	48		
Blood constituents			
Leukocytes	70–100		
Fibrinogen	50		
Platelets	33		
Carbon dioxide		25	
Standard bicarbonate		10	
Proteins		15	
Lipids	33		
Phospholipids	30–40		
Cholesterol	100		
Gastrointestinal system			
Cardiac sphincter tone		X	
Acid secretion		X	
Motility		X	
Gallbladder emptying		X	
Urinary tract			
Renal plasma flow	25–50		
Glomerular filtration rate	50		
Ureter tone		X	
Ureteral motility			X
Metabolism			
Nitrogen stores	X		
Sodium stores	X		
Potassium stores	X		
Calcium stores	X		
Oxygen consumption	14		

*From Danforth DN (ed): *Obstetrics and Gynecology,* ed 4. Philadelphia, Harper & Row, 1982, p 339.

The diaphragm is elevated and the substernal angle is increased as a result of pressure from the enlarging uterus. This change causes the rib cage to flare, with a decrease in the vertical diameter and increases in the anteroposterior and transverse diameters. The circumference of the chest may increase by as much as 6 cm. The increase compensates for the elevated diaphragm, and there is no significant loss of intrathoracic volume. Breathing changes from abdominal to thoracic as pregnancy progresses, and descent of the diaphragm on inspiration becomes less possible.

Nasal "stuffiness" and epistaxis are not uncommon. They occur because of estrogen-induced edema and vascular congestion of the nasal mucosa.

Cardiovascular System

The growing uterus exerts pressure on the diaphragm, pushing the heart upward and to the left and rotating it forward. This lateral displacement makes the heart appear somewhat enlarged on x-ray examination.

Blood volume progressively increases throughout pregnancy, beginning in the first trimester and peaking in the middle of the third trimester at about 45 percent above nonpregnant levels. This increase is due to increases in both plasma and erythrocytes. The exact cause of these increases is not certain, although the increased secretion of aldosterone caused by elevated estrogen levels and the resulting salt and water retention may play a role (Key & Resnik 1986).

During pregnancy organ systems receive additional blood flow according to their increased workload. Thus blood flow to the uterus and kidneys increases, while hepatic and cerebral flow remains unchanged.

The pulse rate frequently increases during pregnancy, although the amount varies from almost no increase to an increase of 10 to 15 beats/min at term. The blood pressure decreases slightly during pregnancy, reaching its lowest point during the second trimester. The blood pressure then gradually increases during the third trimester and is near prepregnant levels at term.

The femoral venous pressure slowly rises as the uterus exerts increasing pressure on return blood flow. There is an increased tendency toward stagnation of blood in the lower extremities, with a resulting dependent edema and tendency toward varicose vein formation in the legs, vulva, and rectum late in pregnancy. The pregnant woman becomes more prone to develop postural hypotension because of the increased blood volume in the lower extremities.

The enlarging uterus may cause pressure on the vena cava when the woman lies supine, resulting in the *vena caval syndrome* or *supine hypotensive syndrome* (Figure 14–1). This pressure interferes with returning blood flow and produces a marked decrease in blood pressure with accompanying symptoms of dizziness, pallor, and clamminess. This may be prevented to a certain extent by the development of collateral circulation in the woman's back and abdominal wall.

The total red blood cell volume increases by 20 percent to 30 percent. This increase is necessary to transport the additional oxygen required during pregnancy (Key & Resnik 1986). Because the plasma volume increase is greater than the erythrocyte increase, the hematocrit, which measures the portion of whole blood that is composed of erythrocytes, decreases by an average of about 7 percent. This apparent decrease is referred to as the *physiologic anemia of pregnancy* (pseudoanemia).

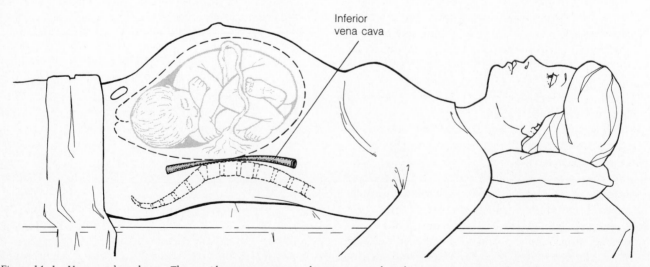

Inferior vena cava

Figure 14–1   Vena caval syndrome. The gravid uterus compresses the vena cava when the woman is supine. This reduces the blood flow returning to the heart and may cause maternal hypotension.

Iron is necessary for hemoglobin formation, and hemoglobin is the oxygen-carrying component of erythrocytes. Thus the increase in erythrocyte levels results in an increased need for iron by the pregnant woman. Even though the gastrointestinal absorption of iron is moderately increased during pregnancy, it is usually necessary to add supplemental iron to the diet to meet the expanded red blood cell and fetal needs.

Leukocyte production equals or is slightly greater than the increase in blood volume. The average cell count is 10,000 to 11,000/mm^3, with an occasional woman developing a physiologic leukocytosis of 15,000/mm^3. During labor and the early postpartum period these levels may reach 25,000/mm^3. Although an estrogen-related cause has been suggested, the reason for this dramatic increase remains unknown.

The fibrin level in the blood is increased by as much as 40 percent at term, and the plasma fibrinogen has been known to increase by as much as 50 percent. The increased fibrinogen accounts for the nonpathologic rise of the sedimentation rate. Although the clotting time of the pregnant woman does not differ significantly from that of the nonpregnant woman, blood factors VII, IX, and X are increased so that pregnancy becomes a somewhat hypercoagulable state. When these changes are coupled with venous stasis in late pregnancy, it becomes obvious that the pregnant woman has an increased risk of developing venous thrombosis.

Gastrointestinal System

Many of the discomforts of pregnancy are attributed to changes in the gastrointestinal system. Nausea and vomiting during the first trimester are associated with the hCG secreted by the nidated ovum and with a change in carbohydrate metabolism that occurs in early pregnancy. Peculiarities of taste and smell are common and can further aggravate gastrointestinal discomfort. Gum tissue may become softened and may bleed when only mildly traumatized. The secretion of saliva may increase or even become excessive (*ptyalism*). Gastric acidity decreases.

During the second half of pregnancy, numerous gastrointestinal symptoms are attributable to the pressure of the growing uterus and smooth muscle relaxation caused by elevated progesterone levels. The intestines are displaced laterally and posteriorly and the stomach superiorly. Heartburn (pyrosis) is caused by the reflux of acidic secretions from the stomach into the lower esophagus as a result of relaxation of the cardiac sphincter. Gastric emptying time and intestinal motility are delayed, leading to frequent complaints of bloating and constipation, which can be aggravated by the smooth muscle relaxation and increased electrolyte and water reabsorption in the large intestine. Hemorrhoids frequently develop if constipation is a prob-

lem or, in the second half of pregnancy, from pressure on vessels below the level of the uterus.

Only minor liver changes occur with pregnancy. Plasma albumin concentrations and serum cholinesterase activity decrease with normal pregnancy as with certain liver diseases.

The emptying time of the gallbladder is prolonged during pregnancy as a result of smooth muscle relaxation from progesterone. Hypercholesterolemia may follow, and it can predispose the woman to gallstone formation.

Urinary Tract

The kidneys, ureters, and bladder undergo striking changes in both structure and function. The growing uterus puts pressure on the bladder and bladder irritation is present until the uterus rises out of the pelvis. Near term, when the presenting part engages in the pelvis, pressure is again exerted on the bladder. This pressure can impair the drainage of blood and lymph from the hyperemic bladder, rendering it more susceptible to infection and trauma. The bladder, normally a convex organ, becomes concave from the external pressure, and its retention capacity is greatly reduced.

Dilation of the kidneys and ureter may occur, most frequently on the right side, above the pelvic brim, due to the lie of the uterus. This dilation is accompanied by elongation and curvature of the ureter. There appears to be no single factor accounting for this anatomic variation but a combination of ureteral atonia and hypoperistalsis, possibly caused by the placental progesterone and by pressure from the enlarging fetus. The same type of hydroureter and bladder relaxation can be produced in the nonpregnant female with massive doses of progesterone.

The glomerular filtration rate (GFR) and renal plasma flow (RPF) increase early in pregnancy. The GFR rises by as much as 50 percent by the beginning of the second trimester and remains elevated until delivery. The increase in RPF is slightly less and decreases somewhat during the third trimester (Pritchard et al 1985). The mechanism for these rises remains unclear, but hPL may play a part as it possesses properties similar to the pituitary growth hormone and has been shown experimentally to produce rises in GFR. Changes in posture definitely affect excretion of sodium and water in late pregnancy. However, the influence of posture on GFR and RPF is unclear, with different studies producing varying and contradictory results (Pritchard et al 1985).

An increased renal tubular reabsorption rate compensates for the increased glomerular activity. Amino acids and water soluble vitamins are excreted in greater amounts than in the nonpregnant woman. Glycosuria is not uncommon or necessarily pathogenic during pregnancy but is merely a reflection of the kidneys' inability to reabsorb all of the glucose filtered by the glomeruli. However, pregnancy can be diabetogenic, so the possibility of diabetes mellitus cannot be disregarded.

The increased renal function during pregnancy results in an increased clearance of urea and creatinine and in a lowering of the blood urea and nonprotein nitrogen values. Because of this, measurement of creatinine clearance provides an accurate test of renal functioning during pregnancy.

Skin

Changes in skin pigmentation commonly occur during pregnancy. These changes are stimulated by elevated levels of melanocyte-stimulating hormone, which may be caused by increased estrogen and progesterone levels.

The pigmentation of the skin increases primarily in areas that are already hyperpigmented: the areola, the nipples, the vulva, the perianal area, and the linea alba. The linea alba refers to the midline of the abdomen from the pubic area to the umbilicus and above. During pregnancy increased pigmentation may cause this area to darken. It is then referred to as the linea nigra (See Color Plate II). Some women also develop facial chloasma or the "mask of pregnancy." This is an irregular pigmentation of the cheeks, forehead, and nose that occurs in approximately 70 percent of women during pregnancy and is accentuated by sun exposure (Creasy & Resnik 1984). Similar changes may occur in women who are taking oral contraceptives. Facial chloasma is more prominent in dark-haired women and is occasionally disfiguring. Fortunately it fades, or at least regresses, soon after delivery when the hormonal influence of pregnancy has stopped. In addition, the sweat and sebaceous glands are frequently hyperactive during pregnancy.

Striae, or stretch marks, are reddish, wavy, depressed streaks that may occur over the abdomen, breasts, and thighs as pregnancy progresses. They are caused by reduced connective tissue strength. While distention may contribute to the formation of abdominal striae, a systemic hormone is also suspected (Creasy & Resnik 1984).

Vascular spider nevi may develop on the chest, neck, face, arms, and legs. They are small bright-red elevations of the skin radiating from a central body. They may be caused by increased subcutaneous blood flow in response to increased estrogen levels. This condition frequently occurs in conjunction with palmar erythema and is of no clinical significance. Both usually disappear shortly after the termination of pregnancy, when there is a decrease in estrogen levels in the tissues.

Hair growth may also be altered during pregnancy due to the effects of estrogen. The rate of hair growth may be decreased, and the number of hair follicles in the resting or dormant phase is also decreased. After delivery the number of hair follicles in the resting phase increases sharply and the woman may notice increased shedding of hair for three to four months. Practically all hair is replaced within six to nine months, however (Key & Resnik 1986).

Skeletal System

No demonstrable changes occur in the teeth of the pregnant woman. No demineralization takes place. The fairly common occurrence of dental caries during pregnancy has led to the myth, "A tooth for every pregnancy." The dental caries that may accompany pregnancy are likely to be caused by inadequate oral hygiene and dental care.

With a well-balanced diet the pregnant woman's calcium and phosphorus requirements of 1.2 g/day can be met. This is an increase of 0.4 g over the needs of the nonpregnant body.

The sacroiliac, sacrococcygeal, and pubic joints of the pelvis relax in the later part of the pregnancy, presumably as a result of hormonal changes. This often causes a waddling gait. A slight separation of the symphysis pubis can often be demonstrated on radiologic examination.

As the pregnant woman's center of gravity gradually changes, the lumbodorsal spinal curve is accentuated and posture changes (Figure 14–2). This posture change compensates for the increased weight of the uterus anteriorly and frequently results in low backache. Late in pregnancy, neck, shoulder, and upper extremity aching may occur from shoulder slumping and anterior flexion of the neck accompanying the lumbodorsal lordosis.

Metabolism

Most metabolic functions accelerate during pregnancy to support the additional demands of the growing fetus and its support system. The expectant mother must meet her own tissue replacement needs, those of the fetus, and those preparatory for labor and lactation. No other event in life induces such profound metabolic changes.

WEIGHT GAIN

The average weight gain during a normal pregnancy is 25 to 30 lb or 11.0 to 13.6 kg. Weight may decrease slightly during the first trimester due to the nausea, vomiting, and food intolerances of early pregnancy. The lost weight is soon regained, and an average increase of 3, 12, and 12 lb occurs in the first, second, and third trimesters, respectively. The total weight gain may be accounted for as follows: fetus, 7½ lb; placenta and membranes, 1½ lb; amniotic fluid, 2 lb; uterus, 2½ lb; breasts, 3 lb; and increased blood volume, 2 to 4 lb. The remaining 4 to 9 lb is extravascular fluid and fat reserves.

Adequate nutrition and weight gain are important during pregnancy. Maternal nutrition is discussed in detail in Chapter 17.

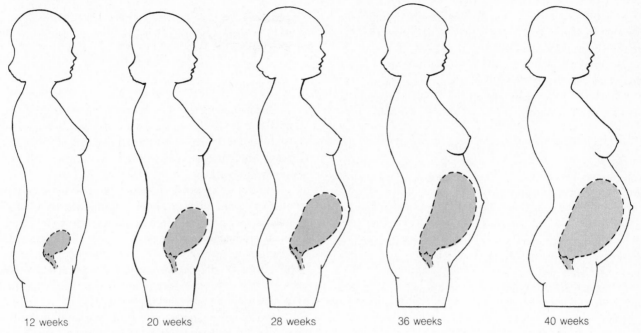

| 12 weeks | 20 weeks | 28 weeks | 36 weeks | 40 weeks |

Figure 14–2   Postural changes during pregnancy

WATER METABOLISM

Increased water retention is one of the basic chemical alterations of pregnancy. Several interrelated factors cause this phenomenon. The increased level of steroid sex hormones affects sodium and fluid retention. The lowered serum protein also influences the fluid balance, as does the increased intracapillary pressure and permeability. The products of conception—fetus, placenta, and amniotic fluid—account for an average increase of 3.5 L of water. Another increase of 3.5 L is contained within the mother's hypertrophied organs and augmented blood volume and interstitial fluids. The extracellular fluid is distributed primarily below the uterus, the area of elevated venous pressure.

NUTRIENT METABOLISM

The fetus makes its greatest protein and fat demands during the last half of gestation; it doubles in weight in the last 6 to 8 weeks. The increased nitrogen (*protein*) retention that begins in early pregnancy is initially used for hyperplasia and hypertrophy of maternal tissues, such as the uterus and breasts. Nitrogen must be stored during pregnancy to maintain a constant level within the breast milk and to avoid depletion of maternal tissues.

Fats are more completely absorbed during pregnancy, resulting in a marked increase in the serum lipids, lipoproteins, and cholesterol and decreased elimination through the bowel. Fat deposits in the fetus increase from about 2 percent at midpregnancy to almost 12 percent at term. The excess nitrogen and lipidemia are considered to be a preparation for lactation.

Carbohydrate needs increase, especially during the last two trimesters. Ketosis can be a problem, especially with the diabetic woman, due to glycosuria, reduced alkaline reserves, and lipidemia. Intermittent glycosuria is not uncommon during pregnancy. When it is not accompanied by a rise in blood sugar levels, glycosuria is a physiologic entity secondary to the increased glomerular filtration rate. Fasting blood sugar levels tend to fall slightly, returning to more normal levels by the sixth postpartal month. The oral glucose tolerance test shows no change with pregnancy.

The possibility of diabetes must not be overlooked during pregnancy. Plasma levels of insulin are increased during pregnancy, and rapid destruction of insulin takes place within the placenta. Insulin production must be increased by the mother, and any marginal pancreatic function quickly becomes apparent. The diabetic woman often experiences increased exogenous insulin demands during pregnancy.

MINERAL AND VITAMIN METABOLISM

The demand for *iron* during pregnancy is accelerated, and the pregnant woman must guard against anemia. Iron is necessary for the increase in erythrocytes, hemoglobin, and blood volume, as well as for the increased tissue demands of both woman and fetus.

Iron transfer takes place at the placenta in only one direction: toward the fetus. It has been demonstrated that approximately five-sixths of the iron stored in the fetal liver has been assimilated during the last trimester of pregnancy. This stored iron in the fetal liver compensates in the first four months of neonatal life for the normal inadequate amounts of iron available in breast milk and non-iron-fortified formulas.

The progressive absorption and retention of *calcium* during pregnancy has been noted. The maternal plasma concentration of bound calcium decreases as the levels of bindable plasma proteins fall. Approximately 30 g of calcium is retained in maternal bone for fetal deposition late in pregnancy.

Pregnancy produces little change in the metabolism of most other minerals other than retention of amounts needed for fetal growth.

Vitamin metabolism does not change appreciably with pregnancy (see Chapter 17 for requirements of minerals and vitamins).

Endocrine System

THYROID

Pregnancy influences the thyroid gland's size and activity. Often a palpable change is noted, which represents an increase in vascularity and hyperplasia of glandular tissue. The accompanying rise in the amount of iodine in the blood is in the form of total thyroxine (T_4), with thyroxine-binding capacity increasing as early as the third week of pregnancy and continuing until 6 to 12 weeks postpartum. Increased thyroxine-binding capacity is represented by the change in serum protein-bound iodine (PBI) from a non-pregnant level of 5 to 12 μg/dL to a pregnant level of 9 to 16 μg/dL. The cause is the increase in circulating estrogens; the same situation can be simulated by the exogenous administration of estrogens, including oral contraceptives, to the nonpregnant woman.

The basal metabolism rate (BMR) rises to a +25 percent level in late pregnancy. Most of the increase in oxygen consumption is a result of fetal metabolic activity. Blood studies and BMR indicate the existence of hyperthyroidism, but is it not present clinically. It should be noted that spontaneous abortion often occurs in the presence of hypothyroidism.

PARATHYROID

The concentration of the hormone secreted by the parathyroids and the size of the glands increase, paralleling the fetal calcium requirements. Parathyroid hormone concentration reaches its highest level of approximately two-

fold between 15 and 35 weeks of gestation, returning to a normal or even subnormal level before parturition.

PITUITARY

During pregnancy, the pituitary gland enlarges somewhat, but it returns to normal size after delivery. There is no significant change in the posterior lobe of the gland, although the anterior lobe increases in weight with each successive pregnancy.

Pregnancy is made possible by the hypothalamic stimulation of the anterior pituitary hormones: FSH, which stimulates ova growth, and LH, which effects ovulation. Pituitary stimulation prolongs the corpus luteal phase of the ovary, which maintains the secretory endometrium for development of the pregnancy. Two additional pituitary hormones, thyrotropin and adrenotropin, alter maternal metabolism to support the pregnancy. Prolactin, also an anterior pituitary secretion, is responsible for initial lactation. (Continued lactation depends on the suckling of the infant.)

The posterior pituitary contains the mechanism for the release of oxytocin and vasopressin, which exert oxytocic, vasopressor, and antidiuretic effects. The main effects of oxytocin are the promotion of uterine contractility and the stimulation of milk ejection from the breasts. Vasopressin causes vasoconstriction, which results in increased blood pressure; it also has an antidiuretic effect and plays an important role in the regulation of water balance. Vasopressin secretion is controlled by changes in plasma osmolarity and blood volume.

ADRENALS

Little structural change occurs in the adrenal glands during a normal pregnancy. Estrogen-induced increases in the levels of circulating cortisol result primarily from lowered renal excretion. The circulating cortisol levels regulate carbohydrate and protein metabolism. A normal level resumes one to six weeks postpartum.

The adrenals secrete increased levels of aldosterone by the early part of the second trimester. The levels of secretion are even more elevated in the woman on a sodium-restricted diet. This increase in aldosterone in a normal pregnancy may be the body's protective response to the increased sodium excretion associated with progesterone (Pritchard et al 1985).

PANCREAS

The pregnant woman has increased insulin needs. The islets of Langerhans are stressed to meet this increased demand, and a latent deficiency may become apparent during pregnancy, producing symptoms of gestational diabetes.

HORMONES IN PREGNANCY

Several hormones are required to maintain pregnancy. Most of these are produced initially by the corpus luteum; production is then assumed by the placenta. The hormones produced during pregnancy are human chorionic gonadotropin, human placental lactogen, estrogen, progesterone, and relaxin. (For an in-depth discussion of placental hormones, see Chapter 13.)

○ *HUMAN CHORIONIC GONADOTROPIN (hCG)* The trophoblast secretes hCG in early pregnancy. HCG stimulates progesterone and estrogen production by the corpus luteum to maintain the pregnancy until the placenta is developed sufficiently to assume that function.

○ *HUMAN PLACENTAL LACTOGEN (hPL)* Also called human chorionic somatomammotropin, hPL is produced by the syncytiotrophoblast. hPL is an antagonist of insulin; it increases the amount of circulating free fatty acids for maternal metabolic needs and decreases maternal metabolism of glucose.

○ *ESTROGEN* Secreted originally by the corpus luteum, estrogen is produced primarily by the placenta as early as the seventh week of pregnancy. Estrogen stimulates uterine development to provide a suitable environment for the fetus. It also helps to develop the ductal system of the breasts in preparation for lactation.

○ *PROGESTERONE* Progesterone, also produced initially by the corpus luteum and then by the placenta, plays the greatest role in maintaining pregnancy. It maintains the endometrium and inhibits spontaneous uterine contractility, thus preventing early spontaneous abortion due to uterine activity. Progesterone also helps develop the acini and lobules of the breasts in preparation for lactation.

○ *RELAXIN* Relaxin is detectable in the serum of a pregnant woman by the time of the first missed menstrual period. Relaxin inhibits uterine activity, diminishes the strength of uterine contractions, aids in the softening of the cervix, and has the long-term effect of remodeling collagen. Its primary source is the corpus luteum, but small amounts are believed to be produced by the placenta and decidua.

PROSTAGLANDINS IN PREGNANCY

Prostaglandins (PGs) are lipid substances that can arise from most body tissues but occur in high concentrations in the female reproductive tract and are present in the decidua during pregnancy. The exact functions of PGs during pregnancy are still unknown, but they play a role in the complex biochemistry that initiates labor.

● Subjective (Presumptive) Changes

The subjective changes of pregnancy are the symptoms the woman experiences and reports. They can be caused by other conditions (Table 14–2) and therefore cannot be considered proof of pregnancy. The following can be diagnostic clues when other signs and symptoms of pregnancy are also present.

Amenorrhea is the earliest symptom of pregnancy. In a healthy woman whose menstrual cycles are regular, missing one or more menstrual periods leads to the consideration of pregnancy.

Nausea and vomiting are experienced by almost half of all pregnant women during the first three months of pregnancy and result from elevated hCG levels and changed carbohydrate metabolism. The woman may feel merely a distaste for food or may suffer extreme vomiting. These symptoms frequently occur in the early part of the

Table 14–2 Differential Diagnosis of Pregnancy—Subjective Changes

Subjective changes	Possible causes
Amenorrhea	Endocrine factors: early menopause; lactation; thyroid, pituitary, adrenal, ovarian dysfunction Metabolic factors: malnutrition, anemia, climatic changes, diabetes mellitus, degenerative disorders, long-distance running Psychologic factors: emotional shock, fear of pregnancy or sexually transmitted disease, intense desire for pregnancy (pseudocyesis), stress Obliteration of endometrial cavity by infection or curettage Systemic disease (acute or chronic), such as tuberculosis or malignancy
Nausea and vomiting	Gastrointestinal disorders Acute infections such as encephalitis Emotional disorders such as pseudocyesis or anorexia nervosa
Urinary frequency	Urinary tract infection Cystocele Pelvic tumors Urethral diverticula Emotional tension
Breast tenderness	Premenstrual tension Chronic cystic mastitis Pseudocyesis Hyperestrinism
Quickening	Increased peristalsis Flatus ("gas") Abdominal muscle contractions Shifting of abdominal contents

day and disappear within a few hours and hence are commonly called *morning sickness.* Some women may complain of nausea or vomiting in late afternoon and evening, especially in association with fatigue. This gastrointestinal disturbance usually appears about the end of the first month of pregnancy and disappears spontaneously six to eight weeks later, although it may be prolonged in some instances. Recent research suggests that women who vomit in early pregnancy have a decreased incidence of spontaneous abortion, stillbirth, or premature labor (Klebanoff et al 1985).

Excessive fatigue may be noted within a few weeks after the first missed menstrual period and may persist throughout the first trimester.

Urinary frequency is experienced during the first trimester. In the early weeks of pregnancy the enlarging uterus is still a pelvic organ and exerts pressure on the bladder. The increased vascularization and pelvic congestion that occurs in each pregnancy can also cause frequent voiding. This symptom decreases during the second trimester, when the uterus is an abdominal organ, but reappears during the third trimester when the presenting part descends into the pelvis.

Changes in the breasts are frequently noted in early pregnancy. Some women report significant breast changes prior to missing their first menses. Engorgement of the breasts due to the hormone-induced growth of the secretory ductal system results in the subjective symptoms of tenderness and tingling, especially of the nipple area.

Quickening, or the mother's perception of fetal movement, occurs about 18 to 20 weeks after the LMP in primigravidas but may occur as early as 16 weeks in multigravidas. Quickening is a fluttering sensation in the abdomen that gradually increases in intensity and frequency.

● **Objective (Probable) Changes**

An examiner can perceive the objective changes that occur in pregnancy. They are more diagnostic than the subjective symptoms. However, their presence does not offer a definite diagnosis of pregnancy (Table 14–3).

Changes in the pelvic organs caused by increased vascular congestion are the only physical signs detectable within the first three months of pregnancy. These changes are noted on pelvic examination. There is a softening of the cervix, called *Goodell's sign. Chadwick's sign* is the deep red to purple or bluish coloration of the mucous membranes of the cervix, vagina, and vulva due to increased vasocongestion of the pelvic vessels. (Pritchard et al [1985] consider Chadwick's sign a presumptive sign, while Danforth and Scott [1986] consider it an objective sign.) *Hegar's sign* is a softening of the isthmus of the uterus, the area between the cervix and the body of the uterus, which

Table 14–3 Differential Diagnosis of Pregnancy—Objective Changes

Objective changes	Possible causes
Changes in pelvic organs	Increased vascular congestion
Goodell's sign	Estrogen-progestin oral contraceptives
Chadwick's sign	Vulvar, vaginal, cervical hyperemia
Hegar's sign	Excessively soft walls of nonpregnant uterus
Uterine enlargement	Uterine tumors
Braun von Fernwald's sign	Uterine tumors
Piskacek's sign	Uterine tumors
Enlargement of abdomen	Obesity, ascites, pelvic tumors
Braxton Hicks contractions	Hematometra, pedunculated, submucous and soft myomas
Uterine souffle	Large uterine myomas, large ovarian tumors, or any condition with greatly increased uterine blood flow
Pigmentation of skin	Estrogen-progestin oral contraceptives
Chloasma	
Linea nigra	Melanocyte hormonal stimulation
Nipples/areola	
Abdominal striae	Obesity, pelvic tumor
Ballottement	Uterine tumors/polyps, ascites
Pregnancy tests	Increased pituitary gonadotropins at menopause, choriocarcinoma, hydatidiform mole
Palpation for fetal outline	Uterine myomas

occurs at six to eight weeks of pregnancy. This area may become so soft that on a bimanual exam there seems to be nothing between the cervix and the body of the uterus (Figure 14–3). *Ladin's sign* is a soft spot anteriorly in the middle of the uterus near the junction of the body of the uterus and cervix (Figure 14–4A). *McDonald's sign* is an ease in flexing the body of the uterus against the cervix.

The uterus assumes an irregular globular shape during the early months of pregnancy. Irregular softening and enlargement at the site of implantation, known as *Braun von Fernwald's sign,* occurs about the fifth week (Figure 14–4B). Occasionally an almost tumorlike asymmetrical enlargement occurs, called *Piskacek's sign* (Figure 14–4C). Generalized enlargement and softening of the body of the uterus are present after the eighth week of pregnancy. The fundus of the uterus is palpable just above the symphysis pubis at approximately 10 to 12 weeks' gestation and at the level of the umbilicus at 20 to 22 weeks' gestation (Figure 14–5).

Enlargement of the abdomen during the childbearing years is usually regarded as evidence of pregnancy, especially if the enlargement is progressive and is accompanied

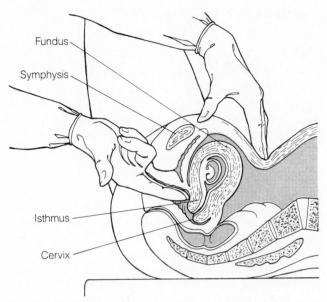

Figure 14–3 Hegar's sign

by a continuing amenorrhea. It is usually more pronounced in a multiparous woman whose abdominal musculature has lost some of its tone.

As mentioned earlier, *Braxton Hicks contractions* are ordinarily painless contractions that occur at irregular intervals throughout pregnancy but are felt more commonly after week 28. As the woman approaches the end of the pregnancy, these contractions may become more uncomfortable and are then often called "false labor."

Uterine souffle may be heard when auscultating the abdomen over the uterus. It is a soft blowing sound at the same rate as the maternal pulse and is due to the increased uterine vascularization and the blood pulsating through the placenta.

Changes in pigmentation of the skin and the *appearance of abdominal striae* are common manifestations in pregnancy. Facial *chloasma* occurs in varing degrees in pregnant women after week 16. The pigmentation of the nipple and areola may darken, especially in primigravidas and dark-haired women. The Montgomery glands of the areola may become enlarged. The skin in the midline of the abdomen may develop a pigmented line, the *linea nigra* (Color Plate II), which may also include the umbilicus and surrounding area. As the uterus enlarges, striae appear on the abdomen and buttocks as the underlying connective tissue breaks down. These changes occur in about one-half of all pregnant women.

The *fetal outline* may be identified by palpation in many pregnant women after 24 weeks of gestation, becoming easier to distinguish as term approaches. *Ballottement* is the passive fetal movement elicited by tapping the cervix with two fingers. This pushes the fetal body up and, as it falls back, the examiner feels a rebound.

Pregnancy tests are based on analysis of maternal blood or urine for the detection of human chorionic gonadotropin (hCG), the hormone secreted by the trophoblast. These tests are not considered positive signs of pregnancy because the similarity of hCG and the pituitary-secreted LH occasionally results in cross-reactions. In addition, certain conditions other than pregnancy can cause elevated levels of hCG.

● **Pregnancy Tests**

Most pregnancy tests in the past were bioassays that used laboratory animals. These tests were time-consuming and subject to error. Consequently they have been replaced by immunoassays and radioreceptor assay tests.

Immunoassay

The immunologic pregnancy tests are based on the antigenic property of hCG. There are three types of tests:

1. *Hemagglutination-inhibition test (Pregnosticon R).* No clumping of cells occurs when the urine of a preg-

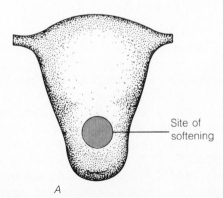

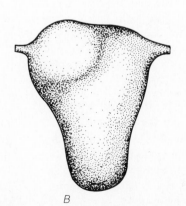

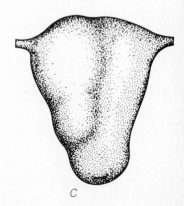

Figure 14–4 Early uterine changes in pregnancy: A Ladin's sign. B Braun von Fernwald's sign. C Piskacek's sign

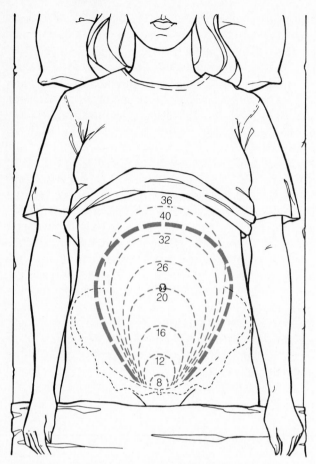

Figure 14–5 *Approximate height of the fundus at various weeks of pregnancy*

nant woman is added to the hCG-sensitized red blood cells of sheep.

2. *Latex agglutination tests* (*Gravindex and Pregnosticon slide test*). Latex particle agglutination is inhibited in the presence of urine containing hCG.

These two tests are approximately 95 percent accurate in diagnosing pregnancy and 98 percent accurate in determining the absence of pregnancy. The tests become positive approximately 10 to 14 days after the first missed menstrual period. The specimen used for the tests is the first early morning midstream urine because it is adequately concentrated for accuracy. The presence of protein substances (such as blood) in the specimen should be avoided because false positive results may occur.

3. *β subunit radioimmunoassay or RIA.* This test uses an antiserum with specificity for the β subunit of hCG in blood plasma. This is the most accurate pregnancy test. It requires about one hour to complete and becomes positive a few days after presumed implantation, thereby permitting earlier diagnosis of pregnancy. This test is also used in the diagnosis of ectopic pregnancy or trophoblastic disease.

Radioreceptor Assay (RRA)

Radioreceptor assay (Biocept-G) uses radio-iodine-labeled hCG. It is a sensitive test and can be quickly performed in one hour, but because it fails to distinguish between hCG and LH, cross-reactions may occur.

Over-the-Counter Pregnancy Tests

Over-the-counter pregnancy tests are available at the local pharmacy or drugstore for approximately $10. These tests, performed on urine, employ the hemagglutination-inhibition or the β subunit antibody principle. The false positive rate of these tests is approximately 5 percent, while the false negative rate is approximately 20 percent. One study of users found the false negative rate to be almost 25 percent. Furthermore, only one-third of the users complied with the test kit instructions (Pritchard et al 1985).

Home pregnancy test instructions are quite explicit and should be followed carefully to get optimum results. Best results are obtained when the first morning-voided clear urine specimen is collected in a new container or in a clean container free of detergents or contaminants. Exact measurements must be made of urine and reagents. The test tube must remain undisturbed for the appropriate time, free of heat, vibration, or direct sunlight, although the newer kits do state that they are not sensitive to vibration. The reading must be made at the appropriate time. The tests vary in their ability to identify a pregnancy, ranging from three to nine days after the expected last menstrual period.

Opinion varies about the advisability of making these tests available to the general public. Proponents suggest that the results will encourage women to seek care earlier in the event of pregnancy. Opponents suggest that once a woman has her pregnancy confirmed she may delay seeking care. They also believe that false results may lead to unnecessary anxiety or, more importantly, a false sense of security or even relief.

● Diagnostic (Positive) Changes

The positive signs of pregnancy are completely objective, cannot be confused with pathologic states, and offer conclusive proof of pregnancy, but they are usually not present until after the fourth month of pregnancy.

The *fetal heartbeat* can be detected with a fetoscope by approximately week 17 to 20 of pregnancy. With the electronic Doppler device, it is possible to detect the fetal heartbeat as early as week 10 to 12. The fetal heart rate is between 120 and 160 beats/min and must be counted and compared with the maternal pulse for differentiation. Auscultation of the abdomen may reveal sounds other than that of the fetal heart. The maternal pulse, emanating from the abdominal aorta, may be unusually loud or a uterine souffle may be heard.

Fetal movements are actively palpable by a trained examiner after about week 18 of pregnancy. They vary from a faint flutter in the early months to more vigorous movements late in pregnancy.

In the past radiologic examination was occasionally used to diagnose pregnancy. This technique is no longer used, however, because of the possibility of causing gonadal damage and genetic abnormalities.

Fetal electrocardiographic evidence has been recorded as early as day 84 of pregnancy and offers proof of a living fetus. Failure to detect fetal cardiac electrical activity does not exclude pregnancy, however, nor does it necessarily indicate the death of a fetus.

Ultrasound is a technique that can be used for a positive diagnosis as early as the sixth week of pregnancy. The gestational sac can be observed by 5 to 6 weeks' gestation (3 to 4 weeks after conception); fetal parts and fetal heart movement can be seen as early as 10 weeks. Fetal movement can be detected with the real-time methods at approximately 12 weeks after the LMP (10 weeks after conception). (See Chapter 20 for further discussion.)

● **Psychologic Response of the Expectant Family to Pregnancy**

Pregnancy is a developmental challenge, a turning point, in a family's life and therefore is accompanied by stress and anxiety whether the pregnancy is desired or not. Pregnancy confirms one's biologic capabilities to reproduce. It is evidence of one's participation in sexual activity and as such is an affirmation of one's sexuality. For beginning families pregnancy is the transition period from childlessness to parenthood. If the pregnancy terminates in the birth of a child, the couple enters a new stage of their life together, one that is irreversible and characterized by awesome responsibilities.

The expectant couple may be unaware of the physical, emotional, and cognitive states peculiar to pregnancy. The couple may anticipate no problem from such a normal event as pregnancy and therefore may be confused and distressed by the feelings and behaviors commonly associated with childbearing.

If the expectant woman is married or has a stable partner, she no longer is only a mate but also must assume the role of mother. Her partner will soon be a father. Career goals and mobility may be altered or thwarted for one or both partners. Each partner begins to see the other in a different light. Their relationship takes on a different meaning to them and within the larger family and community. Their life-style changes. Role reorientation and re-identification are inevitable with each additional pregnancy and

child. The set routines, family dynamics, and interactions are altered again with each pregnancy and require readjustment and realignment.

Even if a pregnant woman is without a stable partner, by design or circumstance, but plans to keep the baby or place it for adoption, she will still experience changes in role identity and psychobiologic maturation. The woman is no longer a separate individual. She must now consider the needs of another being who is totally dependent on her, at least during the pregnancy.

Decisions regarding financial matters also need to be made at this time. Will the woman work during the pregnancy and return to work after the baby is born? If she chooses to return to work, how soon after the birth of the child will she return? Many individuals have strong feelings about men being providers and caretakers of their families. Decisions may also need to be made about the division of tasks within the home. If the woman expects to share household and child-care tasks with the man, but he believes that women take care of home and children and men provide the income, conflicts will inevitably arise. When these differences are discussed openly, needs are identified, and solutions developed mutually, the newly forming family moves toward meeting the needs of its members.

Colman and Colman (1971) undertook a comprehensive study of parents' reactions to pregnancy. They found that, although it is a time of crisis, pregnancy can be a rewarding experience, especially if the couple has formed a trusting alliance and are sincere in their desire to share every aspect of the experience. However, a weak relationship is often in greater jeopardy during pregnancy, especially if the man is forced to become involved in childbirth education classes and to be the woman's coach during labor and her supporter in the delivery room.

The couple must face the realities of labor and delivery before parenthood can be realized. Many nonparents have little idea what labor entails. Their information is frequently based on experiences related to them by family members or friends, and these tales are often fraught with myths and exaggerations. Classes in prepared childbirth can help them overcome much of this lack of information or misinformation.

Labor is threatening in many respects. Pain, disfigurement, disruption of bodily function, and even death are potential threats for the woman. The man faces the potential disfigurement of his wife, impairment of her health, or her death. Both fear that the baby may be ill or disfigured. The expectant couple is subject to anxiety during this period, and no one can reassure them about the outcome.

For some couples pregnancy is more than a developmental stage; it is a crisis. *Crisis* can be defined as a disturbance or conflict in which the individual cannot maintain a state of equilibrium. Habitual problem-solving techniques are inadequate. Any natural turning point (courtship, pregnancy, parenthood, death, or loss of a loved one) that necessitates intrapersonal and interpersonal changes and reorganization can precipitate a crisis.

Pregnancy can be considered a *maturational crisis,* since it is a common event in the normal growth and development of the family. During such a crisis, the individual or family is in disequilibrium. Egos weaken, usual defense mechanisms lose their effectiveness, unresolved material from the past reappears, and relationships shift. The period of disequilibrium and disorganization is characterized by abortive attempts to solve the perceived problems. If the crisis is unresolved, it will result in maladaptive behaviors in one or more family members, and possible disintegration of the family. Families who are able to resolve a maturational crisis successfully will return to normal functioning and can even strengthen the bonds in the family relationship.

Crisis and its potential for successful resolution are affected by the individual or family's (a) present level of organization or disorganization; (b) past experiences of success or failure with crisis, stress, and anxiety; (c) established coping patterns, productive or unproductive; and (d) availability and effectiveness of resources and support persons. What one person considers a crisis may not be perceived as a crisis by another. Previous experience, for example, may alter an individual's perception of the event.

Pregnancy as a Developmental Stage

Pregnancy can be viewed as a developmental stage with its own distinct developmental tasks. Pregnancy can be a time of support or conflict for a couple, depending on the amount of adjustment each is willing to make to maintain the family's equilibrium.

During pregnancy the couple plans together for the first child's arrival, collecting information on how to be parents. At the same time each continues to participate in some separate activities with friends or family members. The availability of social support is an important factor in psychosocial well-being during pregnancy. For example, Cronenwett (1985) found that availability of emotional and material support (financial assistance, gifts, help with housework, etc) is positively associated with postpartum outcomes for couples. During this time relatives tend to dominate a couple's social network. While men derive most emotional support from relatives, however, women derive somewhat less support from relatives and somewhat more support from friends (Cronenwett 1985).

Although individual activities are important, some conflict may arise if the couple's activities become too divergent. Thus they may find it necessary to limit their outside associations.

During pregnancy the expectant mother and father both face significant changes and must deal with major psychosocial adjustments (Table 14–4). Other family members, especially the couple's other children and the grandparents-to-be, must also adjust to the pregnancy.

The Mother

Pregnancy is a condition that alters body image and also necessitates a reordering of social relationships and changes in roles of family members. The way a particular woman meets the stresses of pregnancy is influenced by her emotional makeup, her sociologic and cultural background, and her acceptance or rejection of the pregnancy. Many women manifest similar psychologic and emotional responses during pregnancy, including ambivalence, acceptance, introversion, mood swings, and changes in body image.

AMBIVALENCE

Initially, even if the pregnancy is planned, there is an element of surprise that conception has occurred. This feeling is generally coupled with a feeling that the timing is wrong, that pregnancy is desirable "some day" but "not now" (Rubin 1970). The reasons women cite may vary widely—long-term plans, job commitments, financial stress, the needs of an existing child—but the general feeling is that one is not ready to have a child at this time. This feeling accounts for much of the ambivalence commonly experienced by women during early pregnancy. Ambivalence may also be related to the need to modify personal relationships or career plans, to fear coupled with excitement about assuming a new role, to unresolved emotional conflicts with one's own mother, and to fears about pregnancy, labor, and delivery. Such feelings may be even more pronounced in the event of an unplanned or unwanted pregnancy. Women who feel comfortable addressing the issue of ambivalence tend to focus on two main areas: changed life-style, including the career-motherhood dilemma, and financial security. Indirect evidence of ambivalence includes complaints about depression, physical discomfort, and feeling "ugly" and unattractive (Lederman 1984).

During the early months the pregnant woman may seriously consider the possibilty of an abortion if the pregnancy is unwanted. In the event of religious conflicts about induced abortion, the woman may experience guilt feelings about her thoughts or may tend to focus on the possibility of spontaneous abortion (miscarriage). Even when the pregnancy is consciously planned and desired, thoughts of abortion and miscarriage arise. The idea that the baby might be lost has a certain emotional appeal because it represents the possible relief of fears and ambivalence.

ACCEPTANCE

Acceptance of pregnancy is influenced by many factors. Lower acceptance tends to be related to an unplanned pregnancy and greater evidence of fear and conflict. The woman carrying an unplanned pregnancy tends to experience more physical discomfort and depression. When a pregnancy is well accepted, on the other hand, the woman demonstrates feelings of happiness and pleasure in the pregnancy. She experiences less physical discomfort and shows a high degree of tolerance for the discomforts associated with the third trimester (Lederman 1984).

During the *first trimester,* evidence of pregnancy is limited to amenorrhea and to the word of the care giver that the pregnancy test was positive. In an effort to verify her condition a woman may become minutely conscious of changes in her body that could validate the pregnancy. She closely watches for thickening of her waist, breast development, and weight increase. During the first trimester the woman's baby does not seem real to her and she focuses on herself and her pregnancy (Rubin 1984).

The *second trimester* is relatively tranquil. Morning sickness generally passes, the threat of spontaneous abortion diminishes, and the woman begins to accept the reality of her pregnancy (Figure 14–6). It is not unusual for an enthusiastic primagravida to don maternity clothes at the beginning of this trimester even when it is not truly necessary. The clothing serves as a verification of her pregnant state.

The highlight of the second trimester is quickening, which generally occurs about week 20—midway through the pregnancy. Actual perception of fetal movement frequently produces dramatic changes in the woman. She now perceives her baby as a real person and generally becomes excited about the pregnancy even if she hasn't been prior to this time.

As quickening and her altered physical appearance confirm her pregnant state, the woman adjusts to the idea of change and begins to prepare for her new role and her new set of relationships—with her partner and family, the child-to-be and other children, friends, and loved ones.

Table 14–4 Parental Reactions to Pregnancy

First trimester		Second trimester (continued)	
Mother's reactions	**Father's reactions**	**Mother's reactions**	**Father's reactions**
Informs father secretively or openly	Differ according to age, parity, desire for child, economic stability	Remains regressive and introspective; all problems with authority figures projected onto partner; may become angry as if lack of interest is sign of weakness in him	If he can cope, will give her extra attention she needs; if he cannot cope, will develop a new time-consuming interest outside of home
Feels ambivalent toward pregnancy; anxious about labor and responsibility of child	Acceptance of pregnant woman's attitude or complete rejection and lack of communication	Continues to deal with feelings as a mother and looks for furniture as something concrete	May develop a creative feeling and a "closeness to nature"
Is aware of physical changes; daydreams of possible miscarriage	Is aware of his own sexual feelings; may develop more or less sexual arousal	May have other extreme of anxiety and wait until ninth month to look for furniture and clothes for baby	May become involved in pregnancy and buy or make furniture
Develops special feelings for, renewed interest in mother, with formation of own mother identity	Accepts, rejects, or resents mother-in-law		
	May develop new hobby outside family as sign of stress		

Second trimester		Third trimester	
Mother's reactions	**Father's reactions**	**Mother's reactions**	**Father's reactions**
Feels movement and is aware of fetus and incorporates it into herself	Feels for movement of baby, listens to heartbeat, or remains aloof with no physical contact	Experiences more anxiety and tension, with physical awkwardness	Adapts to alternative methods of sexual contact
Dreams that partner will be killed, telephones him often for reassurance	May have fears and fantasies about himself being pregnant; may become uneasy with this feminine aspect in himself	Feels much discomfort and insomnia from physical condition	Becomes concerned over financial responsibility
Experiences more distinct physical changes; sexual desires may increase or decrease	May react negatively if partner is too demanding; may become jealous of physician and of his/her importance to partner and her pregnancy	Prepares for delivery, assembles layette, picks out names	May show new sense of tenderness and concern; treats partner like doll
		Dreams often about misplacing baby or not being able to deliver it; fears birth of deformed baby	Daydreams about child as if older and not newborn; dreams of losing partner
		Feels ecstasy and excitement; has spurt of energy during last month	Renewed sexual attraction to partner
			Feels ultimately responsible for whatever happens

When the pregnancy is well accepted, the woman takes pleasure in the sensations of pregnancy and attempts to picture her baby in order to know him or her better. The woman may avidly delve into folklore regarding the child's sex and may carefully study photos of herself and her partner to gain some clues about her child's appearance. She may ask her friends about childbirth and seek out other women who are pregnant or have recently given birth. She feels well, is excited, and may exhibit the "glow" so often attributed to pregnant women.

The *third trimester* combines a sense of pride with anxiety about what is to come in order for the child to be born. During this time the special prerogatives of pregnancy may be most marked. As her protruding abdomen proclaims her advanced pregnancy, the woman may find that others become more solicitous, that a chair may be offered in a crowded room, that others may carry her parcels. The woman may actually need this help, she may simply enjoy it as a privilege of pregnancy, or she may reject it if she fears that such gestures indicate she is helpless.

During the final trimester physical discomforts again increase, and adequate rest becomes a necessity. The woman, eager for the pregnancy to end, wonders if her expected date of delivery is accurate. She makes final preparation for the baby and may spend long periods considering names for the child.

Rubin (1970) points out that during this time the woman feels very vulnerable to rejection, loss, or insult. She may worry about a variety of things and hesitate to go out unless accompanied by someone she is certain cares about her. She may withdraw into the security and quiet of her home. Toward the end of this period there is often a burst of energy as the woman prepares the "nest" for her expected infant. Many women report bursts of energy in which they vigorously clean and organize their homes.

INTROVERSION

Introversion, or turning in on one's self, is a common occurrence in pregnancy. An active, outgoing woman may becomes less interested in previous activities and more concerned with needs for rest and time alone. This concentration of attention permits the woman to plan, adjust, adapt, build, and draw strength in preparation for her child's birth (Rubin 1975). As she becomes more aware of herself, her partner may feel she is being overly sensitive. He may perceive her introversion and passivity as exclusion

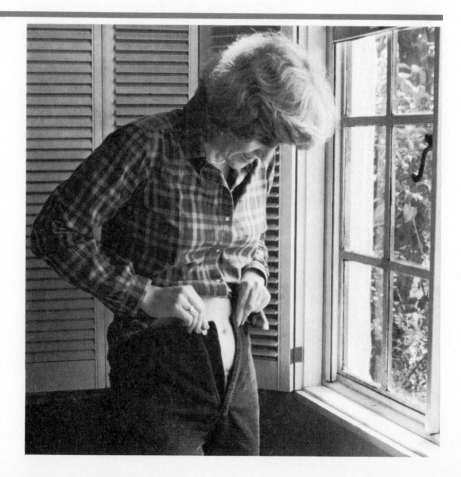

Figure 14–6 During the second trimester the most obvious evidence of pregnancy is the woman's expanding abdomen.

of him and may in turn become unable to interact with her, either verbally or physically, or to provide the affection, support, and consideration she requires (Stickler et al 1978). This change in relationships may result in disequilibrium and stress for the entire family. It is essential that the couple work together to establish new, mutually acceptable patterns of response in order to overcome these blocks to communication.

I don't know if this is really considered a problem or not, but at times it seems like a problem. I'm really subject to drastic mood changes. That, or I'll be extremely emotional. For no reason at all I'll start crying or just laugh until I can hardly breathe. I don't know why; and if I can't understand it, it's twice as hard for John, especially if I'm bummed out or crying. It doesn't seem normal for a person to cry for no reason and I never did it before. (Quoted in *Psychosocial Adaptation to Pregnancy*)

MOOD SWINGS

Throughout pregnancy the emotions of many women are characterized by mood swings, from great joy to deep despair. Frequently the woman will become tearful with little apparent cause. When asked why she is crying, she may find it difficult or impossible to give a reason. The situation is extremely unsettling for the partner, causing him to feel confused and inadequate. Because the man may feel unable to handle the woman's tears, he often reacts by withdrawing and ignoring the problem. Since the pregnant woman needs increased love and affection, she may perceive his reaction as unloving and nonsupportive. Once the couple understands that this behavior is characteristic of pregnancy, it becomes easier for them to deal with it more effectively—although it will be a source of stress to some extent throughout pregnancy.

CHANGES IN BODY IMAGE

Body image refers to the mental image or picture one has of his or her body. It involves personal attitudes, feelings, and perceptions and may be influenced by environmental, cultural, temporal, physiologic, psychologic, and interpersonal factors. Thus it is dynamic and ever changing.

Pregnancy produces marked changes in a woman's body within a relatively short period of time. Women perceive that they require more body space as pregnancy progresses (Fawcett et al 1986). They also experience changes in body image. The degree of this change is related to a certain extent to personality factors, social network responses, and attitudes toward pregnancy. However, research suggests that women tend to feel somewhat negative about their bodies by the third trimester of pregnancy (Strang & Sullivan 1985).

Body boundary is another aspect of body image. It is the boundary that defines self, "containing and demar-cating self as an entity separate from the surroundings" (Rubin 1984, p 17). When the body boundary is definite, the body is seen as firm, strong, and distinct from its environment. Body boundary vulnerability occurs when the body boundary is perceived as delicate, capable of being penetrated, and not readily distinguishable from its environment. The pregnant woman may feel both increased body boundary definitions and body boundary vulnerability during pregnancy, which suggests that the woman may perceive her body as vulnerable and yet as a protective container (Fawcett 1978).

Changes in body image are normal but can be very stressful for the pregnant woman. Explanation of the changes and discussion of the alterations in body image may help both the woman and her partner deal with the stress associated with this aspect of pregnancy.

PSYCHOLOGIC TASKS OF THE MOTHER

Rubin (1984) has identified four major tasks that the pregnant woman undertakes to maintain her intactness and that of her family and at the same time incorporate her new child into the family system. These tasks form the foundation for a mutually gratifying relationship with her infant:

1. *Ensuring safe passage through pregnancy, labor, and birth.* The pregnant woman feels concern for both her unborn child and herself. She seeks competent maternity care to provide a sense of control and wishes to establish a relationship with her nurse-midwife or physician so that they "know" her and her needs. During this time the woman seeks knowledge from literature, observation of other pregnant women and new mothers, and discussion with others who have borne children. In the third trimester, as her movements slow and her body mass increases, she becomes aware of external threats in the environment—a toy on a stair, the awkwardness of an escalator—that pose a threat to her intactness and represent hazards to be overcome. External threats become more significant, and the woman worries if her partner is late or she is home alone. Sleep becomes difficult and she begins to long for delivery even though it, too, is frightening.

2. *Seeking of acceptance of this child by others.* The birth of a child alters a woman's primary support group, her family, and her secondary affiliative groups. During the first trimester, the woman may feel sorrow at the anticipated changes, but in most cases the transition from existing social groupings to newer groupings occurs smoothly. The family generally makes the transition, and the woman slowly and subtly alters her secondary network to meet the needs of her pregnancy. In this adjustment the wom-

an's partner is the most important figure. His support and acceptance influence her completion of her maternal tasks, the formation of her maternal identity, indeed the entire course of her pregnancy. If there are other children in the home the mother also works to ensure their acceptance of the coming child. Accepting the coming change in exclusive relationships—woman and partner or mother and first child—is sometimes stressful, and the woman will often work to maintain some special time with her partner or older child. Achieving social acceptance of the child and herself as mother may be more difficult for the adolescent mother or single woman. The child to come is not always wanted, and the woman often must direct her energies to changing this situation.

3. *Seeking of commitment and acceptance of self as mother to the infant (binding-in).* During the first trimester the child remains a rather abstract concept. With quickening, however, the child begins to become a real person, and the mother begins to develop bonds of attachment. The mother experiences the movement of the child within her in an intimate exclusive way, and out of this experience bonds of love form. The mother develops a fantasy image of her ideal child. This possessive love increases her maternal commitment to protect her fetus now and her child after he or she is born.

4. *Learning to give of oneself on behalf of one's child.* Childbirth involves many acts of giving. The man "gives" a child to a woman; she in turn "gives" a child to the man. Life is given to an infant, a sibling is given to older children of the family. The woman begins to develop a capacity for self-denial and learns to delay immediate personal gratification to meet the needs of another. Baby showers and baby gifts are acts of giving that help the mother's self-esteem while also helping her acknowledge the separateness and needs of the coming baby.

Accomplishment of these tasks helps the expectant woman develop her self-concept as mother. Often the expectant mother turns to her own mother during pregnancy because her mother is a source of information and can serve as a role model (Lederman 1984). A woman's self-concept as mother expands with actual experience and continues to grow through subsequent childbearing and childrearing. Occasionally a woman never accepts the mother role but plays the role of babysitter or older sister.

The Father

Pregnancy is a psychologically stressful time for the expectant father because he, too, is facing the transition from nonparent to parent or from parent of one or more to parent of two or more.

Expectant fathers experience many of the same feelings and conflicts experienced by expectant mothers when the pregnancy has been confirmed. Contradictory feelings may occur when men first become aware of the pregnancy. For example, with most men, there is an initial source of pride in their virility implicit with fertilization whether the pregnancy was planned or not. At the same time feelings of ambivalence are prevalent. The extent of ambivalence depends on many factors, such as whether the pregnancy was planned, his relationship with his partner, his previous experiences with pregnancy, his age, and his economic stability.

The expectant father must establish a fatherhood role just as the woman develops a concept of herself as mother. Fathers who are most successful at this generally like children, are excited about the prospect of fatherhood, are eager to nurture a child, have confidence in their ability to be a parent, and share the experiences of pregnancy and delivery with their partners (Lederman 1984).

FIRST TRIMESTER

After the initial excitement of the announcement of the pregnancy to friends and relatives and their congratulations, an expectant father may begin to feel left out of the pregnancy. He is also often confused by his partner's mood changes and perhaps bewildered by his responses to her changing body. He may resent the attention given to the woman and the need to change their relationship as she experiences fatigue and a decreased interest in sex. Many questions begin to haunt him at this time. A worry he will have throughout the pregnancy is the expense of having a baby. In addition he is concerned about what kind of father he will be and may become involved with many memories of his own father.

Some expectant fathers experience *mitleiden* ("suffering along") and develop symptoms similar to those of the pregnant woman: weight gain, nausea, and various aches and pains. The exact significance of this phenomenon is unknown. It may be a means for the man to identify with his partner and the pregnancy and can be a positive force drawing the couple close together.

SECOND TRIMESTER

The father's role in the pregnancy is still vague in the second trimester, but his involvement can be facilitated by his watching and feeling fetal movement. Many women report that their partner kisses them on the abdomen more in pregnancy than at any other time. Both may find this sexually arousing, and, during the second trimester especially, it can be a facilitator in increasing sexual activity.

Some couples fantasize that the unborn baby is thus bringing them closer together (Bittman & Zalk 1978).

It is helpful if the father, as well as the mother, has the opportunity to hear the fetal heartbeat. That involves a visit to the nurse-midwife's or physician's office. Involvement of fathers in antepartal care is increasing as fathers becomes more comfortable with this new role.

The expectant father needs to confront and resolve some of his own conflicts about the fathering he experienced. He will need to sort out those behaviors in his own fathering that he wants and does not want to imitate. This process usually occurs gradually as the pregnancy progresses. Since a more active involvement in childbirth and parenting by fathers is somewhat new, men may have few role models available to them. Fishbein (1984) suggests that the actual role a father assumes is less important than the process of negotiation between husband and wife to reach agreement on the father's role. Fishbein found that agreement was more important than actual degree of paternal involvement. Agreement between partners tended to increase with age and combined family income.

The middle trimester has been described by some authors as "quietly tumultuous" months for men. They feel that some men may avoid feeling fetal movement initially because of the envy they experience in not being able to carry the pregnancy, a not-so-uncommon feeling but one that is rarely expressed (Bittman & Zalk 1978). Others believe men respond with mixed feelings to palpation of fetal movement—excitement is experienced but so is increased concern about the well-being of the fetus (Colman & Colman 1971).

The woman's appearance begins to change at this time too, and men react differently to the physical change. For some it decreases their sexual interest; for others it may have the opposite effect. A multitude of emotions are experienced by both partners, and it continues to be important for them to communicate and accept each other's feelings and concerns. In situations in which the expectant mother's demands dominate the relationship, the expectant father's resentment may increase to the point that he is spending more time at work, involved in a hobby, or with his friends. The behavior is even more likely if the expectant father did not want the pregnancy and/or if the relationship was not a good one prior to the pregnancy.

THIRD TRIMESTER

If the couple have communicated their concerns and feelings to one another and grown in their relationship, the third trimester is a special and rewarding time. A more clearly defined role evolves at this time for the expectant father, and it becomes more obvious how the couple can prepare together for the coming event. They may become involved in childbirth education classes, and more concrete preparations for the arrival of the baby begin, such as shopping for a crib, car seat, and other equipment. If the expectant father has developed a detached attitude about the pregnancy prior to this time, however, it is unlikely that he will become a willing participant even though his role becomes more obvious.

Concerns and fears may recur. Many men are afraid of hurting the unborn baby during intercourse. Some feel uncomfortable with fetal activity during foreplay or after intercourse, which may make it seem that the unborn baby was an observer. The father may also begin to have anxiety and fantasies about what could happen to his partner and the unborn baby during labor and delivery and feels a great sense of responsibility. The questions asked earlier in pregnancy emerge again. What kind of parents will he and his partner be? Will he really be able to help his partner in labor? Can they afford to have a baby? Is his job really stable?

COUVADE

The term *couvade* refers to the observance of certain rituals and taboos by the male to signify the transition to fatherhood. Acting out these socially acceptable and patterned behaviors establishes the man's new identity for himself and others. Some taboos restrict his actions. For example, he may be forbidden to eat certain foods, to kill certain animals, or to carry certain weapons prior to and immediately after the birth.

With couvade the father plays an active and vital role during the woman's labor. The father's participation in the couvade affirms his psychosocial and biophysical relationship to the woman and child. Recent trends in this country toward a more active role of the father during pregnancy and childbirth may be a couvade in embryonic stage.

Siblings

The introduction of a new baby into the family unit is often the beginning of sibling rivalry. Sibling rivalry results from children's fear of change in the security of their relationships with their parents. Some of the behaviors demonstrating feelings of sibling rivalry may even be directed toward the mother during the pregnancy as she experiences more fatigue and less patience with her toddler. Parents' recognition early in pregnancy of the potential effects of this new relationship and initiation of constructive steps at this time to decrease negative aspects of the interaction help minimize the problems of sibling rivalry.

Preparation for the young child begins several weeks prior to the anticipated birth and is designed according to the age and experience of the child. Because they do not have a clear concept of time, young children should not be told too early about the pregnancy. When the toddler is told, he or she may expect the baby in the next hour, or within a day or two. From the toddler's point of view,

Research Note

In some cultures an expectant father performs rituals of *couvade*, which are socially sanctioned behaviors or restrictions carried out during his partner's pregnancy. In societies where this formal ritual is not practiced, many men suffer from a *couvade syndrome* consisting of various health complaints.

Clifton's descriptive study examined the risk factors for couvade syndrome, and explored the incidence, duration, and perceived severity of associated symptoms. The study compared 81 expectant fathers with 66 nonexpectant men, interviewing them monthly during pregnancy and the postpartum period.

The expectant men complained of a wide variety of symptoms, including headache, irritability, backache, nervousness, weight gain, gas pains, and depression. The men most at risk for developing couvade syndrome were those of ethnic minorities, with previous children, with health problems the year prior to pregnancy, of low income, and/or with a high level of affective involvement in pregnancy.

The results indicate that couvade syndrome is a very real phenomenon that poses a threat to physical and emotional health for expectant fathers. In providing family-centered prenatal care and education, the nurse needs to include ongoing assessments of the expectant father's health in order to give adequate care, anticipatory guidance, and referral.

Clifton F: Expectant fathers at risk for couvade. Nurs Res 1985;35(September/October):290.

"several weeks" is an extremely long time. The mother may let the child feel the baby moving in her uterus, explaining that this is "a special place where babies grow." (Many parents need to be reminded to use the word *uterus* rather than *stomach,* because *stomach* connotes something being eaten and something that can be vomited. Thus some children develop a dread of eating or defecating or become afraid when they see their mother vomiting.) The child can assist in unpacking the baby's clothes and putting them in drawers or in preparing the nursery room or area. The child will probably be interested in trying on the clothes, lying in the crib, and trying out other baby items.

The concept of consistency is important in dealing with young children. They need reassurance that certain people, special things, and familiar places will continue to exist after the new baby arrives. The crib is an important though transient object in a child's life. If it is to be given to the new baby the parents should thoughtfully help the child adjust to this change (Honig 1986). Any move from crib to bed or from one room to another should precede the baby's birth.

If the child is ready for toilet training, it is most effectively done several months before or after the baby's arrival. Parents should know that the older toilet-trained child may regress to wetting or soiling because he or she sees the new baby getting attention for such behavior. The older weaned child may want to drink from a bottle again after the new baby comes. Lack of knowledge of these common occurrences can be frustrating to the new mother and can compound the stress that she feels during the early postpartum days.

During the pregnancy the older child should be introduced to a new baby for short periods to get an idea of what a new baby is like. This introduction dispels fantasies that the new arrival will be big enough to be a playmate.

Pregnant women may also find it helpful to bring their children to a prenatal visit after they have been told about the expected baby. The children are encouraged to become involved in prenatal care and to ask any questions they may have. They are also given the opportunity to hear the baby's heartbeat, either with a stethoscope or with the Doppler. This helps make the baby more real to them.

The school-age child should be involved in the pregnancy. If the pregnancy is viewed as a family affair, the child is not excluded from the experience. Teaching about the pregnancy should be based on the child's level of understanding and interest. Overeager parents may go into lengthier and more in-depth responses than the child is interested in. Some children are more curious than others. Books at their level of understanding can be made available in the home. Involvement in family discussions, attendance at sibling preparation classes, encouragement to feel fetal movement, and an opportunity to listen to the fetal heart supplement the learning process and help make the school-age child feel part of the pregnancy.

The older child may appear to have a sophisticated knowledge base, but it may be intermingled with many misconceptions. One 36-year-old multipara related that when her 14-year-old son was told about her pregnancy, he was concerned about her age and a need for an amniocentesis. He had learned about the association of increased incidence of genetic disease with increased age in his science class at school and was concerned about the fetus. In contrast, however, he was very naive about childbirth itself.

Even after the birth siblings need to feel that they are part of a family affair. Changes in hospital regulations allowing siblings to be present at the birth or to visit their mother and the new baby facilitate this process. On arrival at home siblings can share in "showing off" the new baby.

Preparation of siblings for the arrival of a new baby is essential in minimizing sibling rivalry. Other critical factors, however, are equally important. These include the amount of parental attention focused on the new arrival, amount of parental attention given the older child after the birth of the new arrival, and parental reinforcement of regressive and/or aggressive behavior.

Grandparents

The first relatives told about a pregnancy are usually the grandparents. Although relationships with parents can be very complex, this period in a family's life most often promotes a closer relationship between the expectant couple and their parents. The expectant mother may find she is increasing contact with her mother, and anticipates finding the support she needs from the relationship. The expectant father may find he is doing the same with both of his parents. But how are the expectant grandparents responding to the pregnancy? Usually they become increasingly supportive of the expectant couple, even if disapproval of the couple's marriage and/or other conflicts were previously present.

Grandparents may be unsure about the amount of involvement they are "allowed" during the pregnancy and childbearing process. Most want to be helpful; some may bestow advice and/or gifts unsparingly. Since grandparenting can occur over a wide span of years, people's response to this role can vary considerably. For some this new role may occur at a relatively young age, and the connotation of aging that accompanies the role may affect their response to the pregnancy. The younger grandparent may also be active in work and other activities, and may not demonstrate as much interest as the young couple would like.

It can be difficult for even sensitive grandparents to know how much involvement the couple want. The mood changes of the expectant mother, as well as other complex factors in the relationship, cause her to ask for advice and the next moment turn away. Expectant couples want to feel in control of their new situation, which may be initially difficult in their changing roles. Grandparents find that this factor, as well as changing roles in their own life (for example, retirement, financial concerns, menopause of the expectant grandmother, death of a friend), may contribute to conflicts in the changing family structure. Some parents of expectant couples may already be grandparents and have already developed their own style of grandparenting, which will be an important factor in how they respond to the pregnancy.

Childbearing and childrearing practices are very different for today's childbearing couple. It helps family cohesiveness for young couples to share with interested grandparents what today's practices are and why they feel they are effective. Some couples may even choose to have grandparents attend the birth. At the same time, it is important for young couples to listen to any differences expectant grandparents want to explain. When grandparents give advice, it helps to remember that they care. When their recommendations seem effective, it is significant to grandparents that young couples do listen.

Occasionally young couples feel they are receiving more advice than they can tolerate. Too often they perceive parents' suggestions as criticizing their ability to prepare adequately for the childbearing process, and later as criticism of their care of the newborn. The advice may not be difficult to deal with during the pregnancy, but the situation changes if a grandparent plans to help in the home after the arrival of the newborn. It then becomes essential for the young couple to discuss the problem and agree on a plan of action. The role of the helping grandparents when the new baby is brought home needs to be clarified before the event to ensure a comfortable situation for all.

In some areas classes are available to provide information for grandparents about changes in birth and parenting practices. These classes help familiarize grandparents with new parents' needs and may offer suggestions for ways in which the grandparents can support the childbearing couple (Horn & Manion 1985).

● Cultural Values and Reproductive Behavior

A universal tendency exists to create ceremonial rituals and rites around important life events. Thus pregnancy, childbirth, marriage, and death are often tied to ritual. Scott & Stern (1985) suggest that ritual is passed from one generation to another in three ways:

- *Formal teaching* such as childbirth preparation classes

- *Informal teaching* through role modeling or observation

- *Folktales or stories of advice or warning,* often passed on by the mother or grandmother of the family

The rituals, customs, and practices of a group are a reflection of the group's values. Thus the identification of cultural values is useful in predicting reactions. An understanding of male and female roles, family life-styles, or the meaning of children in a culture may explain reactions of joy or shame. Pregnancy is a joyful event in a culture that values children. In some cultures, however, pregnancy is a shameful event if it occurs outside of marriage.

Health values and beliefs are also important in understanding reactions and behavior. Certain behaviors can be expected if a culture views pregnancy as a sickness, whereas other behaviors can be expected if pregnancy is viewed as a natural occurrence. Prenatal care may not be a priority for women who view pregnancy as a natural phenomenon.

Generalizations about cultural characteristics or cultural values are difficult since these characteristics may not be exhibited by every individual within a culture. Just as variations are seen *between* cultures, variations are also seen *within* cultures. These variations are often related to social and economic factors such as class, income, and education. For this reason a general knowledge of cultural values and practices, in addition to an individual assessment, usually leads to an accurate understanding of a client's behavior.

Variation within a culture is seen in the black community where three classes—upper, middle, and lower—are recognized. Many factors, which are primarily social and economic, influence the way the black woman regards pregnancy. Pregnancy is usually seen as a state of wellness. Acceptance of the pregnancy may depend upon the marital and social situation and whether the pregnancy is planned (Carrington 1978).

Pregnancy, viewed as a natural condition, is usually desired as soon as possible in the traditional Mexican-American family (Kay 1978). The importance of family is one factor influencing this behavior. Moreover, the role of the traditional Mexican-American woman is one of complete devotion to her husband and children (Murillo 1978). Children are an important part of the Mexican-American family; they assure continuation of the family and cultural values.

Machismo, or manliness, is another cultural concept that influences the reproductive behavior in this group. The term *macho* has various definitions, with the most frequent being "virile." Research suggests that male individualism and large family size are evidence of machismo (Tamez 1981).

Traditional practices may change with time. As in the black family, social and economic factors also influence Mexican-American practices. Today middle-class Mexican-American couples are not starting their families right away (Ehling 1978). In addition, a reduced fertility pattern is found among Mexican-American women who participate in the labor force.

Pregnancy and birth are significant events for the Asian family. In the traditional Chinese family the wife's status improves with the birth of a child, especially the birth of a son, because a son assures the continuation of a family name. Pregnancy has been referred to among Asians as "happiness in her body" (Rose 1978). It is considered a normal and natural process, but is also a time of anticipation and anxiety (Char 1981).

Health Beliefs

Two major explanations of illness have been proposed by Foster and Anderson (1978). The first is the view that illness is the result of the intervention of an agent that may be a supernatural, a nonhuman, or a human being. Beliefs in witches, evil spirits, or God as primary factors in health are part of this view. The second explanation conforms to an equilibrium model of health. For example, health may be viewed as a balance between hot and cold. When this equilibrium is disturbed, illness results.

Although pregnancy is perceived as a natural occurrence in many cultures, it may also be viewed as a time of increased vulnerability. In groups that adhere to beliefs in evil spirits, certain protective precautions are often followed. For example, pregnant Vietnamese women are admonished to avoid funerals, places of worship, and streets at noon and five o'clock in the afternoon since spirits are present at these times (Stringfellow 1978). In the Mexican-American culture, the concept of *mal aire* or bad air is sometimes related to evil spirits. It is thought that air, especially night air, may enter the body and cause harm. Preventive measures, such as keeping the windows closed or covering the head, are used.

Most of the taboos stemming from the belief in evil spirits exist for fear of injuring the unborn child. They arise from a general belief that the unborn infant is the weakest of all beings and is at the mercy of the mother's prenatal behavior. Taboos also emanate from the fear that a pregnant woman has evil powers (Brown 1976). For this reason pregnant women are sometimes prohibited from taking part in certain activities. For example, the pregnant Vietnamese woman cannot attend a wedding for fear of bringing bad luck to the newlyweds (Hollingsworth et al 1980).

The equilibrium model of health is based on the concept of balance between light and dark, heat and cold. Oriental belief focuses on the notion of *yin* and *yang*. Yin represents the female passive principle—darkness, cold, wetness—while yang is the masculine, active principle—light, heat, and dryness. When the two are combined, they are all that can be. The hot-cold classification is seen in cultures in Latin America, the Near East, and Asia. The dimensions and meanings of this classification vary, however, and require further investigation (Messer 1981).

Mexican Americans often consider illness to be an excess of either hot or cold. To restore health, imbalances are often corrected by the proper use of foods, medications, or herbs. These substances are also classified as hot or cold. For example, an illness attributed to an excess of coldness will be treated only with hot foods or medications. The classification of foods is not always consistent but it does conform to a general structure of traditional knowledge (Messer 1981). Certain foods, spices, herbs, and medications are perceived to cool or heat the body. These perceptions do not necessarily correspond to the actual temperature; some hot dishes are said to have a cooling quality.

The Vietnamese also consider that pregnancy is a cold state because a great deal of body heat is lost. Therefore they avoid cold drinks and foods following birth (Calhoun 1985).

The concepts of hot and cold are not as important in American Indian or black American beliefs. There are some similarities, however, in all of these groups because of the emphasis on a balance in nature. Black Americans believe that health is a harmony with nature and a balance between good and evil, while the American Indians have traditionally seen health as harmony with nature (Henderson & Primeaux 1981).

Health Practices

Health care practices during pregnancy are influenced by numerous factors, such as the prevalence of traditional home remedies and folk beliefs, the importance of indigenous healers, and the influence of professional health care workers. In an urban setting the age, length of time in the city, marital status, and strength of the family may affect these patterns. Socioeconomic status is also important since modern medical services are more accessible to those who can afford it.

An awareness of alternative health sources is crucial for health professionals since these practices affect health outcomes. Many Mexican-American mothers are strongly influenced by familism and will seek and follow the advice of their mothers or older women in the childbearing period (Tamez 1981).

Indigenous healers are also important to specific cultures. In the Mexican-American culture the healer is called a *curandero*. In some American Indian tribes the medicine man may fulfill the healing role. Herbalists are often found in Asian cultures, and faith healers, root doctors, and spiritualists are sometimes consulted in the black culture.

Cultural Factors and Nursing Care

In recent years people from a variety of cultures have immigrated to the United States. This influx of people has had a significant impact on the health care system. Numerous differences exist in beliefs, values, health care practices and expectations, language, world views, and etiquette between these newly arrived people and the majority of health care providers.

Health care providers are often unaware of the cultural characteristics they themselves demonstrate. Without cultural awareness care givers tend to project their own cultural responses onto foreign-born clients and assume that the clients are demonstrating a specific behavior for the same reason that they would. For example, health care providers sometimes label a pregnant or postpartum Filipino woman as "lazy" because of her rather sedentary lifestyle. In reality this style results from the cultural belief that inactivity is necessary to protect the mother and child (Stern et al 1985). Thiederman (1986) suggests that if health care providers fail to understand the reasons for a person's behavior, it is impossible for them to intervene appropriately and assure cooperation.

To a certain extent most of us are guilty of ethnocentrism, at least some of the time. *Ethnocentrism* "involves the belief that the values and practices of one's own culture are the best ones, and, in some cases, the only ones of any worth" (Thiederman 1986, p 52). Thus the nurse who values stoicism during labor may be uncomfortable with the more vocal response of Hispanic women. Another nurse may be disconcerted by the Vietnamese woman who is so intent on maintaining self-control that she smiles throughout labor (Calhoun 1985).

Health care providers sometimes believe that if members of other cultures do not share Western values, they should adopt them. This is especially difficult for some nurses caring for childbearing families if the nurse is a firm believer in equality of the sexes and women's liberation. The nurse may find it difficult to remain silent if a woman from a Middle Eastern culture defers to her husband in decision making. It is important to remember that pressure to defy cultural values and beliefs can be stressful and anxiety provoking for these women (Thiederman 1986).

Members of minority culture groups are often found living in a certain area of a community. The nurse can begin developing cultural sensitivity by becoming knowledgeable about the cultural practices of local groups. For example, is it considered courteous to avoid eye contact? Should last names be used in conversation as a sign of respect? Are the needs of the family considered more important than the desires of the individual? Is a female health care provider necessary? Are there specific dietary practices that must be followed?

Cultural assessment is an important aspect of prenatal care. It is not necessary to do an in-depth analysis of all aspects of the culture. However, the nurse should identify the main beliefs, values, and behaviors that relate to pregnancy and childbearing. This includes information about ethnic background, amount of affiliation with the ethnic group, patterns of decision making, religious preference, language, communication style, and common etiquette practices (Tripp-Reimer et al 1984). The nurse can also explore the woman's (or family's) expectations of the health care system.

Before considering a nursing intervention, it is necessary to determine the impact of traditional practices on the planned intervention. For example, nutritional counseling will be ineffective unless an effort is made to identify preferred and available foods as well as foods that are commonly avoided.

In planning care the nurse considers the extent to which the woman's personal values, beliefs, and customs are in accord with the values, beliefs, and customs of the woman's identified cultural group, the nurse providing care, and the health care agency. If discrepancies exist, the nurse then considers whether the woman's system is supportive, neutral, or harmful in relation to possible interventions (Tripp-Reimer et al 1984). If the woman's system is supportive or neutral, it can be incorporated into the plan. For example, individual food practices or methods of pain expression may differ from those of the nurse or agency but would not necessarily interfere with the nursing plan. On the other hand, certain cultural practices might pose a threat to the health of the childbearing woman. For example, some Filipinas will not take any medication during pregnancy. The health care provider may consider a certain medication essential to the woman's well-being. In this case the woman's cultural belief may be detrimental to her own health. The nurse then faces two considerations: (1) identifying ways of persuading the woman to accept the proposed therapy; or (2) accepting the woman's rationale for refusing therapy if she is not willing to change her belief system (Tripp-Reimer et al 1984).

KEY CONCEPTS

Virtually all systems of a woman's body are altered in some way during pregnancy.

Blood pressure decreases slightly during pregnancy. It reaches its lowest point in the second trimester and gradually increases to near normal levels in the third trimester.

The enlarging uterus may cause pressure on the vena cava when the woman lies supine. This is called the vena caval syndrome.

A physiologic anemia may occur during pregnancy because the total plasma volume increases more than the total number of erythrocytes. This produces a drop in the hematocrit.

The glomerular filtration rate increases somewhat during pregnancy. Glycosuria may be caused by the body's inability to reabsorb all the glucose filtered by the glomeruli.

Changes in the skin include the development of chloasma; linea nigra; darkened nipples, areola, and vulva; striae; spider nevi; and palmar erythema.

Insulin needs are increased during pregnancy. A woman with a latent deficiency state may respond to the increased stress on the islets of Langerhans by developing gestational diabetes.

The placenta produces four hormones: estrogen, progesterone, human chorionic gonadotropin, and human placental lactogen.

The presumptive signs of pregnancy are those symptoms experienced and reported by the woman, such as amenorrhea, nausea and vomiting, fatigue, urinary frequency, breast changes, and quickening.

The probable signs of pregnancy can be perceived by the examiner but may be caused by conditions other than pregnancy.

The positive signs of pregnancy can be perceived by the examiner and can only be caused by pregnancy.

For many families pregnancy represents a developmental challenge; for some it is a maturational crisis.

During pregnancy the expectant woman may experience ambivalence, acceptance, introversion, emotional lability, and changes in body image.

Rubin (1984) has identified four developmental tasks for the pregnant woman: (1) ensuring safe passage through pregnancy, labor, and birth; (2) seeking acceptance of this child by others; (3) seeking commitment and acceptance of self as mother to the infant; and (4) learning to give of oneself on behalf of one's child.

Fathers also face a series of adjustments as they accept their new role.

Siblings of all ages require assistance in dealing with the birth of a new baby.

Cultural values, beliefs, and behaviors influence a couple's response to childbearing and the health care system.

The equilibrium model of health is based on a balance of yin and yang, cold and hot, dark and light.

Ethnocentrism is the belief that one's own cultural beliefs, values, and practices are the best ones, indeed the only ones worth considering.

A cultural assessment does not have to be exhaustive, but it should focus on factors that will influence the practices of the childbearing family with regard to their health needs.

REFERENCES

Bittman S, Zalk SR: *Expectant Fathers*. New York, Hawthorne Books, 1978.

Brown MS: A cross-cultural look at pregnancy, labor, and delivery. *J Obstet Gynecol Neonat Nurs* 1976;5(September/October):35.

Brown MS: *Normal Development of Body Image*. New York, John Wiley, 1977.

Calhoun MA: The Vietnamese woman: Health/illness attitudes and behaviors. *Health Care Women Internat* 1985; 6:61.

Carrington BW: The Afro American, in **Clark** AL (ed): *Culture, Childbearing, Health Professionals.* Philadelphia, Davis, 1978.

Char EI: The Chinese American, in **Clark** AL (ed): *Culture and Childrearing.* Philadelphia, Davis, 1981.

Colman A, **Colman** L: *Pregnancy: The Psychological Experience.* New York, Herder & Herder, 1971.

Creasy RC, **Resnik** R: *Maternal-Fetal Medicine.* Philadelphia, Saunders, 1984.

Cronenwett LR: Network structure, social support, and psychological outcomes of pregnancy. *Nurs Res* 1985;34(March/April):93.

Danforth DN, **Scott** JR: *Obstetrics and Gynecology,* ed 5. Philadelphia, Lippincott, 1986.

Danforth DN, **Ueland** K: Physiology of uterine action, in **Danforth** DN, **Scott** JR (eds): *Obstetrics and Gynecology,* ed 5. Philadelphia, Lippincott, 1986.

Ehling MB: The Mexican American (el Chicano), in **Clark** AL (ed): *Culture, Childbearing, Health Professionals.* Philadelphia, Davis, 1978.

Fawcett J: Body image and the pregnant couple. *Am J Mat Child Nurs* 1978;3(July/August):227.

Fawcett J, et al: Spouses' body image changes during and after pregnancy: A replication and extension. *Nurs Res* 1986;35(July/August):220.

Fishbein EG: Expectant father's stress—Due to mother's expectations? *J Obstet Gynecol Neonat Nurs* 1984;13 (September/October):325.

Foster GM, **Anderson** BG: *Medical Anthropology.* New York, John Wiley, 1978.

Henderson G, **Primeaux** M: *Transcultural Health Care.* Menlo Park, Calif, Addison-Wesley, 1981.

Hollingsworth AO, et al: The refugees and childbearing: What to expect. *RN* 1980;43(November):45.

Honig JC: Preparing preschool-aged children to be siblings. *MCN* 1986;11(January/February):37.

Horn M, **Manion** J: Creative grandparenting: Bonding the generations. *J Obstet Gynecol Neonat Nurs* 1985;14(May/June):233.

Kay MA: The Mexican American, in **Clark** AL (ed): *Culture, Childbearing, Health Professionals.* Philadelphia, Davis, 1978.

Key TC, **Resnik** R: Maternal changes in pregnancy, in **Danforth** DN, **Scott** JR (eds): *Obstetrics and Gynecology,* ed 5. Philadelphia, Lippincott, 1986.

Klebanoff et al: Epidemiology of vomiting in early pregnancy. *Obstet Gynecol* 1985;66(November):612.

Lederman RP: *Psychosocial Adaptation in Pregnancy.* Englewood Cliffs, NJ, Prentice-Hall, 1984.

Messer E: Hot-cold classification: Theoretical and practical implications of a Mexican study. *Soc Sci Med* 1981;15B:133.

Murillo N: The Mexican American family, in **Martinez** RA (ed): *Hispanic Culture and Health Care.* St Louis, Mosby, 1978.

Pritchard JA, **MacDonald** PC, **Gant** NF: *Williams' Obstetrics,* ed 17. New York, Appleton-Century-Crofts, 1985.

Rose PA: The Chinese American, in **Clark** AL (ed): *Culture, Childbearing, Health Professionals.* Philadelphia, Davis, 1978.

Rubin R: Cognitive style in pregnancy. *Am J Nurs* 1970;70(March):502.

Rubin R: *Maternal Identity and the Maternal Experience.* New York, Springer, 1984.

Rubin R: Maternal tasks in pregnancy. *Am J Mat Child Nurs* 1975;4(Fall):143.

Scott MDS, **Stern** PN: The ethno-market theory: Factors influencing childbearing health practices of northern Louisiana black women. *Health Care Women Internat* 1985;6:45.

Simpson ER, **MacDonald** PC: Endocrine physiology of the placenta. *Ann Rev Physiol* 1981;43:163.

Stern PN, et al: Culturally induced stress during childbearing: The Phillipine-American experience. *Health Care Women Internat* 1985;6:105.

Stickler J, et al: Pregnancy: A shared emotional experience. *Am J Mat Child Nurs* 1978;3(May/June):153.

Strang VR, **Sullivan** PL: Body image attitudes during pregnancy and the postpartum period. *J Obstet Gynecol Neonat Nurs* 1985;14(July/August):332.

Stringfellow L: The Vietnamese, in **Clark** AL (ed): *Culture, Childbearing, Health Professionals.* Philadelphia, Davis, 1978.

Tamez EG: Familism, machismo, and childbearing practices among Mexican Americans. *J Psychiatr Nurs* 1981;19:21.

Thiederman SB: Ethnocentrism: A barrier to effective health care. *Nurse Practitioner* 1986;11(August):52.

Tripp-Reimer T, et al: Cultural assessment: Content and process. *Nurs Outlook* 1984;32(March/April):78.

Vande Wiele RL, et al: Progesterones in pregnancy, in **New** MI, **Fiser** RH (eds): *Diabetes and Other Endocrine Disorders during Pregnancy and in the Newborn.* New York, Alan R. Liss, 1976.

ADDITIONAL READINGS

Brown MA: Social support during pregnancy: A unidimensional or multidimensional construct? *Nurs Res* 1986;35(January/February):4.

Caine ME, **Mueller-Heubach** E: Kell sensitization in pregnancy. *Am J Obstet Gynecol* 1986;154(1):85.

Clapp JF III: Fetal heart rate response to running in midpregnancy and late pregnancy. *Am J Obstet Gynecol* 1985;153:251.

Clinton JF: Expectant fathers at risk for couvade . . . physical and emotional symptoms. *Nurs Res* 1986;35(5):290.

Cornford-Wood LJ: Normal pregnancy. *Nursing (Lond)* 1986;3(1):2.

Daya S: Human chorionic gonadotropin increase in normal early pregnancy. *Am J Obstet Gynecol* 1987;156(2):286.

DiLorio C: First trimester nausea in pregnant teenagers: incidence, characteristics, intervention. *Nurs Res* 1985; 34(November/December):372.

Fawcett J, et al: Pretty big . . . body attitudes during pregnancy. *Health* 1986;18(6):6.

Mercer RT, et al: Theoretical models for studying the effect of antepartum stress on the family. *Nurs Res* 1986;35(November/December):330.

Moore L, et al: Self-Assessment: A personalized approach to nursing during pregnancy. *J Obstet Gynecol Neonat Nurs* 1986;15(July/August):311.

Musey VC, et al: Long term effects of first pregnancy on the hormonal environment: Estrogens and androgens. *J Clin Endocrinol Metab* 1987;64(1):111.

Patterson ET, et al: Reducing uncertainty: Self-diagnosis of pregnancy. *Image* 1986;18(Fall):105.

Poole CJ: Fatigue during the first trimester of pregnancy. *J Obstet Gynecol Neonat Nurs* 1986;15(September/October):375.

Robinson GE, et al: Psychological adaptation to pregnancy in childless women more than 35 years of age. *Am J Obstet Gynecol* 1987;156(2):328.

Sherwen LN: Third trimester fantasies of first-time expectant fathers. *Am J Mat Child Nurs* 1986;15(3):153.

Ventura SJ, **Taffel** SM: Childbearing characteristics of U.S.- and foreign-born Hispanic mothers. *Public Health Rep* 1985;100(November/December):647.

The atmosphere of approval in which I was bathed—even by strangers on the street, it seemed—was like an aura I carried with me . . . this is what women have always done. (Adrienne Rich, Of Woman Born)

Antepartal Nursing Assessment

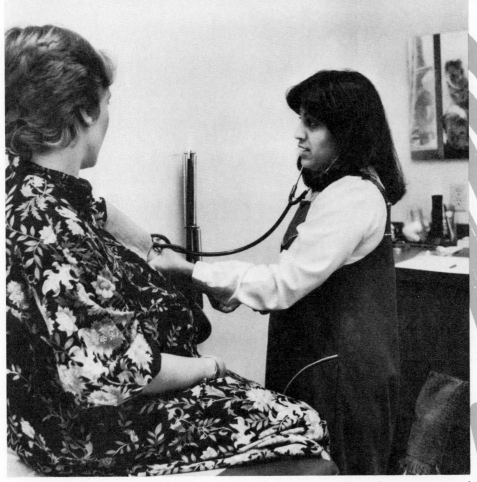

This Indian nurse, herself also pregnant, shares the anticipation and concerns of her pregnant clients.

Chapter Fifteen

OBJECTIVES

- Summarize the essential components of a prenatal history.
- Explain the common obstetric terminology found in the history of a maternity client.
- Identify factors related to the father's health that should be recorded on the prenatal record.
- Describe the normal physiologic changes one would expect to find when performing a physical assessment on a pregnant woman.
- Explain the use of Nägele's rule to determine estimated date of delivery.
- Develop an outline of the essential measurements that can be determined by clinical pelvimetry.
- Describe areas that should be evaluated as part of the initial assessment of psychosocial factors related to a woman's pregnancy.
- Relate the danger signs of pregnancy to their possible causes.

Pregnancy is increasingly viewed as a normal physiologic process and not a disease condition. This view has permitted nurses to assume a more important role in prenatal care, particularly in the area of assessment. The certified nurse-midwife has the education and skill to perform in-depth prenatal assessments. The nurse-practitioner may share the assessment responsibilities with a physician. An office nurse, whose primary role may be to counsel and meet the psychologic needs of the expectant family, performs assessments in those areas.

In the prenatal clinic or obstetrician's office, it is often the nurse who has the first contact with the pregnant woman, as the nurse performs initial assessments such as vital signs and weight. The nurse's attitude toward the woman during this early period can set the tone for the remainder of the visit.

An environment of comfort and open communication should be established with each antepartal visit. The nurse should convey concern for the woman as an individual and availability to listen and discuss the woman's concerns and desires. A supportive atmosphere coupled with the information found in the physical and psychosocial assessment guides in this chapter will enable the nurse to identify needed areas of education and counseling.

If optimum maternal health is to be maintained, a thorough history and physical examination are essential to identify problem areas. The history and physical examination may be done by a nurse, a physician, or both.

● Client History

The course of a pregnancy depends on a number of factors, including the prepregnancy health of the woman, presence of disease states, emotional status, and past health care. Ideally health care before the advent of pregnancy has been adequate, and antenatal care will be a continuation of that established care. One important method of determining the adequacy of a woman's prepregnancy care is a thorough history.

Definition of Terms

The following terms are used in the obstetric history of maternity clients:

Weeks of gestation: The number of weeks since the first day of the last menstrual period (LMP)

Abortion: Delivery that occurs prior to the end of 20 weeks' gestation

Preterm or premature labor: Labor that occurs after 20 weeks but before the completion of 37 weeks of gestation (pregnancy)

Postterm labor: Labor that occurs after 42 weeks of gestation

Gravida: Any pregnancy, regardless of duration, including present pregnancy

Primigravida: A woman who is pregnant for the first time

Multigravida: A woman who is in her second or any subsequent pregnancy

Para: Delivery after 20 weeks of gestation (pregnancy) regardless of whether the fetus is born alive or dead

Nullipara: A woman who has not had a delivery at more than 20 weeks' gestation

Primipara: A woman who has had one delivery at more than 20 weeks' gestation, regardless of whether the infant is born alive or dead

Multipara: A woman who has had two or more deliveries at more than 20 weeks' gestation

Stillbirth: A fetus born dead after 20 weeks of gestation

The terms *gravida* and *para* refer to pregnancies/deliveries, not to the fetus.

The following examples illustrate how these terms are applied in clinical situations:

1. Jean Smith has one child born at 38 weeks and is pregnant for the second time. At her initial prenatal visit, the nurse indicates her obstetric history as "gravida 2 para 1 ab O." Jean Smith's present pregnancy terminates at 16 weeks' gestation. She is now "gravida 2 para 1 ab 1."

2. Liz Alexander is pregnant for the fourth time. She has twins born at 35 weeks at home. She lost one pregnancy at 10 weeks' gestation and delivered another infant stillborn at term. At her prenatal assessment the nurse records Liz Alexander's obstetric history as "gravida 4 para 2 ab 1." Note that twins are considered as one pregnancy (gravida) and one delivery (para).

Because of the confusion that may result from this system when a multiple pregnancy occurs, a more detailed approach is used in some settings. Using the detailed system, gravida keeps the same meaning, while that of para is altered somewhat to focus on the number of infants born rather than the number of deliveries. A useful acronym for remembering the system is TPAL.

First digit, **T**—number of *term* infants born; that is, the number of infants born at 37 weeks' gestation or beyond.

Second digit, **P**—number of *preterm* infants born; that is, the number of infants born before 37 weeks' gestation.

Third digit, **A**—number of pregnancies ending in either spontaneous or therapeutic *abortion.*

Fourth digit, **L**—number of currently *living* children.

CONTEMPORARY DILEMMA

Do I Have a Right to Know?

For thousands of adults the decision to have a child is fraught with uncertainty because they have no knowledge of their family histories. Because they are adopted their decision is a form of medical Russian roulette. This lack of information becomes part of day-to-day existence for adopted people. They learn to live without the information so many of us take for granted—information about potential health problems that form part of a family's history. Would a man watch his diet and exercise program more carefully, for example, if he knew he had a strong family history of heart disease? How would a woman react if she knew her biologic mother, grandmother, and aunt all developed breast cancer? It is impossible to predict.

The problem changes subtly but significantly when the question of conceiving a child arises. People have no control over their genetic inheritance. They can, however, decide whether to pass their genetic inheritance on to a child, but only if they know what that inheritance entails.

Many adopted children are speaking up, urging that family histories be made available so that they can plan their lives more thoughtfully. In the future it is possible that a complete family history will be provided to parents who adopt a child to help them in raising the child and to help the child in adulthood. Unfortunately, unless a form of updating is available, health problems that develop for the biologic parents or their families after the adoption would still be missed.

The problems and concerns that are being raised focus on several issues:

- Is it fair to ask the biologic mother, who made the difficult decision to relinquish her child, to step forward and become involved again? Aren't we "changing the rules" on her and violating her right to privacy and anonymity?

- Ethically, do people have a right to know their history? Does a moral obligation exist to inform family members of possible health problems?

- Should a system of family history reporting be developed? Who would maintain it? How would it be updated?

- Is there a way to meet the needs of adopted people to know their health histories? Should it be left up to the biologic parents to provide significant information for adoption agencies to pass along to the children? Do the children have a right to ask that adoption records be made public so that they can contact their biologic parents? What if the parents refuse to share information?

- What of the rights and needs of children conceived by parents who were adopted? How can they be helped?

Using this approach, Jean Smith (described in the first example) would initially have been classified as "gravida 2 para 1001." Following her abortion she would be "gravida 2 para 1011." Liz Alexander would be described as "gravida 4 para 1212."

Client Profile

The history is essentially a screening tool that identifies the factors that may detrimentally affect the course of a pregnancy. For optimal prenatal care the following information should be obtained for each maternity client at the first prenatal assessment:

1. Current pregnancy:

   a. First day of last normal menstrual period.

   b. Presence of cramping, bleeding, or spotting since last period.

   c. Woman's opinion about when conception occurred and when infant is due.

   d. Woman's attitude toward pregnancy. Is pregnancy planned?

   e. Results of pregnancy test, if it has been done.

   f. Any discomforts since last menstrual period (LMP): nausea, vomiting, frequency, headache, etc.

2. Past pregnancies:

   a. Number of pregnancies.

   b. Number of abortions, spontaneous or induced.

   c. Number of living children.

   d. History of preceding pregnancies: length of pregnancy, length of labor and delivery, type of delivery (vaginal, forceps or silastic cup, cesarean, etc), place of delivery, woman's perception of the experience, complications (antepartal, intrapartal, postpartal).

   e. Perinatal status of previous children: Apgar scores, birth weights, general development, complications, feeding patterns (breast/bottle).

   f. Blood type and Rh factor (if negative—medication after delivery to prevent sensitization).

   g. Prenatal education classes, resources (books).

3. Gynecologic history:

   a. Previous infections: vaginal, cervical, tubal, sexually transmitted.

   b. Previous surgery.

   c. Age of menarche.

   d. Regularity, frequency, and duration of menstrual flow.

   e. History of dysmenorrhea.

   f. Sexual history.

   g. Contraceptive history: If birth control pills were used, did pregnancy immediately follow cessation of pills? If not, how long after?

4. Current medical history:

   a. Weight.

   b. Blood type and Rh factor, if known.

   c. Any medications presently being taken (including nonprescription medications) or taken since the onset of pregnancy.

   d. Previous or present use of alcohol, cigarettes, or caffeine.

   e. Illicit drug use and/or abuse.

   f. Drug allergies.

   g. Potential teratogenic insults to this pregnancy, such as viral infections, medications, x-ray examinations, surgery, live cats in home (possible source of toxoplasmosis).

   h. Presence of disease conditions, such as diabetes, hypertension, cardiovascular disease, renal problems.

   i. Record of immunizations (especially rubella).

   j. Presence of any abnormal symptoms.

5. Past medical history:

   a. Childhood diseases.

   b. Past treatment for any disease condition: Any hospitalizations? History of hepatitis? Rheumatic fever?

   c. Surgical procedures.

   d. Presence of bleeding disorders or tendencies: Has she received blood transfusions?

6. Family medical history:

   a. Presence of diabetes, cardiovascular disease, hypertension, hematologic disorders, tuberculosis, allergies, preeclampsia-eclampsia.

   b. Multiple births.

   c. History of congenital diseases or deformities.

   d. Cesarean deliveries.

7. Religious/cultural history:

a. Does the woman wish to specify a religious preference on her chart? Does she have any religious beliefs or practices that might influence her health care or that of her child, such as prohibition against receiving blood products, dietary considerations, circumcision rites, etc?

b. Are there practices in her culture or that of her partner that might influence her care or that of her child?

8. Occupational history:

a. Occupation.

b. Does she stand all day, or are there opportunities to sit and elevate her legs? Any heavy lifting?

c. Exposure to harmful substances.

d. Opportunity for regular lunch, breaks for nutritious snacks.

e. Provision for maternity leave.

9. Partner's history:

a. Presence of genetic conditions or diseases.

b. Age.

c. Significant health problems.

d. Previous or present alcohol intake, drug use.

e. Blood type and Rh factor.

f. Occupation.

g. Educational level.

h. Attitude toward the pregnancy.

10. Personal information:

a. Cultural patterns that could influence pregnancy, such as dietary practices or self-medication.

b. Regular exercise program: type, frequency, duration.

c. Race or ethnic group (to identify need for prenatal genetic screening or counseling).

d. Stability of living conditions.

e. Economic level.

f. Housing.

g. Any history of emotional or physical deprivation (herself or children).

h. History of emotional problems.

i. Support systems.

j. Overuse or underuse of health care system.

k. Personal preferences about the delivery (plans to attend, expectations of both the woman and her partner, presence of others, and so on).

Obtaining Data

A questionnaire like the one shown in Figure 15–1 is used in many instances to obtain information. The woman should be able to complete the questionnaire in a quiet place with a minimum of distractions.

Further information may be elicited by direct interview. A quiet setting where privacy is assured creates a comfortable environment for the interview process. During the interview the pregnant woman can expand or clarify her responses to the questionnaire and the nurse can begin establishing rapport with the client. This beginning dialogue sets the stage for a relationship in which the woman feels comfortable asking questions of and expressing concerns to the nurse about her pregnancy, and the nurse can be an active educator-counselor to facilitate the woman's understanding of her pregnancy, its influences on her, and how she influences her health care.

The expectant father should be encouraged to attend the initial and subsequent prenatal assessments. He may be able to contribute information to the history. In addition, the interview process may provide him with the opportunity to ask questions and express concerns that may be of particular importance to him.

Prenatal High-Risk Screening

A highly significant part of the prenatal assessment is the screening for high-risk factors. Risk factors are any findings that have been shown to have a negative effect on pregnancy outcome, either for the woman or her unborn child.

Many risk factors can be identified during the initial prenatal assessment; other conditions predisposing to maternal or fetal compromise may be detected by subsequent examinations. The nurse must be aware of these high-risk factors and their implications for a successful completion of pregnancy. It is important that high-risk pregnancies be identified early so that appropriate interventions can be instituted immediately.

All risk factors do not threaten the pregnancy to the same degree. To determine the possible effect of certain variables on the pregnancy, centers that provide prenatal care have devised various scoring tools. These scoring tools can be used to collect data and identify the woman who needs to be observed more closely during the pregnancy.

Some agencies use a risk-scoring sheet, which is initiated at the first visit and becomes a permanent part of the woman's record. Information may be updated throughout the pregnancy as necessary. It is always possible that a pregnancy may begin as low risk and convert to high

Name _____ **Age** _____

Address _____ **Home Telephone** _____

What was the last year of schooling completed? _____

How old were you when your menstrual periods started? _____

How many days does a normal period last? _____

How many days are there between periods? _____

Do you have cramping with your periods? yes___no___

Is the pain: minimal _____

moderate _____

severe _____

What was the date of your last normal menstrual period? _____

Have you had bleeding or spotting
since your last menstrual period? yes___no___

Have you been on birth control pills? yes___no___

If yes, when did you stop taking them? _____

How many previous pregnancies have you had? _____

How many living children do you have? _____

Have you had any abortions or stillbirths? yes___no___

If yes, how many? _____

Were any of your previous babies born prematurely? yes___no___

List the birth weight of all previous children.

1. _____   3. _____

2. _____   4. _____

Did any of your children have problems immediately after birth?
yes___no___

If yes, check the problems that occurred:

Respiratory _____   Feeding _____

Jaundice _____   Heart _____

Bleeding _____

Did you have any problems with:

previous pregnancies? yes___no___

If yes, what was the problem? _____

previous labors? yes___no___

If yes, what was the problem? _____

previous postpartal periods: yes___no___

If yes, what was the problem? _____

Are you Rh negative: yes___no___

Did you receive RhoGam after each pregnancy? yes___no___

What is your present weight? _____

Are you presently taking any prescripton or nonprescription drugs?
yes___no___

If yes, please list medications:

1. _____   3. _____

2. _____   4. _____

Do you smoke? yes___no___

If yes, how many cigarettes per day? _____

How much alcohol do you consume each day? _____

each week? _____

If you have had any of the following diseases,
place a check beside it.

_____ Chickenpox		_____ High blood pressure
_____ Mumps		_____ Heart disease
_____ Measles (3 day)		_____ Respiratory disease
_____ Measles (2 week)		_____ Kidney disease
_____ Asthma		_____ Frequent bladder
		infections

If any of the following diseases is present in your family,
place a check beside the item.

_____ Diabetes	_____ Preeclampsia-eclampsia
_____ Cardiovascular disease	_____ Multiple pregnancies
_____ High blood pressure	_____ Congenital disorder
_____ Breast cancer	

The following questions pertain to the father of this child.

What is the father's age? _____

Does he take prescription or nonprescription drugs? yes___no___

If yes, please list the medications:

1. _____   3. _____

2. _____   4. _____

What is his alcohol intake each day? _____

each week? _____

Figure 15–1   Sample prenatal questionnaire

Table 15–1 System for Determining Risk of Spontaneous Preterm Delivery*

Points assigned	Socioeconomic factors	Previous medical history	Daily habits	Aspects of current pregnancy
1	Two children at home Low socioeconomic status	Abortion × 1 Less than 1 year since last birth	Works outside home	Unusual fatigue
2	Maternal age <20 years or >40 years Single parent	Abortion × 2	Smokes more than 10 cigarettes per day	Gain of less than 5 kg by 32 weeks
3	Very low socioeconomic status Height <150 cm Weight <45 kg	Abortion × 3	Heavy or stressful work Long, tiring trip	Breech at 32 weeks Weight loss of 2 kg Head engaged at 32 weeks Febrile illness
4	Maternal age <18 years	Pyelonephritis		Bleeding after 12 weeks Effacement Dilation Uterine irritability
5		Uterine anomaly Second-trimester abortion DES exposure Cone biopsy		Placenta previa Hydramnios
10		Preterm delivery Repeated second-trimester abortion		Twins Abdominal surgery

*Score is computed by adding the number of points given any item. The score is computed at the first visit and again at 22 to 26 weeks gestation. A total score of 10 or more places the patient at high risk of spontaneous preterm delivery.

Adapted from Creasy RK, Gummer BA, Liggins GC: A system for predicting spontaneous preterm birth. *Obstet Gynecol* 1980;55:692.

risk because of complications. Risk is also assessed intrapartally and postpartally.

Table 15–1 is an example of one risk-scoring protocol that evaluates the woman for factors that increase her risk of spontaneous preterm delivery. The following situation demonstrates how the scoring system is used:

Debbie Williams, a gravida 3, para 2, is ten weeks pregnant when she seeks prenatal care. She works as a legal secretary and smokes about one pack of cigarettes per day. Her children are ages 7 and 4. Her husband is an electrician and has been with the same company for nine years. In assessing Mrs Williams, the nurse notes the following risk factors:

1 point	Two children in the home
1 point	Works outside home
2 points	Smokes more than ten cigarettes/day
4 points	

The nurse determines that at this time Mrs Williams is not at high risk for preterm delivery. The score will be determined again at 22 to 26 weeks' gestation.

Table 15–2 identifies the major risk factors currently recognized. The table describes maternal and fetal/neonatal implications should the risk be present in the pregnancy. In addition to the factors listed, the perinatal health team also needs to evaluate such psychosocial factors as ethnic background; occupation and education; financial status; environment, including living arrangements and location; and the women's and her family's or significant others' concept of health, which might influence her attitude toward seeking health care.

● Initial Physical Assessment

After a complete history is obtained, the woman is prepared for a thorough physical examination.

The Initial Prenatal Physical Assessment Guide beginning on p 346 can be used by the nurse performing the initial prenatal physical examination (see Chapter 14 for a discussion of the diagnosis of pregnancy). The assessment guide is detailed so that maternity nurses using it will be able to use the information pertinent to them in their role, at their level of expertise, and based on the practices and policies of each agency. However, essential components of the assessment have been highlighted to help focus the reader's attention.

The physical examination begins with assessment of vital signs, and proceeds to a complete examination of the woman's body. The pelvic examination is performed last.

Before the examination, the woman should provide a clean voided urine specimen. After emptying her bladder,

(Text continues on page 356.)

Table 15–2 Prenatal High-Risk Factors

Factor	Maternal implication	Fetal/neonatal implication
SOCIAL-PERSONAL		
Low income level and/or low educational level	Poor antenatal care Poor nutrition ↑ risk of preeclampsia	Low birth weight Intrauterine growth retardation (IUGR)
Poor diet	Inadequate nutrition ↑ risk anemia ↑ risk preeclampsia	Fetal malnutrition Prematurity
Living at high altitude	↑ hemoglobin	Prematurity IUGR
Multiparity > 3	↑ risk antepartum/postpartum hemorrhage	Anemia Fetal death
Weight < 100 lb	Poor nutrition Cephalopelvic disproportion Prolonged labor	IUGR Hypoxia associated with difficult labor and delivery
Weight > 200 lb	↑ risk hypertension ↑ risk cephalopelvic disproportion	↓ fetal nutrition
Age < 16	Poor nutrition Poor antenatal care ↑ risk preeclampsia ↑ risk cephalopelvic disproportion	Low birth weight ↑ fetal demise
Age > 35	↑ risk preeclampsia ↑ risk cesarean delivery	↑ risk congenital anomalies ↑ chromosomal aberrations
Smoking one pack/day or more	↑ risk hypertension ↑ risk cancer	↓ placental perfusion → ↓ O_2 and nutrients available Low birth weight IUGR Preterm birth
Use of addicting drugs	↑ risk poor nutrition ↑ risk of infection with IV drugs	↑ risk congenital anomalies ↑ risk low birth weight Neonatal withdrawal Lower serum bilirubin
Excessive alcohol consumption	↑ risk poor nutrition Possible hepatic effects with long-term consumption	↑ risk fetal alcohol syndrome
PREEXISTING MEDICAL DISORDERS		
Diabetes mellitus	↑ risk preeclampsia, hypertension Episodes of hypoglycemia and hyperglycemia ↑ risk cesarean delivery	Low birth weight Macrosomia Neonatal hypoglycemia ↑ risk congenital anomalies ↑ risk respiratory distress syndrome
Cardiac disease	Cardiac decompensation Further strain on mother's body ↑ maternal death rate	↑ risk fetal demise ↑ perinatal mortality
Anemia:* hemoglobin < 9 g/dL (white) < 29% hematocrit (white) < 8.2 g/dL hemoglobin (black) < 26% hematocrit (black)	Iron deficiency anemia Low energy level Decreased oxygen-carrying capacity	Fetal death Prematurity Low birth weight
Hypertension	↑ vasospasm ↑ risk CNS irritability → convulsions ↑ risk CVA ↑ risk renal damage	↓ placental perfusion → low birth weight Preterm birth

Table 15–2 Prenatal High-Risk Factors (continued)

Factor	Maternal implication	Fetal/neonatal implication
Thyroid disorder 　Hypothyroidism	↑ infertility ↓ BMR, goiter, myxedema	↑ spontaneous abortion ↑ risk congenital goiter Mental retardation → cretinism ↑ incidence congenital anomalies
Hyperthyroidism	↑ risk postpartum hemorrhage ↑ risk preeclampsia Danger of thyroid storm	↑ incidence preterm birth ↑ tendency to thyrotoxicosis
Renal disease (moderate to severe)	↑ risk renal failure	↑ risk IUGR ↑ risk preterm delivery
DES exposure	↑ infertility, spontaneous abortion ↑ cervical incompetence	↑ spontaneous abortion ↑ risk preterm delivery
OBSTETRIC CONSIDERATIONS PREVIOUS PREGNANCY		
Stillborn	↑ emotional/psychologic distress	↑ risk IUGR ↑ risk preterm delivery
Habitual abortion	↑ emotional/psychologic distress ↑ possibility diagnostic workup	↑ risk abortion
Cesarean delivery	↑ probability repeat cesarean delivery	↑ risk preterm birth ↑ risk respiratory distress
Rh or blood group sensitization	↑ financial expenditure for testing	Hydrops fetalis Icterus gravis Neonatal anemia Kernicterus Hypoglycemia
CURRENT PREGNANCY		
Rubella (first trimester)		Congenital heart disease Cataracts Nerve deafness Bone lesions Prolonged virus shedding
Rubella (second trimester)		Hepatitis Thrombocytopenia
Cytomegalovirus		IUGR Encephalopathy
Herpesvirus type 2	Severe discomfort Concern about possibility of cesarean delivery, fetal infection	Neonatal herpesvirus type 2 2° hepatitis with jaundice Neurologic abnormalities
Syphilis	↑ incidence abortion	↑ fetal demise Congenital syphilis
Abruptio placenta and placenta previa	↑ risk hemorrhage Bed rest Extended hospitalization	Fetal/neonatal anemia Intrauterine hemorrhage ↑ fetal demise
Preeclampsia/eclampsia	See hypertension	↓ placental perfusion → low birth weight
Multiple gestation	↑ risk postpartum hemorrhage	↑ risk preterm birth ↑ risk fetal demise
Elevated hematocrit* > 41% (white) > 38% (black)	Increased viscosity of blood	Fetal death rate 5 times normal rate
Spontaneous premature rupture of membranes	↑ uterine infection	↑ risk preterm birth ↑ fetal demise

*Data from Garn SM, et al: Maternal hematologic levels and pregnancy outcomes. *Semin Perinatol* 1981;5(April):155.

Initial Prenatal Physical Assessment Guide

Assess/normal findings	Alterations and possible causes*	Nursing responses to data†
VITAL SIGNS		
Blood pressure (BP): 90–140/60–90	High BP (essential hypertension; renal disease; pregestational hypertension; apprehension or anxiety associated with pregnancy diagnosis, exam, or other crises)	BP > 150/90 requires immediate consideration. Establish client's BP. Refer to physician if necessary. Assess woman's knowledge about high BP. Counsel on self- and medical management.
Pulse: 60–90/min Rate may increase 10 beats/min during pregnancy	Increased pulse rate (excitement or anxiety, cardiac disorders)	Count for one full minute. Note irregularities.
Respiration: 16–24/min (or pulse rate divided by four) Pregnancy may induce a degree of hyperventilation; thoracic breathing predominant	Marked tachypnea or abnormal patterns	Assess for respiratory disease.
Temperature: 36.2–37.6C (98–99.6F)	Elevated temperature (infection)	Assess for infection process or disease state if temperature is elevated. Refer to physician.
WEIGHT		
Depends on body build	Weight < 100 or > 200 lb Rapid, sudden weight gain (preeclampsia-eclampsia)	Evaluate need for nutritional counseling. Obtain information on eating habits, cooking practices, foods regularly eaten, income limitations, need for food supplements, pica and other abnormal food habits. Note initial weight to establish baseline for weight gain throughout pregnancy.
SKIN		
Color: Consistent with racial background; pink nail beds	Pallor (anemia) Bronze, yellow (hepatic disease, other causes of jaundice) Bluish, reddish, mottled Dusky appearance or pallor of palms and nail beds in dark-skinned women (anemia)	The following lab tests should be performed: CBC, bilirubin level, urinalysis, and BUN. If abnormal, refer to physician.
Condition: Absence of edema Slight edema of extremities normal during pregnancy	Edema (preeclampsia) Rashes, dermatitis (allergic response)	Counsel on relief measures for slight edema. Initiate preeclampsia assessment. Refer to physician.
Lesions: Absence of lesions	Ulceration (varicose veins, decreased circulation)	Further assess circulatory status. Refer to physician if lesion severe.
Spider nevi common in pregnancy	Petechiae, multiple bruises, ecchymosis (hemorrhagic disorders)	Evaluate for bleeding or clotting disorder.
Moles	Change in size or color	Refer to physician.
Texture: Moderately smooth	Dryness, roughness (dry skin)	Thyroid function tests should be performed.
	Scaliness, broken skin (hypothyroidism, vitamin A deficiency)	Determine usual daily vitamin A intake. Counsel about sources and methods of obtaining necessary vitamin A. If necessary, refer to physician.
Turgor: Skin is elastic and returns to normal shape after pinching	Skin maintains pinched or "tent shape" (dehydration)	Assess for other symptoms of dehydration. Identify ways to control fluid loss and replace necessary fluids. Refer to physician if severe.
Pigmentation: Normal color Café-au-lait spots	Six or more (Albright syndrome or neurofibromatosis)	Consult with physician.
Pigmentation changes of pregnancy include linea nigra, striae gravidarum, chloasma, spider nevi		Assure client that these are normal manifestations of pregnancy and explain the physiologic basis for the changes.
HAIR		
Distribution: Even over entire body	Hirsutism, alopecia (Cushing syndrome, hypothyroidism)	Assess for presence of other symptoms of Cushing's syndrome and hypothyroidism. Refer to physician.

*Possible causes of alterations are placed in parentheses.
†This column provides guidelines for further assessment and initial nursing interventions.

Initial Prenatal Physical Assessment Guide (continued)

Assess/normal findings	Alterations and possible causes*	Nursing responses to data†
Texture: Consistent with racial background	Brittleness, dryness (hypothyroidism, nutritional deficiency)	Evaluate nutritional status. Initiate appropriate dietary education. Evaluate thyroid function.
HEAD		
Size, movement, general appearance: Size appropriate to body; symmetrical; easily supported and moves with smooth control; facial symmetry	Lesions (skin disorders); observable vascularity; drooping of musculature (muscle or nerve disorder); edema; involuntary movement	Do expanded assessment of neurologic function. Refer to physician.
Temporal artery: Able to palpate temporal artery without discomfort to client	Bounding, hard nodules; sensitivity to pressure (high or low carotid pressure)	Assess other pulses. Refer to physician.
Scalp: Normal pattern	Scaliness, excess oiliness, nits or mites (head lice)	Evaluate hygiene. Institute programs to improve hygiene as needed and carry out medical treatment.
	Lumps or tenderness (infection)	Examine for local infection; if none found, refer to physician.
EYES		
Near vision: Able to read print at about 18-in distance	Any deviation from this standard	Refer to physician for further evaluation.
Conjunctiva: Salmon-colored	Pale or infected	The following lab tests should be done: CBC, bilirubin level.
Sclera: White with a few small blood vessels	Localized and/or general hemorrhage; lesions; jaundice; increased vascularity; excess tearing; thick, purulent discharge; opacity of lens; scars; thick pearlike covering over pupil	Refer to physician for further evalution.
Eyelids: Smooth; move easily and close completely; when open, expose pupils equally; lashes full from inner to outer canthus; normal blinking	Exophthalmos (hypothyroidism), loss of elasticity, inflammation, purulent discharge, edema, ptosis, loss of lashes, accentuated or diminished blinking, nystagmus	Thyroid function tests (T_1–T_4) should be performed. Refer to physician.
Pupils: Round and equal; respond briskly to light	Constantly constricted or dilated, abnormal in shape, unresponsive to light	Evaluate for associated ptosis and facial muscle weakness. Refer to physician.
EARS		
External auricle: Size, position, and shape within normal limit for head size	Absence, deformity, lesions, swelling, discharge, foreign bodies	Evaluate for associated problems. Refer to physician.
Inner ear: Cerumen	Golden yellow (fresh cerumen) Darker brownish (older cerumen) Excessive cerumen (difficulty visualizing tympanic membrane)	
Tympanic membrane flat, intact, pearly gray	Bulging, inflammation, tears Exaggerated sound; bulging membrane, reddened membrane (infection)	Refer to physician for further evaluation.
Hearing	Poor perception of sound, no ability to hear	Refer to physician for further evaluation.
JAW		
Temporomandibular joint: Smooth, voluntary opening and closing, full range of motion	Partial movement, pain or tenderness, crepitation, dislocation	Refer to physician for further evaluation.
NOSE		
Patency and symmetry: Partial or fully open, normal contour	Closure or deformity (deviated septum), inflammation, bleeding, discharge, polyps, swelling, rhinitis, folliculitis	Refer to physician for deformities that are bothersome. Treat inflammation or bleeding.
Mucosa: Redder than oral mucosa		
Olfactory ability: In pregnancy, nasal mucosa is edematous in response to increased estrogen, resulting in nasal stuffiness and nosebleeds.	Olfactory loss (first cranial nerve deficit)	Counsel client about possible relief measures for nasal stuffiness and epistaxis. Refer to physician for olfactory loss.

*Possible causes of alterations are placed in parentheses.
†This column provides guidelines for further assessment and initial nursing interventions.

Initial Prenatal Physical Assessment Guide (continued)

Assess/normal findings	Alterations and possible causes*	Nursing responses to data†
SINUSES		
Smooth; normal body temperature	Tenderness; increased temperature; swelling (infection, inflammation)	Assess for other signs of allergy or infection.
MOUTH		
Lips: Even border; pink mucous membrane, free of scaling, lesions; symmetrical shape and opening	Broken areas with mucocutaneous junction swelling, lesions (herpes simplex; benign or malignant lesions)	Discuss comfort measures for herpes. Refer to physician for questionable lesions.
Tongue: Full mobility in mouth; pink color Moderate distribution of papillae over entire tongue Papillae moderately rough	Too large or thick; protuding from oral cavity; smooth; fissured lesions; geographically "hairy"; deviation of tongue from midline	Assess for signs of acromegaly, hypothyroidism, vitamin B_{12} deficiency. Reassure client that some of these signs appear with age.
Mucosa, palate, pharnyx: Pink, unobstructed, moist mucosa; minimal or absent swelling in tonsillar area; hard palate intact	Canker sore; white, curdy patches (thrush) Redness of pharynx; enlarged tonsil and uvula; white patches or gray membrane over throat	Refer if bony tumor not along midline. Culture for thrush and treat. Assess for infections. Counsel regarding seeking prompt health supervision for all infections or colds.
	Deviation of uvula plus soft palate fails to rise when client says "ah" (tenth nerve paralysis)	Refer to physician for further neurologic evaluation.
Gums: May note hypertrophy of gingival papillae because of estrogen	Edema, inflammation (infection); pale (anemia)	Assess hematocrit for anemia. Counsel regarding dental hygiene habits. Refer to physician or dentist if necessary.
NECK		
Nodes: Small, mobile, nontender nodes	Tender, hard, fixed, or prominent nodes (infection, malignancy)	Examine for local infection. Refer to physician.
Trachea: Trachea should be in midline of neck; larynx, trachea, and thyroid rise with swallowing	Deviation to one side or the other; tension on one side or decreased expansion on one side	Chest x-ray examination should be done to identify normal or abnormal lung expansion. Refer to physician if deviation present.
Thyroid: Small, smooth lateral lobes palpable on either side of trachea; slight hyperplasia by third month of pregnancy	Enlargement or nodule tenderness (hyperthyroidism)	Listen over thyroid for bruits, which may indicate hyperthyroidism. Question client about dietary habits (iodine intake). Ascertain history of thyroid problems. Refer to physician.
Major vessels: Easily palpable, good pulse in carotid	Absent or diminished pulses (cardiovascular disease)	Refer to physician.
Jugular veins	Not distended, nonpalpable (low cardiac output)	Assess level of distention with client at 45-degree angle. Refer to physician.
Muscle strength: Able to move head from side to side Resists movement back to midline Equality of strength; able to raise shoulders	Examiner able to return head to midline (weakness of sternocleidomastoid—possible eleventh nerve problem) Unable to elevate shoulders under added pressure (weakness of sternocleidomastoid and trapezius muscles)	Refer for neurologic evaluation.
CHEST AND LUNGS		
Chest: Symmetrical, elliptical, smaller anteroposterior (A-P) than transverse diameter	Increased A-P diameter, funnel chest, pigeon chest (emphysema, asthma, chronic obstructive pulmonary disease, COPD)	Evaluate for emphysema, asthma, pulmonary disease (COPD).
Ribs: Slope downward from nipple line	More horizontal (COPD) Angular bumps Rachitic rosary (vitamin C deficiency)	Evaluate for COPD. Evaluate for fractures. Consult physician. Consult nutritionist
Inspection and palpation: No retraction or bulging of intercostal spaces (ICS) during inspiration or expiration; symmetrical expansion Tactile fremitus	ICS retractions with inspiration, bulging with expiration; unequal expansion (respiratory disease) Tachypnea, hyperpnea, Cheyne-Stokes respirations (respiratory disease)	Do thorough initial assessment. Refer to physician. Refer to physician.
Percussion: Bilateral symmetry in tone	Flatness of percussion, which may be affected by chest wall thickness	Evaluate for pleural effusions, consolidations, or tumor.

*Possible causes of alterations are placed in parentheses.
†This column provides guidelines for further assessment and initial nursing interventions.

Initial Prenatal Physical Assessment Guide (continued)

Assess/normal findings	Alterations and possible causes*	Nursing responses to data†
Low-pitched resonance of moderate intensity	High diaphragm (atelectasis or paralysis), pleural effusion	Refer to physician.
Auscultation: Upper lobes: bronchovesicular sounds above sternum and scapulas; equal expiratory and inspiratory phases	Abnormal if heard over any other area of chest	Refer to physician.
Remainder of chest: vesicular breath sounds heard; inspiratory phase longer (3:1)	Rales, rhonchi, wheezes; pleural friction rub; absence of breath sounds; bronchophony, egophony; whispered pectoriloquy	Refer to physician.
BREASTS		
Supple; symmetry in size and contour; darker pigmentation of nipple and areola; may have supernumerary nipples, usually 5–6 cm below normal nipple line	"Pigskin" or orange-peel appearance; nipple retraction; swelling, hardness (carcinoma); redness, heat, tenderness, cracked or fissured nipple (infection)	Encourage monthly breast checks. Instruct client how to examine own breasts (Procedure 10–1). Refer to physician.
Axillary nodes unpalpable or pellet size	Tenderness, enlargement, hard node; may be visible bump (infection); carcinoma	Refer to physician if evidence of inflammation.
Pregnancy changes: 1. Size increase noted primarily in first 20 weeks. 2. Breasts become nodular. 3. Tingling sensation may be felt during first and third trimester; woman may report feeling of heaviness. 4. Pigmentation of nipples and areolas darkens. 5. Superficial veins dilate and become more prominent. 6. Striae seen in multiparas. 7. Tubercles of Montgomery enlarge. 8. Colostrum may be present after 12 weeks. 9. Secondary areola appears at 20 weeks, characterized by series of washed-out spots surrounding primary areola. 10. Breasts are less firm, old striae may be present in multiparas.		Discuss normalcy of changes and their meaning with the client. Teach and/or institute appropriate relief measures (see Chapter 16). Encourage use of supportive brassiere.
HEART		
Size and placement: Lies in thoracic cavity within mediastinum; upper border lies behind upper portion of sternum; lower border lies at level of third left costal cartilage close to sternum	Enlargement (cardiac disease)	Complete initial cardiac assessment. Refer to physician.
Palpation: PMI 1–2 cm in diameter and located 7–9 cm left of midsternal point in the fourth or fifth intercostal space (may be further left of midsternal line during pregnancy)	Diffuse PMI located farther than 9 cm left of midsternal point (left ventricular hypertrophy or dilatation)	Assess other cardiac findings. Refer to physician if indicated.
Thrills not present Palpitation may occur in pregnancy due to sympathetic nervous system disturbance	Thrills, palpable vibrations that resemble a cat's purr, are associated with cardiac defects; thrusting of chest wall felt during palpation (cardiac disease)	Refer to physician.
Rate and rhythm: Normal rate and rhythm	Gross irregularity or skipped beats	Refer to physician. Twelve-lead EKG may be part of cardiac evaluation process to screen for abnormalities of rhythm or electrical conduction.
Rhythm may vary slightly with respirations	Three heart sounds or gallop rhythm may signal presence of decompensation or carditis	

Possible causes of alterations are placed in parentheses.
†*This column provides guidelines for further assessment and initial nursing interventions.*

Initial Prenatal Physical Assessment Guide (continued)

Assess/normal findings	Alterations and possible causes*	Nursing responses to data†
Sounds: Normal heart sounds No murmurs present (short systolic murmurs that ↑ in held expiration are normal during pregnancy)	Extra or prolonged sounds may signify valvular disease Murmur (obstruction to cardiac blood flow)	Assure client of normalcy of short systolic murmurs in pregnancy. Refer to physician for abnormal sounds.
ABDOMEN Appearance: Skin clear with exception of whitish silver striae of multiparas	Purple striae (Cushing syndrome)	Assess for presence of other symptoms of Cushing syndrome.
Fine venous network	Dilated veins (vena cava obstruction)	
Peristalsis may be visible in very thin women	Increased peristaltic waves (intestinal obstruction)	Refer to physician.
Aortic pulsation may be visible in epigastrium	Increased pulsation (aortic aneurysm)	
Pubic hair limited to pubic area	Hair distribution extending to umbilicus (bilateral polycystic ovary, Cushing ovary, ovarian tumor)	
Umbilicus deeply indented early in pregnancy and more shallow as pregnancy progresses; at end of pregnancy, level with surface or may protrude slightly	Exudate or bleeding from umbilicus (infection, fistula) Herniation or bulging	Evaluate for infection.
Auscultation: Bowel sounds 5–34/min	Hyperactivity (hyperperistalsis)	Discuss dietary habits. Evaluate for stress-related factors. Refer to physician if indicated.
Palpation: Abdomen nontender and relaxed, especially during expiration	Muscle guarding (anxiety, acute tenderness); tenderness, mass (ectopic pregnancy, inflammation, carcinoma)	Evaluate client anxiety level. Refer to physician if indicated.
Diastasis of the rectus muscles late in pregnancy	Excessive separation of muscles	Assure client of normalcy of diastasis. Provide initial information about appropriate postpartum exercises.
Liver nonpalpable	Rebound tenderness (peritoneal inflammation) Liver palpable below right costal margin, tender and/or nodules (suggest malignancy)	Refer to physician.
Absence of pain	Pains in any abdominal quadrants; tenderness above inguinal ligaments (salpingitis)	Refer to physician for evaluation of specific cause.
Size: Flat or rotund abdomen Progressive increase in size of uterus due to pregnancy 10–12 weeks: fundus slightly above symphysis pubis 16 weeks: fundus halfway between symphysis and umbilicus 20–22 weeks: fundus at umbilicus 28 weeks: fundus three finger-breadths above umbilicus 36 weeks: fundus just below ensiform cartilage	Size of uterus inconsistent with length of gestation (IUGR, multiple pregnancy, fetal demise, hydatidiform mole)	Reassess menstrual history regarding pregnancy dating. Evaluate increase in size by measuring fundal height (p. 358). Use ultrasound to establish diagnosis.
Fetal heart beat: 120–160 beats/min May be heard with Doppler at 10–12 weeks' gestation May be heard with fetoscope at 17–20 weeks	Failure to hear fetal heartbeat at 17–20 weeks (fetal demise, hydatidiform mole)	Refer to physician. Administer pregnancy tests. Use ultrasound to establish diagnosis.
Fetal movement: Not felt prior to 20 weeks' gestation by examiner	Failure to feel fetal movements after 20 weeks gestation (fetal demise, hydatidiform mole)	Refer to physician for evaluation of fetal status.
Ballottement: During fourth to fifth month, fetus rises and then rebounds to original position when uterus is tapped sharply	Failure to ascertain ballottement	Refer to physician for evaluation of fetal status.
EXTREMITIES Arms and hands: Hands warm, may be slightly moist; full range of motion; strong grip; good palpable pulses	Hands cold, stiff, tender; enlargement or deflation of phalanges; deviation of ulna or radius; presence of nodules (arthritis)	Evaluate for other symptoms of vascular disease or arthritis. Refer to physician if these are found or if data are questionable.

*Possible causes of alterations are placed in parentheses.
†This column provides guidelines for further assessment and initial nursing interventions.

Initial Prenatal Physical Assessment Guide (continued)

Assess/normal findings	Alterations and possible causes*	Nursing responses to data†
In late pregnancy, may have some edema of hands	Marked edema (preeclampsia)	Initiate follow-up if client mentions that her rings feel tight.
Nails: Pink nail beds, nail base angle 160°, nail base firm	Clubbing (hypoxia); spoon nails (iron-deficiency anemia)	Evaluate for anemia or heart disease.
Legs/feet: Toes pink; femoral, popliteal, posterior tibial, and dorsalis pedis pulses palpable; Homan's sign negative	Unpalpable or diminished pulses (arterial insufficiency); pallor on elevation, cool temperature, skin atrophic and shiny, ulcerations, brown pigmentation around ankles (venous insufficiency, varicose veins)	Discuss prevention and self-treatment measures for varicose veins. Refer to physician if indicated.
MUSCULOSKELETAL SYSTEM		
Full range of motion	Limitation or deviation of joints Swollen, tender, hot joints and subcutaneous nodules (rheumatoid arthritis) Bony enlargement of joints (osteoarthritis) Knock knees, bowlegs, painful swelling of metatarsophalangeal joint (gout)	Determine which joints are involved. Refer to physician.
Spine: Normal spinal curves: concave cervical, convex thoracic, concave lumbar	Abnormal spinal curves: flatness, kyphosis, lordosis	Refer to physician for assessment of cephalopelvic disproportion. May have implications for administration of spinal anethesia.
Dorsal and lumbar spinal curve may be accentuated during pregnancy	Backache	See p. 382 for relief measures.
Shoulders and iliac crests should be even	Uneven shoulders and iliac crests (scoliosis)	Refer very young clients to a physician. Discuss back stretching exercises with older clients.
Vertebras: In straight vertical line Absence of tenderness	Curvature (kyphosis, scoliosis) Tenderness lateral to spine on flexion-extension or pressure	Refer to physician.
	Costovertebral angle tenderness (kidney infection or disease)	Obtain urinalysis. Refer to physician.
Able to do straight leg raises without back pain During advanced pregnancy, hypermotility of pelvic joints and accentuation of dorsal and lumbar curvature	Back pain (disc disease) Separation of symphysis, synchondrosis	Refer to physician.
Reflexes: Reflexes normal and symmetrical	Hyperactivity, clonus (preeclampsia) Asymmetrical, diminished (cerebral or spinal nerve damage)	Evaluate for preeclampsia and cerebral or spinal nerve damage. (See Chapter 19 for specific nursing interventions.)
PELVIC AREA		
External genitalia: Mons pubis covered with hair in shape of inverted triangle: labia majora symmetrical, not adherent or enlarged; vulva appears pink and moist	Lesions, hematomas, cellulitis, varicosities, urethral caruncle, inflammation of Bartholin's gland	Explain pelvic examination procedure (Procedure 15–1 on p 355.). Encourage woman to minimize her discomfort by relaxing her hips. Provide privacy.
Small clitoris not exceeding 2 cm in length and 1 cm in width	Clitoral hypertrophy (masculinization)	
In multiparas, labia majora loose and pigmented	Vulva inflamed, white patches present on mucosa and cervix (carcinoma)	Refer to physician.
Urinary and vaginal orifices visible and appropriately located	Single meatus for urethra and vagina (fistula) Fistulous opening	Refer to physician.
	Urethral irritation and/or discharge (urethritis, foreign body)	Obtain smear, urinalysis. Refer to physician.
Vagina: Pink or dark pink in color	Grayish white patches (carcinoma)	Refer to physician.
No bulging into vagina when woman strains	Bulging into vagina from upper wall (cystocele) Bulging into vagina from posterior wall (rectocele)	

*Possible causes of alterations are placed in parentheses.
†This column provides guidelines for further assessment and initial nursing interventions.

Initial Prenatal Physical Assessment Guide (continued)

Assess/normal findings	Alterations and possible causes*	Nursing responses to data†
Vaginal discharge odorless, nonirritating, thin or mucoid, clear or cloudy	Discharge associated with vaginal infections: 1. Monilial infection: thick, white, curdy 2. Trichomonal infection: profuse, watery, gray or green, frothy, with odor 3. *Gardnerella vaginalis* (bacterial vaginosis): malodorous, gray 4. Gonorrhea: green-yellow discharge, inflamed cervix and vulva 5. Chlamydia: thick mucus discharge, cervix may be inflamed, adnexa may be tender	Obtain vaginal smear See p. 512 for management of infections. Provide understandable verbal and written instructions to facilitate safe and effective treatment. Treat sexual partner if indicated.
In multipara, vaginal folds smooth and flattened, entire vaginal canal widened; may have old episiotomy scar Cervix: (Figure 15–2) Pink color; os closed except in multipara, in whom os admits fingertip	Eversion, reddish erosion, nabothian or retention cysts, cervical polyp; granular area that bleeds (carcinoma of cervix) Red spots on and around cervix (trichomonas vaginitis) Presence of string or plastic tip from cervix (IUD in uterus)	Provide client with a hand mirror and identify genital structures for her. Encourage her to view her cervix. Refer to physician if indicated. Advise client of potential serious risks of leaving an IUD in place during pregnancy. Refer to physician for removal.

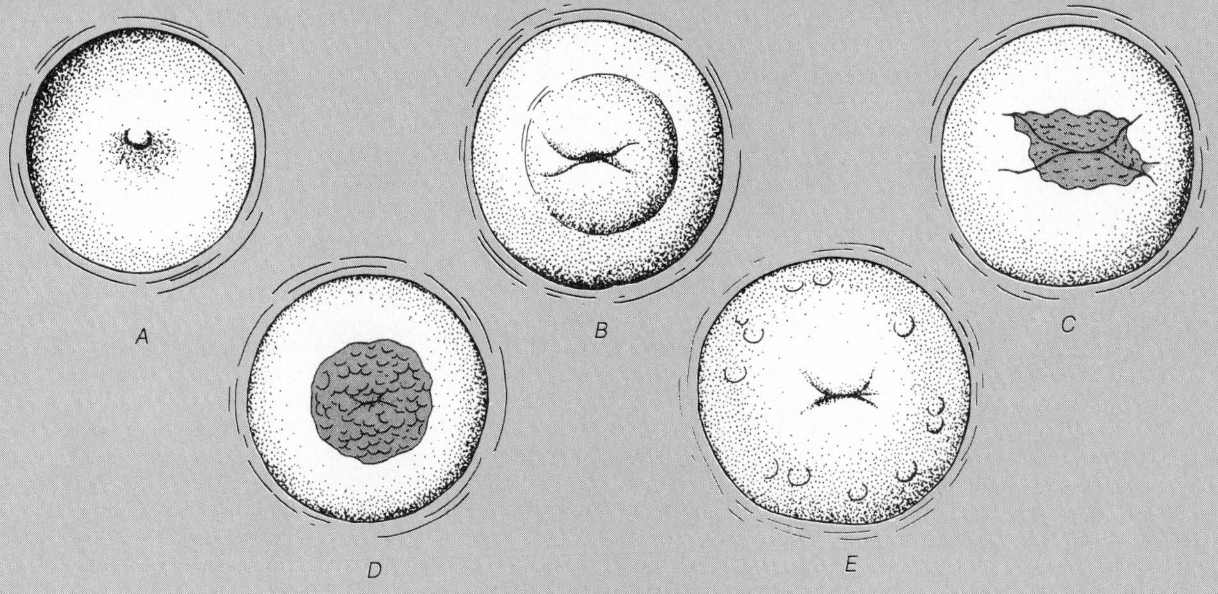

Figure 15–2 Common appearance of cervix on vaginal exam. A Healthy nulliparous cervix. B Lacerated multigravidous cervix. C Everted cervix. D Eroded cervix. E Nabothian cysts.

Pregnancy changes: 1–4 weeks' gestation: enlargement in anteroposterior diameter 4–6 weeks' gestation: softening of cervix (Goodell's sign) and cervicouterine junction (Ladin's sign); softening of isthmus of uterus (Hegar's sign); cervix takes on bluish coloring (Chadwick's sign) 8 weeks' gestation: uterus globular in shape and anteflexed against bladder 8–12 weeks' gestation: vagina and cervix appear bluish violet in color (Chadwick's sign)	Inability to elicit Goodell's sign (inflammatory conditions and carcinomas)	Refer to physician.

*Possible causes of alterations are placed in parentheses.
†This column provides guidelines for further assessment and initial nursing interventions.

Initial Prenatal Physical Assessment Guide (continued)

Assess/normal findings	Alterations and possible causes*	Nursing responses to data†
Uterus: Pear-shaped Located at upper end of vagina Mobile within pelvis Smooth surface	Retroversion, retroflexion Prolapse Fixed (pelvic inflammatory disease) Nodular surface (fibromas)	Discuss appropriate individualized exercises and need for rest. Refer to physician if indicated. Refer to physician.
Ovaries: Small, walnut-shaped, nontender	Pain on movement of cervix (pelvic inflammatory disease) Enlarged or nodular ovaries (cyst, tumor, tubal pregnancy, corpus luteum of pregnancy)	Evaluate adnexal areas. Refer to physician.
Pelvic measurements: Internal measurements: 1. Diagonal conjugate 12.5 cm	Measurement below normal	Vaginal delivery may not be possible if deviations are present. Consider possibility of cesarean delivery. Determine CPD by ultrasound.
2. Obstetric conjugate estimated by subtracting 1.5–2 cm from diagonal conjugate	Disproportion of pubic arch	
3. Inclination of sacrum 4. Motility of coccyx External measurements: intertuberosity diameter >8 cm	Abnormal curvature of sacrum Fixed or malposition of coccyx	
ANUS AND RECTUM		
No lumps, rashes, excoriation, tenderness	Hemorrhoids, rectal prolapse Nodular lesion (carcinoma)	Counsel about appropriate prevention and relief measures. Refer to physician for further evaluation.
Cervix may be felt through rectal wall	Pilonidal cyst or sinus, anorectal fistula, anal fissure, rectal polyps, internal or external hemorroids	Counsel about appropriate relief measures (see Chapter 16).
Stool negative for obvious or occult blood Symmetrical buttocks	Stool positive for blood (intestinal bleeding)	Refer to physician.
LABORATORY EVALUATION		
Hemoglobin: 12–16 g/dL	<12 g/dL (anemia)	Hemoglobin <12 g/dL requires iron supplementation and nutritional counseling.
Women residing in high altitude may have higher levels of hemoglobin		
ABO and Rh typing: Normal distribution of blood types	Rh negative	If Rh negative, check for presence of anti-Rh antibodies. Check partner's blood type. If partner is Rh positive, discuss with client the need for antibody titers during pregnancy, management during the intrapartal period, and possible candidacy for RhoGAM.
Complete blood count (CBC): Hematocrit: 38%–47%	Anemia or blood dyscrasias	Perform WBC and Schilling differential cell count.
Red blood cells: 4.2–5.4 million/μL White blood cells: 4500–11,000/μL	Presence of infection; may be elevated in pregnancy and with labor	Evaluate for other signs of infection.
Differential: Neutrophils 40%–60% Bands up to 5% Eosinophils 1%–3% Basophils up to 1% Lymphocytes 20%–40% Monocytes 4%–8%		
Syphilis tests—STS (serologic test for syphilis); complement fixation test; VDRL (Venereal Disease Research Laboratory test): nonreactive	Positive reaction STS tests may have 25%–45% incidence of biologic false positive results; false results may occur in individuals who have acute viral or bacterial infections, hypersensitivity reactions, recent vaccination, collagen disease, malaria, or tuberculosis	Positive results may be confirmed with the FTA-ABS tests (fluorescent treponemal antibody absorption tests). All tests for syphilis give positive results in the secondary stage of the disease; antibiotic tests may cause negative test results.

*Possible causes of alterations are placed in parentheses.
†This column provides guidelines for further assessment and initial nursing interventions.

Initial Prenatal Physical Assessment Guide (continued)

Assess/normal findings	Alterations and possible causes*	Nursing responses to data†
Gonorrhea culture: Negative	Positive	Refer for treatment
Urinalysis (u/a): Pale golden yellow color	Orange, red, brown hues (porphyria, hemoglobinuria, urobilinuria, or bilirubinemia, treatment with phenazopyridine)	Assess for deviations. Porphyria may be indicated if urine becomes burgundy red on exposure to light.
Specific gravity: 1.015–1.025	<1.015 (renal tubular dysfunction); >1.025 (ADH deficiency)	Refer to physician.
Ph: 4.6–8.0	Alkaline urine (metabolic alkalemia, *Proteus* infections, old specimen)	
Glucose: Negative (small amount of glycosuria may occur in pregnancy)	Glycosuria (low renal threshold for glucose, diabetes mellitus, Cushing disease, pheochromocytoma)	Assess blood glucose. Test urine for ketones.
Protein: Negative	Proteinuria (urine specimen contaminated with vaginal secretions, strenuous physical exercise, fever, kidney disease, postrenal infection, preeclampsia)	Repeat urinalysis. Instruct client in collection technique. If second specimen positive, do further assessment.
Red blood cells: Negative	Blood in urine (calculi, cystitis, glomerulonephritis, neoplasm)	Refer to physician.
White blood cells: Negative	Presence of white blood cells (infection in genitourinary tract)	Assess for other signs of infection. Refer to physician if indicated.
Casts: Negative	Presence of casts (nephrotic syndrome)	
Rubella titer: Hemagglutination-inhibition test (HAI) > 1:10 indicates woman is immune	HAI titer < 1:10	Immunization will be given within 6 weeks after delivery. Instruct client whose titers are < 1:10 to avoid children who have rubella.
Antibody screen: Negative	Positive	For positive results, further testing should be done to identify specific antibodies. Antibody titers may also be done during pregnancy.
Sickle cell screen for black clients: Negative	Positive; test results would include a description of cells	Refer to physician.
Papanicolaou (Pap) test: Negative	Test results that show atypical cells†	Refer to physician. Discuss the meaning of the various classes with the client and importance of follow-up.

*Possible causes of alterations are placed in parentheses.
†This column provides guidelines for further assessment and initial nursing interventions.
†The current trend is to report Pap test results as follows:
1. Negative
2. Atypical (this finding would describe the cells)
Some clinicians may still use Class I to Class V terminology, with Class I being negative and Class V cancer in situ. It is important to know the scoring system used by the laboratory doing the test.

· Procedure 15–1   Assisting with Pelvic Examination ·

Objective	Nursing action	Rationale
Prepare woman	Explain procedure.	Explanation of procedure decreases anxiety.
	Instruct woman to empty her bladder and to remove clothing below waist. She may be encouraged to keep her shoes on and may be given a disposable drape to hold in front of herself.	Comfort is promoted during internal examination. She may feel more comfortable with shoes on rather than supporting her weight with bare heels against cold stirrups.
	Position woman in lithotomy position with thighs flexed and adducted. Place her feet in stirrups. Buttocks should extend slightly beyond end of examining table (Figure 15–3).	
	Drape woman with a sheet, leaving flap so perineum can be exposed.	
Ensure smooth accomplishment of procedure	Prepare and arrange following equipment so that they are easily accessible:	Examination is facilitated.
	1. Various-sized vaginal specula, warmed prior to insertion.	Warmed speculum assists in lubrication and facilitates initial insertion when culture and smears are to be taken; many standard lubricants cannot be utilized.
	2. Glove.	
	3. Lubricant.	
	4. Pelvimeter.	
	5. Materials for Pap smear and gonorrhea culture.	
	6. Good light source.	
Provide support to woman as physician or nurse practitioner carries out examination	Explain each part of examination as it is performed: inspection of external genitals, vagina, and cervix: bimanual examination of internal organs. Instruct woman to relax and breathe slowly.	Relaxation is promoted.
	Advise woman when speculum is to be inserted and ask her to bear down.	When speculum is inserted, woman may feel intravaginal pressure. Bearing down helps open vaginal orifice and relax perineal muscles.
	Lubricate examiner's finger well prior to bimanual examination.	
Provide for woman's comfort at end of examination	Assist woman to sitting position.	Supine position may create postural hypotension.
	Provide tissues to wipe lubricant from perineum.	Upon assuming sitting position, vaginal secretions along with lubricant may be discharged.
	Provide privacy for woman to dress.	Comfort and sense of privacy is promoted.

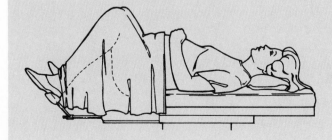

Figure 15–3   Woman in lithotomy position and draped for a pelvic examination

she is asked to disrobe and is given a gown and a sheet or some other protective covering. The woman who has emptied her bladder will be more comfortable during the pelvic examination, and the examiner will be able to palpate the abdominal organs more easily.

The physical examination is facilitated when the woman is at ease and comfortable.

As a result of basic education programs or physical assessment or practitioner courses, increasing numbers of nurses are prepared to perform physical examinations. The nurse who has not yet fully developed specific assessment skills assesses the woman's vital signs, explains the pro-

Research Note

Many women find a pelvic exam an unpleasant experience and delay gynecologic care to avoid it. Early cervical cancer detected by PAP smear during routine gynecologic care is curable, yet 6800 American women died of the disease in 1985. Willard and Heaberg looked at whether a new approach to the pelvic exam would give women a more positive attitude toward this part of their gynecologic care.

The study used a convenience sample of 213 women who were randomly assigned to have either a traditional pelvic exam or an educational pelvic exam. The examiners attempted to establish a warm relationship with women in both groups, but in the educational group the women were positioned and draped to allow eye contact with the examiner, were offered a mirror to hold and watch the exam, and were encouraged to participate by asking questions. Pre- and postexam questionnaires were used to elicit data.

The researchers found that while both groups had similar preexisting attitudes about pelvic exams, the educational group had a significantly more positive attitude about this exam than the control group, were more physically comfortable, and felt that they learned more.

The nurse can play an important role in improving a woman's experience of a pelvic exam by incorporating the aspects of the educational pelvic exam when performing or assisting with the exam. While 80% of the women said that they would like to look in the mirror in their next exam, only 47% said that they would actually ask for one. It seems that the nurse needs to take the initiative in offering a mirror, pointing out anatomic parts, draping to allow eye contact, and encouraging the client to ask questions.

Willard MD, Heaberg GL, Pack JB: *The educational pelvic exam: Women's responses to a new approach. J Obstet Gynecol Neonat News* 1986;15(March/April):135–140.

cedures to allay apprehension, positions her for examination, and assists the examiner as necessary.

Each nurse is responsible for operating at the expected standard for someone with that individual nurse's skill and knowledge base. The following situation demonstrates this expectation.

Margo Cole is being seen in the clinic at 36 weeks' gestation. She began prenatal care at 12 weeks and her pregnancy to date has been uneventful. Pam Forbes graduated from her nursing program 9 months ago without having received any formal classes in physical assessment. Ms Forbes is doing the initial routine assessments for Ms Cole and observes that her weight gain has been excessive. When checking the vital signs Ms Forbes also notes a significant increase in Ms Cole's blood pressure. At this point Ms Forbes should be considering the possibility that Ms Cole may be developing preeclampsia. Ms Forbes would continue her assessment by using a dipstick to check the urine for the presence of protein, query Margo Cole about any recent problems with swelling, and do at least an initial check for any edema. Ms Forbes is not expected to diagnose the condition, but her charting should reflect her findings in a logical manner so that the clinician will be alerted, an in-depth assessment will be made, and treatment initiated if necessary.

Thoroughness and a systematic procedure are the most important considerations when performing a physical exam. To promote completeness the assessment guide is organized into three columns: area to be assessed/normal findings, alterations and possible causes of the alterations, and nursing response to data. The nurse should be aware that certain organs and systems are assessed concurrently with other systems.

Nursing interventions based on assessment of the normal physiologic and psychologic changes associated with pregnancy and client teaching and counseling needs that have been mutually defined are discussed in more detail in Chapter 16.

● Determination of Delivery Date

Childbearing families generally want to know the "due date," or the date around which delivery will occur. Historically the delivery date has been called the estimated date of confinement (EDC). The concept of confinement is, however, rather negative, and there is a trend in the literature to avoid it by referring to the delivery date as the EDD or *estimated date of delivery*.

To calculate the EDD it is helpful to know the first day of the woman's last menstrual period (LMP). However, some women have episodes of irregular bleeding or fail to keep track of menstrual cycles. Thus other techniques also help to determine how far along a woman is in her pregnancy, that is, at how many weeks gestation she is. Other techniques that can be used include evaluating uterine size, determining when quickening occurs, and auscultating fetal heart rate with a fetoscope.

Nägele's Rule

The most common method of determining the EDD is Nägele's rule. To use this method, one begins with the first day of the last menstrual period, subtracts three months, and adds seven days. For example:

First day of LMP	November 21
Subtract 3 months	− 3 months
	August 21
Add 7 days	+ 7 days
EDD	August 28

A simpler method is to change the months to numerical terms:

November 21 becomes	11–21
Subtract 3 months	− 3
	8–21
Add 7 days	+ 7
EDD	August 28

If a woman with a history of menses every 28 days remembers her LMP and was not taking oral contraceptives prior to becoming pregnant, Nägele's rule may be a fairly accurate determiner of her predicted delivery date. However, if her cycle is irregular or 35 to 40 days in length, the time of ovulation may be delayed by several days. If she has been on oral contraceptives, ovulation may be delayed several weeks following her last menses. Ovulation usually occurs 14 days before the onset of the next menses, not 14 days after the previous menses.

A gestation calculator or "wheel" permits the care giver to calculate the EDD even more quickly (Figure 15–4). The arrow that is labeled "last menses began" is rotated until it is lined up on the date of the first day of the woman's LMP. The EDD is found by reading the date at the end of the arrow marked 40. This is called the term arrow. Postpartally the woman's actual length of gestation can be determined by aligning the term arrow with the EDD and then reading the weeks of gestation that aligns with the actual delivery date. For example, if the EDD is August 28, but the woman delivers on September 7, her gestation was 41 and 3/7 weeks, or approximately 41½ weeks. This information is useful when calculating the newborn's gestational age (see Chapter 28).

Uterine Assessment

PHYSICAL EXAMINATION

When a woman is examined in the first 10 to 12 weeks of her pregnancy and the nurse practitioner or phy-

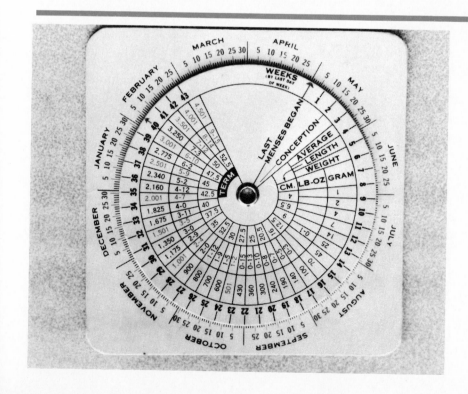

Figure 15–4 The EDD wheel can be used to calculate delivery date.

sician thinks that her uterine size is compatible with her menstrual history, uterine size may be the single most important clinical method for dating her pregnancy. In many cases, however, women do not seek obstetric attention until well into their second trimester, when it becomes much more difficult to evaluate specific uterine size. In the case of the obese woman, it is most difficult to determine uterine size early in a pregnancy.

FUNDAL HEIGHT

Fundal height may be used as an indicator of uterine size, although this cannot be used late in pregnancy. A centimeter tape measure is used to measure the distance abdominally from the top of the symphysis pubis over the curve of the abdomen to the top of the uterine fundus (McDonald's method) (Figure 15–5). Fundal height in centimeters (when determined after the woman has emptied her bladder) correlates well with weeks of gestation between 20 and 31 weeks. At 26 weeks gestation, for example, fundal height is probably about 26 cm. At 20 weeks gestation the fundus is about 20 cm and at the level of the umbilicus in an average female. If the woman is very tall or very short, however, fundal height will differ. In the third trimester variations in fetal weight decrease the accuracy of fundal height measurements.

Measurements of fundal height from month to month and week to week may give indications of intrauterine growth retardation (IUGR) if there is a lag in progression, or indications of the presence of twins or hydramnios if there is a sudden increase in height. Unfortunately this method of dating a pregnancy can be quite inaccurate in obese women, in women with uterine fibroids, and in mothers who develop hydramnios.

QUICKENING

Fetal movements felt by the mother may give some indications that the fetus is nearing 20 weeks' gestation. However, quickening may be experienced between 16 and 22 weeks' gestation, so this is not a completely accurate method. One can begin to listen for a fetal heartbeat weekly after the woman experiences quickening and can use this indication to assist documentation for a delivery date. Because multiparous women have experienced quickening before, they often report it earlier than a primigravida does.

FETAL HEARTBEAT

The fetal heartbeat can be detected as early as week 16 and almost always by 19 or 20 weeks of gestation with an ordinary fetoscope. In the case of twins or the obese woman, it may be later than this before the fetal heartbeat can be detected. Fetal heartbeat may be detected with the ultrasonic Doppler device (Figure 15–6) at about 10 to 12 weeks' gestation.

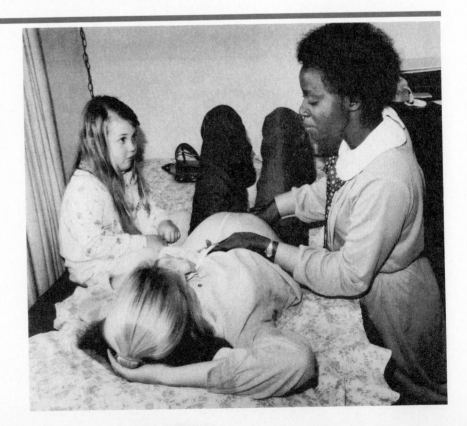

Figure 15–5   The nurse measures fundal height using McDonald's method.

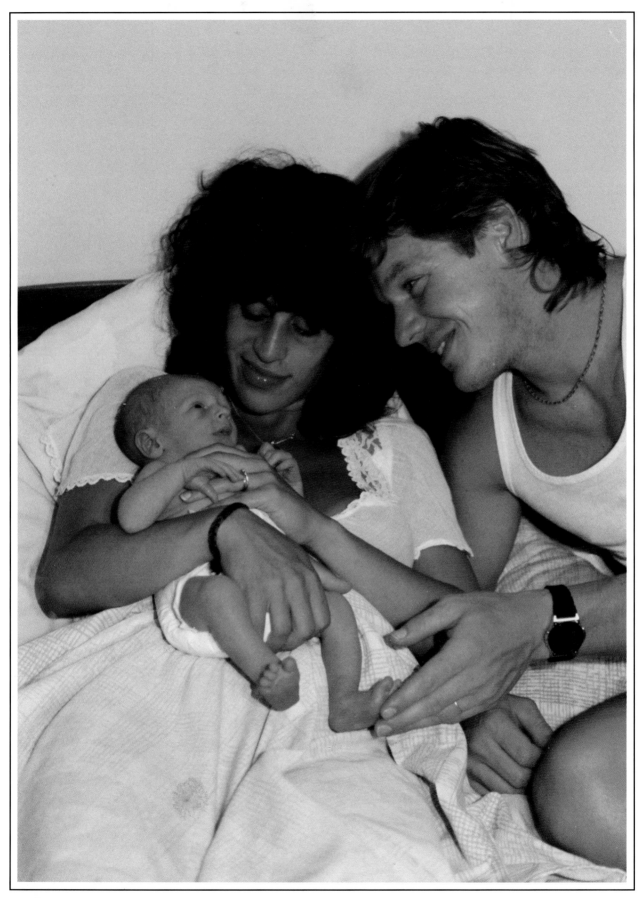

Plate I   Beginnings . . .

Development is rapid; heart begins to pump blood; limb buds are well developed. Facial features and major divisions of the brain are discernible. Ears develop from skin folds; tiny bones and muscles are formed beneath the thin skin.

Embryo becomes a fetus, its beating heart discernible by ultrasound. Assumes a more human shape as lower body develops. At week 12, first movements begin. Sex is determinable. Kidneys produce urine.

Musculoskeletal system has matured; nervous system begins to exert control. Blood vessels rapidly develop. Fetal hands can grasp; legs kick actively. All organs begin to mature and grow. Fetus weighs about 7 oz (½ lb). FHT discernible with Doppler. Pancreas produces insulin.

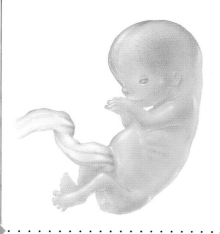

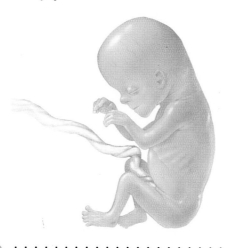

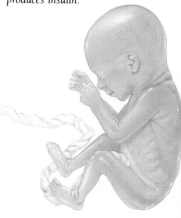

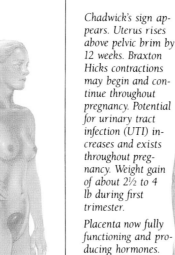

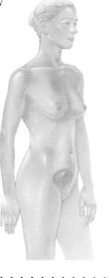

Morning sickness, may persist to 12 weeks. Uterus changes from pear to globular shape. Hegar's, Goodell's and Piskacek's signs appear. Cervix flexes; leukorrhea increases. Surprise and ambivalence about pregnancy may occur. No noticeable weight gain.

Chadwick's sign appears. Uterus rises above pelvic brim by 12 weeks. Braxton Hicks contractions may begin and continue throughout pregnancy. Potential for urinary tract infection (UTI) increases and exists throughout pregnancy. Weight gain of about 2½ to 4 lb during first trimester.

Placenta now fully functioning and producing hormones.

Fundus halfway between symphysis and umbilicus. Woman gains slightly less than 1 lb per wk for remainder of pregnancy. May feel more energetic. BPD measurement on ultrasound. Vaginal secretions increase. Itching, irritation, malodor suggest infection. Woman may begin wearing maternity clothes. Pressure on bladder lessens and urinary frequency decreases.

Eat dry crackers before arising; try frequent small, dry, low-fat meals with fluids taken between meals. Avoid use of hot tubs, saunas, and steam rooms throughout pregnancy.

Discuss attitudes toward pregnancy. Discuss value of early pregnancy classes that focus on what to expect during pregnancy. Provide information about childbirth preparation classes.

Adequate fluid intake and frequent voiding (every 2 hr while awake) help prevent UTI. Also helpful to void following intercourse. Wipe from front to rear.

Discuss nutrition and appropriate weight gain. Stress value of regular physical exercise, especially non-weightbearing activities or walking. Discuss possible effects of pregnancy on sexual relationship.

Daily shower or bath and thorough drying of vulva helpful; avoid douching during pregnancy. Consult caregiver if infection suspected; use only prescribed medications.

Review danger signs of pregnancy. Discuss infant feeding options; provide information on the value of breastfeeding. Provide information about clothing, shoes.

FETAL DEVELOPMENT

MATERNAL CHANGES

CLIENT TEACHING/
ANTICIPATORY GUIDANCE

The sperm fertilizes the ovum, which then divides and burrows into the uterus.

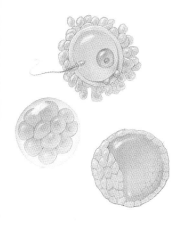

From the embryonic disk (ect‍derm, entoderm, mesoderm), first body segments appear th‍will eventually become the sp‍brain, and spinal cord. Heart‍blood circulation, and digesti‍tract take shape. Embryo is le‍than a quarter-inch long.

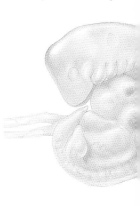

Mother misses first period; breasts become tender, may enlarge. Chronic fatigue and urin‍ary frequency be‍gin, may persist for three or more months. hCG in urine and serum 9 days after conception.

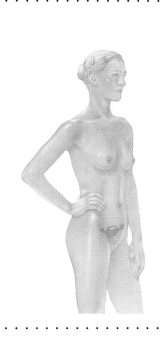

Supportive bra may ease disc‍fort. Increased rest and relax‍necessary now and throughou‍pregnancy. Increase fluids du‍the day; decrease fluid intake‍at night to help prevent noctu‍sleep on side to decrease pres.‍on bladder. Avoid using any r‍cations unless prescribed. Avo‍use of social drugs; check wit‍caregiver before using any OT‍preparations.

Plate II Linea nigra

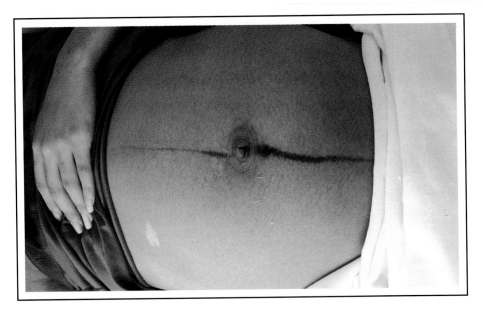

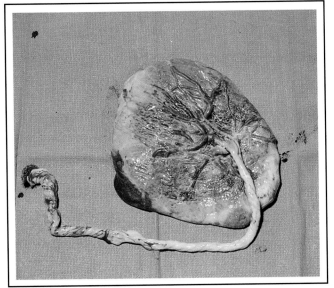

Plate III Fetal side of placenta

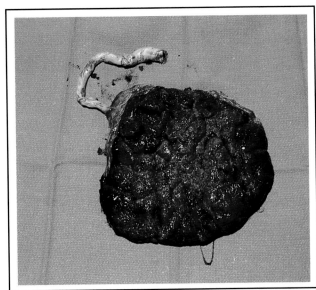

Plate IV Maternal side of placenta

Plate V Acrocyanosis

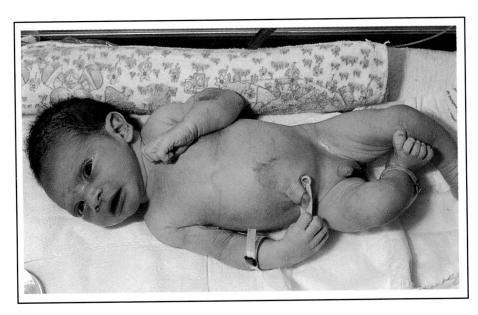

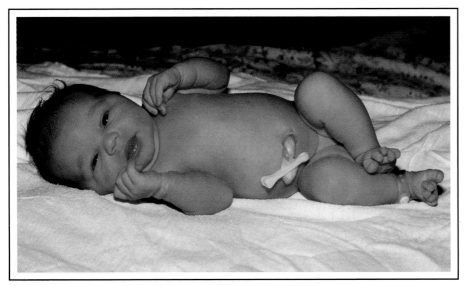

Plate VI   Normal newborn

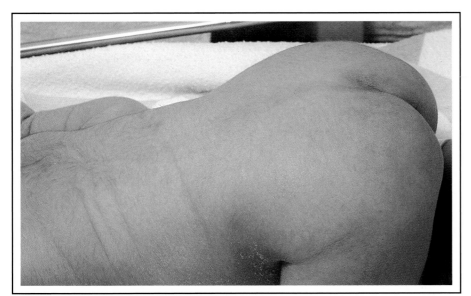

Plate VII   Mongolian spots

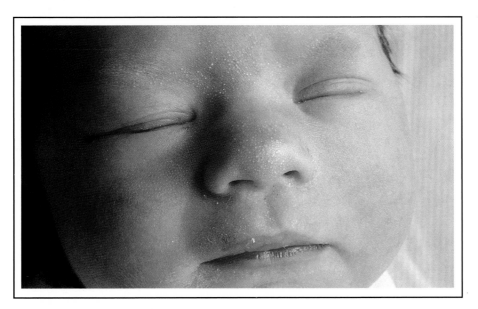

Plate VIII   Facial milia

Brown fat deposits are developing beneath the skin to insulate the baby following birth. Baby has grown to about 15–17 in. Begins storing iron, calcium, and phosphorus.

The entire uterus is occupied by the baby, thus restricting its activity. Maternal antibodies are transferred to the baby. This provides immunity for about 6 months until the infant's own immune system can take over.

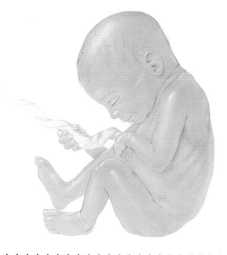

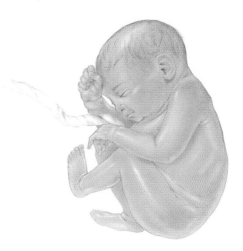

Fundus reaches xyphoid process; breasts full and tender. Urinary frequency may return. Swollen ankles and sleeping problems may develop. Dyspnea may develop.

The fetus descends deeper into the mother's pelvis (lightening). The placenta is nearly 4 times as thick as it was 20 weeks ago, weighing nearly 20 oz. Mother is eager for birth, may have final burst of energy. Backaches, urinary frequency increase. Braxton Hicks contractions intensify as cervix and lower uterine segment prepare for labor. Couple may tour labor and delivery area.

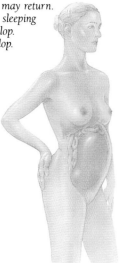

Wear well-fitting supportive bra. Elevate legs once or twice daily for an hour or so. Sleep on left side if possible. Use naturally occurring diuretics such as 2 tbsp lemon juice in 1 cup water or a generous serving of watermelon if available. Avoid most diuretics unless specifically prescribed. Maintain proper posture; use extra pillows at night for severe dyspnea. Following culture and personal preference, may begin preparing nursery now.

Review signs of labor. Discuss plans for other children (if any), transportation to agency.

Continue pelvic tilt exercises. Wear low-heeled shoes or flats. Avoid heavy lifting. Sleep on side to relieve bladder pressure. Urinate frequently. Avoid all analgesics except acetaminophen. Pack suitcase for delivery.

Discuss postpartum period including decisions such as circumcision, rooming-in. Discuss common postpartum discomforts; mention postpartum blues. Discuss family planning methods, infant care. Stress need for adequate rest postpartally. Provide support, especially if baby is overdue.

© 1987 Addison-Wesley Publishing Company

Illustrations by Charles W. Hoffman, MA, AMI
Design by Rudy Zehntner, The Belmont Studio
From Olds et al, **Maternal-Newborn Nursing,** Third Edition

ADDISON-WESLEY PUBLISHING COMPANY
Health Sciences Division, Menlo Park, California
Reading, Massachusetts • Menlo Park, California • New York
Don Mills, Ontario • Wokingham, England • Amsterdam • Bonn
Sydney • Singapore • Tokyo • Madrid • Bogota • Santiago • San Juan

x protects the body; fine hair
go) covers the body and keeps the
the skin. Eyebrows, eyelashes,
ead hair develop. Fetus develops
ular schedule of sleeping, sucking
kicking.

Skeleton develops rapidly as bone-forming
cells increase activity. Respiratory movements
begin. Fetus weighs about 1 lb, 10 oz.

Fetus can breathe, swallow, regulate temperature. Surfactant forms in lungs. Eyes begin to
open and close. Baby is ⅔ the size it will be
at birth.

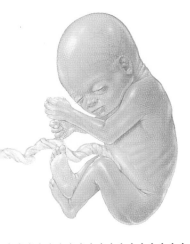 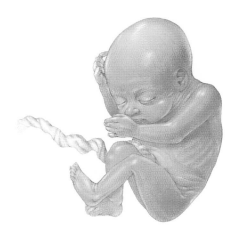 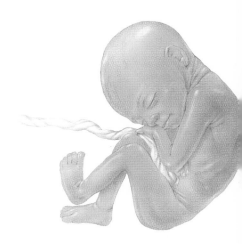

us reaches level
mbilicus. Breasts
secreting co-
um. Amniotic
olds about
nL fluid.
ness and diz-
s may occur,
ially with sud-
osition changes.
ose veins may
to develop.
an experiences
movement, and
ancy may sud-
seem more
." Areola
en. Nasal stuff-
may develop.
ramps may
to occur. Con-
ion may
op.

Fundus above umbilicus.
Backache and leg cramps
may begin. Skin changes
can include striae grav-
idarum, chloasma, linea
negra, acne, redness on
palms of hands and soles of
feet. Nosebleeds can occur.
May experience abdominal
itching as uterus enlarges;
will continue until end
of pregnancy.

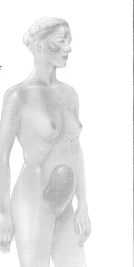

Fundus halfway between
umbilicus and xyphoid
process. May develop hem-
orrhoids. Thoracic breathing
replaces abdominal breathing. Fetal outline palpable.
May be tired of pregnancy
and eager for the mothering
role. Heartburn may begin
to occur. May begin taking
childbirth preparation
classes with partner or
support person.

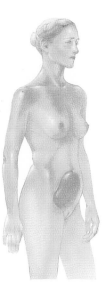 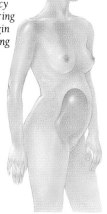

ith feet elevated when possible;
slowly and carefully. Avoid pres-
on lower thighs. Support stockings
be helpful. Cool-air vaporizer
help. Eat foods containing fiber,
as raw fruits, vegetables, cereals
bran; drink liquids and exercise
ently.

uss breast care. Discuss dorsiflex-
f foot to relieve cramps; heat to
ted muscle.

Assure woman that skin changes generally
subside soon after birth. Discuss specific exercises such as pelvic tilt to help strengthen
back and abdominal muscles, and stress importance of good body mechanics. Reiterate
importance of avoiding medications, caffeine,
alcohol and smoking.

Woman may choose to apply petroleum jelly
in nostrils to relieve nosebleeds. Cool vaporizer may also help. Lanolin-based cream can
relieve itching. Mild soap can remove excess
oil associated with acne.

Avoid constipation; use sitz baths, gentle reinsertion of hemorrhoids with a fingertip as
necessary. Topical anesthetic agents may offer
relief of hemorrhoids. Stool softeners may be
prescribed by caregiver. Elevate legs and assume sidelying position when resting. Eat
small, more frequent meals; avoid fatty foods,
lying down after eating. Maalox or mylanta
may be helpful; Avoid sodium bicarbonate.
Discuss expectations about labor and delivery, caring for an infant.

Plate IX   Stork bites

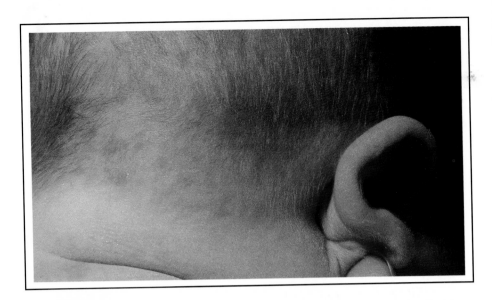

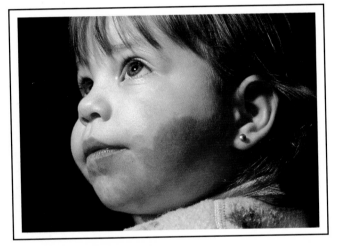

Plate X   Portwine stain

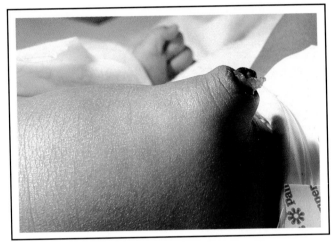

Plate XI   Umbilical hernia

Plate XII   Erythema toxicum

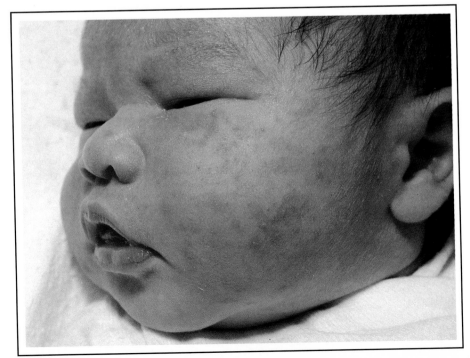

Ultrasound

In the first trimester, ultrasound scanning can detect a gestational sac as early as 5 to 6 weeks after the LMP, fetal heart activity by 9 to 10 weeks and occasionally earlier, and fetal breathing movement by 11 weeks of pregnancy. Crown-to-rump measurements can be made for assessment of fetal age until the fetal head can be defined. Biparietal diameter measurements can be made by approximately 12 to 13 weeks, and are most accurate between 20 and 30 weeks, when rapid growth in biparietal diameter occurs. (See Chapter 20 for an in-depth discussion of ultrasound scanning of the fetus.)

● Assessment of Pelvic Adequacy

The pelvis is assessed vaginally to determine whether its size is adequate for a vaginal delivery. Nurses with special preparation may perform the vaginal assessment and interpret pelvimetry findings. This is sometimes referred to as clinical pelvimetry. (X-ray pelvimetry is used only rarely in modern maternity care because of the risks associated with radiation.)

Pelvic Inlet

The important anteroposterior diameters of the inlet for childbearing are the diagonal conjugate, the obstetric conjugate, and the conjugata vera or true conjugate (Figure 15–7). Others are the transverse (13.5 cm) and the oblique diameters (12.5 cm).

The anteroposterior diameter of the pelvic inlet may be assessed by attempting to reach from the lower border of the symphysis pubis to the sacral promontory with the middle finger. The clinician should determine the length of the finger before attempting this. The diagonal conjugate can then be measured by marking the place where the proximal part of the hand makes contact with the pubis (Figure 15–8). Then the distance is measured (about 12.5 cm). The obstetric conjugate can be estimated by subtracting 1.5 from the length of the diagonal conjugate. At about 11 cm in length, it is the smallest and thus the most important anteroposterior diameter through which the fetus must pass. It is measured by x-ray examination from the sacral promontory to the upper inner point on the symphysis that extends farthest back into the pelvis. The true conjugate extends from the upper border of the symphysis pubis to the sacral promontory. It can be determined by subtracting 1.0 cm from the diagonal conjugate.

Pelvic Cavity (Midpelvis)

Important midpelvic measurements include the plane of greatest dimension, or midplane (12.75 cm), and the planes of least dimension (anteroposterior diameter, 11.5–12.0 cm; posterior sagittal diameter, 4.5–5.0 cm; and transverse diameter, 10.5 cm). These latter diameters can be measured digitally.

Location of the sacrospinous ligament, a firm ridge of tissue, makes location of the ischial spines easier. When this ligament is located, the examiner should run the fingers along it laterally toward the anterior portion of the pelvis. The spines may range from a small firm bump like the knuckle of a finger (termed *not encroaching*) to a very prominent bone. The space between the ischial spines

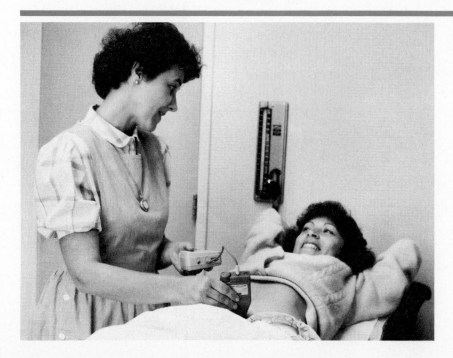

Figure 15–6   Listening to fetal heartbeat with Doppler device

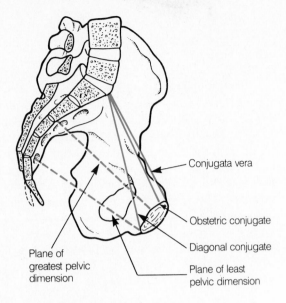

Figure 15-7   Anteroposterior diameters of the pelvic inlet and their relationship to the pelvic planes

(transverse diameter) is estimated according to the prominence of the spines.

The sacrosciatic notch should admit two fingers. A wide notch means that the sacrum curves posteriorly, giving the anteroposterior diameter of the midpelvis a greater length. A narrow notch indicates a decreased diameter. The width of the sacrosciatic notch is more accurately evaluated through x-ray examination but can be estimated through vaginal examination.

The length of the sacrospinous ligament is measured by tracing the ligament from its origin on the ischial spines to its insertion on the sacrum. It is usually 4 cm or two to three finger breadths long.

The capacity of the cavity can be assessed by sweeping the fingers down the side walls bilaterally to evaluate the shape of the pelvic side walls—whether convergent, divergent, or straight. The curvature, inclination, and hollowness of the sacrum help indicate the capacity of the posterior pelvis. It is estimated digitally by palpating the

Figure 15-8   Manual measurement of inlet, midpelvis, and outlet: A Estimation of diagonal conjugate, which extends from lower border of symphysis pubis to sacral promontory. B Estimation of anteroposterior diameter of the outlet, which extends from the lower border of the symphysis pubis to the tip of the sacrum. C Methods that may be used to check manual estimation of anteroposterior measurements.

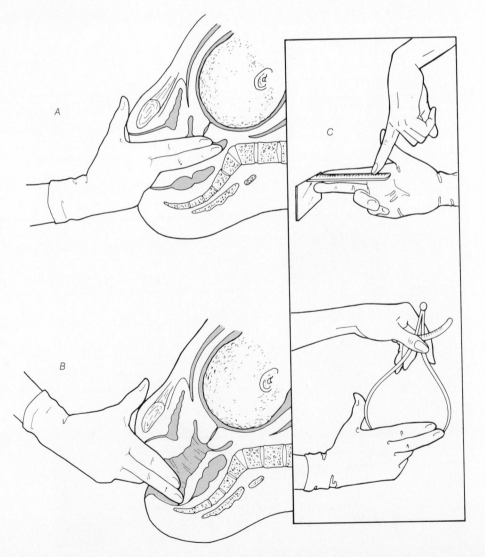

sacrococcygeal junction and by inching up toward the promontory. The examiner then estimates the hollowness of the sacrum, which is normally hollow.

Pelvic Outlet

The anatomic anteroposterior diameter of the pelvic outlet, which is normally 9.5 cm, can be measured digitally (Figure 15–9). The mobility of the coccyx is determined by pressing down on it with the forefinger and middle finger during the initial vaginal exam. An immobile coccyx can decrease the diameter of the outlet. The obstetric anteroposterior diameter of the outlet is normally 11.5 cm.

The transverse diameter of the outlet is measured by placing the fist between the ischial tuberosities. The transverse diameter normally measures 8 cm.

The subpubic angle is estimated by palpating the bony structure externally. It should be 85° to 90°. The subpubic angle is estimated by placing two fingers side by side at the border of the symphysis (Figure 15–10). It is probably reduced if the examiner cannot separate his or her fingers.

The length and shape of the pubic rami affect the transverse diameter of the outlet. The pubic ramus is expected to be short and concave inward, as opposed to straight and long.

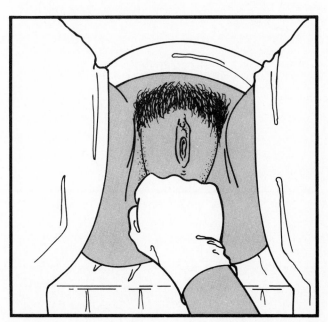

Figure 15–9   Use of closed fist to measure outlet. Examiner should know distance between first and last proximal knuckles.

Figure 15–10   Evaluation of outlet: A Estimation of subpubic angle. B Estimation of length of pubic ramus. C Estimation of depth and inclination of pubis. D Estimation of contour of subpubic angle. ⟶

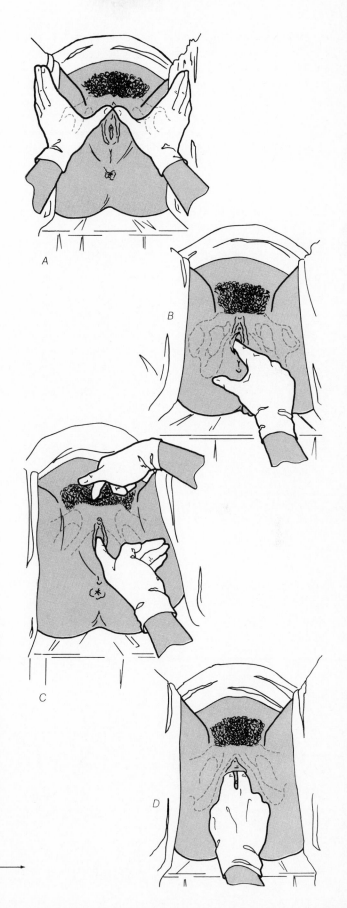

The height and inclination of the symphysis pubis are measured, and the contour of the pubic arch is estimated. Excessively long or angulated bone structure shortens the diameter of the obstetric conjugate. Height can be determined by placing the index finger of the gloved hand up to the superior border of the symphysis. The examiner should measure the length of the first phalanx of the index finger (normally about 2.5 cm). Inclination can be determined by externally placing one finger on the top of the symphysis while the internal finger palpates the internal margin. An imaginary line is drawn between the fingers and the angle is estimated.

A posterior inclination with the lower border of the pubis slanting inward decreases the anteroposterior diameter. The anteroposterior sagittal diameter is the most significant diameter of the outlet, as it is the shortest diameter through which the infant must pass. Estimating the contour of the pubic arch provides information on the width of the angle at which these bones come together. The pubic arch has obstetric importance; if it is narrow the infant's head

Initial Psychosocial Assessment Guide

Assess/normal findings	Alterations and possible causes*	Nursing responses to data†
PSYCHOLOGIC STATUS		
Excitement and/or apprehension; ambivalence	Marked anxiety (fear of pregnancy diagnosis, fear of medical facility)	Establish lines of communication. Active listening is useful. Establish trusting relationship. Encourage woman to take active part in her care.
	Apathy Display of anger with pregnancy diagnosis	Establish communication and begin counseling. Use active listening techniques.
EDUCATIONAL NEEDS		
May have questions about pregnancy or may need time to adjust to reality of pregnancy		Establish educational, supporting environment that can be expanded throughout pregnancy.
SUPPORT SYSTEMS		
Can identify at least two or three individuals with whom woman is emotionally intimate (partner, parent, sibling, friend, etc.)	Isolated (no telephone, unlisted number); cannot name a neighbor or friend whom she can call upon in an emergency; does not perceive parents as part of her support system	Institute support system through community groups. Develop trusting relationship with health care professionals.
CULTURAL OR RELIGIOUS CONSIDERATIONS		
Any cultural or religious beliefs or practices that might influence pregnancy. Is able to express her personal preferences and beliefs about the childbearing experience. Identifies any people (mother, curendara, tribal healer, etc) that influence her.	Language barriers that prevent effective communication Cultural beliefs or practices that might endanger her health or that of fetus	Work with knowledgeable translator to provide information and answer questions. Have information printed in the language of different cultural groups that live in the area. Work with significant people to meet woman's health needs.
FAMILY FUNCTIONING		
Emotionally supportive Communications adequate Mutually satisfying Cohesiveness in times of trouble	Long-term problems or specific problems related to this pregnancy, potential stressors within the family, pessimistic attitudes, unilateral decision making, unrealistic expectations of this pregnancy and/or child	Help identify the problems and stressors, encourage communication, discuss role changes and adaptations.
ECONOMIC STATUS		
Source of income is stable and sufficient to meet basic needs of daily living and medical needs	Limited prenatal care Poor physical health Limited use of health care system Unstable economic status	Discuss available resources for health maintenance and delivery. Institute appropriate referral for meeting expanding family's needs—food stamps, etc.
STABILITY OF LIVING CONDITIONS		
Adequate, stable housing for expanding family's needs	Crowded living conditions Questionable supportive environment for newborn	Refer to appropriate community agency. Work with family on self-help ways to improve situation.

*Possible causes of alterations are placed in parentheses.
†This column provides guidelines for further assessment and initial nursing interventions.

may be pushed backward toward the coccyx, making extension of the head difficult.

● Initial Psychosocial Assessment

At the initial visit the woman may be most concerned wtih the diagnosis of pregnancy. However, during this visit she (and her partner, if he is present) is also evaluating the health team that she has chosen. The establishment of the nurse–client relationship will help the woman evaluate the health team and also provides the nurse with a basis for an atmosphere that is conducive to interviewing, support, and education. A psychosocial assessment is difficult to obtain if the woman does not feel free to talk.

Many women are excited and anxious on the initial visit. Because of this, the initial psychosocial assessment is general and the goal is to set the foundation for a trusting nurse–client relationship.

As part of the initial psychosocial assessment the nurse discusses with the woman any cultural factors that influence the woman's expectations about the childbearing experience. It is especially helpful if the nurse is familiar with common practices of various cultural groups that reside in the community. If the nurse gathers this data in a tactful, caring way it can help make the childbearing woman's experience a positive one.

Religious practices also require consideration. If the woman is a Jehovah's Witness, she may be opposed to receiving blood products should the need arise. Other religious influences can also be discussed. What does the woman's religion teach about the role of children? Of parents? Of boys or girls? Are there any religious ceremonies or practices that are generally performed during pregnancy or the postpartum period?

The Initial Psychosocial Assessment Guide on the opposite page can be used as a basis for evaluating the woman's needs for education and support.

● Subsequent Client History

At subsequent prenatal visits the nurse continues to gather data about the course of the pregnancy to date. The nurse asks specifically whether the woman has experienced any discomfort, especially the kinds of discomfort that are often seen at specific times during a pregnancy. Thus in the first trimester the nurse would consider discomforts such as nausea, vomiting, frequency, breast tenderness, and so forth. The nurse inquires about physical changes that relate directly to the pregnancy, such as fetal movement. The nurse also asks about any of the danger signs of pregnancy (see Box 15–1).

Other pertinent information includes: any exposure to contagious illnesses; medical treatment and therapy prescribed for nonpregnancy problems since the last visit; any

---

Box 15–1   Danger Signs in Pregnancy

The woman should report the following danger signs in pregnancy immediately:

Danger sign	Possible cause
1. Sudden gush of fluid from vagina	Premature rupture of membranes
2. Vaginal bleeding	Abruptio placentae, placenta previa Lesions of cervix or vagina, "Bloody show"
3. Abdominal pain	Premature labor, abuptio placentae
4. Temperature above 38.3C (101F) and chills	Infection
5. Dizziness, blurring of vision, double vision, spots before eyes	Hypertension, preeclampsia
6. Persistent vomiting	Hyperemesis gravidarum
7. Severe headache	Hypertension, preeclampsia
8. Edema of hands, face, legs, and feet	Preeclampsia
9. Muscular irritability, convulsions	Preeclampsia, eclampsia
10. Epigastric pain	Preeclampsia—ischemia in major abdominal vessels
11. Oliguria	Renal impairment, decreased fluid intake
12. Dysuria	Urinary tract infection
13. Absence of fetal movement	Maternal medication, obesity, fetal death

---

prescription or over-the-counter medications that were not prescribed as part of the woman's prenatal care.

The early possible danger signs of pregnancy are generally discussed with the woman during her initial prenatal visit. However, the woman may feel overwhelmed by information during the first visit. It is advisable to review carefully the danger signs that a woman should report immediately when she comes for her second prenatal visit. In most cases she is calmer and better able to absorb the information at that time. Many care givers also provide printed information on the subject that is written in lay

Subsequent Physical Assessment Guide

Assess/normal findings	Alterations and possible causes*	Nursing responses to data†
VITAL SIGNS Temperature: 36.2–37.6C (98–99.6F)	Elevated temperature (infection)	Evaluate for signs of infection. Refer to physician.
Pulse: 60–90/min Rate may increase 10 beats/min during pregnancy	Increased pulse rate (anxiety, cardiac disorders)	Note irregularities. Evaluate anxiety and stress.
Respiration: 16–24/min	Marked tachypnea or abnormal patterns (respiratory disease)	Refer to physician.
Blood pressure: 90–140/60–90 (falls in second trimester)	> 140/90 or increase of 30 mm systolic and 15 mm diastolic (preeclampsia)	Assess for edema, proteinuria, hyperreflexia. Refer to physician. Schedule appointments more frequently.
WEIGHT GAIN First trimester: 2–4 lb Second trimester: 12 lb Third trimester: 12 lb	Inadequate weight gain (poor nutrition, nausea, IUGR) Excessive weight gain (excessive caloric intake, edema, preeclampsia)	Discuss appropriate weight gain. Provide nutritional counseling. Assess for presence of edema or anemia.
EDEMA Small amount of dependent edema, especially in last weeks of pregnancy	Edema in hands, face, legs, feet (preeclampsia)	Identify any correlation between edema and activities, blood pressure, or proteinuria. Refer to physician if indicated.
UTERINE SIZE See Initial Physical Assessment Guide for normal changes during pregnancy	Unusually rapid growth (multiple gestation, hydatidiform mole, hydramnios, miscalculation of EDD)	Evaluate fetal status. Determine height of fundus (p. 358). Use diagnostic ultrasound.
FETAL HEARTBEAT 120–160/min Funic souffle	Absence of fetal heartbeat after 20 weeks' gestation (maternal obesity, fetal demise)	Evaluate fetal status.
LABORATORY EVALUATION Hemoglobin: 12–16 g/dL Pseudoanemia of pregnancy	< 12 g/dL (anemia)	Provide nutritional counseling. Hemoglobin is repeated at 7 months' gestation. Women of Mediterranean heritage need a close check on hemoglobin because of possibility of thalassemia.
Antibody screen: Negative	Positive	Refer for further testing to identify specific antibodies. Titers may be indicated. If negative repeat at 7 months.
50 g, one-hour glucose screen (done between 24 and 28 weeks' gestation)	Plasma glucose level > 140 mg/dL (gestational diabetes mellitus [GDM])	Discuss implications of GDM. Refer for a diagnostic glucose tolerance test.
Urinalysis: See Initial Prenatal Physical Assessment Guide (p. 346) for normal findings	See Initial Prenatal Physical Assessment Guide (p. 346) for deviations	Repeat urinalysis at 7 months' gestation. Dipstick test at each visit.
Protein: Negative	Proteinuria, albuminuria (contamination by vaginal discharge, urinary tract infection, preeclampsia)	Obtain dipstick urine sample. Refer to physician if deviations are present.
Glucose: Negative Note: Glycosuria may be present due to physiologic alterations in glomerular filtration rate and renal threshold	Persistent glycosuria (diabetes mellitus)	Refer to physician.

*Possible causes of alterations are placed in parentheses.
†This column provides guidelines for further assessment and initial nursing interventions.

terms. Box 15–1 identifies the danger signs of pregnancy and possible causes for each.

● Subsequent Physical Assessment

The recommended frequency of prenatal visits is as follows

- Every 4 weeks for the first 28 weeks of gestation
- Every 2 weeks to week 36
- After week 36, every week until delivery

The Subsequent Physical Assessment Guide on the opposite page provides a systematic approach to the regular physical examinations that the pregnant woman should undergo for optimal prenatal care.

● Subsequent Psychosocial Assessment

Periodic prenatal examinations offer the nurse an opportunity to assess the childbearing woman's psychologic needs and emotional status. If the woman's partner attends the prenatal visits, his needs and concerns can also be identified.

The interchange between the nurse and woman will be facilitated if it takes place in a friendly, trusting environment. The woman should be given sufficient time to ask questions and to air concerns. If the nurse provides the time and demonstrates genuine interest, the woman will feel more at ease bringing up questions that she may believe are silly or concerns that she has been afraid to

verbalize. The nurse who has an accurate understanding of all the changes of pregnancy is most able to answer questions and provide information. See the foldout color chart, "Maternal–Fetal Development," for vivid illustrations of some of this information.

During the prenatal period, it is essential to begin assessing the ability of the woman (and her partner, if possible) to assume their responsibilities as parents successfully. Table 15–3 identifies areas for assessment and provides some sample questions the nurse might use to obtain necessary information. If the woman's responses are primarily negative, interventions can be planned for the prenatal and postpartal periods.

During the subsequent psychologic assessments, a woman may exhibit psychologic problems such as the following:

- Increasing anxiety
- Inability to establish communication
- Inappropriate responses or actions
- Denial of pregnancy
- Inability to cope with stress
- Failure to acknowledge quickening
- Failure to plan and prepare for the baby (for example, living arrangements, clothing, feeding methods)

If the woman appears to have these or other critical psychologic problems, the nurse should refer her to appropriate professionals.

The Subsequent Psychosocial Assessment Guide on this page provides a model for the evaluation of both the pregnant woman and the expectant father.

Subsequent Psychosocial Assessment Guide

Assess/normal findings	Alterations and possible causes*	Nursing responses to data†
EXPECTANT MOTHER Psychologic status: First trimester: incorporates idea of pregnancy; may feel ambivalent, especially if she must give up desired role; usually looks for signs of verification of pregnancy, such as increase in abdominal size, fetal movement, etc. Second trimester: baby becomes more real to woman as abdominal size increases and she feels movement; she begins to turn inward, becoming more introspective Third trimester: begins to think of baby as separate being; may feel restless and may feel that time of labor will never come; remains self-centered and concentrates on preparing place for baby	Increasing stress and anxiety Inability to establish communication; inability to accept pregnancy; inappropriate response or actions; denial of pregnancy; inability to cope	Encourage woman to take an active part in her care. Establish lines of communication. Establish a trusting relationship. Counsel as necessary. Refer to appropriate professional as needed.

(continued)

Subsequent Psychosocial Assessment Guide (continued)

Assess/normal findings	Alterations and possible causes*	Nursing responses to data†

Educational needs:
Self-care measures and knowledge about following:
   Breast care
   Hygiene
   Rest
   Exercise
   Nutrition
   Relief measures for common discomforts of pregnancy
   Danger signs of pregnancy (Box 15–1)
	Inadequate information	Teach and/or institute appropriate relief measures (see Chapter 16).

Sexual activity: Woman knows how pregnancy affects sexual activity	Lack of information about effects of pregnancy and/or alternative positions during sexual intercourse	Provide counseling.
Preparation for parenting: Appropriate preparation; See Table 15–3	Lack of preparation (denial, failure to adjust to baby, unwanted child) See Table 15–3	Counsel. If lack of preparation is due to inadequacy of information, provide information (see Chapter 16).
Preparation for childbirth: Client aware of following: 1. Prepared childbirth techniques 2. Normal processes and changes during childbirth		If couple chooses particular technique, refer to classes (see Chapter 18 for description of childbirth preparation techniques). Encourage prenatal class attendance. Educate woman during visits based on current physical status. Provide reading list for more specific information.
3. Problems that may occur as a result of drug and alcohol use and of smoking	Continued abuse of drugs and alcohol; denial of possible effect on self and baby	Review danger signs that were presented on initial visit.
Woman has met other physician and/or nurse-midwife who may be attending her delivery in the absence of primary care giver	Introduction of new individual at delivery may increase stress and anxiety for woman and partner	Introduce woman to all members of group practice.
Impending labor: Client knows signs of impending labor: 1. Uterine contractions that increase in frequency, duration, intensity 2. Bloody show 3. Expulsion of mucous plug 4. Rupture of membranes	Lack of information	Provide appropriate teaching, stressing importance of seeking appropriate medical assistance.
EXPECTANT FATHER Psychologic status: First trimester: may express excitement over confirmation of pregnancy and of his virility; concerns move toward providing for financial needs; energetic; may identify with some discomforts of pregnancy and may even exhibit symptoms	Increasing stress and anxiety Inability to establish communication Inability to accept pregnancy diagnosis Withdrawal of support Abandonment of the mother	Encourage expectant father to come to prenatal visits. Establish lines of communication. Establish trusting relationship.
Second trimester: may feel more confident and be less concerned with financial matters; may have concerns about wife's changing size and shape, her increasing introspection		Counsel. Let expectant father know that it is normal for him to experience these feelings.
Third trimester: may have feelings of rivalry with fetus, expecially during sexual activity; may make changes in his physical appearance and exhibit more interest in himself; may become more energetic; fantasizes about child but usually imagines older child; fears of mutilation and death of woman and child arise		Include expectant father in pregnancy activities as he desires. Provide education, information, and support. Increasing number of expectant fathers are demonstrating desire to be involved in many or all aspects of prenatal care, education, and preparation.

*Possible causes of alterations are placed in parentheses.
†This column provides guidelines for further assessment and initial nursing interventions.

Table 15–3 Prenatal Assessment of Parenting Guide*

Areas assessed	Sample questions
I. PERCEPTION OF COMPLEXITIES OF MOTHERING	1. Did you plan on getting pregnant?
A. Baby is desired for itself.	2. How do you feel about being pregnant?
Positive:	3. Why do you want this baby?

I. PERCEPTION OF COMPLEXITIES OF MOTHERING

A. Baby is desired for itself.
Positive:
   1. Feels positive about pregnancy.
Negative:
   1. Wants baby to meet own needs such as someone to love her, someone to get her out of unhappy home.
B. Expresses concern about impact of mothering role on other roles (wife, career, school).
Positive:
   1. Realistic expectations of how baby will affect job, career, school, and personal goals.
   2. Interested in learning about child care.
Negative:
   1. Feels pregnancy and baby will make no emotional, physical, or social demands on self.
   2. No insight that mothering role will affect other roles or lifestyle.
C. Gives up routine habits because "not good for baby"; e.g., quits smoking, adjusts time schedule, etc.†
Positive:
   1. Gives up routines not good for baby: quits smoking, adjusts eating habits, etc.

1. Did you plan on getting pregnant?
2. How do you feel about being pregnant?
3. Why do you want this baby?

1. What do you think it will be like to take care of a baby?
2. How do you think your life will be different after you have your baby?
3. How do you feel this baby will affect your job, career, school, and personal goals?
4. How will the baby affect your relationship with boyfriend or husband?
5. Have you done any reading, babysitting, or made any things for a baby?

II. ATTACHMENT

A. Strong feelings regarding sex of baby.
   Why?
Positive:
   1. Verbalizes positive thoughts about the baby.
Negative:
   1. Baby will be like negative aspects of self and partner.
B. Interested in data regarding fetus, e.g., growth and development, heart tones, etc.
Positive:
   1. As above.
Negative:
   1. Shows no interest in fetal growth and development, quickening, and fetal heart tones.
   2. Negative feelings about fetus expressed by rejection of counseling regarding nutrition, rest, hygiene.
C. Fantasies about baby.
Positive:
   1. Follows cultural norms regarding preparation.
   2. Time of attachment behaviors appropriate to her history of pregnancy loss.
Negative:
   1. Bonding is conditional depending on sex, age of baby, and/or labor and delivery experience.
   2. Patient only considers own needs when making plans for baby.
   3. Exhibits no attachment behaviors after critical period of previous pregnancy.
   4. Failure to follow cultural norms regarding preparation.

1. Why do you prefer a certain sex? (Is reason inappropriate for a baby?)
2. Note comments client makes about baby not being normal and why client feels this way.

1. What did you think or feel when you first felt the baby move?
2. Have you started preparing for the baby?
3. What do you think your baby will look like—what age do you see your baby at?
4. How would you like your new baby to look?

III. ACCEPTANCE OF CHILD BY SIGNIFICANT OTHERS

A. Acknowledges acceptance by significant other of the new responsibility inherent in child.
Positive:
   1. Acknowledges unconditional acceptance of pregnancy and baby by significant others.
   2. Partner accepts new responsibility inherent with child.
   3. Timely sharing of experience of pregnancy with significant others.
Negative:
   1. Significant others not supportively involved with pregnancy.

1. How does your partner feel about pregnancy?
2. How do your parents feel?
3. What do your friends think?
4. Does your partner have a preference regarding the baby's sex? Why?
5. How does your partner feel about being a father?
6. What do you think he'll be like as a father?
7. What do you think he'll do to help you with child care?
8. Have you and your partner talked about how the baby might change your lives?
9. Who have you told about your pregnancy?

(continued)

Table 15–3 Prenatal Assessment of Parenting Guide (continued)

Areas assessed	Sample questions
2. Conditional acceptance of pregnancy depending on sex, race, age of baby. 3. Decision making does not take in needs of fetus; e.g., spends food money on new car. 4. Takes no/little responsibility for needs of pregnancy, woman/fetus. B. Concrete demonstration of acceptance of pregnancy/baby by significant others; e.g., baby shower, significant other involved in prenatal education.† Positive: 　1. Baby shower. 　2. Significant other attends prenatal class with client.	1. Note if partner attends clinic with client (degree of interest); e.g., listens to heart tones, etc. Significant other plans to be with client in labor and delivery. 2. Is your partner contributing financially?
IV. ENSURES PHYSICAL WELL-BEING A. Concerns about having normal pregnancy, labor and delivery, and baby. Positive: 　1. Client preparing for labor and delivery, attends prenatal classes, interested in labor and delivery. 　2. Client aware of danger signs of pregnancy. 　3. Seeks and uses appropriate health care: e.g., time of initial visit, keeps appointments, follows through on recommendations. Negative: 　1. Denial of signs and symptoms that might suggest complications of pregnancy. 　2. Verbalizes extreme fear of labor and delivery—refuses to talk about labor and delivery. 　3. Fails appointments, failure to follow instructions, refuses to attend prenatal classes. B. Family/client decision reflect concern for health of mother and baby; e.g., use of finances, time.† Positive: 　1. As above.	1. What have you heard about labor and delivery? 2. Note data about client's reaction to prenatal class.

†When "Negative" is not listed in a section, the reader may assume that negative is the absence of positive responses.

*Modified and used with permission of the Minneapolis Health Dept., Minneapolis, MN.

KEY CONCEPTS

A complete history forms the basis of prenatal care and is reevaluated and updated as necessary throughout the pregnancy.

Screening for risk factors is an ongoing process beginning at the first prenatal visit.

The initial prenatal physical assessment is a careful and thorough physical examination designed to identify physical variations and potential risk factors.

Laboratory tests completed at the initial visit, such as a complete blood count, ABO and Rh typing, urinalysis, Pap smear, gonorrhea culture, rubella titer, and various blood screens, provide information about the woman's health during early pregnancy and also help detect potential problems.

The estimated date of delivery (EDD) can be calculated using Nägele's rule. Using this approach, one begins with the first day of the last menstrual period (LMP), subtracts three months, and adds seven days. A "wheel" may also be used to calculate the EDD.

Accuracy of the EDD may be evaluated by physical examination to assess uterine size, measurement of fundal height, and ultrasound. Perception of quickening and auscultation of fetal heartbeat are also useful tools in confirming the gestation of a pregnancy.

The pelvis can be assessed vaginally to determine whether its size is adequate to permit vaginal delivery.

The diagonal conjugate is the distance from the lower posterior border of the symphysis pubis to the sacral promontory. The obstetric conjugate is estimated by subtracting 1.5 from the length of the diagonal conjugate.

As part of the assessment of the pelvic cavity (midpelvis) the prominence of the ischial spines is assessed, the sacrosciatic notch and the length of the sacrospinous ligament are measured, and the shape of the pelvic side walls is evaluated. Finally, the hollowness of the sacrum is determined.

The anteroposterior diameter of the pelvic outlet is determined, the mobility of the coccyx is assessed, the suprapubic angle is estimated, and the contour of the pubic arch is evaluated to assess the adequacy of the pelvic outlet.

The nurse begins evaluating the woman psychosocially during the initial prenatal assessment. This assessment continues and is modified throughout the pregnancy.

Cultural and ethnic beliefs may strongly influence the woman's attitudes and apparent compliance with care during pregnancy.

REFERENCES

Garn SM, et al: Maternal hematologic levels and pregnancy outcomes. *Semin Perinatol* 1981;5(April):155.

Oxorn H: *Human Labor and Birth,* ed 5. Norwalk, Conn, Appleton-Century-Crofts, 1986.

ADDITIONAL READINGS

Brooten D, et al: A survey of nutrition, caffeine, cigarette and alcohol intake in early pregnancy in an urban clinic population. *J Nurs-Midwifery* 1987;32(2):85.

Danforth D, Scott J: *Obstetrics and Gynecology,* ed 5. Philadelphia, Lippincott, 1986.

Engstrom JL: Quickening and auscultation of fetal heart tones as estimators of the gestational interval: A review. *J Nurs-Midwifery* 1985;30(1):25.

Kemp VH, et al: Health assessment in high-risk pregnancies. *Fam Commun Health* 1986;8(4):10.

Lederman RP: Maternal anxiety in pregnancy: Relationship to fetal and newborn health status. *Annu Rev Nurs Res* 1986;4:3.

Malasanos L, et al: *Health Assessment,* ed 3. St Louis, Mosby, 1986.

Marquette GP, Skoll MA: How should you screen for gestational diabetes? *Contemp OB/GYN* 1986;27(4):67.

Methven R: Out-patient nursing: Mother knows best . . . recording an obstetric history part 4. *Nurs Mirror* 1985;160(January):38.

Miller SJ: Prenatal nursing assessment of the expectant family. *Nurse Pract* 1986;11(5):40.

Nichols CW: Clinical management of size/dates discrepancy. *J Nurs-Midwifery* 1985;30(1):15.

Wawrzyniak MN: The painless pelvic. *Am J Mat Child Nurs* 1986;11(3):178.

Willard MD, et al: The educational pelvic examination: Women's responses to a new approach. *J Obstet Gynecol Neonat Nurs* 1986;15(2):135.

Pregnancy is not bad for me at all, and I'm having an easy time, but I know that I would feel more energetic and . . . more comfortable in the summer if I wasn't pregnant. It's funny because it's not an ordeal, but I'm not enjoying pregnancy . . . I don't hate the idea of being pregnant. I haven't cried because of it or been depressed because of it. It's just that afterwards you think about having to lose weight and exercise and get yourself back in shape, and that's a lot of energy. (RP Lederman, Psychosocial Adaptation in Pregnancy)

The Expectant Couple: Needs and Care

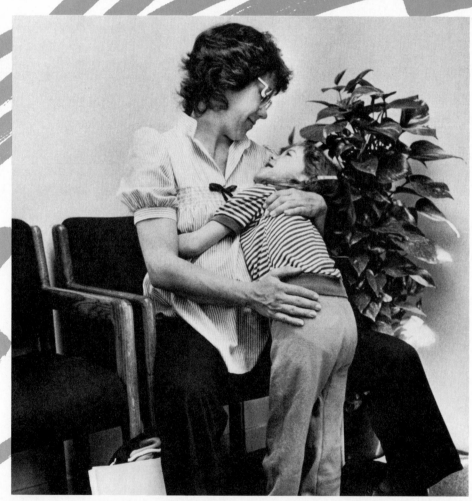

Supporting the psychologic needs of each member of the expectant family is critical to everyone's well-being.

Chapter Sixteen

OBJECTIVES

- Summarize the areas of assessment important in establishing a comprehensive data base for the expectant woman and her family.

- Describe communication skills that nurses can use to enhance effectiveness in nursing assessments and implementation of care.

- Explain the causes of the common discomforts of pregnancy and appropriate measures to alleviate these discomforts.

- Develop a plan of care incorporating anticipatory guidance of the pregnant woman and her family to maintain and promote well-being for each trimester of pregnancy.

- Discuss the significance of cultural considerations in managing nursing care during pregnancy and common practices of specific cultures.

- Discuss the significance of using the nursing process to promote health in the woman and her family during pregnancy.

- Compare similarities and differences in the needs of expectant women in various age groups.

From the moment a woman finds out that she is pregnant, she faces a future marked by dramatic changes. Her appearance will be altered drastically. Her relationships will change. She will experience a variety of unique physical changes throughout the pregnancy. Even her psychologic state will be affected.

Her family must also adjust to the pregnancy. Roles and responsibilities of family members will be altered as the woman's ability to perform certain activities changes. They too must adapt psychologically to the situation.

The expectant woman and her family will probably have many questions about the pregnancy and its impact on her and the other members of the family. Common questions include: "How will our life-style be affected? What adjustments will we have to make? What risks are involved?" In addition, the daily activities and health care practices of the woman become of great concern when she and her family realize that the well-being of the unborn child can be affected by what she does.

The nurse often assumes the dual roles of teacher and counselor for expectant families who desire information about pregnancy and the adjustments they must make. In particular the nurse teaches the pregnant woman about the physical discomforts that may occur and the self-care measures that the woman can use to obtain relief.

This chapter provides the information necessary for nurses to teach and counsel pregnant women and their families. It describes the common discomforts of pregnancy, their causes, and self-care measures. The chapter also contains information and advice on general health practices and other activities that may affect, or be affected by, pregnancy.

Using the Nursing Process During the Antepartal Period

Pregnancy is a healthy process for most women. Thus antepartal nursing care primarily involves anticipatory guidance and education. The nursing process provides a framework for the nurse to identify and meet the needs of the expectant woman and her family.

Nursing Assessment

In many areas of nursing, assessment involves gathering data about symptoms that reflect a health problem or complication. Because most pregnant women are healthy, however, the purpose of assessment during pregnancy is to ensure that everything is progressing normally and to identify potential problems that may affect the woman's or fetus's well-being.

The nurse must assess not only the woman's physical condition but also the psychosocial factors that affect her pregnancy experience. The population of pregnant women is diverse in age, life experiences, cultural beliefs, educational background, health practices, family structure, attitudes, and interests. Each of these factors need to be assessed so that the nurse can develop a plan of care that considers the woman's specific needs and concerns. A plan of care that does not acknowledge a woman's uniqueness will not be effective.

The accuracy of the nurse's assessment often depends on the nurse's ability to develop rapport with the woman and use communication skills effectively. The nurse's comfort level in dealing with the concerns expressed by the pregnant woman and her family is also important. The concerns expressed during pregnancy are frequently very personal. Some nurses hesitate to assess the woman's needs in these areas due to their own discomfort or lack of clarity about the purpose of their data collection. For example, a nurse may feel uncomfortable assessing a woman's concerns about intercourse during pregnancy or use of alcohol or other drugs. A nonjudgmental approach and knowledge about health promotion behaviors during pregnancy are essential. The nurse must remember that promotion of maternal well-being and optimum fetal outcome is the purpose of care. With this thought in mind, personal concerns should not be as difficult to assess.

Analysis and Nursing Diagnosis

The nurse may see a specific woman only once every three to four weeks at the beginning of pregnancy. As a result, a written plan of care that incorporates the data base, nursing diagnoses, and goals is essential for continuity of care.

The American Nurses' Association's *Standards of Maternal and Child Health Nursing Practice* (ANA 1983) encourages the use of nursing diagnoses. It is difficult, however, to use nursing diagnoses accepted by the National Conference Group for Nursing Diagnoses because they are oriented to illness or prevention of complications. As a result, maternity nurses may tend to avoid using nursing di-

agnoses since they are caring for essentially healthy individuals (Stolte 1986). A more positive and ultimately more useful approach is for maternity nurses to increase their input to the National Conference Group for Nursing Diagnoses and apply their experience in the area of health promotion to the development of nursing diagnoses oriented to health promotion.

Several existing nursing diagnoses may apply to a woman with a healthy pregnancy. Examples of applicable nursing diagnoses include:

- Knowledge deficit related to the use of medication during pregnancy

- Noncompliance with prenatal appointment schedule related to a lack of understanding about the importance of prenatal care

- Alteration in bowel elimination: constipation related to the physiologic effects of pregnancy

- Altered sexuality patterns related to changed sexual activity during pregnancy

Nursing Plan and Implementation

Once nursing diagnoses have been identified, the next step is to establish priorities of nursing care. Sometimes priorities of care are based on the most immediate needs or concerns perceived by the woman. For example, during the first trimester, when a woman is experiencing nausea or is concerned about sexual intimacy with her partner, she is not likely to be ready to hear about labor and delivery.

The woman's priorities may not always be the same as the nurse's. If the safety of the woman or her fetus is at issue, however, that takes priority over other concerns of the woman or her family. It is the responsibility of the medical and nursing professions to help the woman and her family understand the significance of a problem and to assess why potential noncompliance may occur. Suppose, for example, a woman with early signs of preeclampsia is advised to enter the hospital immediately to begin bedrest. If she does not have hospital insurance, however, and there is no one to care for her young children, compliance with the treatment advice may be impossible. As a result, the signs of preeclampsia may become more severe. It is important for the nurse to assess the causes of noncompliance and plan care accordingly.

The intervention methods most used by nurses in caring for the expectant woman and her family are communication techniques and teaching-learning strategies. These intervention methods are most obvious when used in groups, such as early pregnancy classes and childbirth education classes, but the nurse in the prenatal setting often applies these techniques on an individual basis.

The value of providing a primary care nurse to coordinate care for each childbearing family is beginning to be recognized (Mahan and McKay 1984). The nurse in a clinic or HMO may be the only source of continuity for the woman, who may see a different physician or nurse-midwife at each visit. The nurse can be extremely effective in working with the expectant family by providing them with necessary and complete information about pregnancy, self-care measures, and community resources or referral agencies that may be of help to them. Such education allows the family to assume equal responsibility with health care providers in working toward their common goal of a positive childbearing experience.

Evaluation

Evaluation is an ongoing process. At each prenatal visit the nurse evaluates the effectiveness of previous teaching by using information obtained from the woman and from various assessment tools. For instance, the woman's pattern of weight gain, her vital signs, her degree of comfort, and her success in implementing previously discussed strategies provide information about the success of previous nursing interventions. When the woman has been unable to follow an established treatment plan, it may be due to factors in the woman's environment that were not previously known. Thus the cycle of the nursing process begins again with assessment as the nurse collects further data.

● Care of the Expectant Couple

Nursing Assessment

As described in Chapter 15, during the initial contact with the expectant mother or couple, the nurse obtains a client profile that includes information about the following:

- The family's environment, life-style, habits, and relationships

- The family's sources and adequacy of income

- The family's race and/or culture

- The woman's temperament and usual way of coping with stressful situations

- An average day in the life of the family

- The impact of the pregnancy on the mother, the family, and significant others

- Personal habits relevant to pregnancy (patterns of diet, sleep, and sexual activity; exercise; hobbies; and use of alcohol, tobacco, caffeine, and other drugs)

- The woman's health history

- A family history to determine expected support of family members

The data base is completed with a description of body functioning, a complete physical examination, laboratory tests, and a psychologic evaluation (Chapter 15).

During subsequent visits, the nurse may ask the woman what *mother* means to her, what she thinks an average day with the baby will be like, and what she expects from the father. The nurse can ask the father similar questions about his expectations of himself and his partner as parents. The couples' answers will provide information about their progress in accomplishing the developmental tasks of pregnancy and will help the nurse determine whether their expectations are realistic.

Many nonparents are not prepared for the sleep and feeding patterns of newborns. They have not considered their feelings about the inevitable crying of the newborn and what they will do when the baby cries. Many couples are surprised to discover the sometimes extreme disparity between their views of parenthood. Guided discussion of these topics allows parents-to-be to attack problems, arrive at compromises, and appreciate each other's uniqueness.

From the health assessment, the nurse develops an initial plan for interventions during the couple's preparation for childbearing and childrearing. The plan anticipates the need for information, guidance, and physical care. Interventions are timed to coincide with the woman's (couple's) readiness and needs. Box 16–1 identifies areas the nurse will discuss with the childbearing woman to provide pertinent anticipatory guidance.

Once the data base is established and the nurse has completed an initial assessment of the childbearing family, the nurse will identify the following goals:

- To promote family adaptation

- To provide anticipatory guidance for the puerperium

- To integrate cultural factors influencing pregnancy

- To relieve the common discomforts of pregnancy

- To promote maternal and fetal well-being during pregnancy

- To teach the pregnant woman how to monitor fetal activity

Nursing Goal: Promotion of Family Adaptation

Any crisis makes the involved parties not only more vulnerable but also more accepting of intervention. The nurse is often in a good position to intervene therapeutically. Two primary functions of the nurse caring for the expectant family are (1) to support the family unit and (2) to provide prenatal education. If these functions are per-

Box 16–1 Anticipatory Guidance with the Healthy Pregnancy

All three trimesters:	Discomforts of pregnancy (see Table 16–3)
	Nutrition and weight gain
	Sexual activity
	Sibling preparation

First trimester

Attitude toward pregnancy

Exercise and rest

Smoking; use of alcohol and other drugs

Traveling

Fetal growth and development

Danger signals associated with spontaneous abortion

Employment

Early pregnancy classes

Second trimester

Concerns related to changes in body

Fetal growth and development

Fetal movement

Clothing

Care of skin and breasts

Beginning preparation for care of the infant (equipment and room)

Decisions about infant feeding

Third trimester

Exercise and rest

Traveling

Danger signals

Preparation for labor and delivery

Completion of preparation in home for new baby

Decisions about the infant (circumcision, method of feeding, etc.)

Decision making for the early postpartum period

Education about psychologic and physical expectations in the early postpartum period

---

formed well, family members may gain greater problem-solving ability, self-esteem, self-confidence, and ability to participate in health care. Parents who feel good about themselves also have a solid foundation on which to build meaningful relationships with their children.

The problems and concerns of the pregnant woman, the relief of her discomforts, and the maintenance of her physical health receive much attention. However, her well-being also depends on the well-being of those closest to her. The nurse must help meet the needs of the woman's family to maintain the integrity of the family unit.

As discussed in Chapter 3, however, there are many variations in family structure today. One of the initial assessments involving the family will be about the family structure. Although the father of the baby is present in most cases, his presence cannot be assumed. If he is not a part of the family structure, it is important to assess the woman's support system to determine what significant persons in her life will play a major role during this childbearing experience.

FATHER

When the father is part of the family or support system, providing anticipatory guidance to him is a necessary part of any plan of care. He may need information about the anatomic, physiologic, and emotional changes that occur during pregnancy and postpartum, the couple's sexuality and sexual response, and the reactions that he may experience. He may wish to express his feelings about breast- versus bottle-feeding, the sex of the child, and other topics. If it is culturally acceptable to the couple and personally acceptable to him, the nurse refers the couple to expectant parents' classes for further information and support from other couples.

The nurse assesses the father's intended degree of participation during labor and delivery and his knowledge of what to expect. If the couple prefers that the father's participation be minimal or restricted, the nurse supports their decision. With this type of consideration and collaboration, the father is less apt to develop feelings of alienation, helplessness, and guilt during the intrapartal period. The relationship between the couple may be strengthened and his self-esteem raised. He is then better able to provide physical and emotional support to his partner during labor and delivery.

SIBLINGS

The nurse incorporates in the plan for prenatal care a discussion about the negative feelings that older children may have. Parents may be distressed to see an older child become aggressive toward the newborn. Parents who are unprepared for the older child's feelings of anger, jealousy, and rejection may respond inappropriately in their con-

Research Note

Lederman's review of the literature examined human and animal studies that investigate the effect of maternal anxiety on delivery outcome and infant development. The report focused on psychosocial conditions, relationships, and developmental conflicts that cause maternal anxiety, which in turn adversely affects intrauterine environment and fetal and newborn development.

Various studies have demonstrated that maternal stress can cause a decrease in fetal heart rate, fetal arterial oxygenation, and fetal blood flow. Such factors as overcrowding, geographical moves during pregnancy, disturbed personal relationships, and economic instability have been shown to increase maternal stress and to affect neonatal well-being. Maternal prenatal stress has been associated with an increased incidence of prematurity, stillbirth, congenital malformations, and neonatal deaths, as well as with abnormal labor patterns and perinatal complications.

The nurse is in a unique position to evaluate prenatal anxiety and provide counseling or referral to help clients minimize stress. Appreciation of the impact of stress on fetal and newborn development can guide interventions as the nurse provides comprehensive psychosocial and physical care throughout the maternity cycle.

Lederman R: Maternal anxiety in pregnancy: Relationship to fetal and newborn health status. Annu Rev Nurs Res 1986;4:3–15.

fusion and surprise. The nurse emphasizes that open communication between parents and children (or acting out feelings with a doll if the child is too young to verbalize) helps children master their feelings and may prevent them from hurting the baby when they are unsupervised. Children may feel less neglected and more secure if they know that their parents are willing to help with their anger and aggressiveness.

Parents may be encouraged to bring their children to antepartal visits. Seeing what is involved and listening to the fetal heartbeat may make the pregnancy more real to siblings. Many agencies also provide sibling classes geared to different ages and levels of understanding.

Nursing Goal: Provision of Anticipatory Guidance for the Puerperium

The nurse provides informal and formal education to the childbearing family throughout the prenatal period. This education is designed to help the family carry out self-care when appropriate and to report changes that may in-

dicate a possible health problem. The nurse also provides anticipatory guidance to help the family plan for changes that will occur following childbirth. Issues that could be possible sources of postpartal stress should be discussed by the expectant couple. Some issues to be resolved beforehand may include the sharing of infant and household chores, help in the first few days, options for babysitting to allow the mother and couple some free time, the mother's return to work after the baby's birth, and sibling rivalry. Couples resolve these issues in different ways; however, postpartal adjustment is easier for a couple who agree on the issues beforehand than for a couple who do not confront and resolve these issues.

Nursing Goal: Integration of Cultural Beliefs Influencing Pregnancy

As discussed in Chapter 14 specific actions during pregnancy are often determined by cultural beliefs. Some beliefs that have been passed down from generation to generation may be called "old wives' tales." These beliefs certainly had some meaning at one time, but the meanings have often been lost with the passing of time. Other beliefs have definite meanings that are retained. Tables 16–1 and 16–2 present activities prescribed and proscribed by certain cultures. The tables are not meant to be all-inclusive; they offer a few examples of cultural activities encouraged or proscribed during the prenatal period.

In working with clients of another culture, the health professional should be as open as possible to other beliefs. If certain activities are not harmful, there is no need to impose one's beliefs and practices upon a person of another culture. If the activities are harmful, the nurse can consult or work with someone within the culture or someone aware of cultural beliefs and values to help modify a client's behavior.

Nursing Goal: Relief of the Common Discomforts of Pregnancy

Common discomforts of pregnancy are often referred to as minor discomforts by health care professionals. These discomforts, however, are not minor to the pregnant woman.

Most of the discomforts of pregnancy are a result of physiologic and anatomic changes and are fairly specific to each of the three trimesters. Some preexisting problems, such as hemorrhoids and varicose veins, are aggravated during pregnancy. These discomforts worsen with enlargement of the gravid uterus; they may appear in the second trimester and become intensified in the third trimester. For women who do not have these preexisting conditions, the second trimester of pregnancy may be a relatively comfortable time. The discomforts caused by the enlarging

Table 16–1 Activities or Rituals During Pregnancy

Culture	Activity	Cultural meaning or belief	Nursing intervention
Mexican American	Certain clothing worn (muneco-cord worn beneath the breasts and knotted over the umbilicus; Brown 1976)	Ensures a safe delivery	If practice does not cause any danger, do not interfere with it.
	Use of spearmint or sassafras tea or benedictine (Brown 1976)	Eases morning sickness	Assess use of herbs and determine safety of their use.
	Use of cathartics during the last month of pregnancy (Brown 1976)	Ensures a good delivery of a healthy boy	Assess use of cathartics. Provide teaching about dangers of the practice and explore culturally acceptable means of resolving constipation (high-fiber foods).
Black American	Use of self-medication for many discomforts of pregnancy (Epsom salts, castor oil for constipation; herbs for nausea and vomiting; vinegar and baking soda for heartburn) (Carrington 1978)	Improves health and builds resistance	Assess use of self-medication; discourage those practices that may present problems.
American Indian (selected examples)	*Navajo* Meeting with medicine man 2 months prior to delivery (Farris 1976)	Prayers ensure safe delivery and healthy baby	Encourage the use of support systems.
	Exercise during pregnancy; concentrating on good thoughts, and being joyful (Farris 1976)	"Produce[s] efficiency and promote[s] joy" (Sevcovic 1979, p 39)	Encourage exercise as tolerated.
	Muckeshoot Indians Keeping busy and walking a lot (Horn 1982)	Makes baby be born earlier, and labor and delivery easier	Encourage walking as tolerated.
	Tonawanda Seneca Eating sparingly and exercising freely (Evaneshko 1982)	Makes delivery easier	Assess nutritional patterns and provide teaching if needed.
Vietnamese	Consuming ginseng tea Conversing with and counseling fetus (Hollingsworth et al 1980)	Gives strength	Assess use and be certain it is not taken to the exclusion of necessary nutrients.
White American	Certain clothing worn Self-medication for discomforts of pregnancy Seeks obstetric care	Promotes comfort Improves health Ensures safe pregnancy and delivery	Counsel regarding effect of drugs on fetus.
	Attends classes, reads books, attempts to gain more knowledge	Increases knowledge	Assist with pertinent books and topics.
	Concerned that maternity clothes make her look fat	Self-image	
	Oils & creams applied to avoid stretch marks	Self-image	Provide information regarding skin care.

uterus do not affect them until the last trimester or even until the last month.

The nurse knows appropriate interventions to help relieve these discomforts and works with the childbearing woman to plan and implement appropriate self-care measures. If these methods are not effective, the nurse must determine why. Are they ineffective because the source of discomfort was incorrectly assessed or because the woman did not receive sufficient instruction? After the situation is reevaluated, nursing interventions and client education can be changed as necessary to meet the woman's comfort and safety needs.

Table 16–3 identifies the common discomforts of pregnancy, influencing factors, and self-care measures the woman may implement.

FIRST TRIMESTER

○ *NAUSEA AND VOMITING*   Nausea and vomiting are early symptoms in pregnancy. Some degree of nausea occurs in the majority of pregnant women. These symptoms appear sometime after the first missed menstrual period and usually cease by the fourth missed menstrual period.

Table 16–2 Proscribed Activities

Culture	Activity	Rationale
Mexican American	Pregnant woman should not look at the full moon (Brown 1976)	It will cripple or deform the unborn child
	She should not hang laundry or reach high	This will cause knots in the umbilical cord
	Baby showers should not be planned until delivery time (Kay 1978)	Earlier would invite bad luck or the "evil eye"
	The woman should not allow herself to quarrel or express anger (Kay 1978)	Consequences are spontaneous abortion, premature labor, or knots in the cord
Black American	Avoid any emotional fright (Carrington 1978)	Baby will have a birthmark
	Avoid reaching up	The umbilical cord may wrap around the baby's neck
American Indian (selected examples)	*Navajo*	
	Rug weaving is forbidden; carrying and lifting also avoided (Sevcovic 1979)	Puts unnatural strain on the body
	Avoid funerals or looking at dead animals (Sevcovic 1979)	Exposes the baby to the realm of the dead and may cause later illness to the baby
	Laguna Pueblo	
	Do not sew with a bone or a needle (Farris 1976)	This will have an unkind effect on the baby
Vietnamese	Do not attend weddings or funerals (Hollingsworth et al 1980)	Bad luck for the newlyweds; the baby may cry
White American	Don't reach above head	Umbilical cord will wrap around baby's neck
	If frightened by snakes or other animals	May cause birthmark
	Don't lift heavy objects	May cause separation of the placenta

Some women develop an aversion only to specific foods, many experience nausea upon arising in the morning, and others experience nausea throughout the day or in the evening. Vomiting does not occur in the majority of these women.

Although the specific cause of nausea and vomiting in early pregnancy is not known, various theories have been proposed. A common theory attributes the nausea to hormonal changes related to hCG levels in the body. hCG begins to be present in the body at about the time that symptoms of morning sickness usually begin, and hCG levels are subsiding when the discomfort of nausea and vomiting usually ends.

Another theory suggests that changes in carbohydrate metabolism may create a slight decrease in blood glucose levels in early pregnancy. Nausea may occur as the result of intense hunger. Still another theory suggests that feelings of nausea may be related to episodes of maternal hypotension. Some authorities consider emotional factors to have a role in the experience of nausea and vomiting (Pritchard et al 1985).

Education for Self-Care   Treatment of nausea and vomiting is not always successful, but the symptoms can be reduced. The nurse must assess when the nausea and/or vomiting occurs to be helpful in suggesting methods of relief. For some women, nausea may be relieved simply by avoiding the odor of certain foods or other conditions that precipitate the problem. If nausea occurs most frequently during early morning, the woman may find it helpful to eat dry crackers or toast before arising slowly. Arising slowly and avoiding sudden position changes throughout the day may also help prevent nausea due to hypotensive episodes.

It is generally helpful to eat small, frequent meals (sometimes as often as every two hours) throughout the day and to avoid greasy or highly seasoned foods. Eating dry meals and taking all liquids, including soups, between meals may help some women. Sudden changes in blood sugar levels can be avoided if the small meals are high in protein or complex carbohydrates. While health care providers are reluctant to prescribe any medication during pregnancy, some women find a 10 mg vitamin B_6 supplement taken at bedtime is also helpful.

Although some nausea is common, the woman who suffers from extreme nausea coupled with vomiting requires additional assessment. She should be advised to contact her health care provider if she vomits more than once per day or shows signs of dehydration such as dry mouth, decreased amounts of highly concentrated urine, and the like. In such cases the physician may order antiemetics. However, antiemetics should be avoided if at all possible during the first trimester because of the danger of teratogenic effects on embryo development.

Nausea and vomiting generally cease by the fourth month of pregnancy. If they do not, hyperemesis gravidarum (a complication of pregnancy discussed in Chapter 19) may develop.

Table 16–3   Self-Care Measures for Common Discomforts of Pregnancy

Discomfort	Influencing factors	Self-care measures
FIRST TRIMESTER		
Nausea and vomiting	Increased levels of hCG Changes in carbohydrate metabolism Emotional factors Fatigue	Avoid odors or causative factors. Eat dry crackers or toast before arising in morning. Have small but frequent meals. Avoid greasy or highly seasoned foods. Take dry meals with fluids between meals. Drink carbonated beverages.
Urinary frequency	Pressure of uterus on bladder in both first and third trimester	Void when urge is felt. Increase fluid intake during the day. Decrease fluid intake *only* in the evening to decrease nocturia.
Breast tenderness	Increased levels of estrogen and progesterone	Wear well-fitting supportive bra.
Increased vaginal discharge	Hyperplasia of vaginal mucosa and increased production of mucus by the endocervical glands due to the increase in estrogen levels	Promote cleanliness by daily bathing. Avoid douching, nylon underpants, and pantyhose; cotton underpants are more absorbent; powder can be used to maintain dryness if not allowed to cake.
Nasal stuffiness and epistaxis	Elevated estrogen levels	May be unresponsive but cool air vaporizer may help; avoid use of nasal sprays and decongestants.
Ptyalism	Specific causative factors unknown	Use astringent mouthwashes, chew gum, or suck hard candy.
SECOND AND THIRD TRIMESTERS		
Heartburn (pyrosis)	Increased production of progesterone; decreasing gastrointestinal motility and increasing relaxation of cardiac sphincter; displacement of stomach by enlarging uterus; thus regurgitation of acidic gastric contents into esophagus	Eat small and more frequent meals. Use low sodium antacids. Avoid overeating, fatty and fried foods, lying down after eating, and sodium bicarbonate.
Ankle edema	Prolonged standing or sitting Increased levels of sodium due to hormonal influences Circulatory congestion of lower extremities Increased capillary permeability Varicose veins	Practice frequent dorsiflexion of feet when prolonged sitting or standing is necessary. Elevate legs when sitting or resting. Avoid tight garters or restrictive bands around the legs.
Varicose veins	Venous congestion in the lower veins that increases with pregnancy Hereditary factors (weakening of walls of veins, faulty valves) Increased age and weight gain	Elevate legs frequently. Wear supportive hose. Avoid crossing legs at the knees, standing for long periods, garters, and hosiery with constrictive bands.
Hemorrhoids	Constipation (see following discussion) Increased pressure from gravid uterus on hemorrhoidal veins	Avoid constipation. Apply ice packs, topical ointments, anesthetic agents, warm soaks, or sitz baths; gently reinsert into rectum as necessary.
Constipation	Increased levels of progesterone, which cause general bowel sluggishness Pressure of enlarging uterus on intestine Iron supplements Diet, lack of exercise, and decreased fluids	Increase fluid intake, fiber in the diet, exercise. Develop regular bowel habits. Use stool softeners as recommended by physician.
Backache	Increased curvature of the lumbosacral vertebras as the uterus enlarges Increased levels of hormones, which cause softening of cartilage in body joints Fatigue Poor body mechanics	Use proper body mechanics. Practice the pelvic tilt exercise. Avoid uncomfortable working heights, high-heeled shoes, lifting heavy loads, and fatigue.
Leg cramps	Imbalance of calcium/phosphorus ratio Increased pressure of uterus on nerves Fatigue Poor circulation to lower extremities Pointing the toes	Practice dorsiflexion of feet in order to stretch affected muscle. Evaluate diet. Apply heat to affected muscles.

Table 16–3   Self-Care Measures for Common Discomforts of Pregnancy (continued)

Discomfort	Influencing factors	Self-care measures
Faintness	Postural hypotension Sudden change of position causing venous pooling in dependent veins Standing for long periods in warm area Anemia	Arise slowly from resting position. Avoid prolonged standing in warm or stuffy environments. Evaluate hematocrit/hemoglobin.
Dyspnea	Decreased vital capacity from pressure of enlarging uterus on the diaphragm	Use proper posture when sitting and standing. Sleep propped up with pillows for relief if problem occurs at night.

○   *NASAL STUFFINESS AND EPISTAXIS*   Once pregnancy is well established, elevated estrogen levels may produce edema of the nasal mucosa resulting in nasal stuffiness, nasal discharge, and obstruction. Epistaxis may also result.

Education for Self-Care   Cool air vaporizers and normal saline nose drops may be helpful. However, the problem is often unresponsive to treatment. Women experiencing these problems find it difficult to sleep and may resort to nasal sprays and decongestants to relieve the problem. Such interventions can exaggerate the nasal stuffiness, and create other discomforts. The use of any medication in pregnancy should be avoided if possible.

○   *URINARY FREQUENCY AND URGENCY*   Two common discomforts of pregnancy are urinary frequency and urgency. They occur early in pregnancy because of the pressure of the enlarging uterus on the bladder. This condition subsides for a while when the uterus moves out of the pelvic area into the abdominal cavity around the twelfth week. Although the glomerular filtration rate increases in pregnancy, it does not cause a significant increase in urine output. Frequency recurs in the last trimester as the enlarging uterus begins to press on the bladder again. Coughing or sneezing in the last month may even cause leakage of urine.

As long as other symptoms of urinary tract infection do not appear, frequency and urgency of urination are considered normal during the first and third trimesters.

Education for Self-Care   There are no methods of decreasing the frequency and urgency of urination in pregnancy. Fluid intake should never be decreased to prevent frequency. The woman should be encouraged to maintain an adequate fluid intake: at least 2000 mL/day. She should also be encouraged to empty her bladder frequently. Efforts directed toward "holding" her urine may result in problems such as urinary tract infection.

Frequent bladder emptying helps decrease the incidence of leakage of urine. Since frequency often results in several trips to the bathroom each night, it is important to remind the woman to consider safety factors in the home such as a clear path to the bathroom, the use of a night light, and the like. The woman who leaks urine may choose to wear pantyliners during the day. If she does, she should understand the importance of changing them as soon as they become damp to avoid perineal excoriation and to avoid contamination of the perineum from the rectal area if the pads move back and forth as she walks. Tightening of the pubococcygeus muscle, which supports the internal organs and controls voiding, can help maintain good perineal tone. This procedure, known as Kegel's exercise, is discussed on page 390.

Research Note

DiIorio investigated the incidence and characteristics of nausea and vomiting of pregnancy (NVP) among teenagers, the measures they used to control NVP, and the effectiveness of the measures. Of the 78 subjects who responded to questionnaires, 74% were black, 70% were unmarried, and 21% had planned pregnancies.

Of the 56% of the subjects who experienced NVP, 47% were nauseous every day (most commonly in the early morning, although 20% reported evening nausea and 27% reported nausea all the time). Most subjects said that episodes of NVP lasted from two to four hours and that NVP was limited to three months or less. It was more common among white teenagers (contrary to data from previous studies) and among girls who wanted to become pregnant. The most common measure used to control NVP and the remedy rated as most helpful was "lying down." DiIorio pointed out that this makes sense in terms of the theory that NVP is related to postural hypotension.

DiIorio cautioned that controlled studies are needed before generalizing the data or basing care on these results. She suggested that because so few studies have been done on NVP, this condition offers fertile ground for nursing research.

DiIorio C: First trimester nausea in pregnant teenagers: Incidence, characterisitics, intervention. Nurs Res 1985;34(November/December):372–374.

While urgency and frequency are considered normal during the first and third trimesters, signs of bladder infection, such as pain, burning with voiding, or blood in the urine, should be reported to the woman's health care provider. If the woman has a history of frequent urinary tract infections, she may be advised to drink up to a quart of cranberry juice each day as a prophylactic measure.

○ *BREAST TENDERNESS* Sensitivity of the breasts occurs early and continues throughout the pregnancy. Increased levels of estrogen and progesterone play large roles in the soreness and tingling sensation felt in the breasts and in the increased sensitivity of the nipples.

Education for Self-Care A well-fitting supportive brassiere gives the most relief for this discomfort. The qualities of a proper supportive brassiere are discussed in the section on breast care (p 385).

○ *PTYALISM* Ptyalism is a rare discomfort of pregnancy in which excessive, often bitter saliva is produced. Causal theories are vague, and effective treatments are limited.

Education for Self-Care Astringent mouthwashes, chewing gum, or sucking on hard candy may minimize the problem of ptyalism.

○ *INCREASED VAGINAL DISCHARGE* Increased vaginal discharge (leukorrhea) is common in pregnancy. The discharge is usually whitish and consists of mucus and exfoliated vaginal epithelial cells. It occurs as the result of hyperplasia of vaginal mucosa and increased production of mucus by the endocervical glands. In addition, an accompanying reduction in the acidity of the secretions allows organisms to grow more easily.

Education for Self-care Cleanliness is important in preventing excoriation and vaginal infections. Daily bathing should be adequate, and douching should be avoided during pregnancy if vaginal infections do not occur. Nylon underpants and pantyhose retain heat and moisture in the genital area; absorbent cotton underpants should be worn to help prevent problems. Bath powder is also helpful in maintaining dryness and promoting comfort. The pregnant woman should be encouraged to report any change in vaginal discharge and any irritation in the perineal area. These changes frequently indicate vaginal infections.

SECOND AND THIRD TRIMESTERS

It is more difficult to classify discomforts as specifically occurring in the second or third trimester, since many problems are due to individual variations in women, such as number of previously existing conditions. The symptoms discussed in this section usually do not appear until the third trimester in primigravidas but occur earlier with each succeeding pregnancy.

○ *HEARTBURN (PYROSIS)* Heartburn is the regurgitation of acidic gastric contents into the esophagus. It creates a burning or irritating sensation in the esophagus and radiates upward, sometimes leaving a bad taste in the mouth. Heartburn appears to be primarily a result of the displacement of the stomach by the enlarging uterus. The increased production of progesterone in pregnancy, decreases in gastrointestinal motility, and relaxation of the cardiac sphincter also contribute to heartburn.

Education for Self-Care Activities that aggravate heartburn are overeating, ingesting fatty and fried foods, and lying down soon after eating. These situations should therefore be avoided. The woman should be encouraged to drink an adequate amount of fluid (6 to 8 glasses) each day and to eat smaller and more frequent meals to accommodate the decreased size of her stomach. Antacids such as aluminum hydroxide (Amphojel) or a combination of aluminum hydroxide and magnesium hydroxide (Maalox) can be recommended. However, common household remedies containing sodium bicarbonate (baking soda) should never be used for heartburn during pregnancy because of the potential for electrolyte imbalance.

○ *ANKLE EDEMA* Most woman experience ankle edema in the last part of their pregnancy because of the increasing difficulty of venous return from the lower extremities. Prolonged standing or sitting and warm weather increase the edema. It is also associated with varicose veins. Ankle edema becomes a concern only when accompanied by hypertension or proteinuria or when the edema is not postural in origin.

Education for Self-Care The aggravating conditions just mentioned should be avoided. If the woman has to sit or stand for long periods, frequent dorsiflexion of her feet will help contract muscles, thereby squeezing the fluid back into circulation. The pregnant woman should not wear tight garters or other restrictive bands around her legs. During rest periods, the woman should elevate her legs and hips as described in the following section on varicose veins.

○ *VARICOSE VEINS* Varicose veins are a result of weakening of the walls of veins or faulty functioning of the valves. Poor circulation in the lower extremities predisposes to varicose veins in the legs and thighs. With poor circulation, the valves of the veins prevent the blood from going downward, and stasis of the blood exerts pressure, which gradually weakens the walls of the veins and causes varicosities. In other cases faulty functioning of the valves causes pooling of blood in the lower extremities with concomitant pressure on the vein walls.

Pregnancy significantly increases the conditions that cause varicose veins. The weight of the gravid uterus in the pelvis aggravates the development of varicosities in the legs and pelvic area by preventing good venous return. Most women who do not have other predisposing factors can avoid the development of varicose veins in pregnancy with good preventive measures. Some women, however, experience obvious changes in the veins of their legs. Increased maternal age, excessive weight gain, a large fetus, and multiple pregnancy can all contribute to the problem.

Women with leg varicosities experience aching and tiredness in the lower extremities, with the discomfort increasing throughout the day. They frequently become discouraged by the discoloration in the veins of their legs and by obvious blemishes. Prevention or relief of the discomfort occurs when good venous return from the lower extremities is restored.

Vulvar varicosities may also be a problem in pregnancy, although they are less common. Varicosities in the vulva and perineum cause aching and a sense of heaviness. Support in these areas promotes relief.

Treatment of varicose veins by surgery or the injection method is not recommended during pregnancy. The woman should be aware that treatment may be needed after pregnancy because the problem will be aggravated by a succeeding pregnancy.

Phlebothrombosis and thrombophlebitis are possible complications of varicose veins, but they usually do not occur in a healthy pregnant woman. If these complications occur, the cause is often a local injury.

Education for Self-Care   The nurse plays an important role in teaching pregnant women how to help prevent the development of varicose veins. Regular exercise, such as swimming, cycling, or walking, promotes venous return, which helps prevent varicosities. Avoiding factors that contribute to venous stasis also helps prevent the development of varicose veins. The pregnant woman should avoid standing or sitting for prolonged periods. She should also avoid crossing her legs at the knees because of the pressure on her veins. She should not wear garters or hosiery with constricting bands, such as knee-high hose. However, supportive hose or elastic stockings may be extremely helpful, depending on the amount of discomfort. Supportive hose should be put on in the morning and should be washed daily with soap and warm water to help retain elasticity.

One important habit that the pregnant woman can develop is always to elevate her legs level with her hips when she sits. Comfort is enhanced if she supports the entire leg rather than simply propping her feet up on a stool, which may lead to hyperextension of the knees. The woman who sits or stands for long periods should walk around frequently to promote venous return to the heart. Venous return is most effectively promoted if the woman lies down with her feet elevated several times a day. To avoid difficulty related to pressure of the uterus on the vena cava, the woman can lie with her legs elevated on pillows and a pillow placed under one hip to displace the uterus to one side (Figure 16–1).

Support for vulvar varicosities can be provided by wearing two sanitary pads inside the underpants. Elevation of only the legs aggravates vulval varicosities by creating

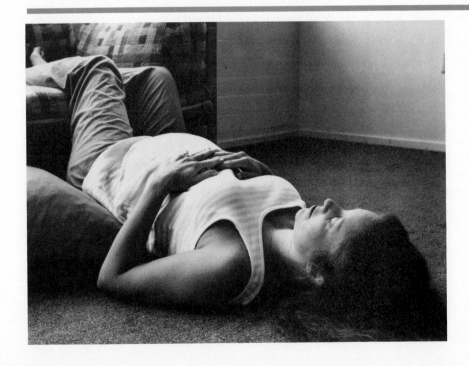

Figure 16–1   Swelling and discomfort from varicosities can be decreased by lying down with the legs and one hip elevated (to avoid compression of the vena cava).

stasis of blood in the pelvic area. Therefore, it is important that the pelvic area also be elevated to promote venous drainage into the trunk of the body. More than one firm pillow under the hips may be needed to accomplish this elevation. Near the end of pregnancy, this position may be extremely awkward; the woman may best relieve uterine pressure on the pelvic veins by resting on her side. Blocks may also be placed under the foot of her bed to elevate it slightly.

○　HEMORRHOIDS　　　Hemorrhoids are varicosities of the veins around the lower end of the rectum and anus. In the nonpregnant state, hemorrhoids are usually caused by the straining that occurs with constipation. When a woman becomes pregnant, the gravid uterus creates pressure on the veins and thus interferes with venous circulation. As the pregnancy progresses and the fetus grows, greater pressure on the veins and displacement of intestines occur, increasing the problem of constipation and often resulting in hemorrhoids.

Some women may not be aware of hemorrhoids in pregnancy until the second stage of labor, when the hemorrhoids appear as they push. Hemorrhoids that occur in pregnancy or at delivery usually subside, and they become asymptomatic after the early postpartal period.

Women who have hemorrhoids prior to pregnancy probably experience more difficulties with them during pregnancy because of the aggravating conditions just discussed.

Symptoms of hemorrhoids include itching, swelling, and pain, as well as hemorrhoidal bleeding. Internal hemorrhoids are located above the anal sphincter and are responsible for bleeding, usually with defecation. They are not usually painful unless they protrude from the anus. External hemorrhoids are located outside the anal sphincter. They are not usually the source of bleeding or pain; however, thrombosis of these hemorrhoids can occur, and in that case they become extremely painful. The thrombosis may resolve itself in 24 hours, or it can be treated in the physician's office by incising and evacuating the blood clot.

Education for Self-Care　　Relief can be achieved by gently reinserting the hemorrhoid. Reinsertion is aided by gravity; it is more successful if the woman lies on her side or in the knee to chest position. She places some lubricant on her finger and presses against the hemorrhoids, pushing them inside. She holds them in place for 1 to 2 minutes and then gently withdraws her finger. The anal sphincter should then hold them inside the rectum. The woman will find it especially helpful if she can then maintain a side-lying position for a time, so this procedure is best done before bed or prior to a daily rest period.

Avoidance of constipation is an important factor in preventing and/or relieving the discomfort of hemorrhoids. Relief measures for existing hemorrhoid symptoms include

ice packs, use of topical ointments and anesthetic agents, and warm soaks.

The woman should contact her health care provider if the hemorrhoids become hardened and noticeably tender to touch. Rectal bleeding that is more than spotting following defecation should also be reported.

○　CONSTIPATION　　Conditions in pregnancy that predispose the woman to constipation include general bowel slugglishness caused by increased progesterone and steroid metabolism; displacement of the intestines, which increases with the growth of the fetus; and oral iron supplements, which may be needed by the pregnant woman.

Education for Self-Care　　Increased fluid intake (at least 2000 mL/day), adequate roughage or bulk in the diet, regular bowel habits, and adequate daily exercise can often maintain good bowel function in women who have not had previous problems. Some women find it helpful to drink a warm beverage or glass of prune juice in the morning. Women should leave sufficient time following breakfast so that the natural action of the body will produce defecation. Some women, rushing to leave for work or school, ignore or suppress the urge to defecate.

Women who try to develop good bowel habits during pregnancy will be prepared to maintain good bowel function after delivery; meanwhile, they may need to use mild laxatives, stool softeners, and suppositories as recommended by their care giver. The nurse should help women with constipation to develop good daily bowel habits and to avoid becoming dependent on laxatives during pregnancy, a habit that may continue after delivery.

○　BACKACHE　　Many pregnant women experience backache. As the uterus enlarges, increased curvature of the lumbosacral vertebras occurs. Circulating steroid hormones cause a softening and relaxation of pelvic joints, the growing uterus stretches the abdominal muscles, and the increasing weight creates a gradual tilt of the anterior portion of the pelvis. As the anterior portion of the pelvis tilts downward, the spinal curvature increases. If the woman does not learn how to correct this curvature, the strain on the muscles and ligaments will cause backache.

Education for Self-Care　　An exercise called the *pelvic tilt* can help restore proper body alignment. As the anterior pelvis is tilted upward, the curvature of the back is automatically decreased, relieving much of the discomfort. If proper body alignment is maintained throughout pregnancy, backaches can be relieved or even prevented. See discussion on exercises, page 388.

The use of proper posture and good body mechanics throughout pregnancy is also important. The pregnant woman should not curve her back by bending over to lift or pick up items from the floor. The strain is felt in the muscles of the back. Leg muscles should be used to do the work instead. The woman can keep her back straight by bending her knees to lower her body into the squatting position (Figure 16–2). Her feet should be placed 12 to 18 inches apart to maintain body balance. When lifting heavy objects such as a child, she should place one foot flat on the floor, slightly in front of the other foot, and lower herself to the other knee. The object is held close to her body for lifting. This same principle of keeping the back straight and bending the knees applies when the woman sits down or gets out of a chair.

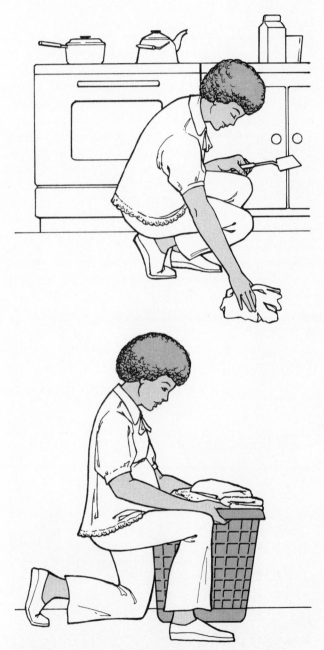

Figure 16–2 Proper body mechanics must be used by the pregnant woman when picking up objects from floor level or when lifting objects.

Work heights that require constant bending of the back can contribute to backache and therefore should be adjusted as necessary. Women who do not experience backache in pregnancy may become aware of it later as they bend to change a newborn's diaper.

A pendulous abdomen contributes to backache by increasing the curvature of the spine. The use of a good supportive maternity girdle is discussed in the section on clothing, as is the role of high-heeled shoes in increasing the lumbosacral curvature (p 386).

○ *LEG CRAMPS* Leg cramps are painful muscle spasms in the gastrocnemius muscles. They occur most frequently at night after the woman has gone to bed but may occur at other times. Extension of the foot can often cause leg cramps, so the pregnant woman should be warned not to do so while doing exercises for childbirth preparation or when she is resting.

The exact cause of leg cramps is not known. Proposed contributing factors include an inadequate calcium intake, an imbalance in the calcium/phosphorus ratio, pressure of the enlarged uterus on the pelvic nerves leading to the legs, or pressure on the pelvic vessels causing impaired circulation.

Leg cramps are more common in the third trimester because of increased weight of the uterus on the nerves supplying the lower extremities. Fatigue and poor circulation in the lower extremities contribute to this problem.

Education for Self-Care Immediate relief of the muscle spasm is achieved by stretching the muscle. This is most effectively done with the woman lying on her back and another person pressing the woman's knee down to straighten her leg while pushing her foot toward her leg (Figure 16–3). Foot flexion techniques, massage, and warm packs can be used to alleviate discomfort from leg cramps.

The physician may recommend that the woman drink no more than a pint of milk daily and take calcium lactate, or the physician may suggest a quart of milk daily and prescribe aluminum hydroxide gel. Aluminum hydroxide gel stops the action of phosphorus on calcium by absorbing the phosphorus and eliminating it directly through the intestinal tract. The treatment recommendations depend on the frequency of the leg cramps.

When planning a treatment regimen, one must be careful not to totally exclude milk from the woman's diet because it is an excellent source of other essential nutrients.

○ *FAINTNESS* Faintness is experienced by many pregnant women, especially in warm, crowded areas. The cause of faintness is a combination of changes in the blood volume and postural hypotension due to venous pooling of blood in the dependent veins. Sudden change of position or standing for prolonged periods can cause this sensation, and fainting can occur.

Education for Self-Care The nurse should first be certain that the pregnant woman understands the symptoms of faintness. These include slight dizziness, a "swirling" or "floating" sensation, and a decreased ability to hear or focus attention. If faintness is experienced from prolonged standing or being in a warm, crowded room, the woman should sit down, and lower her head between her legs. If this procedure does not help, the woman should be assisted to an area where she can lie down and get fresh air. When arising from a resting position, she should move slowly.

○ SHORTNESS OF BREATH Shortness of breath occurs as the uterus rises into the abdomen and causes pressure on the diaphragm. This problem worsens in the last trimester as the enlarged uterus presses directly on the diaphragm, decreasing vital capacity. When lightening occurs in the last few weeks of pregnancy in the primigravida, the fetus and uterus move down in the pelvis, engagement occurs, and the woman experiences considerable relief. Because the multigravida does not usually experience lightening until labor, shortness of breath will continue throughout her pregnancy.

Education for Self-Care During the day relief can be found by sitting straight in a chair and using proper posture when standing. If distress is great at night, the woman can sleep propped up in bed, with several pillows behind her head and shoulders.

○ DIFFICULTY SLEEPING Although the pregnant woman may experience difficulty sleeping for many of the same psychologic reasons as the nonpregnant woman, many physical factors also contribute to this problem. The enlarged uterus may make it difficult to find a comfortable position for sleep, and an active fetus may aggravate the problem. The other discomforts of pregnancy such as urinary frequency, shortness of breath, and leg cramps may also be contributing factors.

Education for Self-Care The pregnant woman may find it helpful to drink a warm (caffeine-free) beverage before bed and may benefit from a soothing backrub given by her partner or a family member. Pillows may be used to provide support for her back, between her legs, or for her upper arm when she lies on her side. Relaxation techniques may also help. The woman should avoid caffeine products, stimulating activity, and sleeping medication.

○ ROUND LIGAMENT PAIN As the uterus enlarges during pregnancy, the round ligaments stretch, hypertrophy, and lengthen as the uterus rises up in the abdomen. Round ligament pain is attributed to this stretching.

Education for Self-Care The woman may feel concern when she first experiences round ligament pain because it is often intense and causes a "grabbing" sensation in the lower abdomen and inguinal area. The nurse should warn women of this possible discomfort. Few treatment

Figure 16–3 The expectant father can help relieve the woman's painful leg cramps by dorsiflexing the foot while holding her knee flat.

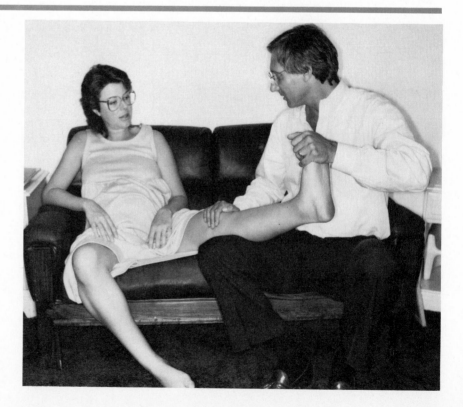

measures really alleviate this discomfort, but understanding the cause will help decrease anxiety. Once the care giver has ascertained that the cause of the discomfort is not related to a medical complication such as appendicitis or gall bladder disease, the woman may find that a heating pad applied to the abdomen brings some relief.

Nursing Goal: Promotion of Maternal and Fetal Well-Being During Pregnancy

The pregnant woman is faced with the important responsibility of maintaining her health not only for her sake but also for the sake of her unborn child. Nurses can help promote maternal and fetal well-being by providing expectant couples with accurate and complete information about health behaviors that can affect pregnancy and childbirth. These health behaviors include hygienic practices, potentially harmful habits such as smoking, and practices that help prepare the woman for the physical demands of childbirth and breast-feeding.

BREAST CARE

Whether the pregnant woman plans to bottle- or breast-feed her infant, proper support of the breasts is important to promote comfort, retain breast shape, and prevent back strain, particularly if the breasts become large and pendulous. The sensitivity of the breasts in pregnancy is also relieved by good support.

A well-fitting, supportive brassiere has the following qualities:

- The straps are wide and do not stretch (elastic straps soon lose their tautness due to the weight of the breasts and frequent washing).

- The cup holds all breast tissue comfortably.

- The brassiere has tucks or other devices that allow it to expand, thus accommodating the enlarging chest circumference.

- The brassiere supports the nipple line approximately midway between the elbow and shoulder. At the same time, the brassiere is not pulled up in the back by the weight of the breasts.

Cleanliness of the breasts is important, especially as the woman begins producing colostrum. Colostrum that crusts on the nipples should be removed with warm water. The woman planning to breast-feed should not use soap on her nipples because of its drying effect.

Nipple preparation, begun during the third trimester, may help the breast-feeding mother by decreasing the amount of nipple soreness she experiences during the early days of breast-feeding. Nipple preparation is aimed at promoting distribution of the natural lubricants produced by Montgomery's tubercles, stimulating blood flow to the breast, and developing the protective layer of skin over the nipple. Women who are planning to nurse can begin by going braless when possible and by exposing their nipples to sunlight and air. Rubbing the nipples removes protective lubrication and should be avoided, but tugging and rolling the nipple may be beneficial. This is done by grasping the nipple between thumb and forefinger and gently rolling and pulling on it. A woman with a history of preterm labor is advised not to do this because nipple stimulation triggers the release of oxytocin. (See Chapter 25 for further discussion.)

Nipple-rolling is more difficult for women with flat or inverted nipples, but it is still a useful preparation for breast-feeding. Nipple inversion is usually diagnosed during the initial antepartal assessment. When a nipple is truly inverted, pressure on the alveoli with the examiner's thumb and finger causes the nipple to retract. The normal or flat nipple protrudes when this is done (Figure 16–4).

The woman with nipple inversion can increase nipple protractility by performing Hoffman's exercises (Figure 16–5) (Hoffman 1953). If the nipple is truly inverted, she can wear special breast shields (such as Woolrich or Eschmann shields) for the last three or four months of pregnancy (Figure 16–6). These shields tend to absorb moisture so

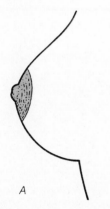
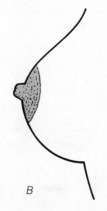
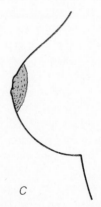

A   B   C

Figure 16–4   A When not stimulated, normal and inverted nipples look alike. B When stimulated, the normal nipple protrudes. C When stimulated, the inverted nipple retracts.

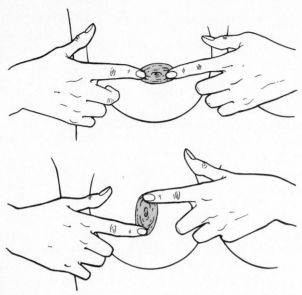

Figure 16–5 Hoffman's exercises are designed to increase nipple protractility. The woman is instructed to place her thumbs or index fingers opposite each other near the edge of the areola. She then presses into the breast and stretches outward to break any adhesions. This is done both horizontally and vertically.

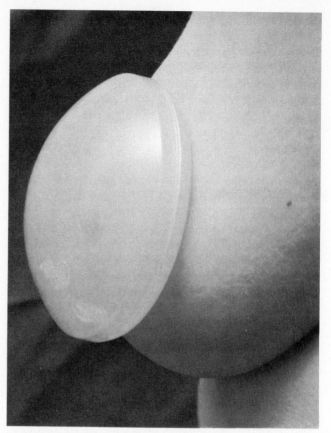

Figure 16–6 This breast shield is designed to increase the protractility of inverted nipples. These shields, worn the last three to four months of pregnancy, exert gentle pulling pressure at the edge of the areola, gradually forcing the nipple through the center of the shield. They may be used after delivery if still necessary.

they should not be worn more than a few hours at a time. Breast shields appear to be the only measure that really helps women with inverted nipples.

Oral stimulation of the nipple by the woman's partner during sex play is also an excellent technique for toughening the nipple in preparation for breast-feeding. The couple who enjoys this stimulation should be encouraged to continue it throughout the pregnancy.

CLOTHING

Maternity clothes are constructed with fuller lines to allow for the increase in abdominal size during pregnancy. Skirts and slacks have soft elastic waistbands and a stretchable panel over the abdominal area. Maternity clothes keep pace with fashion trends, enabling the woman to feel stylish whether in casual clothes, sporting clothes, or business wear. Maternity clothes are expensive, and if they are seasonal in style or fabric, a pregnant woman may not be able to wear them during subsequent pregnancies. Women can economize by sharing clothes with friends, sewing their own garments, or buying used maternity clothing.

Clothing affects a woman's general comfort during pregnancy. Clothing should be loose and nonconstricting both for general comfort and to prevent some of the specific discomforts of pregnancy. For example, restricting bands around the waist can be uncomfortable; those around the lower extremities, such as garters, can interfere with venous circulation and predispose to varicose veins or aggravate existing ones.

Maternity girdles are seldom worn today and many young women have never seen a girdle. They are sometimes used by women athletes, such as runners, dancers, or gymnasts, who maintain a light workout schedule during pregnancy. Women with large pendulous abdomens may also benefit considerably from a well-fitting supportive girdle. Without this support, the pendulous abdomen increases the curvature of the back and is a source of backache and general discomfort. Tight leg bands on girdles should be avoided.

High-heeled shoes aggravate back discomfort by increasing the curvature of the back and should not be worn if the woman experiences backache or problems with balance. Shoes should fit properly and feel comfortable.

BATHING

Because of the increased perspiration and mucoid vaginal discharge that occurs in pregnancy, daily bathing is important. The woman may generally take either a shower or a tub bath according to her preference. Caution is needed during tub baths because balance becomes a problem as pregnancy advances. Rubber mats in the tub and hand grips are valuable safety devices. *To avoid introducing infection, tub baths are contraindicated in the presence of vaginal bleeding or when the membranes are ruptured.*

Women are advised to avoid hot tubs or prolonged immersion in a very hot bath because of the possible harmful effects on the fetus when the maternal core temperature is elevated.

EMPLOYMENT

Fetotoxic hazards in the environment, overfatigue, excessive physical strain, and medical or pregnancy complications are the major deterrents to employment during pregnancy. Employment involving balance should be adjusted during the last half of pregnancy to protect the mother.

Fetotoxic hazards in the environment are always a concern to the expectant couple. If the pregnant woman or the woman contemplating pregnancy is working in industry, she should contact her company physician or nurse about possible hazards in her work environment and should do her own reading and research on environmental hazards. Some industrial products, such as turpentine and lead paint (which are also occasionally found in the home), are considered toxic substances during pregnancy. (See also Chapter 4 for a discussion of environmental hazards.)

TRAVEL

Pregnant women often have many questions about the effects of travel on them and the fetus. If medical or pregnancy complications are not present, there are no restrictions on travel.

Travel by automobile can be especially fatiguing, aggravating many of the discomforts of pregnancy. The pregnant woman needs frequent opportunities to get out of the car and walk. A good pattern to follow is to stop every 2 hours and walk around for approximately 10 minutes.

Seat belts should be worn, including both lap and shoulder belts. The lap belt should fit snugly and be positioned under the abdomen. The most frequent cause of fetal loss in car accidents is maternal death, and the importance of seat belts in preventing death in the general population is well known and documented (Krozy & McColgan 1985). The second leading cause of fetal loss in car accidents is placental separation believed to occur as a result of uterine distortion. Researchers suggest that use of the shoulder belt decreases the risk of traumatic flexion of the woman's body, thus decreasing risk of placental separation (Krozy & McColgan 1985; Crosby 1983).

As pregnancy progresses, flying or travel by train is recommended for long-distance traveling. The availability of medical care at one's destination also becomes an important factor for the near-term pregnant woman who is traveling.

ACTIVITY AND REST

Normal participation in exercise can continue throughout an uncomplicated pregnancy. The woman should check with her physician or nurse-midwife about taking part in strenuous sports, such as skiing, diving, and horseback riding. In general, however, the skilled sportswoman is no longer discouraged from participating in these activities if her pregnancy is uncomplicated. Pregnancy, however, is not the appropriate time to learn strenuous sports.

With the emphasis on physical fitness in our society, increasing numbers of women jog routinely as a part of a physical fitness program prior to pregnancy. There are many questions about continuing this activity during pregnancy. Concerns in the latter part of pregnancy are related to balance and the jarring effect on breasts and abdomen. A few small studies have recently been done on the effect of this type of exercise on the fetus and uterine activity in the last trimester of pregnancy. None of these studies noted any increase in uterine activity (Veille et al 1985) or interference with the well-being of the fetus (Collings & Curet 1985). It is generally believed, however, that as pregnancy progresses, non-weight-bearing activities, such as swimming and bicycling, are safer and provide fitness as well as comfort. They eliminate the bouncing associated with other exercise and are well tolerated physically (Ketter & Shelton 1984). More research needs to be done on the effect jogging during late pregnancy may have on the musculoskeletal system.

The nurse may find the following guidelines useful in counseling pregnant women about exercise during pregnancy.

- Exercise for shorter intervals. By exercising for 10 to 15 minutes, resting for a few minutes, and then exercising for an additional 10 to 15 minutes the woman decreases potential problems that may be associated with the shunting of blood to the musculoskeletal system and away from organs such as the uterus.

- As pregnancy progresses, decrease the intensity of the exercise. This helps compensate for the decreased cardiac reserve, increased respiratory effort, and increased weight of the pregnant woman.

- Avoid prolonged overheating. Strenuous exercise, especially in a humid environment, can raise the core body temperature. Prolonged maternal hyperthemia, especially in the first trimester, may increase the risk of teratogenesis. By the same token the woman should avoid hot tubs and saunas.

- As pregnancy progresses, avoid high-risk activities such as skydiving, mountain climbing, racquetball, and surfing. Such activities require balance and coordination but the woman's changed center of gravity and softened joints may decrease coordination.

- Warm up and stretch to help prepare the joints for activity, and cool down with a period of mild activity to help restore circulation while avoiding pooling of blood.

- After exercising, lie on the left side for ten minutes to rest. This improves return of circulation from the extremities and promotes placental perfusion.

- Wear supportive shoes and a supportive bra.

- Stop exercising and contact the care giver if dizziness, shortness of breath, tingling, numbness, vaginal bleeding, or abdominal pain occur.

- Reduce exercise significantly during the last four weeks of pregnancy. Some evidence suggests that strenuous exercise near term increases the risk of low birth weight, stillbirth, and infant death (Paolone & Worthington 1985).

Exercise helps to prevent constipation, condition the body, and maintain a healthy mental state. However, an important rule to follow, especially during pregnancy, is not to overdo.

Adequate rest in pregnancy is important for both physical and emotional health. Women need more sleep throughout pregnancy, particularly in the first and last trimesters, when they tire easily. Without adequate rest, pregnant women have less resilience.

Finding time to rest during the day may be difficult for women who work or have small children. The nurse can help the expectant mother examine her daily schedule to develop a realistic plan for short periods of rest and relaxation.

Sleeping becomes more difficult during the last trimester because of the enlarged abdomen, increased frequency of urination, and greater activity of the fetus. Finding a comfortable position becomes difficult for the pregnant woman.

Figure 16–7 shows a position most pregnant women find comfortable. Progressive relaxation techniques similar to those taught in prepared childbirth classes can help prepare the woman for sleep.

EXERCISES TO PREPARE FOR CHILDBIRTH

Certain exercises help strengthen muscle tone in preparation for delivery and promote more rapid restoration of muscle tone after delivery. Some physical changes of pregnancy can be reduced considerably by faithfully practicing prescribed body-conditioning exercises early in the prenatal period, as well as during the puerperium. A great variety of body-conditioning exercises are taught, but only a few are discussed here.

The pelvic tilt, or pelvic rocking, helps prevent or reduce back strain and strengthens abdominal muscle tone. To do the pelvic tilt, the pregnant woman lies on her back and puts her feet flat on the floor. This bent position of the knees helps prevent strain and discomfort (Figure 16–8). She decreases the curvature in her back by pressing her spine toward the floor. With her back pressed to the floor, the woman tightens her buttocks and abdominal muscles as she tucks in her buttocks. The pelvic tilt can also be performed on hands and knees, while sitting in a chair, or while standing with the back against a wall. The body alignment achieved when the pelvic tilt is correctly done should be maintained as much as possible throughout the day.

Figure 16–7 Position for relaxation and rest as pregnancy progresses

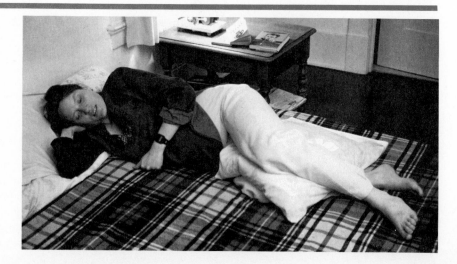

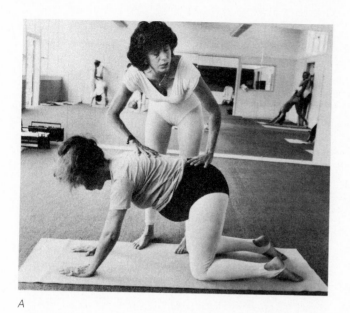

A

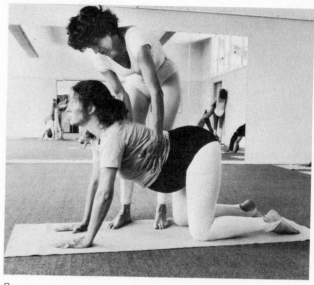

B

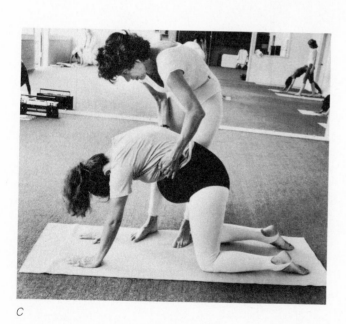

C

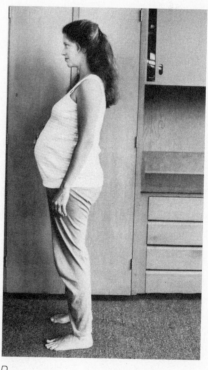

D

Figure 16–8A   Starting position when the pelvic tilt is done on the hands and knees. The back is flat and parallel to the floor, the hands are under the head, and the knees are directly under the buttocks. B A prenatal yoga instructor offers pointers for proper positioning for the first part of the tilt: head up, neck long and separated from the shoulders, buttocks up and pelvis thrust back, allowing the back to drop and release on an inhaled breath. C The instructor assists the woman in assuming the correct position for the next part of the tilt. It is done on a long exhalation, allowing the pregnant woman to arch her back, drop her head loosely, push away from her hands, and draw in the muscles of her abdomen to strengthen them. Note that in this position the pelvis and buttocks are tucked under and the buttock muscles are tightened. D Proper posture. The knees are not locked but slightly bent, the pelvis and buttocks are tucked under, thereby lengthening the spine and helping to support the weighty abdomen. With her chin tucked in, this woman's neck, shoulders, hips, knees, and feet are all in a straight line perpendicular to the floor. Her feet are parallel. This is also the starting position for doing the pelvic tilt while standing.

○   *ABDOMINAL EXERCISES*   A basic exercise to increase abdominal muscle tone is tightening abdominal muscles in synchronization with respirations. It can be done in any position, but it is best learned while the woman lies supine. With knees flexed and feet flat on the floor, the woman expands her abdomen and slowly takes a deep breath. As she slowly exhales, she gradually pulls in her abdominal muscles until they are fully contracted. She relaxes for a few seconds, and then repeats the exercise.

Partial sit-ups strengthen abdominal muscle tone and are done according to individual comfort levels. When doing a partial sit-up, the woman lies on the floor as described above (Figure 16–9). It is imperative that this exercise be done with the knees bent and the feet flat on the floor to avoid undue strain on the lower back. She stretches her arms toward her knees as she slowly pulls her head and shoulders off the floor to a comfortable level. (If she has poor abdominal muscle tone, she may not be able to pull up very far.) She then slowly returns to the starting position, takes a deep breath, and repeats the exercise. To strengthen the oblique abdominal muscles, she repeats the process, but stretches the left arm to the side of her right knee, returns to the floor, takes a deep breath, and then reaches with the right arm to the left knee.

These exercises can be done approximately five times in a sequence, and the sequence can be repeated at other times during the day as desired. It is important to do the exercises slowly to prevent muscle strain and overtiring.

○   *PERINEAL EXERCISES*   Perineal muscle tightening, also referred to as *Kegel's exercises,* strengthens the pubococcygeus muscle and increases its elasticity (Figure 16–10).

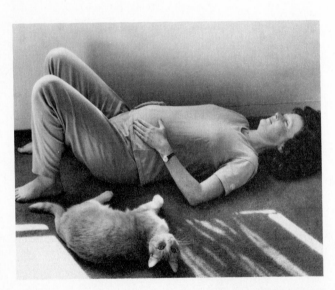

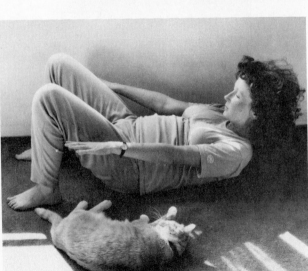

Figure 16–9   The pregnant woman can strengthen her abdominal muscles by doing partial sit-ups.

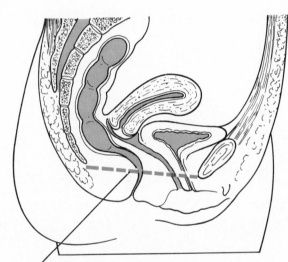

Pubococcygeus muscle with good tone

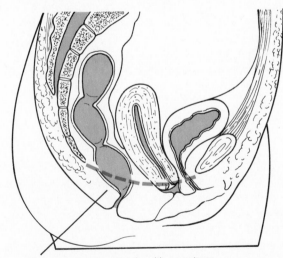

Pubococcygeus muscle with poor tone

Figure 16–10   Kegel's exercises. The woman learns to tighten the pubococcygeus muscle, which improves support to the pelvic organs.

The woman can feel the specific muscle group to be exercised by stopping urination midstream. However, doing Kegel's exercises while urinating is discouraged because this practice has been associated with urinary stasis and urinary tract infection.

Childbirth educators sometimes use the following technique to teach Kegel's exercises. They tell the woman to think of her perineal muscles as an elevator. When she relaxes, the elevator is on the first floor. To do the exercises, she contracts, bringing the elevator to the second, third, and fourth floors. She keeps the elevator on the fourth floor for a few seconds, and then gradually relaxes the area (Fenlon et al 1986). If the exercise is properly done, the woman does not contract the muscles of the buttocks and thighs.

Kegel's exercises can be done at almost any time. Some women use ordinary events—for instance, stopping at a red light—as a cue to remember to do the exercise. Others do Kegel's exercises while waiting in a checkout line, talking on the telephone, or watching television.

○ *INNER THIGH EXERCISES* The pregnant woman should assume a cross-legged sitting position whenever possible. The *tailor sit* stretches the muscles of the inner thighs in preparation for labor and delivery.

SEXUAL ACTIVITY

As a result of the physiologic, anatomic, and emotional changes of pregnancy, the couple usually has many questions and concerns about sexual activity during pregnancy. Often these questions are about possible injury to the baby or the woman during intercourse and about changes in the desire each partner feels for the other.

In the past, couples were frequently warned to avoid sexual intercourse during the last 6 to 8 weeks of pregnancy to prevent complications such as infection or premature rupture of the membranes. However, these fears seem to be unfounded. In a healthy pregnancy there is no valid reason to limit sexual activity (Reamy & White 1985). Intercourse is contraindicated only when bleeding is present, membranes are ruptured, or there are other complications that might lead to preterm delivery.

The expectant mother may experience changes in sexual desire and response. Often these are related to the various discomforts that occur throughout pregnancy. For instance, during the first trimester, fatigue or nausea and vomiting may decrease desire, while breast tenderness may make the woman less responsive to fondling of her breasts. During the second trimester, many of the discomforts have lessened, and, with the vascular congestion of the pelvis, the woman may experience even greater sexual satisfaction than she experienced prior to pregnancy.

During the third trimester, interest in coitus may again decrease as the woman becomes more uncomfortable and fatigued. In addition, shortness of breath, painful pelvic ligaments, urinary frequency, and decreased mobility may lessen sexual desire and activity (Swanson 1980). If they are not already using them, the couple should consider coital positions other than male superior, such as side-by-side, female superior, and vaginal rear entry.

The pregnant woman may be alarmed by orgasmic changes in the last trimester. Instead of the rhythmic contractions of orgasm, she may experience longer contractions that may be followed by cramps and backache. Masturbation often creates a more intense contraction than occurs with intercourse (Masters and Johnson 1966). There is no evidence, however, that these contractions cause preterm labor in the large majority of pregnant women (Klebanoff et al 1984).

Sexual activity does not have to include intercourse. Many of the nurturing and sexual needs of the pregnant woman can be satisfied by cuddling, kissing, and being held. The warm, sensual feelings that accompany these activities can be an end in themselves. Her partner, however, may need to masturbate more frequently than before.

The sexual desires of men are also affected by many factors in pregnancy. These include the previous relationship with the partner, acceptance of the pregnancy, attitudes toward the partner's change of appearance, and concern about hurting the expectant mother or baby. Some men may withdraw from sexual contact because of a belief that sex with a pregnant woman is immoral. This may be especially true for the couple whose religious beliefs teach that sexual intercourse is only for procreation. Some men find it difficult to view their partners as sexually appealing while they are adjusting to the concept of her as a mother. On the other hand, some men find their partner's pregnancy arousing and experience feelings of increased happiness, intimacy, and closeness (Reamy & White 1985).

The expectant couple should be aware of their changing sexual desires, the normality of these changes, and the importance of communicating these changes to each other so that they can make nurturing adaptations. The nurse has an important role in helping the expectant couple adapt. It is essential that nurses feel comfortable about their own sexuality and be well informed about the subject. When nurses counsel expectant couples, an accepting and nonjudgmental attitude is important. The couple must feel free to express concerns about sexual activity, and the nurse must be able to respond and give anticipatory guidance in a comfortable manner.

Occasionally a woman initiates discussion about her sexual concerns, especially if she has good rapport with the nurse. More often, the nurse must broach the subject.

A statement such as "Many couples experience changes in sexual desire during pregnancy" can initiate the discussion. This generalization can be followed by an exploration of the couple's personal experience. The question "What kind of changes have you experienced?" stimulates discussion more effectively than "Have you experienced any changes?"

The presence of both partners during sexual counseling is most effective in fostering communication between them.

DENTAL CARE

Proper dental hygiene is important in pregnancy. In spite of such discomforts as nausea and vomiting, gum hypertrophy and tenderness, possible ptyalism, and heartburn, regular oral hygiene must not be neglected.

The pregnant woman is encouraged to have a dental checkup early in her pregnancy. Women who neglect to obtain dental care prior to pregnancy become aware of dental problems during this time and thus may associate these problems with pregnancy. General dental repair and extractions can be done during pregnancy, preferably under local anesthetic. The woman should inform her dentist of her pregnancy so that she is not exposed to teratogenic substances. Dental x-ray examinations and extensive dental work should be delayed when possible until after delivery. Extensive dental care during pregnancy requires consultation between the dentist and the maternal health care professional.

IMMUNIZATIONS

All women of childbearing age need to be fully aware of the risks of receiving specific immunizations if pregnancy is possible. Expectant women, especially those who intend to travel throughout the world, should be aware of the immunizations that are contraindicated during pregnancy. In addition, it is important that expectant women clearly understand the recommendations that are made regarding other immunizations, such as those for influenza epidemics.

Immunizations with attenuated live viruses, such as rubella vaccine, should not be given in pregnancy because of the possible harmful effect of the live viruses on the developing embryo. Vaccinations using killed viruses can be used. Recommendations for immunizations during pregnancy are given in Table 16–4.

TERATOGENIC SUBSTANCES AND FACTORS

Substances that adversely affect the normal growth and development of the fetus are called *teratogens*. Many of these effects are readily apparent at birth, but others may not be identified for years. A well-known example is the development of cervical cancer in adolescent females whose mothers took diethylstilbestrol (DES) during pregnancy.

Many suspected teratogenic substances exist. The harmful effects of others, such as some pesticides and ex-

Table 16–4 Recommendations of American College of Obstetricians and Gynecologists (1982) for Specific Immunizations During Pregnancy

Immunizations	Notes
Tetanus-diphtheria	Allowed if no primary series or no booster in 10 years
Poliomyelitis	Not recommended routinely for adults but mandatory in epidemics
Measles	Contraindicated
Mumps	Contraindicated
Rubella	Contraindicated
Influenza	Evaluate according to same criteria as applied to other persons
Typhoid	Recommended if traveling in endemic region
Smallpox	Not needed; smallpox eradicated
Yellow fever	Recommended before travel to high-risk area; risk of yellow fever to mother and fetus greater than risk from immunization
Cholera	Recommended only to meet travel requirements
Rabies	Evaluated by same criteria as nonpregnant persons
Hepatitis-A	Recommended after exposure or before travel in developing countries
Plague	Used only if substantial risk of infection
Varicella	Varicella-zoster immune globulin allowed

*Source: Pritchard J, MacDonald PC, Gant NF: *Williams Obstetrics*, Ed 17. New York, Appleton-Century-Crofts, 1985, p 250.

posure to radiation (x rays, radioactive iodine, and atomic fallout) in the first trimester of pregnancy, have been documented.

Some environmental factors are also suspected to be teratogenic, but due to the complexities of the environment, causal relationships are difficult to demonstrate. Nevertheless, some definitive research has been done. For example, studies conducted on pesticides resulted in some pesticides being withdrawn from the market as potential causative factors in increased spontaneous abortion in areas where their use was widespread. In contrast, insecticide levels have been found in maternal and fetal circulatory systems without associated teratogenic problems (Hayes 1981). Moreover, expectant women who live in high-altitude areas have been found to have an increased incidence of small-for-gestational-age babies.

Medications are perhaps the most likely documented teratogens, but other factors can also harm the fetus, including certain infections such as rubella, syphilis, herpesvirus type 2, and toxoplasmosis. Hyperthermia (temperature greater than 39.4C [102.9F]) lasting 5 hours or more, especially if it occurs in the critical period of organ development from 18 to 28 days postconception, can cause CNS disorders such as anencephaly and meningomyelocele (Shepard 1984).

During pregnancy, women need to have adequate information available and a realistic perspective on potential environmental hazards. Factors that are suspected to be hazardous to the general population should obviously be avoided if possible. The expectant woman must remember that factors present in the environment for lengthy periods of time, such as pollution, have not resulted in epidemics of newborn defects.

Much research is being conducted on medications, alcohol, and cigarettes, and their roles as teratogenic substances. This information is discussed in the following sections.

MEDICATIONS

The prevalent use of medication in pregnancy is of great concern. Studies have demonstrated that the average pregnant woman takes many more medications than commonly believed, including over-the-counter drugs as well as prescription drugs. Medications sold over the counter (OTC) can be as dangerous as prescription drugs.

For example, aspirin is known to inhibit prostaglandin synthesis. This may result in prolonged pregnancy or labor if the woman has used aspirin regularly. Because aspirin crosses the placenta easily, it may result in bleeding problems for both mother and fetus, especially if taken within a week of delivery (Rayburn 1984).

Over-the-counter cold and allergy preparations often contain a mixture of ingredients that may include an antipyretic, a cough suppressant, an expectorant, a decongestant, an antihistamine, an anticholinergic, and an atopical anesthetic! When medication is needed, careful practitioners recommend preparations containing the fewest possible ingredients.

A major difficulty, even for women who attempt to eliminate all medication in pregnancy, involves ingestion of potential teratogenic medications for therapeutic purposes before pregnancy is diagnosed. It can be a problem for any woman, but especially for those with irregular menstrual cycles or for those who, because of great faith in their method of contraception, do not anticipate pregnancy. Although it is generally felt that the process of teratogenesis does not occur until 11 or 12 days after fertilization, this leaves enough time for damage to be done before a woman's first missed menstrual period—given a regular cycle and nonexpectations of a pregnancy. Table 16–5 identifies possible effects of selected drugs on the fetus or neonate.

An example of this problem is the use of isotretinoin (Accutane), which is given orally for severe acne. This medication came on the market in the fall of 1982 with warnings from the FDA that it not be used by women who were pregnant. These warnings were based on malformations in animals who were exposed to isotretinoin in early gestation (Benke 1984). By late summer of 1983, several reports had been made to the FDA of birth defects and spontaneous abortions with women who had used isotretinoin. Warnings were again sent to all physicians, and new labels were put on boxes containing this medication, with the warnings including women with any immediate plans to become pregnant (Marwick 1984).

As previously indicated, the greatest concern for gross structural defects in the fetus is during the first trimester when organ development is occurring. Innumerable factors determine if a fetus in utero will have gross structural defects when the mother has taken a known teratogenic substance in this period. The medication dosage and timing of ingestion correlated with the specific period of organ development is critical. Other factors about the subtance and a variety of individual metabolic and circulatory factors in the mother, placenta, and fetus are also influential.

Although the first trimester is the critical period for teratogenesis, some medications are known to have teratogenic effects when ingested in the second and third trimesters. Two examples of prescription drugs include tetracycline and sulfonamides. Tetracycline taken in late pregnancy is commonly associated with staining of teeth in children and has been shown to retard limb growth in premature infants; ingestion should be avoided during pregnancy. Sulfonamides taken in the last few weeks of pregnancy are known to compete with bilirubin attachment of protein-binding sites, resulting in jaundice in the newborn (Knothe & Dette 1985).

Other medications affect the fetus in much the same way that an adult is affected by an overdose. For example, the use of anticoagulants to treat thromboembolism in the mother can interfere with clotting factors in the fetus. However, this risk is lessened by frequent monitoring of prothrombin time in the mother, accompanied by appropriate changes in dosages of the anticoagulants. Heparin taken early in pregnancy is associated with a high rate of spontaneous abortion (Brill 1986). However, since it does not cross the placenta, it is probably safer for the fetus than warfarin (Coumadin) and other anticoagulants. Moreover, warfarin is associated with multiple congenital anomalies when taken in early pregnancy (Rao & Arulappu 1981).

Many pregnant women need medication for definitive therapeutic purposes, such as the treatment of infections, allergies, or multiple other pathologic processes. In these situations, the problem can be extremely complex. Known teratogenic agents are not prescribed and usually can be replaced by medications considered safe.

All medication should be avoided if possible. If no alternative exists, the following guidelines should be fol-

Table 16–5 Possible Effects of Selected Drugs on the Fetus and Neonate*

Maternal drug	Effects on fetus and neonate
Risk outweighs benefits if the following drugs are given in the first trimester:	
Thalidomide	Limb, auricle, eye, and visceral malformations
Tolbutamide (Orinase)	Increase of anomalies
Streptomycin	Eighth nerve damage; multiple skeletal anomalies
Tetracycline	Inhibition of bone growth, syndactyly, discoloration of teeth
Iodide	Congenital goiter; hypothyroidism; mental retardation
Methotrexate	Multiple anomalies
Diethylstilbestrol	Clear-cell adenocarcinoma of the vagina and cervix; genital tract anomalies
Warfarin (Coumadin)	Skeletal and facial anomalies; mental retardation
Risk vs. benefits uncertain in the first trimester:	
Gentamicin	Eighth cranial nerve damage
Kanamycin	Eighth cranial nerve damage
Lithium	Goiter; eye anomalies; cleft palate
Barbiturates	Increase of anomalies
Quinine	Increase of anomalies
Septra or Bactrim	Cleft palate
Cytotoxic drugs	Increase of anomalies
Benefit outweighs risk in the first trimester:	
Clomiphene (Clomid)	Increase of anomalies; neural tube defects; Down syndrome
Glucocorticoids	Cleft palate; cardiac defects
General anesthesia	Increase of anomalies
Tricyclic antidepressants	CNS and limb malformations
Sulfonamides	Cleft palate; facial and skeletal defects
Antacids	Increase of anomalies
Salicylates	Central nervous system, visceral, and skeletal malformations
Acetaminophen	None
Heparin	None
Terbutaline	None
Phenothiazines	None
Insulin	Skeletal malformations
Penicillins	None
Chloramphenicol	None
Isoniazid (INH)	Increase of anomalies

*Adapted from Howard FM, Hill JM: *Obstet Gynecol Surv* 1979;34:643. Modified and used with permission from Danforth DN: *Obstetrics and Gynecology*, ed 4. Philadelphia, Harper & Row, 1982, p 496.

lowed when medication is prescribed (Whipkey et al 1984):

● Select well-known medications rather than newer drugs whose potential teratogenic effects may not be known.

● Reduce the effects of fetal exposure by using the lowest possible therapeutic dose for the shortest time possible.

● When possible, use the oral form of a medication.

● Carefully consider the multiple components of the medication.

Consumers today are more aware of the potential risk of taking medications during pregnancy. They are asking for information and physicians are being held accountable to provide it. Skolnick (1985) reports that in the recent case of *Harbeson v Parke-Davis* the court ruled that the physicians caring for Ms Harbeson breached their duties

to her because they did not satisfactorily answer her questions about the possible effects on her pregnancy of taking the anticonvulsive medication Dilantin even though information on it is available. The court pointed out that the physicians should have reviewed the literature or sought additional opinions.

A woman clearly has a right to the most comprehensive information available concerning medications. The nurse can assist her by suggesting appropriate references and helping her research information. Some fine reference books on drugs and pregnancy are currently available and should be part of the library of every office and clinic that provides prenatal care.

The nurse should also remind the woman of the importance of checking with her physician about medications she was taking when pregnancy occurred and about any nonprescription drugs she is contemplating using. A good rule to follow is that the advantage of using a particular medication must outweigh the risks. Any medication with possible teratogenic effects must be avoided.

SMOKING

Many studies in the last several years have shown that infants of mothers who smoke have a lower birth weight than infants of mothers who do not smoke. In addition, many studies have found that intrauterine growth retardation (IUGR) increases as the number of cigarettes increases; IUGR was minimal or eliminated when smokers stopped smoking early in the pregnancy (Naeye 1981). Smoking may also be related to an increased incidence of preterm delivery (Shiono et al 1986).

The specific mechanism of smoking's effect on fetuses is not known, but various theories have been proposed. Many authorities theorize that passage of carbon monoxide through the placenta produces intrauterine hypoxia. The carbon monoxide blood levels are increased in smoking women and cross the placental barrier. The carbon monoxide attaches to hemoglobin before oxygen does, thus decreasing perfusion of oxygen to fetal tissues. Others suggest that the nicotine in tobacco has a direct effect on the fetus through its vasoconstrictive actions and/or indirect action by impairment of placental perfusion (Mochizuki et al 1984).

As smoking continues to be the focus of intensive research, some interesting findings offer positive information that nurses can use in providing prenatal care. Fewer women smoke today than did 20 years ago, presumably due to the intensive antismoking campaigns that have become common. Women who do smoke significantly reduce their smoking once pregnancy is diagnosed. Moreover, intervention programs designed to reduce smoking during pregnancy have been surprisingly successful and the results have been continued during the postpartum period (Kruse et al 1986). As primary client educator, the prenatal nurse has a wonderful opportunity to provide teaching, either individually or in classes, to help pregnant women reduce their smoking. The strong motivation of a pregnant woman to protect her unborn child may increase the woman's motivation dramatically.

Hundreds of chemical compounds are found in tobacco smoke. It may be some time before the mechanisms actually causing IUGR are known. Studies are demonstrating, however, that any decrease in smoking during pregnancy will result in better fetal outcome. Pregnancy may be a difficult time for a woman to stop smoking, but she should be encouraged to reduce the number of cigarettes she smokes daily. The need to protect her unborn baby can increase her motivation.

ALCOHOL

In 1968 the medical literature contained the first report recognizing alcohol as a teratogenic substance during pregnancy (Lemoine et al 1968). At that time newborns with a specific combination of characteristics became as-sociated with the common factor of heavy alcohol consumption by their mothers during the pregnancy. Since that time, much research has been done to validate this association.

Fetuses of women who consume large amounts of alcohol are at risk for developing *fetal alcohol syndrome* (FAS), which is characterized by IUGR and various congenital anomalies (see Chapter 31).

Most of the research reported to date demonstrates that heavy consumption of alcohol in pregnancy increases the risk of FAS, but the effect of moderate consumption of alcohol in pregnancy is still not clear. Although moderate consumption may not produce FAS, some research has indicated increased association with spontaneous abortion, mental retardation, and behavioral problems including attention deficit disorder (Kruse et al 1986). General conclusions are that the risk of teratogenic effects increases proportionally with increase in average daily intake of alcohol. Pregnant women who have an occasional drink should not be unduly alarmed about the effect it will have on the fetus.

Once women are aware of the pregnancy, most decrease their alcohol consumption because of concern for the fetus. In fact, women who consume alcohol reduce their drinking proportionately more than women who smoke reduce their smoking. This may be due to the habit-forming nature of smoking and to the fact that the fetal alcohol syndrome has been so widely publicized (Rubin et al 1986).

The alcohol consumption immediately after conception and prior to the awareness of the pregnancy may be of greatest concern. Not only is this a critical period, but the problem is doubly critical as alcohol consumption and abuse are rapidly increasing among women in the childbearing age. Some feel the occasional binge, in which the woman becomes highly intoxicated, can be as harmful as heavy daily consumption, particularly if binges occur during the critical periods of organ formation. Alcohol should always be considered foremost as a drug and not just as a beverage. Alcohol passes the placental barrier within minutes after consumption, with the potential alcohol blood levels in the fetus becoming equivalent to maternal alcohol blood levels.

Increased research is needed to determine the results of alcohol consumption at various stages of pregnancy. Awareness of the critical period of rapid development of brain cells in the fetus during the last trimester has created concerns about the effect of alcohol consumption during this period. Decreased consumption of alcohol in mid-pregnancy is associated with fewer incidents of growth retardation.

Some believe that maternal malnutrition in conjunction with chronic alcoholism is the cause of the growth retardation. It has been found that alcohol interferes with the passage of amino acids across the placental barrier, thus interfering with availability of nutritious elements to the fetus; therefore, the nutrition and alcohol factors may play important roles (Lin and Maddatu 1980).

Assessment of a woman's alcoholic intake should be a chief part of each woman's medical history, with questions asked in a direct and nonjudgmental manner. All women should be counseled about the role of alcohol in pregnancy. When pregnant women become aware of the risk of alcohol to the fetus, most usually attempt to modify their alcoholic consumption. If heavy consumption is involved, these women should be referred early to an alcoholic treatment program. Since the drug disulfiram (Antabuse), often used in conjunction with alcohol treatment, is suspected as a teratogenic agent, counselors in these programs need to be aware of a woman's pregnancy.

Counseling about the effects of alcohol during pregnancy has been effective and should, of course, continue. Since the most profound impact of alcohol occurs in the first weeks after conception, nurses and other health care providers will see the most dramatic decrease in the effects of alcohol during pregnancy by increasing their teaching efforts in the period prior to conception. Teaching must take place in family-planning clinics, in preconception clinics, and during regular health care maintenance (Wright & Toplis 1986).

MARIJUANA

The prevalence of marijuana use in our society raises many concerns about its effect on the fetus. Doing research on marijuana use in pregnancy is difficult, however, because it is an illegal drug. Unreliability of reporting, lack of a representative population, inability to determine strength or composition of the marijuana used, presence of herbicides, and use of other drugs at the same time are major factors complicating the research being done (Fried et al 1983). A few studies have been attempted without conclusive results. Some suggest that infants of mothers who use marijuana are small either as a result of IUGR or decreased length of gestation, and may even have increased risk of having features similar to those identified with FAS (Fried et al 1984, Hingson et al 1982).

It is known that women who smoke or consume alcohol decrease their smoking or alcohol consumption once pregnancy is diagnosed. A recent study also included a comparison of heavy marijuana users with those who smoke and consume alcohol. Even though the women in the study were volunteers, the heavy marijuana users did not alter their pattern of use during pregnancy. The women who were cigarette smokers and consumed alcohol followed the trend that has been demonstrated in other studies (Fried et al 1985). Perhaps the lack of conclusive results about the effects of marijuana in pregnancy lends a false sense of security.

COCAINE

Research about the impact of cocaine on pregnancy is still rather limited. Physiologically, cocaine acts to block norepinephrine uptake in the peripheral nerves. This leads to increased norepinephrine levels, which cause vasoconstriction, tachycardia, and a rise in blood pressure. The pregnant woman who uses cocaine has decreased blood flow to the placenta because of the vasoconstriction. Uterine contractability also increases. Some research suggests that the rate of spontaneous abortion is higher in cocaine-addicted women, and that finding seems logical in light of the physiologic effects of the drug.

Cocaine use during pregnancy is associated with various problems in the newborn. Infants exposed to cocaine in utero are less able to respond well to environmental stimuli and show signs of depressed interactive behavior (Chasnoff et al 1985). Others report more dramatic symptoms in the newborn including poor feeding, increased respiratory and heart rates, irritability, irregular sleep patterns, and diarrhea (Newald 1986).

As cocaine becomes more widely used by women of childbearing age, health care providers must become alert to early signs of cocaine use. It is often difficult for a nurse or physician to face the fact that a woman with whom they have a relationship may be using cocaine, but ongoing alertness and an open, nonjudgmental approach are important in early detection. Urine screening for cocaine is not presently available in all agencies, but urine screening may become a useful tool in early detection.

Nursing Goal: Teaching the Pregnant Woman How to Monitor Fetal Activity

Measuring of fundal height at each prenatal visit is considered one of many assessments of fetal well-being. Most assessments of this nature are done by the clinician who manages the care of the pregnant woman. The woman who wants to increase her involvement can learn maternal assessment of fetal activity. This method of fetal assessment does not involve any equipment or expense, but it is a valid tool in assessing the health status of the fetus.

When teaching any pregnant woman about fetal activity, she must be reassured that there are times when minimal or no fetal movement may occur with the healthy fetus.

Some movements are not felt by the woman. Ultrasound observations have revealed fetuses performing stretching, rolling, and limb movements that were not perceived by the woman.

Most women are aware when the activity of their fetus changes drastically and will report this if they have been told to be cognizant of it. Some clinicians have clients use fetal movement records (FMR) or a fetal activity diary (FAD). Keeping a written record of movements at particular intervals during the day makes the woman more aware of her fetus's activity. Otherwise a busy and active pregnant woman may be concerned about perceived decreased fetal activity. With the existence of a fetal activity diary and conscious assessment of her fetus, she can be assured by her own assessment that no problems exist, which will usually be the situation with the low-risk pregnancy. On the other hand, if overt decreased fetal activity has occurred, she can contact her physician with documentation for the need of further testing, which may prevent an intrauterine death.

Factors that affect fetal activity include drugs, cigarette smoking, sleep status of the fetus, glucose levels, and time of day. The expectant mother's perception of fetal movements and accuracy in documentation may also be influenced by many factors.

Authorities differ on how many fetal movements indicate health in the fetus. Freeman and Garite (1981) report that two or more movements per hour are reassuring, while fewer than two should be reported to the clinician for evaluation with a nonstress test. Chez and Sadovsky (1984) recommend that beginning at 27 weeks the woman count fetal movements twice daily for 20 to 30 minutes. Five to six movements during each counting session is a reassuring sign. If fewer than three movements are noted in the session, the counting time is extended to one hour. If there are fewer than ten movements in a 12 hour period of counting, the clinician should be notified. The use of maternal assessment of fetal activity as a component of the fetal biophysical profile is discussed in Chapter 20.

Case Study

Pamela Paulson is a 24-year-old gravida 2 para 0, whose first pregnancy ended in spontaneous abortion a year ago. Pam is a secretary for a construction firm and plans to continue working as long as possible. Her husband, Steve, is an electrician and has a fairly stable year-round income. Mrs Paulson was first seen in the clinic when she was nine weeks pregnant. Her first contact was Marie Carlson, an RN. Ms Carlson checked Mrs Paulson's vital signs, weight, and urine specimen; drew blood for laboratory tests; and completed the health history. She then asked Mrs Paulson if she had any questions or concerns. Mrs Paulson revealed that her pregnancy had been planned, and both she and her husband were eager to have a baby. However, she was constantly afraid that she would do something that might result in another miscarriage. Ms Carlson reassured her that it was not unusual for a woman to have one miscarriage. She then asked Mrs Paulson if there was anything in her life-style or environment that might be a risk factor. Mrs Paulson stated she was an avid swimmer and generally stopped at the YWCA on her way home from work to swim. However, she had given that up once she suspected she was pregnant for fear of causing another miscarriage. Ms Carlson reassured her that as long as she was not having any bleeding or other problems that might interfere, swimming was a wonderful exercise that she certainly could continue. She was advised to monitor her level of fatigue to avoid overdoing it. They discussed Mrs Paulson's lifestyle further, and the nurse was able to reassure her that it was a healthy one. The remainder of the visit went well. Mrs Paulson's physician, Warren Lindsey, reported that her physical exam was normal and her pelvis appeared large enough for successful vaginal delivery. She was started on a vitamin and iron supplement; the warning signs of potential problems in pregnancy were reviewed; and she left with literature to read about all other aspects of pregnancy.

The early months of Mrs Paulson's pregnancy went smoothly. She did not suffer from nausea, and the urinary frequency she experienced eased in her fourth month. She continued prenatal visits every four weeks. As Mrs Paulson began wearing maternity clothes, her fear of miscarriage abated.

Mrs Paulson felt the first flutterings of fetal movement at 19 weeks, and the fetal heart tones (FHT) were auscultated a week later. She persuaded her husband to accompany her on a prenatal visit, and he obviously enjoyed hearing the FHT with the Doppler.

In her seventh month, Mrs Paulson began to develop varicose veins in her legs and had problems with hemorrhoids. Ms Carlson and Mrs Paulson discussed her schedule and habits, identifying some changes she might make to ease her discomfort. Mrs Paulson began wearing maternity support hose to work and walking around her office every hour. During her breaks and at lunch, she lay on her side in the staff lounge with her feet elevated. She continued her evening swims. A review of Mrs Paulson's diet showed it had sufficient fiber, fresh fruit, and vegetables. She also drank several glasses of water every day. Nevertheless, constipation was still a problem. Ms Carlson reported these findings to Dr Lindsey, and he prescribed a mild stool softener. Mrs Paulson continued to follow this regimen, and her symptoms eased.

At 37 weeks, Mrs Paulson began experiencing urinary frequency again, and physical assessment showed that lightening had occurred. Mrs Paulson reported to Ms Carlson that the nursery was ready and her suitcase was packed. She and her husband had taken the childbirth preparation classes offered at the clinic, and she felt well prepared.

Mrs Paulson and Ms Carlson spent some time talking about what being a parent meant, and Ms Carlson gave Mrs Paulson some interesting articles on adjusting to a new baby. They also spoke about some of the sexual changes Mrs Paulson might experience. At the end of the conversation, Mrs Paulson said, "I'm so glad you brought this up. I wondered what sex would be like afterward but felt a little embarrassed about asking."

One day before her EDD, Mrs Paulson went into labor and, following a 12-hour labor, successfully delivered a 7 lb 2 oz son—Ryan Erik Paulson.

● Care of the Pregnant Adolescent

Pregnancy is a developmental challenge no matter what the age of the individual involved. However, many factors make it more complicated for the adolescent. Her physical development is incomplete; she has not yet completed the psychologic development tasks of adolescence; and her available support systems may be limited. In addition, her education is unfinished and plans for its completion may be jeopardized.

The teenage pregnancy rate has continued to increase during the last decade, with at least one in 10 young women becoming pregnant each year (Alan Guttmacher Institute 1981). Although contraceptive use has increased among adolescents, it has not kept pace with increasing sexual activity.

Adolescent pregnancy has been a concern of the health profession for some time. That it is also becoming a concern of the general population is reflected by the growing coverage of the problem in the media. According to one source, this tremendous increase in media attention began with the release of the results of a study done by Alan Guttmacher Institute (Wallis 1985). The study compared teenage birthrates in 37 countries and abortion rates in 13 other countries. The results demonstrated that the number of births per 1000 women under 20, as well as the incidence of abortion in the same age group, were significantly higher in the United States than in other developed countries in the study. In contrast the incidence of women having sexual intercourse during the teenage years is comparable, except in Sweden where it is higher (Jones et al 1985).

Authorities believe that many factors contribute to the increased incidence of adolescent pregnancy in the United States. There has been a trend in all age groups toward increased premarital or extramarital sexual activity and cohabitation, which is often perceived as socially acceptable. Sexual innuendo permeates every aspect of the popular media. As a result of these trends sexual activity occurs at a younger age and is encouraged by peer pressure in the adolescent population. At the same time there is great controversy about sex education in the schools and availability of contraception to adolescents.

With menarche and first sexual intercourse occurring at an earlier age, it is not surprising that a greater number of younger teenagers are getting pregnant. In contrast the statistics indicate a decrease in older teenage pregnancy (Ventura & Hendershot 1984).

Some pregnant adolescents are continuing to go to school, thus increasing their visibility in the community. Twenty years ago, pregnant adolescents were expelled from school and generally not seen for nine months. Fewer young women are choosing to "legitimize" their newborns by marriage, and more of them are choosing to keep their newborns rather than relinquish them for adoption.

Even though the incidence of adolescent pregnancy has increased, the birth rate is declining, partially because of the availability of legal abortion services. Nevertheless, adolescents are becoming pregnant in greater numbers, and the consequences must be addressed by the health care professions.

Overview of the Adolescent Period

PHYSICAL CHANGES

Menarche usually occurs in adolescents between 12 and 13 years of age (Goldsmith & Weiss 1986). The major physical changes of puberty include a height spurt, weight change, and the appearance of secondary sex characteristics.

The first menstrual cycles are irregular and usually anovulatory. The hypothalamic–pituitary–ovarian axis takes up to five years to complete maturation (Lemarchand-Beraud et al 1982). Long bone growth is also incomplete until well after menarche.

Nutritional status is an important determinant of menarche. Undernourished girls tend to have a later menarche. Anemia can be a problem for adolescents, especially during the growth spurt that precedes menarche.

PSYCHOSOCIAL DEVELOPMENT

The period of adolescence is marked by joy and stress. The stress lies in dealing with body changes and social and family relationship changes; the joy lies in new discoveries, independence, and responsibilities. The struggle to become an adult while still needing the security of childhood creates a turbulent era for the entire family.

Developmental tasks of the adolescent have been described by many writers. Mercer (1979) enumerated six tasks:

- Acceptance and achievement of comfort with body image

- Determination and internalization of sexual identity and role

- Development of a personal value system

- Preparation for productive citizenship

- Achievement of independence from parents

- Development of an adult identity

These tasks are overwhelming for many adolescents; the guidance, nurturing, and support offered by the family and community play a large part in successful integration.

Adolescent rebellion is a means by which young people work at accomplishing these tasks. Rebellion permits them to make the transition to adult social roles.

The early adolescent (under age 15) still sees authority in the parents. During these years she is working to become comfortable with her changing body and her body image. She is a concrete thinker. The early adolescent has only minimal ability to see herself in the future or foresee the consequences of her behavior. She perceives her focus of control as external; that is, her destiny is controlled by others such as parents and school authorities.

Middle adolescence (15 to 17 years) is the time for challenging: Experimenting with drugs, alcohol, and sex is a common avenue for rebellion. The middle adolescent seeks independence and turns increasingly to her peer group. She wants to be treated as an adult. However, fear of adult responsibility may cause fluctuation in behavior. At times she seems like a child, while at other times she is surprisingly mature. She is beginning to move from concrete thinking to formal operational thought but is not yet able to anticipate the long-term implications of all her actions.

In late adolescence (17 to 19 years) the young woman is more at ease with her individuality and decision-making ability. She can think abstractly and anticipate consequences. During this time she becomes more confident of her personal identity. The experiences of middle adolescence assist her in completing her developmental tasks. The late adolescent is capable of formal operational thought. She is learning to solve problems, to conceptualize, and to make decisions. These abilities help her see herself as having control, which leads to the ability to understand and accept the consequences of her behavior.

The Adolescent Mother

The psychologic rationales for adolescent pregnancy have received major attention in the literature. One school of thought suggests that if the young woman's mother has been an inconsistent nurturer, the daughter may enter adolescence with deficits in her sense of time, reality testing, and ability to handle frustration. These deficits make it difficult for her to accomplish her developmental tasks (Spain 1980).

Deficits in ego functioning have been cited as reasons for sexual acting out. Young women with poor ego integrity have little sense of self-worth and some hopelessness regarding their future. Other psychologic rationales for adolescent pregnancy include unstable family relationships; needing someone to love; competition with the mother; punishment of the father and/or mother; emancipation from an undesirable home situation; and attention getting. Pregnancy may be a young woman's form of delinquency because this is one area that parents cannot control.

Cultural values may also cause a young woman to desire pregnancy. Many cultures equate evidence of fertility with adult status. Thus the young woman who sees being a mother as her primary adult role has little motivation to delay having a child (Moore et al 1984).

Another school of thought suggests that pregnancy is a result of unmotivated accidents. The adolescent, who is not yet capable of thinking abstractly, is unable to perceive the consequences of her sexual activity. She has sex infrequently, often not planning to have it, and therefore does not consider contraception. She may have guilt feelings about sex and may not be able to admit she is sexually active. Being contraceptively prepared is an admission of sexuality. She is incapable of understanding how pregnancy will affect her future. Her rationale may include comments such as, "I'm too young to get pregnant," "I don't have intercourse often enough," or "It was the safe time of the month." Most young people have no idea of when they ovulate and how they conceive.

PHYSIOLOGIC RISKS

Previous research demonstrated that adolescents were more at risk than older women for a myriad of problems during pregnancy. New studies that control for age, race, socioeconomic status, and prenatal care show that adolescents over 15 years old who receive early, thorough prenatal care have no greater risk than women over 20 years old (Brucker & Mueller 1985, Piechnik & Corbett 1985). It is the young adolescent (under age 15) who remains at risk for premature births; low-birth-weight (LBW) infants; pregnancy-induced hypertension (PIH) and its sequela; cephalopelvic disproportion (CPD); and iron deficiency anemia (Carey et al 1981). In this age group, prenatal care is the critical factor that most influences pregnancy outcome.

Pregnancy-induced hypertension represents the most prevalent medical complication in adolescents; the incidence of PIH is higher in teens than among older women. The etiology of PIH remains unclear, but hypotheses point to uterine ischemia, nutritional factors, and immunologic variances that appear to affect adolescents. There may be a suboptimal development of the uterine vasculature in the very young adolescent that predisposes them to PIH (Chesley 1978).

Iron deficiency anemia is a problem in all pregnant women. The adolescent who begins her pregnancy already anemic, however, is at increased risk and must be followed closely and carefully counseled regarding nutrition during pregnancy.

Teenagers 15 to 19 years old have the second highest incidence of sexually transmitted diseases in the United States. The presence of herpes virus or gonorrhea during a pregnancy increases the dangers greatly. The incidence of chlamydial infection also increases (Osofsky 1985). Other problems seen in adolescents are cigarette smoking and drug use. The damage may be already done to the

Table 16–6 Developmental Tasks of Adolescence and Their Implications During Pregnancy

Developmental tasks of adolescence (Mercer 1979)	Impact on pregnant adolescent	Nursing role
Acceptance and comfort with body image	Must learn to deal with changing body: enlarging breasts and abdomen, striae, chloasma, weight gain; may not have yet incorporated the changes of puberty	Assist the client in determining what the changes of puberty meant to her; how she feels about the changes of pregnancy. Help her think of ways in which she can feel good about herself.
	May be reticent about wearing maternity clothes	Assess at what point in the pregnancy she begins to wear maternity clothes; ask why if she is not wearing them at the appropriate time.
	May try fad diets or eat junk food, due to peer pressure and the slender image society has of women; does not want to get fat	Give nutrition counseling to every adolescent. Emphasize that pregnant women do not diet, she can lose the weight later; give exercises for pregnant women.
	Must learn to cope with looking different from her peers	Elicit feelings about how she is coping with this; support from friends, family.
Determination and internalization of sexual role and identity	May not be able to perceive of herself as a sexual being (pregnancy confers overt sexuality)	Elicit feelings about sexuality.
	Must learn to incorporate the concept of becoming a mother	Find out what motherhood means to the client.
	Must cope with possible changes in relationships with friends, boyfriend, and family	Ask how she sees relationships changing. How she is dealing with it.
	May see her role as solely procreator, other opportunities for development of other female roles may be temporarily abandoned	Ask what other roles she sees for herself now. In 5 years.
Development of a personal value system	Must cope with and adjust to the fact that she became pregnant; is this in conflict with her self-ideal of chastity? Adjust to premature motherhood and inherent responsibilities	Discuss her feelings of conflict, if any: Is she living up to her expectations and how can she do so? Explore the value the client places on becoming a mother and having children. How does she see her relationship with her newborn, now and 5 years from now?
	Incorporate problem-solving skills and decision-making skills	Explore values regarding career, school, marriage. Apply reality test: "Tell me how you see a typical day with a two-month-old infant."
Preparation for productive citizenship	Adjust to interruption of school May see school as unnecessary or postpone indefinitely	Explore provisions for school while pregnant: When can she return? Refer to Social Service; discuss importance of education regarding her career and future.
	Incorporate career goals with parenting; may not consider working important	Discuss future economic consolidation. Assist problem solving in this area.
Achievement of independence from parents	Cope with realities of pregnancy, and dependence on family (or someone) for financial help	Elicit what changes she perceives and how she feels about them. Discuss the reality of her situation (reality testing is constructive): How can she adjust? How can she plan independence? Living at home may be out of the question; she may end up on welfare. Check her home and family situation often during the pregnancy.
	Adjust to need for financial assistance until she can earn her own living	Ask what role the father of the child will play. If she does not live at home, who will support her?
Development of an adult identity	Learn to accept the responsibilities of adulthood and parenthood Learn to accept the responsibilities for her actions Learn to plan for her future	Encourage prenatal classes, parenting classes. Discuss prenatal care and the effects on her pregnancy. Explore options through all of the above.

fetus by smoking or drug use by the time pregnancy is confirmed in young women.

PSYCHOLOGIC RISKS

The most profound psychologic risk to the pregnant adolescent is the interruption of work on her developmental tasks. Although adolescents have become sexually active at an earlier age and the incidence of pregnancy has increased, the developmental tasks of this age group remain the same. Add to this the tasks of pregnancy, and the young woman has an overwhelming amount of psychologic work to do, the success of which will affect her own and her newborn's future.

The successful achievement of developmental tasks in the various life stages preclude completion of the next set of tasks. Unless one is able to complete the tasks of adolescence and incorporate an adult identity, the adult tasks will be difficult to attain. These tasks are building blocks to maturation and positive self-growth.

Table 16–6 lists adolescent developmental tasks (as identified by Mercer 1979), the impact on the pregnant

adolescent, and nursing implications. Tasks of pregnancy are included in Table 16–7.

Through the nursing process, the nurse should assist the woman in meeting these tasks during prenatal visits. An interdisciplinary approach, utilizing the social worker, nutritional counselor, and school counselor will benefit the adolescent.

SOCIOLOGIC RISKS

The adolescent pregnancy affects not only the adolescent but also society. Waters (1969) describes the sequence of events for which the adolescent continues to be at risk in the 1980s, and the brunt of which society must bear. This includes:

- Failure to fulfill the functions of adolescence
- Failure to remain in school
- Failure to limit family size
- Failure to establish stable families

Table 16–7 Tasks of Pregnancy and the Adolescent

Task	Impact on adolescent	Nursing role
Acceptance of pregnancy	May deny until well into pregnancy, thus having no alternative but to carry pregnancy	Counsel or refer for counseling regarding whether she will keep or relinquish her newborn. Discuss importance of early prenatal care. Elicit feelings about pregnancy (see Table 16–6, first developmental task).
	May have difficulty bonding with fetus, which may carry over to unresponsiveness to newborn	
Acceptance of termination of pregnancy	Toward end of pregnancy may focus on "wanting it to be over"; may have trouble individuating fetus	Elicit why she has these feelings. Assist with coping mechanisms. Discuss preferred sex, names, showers, and readiness for newborn's arrival.
Acceptance of mother role	May not perceive of newborn as being her own, especially if her mother will be caring for the newborn; may think of newborn as a doll or sister	Discuss plans for newborn, include client's mother as indicated. Elicit client's perception of motherhood (see Table 16–6, second developmental task). Discuss dreams, role playing, fantasies that she experiences. Does she know any new mothers? Encourage prenatal classes.
Resolution of fears about childbirth	May focus on labor and delivery as mutilating to her body	Encourage attendance at prenatal classes, childbirth education. Offer literature or references for reading.
	May not see childbirth education as necessary for coping and learning	Elicit expectations, knowledge, and fears about childbirth. Discuss analgesia, labor process; offer tour of facilities.
	May have fantasies, dreams, or nightmares about childbirth	Reinforce that fantasies or dreams are normal. Encourage support person to attend classes with client.
Bonding	May feel ambivalent about pregnancy and motherhood	Assess all parameters of feelings about pregnancy in other developmental tasks and tasks of pregnancy. Refer for counseling if there is any sign of maladjustment to pregnancy.

- Failure to be self-supporting

- Failure to have healthy infants

The frustration of being forced into adult roles before completing adolescent developmental tasks causes a negative series of events that affects the adolescent's entire life.

Many adolescents who become pregnant drop out of school and never complete their education. Lack of education reduces the quality of jobs available to these individuals. Programs for pregnant adolescents and adolescent mothers may help decrease this problem.

Although adolescent mothers are more immediately affected by a pregnancy, adolescent fathers are also adversely affected in that they tend to pursue less prestigious careers, earn less income, and have less job satisfaction than men who marry at an older age.

Failure to limit family size is another element of the syndrome. The younger the adolescent at her first pregnancy, the more likely she is to become pregnant again while still an adolescent. These young women frequently fail to establish a stable family. Their family structure tends to be single parent and matriarchal, often the same family structure in which the adolescent was raised. If such women do marry, their divorce rate is the highest of any age group in the United States. Certainly poverty aggravates this problem.

Failure to be self-supporting logically follows lack of education and lost career goals. Many adolescents with children end up on welfare.

Finally, adolescents are at risk for having unhealthy babies because of potential complications and lack of prenatal care.

The Adolescent Father

The unwed adolescent father historically has been met with less-than-supportive services. His stresses, concerns, and needs have been ignored by society.

The adolescent father is usually about the same age (within 3 to 4 years) as the adolescent mother. They are generally from similar socioeconomic backgrounds and have similar education.

Adolescent fathers do become sexually active at an earlier age than adolescent mothers, but, somewhat surprisingly, their knowledge of sexuality and reproduction is no greater than that of their nonfather peers (Barret & Robinson 1985). In an earlier study Barret and Robinson (1982) learned that most adolescent fathers seldom talked about the possibility of pregnancy and only a few used contraception. When asked to respond to the sentence "I did not think she would get pregnant because . . . ," their comments included: "She didn't look like the type." "We only had sex once a week." "She had such little breasts."

Obviously adolescent fathers need more information about human sexuality. The boy who has a good relationship with his own father or a supportive adult may obtain information, but the only ongoing source of accurate information for many adolescents has been the schools. Because of funding issues and the ongoing controversy over the best place for sex education, many adolescent fathers are not receiving the information they need.

Psychologic and sociologic risks to the adolescent father are in many ways similar to the adolescent mother's risks. Card and Wise (1978) found that adolescent fathers achieve less formal education than older fathers, and they enter the labor force earlier with less education. They also found that adolescent fathers marry at a younger age and have larger families than older fathers. The divorce rate of adolescent fathers is two to four times greater than that of couples who postpone childbearing and marriage.

Psychologically the adolescent father's developmental tasks will be interrupted. Because he is not yet mature his level of cognitive development and decision-making skills will influence whether he remains supportive or flees the situation. Certainly he will be more vulnerable to emotional stressors than an adult man.

The stresses of pregnancy on the adolescent male come from many sources. He faces negative reactions from people in his environment, including his own family and the family of the young woman. Feelings of anger, shame, and disappointment will be aimed at him. Although both young people were involved in the act of intercourse, the young man is usually considered the guilty party. He will feel isolated and alone, and if the young woman's parents refuse to allow him to see her, his sole emotional support may be gone.

Another source of stress arises from changes in his life. His educational and career goals may be threatened as he anticipates marriage or quitting school to support the young woman and his forthcoming child. His relationship with his peers may be altered as well.

A third stressor will be his concerns regarding the health of the young woman and the fetus. He may be protective yet may not understand the physical and psychologic changes of pregnancy.

The adolescent father faces a serious situation, which may be overwhelming for him. The unresolved stress may lead to a severe crisis, manifested by abnormal adaptive behavior, marked depression, somatic symptoms, sexually deviant behavior, or even acute psychosis.

The implications for the health care team are important. Even if the couple has severed their relationship, the father should be sought to assess how he is coping and to offer him counseling. He may not understand why he needs to come to the clinic, and the nurse must let him know that the staff would like to help him, too.

Many adolescent fathers are involved in meaningful relationships. They want to participate in decision making, and they feel frustrated when excluded. Barret and Robinson (1986) state that "For many, the pregnancies were their first opportunities to function in the adult world. Being excluded only increased their sense of alienation and helplessness. Yet their participation demands a tremendous initiative on the part of both adolescent mothers and health care agencies" (p 275).

The father should be told that his participation is important, that he is an excellent support person for the young woman, and that he is welcome to attend clinic and classes. Many clinics interview the couple routinely on the first prenatal visit.

The young man will need education regarding pregnancy, childbirth, childcare, and parenting. Some clinics have couples attend classes together; others offer "father" classes. In becoming parents, men need to learn rates of growth and development so they understand their newborn's potential and do not become frustrated and dissatisfied with the child's behavior.

As part of his counseling, the nurse should assess the young man's stressors, his support systems, his plans for involvement in the pregnancy and childrearing, his future plans, and his health care needs. He should be referred to social services for an opportunity to be counseled regarding his educational and vocational future. When the father is involved in the pregnancy, the young mother feels less deserted, more confident in her decision making, and better able to discuss her future.

Parents' Reactions to Adolescent Pregnancy

Perhaps the first, most intense crisis of the pregnant adolescent is telling her parents that she is pregnant. The young woman may not talk about her pregnancy until it is obvious. Her mother is usually the first to find out and often attempts to protect the young woman's father from discovering his daughter is pregnant. Little research is available on the reactions of these fathers, however.

Parents' initial reactions to the news are usually shock, anger, shame, guilt, and sorrow. The angry mother may accompany her daughter to the clinic. The nurse must assess the disharmony that is occurring and explain the process of adaptation that follows.

The stereotype of the poor family accepting the pregnant daughter and her newborn unequivocally is not true. Studies of poor black families found that the mother was often angry and disappointed. These mothers had high aspirations, hoping that their daughters would fare better in life than they had.

Mothers frequently feel guilty about their daughters' pregnancies. They wonder what they have done wrong and feel they have been inadequate parents. They are also angry because they are concerned about themselves. Just as their children are growing up and they see a new sense of freedom coming, they now have the responsibility of helping their daughters deal with a crisis. They may also feel angry

at "being made a grandmother," perhaps at a young age. Once these reactions are dealt with, the atmosphere begins to return to normal. The mother becomes involved in decision making regarding abortion, adoption, marriage, and dealing with the father-to-be and his family. Family input in these matters is important in the adolescent's decision making. If the pregnant adolescent is encouraged by her family to carry and keep the newborn, she is unlikely to disregard her family's wishes and seek an abortion. On the other hand, if the adolescent is not allowed to remain at home because of her pregnancy, she is more likely to seek abortion or relinquish her newborn.

As the pregnancy progresses the mother begins to take on the grandmother role. She may begin to buy presents for the newborn and plan for the future. She may participate in prenatal care and classes and can be an excellent support system for her daughter. She should be encouraged to participate if the mother-daughter relationship is positive. The mother should be updated on obstetrical practice to clarify any misconceptions she might have. During labor and delivery, the mother will be a key figure for her daughter. Drawing on her own experience, she can offer reassurance and instill confidence in the adolescent.

The last stages of a mother's acceptance occur after her daughter's child is born. As the mother attempts to integrate her role of grandmother, an initial blurring of roles occurs. The grandmother now sees her daughter as a mother, and the daughter begins to identify herself as a mother. Role confusion may develop and sometimes continues for years—the grandmother may essentially do all the mothering and caretaking activities for the newborn, while the daughter remains only a daughter and becomes a sibling of her newborn. Until the daughter is able to internalize her role as mother, the grandmother will be unable to identify completely as a grandmother.

This new role development is clouded by the adolescent's struggle to complete her tasks of adolescence. The wise mother will gently encourage a balance between helping her daughter parent and allowing her to complete the tasks of adolescence. As her daughter becomes more confident in the role of parent, the grandmother can gradually encourage more independence for the daughter.

The Nursing Process and Adolescent Pregnancy

NURSING ASSESSMENT

The nurse must establish a data base to plan interventions for the adolescent mother-to-be. Areas of assessment include a history of family and personal physical health, developmental level and impact of pregnancy, and a thorough assessment of emotional and financial support.

○ *PHYSICAL HEALTH* As with all pregnant women, it is important prenatally to have information on general physical health. This may be the first time many adolescents have ever provided a health history. The nurse may find it helpful to ask very specific questions and give examples if the young woman appears confused about a question.

The following areas should be assessed:

Family and personal history. Family diseases such as diabetes, cardiovascular diseases, epilepsy, blood dyscrasia, hereditary diseases, congenital anomalies, tuberculosis, or mental illness; multiple pregnancies; cultural influences; relationship within the family and with significant others; previous sexual experience and sex education.

Medical history. The adolescent's general health; past or current heart disease, diabetes mellitus, epilepsy, rheumatic fever, childhood diseases, blood dyscrasia, tuberculosis, urinary tract disease, drug sensitivity, or allergies; immunization; recent viral diseases; and exposure to drugs or pollutants.

Menstrual history. Onset of menses, regularity and duration of menses, and any problems with menses.

Obstetric history. Number of pregnancies, interrupted pregnancies, abortions, premature deliveries, and viable births; health status of any living children; neonatal complications and/or stillbirths; previous pregnancy complications; experience with contraceptive methods.

○ *DEVELOPMENTAL LEVEL AND THE IMPACT OF PREGNANCY* The developmental tasks common to adolescence and implications of pregnancy are listed in Table 16–7. Within any age group, however, the maturational level varies from one individual to another. In planning nursing care, it is important to assess the maturational level of each individual. Assessment of the adolescent's developmental level and the impact of pregnancy is reflected in the degree of recognition of the realities and responsibilities involved in teenage pregnancy and parenting. The mother's self-concept (including body image), her relationship with the significant adults in her life, her attitude toward her pregnancy, and her coping methods in the situation are just a few of the significant factors that need to be assessed.

○ *SUPPORT SYSTEMS* As noted previously, early and thorough prenatal care plays a significant role in decreasing physical risks in adolescent pregnancies and promoting healthy outcomes. The socioeconomic status of the pregnant adolescent, however, often places the baby at risk throughout life, beginning with conception. It is essential also to assess emotional and financial support systems. The nursing response to this data base usually requires referral of pregnant teenagers to social service programs and other community support programs for the pregnant teenager. A multidisciplinary team approach is the most effective in dealing with complex problems created by the socioeconomic needs of this age group.

Adolescent life-styles and support systems vary tremendously. It is imperative that the interdisciplinary health team have information regarding the expectant adolescents' feelings and perceptions about themselves, their sexuality, and the coming baby; their knowledge of, attitude toward, and anticipated ability to care for and support the infant; and their maturational level and needs.

NURSING DIAGNOSIS

Nursing diagnoses that may apply to the pregnant adolescent will vary according to the age, support systems, health, and maturity of the young woman. The following nursing diagnoses might be applicable depending on the circumstances:

- Altered growth and development related to adolescent pregnancy
- Alteration in family process related to parents' refusal to accept their daughter's pregnancy
- Knowledge deficit related to adequate nutrition during pregnancy
- Noncompliance with prenatal appointments related to lack of understanding of the value of prenatal care
- Ineffective individual coping related to inadequate psychologic reserves to deal with the stress of being pregnant as a single woman

Unfortunately, these nursing diagnoses tend to focus on areas of concern or problems. Areas of strength also deserve recognition. Maternal-infant nurses may have to modify the format until more appropriate nursing diagnoses have been developed in this area. Possible examples include:

- Excellent personal coping related to strong sense of satisfaction about the birth of a daughter
- Continuity of family process related to parental support for pregnant daughter

NURSING PLAN AND IMPLEMENTATION

Early, thorough prenatal care is the strongest and most critical determinant for reducing risk for the adolescent mother and her newborn. This point cannot be overemphasized. The nurse must understand the special needs of the adolescent mother to meet this challenge successfully. In providing care to the pregnant adolescent the major nursing goals are:

- To develop a trusting relationship with the adolescent

- To promote the adolescent's self-esteem and decision-making and problem-solving skills

- To promote the adolescent's physical well-being

- To promote family adaptation

- To facilitate the adolescent's prenatal education

EVALUATION

In evaluating the effectiveness of nursing care for the pregnant adolescent it is necessary to differentiate short-term and long-term outcomes.

In the short term, care has been effective if the adolescent receives regular prenatal care, has a successful labor and delivery experience free of complications, and has an uneventful postpartum recovery. It is also effective if the young woman is comfortable in whatever decision she makes about keeping or relinquishing her infant. If she keeps her child, care is successful if she bonds well.

In the long term, care is effective if the adolescent develops effective parenting skills, avoids a subsequent adolescent pregnancy, and establishes a life that is satisfying and healthy for her.

Nursing Goal: Development of a Trusting Relationship With the Pregnant Adolescent

The nurse must be attentive to the special problems of adolescents. The first visit to the clinic or office will be fraught with extreme anxiety on the part of the young woman. Not only will she be nervous because of her situation, but also this may well be her first exposure to the health care system since childhood. Making this first experience as positive as possible will encourage her compliance in returning for follow-up care and ensure a favorable attitude toward the importance of health care for her and her newborn.

Depending on how young the adolescent is, this may be her first pelvic examination, an anxiety-provoking experience for any woman. A thorough explanation of the procedure is a must. A gentle and thoughtful examination technique will put the young woman at ease. A mirror is helpful in allowing the client to see her cervix, educating her about her anatomy, and giving her a part in the exam. If she is extremely anxious, she may even take part in speculum insertion; she should be told to insert it as she does a tampon.

Clinical pelvimetry is an essential tool in determining spacial capacity as a predictor for CPD. If the adolescent is nervous and uncomfortable during the first pelvic exam, the pelvimetry may be deferred until a later visit, since it tends to be an uncomfortable procedure.

Developing a trusting relationship with the pregnant adolescent is critical to compliance. Honesty and respect for the individual and a caring attitude promote self-esteem. A verbal contract at the first visit will enable the woman to begin to take responsibility for health and care during pregnancy. As a role model the nurse's attitudes about self-care and responsibility affect the adolescent's maturation process.

Nursing Goal: Promotion of Self-Esteem and Decision-Making and Problem-Solving Skills

The nurse assists the adolescent in her decision-making and problem-solving skills so that she may proceed with her developmental tasks and begin to assume responsibility for her life as well as her newborn's life. An overview of what the young woman will experience over the prenatal course, along with thorough explanations and rationale for each procedure as it occurs, will foster the adolescent's understanding and give her some measure of control. Actively involving the young woman in her care will give her a sense of participation and responsibility (Figure 16–11).

Adolescents tend to be egocentric, and even the realization that their health and habits affect the fetus may not be regarded as important by them. It is often helpful to emphasize the effects of these practices on the client herself. Because of their immature cognitive development, the nurse must assist young women in problem solving and help them begin to visualize themselves in the future and imagine what the consequences of their actions might be. This can be accomplished by various introspective techniques. In addition, the nurse must understand that the developmental tasks of pregnancy must be met by the adolescent in addition to the stage-related developmental tasks she is already coping with. Table 16–7 identifies the tasks of pregnancy and their impact on the adolescent.

Nursing Goal: Promotion of Physical Well-Being

Baseline weight and blood pressure measurements will be valuable in assessing weight gain and predisposition to pregnancy-induced hypertension (PIH). The adolescent may be encouraged to take part in her care by measuring and recording her weight. The nurse may use this time as an opportunity for assisting the young woman in problem solving: "Have I gained too much or too little weight?" "What influence does my diet have on my weight?" "How can I change my eating habits?"

Another way to introduce the subject of nutrition is during measurement of baseline and subsequent hemoglobin and hematocrit values. Since the adolescent is at risk for anemia, she will need education regarding the importance of iron in her diet.

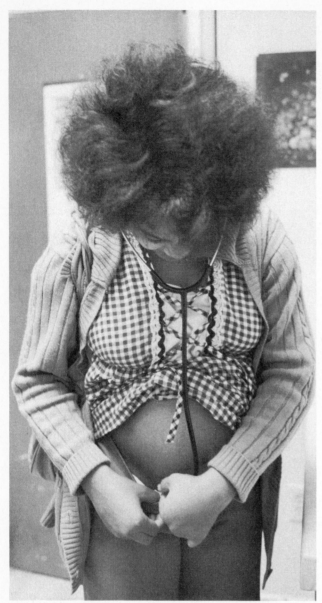

Figure 16–11   The nurse provides this young mother with an opportunity to listen to her baby's heartbeat.

The nurse must keep in mind that adolescents may fear laboratory tests, which can evoke early childhood memories of being "stuck" with needles or hurt. Explanations help ease nerves, and coordination of services will avoid multiple venous punctures.

A nutritional consultation is indicated for all adolescents. Group classes are helpful because peer pressure is strong among this age group.

Pregnancy-induced hypertension represents the most prevalent medical complication of pregnant adolescents. The criteria of blood pressure readings of 140/90 mm Hg are not acceptable as the determinant of PIH in adolescents. Women aged 14 to 20 years without evidence of high blood pressure usually have diastolic readings between 50 and 66

mm Hg. Gradual increases from the prepregnant diastolic readings, along with excessive weight gain, must be evaluated as precursors to PIH. This is one reason why early prenatal care is vital to management of the adolescent.

As mentioned earlier, adolescents have an increased incidence of sexually transmitted diseases. The initial prenatal examination should include a gonococcal culture and wet prep for *Candida, Trichomonas,* and *Gardnerella.* Tests for syphilis should also be done. Education about sexually transmitted disease is important, as is careful observation of herpetic lesions or other symptoms throughout the young woman's pregnancy.

Substance abuse should be discussed with adolescents. It is important to review the risks associated with the use of cigarettes, caffeine, drugs, and alcohol with the young woman. She should be aware of the effects of these substances on her development as well as on the development of the fetus.

Ongoing care should include the same assessments that the older woman receives. Special attention should be paid to evaluating fetal growth by measurement of fundal height, fetal heart tones, quickening, and fetal movement. The corresponding dates of auscultating fetal heart tones with the date of last menstrual period and quickening can be helpful in determining correct estimations of delivery time. If there is a question of size—date discrepancy by 2 cm either way, an ultrasound is warranted to establish fetal age so that instances of IUGR may be diagnosed and treated early.

Nursing Goal: Promotion of Family Adaptation

The nurse must assess the family situation during the first prenatal visit. She should find out the level of involvement the adolescent desires from each of her family members. A sensitive approach to daughter-mother relationships helps motivate their communication. If the mother and daughter agree, the mother should be included in the client's care. Encouraging the mother to become part of the maternity team, to join grandmother crisis support groups, and to obtain counseling aids the mother in adapting to her role and in supporting her daughter.

The nurse should also help the mother assess her daughter's needs and assist her in meeting them. Some adolescents become more dependent during pregnancy, and some become more independent. The mother can ease and encourage her daughter's self-growth by understanding how best to respond and support the adolescent.

Nursing Goal: Facilitation of Prenatal Education

Prenatal education is crucial in the care of the pregnant adolescent. An important challenge to health professionals is to develop prenatal classes that meet the special needs of this age group (Figure 16–12). Prenatal education programs should include the clinic and the school system.

Many adolescents cite the school as the preferred agency for education during pregnancy and early parenting. School systems are currently attempting to meet this need in a variety of ways. The most effective method appears to be mainstreaming the pregnant adolescent in academic classes with her peers and adding classes appropriate to her needs during pregnancy and early parenting. Classes about growth and development beginning with the newborn and early infancy can help teenage parents have more realistic expectations of their infants and may help decrease child abuse. Mainstreaming pregnant adolescents in school is also an ideal way to help them complete their education while learning the skills they need to cope with childbearing and parenting. Vocational guidance in this setting is also most beneficial to their future.

Regardless of the sponsorship or setting of prenatal classes for pregnant teenagers and adolescent fathers, the developmental tasks of the adolescent must be considered. For example, the methods of teaching this age group should be somewhat different from regular prenatal classes. The younger adolescent tends to be a more concrete thinker than the older and more mature pregnant adult. Increased use of audiovisuals that are appropriate to their social situation and age is helpful. More demonstrations may be required, and they need to be simple and direct. For example, one group finds that teaching about formula preparation is most effective when demonstrating each step involved, including adequate rinsing of bottles (Westman 1984).

Other variations in methods of teaching specific content are based on recognizing typical adolescent behavior. The approach to teaching nutrition in these groups must have significance to promote compliance. Teaching might include how to select a balanced meal at a fast food restaurant. Some groups have adolescents complete nutritional assessments and discuss the significance of good nutrition in pregnancy and appropriate newborn feeding practices as well as food budgeting. To emphasize good nutrition, the groups serve juice and nourishing snacks (Ortega et al 1984).

Ideally, prenatal classes for the adolescent are oriented to more than just pregnancy, childbirth, and immediate newborn care. The goals of many of these classes are expanding to deal with more complex social issues that result from adolescent pregnancies. A multidisciplinary team approach is important in planning and implementing these classes. Goals for many of these classes now include promoting self-esteem; helping participants identify the problems and conflicts of teenage parenting and how to prepare for them; educating participants about sexuality, relationships, and contraception to deter unwanted pregnancies; teaching participants parenting skills, which includes information about community resources and other resources available to teenage parents; and helping participants develop more adaptive coping skills.

● Care of the Older Expectant Couple

Not too many years ago, women who were 30 years old or older and pregnant with their first baby were labeled "elderly primiparas" by the medical profession. A person who is 30 years old is certainly not elderly, but until recently most women married young and had their first children soon after marriage. It was unusual for a woman to have her first baby after the age of 30. The woman who

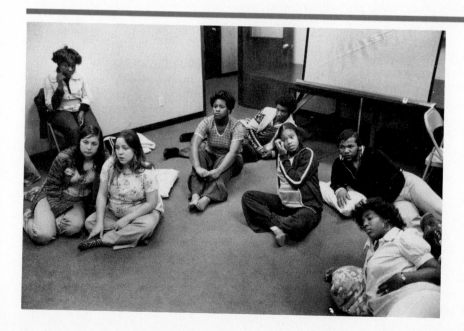

Figure 16–12 *Prenatal classes designed for young adolescents*

did have her first baby after the age of 30 was one of the relatively few women who got married later than expected or who had fertility problems that had been overcome.

Today an increasing number of women are choosing to have their first baby after the age of 30. Some are even waiting until after the age of 35. Many factors have contributed to this trend. The development of effective birth control methods has been a significant factor. Equally important has been the women's liberation movement and its position that women can perform other roles besides those of wife and mother.

Women are obtaining advanced education and seeking careers that had previously been considered appropriate only for men. Because of the commitment of time and energy that professional advancement requires, many women are delaying childbearing until they achieve their professional goals. In 1980, 90 percent of the women who had their first child over the age of 30 were employed, and more than half were in professional occupations (Ventura & Hendershot 1984).

Other factors contributing to the growing number of pregnancies of older women are the increases in later marriages and second marriages. The high cost of living is also contributing to this trend; many young couples delay childbearing because they feel that they cannot afford to have a child at this time in their lives.

One factor that is sometimes overlooked is that the population of women in this age group is growing. It has been projected that in the 1980s the number of women between the ages of 35 and 40 will increase 42 percent in the United States. The number of births to women in this age group is expected to increase 37 percent in this decade (Kirz et al 1985).

There are advantages to having a first baby after the age of 30. Couples who delay childbearing until they are older tend to be well educated and financially secure. Usually their decision to have a baby was deliberately and thoughtfully made. Given their greater life experiences, they are much more aware of the realities of having a child and what it means to have a baby at their age. Many of the women have experienced fulfillment in their careers and feel secure enough to take on the added responsibility of a child. Some women are ready to make a change in their lives, desiring to stay home with a new baby. Those who plan to continue working are able to afford good child care.

Medical Risks

Medical professionals consider that women who are over 30, especially those who are 35 or older, at the time of their first pregnancy are at a higher risk for maternal or fetal complications than younger women. The risk of conceiving a child with Down syndrome increases significantly with age (see Table 9–6 on p 190). In addition, the in-

cidence of medical conditions such as diabetes and hypertension, which can be serious complications during pregnancy, increases for women over the age of 35.

Medical conditions associated with the reproductive organs, such as uterine fibroids, occur with greater frequency in women in their late thirties. Decreased fertility is also a concern of women as they grow older.

Although statistically a woman in her thirties and early forties is at greater risk for certain conditions than a younger woman, most women in their thirties and early forties are in good health. Recent studies compared healthy pregnant women over 35 years of age with healthy younger pregnant women. These studies suggest that preexisting medical problems play a more significant role than age in maternal well-being and outcome of pregnancy (Kirz et al 1985, Stein 1983).

For women who are concerned that their age may adversely affect the well-being of their offspring, technological advances permit the detection of several chromosomal abnormalities. Legalized abortion provides the opportunity to terminate the pregnancy if desired.

Special Concerns of the Older Expectant Couple

No matter what their age, most expectant couples have concerns regarding the well-being of the fetus and their ability to parent. The older couple has additional concerns related to their age, especially the closer they are to 40.

Some couples are concerned about whether they will have enough energy to care for a new baby. Of greater concern is their ability to deal with the needs of the child in ten years when they, too, are ten years older.

The financial concerns of the older couple are usually different from those of the younger couple. The older couple is generally more financially secure than the younger couple. However, when their "baby" is ready for college, the older couple may be close to retirement, when they might not have the means to provide for their child.

While considering their financial future and future retirement, the older couple may be forced to face their own mortality. Certainly this is not uncommon in midlife, but instead of confronting this issue at 40 to 45 years of age or later, the older expectant couple may confront the issue several years earlier as they consider what will happen as their child grows.

The older expectant couple may find themselves somewhat isolated socially. They may feel "different" because they are often the only couple in their peer group expecting their first baby. In fact, many of their peers are parents of adolescents or young adults and may be grandparents as well. The 40-year-old woman holding a newborn is more often assumed to be the grandmother of the baby than the new mother.

Health care professionals may also treat the older expectant couple differently than they would a younger couple. As mentioned earlier, the medical profession tends to view the older pregnant woman as a high-risk client. Older women may be asked to submit to more medical procedures, such as amniocentesis and ultrasound, than younger women. An older woman may be prevented from using a birthing room or birthing center even if she is healthy because her age is considered to put her at risk.

The woman who has delayed pregnancy may be concerned about the limited amount of time that she has to bear children. When pregnancy does not occur as quickly as she hoped, the older woman may become increasingly anxious as time slips away on her "biological clock." When an older woman becomes pregnant but experiences a spontaneous abortion, her grief for the loss of her unborn child is exacerbated by her anxiety about her ability to conceive again in her remaining time.

The goals of nursing care discussed on pages 373 to 397 also apply to the older expectant couple. In addition, the expectant couple has unique needs. Nursing goals to meet these needs are:

- To promote adaptation to pregnancy

- To support the couple if amniocentesis is advised

Nursing Goal: Promotion of Adaptation to Pregnancy

Once an older couple has made the decision to have a child, it is the responsibility of the health care professional to respect and support the couple in this decision. As with any client, risks need to be discussed, concerns need to be identified, and strengths need to be promoted. The woman's age should not be made an issue. Reminding a woman that she and her fetus are at increased risk because of her age does not promote a sense of well-being but a sense of anxiety and fear. To promote a sense of well-being, the care giver should treat the pregnancy as "normal" unless specific health risks are identified.

As the pregnancy continues the nurse should identify and discuss concerns the woman may have related to her age or to specific health problems. The older woman who has made a conscious decision to become pregnant often has carefully thought through potential problems and may actually have fewer concerns than a younger woman or one with an unplanned pregnancy.

Childbirth education classes are important in promoting adaptation to the event of childbirth for expectant couples of any age. However, older expectant couples, who are still in the minority, often feel uncomfortable in classes where the majority of participants are much younger. Because of the differences in age and life experiences, many of the needs of the older couple may not be met in the class. The nurse teaching a childbirth education class should try to anticipate the informational needs of the older couple. At the same time, the nurse should not make the couple feel any more uncomfortable by drawing attention to their age. As the number of expectant older couples increases, the nurse may find it useful to offer an "over 30" childbirth education class to accommodate the specific needs of older couples. Such classes are being developed in some of the larger urban areas.

Couples who are over 30 years of age are often better educated than other health care consumers. These clients frequently know the kind of care and services they want and are assertive in their interactions with the health care system. The nurse should neither be intimidated by these individuals nor assume that anticipatory guidance and support are not needed. Instead the nurse should support the couple's strengths and be sensitive to their individual needs.

Nursing Goal: Support of Couple if Amniocentesis Is Advised

In working with older expectant couples, the nurse must be sensitive to their special needs. A particularly difficult issue these couples face is the possibility of bearing an unhealthy child. Because of the risk of Down syndrome in these families, amniocentesis is often suggested. The decision to have amniocentesis can be difficult to make merely on the basis of its possible risks to the fetus. But that becomes almost a minor concern when the couple thinks of the implications of the possible findings of Down syndrome or other chromosomal abnormalities. The finding of abnormalities means that the couple may be faced with an even more difficult decision about continuing the pregnancy.

A couple's decision to have amniocentesis is usually related to their beliefs and attitudes about abortion. Amniocentesis is usually not even considered by couples who are strongly opposed to abortion for any reason. Health professionals must respect their decision and take a nonjudgmental approach to their continued care.

Other couples may be opposed to abortion but also concerned about their ability to care for a seriously limited child as times passes. How will they care for this child when he or she becomes an adult and they are elderly? What will happen to this child when they die? Such questions may cause the couple to permit amniocentesis to be performed. The results of the procedure may force the couple to make the painful decision to terminate the pregnancy.

The decision to have an abortion is a painful one even when couples are not opposed to abortion on political or philosophical grounds. Even though the couple may believe that terminating a high-risk pregnancy is right for their family, they may feel a great deal of ambivalence about amniocentesis. If the results are such that the couple elects to have an abortion, they will feel much grief for their loss.

Many health professionals assume that the couple who agrees to amniocentesis will also elect to have an abortion if Down syndrome or another condition is diagnosed. This is not necessarily the case. Some couples choose not to have an abortion after being informed that their unborn child has genetic abnormalities.

For the couple who agrees to amniocentesis, the first few months of pregnancy is a difficult time. Amniocentesis cannot be done until 14 weeks of pregnancy and the chromosomal studies take roughly two weeks to complete. For almost 16 weeks, until the woman is in her second trimester, the couple is "on hold," not knowing if their unborn child is healthy or not. Their fear that the fetus is at risk may delay the successful completion of the psychological tasks of early pregnancy.

The nurse can support couples who decide to have amniocentesis in several ways:

1. The nurse should make sure that the couple is aware of the risks of amniocentesis and why it is being performed.

2. The nurse who is present during the amniocentesis procedure can offer comfort and emotional support to the expectant woman. The nurse can also provide information about the procedure as it is being performed.

3. The nurse can facilitate a support group for women during the difficult waiting period between the procedure and the results.

4. If the results indicate that the fetus has Down syndrome or another genetic abnormality, the nurse can ensure that the couple has complete information about the condition, its range of possible manifestations, and its developmental implications.

5. The nurse can support the couple in their decision about continuing or terminating the pregnancy. It is essential that the nurse and other health professionals involved with the couple not impose their philosophical or political beliefs about abortion on the couple. The decision is the couple's, and it should be based on their belief system and a nonbiased presentation of risks and choices from care givers.

KEY CONCEPTS

The nursing process can be used effectively to plan and provide care to women during pregnancy.

Provision of anticipatory guidance about childbirth, the puerperium, and childrearing is a primary responsibility of the nurse caring for women in an antepartal setting.

The nurse assesses the expectant father's knowledge level and intended degree of participation and then works with the couple to help ensure a satisfying experience.

Culturally based practices and proscribed activities may have a major impact on the childbearing family.

The common discomforts of pregnancy occur as a result of physiologic and anatomic changes. The nurse provides the woman with information about self-care activities aimed at reducing or relieving discomfort.

To make appropriate self-care choices and ensure healthful habits, a pregnant woman requires accurate information about a range of subjects from exercise to sexual activity, from bathing to immunizations.

Teratogenic substances are substances that adversely affect the normal growth and development of the fetus.

A pregnant woman should avoid taking medications or using over-the-counter preparations during pregnancy.

Evidence exists that smoking or consuming alcohol during pregnancy may be harmful to the fetus.

Maternal assessment of fetal activity keeps the woman "in touch" with her fetus and provides ongoing assessment of fetal status.

Adolescent pregnancy is a major health concern that has profound physical, social, psychologic, and economic implications.

Childbirth among women over age 30 is becoming increasingly common. It poses fewer health risks than previously believed and offers definite advantages for the woman or couple who make the choice.

REFERENCES

The Alan Guttmacher Institute. *Teen Pregnancy: The Problem That Hasn't Gone Away.* New York, the institute, 1981.

American Nurses' Association: *Standards of Maternal and Child Health Nursing Practice.* Pub. No. MCH-3. Kansas City, Mo, the association, 1983.

Barret RL, **Robinson** BE: A descriptive study of teenage expectant fathers. *Fam Relat* 1982;31:349.

Barret RL, **Robinson** BE: Adolescent fathers: Often forgotten fathers. *Pediatr Nurs* 1986;12(July/August):273.

Barret RL, **Robinson** BE: The adolescent father, in **Hanson** S, **Bozett** F (eds): *Dimensions of Fatherhood*. Beverly Hills, Calif, Sage Publications, 1985.

Benke PJ: The isotretinoin teratogen syndrome. *JAMA*. 1984;251:3267.

Brill JC: Drugs in pregnancy. *Top Emerg Med* 1986;8(April):84.

Brown MS: A cross-cultural look at pregnancy, labor and delivery. *J Obstet Gynecol* 1976;5(September/October):35.

Brucker MC, **Mueller** M: Nurse-midwifery care of adolescents. *J Nurs-Midwife* 1985;30:277.

Card JJ, **Wise** LL: Teenage mothers and teenage fathers: The impact of early childbearing on the parent's personal and professional lives. *Fam Plan Perspect* 1978;10(July/August):199.

Carey WB, et al: Adolescent age and obstetric risk. *Semin Perinatol* 1981;5(January):9.

Carrington BW: The Afro American, in **Clark** AL (ed): *Culture, Childbearing, Health Professionals*. Philadelphia: Davis, 1978.

Chasnoff IJ, et al: Cocaine use in pregnancy. *N Engl J Med* 1985;313:666.

Chesley LC: *Hypertensive Disorders in Pregnancy*. New York, Appleton-Century-Crofts, 1978.

Chez RA, **Sadovsky** E: Teaching patients how to record fetal movements. *Contemp OB/GYN* 1984;24(October):85.

Collings C, **Curet** LB: Fetal heart response to maternal exercise. *Am J Obstet Gynecol* 1985;151(February):498.

Crosby WM: Traumatic injuries during pregnancy. *Clin Obstet Gynecol* 1983;26(4):902.

Dorfman SF: Age as a factor in pregnancy. *Contemp OB/GYN* 1986;27(February):64.

Evaneshko V: Tonawanda Seneca childbearing culture, in **Kay** MA (ed): *Anthropology of Human Birth*. Philadelphia, Davis, 1982.

Facts about Down Syndrome, NIH Publication. US Department of Health and Human Services, 1984.

Farris LS: Approaches to care for the American Indian maternity patient. *Am J Mat Child Nurs* 1976;1(March/April):81.

Fenlon A, et al: *Getting Ready for Childbirth*. ed 2. Boston, Little, Brown, 1986.

Freeman RK, **Garite** TJ: *Fetal Heart Rate Monitoring*. Baltimore, Williams & Wilkins, 1981.

Fried PA, et al: Soft drug use after pregnancy compared to use before and during pregnancy. *Am J Obstet Gynecol* 1985;151(March):787.

Fried PA, et al: Marijuana use during pregnancy and perinatal risk factors. *Am J Obstet Gynecol* 1983;146:992.

Fried PA, et al: Marijuana use during pregnancy and decreased length of gestation. *Am J Obstet Gynecol* 1984;150(September):23.

Goldsmith LT, **Weiss** G: Puberty, adolescence, and the clinical aspects of normal menstruation, in **Danforth** DN, **Scott** JR (eds): *Obstetrics and Gynecology,* ed 5. Philadelphia, Lippincott, 1986.

Hayes D: Teratogenesis: a review of the basic principles with a discussion of selected agents: Part III. *Drug Intell Clin Pharm* 1981;15(September):639.

Hingson R, et al: Effects of maternal drinking and marijuana use on fetal growth and development. *Pediatr* 1982;70:539.

Hoffman JB: A suggested treatment for inverted nipples. *Am J Obstet Gynecol* 1953;66:346.

Hollingsworth AO, et al: The refugees and childbearing: What to expect. *RN* 1980;43(November):45.

Horn BM: Northwest coast Indians: The Muckleshoot, in **Kay** MA (ed): *Anthropology of Human Birth*. Philadelphia, Davis, 1982.

Jones EF, et al: Teenage pregnancy in developed countries: Determinants and policy implications. *Fam Plan Perspect* 1985;17(March/April):53.

Kay MA: The Mexican American, in **Clark** AL (ed): *Culture, Childbearing, Health Professionals*. Philadelphia, Davis, 1978.

Ketter DE, **Shelton** BJ: Pregnant and physically fit, too. *Am J Mat Child Nurs* 1984;9(March/April):120.

Kirz DS, et al: Advanced maternal age: The mature gravida. *Am J Obstet Gynecol* 1985;152(May):7.

Klebanoff MA, et al: Coitus during pregnancy: Is it safe? *Lancet* 1984;2(October):914.

Knothe H, **Dette** GA: Antibiotics in pregnancy: Toxicity and teratogenicity. *Infection* 1985;13:49.

Krozy RE, **McColgan** JJ: Auto safety . . . Pregnancy and the newborn. *J Obstet Gynecol Neonat Nurs* 1985;14(January/February):11.

Kruse J, et al: Changes in smoking and alcohol consumption during pregnancy: A population-based study in a rural area. *Obstet Gynecol* 1986:67(5):627.

Lemarchand-Beraud T, et al: Maturation of the hypothalmo-pituitary-ovarian axis in adolescent girls. *J Clin Endocrinol Metabol* 1982;54(February):241.

Lemoine P, et al: Children of alcoholic parents, observed anomalies (127 cases). *Quest Med* 1968;21:476.

Lin GWJ, **Maddatu** AP: Effects of ethanol feeding during pregnancy on maternal-fetal transfer of α-aminosobutyric acid in the rat (abstract). *Alcoholism: Clin Exp Res* 1980;4:222.

Linn S, et al: The association of marijuana use with outcome of pregnancy. *Am J Pub Health* 1983;73:1161.

Longo D: The biological effect of carbon monoxide on the pregnant woman, fetus and newborn infant. *Am J Obstet Gynecol* 1977;129:69.

Mahan CS, **McKay** S: Let's reform our antenatal care methods. *Contemp ON/GYN* 1984;23(May):147.

Marks MA, **Pfeffer** C: Over-thirty childbirth preparation. *Genesis* 1985;7(June/July):20.

Marwick C: Medical news. *JAMA* 1984;251:3208.

Masters WH, **Johnson** VE: *Human Sexual Response.* Boston, Little, Brown, 1966.

Mercer R: *Perspectives on Adolescent Health Care.* New York, Lippincott, 1979.

Mochizuki M, et al: Effects of smoking on fetoplacental-maternal systems during pregnancy. *Am J Obstet Gynecol* 1984;149(June):413.

Moore DS, et al: Adolescent pregnancy and parenting: The role of the nurse. *Top Clin Nurs* 1984;6(October):72.

Naeye RL: Influence of maternal cigarette smoking during pregnancy on fetal and childhood growth. *Obstet Gynecol* 1981;57(1):18.

Newald J: Cocaine infants: A new arrival at hospitals' step? *Hospital,* April 5, 1986, p 96.

O'Brien TE, **Balmer** JA: Drugs and the human fetus. *US Pharmacist,* March 1981, p 44.

Ortega EA, et al: The multidisciplinary team approach to perinatal care of adolescents, in *Nursing Care Models for Adolescent Families.* Kansas City, Mo, American Nurses' Association, 1984.

Osofsky HJ: Mitigating the adverse effects of early parenthood. *Contemp OB/GYN* 1985;25(January):57.

Paolone AM, **Worthington** S: Cautions and advice on exercise during pregnancy. *Contemp OB/GYN* 1985; 25(May):150.

Piechnik SL, **Corbett** MA: Reducing low birth weight among socioeconomically high-risk adolescent pregnancies: Successful intervention with certified nurse-midwife-managed care and a multidisciplinary team. *J Nurs-Midwife* 1985;30:88.

Pritchard J, **MacDonald** PC, **Gant** NF: *Williams Obstetrics,* ed 17. New York, Appleton-Century-Crofts, 1985.

Rao JM, **Arulappu** R: Drug use in pregnancy: How to avoid problems. *Drugs* 1981;22:409.

Rayburn WF: OTC drugs and pregnancy. *Perinatol Neonatol* 1984;8(September/October):21.

Reamy K, **White** SE: Sexuality in pregnancy and the puerperium: A review. *Obstet Gynecol* 1985;40(1):1.

Rubin PC, et al: Prospective survey of use of therapeutic drugs, alcohol, and cigarettes during pregnancy. *Br Med J* 1986;292(January):81.

Sevcovic: Traditions of pregnancy which influence maternity care of the Navajo people, in **Leininger** M (ed): *Transcultural Nursing.* New York, Masson, 1979.

Shepard TH: Teratogens: An update. *Hosp Pract,* January 1984, p 191.

Shiono PH, et al: Smoking and drinking during pregnancy. *JAMA* 1986;255(January):82.

Skolnick M: Expanding physician duties and patients' rights in wrongful life: Harbeson v Parke-Davis. *Med Law* 1985;4:283.

Spain J: Psychological aspects of contraceptives use in teenage girls, in **Blum** GL (ed): *Psychological Aspects of Pregnancy, Birthing and Bonding.* New York, Human Sciences Press, 1980.

Stein Z: Pregnancy in gravidas over age 35. *J Nurs-Midwife* 1983;28(January/February):17.

Stolte K: Nursing diagnosis and the childbearing woman. *Am J Mat Child Nurs* 1986;13(January/February):13.

Swanson J: The marital sexual relationship during pregnancy. *J Obstet Gynecol Neonatal Nurs* 1980;9:267.

Veille JC, et al: The effect of exercise on uterine activity in the last eight weeks of pregnancy. *Am J Obstet Gynecol* 1985;15(March):727.

Ventura SJ, **Hendershot** GE: Infant health consequences of childbearing by teenagers and older mothers. *Pub Health Rep* 1984;99(March/April):138.

Wallis C: Children having children: Teen pregnancy in America. *Time* 1985;126(December):78.

Waters JL: Pregnancy in young adolescents: A syndrome of failure. *South Med J* 1969;62(June):655.

Westman DL: Teaching pregnant adolescents and their helpers: Keep it simple, make it fun, in *Nursing Care Models for Adolescent Families.* Kansas City, Mo, American Nurses' Association, 1984.

Whipkey RR, et al: Drug use in pregnancy. *Ann Emerg Med* 1984;13:346.

Wright JT, **Toplis** PJ: Alcohol in pregnancy. *Br J Obstet Gynaecol* 1986;93(March):201.

ADDITIONAL READINGS

Alley NM: Morning sickness: The client's perspective. *J Obstet Gynecol Neonat Nurs* 1984;13(May/June):185.

Becerea RM, et al: Pregnancy and motherhood among Mexican-American adolescents. *Health Soc Work* 1984; 9(Spring):106.

Brooten D, et al: A survey of nutrition, caffeine, cigarette and alcohol intake in early pregnancy in an urban clinic population. *J Nurs-Midwife* 1987;32(2):85

Burt MR: Estimating the public costs of teenage childbearing. *Fam Plan Perspect* 1986;18(5):221.

Clark J, **Britton** K: Factors contributing to client nonuse of the Cardiff count-to-ten fetal activity chart. *J Nurs-Midwife* 1985;30(December):320.

Davis L: Daily fetal movement counting: A valuable assessment tool. *J Nurs-Midwife* 1987;32(1):11.

de la Luz Alvarez M, et al: Sociocultural characteristics of pregnant and nonpregnant adolescents of low socioeconomic status: A comparative study. *Adolescence* 1987; 22(Spring):149.

Drinville-Shank G: The pregnant OR employee: Ensuring maternal health, part I. *AORN J* 1987;45(2):404.

Goldberg BD, et al: Teen pregnancy service: An interdisciplinary health care delivery system utilizing certified nurse-midwives. *J Nurs-Midwife* 1986;31(6):263.

Horan M: Discomfort and pain during pregnancy. *Am J Mat Child Nurs* 1984;9(July/August):267.

Knothe H, **Dette** GA: Antibiotics in pregnancy: Toxicity and teratogenicity. *Obstet Gynecol Surv* 1986; 41(January):31.

Luke B: Does caffeine influence reproduction? *Am J Mat Child Nurs* 1985;7(July/August):24.

Maloni JA, et al: Expectant grandparents class. *J Obstet Gynecol Neonat Nurs* 1987;16(1):26.

Mueller LS: Pregnancy and sexuality. *J Obstet Gynecol Neonatal Nurs* 1985;14(July/August):289.

Poole CJ: Fatigue during the first trimester of pregnancy. *J Obstet Gynecol Neonat Nurs* 1986; 15(September/October):375.

Proctor SE: A developmental approach to pregnancy prevention with early adolescent females. *J Sch Health* 1986;56(8):313.

Robinson GE, et al: Psychological adaptation to pregnancy in childless women more than 35 years of age. *Am J Obstet Gynecol* 1987;156(2):328.

Robinson J, **Sachs** B: *Nursing Models for Adolescent Families.* Kansas City, Mo, American Nurses' Association Division on Maternal and Child Health Nursing Practice, 1984.

Srisuphan W, **Bracken** MB: Caffeine consumption during pregnancy and association with late spontaneous abortion. *Am J Obstet Gynecol* 1986;154(January):14.

Wallace AM, et al: Aerobic exercise, maternal self-esteem, and physical discomforts during pregnancy. *J Nurs-Midwife* 1986;31(6):255.

Zdanuk JM, et al: Adolescent pregnancy and incest: The nurse's role as counselor. *J Obstet Gynecol Neonat Nurs* 1987;16(2):99.

Talk about subtle messages from potential grandparents! My parents were really eager to become grandparents. Every once in a while, when they felt they couldn't stand it any longer, they would mention how much fun it would be to have grandchildren. But mostly they showed magnificent restraint.

One evening we got a call to come over to their house. When we got there we found packages piled up, all decorated with bright ribbons. Not being shy, we piled into them. First there was a delicate little yellow dress with ribbons and lace. Next came a tiny blue suit with knee pants and a striped hankerchief tucked in a pocket. These were followed by a blue-and-pink rattle and diaper pins and diapers and soft flannel blankets with kittens and ducks. My parents watched all this and then proudly proclaimed, "We're ready." Their timing was great, because so were we. They made such proud grandparents.

Maternal Nutrition

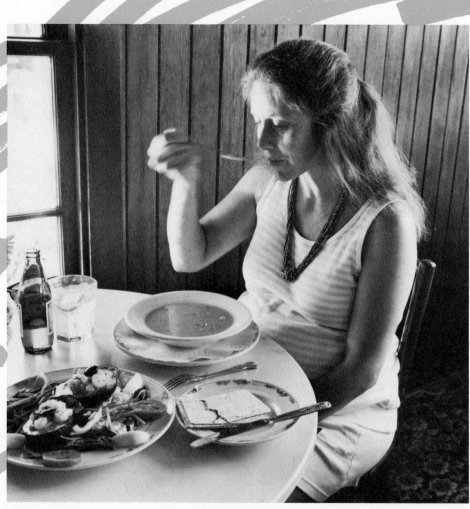

Pregnant women can feel happier and more confident about what they eat through the support and guidance of an understanding nurse.

Chapter Seventeen

OBJECTIVES

- **Identify the role of specific nutrients in the diet of the pregnant woman.**

- **Compare nutritional needs during pregnancy and lactation with nonpregnant requirements.**

- **Evaluate adequacy and pattern of weight gain during different stages of pregnancy.**

- **Plan adequate prenatal vegetarian diets based on nutritional requirements of pregnancy.**

- **Describe ways in which various physical, psychosocial, and cultural factors can affect nutritional intake and status.**

- **Compare recommendations for weight gain and nutrient intakes in the pregnant adolescent with those for the mature pregnant adult.**

- **Describe basic factors a nurse should consider when offering nutritional counseling to a pregnant adolescent.**

- **Assess prenatal and postpartal nutritional status based on anthropometric, biochemical, clinical, and dietary data.**

- **Compare nutritional counseling issues for nursing and nonnursing mothers.**

- **Formulate a nutritional care plan for pregnant women based on a diagnosis of nutritional problems.**

$\mathbf{A}$ woman's nutritional status prior to and during pregnancy can significantly influence her health and that of her unborn child. In most prenatal clinics and offices, nurses offer nutritional counseling directly or work closely with the nutritionist in providing necessary nutritional assessment and teaching.

This chapter focuses on the nutritional needs of a normal pregnant woman. Special sections consider the nutritional needs of the pregnant adolescent and the woman after delivery.

Good prenatal nutrition is the result of proper eating for a lifetime, not just during pregnancy. Many factors influence the ability of a woman to achieve good prenatal nutrition:

- *General nutritional status prior to pregnancy.* Nutritional deficits at the time of conception and the early prenatal period may influence the outcome of the pregnancy.

- *Maternal age.* An expectant adolescent must meet her own growth needs in addition to the nutritional needs of pregnancy. This may be especially difficult because teenagers often have nutritional deficiencies.

- *Maternal parity.* The mother's nutritional needs and the outcome of the pregnancy are influenced by the number of pregnancies she has had and the interval between them.

A mother's nutritional status does affect her fetus. Factors influencing fetal well-being are interrelated, but research suggests that nutrient deficiency can produce measurable effects on cell and organ growth.

Fetal growth occurs in three overlapping stages: (1) growth by increase in cell number, (2) growth by increase in cell number and cell size, and (3) growth by increase in cell size alone. It is now thought that nutritional problems that interfere with cell division may have permanent consequences. If the nutritional insult occurs when cells are mainly enlarging, the changes are reversible when normal nutrition occurs.

Growth of fetal and maternal tissues requires increased quantities of essential dietary components. Table 17–1 compares the *recommended dietary allowances (RDA)* for nonpregnant females with those for pregnant and lactating teenage and adult women.

Most of the recommended nutrients can be obtained by eating a well-balanced diet each day. The basic food

415

Table 17–1 Recommended Dietary Allowances for Women 11 to 40 Years of Age

Nutrient	(11–14 years)	(15–18 years)	Nonpregnant (19–22 years)	(23–40 years)	Pregnant	Lactating
Energy, calories	2200	2100	2100	2000	+300	+500
Protein (g)	46	46	44	44	+30	+20
Vitamin A (μg RE)	800	800	800	800	+200	+400
Vitamin D (μg)	10	10	7.5	5	+5	+5
Vitamin E (IU)	8	8	8	8	+2	+3
Ascorbic acid (mg)	50	60	60	60	+20	+40
Folacin (μg)	400	400	400	400	+400	+100
Niacin (mg)	15	14	14	13	+2	+5
Riboflavin (mg)	1.3	1.3	1.3	1.2	+0.3	+0.5
Thiamine (mg)	1.1	1.1	1.1	1.0	+0.4	+0.5
Vitamin B_6 (mg)	1.8	2.0	2.0	2.0	+0.6	+0.5
Vitamin B_{12} (μg)	3.0	3.0	3.0	3.0	+1.0	+1.0
Calcium (mg)	1200	1200	800	800	+400	+400
Phosphorus (mg)	1200	1200	800	800	+400	+400
Iodine (μg)	150	150	150	150	+25	+50
Iron (mg)	18	18	18	18	*	*
Magnesium (mg)	300	300	300	300	+150	+150
Zinc (mg)	15	15	15	15	+5	+10

*This iron requirement cannot be met by ordinary diets. Therefore, the use of 30–60 mg supplemental iron is recommended.

Source: Food and Nutrition Board: *Recommended Dietary Allowances.* Washington, DC, National Academy of Sciences, National Research Council, 1980.

groups and recommended amounts during pregnancy and lactation are presented in Table 17–2.

● **Maternal Weight Gain**

The best assurance of an adequate caloric intake during pregnancy is a satisfactory weight gain over time. The optimal weight gain depends on the woman's height, bone structure, and prepregnant nutritional state. However, maternal weight gains averaging 10 to 12.7 kg (22 to 28 lb) are associated with the best reproductive outcomes (Gordon 1981).

The pattern of weight gain is also important. The ideal pattern of weight gain during pregnancy consists of a gain of 1 to 2 kg (2 to 4.4 lb) during the first trimester, followed by an average gain of 0.4 kg (slightly less than a pound) per week during the last two trimesters. During the second trimester, most of the weight gain reflects an increase in blood volume; enlargement of breasts, uterus, and associated tissue and fluid; and deposit of maternal fat. In the last trimester, the weight gain is mainly that of the conceptus (fetus, placenta, and amniotic fluid). Figure 17–1 is an approximate breakdown of where and when the weight gain occurs.

A 25 lb weight gain would be distributed as follows:

11 lb	Fetus, placenta, amniotic fluid
2 lb	Uterus and breasts
4 lb	Increased blood volume
3 lb	Tissue fluid
5 lb	Maternal stores

Inadequate gains (less than 1.0 kg [2.2 lb] per month during the second and third trimesters of pregnancy) or excessive gains (more than 3 kg [6.6 lb] per month) should be evaluated and the need for nutritional counseling considered. Inadequate weight gain has been associated with low-birth-weight infants. Sudden sharp increases (weight

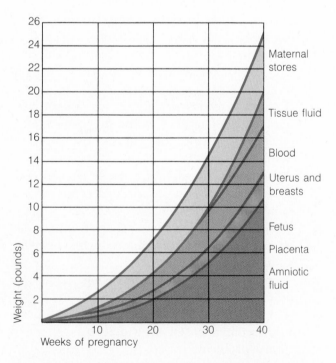

Figure 17–1 Composition of weight gain during pregnancy (From Karls L: *Nutrition for Pregnancy.* Madison, Wis, Jackson Clinic, 1983)

Table 17–2 Daily Food Plan for Pregnancy and Lactation*

Food group	Nutrients provided	Food source	Recommended daily amount during pregnancy	Recommended daily amount during lactation
Dairy products	Protein; riboflavin; vitamins A, D, and others; calcium; phosphorus; zinc; magnesium	Milk—whole, 2%, skim, dry, buttermilk Cheeses—hard, semisoft, cottage Yogurt—plain, low-fat Soybean milk—canned, dry	Four 8 oz cups (five for teenagers) used plain or with flavoring, in shakes, soups, puddings, custards, cocoa Calcium in 1 c milk equivalent to 1½ c cottage cheese, 1½ oz hard or semisoft cheese, 1 c yogurt, 1½ c ice cream (high in fat and sugar)	Four 8 oz cups (five for teenagers); equivalent amount of cheese, yogurt, etc
Meat group	Protein; iron; thiamine, niacin, and other vitamins; minerals	Beef, pork, veal, lamb, poultry, animal organ meats, fish, eggs; legumes; nuts, seeds, peanut butter, grains in proper vegetarian combination (vitamin B$_{12}$ supplement needed)	Three servings (one serving = 2 oz) Combination in amounts necessary for same nutrient equivalent (varies greatly)	Two servings
Grain products, whole grain or enriched	B vitamins; iron; whole grain also has zinc, magnesium, and other trace elements; provides fiber	Breads and bread products such as cornbread, muffins, waffles, hot cakes, biscuits, dumplings, cereals, pastas, rice	Four servings daily: one serving = one slice bread, ¾ c or 1 oz dry cereal, ½ c rice or pasta	Four servings
Fruits and fruit juices	Vitamins A and C; minerals; raw fruits for roughage	Citrus fruits and juices, melons, berries, all other fruits and juices	Two to three servings (one serving for vitamin C): one serving = one medium fruit, ½–1 c fruit, 4 oz orange or grapefruit juice	Same as for pregnancy
Vegetables and vegetable juices	Vitamins A and C; minerals; provides roughage	Leafy green vegetables; deep yellow or orange vegetables such as carrots, sweet potatoes, squash, tomatoes; green vegetables such as peas, green beans, broccoli; other vegetables such as beets, cabbage, potatoes, corn, lima beans	Two to three servings (one serving of dark green or deep yellow vegetable for vitamin A): one serving = ½–1 c vegetable, two tomatoes, one medium potato	Same as for pregnancy
Fats	Vitamins A and D; linoleic acid	Butter, cream cheese, fortified table spreads; cream, whipped cream, whipped toppings; avocado, mayonnaise, oil, nuts	As desired in moderation (high in calories): one serving = 1 Tbsp butter or enriched margarine	Same as for pregnancy
Sugar and sweets		Sugar, brown sugar, honey, molasses	Occasionally, if desired	Same as for pregnancy
Desserts		Nutritious desserts such as puddings, custards, fruit whips, and crisps; other rich, sweet desserts and pastries	Occasionally, if desired (high in calories)	Same as for pregnancy
Beverages		Coffee, decaffeinated beverages, tea, bouillon, carbonated drinks	As desired, in moderation	Same as for pregnancy
Miscellaneous		Iodized salt, herbs, spices, condiments	As desired	Same as for pregnancy

*The pregnant woman should eat regularly, three meals a day, with nutritious snacks of fruits, cheese, milk, or other foods between meals if desired. (More frequent but smaller meals are also recommended.) Four to six glasses (8 oz) of water and a total of eight to ten cups (8 oz) total fluid should be consumed daily. Water is an essential nutrient.

gains of 1.4 to 2.3 kg [3 to 5 lb] in a week) result from fluid retention and require further evaluation because they may indicate that the woman is developing preeclampsia.

Because of the association between inadequate weight gain and low-birth-weight infants, most care givers pay particular attention to weight gain during pregnancy. A woman should generally gain 10 lb by 20 weeks' gestation. Failure to do so puts the woman at risk for intrauterine growth retardation and requires further evaluation and possible nutritional counseling.

Sometimes a woman will gain excessively during the first two-thirds of her pregnancy because of overeating. Dieting is not advised at this time, however, because the third trimester is the time of maximum fetal growth. Consequently nutritional counseling is directed toward helping the woman plan her diet to gain up to a pound per week. Calorie intake should focus on the RDA guidelines.

Monitoring the weight gain of the obese woman (one who weighs 20 percent or more above her recommended prepregnant weight) during pregnancy may be difficult. Obese women may have diets that are high in energy (from carbohydrates and fats) but low in protein, vitamins, and minerals. Thus weight gain alone does not guarantee adequate nutrition. Pregnancy is not a time for dieting, and severe weight restriction during pregnancy can result in maternal ketosis, a threat to fetal well-being. Although obesity is a complex problem, pregnancy is a practical time for the obese woman to evaluate the quality of her diet.

Counseling for the obese pregnant woman usually focuses on encouraging her to eat according to the RDA for pregnancy. Less emphasis is placed on the amount of weight gain and more emphasis is placed on the quality of her intake (Anderson 1986).

Women who are 10 percent or more below their recommended weight prior to conception have an increased risk of delivering a low-birth-weight infant and may have an increased risk of developing preeclampsia as well (Pitkin 1986). Merely advocating the traditional weight gain is not adequate counseling for the underweight woman who is pregnant. The nurse first assesses why the woman is underweight. Is it due to the woman's belief that she looks best at this weight? Does she have a chronic illness? Is she anorexic? Does she participate in strenuous activity at work or in her exercise program? Does she have a small appetite? Has she had a recent weight loss? Is she experiencing severe nausea and vomiting? Once the cause is determined, intervention can be planned with the woman. The underweight woman is usually advised to increase her caloric intake by 500 kcal above the nonpregnant RDA (as opposed to the 300 kcal usual increase). She should also consume 20 g additional protein. Her ideal weight gain is a combination of the amount she is underweight plus a 25 lb gain (Anderson 1986). This is often difficult for the underweight woman, especially if she has a small appetite, and she will require support and encouragement.

Research Note

Taffel examined the association between maternal weight gain and pregnancy outcomes using information from the 1980 National Natality and Fetal Mortality Surveys conducted by the National Center for Health Statistics. Taffel found that women who have a high prepregnancy weight, are 35 years old or older, are black, have under nine years of school, have a low family income, or smoke during pregnancy are most likely to gain less than 16 pounds and least likely to gain 26 pounds or more during pregnancy. A low prepregnancy weight combined with a small weight gain is associated with the highest risk of delivering a low-birth-weight infant, and regardless of prepregnancy weight there is a declining risk of low birth weight as a woman's weight gain increases.

Taffel also found that after controlling for prepregnant weight, age, education, period of gestation, live birth order, and sex, a mother who gains less than 21 pounds is 2.3 times more likely to bear a low-birth-weight infant than a mother who gains at least 21 pounds. Women gaining less than 21 pounds were 1.5 times more likely to have a fetal death than women who gained more. The incidence of fetal death decreased with increased weight gain up to 35 pounds.

This study documents the crucial role of adequate pregnancy weight gain in preventing low-birth-weight infants and fetal death. Nurses must provide thorough nutritional counseling during pregnancy and counter the common misconception that weight gain is detrimental during pregancy. This study demonstrates that an ideal gain is somewhere in the range of 21 to 35 pounds and that "too much" will probably result in a better outcome than "too little."

Taffel M: Association between maternal weight gain and outcome of pregnancy. *J Nurs-Midwife* 1986;31(March/April): 78–86.

● Nutritional Requirements

The RDA (Table 17–1) for all nutrients increase during pregnancy. However, the amount of increase varies with each nutrient. The needs for protein, iron, folacin, vitamin D, calcium, phosphorus, and magnesium increase by 50 percent or more. Recommended increases for other nutrients range from 15 percent to 50 percent (see Figure 17–2).

As the percentage increase for energy is lower (only 15 percent) than the percentage increase for most nutrients, nutrient density becomes very important for the pregnant woman. This means that the woman should select foods

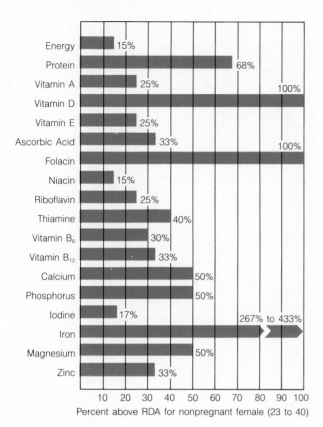

Figure 17–2 Recommended nutrient increases for adult pregnancy (From Food and Nutrition Board: *Recommended Dietary Allowances.* Washington, DC, National Academy of Sciences, National Research Council, 1980)

that are rich sources of protein, vitamins, or minerals for each kcal of energy they provide.

Calories

The term *calorie* (cal) stands for the amount of heat required to raise the temperature of 1 g of water 1C. The *kilocalorie* (kcal) is equivalent to 1000 cal and is the unit used to express the energy value of food.

Considering the amount of protein and fat accumulated by the mother and fetus and the additional metabolic costs incurred by these tissues, the total energy cost of an "average" pregnancy is about 80,000 cal. This is an average of about 300 cal a day above prepregnancy needs. The actual increment is less than 300 cal per day early in pregnancy and may be more later on, near term. Late in pregnancy, however, this increased caloric need may be partially offset by decreased physical activity.

For this reason, weight gains should be monitored regularly, and diets should be individualized for caloric

needs. Prepregnant weight, height, maternal age, activity, and health status all affect caloric needs.

As body size varies, the Food and Nutrition Board suggests that individual caloric needs be calculated by allowing at least 36 cal per kilogram (kg) of pregnant body weight as a starting point. Moderately active pregnant women and underweight women require more calories: approximately 40 cal per kg. Therefore, a moderately active 60 kg (132 lb) woman in her second trimester needs about 2400 cal per day.

Protein

During pregnancy protein is needed in increased amounts to provide amino acids for fetal development, blood volume expansion, and growth of other maternal tissues such as breasts and uterus. Protein also contributes to the body's overall energy metabolism. In the absence of the preferred energy source, carbohydrate, about 58 percent of total dietary protein may become available as glucose and is oxidized as such to yield energy.

Nitrogen balance studies suggest 30 g of protein should be added to daily prepregnancy protein allowances (see Table 17–1). Suggested protein requirements during pregnancy range from 74 to 76 g/day. However, since protein needs also vary with body size, a more appropriate protein level may be calculated by allowing 1.3 g of protein per kg of nonpregnant desirable body weight.

An important source of protein is milk. A quart of milk supplies 32 g of protein, almost half the average daily protein requirement. (See Table 17–1 on p 417.)

Milk can be incorporated into the diet in a variety of dishes, including soups, puddings, custards, sauces, and yogurt. Beverages such as hot chocolate and milk-and-fruit drinks can also be included, but they are high in calories. Various kinds of hard and soft cheeses and cottage cheese are excellent protein sources, although cream cheese is categorized as a fat source only. Table 17–3 provides information on the protein content of commonly used foods.

Women who have allergies to milk (lactose intolerance) or who practice vegetarianism may find dried or canned soy milk acceptable. It can be used in cooked dishes or as a beverage. Tofu, or soybean curd, can replace cottage cheese. Those who are allergic to cow's milk can sometimes tolerate goat's milk and cheese. Frequently, cooked milk can also be tolerated.

Meat, poultry, fish, eggs, and legumes are good sources of protein. Small amounts of complete animal protein can be combined with partially complete plant protein for an excellent, easily used supply of protein. Several examples of complementary proteins are eggs and toast, tuna and rice, cereal and milk, spaghetti and meat sauce, macaroni and cheese, and peanut butter and bread. Except in unusual medical situations, dietary protein should be obtained through natural foods, and the use of protein supplements should be avoided (Johnstone 1984).

Fat

Fats are valuable sources of energy for the body. Fats are more completely absorbed during pregnancy, resulting in a marked increase in serum lipids, lipoproteins, and cholesterol and decreased elimination of fat through the bowel. Fat deposits in the fetus increase from about 2 percent at midpregnancy to almost 12 percent at term.

Carbohydrates

Carbohydrates provide protective substances, bulk, and energy. Carbohydrates contribute to the total caloric intake required. If the total caloric intake is not adequate, the body uses protein for energy. Protein then becomes unavailable for growth needs. In addition, protein breakdown leads to ketosis. Ketosis can be a problem, especially in diabetic women, due to glycosuria, reduced alkaline reserves, and lipidemia.

The carbohydrate and caloric needs of the pregnant woman increase, especially during the last two trimesters. Carbohydrate intake promotes weight gain and growth of the fetus, placenta, and other maternal tissues. Milk, fruits, vegetables, and whole-grain cereals and breads all contain carbohydrates and other important nutrients.

Minerals

Increased minerals needed for the growth of new tissue during pregnancy are obtained by improved mineral absorption and an increase in mineral allowances.

CALCIUM AND PHOSPHORUS

Calcium and phosphorus are involved in mineralization of fetal bones and teeth, energy and cell production, and acid-base buffering. Calcium is absorbed and used more efficiently during pregnancy. Some calcium and phosphorus are required early in pregnancy, but most of the fetus's bone calcification occurs during the last two or three months. Teeth begin to form at about eight weeks' gestation and are formed by birth. The six-year molars begin to calcify just before birth. This means that calcium is particularly important as a structural element. At term the fetus contains about 28 g of calcium. Additional calcium is stored in the maternal skeleton as a reserve for lactation.

The RDA of calcium for the adult woman is set at 800 mg/day, with an additional 400 mg/day during pregnancy. If calcium intakes are low, fetal needs will be met at the mother's expense by demineralization of maternal bone.

Table 17–3 Levels of Protein in Commonly Used Foods

Food	Grams protein
MILK	
Milk, 8 oz	8
Cheese, cheddar, swiss, etc, 1 oz	7
Cottage cheese, ¼ c	7
MEAT GROUP	
Meat, fish, poultry, 1 oz	7
Egg, 1	7
Cooked dry beans & peas, ½ c	7
Cooked soybeans, ½ c	11
Peanut butter, 2 Tbsp	7
Peanuts (3 Tbsp), cashews/almonds (5 Tbsp)	7
BREADS AND CEREALS	
Bread, 1 slice	2
Buns, biscuits, muffins, 1	2
Cooked cereals & grain, ½ c	2
Breakfast cereal, 1 oz	2
VEGETABLES AND FRUITS	
Vegetables, ½ c	0.5–1
Fruits & juices, ½ c	0.5

A diet that includes 4 cups of milk or an equivalent dairy alternate (see Table 17–2) will provide sufficient calcium. Smaller amounts of calcium are supplied by legumes, nuts, dried fruits, and dark green leafy vegetables (such as kale, cabbage, collards, and turnip greens). It is important to remember that some of the calcium in beet greens, spinach, and chard is bound with oxalic acid, which makes it unavailable to the body.

The RDA for phosphorus is the same as the RDA for calcium: 800 mg/day with an extra 400 mg/day during pregnancy. Phosphorus is readily supplied through calcium- and protein-rich foods, especially milk, eggs, and meat.

As phosphorus is so widely available in foods, the dietary intake of phosphorus frequently exceeds calcium intake. An excess of phosphorus can result in a disturbance of the calcium-phosphorus ratio in the body, decreased calcium absorption, and increased excretion of calcium. Excess phosphorus can be reduced by avoiding the snack foods, processed meats, and cola drinks in which it abounds. However, if vitamin D and magnesium are adequate, most adults can tolerate relatively wide variations in dietary calcium-phosphorus ratios.

IODINE

Inorganic iodine is excreted in the urine during pregnancy. Enlargement of the thyroid gland may occur if iodine is not replaced by adequate dietary intake or additional supplement. Moreover, cretinism may occur in the infant if the mother has a severe iodine deficiency.

The iodine allowance of 175 μg/day can be met by using iodized salt. When sodium is restricted, the physician may prescribe an iodine supplement.

Excessive intake of iodine may result in neonatal hypothyroidism and congenital goiter. The iodine found in iodized salt and prenatal vitamins does not generally pose a threat. Women should be advised, however, to avoid ingestion of kelp tablets (0.2 mg iodine in each) and to refrain from using cough preparations containing iodide (Cruikshank 1986).

SODIUM

The sodium ion is essential for proper metabolism. Sodium intake in the form of salt is never entirely curtailed during pregnancy, even when hypertension or PIH is present. Food may be seasoned to taste during cooking but the use of extra salt at the table is avoided. Salty foods such as potato chips, ham, sausages, and sodium-based seasonings can be eliminated to avoid excessive intake.

ZINC

Zinc was recognized as a nutrient factor affecting growth in 1974. The RDA during pregnancy is 20 mg. Sources include milk, liver, shellfish, and wheat bran.

MAGNESIUM

Magnesium is essential for cellular metabolism and structural growth. The RDA for pregnancy is 450 mg. Sources include milk, whole grains, beet greens, nuts, legumes, and tea.

IRON

Anemia in pregnancy is mainly caused by low iron stores, although it may also be caused by inadequate intake of other nutrients, such as vitamins B_6 and B_{12}, folic acid, ascorbic acid, copper, and zinc. Anemia is probably the most common problem in pregnancy, because nutritional anemia occurs frequently in nonpregnant women and the risk of anemia is increased by the normal physiologic changes of pregnancy. Women with poor diet histories, frequent conceptions, or records of prior iron depletion are particularly at risk.

Anemia is generally defined as a decrease in the oxygen-carrying capacity of the blood. This significantly reduces the hemoglobin per decaliter of blood, the volume of packed red cells per decaliter of blood (hematocrit), or the number of erythrocytes.

The normal hematocrit in the nonpregnant woman is 38 percent to 47 percent. In the pregnant woman, the level may drop as low as 34 percent, even when nutrition is adequate. This condition is called the *physiologic anemia of pregnancy*. During pregnancy the number of red blood cells increases, but the plasma volume increases even more. This increased plasma volume dilutes the blood and causes a drop in hematocrit level between 24 and 32 weeks' gestation.

Fetal demands for iron further contribute to symptoms of anemia in the pregnant woman. The fetal liver stores iron, especially during the third trimester. The infant needs this stored iron during the first four months of life to compensate for the normally inadequate levels of iron in breast milk and non–iron-fortified formulas.

To prevent anemia, the woman must balance iron requirements and intake. This is a problem for nonpregnant women and a greater one for pregnant ones.

By carefully selecting foods high in iron, the woman can increase her daily iron intake considerably. Lean meats, dark green leafy vegetables, eggs, and whole-grain and enriched breads and cereals are the foods usually depended on for their iron content. Other iron sources include dried fruits, legumes, shellfish, and molasses.

Iron absorption is generally higher for animal products than for vegetable products. However, absorption of iron from nonmeat sources may be enhanced by combining them with meat or a good vitamin C source.

The most iron that can reasonably be obtained from the diet is about 15 to 18 mg per day. Thus, during pregnancy a supplement of simple iron salt, such as ferrous gluconate, ferrous fumarate, or ferrous sulfate (30 to 60 mg daily) is needed. Supplements may not be given during the first trimester because the increased demand is still minimal, and iron may increase the woman's nausea.

Vitamins

Vitamins are organic substances necessary for life and growth. They are found in small amounts in specific foods and generally cannot be synthesized by the body.

Vitamins are grouped according to solubility. Those vitamins that dissolve in fat are A, D, E, and K; those soluble in water include C and the B complex. An adequate intake of all vitamins is essential during pregnancy; however, several are required in larger amounts to fulfill specific needs.

Many food faddists and people who are concerned about nutrition have become involved in the practice of taking exceptionally large doses—megadoses—of vitamins. However, in vitamin therapy more is not necessarily better. Megadoses of vitamins, especially vitamins A, D, C, and B_6, have had a negative effect on the fetus. Furthermore, excessive intake of one vitamin may interfere with the body's use of another vitamin. For example, excessive intake of vitamin C may block the body's use of vitamin B_{12}, while the body's use of vitamin B_2 (riboflavin) may be altered by megadoses of vitamin B_6 (Luke 1985). Consequently, while it is important to meet the RDA of vitamins during pregnancy, megadoses are best avoided.

FAT-SOLUBLE VITAMINS

The fat-soluble vitamins A, D, E, and K are stored in the liver and thus are available should the dietary intake become inadequate. The major complication related to these vitamins is not deficiency but toxicity due to overdose because excess amounts of A, D, E, and K are not excreted in the urine. Symptoms of vitamin toxicity include nausea, gastrointestinal upset, dryness and cracking of the skin, and loss of hair.

Vitamin A is involved in the growth of epithelial cells, which line the entire gastrointestinal tract and compose the skin. Vitamin A plays a role in the metabolism of carbohydrates and fats. The body cannot synthesize glycogen in the absence of vitamin A, and the body's ability to handle cholesterol is also affected. The protective layer of tissue surrounding nerve fibers does not form properly if vitamin A is lacking.

Probably the best-known function of vitamin A is its effect on vision in dim light. A person's ability to see in the dark depends on the eye's supply of retinol, a form of vitamin A. In this manner, vitamin A prevents night blindness. Vitamin A is associated with the formation and development of healthy eyes in the fetus.

If maternal stores of vitamin A are adequate, the overall effects of pregnancy on the woman's vitamin A requirements are not remarkable. The blood serum level of vitamin A decreases slightly in early pregnancy, rises in late pregnancy, and falls before the onset of labor.

Excessive intake of preformed vitamin A is toxic to both children and adults. There are indications that excessive intake of vitamin A in the fetus can cause eye, ear, and bone malformation, cleft palate, possible renal anomalies, and central nervous system damage (Luke 1985).

Rich plant sources of vitamin A include deep green and yellow vegetables; animal sources include liver, liver oil, kidney, egg yolk, cream, butter, and fortified margarine.

Vitamin D is best known for its role in the absorption and utilization of calcium and phosphorus in skeletal development. To supply the needs of the developing fetus, the woman should increase vitamin D intake by 5 μg/day.

A deficiency of vitamin D results in rickets, a condition caused by improper calcification of the bones. It is treated with relatively large doses of vitamin D under a physician's direction.

Main food sources of vitamin D include fortified milk, margarine, butter, liver, and egg yolks. Drinking a quart of milk daily provides the vitamin D needed during pregnancy.

Excessive intake of vitamin D is not usually a result of eating but of taking high-potency vitamin preparations.

Overdoses during pregnancy can cause hypercalcemia or high blood calcium levels due to withdrawal of calcium from the skeletal tissue. In the fetus, cardiac defects, especially aortic stenosis, may occur (Luke 1985). Continued overdose can also cause hypercalcemia and eventually death, especially in young children. Symptoms of toxicity are excessive thirst, loss of appetite, vomiting, weight loss, irritability, and high blood calcium levels.

The major function of *vitamin E,* or tocopherol, is as an antioxidant. Vitamin E takes on oxygen, thus preventing another substance from undergoing chemical change. For example, vitamin E helps spare vitamin A by preventing its oxidation in the intestinal tract and the tissues. It decreases the oxidation of polyunsaturated fats, thus helping to retain the flexibility and health of the cell membrane. In protecting the cell membrane, vitamin E affects the health of all cells in the body. Its role during pregnancy is not known.

Vitamin E is also involved in certain enzymatic and metabolic reactions. It is an essential nutrient for the synthesis of nucleic acids required in the formation of red blood cells in the bone marrow. Vitamin E is beneficial in treating certain types of muscular pain and intermittent claudication, in surface healing of wounds and burns, and in protecting lung tissue from the damaging effects of smog. These functions may help explain the abundant claims and cures attributed to vitamin E, many of which have not been scientifically proved.

The newborn's need for vitamin E has been widely recognized. Human milk provides adequate vitamin E, whereas cow's milk is lower in E content. Deficiency symptoms of vitamin E are related to long-term inability to absorb fats. In humans, malabsorption problems exist in cases of cystic fibrosis, liver cirrhosis, postgastrectomy, obstructive jaundice, pancreatic problems, and sprue.

The recommended intake of vitamin E increases from 8 IU for nonpregnant females to 10 IU for pregnant women. The vitamin E requirement varies with the polyunsaturated fat content of the diet. Vitamin E is widely distributed in foodstuffs, especially vegetable fats and oils, whole grains, greens, and eggs.

Some pregnant women use vitamin E oil on the abdominal skin to make it supple and possibly prevent permanent stretch marks. It is questionable whether taking high doses internally will accomplish this goal or satisfy any other claims related to vitamin E's role in reproduction or virility. In addition, excessive intake of vitamin E has been associated with abnormal coagulation in the newborn.

Vitamin K, or menadione as used synthetically in medicine, is an essential factor for the synthesis of prothrombin; its function is thus related to normal blood clotting. Synthesis occurs in the intestinal tract by the *Escherichia coli* bacteria normally inhabiting the large intestine. These organisms generally provide adequate vitamin K.

Newborn infants, having a sterile intestinal tract and receiving sterile feeding, lack vitamin K. Thus newborns often receive a dose of menadione as a protective measure.

Intake of vitamin K is usually adequate in a well-balanced prenatal diet; an increased requirement has not been identified. Secondary problems may rise if an illness is present that results in malabsorption of fats or if antibiotics are used for an extended period, which would inhibit vitamin K synthesis.

WATER-SOLUBLE VITAMINS

Water-soluble vitamins are excreted in the urine. Only small amounts are stored, so there is little protection from dietary inadequacies. Thus, adequate amounts must be ingested daily. During pregnancy, the concentration of water-soluble vitamins in the maternal serum falls, whereas high concentrations are found in the fetus.

The requirement for *vitamin C* (ascorbic acid) is increased in pregnancy from 60 to 80 mg. The major function of vitamin C is to aid the formation and development of connective tissue and the vascular system. Ascorbic acid is essential to the formation of collagen. Collagen is like a cement that binds cells together, just as mortar holds bricks together. If the collagen begins to disintegrate due to a lack of ascorbic acid, cell functioning is disturbed and cell structure breaks down, causing muscular weakness, capillary hemorrhage, and eventual death. These are symptoms of scurvy, the disease caused by vitamin C deficiency. Infants fed mainly cow's milk become deficient in vitamin C, and they constitute the main population group that develops these symptoms (Food and Nutrition Board 1980). Surprisingly, newborns of women who have taken megadoses of vitamin C may experience a rebound form of scurvy (Anderson 1986).

Maternal plasma levels of vitamin C progressively decline throughout pregnancy, with values at term being about half those at midpregnancy. It appears that ascorbic acid concentrates in the placenta; levels in the fetus are 50 percent or more above maternal levels.

A nutritious diet should meet the pregnant woman's needs for vitamin C without additional supplementation. Common food sources of vitamin C include citrus fruit, tomatoes, cantaloupe, strawberries, potatoes, broccoli, and other leafy greens. Ascorbic acid is readily destroyed by oxidation. Therefore, foods containing vitamin C must be stored and cooked properly.

The *B vitamins* include thiamine (B_1), riboflavin (B_2), niacin, folic acid, pantothenic acid, vitamin B_6, and vitamin B_{12}. These vitamins serve as vital coenzyme factors in many reactions, such as cell respiration, glucose oxidation, and energy metabolism. The quantities needed, therefore, invariably increase as caloric intake increases to meet the metabolic and growth needs of the pregnant woman.

The *thiamine* requirement increases from the pre-pregnant level of 1.1 mg/day to 1.5 mg/day. Sources include pork, liver, milk, potatoes, enriched breads, and cereals.

Ribloflavin deficiency is manifested by cheilosis and other skin lesions. During pregnancy, women may excrete less riboflavin and still require more, because of increased energy and protein needs. An additional 0.3 mg/day is recommended. Sources include milk, liver, eggs, enriched breads, and cereals.

An increase of 2 mg daily in *niacin* intake is recommended during pregnancy and 5 mg during lactation, although no information on the niacin requirements of pregnant and nursing women is available. Sources of niacin include meat, fish, poultry, liver, whole grains, enriched breads, cereals, and peanuts.

Folic acid promotes adequate fetal growth and prevents the macrocytic, megaloblastic anemia of pregnancy. Folic acid is directly related to the outcome of pregnancy and to maternal and fetal health. Folate deficiency has been associated with abortion, fetal malformation, abruptio placentae, and other late bleeding complications. Severe maternal folate deficiency may have other unrecognized effects on the fetus and newborn. Hemorrhagic anemia in the newborn is attributed to this deficiency.

Megaloblastic anemia due to folate deficiency is rarely found in the United States, but those caring for pregnant women must be aware that it does occur. Folate deficiency can also be present in the absence of overt anemia.

The RDA for folic acid increases by 100 percent—from 400 μg to 800 μg—during pregnancy. Many women have problems ingesting this amount since good dietary sources of folic acid are limited (see Table 17–4). For this reason, a supplement of 0.4 mg (400 μg) of folic acid daily is recommended. Due to the risks associated with deficiency during pregnancy, folic acid supplementation often begins with the onset of pregnancy or even before.

Normal serum folic acid levels in pregnancy range from 3 to 15 mg/ml; less than 3 mg/ml constitutes acute deficiency. If no other complications are present, this deficiency can be easily remedied with folic acid therapy. After the baby is born, a routine nutritious diet generally provides adequate folic acid to alleviate the woman's symptoms; however, it is wise to give additional folate therapy to build up stores and promote rapid hematologic changes.

Women on phenytoin (Dilantin) for the control of seizures and women carrying twins are also especially susceptible to folic acid deficiency. Daily supplements of 0.8 to 1.0 mg folic acid are indicated for these women (Cruikshank 1986).

The best food sources of folates are fresh green leafy vegetables, kidney, liver, food yeasts, and peanuts. As indicated by the list of food sources in Table 17–4, many foods contain small amounts of folic acid. Cow's milk contains a small amount of folic acid, but goat's milk contains

Table 17–4 Folic Acid Content of Selected Foods

Food	Amount	Folic acid (μg)	Food	Amount	Folic acid (μg)
Yeast, torula	1 Tbsp	240.0	Chocolate	1 oz	28.1
Beef liver, cooked	2 oz	167.6	Corn, fresh	3½ oz	28.0
Yeast, brewer's	1 Tbsp	161.8	Snap beans, green fresh	3½ oz	27.5
Cowpeas, cooked	½ c	140.5	Peas, green, fresh	3½ oz	25.0
Pork liver, cooked	2 oz	126.0	Shredded wheat cereal	1 biscuit	16.5
Asparagus, fresh	3½ oz	109.0	Figs, fresh	3 small	16.0
Wheat germ	1 oz	91.5	Sweet potatoes, fresh	½ medium	12.0
Spinach	3½ oz	75.0	Walnut halves, raw	8–15	11.5
Soybeans, cooked	½ c	71.7	Oysters, canned	3½ oz	11.3
Wheat bran	1 oz	58.5	Pork (ham)	3½ oz	10.6
Kidney beans, cooked	½ c	57.6	Banana, fresh	1 medium	9.7
Broccoli, fresh	⅔ c	53.5	Cantaloupe, diced, fresh	⅔ c	9.0
Brussels sprouts, fresh	3½ oz	49.0	Cottage cheese	1 oz	8.8
Whole-wheat flour	1 c	45.6	White flour	1 c	8.8
Garbanzos, cooked	½ c	40.0	Peanut butter	1 Tbsp	8.5
Wheat bran cereal	1 c	35.0	Blueberries, fresh	⅔ c	8.0
Beans, lima, fresh	3½ oz	34.0	Turkey	3½ oz	7.5
Asparagus, green, fresh	3½ oz	32.4	Celery, diced, fresh	1 c	7.0

Source: Modified from Hardinga MG, Crooks HN: *Lesser known vitamins in food.* ©The American Dietetic Association. Reprinted by permission from *J Am Diet Assoc* 1961;38:240.

none. Therefore, infants and children who are given goat's milk must receive a folate supplement to prevent a deficiency.

Folic acid content of foods can be altered by preparation methods. Since folic acid is a water-soluble nutrient, care must be taken in cooking. Loss of the vitamin from vegetables and meats can be considerable when they are cooked in large amounts of water.

No allowance has been set for *pantothenic acid* in pregnancy. Some studies suggest that it is advisable to supplement the diet with 5 to 10 mg of pantothenic acid daily. Sources include liver, egg yolk, yeast, and whole-grain cereals and breads.

Vitamin B_6 (pyridoxine) has long been associated biochemically with pregnancy. The RDA for vitamin B_6 during pregnancy is 2.6 mg, an increase of 0.6 mg over the allowance for nonpregnant women. Since pyridoxine is associated with amino acid metabolism, a higher-than-average protein intake requires increased pyridoxine intake. The slightly increased need can generally be supplied by dietary sources, which include wheat germ, yeast, fish, liver, pork, potatoes, and lentils.

Vitamin B_{12}, or cobalamin, is the cobalt-containing vitamin found only in animal sources. Rarely is B_{12} deficiency found in women of reproductive age. Vegetarians can develop a deficiency, however, so it is essential that their dietary intake be supplemented with this vitamin. Occasionally vitamin B_{12} levels decrease during pregnancy but

increase again after delivery. The RDA during pregnancy is 4 μg/day, an increase of 1 μg.

A deficiency may be due to inability to absorb vitamin B_{12}. Pernicious anemia results; infertility is a complication of this type of anemia.

Folic acid and iron are the only nutritional supplements generally recommended during pregnancy. The increased need for other vitamins and minerals can be met with an adequate diet. To avoid possible deficiencies, however, many care givers also recommend a daily vitamin supplement.

● Vegetarianism

Vegetarianism is the dietary choice of many people, for religious (Seventh-Day Adventists), health, and ethical reasons. There are several types of vegetarians. *Lacto-ovo-vegetarians* include milk, dairy products, and eggs in their diet. Occasionally fish, poultry, and liver are consumed. *Lactovegetarians* include dairy products but no eggs in their diet. *Vegans* are "pure" vegetarians who will not eat any food from animal sources.

Whether her family is currently practicing vegetarianism or is considering it as an alternative, it is vital that the expectant woman eat the proper combination of foods to obtain adequate nutrients. If her diet allows, a woman can obtain ample and complete proteins from dairy products and eggs. Plant protein quality may be improved if consumed with these animal proteins at the same meal. If the diet contains less than four servings of milk and milk products, calcium supplementation may be necessary.

If a "pure" vegetarian diet is followed, careful planning is necessary to obtain sufficient calories and complete proteins. Obtaining sufficient calories to achieve adequate weight gains can be quite difficult. Low prepregnancy weight and optimum pregnancy weight gains are often a problem. Supplementation with energy-dense foods helps provide increased energy intake to prevent the body from using protein for calorie needs.

If energy needs are adequate, protein needs can usually be met if recommendations for complementing proteins are followed. An adequate pure vegetarian diet contains protein from unrefined grains (brown rice and whole wheat), legumes (beans, split peas, lentils), nuts in large quantities, and a variety of cooked and fresh vegetables and fruits. Complete protein may be obtained by eating any of the following food combinations at the same meal: legumes and whole-grain cereals, nuts and whole-grain cereals, or nuts and legumes. Seeds may be used in the vegetarian diet if the quantity is large enough.

Because vegans use no animal products, a daily supplement of 4 μg of vitamin B_{12} is necessary. If soy milk is used, only partial supplementation may be needed. If no soy milk is taken, daily supplements of 1200 mg of calcium and 10 μg of vitamin D are needed.

As the best sources of iron and zinc are found in animal products, strict vegetarian diets are also low in these minerals. In addition, a high fiber intake may reduce mineral (calcium, iron, and zinc) bioavailability. Emphasis should be placed on use of foods containing these nutrients.

Sample vegetarian menus that meet the requirements of good prenatal nutrition are given in Table 17–5.

● Factors Influencing Nutrition

Besides having knowledge of nutritional needs and food sources, the nurse needs to be aware of other factors that affect a client's nutrition. What is the age, life-style, and culture of the pregnant woman? What food beliefs and habits does she have? What a person eats is determined by availability, economics and symbolism. These factors and others influence the expectant mother's acceptance of the nurse's intervention.

Lactose Intolerance

Some individuals have difficulty digesting milk and milk products. This condition, known as lactose intolerance, results from an inadequate amount of the enzyme lactase, which breaks down the milk sugar lactose into smaller digestible substances.

Lactose intolerance is found in many blacks, Mexican Americans, American Indians, Ashkenazic Jews, and Orientals. Symptoms include abdominal distention, discomfort, nausea, vomiting, loose stools, and cramps.

In counseling pregnant women who might be intolerant of milk and milk products, the nurse should be aware of the following:

● Even one glass of milk can produce symptoms. Tolerances vary with the individual.

● Milk is sometimes tolerated in cooked form, such as in custards.

● Fermented dairy products, such as cheese and yogurt, are sometimes tolerated.

● In some instances, the enzyme lactase may be used to alleviate the problem. It is available in several forms: as a tablet to be chewed before ingesting milk or milk products and as a liquid to add to milk itself. Lactase-treated milk is also available commercially in some grocery stores.

Pica

Pica is the eating of substances that are not ordinarily considered edible or to have nutritive value. Most women who practice pica in pregnancy eat such substances only during that time. Women usually explain this practice by saying it relieves various discomforts of pregnancy or that it ensures a beautiful baby (Curda 1977).

Pica is most commonly practiced in poverty-stricken areas, where diets tend to be inadequate, but may also be found at other socioeconomic levels. The substances most commonly ingested in this country are dirt, clay, starch, and freezer frost. Iron-deficiency anemia is the most common concern in pica. Studies indicate that ingestion of laundry starch or certain types of clay may contribute to iron deficiency by interfering with iron absorption. The ingestion of large quantities of clay could fill the intestine and cause fecal impaction, while the ingestion of starch may be associated with excessive weight gain (Pritchard et al 1985).

Nurses should be aware of pica and its implications for the woman and her fetus. Often pica is part of the tradition of certain communities or families. Assessment for pica is an important part of the nutritional history. However, women may be embarrassed about their cravings or reluctant to discuss them for fear of criticism. It is helpful if the nurse uses a nonjudgmental approach. The nurse can seek information about pica by saying, "Many women have cravings during pregnancy for things like starch, clay, or freezer frost. Have you experienced any cravings like that?" The nurse can then determine the amount the woman is

Table 17–5 Suggested Menus for Adequate Prenatal Vegetarian Diets

Meal pattern	Mixed diet	Lacto-ovovegetarian	Lactovegetarian	Seventh-Day Adventist	Vegan
BREAKFAST					
Fruit	¾ c orange juice	Same as mixed diet	Same	Same	Same
Grains	½ c granola, 1 slice whole wheat toast				1 c granola, 1 slice whole grain toast
Meat group	1 scrambled egg with cheese		1 oz cheese melted over toast (no egg)		
Fat	1 tsp butter		Same		1 tsp sesame butter
Milk	½ c milk				1 c soy milk
MIDMORNING					
Milk	1 c hot chocolate				1 c protein drink*
LUNCH					
Meat group/vegetable	1 c lentil chowder† (made with ground beef)	1 c lentil chowder† (no ground beef)	1 c lentil chowder† (no ground beef)	1 c lentil chowder† (made with vegeburger)‡	1½ c lentil chowder† (1 Tbsp torula yeast, wheat germ added)
Grains	1 corn muffin	Same	Same	Same	2 corn muffins§
Fat	1 tsp butter, honey				2 tsp margarine, honey
Fruit/dessert	½ peach, ½ c cottage cheese salad				½ peach, ½ c tofu salad
Tea	1 c tea			Decaffeinated or herbal tea	Same as Seventh-Day Adventist
MIDAFTERNOON					
Milk	¾ c vanilla pudding			Same	1 c pudding (soy milk)
Fruit	¼ c sliced banana				½ banana

*Protein drink recipe is: 3 c cow's or goat's milk, ½ c nonfat soy milk powder, 2 Tbsp wheat germ, 2 Tbsp brewer's yeast, fruit, and vanilla. Vegans may make the drink with soy milk in place of cow's or goat's milk.
†Lentil chowder is make from lentils, celery, carrots, potatoes, onion, and tomatoes.
‡Vegeburger is made from meat analogs.
§Wheat germ and soy flour are added to corn muffin mixture.

consuming and discuss her feelings about the practice. Reeducation of the expectant woman is important in helping her to decrease or eliminate this practice.

Food Myths

The relationship of food to pregnancy is reflected in some common beliefs or sayings. Nurses frequently hear that the pregnant woman must eat for two or that the fetus takes from the mother all the nutrients it needs. The practice of pica, for example, has roots in myth. Common beliefs regarding pica include (a) that laundry starch will make the newborn lighter in color, and (b) that the baby will "slide out" more easily during delivery (Curda 1977).

Cultural, Ethnic, and Religious Influences

Cultural, ethnic, and occasionally religious background determines one's experiences with food and influences food preferences and habits (Figure 17–3). People of different nationalities are accustomed to eating different foods because of the kinds of foodstuffs available in their countries of origin. The way food is prepared varies, depending on the customs and traditions of the ethnic and cultural group. In addition, the laws of certain religions sanction particular foods, prohibit others, and direct the preparation and serving of meals.

In each culture, certain foods have symbolic significance. Generally, these symbolic foods are related to major life experiences such as birth, death, or developmental milestones. (General food practices of different cultural and ethnic groups are presented in Table 17–6. Sample daily menus that meet minimal nutritional requirements for differing cultural groups during pregnancy are presented in Table 17–7.) For example, Navajo Indian women believe that eating raisins will cause brown spots on the mother or baby. Many black Americans believe that craving one food excessively can cause the baby to be "marked"; some

Table 17–5 Suggested Menus for Adequate Prenatal Vegetarian Diets (continued)

Meal pattern	Mixed diet	Lacto-ovovegetarian	Lactovegetarian	Seventh-Day Adventist	Vegan
Grain	1 graham cracker	↓		↓	↓ 1 graham cracker with peanut butter
DINNER					
Meat group/vegetable	¾ c meat sauce (onion, celery, carrot, tomato, mushroom in sauce), parmesan cheese	¾ c tomato sauce (same vegetables as in mixed diet), ¼ c cheese	Same as lacto-ovo-vegetarian	Same (add vegeburger‡ to tomato sauce)	Same (use tofu instead of cheese)
Grains	¾ c spaghetti, bread	1 c whole-wheat spaghetti, 1 slice French bread	↓		↓
Vegetable	Mixed vegetable salad	Mixed vegetable salad with ¼ c sprouts, ½ egg, ½ oz cheese, ¼ c kidney beans added	(No egg in salad)		(Add tofu; no egg in salad)
Fat	Oil-vinegar dressing, ½ tsp butter	Same as mixed diet	Same		1 tsp margarine
Fruit	Fresh pear or baked pear half				Same as mixed diet
Tea	1 c tea			Decaffeinated or herbal tea	Same as Seventh-Day Adventist
BEDTIME					
Milk	1 c milk			Same	
Meat group/vegetable	2 tsp peanut butter on celery or on wheat crackers				1 c protein drink*
Grain		↓	↓	↓	Corn muffins§

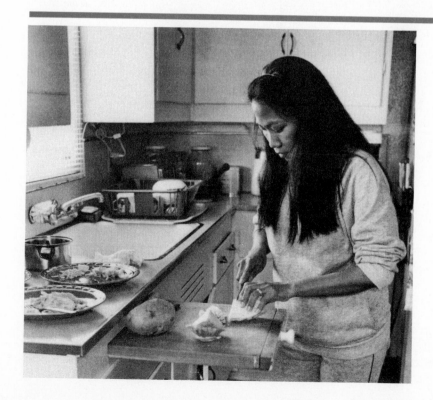

Figure 17–3 Food preferences and habits are affected by cultural factors.

Table 17-6 Food Practices of Various Ethnic and Religious Groups

Cultural group	Staple foods	Prohibitions or foods not used	Food preparation
Jewish Orthodox	Meat: Forequarter of cattle, sheep, goat, deer Poultry: chicken, pheasant, turkey, goose, duck Dairy products	No blood may be eaten in any form Combining milk and meat at meal not allowed; milk and cheese may be eaten before meal, but must not be eaten for 6 hours after meal containing meat No shellfish or eels	Animal slaughter must follow certain rules, including minimal pain to animal and maximal blood drainage Two sets of dishes are used: one for meat, one for milk meals
	Fish with fins and scales No restrictions on cereals, fruits, or vegetables		
Mexican American	Main vegetables: corn (source of calcium) and chili peppers (source of vitamin C); pinto beans or calice beans; potatoes Coffee and eggs Grain products: corn is basic grain; tortillas from enriched flour made daily	Milk rarely used	Chief cooking fat is lard Usually beans are served with every meal
Chinese	Rice is staple grain and used at most meals Traditional beverage is green tea Most meats are used, but in limited amounts Fruits are usually eaten fresh	Milk and cheese rarely used Meat considered difficult to chew, so may be eliminated from child's diet	Foods are kept short time and are cooked quickly at high temperature so that natural flavors are enhanced and texture and color maintained Chief cooking fat is lard or peanut oil.
Japanese	Seafood (raw fish) eaten frequently Most meats; large variety of vegetables and fresh fruits Rice is staple grain, but corn and oats also used	Milk and cheese rarely used	Chief cooking fat is soybean oil

say the shape of the birthmark echoes the shape of the food the mother craved during pregnancy. This belief is also held by some Mexican-American women. Some Mexican Americans believe drinking milk makes their babies too big, thereby causing difficult deliveries.

The traditional Chinese classify food as either hot or cold, and these classifications are related to the balance of forces for good health. Since childbirth is considered a cold condition, it must be treated with hot foods, such as chicken, squash, and broccoli. Vietnamese women believe that eating "unclean foods," such as beef, dog, and snake,

during pregnancy will cause the baby to be born an imbecile. Cabbage is also avoided because it is believed to produce flatulence that might bring on false labor (Clark 1978).

Psychosocial Factors

Sharing food has long been a symbol of friendliness, warmth, and social acceptance in many cultures. Food is also symbolic of motherliness; that is, taking care of the family and feeding them well is a part of the traditional

Table 17–7 Sample Menus for Adequate Prenatal Diet for Various Cultural Groups*

Caucasian	Mexican-American	Southern U.S.	Oriental	Jewish	Italian
BREAKFAST					
Peaches Oatmeal/milk Toast with peanut butter Milk	Peaches Oatmeal/milk Corn tortilla Refried beans Milk	Peaches Oatmeal/milk Cornbread with molasses Milk	Peaches Steamed rice/milk (soy) Rice cracker Tea	Peaches Oatmeal/milk Bagel with unsalted butter Milk	Peaches Oatmeal/milk Bread with butter Cheese Coffee/milk
MIDMORNING					
Fruit/juice	Fruit/juice	Fruit	Fruit	Fruit	Fruit/juice
LUNCH					
Cheese omelet and vegetables Whole grain muffin with butter Lettuce and tomato salad Raw apple Milk	1 fried egg Refried beans with cheese Corn tortilla Fresh tomato and chilies Banana Milk	1 fried egg Black-eyed peas and salt pork Cornbread with molasses Turnip greens Ice cream	Miso soup Chinese omelet (with bean sprouts, pepper, green onion, mushroom) and fried rice Spinach Tea	Cheese omelet Brown rice Lettuce and tomato salad Honey cookie Milk	Cheese omelet Zucchini, green salad Grapes/cheese Milk
MIDAFTERNOON					
Fruit Cottage cheese	Fruit Cottage cheese	Fruit	Fruit Tofu	Fruit	Fruit Cheese
DINNER					
Roast beef and gravy Whole grain roll with butter Parsley, carrots, cabbage slaw Banana cream pie Tea	Refried beans with cheese Fried macaroni Tortilla Carrots, steamed tomato, chilies Corn pudding milk	Beef stew with vegetables (carrots, greens) Dumplings Steamed potato, cabbage slaw Corn pudding	Beef strips with pan-fried vegetables Brown rice, steamed Milk custard	Beef stew with vegetables Barley pilaf Cooked cabbage Unsalted butter Coffeecake Fruit/juice	Spaghetti and meatballs with tomato sauce Italian bread with butter Sauteed eggplant, cabbage, salad Fruit Coffee/milk
BEDTIME					
Milk Wheat crackers 1 oz cheese	Milk Tortilla with beans Cheese	Milk Corn pudding	Ice cream	Ice cream	Ice cream

*Modified from American Dietetic Association. Cultural food patterns in the U.S.A.

mothering role. The mother influences her children's likes and dislikes by what she prepares and by her attitude about foods. Certain foods are assigned positive or negative values, as reflected in the statements "Milk helps you grow" and "Coffee stunts your growth."

Some foods and food-related practices are associated with status. Some foods are prepared "just for company." Other foods are served only on special occasions—for example, holidays such as Thanksgiving.

SOCIOECONOMIC FACTORS

Socioeconomic level may be a determinant of nutritional status. Poverty-level families are unable to afford the same foods that higher-income families can. Thus, pregnant women with low incomes are frequently at risk for poor nutrition.

EDUCATION

Knowledge about the basic components of a balanced diet is essential. Often educational level is related to economic status, but even people on very limited incomes can prepare well-balanced meals if their knowledge of nutrition is adequate.

PSYCHOLOGIC FACTORS

Emotions affect nutritional well-being directly. For example, anorexia nervosa, a psychologic disorder that occurs primarily in adolescent girls, is due chiefly to self-inflicted starvation, resulting in malnutrition and ultimately death if not treated. Loss of appetite is also a common symptom of serious depression.

The expectant woman's attitudes and feelings about her pregnancy influence her nutritional status. The woman who is depressed or who does not wish to be pregnant may manifest these feelings by loss of appetite or by improper food practices, such as overindulgence in sweets or alcohol.

The Pregnant Adolescent

Nutritional care of the pregnant adolescent is of particular concern to health care professionals. Many adolescents are nutritionally at risk due to a variety of complex and interrelated emotional, social, and economic factors that may adversely affect dietary intake.

Nutritional Concerns

GENERAL CONCERNS

In determining nutrient needs for pregnant adolescents, it is important to consider gynecological age: the number of years that have passed since menstruation began. Those who have reached a gynecological age of 4 years are considered physiologically mature, as linear growth is usually completed by this time (Marino & King 1980). Their nutritional needs would be similar to other "adult" women.

Adolescents who become pregnant at a gynecological age of less than 4 years, however, are at a high biological risk due to their physiological and anatomical immaturity. Nutritional needs for these young women (who are most likely to be growing) will be higher than for those whose growth has been completed.

Very little information is currently available on the nutritional needs of adolescents. Estimates are usually obtained by using the RDA for nonpregnant teenagers (age 11 to 14 or 15 to 18) and adding nutrient amounts recommended for all pregnant women (see Table 17–1). Although the RDA are based on chronological age, they are probably the best available figures to use if the pregnant female is still growing. However, if mature, the pregnant adolescent's nutritional needs would approach those reported for pregnant adults.

WEIGHT GAIN

Preliminary studies have confirmed that adolescents tend to gain a greater amount of weight during pregnancy than adults (Meserole 1984). In addition, it has been shown that young adolescents (13 to 15 years) needed to gain more weight than older adolescents (16 years or older) to produce babies of equal size (Frisancho et al 1983). In determining the optimum weight gain for the pregnant adolescent, it is important to consider the following factors:

● Recommended weight gain for a normal pregnancy

● Amount of weight gain expected during the postmenarcheal year during which the pregnancy occurs

The issue of recommended weight gains during pregnancy was addressed earlier (see the section entitled Maternal Weight Gain). Frisch (1976) defined the amount of expected weight gain due to growth according to the number of years postmenarche. These weight gains are reported in Table 17–8.

The weight gain for a normal pregnancy and the expected weight gain due to growth would be added together to obtain a recommended weight gain for the pregnant adolescent. If the teenager is underweight, additional weight gain is recommended to bring her to a normal weight for her height.

SPECIFIC NUTRIENT CONCERNS

Caloric needs of pregnant adolescents will vary widely. Major factors in determining calorie needs include whether growth has been completed and the amount of physical activity. Figures as high as 50 cal per kg have been suggested for young, growing teens who are very active physically. A satisfactory weight gain will confirm adequacy of caloric intake in most cases.

In order to promote optimal physical development of the pregnant adolescent, the Food and Nutrition Board recommends a higher protein intake for the younger pregnant female. Girls 15 to 18 years of age should consume about 1.5 g/kg of body weight. Those who are 11 to 14 years old should consume about 1.7 g/kg of body weight. As mentioned earlier, if growth has been completed, needs approach that of the pregnant adult female (1.3 g/kg).

Inadequate iron intake is a main concern with the adolescent diet. Estimates suggest that 20 percent of the adolescent population is at risk of iron deficiency anemia

Table 17–8 Expected Weight Gain Due to Growth After Menarche

Postmenarcheal year	Pounds gained each year
1	10.12
2	6.16
3	2.42
4 and 5	1.76

Source: Frisch RE: Fatness of girls from menarche to age 18 years, with a nomogram. *Hum Biol* 1976;48:353.

(Mellendick 1983). Iron needs are high for the pregnant teen due to the requirement for iron by the enlarging muscle mass and blood volume. Iron supplements—providing between 30 to 60 mg of elemental iron—are definitely indicated.

Calcium is another nutrient that demands special attention from pregnant adolescents. Inadequate intake of calcium is frequently a problem in this age group. Adequate calcium intake is needed to support normal growth and development of the fetus as well as growth and maintenance of calcium stores in the adolescent. To provide for these needs, an intake of 1600 mg/day of calcium is recommended (see Table 17–1). This is 400 mg/day more than the recommended amount for pregnant adults. An extra serving of dairy products is usually suggested for teenagers (see Table 17–2). Calcium supplementation is indicated for teens with an aversion to milk, unless other dairy products or significant calcium sources are consumed in sufficient quantities.

As folic acid plays a role in cell reproduction, it is also an important nutrient for pregnant teens. As previously indicated, a supplement is usually suggested for all pregnant females, whether adult or teenager.

Other nutrients and vitamins must be considered when evaluating the overall nutritional quality of the teenager's diet. Nutrients that have frequently been found to be deficient in this age group include zinc and vitamins A, D, and B_6. Inclusion of a wide variety of foods—especially fresh and lightly processed foods—is helpful in obtaining adequate amounts of trace minerals, fiber, and other vitamins.

DIETARY PATTERNS

Healthy adolescents often have irregular eating patterns. Many skip breakfast, and most tend to be frequent snackers. Teens rarely follow the traditional three-meals-a-day pattern; their day-to-day intake often varies drastically; and they eat food combinations that may seem bizarre to adults. Despite this, adolescents usually achieve a better nutritional balance than most adults would expect.

In assessing the diet of the pregnant adolescent, the nurse should consider the eating pattern over time, not simply a single day's intake. This pattern is critical because of the irregularity of most adolescent eating patterns. Once the pattern is identified, counseling can be directed toward correcting deficiencies.

Counseling Issues

Nutritional counseling of the pregnant teenager is very challenging. Social, emotional, and physical factors that accompany teenage pregnancy may make it difficult for the adolescent to concentrate on dietary issues.

A positive approach is more effective than a negative one. The nurse must be ready to suggest valuable foods that pregnant teens can choose in many places and at any time. Establishment of a traditional meal pattern is not necessary if the nurse can give suggestions for specific foods for particular times during the day. If the adolescent's mother does most of the meal preparation, it may be useful to include her in the discussion if the adolescent agrees.

The pregnant teenager will soon become a parent, and her understanding of nutrition will influence not only her well-being but also that of her child. However, teens tend to live in the present, and counseling that stresses long-term changes may be less effective than more concrete approaches. In many cases, group classes are effective, especially those with other teens. In a group atmosphere, adolescents often work together to plan adequate meals including foods that are special favorites.

● Postpartum Nutrition

Nutritional needs will change following delivery. Nutrient requirements will vary depending on whether the mother decides to breast-feed. An assessment of postpartal nutritional status is necessary before nutritional guidance is given.

Postpartal Nutritional Status

Determination of postpartal nutritional status is based primarily on the following factors: anthropometric data, biochemical data, clinical signs, and dietary information obtained from the mother.

Anthropometric data are gathered by evaluating the mother's weight. As previously discussed, an ideal weight gain during pregnancy is between 22 and 28 pounds. Upon delivery, there is a weight loss of approximately 10 to 12 pounds. Additional weight loss will be most rapid during the first few weeks after delivery, as the uterus returns to normal size, tissue fluids are released, and blood volume returns to normal. The mother's weight will then begin to stabilize. Some women reach their prepregnancy weight several weeks after delivery; some reach this weight after several months. If excessive weight was gained during pregnancy, returning to prepregnancy weight will take longer.

It is important to evaluate the mother's current weight, ideal weight for her height, weight before pregnancy, and weight before delivery. Women who are interested in weight reduction should be referred to the dietitian. Different guidelines for weight loss are used for nursing mothers and nonnursing mothers.

Biochemical data include evaluations of various blood values, especially hemoglobin and hematocrit. Hemoglobin and erythrocyte values vary after delivery, but they should return to normal levels within two to six weeks. Hematocrit levels should rise gradually due to hemoconcentration as extracellular fluid is excreted. The hematocrit is usually checked at the postpartum visit to detect any anemia. Iron supplements are generally prescribed for two to three months following delivery to replenish supplies depleted by pregnancy.

Clinical symptoms the new mother may be experiencing are assessed. Constipation, in particular, is a common problem following delivery. The nurse can encourage the woman to maintain a high fluid intake to keep the stool soft. Dietary sources of fiber, such as whole grains, fruits, and vegetables, are also helpful in preventing constipation.

Specific information on dietary intake and eating habits is obtained directly from the woman. Visiting the mother during mealtimes provides an opportunity for unobtrusive nutritional assessment. Which foods has a woman selected? Has she avoided fruits and vegetables? Is her diet mainly carbohydrates and fats? Is her diet nutritionally sound? A comment focusing on a positive aspect of her meal selection may initiate a discussion of nutrition.

The dietitian should be informed of any woman whose cultural or religious beliefs require specific foods. Appropriate meals can then be prepared for her. The nurse may also refer women with unusual eating habits or numerous questions about good nutrition to the dietitian. In all cases, the nurse should provide literature on nutrition so that the woman will have a source of appropriate information at home.

Nutritional Care of Nonnursing Mothers

After delivery, the nonnursing mother's dietary requirements return to prepregnancy levels (see Table 17–1). If the mother has a good understanding of nutritional principles, it is sufficient to advise her to reduce her daily caloric intake by about 300 kcal and to return to prepregnancy levels for other nutrients.

If the mother has a poor understanding of nutrition, now is the time to teach her the basic principles and the importance of a well-balanced diet. Her eating habits and dietary practices will eventually be reflected in the diet of her child.

If the mother has gained excessive weight during pregnancy (or perhaps was overweight before pregnancy), a referral to the dietitian is appropriate. The dietitian can design weight-reduction diets to meet nutritional needs and food preferences. Weight loss goals of 1 to 2 lb/week are usually suggested.

In addition to meeting her own nutritional needs, the new mother will be interested in learning how to provide for her infant's nutritional needs. A discussion on infant feeding, which includes topics such as selecting infant formulas, formula preparation, and vitamin/mineral supplementation, is appropriate and generally well accepted.

Nutritional Care of Nursing Mothers

NUTRIENT NEEDS

Nutrient needs are increased during breast-feeding. Table 17–1 lists the RDA during breast-feeding for specific nutrients. Table 17–2 provides a sample daily food guide for lactating women. A few key nutrients need further discussion.

○   *CALORIES*   One of the most important factors in the diet while breast-feeding is calories. An inadequate caloric intake can reduce milk volume. However, milk quality generally remains unaffected.

The nursing mother should increase her caloric intake by 200 kcal over the pregnancy requirement (that is, a 500 kcal increase from her prepregnancy requirement). This results in a total of about 2500 to 2700 kcal per day for most women.

A good tool for the nursing mother to use in assessing the adequacy of her caloric intake is her weight. After weight stabilizes several weeks following delivery, weight loss should not exceed more than 1 lb/week for nursing mothers.

○   *PROTEIN*   As protein is an important ingredient in breast milk, an adequate intake while breast-feeding is essential. A 20 g/day increase in protein over nonpregnant needs is recommended: a total of 64 to 66 g/day. (This is 10 g/day less than is needed for pregnancy.) As in pregnancy, it is important to consume adequate nonprotein calories in order to prevent the use of protein as an energy source.

○   *CALCIUM*   Calcium is also an important ingredient in milk production, and increases over nonpregnancy needs are expected. Requirements during breast-feeding remain the same as requirements during pregnancy: an additional 400 mg/day. An inadequate intake of calcium from food sources necessitates the use of calcium supplements.

○   *IRON*   As iron is not a principal mineral component of milk, needs during lactation are not substantially different from those of nonpregnant women. However, as previously mentioned, continued supplementation of the mother for two to three months after parturition is advisable in order to replenish stores depleted by pregnancy.

○   *FLUIDS*   Liquids are especially important during lactation, since inadequate fluid intake may decrease milk volume. Fluid recommendations while breast-feeding are 8 to 10 glasses daily, including water, juice, milk, soups, etc.

COUNSELING ISSUES

In addition to counseling nursing mothers on how to meet their increased nutrient needs during breast-feeding, it is important to discuss a few issues related to infant feeding.

For example, many mothers are concerned about how specific foods they eat will affect their babies during breast-feeding. Generally there are no foods the nursing mother must avoid except those to which she might be allergic. Occasionally, however, some nursing mothers find that their babies are affected by certain foods. Onions, turnips, cabbage, chocolate, spices, and seasonings are commonly listed as offenders. The best advice to give the nursing mother is to avoid those foods she suspects cause distress in her infant. For the most part, however, she should be able to eat any nourishing food she wants without fear that her baby will be affected.

Other infant-feeding topics that should be explored include: vitamin/mineral supplementation, feeding schedules, and successful breast-feeding management. For further discussion of successful infant feeding see Chapter 30.

● The Nurse's Role

As a member of the health care team, the nurse can play an important role in the nutritional care of the pregnant woman. By following the steps outlined below, the nurse will be able to assess and improve the nutritional status of pregnant women.

Nursing Assessment

Assessment of nutritional status must be made by the health care team to facilitate planning an optimal diet with each woman. Data may be gathered from the medical record and by interviewing the woman. Information is obtained in four areas: anthropometric, biochemical, clinical, and dietary.

Assessment of anthropometric data involves pertinent information related to the woman's weight and height. For example:

- Usual nonpregnant weight (or weight before pregnancy)

- Current weight

- Height

- Weight gain during previous pregnancies

Assessment of biochemical data involves reviewing pertinent blood values, such as hematocrit and hemoglobin.

Clinical signs that are most frequently found in pregnancy include: anorexia, nausea, vomiting, constipation, and heartburn. The nurse should take note of these and other signs that may have nutritional implications.

Each person's view of nutrition and its relationship to pregnancy depends on previous teaching and dietary habits. A complete diet history is obtained to evaluate these views, as well as the specific nutrient intake of the woman. A diet history may be obtained by asking the woman to complete a 24-hour diet recall. To do this she is asked to list everything consumed in the previous 24 hours, including foods, fluids, and any supplements.

Another method of evaluating diet involves the use of a food summary. The woman is given a list of common categories of foods and asked how frequently she consumes foods from the list in a day (or week). Common categories include: vegetables, fruits, milk or cheese, meat or poultry, fish, desserts or sweets, coffee or tea, alcoholic beverages, etc. This method may be less reliable because it requires the individual to be accurate in generalizing about her intake.

In some instances the nurse will ask the woman to keep a food record or diary of everything she eats for a specified period of time (such as a week). This provides a clearer picture of nutritional patterns and may prompt the woman to make changes if the diary reveals areas of deficiency or excess.

During the data-gathering process the nurse has an opportunity to discuss important aspects of nutrition in the context of the family's needs and life-style. The nurse also seeks information about psychologic, cultural, and socio-economic factors that may influence food intake.

The nurse can use a nutritional questionnaire such as the one shown in Figure 17–4 to gather and record important facts. This information provides a data base the nurse can use to develop an intervention plan to fit the woman's individual needs. The sample questionnaire has been filled in to demonstrate this process.

Analysis and Nursing Diagnosis

Once all necessary data are obtained, the nurse begins to analyze the information and formulate appropriate nursing diagnoses. For a woman during the first trimester, for example, the diagnosis may be "Alteration in nutrition: less than body requirements related to nausea and vomiting." In many cases the diagnosis may be related to excessive weight gain. In such cases the diagnosis might be "Alteration in nutrition: more than body requirements related to excessive intake of calories." Although these diagnoses are broad, the nurse must be specific in addressing issues such as inadequate intake of nutrients such as iron, calcium, or folic acid; problems with nutrition due to a limited food budget; problems related to physiologic al-

NUTRITIONAL QUESTIONNAIRE

Name Susan Longmont   **Date** 12-16-87

Age 20

Ethnic group white middle class

Religion Protestant

Gravida 1̇   **Para** 0̇   **EDC** 7-7-88

Age of youngest child? NA

Birth weights of previous children? NA

Usual nonpregnant weight 115   **Present weight** 125

Weight gain during last pregnancy? NA

Vitamin supplements? none

Current medications? aspirin for headache

Do you smoke? yes   **How much per day?** 1-1½ packs

Eating patterns:

1. **How many meals per day?** 2 **when** 12:30 pm 6:30 pm

2. **How many snacks per day?** 3 **when** 10:30 am 4:00 pm 10:00 pm

3. **What other foods are important to your usual diet?** chocolate and candy bars

4. **Amount per day** 4 bars/week

5. **Do you have any different food preferences now?** no

6. **Do you eat nonfoods such as:**

		Amount
laundry starch	no	NA
ice	yes	10 cubes/day
other (name)	no	NA

7. **What foods do you dislike or do not eat?** spinach and dried beans

8. **For added information complete a typical daily intake (24 hour recall is suggested).**

Do you have special problems in food preparation such as:

1. Physical disability	yes	no ✓	Explain
2. Cooking appliances	yes	no ✓	Explain
3. Refrigeration of food	yes	no ✓	Explain

Who does the meal planning? I do.   **shopping?** We both do.

cooking? I do most of the time but my husband likes to help.

Are there transportation problems? We have only one car but we go in the evening.

Financial situation: My husband is working and going to school.

  I am not working.   **Foodstamps** yes   **w/c** no

Do you have any previous nutritional problems? No. I have never paid much attention

to food before, but now I have a lot of questions.

Are there any problems with this pregnancy? Nausea Yes, in the morning.

Constipation No   **Other** NA

Assessment by the nurse following the completion of the questionnaire.

Basic estimated nutrient and caloric value of typical daily intake.

Please circle one of the following:

Protein intake was	low	adequate	high
Caloric intake was	low	adequate	⟨high⟩
Calcium intake was	⟨low⟩	adequate	high
Iron intake was	⟨low⟩	adequate	high
Vitamin C intake was	low	⟨adequate⟩	high

Figure 17–4 Sample nutritional questionnaire used in nursing management of a pregnant woman

terations such as anorexia, heartburn, or nausea; and behavioral problems related to excessive dieting, anorexia nervosa, etc. In some instances the category "Knowledge deficit" may seem most appropriate.

Planning and Implementation

After the nursing diagnosis is made, the nurse can plan an approach to correct any nutritional deficiencies or improve the overall quality of the diet. To be truly effective, this plan must be made in cooperation with the pregnant woman. The following examples demonstrate ways in which the nurse can plan with the woman based on the nursing diagnosis.

EXAMPLE 1

Diagnosis: Alteration in nutrition: less than body requirements related to low intake of calcium

Implementation:

1. Plan with the woman additional milk or dairy products that can reasonably be added to the diet (specify amounts).

2. Encourage the use of other calcium sources such as leafy greens and legumes.

3. Plan for the addition of powdered milk in cooking and baking.

4. If none of the above are realistic or acceptable, consider the use of calcium supplements.

EXAMPLE 2

Diagnosis: Alteration in nutrition: more than body requirements related to excessive intake of high potency vitamins

Implementation:

1. Review need for vitamin supplements during pregnancy.

2. Discuss harmful effects to both mother and fetus of oversupplementation.

3. Recommend appropriate supplements.

EXAMPLE 3

Diagnosis: Alteration in nutrition: less than body requirements related to nausea and vomiting

Implementation:

1. Plan six or eight small meals per day.

2. Suggest foods high in carbohydrate (such as toast, dry crackers, cereal); add small serving of protein source to each snack.

3. Suggest that fluids be consumed between meals rather than with food.

4. Advise the woman to discuss with her family ways in which she can avoid situations that trigger episodes of nausea (such as the smell of frying food).

Evaluation

Once a plan has been developed and implemented, the nurse and client may wish to identify ways of evaluating its effectiveness. Evaluation may involve keeping a food journal, writing out weekly menus, returning for weekly weigh-ins, and the like. If anemia is a special problem, periodic hematocrit assessments are also indicated.

Women with serious nutritional deficiencies are referred to a nutritionist. The nurse can then work closely with the nutritionist and the client to improve the pregnant woman's health by modification of her diet.

Case Study

Mrs Jennifer Snow, age 26, is a slender and well-groomed woman. The Snows have been married for eight months. Mrs Snow is employed as a postal clerk in her hometown.

Mrs Snow is weight conscious and has attempted many fad diets to lose weight. She describes herself as having a small appetite at mealtime. She does not drink milk. Breakfast usually consists of a glass of orange juice and a piece of toast. At noon she eats a slice of cheese or hard-cooked egg plus a piece of fresh fruit. However, after work she is famished and snacks on soda pop and cookies. Mrs Snow eats a late dinner of meat, potatoes, vegetable, and a green salad. Portions are small. Before retiring for the evening, the Snows snack on potato chips, pretzels, and soda pop.

Recently, Mrs Snow has felt queasy in the morning before breakfast. After she missed her menstrual period, a pregnancy test confirmed she was two months pregnant.

The medical history and physical examination were unremarkable. A year ago, she weighed 50 kg (110 lbs). Currently she is 46 kg (101 lbs) and 164 cm (65 in) tall. Laboratory test results were: hemoglobin, 12 g/100 ml; hematocrit, 36 percent; and albumin 3.1 g/100 ml. There was no evidence of glucose, protein, or ketones in her urine.

The nurse noted a concern about Mrs Snow's weight and history of weight loss attempts. She talked with Mrs Snow about the importance of a well-balanced diet during pregnancy. Mrs Snow was given a prescription for a vitamin and iron supplement and a pamphlet on nutrition and pregnancy. An appointment was scheduled for one month later. Mrs Snow was instructed to bring the nurse a three-day food record.

During the consultation one month later, the nurse learned that Mrs Snow had not followed the diet described in the pamphlet. Her intake was approximately 1200 calories. Mrs Snow feared she would gain too much weight and lose her figure. She had gained ½ lb and reported continued nausea.

The nurse recognized that her client's concerns about weight gain were interfering with her ability to make appropriate nutritional choices. The nurse consulted with the staff dietitian who had had some experience working with this type of client. Together they met with Mrs Snow to express their concerns and to plan a nutritional approach that would accomplish the following:

1. Develop a diet that was higher in calories, protein, and essential nutrients such as calcium, while limiting fat.

2. Arrange for ongoing nutrition education and counseling for Mrs Snow, especially involving topics of interest to her.

To accomplish these goals, the nutritionist agreed to work closely with Mrs Snow following delivery to assist her in losing any remaining weight. Mrs Snow agreed to keep a food diary and to practice evaluating the nutritional content of the food she consumed. In addition to her prenatal vitamin and iron supplements, Mrs Snow began taking a calcium supplement. The nurse and dietitian discussed with Mrs Snow several approaches to relieve her nausea.

It was very difficult for Mrs Snow to change her eating habits, but she was eager to do what she could for her unborn child. She made a conscious effort to improve the nutritional quality of the foods she chose and to avoid an excessive intake of fatty convenience snack foods.

The nurse did not want Mrs Snow to begin feeling that her eating was the entire focus of each visit, so she made certain that all aspects of good prenatal care were discussed. She encouraged Mrs Snow to attend childbirth preparation classes with her husband. At one of the classes a nursing mother spoke about breast-feeding. This mother was fit and slender. Mrs Snow was able to relate to the woman and accept her advice about the importance of an adequate diet and sufficient fluid intake for successful breast-feeding.

Although it was difficult at times, Mrs Snow did improve her eating habits. She rode her bicycle several times a week and did prenatal exercises to keep toned. At term she had gained 26¼ lb. Her baby, a son, weighed 6 lb 14 oz and did well after birth. In the weeks following her delivery, Mrs Snow followed the guidelines for intake for a nursing mother. To help with weight loss she also attended postpartum exercise classes. With the advice of the nurse and dietitian and the support of her husband, Mrs Snow stabilized her weight at 112 lb. Both the Snows agreed that although they occasionally "splurged on junk food," they were far more conscious about nutrition and planned to remain so to set a good example for their young son.

KEY CONCEPTS

Maternal weight gains averaging 22 to 28 lb are associated with the best reproductive outcomes.

If the diet is adequate, folic acid and iron are the only supplements generally recommended during pregnancy.

Caloric restriction to reduce weight should not be undertaken during pregnancy.

Pregnant women should be encouraged to eat regularly and to eat a wide variety of foods, especially fresh and lightly processed foods.

Taking megadoses of vitamins during pregnancy is unnecessary and potentially dangerous.

In vegetarian diets, special emphasis should be placed on obtaining ample complete proteins, calories, calcium, iron, vitamin D, vitamin B$_{12}$, and zinc through food souces or supplementation if necessary.

Evaluation of physical, psychosocial, and cultural factors that affect food intake is essential before nutritional status can be determined and nutritional counseling planned.

Adolescents who become pregnant at a gynecological age of less than 4 years have higher nutritional needs and are considered to be at a high biological risk.

Weight gains during adolescent pregnancy must accommodate recommended gains for a normal pregnancy plus necessary gains due to growth.

After delivery, the nonnursing mother's dietary requirements return to prepregnancy levels.

Nursing mothers require an adequate calorie and fluid intake to maintain ample milk volume.

Anthropometric, biochemical, clinical, and dietary data all need to be considered when determining prenatal and postpartal nutritional status.

REFERENCES

Anderson GD: Nutrition in pregnancy, in **Sciarri** JJ (ed): *Gynecology and Obstetrics.* Philadelphia, Harper & Row, 1986, vol 2.

Clark AL (ed): *Culture, Childbearing, Health Professionals.* Philadelphia, Davis, 1978.

Cruikshank DP: Don't overdo nutritional supplements during pregnancy. *Contemp OB/GYN* 1986;27 (February):101.

Curda LR: What about pica? *J Nurs-Midwife* Spring 1977;23:8.

Food and Nutrition Board: *Recommended Dietary Allowances.* Washington, DC, National Academy of Sciences, National Research Council, 1980.

Frisancho AR, et al: Maternal nutritional status and adolescent pregnancy outcome. *Am J Clin Nutr* 1983;38:739.

Frisch RE: Fatness of girls from menarche to age 18 years, with a nomogram. *Hum Biol* 1976;48:353.

Gordon AN: *Nutritional Management of High Risk Pregnancy.* Society for Nutrition Education, 1981.

Johnstone FD: Nutrition intervention and pregnancy: What are clinicians' choices? *Contemp OB/GYN* 1984;23(January):211.

Karls L: *Nutrition for Pregnancy.* Madison, Wis, Jackson Clinic, 1983.

Luke B: Megavitamins and pregnancy: A dangerous combination. *Am J Mat Child Nurs* 1985;10(January/February):18.

Marino DD, **King** JC: Nutrition concerns during adolescence. *Pediatr Clin North Am* 1980;27:25.

Mellendick GJ: Nutritional issues in adolescence, in **Hofmann** AD (ed): *Adolescent Medicine.* Menlo Park, Calif, Addison-Wesley, 1983.

Meserole LP, et al: Prenatal weight gain and postpartum weight loss patterns in adolescents. *J Adolescent Health* 1984;5:21.

Pitkin RL: Nutrition in obstetrics and gynecology, in **Danforth** DN, **Scott** JR (eds): *Obstetrics and Gynecology,* Ed 5. Philadelphia, Lippincott, 1986.

Pritchard JA, **MacDonald** PC, **Gant** NF: *Williams' Obstetrics,* ed 17. New York, Appleton-Century-Crofts, 1985.

Cann B, et al: Benefits associated with WIC supplemental feeding during the interpregnancy interval. *Am J Clin Nutr* 1987;45(1):29.

Catanzarite VA, et al: Malnutrition during pregnancy? Consider parenteral feeding. *Contemp OB/GYN* 1986; 27(June):110.

Cerrato PL: When your patient is eating for two. *RN* 1986;49(6):67.

Corbett MA, et al: Nutritional interventions in pregnancy. *J Nurse-Midwife* 1983;28(July/August):23.

Franz MJ, et al: Exchange lists: Revised 1986. *J Am Diet Assoc* 1987;87(1):28.

Hillard PA: Preparing for pregnancy. *Parents* 1986; 61(11):238.

Rudman D, **Williams** PJ: Megadose vitamins: Use and abuse. *N Engl J Med* 1983;309(August 25):488.

Seifer DB, et al: Total parenteral nutrition in obstetrics. *JAMA* 1985;253:2073.

Stevenson DK, et al: Overfeeding and underfeeding the fetus: The plight of a vulnerable guest. *Perinat Neonat* 1985;9(6):10.

Suter CB, et al: Maternal and infant nutrition recommendations: A review. *J Am Diet Assoc* 1984;84(May):572.

Viegas OA, et al: Impaired fat deposition in pregnancy: An indicator for nutritional intervention. *Am J Clin Nutr* 1987;45(1):23.

Winick M: Maternal nutrition and fetal growth. *Perinat Neonat* 1986;10(5):28.

Wolf DM, et al: The consulting nutritionist in perinatal health care. *J Perinat* 1986;6(Fall):335.

ADDITIONAL READINGS

Allard JP: Maternal nutrition for clients in the private sector. *J Am Diet Assoc* 1986;86(8):1069.

Bull N, et al: Food habits of 15–25 year olds: Dietary patterns and nutrient intakes of young women. Part 1. *Health Visit* 1984;57(March):84.

I couldn't believe the sight of myself, belly protruding and breasts huger than they had ever been, with nipples which had suddenly doubled their size. No one had ever told me to expect such things. I was outraged. (Jane Lazarre, *The Mother Knot*)

Preparation for Parenthood

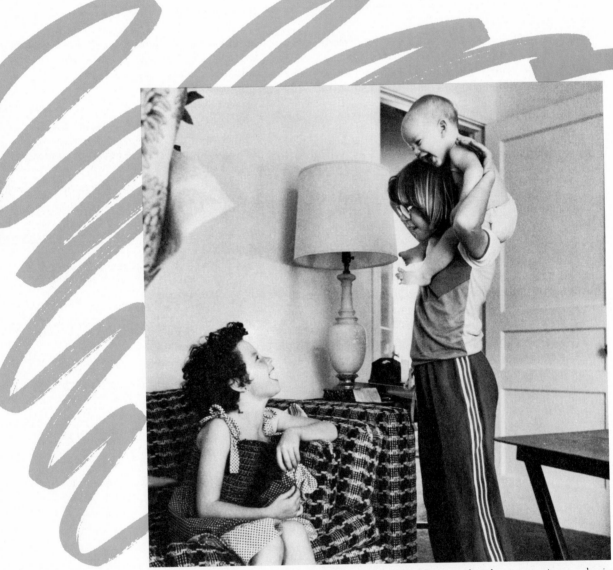

The development of healthy attitudes about parenting can begin
at an early age.

Chapter Eighteen

OBJECTIVES

- Identify the various issues related to pregnancy, labor, and delivery that require decision making by the parents.
- Discuss the basic goals of childbirth education.
- Describe the types of antepartal education programs available to expectant couples and their families.
- Discuss ways of making group teaching effective for maternity clients.
- Compare methods of childbirth preparation.

A person's preparation for parenthood begins with his or her own birth into a family. An individual's attitudes, feelings, and fears about parenthood are molded by the relationship that he or she had with his or her parents as well as observations of and encounters with other children and parents.

A person's experiences with parenting or children may have been pleasant or uncomfortable. The information an individual has about parenthood and related areas may or may not be accurate. Since people bring their beliefs

and fears with them to the childbearing period, the nurse can do much to correct misconceptions and calm fears regarding pregnancy, childbirth, and parenthood in general.

One way that a couple can cope with feelings about impending parenthood is to assume an active, participatory role during the antepartal and intrapartal periods. An active role involves the parents-to-be. It enables them to be involved in many of the decisions regarding the conduct of the birth. It offers them a degree of control over what could be an overwhelming experience.

Some of the decisions that the childbearing family must consider are presented in this chapter. The chapter addresses issues such as the choice of care provider, type of childbirth preparation, place of birth, activities during the birth, method of infant feeding, and choices surrounding treatment of the newborn. It also considers the role of the nurse, who provides information that enables the couple to make informed decisions.

Using the Nursing Process With Couples Preparing for Parenthood

Nursing Assessment

The nurse assesses the couple's information base and need for additional information. Cultural factors and developmental needs are also assessed so that the nursing plan of care can deal with the couple holistically.

Analysis and Nursing Diagnosis

After analysis of the learning needs of the couple or family, the nurse establishes appropriate nursing diagnoses. A common nursing diagnosis would be "Knowledge deficit related to informational and care needs during pregnancy and childbirth." The nurse knows that the knowledge base will affect the many decisions that face the childbearing couple.

Nursing Plan and Implementation

The nurse devises a plan to clarify learning needs and factors that may affect the learning process. The nurse assists the couple in identifying learning goals and helps the family gather information so that the decisions they make during this time are based on thorough, accurate information.

Another important nursing action is to be an advocate for the childbearing couple. As parent advocates and supporters, nurses need to provide information that reflects respect for the dignity and rights of the couple and promotes the safety of the mother and fetus. The health care information given should focus on:

- The right of the woman to know her own personal health status and the health status of her baby

- The parents' options

- Their participation in decision-making

- Responsibilities for self-care

- Treatments and their rationale

- Maintenance of family support systems

- Consideration and respect of each individual's needs

Finally, the nurse needs to operate from a sound knowledge base in order to be able to assist the parents in gaining desired information. Parent education literature and conversations with parents help the nurse stay abreast of parental concerns and trends in childbearing.

Evaluation

In the evaluation process the nurse assesses not only the success of specific teaching situations but also the adequacy of the overall nursing diagnosis. Does the couple have the knowledge base that they need? Have unknown factors interfered with the learning process? Does the couple feel confident in making the needed decisions during pregnancy, childbirth, and newborn care?

● Childbearing Decisions

When a man and woman decide to have a child or learn that they are pregnant, they are faced with many decisions. For instance, they must make decisions about who will provide health care, where their child will be born, who will attend the birth, and whether to attend prepregnancy or prenatal classes (Figure 18–1). The woman must also make decisions about whether to allow analgesia, perineal preparation, an enema, or the use of stirrups; what position to use during labor and delivery; and whether to breast-feed her child.

Some parents deal with the numerous decisions regarding childbirth by devising a birth plan. In this plan

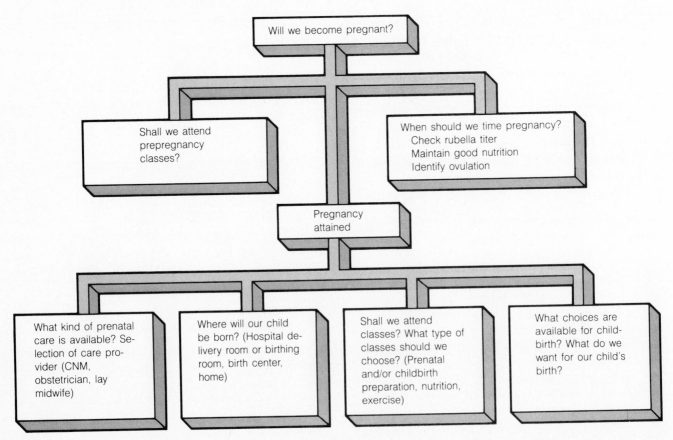

Figure 18–1 Pregnancy decision tree

they identify aspects of the childbearing experience that are most important to them. The birth plan helps identify options that may be available, and it becomes a tool for communication between the couple, the health care providers, and the birth setting. The plan helps the couple set priorities for activities that they want. A sample birth plan is presented in Figure 18–2. Once the couple has used the plan to identify their priorities, the birth plan can be shared with health care providers and can also be taken to the birth setting.

The birth plan identifies many factors associated with childbirth. One of the first decisions that the woman or couple needs to make is the type of care provider to use and how to choose that health care provider. The choice of care provider and place of birth frequently go hand in hand.

As the couple seeks information, nurses can assist in the decision-making process. The nurse can discuss various types of care providers so that the couple knows what to expect from each type. The couple needs to know the differences between the educational preparation, skill level, and general philosophy of certified nurse-midwives, obstetricians, family practice physicians, and lay midwives. The nurse also provides information about different types of birth settings and assists the couple in obtaining further information through tours of facilities and reading. Questions regarding the care provider's credentials, basic and special education and training, fee schedule, and availability for new patients can be answered by telephoning a receptionist in the office. As the couple prepares to interview different care providers, they may want to develop a list of questions so that they will learn the desired information during the interview process. Sample questions may include:

- Who is in practice with you, or who covers for you when you are off?

- How do your partners' philosophies compare to yours?

- What are your feelings about my partner (or other children) coming to the prenatal visits?

- What weight gain do you recommend and why?

- How many of your parents attend prenatal and/or childbirth preparation classes, and what type do they choose?

- What are your feelings about (add in special desires for the birth event, such as, different positions during labor, episiotomy, induction of labor, other people being present during birth, breast-feeding immedi-

Figure 18–2 Birth plan for childbirth choices ⟶

Choice	I would like to have		Available	
	Yes	No	Yes	No
Care provider				
Certified nurse-midwife	——	——	——	——
Obstetrician	——	——	——	——
Lay midwife	——	——	——	——
Birth setting				
Hospital:				
Birthing room	——	——	——	——
Delivery room	——	——	——	——
Birth center	——	——	——	——
Home	——	——	——	——
Partner present				
During labor	——	——	——	——
During birth	——	——	——	——
During cesarean	——	——	——	——
During whole postpartum period	——	——	——	——
During labor				
Ambulate as desired	——	——	——	——
Shower if desired	——	——	——	——
Wear own clothes	——	——	——	——
Use hot tub	——	——	——	——
Use own rocking chair	——	——	——	——
Have perineal prep	——	——	——	——
Have enema	——	——	——	——
Electronic fetal monitor	——	——	——	——
Membranes:				
Rupture naturally	——	——	——	——
Amniotomy if needed	——	——	——	——
Labor stimulation if needed	——	——	——	——
Medication:				
Identify type desired	——	——	——	——
Fluids or ice as desired	——	——	——	——
Music during labor and birth	——	——	——	——
During birth				
Position:				
On side	——	——	——	——
Hands and knees	——	——	——	——
Kneeling	——	——	——	——
Squatting	——	——	——	——
Birthing chair	——	——	——	——
Birthing bed	——	——	——	——
Other:	——	——	——	——
Family present (sibs)	——	——	——	——
Filming of birth	——	——	——	——
Leboyer	——	——	——	——
Episiotomy	——	——	——	——
No sterile drapes	——	——	——	——
Partner to cut umbilical cord	——	——	——	——
Hold baby immediately after birth	——	——	——	——
Breast-feed immediately after birth	——	——	——	——
No separation after birth	——	——	——	——
Save the placenta	——	——	——	——
Newborn care:				
Eye treatment for the baby	——	——	——	——
Vitamin K injection	——	——	——	——
Breast-feeding	——	——	——	——
Formula feeding	——	——	——	——
Glucose water	——	——	——	——
Circumcision	——	——	——	——
Feeding on demand	——	——	——	——
Postpartum care:				
Rooming-in	——	——	——	——
Short stay	——	——	——	——
Sibling visitation	——	——	——	——
Infant care classes	——	——	——	——
Self-care classes	——	——	——	——
Other:				

Research Note

The home birth movement of the 1970s was accompanied by increased consumer demands for in-hospital childbirth alternatives. Chute compared the expectations and actual experiences of clients who chose a nurse-midwife for their care provider with clients who chose a more traditional physician care provider. Chute gave 15 nurse-midwife clients and 18 physician clients a pre- and postdelivery questionnaire to evaluate physical activities, decision making, and focus of attention during labor and delivery.

The predelivery questionnaires revealed that clients of nurse-midwives expected to take more active roles in their birth experiences, and the postdelivery questionnaires revealed that they actually did take more active roles than the physician clients. However, women in the nurse-midwife group reported a greater discrepancy between predelivery expectations and actual delivery experience than the physician group. The questionnaires also indicated that nurse-midwife clients saw themselves and their partners as the most important individuals contributing to the satisfaction of the experience, while the physician clients more often viewed the infant as most important.

Chute pointed out that until birth options become more widely available, nurses need to encourage in-depth collaborative planning with clients, especially in areas where participation is important to the client, in order to facilitate satisfying birth experiences.

Chute GE: Expectation and experience in alternative and conventional birth. *J Obstet Gynecol Neonat Nurs* 1985;14(January/Febuary):61–66.

ately after delivery, no separation of infant and parents following birth, and so on).

- If a cesarean is necessary could my partner be present?

The couple will also need to discuss the qualities that they want in a care provider for their newborn. They will probably want to visit with care providers prior to birth in order to select one who meets their needs.

Choosing a care provider is just one of the myriad of choices and decisions with which the couple is faced (see Table 18–1). Another area of decision making is demonstrated in the following situation.

Mr and Mrs Cline were discussing newborn care with Ms Gayle, the clinic nurse during one of their prenatal appointments. The Cline's had been gathering information about the clothes that are needed and about infant feeding but had not yet considered whether to use cloth or disposable diapers. They wanted some help in getting information. Ms Gayle suggested that they collect information from a variety of sources. Together they devised a plan to obtain information regarding cost, convenience, and any implications for their baby. They called a number of stores to determine the prices for cloth and disposable diapers. They investigated the cost of diaper service, as well as the cost of laundering their own diapers. They found that laundering their own diapers was the least expensive, but having a diaper service was only about a dollar more a week, and the convenience was important because of the work schedule that both the Cline's would have to keep even after the baby was born. Disposables were the most expensive and were almost double the cost of laundering their own diapers (Martin 1985). They had seen coupons for disposables and knew that that would affect the price, but they anticipated having a storage problem with the boxes if they purchased many at once. They reviewed current literature regarding implications for their baby and found comments regarding health care concerns (Solomon 1986) and the possibility of foreign body hazards (Johnson 1985) with disposables.

The Clines were surprised at the amount of information they were gathering. One other concern began to surface due to their concerns for ecology. They noted that they needed to consider the implications of a natural product (cotton cloth diapers) vs. the use of natural resources (trees) to create disposable diapers. They were also concerned when they learned that 1 million plastic diapers are discarded every day and do not decompose (Nat'l Assoc of Diaper Services 1986). The Clines studied all the information and—based on cost, convenience, identified concerns for their baby, and ecological concerns—decided to have a diaper service. They shared their information with Ms Gayle and put together a packet for other parents to review if they wanted to.

The Clines felt they had investigated the questions thoroughly and were able to make an informed decision.

Although most birth experiences are very close to the desired experience, at times the expectations cannot be met. This may be due to unavailability of some choices in the couple's community or the presence of unexpected problems during pregnancy or birth. It is important for nurses to help expectant parents keep sight of what is realistic and possible and to help them understand that when choices are made alternatives may be needed (Sandelowski 1984).

● Birthing Environments: Choices

The maternity nurse needs to be aware of all birthing settings and their similarities and differences. Until recently the most prevalent setting for labor and delivery was a hospital labor unit, composed of separate labor rooms, delivery rooms, and recovery area, and a different unit for the remaining hospital stay. This type of unit is still available in some hospitals. However, many hospitals have

Table 18–1 Some Consumer Decisions During Pregnancy and Labor and Delivery

Issue	Benefits	Risks
Breast-feeding	No additional expense Contains maternal antibodies Decreases incidence of infant otitis media, vomiting, and diarrhea Easier to digest than formula Immediately after delivery, promotes uterine contractions and decreases incidence of postpartum hemorrhage	Transmission of pollutants to newborn Irregular ovulation and menses can cause false sense of security and nonuse of contraceptives. Increased nutritional requirement in mother
Perineal prep	May decrease risk of infection Facilitates episiotomy repair	Nicks can be portal for bacteria Discomfort as hair grows back
Enema	May facilitate labor Increases space for infant in pelvis May increase strength of contractions May prevent contamination of sterile field	Increases discomfort and anxiety
Ambulation during labor	Comfort for laboring woman May assist in labor progression by: a. Stimulating contractions b. Allowing gravity to help descent of fetus c. Giving sense of independence and control	Cord prolapse with ruptured membranes unless engagement has occurred Delivery of infant in undesirable situations
Electronic fetal monitoring	Helps evaluate fetal well-being Helps diagnose fetal distress Useful in diagnostic testing Helps evaluate labor progress	Supine postural hypotension Intrauterine perforation (with internal monitoring) Infection (with internal monitoring) Decreases personal interaction with mother because of attention paid to the machine Mother is unable to ambulate or change her position freely
Oxytocin	Decreases incidence of cesarean birth with augmentation of labor Restimulates labor in cases of slowing contractions resulting from epidural blocks or uterine atony	Hyperstimulated contractions interfere with oxygenation of fetus Uterine rupture Early placental separation
Analgesia	Maternal relaxation facilitates labor	All drugs reach the fetus in varying degrees and with varying effects
Delivery position (lithotomy) (see Chapter 23 for further discussion of positions)	Ease of visualization of perineum by birth attendant Facilitates elective operative intervention, if necessary	Increases need for episiotomy May decrease normal intensity of contractions
Stirrups	Assist in positioning for pushing (can be used in side-lying position) Comfortable for some women Convenient for the person delivering the baby	Supine postural hypotension Uncomfortable for some women Leg cramping and/or palsy Increased chance of tearing the perineum Thrombophlebitis Prolonged 2nd stage due to ineffective positioning for pushing
Episiotomy	Decreases irregular tearing of perineum May decrease stretch and loss of sexual pleasure after pregnancy	Painful healing May spasm during sexual intercourse due to poor repair Permanent scarring with certain episiotomies Infection

Sources: Burst H: The influence of consumers on the birthing movement. *Topics Clin Nurs* 1983;5(October):42, Hotchner T: *Pregnancy and Childbirth: A Complete Guide for a New Life.* New York, Avon Books, 1979.

changed their labor and delivery units to reflect the philosophy of family-centered care. In the newer units, the woman is not moved from room to room during labor and delivery.

Couples in some communities also have the option of delivering in a free-standing birth center. These facilities have been created in answer to consumer demand for a more homelike, natural setting for their childbearing experience. The childbearing consumer wants to know what is happening, to maintain a sense of dignity, and to maintain control over what the childbearing experience will be (Burst 1983).

For the small number of couples who feel that even the family-centered hospital setting or a free-standing birth center do not offer them enough control, home birth is another possibility.

Choices are important. They determine how you experience giving birth and how your baby enters the world. They must be made in the present and lived with in the future. (*Pregnant Feelings*)

The Hospital Setting

Hospitals' initial responses to criticism about the traditional hospital labor unit previously described has resulted in the development of *single-purpose units*. In these units, the woman stays in the same room for labor, delivery, and recovery. The rooms have various names, but most commonly they are called birthing rooms. To decrease confusion about what happens in these rooms, however, hospital staff may call them LDR rooms (labor, delivery, recovery).

More recently, maternity wards in some hospitals are converting some or all of their rooms so that the woman remains in one room throughout her hospitalization. Thus the woman remains in the same room from admission for labor until her postpartum discharge. The healthy newborn baby may remain continuously at the bedside of the mother if she desires. Flexibility in rules and regulations, however, varies from one hospital to another and seems to be directed by the philosophy of the hospital and birthing unit. When the philosophy is truly family centered there is a working framework of humanistic care in which the childbearing woman is treated with respect and is viewed as a full participant in the childbearing experience (Chute 1985).

The physical environment for these units varies tremendously. The units usually provide a bathroom and family sitting area. More extensive environmental changes may include additional room for the family sitting area and a kitchenette (Young 1982). Whatever the physical layout, a nonmedical environment is promoted, which includes keeping all required equipment out of view until needed (Young 1982). Hospitals refer to these units as family birthing centers, but the staff may refer to them as LDRPP units (labor, delivery, recovery, and postpartum) to clarify their function.

Changes in the hospital environment alone cannot ensure family-centered childbirth. The philosophy of the health team is significant in promoting the concept of family-centered care. It is possible, for example, that the only difference between these new units and the traditional labor and delivery units is that the woman remains in the same unit throughout her hospitalization. In this case, the only acceptable position for delivery would be supine with the woman's legs in stirrups. The health team would wear caps and masks; the birth attendant would wear full sterile attire and use abdominal and leg drapes. Immediately after birth, the newborn would be placed in the radiant-heat unit until the birth attendant had finished interventions needed to complete the birthing process. In other words, a more medically oriented environment would prevail.

If the health team truly supported the changing concepts of family-centered care, however, the scene at delivery would be very different from the previous description. Stirrups would not be used in positioning the woman for delivery. The woman would be encouraged to use alternative positions that promoted her comfort. Members of the health team would not wear caps and masks; the birth attendant would not wear a sterile gown; and the use of sterile drapes would be minimal. The baby would be placed in the mother's arms immediately after delivery, and siblings and/or other family members would be present, in addition to the support person. In short, a more relaxed, natural, and homelike atmosphere would be provided.

Nurses can help promote a family-centered approach to hospital births, but to do so the traditional approach to staffing must be modified. In traditional hospital units, there are labor and delivery nurses, postpartal nurses, and newborn nursery nurses; each type of nurse has different responsibilities. In LDR and LDRPP units, a nurse needs to be knowledgeable about and deliver care during all phases of the childbearing experience. For example, the nurse who previously functioned as a labor and delivery nurse will be expected to incorporate the knowledge and skills of the postpartal and newborn nurse in the repertoire of nursing responsibilities.

Thus, for family-centered care to become a reality in many hospitals, nurses may require further education and preparation. There must also be education, communication, and cooperation among different medical specialties if family-centered maternity care is to be fully implemented (May and Ditolla 1984).

Free-Standing Birth Centers

Care in free-standing birth centers is given by certified nurse-midwives, labor and delivery nurses, nurse practitioners, physicians, nonmedical assistants, public health nurses, families themselves, or any combination of these. *Birth centers* require families to take more responsibility for the birth experience than usual while at the same time providing a more flexible and less costly way to give birth.

Birth centers strive for a warm, homelike atmosphere, with birthing rooms similar to typical bedrooms. The room is generally furnished with a bed, in which the woman labors and delivers, comfortable chairs for the father and other relatives or friends, a cradle, and private bath and/or shower. Some free-standing centers also have play rooms for siblings, kitchens where families may keep food or beverages, and other amenities. Most free-standing centers encourage children to participate to whatever extent they choose. Many hospital-based centers are somewhat more reluctant to allow total participation by siblings.

Birth centers meet criteria for maintaining safety in out-of-hospital births. These criteria include: attendance by qualified health care professionals, screening and transfer criteria, a transport system immediately available, and a readily accessible backup physician and hospital facility (Burst 1983).

In keeping with the concept of birth as a normal event, most birth center settings are set up for nurse-midwife management of labor and delivery rather than for obstetric technology and treatment. Therefore, these centers are not appropriate for high-risk deliveries. Couples intending to use the centers are screened during pregnancy for high-risk factors (see Chapter 19). The presence of any one factor does not automatically exclude the woman from delivering in a birth center, but it does mean that careful and continuous assessment is needed.

...what I've seen time and again is that the technology of the hospital overwhelms patients' natural instincts; they are intimidated, afraid of appearing stupid or clumsy or sentimental in a surrounding that seems too efficient and immaculate and intelligent. (A Midwife's Story)

Each center also has policies about various circumstances that would require the woman to be transferred to a hospital labor and delivery setting. These may include, but are not limited to, the following:

- An increase in maternal temperature to over 100.4F (37.8C)

- A significant change in blood pressure

- Meconium-stained amniotic fluid

- Prolonged true labor

- Significant vaginal bleeding

- Prolonged second stage of labor (more than two hours for a nullipara and more than one hour for a multipara)

- Indications of fetal distress

The couple is usually required to attend prenatal classes to prepare for childbirth. They are also encouraged to meet birthing center personnel and to discuss their desires and preferences.

Traditional obstetric procedures are frequently not used. Episiotomies are not routine, forceps are not used, and in many centers the woman may deliver in the position of her choice. After delivery, physical contact between the parents and newborn is encouraged. The mother may breast-feed immediately. Siblings and accompanying support persons are also encouraged to interact with the newborn as they choose.

In most instances, rooming-in is immediate, and healthy newborns and their families are never separated. The initial pediatric examination is conducted in the presence of the family. The mother and newborn are monitored for 2 to 24 hours after delivery and then discharged.

Birth center personnel usually perform a home visit after discharge. The home visit provides an opportunity to see the family in their home setting, to make assessments of the mother and newborn, to answer questions, and to provide information and support.

Home Births

Another alternative to the traditional hospital delivery is home birth. Couples who choose home birth generally have strong beliefs about their rights to make their own birth choices. Couples choosing home births believe that the responsibility for the birth outcome is theirs. Furthermore, they do not believe the hospital is necessarily the safest place to give birth, and they see standard medical practice as frequently involving unnecessary trauma and intervention. Some women may feel that hospital routines and expectations will not allow them to conform to their cultural norms for childbearing behavior (Brackbill et al 1984).

In making the choice between home and hospital birth, medical risk is only one issue. The effect on the family unit is another issue. Parents who take responsibility for a home delivery feel that it is a warm, close, loving experience under their control. The newborn is immediately incorporated into the family, and the continuous contact between the newborn and the family helps to bond the family as a unit. Siblings present during delivery are able to welcome the newborn into the family and are participants in an exciting and beautiful experience.

The safety of any home birth is maximized by thorough planning, careful prenatal care and screening, skilled physicians or nurse-midwives, and an organized and tested transport system to a facility where accepting care givers are available. However, adequate medical backup care is frequently unobtainable. Obstetricians as a group are particularly vocal opponents of home birth. Their opposition is often based on memories of serious emergencies they have witnessed at the time of birth. Therefore, they usually view home birth as a backward step in maternal child care. For the small number of physicians who would participate in home births, the increase in malpractice insurance is prohibitive.

An unfortunate side-effect of physician opposition has been that home births, when they do occur, are even less safe (Zimmerman 1980). Physicians may refuse to supervise the prenatal care of a couple planning a home birth or may refuse to attend one. Many physicians also refuse to act as backup caregivers for home births. Hospital personnel in general also tend to oppose home birth. They may manifest this disapproval through punishing attitudes when couples unable to complete birth at home come to the hospital. Despite the opposition, however, the trend toward home births seems to be growing rather than slowing.

Some religious groups plan and carry out home births without any prenatal care or trained attendants at birth. In this case maternal and perinatal mortality are far beyond the national statistics (Kaunitz et al 1984).

Home deliveries may be attended by a certified nurse-midwife (contingent upon the laws of respective states) or physician, but most often the birth attendant is a lay midwife. Certified nurse-midwives are well educated, skilled practitioners whose scope of practice is closely regulated by state nurse practice acts, but CNM attendance at home birth is a controversial issue even within the profession. Lay midwives may or may not have formal education; some states have a program of certification, and others consider their practice unlawful.

Choosing the Birth Setting

Information regarding the birth setting can be obtained from tours of the facilities and from talking with nurses and recent parents. Expectant couples may ask the parents the following questions:

- What kind of support did you receive during labor? Was it what you wanted?

- If the setting has both labor and delivery rooms and birthing rooms, was a birthing room available when you wanted it?

- Were you encouraged to be mobile during labor or to do what you wanted to do (walking, sitting in a rocking chair, remaining in bed, sitting in a hot tub, standing in a shower, and so on)?

- Was your labor partner or coach treated well?

- Was your birth plan respected? Did you share it with the facility before the birth? If something didn't work, why do you think there were problems?

- How were medications handled during labor? Were you comfortable with it?

- Were siblings welcomed in the birth setting? After the birth?

- Was the nursing staff helpful after the baby was born? Did you receive self-care and infant care information? Was it in a usuable form? Did you have a choice about what information you got? Did they let you decide what information you needed?

The prospective parents have many choices of birth settings available to them. It is important to ascertain the care providers' philosophy early in the pregnancy as it may affect the possibility of using some birth settings.

● Siblings at Birth

More couples are choosing to extend the family-centered concept beyond mother, father, and newborn by including their other children in the birth experience. Many hospitals have yet to develop programs that allow siblings to visit the baby; having siblings attend a birth is an even rarer option. However, families who strongly wish their children to attend will probably find a way, even if they must create their own birthing situation.

The decision to have children present at birth is a personal and individual one. Children who will attend a birth can be prepared through books, audiovisual materials, models, and parental discussion. Nurses can assist parents with sibling preparation by helping them understand the stresses a child may experience. For example, the child may feel left out when there is a new child to love, or a brother may come when a sister was expected (MacLaughlin & Johnston 1984). (For further discussion of sibling preparation, see p. 449.)

It is highly recommended that the child have his or her own support person or coach whose sole responsibility is tending to the needs of the child. The support person should be well known to the child, warm, sensitive, flexible, knowledgeable about the birth process, and comfortable with sexuality and birth. This person must be prepared to interpret what is happening to the child and intervene when necessary (Daniels 1983).

The child should be given the option of relating to the birth in whatever manner he or she chooses as long as it is not disruptive. Children should understand that it is their own choice to be there and that they may stay or leave the room as they choose. To help the child meet his or her goal, the nurse may wish to elicit from the child exactly what he or she expects from the experience. The child needs to feel free to ask questions and express feelings (Daniels 1983).

Many agencies are concerned about neonatal infection when siblings are present. However, recent studies have demonstrated that sibling contact with newborns does not increase bacterial colonization rates in the newborn (Kowba & Schwirian 1985, Wranesh 1982). Parents are requested not to bring children who are obviously ill. Children are requested to perform an antiseptic scrub and put on a cover gown. In agencies that allow siblings to visit only after the birth, infection has not been an issue.

In general, the presence of siblings at birth engenders feelings of interest and the desire to nurture "our" baby, as opposed to jealousy and rivalry directed at "Mom's" baby. The mother does not disappear mysteriously to the hospital and return with a demanding outsider. Instead, the family attending delivery together finds a new opportunity for closeness and growth by sharing in the birth of a new member. In a study by Krutsky (1985), parents viewed the children's presence as positive, felt it added to family unity, and would have the children present again. Another group of parents who had siblings present at birth felt that sharing the birth experience brought the family closer together. In addition, the parents thought that the event was a good learning experience and taught the child that birth was normal. Finally, the parents felt that the

Research Note

This researcher explores clients' expectations of childbirth classes and differences in male and female expectations. Two groups of 50 clients were selected for study: one group who had not yet begun classes, and one group who were one month postdelivery. The pre-class group was asked by questionnaire why they had enrolled in classes, their interest level in specified topics, and their expectations of the classes. The postdelivery group was asked reasons for enrolling, the usefulness of specified topics, and the usefulness of the classes.

Responses showed that, while all subjects were interested in the same general topics, men were more interested in factual information about labor and childbirth, infant development and child care, and women were more interested in gaining confidence and in improving their ability to cope. Pre-class clients expressed a greater interest in learning about the signs and symptoms of pregnancy, while postdelivery clients thought the hospital tour and breathing and relaxation techniques were most useful. Both groups agreed that information about electronic monitoring, cesarean birth, and new tests and procedures were of least importance. Of the postdelivery group, 53 percent of the men and 64 percent of the women felt the classes met their expectations or exceeded them.

This author suggests that a flexible approach to childbirth classes would best meet the needs of a particular group of clients and that the traditional 6- to 10-week course may be too short to cover topics of interest in adequate depth. She suggests that regular childbirth education classes only deal with incidental questions on topics of low interest, and that additional reading and supplementary classes on these topics be made available to those clients with a specific interest.

Maloney R: Childbirth education classes: Expectant parents' expectations. *J Obstet Gynecol Neonat Nurs* 1985;14(May/June):245–48.

presence of the siblings made the baby feel welcome and provided memories that the family could share for many years (Clark 1986).

● Classes for Family Members During Pregnancy

Prenatal Education

Antepartal educational programs vary in their goals, content, leadership techniques, and method of teaching. The content of a class is generally dictated by its goals. For example, if the goal of a class is to prepare the couple for childbirth, it does not address the discomforts of pregnancy and the care of the newborn. Other classes may focus only on pregnancy, not labor and delivery. Special classes are also available for couples who know that the woman will be having a cesarean delivery. Nurses should be aware of couples' goals before directing them to specific classes.

ONE-TO-ONE TEACHING

Teaching on an individual basis occurs when the woman needs it. Anticipatory guidance is also a positive part of teaching and is useful for discussing such topics as care of the breasts in pregnancy, sexual activity, and preparation for labor and delivery.

The nurse makes use of teaching strategies that enhance the learning process. DiFloria and Duncan (1986) have identified several components of the teaching process that can make the nurse a more effective teacher. Some of these components are:

1. Identification of an instructional goal: What does the educator want the couple to know, or what does the learner want to know?

2. Analysis of the characteristics of the learner and the information that needs to be learned.

3. Identification of behavioral objectives: What will the learner learn, or what behavior will be demonstrated?

4. Selection of teaching strategies: What method will be most appropriate for the situation?

5. The actual teaching situation with presentation of information.

6. Evaluation of the teaching session. Does the couple have the information they needed? Do they feel they can make informed decisions? Do they know where to seek further information?

7. Revision of the teaching plan to address components identified in the evaluation process.

Incorporating these components helps the nurse be more successful in teaching situations.

Nurses' teaching skills improve as they broaden their base of knowledge and become more aware of the needs of expectant families. A continuous evaluation of the effectiveness of one's teaching is essential in developing these skills.

GROUP TEACHING

Group discussion is a useful teaching method. In group teaching, the nurse asesses the needs of the group instead of the needs of an individual. Skill in dealing with groups is essential. Skill in teaching groups can be developed in several ways, including professional reading on the subject, attendance at workshops or courses, and ongoing practice. The following guidelines identify some basic principles of effective group teaching:

- Groups of couples should contain no more than 20 individuals.

- Groups of mothers only should be smaller.

- The environment should be informal and friendly.

- Members should be encouraged to attend consistently, and other activities should be encouraged to increase group cohesiveness.

Helping the group to set an agenda at the initial session is one way of assessing members' needs. The individuals in the group must become comfortable with each other so that they feel free to share concerns, questions, and information.

Nursing intervention during group discussion takes many forms and frequently overlaps with assessment and evaluation as specific interests and concerns are clarified. The nurse may need to draw other members into the discussion or to clarify information. However, most prenatal classes are not purely discussion groups but include films, tours of maternity wards, demonstrations, and lengthy explanations. In classes concerned with selected methods of childbirth preparation, many group members may have read extensively on the subject and can contribute considerably to the discussion. Other members may know nothing about the topic and thus require more explanations and demonstrations by the nurse. In situations where group members know little about the method, a more structured approach to discussion and exercises may be useful.

Evaluation of the teaching-learning process is continuous and difficult. For example, checking each individual's performance after demonstration of an exercise is the most concrete way to evaluate learning. Evaluating members' changes in attitude or misconceptions is more difficult. A general evaluation of the series may be conducted in the last class, or the nurse can give group members evaluation forms to return by mail (Whitley 1985).

Class Content

Childbirth preparation classes usually contain information regarding changes in the woman and the developing baby.

From the expectant parents' point of view, class content is best presented in chronology with the pregnancy. While both parents expect to learn breathing and relaxation techniques and infant care, fathers usually expect facts and mothers expect coping strategies (Maloney 1985).

Overall, the content areas of most classes include:

Prenatal care and planning

- Obtaining the type of care desired (birth setting and care provider)

- Nutritional, exercise, and rest needs

- Prenatal discomforts and self-care measures

Fetal developmental concerns

- Drugs

- Inadequate diet

- Environmental hazards

Impact of pregnancy and new baby on the family

- Developmental tasks

- Introduction to parenting skills and information

- Dealing with sibling rivalry

Childbirth

- Preparation for childbirth through exercises, relaxation techniques, breathing techniques

- Information regarding labor and delivery

- Information about the possibility of a cesarean delivery and specific coping mechanisms

Postpartum care

- Self-care

- Infant care

- Feeding methods

At times prenatal classes are divided into early and late classes.

Early Classes: First Trimester

Early prenatal classes should include both couples in early pregnancy and prepregnant couples. The classes contain information regarding early gestational changes, self-care during pregnancy, fetal development and environmental dangers for the fetus, sexuality in pregnancy, birth settings and types of care providers, nutrition, rest and exercise suggestions, common discomforts of pregnancy and relief measures, psychological changes in pregnancy for the woman and man, and information needed to get the pregnancy off to a good start. Early classes should provide information about factors that place the woman at risk for preterm labor and recognition of possible signs and symptoms of preterm labor. Early classes should also include information on advantages and disadvantages of breast- and bottle feeding. Studies indicate that the majority of women (50 percent to 80 percent) have made their infant feeding decision before the sixth month of pregnancy, so information in an early prenatal class would be helpful (Aberman & Kirchoff 1985).

Later Classes: Second and Third Trimesters

The later classes focus on preparation for the birth, infant care and feeding, postpartum self-care, birth choices (episiotomy, medications, fetal monitoring, perineal prep, enema, and so forth). Safety issues regarding the newborn should also be included. One of the first issues the new parents encounter is use of a car seat. Since many parents purchase the car seat prior to birth, later classes should include information regarding how car seats work, the importance of car seats, and how to select an approved car seat (Davis 1985).

Adolescents have special content learning needs during pregnancy. In a recent study by Levenson, Smith, and Morrow (1986), teens identified informational needs according to priority. The most important areas of concern were: how to be a good parent, how to care for the new baby, health dangers to the baby, and healthy foods to eat during pregnancy. The teens stated that the need for information about these areas continues after the birth of the baby. Howard and Sater (1985) found that informational needs are relatively consistent after birth. Teens in their study identified the highest priority items as how to recognize when the baby is sick, take care of the baby, protect the baby from accidents, and make the baby feel happy and loved.

Breast-Feeding Programs

Programs offering prenatal and postpartal information on breast-feeding are becoming more numerous. For many years, the primary source of information has been La Leche League. However, information can also be obtained from birthing centers, hospitals, health clinics, and individuals such as lactation consultants (Edwards 1985). Informational content seems to be similar and includes advantages-disadvantages, techniques of breast-feeding, and

methods of breast preparation (Lauwers & Woessner 1983). The father is being included in the educational programs more frequently as his support and encouragement is vital and it is important to include him in decision making. Some fathers feel negative and resentful about breast-feeding and need opportunities in the prenatal period for discussion and sharing of information (Jordan 1986).

Prepared Sibling Programs

The birth of a new sibling is a significant event in a child's life. It may be associated with negative behavior toward the newborn, withdrawal, and sleep problems. More positively, the child seems to increase in developmental maturity after the birth of a sibling (Marecki et al 1985). With increased emphasis on family-centered birth, siblings are now being included in the birthing process. Their involvement may include visiting during labor, being present at birth, and/or visiting in the postpartal period.

Classes that prepare the sibling for attendance at labor and/or delivery are becoming more prevalent. Such classes may have from one to four or more sessions.

Classes for siblings usually involve a tour of the maternity ward where the children will visit their mothers. Children usually show interest in such items as television sets, electric beds, and telephones the mothers will use to call them. The youngsters can climb on footstools at the nursery window to see the new babies. Most tours involve a visit to a birthing room, but not to delivery rooms. After the tour, the children have an opportunity to see and hear more about what happens to the parents and newborn in the hospital, how babies are born, and what babies are like. This teaching usually involves a combination of books, audiovisual materials, models, parental discussion, formal classes, and play experiences. Children also have the opportunity to discuss their feelings about having a new baby in the family (MacLaughlin & Johnston 1984). Discussion sessions may be divided into two age groups if the ages of the attending children vary greatly.

After the class, parents usually receive additional resources that tell how to prepare children for a baby in the family. Some programs award certificates to the children who attended, offer refreshments to the children and their parents, and give gift packets with articles similar to those new mothers receive (lotion, diapers for the new baby, etc).

Classes that prepare children for attendance at birth vary. It is important that the children be at least familiar with what to expect during the labor and delivery: how the parents will act, especially the sounds and faces the mother may make; what they will see, including the messiness, blood, and equipment; and how the baby will look and act at birth. In addition, parents are encouraged to involve the child early in the pregnancy, including taking the child on a prenatal visit to see the birth attendant and listen to the fetal heart beat. Most advocates feel the child also needs to be comfortable with seeing the mother without clothes prior to seeing her during labor and delivery.

Classes for Grandparents

Grandparents are an important source of support and information for prospective and new parents. They are now being included in the birthing process more frequently. Prenatal programs for grandparents can be an important source of information regarding current beliefs and practices in childbearing. The most useful content may include changes in birthing and parenting practices and helpful tips for being a supportive grandparent. Some grandparents are integral members of the labor and birth experience and also need information on being a coach (Horn & Manion 1985).

● Education of the Family Having Cesarean Birth

Preparation for Cesarean Birth

Cesarean birth is an alternative method of delivery. Since one out of every five deliveries is a cesarean, preparation for this possibility should be an integral part of every childbirth education curriculum. The instructor should present factual information that will allow a couple to make choices and participate in their birth experience. The instructor can emphasize the similarities between cesarean and vaginal births to minimize undertones of "normal" versus "abnormal" delivery (Affonso 1981). This will diminish feelings of anger, loss, and grief.

Fawcett and Burritt (1985) investigated the effectiveness of a prenatal education program regarding cesarean birth. The couples were given a pamphlet containing information about cesarean birth: What happens during a cesarean birth, what the parents will feel, and what the parents can do. The pamphlet was followed by a home visit or telephone call to emphasize the information and provide time for questions. Their findings indicated that parents found the program very helpful and useful.

All couples should be encouraged to discuss with their physician or nurse-midwife what the approach would be in the event of a cesarean. They can also discuss their needs and desires. Their preferences may include the following:

- Participating in the choice of anesthetic

- Father (or significant other) being present during the procedure

Preparation for Repeat Cesarean Birth

When a couple is anticipating a repeat cesarean birth, they have time to analyze and synthesize the information and to prepare for some of the specifics. Many hospitals or local groups (such as C/Sec, Inc) provide preparation classes for cesarean birth. Couples who have had previous negative experiences need an opportunity to describe what they felt contributed to their feelings. They should be en-

Table 18–2 Summary of Selected Childbirth Preparation Methods

Method	Characteristics	Breathing techniques
Lamaze	See narrative discussion.	
Read	First of the 'natural' childbirth methods. Method utilizes information on progressive relaxation techniques and on abdominal breathing.	Primarily abdominal. Woman concentrates on forcing the abdominal muscles to rise. Works on slowing number of respirations per minute so that she can take one breath/ minute (30 sec inhalation and 30 sec exhalation). Slow abdominal breathing used during first stage. Rapid chest breathing used toward end of labor if abdominal breathing not sufficient; panting is used to prevent pushing until needed.
Bradley	Frequently referred to as partner- or husband-coached natural childbirth. The exercises used to accomplish relaxation and slow controlled breathing are basically those used in the Read method.	Primarily abdominal as in Read method.
Kitzinger	Uses sensory memory to help the woman understand and work with her body in preparation for birth. Incorporates the Stanislavsky method of acting as a way to teach relaxation.	Uses chest breathing in conjunction with abdominal relaxation.
Hypnosis	Basic technique of hypnosis used in obstetrics is called hypnoreflexogenous method and is a combination of hypnosis and conditioned reflexes. Specific techniques of producing anesthesia and analgesia are not taught, but they are believed to be by-products of the method (Werner et al 1982).	Normal breathing pattern.

couraged to identify what they would like to change and to list interventions that would make the experience more positive. Those who have had positive experiences need reassurance that their needs and desires will be met in the same manner. In addition, couples need an opportunity to discuss any fears or anxieties.

A specific concern of the woman facing a repeat cesarean is anticipation of the pain. She needs reassurance that subsequent cesareans are often less painful than the first. If her first cesarean was preceded by a long or strenuous labor, she will not experience the same fatigue. This information will help her cope more effectively with stressful stimuli, including pain. The nurse can remind the woman that she has already had experience with how to prevent, cope with, and alleviate painful stimuli.

Preparation for Couples Desiring Vaginal Birth After Cesarean Birth

Couples who have had a cesarean birth and are now anticipating a vaginal birth have different needs from other couples. Because they may have unresolved questions and concerns about the last birth, it is helpful to begin the series of classes with an informational session. During this session, couples can ask questions, share experiences, and begin to form bonds with each other. The nurse can supply information regarding the criteria necessary to attempt a trial of labor and identify decisions regarding the birth experience. Some childbirth educators find it is helpful to have the couples prepare two birth plans: one for vaginal birth and one for cesarean birth. The preparation of the birth plans seems to assist the couple in taking more control of the birth experience and tends to increase the positive aspects of the experience (Austin 1986).

After an informational session, the classes may be divided depending on the needs of the couple. Those with recent coached childbirth experience may only need refresher classes while other couples may need complete training. Some couples may choose to attend regular classes after obtaining the beginning information in the informational session.

● Selected Methods of Childbirth Preparation

Various methods of childbirth preparation are taught in North America. Some antepartal classes are more specifically oriented to preparation for labor and delivery, have a name indicating a theory of pain reduction in childbirth, and teach specific exercises to reduce pain. The three most common methods of this type are the Read (natural childbirth), the Lamaze (psychoprophylactic), and the Bradley (partner-coached childbirth) methods. Hypnosis is also discussed here because it is sometimes used to help the ex-

pectant mother reduce or even eliminate pain in labor and delivery. Each of these methods is designed to provide the woman with self-help measures so that her pregnancy and delivery are healthy and happy events in which she participates.

Expectant parents are taught that childbirth exercises and preparation for childbirth do not exclude the use of analgesics but that they often reduce the amount necessary. Some women will not choose medication. Unfortunately, some groups teach that painless childbirth is the desired goal, which makes women who experience discomfort and accept pain medication feel like failures. This feeling can be extremely destructive to the woman's self-concept at a time when she needs positive reinforcement about her abilities to achieve and perform competently. Fortunately, current thinking recognizes that individuals vary in their responses to stress, that the character of individual labor differs, and that pain medication used judiciously may enhance the woman's ability to use relaxation techniques.

The programs in prepared childbirth have some similarities. All have an educational component to help eliminate fear (Peterson 1983). The classes vary in the amount of coverage of various subjects related to the maternity cycle, but they all teach relaxation techniques and all prepare the participants for what to expect during labor and delivery. Except for hypnosis, these methods also feature exercises to condition muscles and breathing patterns to use in labor. The greatest differences among the methods lie in the theories of why they work and in the relaxation techniques and breathing patterns they teach (see Table 18–2).

The advantages of these methods of childbirth preparation are several. The most important is that the baby may be healthier because of the reduced need for analgesics and anesthetics. Another advantage is the satisfaction of the couples for whom childbirth becomes a shared and profound emotional experience. In addition, proponents of each method claim that it shortens the labor process, a claim that has been clinically validated.

All maternity nurses must know how these methods differ so that they can support each couple in their chosen method. It is important to assess the couple's emotional resources and their expectations so that the nurse can help them achieve their goals more effectively.

Psychoprophylactic (Lamaze) Method

The terms *psychoprophylactic* and *Lamaze* are used interchangeably. *Psychoprophylactic* means "mind prevention," and Dr. Fernand Lamaze, a French obstetrician, was the first person to introduce this method of childbirth preparation to the Western world. Psychoprophylaxis actually originated in Russia and is based on Pavlov's research with conditioned reflexes. Pavlov found that the cortical centers of the brain can respond to only one set of signals at a time and that they accept only the strongest signal; the weaker signals are inhibited. Pavlov's research also demonstrated that verbal representation of a stimulus can create a response. When the real stimulus is substituted, the conditioned response continues to be produced. This theory was successfully applied to preparation for childbirth by Russian physicians.

Lamaze first became familiar with the psychoprophylaxis method when attending a conference in Russia. He introduced the method in France in 1951, adding innovations of his own. It was popularized soon after in this country through Marjorie Karmel's book *Thank You, Dr. Lamaze* (1965). The method was called "painless childbirth" and was much resisted by the medical profession in this country, many of whom believed that pain in childbirth is inevitable. Also, with the development of many analgesics and anesthetics, it did not seem necessary to condition women for childbirth.

Proponents of the method gradually organized and in 1960 formed a nonprofit group called the American Society for Prophylaxis in Obstetrics (ASPO). Two of the founders were Marjorie Karmel and Elizabeth Bing, a physical therapist who had also written about childbirth preparation using this method (Bing 1967). This organization helped establish many programs throughout the country for what has become one of the most popular methods of childbirth education.

The two components of Lamaze classes are education and training. Class content was originally confined to exercises, relaxation, breathing techniques, and the normal labor and delivery experience. Childbirth educators have recently added information on prenatal nutrition, infant feeding, cesarean birth, and other variations from usual labor as well as discussions of sexuality, early parenting, and coping skills for the postpartum period.

Instructors teaching the method in this country have modified many of the original exercises, but the basic theory of conditioned reflex remains the same. Women are taught to substitute favorable conditioned responses for unfavorable ones. Rather than restlessness and loss of control in labor, the woman learns to respond to contractions with conditioned relaxation of the uninvolved muscles and a learned respiratory pattern. Exercises taught in these classes include proper body mechanics and body conditioning, breathing techniques for labor, and relaxation.

Another major modification in the Lamaze method involves the goals of expectant couples. Lamaze and his supporters implied that specific criteria must be met if the childbirth experience was to be successful (painless with no anesthetic). Couples using this method are now encouraged to set their own goals for success. Lamaze childbirth education in this country supplies couples with the tools to accomplish their goals. The couple is encouraged to discuss goals with the care provider and maternity nursing personnel in labor and delivery units. The nursing staff

who knows the couple's goals and resources is able to offer effective support.

TONING EXERCISES

Some of the body conditioning exercises, such as the pelvic tilt, pelvic rock, and Kegel's exercises, are similar to those taught in other childbirth preparation classes. Other exercises strengthen the abdominal muscles for the expulsive phase of labor. (See Chapter 16 for a description of recommended exercises.)

RELAXATION EXERCISES

Relaxation during labor allows the woman to conserve energy and allow the uterine muscles to work more efficiently. Without practice it is very difficult to relax the whole body in the midst of intense uterine contractions. Many people are familiar with progressive relaxation exercises such as those taught to aid relaxation and induce sleep. One example follows:

> Lie down on your back or side. (The left side position is best for pregnant women.) Tighten your muscles in both feet. Hold the tightness for a few seconds and then relax the muscles completely, letting all the tension drain out. Tighten your lower legs, hold for a few seconds, and then relax the muscles letting all the tension drain out. Continue tensing and relaxing parts of your body, moving up the body as you do so.

Another type of relaxation exercise requires cooperation between the woman and her coach. It is particularly useful in learning how to work together during labor. See Box 18–1.

An additional exercise specific to Lamaze is disassociation relaxation. This pattern of active relaxation is in contrast to the Read method of passive relaxation. The woman is taught to become familiar with the sensation of contracting and relaxing the voluntary muscle groups throughout her body. She then learns to contract a specific muscle group and relax the rest of her body. This process of isolating the action of one group of voluntary muscles from the rest of the body is called *neuromuscular disassociation* and is basic to the psychoprophylaxis method of prepared childbirth. The exercise conditions the woman to relax uninvolved muscles while the uterus contracts. See Box 18–2.

In order to practice the relaxation exercises in a more realistic setting, the coach may use two methods to induce some discomfort:

1. The coach places both hands in a grasping position firmly on the upper arm and turns them in opposite directions to create a burning sensation. This is begun slowly and gently and increased at the direction of the woman as she continues to practice relaxation

Box 18–1   Touch Relaxation

Practice is vital to the following exercises, which require that the pregnant woman and her partner work very closely together. Tell the woman, "With practice you will train yourself to release not only in response to your partner's touch but also to the touch of doctors or nurses as they examine you. This technique will also help you to be more comfortable with your own body."

Goals:

(For her) To recognize and release tension in response to partner's touch; to be able to do this automatically and spontaneously.
(For partner) To recognize her tension in its very early stages; to learn how to touch in a firm yet sensitive way; to concentrate on her problem areas.

Tools:

(For her) Conscious relaxation, comfortable positioning, and trust.
(For him) Sensitivity, patience, and warm hands!

Procedure:

She tenses.
Partner touches.
She immediately releases towards touch.
Partner strokes, "drawing" tension from her.
She releases all residual tension.

Sequence:

- Contract muscles of the scalp and raise eyebrows. Partner cups hands on either side of the scalp. Immediately release tension in response to the pressure of your partner's touch. Then release any residual tension as your partner strokes your head.

- Frown, wrinkle nose, and squeeze eyes shut. Partner rests hands on brow and then strokes down over temples. Release.

- Grit teeth and clench jaw. Partner rests hands on either side of jaw. Release.

- Press shoulder blades back. Partner rest hands on front of shoulders. Release.

- Pull abdominal wall towards spine. Partner rests hands on sides of abdomen and then strokes down over hips. Partner might also stroke the lower curve of abdomen across pubic symphysis. Release.

- Press thighs together. Partners touches outside of each leg. Relax and let legs move apart. Partner strokes firmly down outside of leg with light strokes up on inner thigh.

- Press legs outward, still flexed but forcing thighs apart. Partner rests hands with fingers pointing downward, on inner thighs. Firmly stroke down to knees, then lightly stroke upward on outside of leg. Release.

- Tense arm muscles. Partner places hands on the upper arm and shoulder area, one on the inside and one on the outside of the arm. Stroke down to the elbow and then down forearm to wrist, and over fingertips. Release. Repeat with other arm.

- Tighten leg muscles, being careful not to cramp them. Partner touches foot around the instep, firmly without tickling. Release whole leg. Partner moves hands up, placing one on either side of the thigh, stroking down to the knee then down the calf to the foot and over the toes. Release. Repeat with other leg.

- Change to the Sims lateral or side-lying position. Raise chin, contracting the muscles at the back of the neck. Partner rests hand on nape of neck and massages. Release.

- Curl into fetal position, drawing shoulders forward. Partner applies pressure to back of shoulders. Stroke upper back. Release.

- Hollow the small of back by arching back. Partner rests hands against either side of spine and follows with stroking down over buttocks. Release.

- Press buttocks together. Partner rests one hand on each buttock. After initial release, stroke down toward thighs.

Source: O'Halloran S: *Pregnant and Prepared: A Guide to Preparing for Childbirth.* Wayne, NJ, Avery, 1984, pp 43–44. Courtesy of NACE: The Nashua Association for Childbirth Education.

Box 18–2   Disassociation Relaxation

The uterus, an involuntary muscle over which you have no control, will work most efficiently and effectively when the rest of your body is free from tension. The following exercises will give you further practice in conscious release. They will also give you and your partner a way to evaluate your progress.

Goals:

During pregnancy, disassociation relaxation will teach you consciously to release certain sets of muscles, while contracting others, and to disassociate yourself from voluntary tension.

During labor, this technique will release all voluntary muscles of your body at will, while the uterus contracts. This conserves energy and fights fatigue.

Tools:

Body awareness, touch release, and concentration.

Procedure:

Partner gives consistent suggestions.
Partner checks relaxation using touching.

Example:

Partner: "Contraction begins."
Mother: Relaxation breath (following with a comfortable rate of breathing).
Partner: See suggested patterns below.
Mother: Relaxation breath.

Sequence:

"Contract right arm. Hold. Release."
"Contract left arm. Hold. Release."
"Contract right leg. Hold. Release."
"Contract left leg. Hold. Release."
"Contract both arms. Hold. Release."
"Contract both legs. Hold. Release."
"Contract right side (arm and leg). Hold. Release."
"Contract left side (arm and leg). Hold. Release."
"Contract right arm and left leg. Hold. Release."
"Contract left arm and right leg. Hold. Release."

For Variety:

- Contract right arm and left leg.
- Release left leg. Contract right leg. Release right arm. Contract left arm.
- Release.

Source: O'Halloran S: *Pregnant and Prepared: A Guide to Preparing for Childbirth.* Wayne, NJ, Avery, 1984, pp 45–46. Courtesy of NACE: The Nashua Association for Childbirth Education.

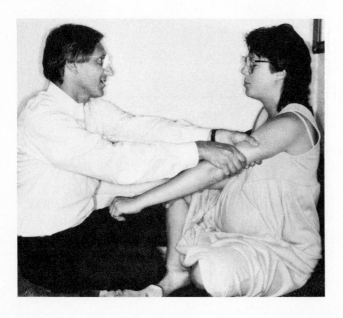 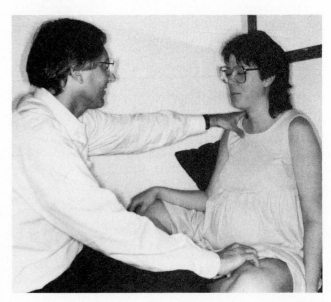

Figure 18–3   To practice relaxing in the presence of discomfort, the coach can induce discomfort by "twisting" the skin of the woman's upper arm or by pinching her inner thigh.

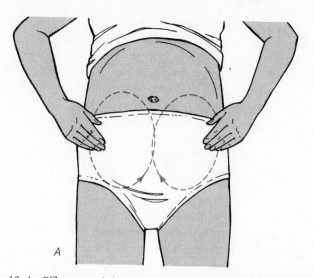
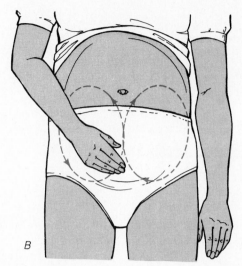

Figure 18–4 Effleurage is light stroking of the abdomen with the fingertips. A Starting at the symphysis, the woman lightly moves her fingertips up and around in a circular pattern. B An alternative approach involves the use of one hand in a figure-eight pattern.

and/or practices the breathing techniques (Figure 18–3).

2. The coach places a hand on the woman's inner thigh just above the knee and pinches the area.

While practicing, the coach checks the woman's neck, shoulders, arms, and legs for relaxation. As tense areas are found, the coach encourages the woman to relax that particular body part. The woman learns to respond to her own perceptions of tense muscles and also to the suggestion from others. The suggestion can come verbally or from touch. The exercises are usually practiced each day so that they become comfortable and easy to do.

A specific type of cutaneous stimulation used prior to the transitional phase of labor is known as *abdominal effleurage* (Figure 18–4). This light abdominal stroking is used in the Lamaze method of childbirth preparation. It effectively relieves mild to moderate pain, but not intense pain. Deep pressure over the sacrum is more effective for relieving back pain. In addition to the measures just described, the nurse can promote relaxation by encouraging and supporting the client's controlled breathing.

BREATHING TECHNIQUES

The breathing techniques use three levels of chest breathing. Proponents of the Lamaze method believe that the variety of chest breathing patterns helps keep the pressure of the diaphragm off the contracting uterus. The patterns of breathing taught in different classes vary. The woman is taught to use one pattern until it is no longer effective rather than in conjunction with the phases of labor.

Regardless of the level of breathing used, a cleansing breath begins and ends each pattern. A cleansing breath involves only the chest. It consists of inhaling through the nose and exhaling through pursed lips (as if blowing on a spoonful of hot food).

○   *FIRST LEVEL*   This pattern may also be called slow, deep breathing or slow-paced breathing. During the breathing movements only the chest is moved. The woman inhales slowly through her nose. She lifts her chest up and out during the inhalation. She exhales through pursed lips. The breathing rate is six to nine breaths a minute (or two breaths every 15 seconds). When the first level is no longer effective, the second level is used (see Figure 18–5).

○   *SECOND LEVEL*   This pattern may also be called shallow breathing or modified paced breathing. The woman begins with a cleansing breath and at the end of the cleansing breath she pushes out a short breath. She then inhales and exhales through the mouth at a rate of about four breaths every five seconds. She keeps her jaw relaxed and her mouth slightly open. The air should move in and out smoothly and silently, and the breathing should be mouth centered.

This pattern can be altered into a more rapid rate that does not exceed 2 to 2½ breaths every second. During the second level it is important for the whole body to be relaxed. It may help for the woman to count silently to pace the breathing (eg, count "one and two and three and. . . ." Inhalations occur on the *number* and exhalations on the *and*). Slow and rapid shallow breathing may be combined during the contraction. The more rapid rate is usually used at the height of the contraction.

○   *THIRD LEVEL*   This is also called pant-blow or pattern-paced breathing. This pattern is very similar to the rapid shallow breathing except the breathing is punctuated every

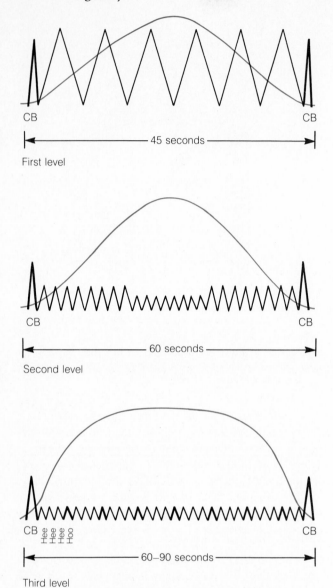

Figure 18–5   Lamaze breathing patterns. Each diagram represents a different breathing pattern. The curved line represents the uterine contraction. The peaked lines represent the breaths taken during the contraction. Each pattern begins and ends with a cleansing breath.

few breaths by a forceful exhalation through pursed lips. A variation of this pattern consists of drawing the lips back to the teeth and making a "Hee" sound with the exhalations. The forceful exhalation is through more pursed lips making a "Hoo" sound (Green & Naab, 1985).

A pattern of 4 breaths may be used to begin. All breaths are kept equal and rhythmical. As the contraction becomes more intense, the pattern may be changed to 3:1, 2:1, and finally 1:1 as it is important for the woman to adjust the pattern as needed. Thus the pattern evolves as Hee-Hee-Hee-Hoo (3:1), Hee-Hee-Hoo (2:1), or Hee-Hoo, depending on the count used.

In the second stage of labor, the woman may assume any comfortable physiologic position (a 35° semisitting, squatting, or side-lying position), take several deep breaths, then hold her breath, bulge abdominal muscles, relax the perineum, and push out through the vagina. This pushing effort is repeated throughout the contraction, timed and coached by the partner (Green & Naab 1985).

○   *POSSIBLE PROBLEMS AND SOLUTIONS*   During the breathing patterns the woman's mouth may become dry. To help correct this she may put her tongue up behind the front top teeth during breathing. She may suck on ice chips or a sucker at intervals. Small sips of water can be swished around the mouth to moisten mucous membranes. The woman may begin to feel tingling in her fingers and toes, which proceeds to numbness and a feeling of dizziness. These feelings are caused by hyperventilation (breathing at a rate that is too rapid or deep), which brings in more oxygen than is needed. The woman may cup her hands over her mouth, breathe through a washcloth, or breathe into a paper bag. These interventions increase the carbon dioxide content of the inhaled air and usually relieve the symptoms of hyperventilation very efficiently. At times it is also necessary to talk the woman through her breathing and to count out loud so that she can slow the rate. As the nurse or coach does this, it is important to maintain eye contact. If it is during the early stages of labor, touching her hand or shoulder may also be comforting. Even though she is hyperventilating, the woman often feels that she cannot get enough air and must breathe faster and deeper. It is important for the nurse to reiterate that she or he understands what is happening and how the woman feels. The nurse provides reassurance that as the woman slows her breathing, she will feel better, and the feeling that she cannot get her breath will lessen and then go away.

KEY CONCEPTS

Antepartal education programs vary in their goals, content, leadership techniques, and method of teaching.

Antepartal classes may be offered early and/or late in the gestational period. The class content varies depending on the type of class and the individual offering it. Expectant parents tend to want information in chronological sequence with the pregnancy. Adolescents have special content learning needs.

Breast-feeding programs are offered in the prenatal period. Siblings are now being included in the whole birthing process, and classes for them are available from many sources.

Grandparents have unique needs for information in grandparents' classes.

Information regarding cesarean birth is included in antepartal classes to help prepare parents.

The major types of childbirth preparation methods are Bradley, Read, Kitzinger, hypnosis, and Lamaze.

Lamaze is a type of psychoprophylactic method. The classes include information on toning exercises, relaxation exercises and techniques, and breathing methods for labor.

REFERENCES

Aberman S, **Kirchoff** KT: Infant-feeding practices: mothers' decision making. *J Obstet Gynecol Neonat Nurs* 1985; 14(September/October):394.

Affonso DD: *Impact of Cesarean Childbirth.* Philadelphia, Davis, 1981.

Austin SEJ: Childbirth classes for couples desiring VBAC. *Am J Mat Child Nurs* 1986;11:250.

Bing E: *Six Practical Lessons for an Easier Childbirth.* New York, Bantam Books, 1967.

Brackbill Y, et al: Characteristics related to drug consumption of women choosing between nontraditional birth alternatives. *J Nurs-Midwife* 1984;29(May/June):177.

Bradley RA: *Husband-Coached Childbirth,* ed 3. New York, Harper & Row, 1981.

Burst H: The influence of consumers on the birthing movement. *Topics Clin Nurs* 1983;5(October):42.

Clark L: When children watch their mothers deliver. *Contemp OB/GYN* 1986;28(August):69.

Chute GE: Expectation and experience in alternative and conventional birth. *J Obstet Gynecol Neonat Nurs* 1985;14(January/February):61.

Daniels MB: The birth experience for the sibling: Description and evaluation of a program. *J Nurs-Midwife* 1983;28(September/October):15.

Davis DJ: Infant care safety: The role of perinatal caregivers. *Birth Suppl* 1985;12(Fall):21.

Dick-Read G: *Childbirth Without Fear,* ed 2. New York, Harper & Row, 1959.

DiFloria IA, **Duncan** PA: Design for successful patient teaching. *Am J Mat Child Nurs* 1986;11:246 .

Edwards M: The lactation consultant: A new profession. *Birth Suppl* 1985;12(Fall):9

Fawcett J, **Burritt** J: An exploratory study of antenatal preparation for cesarean birth. *J Obstet Gynecol Neonat Nurs* 1985;14(May/June):224.

Green M, **Naab** M: *Lamaze Is for Chickens: A Guide for Prepared Childbirth.* Wayne, NJ, Avery, 1985.

Hartman R: *Exercises for True Natural Childbirth.* New York, Harper & Row, 1959.

Hassid P: *Textbook for Childbirth Educators.* Philadelphia, Lippincott, 1984.

Horn M, **Manion** J: Creative grandparenting: Bonding the generations. *J Obstet Gynecol Neonat Nurs* 1985;14(May/June):233.

Hotchner T: *Pregnancy and Childbirth: A Complete Guide for a New Life.* New York, Avon Books, 1979.

Howard JS, **Sater** J: Adolescent mothers: Self-perceived health education needs. *J Obstet Gynecol Neonat Nurs* 1985;14(September/October):399.

Johnson CM: Disposable diapers: A foreign body hazard. Department of Otolaryngology/Head and Neck Surgery, The University of Virginia Medical Center, Charlottesville, Virginia, 1985.

Jordan PL: Breast-feeding as a risk factor for fathers, the marital relationship, breast-feeding success and father-infant attachment. *J Obstet Gynecol Neonat Nurs* 1986; 15(March/April):94.

Karmel M: *Thank You, Dr. Lamaze.* New York, Doubleday, 1965.

Kaunitz AM, et al: Perinatal and maternal mortality in a religious group avoiding obstetric care. *Am J Obstet Gynecol* 1984:150(December):826.

Kitzinger S: *The Experience of Childbirth.* Harmondsworth, England, Penguin, 1984.

Kowba MD, **Schwirian** PM: Direct sibling contact and bacterial colonization in newborns. *J Obstet Gynecol Neonat Nurs* 1985;14(September/October):412.

Krutsky CD: Siblings at birth: Impact on parents. *J Nurs-Midwife* 1985;30(September/October):269.

Leonard CH, et al: Preliminary observations on the behavior of children present at the birth of a sibling. *Pediatrics* 1979;64:950.

Lauwers J, **Woessner** C: *Counseling the Nursing Mother.* Wayne, NJ, Avery, 1983.

Levenson PM, **Smith** PB, **Morrow** JR: A comparison of physician-patient views of teen prenatal information needs. *J Adolesc Health Care* 1986;7:6.

MacLaughlin SM, **Johnston** KB: The preparation of young children for the birth of a sibling. *J Nurs-Midwife* 1984;29(November/December):371.

Maloney R: Childbirth education classes: Expectant parents' expectations. *J Obstet Gynecol Neonat Nurs* 1985; 14(May/June):245.

Marecki M, et al: Early sibling attachment period. *J Obstet Gynecol Neonat Nurs* 1985;14(September/October):418.

Martin D: Diapering alternatives. *Baby Talk* 1985; 22(April):18.

May KA, **Ditolla** K: In hospital alternative birth centers: where do we go from here? *Am J Mat Child Nurs* 1984;9(January/February):48.

National Association of Diaper Services. *Fact Sheet.* 1987.

O'Halloran S: *Pregnant and Prepared: A Guide to Preparing for Childbirth.* Wayne, NJ, Avery, 1984.

Parma S: A family centered event? Preparing the child for sharing in the experience of childbirth. *J Nurs-Midwife* 1979;24:6.

Peterson G: Addressing complications of childbirth in the prenatal setting. *J Nurs-Midwife* 1983:28(March/April):25.

Roig-Garcia S: The hypnoreflexogenous method: A new procedure in obstetrical psychoanalgesia. *Am J Clin Hypnosis* 1961;4(July):1.

Sandelowski M: Expectations for childbirth versus actual experiences: The gap widens. *Am J Mat Child Nurs* 1984:9:237.

Solomon J: Superabsorbent diapers: Marketers seek doctors support amid health concerns. *Wall Street Journal,* September 5, 1986.

Tinterow MM: Techniques of hypnosis, in **Bonica** JJ (ed): *Obstetric Analgesia and Anesthetics.* Philadelphia, Davis, 1972.

Werner ME, et al: An argument for the revival of hypnosis in obstetrics. *Am J Clin Hypnosis* 1982;24(January):149.

Whitley N: *Clinical Obstetrics.* Philadelphia, Lippincott, 1985.

Wranesh BL: The effect of sibling visitation on bacterial colonization rate in neonates. *J Obstet Gynecol Neonat Nurs* 1982;11(July/August):211.

Young D: *Changing Childbirth.* Rochester, NY, Childbirth Graphics, 1982.

Zimmerman BN: Human questions vs. human hurry. *Am J Nurs* 1980;80(April):719.

Brucker MC, et al: Delivery scripts: Fantasy vs. reality. *Point View* 1987;24(January):20.

Cohen J: Reaching out in childbirth education. *NZ Nurs J* 1986;79(January):26.

Giblin PT, et al: Pregnant adolescents' health-information needs: Implications for health education and health seeking. *J Adolesc Health Care* 1986;7(May):168.

Fawcett J, et al: Antenatal education for cesarean birth: Extension of a field test. *J Obstet Gynecol Neonat Nurs* 1987;16(January/February):61.

Flanagan JA: Childbirth in the 80's: What next? When alternatives become mainstream. *J Nurs-Midwife* 1986; 31(July/August):194.

Hammond N, et al: Doing away with "us and them" parentcraft classes. *Midwives Chron* 1986;99(February):42.

Geden E, et al: Self report and psychophysiological effects of Lamaze preparation: An analogue of labor pain. *Res Nurs Health,* June 1985, p 155.

Glover JF, et al: A survey of postnatal educational hospitals. *Can Nurse* 1985;81(December):54.

Jamieson L: Education for parenthood. *Nursing* (London) 1986;79(January):13.

Lesko W: The birth chart . . . 21 ways to have a baby. *Good Housekeep* 1986;202(June):123.

Maloni JA, et al: Expectant grandparents class. *J Obstet Gynecol Neonat Nurs* 1987;16(January/February):26.

Romito P: The humanizing of childbirth: The response of medical institutions to women's demands for change. *Midwifery* 1986;2(September):135.

Zander LI: Maternity care: An international perspective. *J Nurs-Midwife* 1986;31(September/October):227.

ADDITIONAL READINGS

Austin SEJ: Childbirth classes for couples desiring VBAC . . . vaginal birth after cesarean. *Am J Mat Child Nurs* 1986;11(July/August):250.

Broome ME, et al: Childbirth education: A review of the effects on the woman and her family. *Fam Community Health* 1986;9(May):33.

Birth is something that you go through . . . into parenting. Although significant and intense, it usually lasts only a short time in comparison with the nine months of pregnancy and the decades of parenting. It is not to be focused on primarily for itself, but as a means through which your baby enters the world. (Pregnant Feelings)

Pregnancy at Risk

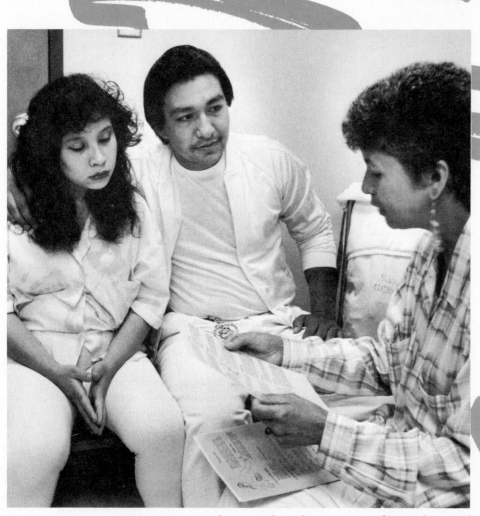

A Latina nurse educator explains the importance of prenatal care and proper exercise and nutrition to a 19-year-old Mexican-American man and his 16-year-old Nicaraguan-American wife, who is 5 months pregnant.

Chapter Nineteen

OBJECTIVES

- Compare the effects of different preexisting medical conditions on pregnancy.
- Discriminate among the bleeding problems associated with pregnancy.
- Describe the development and course of hypertensive disorders associated with pregnancy.
- Explain the cause and prevention of Rh hemolytic disease of the newborn.
- Describe the effects of surgical procedures on pregnancy, and how pregnancy may complicate diagnosis.
- Discuss some common infections that may be contracted during pregnancy or may coexist with pregnancy.
- Discuss possible teratogenic effects of infections and drugs.
- Discuss drug use and abuse during pregnancy.

Even though it is a normal process, pregnancy is biologically, physiologically, and psychologically stressful. For some women, pregnancy may even be a life-threatening event. Prenatal care is aimed toward identification, assessment, and management of women whose pregnancies are at risk because of potential or existing complications.

Disruptive conditions that arise during the gestational period are the result of many high-risk factors, such as age, blood type, socioeconomic status, parity, psychologic well-being, and predisposing chronic illnesses. The major thrust of prenatal nursing care should be toward screening women for these complications and developing supportive therapies that will promote optimal health for mother and fetus.

Whether the woman at risk remains ambulatory or is hospitalized, she and her family have needs that the nurse is specifically prepared to meet. This is especially true of the family's emotional needs. In the teaching role, the nurse fulfills a crucial need by providing information about the risk factors affecting the pregnant woman and about how the woman and her family can meet many of her health care needs.

In this chapter the discussion focuses on women with pregestational medical disorders, as well as specific disorders that develop as a result of pregnancy, and the possible effects of these disorders on the outcome of pregnancy. Surgical procedures, accidents and trauma, and infectious processes that may influence maternal and fetal well-being are also described.

● Using the Nursing Process With Pregnant Women at Risk

Nursing Assessment

Often the initial prenatal nursing assessment enables the nurse to identify factors in a woman's history that place her at risk during a pregnancy. Once these risk factors are identified, the nurse can plan appropriate care with the woman and her family. In other cases a woman enters a pregnancy with a preexisting condition such as heart disease or diabetes. In these cases the nurse assesses the course of the pregnancy, the impact of the condition on the pregnancy and the effects of pregnancy on the existing condition. In all cases the nurse assesses the woman's physical condition and her psychosocial response, taking a holistic view of the woman and her family.

Analysis and Nursing Diagnoses

Once the nurse has assessed the woman, it is necessary to analyze the data, draw some conclusions, and formulate nursing diagnoses. For example, for a woman with herpesvirus type 2, a possible nursing diagnosis might be "Knowledge deficit related to the impact of the presence of herpes lesions on the method of delivery."

For a woman with preexisting heart disease who has no limitation of activity prior to pregnancy, a possible nursing diagnosis might be "Noncompliance with rest schedule due to lack of understanding of the strain pregnancy places on the heart."

The nursing diagnosis helps focus and guide the development of the plan of care. Once suitable, validated diagnoses are formulated, the nurse can apply the remaining steps of the nursing process.

Nursing Plan and Implementation

The nursing plan and its implementation should follow logically from assessment, analysis, and nursing diagnoses. The plan reflects the nurse's understanding of the woman's pregnancy and the risk factors that affect it. In some instances the plan will include provisions for ongoing assessment of the woman's health status. Implementation of the plan is best accomplished when the nurse has established an effective relationship with the woman and her family. The plan should reflect the nurse's awareness of the woman's needs, personal preferences, cultural focus, and beliefs. For example, dietary counseling for a woman who develops gestational diabetes will not be very effective if the food choices identified as appropriate do not reflect cultural food preferences. Thus, in many instances, implementation of the plan is a joint effort by nurse and client.

Evaluation

Evaluation requires that the nurse critically review the plan and its implementation to determine whether it was effective. If the plan was effective, the nurse determines whether it can continue or if changes in the woman's situation require modifications. If it was not effective, the nurse must try to determine why. Were the data inadequate? Did the situation change? Did the nurse fail to consider certain aspects of the available information? The nurse then makes necessary additional assessments and modifies the plan accordingly. The goal in all cases is to provide effective nursing care.

● Care of the Woman With Heart Disease

A healthy woman with a normal heart has adequate cardiac reserve to adjust to the demands of pregnancy with little difficulty. The woman with heart disease has decreased cardiac reserve because of the higher workload that her heart must assume just to accommodate her body needs. The demands of pregnancy may threaten this woman's well-being.

Approximately 0.5 percent to 1.0 percent of pregnant women are at risk because of preexisting heart disease. Rheumatic heart disease formerly accounted for the great majority of cases but is now responsible for only about half the cases. Congenital heart defects are responsible for most of the remaining half (Cruikshank 1986). Other, less common causes of heart disease in pregnancy include syphilis; arteriosclerosis; coronary occlusion; and renal, pulmonary, and thyroid disorders.

The pathophysiology found in a pregnant woman with heart disease varies with the type of disorder. More-common conditions are discussed briefly here.

Rheumatic heart disease has declined rapidly in the last three decades, primarily because of prompt identification and treatment of pharyngeal streptococcal infection. Although mitral stenosis is the most common lesion seen when rheumatic endocarditis occurs, the aortic or tricuspid valves may also be affected. Recurrent acute inflammation from bouts of rheumatic fever causes scar tissue formation on the valves. The scarring results in either stenosis (failure to open completely) or regurgitation due to failure to close completely, or a combination of both effects. Stenosis causes a decrease in blood flow through the valve, and therefore causes an increase in work load on the heart chamber just before the stenotic valve. A regurgitant (incompetent) valve allows blood to leak through when it is closed. Leaking increases the work load on the heart chambers on either side of the diseased valve.

The increased blood volume of pregnancy, coupled with the pregnant woman's need for increased cardiac output, stresses the heart of a woman with mitral stenosis and increases her risk of developing congestive heart failure. Even the woman who has no symptoms at the onset of her pregnancy is at risk.

Congenital heart defects have become a more common finding in pregnant women as improved surgical techniques enable females born with heart defects to live to childbearing age. The exact pathology depends on the specific defect in the septa, valves, or conduction system. Congenital defects commonly seen in pregnant women include atrial septal defect, ventricular septal defect, patent ductus arteriosus, pulmonary stenosis, coarctation of the aorta, and tetralogy of Fallot. When surgical repair can be accomplished with no remaining evidence of organic heart disease, pregnancy may be undertaken with confidence. In such cases antibiotic prophylaxis is recommended to prevent subacute bacterial endocarditis at the time of delivery. When congenital heart disease is associated with cyanosis, whether the defect was originally uncorrected or whether the correction failed to relieve the cyanosis, the woman should be counseled to avoid pregnancy because the risk to both her and the fetus would be high.

Mitral valve prolapse (MVP) is a usually asymptomatic condition that is found in about 6 percent to 10 percent of women of childbearing age (Cruikshank 1986). The condition is more common in women than in men and seems to run in families. In MVP the mitral valve leaflets tend to prolapse into the right atrium during ventricular systole because the chordae tendineae that support them are long and thin. As a result, some mitral regurgitation may occur.

Women with MVP usually tolerate pregnancy well, and the prognosis is excellent. Most women require assurance that they can continue with normal activities. A few women experience symptoms—primarily palpitations, chest pain, and dyspnea—which are usually due to arrhythmias. They are often treated with propranolol hydrochloride (Inderal). Limiting caffeine intake also helps decrease palpitations. Antibiotics are given prophylactically at the time of delivery to prevent bacterial endocarditis.

Peripartum cardiomyopathy is a dysfunction of the left ventricle that occurs in the last month of pregnancy or the first five months postpartum in a woman with no previous history of heart disease. The symptoms are related to congestive heart failure: dyspnea, orthopnea, chest pain, palpitations, weakness, and edema. The cause is unknown. Treatment includes digitalis, diuretics, anticoagulants, and bed rest. The condition may resolve with bed rest as the heart gradually returns to normal size. Subsequent pregnancy is strongly discouraged because the disease tends to recur during pregnancy.

Medical Therapy

The primary goal of medical management is early diagnosis and ongoing management of the woman with cardiac disease. Echocardiogram, chest x ray, and auscultation of heart sounds are essential for establishing the type and severity of the heart disease. The severity of heart disease can also be determined by the individual's ability to perform ordinary physical activity. The following classification of functional capacity has been standardized by the Criteria Committee of the New York Heart Association (1955):

- Class I. No limitation of physical activity. Ordinary physical activity causes no discomfort; anginal pain is not present.

- Class II. Slight limitation of physical activity. Ordinary physical activity causes fatigue, dyspnea, palpitation, or anginal pain.

- Class III. Moderate to marked limitation of physical activity. During less than ordinary physical activity, the person experiences excessive fatigue, dyspnea, palpitation, or anginal pain.

- Class IV. Inability to carry on any physical activity without experiencing discomforts. Even at rest, the person experiences symptoms of cardiac insufficiency or anginal pain.

Women in classes I and II usually experience a normal pregnancy and have few complications, whereas those in classes III and IV are at risk for more severe complications.

DRUG THERAPY

Besides the iron and vitamin supplements prescribed during pregnancy, the pregnant woman with heart disease may need additional drug therapy to maintain health. If the woman develops coagulation problems, the anticoagulant heparin may be used. Heparin offers the greatest safety to the fetus because it does not cross the placenta. The thiazide diuretics and furosemide (Lasix) may be used to treat congestive heart failure if it develops. Digitalis glycosides and common antiarrhythmic drugs may be used to treat cardiac failure and arrhythmias. These agents do cross the placenta but have no reported teratogenic effect. Penicillin is used to protect against infection if not contraindicated by allergy.

DELIVERY

Use of low forceps provides the safest method of delivery, with a regional anesthetic to reduce the stress of pushing. Cesarean delivery is used only if fetal or obstetric indications exist, not on the basis of heart disease alone.

Nursing Assessment

The stress of pregnancy on the functional capacity of the heart is assessed during every antepartal visit. The nurse notes the category of functional capacity assigned to the woman, takes the woman's pulse, respirations, and blood pressure, and compares them to the normal values expected during pregnancy. The nurse then determines the woman's activity level, including rest, and any changes in the pulse and respirations that have occurred since previous visits. The nurse also identifies and evaluates other factors that would increase strain on the heart. These might include anemia, infection, anxiety, lack of a support system, and insufficient household help.

The following symptoms, if they are progressive, are indicative of congestive heart failure, the heart's signal of its decreased ability to meet the demands of pregnancy.

- Cough (frequent, with or without hemoptysis)

- Dyspnea (progressive, upon exertion)

- Edema (progressive, generalized, including extremities, face, eyelids)

- Heart murmurs (heard on auscultation)

- Palpitations

- Rales (auscultated in lung bases)

It should be noted that this cycle is *progressive*, because some of these same behaviors are seen to a minor degree in a pregnancy without cardiac problems.

Nursing Diagnosis

Nursing diagnoses that might apply to the pregnant woman with heart disease include:

- Alteration in cardiac output: easy fatigability

- Knowledge deficit related to the cardiac condition and requirement to alter self-care activities

- Fear related to the effects of the maternal cardiac condition on fetal well-being

Nursing Care During the Antepartal Period

Nursing actions are directed toward meeting the physiologic and psychosocial needs of the pregnant woman with heart disease. The priority of nursing actions varies, depending on the severity of the disease process.

NURSING GOAL: PROMOTION OF ADEQUATE NUTRITION

A diet should be instituted that is high in iron, protein, and essential nutrients and low in sodium and calories. Such a diet is needed to meet the demands of pregnancy for increased blood volume and oxygen.

NURSING GOAL: PROMOTION OF REST

Rest is necessary to reduce the work load of the heart. Eight to ten hours of sleep are essential, with frequent daily rest periods. The nurse should help the woman understand the absolute necessity for this rest.

NURSING GOAL: PROTECTION FROM INFECTION

The woman must be informed about the importance of protecting herself from infections, especially upper respiratory infections. These place additional stress on the heart. If the heart's reserve capacity is overloaded, cardiac failure may result.

NURSING GOAL: PROMOTION OF CLIENT ACCEPTANCE OF THE NEED TO RESTRICT ACTIVITY

Decreased exertion reduces fatigue, thereby promoting adequate ventilation and preservation of cardiac reserves. To ensure this, the couple may require additional household help. The nurse can make suggestions about ways of obtaining assistance.

NURSING GOAL: MONITORING OF CARDIAC STATUS

During the first half of pregnancy the woman is seen approximately every two weeks to assess cardiac status. During the second half of pregnancy the woman is seen weekly. These assessments are especially important between weeks 28 and 30 when the blood volume reaches maximum amounts. If symptoms of cardiac decompensation occur, prompt medical intervention is indicated to correct the cardiac problem.

NURSING GOAL: EDUCATION FOR SELF-CARE

The woman should have a thorough understanding of her condition, signs of decompensation, any medication she is taking, and reasons for the need to decrease activity if symptoms occur. When the woman receives thorough explanations, printed material, and an opportunity to ask questions and discuss concerns, she is better able to meet her own health care needs and seek assistance appropriately.

NURSING GOAL: PROMOTION OF FAMILY ADAPTATION

The woman and her family are provided with information concerning her condition and management. This will increase their understanding and decrease anxiety. The nurse can counsel them regarding their preparation for childbirth, offer them encouragement to boost their morale, and put them in contact with self-help or support groups for at-risk pregnancies.

Nursing Care During the Intrapartal Period

Labor and delivery exert tremendous stress on the woman and the unborn fetus. This stress could be fatal to the fetus of a woman with cardiac disease because of the possible decreased oxygen and blood supply to it. To prevent the negative effects of this stress, the intrapartum management of a woman with cardiac disease is aimed at reducing the amount of physical exertion and accompanying fatigue.

NURSING GOAL: MONITORING OF MATERNAL AND FETAL VITAL SIGNS

The nurse frequently assesses maternal blood pressure, pulse, and respirations to evaluate the woman's response to labor. A pulse rate greater than 100 beats/min or respirations greater than 25/min require careful evaluation to detect early signs of cardiac decompensation. Continuous electronic fetal monitoring is generally used to provide ongoing assessment of the fetus's response to labor. Maternal contractions are also monitored because they provide information about the status of labor.

NURSING GOAL: PROMOTION OF OPTIMUM CARDIAC FUNCTIONING THROUGH PROPER POSITIONING

Side-lying and semi-Fowler's positions are the positions of choice because they help assure cardiac emptying, proper oxygenation, and maximum utero–placental blood flow.

NURSING GOAL: MONITORING PULMONARY FUNCTION

The nurse auscultates the woman's lungs frequently for evidence of rales. Dyspnea and coughing are additional signs of pulmonary decompensation and require careful assessment.

NURSING GOAL: IMPLEMENTATION OF SUPPORTIVE THERAPIES

Supportive measures include the use of prophylactic antibiotics; oxygen by mask if dyspnea occurs; and administration of diuretics, sedatives, analgesics, and digitalis as indicated.

NURSING GOAL: REDUCTION OF PHYSICAL EXERTION DURING LABOR AND DELIVERY

The nurse provides as much assistance to the woman as possible during labor to avoid overexertion and accompanying fatigue. Encouraging relaxation and sleep between contractions, supporting the woman emotionally so that she is less anxious, and alleviating discomfort during contractions may reduce stress. The nurse guards the woman against overexertion during pushing by coaching her to use shorter, more moderate, open glottis pushes, with complete relaxation between pushes. Vital signs are monitored closely during the second stage. A semi-Fowler's position may be maintained.

NURSING GOAL: PROVISION OF PSYCHOLOGIC SUPPORT

The nurse needs to maintain an atmosphere of calm to lessen the anxiety of the woman and her family. The nurse remains with the woman to support and encourage her. The nurse keeps the woman and her family informed of labor progress and management, collaborating with the couple to fulfill their wishes for the birth experience as much as possible.

Nursing Care During the Postpartal Period

The postpartal period is a most significant time for the woman with heart disease. After delivery, the intraabdominal pressure is reduced significantly, venous pressure is reduced, the splanchnic vessels engorge, and blood flow to the heart increases. The extravascular fluid moves into the bloodstream. This mobilization of fluid can place a great strain on the heart if excess interstitial fluid is present. Such stress on the heart could lead to cardiac decompensation, especially during the first 48 hours postpartum or as late as the sixth postpartal day. To permit careful assessment and allow recovery of cardiac function, the woman generally remains hospitalized for about a week.

NURSING GOAL: PROMOTION OF RECOVERY

Frequent assessment permits early detection of potential complications. Vital signs are monitored regularly, and the woman is assessed for any signs of cardiac decompensation. The nurse continues to maintain the woman in semi-Fowler's and side-lying positions, with elevation of the head and shoulders to assist respiratory and cardiac functioning. The woman resumes activity gradually and progressively, based on nursing assessment of her status. The woman is often on bed rest initially, and the nurse performs many of the activities of daily living. As her tolerance for activity improves, the woman can assume responsibility for more of her own care and begin a program of progressive ambulation. To facilitate bowel elimination without strain, nursing interventions include the use of diet and stool softeners to prevent constipation.

NURSING GOAL: PROVISION OF PSYCHOLOGIC SUPPORT

The nurse gives the woman opportunities to discuss her birth experience and helps her deal with any feelings or concerns that cause her distress. The nurse also encourages maternal-infant attachment by providing frequent opportunities for the mother to interact with her child.

NURSING GOAL: EDUCATION AND ASSISTANCE IN NEWBORN CARE

For the first few days, as determined by cardiac status, the nurse will provide care for the newborn. This is best done at the mother's bedside to increase her contact with her newborn and to provide teaching opportunities. If the mother's cardiac condition is class I or class II, she may breast-feed her baby in bed. The nurse can assist her to a comfortable side-lying position with her head moderately elevated or to a semi-Fowler's position. The nurse should position the newborn at the breast and be available to burp the baby and reposition him or her at the other breast.

The advisability of breast-feeding for the woman with class III or class IV cardiac disease must be evaluated carefully. In many cases, because of the excessive fatigue factor and because the mother may be taking several medications that pass into the breast milk, breast-feeding may not be appropriate.

NURSING GOAL: PREPARATION FOR DISCHARGE

The woman will need education, referrals, and support for her care and that of her newborn.

1. Determine whether there are significant others to assist the mother at home in caring for herself and the baby. Ensure that the woman's needs are clearly communicated to the care provider so that realistic home care plans can be made. Refer the woman to community homemaking services if needed.

2. Plan with the woman an activity schedule that is gradual, progressive, and appropriate to her needs and home environment.

3. Give appropriate information regarding sexual relations and contraception.

4. Ensure that the woman understands signs and symptoms that indicate possible problems from her heart disease or from other postpartal complications.

Evaluative Outcome Criteria

Anticipated outcomes of nursing care include the following:

- The woman clearly understands her condition and its possible impact on pregnancy, labor and delivery, and the postpartal period.

- The woman participates in developing an appropriate health care regimen and follows it throughout her pregnancy.

- The woman successfully delivers a healthy infant.

- The woman avoids congestive heart failure.

- The woman is able to identify signs and symptoms of possible complications postpartally.

- The woman is comfortable caring for her newborn infant.

● Care of the Woman With Diabetes Mellitus

Diabetes mellitus complicates 2 percent to 3 percent of pregnancies (Gabbe 1986). It is an endocrine disorder of carbohydrate metabolism that results from inadequate production or utilization of insulin. Insulin is a powerful hypoglycemic agent, normally produced by the β cells of the islets of Langerhans in the pancreas. It lowers blood glucose levels by enabling the glucose to move from the blood into muscle and adipose tissue cells.

Carbohydrate Metabolism in Pregnancy

The changes in carbohydrate, protein, and fat metabolism in normal pregnancy are profound. Carbohydrate metabolism is affected early in pregnancy by a rise in serum levels of estrogen and progesterone. These hormones stimulate increased insulin production by the maternal pancreatic β cells, and increased tissue response to insulin early in pregnancy. Therefore an anabolic state exists during the first half of pregnancy with storage of glycogen in the liver and other tissues.

The second half of pregnancy is characterized by increased resistance to insulin, which appears to be due to secretion of human placental lactogen (hPL) and elevated levels of estrogen, progesterone, and other hormones (Hollingsworth 1985). This diminished effectiveness of insulin results in a catabolic state during fasting periods (eg, during the night and after meal absorption). Fat is metabolized at these times much more readily than in a nonpregnant person, a process called *accelerated starvation*. Ketones may be present in the urine as a result of lipolysis.

A rise in the glomerular filtration rate in the kidneys in conjunction with decreased tubular glucose reabsorption results in glycosuria. A decrease in the normal fasting blood glucose occurs in pregnancy, but free fatty acids and ketones are increased. The fed state is also altered by a more pronounced and prolonged elevation in plasma glucose (Freinkel et al 1985).

In summary, the delicate system of checks and balances that exists between glucose production and glucose utilization is stressed by the growing fetus, who derives energy from glucose taken solely from maternal stores. This stress is referred to as the *diabetogenic effect* of pregnancy. Thus any preexisting disruption in carbohydrate metabolism is augmented by pregnancy, and any diabetic potential may precipitate *gestational diabetes*.

Pathophysiology of Diabetes Mellitus

In diabetes mellitus, the pancreas does not produce sufficient amounts of insulin to allow necessary carbohydrate metabolism. With inadequate amounts of insulin, glucose cannot enter the cells but remains outside in the blood. The body cells become energy depleted, while the blood glucose level remains elevated. Fats and proteins in the body tissues are then oxidized by the cells as a source of energy. This results in wasting of fat and muscle tissue of the body, negative nitrogen balance due to protein breakdown, and ketosis due to fat metabolism. The strong osmotic force of the glucose concentration in the blood pulls water from the cells into the blood, which results in cellular dehydration. The high level of glucose in the blood eventually spills over into the urine, producing glycosuria. Osmotic pressure of the glucose in the urine prevents reabsorption of water into the kidney tubules, causing extracellular dehydration.

These pathologic developments cause the four cardinal signs and symptoms of diabetes mellitus: polyuria, polydipsia, weight loss, and polyphagia. *Polyuria* (frequent urination) results because water is not reabsorbed by the renal tubules due to the osmotic activity of glucose. *Polydipsia* (excessive thirst) is caused by dehydration from polyuria. *Weight loss* (seen in insulin-dependent diabetes, also called type I diabetes) is due to the use of fat and muscle tissue for energy. *Polyphagia* (excessive hunger) is caused by tissue loss and a state of starvation, which results from the inability of the cells to utilize the blood glucose. Diagnosis of diabetes is based on the presence of clinical symptoms and laboratory tests showing elevated glucose levels in the blood and urine.

Classification of Diabetes Mellitus

States of altered carbohydrate metabolism have been classified several different ways. Table 19–1 shows the current accepted classification, a result of the 1979 report of a special committee of the National Institutes of Health (National Diabetes Data Group 1979). This classification contains three main categories: diabetes mellitus (DM), impaired glucose tolerance (IGT), and gestational diabetes mellitus (GDM). The DM group is subdivided into three types:

1. *Type I or insulin-dependent diabetes mellitus (IDDM).* Type I formerly was called juvenile-onset diabetes, ketosis-prone diabetes, or unstable or brittle diabetes. Insulin-dependent diabetes can occur at any age but is usually seen in young persons. Little or no insulin is produced by the pancreas in type I diabetes.

2. *Type II or noninsulin-dependent diabetes mellitus (NIDDM).* Type II has been called maturity-onset diabetes, but it can occur in children. Persons with type II diabetes are not ketosis prone. Type II is further subdivided into obese and nonobese groups. Ideally, the type II disease is controlled by diet alone.

3. *Secondary diabetes.* The third, rather rare, type of diabetes is called secondary diabetes because it arises from another condition such as pancreatic disease (for example, pancreatitis or cystic fibrosis), hormonal disorder (for example, acromegaly or Cushing syndrome), drug-induced conditions (for example,

Table 19–1 Classification of Diabetes Mellitus (DM) and Other Categories of Glucose Intolerance

1. Diabetes mellitus
    a. Type I, insulin-dependent (IDDM)
    b. Type II, noninsulin-dependent (NIDDM)
        (1) Nonobese NIDDM
        (2) Obese NIDDM
    c. Secondary diabetes
2. Impaired glucose tolerance (IGT)
3. Gestational diabetes (GDM)

Source: National Diabetes Data Group of National Institutes of Health, 1979. *Diabetes* 1979;28:1039. Adapted with permission from the American Diabetes Association Inc.

from steroids or birth control pills), or insulin-receptor abnormalities.

In the IGT category are persons whose fasting plasma glucose level is normal or only slightly elevated (140 mg/dL) but whose glucose tolerance tests show abnormal values. These persons are asymptomatic. This condition was formerly called chemical diabetes, borderline diabetes, or latent diabetes.

In GDM, the diabetes has its onset or is first diagnosed during pregnancy. Except for an impaired tolerance to glucose, the woman may remain asymptomatic or may have a mild form of the disease. Diagnosis of GDM is very important, however, because even mild diabetes causes increased risk for perinatal morbidity and mortality. After pregnancy, women with GDM need to be reclassified as either type I, type II, IGT, or previously IGT, as determined by postpartal testing. Most women will revert to normal and can be reclassified as previously IGT.

Table 19–2 shows White's classification of diabetes in pregnancy. This classification is still used in many agencies.

Influence of Pregnancy on Diabetes

Pregnancy can affect diabetes significantly. First, the physiologic changes of pregnancy can drastically alter insulin requirements. Second, pregnancy may accelerate the progress of vascular disease secondary to diabetes.

Table 19–2 White's Classification of Diabetes in Pregnancy

Class	Criterion
A	Chemical diabetes
B	Maturity onset (age over 20 years), duration under 10 years, no vascular lesions
C_1	Age 10 to 19 years at onset
C_2	10 to 19 years' duration
D_1	Under 10 years at onset
D_2	Over 20 years' duration
D_3	Benign retinopathy
D_4	Calcified vessels of legs
D_5	Hypertension
E	No longer sought
F	Nephropathy
G	Many failures
H	Cardiopathy
R	Proliferating retinopathy
T	Renal transplant (added by Tagatz and colleagues of the University of Minnesota)

Source: From White P: Classification of obstetric diabetes. *Am J Obstet Gynecol.* 1978;130:228.

The disease may be more difficult to control during pregnancy, because insulin requirements are changeable. Insulin need frequently decreases early in the first trimester. Levels of hPL, an insulin antagonist, are low, energy demands of the embryo are minimal, and the woman may be consuming less food due to nausea and vomiting. Nausea and vomiting may also cause dietary fluctuations, which can increase the risk of hypoglycemia or insulin shock. Insulin requirements begin to rise late in the first trimester as glucose use and glycogen storage by the woman and fetus are increased. As a result of placental maturation and production of hPL and other hormones, insulin requirements may double or quadruple by the end of pregnancy.

Increased energy needs during labor may require more insulin to balance intravenous glucose. After delivery of the placenta, insulin requirements usually decrease abruptly with loss of hPL in the maternal circulation.

Other factors contribute to the difficulty in controlling the disease. As pregnancy progresses, the renal threshold for glucose decreases. There is also an increased risk of ketoacidosis, which may occur at lower serum glucose levels in the pregnant woman with diabetes. The vascular disease that accompanies diabetes may progress during pregnancy. Hypertension may occur. Nephropathy may result from renal impairment, and retinopathy may also occur.

The primary concern for the pregnant woman who has diabetes is control of circulating blood glucose levels. If control can be achieved and maintained, diabetes generally does not worsen during pregnancy. The woman's health status may even improve due to close medical supervision.

Influence of Diabetes on Pregnancy Outcome

The discovery of insulin in 1922 allowed women with diabetes to survive to adulthood and bear children. Since then maternal mortality from diabetes has been minimal. However, the pregnancy of a woman who has diabetes carries a higher risk of complications, especially perinatal mortality. The risk of perinatal mortality has been reduced by the recent recognition of the importance of tight metabolic control (glucose between 70 mg/dL and 120 mg/dL). New techniques for monitoring blood glucose, delivering insulin, and monitoring the fetus have also reduced perinatal mortality in major medical centers to between 2 percent and 4 percent (Hollander & Maeder 1985) or less.

MATERNAL RISKS

Maternal health problems from diabetic pregnancy have been greatly reduced with the team approach to early prenatal care and emphasis on maintaining control of blood glucose levels. The prognosis for the pregnant woman with gestational, type I, or type II diabetes that has not resulted in significant vascular damage is positive. However, diabetic pregnancy still carries higher risks for complications than normal pregnancy.

Hydramnios, or an increase in the volume of amniotic fluid, occurs in 10 percent of pregnant diabetics (Gilbert & Harmon 1986). The exact mechanism causing the increase is unknown. Premature rupture of membranes and onset of labor may result, but only occasionally does this pose a threat. Amniocentesis may be used to decrease fluid volume; however, this procedure predisposes the woman to infection, initiation of premature labor, premature separation of the placenta due to manipulation, and hemorrhage due to placental laceration.

Pregnancy-induced hypertension occurs more often in diabetic pregnancies, especially when diabetes-related vascular changes already exist.

Hyperglycemia due to insufficient amounts of insulin can lead to *ketoacidosis* as a result of the increase in ketone bodies (which are acidic) in the blood released in metabolism of fatty acids. Ketoacidosis usually develops slowly, but it may develop more rapidly in the pregnant woman because of the hyperketonemia associated with accelerated starvation in the nonfed state. The tendency for higher postprandial glucose levels because of decreased gastric motility and the contrainsulin effects of hPL also predispose the woman to ketoacidosis. If the ketoacidosis is not treated, it can lead to coma and death of both mother and fetus.

In pregnancy, particularly in the presence of prolonged vomiting, carbohydrate deficiency may lead to ketosis as fat cells are metabolized for energy needs. Measurement of blood glucose levels will easily differentiate starvation ketosis (a hypoglycemic state treated with glucose solution) from diabetic ketoacidosis (a hyperglycemic state treated with insulin).

Another risk to the pregnant woman with diabetes is dystocia, caused by feto-pelvic disproportion if fetal macrosomia exists. Anemia may develop as a result of vascular involvement and poor nutritional intake. Infections, particularly monilial vaginitis and urinary tract infections, may develop if glycosuria persists. Intrauterine fetal death may occur if maternal glucose levels are not well controlled.

FETAL-NEONATAL RISKS

Maintaining maternal glucose in the normal range has resulted not only in decreased perinatal mortality but also in reduced perinatal morbidity. It is now clear that many of the problems of the neonate result directly from high maternal plasma glucose levels (Steel 1985).

Macrosomia and *hypoglycemia* in the neonate are due to high levels of fetal production of insulin, stimulated by the high levels of glucose crossing the placenta from the mother. Sustained fetal hyperinsulinism and hyperglycemia ultimately lead to excessive growth and deposition of fat. After birth the umbilical cord is severed, and thus the generous maternal blood glucose supply is eliminated. However, continued islet cell hyperactivity leads to excessive insulin levels and depleted blood glucose (hypoglycemia) in 2 to 4 hours. Macrosomia can be significantly reduced by tight maternal blood glucose control before 32 weeks' gestation (Lin et al 1986).

Infants of mothers with advanced diabetes may demonstrate intrauterine growth regardation (IUGR). This occurs because vascular changes in the diabetic woman decrease the efficiency of placental perfusion and the infant is not as well sustained in utero.

Respiratory distress syndrome appears to result from inhibition, by high levels of fetal insulin, of some fetal enzymes necessary for surfactant production. *Polycythemia* in the neonate is due primarily to the diminished ability of glycosylated hemoglobin in the mother's blood to release oxygen. *Hyperbilirubinemia* is a direct result of the inability of immature liver enzymes to metabolize the increased bilirubin resulting from the polycythemia.

In the presence of untreated maternal ketoacidosis, the risk of fetal death increases to between 50 percent and 90 percent (Brumfield & Huddleson 1984). The fetal enzymes systems cease functioning in an acidic environment.

Despite the reduction in perinatal mortality and morbidity, the incidence of *congenital anomalies* in diabetic pregnancies remains at least four times the rate in nondiabetic pregnancy (Steel 1985). Most of the anomalies involve the heart, central nervous system, and skeletal system and occur in the presence of high glucose levels during organogenesis prior to seven weeks' gestation. To reduce the incidence of congenital anomalies there is a clear need for diabetic control well before conception.

Medical Therapy

Screening for the detection of diabetes is a standard part of prenatal care. If the possibility of diabetes is suspected, further testing is undertaken for diagnosis.

DETECTION AND DIAGNOSIS

Two screening tests are commonly administered to pregnant women:

1. *Urine testing.* The pregnant woman's urine is tested for glucose at her first prenatal visit and again on subsequent visits. Glycosuria is not diagnostic of diabetes mellitus, but the presence of glycosuria is indication for glucose tolerance testing. In the nonpregnant adult, glucose is not generally spilled into the urine until the blood sugar level is 180 mg/dL

or greater. In the presence of pregnancy the renal threshold is lower, and glucose may spill into the urine when blood glucose levels are 130 mg/dL.

Tes-Tape and Diastix are methods of choice in urine testing. They are specific for glucose and do not show positive readings in the presence of lactose or fructose. Single-specimen urine tests are used in routine screening each antenatal visit.

Urine is also tested for ketones. Ketostix is specific for acetoacetic acid, the first by-product of fat oxidation, while Acetest is specific for both acetone and acetoacetic acid. Both are simple tests for detecting ketones in the urine and are usually done routinely for type I (ketosis-prone) diabetes.

2. *50 g, 1-hour diabetes screening test.* It has become common practice to screen all pregnant women for gestational diabetes between 24 and 28 weeks' gestation. To do this test, the woman ingests a 50 g oral glucose solution. One hour later a blood sample is obtained. If the plasma glucose level exceeds 140 mg/dL, a diagnostic glucose tolerance test (GTT) is necessary. The 50 g screen test is convenient because the woman does not need to be fasting, and the test does not need to be done following a meal (Coustan & Carpenter 1985).

During pregnancy gestational diabetes mellitus is diagnosed using a 100 g oral glucose tolerance test. To do this test the woman eats a high-carbohydrate (greater than 200 g carbohydrate daily) diet for two days prior to her scheduled test. She then fasts from midnight on the day of the test. A fasting plasma glucose level is obtained, and the woman ingests 100 g oral glucose solution. Plasma glucose levels are determined at one, two, and three hours. Gestational diabetes is diagnosed if two or more of the following values are equaled or exceeded (Gabbe 1986):

Fasting	105 mg/dL
1 hr	190 mg/dL
2 hr	165 mg/dL
3 hr	145 mg/dL

If the woman presents with any of the following, the screen is omitted and she is given a three-hour glucose tolerance test:

● The cardinal signs of DM (polyuria, polydipsia, polyphagia, weight loss)

● Obesity

● Family history of DM

● Obstetric history that includes a large-for-gestational-age (LGA) neonate, hydramnios, unexplained stillbirth, or congenital anomalies

LABORATORY ASSESSMENT OF LONG-TERM GLUCOSE CONTROL

○ *GLYCOSYLATED HEMOGLOBIN* This test reflects glucose control over the previous 4 to 12 weeks (Cousins et al 1985). It measures the percentage in the blood of glycohemoglobin (HbA_{1c}, hemoglobin to which a glucose molecule is attached). Because glycosylation is a rather slow and essentially irreversible process, the level of HbA_{1c} gives an indication of previous average serum glucose concentrations.

Normally 6 percent to 8 percent of hemoglobin is glycosylated. An elevation of glycohemoglobin in pregnancy is associated with increased incidence of congenital anomalies (Miller et al 1981). Further studies have shown that spontaneous abortions increase with glycosylated hemoglobin concentrations over 12 percent (Miodovnik et al

Research Note

Antepartal medical management of diabetes requires frequent physician visits, diet control, monitoring of blood glucose levels, urine testing, ultrasound, nonstress testing, and sometimes insulin injections and amniocentesis. The purpose of this survey was to identify which aspects of the regimen are most stressful to pregnant women, and to determine if the regimen is more stressful to the woman with gestational diabetes who is unfamiliar with it than to the woman with chronic diabetes who has experienced many parts of the regimen before pregnancy.

Questionnaires were completed by 20 gestational diabetic women and 18 women with chronic diabetes. The responses indicated that amniocentesis was most stressful for both groups, and ultrasound and nonstress tests were least stressful. The more invasive procedures, i.e., blood tests, amniocentesis, and insulin administration, were more stressful to women with gestational rather than chronic diabetes. Diet and urine tests were more stressful to women with chronic diabetes.

Nurses need to be aware that a diabetic woman experiences pregnancy as both a maturational and situational crisis.

The related stress, validated in this study, can decrease learning ability, so these women may need repeated instruction as well as realistic positive support during pregnancy.

Zigrossi, ST, Riga-Ziegler, M: The stress of medical management on pregnant diabetics. Am J Mat Child Nurs 1985;11(September/October):320–23.

1985). Neonatal macrosomia and hyperbilirubinemia are associated with maternal levels over 7 percent. For a woman who is a known diabetic, this test should be done at preconception counseling, again at the first prenatal visit, and once each succeeding trimester.

MANAGEMENT OF PREGESTATIONAL DIABETES MELLITUS

The major goals of medical care for a pregnant woman with diabetes are: (a) to maintain a physiologic equilibrium of insulin availability and glucose utilization during pregnancy, and (b) to deliver an optimally healthy mother and newborn. To achieve these goals, good prenatal care using a team approach must be a top priority. This care is best accomplished at a medical center. The team consists of an obstetrician, an endocrinologist, a perinatologist, a nurse-diabetes educator, a perinatal nurse, a nutritionist, a social worker, and, most importantly, the diabetic woman and her partner. Education of the couple and their active involvement in managing her care are essential for a good outcome (McCoy & Oswald 1983).

○ ANTEPARTAL PERIOD During the antepartal period, medical therapy focuses on several aspects including the following:

- *Dietary regulation.* In early pregnancy the recommended daily calorie intake does not increase but remains at 30 to 35 kcal/kg body weight. During the second and third trimesters daily intake is increased to 200 kcal/day over prepregnancy intake. Approximately 45 percent of the calories should come from complex carbohydrates with adequate fiber to slow down absorption, about 20 percent of calories (or 1.5 g/kg body weight) should be protein, and 30 percent to 35 percent should be fat (Gabbe 1985). This food is divided among three meals and three snacks. Usually 25 percent of the calories are taken at breakfast, 30 percent at lunch, 30 percent at dinner, and 15 percent divided among snacks (Gabbe 1985). The prebedtime snack is the most important and must include both protein and complex carbohydrates to prevent hypoglycemia at night. Because it is so important that the pregnant woman follow these guidelines, a nutritionist works out meal plans based on the woman's life-style, culture, and food preferences and teaches her food exchanges so she can vary and plan her own meals. Cookbooks for diabetics are available and can be a great help.

- *Glucose monitoring.* Home monitoring of blood glucose levels is the most accurate and convenient method for determining insulin dose and assessing glucose control. A drop of capillary blood, obtained by finger puncture, is placed on a glucose oxidase-impregnated reagent strip. The strip changes or intensifies color in proportion to the glucose concentration in the blood. Depending on the brand, the color on the strip is compared to a color chart on the bottle label for a semiquantitative estimation of glucose level or is used with a glucose reflectance meter, which gives a digital reading of the glucose value.

- *Insulin administration.* Insulin is given either in multiple injections or by continuous subcutaneous infusion. Multiple injections are used more commonly, and with excellent results. A mixture of intermediate-acting (NPH) and short-acting (regular) insulin is taken twice a day. Usually two-thirds of the total insulin dose is taken with breakfast in a ratio of NPH to regular of 2:1. The remaining third is taken with supper in a 1:1 ratio (Granados 1984).

- *Evaluation of fetal status.* Information regarding the well-being and maturation of the fetus is important for planning the course of pregnancy and the timing of delivery. Biophysical methods of fetal surveillance, such as the nonstress test (NST), serial ultrasounds, fetal movement counts, and contraction stress tests (CST), have proved more valuable than biochemical tests (Gabbe 1985). Serial estriol levels are less accurate and more expensive than biophysical methods and are sometimes difficult and slow to interpret.

  Nonstress testing is usually begun weekly at about 28 weeks and increased to twice weekly at about 34 weeks. If the woman requires hospitalization (eg, to control glycemia, for PIH, or hydramnios), nonstress testing is done daily (Granados 1984).

  Maternal evaluation of fetal activity is effective, simple to perform, and begun at about 28 weeks. The woman is taught a particular method for counting fetal movements (see Chapter 20). She is given a card on which to record movements and brings the card to each subsequent office visit.

- *Ultrasound* early in pregnancy establishes gestational age and diagnoses multiple pregnancy or congenital anomalies. Later in pregnancy repeated ultrasound can monitor fetal growth for IUGR or macrosomia (Granados 1984).

- *Contraction stress testing* is used primarily if there is a nonreactive NST or if some variable decelerations are seen on the tracing (see Chapter 20).

○ INTRAPARTAL PERIOD During the intrapartal period, medical therapy includes:

- *Timing of delivery.* In most diabetic pregnancies, pregnancy is allowed to go to term, with spontaneous labor, thereby decreasing the risk of respiratory distress in the neonate. In pregnancies in which there is evidence of fetal macrosomia, fetal compromise, or elevated maternal HbA$_{1c}$, amniocentesis is done for lecithin/sphingomyelin ratio and the presence of the phospholipid phosphatidylglycerol (PG). If the L/S ratio is ≥2.0 and PG is present, the fetal lungs are considered mature and delivery can be undertaken by induction or cesarean.

● *Labor management.* The degree of prenatal maintenance of normal maternal glucose levels (euglycemia) and the maintenance of maternal euglycemia during labor are important in preventing neonatal hypoglycemia (Gabbe 1986). A 5 percent dextrose solution is given by intravenous infusion covered by subcutaneous or IV insulin. Maternal glucose levels are measured every one or two hours to determine insulin dosage. It has been found that insulin clings to the plastic intravenous bag and tubing. To ensure that the woman receives the desired dose, the intravenous tubing must be flushed with insulin before the prescribed amount is added to the intravenous bag of dextrose and water. During the second stage of labor and the immediate postdelivery period, the woman may not need additional insulin. The intravenous insulin is discontinued with the completion of the third stage of labor.

○ **POSTPARTAL PERIOD** Postpartally maternal insulin requirements fall significantly. This occurs because the levels of hPL, progesterone, and estrogen fall after placental separation and their anti-insulin effect ceases, resulting in decreased blood glucose levels. The diabetic mother may require no insulin for the first 24 hours or only one-fourth to one-half her previous dose. Then reestablishment of insulin needs based on blood sugar testing is necessary. Diet and exercise levels must also be redetermined.

Diabetic control and the establishment of parent-child relationships in light of neonatal needs are the priorities of this period. If her newborn must be cared for in a special care nursery, the mother needs support and information about the baby's condition. Every effort must be made to provide as much contact as possible between the parents and their newborn.

Other components of postpartal care include:

● *Breast-feeding.* Breast-feeding is encouraged as beneficial to both mother and baby. Blood glucose levels may be lower because glucose is transferred from serum to breast to be converted to lactose, and energy is expended in milk production. Therefore calorie needs increase during lactation, and insulin must be adjusted accordingly. Home blood glucose monitoring should continue for the insulin-dependent diabetic.

● *Contraception.* Combined estrogen/progesterone oral contraceptives are not recommended for insulin-dependent diabetic women because of the increased risk of thromboembolic disease and vasculopathy (Gabbe 1985). The progesterone-only pill carries a higher failure rate but is otherwise safer. The IUD remains controversial. Barrier methods are safe but have a slightly higher failure rate. Elective sterilization is often discussed with the couple who have completed their family.

MANAGEMENT OF GESTATIONAL DIABETES

Gestational diabetes most often develops in the third trimester. Therefore women should be screened for diabetes at approximately 24 to 28 weeks' gestation with the 50 g oral glucose test. Most gestational diabetics can be controlled by diet, but about 10 percent to 15 percent will need supplemental insulin, as evidenced by a fasting plasma glucose level >105 mg/dL or a postprandial (two hours after breakfast) plasma glucose level >120 mg/dL. For these women a highly purified porcine insulin or human insulin should be used to reduce the risk of antibody formation (Gabbe 1985). Oral hypoglycemics are never used during pregnancy as they are considered teratogenic. Fetal surveillance, usually by NST, is important during the last two months of pregnancy to ensure optimal timing of delivery.

Nursing Assessment

Whether diabetes (usually type I) has been diagnosed before pregnancy occurs or the diagnosis is made during pregnancy (GDM), careful assessment of the disease process and the woman's understanding of diabetes is important. Thorough physical examination, including assessment for vascular complications of the disease, any signs of infectious conditions, and urine and blood testing for glucose, is essential on the first antenatal visit. Follow-up visits are usually scheduled twice a month during the first two trimesters and once a week during the last trimester.

Assessment is also needed to yield information about the woman's ability to cope with the combined stress of pregnancy and diabetes, and her ability to follow a recommended regimen of care. Determination of the woman's knowledge about diabetes and self-care is needed before formulating a teaching plan.

Nursing Diagnosis

Nursing diagnoses that may apply are included in the nursing care plan beginning on p 472.

Nursing Care Plan: Diabetes Mellitus

Roxie Williams is a G2 P1 woman who is 23 weeks pregnant. During her first pregnancy Mrs Williams developed gestational diabetes and mild preeclampsia. Her son weighed 4150 g and had some difficulty with low Dextrostix readings. Mrs Williams's maternal grandmother was an insulin-dependent diabetic who died of complications of the disease. Mrs Williams's FPG and 3-hour OGTT were abnormally high, and she was admitted to the hospital to stabilize her diabetes. Mrs Williams experienced monilial vaginitis early in her pregnancy. Mrs Williams's husband was not able to get much time off from work, but her mother is caring for their son, Dean.

Assessment

NURSING HISTORY

Identification of predisposing factors including:
a. Previous history gestational diabetes mellitus
b. History of preeclampsia
c. Previous LGA infant (>4000 gm)
d. Family history of DM

PHYSICAL EXAMINATION

a. Frequent urination beyond first trimester and prior to third
b. Presence of monilial vaginitis on examination
c. Fundal height greater than expected for length of gestation (twins previously R/O by ultrasound)

LABORATORY EVALUATION

a. Elevated fasting plasma glucose (FPG)
b. Elevated 3-hour OGTT
c. Monilial vaginitis confirmed with wet mount

NURSING PRIORITIES

a. Observe for signs of hypoglycemia, hyperglycemia, preeclampsia
b. Test blood regularly for glucose levels
c. Implement insulin and dietary regulation as needed
d. Assess knowledge level of client relative to disease

Nursing Diagnosis and Goals	Nursing Interventions	Rationale
NURSING DIAGNOSIS: Alteration in nutrition: more than body requirements related to imbalance between intake and available insulin	Maintain strict diet: 1. 30–35 kcal/kg 2. 150–200 g carbohydrate 3. 125 g protein 4. 60–80 g fat to provide approximately 35% of fetal stores 5. Sodium intake may be restricted	Maintain ideal weight in first trimester and average gain in last two trimesters (no more than 3–3.5 lb/month).
SUPPORTING DATA: Mrs Williams has already gained 24 lb. Ultrasound reveals that her fetus is already showing evidence of being LGA.	Assess insulin needs: 1. Check lab results of FPG and 2-hour postprandial. 2. Test blood four times daily using Dextrostix. 3. Teach use of home blood glucose monitoring device. Determine amount of insulin based on sliding scale. 4. Adminster regular or NPH insulin, or combination, as ordered.	Sufficient insulin must be present to enable proper carbohydrate metabolism to take place; pregnancy requires a marked increase in circulating insulin to maintain normal blood glucose. Fasting glucose level tends to be lower than nonpregnant value. Effectiveness of insulin may be reduced by presence of hPL. Insulin requirements fluctuate widely during pregnancy because of factors mentioned in text and because of lowered glucose tolerance, especially in second half of pregnancy, and fluctuate during intrapartal period because of depletion of glycogen stores during labor; fluctuations during puerperium are a result of involuntary process; in addition, conversion of blood glucose into lactose during lactation may cause marked changes in glucose tolerance and/or hypoglycemia.
CLIENT GOALS: Mrs Williams will be able to describe her prescribed diet and agree to follow it. Mrs Williams will be able to explain her insulin dosage routine.		

Nursing Care Plan: Diabetes Mellitus (continued)

Nursing Diagnosis and Goals	Nursing Interventions	Rationale

NURSING DIAGNOSIS:
 	
Potential for injury related to possible complications secondary to hypoglycemia
	1. Teach early signs of hypoglycemia and treatment.
	2. Observe for signs of hypoglycemia (see Table 19–3).
	3. Treat within minutes of onset if hypoglycemia develops.
	  a. Obtain immediate blood samples for testing.
	  b. If Mrs Williams is alert give half a glass of orange juice or other liquid containing sugar; notify physician.
	  c. If Mrs Williams is not alert enough to swallow, give 1 mg glucagon subcutaneously or intramuscularly; notify physician.
	  d. If Mrs Williams is in labor with intravenous lines in place, 10–20 mL of 50% dextrose may be given IV.
	Standing order should be available; notify physician.
		Self-care at home is a preventive measure so hypoglycemia will not become serious.
		
		Correction of hypoglycemia and maintenance of controlled state provide optimal fetal health
		
		Rapid treatment of hypoglycemia is essential to prevent brain damage as the brain requires glucose to function (skeletal and heart muscles can derive energy from ketones and free fatty acids).

SUPPORTING DATA: Mrs Williams developed signs of hypoglycemia twice while attempting to determine appropriate insulin dosage.		Baseline information is needed on glucose levels. Liquids are absorbed from the GI tract faster than solids; 10 g of glucose, which will reverse most hypoglycemic reactions, is the amount found in one-half glass orange juice, 2 tsp sugar, or 1 or 2 hard candies.
CLIENT GOAL: Mrs Williams will identify signs of hypoglycemia and will be able to describe appropriate self-treatment		Glucagon triggers the conversion of glycogen stored in the liver to glucose.

NURSING DIAGNOSIS:
 	
Potential for injury related to possible complications secondary to hyperglycemia.
	1. Teach Mrs Williams early signs of hyperglycemia and treatment.
	2. Observe for signs of hyperglycemia (see Table 19–3); administer treatment; notify physician.
	  a. Obtain frequent measurement of blood and urine glucose; measure urine acetone.
	  b. Administer prescribed amount regular insulin subcutaneously or intravenously, or combination of routes.
	  c. Replace fluids IV, orally, or both.
	  d. Measure intake and output.
	  e. Observe for symptoms of circulatory collapse; monitor BP and pulse.
		Client can recognize signs and administer self-treatment.
		
		Client can also report any symptoms that may occur.
		
		Administer insulin to restore body's normal metabolism of carbohydrate, protein, and fat.

SUPPORTING DATA: Mrs Williams was mildly hyperglycemic when admitted to the hospital. Because her diabetes requires insulin she should be familiar with the signs of this common complication.		Need to establish a baseline and to determine additional insulin dosage and prevent overtreatment; urine acetone indicates development of ketoacidosis. Regular insulin used because it acts immediately and is of short duration.
CLIENT GOAL: Mrs Williams will be able to identify signs of hyperglycemia and describe appropriate interventions if it occurs.		Fluids are depleted in the process of ketoacidosis; hypotension can result from decreased blood volume due to dehydration. Polyuria is an early sign of hyperglycemia; oliguria develops with hypotension and decreased blood flow to kidneys. Circulatory collapse can result from hypotension.

Nursing Care Plan: Diabetes Mellitus (continued)

Nursing Diagnosis and Goals	Nursing Interventions	Rationale
NURSING DIAGNOSIS: Possible alteration in comfort: acute itching and burning related to monilial vaginitis	Observe for symptoms of burning, itching, and leukorrhea; obtain vaginal smear; treat with prescription based on the causative organism and gestation.	Vaginitis is more common in the woman with diabetes; treatment is specific to the organism.
SUPPORTING DATA: Mrs Williams has a history of monilial vaginitis and is more susceptible to recurrence due to DM and pregnancy	Discuss self-care measures Mrs Williams can use to help avoid recurrence.	Self-care measures enable the woman to meet her own health needs at home and enable her to function independently.
CLIENT GOALS: 1. Mrs Williams will be able to describe appropriate self-care measures to avoid recurrence of infection. 2. Mrs Williams will identify early symptoms of monilial vaginitis.		
NURSING DIAGNOSIS: Knowledge deficit about the disease, its treatment, its implications for her and her fetus and for the birth process.	Support and encourage Mr and Mrs Williams: 1. Explain procedures. 2. Allow them to ask questions. 3. Develop a teaching plan to discuss and provide opportunities to practice administering insulin. Provide written information. Include Mr Williams so he can administer insulin if necessary. 4. Assess their level of knowledge of childbirth and use this to teach about what is happening. 5. Provide information about possible changes to expect during L & D due to DM. Explain about IV insulin, continuous monitoring of fetal status. Stress unchanged aspects of the experience.	Decreasing fear and increasing knowledge will make the client a more-effective member of the antepartal-intrapartal health team.
SUPPORTING DATA: Mrs Williams stated, "It seems like so much. I don't know if I'll ever understand everything or be able to give myself insulin." Mrs Williams stated, "This will change everything about delivery, won't it?"		Anticipatory guidance helps the couple prepare for the upcoming experience.
CLIENT GOALS: 1. Mrs Williams and her partner will be able to demonstrate correct procedure for administering insulin. 2. Mrs Williams will be able to discuss the possible impact of DM on her delivery.		

Nursing Care Plan: Diabetes Mellitus (continued)

Nursing Diagnosis and Goals	Nursing Interventions	Rationale
NURSING DIAGNOSIS: Potential for fetal injury related to effects of DM on uteroplacental functioning.	Periodic assessments: 1. Level of plasma and/or urine estriol	Continued slow rise of estriol indicates adequate functioning of maternal system, placental function, and fetal status, because estriol and creatinine require interplay of all three systems.
	2. Creatinine clearance	It is necessary to assess fetal growth.
	3. Regular assessment of fetal size 4. Ultrasonographs 5. L/S ratio, or phosphatidylgycerol or phosphatidylinositol levels 6. NST or CST	It is necessary to evaluate fetal size. A 2:1 ratio usually indicates fetal lung maturity sufficient to sustain infant in extrauterine environment. In one-third of insulin-dependent women, L/S ratio fails to show a terminal rise; others show early excessive rise.
SUPPORTING DATA: Mrs Williams's history with first pregnancy Confirmation of IDDM in this pregnancy		
CLIENT GOAL: 1. Mrs Williams will be able to discuss the importance of scrupulous control of her diabetes and the need to monitor fetal activity to ensure the delivery of a healthy baby.		
NURSING DIAGNOSIS: Alterations in family process related to Mrs Williams's DM and the need for hospitalization	Provide Mrs Williams with frequent opportunities to see her son, Dean, including day passes. Discuss with Mrs Williams, her mother, and Mr Williams their plans for coping when Mrs Williams is discharged.	Illness in one family member impacts the entire family. Sometimes outside support is necessary to help the family deal with feelings and identify ways of dealing with the illness of a member.
SUPPORTING DATA: Mr Williams stated, "Dean really seems to miss you and, boy, I sure do, too." Mrs Williams stated, "How are we going to manage when Mother leaves?"	Arrange for social services to visit or for homemaker assistance if necessary following discharge. Give the family members information about the frustration that can occur when a family member is ill. Provide opportunities for them to discuss their feelings. Offer suggestions for coping.	
CLIENT GOALS: 1. Mr and Mrs Williams will work out a plan that is acceptable to both. 2. The couple will discuss their feelings with each other in an open, caring way.		

Epilogue

Mrs Williams was discharged after six days. She was readmitted once at 32 weeks for problems with hypoglycemia, and her insulin dosage was again stabilized. Mrs Williams followed her diet faithfully and monitored her glucose levels at home with a glucometer. Mr Williams accompanied her for her NSTs when he was able. On other occasions a close friend came with her. Mrs Williams had no recurrence of monilial vaginitis and never developed signs of preeclampsia. She went into labor spontaneously at 39 weeks and delivered an 8 lb 5 oz daughter. Postpartally all did well.

Nursing Goal: Provision of Prepregnancy Counseling

This counseling may be provided by a nurse and a physician, using a team approach.

Ideally the couple is seen prior to pregnancy so that the diabetes can be assessed by ophthalmologic evaluation, electrocardiographic study, and a 24-hour urine collection for creatinine clearance and protein excretion. This will determine the woman's suitability for pregnancy (Gabbe 1985). If the diabetes is of recent onset without vascular complications, the outcome of pregnancy should be good if glucose levels can be controlled. The couple is given education regarding nutrition, insulin administration, home glucose monitoring, exercise, and the importance of maintaining good glucose control for a positive perinatal outcome. They need to have time to incorporate these teachings into their lives.

Nursing Goal: Promotion of Effective Insulin Use

The nurse ensures that the couple understands the purpose of the insulin, the types of insulin the woman is to use, and the correct procedure for its administration. The woman's partner is also instructed about insulin administration in case it should be necessary for him to give it.

For some highly motivated women whose glucose levels are not well controlled with multiple injections, the continuous insulin infusion pump offers the best control (Granados 1984). A needle is secured in the subcutaneous tissue of the anterior abdominal wall and connected by cannula to a syringe filled with regular insulin. A pump that automatically resets to the basal infusion rate after giving the preprandial bolus is important for preventing problems of hypoglycemia (Landon & Gabbe 1985). The woman needs to learn to use the insulin pump and become confident in coordinating the dosages with her glucose readings to achieve euglycemia. The nurse-diabetes educator works with her to achieve these goals.

As part of the woman's ongoing care she is taught to monitor her blood glucose levels at home. The information this monitoring provides is used to regulate insulin dosage. The nurse works with the woman to teach her the correct method for home glucose monitoring (Figure 19–1). Spring devices are available for sticking the finger to obtain blood samples. These devices make the procedure easier and less painful. The woman should be taught to use the sides of her fingertips rather than the more sensitive tips themselves. She should be taught to cleanse the area before sticking to avoid infection. The reagent strip container should be kept tightly closed when not being used. Once the specimen of blood has been obtained and is placed on the reagent strip, directions for timing and for washing or wiping the blood off should be followed exactly to ensure accurate readings.

Nursing Goal: Promotion of a Planned Exercise Program

The nurse-diabetes educator and the nutritionist, collaborating with the physician, work out a regular, appropriate, and satisfactory exercise plan with the woman.

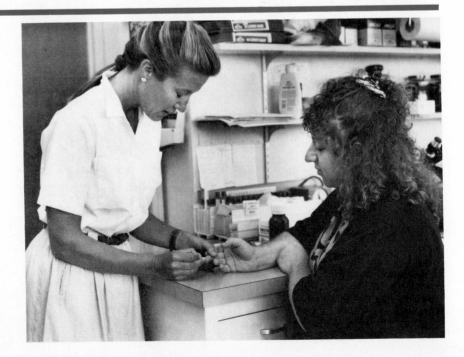

Figure 19–1   The nurse teaches the mother how to do home glucose monitoring.

Exercise is encouraged for the woman's overall well-being. If she is used to a regular exercise program, she is encouraged to continue, following the guidelines in Box 19–1. If not, she is encouraged to begin gradually, with a plan structured around (1) the desired effects of exercise; (2) preferences for type of exercise, location, time of day, duration, and company; and (3) any medical or physical limitations to exercise (McCoy & Oswald 1983). Due to alterations in metabolism with exercise, the woman's blood glucose should be well controlled before she begins an exercise program.

Nursing Goal: Education for Self-Care

The nurse provides appropriate information to the pregnant woman and her family so that the woman can meet her own health care needs as much as possible. Such health teaching should include information on the following.

SYMPTOMS OF HYPOGLYCEMIA AND KETOACIDOSIS

It is essential that the pregnant diabetic woman recognize symptoms of changing glucose levels and take appropriate action (see Table 19–3). She needs to know fast sources of glucose (simple carbohydrates) that she can use to treat an insulin reaction. The woman should also be informed about foods containing complex carbohydrates and protein, which provide the type of glucose needed to prevent nocturnal hypoglycemia (Ceresa & Theiss 1983).

Because the pregnant diabetic is more prone to ketoacidosis than the nonpregnant diabetic, she and her partner need to know its symptoms, monitor blood glucose levels, and notify the physician if symptoms occur.

SMOKING

Smoking is contraindicated for both pregnancy and diabetes. Smoking has harmful effects on both the maternal vascular system and the developing fetus.

TRAVEL

Insulin can be kept at room temperature while traveling. Small travel kits are available for carrying insulin, syringes, and glucagon. These items should always be carried on the person rather than in luggage in a baggage compartment. A diabetic person should always wear an identification bracelet or necklace stating that she is diabetic. Meals can be arranged with airlines a few days before traveling and exchange lists can be carried. The woman should learn to say *diabetes* in a few foreign languages. She should check with her physician for any instructions, prescriptions, or advice before leaving.

Box 19–1 Guidelines for Prevention of Hypoglycemia From Exercise

1. Exercise after a meal, not when blood sugar may be low.

2. Do not administer insulin into an extremity that will be immediately used in the exercise.

3. Carry simple sugar carbohydrate with you when exercising, eg, Lifesavers or hard candy.

4. Wear diabetic identification.

5. Eat after prolonged exercise.

6. Monitor your blood glucose to determine its variations with exercise.

Modified from McCoy D, Oswald J: An interactive model program of care for diabetic women before and during pregnancy. *Diabetes Educator* 1983;9(Summer suppl):11s.

HOSPITALIZATION

Hospitalization may become necessary during the pregnancy to evaluate blood glucose levels and adjust insulin requirements.

SUPPORT GROUPS

Many communities have diabetes support groups or education classes, which can be most helpful to women with newly diagnosed diabetes. Learning that others have faced a similar situation and hearing how they managed are great aids in trying to cope with a chronic disease.

CESAREAN BIRTH

Chances for a cesarean birth are increased if the pregnant woman is diabetic. This possibility should be anticipated—enrollment in cesarean birth preparation classes may be suggested. Many hospitals offer classes, and information is available through organizations such as Cesarean/Support Education and Concern (C/Sec, Inc); Cesarean Birth Council; or the Cesarean Association for Research, Education, Support and Satisfaction in Birthing (CARESS). The couple may prefer simply to discuss cesarean birth with the nurse and their obstetrician and read some books on the topic.

Evaluative Outcome Criteria

Anticipated outcomes of nursing care include the following:

• The woman clearly understands her condition and

Table 19–3   Comparison of Hypoglycemia and Hyperglycemia

	Hypoglycemia	Hyperglycemia
Causes	Too much insulin Too little food Increased exercise without increased food	Too little insulin Too much food (especially carbohydrate) Emotional stress Infection
Onset	Usually sudden (minutes to half-hour)	Slow (days)
Symptoms in general order of appearance	Nervousness Shakiness Weakness Hunger Sweatiness Cool clammy skin Pallor Blurred or double vision Headache Disorientation Shallow respirations Irritability Convulsions Coma	Polyuria Polydipsia Dry mouth Increased appetite Tiredness Nausea Hot flushed skin Abdominal cramps Abdominal rigidity Rapid deep breathing Acetone breath Paralysis Headache Soft eyeballs Drowsiness Oliguria or anuria Depressed reflexes Stupor Coma
Laboratory findings: Urine	Glucose—negative Acetone—usually negative	Glucose—positive Acetone—positive
Blood	Glucose—60 mg/dL or lower Acetone—negative	Glucose—±250 mg/dL Acetone—usually positive

Treatment: See Nursing Care Plan for Diabetes Mellitus

Other comas: Hyperosmolar coma is most often seen in persons over 60 years of age with type II diabetes. Lactic acidosis coma occurs in advanced stages of diabetes, especially in persons with uremia, arteriosclerotic heart disease, pneumonia, acute pancreatitis, chronic alcoholism, and bacterial infection.

Adapted from Guthrie DW, Guthrie RA: *Nursing Management of Diabetes Mellitus,* ed 2. St Louis, Mosby, 1982.

its possible impact on her pregnancy, labor and delivery, and postpartal period.

● The woman cooperates and participates in developing a health care regimen to meet her needs and follows it throughout her pregnancy.

● The woman successfully delivers a healthy newborn.

● The woman avoids developing hypoglycemia or hyperglycemia.

● The woman is able to care for her newborn.

● **Care of the Woman With Anemia**

Anemias in pregnancy may be due specifically to the pregnancy, or they may exist coincidentally with the pregnancy. For example, iron deficiency anemia and folic acid deficiency anemia may be caused by pregnancy. Anemias that are not induced by pregnancy but are acquired or hereditary, such as sickle cell anemia, may be exacerbated by pregnancy.

Iron Deficiency Anemia

Dietary iron is needed to synthesize hemoglobin. Since hemoglobin is necessary for the transport of oxygen, a deficiency of iron leads to a decrease in hemoglobin and may affect the body's transport of oxygen.

Iron deficiency anemia is the most common medical complication of pregnancy, affecting between 15 percent and 50 percent of all pregnant women in the United States (Troy & Wisch 1985). Approximately 200 mg of iron will be conserved due to the functional amenorrhea of pregnancy, but a pregnant woman needs approximately 1000 mg more iron intake during the pregnancy. Between 300 and 400 mg of iron is transferred to the fetus; 500 mg is needed for the increased red blood cell mass in the woman's own increased circulating blood volume; another 100 mg is needed for the placenta; and about 280 mg is needed to replace the 1 mg of iron lost daily through feces, urine, and sweat.

The greatest need for increased iron intake is in the second half of pregnancy. When the iron needs of pregnancy are not met, hemoglobin (Hb) falls below 11 g/dL.

Serum ferritin levels, indicating iron stores, are below 12 μg/L.

Many women begin pregnancy in a slightly anemic state. In pregnancy mild anemia can rapidly become more severe; therefore it needs immediate treatment.

MATERNAL RISKS

The woman with iron deficiency anemia is more susceptible to infection, tires easily, has an increased chance of postpartal hemorrhage, and tolerates poorly even minimal blood loss during delivery. If the anemia is severe (Hb less than 6 g/dL), cardiac failure may ensue.

FETAL-NEONATAL RISKS

The incidence of stillbirth and SGA neonates is increased with severe anemia. Fetal iron stores are not significantly impaired. The fetus may be hypoxic during labor due to impaired uteroplacental oxygenation.

MEDICAL THERAPY

The first goal of health care is to prevent iron deficiency anemia. If it occurs, the goal is to return low iron and hemoglobin levels to normal.

Iron supplements are essential during pregnancy because dietary sources cannot meet the extra requirements. Oral doses of a ferrous salt such as ferrous sulfate 300 mg (60 mg of elemental iron) are taken daily to prevent anemia. The dose is increased to three times daily to treat deficiency and restore hemoglobin to 12 g/dL. With a twin pregnancy a larger dose is needed. If a large dose causes vomiting and diarrhea, or if the anemia is discovered late in pregnancy, parenteral iron may be needed.

NURSING ASSESSMENT

The main presenting symptom of iron deficiency anemia may be fatigue. Nutritional history usually gives evidence of poor dietary intake of iron. Physical examination reveals pallor of skin and conjunctiva. Laboratory studies show Hb values below 11 mg/dL, serum ferritin levels below 12 μg/L, and possibly microcytic and hypochromic red blood cells (a late finding).

NURSING DIAGNOSIS

Nursing diagnoses that might apply to a pregnant woman with iron deficiency anemia include:

- Alteration in nutrition: less than body requirements related to inadequate intake of iron-containing foods

- Alteration in bowel elimination: constipation related to daily intake of iron supplements

NURSING GOAL: EDUCATION FOR SELF-CARE

The woman is taught to take iron tablets with meals to decrease adverse gastrointestinal symptoms, and with vitamin C (orange juice etc) to increase absorption. She is informed that her stool will turn black and may be more formed. She is also advised to keep the tablets out of the reach of children.

EVALUATIVE OUTCOME CRITERIA

Anticipated outcomes of nursing care include the following:

- The woman is able to identify the risks associated with iron deficiency anemia during pregnancy.

- The woman takes her iron supplements as recommended.

- The woman's hemoglobin levels remain normal or return to normal levels (if she was anemic at the start of pregnancy) during her pregnancy.

Folic Acid Deficiency Anemia (Megaloblastic Anemia)

Folate deficiency is the most common cause of megaloblastic anemia during pregnancy, affecting between 1 percent and 4 percent of pregnant women in the United States. It is more prevalent with twin pregnancies.

Folic acid is needed for the DNA and RNA synthesis necessary for the normal division of red blood cells. In its absence, immature red blood cells fail to divide, become enlarged (megaloblastic), and are fewer in number. With the tremendous cell multiplication that occurs in pregnancy an adequate amount of folic acid is crucial. However, increased folic acid metabolism during pregnancy and lactation can rapidly result in folic acid deficiency. It is usually diagnosed late in pregnancy or early puerperium. Hemoglobin levels as low as 3 to 5 g/dL may be found.

MEDICAL THERAPY

Diagnosis of folic acid deficiency anemia may be difficult. Serum folate levels typically fall as pregnancy progresses. Even though folate levels are lower with deficiency, they will fluctuate with diet. Measurement of erythrocyte folate status is more reliable but indicates folate status of several weeks previously (Troy & Wisch 1985). Bone marrow biopsy is diagnostic but should rarely be used due to the discomfort it causes the woman.

Folic acid deficiency during pregnancy is prevented by a daily supplement of 0.4 mg of folate. Treatment of deficiency consists of 1 mg folic acid supplement. Iron deficiency anemia almost always coexists with folic acid deficiency, and therefore the woman would also need iron supplements.

NURSING GOAL: EDUCATION FOR SELF-CARE

The nurse can help the pregnant woman avoid megaloblastic anemia by teaching her food sources of folic acid and cooking methods for preserving folic acid. The best sources are fresh leafy green vegetables, red meats, fish, poultry, and legumes. As much as 50 percent to 90 percent of folic acid can be lost by cooking in large volumes of water. Microwave cooking destroys more folic acid than conventional cooking.

Sickle Cell Anemia

Sickle cell anemia is a recessive autosomal disorder characterized by acute, painful, recurring vasoocclusive attacks and manifested by abnormal red blood cells. Individuals manifesting the disorder are homozygous for the trait (HbS), inheriting it from each parent. Carriers, who are usually asymptomatic, are heterozygous for the disorder, with one normal HbA gene and one HbS gene. The sickle cell trait is carried by 8 percent of American blacks, while approximately 1 in 600 blacks have the anemia itself.

The abnormal red blood cells, which are sickle or crescent shaped, are due to an alteration in a polypeptide chain in the hemoglobin protein. The amino acid valine is substituted for glutamic acid in the polypeptide chain. This single substitution, out of 509 amino acids, causes the anemia. The result of the substitution is low solubility of the hemoglobin in the presence of decreased oxygenation. The red blood cells become distorted, rigid, and interlocked with one another. This causes vascular obstruction in the capillaries, particularly in organs characterized by slow flow and high oxygen extraction, such as the spleen, bone marrow, and placenta (Martin & Morrison 1984). This phenomenon is called *sickling,* and varies in frequency by the amount of the S hemoglobin in the red blood cells (there is seldom a crisis with levels below 40 percent) and other hemoglobin factors. Diagnosis is confirmed by hemoglobin electrophoresis or a test to induce sickling in a blood sample.

MATERNAL RISKS

Low oxygen pressure—caused by high temperature, dehydration, infection, or acidosis, for example—may precipitate a vasoocclusive crisis. The crisis produces sudden attacks of pain that may be general or localized in bones or joints, lungs, abdominal organs, or the spinal cord. Vasoocclusive crises are most apt to occur in the second half of pregnancy.

The woman with sickle cell anemia has increased susceptibility to certain infections due to impaired immune functioning. Congestive heart failure or acute renal failure may also occur.

FETAL-NEONATAL RISKS

The incidence of fetal death during and immediately following an attack is high but has decreased greatly in recent years. Prematurity and intrauterine growth retardation (IUGR) are also associated with sickle cell anemia.

MEDICAL THERAPY

Vasoocclusive crisis is best treated by a perinatal team in a medical center. Partial exchange transfusion of HbA (normal adult hemoglobin) for HbS red cells is most important. With erythrocytophoresis, the woman's blood is removed, the HbS is separated out, and the woman's plasma and other blood factors are returned to her through another vein (Martin & Morrison 1984). The crisis and pain subsides much more quickly with this new technique.

Rehydration with intravenous fluids, administration of antibiotics and analgesics, and fetal heart rate monitoring are also important aspects of therapy. Antiembolism stockings are used postpartally.

If vassoocclusive crisis occurs during labor the previous therapies are instituted. The woman is also given oxygen and kept in a left lateral position. Oxytocics may be used if needed. Episiotomy and outlet forceps are recommended to shorten the second stage.

Several antisickling agents are being extensively researched and in the future sickle cell crisis may be prevented.

NURSING ASSESSMENT

The woman with sickle cell anemia usually relates a history of frequent illnesses and recurrent abdominal and joint pains, and is found to be extremely anemic. The woman may appear undernourished and have long, thin extremities. Ulcers are often present on ankles. Anemia may be severe.

A diagnosis of sickle cell anemia is confirmed by hemoglobin electrophoresis, or a test to induce sickling in a blood sample. The woman should be assessed for infection, which is associated with one-third of sickle cell crises in adults. Those most commonly seen during pregnancy or postpartum are pneumonia, urinary tract infections, puerperal endomyometritis, and osteomyelitis (Martin & Morrison 1984).

Fetal status is assessed during a crisis by electronic fetal monitoring.

During labor the woman's vital signs and FHTs are assessed frequently. Compatible blood should be available for transfusion. Oxygen is administered if necessary. The woman is assessed for joint pains and other signs of sickle cell crisis.

NURSING DIAGNOSIS

Nursing diagnoses that might apply to the pregnant woman with sickle cell anemia include:

- Alteration in comfort: acute pain related to the effects of a sickle cell crisis

- Knowledge deficit related to the need to avoid exposure to infection secondary to the risk of a sickle cell crisis

NURSING GOAL: EDUCATION FOR SELF-CARE

The nursing goal when working with a pregnant woman with sickle cell disease is to provide effective health teaching to help prevent a sickle cell attack (crisis), improve the anemia, and prevent infection. The woman is taught to increase hydration, use good hygiene practices, avoid people with infections, and take folic acid supplements. Folic acid is important because of its role in red blood cell production. The woman with sickle cell anemia maintains her hemoglobin levels by intense erythropoiesis and thus requires folic acid supplements. Bed rest is sometimes recommended to decrease the chance of preterm labor. Other nursing interventions are aimed at facilitating the medical therapy and alleviating anxiety through support and education.

Genetic counseling is recommended when both parents are known carriers or have the disease.

EVALUATIVE OUTCOME CRITERIA

Anticipated outcomes of nursing care include the following:

- The woman is able to describe her condition and identify its possible impact on her pregnancy, labor and delivery, and postpartal period.

- The woman takes appropriate health care measures to avoid a sickle cell crisis.

- The woman successfully delivers a healthy infant.

- The woman and her care givers quickly identify and successfully manage any complications that arise.

● Care of the Woman With Hyperemesis Gravidarum

Hyperemesis gravidarum, a relatively rare condition, is pernicious vomiting during pregnancy. Hyperemesis can progress to a point at which the woman not only vomits everything she swallows but retches between meals. Dehydration, starvation, and, eventually, death are the result of untreated hyperemesis.

The cause of hyperemesis during pregnancy is still unclear but may be related to trophoblastic activity and gonadotropin production and may sometimes be stimulated or exaggerated by psychologic factors. The pathology of hyperemesis in extreme cases begins with dehydration. This leads to fluid-electrolyte imbalance, and alkalosis from the loss of hydrochloric acid. More prolonged vomiting can result in loss of predominantly alkaline intestinal juices and occurrence of acidosis. Hypovolemia from dehydration leads to hypotension and increased pulse rate, with increased hematocrit and blood urea nitrogen levels and decreased urine output. Severe potassium loss (hypokalemia) interferes with the ability of the kidneys to concentrate urine, and disrupts cardiac functioning. Starvation causes severe protein and vitamin deficiencies.

Characteristic symptoms include jaundice and hemorrhage due to deficiencies of vitamin C and B-complex vitamins and bleeding from mucosal areas due to hypothrombinemia.

The differential diagnosis may involve infectious diseases such as encephalitis or viral hepatitis, intestinal obstruction, hydatidiform mole, or peptic ulcer.

Fetal or embryonic death may result, and the woman may suffer irreversible metabolic changes or death.

Medical Therapy

The goals of treatment include control of vomiting, correction of dehydration, restoration of electrolyte balance, and maintenance of adequate nutrition. Initially, the woman with hyperemesis gravidarum is given nothing orally, with administration of intravenous fluids of at least 3000 mL in the first 24 hours. This therapy provides fluid, glucose, vitamin (B-complex, C, A, and D), and electrolyte replacement. Desired urine output is a minimum of 1000 mL/24 hours. Intake and output are measured. Oral hygiene is especially important as the mouth is very dry and may be irritated from the vomitus. Use of promethazine (Phenergan) parenterally in a continuous low dose may be helpful in controlling nausea and vomiting (Cruikshank 1986).

Usually nothing is given by mouth for 48 hours. IV therapy is continued until all vomiting ceases and the woman's condition improves sufficiently to begin oral feedings. Six small dry feedings followed by clear liquids is one treatment of choice. Another method is 1 oz of water offered each hour, followed as tolerated by clear, then nourishing liquids, progressing on succeeding days to low-fat soft and general diets.

Nursing Assessment

When a woman is hospitalized for control of vomiting, the nurse must regularly assess the amount and character of further emesis, intake and output, fetal heart tones, evidence of jaundice or bleeding, and the woman's emotional state.

Nursing Diagnosis

Nursing diagnoses that may apply to the woman with hyperemesis gravidarum include:

- Alteration in nutrition: less than body requirements related to persistent vomiting secondary to hyperemesis.

- Fear related to the effects of hyperemesis on fetal well-being.

- Potential alteration in health maintenance related to inability to retain adequate food and fluid intake.

Nursing Goal: Reduction of Stress

Nursing care should be supportive and directed at maintaining a relaxed, quiet environment. Because emotional factors have been found to play a major role in this condition, psychotherapy may be recommended. With proper treatment, prognosis is favorable.

Evaluative Outcome Criteria

Anticipated outcomes of nursing care include the following:

- The woman is able to explain hyperemesis gravidarum, its therapy, and its possible effects on her pregnancy.

- The woman's condition is corrected and possible complications are avoided.

● Care of the Woman With a Bleeding Disorder

During the first and second trimesters of pregnancy, the major cause of bleeding is *abortion*. This is defined as the termination of a pregnancy prior to viability of the fetus, which now occurs at about 26 weeks' gestation. Abortions are either *spontaneous,* occurring naturally, or *in-*

duced, occurring as a result of artificial or mechanical interruption. Early spontaneous abortions occur prior to 16 weeks; late abortions occur after 16 weeks. *Miscarriage* is a lay term applied to spontaneous abortion.

Other complications that can cause bleeding in the first half of pregnancy are ectopic pregnancy and hydatidiform mole. In the second half of pregnancy, particularly in the third trimester, the two major causes of bleeding are placenta previa and abruptio placentae.

General Principles of Nursing Intervention

Spotting is relatively common during pregnancy and usually occurs following sexual intercourse or exercise due to trauma to the highly vascular cervix. However, the woman is advised to report any spotting or bleeding that occurs during pregnancy so that it can be evaluated.

It is often the nurse's responsibility to make the initial assessment of bleeding. In general, the following nursing measures should be implemented for pregnant women being treated for bleeding disorders:

- Monitor vital signs of blood pressure and pulse constantly.

- Observe woman for behaviors indicative of shock, such as pallor, clammy skin, perspiration, dyspnea, or restlessness.

- Count pads to assess amount of bleeding over a given time period; save any tissue or clots expelled.

- If pregnancy is of 12 weeks' gestation or beyond, assess fetal heart tones with a Doppler.

- Prepare for intravenous therapy.

- Prepare equipment for examination.

- Have oxygen therapy available.

- Collect and organize all data, including antepartal history, onset of bleeding episode, laboratory studies (hemoglobin, hematocrit, and hormonal assays).

- Assess coping mechanisms of woman in crisis. Give emotional support to enhance her coping abilities by continuous, sustained presence, by clear explanation of procedures, and by communicating her status to her family. Most important, prepare the woman for possible fetal loss. Assess her expressions of anger, denial, silence, guilt, depression, or self-blame.

Spontaneous Abortion

Many pregnancies are lost in the first trimester as a result of spontaneous abortion. Statistics are inaccurate because some woman may have aborted without being aware that they were pregnant during the first early weeks of gestation (through week 8). The bleeding is seen as a heavy menstrual period.

Approximately 82 percent of spontaneous abortions occur in the first trimester, with only 18 percent in the second. The overall figures range from 15 percent to 20 percent of all pregnancies (Borg & Lasker 1981).

When a spontaneous abortion occurs, the woman and her family may search for a cause so that they may plan knowledgeably for future family expansion. However, even with current technology and medical advances, a direct cause cannot always be determined.

About 60 percent of early spontaneous abortions are related to chromosomal abnormalities. Other causes include teratogenic drugs, faulty implantation due to abnormalities of the female reproductive tract, a weakened cervix, placental abnormalities, chronic maternal diseases, endocrine imbalances, and maternal infections from the TORCH group. It is believed by some that psychic trauma and accidents are a primary cause of abortion, but statistics do not support this belief.

The pathophysiology of spontaneous abortion differs according to the cause. In most cases embryonic death occurs, which results in loss of hCG and decreased progesterone and estrogen levels. The uterine decidua is then sloughed off (vaginal bleeding) and the uterus becomes irritable, contracts, and usually expels the embryo/fetus. In late spontaneous abortion the cause is usually a maternal factor, for example, incompetent cervix or maternal disease, and fetal death may not precede the onset of abortion.

Abortion can be extremely distressing to the couple desiring a child. For a woman who has already lost a fetus in a previous pregnancy, the crucial time is the month corresponding to the time of the previous abortion. She may become more upset and fearful at that time (Weil 1981). Chances for carrying the next pregnancy to term after one spontaneous abortion are as good as they are for the general population. Thereafter, however, chances of successful pregnancy decrease with each succeeding abortion.

CLASSIFICATION

Spontaneous abortions are subdivided into the following categories so that they can be differentiated clinically:

1. *Threatened abortion.* The fetus is jeopardized by unexplained bleeding, cramping, and backache. Bleeding may persist for days. The cervix is closed. It may be followed by partial or complete expulsion of pregnancy (Figure 19–2).

2. *Imminent abortion.* Bleeding and cramping increase. The internal cervical os dilates. Membranes may rupture. The term *inevitable abortion* applies.

3. *Complete abortion.* All the products of conception are expelled.

4. *Incomplete abortion.* Part of the products of conception are retained, most often the placenta. The internal cervical os is dilated and will admit one finger.

5. *Missed abortion.* The fetus dies in utero but is not

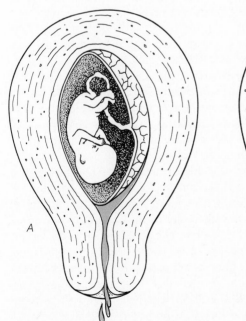
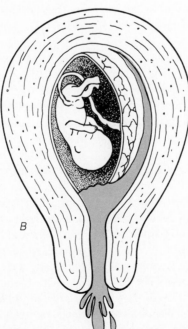
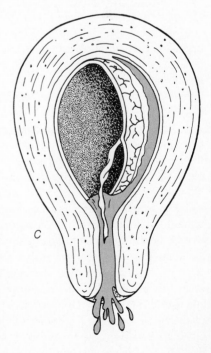

Figure 19–2   Types of spontaneous abortion: A Threatened. B Imminent. C Incomplete.

expelled. Uterine growth ceases, breast changes regress, and the woman may report a brownish vaginal discharge. The cervix is closed. Diagnosis is made based on history, pelvic examination, a negative pregnancy test, and may be confirmed by ultrasound if necessary. If the fetus is retained beyond six weeks, fetal autolysis results in the release of thromboplastin and disseminated intravascular coagulation (DIC) may develop.

6. *Habitual abortion.* Abortion occurs consecutively in three or more pregnancies.

MEDICAL THERAPY

Medical goals in the care of the woman who presents with signs of spontaneous abortion include (1) an attempt to prevent the pregnancy loss if she has not progressed beyond the threatened abortion stage, (2) control of blood loss and successful removal of all fragments of the products of conception, (3) uncomplicated postsurgical recovery, (4) education and support concerning the loss of the pregnancy.

Because 20 percent to 25 percent of pregnant women have episodes of spotting or bleeding during early pregnancy, it is important to determine whether vaginal bleeding is related to spontaneous abortion or other factors (Scott 1986b). One of the more reliable indicators is the presence of pelvic cramping and backache. These symptoms are usually absent in bleeding caused by polyps, ruptured cervical blood vessels, or cervical erosion.

Laboratory evaluations to help determine the cause of vaginal bleeding include ultrasound scanning for presence of gestational sac, and hCG level. The latter can confirm a pregnancy, but because hCG level falls slowly after fetal death, it cannot confirm a live embryo/fetus. Hemoglobin and hematocrit levels are obtained to assess blood loss. Blood is typed and cross-matched for possible replacement needs.

The therapy prescribed for the pregnant woman with bleeding is abstinence from coitus, and perhaps sedation. If bleeding persists and abortion is imminent or incomplete, the woman is hospitalized, intravenous therapy or blood transfusions may be started to replace fluid, and dilation and curettage or suction evacuation is performed to remove the remainder of the products of conception. If the woman is Rh negative and not sensitized, Rh_0 (D) immune globulin (RhoGAM) is given within 72 hours.

In missed abortions, the products of conception eventually are expelled spontaneously. If this does not occur within one month to six weeks after fetal death, hospitalization is necessary. Suction evacuation or dilation and curettage is done if the pregnancy is in the first trimester. Beyond 12 weeks' gestation, induction of labor by intravenous oxytocin and prostaglandins may be used to expel the dead fetus.

NURSING ASSESSMENT

The nurse assesses the responses of the woman and her family to this crisis and evaluates their coping mechanisms and ability to comfort each other.

My miscarriage was the last straw that broke up my marriage. If the baby had lived, I'm sure I would still be married. But my husband just didn't care about what was happening, and he couldn't understand how I felt. It made me see him as he really is, and later I decided to leave him. (*When Pregnancy Fails*)

NURSING DIAGNOSIS

Nursing diagnoses that may apply include:

- Fear related to possible pregnancy loss

- Alteration in comfort: acute pain related to abdominal cramping secondary to threatened abortion

- Grieving related to fetal loss

NURSING GOAL: PROVISION OF PSYCHOLOGIC SUPPORT

Providing emotional support is an important task for nurses caring for women who have aborted because the attachment process already begun is disrupted (Wall-Haas 1985). Feelings of shock or disbelief are normal at first. Couples who approached the pregnancy with feelings of joy and a sense of expectancy now feel grief, sadness, and possibly anger.

Since many women, even with planned pregnancies, feel some ambivalence initially, guilt is a common emotion. These feelings may be even stronger for women who were negative about their pregnancies. The woman may harbor negative feelings about herself, ranging from lowered self-esteem, resulting from a belief that she is lacking or abnormal in some way, to a notion that the abortion may be a punishment for some wrongdoing.

The nurse can offer invaluable psychologic support to the woman and her family by encouraging them to verbalize their feelings, allowing them the privacy to grieve, and listening sympathetically to their concerns about this pregnancy and future ones. The nurse can aid in decreasing any feelings of guilt or blame by supplying the woman and her family with information regarding the causes of spontaneous abortion and possibly referring them to other health care professionals for additional help, such as a genetic counselor if there is a history of habitual abortions.

The grieving period following a spontaneous abortion usually lasts 6 to 24 months (Borg & Lasker 1981). Many couples can be helped during this period by an organization or support group established for parents who have lost a fetus or newborn.

We lost our baby together. I know, you could say I never really had a baby, except during those few hours when it was already over and done with, but I guess these things aren't entirely logical. I loved my baby. . . . absorbed in pain and self-pity, still I was flooded with adoration for this tiny, not yet shaped baby who had lived in me. (A Midwife's Story)

NURSING GOAL: PROMOTION OF PHYSICAL WELL-BEING

The physical pain of the cramps and the amount of bleeding may be more severe than a couple anticipates, even when they are prepared for the possibility of an abor-

Research Note

Fifteen to twenty percent of all pregnancies end in spontaneous abortion. Because this is usually not life threatening to the woman, and because treatment is relatively simple and physical recovery is rapid, medical and nursing personnel may treat this as a routine occurrence without considering the profound and long-term consequences this event may have for the woman. The intent of this study was to better understand the complexity of women's responses to first trimester spontaneous abortions.

Nine women, ranging in age from 18 to 33 and representing a variety of educational levels and obstetric histories, were asked to fill out a short questionnaire relating their experiences. Although five of the women indicated that this pregnancy was unplanned, eight were pleased to some degree about being pregnant.

Most of the women in this study denied having problems with somatic responses (sleeping or eating disturbances), however they did complain of sadness, preoccupation, thinking and dreaming about the baby, irritability, and anger. Eight of the women experienced depression.

At the end of the questionnaire the women were invited to add comments about their experiences with miscarriage. The responses clearly indicate that the women were affected by the spontaneous abortions, and attempts by health care personnel and friends to minimize the loss were not helpful. Nurses can be most effective in helping these women by active listening and by arranging follow-up care.

Wall-Haas, CL: Women's perceptions of first trimester spontaneous abortion. J Obstet Gynecol Neonat Nurs 1985;14(January/February)50.

tion. Nurses need to be aware that couples feel unprepared for their first experience of spontaneous abortion (Borg & Lasker 1981). Nurses should offer support in dealing with the physical experience by explaining why the discomfort is occurring and by providing analgesics for pain relief.

I lay in my bed moaning while great boulders of pain rolled back and forth over my abdomen. I stayed there in torment for several hours before I finally realized what was happening. I was having a miscarriage. . . . I used to say to my patients that miscarriage—that far along (three months)—was often said to be more painful than normal labor. I say it with greater conviction now. (A Midwife's Story)

NURSING GOAL: EDUCATION FOR SELF-CARE

The pregnant woman is informed that she should report all episodes of bleeding to her health care provider. The woman hospitalized for spontaneous abortion may require information about possible causes of the loss and the chances of recurrence with a future pregnancy. She may also require information about the grief process so she is prepared for it when she goes home. She should also receive information about available resources if needed.

EVALUATIVE OUTCOME CRITERIA

Anticipated outcomes of nursing care include the following:

- The woman is able to explain spontaneous abortion, the treatment measures employed in her care, and long-term implications for future pregnancies.

- The woman suffers no complications.

- The woman and her partner are able to begin verbalizing their grief and recognize that the grieving process usually lasts several months.

Ectopic Pregnancy

Ectopic pregnancy is an implantation of the blastocyst in a site other than the endometrial lining of the uterine cavity. It may result from a number of different causes, including tubal damage caused by pelvic inflammatory disease, previous pelvic or tubal surgery, hormonal factors that impede ovum transport and mechanically stop the forward motion of the egg in the fallopian tube, congenital anomalies of the tube, and blighted conceptus.

The incidence of ectopic pregnancy has increased dramatically in the past several years. In 1970 the rate was 4.5 per 1000 reported pregnancies. By 1983 the rate had more than doubled to 14 per 1000 reported pregnancies. This increased incidence may be related to improved diagnostic technology and to the parallel increase in the incidence of pelvic inflammatory disease (Dorfman 1987).

Some authorities suggest an association between IUD use and ectopic pregnancy, but this is not universally accepted. Although IUDs prevent intrauterine pregnancies they offer no protection against tubal pregnancies. Thus, women who use IUDs have a greater risk of ectopic pregnancy than women who use oral contraceptives. However, they have about the same risk as women who use traditional contraceptives (Russell 1987).

While ectopic pregnancy still accounts for 12.8 percent of all maternal deaths in the United States, and is second only to PIH as a cause of maternal mortality, the actual death rate has decreased dramatically even as the condition itself has increased. This reduction is due primarily to earlier detection and treatment (Queenan 1987).

The actual pathogenesis of ectopic pregnancy occurs when the fertilized ovum is prevented or slowed in its progress down the tube.

The fertilized ovum either implants in the fallopian tube or in the ovary, peritoneal cavity, cervix, or uterine cornua (see Figure 19–3). The most common location for implantation of an ectopic pregnancy is the ampulla of the tube. Other tubal sites are the isthmus, infundibulum, fimbria, and interstitium. Ectopic pregnancies comprise 97.7 percent tubal, 1.3 percent abdominal, and 0.15 percent ovarian pregnancies. Most abdominal pregnancies are believed to be secondary to a tubal pregnancy that has been expelled out the end of the tube or expelled by rupture of the tube (Weckstein 1985).

Initially the normal symptoms of pregnancy may be present, specifically amenorrhea, breast tenderness, and nausea. The hormone hCG is present in the blood and urine.

The chorionic villi grow into the wall of the tube or site of implantation and a blood supply is established.

In the tube the implanted ovum quickly ruptures out of the tiny tubal lumen and grows in the connective tissues between layers of the tube. Bleeding occurs out of this space into the abdominal cavity (Weckstein 1985). When the embryo outgrows this space, the tube ruptures and there is further bleeding into the abdominal cavity. This irritates the peritoneum, causing the characteristic symptoms of sharp, one-sided pain, syncope, and referred shoulder pain as the abdomen fills with blood. The woman may also experience lower abdominal pain and faintness.

Vaginal bleeding, a common finding with ectopic pregnancy, occurs with the death of the embryo and sloughing off of the uterine decidua, which has built up in response to the normal hormones of pregnancy.

In many instances, the symptoms are not obvious. One-fourth of ectopic pregnancies may involve uterine enlargement. Physical examination usually reveals adnexal tenderness; an adnexal mass is palpable in approximately one-half of the cases.

If internal hemorrhage is profuse, the woman rapidly develops signs of hypovolemic shock. More commonly the bleeding is slow (chronic), and the abdomen gradually becomes rigid and very tender. If bleeding into the pelvic cavity has been extensive, vaginal examination causes extreme pain and a mass of blood may be palpated in the cul-de-sac of Douglas.

Laboratory tests may reveal low hemoglobin and hematocrit levels and rising leukocyte levels. The hCG titers are lower than in intrauterine pregnancy.

MEDICAL THERAPY

The goal of medical management is to establish the diagnosis of ectopic pregnancy, control blood loss, remove the products of conception, and take appropriate steps to preserve childbearing function if the woman wishes.

It is important to differentiate an ectopic pregnancy from other disorders with similar clinical presenting pic-

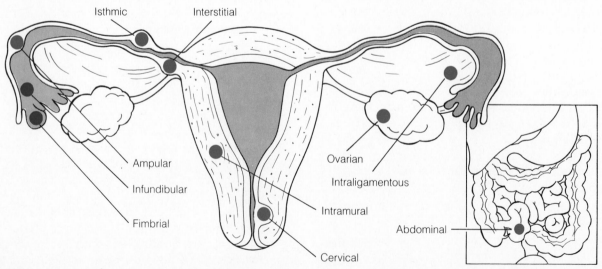

Figure 19–3   Various implantation sites in ectopic pregnancy

tures. Consideration must be given to possible uterine abortion, ruptured corpus luteum cyst, appendicitis, salpingitis, torsion of the ovary, ovarian cysts, and urinary tract infection.

The following measures are used to establish the diagnosis of ectopic pregnancy and assess the woman's status:

- A careful assessment of menstrual history, particularly the LMP.

- Careful pelvic exam to identify any abnormal pelvic masses and tenderness.

- Culdocentesis. The woman is positioned with her legs in stirrups, and a needle is inserted through the posterior vaginal vault into the cul-de-sac of Douglas. If nonclotting blood (blood that was clotted and then fibrinolysed) is aspirated, it is indicative of ectopic pregnancy.

- Laparoscopy, which may reveal an extrauterine pregnancy and is especially helpful in diagnosing an unruptured tubal pregnancy. If culdocentesis reveals free abdominal blood, laparoscopy is not necessary.

- Ultrasound, which may be useful in identifying a gestational sac in an unruptured tubal pregnancy. Its most common value is in confirming an intrauterine pregnancy, which usually rules out an ectopic one.

- Laparotomy, which will give a confirmed diagnosis and allow opportunity for immediate treatment.

Once the diagnosis of ectopic pregnancy has been made, surgery is necessary. Conservative management by linear salpingostomy is the treatment of choice when this is possible (Weckstein 1985). Using this method, a linear incision is made in the tube and the products of conception are gently removed, usually by washing. The surgical incision in the tube is left open and allowed to close by secondary intention (Droegemueller 1986). If the tube is badly damaged, a total salpingectomy is performed, leaving the ovary in place unless it is damaged. If massive infection is found, a complete removal of uterus, tubes, and ovaries may be necessary.

Intravenous therapy and blood transfusion are used to replace fluid loss. During surgery the most important risk to be considered is potential hemorrhage. Bleeding must be controlled and replacement therapy should be on hand. The Rh negative nonsensitized woman is given $Rh_0(D)$ immune globulin to prevent sensitization.

NURSING ASSESSMENT

When the woman with a suspected ectopic pregnancy is admitted to the hospital, the nurse assesses vaginal bleeding for appearance and amount. The nurse also monitors vital signs, particularly blood pressure and pulse, for evidence of developing shock.

It is also the nurse's responsibility to assess the woman's emotional status and coping abilities and to evaluate the couple's informational needs.

If surgery is necessary, the nurse performs the ongoing assessments appropriate for any client postoperatively.

NURSING DIAGNOSIS

Nursing diagnoses that might apply for a woman with an ectopic pregnancy include:

- Grief related to the loss of the anticipated infant

- Fear related to uncertainty of the effects of the ectopic pregnancy on future childbearing

- Alteration in comfort: acute pain related to severe abdominal bleeding secondary to tubal rupture

NURSING GOAL: PROVISION OF EMOTIONAL SUPPORT

The woman and her family will need emotional support during this difficult time. Their feelings and responses to this crisis will probably be similar to those that occur in cases of spontaneous abortion. As a result, similar nursing actions are required for these women.

NURSING GOAL: EDUCATION FOR SELF-CARE

Teaching is an important part of the nursing care. The woman may want procedures and the ectopic condition explained. She may need instruction regarding self-care measures to prevent further infections, symptoms to report (pain, bleeding, fever), and her follow-up visit.

EVALUATIVE OUTCOME CRITERIA

Anticipated outcomes of nursing care include the following:

- The woman is able to explain ectopic pregnancy, treatment alternatives, and implications for future childbearing.

- The woman and her care givers detect possible complications of therapy early and manage them successfully.

- The woman and her partner are able to begin verbalizing their loss and recognize that the grieving process usually lasts several months.

Gestational Trophoblastic Disease

Gestational trophoblastic disease (GTD) has been categorized into benign (hydatidiform mole) and malignant (nonmetastatic and metastatic) components (Runowicz 1985).

Hydatidiform mole (molar pregnancy) is a disease in which (1) the chorionic villi of the placenta become swollen, fluid-filled (hydropic) grapelike clusters, while a central fluid-filled space forms in the placenta (central cistern formation); and (2) the trophoblastic tissue proliferates. The significance of this disease for the woman who has it is the loss of the pregnancy and the possibility, though remote, of developing choriocarcinoma from the trophoblastic tissue.

Molar pregnancies are classified into two types, complete and partial, both of which meet the above criteria. Little is known about the cause of either type, but some of the pathophysiology has been clarified. The complete mole develops from an ovum that contains no maternal genetic material, an "empty" egg. How the maternal chromosomes are lost is not known. In most cases a haploid sperm, 23X, fertilizes the egg and duplicates before the first cell division. The conceptus then contains a 46XX chromosomal set in its cells, of totally paternal origin (Szulman & Surti 1984). The embryo dies very early, when just a few millimeters long and before embryo-placental circulation has been established. Therefore, the villous hydropic vesicles are avascular in the complete mole. No embryonic-fetal tissue or membranes are found. The vesicular swelling is of all the villi. Choriocarcinoma seems to be associated exclusively with the complete mole.

The partial mole has a triploid karyotype; ie, 69 chromosomes. Most often a normal ovum with 23 chromosomes is fertilized by a sperm that has failed to undergo the first meiosis and therefore contains 46 chromosomes. In about one fourth or less of the cases the ovum did not undergo reduction division, so it contains 46 chromosomes and is fertilized by a normal sperm (Szulman & Surti 1984).

In partial molar pregnancy there may be a fetal sac or even a fetus with fetal heart sounds. The fetus has congenital anomalies associated with triploidy and little chance for survival. The villi are often vascularized and may be hydropic in only sections of the placenta rather than universally as with complete mole. Twin pregnancies sometimes carry one normal placenta and the other a partial or complete mole (Kohorn 1984). The ratio of partial to complete moles is about 2:1 (Buckley 1984).

Incidence of hydatidiform moles varies greatly throughout the world with a high of 1 out of 85 pregnancies in one study in Indonesia. The incidence was 1 out of 923 in a broad population-based U.S. study (Buckley 1984).

Incidence of molar pregnancy increases with advanced maternal age and has a familial tendency, especially if the mother or sisters had a molar pregnancy. Although a repeat molar pregnancy is rare, the chances are increased after the first one (Buckley 1984).

MEDICAL THERAPY

Diagnosis of hydatidiform mole is often suspected in the presence of the following signs:

● Vaginal bleeding is almost universal with molar pregnancies, and may occur as early as the fourth week, or as late as the second trimester. It is often brownish "like prune juice" due to liquefaction of the uterine clot, but it may be bright red.

● Anemia occurs frequently due to the loss of blood.

● Hydropic vesicles may be passed, and if so are diagnostic (Figure 19–4). With a partial mole the vesicles are often smaller and may not be noticed by the woman.

● Uterine enlargement greater than expected for gestational age is a classic sign, present in about 50 percent of cases. In the remainder, the uterus is appropriate or small for the gestational stage. Enlargement is due to the proliferating trophoblastic tissue and to a large amount of clotted blood.

● Absence of fetal heart sounds in the presence of other signs of pregnancy is a classic sign of molar preg-

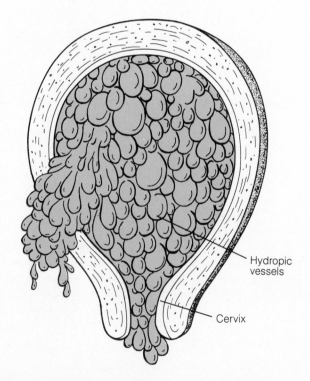

Figure 19–4   Hydatidiform mole

nancy. Only rarely has a viable fetus been born in a molar pregnancy.

- Elevated serum hCG is associated with molar pregnancies but is more clinically significant following evacuation of the mole than during pregnancy.

- Hyperemesis is considered a classic symptom of molar pregnancy but is found in only 20 percent to 25 percent of reported studies (Kohorn 1984).

- Pregnancy-induced hypertension may be seen in approximately 25 percent of cases, less if the molar pregnancy is diagnosed early. However, since PIH is a late pregnancy disease, if symptoms of PIH occur in the first half of pregnancy, molar pregnancy must be considered as the first diagnosis.

Ultrasound is the primary means of diagnosing a molar pregnancy, usually after six to eight weeks, when the vesicular enlargement of the villi can be identified. In some cases a molar pregnancy may not be recognized until after spontaneous abortion of the uterine contents and examination of the placenta. This examination is important for correct diagnosis and medical follow-up.

Therapy begins with evacuation of the mole and curettage of the uterus to remove all fragments of the placenta. Early evacuation decreases the possibility of other complications (Runowicz 1985). If the woman is older and therefore at increased risk of malignant sequelae, or if there is excessive bleeding, hysterectomy may be the treatment of choice.

Complications associated with hydatidiform mole that require medical recognition and therapy include:

- Anemia

- Thyrotoxicosis (rare)

- Infection, usually seen with late diagnosis and spontaneous abortion of the mole

- Disseminated intravascular coagulation

- Trophoblastic embolization of the lung, usually seen after molar evacuation of a significantly enlarged uterus (this creates a cardiorespiratory emergency)

- Theca-lutein cysts, which may be small or large enough to displace the uterus (Kohorn 1984).

Follow-up is an essential aspect of care. It is necessary to monitor serum hCG levels in all women who have had a hydatidiform mole. This consists of weekly measurements of hCG levels until they have been normal for three weeks, monthly measurements until they have been normal for six months, and then bimonthly measurements for six more months.

Continued high or rising hCG levels are found in 2 percent to 3 percent of women who have had molar preg-

nancy and are indicative of choriocarcinoma. Hospitalization is required for thorough evaluation including endometrial curettage. This is followed by chemotherapy, which is usually highly effective.

Because choriocarcinoma is very malignant if not treated, thorough evaluation for metastasis is necessary, including chest x ray, which is obtained at diagnosis and repeated if hCG serum levels plateau or rise (Runowicz 1985). The hCG levels are monitored closely after treatment although the exact schedule may vary. One follow-up protocol involves monitoring hCG levels weekly until normal, then every other week for three to four months, and then monthly for a year (Gestational trophoblastic disease 1987).

NURSING ASSESSMENT

It is important for nurses involved in antepartal care to be aware of symptoms of hydatidiform mole and observe for these at each antepartal visit. The classic symptoms used to diagnose molar pregnancy are found more frequently with the complete than with the partial mole. The partial mole may be difficult to distinguish from a missed abortion prior to evacuation.

When the woman is hospitalized for evacuation of the mole, the nurse must monitor vital signs and vaginal bleeding for evidence of hemorrhage. In addition, the nurse determines whether abdominal pain is present and assesses the woman's emotional state and coping ability.

NURSING DIAGNOSIS

Nursing diagnoses that may apply to a woman with a hydatidiform mole include:

- Fear related to the possible development of choriocarcinoma

- Knowledge deficit related to a lack of understanding of the need for regular monitoring of hCG levels

- Grief related to the loss of the anticipated infant

NURSING GOAL: PROVISION OF EMOTIONAL SUPPORT

When molar pregnancy is suspected, the woman needs support. The nurse can relieve some of the woman's anxiety by answering questions about the disease process and explaining what ultrasound and other diagnostic procedures will entail. If a molar pregnancy is diagnosed, the nurse supports the childbearing family as they deal with their grief about the lost pregnancy. The hospital chaplain or their own clergy may be of assistance in helping them deal with this loss.

The woman may need information and support to deal with her fears about the potential for carcinoma after molar pregnancy. She will probably also fear the outcome of future pregnancies.

NURSING GOAL: EFFECTIVE PERIOPERATIVE CARE

When the woman is hospitalized for evacuation of the mole, explanation of the curettage procedure is necessary. Although the physician is responsible for providing this explanation, the woman and her partner may have many questions and concerns that the nurse can discuss with them. The nurse may also clarify areas of confusion or misunderstanding.

Typed and cross-matched blood must be available for surgery because of previous blood loss and the potential for hemorrhage. Oxytocin is administered to keep the uterus contracted and prevent hemorrhage.

Following surgery the nurse carefully observes the woman's urinary output because of the antidiuretic effects of oxytocin. The nurse also watches for further bleeding, and for any signs of infection. If the woman is Rh negative and not sensitized, she is given $Rh_0(D)$ immune globulin to prevent antibody formation.

NURSING GOAL: EDUCATION FOR SELF-CARE

The woman needs to know the importance of the follow-up visits. She is advised to delay becoming pregnant again until after the follow-up program is completed. She should be advised against using an intrauterine contraceptive device because of bleeding irregularities associated with it. Oral contraceptives are considered ideal as they are highly effective and suppress the midcycle LH surge (Runowicz 1985).

EVALUATIVE OUTCOME CRITERIA

Anticipated outcomes of nursing care include the following:

- The woman has a smooth recovery following successful evacuation of the mole.

- The woman is able to explain GTD, its treatment, follow-up, and long-term implications for pregnancy.

- The woman and her partner are able to begin verbalizing their grief at the loss of their anticipated child.

- The woman understands the importance of follow-up assessment and indicates her willingness to cooperate with the regimen.

Placenta Previa

In placenta previa, the placenta is improperly implanted in the lower uterine segment, perhaps on a portion of the lower segment or over the internal os. As the lower uterine segment contracts and the cervix dilates in the later weeks of pregnancy, the placental villi are torn from the uterine wall, thus exposing the uterine sinuses at the placental site. Bleeding begins, but because its amount depends on the number of sinuses exposed, it may initially be either scanty or profuse. The classic symptom is painless vaginal bleeding usually occurring after 20 weeks' gestation. See Chapter 25 for an in-depth discussion of placenta previa.

Abruptio Placentae

Abruptio placentae is the premature separation of the placenta from the uterine wall. It occurs prior to delivery, usually during the labor process. See Chapter 25 for an in-depth description of abruptio placentae.

● Care of the Woman With an Incompetent Cervix

Cervical incompetence is the premature dilatation of the cervix, usually about the fourth or fifth month of pregnancy. It is associated with repeated second trimester abortions. A possible cause is cervical trauma associated with previous surgery or delivery, or congenital cervical structural defects.

Diagnosis is established by eliciting a positive history of repeated, relatively painless and bloodless second trimester abortions. Serial pelvic exams early in the second trimester reveal progressive effacement and dilatation of the cervix and bulging of the membranes through the cervical os.

Incompetent cervix is managed surgically with a Shirodkar-Barter operation (cerclage), or a modification of it by McDonald, which reinforces the weakened cervix by encircling it at the level of the internal os with suture material. A purse-string suture is placed in the cervix between 14 and 18 weeks of gestation. The procedure should not be done if any of the following conditions exists: The diagnosis is in doubt, membranes are ruptured, vaginal bleeding and cramping exists, or the cervix is dilated beyond 3 cm. Once the suture is in place, a cesarean delivery may be planned (to prevent repeating the procedure in subsequent pregnancies), or the suture may be released at term and vaginal delivery permitted. The woman must understand the importance of contacting her physician immediately if her membranes rupture or labor begins. The physician can remove the suture to prevent possible complications. The success rate for carrying the pregnancy to term is 80 percent to 90 percent.

Nursing Care Plan: PIH

Debbie Martin is a 35-year-old G 1 P 0 who is 36 weeks pregnant. Both Mrs Martin and her husband were initially overwhelmed by the pregnancy, but they are now looking forward to the birth. Mrs Martin's mother developed preeclampsia with her first pregnancy and was concerned when Debbie began having symptoms. Initially Mrs Martin had a slight increase in blood pressure (from 118/68 to 144/84) and noticed that her ankles and hands seemed puffy. Her physician discussed PIH with her and described home therapy. Mrs Martin, a freelance graphic artist, freed her schedule and cooperated with the rest periods, ate a high protein diet, and kept a fetal activity diary. At her prenatal exam yesterday, Mrs Martin's blood pressure was 154/96. She had 2+ proteinuria and a weight gain of 2 kg (4.4 lb) over the previous week. Her reflexes were 3+. Mrs Martin was admitted to the antepartal unit for treatment of her PIH.

Assessment

NURSING HISTORY

Identification of predisposing factors including:
a. Primigravida
b. Older maternal age
c. Family history of PIH

PHYSICAL EXAMINATION

a. Blood pressure elevated
b. Presence of edema as indicated by weight gain, puffy hands and feet; requires ongoing observation for development of facial or periorbital edema
c. Presence of hyperreflexia
d. Presence of visual disturbances, headache, drowsiness, epigastric pain

LABORATORY EVALUATION

1. Urine for urinary protein: 1 g protein/24 hr = 1–2+; 5 g protein/24 hr = 3–4+.
2. Hematocrit: Elevation of hematocrit implies hemoconcentration, which occurs as fluid leaves the intravascular space and enters the extravascular space.
3. BUN: Not usually elevated except in women with cardiovascular or renal disease.
4. Blood uric acid appears to correlate well with the severity of the preeclampsia-eclampsia (Note: thiazide diuretics can cause significant increases in uric acid levels).

NURSING PRIORITIES

1. Carefully monitor client status, especially vital signs, urinary output, hyperreflexia.
2. Evaluate fetal status.
3. Discuss the significance of PIH and its treatment for the health of Mrs Martin and her fetus.
4. Observe for signs of worsening condition:
   a. Increase in BP
   b. Decrease in hourly urine output ≤30 mL/hr
   c. Increased drowsiness
   d. Increased hyperreflexia
   e. Development of severe headache
   f. Visual disturbances
   g. Epigastric pain
   h. Convulsion

Nursing Diagnosis and Goals	Nursing Interventions	Rationale

NURSING DIAGNOSIS:
 	
Fluid volume excess: edema related to sodium and water retention.
	Weigh daily; gain of 1 kg/wk or more in second trimester or ½ kg/wk or more in third trimester is suggestive of PIH.
	
	Assess edema:
	
	    +(1+) Minimal; slight edema of pedal and pretibial areas
	
	    ++(2+) Marked edema of lower extremities
	
	    +++(3+) Edema of hands, face, lower abdominal wall, and sacrum
	
	    ++++(4+) Anasarca with ascites
	
	Maintain on bed rest.
	
	Maintain normal salt intake (4–6 g/24 hr).
		Weight gain and edema are due to sodium and water retention.

Nursing Care Plan: PIH (continued)

Nursing Diagnosis and Goals	Nursing Interventions	Rationale
SUPPORTING DATA: Mrs Martin stated: "My hands are so puffy I can't wear my rings." Weight gain of 2 kg in one week Peripheral edema Blood pressure 154/96		Decreased renal plasma flow and glomerular filtration contribute to retention; actual mechanisms are not clear. Bed rest produces an increase in GFR. Normal salt intake is now advised, but excessive salt intake may make the condition worse.
CLIENT GOALS: Mrs Martin will be able to discuss the significance of edema in PIH. Mrs Martin will be able to describe the purpose of the ongoing assessments and treatment plan and will demonstrate her understanding by following the prescribed routine.	Assess BP every 1–4 hr, using same arm, with Mrs Martin in same position.	Blood pressure can fluctuate hourly; BP increases as a result of increased peripheral resistance due to peripheral vasoconstriction and arteriolar spasm. Diastolic pressure is a better indicator of severity of condition.
NURSING DIAGNOSIS: Potential fluid volume deficit (intravascular) related to protein loss and fluid shifts to the extravascular space.	Provide adequate protein: 1.5 g/kg/24 hr for incipient and mild preeclampsia.	Plasma proteins affect movement of intravascular and extravascular fluids.
SUPPORTING DATA: Proteinuria Oliguria Elevated hematocrit	Obtain clean voided urine specimen. Test urine for proteinuria, hourly and/or daily.	Urine contaminated with vaginal discharge or red cells may test positive for protein. Helps evaluate severity and progression of preeclampsia. Proteinuria results from swelling of the endothelium of the glomerular capillaries. Escape of protein is enhanced by vasospasm in afferent arterioles.
CLIENT GOALS: Mrs Martin will be able to explain the need to monitor urine for protein and the purpose of the high protein diet. Mrs Martin will demonstrate an understanding of the need to monitor urinary output by saving all voidings so they can be measured.	Determine hourly urine output; notify physician if urine output ≤30 mL/hr. Insert indwelling catheter if necessary.	Increasing oliguria signifies a worsening condition. Catheter facilitates hourly urine assessment. Renal plasma flow and glomerular filtration are decreased.

Nursing Care Plan: PIH (continued)

Nursing Diagnosis and Goals	Nursing Interventions	Rationale
NURSING DIAGNOSIS: Potential for injury related to possibility of convulsion secondary to cerebral vasospasm or edema.	Assess knee, ankle, and biceps reflexes. Promote bed rest. Encourage Mrs Martin to rest quietly in a darkened, quiet room. Limit visitors. Administer magnesium sulfate per physician order: 1. IV dose: 3–4 g loading dose MgSO₄ followed by continuous infusion at a rate of 1–2 g/hr. 2. IM dose: 10 g of 50% MgSO₄ injected deep IM (½ in the upper outer quadrants of each buttock) using a 20 gauge, 3-inch needle. (1.0 mL of 2% lidocaine may be added to the syringe to decrease the discomfort.) Monitor magnesium levels frequently to prevent overdose (either 2 hours after beginning infusion or prior to next IM dose).	Assessing reflexes helps determine level of muscle and nerve irritability. Rest reduces external stimuli.
SUPPORTING DATA: Mrs Martin shows evidence that her PIH is worsening: 1. BP 154/96 2. 3+ DTRs 3. Increased edema Because PIH can be progressive, all women who develop severe PIH are considered at risk for convulsion. **CLIENT GOAL:** Mrs Martin will demonstrate understanding of possible complications associated with PIH by cooperating with therapy so that seizures are avoided.	Before administering subsequent doses of magnesium sulfate, check reflexes (knee, ankle, biceps). Check respirations and measure urine output. Do not give magnesium sulfate if: 1. Reflexes are absent 2. Respirations are <12/min 3. <100 mL urine output in past 4 hours Have calcium gluconate available.	Magnesium sulfate is cerebral depressant; it also reduces neuromuscular irritability and causes vasodilatation and drop in BP. Therapeutic blood level is 4–7 mEq/L Knee jerk disappears when magnesium sulfate blood levels are 7 to 10 mEq/L. Toxic signs and symptoms develop with increased blood levels; respiratory arrest can be associated with blood levels of 10 to 15 mEq/L. Cardiac arrest can occur if blood levels are 30 mEq/L (Worley 1986). Kidneys are only route for excretion of magnesium sulfate. Calcium gluconate is antidote for magnesium sulfate.
	Maintain seizure precautions: 1. Keep room quiet, darkened. 2. Have emergency equipment available— O₂, suction, padded tongue blade. 3. Pad side rails. 4. Educate other care givers regarding the possibility of convulsions and appropriate actions.	Quiet reduces stimuli. Padding protects client.

Once Mrs Martin's magnesium levels reach therapeutic range, her physician decided to induce labor by administering oxytocin.

Nursing Care Plan: PIH (continued)

Nursing Diagnosis and Goals	Nursing Interventions	Rationale
NURSING DIAGNOSIS: Potential for injury to the fetus related to inadequate placental perfusion secondary to vasospasm or possible abruptio placentae. **SUPPORTING DATA:** Mrs Martin's fetus shows evidence of intrauterine growth retardation (IUGR) when assessed by ultrasound. **CLIENT GOAL:** Mrs Martin will tolerate the stress of labor without signs of fetal distress.	1. Continue fetal monitoring throughout labor. 2. Observe for evidence of late decelerations (see Chapter 21) and intervene as necessary. Assess for signs of abruptio placentae: 1. Vaginal bleeding 2. Uterine tenderness 3. Change in fetal activity 4. Change in fetal heart rate 5. Sustained abdominal pain	Vasospasm may result in poor placental perfusion. This may decrease the fetus' ability to tolerate the stress of labor, and cesarean delivery may be necessary. A woman with severe preeclampsia is predisposed to abruptio placentae.
Epilogue		
Mrs Martin successfully delivered a 5 lb 2 oz girl. Following delivery Mrs Martin was maintained on magnesium sulfate for 24 hours. Her daughter, Kerry, did well. Mr Martin and Mrs Martin's mother were	both delighted with Kerry and relieved that things had gone so well. Mrs Martin was discharged on her third postpartum day.	

● Care of the Woman With a Hypertensive Disorder

In the past several years Gant and Worley (1980) and then Worley alone (1984) have attempted to develop a classification for related yet distinct conditions characterized by hypertension that can occur in pregnancy. The following is the current classification of the hypertensive disorders of pregnancy:

1. Pregnancy-induced hypertension (PIH)

   a. Preeclampsia

   b. Eclampsia

2. Chronic hypertension preceding pregnancy

3. Chronic hypertension with superimposed pregnancy-induced hypertension

   a. Superimposed preeclampsia

   b. Superimposed eclampsia

4. Transient hypertension

Pregnancy-Induced Hypertension

Pregnancy-induced hypertension (PIH) is the most common hypertensive disorder in pregnancy—up to two-thirds of the cases. It is characterized by the development of hypertension, proteinuria, and edema. Because only hypertension may be present early in the disease process, that finding is therefore the basis for diagnosis.

The definition of PIH is a blood pressure of 140/90 mm Hg during the second half of pregnancy in a previously normotensive woman. An increase in systolic blood pressure of 30 mm Hg and/or of diastolic of 15 mm Hg over baseline also defines PIH. These blood pressure changes must be noted on at least two occasions six hours or more apart for the diagnosis to be made (Worley 1984).

The cause of PIH remains unknown, despite much research over many decades. It has been called "the disease of theories" because so many theories have been proposed for its etiology. The condition's former name, "toxemia of pregnancy," was based on a theory that a toxin produced in a pregnant woman's body caused the disease. The term has fallen into disuse because the theory has not been substantiated.

Preeclampsia and eclampsia are types of PIH. *Preeclampsia* indicates that this is a progressive disease unless there is intervention to control it. *Eclampsia* means "convulsion." If a woman has a convulsion she is considered "eclamptic." Most often PIH is seen in the last ten weeks of gestation, during labor, or in the first 48 hours after delivery. Although delivery of the fetus is the only known cure for PIH, it can be controlled with early diagnosis and careful management.

Although PIH occurs in 7 percent of all pregnancies, the incidence of superimposed PIH among women with chronic hypertension is 15 percent to 30 percent (DeVoe & O'Shaughnessy 1984). It is seen more often in primigravidas; teenagers of lower socioeconomic class; and women over 35, especially if they are primigravidas. Women with a family history of PIH are at higher risk for it, as are women with a large placental mass associated with multiple gestation, hydatidiform mole, Rh incompatibility, and diabetes mellitus.

Today PIH seldom progresses to the eclamptic state due to early diagnosis and careful management. Eclampsia is, however, the leading cause of maternal death in the United States.

NORMAL PHYSIOLOGIC CHANGES IN PREGNANCY

The following are physiologic changes that occur normally, allowing for a healthy adaption to pregnancy:

Blood volume increases 30 percent to 50 percent. Peripheral vascular resistance decreases, and pregnancy-induced arterial dilation occurs.

The increased blood volume is necessary to perfuse the placenta and the increased tissue mass of the uterus and breasts. The higher blood volume also helps protect the fetus from impaired circulation due to maternal supine position, and it compensates for blood loss during delivery.

The lowered peripheral vascular resistance results in lower blood pressure from the middle of the first trimester through the second trimester. Whether blood pressure should slowly return to the woman's normal in the third trimester or remain slightly below normal is still unsettled.

Pregnancy stimulates the increased production of various hormones and enzymes, which have varying and sometimes opposing effects. Plasma levels of the enzyme renin are elevated three to four times over nonpregnant levels. Renin is involved in the formation of angiotensin I, which is converted to angiotensin II. The plasma level of angiotensin II, an active vasoconstrictor, which stimulates a rise in blood pressure, is therefore also elevated. But blood pressure does not rise in normal pregnancy, because the pregnant woman develops a resistance to the pressor effects of angiotensin II by ten weeks' gestation that lasts throughout the pregnancy. This resistance is thought to be due to vasodilator prostaglandins, particularly prostacyclin, which increases during pregnancy (Worley 1984).

Aldosterone, a potent mineralcorticoid hormone secreted by the adrenal cortex, stimulates the kidney tubules to reabsorb sodium and water. Progesterone blocks the effect of aldosterone. Progesterone levels are elevated early in pregnancy and remain so until term. The result is sodium loss by the renal tubules.

The glomerular filtration rate increases 50 percent. This results in faster clearance and decreased plasma levels of creatinine, urea, and uric acid and increased urine levels of these chemicals. Thus values that are considered normal for nonpregnant women may be pathologic in pregnancy.

Physiologic edema, located primarily in the ankles, is a normal occurrence during pregnancy. It is caused by the increased movement of fluid out of the intravascular hemodiluted blood, with its decreased colloid osmotic pressure, into extracellular spaces. This movement is aided by increased hydrostatic pressure in the venous capillaries of the dependent limbs, due to pressure of the gravid uterus on the inferior vena cava.

Clotting factors show some change with normal pregnancy. Platelets remain in the normal range of 150,000/μL to 400,000/μL. Fibrinogen is increased, as are most other clotting factors. However, factor XIII (fibrin stabilizing factor) is decreased due to placental enzymes, which prevents an otherwise hypercoagulable state in pregnancy.

PATHOPHYSIOLOGY OF PIH

The following pathophysiologic changes are associated with PIH (see also Figure 19–5).

Blood pressure begins to rise after 20 weeks of pregnancy, probably due to a gradual loss of the normal pregnancy resistance to angiotensin II.

A finding that is probably related is that synthesis of the prostaglandin PGE$_2$ and prostacyclin (PGI$_2$) is decreased in women with PIH. The cause of this deficiency is being carefully investigated. Both PGE$_2$ and PGI$_2$ are potent vasodilators. It may be that decreases in these factors are responsible for increased sensitivity to angiotensin II and thereby responsible for most or all of the pathology associated with PIH.

The loss of normal vasodilation of uterine arterioles results in decreased placental perfusion (Figure 19–6). Fibrin deposits and ischemic areas may also be found in the placenta. The effect on the fetus may be growth retardation, decrease in fetal movement, and chronic hypoxia or fetal distress.

Decreased renal perfusion is associated with PIH. With a reduction in GFR, serum levels of creatinine, BUN, and uric acid begin to rise from normal pregnant levels, while urine output diminishes. For each 50 percent decrease in GFR, serum creatinine and BUN plasma levels double, while sodium is retained in increased amounts. Sodium retention results in increased extracellular volume and increased sensitivity to angiotensin II. The typical kid-

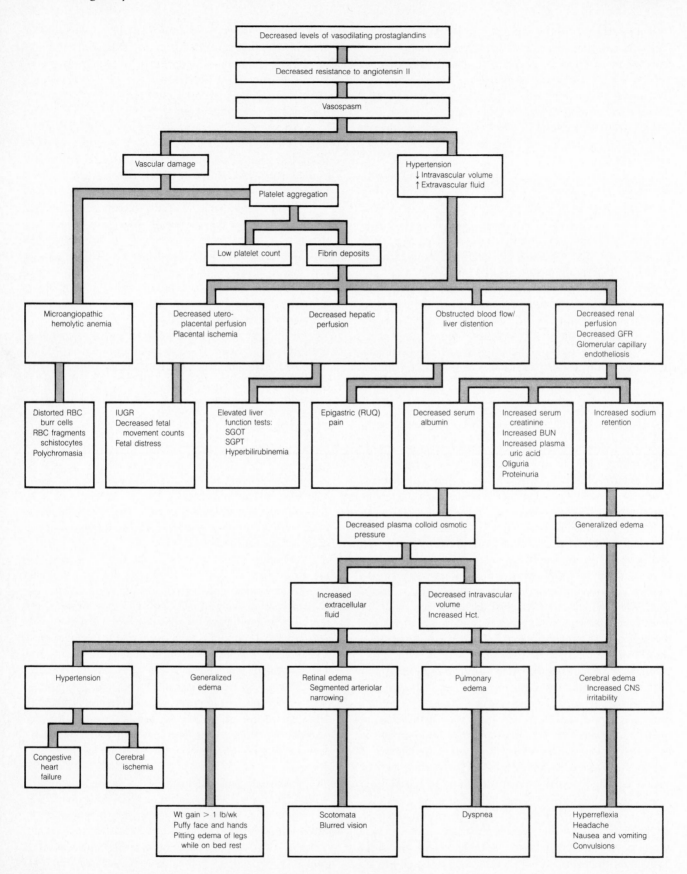

Figure 19–5   Clinical manifestations and possible pathophysiology of PIH

ney lesion of PIH is swollen glomerular capillary endothelial cells containing fibrin deposits. Stretching of the capillary walls allows the large protein molecules, primarily albumin, to escape into the urine, decreasing serum albumin.

Edema is usually more profound in PIH than in normal pregnancy. Its pathological basis is twofold:

1. The higher salt retention draws out intravascular fluid.
2. Plasma colloid osmotic pressure decreases, which causes fluid movement to extracelluar spaces, due to decreased serum albumin.

The decreased intravascular volume causes increased viscosity of the blood and a corresponding rise in hematocrit.

MATERNAL RISKS

Increased intraocular pressure due to PIH can cause retinal detachment, but there is usually spontaneous reattachment with reduction in blood pressure and diuresis.

Central nervous system changes associated with PIH are hyperreflexia, headache, and convulsions. Hyperreflexia may be due to increased intracellular sodium and decreased intracellular potassium levels. Headaches are usually frontal and occipital, may be constant, and are caused by cerebral vasospasm. Cerebral edema and vasoconstriction are responsible for convulsions, while cerebral hemorrhage—either petechial or large hematoma—is the most common cause of death (Burrow & Ferris 1982) following eclampsia.

A syndrome called HELLP has been described (Weinstein 1982, 1985) in association with severe preeclampsia. It is an acronym for hemolysis, elevated liver function tests, and low platelet count. These findings are also associated with mild DIC and therefore may not be a separate entity (Greer et al 1985). The hemolysis is termed *microangiopathic hemolytic anemia*. It is thought that red blood cells are distorted or fragmented during passage through small, damaged blood vessels. Elevated liver enzymes occur from blood flow that is obstructed due to fibrin deposits. Hyperbilirubinemia and jaundice may also be seen. Liver distension causes epigastric pain. Thrombocytopenia is a frequent finding in PIH. Vascular damage is associated with vasospasm, and platelets aggregate at sites of damage, resulting in low platelet count (less than 150,000).

FETAL-NEONATAL RISKS

Infants of women with hypertension during pregnancy tend to be small-for-gestational-age (SGA). The cause is related specifically to maternal vasospasm and hypovolemia, which result in fetal hypoxia and malnutrition. In

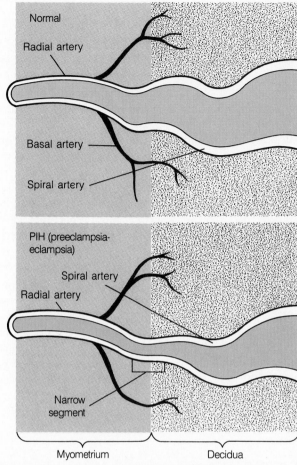

Figure 19–6 *In normal pregnancy the passive quality of the spiral arteries permits increased blood flow to the placenta. In preeclampsia vasoconstriction of the myometrial segment of the spiral arteries occurs.*

addition, the newborn may be premature because of the necessity for early delivery.

Perinatal mortality associated with preeclampsia is approximately 10 percent, and that associated with eclampsia is 20 percent. When preeclampsia is superimposed on chronic hypertension perinatal mortality may be higher.

At the time of delivery, the neonate may be oversedated because of medications administered to the woman. The newborn may also have hypermagnesemia due to treatment of the woman with large doses of magnesium sulfate.

MEDICAL THERAPY

The goals of medical management are prompt diagnosis of the disease; prevention of convulsion, hematologic complications, and renal and hepatic diseases; and delivery of an uncompromised newborn as close to term as possible. Reduction of elevated blood pressure is essential in accomplishing these goals.

Mild Preeclampsia The diagnosis of mild preeclampsia is made based on the following blood pressure findings: a rise in systolic blood pressure of 30 mm Hg or more, and/or a rise in diastolic blood pressure of 15 mm Hg or more above the baseline on two occasions at least six hours apart. Blood pressure between 120/80 and 140/90 forms the lower range for mild preeclampsia. A blood pressure of 150/100 is sometimes designated as moderate preeclampsia. Generalized edema is often present in the woman with mild preeclampsia. It is seen as puffy face, hands, and dependent areas such as the ankles. However, 18 percent of pregnant woman manifest generalized edema without becoming preeclamptic, while 70 percent to 80 percent of pregnant women have dependent edema without developing PIH. Edema is identified by a weight gain of more than 1.5 kg/month in the second trimester or more than 0.5 kg/week in the third trimester. Edema is assessed on a 1+ to 4+ scale. Proteinuria is often a late sign of preeclampsia. It may not be present until the disease has progressed to the severe or eclamptic stage. If proteinuria is present with mild preeclampsia, protein is generally between 300 mg/L (1+ dipstick) and 1 g/L (2+ dipstick). This is measured in a midstream clean-catch or catheter-derived urine specimen. Over a 24-hour period less than 5 g of protein would be lost in the urine.

Severe Preeclampsia Severe preeclampsia may develop suddenly. The following clinical signs are often present:

- Blood pressure of 160/110 or higher on two occasions at least six hours apart while the woman is on bed rest.

- Proteinuria ≥5 g/24 hours

- Oliguria: urine output ≤400 mL/24 hours

- Changes in laboratory values associated with severe preeclampsia. See Figure 19–5.

Other signs or symptoms that may be present include: headache, blurred vision or scotomata (spots before the eyes), narrowed segments on the retinal arterioles when examined with an ophthalmoscope, retinal edema (retinas appear wet and glistening) on fundoscopy, dyspnea due to pulmonary edema, moist breath sounds on auscultation, pitting edema of lower extremities while on bed rest, epigastric pain, hyperreflexia, nausea and vomiting, irritability, and emotional tension.

Eclampsia The grand mal seizure of eclampsia may be preceded by an elevated temperature as high as 38.4C (101.0F), or the temperature may remain normal. If the temperature spikes as high as 39.4C to 40.0C (103F to 104F), it is a very serious sign. The seizure begins with facial twitching. The woman's eyes are usually wide open and staring, with dilated pupils. The convulsion has three phases. The first phase is a tonic phase. All the woman's muscles contract, her back arches, her arms and legs stiffen, and her jaw snaps shut, sometimes causing her to bite her tongue. Her respirations cease due to thoracic muscles held in contraction, and she becomes cyanotic. The tonic phase lasts 15 to 20 seconds, then the woman enters the clonic phase. Alternating forceful contraction and relaxation of all muscles causes the woman to thrash about wildly. She may remain apneic or inhale and exhale irregularly as thoracic muscles contract and relax. Saliva and blood collected in her mouth may foam out. She remains cyanotic. Incontinence of urine and feces may occur. After about a minute the convulsive movements gradually cease and she slips into the third phase, a motionless coma that may last for less than an hour or for several hours. Respirations increase up to 50/min, and may be noisy and forceful. If the woman is not treated, the coma phase may be quite brief, and convulsions may recur in a few minutes.

Some women experience only one convulsion, especially if it occurs late in labor or during the postpartal period. Others may have from 2 to 20 or more. Unless they occur extremely frequently, the woman often regains consciousness between convulsions.

○ ANTEPARTAL MANAGEMENT The medical therapy for PIH depends on the severity of the disease.

Mild Preeclampsia The woman is placed on bed rest, primarily in the left lateral recumbent position, to decrease pressure on the vena cava, thereby increasing venous return, circulatory volume, and placental and renal perfusion. Improved renal blood flow helps decrease angiotensin II levels, promotes diuresis, and lowers blood pressure.

Diet should be well balanced and moderate to high in protein (80 to 100 g/day, or 1.5 g/kg/day) to replace protein lost in the urine. Sodium intake should be moderate, not to exceed 6 g/day. Excessively salty foods should be avoided, but sodium restriction and diuretics are no longer used in treating PIH.

Physicians are often wary about managing even mild preeclampsia on an outpatient basis because it can rapidly progress to severe preeclampsia. The woman whose blood pressure is at the lower end of the range for mild preeclampsia and who has no proteinuria may try home management. The woman and her family must understand the importance of bed rest. In such cases the woman is generally seen every one to two weeks and is carefully instructed about signs that her condition is worsening.

Tests to evaluate fetal status are done more frequently as a pregnant woman's PIH progresses. Monitoring fetal well-being is essential to achieving a safe outcome for the fetus. The following tests are used:

- Fetal movement record.

- Nonstress test.

- Ultrasonography for serial determination of growth.

- Contraction stress test.

- Estriol and creatinine determinations. Estriol (serum or urine) is being used less as a test for fetal wellbeing than formerly because of the lag time between fetal problem and test result, difficulty in interpretation, and expense.

- Amniocentesis to determine fetal lung maturity.

These tests are described in detail in Chapter 20.

Severe Preeclampsia If the uterine environment is considered detrimental to fetal growth and maturation, delivery may be the treatment of choice for both mother and fetus even if the fetus is immature (Sibai et al 1985).

Other medical therapies for severe preeclampsia include the following:

- *Bed rest.* Bed rest must be complete. Stimuli that may bring on a convulsion should be reduced.

- *Diet.* A high-protein, moderate-sodium diet is given as long as the woman is alert and has no nausea or indication of impending convulsion.

- *Anticonvulsants.* Magnesium sulfate (MgSO$_4$) is the treatment of choice for convulsions. Its CNS-depressant action reduces possibility of convulsion. Blood levels of MgSO$_4$ should be maintained at therapeutic levels (levels vary according to laboratory). Excessive blood levels may produce respiratory paralysis and/or cardiac arrest. (See Drug Guide for magnesium sulfate.)

- *Fluid and electrolyte replacement.* The goal of fluid intake is to achieve a balance between correcting hypovolemia and preventing circulatory overload. Fluid intake may be oral or supplemented with intravenous therapy. Intravenous fluids may be started "to keep lines open" in case they are needed for drug therapy even when oral intake is adequate. Criteria vary for determining appropriate fluid intake. Electrolytes are replaced as indicated by daily serum electrolyte levels.

- *Medication.* A sedative, such as diazepam (Valium) or phenobarbital is sometimes given to encourage quiet bed rest.

- *Antihypertensives.* The drug of choice is the vasodilator hydralazine (Apresoline) (Worley 1986). It ef-

fectively lowers blood pressure without adverse fetal effects. Hydralazine is generally given when the diastolic pressure is higher than 110 mm Hg. It may be administered either by slow intravenous push or drip methods. Hydralazine produces tachycardia; therefore the woman's pulse must be monitored with her blood pressure when she is receiving hydralazine. Blood pressure is measured every two to three minutes after the initial dose, and then every five to ten minutes thereafter. The diastolic pressure reading is maintained at 90 to 100 mm Hg to ensure adequate uteroplacental flow. The fetal heart tones are monitored continuously during hydralazine therapy. Hydralazine is not intended for long-term use.

Eclampsia An eclamptic seizure is an emergency situation that requires immediate, effective treatment. Therapy is aimed at controlling the convulsions, correcting any hypoxia and acidosis, lowering the blood pressure, and accomplishing delivery once the mother is stabilized (Pritchard et al 1985).

Magnesium sulfate is given intravenously to control the convulsions. Sedatives such as diazepam or amobarbital sodium are used only if the convulsions are not controlled by the magnesium sulfate. Because of their depressant effect on the fetus, they should not be given if delivery is expected within an hour or two.

The lungs are auscultated for pulmonary edema. The woman is watched for circulatory and renal failure and for signs of cerebral hemorrhage. Furosemide (Lasix) may be given for pulmonary edema; digitalis for circulatory failure. Urinary output is monitored. The woman is observed for signs of placental separation (see Chapter 25). She should be checked every 15 minutes for vaginal bleeding, which may or may not be present with abruptio placentae. The abdomen is palpated for uterine rigidity. While she is still unconscious, the woman should be observed for onset of labor. Convulsions increase uterine irritability and labor may ensue. While the woman is comatose, she is kept on her side with the side rails up.

Often the woman is cared for in an intensive care unit until labor begins or is induced. Invasive hemodynamic monitoring of either central venous pressure (CVP) or pulmonary artery wedge pressure (PAWP) may be instituted using a Swan-Ganz catheter. Both these procedures carry risk to the woman and the decision to use them should be made judiciously.

When the woman's vital signs have stabilized, urinary output is good, and the maternal and fetal hypoxic and acidotic state alleviated, delivery of the fetus should be considered. Delivery is the only known cure for PIH. If the neonate will be preterm, it may be necessary to transfer the woman to a perinatal center for delivery. The woman and her partner deserve careful explanation about the status of the fetus and woman, and the treatment they are

Drug Guide   Magnesium Sulfate (MgSO₄)

Overview of Obstetric Action

MgSO₄ acts as a CNS depressant by decreasing the quantity of acetylcholine released by motor nerve impulses and thereby blocking neuromuscular transmission. This action reduces the possibility of convulsion, which is why MgSO₄ is used in the treatment of preeclampsia. Because magnesium sulfate secondarily relaxes smooth muscle, it may decrease the blood pressure, although it is not considered an antihypertensive, and may also decrease the frequency and intensity of uterine contractions.

Route, Dosage, Frequency
MgSO₄ is generally given intravenously to control dosage more accurately and prevent overdosage. An occasional physician still prescribes intramuscular administration. However it is painful and irritating to the tissues and does not permit the close control that IV administration does.

IV: The intravenous route allows for immediate onset of action and avoids the discomfort associated with IM administration. It must be given by infusion pump for accurate dosage.

Loading Dose: 3–4 g MgSO₄ in D₅W (5 percent dextrose in water) is administered over a 15–20 minute period. (One authority recommends a loading dose of 6 g MgSO₄ in 100 mL D₅W infused over a 15 minute period [Sibai 1987]).

Maintenance Dose: Based on serum magnesium levels and deep tendon reflexes, 1–2 g/hr is administered.

Maternal Contraindications
Extreme care is necessary in administration to women with impaired renal function because the drug is eliminated by the kidneys and toxic magnesium levels may develop quickly.

Maternal Side Effects
Most maternal side effects are related to magnesium toxicity. Sweating, a feeling of warmth, flushing, nausea, slurred speech, depression or absence of reflexes, muscular weakness, hypothermia, oliguria, confusion, circulatory collapse, and respiratory paralysis are all possible side effects. Rapid administration of large doses may cause cardiac arrest.

Effects on Fetus/Neonate
The drug readily crosses the placenta. Some authorities suggest that transient decrease in FHR variability may occur, while others report that no change occurred. Similarly some report low Apgar scores, hypotonia, and respiratory depression in the newborn, while others report no ill effects. Sibai (1987) suggests that the majority of ill effects observed in the newborn may actually be related to fetal growth retardation, prematurity, or perinatal asphyxia.

Nursing Considerations

1. Monitor the blood pressure closely during administration.
2. Monitor respirations closely. If the rate is less than 14–16/min, magnesium toxicity may be developing, and further assessments are indicated. Many protocols require stopping the medication if the respiratory rate falls below 12/min.
3. Assess knee jerk (patellar tendon reflex) for evidence of diminished or absent reflexes. Loss of reflexes is often the first sign of developing toxicity.
4. Determine urinary output. Output less than 100 mL during the preceding 4-hour period may result in the accumulation of toxic levels of magnesium.
5. If the respirations or urinary output fall below specified levels or if the reflexes are diminished or absent, no further magnesium should be administered until these factors return to normal.
6. The antagonist of magnesium sulfate is calcium. Consequently an ampule of calcium gluconate should be available at the bedside. The usual dose is 1 g given IV over a period of about 3 minutes.
7. Monitor fetal heart tones continuously with IV administration.
8. Continue MgSO₄ infusion for approximately 24 hours after delivery as prophylaxis against postpartum seizures.

Note: Protocols for magnesium sulfate administration may vary somewhat according to agency policy. Consequently individuals are referred to their own agency protocols for specific guidelines.

receiving. Plans for delivery and further treatment must be discussed with them.

○   *INTRAPARTAL MANAGEMENT*   If PIH was previously diagnosed, the labor may be induced by intravenous oxytocin when there is evidence of fetal maturity and cervical readiness. In very severe cases, cesarean delivery may be necessary regardless of fetal maturity.

The woman may receive both intravenous oxytocin and MgSO₄ simultaneously. The woman in labor who develops a blood pressure higher than 160/110 may be given MgSO₄ intravenously. Because MgSO₄ has depressant action on smooth muscle, uterine contractions may diminish and labor may be augmented with oxytocin. Another method of inducing labor in the woman with PIH is to administer oxytocin intravenously and then during the course of labor give intravenous MgSO₄. Equipment and intravenous lines for both fluids must be checked frequently to ensure that they are being administered at the proper rate. Infusion pumps should be used to guarantee accuracy. Bags and tubings must be labeled carefully.

Meperidine (Demerol) or fentanyl may be given intravenously for labor. A pudendal block is often used for delivery. An epidural block may be used if it is administered by a skilled anesthesiologist who is knowledgeable about PIH (Worley 1986).

Delivery in the Sims' or semi-sitting position should be considered. If the lithotomy position is used, a wedge should be placed under the right buttock to displace the uterus. The wedge should also be used if delivery is by cesarean. Oxygen is administered to the woman during labor if need is indicated by fetal response to the contractions.

A pediatrician or neonatal nurse practitioner must be available to care for the newborn at delivery. This care giver must be aware of all amounts and times of medication the woman has received during labor.

○ *POSTPARTUM MANAGEMENT* The woman with PIH usually improves rapidly after delivery, although seizures can still occur during the first 48 hours postpartum. For this reason, when the hypertension is severe the woman may continue to receive hydralazine or magnesium sulfate postpartally.

NURSING ASSESSMENT

An essential part of nursing assessment is to obtain a baseline blood pressure early in pregnancy.

Arterial blood pressure varies with position, being highest when the woman is sitting, intermediate when she is supine, and lowest when she is in the left lateral recumbent position. Therefore it is important that the woman be in the same position each visit when the blood pressure is measured. For accuracy the cuff must be the proper size, the same arm should be used for comparison, and the blood pressure reading should be taken at approximately the same time of day. Both phases IV and V of Korotkoff's sounds (muffling and disappearance) should be recorded, because phase V is very low in many pregnant women.

Blood pressure is taken and recorded each antepartal visit. If the blood pressure rises or even if the normal slight decrease in blood pressure expected between 8 and 28 weeks of pregnancy does not occur, the woman should be followed closely.

When blood pressure and other signs indicate that the PIH has become severe, hospitalization is necessary to monitor the woman's condition closely. The nurse then assesses the following:

- *Blood pressure.* Blood pressure should be determined every two to four hours, more frequently if indicated by medication or other changes in the woman's status.

- *Temperature.* Temperature should be determined every 4 hours; every 2 hours if elevated.

- *Pulse and respirations.* Pulse rate and respiration should be determined along with blood pressure.

- *Fetal heart rate.* The fetal heart rate should be determined with the blood pressure or monitored continuously with the electronic fetal monitor if the situation indicates.

- *Urinary output.* Every voiding should be measured. Frequently, the woman will have an indwelling catheter. In this case, hourly urine output can be assessed. Output should be 700 mL or greater in 24 hours or at least 30 mL per hour.

- *Urine protein.* Urinary protein is determined hourly if an indwelling catheter is in place or with each voiding. Readings of 3+ or 4+ indicate loss of 5 g or more of protein in 24 hours.

- *Urine specific gravity.* Specific gravity of the urine should be determined hourly or with each voiding. Readings over 1.040 correlate with oliguria and proteinuria.

- *Edema.* The face (especially eyelids and cheekbone area), fingers, hands, arms (ulnar surface and wrist), legs (tibial surface), ankles, feet, and sacral area are inspected and palpated for edema. The degree of pitting is determined by pressing over bony areas.

- *Weight.* The woman is weighed daily at the same time, wearing the same robe or gown and slippers. Weighing may be omitted if the woman is to maintain strict bed rest.

- *Pulmonary edema.* The woman is observed for coughing. The lungs are auscultated for moist respirations.

- *Deep tendon reflexes.* The woman is assessed for evidence of hyperreflexia in the brachial, wrist, patellar, or Achilles tendons (Table 19–4). The patellar reflex is the easiest to assess. Clonus should also be assessed

Table 19–4 Deep Tendon Reflex Rating Scale

Rating	Assessment
4+	Hyperactive; very brisk, jerky, or clonic response; abnormal
3+	Brisker than average; may not be abnormal
2+	Average response; normal
1+	Diminished response; low normal
0	No response; abnormal

by vigorously dorsiflexing the foot while the knee is held in a fixed position. Normally no clonus is present. If it is present it is measured as one to four beats and is recorded as such.

- *Placental separation.* The woman should be assessed hourly for vaginal bleeding and/or uterine rigidity.

- *Headache.* The woman should be questioned about the existence and location of any headache.

- *Visual disturbance.* The woman should be questioned about any visual blurring or changes, or scotomata. The results of the daily fundoscopic exam should be recorded on the chart.

- *Epigastric pain.* The woman should be asked about any epigastric pain. It is important to differentiate it from simple heartburn, which tends to be familiar and less intense.

- *Laboratory blood tests.* Daily tests of hematocrit to measure hemoconcentration; blood urea nitrogen, creatinine, and uric acid levels to assess kidney function; serum estriol determinations to assess fetal status; clotting studies for any indication of thrombocytopenia or DIC, and electrolyte levels for deficiencies are all indicated.

- *Level of consciousness.* The woman is observed for alertness, mood changes, and any signs of impending convulsion or coma.

- *Emotional response and level of understanding.* The woman's emotional response should be carefully assessed, so that support and teaching can be planned accordingly.

In addition, the nurse continues to assess the effects of any medications administered. Since the administration of prescribed medications is an important aspect of care, the nurse is, of course, familiar with the more commonly used medications, their purpose, implications, and associated untoward or toxic effects.

NURSING DIAGNOSIS

Examples of nursing diagnoses that might apply are included in the care plan beginning on p 491.

NURSING GOAL: PROVISION OF SUPPORT AND TEACHING

A woman with PIH has several major concerns. The first is fear of losing the fetus. Sexual relations are another concern: she and her partner may be afraid to have intercourse for fear it might harm the baby. They may feel resentment because of this fear. A third worry concerns finances—health insurance does not always cover all the

tests, prolonged hospitalization, and so on that may be associated with complications during pregnancy. Finally, the woman's partner may not understand her need for bed rest and may become resentful or feel neglected. The couple's normal social life is interrupted. The woman may be depressed or resentful about being left alone or may feel bored. She may resist asking people to do simple things for her. If she has small children she will have difficulty providing for their care. The woman who does not have children may worry that she never will.

The nurse should identify and discuss each of these areas with the couple. It is necessary to explain to them the reasons for bed rest. A woman with mild preeclampsia may feel very well and be unable to see the need for resting even a few hours a day. The nurse can refer them to many community resources such as homemaking services, a support group for the partner, or a hot-line. Arrangements may be made for the partner to attend childbirth classes if both are not able to, or a nurse may be found to teach the classes privately.

The woman needs to know which symptoms are significant and should be reported at once. Usually the woman with mild preeclampsia is seen every one to two weeks, but she may need to come in earlier if symptoms indicate the condition is progressing. She must understand her diet plan, which must match her culture, finances, and life-style.

The development of severe preeclampsia is a cause for increased concern to the woman and her family. Increased stress can elevate blood pressure. One nursing goal is to decrease anxiety and provide an atmosphere of confidence and calm.

The woman's and her partner's most immediate concerns usually are about the prognosis for herself and the fetus. The nurse can offer honest and hopeful information. She can explain the plan of therapy and the reasons for procedures to the extent that the woman or her partner are interested. Understanding the reason for a procedure such as complete bed rest increases cooperation. The nurse should keep the couple informed of the fetal status. Eye contact, voice, and manner can show that the nurse cares and can encourage the couple to express feelings and ask questions. The woman might worry or feel guilty, thinking that she may have brought on the preeclampsia. Concerns about family at home or financial concerns and questions about the length of her hospital stay may also be expressed. The nurse provides as much information as possible and seeks other sources of information or aid for the family as needed. Nurses can offer to contact a minister or hospital chaplain for additional support if the couple so chooses.

NURSING GOAL: PREVENTION OF CONVULSION

The nurse should maintain a quiet, low-stimulus environment for the woman. The woman should be placed in a private room in a quiet location where she can be watched closely. Visitors are limited to close family or main support persons. The woman should maintain the left lateral recumbent position most of the time, with side rails up for her protection. She should not receive phone calls because the phone ringing may be too jarring.

NURSING GOAL: PROVISION OF EFFECTIVE CARE AND SUPPORT IF ECLAMPSIA DEVELOPS

The occurrence of a convulsion is frightening to any family members who may be present, although the woman will not be able to recall it when she becomes conscious. Therefore, offering explanations to the family member, and to the woman herself later, is essential.

When the tonic phase of the contraction begins, the woman should be turned to her side (if she is not already in that position) to aid circulation to the placenta. Her head should be turned face down to allow saliva to drain from her mouth. Attempting to insert a padded tongue blade has been questioned, but if it can be done without force, injury may be prevented to the woman's mouth. The side rails should be padded, or a pillow put between the woman and each side rail.

After 15 to 20 seconds the clonic phase starts. When the thrashing subsides, intensive monitoring and therapy begin. An oral airway is inserted, the woman's nasopharynx is suctioned, and oxygen administration is begun by nasal catheter. Fetal heart tones are monitored continuously. Maternal vital signs are monitored every 5 minutes until they are stable, then every 15 minutes.

NURSING GOAL: PROMOTION OF MATERNAL-FETAL WELL-BEING DURING LABOR AND DELIVERY

The plan of care for the woman with PIH in labor depends on both maternal and fetal condition. The woman may have mild or severe preeclampsia, may become eclamptic during labor, or may have been eclamptic before onset of labor. Therefore, careful monitoring of blood pressure and checking for edema and proteinuria are necessary for all women in labor. The prenatal record should be obtained so that current blood pressure readings may be compared with the baseline reading.

The laboring woman with PIH must receive all the care and precautions needed for normal labor as well as those required for managing PIH.

The woman with PIH in labor is kept in the left lateral recumbent position for most of labor, turning to the right side only when needed. As mentioned previously, the aorta and inferior vena cava are compressed when the woman is in the supine position.

Both woman and fetus are monitored carefully throughout labor. Signs of progressing labor are noted. In addition, the nurse must be alert for indications of worsening PIH, placental separation, pulmonary edema, circulatory renal failure, and fetal distress; all are more likely in a woman with PIH than in the normotensive client.

During the second stage of labor the woman is encouraged to push while lying on her side. If she is unable to do so comfortably or effectively, she can be helped to a semisitting position for pushing and to resume the lateral position between each contraction. Delivery in Sims' or semisitting position should be considered. If the lithotomy position is used, a wedge should be placed under the right buttock to displace the uterus. If a cesarean birth is indicated due to fetal distress, the wedge is also placed under the right buttock to prevent pressure on the vena cava. Oxygen is administered to the woman during labor as indicated by fetal response to contractions.

NURSING GOAL: PROMOTION OF MATERNAL PSYCHOLOGIC WELL-BEING DURING LABOR AND DELIVERY

A family member is encouraged to stay with the woman as long as possible throughout labor and delivery. This is especially needed if the woman has been transferred to a high-risk center from another facility. The woman in labor and the family member or support person should be oriented to the new surroundings and kept informed of progress and plan of care. The woman should be cared for by the same nurses throughout her hospital stay.

NURSING GOAL: PROMOTION OF MATERNAL WELL-BEING DURING THE POSTPARTAL PERIOD

The amount of vaginal bleeding should be noted carefully. Because the woman with PIH is hypovolemic, even normal blood loss can be serious. Rising pulse rate and falling urine output are indications of excessive blood loss. The uterus should be palpated frequently and massaged when needed to keep it contracted.

Blood pressure and pulse are checked every 4 hours for 48 hours. Hematocrit may be measured daily. The woman is instructed to report any headache or visual disturbance. No ergot products are given, as they have a hypertensive effect. Intake and output recordings are continued for 48 hours postpartum. Increased urinary output within 48 hours after delivery is a highly favorable sign. With the diuresis, edema recedes and blood pressure returns to normal.

Postpartal depression can develop after the long ordeal of the difficult pregnancy. Family members are urged to visit, and as much mother-infant contact as possible should be allowed. There may be fears about a future pregnancy. The couple needs information about the chance of PIH occurring again. They also should be given family-planning information. Oral contraceptives may be used if the woman's blood pressure has returned to normal by the time they are prescribed (usually four to six weeks postpartum) (Worley 1986).

EVALUATIVE OUTCOME CRITERIA

Anticipated outcomes of nursing care include the following:

- The woman is able to explain PIH, its implications for her pregnancy, the treatment regimen, and possible complications.

- The woman suffers no eclamptic convulsions.

- The woman and her care givers detect evidence of increasing severity of the PIH or possible complications early so that appropriate treatment measures can be instituted.

- The woman successfully delivers a healthy newborn.

Chronic Hypertensive Disease

Chronic hypertension exists when the blood pressure is 140/90 or higher before pregnancy, or before the twentieth week of gestation and persists indefinitely following delivery. If the diastolic blood pressure is greater than 80 mm Hg during the second trimester, chronic hypertension should be suspected (Zuspan 1984). The cause of chronic hypertension has not been determined. For the majority of chronic hypertensive women the disease is mild.

The chronically hypertensive woman who is considering becoming pregnant would benefit from counseling on what to expect should she become pregnant. She should have a basic understanding of the disease process, and then she can be taught to take her own blood pressure, the importance of good nutrition, and the need for daily rest periods.

MEDICAL THERAPY

The goal of medical therapy is to prevent the development of preeclampsia and to ensure normal growth of the fetus. When a woman with known hypertension becomes pregnant, she should start prenatal care as soon as possible. She will need to visit her health care provider at least every two weeks during pregnancy. During the woman's initial visit the usual prenatal assessment and laboratory tests are done. Additional laboratory tests include baseline serum creatinine, BUN, serum electrolytes, urine protein, and urine culture. If the hypertension is significant, an ECG and chest x ray are done to obtain baseline values.

Ultrasound is done at 10 to 14 weeks to date the pregnancy as accurately as possible. It is done again between 20 and 26 weeks, and at 32 weeks to diagnose IUGR. Creatinine clearance is determined early in pregnancy and repeated every two months if renal disease is suspected.

In addition to these ongoing assessments, the following interventions are usually instituted:

- *Bed rest.* The woman rests for two one-hour periods, one at noon and one in the late afternoon. Bed rest, primarily in the left lateral recumbent position, is the single most important part of management of the chronic hypertensive woman during pregnancy (Zuspan 1984).

- *Diet.* Protein intake of 1.5 g/kg body weight/day is recommended if proteinuria is significant. Moderate salt intake is acceptable.

- *Medication control.* Diuretic medication is gradually eliminated if the woman was on it prior to pregnancy. Antihypertensive medication may be continued, primarily to prevent maternal complications. The drug of choice and the only one tested in a random study is methyldopa (Aldomet) (Zuspan 1984).

- *Blood pressure.* The woman or her partner can monitor her blood pressure regularly and maintain a record. Home monitoring is often more accurate because the woman is more relaxed in a familiar environment.

NURSING GOAL: EDUCATION FOR SELF-CARE

The primary nursing goal is to provide sufficient information so that the woman is able to meet her self-care needs. The woman is given information about any medications prescribed and receives adequate counseling regarding dietary changes. She is taught to take her own blood pressure three times a week at home and is advised to keep a record of fetal movement during rest periods. She is also informed of the importance of resting in the left lateral recumbent position.

Chronic Hypertension With Superimposed PIH

Preeclampsia may develop in a woman previously found to have chronic hypertension. When elevations of systolic blood pressure 30 mm Hg above the baseline or of diastolic blood pressure 15 to 20 mm Hg above the baseline are discovered on two occasions at least 6 hours apart, proteinuria develops, or edema occurs in the upper half of the body (Gant & Worley 1980), the woman needs close monitoring and careful management. Her condition often progresses quickly to eclampsia, sometimes before 30 weeks of pregnancy.

Late or Transient Hypertension

Late hypertension exists when transient elevation of blood pressure occurs during labor or in the early post-partal period, returning to normal within 10 days postpartum (Gant & Worley 1980).

● Care of the Woman at Risk for Rh Sensitization

Rh sensitization results from an antigen-antibody immunologic reaction within the body. Sensitization most commonly occurs when an Rh negative woman carries an Rh positive fetus, either to term or terminated by spontaneous or induced abortion. It can also occur if an Rh negative nonpregnant woman receives an Rh positive blood transfusion.

The red blood cells from the fetus invade the maternal circulation, thereby stimulating the production of Rh antibodies. Because this usually occurs at delivery, the first offspring is not affected. However, in a subsequent pregnancy Rh antibodies cross the placenta and enter the fetal circulation, causing severe hemolysis. The destruction of fetal red blood cells causing anemia in the fetus is proportional to the extent of maternal sensitization (Figure 19–7).

Several forms of Rh antigen exist. The factors implicated in pathogenesis, in order of antigenic potential, are D, C, E, c, e, and, hypothetically, d (d has never been demonstrated but is thought to exist). There are many genetic combinations (genotypes) possible, such as CDE, cDe, Cde, and so forth. The D antigen is most significant clinically in that it provides the strongest stimulus to antibody formation in Rh negative people. Therefore, individuals who are homozygous for the D antigen (DD) or heterozygous (Dd) are Rh positive; those whose genotype is dd are Rh negative.

Approximately 85 percent of white, 93 percent of black, and 99 percent of Oriental populations are Rh positive (Pritchard et al 1985). An Rh negative woman who delivers an Rh positive, ABO compatible infant has a 16 percent risk of becoming sensitized as a result of her pregnancy (Bowman 1985).

Fetal-Neonatal Risks

Although maternal sensitization can now be prevented by appropriate administration of RhoGAM, infants still die of Rh hemolytic disease. If treatment is not initiated, the anemia resulting from this disorder can cause marked fetal edema, called *hydrops fetalis*. Congestive heart failure may result, as well as marked jaundice (called *icterus*

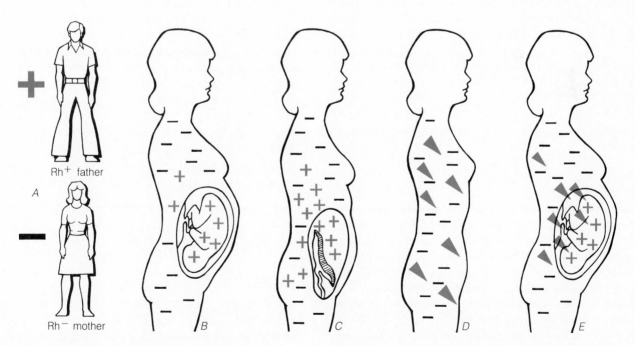

Figure 19–7   Rh isoimmunization sequence. A Rh positive father and Rh negative mother. B Pregnancy with Rh positive fetus. Some Rh positive blood enters the mother's blood. C As the placenta separates, the mother is further exposed to Rh positive blood. D The mother is sensitized to Rh positive blood; anti–Rh positive antibodies are formed. E In subsequent pregnancies with an Rh positive fetus, Rh positive red blood cells are attacked by the anti–Rh positive maternal antibodies causing hemolysis of red blood cells in the fetus.

gravis), which can lead to neurologic damage (kernicterus). This severe hemolytic syndrome is known as *erythroblastosis fetalis.*

The possibility also exists that an Rh negative female fetus carried by an Rh positive mother may become sensitized in utero. This female would not demonstrate signs of hemolytic disease, but since she would be sensitized before even becoming pregnant she would have a positive indirect Coombs' test when receiving prenatal care with her first Rh positive fetus.

Rh sensitization and the resultant hemolytic disease of the newborn are less common today because of the development of RhoGAM. See Chapter 32 for treatment of the neonate.

Screening for Rh Incompatibility and Sensitization

At the first prenatal visit (1) a history is taken of previous sensitization, abortions, blood transfusions, or children who developed jaundice or anemia during the neonatal period; (2) maternal blood type (ABO) and Rh factor are determined and a routine Rh antibody screen is done; and (3) presence of other medical complications such as diabetes, infections, or hypertension are identified.

If the woman is Rh negative (dd), the father of the unborn child is asked to come into the clinic or physician's office to be assessed for his Rh factor and blood type. If he is homozygous for Rh positive (DD), all his offspring will be Rh positive. If he is heterozygous (Dd), 50 percent of his offspring can be Rh negative and 50 percent heterozygous for Rh positive. If the father is Rh negative, all their children will be Rh negative, and no Rh incompatibility with the mother will occur. If the father is Rh positive or the mother is known to have previously carried an Rh positive fetus, further testing and careful management are needed.

When assessment has identified the Rh negative woman who may be pregnant with an Rh positive fetus, an antibody screen (indirect Coombs' test) is done to determine if the woman is sensitized (has developed isoimmunity) to the Rh antigen. The indirect Coombs' test measures the number of antibodies in the maternal blood. A specimen of maternal blood is diluted to specific concentrations. Rh positive red blood cells are added to the maternal blood sample. If the woman's serum contains antibodies, the Rh positive red blood cells will agglutinate (clump) when rabbit immune antiglobulin is added. The titer (the number or level of antibodies) is determined by the dilution at which the Rh positive red blood cells clumped.

Titers should be determined monthly during the first and second trimesters, biweekly during the third trimester, and the week before the due date. If the test shows a ma-

ternal antibody titer of 1:16 or greater early in pregnancy, a Delta optical density (ΔOD) analysis of the amniotic fluid is performed at 26 weeks. If the titer is 1:16 or less late in pregnancy, delivery at 38 weeks or spontaneous labor at term can be anticipated.

Negative antibody titers can consistently identify the fetus *not* at risk. However, the titers cannot reliably point out the fetus in danger, since the level of the titer does not correlate with the severity of the disease. For instance, in a severely sensitized woman, antibody titers may be moderately high and remain at the same level although the fetus is being more and more severely affected. Conversely, a woman sensitized by previous Rh positive fetuses may show a high fixed antibody titer during a pregnancy in which the fetus is Rh negative.

Ultrasound scanning can help determine the fetal condition. It would demonstrate an increase in fetal heart size, ascites, hydramnios, and subcutaneous edema. Placental size and texture are also indicators of fetal condition (Queenan 1982).

The most valuable indicator of fetal status is the ΔOD analysis. Amniotic fluid, obtained by transabdominal amniocentesis, is separated from its cellular components by centrifuge. The amount of pigment from the degradation of red blood cells can be measured in the amniotic fluid. The fluid is subjected to spectrophotometric studies to determine the severity of the fetal hemolytic process and the obstetric-pediatric management.

If the spectrophotometric readings are in zone I (A) ΔOD at 450 nm, a normal or mildly anemic neonate may be anticipated and delivery at term may be permitted. Prognosis for this newborn is good, but phototherapy or exchange transfusion may be necessary. A reading in zone II (B) ΔOD at 450 nm indicates a moderately anemic fetus who may be hydropic or stillborn if delivered at term. Once the fetus reaches viability, induced vaginal or cesarean delivery is indicated. A fair prognosis and possible need for exchange transfusion is anticipated. Readings within zone III (C) ΔOD at 450 nm indicate a severely affected fetus who may require intrauterine transfusion every 1 to 2 weeks between weeks 26 and 32 until viability is reached, followed by delivery, usually cesarean. Neonatal exchange transfusion is anticipated. Prognosis is guarded.

Medical Therapy

The goal of medical management is the delivery of a mature fetus who has not developed severe hemolysis in utero. This requires early identification and treatment of maternal conditions that predispose to hemolytic disease, identification and evaluation of the Rh-sensitized woman, coordinated obstetric-pediatric treatment for the seriously affected neonate, and prevention of Rh sensitization if none is present.

ANTEPARTAL MANAGEMENT

Two primary interventions are used by the physician to aid the fetus whose blood cells are being destroyed by maternal antibodies: early delivery of the fetus and intrauterine transfusion, both of which carry risks. Ideally, delivery should be delayed until fetal maturity is confirmed at about 36 to 37 weeks. This is possible for most pregnancies with spectrophotometric readings in zones I and II (A and B).

Intrauterine transfusion is done to correct the anemia produced by the red blood cell hemolysis. The woman is admitted to the hospital, sedated, and taken to the x-ray department. The location of the placenta and the fetal position are determined by ultrasound. With the woman under local anesthesia and using fluoroscopy, a plastic catheter (threaded through a 15 gauge, 18-cm, Touhy needle) is introduced through the abdomen and the intrauterine space into the fetal peritoneal cavity. A small air bubble is injected to verify that the needle is in the fetal abdomen. About 100 mL of type O, Rh negative, packed red blood cells, which has been cross-matched against the mother's serum, is transfused into the fetus. Diaphragmatic lymphatics absorb the red blood cells into the fetal circulation. Repeat transfusions can be scheduled as necessary until the fetus is sufficiently mature to tolerate delivery.

About 92 percent of transfused fetuses survive. The procedure is hazardous to the fetus, however (Pritchard et al 1985). In addition to the 8 percent possibility of fetal death, direct trauma to the fetus with the needles and catheter is possible. Maternal complications are few; those that occur are usually due to bleeding or infection. Delivery is delayed until at least 32 weeks' gestation if possible. Premature newborns are generally more susceptible to damage from hemolytic disease. They often require exchange transfusion, and usually require intensive nursery care.

Only fetuses between 23 and 32 weeks with a prognosis of death as indicated by the OD450 nm amniotic readings should be given intrauterine transfusion (Pritchard et al 1985). The procedure should be done before hydrops develops because the red blood cells injected into the fetal peritoneal cavity will be absorbed more slowly by the hydropic fetus. However, if ascites has already developed, the fetus should still be transfused since it has a better chance of survival with the transfusion than without it (Bowman 1981).

POSTPARTAL MANAGEMENT

The goals of postpartal care are to prevent sensitization in the as-yet-unsensitized pregnant woman and to treat the isoimmune hemolytic disease in the newborn.

The Rh negative mother who has no titer (indirect Coombs' negative, nonsensitized) and who has delivered an Rh positive fetus (direct Coombs' negative) is given an intramuscular injection of 300 μg anti-Rh$_0$ (D) gamma globulin (RhoGAM) within 72 hours so that she does not have time to produce antibodies to fetal cells that entered her bloodstream when the placenta separated. The anti-Rh$_0$ (D) gamma globulin works to destroy the fetal cells in the maternal circulation before sensitization occurs, thereby blocking maternal antibody production. This provides temporary passive immunity for the mother, which prevents the development of permanent active immunity (antibody formation).

The normal dose of RhoGAM should suppress the immune response to approximately 30 mL Rh positive whole blood. However, if a larger fetomaternal bleed may have occurred, a Betke-Kleihauer test can be performed. This test is used to obtain an estimate of the size of a fetomaternal bleed. Based on the findings, an additional 300 μg of RhoGAM is given for every 25 mL of fetal blood in the woman's circulation. Thus a 300 μg dose should be given every 12 hours until the total necessary dose is given (Bowman 1985).

When the woman is Rh negative and not sensitized and the father is Rh positive or unknown, RhoGAM is also given after each abortion, ectopic pregnancy, or amniocentesis. By 11 weeks' gestation, the D antigen is often present and can stimulate maternal isoimmunization, which would jeopardize the next Rh positive fetus. Since transplacental hemorrhage is possible during pregnancy, RhoGAM is generally administered prophylactically at 28 weeks' gestation to prevent sensitization. RhoGAM is not given to the neonate or the father. It is not effective for and should not be given to a previously sensitized woman. However, sometimes after delivery or an abortion, the results of the blood test do not clearly show whether the mother is already sensitized to the Rh antigen or not. In such cases, the anti-Rh$_0$(D) immunoglobulin should be given as it will cause no harm. Box 19–2 summarizes the major considerations in caring for an Rh negative woman. The treatment of the newborn with isoimmune hemolytic disease is discussed in Chapter 32.

Nursing Assessment

As part of the initial prenatal history the nurse asks the mother if she knows her blood type and Rh factor. Many women are aware that they are Rh negative and that this status has implications for pregnancy. If the woman knows she is Rh negative, the nurse can assess the woman's knowledge of what that means. The nurse can also ask the woman if she has ever received RhoGAM, if she has had any previous pregnancies and their outcome, and if she knows her partner's Rh factor. Should the partner be Rh negative, there is no risk to the fetus, who will also be Rh negative.

Box 19–2 Rh Sensitization

When trying to work through Rh problems, the nurse should remember the following:

- A potential problem exists when an Rh⁻ mother and an Rh⁺ father conceive a child that is Rh⁺.
- In this situation, the mother may become sensitized or produce antibodies to her fetus's Rh⁺ blood.

The following tests are used to detect sensitization:

- Indirect Coombs' tests—done on the mother's blood to measure the number of Rh⁺ antibodies.
- Direct Coombs' test—done on the infant's blood to detect antibody-coated Rh⁺ RBCs.

Based on the results of these tests, the following may be done:

- If the mother's indirect Coombs' test is negative and the infant's direct Coombs' test is negative, the mother is given RhoGAM within 72 hours of delivery.
- If the mother's indirect Coombs' test is positive and her Rh⁺ infant has a positive direct Coombs' test, RhoGAM is *not* given; in this case, the infant is carefully monitored for hemolytic disease.
- It is recommended that RhoGAM be given at 28 weeks antenatally to decrease possible transplacental bleeding concerns.
- RhoGAM is also administered after each abortion (spontaneous or therapeutic), ectopic pregnancy, or amniocentesis.

If the woman does not know what Rh type she is, intervention cannot begin until the initial laboratory data are obtained. Once that is done, the nurse plans interventions based on the findings.

If the woman becomes sensitized during her pregnancy, nursing assessment focuses on the knowledge level and coping skills of the woman and her family. The nurse also provides ongoing assessment during procedures to evaluate fetal well-being, such as ultrasound and amniocentesis.

Postpartally, the nurse reviews data about the Rh type of the fetus. If the fetus is Rh positive, the mother is Rh negative, and no sensitization has occurred, nursing assessment reveals the need to administer RhoGAM.

Nursing Diagnosis

Nursing diagnoses that might apply include:

- Knowledge deficit related to a lack of understanding of the need to receive RhoGAM and when it should be administered
- Ineffective individual coping related to depression secondary to the development of indications of the need for fetal exchange transfusion
- Potential disturbance in self-concept related to the woman's feelings of guilt that she is responsible for her fetus's sensitization

Nursing Goal: Effective Prenatal Education

During the antepartal period the nurse explains the mechanisms involved in isoimmunization and answers any questions the woman and her partner may have. It is imperative that the woman understand the importance of receiving RhoGAM after every spontaneous or therapeutic abortion or ectopic pregnancy. The nurse also explains the purpose of the RhoGAM administered at 28 weeks if the woman is not sensitized.

Nursing Goal: Provision of Psychologic Support

If the woman is sensitized to the Rh factor, it poses a threat to any Rh positive fetus she carries. The nurse provides emotional support to the family to help them deal with their grief and any feelings of guilt about the infant's condition. Should an intrauterine transfusion become necessary, the nurse continues to provide emotional support while also assuming his or her responsibilities as part of the health care team.

Nursing Goal: Successful Administration of RhoGAM

During labor the nurse caring for an Rh negative woman who has not been sensitized ensures that the woman's blood is assessed for any antibodies and also has been cross-matched for RhoGAM. On the postpartum unit the nurse generally is responsible for administering the RhoGAM.

When administering RhoGAM, the nurse must follow the instructions on the packet of RhoGAM carefully. The used packet containing the vial of drug cross-matched to the woman's serum is returned to the pharmacy or laboratory where it is saved. The woman is observed for possible symptoms of blood transfusion reaction.

Occasionally, the coating of maternal antibodies on fetal cells blocks an accurate typing of cord blood; that is, an Rh positive fetus is erroneously typed as Rh negative. Consequently, the RhoGAM will not be given, and the woman may become sensitized.

Evaluative Outcome Criteria

Anticipated outcomes of nursing care include the following:

- The woman is able to explain the process of Rh sensitization and its implications for her unborn child and for subsequent pregnancies.

- If the woman has not been sensitized, she is able to explain the importance of receiving RhoGAM when necessary and cooperates with the recommended dosage schedule.

- The woman successfully delivers a healthy newborn.

- If complications develop for the fetus (or newborn) they are detected quickly and therapy is instituted.

● Care of the Woman at Risk Due to ABO Incompatibility

ABO incompatibility is rather common (occurring in 12 percent of pregnancies) but rarely causes significant hemolysis. In most cases ABO incompatibility is limited to type O mothers with a type A or B fetus. The group B fetus of an A mother and the group A fetus of a B mother are only occasionally affected. Group O infants, because they have no antigenic sites on the red blood cells, are never affected regardless of the mother's blood type. The incompatibility occurs as a result of the maternal antibodies present in her serum and interaction between the antigen sites on the fetal red blood cells.

Anti-A and anti-B antibodies are naturally occurring; that is, women are naturally exposed to the A and B antigens through the foods they eat and through exposure to infection by gram negative bacteria. As a result, some women have high serum anti-A and anti-B titers before they become pregnant. Once the woman becomes pregnant, the maternal serum anti-A and anti-B antibodies cross the placenta and produce hemolysis of the fetal red blood cells. With ABO incompatibility the first infant is frequently involved, and no relationship exists between the appearance of the disease and repeated sensitization from one pregnancy to the next.

Unlike Rh incompatibility, treatment is never warranted antepartally. As part of the initial assessment, however, the nurse should note whether the potential for an ABO incompatibility exists. This alerts care givers so that following delivery the newborn can be assessed carefully for the development of hyperbilirubinemia (see Chapter 32).

● Care of the Woman Requiring Surgery During Pregnancy

While elective surgery should be delayed until the postpartal period, essential surgery can generally be undertaken during pregnancy. Surgery does pose some risks. The incidence of spontaneous abortion is increased for women who have surgery in the first trimester. There is also an increased incidence of fetal mortality and of low-birth-weight (less than 2500 gm) infants. Finally, when pelvic surgery is necessary the incidence of premature labor increases (Triolo 1985).

Medical Therapy

Although general preoperative and postoperative care is similar for gravid and nongravid women, special considerations must be kept in mind whenever the surgical client is pregnant. The early second trimester is the best time to operate because there is less risk of causing spontaneous abortion or early labor, and the uterus is not so large as to impinge on the abdominal field.

The preoperative chest radiograph and electrocardiogram, which are routine for persons over age 40, should be done on the same basis for the pregnant woman. If a chest radiograph is done, the fetus should be shielded from the radiation. Because of decreased intestinal motility and decreased free gastric acid secretion during pregnancy, stomach emptying time is delayed, which increases risk of vomiting during induction of anesthesia and during the postoperative period. Therefore, a nasogastric tube is recommended prior to major surgery. An indwelling urinary catheter prevents bladder distention, decreases risk of injury to the bladder, and promotes ease of monitoring output. Support stockings during and after surgery help prevent venous stasis and the development of thrombophlebitis. Fetal heart tones must be monitored before, during, and after surgery.

Pregnancy causes increased secretions of the respiratory tract and engorgement of the nasal mucous membrane, often making breathing through the nose difficult. Because of this pregnant women often need an endotracheal tube for respiratory support during surgery. Care givers must guard against maternal hypoxia during surgery as uterine circulation will be decreased and fetal oxygenation can decline very quickly. During surgery and the recovery period the woman is positioned to allow optimal utero–placental–fetal circulation. A wedge is placed under her hip to tip the uterus and thereby avoid pressure by the fetus on the maternal vena cava.

Spinal or epidural anesthesia may produce hypotension and respiratory apnea in the pregnant woman. The frequency and degree of the hypotension increase with higher anesthetic levels. This can be prevented in many cases with a preanesthetic infusion of 900 to 1000 mL of fluid.

Blood loss during surgery is monitored carefully. Measurement of fetal heart tones gives the best indication of blood loss. Because of the normal increased blood volume of pregnancy, uterine blood flow may be reduced significantly before the maternal blood pressure begins to fall. Fluid replacement should be done with balanced electrolyte solution, and whole blood if needed.

Nursing Assessment

During the preoperative period the nurse assesses the pregnant woman's health status in the same way that any preoperative client is assessed. Is there any sign of respiratory infection, fever, urinary tract infection, or anemia? Are laboratory values all within normal limits for surgery (except in the case of emergency surgery, which may, of necessity, be done even with abnormal laboratory values)? Do the woman and her family understand the surgical procedure? Do they know what to expect postoperatively? Do they have any questions or concerns?

The nurse also considers the impact of surgery on the woman's pregnancy. Is the fetal heart rate normal? Does the woman understand the implications of surgery with regard to her pregnancy? How is she coping?

Postoperatively the nurse completes all necessary postoperative assessments and also continues to assess fetal status, primarily by monitoring the fetal heart rate.

Nursing Diagnosis

Nursing diagnoses that might apply to the pregnant woman who requires surgery include:

- Potential alteration in tissue perfusion (fetal) related to the effects of general anesthesia on fetal oxygenation

- Knowledge deficit related to a lack of understanding of what to expect postoperatively

Nursing Goal: Provision of Effective Perioperative Care

Much of the nurse's care during the preoperative period is directed toward the educational needs of the woman and her family. The nurse plans time to review the procedure and answer any questions of the family. The nurse recognizes that the need for surgery during the woman's pregnancy is probably very distressing for the family. The nurse works to help decrease their anxiety by providing information and emotional support.

Postoperatively the nurse is caring for two clients: the mother and her unborn child. In addition to monitoring the status of both, the nurse considers both in providing care. If surgery is done in the first trimester, the nurse should be aware of the potential teratogenic effect of any medications prescribed and should discuss the implications with the surgeon and obstetrician. During the third trimester the nurse, recognizing the potential for vena caval syndrome if the woman lies flat on her back, helps the woman maintain a side-lying position. To avoid inadequate oxygenation the nurse also encourages the woman to turn, deep breathe, and cough regularly and also to use any ventilation therapy, such as Spirocare, to avoid developing pneumonia. The pregnant woman is also at increased risk for thrombophlebitis, so the nurse applies antiembolism stockings, encourages leg exercises while the woman is confined to bed, and begins ambulation as soon as possible. The nurse also encourages the woman to maintain or resume an adequate diet as soon as possible. If cultural factors influence the woman's dietary practices, the nurse and dietitian should work together to meet the woman's needs.

Discharge teaching is especially important. The woman and her family should have a clear understanding of what to expect regarding activity level, discomfort, diet, medications, and any special considerations. In addition they should know any warning signs that they should report to their physician immediately.

Evaluative Outcome Criteria

Anticipated outcomes of nursing care include the following:

- The woman is able to explain the surgical procedure, its risks and benefits, and its implications for her pregnancy.

- Care givers maintain adequate oxygenation throughout surgery and postoperatively.

- Potential complications are avoided or detected early and treated successfully.

- The woman is able to describe any necessary post-discharge activities, limitations, and follow-up and agrees to cooperate with the recommended regimen.

- The woman maintains her pregnancy successfully.

● Care of the Woman Suffering Trauma From an Accident

Accidents and injury are not uncommon during pregnancy. Accidental injury may complicate 6 percent to 7 percent of all pregnancies (Patterson 1984). In early pregnancy body changes increase the potential for injury through fatigue, fainting spells, and hyperventilation. Late in pregnancy the woman has less balance and coordination and may fall. Her protruding abdomen is vulnerable to a variety of minor injuries. The fetus is usually well protected by the amniotic fluid, which distributes the force of a blow equally in all directions, and by the muscle layers of the uterus and abdominal wall. In early pregnancy, while the uterus is still in the pelvis it is shielded from blows by the surrounding pelvic organs, muscles, and bony structures. Trauma that causes concern includes blunt trauma, from an automobile accident, for example; penetrating abdominal injuries, such as knife and gunshot wounds; and the complications of maternal shock, premature labor, and spontaneous abortion.

Maternal mortality most often occurs from head trauma or hemorrhage. Uterine rupture may result from strong deceleration forces in an automobile accident with or without seat belts. Traumatic separation of the placenta can occur; it results in a high rate of fetal mortality. Premature labor is another serious hazard to the fetus, often following rupture of membranes during an accident. Premature labor can ensue even if the woman is not injured.

Maternal fractures, even of the pelvis, are tolerated well. However, ruptured bladder, retroperitoneal hemorrhage, and shock are complications to watch for with a fractured pelvis.

Fetal or placental injury occurs in 89 percent of gunshot wounds to the abdomen, with a 66 percent perinatal mortality (Taylor & Slate 1981). Stab wounds tend to cause less damage than bullet wounds.

Medical Therapy

The goal of medical therapy is to stabilize the injury and promote well-being for both mother and fetus. Thus medical therapy initially focuses on ensuring airway adequacy, maintaining ventilation and adequate circulatory volume, controlling acute bleeding, and splinting fractures to prevent vascular or tissue injury.

Care must be taken at the scene of the injury to avoid the development of supine hypotensive syndrome. A wedge is generally placed under the woman's right hip. A neck brace is used if a neck injury is suspected, or the woman is placed on a backboard and the entire board is tilted to displace the uterus (O'Keeffe 1985). Prompt treatment of maternal hypotension or hypovolemia also averts poor fetal oxygenation. Obstetric consultation is necessary to ensure that the needs of both mother and fetus are met. If the mother does not survive, and the fetus is more than 28 weeks' gestation, a rapid cesarean delivery may result in the birth of a live child.

Nursing Assessment

Each individual must be assessed according to the type and extent of her injuries. As with all trauma victims, initial assessments focus on adequacy of the airway, evidence of breathing, existence of cardiovascular stability, and extent of injury. When an injured woman is pregnant,

it is necessary to assess fetal status as well in order to avoid fetal hypoxia. Frequent maternal blood gas determinations are indicated if respiratory function is compromised.

Assessment should include a review of the specific history of past and present pregnancies to avoid incorrect interpretation of vital signs. Care givers do diagnostic tests as necessary, avoiding radiology in favor of ultrasonography whenever possible.

Ongoing assessments include evaluation of intake and output and other indicators of shock, determination of neurologic status, and assessment of mental outlook and anxiety level.

Nursing Diagnosis

Nursing diagnoses that might apply include:

● Alteration in comfort: acute pain related to the effects of the trauma experienced

● Alteration in bowel elimination: constipation related to immobility secondary to the effects of the accident

● Fear related to the effects of the trauma on fetal well-being

Nursing Goal: Provision of Psychologic Support

As a member of the health care team the nurse is actively involved in the ongoing assessment of the status of the woman and fetus. The nurse also has a primary responsibility to assess the childbearing woman's emotional state. The trauma victim must be oriented to her situation and receive explanation and reinforcement as necessary to help her understand any interventions. Family members should be involved as appropriate. The nurse also gives the pregnant woman an opportunity to discuss her feelings and concerns.

Evaluative Outcome Criteria

Anticipated outcomes of nursing care include the following:

● The woman and her family are able to understand the effects of the trauma on her and on her unborn child.

● Adequate oxygenation is maintained to promote fetal well-being.

● The woman's pain is adequately relieved and her trauma is treated.

● Potential complications are quickly identified and appropriate interventions are instituted.

● The woman successfully delivers a healthy newborn.

- If the trauma results in fetal demise, the woman is able to verbalize her feelings and begin working through the grief process.

Care of the Battered Pregnant Woman

There are conflicting opinions about whether family violence increases or decreases during pregnancy. It is important to realize that it does exist and can be a serious problem for the pregnant woman and her unborn child. Women who have been abused are usually at risk for abuse during pregnancy (Hillard 1985). The first step toward helping the battered woman is to identify her. She needs support, confidence in her decision making, and the recognition that she can help herself.

Chronic psychosomatic symptoms can be an indicator of abuse. The woman may have nonspecific or vague complaints. It is important to assess old scars around the head, chest, arms, abdomen, and genitalia. Any bruising or evidence of pain is also evaluated. Other indicators include a decrease in eye contact, silence when the partner is in the room, and a history of nervousness, insomnia, drug overdose, or alcohol problems. Frequent visits to the emergency room and a history of accidents without understandable causes are possible indicators of abuse.

The goals of treatment are to identify the woman at risk, increase her decision-making abilities to decrease the potential for further abuse, and provide a safe environment for the pregnant woman and her unborn child.

It is important to provide an environment that is private, accepting, and nonjudgmental so the woman can express her concerns. She needs to be aware of community resources available to her, such as emergency shelters; police, legal, and social services; and counseling (Hillard 1985). For further discussion refer to Chapter 12.

Care of the Woman With an Infection

A major factor contributing to risk during pregnancy is the presence of maternal infection, whether contracted prior to conception or during the pregnancy. Spontaneous abortion is frequently the result of a severe maternal infection.

Evidence exists that links infection and prematurity. In addition, if the pregnancy is carried to term in the presence of infection, the risk of maternal and fetal morbidity and mortality increases. In many instances of fetal risk due to infection, the woman presents few or no signs or symptoms. It is essential to maternal and fetal health that diagnosis and treatment be prompt.

Urinary tract, vaginal, and sexually transmitted infections are discussed in detail in Chapter 10. Table 19–5 provides a summary of these infections and their implications for pregnancy.

TORCH

The TORCH group of infectious diseases are those identified as causing serious harm to the embryo-fetus. These are: toxoplasmosis (*TO*), rubella (*R*), cytomegalovirus (*C*), and herpesvirus type 2 (*H*). (Some sources identify the *O* as "other infections.") The TORCH identification assists health team members to assess quickly the potential risk to each woman in pregnancy.

The importance of understanding what these infections are and identifying risk factors cannot be overemphasized. Exposure of the woman during the first 12 weeks of gestation may cause developmental anomalies. The three major viral infections are rubella, cytomegalovirus, and herpesvirus type 2. Toxoplasmosis is a protozoal infection.

TOXOPLASMOSIS

Toxoplasmosis is caused by the protozoan *Toxoplasma gondii*. It is innocuous in adults, but when contracted in pregnancy, can profoundly affect the fetus. The pregnant woman may contract the organism by eating raw or poorly cooked meat or by contact with the feces of infected cats, either through the cat litter box or by gardening in areas frequented by cats.

○ *FETAL-NEONATAL RISKS* The incidence of abortion, prematurity, stillbirths, neonatal deaths, and severe congenital anomalies is increased in the affected fetus and neonate. In very mild cases, retinochoroiditis may be the only recognizable damage, and it and other manifestations may not appear until adolescence or young adulthood. Severe neonatal disorders associated with congenital infection include convulsions, coma, microcephaly, and hydocephalus. The infant with a severe infection may die soon after birth. Survivors are often blind, deaf, and severely retarded.

○ *MEDICAL THERAPY* The goal of medical treatment is to identify the woman at risk for toxoplasmosis and to treat the disease promptly if diagnosed. Diagnosis can be made by serologic testing, including the IgM fluorescent antibody test. Elevated titers peak one month after infection and are usually present for four to eight months, although they may persist for a year. Other tests include the Sabin-Feldman dye test and the indirect fluorescent antibody test.

If diagnosis can be established by physical findings, history, and positive serological results, the woman may be treated with sulfadiazine and pyrimethamine. If toxoplasmosis is diagnosed before 20 weeks' gestation, therapeutic abortion should be considered because damage to the fetus is generally more severe than if the disease is acquired later in the pregnancy.

○ *NURSING ASSESSMENT* The incubation period for the disease is ten days. The woman with acute toxoplasmosis

Table 19–5 Infections That Put Pregnancy at Risk

Condition and causative organism	Signs and symptoms	Treatment	Implications for pregnancy
URINARY TRACT INFECTIONS			
Asymptomatic bacteriuria (ASB): *E. coli, Klebsiella, Proteus* most common.	Bacteria present in urine on culture with no accompanying symptoms.	Oral sulfonamides early in pregnancy, ampicillin and nitrofurantoin (Furadantin) in late pregnancy.	Women with ASB in early pregnancy may go on to develop cystitis or acute pyelonephritis by third trimester if not treated. Oral sulfonamides taken in the last few weeks of pregnancy may lead to neonatal hyperbilirubinemia and kernicterus.
Cystitis (Lower UTI): Causative organisms same as ASB.	Dysuria, urgency, frequency; low-grade fever and hematuria may occur. Urine culture (clean catch) show ↑ leukocytes. Presence of 10^5 (100,000) or more colonies bacteria per mL urine.	Same.	If not treated, infection may ascend and lead to acute pyelonephritis.
Acute pyelonephritis: Causative organisms same as ASB.	Sudden onset. Chills, high fever, flank pain. Nausea, vomiting, malaise. May have decreased urine output, severe colicky pain, dehydration. Increased diastolic BP, positive FA-test, low creatinine clearance. Marked bacteremia in urine culture, pyuria, WBC casts.	Hospitalization; IV antibiotic therapy. Other antibiotics safe during pregnancy include carbenicillin, methenamine, cephalosporins. Catheterization if output is ↓. Supportive therapy for comfort. Follow-up urine cultures are necessary.	Increased risk of premature delivery and IUGR. These antibiotics interfere with urinary estriol levels and can cause false interpretations of estriol levels during pregnancy.
VAGINAL INFECTIONS			
Monilial (yeast infection): *Candida albicans.*	Often thick, white, curdy discharge, severe itching, dysuria, dyspareunia. Diagnosis based on presence of hyphae and spores in a wet mount preparation of vaginal secretions.	Intravaginal insertion of miconazole or clotrimazole suppositories at bedtime for 1 week. Cream may be prescribed for topical application to the vulva if necessary.	If the infection is present at delivery and the fetus is delivered vaginally, the fetus may contract thrush.
Bacterial vaginosis: *Gardnerella vaginalis*	Thin, watery, yellow-gray discharge with foul odor often described as "fishy." Wet mount preparation reveals "clue cells." Application of KOH (potassium hydroxide) to a specimen of vaginal secretions produces a pronounced fishy odor.	Nonpregnant women treated with metronidazole (Flagyl). Pregnant women treated with ampicillin, at least during the first half of pregnancy.	Metronidazole has potential teratogenic effects.
Trichomoniasis: *Trichomonas vaginalis*	Occasionally asymptomatic. May have frothy greenish gray vaginal discharge, pruritus, urinary symptoms. Strawberry patches may be visible on vaginal walls or cervix. Wet mount preparation of vaginal secretions shows motile flagellated trichomonads.	During early pregnancy symptoms may be controlled with clotrimazole vaginal suppositories. Both partners are treated.	Metronidazole has potential teratogenic effects.
SEXUALLY TRANSMITTED INFECTIONS			
Chlamydial infection: *Chlamydia trachomatis*	Women are often asymptomatic. Symptoms may include thin or purulent discharge, burning and frequency with urination, or lower abdominal pain. Lab test available to detect monoclonal antibodies specific for *Chlamydia.*	Although nonpregnant women are treated with tetracycline, it may permanently discolor fetal teeth. Thus, pregnant women are treated with erythromycin ethyl succinate.	Infant of woman with untreated chlamydial infection may develop newborn conjunctivitis, which can be treated with erythromycin eye ointment (but not silver nitrate). Infant may also develop chlamydial pneumonia. May be responsible for premature labor and fetal death.

Table 19-5　Infections That Put Pregnancy at Risk (continued)

Condition and causative organism	Signs and symptoms	Treatment	Implications for pregnancy
Syphilis: *Treponema pallidum*, a spirochete	Primary stage: chancre, slight fever, malaise. Chancre lasts about 4 weeks, then disappears. Secondary stage: occurs 6 weeks to 6 months after infection. Skin eruptions (condyloma lata); also symptoms of acute arthritis, liver enlargement, iritis, chronic sore throat with hoarseness. Diagnosed by blood tests such as VDRL, RPR, FTA-ABS. Dark field examination for spirochetes may also be done.	For syphilis less than 1 year in duration: 2.4 million U benzathine penicillin G IM. For syphilis of more than 1 year's duration: 2.4 million U benzathine penicillin G once a week for 3 weeks.	Syphilis can be passed transplacentally to the fetus. If untreated, one of the following can occur: second trimester abortion, stillborn infant at term, congenitally infected infant, uninfected live infant.
Gonorrhea: *Neisseria gonorrhoeae*	Majority of women asymptomatic; disease often diagnosed during routine prenatal cervical culture. If symptoms are present they may include purulent vaginal discharge, dysuria, urinary frequency, inflammation and swelling of the vulva. Cervix may appear eroded.	Nonpregnant women are treated with tetracycline. Pregnant women are treated with aqueous procaine penicillin G 4.8 million U IM with 1.0 g probenicid by mouth. If the woman is allergic to penicillin, spectinomycin is used. All sexual partners are also treated.	Infection at time of delivery may cause ophthalmia neonatorum in the newborn.
Condyloma accuminata: caused by a papovirus	Soft, grayish-pink lesions on the vulva, vagina, cervix, or anus.	Podophyllin not used during pregnancy. Trichloroacetic acid, liquid nitrogen, or cryocautery; CO_2 laser therapy done under colposcopy is also successful (Eschenbach 1986).	Possible teratogenic effect of podophyllin. Large doses have been associated with fetal death.

may be asymptomatic, or she may develop myalgia, malaise, rash, splenomegaly, and enlarged posterior cervical lymph nodes. Symptoms usually disappear in a few days or weeks.

○　*NURSING DIAGNOSIS*　Nursing diagnoses that might apply to the pregnant woman with toxoplasmosis include:

- Knowledge deficit related to a lack of understanding of the ways in which a pregnant woman can contract toxoplasmosis.

- Grieving related to potential effects on infant of maternal toxoplasmosis.

○　*NURSING GOAL: EDUCATION FOR SELF-CARE*　The nurse caring for women during the antepartal period has the primary opportunity to discuss methods of prevention of toxoplasmosis with the childbearing woman. The woman must understand the importance of avoiding poorly cooked meat, especially pork, beef, and lamb. She should avoid contact with the cat litter box by having someone else clean it. In addition, since it takes approximately 48 hours for the cat's feces to become infectious, the litter should be cleaned frequently. The nurse should also discuss the importance of wearing gloves to garden and of avoiding garden areas frequented by cats.

○　*EVALUATIVE OUTCOME CRITERIA*　Anticipated outcomes of nursing care include the following:

- The woman is able to discuss toxoplasmosis, its methods of transmission, the implications for her fetus, and measures she can take to avoid contracting it.

- The woman implements health measures to avoid contracting toxoplasmosis.

- The woman successfully delivers a healthy newborn.

RUBELLA

The effects of rubella (German measles) are no more severe, nor are there greater complications in pregnant women than in nonpregnant women of comparable age. But the effects of this infection on the fetus and neonate are great, because rubella causes a chronic infection that begins in the first trimester of pregnancy and may persist for months after birth.

○ **FETAL-NEONATAL RISKS** The period of greatest risk for the teratogenic effects of rubella on the fetus is during the first trimester. If infection occurs during the first 4 weeks of pregnancy, damage or death occurs in 50 percent of the embryos. In the second month, 25 percent of affected fetuses may have serious defects, and if infection occurs in the third month, 15 percent of fetuses are affected (Pritchard et al 1985). If infection occurs early in the second trimester, the resultant fetal effect is most often permanent hearing impairment.

Clinical signs of congenital infection are congenital heart disease, IUGR, and cataracts. Cardiac involvements most often seen are patent ductus arteriosus and narrowing of peripheral pulmonary arteries. Cataracts may be unilateral or bilateral and may be present at birth or develop in the neonatal period. A petechial rash is seen in some infants, and hepatosplenomegaly and hyperbilirubinemia are frequently seen. Other abnormalities, such as mental retardation or cerebral palsy, may become evident in infancy. Diagnosis in the neonate can be conclusively made in the presence of these conditions and with an elevated rubella IgM antibody titer at birth.

Infants born with congenital rubella syndrome are infectious and should be isolated. These infants may continue to shed the virus for months.

The expanded rubella syndrome relates to effects that may develop for years after the infection. These include an increased incidence of insulin-dependent diabetes mellitus; sudden hearing loss; glaucoma; and a slow, progressive form of encephalitis.

○ **MEDICAL THERAPY** The best therapy for rubella is prevention. Live attenuated vaccine is available and should be given to all children. Women of childbearing age should be tested for immunity and vaccinated if susceptible and if it is established that they are not pregnant. Health counseling in high school and in premarital clinic visits can emphasize the importance of screening prior to planning a pregnancy.

As part of the prenatal laboratory screen the woman is evaluated for rubella using hemagglutination inhibition (HAI), a serology test. The presence of a 1:16 titer or greater is evidence of immunity. A titer less than 1:8 indicates susceptibility to rubella.

Because the vaccine is made with attenuated virus, pregnant women are not vaccinated. However, it is considered safe for newly vaccinated children to have contact with pregnant women.

If a woman who is pregnant becomes infected during the first trimester, therapeutic abortion is an alternative.

○ **NURSING ASSESSMENT** A woman who develops rubella during pregnancy may be asymptomatic or may show signs of a mild infection including a maculopapular rash, lymphadenopathy, muscular achiness, and joint pain. The presence of IgM antirubella antibody is diagnostic of a recent infection. These titers remain elevated for approximately one month following infection.

○ **NURSING DIAGNOSIS** Nursing diagnoses that may apply to the woman who develops rubella early in her pregnancy include:

- Ineffective family coping due to an inability to accept the possibility of fetal anomalies secondary to maternal rubella exposure

- Knowledge deficit about the importance of rubella immunization prior to becoming pregnant

○ **NURSING GOAL: PROVISION OF INFORMATION AND EMOTIONAL SUPPORT** Nursing support and understanding are vital for the couple contemplating abortion due to a diagnosis of rubella. Such a decision may initiate a crisis for the couple who have planned their pregnancy. They need objective data to understand the possible effects on their unborn fetus and the prognosis for the offspring.

○ **EVALUATIVE OUTCOME CRITERIA** Anticipated outcomes of nursing care include the following:

- The woman is able to describe the implications of rubella exposure during the first trimester of pregnancy.

- If exposure occurs in a woman who is not immune, she is able to identify her options and make a decision about continuing her pregnancy that is acceptable to her and her partner.

- A nonimmune woman agrees to receive the rubella vaccine during the early postpartal period.

- The woman successfully delivers a healthy infant.

CYTOMEGALOVIRUS

Cytomegalovirus (CMV) belongs to the herpesvirus group and causes both congenital and acquired infections referred to as *cytomegalic inclusion disease* (CID). The significance of this virus in pregnancy is related to its ability to be transmitted by asymptomatic women across the placenta to the fetus or by the cervical route during delivery.

CID is probably the most prevalent infection in the TORCH group. Nearly half of adults have antibodies for the virus. The virus can be found in urine, saliva, cervical mucus, semen, and breast milk. It can be passed between humans by any close contact such as kissing, breast-feeding, and sexual intercourse. Asymptomatic CMV infection is particularly common in children and gravid women. It is a chronic, persistent infection in that the individual may shed the virus continually over many years. The cervix can habor the virus, and an ascending infection can develop after delivery. While the virus is usually innocuous in adults and children, it may be fatal to the fetus.

Accurate diagnosis in the pregnant woman depends on the presence of CMV in the urine, a rise in IgM levels, and identification of the CMV antibodies within the serum IgM fraction. At present, no treatment exists for maternal CMV or for the congenital disease in the neonate.

○   *FETAL-NEONATAL RISKS*   The cytomegalovirus is the most frequent agent of viral infection in the human fetus. It infects 0.5 percent to 2.0 percent of neonates, and of these about 10 percent develop serious manifestations (Pritchard et al 1985). Subclinical infections in the newborn are capable of producing mental retardation and auditory deficits, sometimes not recognized for several months, or learning disabilities not seen until childhood. CMV may be the most common cause of mental retardation.

For the fetus, this infection can result in extensive intrauterine tissue damage that is incompatible with life; in survival with microcephaly, hydrocephaly, cerebral palsy, or mental retardation; or in survival with no damage at all.

The infected neonate is often SGA. The principal tissues and organs affected are the blood, brain, and liver. However, virtually all organs are potentially at risk. Hemolysis leads to anemia and hyperbilirubinemia. Thrombocytopenia and hepatosplenomegaly may also develop.

HERPES GENITALIS (HERPESVIRUS TYPE 2)

Herpesvirus type 2 is a viral infection that can cause painful lesions in the genital area. Lesions may also develop on the cervix. This condition and its implications for non-pregnant women are discussed in Chapter 10. However, because the presence of herpes lesions in the genital tract may profoundly affect the fetus, herpes infection as it relates to a pregnant woman is discussed here as part of the TORCH complex of infections.

○   *FETAL-NEONATAL RISKS*   Transmission of herpesvirus type 2 to the fetus almost always occurs after the membranes rupture, as the virus ascends from active lesions. It also occurs during vaginal delivery, when the fetus comes in contact with genital lesions. Transplacental infection is rare.

If active herpesvirus type 2 infection occurs during the first trimester there is a 20 percent to 50 percent rate of spontaneous abortion or stillbirth (Stagno & Whitley 1985). Infection after 20 weeks of gestation is associated with an increased risk of preterm labor.

Approximately 54 percent of all infants who are born vaginally when the mother is shedding herpesvirus type 2 in her vagina or cervix develop some form of herpes infection. Of these infants, approximately 70 percent will die

if untreated, while 83 percent of the survivors will have permanent brain damage (Harger 1985).

The infected infant is often asymptomatic at birth but after an incubation period of 2 to 12 days develops symptoms of fever (or hypothermia), jaundice, seizures, and poor feeding. Approximately one-half of infected infants develop the characteristic vesicular skin lesions. Vidarabine has been useful in decreasing serious effects from neonatal herpes, but no definitive treatment exists as yet (Corey & Spear 1986).

○   *MEDICAL THERAPY*   Although the vesicular lesions of herpes have a characteristic appearance, they rupture easily. Thus definitive diagnosis is made by culturing active lesions. Because cultures are expensive and not always available, many care givers obtain a discharge from the lesion and prepare a slide as for a Pap test. The presence of multinucleated giant cells indicates herpes.

Treatment is directed first toward relieving the woman's vulvar pain. If the attack is severe, walking, sitting, and even wearing clothing may be painful. The woman may be most comfortable in bed during the peak of the infection. Sitz baths three to four times daily, followed by drying of the vulva with a hair dryer or light bulb, may promote healing and help prevent secondary infection. Cotton underwear helps keep the genital area dry.

Acyclovir (Zovirax) was approved by the FDA in 1982. It does not cure the infection or prevent recurrence. Acyclovir does reduce healing time of the initial attack and shortens the time that the live virus is in the lesions, thereby reducing the infectious period. Its effects during pregnancy are not yet known.

Herpesvirus type 2 has not been found in breast milk. Present experience shows that breast-feeding is acceptable if the mother washes her hands well to prevent any direct transfer of the virus.

Because most infants become infected when they pass through a birth canal containing herpesvirus it is necessary to determine whether the woman is shedding virus at the time of delivery. If virus is present, the woman is delivered by cesarean; if no virus is present, a vaginal delivery is possible.

To determine whether herpesvirus type 2 is present, the cervix is cultured weekly, beginning four to eight weeks before the due date. Because some women remain asymptomatic while shedding the virus, reports of symptoms are not sufficient to determine delivery method. The following guidelines are generally used to decide the route for delivery. Vaginal delivery is possible if (Harper 1985):

● The two most recent cultures for genital herpes are negative (cultures must have been incubated at least three days).

● The woman is experiencing no symptoms of herpesvirus type 2.

- No lesions are visible on inspection of the vulva and vagina.

- During her pregnancy the woman has had no more than one positive culture, during which she was symptom free.

If the woman has a genital herpes lesion but her membranes rupture, she is at risk for an ascending herpes infection. Then the most appropriate delivery method is less clear. Many physicians recommend a cesarean delivery if the membranes have been ruptured less than four hours.

○ *NURSING ASSESSMENT* During the initial prenatal visit it is important to learn whether the woman or her partner have had previous herpes infections. If so, ongoing assessment by means of cervical cultures is indicated as pregnancy progresses.

○ *NURSING DIAGNOSIS* Nursing diagnoses that may apply to the pregnant woman with herpesvirus type 2 include:

- Sexual dysfunction related to unwillingness to engage in sexual intercourse secondary to the presence of active herpes lesions

- Ineffective individual coping related to depression secondary to the risk to the fetus if herpes lesions are present at delivery

○ *NURSING GOAL: EDUCATION FOR SELF-CARE* Nurses must be particularly concerned with client education about this fast-spreading disease. Women must be informed of the association of genital herpes with spontaneous abortion, neonatal mortality and morbidity, and the possibility of cesarean delivery. A woman needs to inform her future health care providers of her infection. She also should know of the possible association of genital herpes with cervical cancer and the importance of a yearly Pap smear.

○ *NURSING GOAL: PROVISION OF EMOTIONAL SUPPORT* The woman who feels she acquired herpesvirus type 2 as an adolescent may be devastated as a mature young adult who wants to have a family. Clients may be helped by counseling that allows expression of the anger, shame, and depression so often experienced by the herpes victim. Literature may be helpful and is available from Planned Parenthood and many public health agencies. The American Social Health Association has established the HELP program to provide information and the latest research results on genital herpes. The Association has a quarterly journal, *The Helper,* for nurses and herpes clients.

○ *EVALUATIVE OUTCOME CRITERIA* Anticipated outcomes of nursing care include the following:

- The woman is able to describe her infection with

regard to its method of spread, therapy and comfort measures, implications for her pregnancy, and long-term implications.

- The woman has appropriate cultures done as recommended throughout her pregnancy.

- The woman successfully delivers a healthy infant.

Acquired Immunodeficiency Syndrome

Acquired immunodeficiency syndrome (AIDS) is one of today's major health concerns. It was discovered in early 1980 and has spread rapidly since that time. According to the Centers for Disease Control, 54,723 people were diagnosed with AIDS between June 1, 1981, and February 29, 1988; 865 of these cases were children. Of the reported cases, over 56 percent of the adults and 59 percent of the children have died (AWSR, 1988).

The persons at risk for AIDS are homosexual or bisexual men, heterosexual partners of persons with AIDS, heterosexual drug users, recipients of blood transfusions, hemophiliacs, Haitians, Africans in Zaire, and fetuses of mothers at risk (perinatal transmission).

There is a possibility of maternal transmission in utero (Cowen et al 1984) as well as a report on the potential transmission via breast milk of a mother who had a blood transfusion after delivery (Ziegler et al 1985). Therefore, the concern and need to recognize the population at risk is crucial in antenatal care.

Acquired immune deficiency is caused by a virus, human T-lymphotropic retrovirus (HTLV-III) or human immunodeficiency virus (HIV). It enters the body through blood, blood products, or sexual contact (semen) and affects specific T-cells, which decrease the body's immune responses. This makes the affected person susceptible to opportunistic organisms such as cytomegalovirus, herpes simplex and zoster, candidas, *Pneumocystis carinii,* and *Toxoplasma gondii.* These organisms do not usually cause life-threatening illness, but in the case of helper T-cell destruction they can be fatal. The loss of T-helper cells increases the potential for Kaposi's sarcoma as well.

Opportunistic infections are the cause of most fatalities from AIDS; Kaposi's sarcoma is rarely the direct cause. *Pneumocystis carinii* pneumonia is the most common opportunistic infection. The pneumonia creates dyspnea with progressive hypoxemia.

The incubation period for AIDS can be as long as five to seven years. Thus an infant born to a woman with AIDS is not necessarily free of the disease even if he or she shows no symptoms at birth.

FETAL-NEONATAL RISKS

While AIDS may develop in the infants of mothers who are seropositive, transmission does not always occur.

Currently less than half the infants born to women with a positive HIV result have acquired the disease (Scott et al 1985). The signs of AIDS in infants may include: failure to thrive, hepatosplenomegaly, interstitital pneumonia, recurrent infections, cell-mediated immunodeficiency, evidence of Epstein-Barr virus, and neurologic abnormalities (Cowen et al 1984). These infants are also likely to be SGA at birth.

Apparently infection can occur early in fetal development. Facial characteristics that may indicate that the infant has been infected with the AIDS virus include: microcephaly; patulous lips; prominent, boxlike forehead; increased distance between the inner canthus of the eyes; a flattened nasal bridge; and a mild obliquity of the eyes. The mortality rate for these infants is especially high: Of the children who were diagnosed with AIDS more than two years ago, 81 percent have died (Klug 1986).

MEDICAL THERAPY

Currently there is no definitive treatment for AIDS. The goal for antenatal care is identification of the pregnant woman at risk and education of the public about the transmission of AIDS to decrease its potential spread. Following recommended techniques to decrease nosocomial transmission of AIDS in a hospital setting can decrease the potential risk to health workers. It is very important to decrease exposure to contaminated blood and body fluids, which may harbor potential infectious agents, especially during labor and delivery.

Routine laboratory tests appear to be of little value in diagnosing AIDS. Findings include leukopenia, anemia, elevated transaminase and alkaline phosphate, and low serum albumin (LaCamera 1985).

NURSING ASSESSMENT

Based on the recommendations of the Centers for Disease Control, the following women should be screened for a positive HIV (MMWR 1985):

- Women who have engaged in prostitution
- Women who use drugs intravenously
- Women whose current or previous sexual partners have been bisexual, abused intravenous drugs, have hemophilia, or test positive for HIV
- Women from countries where heterosexual transmission is common

A woman who already has AIDS may present with any of the following signs or symptoms: malaise, progressive weight loss, lymphadenopathy, diarrhea, fever, neurologic dysfunction, cell-mediated immunodeficiency, or evidence of Kaposi's sarcoma (purplish, reddish brown lesions either internally or externally).

NURSING DIAGNOSIS

Nursing diagnoses that might apply to a pregnant woman who is immunopositive for AIDS include:

- Potential for infection related to altered immunity secondary to AIDS
- Ineffective family coping related to the implications of the diagnosis of AIDS on the health of the woman, her partner, and their unborn child

NURSING GOAL: PROVISION OF ANTICIPATORY GUIDANCE

It is recommended that women at risk for AIDS should have premarital and prenatal screening for HIV before considering a pregnancy (Curran 1985). The nurse can advise the woman to postpone or avoid pregnancy to prevent in vitro transmission.

NURSING GOAL: REDUCTION OF RISK OF TRANSMISSION

The nurse is faced with the important task of taking the necessary precautions to protect staff, other clients, and families while at the same time meeting the needs of the childbearing woman with AIDS.

Nurses caring for a pregnant woman with suspected or previously diagnosed AIDS should take appropriate precautions. The Centers for Disease Control recommendations include the following:

- When hospitalized the woman is placed on blood and secretion precautions.
- Care givers should wear disposable gloves and a protective apron or gown when having direct contact with the woman's body fluids such as amniotic fluid, excretions, lab specimens, dishes, linen, dressings.
- Care should be taken when handling syringes and needles. They are disposed of in a special container in the woman's room. Needles are not broken, bent, or even returned to their protective cap because that is when most inadvertent punctures occur.
- During labor and delivery, care should be taken to avoid splattering of blood or amniotic fluid. The woman should be admitted to an isolation room where she can labor and deliver vaginally.
- The woman's hygiene should be carefully maintained, following necessary precautions.
- At delivery the newborn should be suctioned with a disposable bulb syringe. DeLee mucus traps are not used because of the risk of inadvertently ingesting secretions.

- Following delivery the room should be cleaned according to CDC guidelines.

- Postpartally, a private room is desirable and permits easier handling of the woman's equipment and secretions (such as lochia).

- In the nursery, blood and secretion precautions are necessary for the infant. If their conditions permit, rooming-in is a fine alternative for the mother and her child because it promotes the development of attachment and facilitates precautions and teaching (Loveman et al 1986).

NURSING COAL: PROVISION OF EMOTIONAL SUPPORT

The psychologic implications of AIDS for the childbearing family are staggering. The woman is faced with the knowledge that she and her newborn have decreased chances for survival. The couple must deal with the impact of the illness on the partner, who may or may not be infected, and other children. Dealing with the tasks and responsibilities of a newborn may be especially difficult if the woman is physically depleted or if she is trying to come to grips with the long-term implications of her condition.

Nurses can help ensure that the woman receives complete, accurate information about her condition and ways she might cope. This usually involves a referral to social services for follow-up care. The hospitalized woman will often welcome the opportunity to talk with someone about her fears and desires.

EVALUATIVE OUTCOME CRITERIA

Anticipated outcomes of nursing care include the following:

- The women is able to discuss the implications of her positive HIV antibody screen (or diagnosis of AIDS), its implications for her unborn child and for herself, method of transmission, and treatment options.

- The woman agrees to a social services (or other agency) referral for follow-up assistance and counseling.

- The woman is able to begin to verbalize her feelings about her condition and its implications in an atmosphere she finds supportive.

Care of the Woman Practicing Substance Abuse

As discussed in Chapter 16, drugs adversely affecting fetal growth and development are called *teratogens*. They act on the developing organs to retard growth at crucial stages of organogenesis during the first trimester. Other drugs ingested by the expectant woman at other times during the pregnancy may negatively influence the well-being of the fetus and produce critical problems in the neonate. Table 19–6 identifies common addictive drugs and their effects on the fetus and neonate. (Use of normal therapeutic drugs during pregnancy is discussed in Chapter 16.)

Drugs that are commonly misused include alcohol, amphetamines, barbiturates, hallucinogens, cocaine, crack, and heroin and other narcotics. Abuse of these drugs constitutes a major threat to the successful completion of pregnancy.

Drug Addiction

Indiscriminate drug use during pregnancy, particularly in the first trimester, may adversely affect the health of the woman and the growth and development of the fetus. Originally it was thought that the placenta acted as a protective barrier to keep the drugs ingested by the woman from reaching the fetal system. This is not true. The degree to which a drug is passed to the fetus depends on the drug's chemical properties, including molecular weight, and on whether it is administered alone or in combination with other drugs.

MATERNAL RISKS

Drug addiction has an adverse effect on the expectant woman. It affects her state of health, nutritional status, susceptibility to infection, and psychosocial condition. A majority of drug abusing pregnant women are malnourished and receive little or no antepartal care. Heroin-addicted pregnant women have two to six times the risk of PIH, malpresentation, third trimester bleeding, and puerperal morbidity. In addition, the risk of drug toxicity is present. In general, the woman's psychologic and physiologic ability to handle the stress of pregnancy is severely reduced.

Cocaine use in pregnancy has sharply increased in recent years. Cocaine causes vasoconstriction, tachycardia, and increased blood pressure. This increases a woman's risk of spontaneous abortion in the first or second trimester. In the third trimester it leads to increased uterine contractility, placental vasoconstriction, increased incidence of meconium staining, fetal tachycardia, and the potential for abruptio placentae (Chasnoff et al 1986).

FETAL-NEONATAL RISKS

The fetus of a pregnant addict is at risk in the following ways:

- The drug may cause chromosomal aberrations or may have a teratogenic effect on the fetus, resulting in congenital anomalies such as limb abnormalities.

Table 19–6　Possible Effects of Selected Drugs of Abuse/Addiction on Fetus and Neonate

Maternal drug	Effect on fetus/neonate
I. Depressants	
A. Alcohol	Cardiac anomalies, IUGR, potential teratogenic effects, FAS, FAE
B. Narcotics	
1. Heroin	Withdrawal symptoms, convulsions, death, IUGR, respiratory alkalosis, hyperbilirubinemia
2. Methadone	Fetal distress, meconium aspiration; with abrupt termination of the drug, severe withdrawal symptoms, neonatal death
C. Barbiturates	Neonatal depression, increased anomalies; teratogenic effect(?); withdrawal symptoms, convulsions, hyperactivity, hyperreflexia, vasomotor instability
1. Phenobarbital	Bleeding (with excessive doses)
D. "T's and Blues" (combination of the following)	
1. Talwin (narcotic)	Safe for use in pregnancy; depresses respiration if taken close to time of birth
2. Amytal (barbiturate)	See barbiturates
E. Tranquilizers	
1. Phenothiazine derivatives	Withdrawal, extrapyramidal dysfunction, delayed respiratory onset, hyperbilirubinemia, hypotonia or hyperactivity, decreased platelet count
2. Diazepam (Valium)	Hypotonia, hypothermia, low Apgar score, respiratory depression, poor sucking reflex, possible cleft lip
F. Antianxiety drugs	
1. Lithium	Congenital anomalies; lethargy and cyanosis in the newborn
II. Stimulants	
A. Amphetamines	
1. Amphetamine sulfate (Benzedrine)	Generalized arthritis, learning disabilites, poor motor coordination, transposition of the great vessels, cleft palate
2. Dextroamphetamine sulfate (dexedrine sulfate)	Congenital heart defects, hyperbilirubinemia
B. Cocaine	Learning disabilities, poor state organization, decreased interactive behavior
C. Caffeine (more than 600 mg/day)	Spontaneous abortion, IUGR, increased incidence of cleft palate; other anomalies suspected
D. Nicotine (half to one pack cigarettes/day)	Increased rate of spontaneous abortion, increased incidence placental abruption, SGA, small head circumference, decreased length
III. Psychotropics	
A. PCP ("angel dust")	Flaccid appearance, poor head control, impaired neurologic development
B. LSD	Chromosomal breakage?
C. Marijuana	IUGR, potential impaired immunologic mechanisms

- The drug may induce physiologic and psychologic changes in the pregnant woman, resulting in placental dysfunction or fetal hypoxia or depression.

- IUGR, increased rate of prematurity, and higher perinatal mortality are associated with maternal heroin addiction.

- The Brazelton Neonatal Behavioral Assessment Scale indicated that infants exposed to cocaine had poor state organization and decreased interactive behaviors (Chasnoff et al 1985).

- About 50 percent of newborns of addicted mothers experience withdrawal symptoms severe enough to require treatment. (See Chapter 31).

- Taking a mixture of drugs may lead to maternal death and thus fetal death.

- If the pregnant woman has periods of drug withdrawal, the fetus also appears to experience withdrawal as noted by increased fetal activity. Increased oxygen is needed by the fetus at these times. If the increased oxygen requirement is not met, for example, during labor, fetal distress with meconium-stained amniotic fluid will occur. Meconium aspiration is then a possibility.

MEDICAL THERAPY

Antepartal care of the pregnant addict involves medical, socioeconomic, and legal considerations. The use of a team approach allows for the comprehensive management necessary to provide safe labor and delivery for woman and fetus.

The management of heroin addiction includes the use of methadone, the current agent of choice in the treatment or prevention of withdrawal symptoms. Dosage must be less than 20 mg/day to prevent severe withdrawal symptoms in the newborn. Hospitalization is necessary to initiate detoxification. "Cold turkey" withdrawal is not advisable during pregnancy because of potential risk to the fetus. Maintenance and support therapy are given during weekly prenatal visits.

Urine screening is also done regularly throughout pregnancy if the woman is a known or suspected substance abuser. This testing is helpful in identifying the type and amount of medication being abused.

NURSING ASSESSMENT

Nursing assessment of a substance abuser who is pregnant focuses on the woman's general health status, with specific attention to skin abscesses and infections, as well as evaluation of other body systems.

The nurse also assesses the woman with regard to her drug addiction. Some women are reluctant to discuss their drug habit, while others are quite open about it. Once the nurse establishes a relationship of trust, he or she can gain information that can be used to plan the woman's ongoing care.

NURSING DIAGNOSIS

Nursing diagnoses that may apply to the pregnant woman who is addicted to drugs include:

- Noncompliance with treatment related to an inability to give up drugs

- Potential alteration in parenting: neglect related to maternal substance abuse.

NURSING GOAL: PREPARATION FOR LABOR AND DELIVERY

Preparation for labor and delivery should be part of the prenatal planning. Analgesic use should be avoided if possible, although it is not necessarily contraindicated. Relief of fear, tension, or discomfort may be achieved through nonnarcotic psychologic support and careful explanation of the labor process. Preferred methods of pain relief include the use of psychoprophylaxis and regional or local anesthetics such as pudendal block and local infiltration.

These techniques are preferred to decrease risk of additional fetal respiratory depression. Immediate intensive care should be available for the newborn, who will probably be depressed, SGA, and premature. For care of the addicted newborn, see Chapter 31.

EVALUATIVE OUTCOME CRITERIA

Anticipated outcomes of nursing care include the following:

- The woman is able to describe the impact of her substance abuse on herself and her unborn child.

- The woman successfully participates in a drug therapy program.

- The woman successfully delivers a healthy infant.

- Care givers detect potential complications early and institute appropriate therapy

- The woman agrees to cooperate with a referral to social services (or another appropriate community agency) for follow-up care after discharge.

● Other Medical Conditions and Pregnancy

A woman with a preexisting medical condition should be aware of the possible impact of pregnancy on her condition, as well as the impact of her condition on the successful outcome of her pregnancy. Table 19–7 discusses some of the less common medical conditions vis a vis pregnancy.

Table 19–7 Less Common Medical Conditions and Pregnancy

Condition	Brief description	Maternal implications	Fetal-neonatal implications
Arthritis	Chronic inflammatory disease believed to be caused by a genetically influenced antigen-antibody reaction (Harris 1985). Symptoms include fatigue, low-grade fever, pain and swelling of joints, morning stiffness, pain on movement. Treated with salicylates, physical therapy, and rest. Corticosteroids used cautiously if not responsive to above.	Usually there is remission of rheumatoid arthritis symptoms during pregnancy, often with a relapse postpartum. Anemia may be present due to blood loss from salicylate therapy. Mother needs extra rest, particularly to relieve weight-bearing joints, but needs to continue range-of-motion exercises. If in remission, may stop medication during pregnancy. Oral contraception acceptable.	Possibility of prolonged gestation and longer labor with heavy salicylate use due to interference with prostaglandin synthesis (Mor-Yosef et al 1984). Possible teratogenic effects of salicylates.

Table 19–7 Less Common Medical Conditions and Pregnancy (continued)

Condition	Brief description	Maternal implications	Fetal/neonatal implications
Epilepsy	Chronic disorder characterized by seizures; may be idiopathic or secondary to other conditions, such as head injury, metabolic and nutritional disorders such as PKU or vitamin B_6 deficiency, encephalitis, neoplasms, or circulatory interferences. Treated with anticonvulsants.	Seizure frequency often increases during pregnancy, with slightly higher incidence of hyperemesis gravidarum, preeclampsia, and vaginal hemorrhage. A woman who has been seizure free for a year should be withdrawn from medication prior to conception; a woman who requires medication has a 90% chance of having a normal child; women who seek advice after the first trimester should be maintained on their medication.	Higher incidence of major congenital anomalies and perinatal mortality. Certain anticonvulsant medications have teratogenic effects.
Hepatitis B	Hepatitis B is caused by the hepatitis B virus (HBV). Although HBV can theoretically be transmitted by all body fluids, it is primarily blood-borne or sexually transmitted. Groups at risk include women from areas with a high incidence (primarily developing countries), illegal IV drug users, prostitutes, and women with multiple sexual partners. Symptoms range from none to mild flulike symptoms to fulminating illness. No specific treatment is available. Supportive care is indicated. A vaccine is available for women in high-risk groups and for health care workers.	Hepatitis B does not usually affect the course of pregnancy. Pregnant women have no higher incidence of complications than the general population (Shaw & Maynard 1986). Women in the high-risk groups should be screened for hepatitis antibodies antepartally but close to the EDD. A woman who is negative may be given hepatitis vaccine. If she is positive the infant should receive prophylactic treatment.	The incidence of fetal malformation is not influenced by maternal infection with hepatitis. Infected newborns have 80% to 90% risk of becoming carriers and may remain infected indefinitely. The newborn who becomes a carrier faces a 1 in 4 risk of dying from liver-related disease (Shaw & Maynard 1986). The infant born to a woman with hepatitis can be treated prophylactically with a dose of hepatitis B immunoglobulin given within the first 12 hours after birth, followed by a series of injections of vaccine, the first during the first week of life, the second at one month, and the third at six months.

Table 19–7 Less Common Medical Conditions and Pregnancy (continued)

Condition	Brief description	Maternal implications	Fetal-neonatal implications
Hyperthyroidism (thyrotoxicosis)	Enlarged, overactive thyroid gland; increased T4:TBG ratio and increased BMR. Symptoms include muscle wasting, tachycardia, excessive sweating, and exophthalmos. Treatment by antithyroid drug propylthiouracil (PTU) while monitoring free T4 levels (Davies & Cobin 1985). Surgery used only if drug intolerance exists.	Mild hyperthyroidism is not dangerous (Davies & Cobin 1985). Increased incidence of PIH and postpartum hemorrhage if not well controlled. Serious risk related to thyroid storm characterized by high fever, tachycardia, sweating, and congestive heart failure. Now occurs rarely. When diagnosed during pregnancy may be transient or permanent.	Neonatal thyrotoxicosis is rare. Even low doses of antithyroid drug in mother may produce a mild fetal-neonatal hypothyroidism; higher dose may produce a goiter or mental deficiencies. Fetal loss not increased in euthyroid women. If untreated, rates of abortion, intrauterine death, and stillbirth increase. Breast-feeding contraindicated for women on antithyroid medication because it is excreted in the milk (may be tried by woman on low dose if neonatal T4 levels are monitored).
Hypothyroidism	Characterized by inadequate thyroid secretions (decreased T4:TBG ration), elevated TSH, lowered BMR, and enlarged thyroid gland (goiter). Symptoms include lack of energy, excessive weight gain, cold intolerance, dry skin, and constipation. Treated by thyroxine replacement therapy.	Long-term replacement therapy usually continues at same dosage during pregnancy as before. Weekly NST after 35 weeks' gestation.	If mother untreated, fetal loss 50%; high risk of congenital goiter or true cretinism. Therefore newborns are screened for T4 level. Mild TSH elevations present little risk since it does not cross the placenta.
Maternal phenylketonuria (PKU) (hyperphenylalaninemia)	Inherited recessive single gene anomaly causing a deficiency of the liver enzyme needed to convert the amino acid phenylalanine to tyrosine resulting in high serum levels of phenylalanine. Brain damage and mental retardation occur if not treated early.	Low phenylalanine diet is mandatory prior to conception and during pregnancy. The woman should be counseled that her children will either inherit the disease or be carriers depending on the zygosity of the father for the disease. Treatment at a PKU center is recommended.	Risk to fetus if maternal treatment not begun preconception. In untreated women, increased incidence of mental retardation, microcephaly, congenital heart defects, and growth retardation. Fetal phenylalanine levels are approximately 50% higher than maternal levels (Lenke 1985).

Table 19-7 Less Common Medical Conditions and Pregnancy (continued)

Condition	Brief description	Maternal implications	Fetal/neonatal implications
Multiple sclerosis	Neurologic disorder characterized by destruction of the myelin sheath of nerve fibers. The condition occurs primarily in young adults, is marked by periods of remission, progresses to marked physical disability in 10 to 20 years.	Associated with remission during pregnancy, but with increased rate of exacerbation postpartum (Korn-Lubetzki et al 1984). Rest is important; help with child care should be planned. Uterine contraction strength is not diminished, but because sensation is frequently lessened labor may be almost painless.	Increased evidence of a genetic causal effect (Sadovnik & Baird 1985). Therefore reproductive counseling is recommended.
Systemic lupus erythematosus (SLE)	Chronic autoimmune collagen disease, characterized by exacerbations and remissions; symptoms range from characteristic rash to inflammation and pain in joints, fever, nephritis, depression, cranial nerve disorders, and peripheral neuropathies	Mild cases—little risk to mother or fetus. Severe cases—because of extra burden on the kidneys, therapeutic abortion may be indicated. Woman must be careful to avoid fatigue, infection, strong sunlight, and so on. Acute postpartum exacerbation is common and often severe.	Increased incidence of spontaneous abortion, stillbirth, prematurity, and SGA neonates. Rarely, the neonate shows manifestations of the disease that respond to steroids and disappear within three months.
Tuberculosis (TB)	Infection caused by *Mycobacterium tuberculosis*; inflammatory process causes destruction of lung tissue, increased sputum, and coughing. Associated primarily with poverty and malnutrition and may be found among refugees from countries where TB is prevalent. Treated with isoniazid and either ethambutol or rifampin or both.	If TB inactive due to prior treatment, relapse rate no greater than for nonpregnant women. When isoniazid is used during pregnancy, the woman should take supplemental pyridoxine (vitamin B₆). Extra rest and limited contact with others is required until disease becomes inactive.	If maternal TB is inactive, mother may breast-feed and care for her infant. If TB is active, neonate should not have direct contact with mother until she is noninfectious. Isoniazid crosses the placenta, but most studies show no teratogenic effects. Rifampin crosses the placenta. Possibility of harmful effects still being studied.

KEY CONCEPTS

The diagnosis of high-risk pregnancy can shock an expectant couple. Providing emotional support, teaching about the condition and prognosis, and educating for self-care are important nursing measures that help the client cope.

Cardiac disease during pregnancy requires careful assessment, limitation of activity, and knowing and reporting signs of impending cardiac decompensation by both client and nurse.

The key point in the care of the pregnant diabetic is scrupulous maternal plasma glucose control. This is best achieved by home blood glucose monitoring, multiple daily insulin injections, and a careful diet. To reduce incidence of congenital anomalies and other problems in the neonate, the woman should be euglycemic prior to conception and throughout the pregnancy. Diabetics more than most other clients need to be educated about their condition and involved with their own care.

Almost any health problem that a person can have when not pregnant can coexist with pregnancy. Some problems, such as anemias, may be exacerbated by pregnancy. Others, such as collagen disease, may go into temporary remission with pregnancy. Regardless of the health probem, careful health care is needed throughout pregnancy to improve the outcome for mother and fetus.

Several health problems associated with bleeding arise from the pregnancy itself, such as spontaneous abortion, ectopic pregnancy, and gestational trophoblastic disease. The nurse needs to be alert to early signs of these situations, to guard the woman against heavy bleeding and shock, to facilitate the medical treatment, and to provide educational and emotional support.

Hypertension may exist prior to pregnancy or, more often, may develop during pregnancy. Pregnancy-induced hypertension can lead to growth retardation for the fetus, and if untreated may lead to convulsions (eclampsia) and even death for the mother and fetus. A woman's understanding of the disease process helps motivate her to maintain the required rest periods in the left lateral position. Antihypertensive or anticonvulsive drugs may be part of the therapy.

Rh incompatibility can exist when an Rh⁻ woman and an Rh⁺ partner conceive a child that is Rh⁺. The use of RhoGAM has greatly decreased the incidence of severe sequelae due to Rh because the drug "tricks" the body into thinking antibodies have been produced in response to the Rh antigen.

The impact of surgery, trauma, or battering on the pregnant woman and her fetus is related to timing in the pregnancy, seriousness of the situation, and other factors influencing the situation.

Urinary tract infections are a common problem in pregnancy. If untreated the infection may ascend, causing more serious illness for the mother. Urinary tract infections are also associated with an increased risk of premature labor.

TORCH is an acronym standing for toxoplasmosis, rubella, cytomegalovirus, and herpes, all of which pose a grave threat to the fetus.

Sexually transmitted diseases pose less threat to the fetus if detected and treated as soon as possible.

Substance abuse (either drugs or alcohol) not only is detrimental to the mother's health but also may have profound lasting effects on the fetus.

REFERENCES

AIDS Weekly Surveillance Report (AWSR)—United States. AIDS Program, Center for Infectious Diseases, Centers for Disease Control, February 29, 1988.

Berkowitz RL, et al: *Handbook for Prescribing Medication During Pregnancy.* Boston, Little, Brown, 1981.

Borg S, **Lasker** J: *When Pregnancy Fails.* Boston, Beacon Press, 1981.

Bowman JM: Blood group incompatibilities, in **Iffy** L, **Kaminetzky** HA (eds): *Principles and Practice of Obstetrics and Perinatology.* New York, Wiley, 1981.

Bowman JM: Controversies of Rh prophylaxis: Who needs Rh immunoglobulin and when should it be given? *Am J Obstet Gynecol* 1985;151(3):289.

Bragonier JR, et al: Social and personal factors in the etiology of preterm birth, in **Fuchs** F, **Stubblefield** PG (eds): *Preterm Birth: Causes, Prevention and Management.* New York, Macmillan, 1984.

Brumfield C, **Huddleson** J: The management of ketoacidosis in pregnancy. *Clin Obstet Gynecol* 1984;27(March):50.

Buckley J: The epidemiology of molar pregnancy and choriocarcinoma. *Clin Obstet Gynecol* 1984;27(March):153.

Burrow G, **Ferris** T: *Medical Complications during Pregnancy.* Philadelphia, Saunders, 1982.

Ceresa C, **Theiss** T: Nutritional aspects of diabetes care and pregnancy. *Diabetes Educator* 1983;9(Summer):21s.

Chasnoff IJ, et al: Cocaine use in pregnancy. *N Engl J Med* 1985;313(11):666.

Chasnoff IJ, et al: Perinatal cerebral infarction and maternal cocaine use. *J Pediatr* 1986;109:456.

Corey L, **Spear** PG: Infections with herpes simplex. *N Engl J Med* 1986;314(11):686.

Cousins L, et al: Screening for carbohydrate intolerance in pregnancy: A comparison of two tests and reassessment of a common approach. *Am J Obstet Gynecol* 1985;153 (October):381.

Coustan D, **Carpenter** M: Detection and treatment of gestational diabetes. *Clin Obstet Gynecol* 1985;28 (September):507.

Cowen MJ, et al: Maternal transmission of acquired immune deficiency syndrome. *Pediatr* 1984;73:382.

Criteria Committee of the New York Heart Association: *Nomenclature and Criteria for Diagnosis of Diseases of the Heart and Blood Vessels,* ed 5. New York, 1955.

Cruikshank DP: Diseases of the alimentary tract, in **Danforth** DN, **Scott** JR (eds): *Obstetrics and Gynecology,* ed 5. Philadelphia, Lippincott, 1986.

Curran JW: The epidemiology and prevention of acquired immunodeficiency syndrome. *Ann Intern Med* 1985; 103:657.

Davies T, **Cobin** R: Thyroid disease in pregnancy and the postpartum period. *Mt Sinai J Med* 1985;52(January):59.

DeVoe S, **O'Shaughnessy** R: Clinical manifestations and diagnosis of pregnancy-induced hypertension. *Clin Obstet Gynecol* 1984;27(December):836.

Dorfman SF: Epidemiology of ectopic pregnancy. *Clin Obstet Gynecol* 1987;30(March):173.

Droegemueller W: Ectopic pregnancy, in **Danforth** DN, **Scott,** JR (eds): *Obstetrics and Gynecology,* ed 5. Philadelphia, Lippincott, 1986.

Eschenbach DA: Pelvic infections, in **Danforth** DN, **Scott** JR (eds): *Obstetrics and Gynecology,* ed 5. Philadelphia, Lippincott, 1986.

Freinkel N, et al: Care of the pregnant woman with insulin-dependent diabetes mellitus. *N Engl J Med* 1985;313(2):96.

Funkhouser JE, **Denniston** RW. Preventing alcohol-related birth defects: Suggestions for action. *Alcohol Health Res World* 1985;10(Fall):54.

Gabbe SG: Diabetes mellitus, in **Danforth** DN, **Scott** JR (eds): *Obstetrics and Gynecology,* ed 5. Philadelphia, Lippincott, 1986.

Gabbe SG: Management of diabetes mellitus in pregnancy. *Am J Obstet Gynecol* 1985;153(December):824.

Gant N, **Worley** R: *Hypertension in Pregnancy: Concepts and Management.* New York, Appleton-Century-Crofts, 1980. Gestational trophoblastic disease. *Contemp OB/GYN* 1987; 29(January):199.

Gilbert ES, **Harmon** JS: *High Risk Pregnancy and Delivery: Nursing Perspectives.* St Louis, Mosby, 1986.

Granados JL: Recent developments in the outpatient management of insulin-dependent diabetes mellitus during pregnancy. *Obstet Gynecol Annal* 1984;13:83.

Greer I, et al: HELLP syndrome: pathologic entity or technical inadequacy?, letter. *Am J Obstet Gynecol* 1985;152(May 1):113.

Guthrie DW, **Guthrie** RA: *Nursing Management of Diabetes Mellitus,* ed 2. St Louis, Mosby, 1982.

Harger JH: Improving the care of pregnant women with genital herpes. *Contemp OB/GYN* 1985;26(4):85.

Harris C: Pregnancy can offer a welcome relief from the chronic inflammation of arthritis. *Am J Nurs* 1985;85(April):415.

Hawkins G, **Whalley** PJ: Acute urinary tract infections in pregnancy. *Clin Obstet Gynecol* 1985;28(2):266.

Hillard PJA: Physical abuse in pregnancy. *Obstet Gynecol* 1985;66:185.

Hollander P, **Maeder** E: Diabetes in pregnancy: no longer a barrier to successful outcome. *Postgrad Med* 1985;77(February):137.

Hollingsworth DR: Maternal metabolism in normal pregnancy and pregnancy complicated by diabetes mellitus. *Clin Obstet Gynecol* 1985;28(September):457.

Klug RM: Children with AIDS. *Am J Nurs* 1986;86(October):1127.

Kochenour NK: Course and conduct of normal pregnancy, in **Danforth** DN, **Scott** JR (eds): *Obstetrics and Gynecology,* ed 5. Philadelphia, Lippincott, 1986.

Kohorn EI: Molar pregnancy: presentation and diagnosis. *Clin Obstet Gynecol* 1984;27(March):181.

Korn-Lubetzki I, et al: Activity of multiple sclerosis during pregnancy and puerperium. *Ann Neurol* 1984;16:229.

LaCamera D: The acquired immunodeficiency syndrome. *Nurs Clin North Am* 1985;20(1):241.

Landon M, **Gabbe** S: Glucose monitoring and insulin administration in the pregnant diabetic patient. *Clin Obstet Gynecol* 1985;28(September):496.

Lenke RR: Maternal hyperphenylalaninemia, in **Gleicher** N (ed): *Principles of Medical Therapy in Pregnancy.* New York, Plenum, 1985.

Lin C, et al: Good diabetic control early in pregnancy and favorable fetal outcome. *Obstet Gynecol* 1986;67 (January):51.

Little RE, et al: An evaluation of the pregnancy and health program. *Alcohol Health Res World* 1985;19(Fall):44.

Loveman A, et al: AIDS in pregnancy. *J Obstet Gynecol Neonat Nurs* 1986;15(2):91.

Martin J, **Morrison** J: Managing the parturient with sickle cell crisis. *Clin Obstet Gynecol* 1984;27(March):39.

McCoy D, **Oswald** J: An interactive model program of care for diabetic women before and during pregnancy. *Diabetes Educator* 1983;9(Summer suppl):11s.

Miller E, et al: Elevated maternal hemoglobin A in early pregnancy and major congenital anomalies in infants of diabetic mothers. *N Engl J Med* 1981;304:1331.

Miodovnik M, et al: Elevated maternal glycohemoglobin in early pregnancy and spontaneous abortion among insulin-dependent diabetic women. *Am J Obstet Gynecol* 1985;153(October 15):439.

MMWR (Morbidity and Mortality Weekly Reports): Recommendation for assisting in the prevention of perinatal transmission of human-T-lymphotropic virus type III/lymphadenopathy-associated virus and acquired immunodeficiency syndrome. 1985;34(December):721.

Mor-Yosef S, et al: Collagen diseases in pregnancy. *Obstet Gynecol Surv* 1984;39(February):67.

National Diabetes Data Group: *Classification of Diabetes Mellitus and Other Categories of Glucose Intolerance*. Washington, DC, NIH, 1979.

O'Keeffe DF: When the accident victim is pregnant. *Contemp OB/GYN* 1985;26(1):148.

Osborne NG, **Pratson** L: Sexually transmitted diseases and pregnancy. *J Obstet Gynecol Neonat Nurs* 1984;13 (January/February):9.

Patterson RM: Trauma in pregnancy. *Clin Obstet Gynecol* 1984;27:1.

Pritchard JA, **MacDonald** P, **Gant** NF: *Williams Obstetrics*, ed 17. New York, Appleton-Century-Crofts, 1985.

Queenan JT: Current management of the Rh-sensitized patient. *Clin Obstet Gynecol* 1982;(2)25.

Queenan JT: Losing the battle and winning the war on ectopics. *Contemp OB/GYN* 1987;29(January):9.

Rubenstein A, et al: Acquired immunodeficiency with reversed T_4/T_8 ratios in infants born to promiscuous and drug-addicted mothers. *JAMA* 1983;249:2350.

Runowicz CD: Clinical aspects of gestational trophoblastic disease. *Mt Sinai J Med* 1985;52(January):35.

Russell JB: The etiology of ectopic pregnancy. *Clin Obstet Gynecol* 1987;30(March):181.

Sadovnik A, **Baird** P: Reproductive counseling for multiple sclerosis patients. *Am J Med Genetics* 1985;20:349.

Schachter J, et al: Experience with routine use of erythromycin for chlamydial infections in pregnancy. *N Engl J Med* 1986;314:276.

Scott GB, et al: Mothers of infants with acquired immunodeficiency syndrome. *JAMA* 1985;253(January 18):363.

Scott JR: Isoimmunization in pregnancy, in **Danforth** DN, **Scott** JR (eds): *Obstetrics and Gynecology*, ed 5. Philadelphia, Lippincott, 1986a.

Scott JR: Spontaneous abortion, in **Danforth** DN, **Scott** JR (eds): *Obstetrics and Gynecology*, ed 5. Philadelphia, Lippincott, 1986b.

Sharp HC: Reproductive tract disorders, in **Danforth** DN, **Scott** JR (eds): *Obstetrics and Gynecology*, ed 5. Philadelphia, Lippincott, 1986.

Shaw FE, **Maynard** JE: Hepatitis B: Still a concern for you and your patients. *Contemp OB/GYN* 1986;27(March):27.

Sibai BM: MgSO$_4$ for preeclampsia-eclampsia. *Contemp OB/GYN* 1987;29(January):155.

Sibai BM, et al: Maternal and perinatal outcome of conservative management of severe preeclampsia in midtrimester. *Am J Obstet Gynecol* 1985;152(May 1):32.

Stagno S, **Whitley** RJ: Herpesvirus infections of pregnancy. Part I: Cytomegalovirus and Epstein-Barr virus infections. *N Engl J Med* 1985;313:(20):1270.

Stagno S, **Whitley** RJ: Herpesvirus infections of pregnancy. Part II: Herpes simplex virus and varicella-zoster virus infections. *N Engl J Med* 1985;313:(21):1327.

Steel JM: Pre-pregnancy counseling and contraception in the insulin-dependent diabetic patient. *Clin Obstet Gynecol* 1985;28(September):553.

Streissguth AP, **LaDue** RA. Psychological and behavioral effects in children prenatally exposed to alcohol. *Alcohol Health Res World* 1985;10(Fall):6.

Sweet RL, et al: Chlamydial infections in obstetrics and gynecology. *Clin Obstet Gynecol* 1983;26(1):143.

Szulman A, **Surti** U: The syndromes of partial and complete molar gestation. *Clin Obstet Gynecol* 1984;27(March):172.

Taylor HW, **Slate** WG: Trauma and diseases requiring surgery during pregnancy, in **Iffy** L, **Kaminetzky** HA (eds): *Principles and Practice of Obstetrics and Perinatology*. New York, Wiley, 1981.

Triolo PK: Nonobstetric surgery during pregnancy. *J Obstet Gynecol Neonatal Nurs* 1985;14(3):179.

Troy K, **Wisch** N: Anemia and pregnancy, in **Cherry** S, **Berkowitz** R, **Kase** N (eds): *Rovinsky and Guttmacher's Medical, Surgical, and Gynecologic Complications of Pregnancy*, ed 3. Baltimore, Williams & Wilkins, 1985.

Wall-Haas C: Women's perceptions of first trimester spontaneous abortion. *J Obstet Gynecol Neonat Nurs* 1985; 14(January/February):50.

Warren K: Alcohol-related birth defects: Current trends in research. *Alcohol Health Res World* 1985;10(Fall):4.

Weckstein L: Current perspectives on ectopic pregnancy. *Obstet Gynecol Surv* 1985;40(5):259.

Weil SG. The unspoken needs of families during high-risk pregnancies. *Am J Nurs* 1981;81(11):2047.

Weinstein L: Preeclampsia/eclampsia with hemolysis, elevated liver enzymes, and thrombocytopenia. *Obstet Gynecol* 1985;66(November):657.

Weinstein L: Syndrome of hemolysis, elevated liver enzymes, and low platelet count: A severe consequence of hypertension in pregnancy. *Am J Obstet Gynecol* 1982;142(January 15):159.

Whalley PJ: Value of treating UTI during pregnancy. *Contemp OB/GYN* 1986;27(5):134.

Wheeler L, **Jones** MB: Pregnancy-induced hypertension. *J Obstet Gynecol Neonat Nurs* 1981;10(3):212.

White P: Classification of obstetric diabetes. *Am J Obstet Gynecol* 1978;130:228.

Worley RJ: Pathophysiology of pregnancy-induced hypertension. *Clin Obstet Gynecol* 1984;27(December):821.

Worley RJ: Pregnancy-induced hypertension, in **Danforth** DN, **Scott** JR (eds): *Obstetrics and Gynecology*, ed 5. Philadelphia, Lippincott, 1986.

Ziegler JB, et al: Postnatal transmission of AIDS-associated retrovirus from mother to infant. *Lancet* 1985; 1(April):896.

Zuspan FP: Chronic hypertension in pregnancy. *Clin Obstet Gynecol* 1984;27(December):854.

ADDITIONAL READINGS

Anderson GD: A systematic approach to eclamptic convulsion. *Contemp OB/GYN* 1987;29(March):65.

Babin V, et al: The impact of chlamydial infections on teen mothers and their children. *J Sch Health* 1986;56 (January):17.

Beall MH: Breastfeeding: Some drug admonitions. *Contemp OB/GYN* 1987;29(February):49.

Bergman A, et al: Cervical cryotherapy for condyloma accuminata during pregnancy. *Obstet Gynecol* 1987;69 (January):47.

Bremer C, et al: Trauma in pregnancy. *Nurs Clin North Am* 1986;21(December):705.

Chez RA, et al: Ketonuria in normal pregnancy. *Obstet Gynecol* 1987;69(February):272.

DeVore N, et al: Ectopic pregnancy on the rise. *Am J Nurs* 1986;86(June):674.

Hutto C, et al: Intrauterine herpes simplex virus infections. *J Pediatr* 1987;110(January):97.

Krebs LU: Pregnancy and cancer. *Semin Oncol Nurs* 1985;1(February):35.

Landers D, et al: Acute cholecystitis in pregnancy. *Obstet Gynecol* 1987;69(January):131.

Levin J: Will all addicted pregnant women have their babies taken into care? *Lancet* 1987;8526(January 24):230.

Minkoff H: Acquired immunodeficiency syndrome. *J Nurse-Midwife* 1986;31(July/August):189.

McGregor JA: Preventing preterm birth caused by infection. *Contemp OB/GYN* 1987;29(April):33.

O'Brien ME, **Gibson** G: Detection and management of gestational diabetes in an out-of-hospital birth center. *J Nurse-Midwife* 1987;32(March/April):79.

Osguthorpe NC: Ectopic pregnancy. *J Obstet Gynecol Neonat Nurs* 1987;16(January/February):36.

Pierson R, et al: Penetrating abdominal wounds in pregnancy. *Ann Emerg Med* 1986;15(October):1232.

Quaggin AL: Get prepared for more cases of AIDS during pregnancy. *Can Med Assoc J* 1987;136(January 15):192.

Rayburn WF, et al: Drug prescribing for chronic medical disorders during pregnancy: An overview. *Am J Obstet Gynecol* 1986;155(September):565.

Ribiero G, et al: Carcinoma of the breast associated with pregnancy. *Br J Surg* 1986;73(August):607.

Steinmetz KS: Gardnerella vaginalis vaginitis: A guide to identification and management for the practitioner. *J Nurse-Midwife* 1986;31(March/April):87.

Sutherland HW, et al: Increased incidence of spontaneous abortions in pregnancies complicated by maternal diabetes mellitus. *Am J Obstet Gynecol* 1987;156(January):135.

Williams ML: Long-term hospitalization of women with high-risk pregnancies: A nurse's viewpoint. *J Obstet Gynecol Neonat Nurs* 1986;15(January/February):17.

Zigrossi ST, et al: The stress of medical management on pregnant diabetics. *Am J Mat Child Nurs* 1986;11 (September/October):320.

The darkness seemed blacker than the background. It had the dense darkness of blood, of a fleshly thing. This was the vessel that would become my baby's heart. Tiny as it was, its pulse was steady and measured. (Suzannah Lessard, *The New Yorker*)

Diagnostic Assessment of Fetal Status

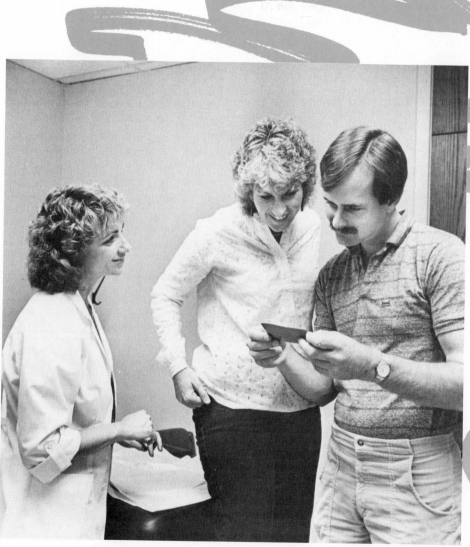

This expectant couple and their nurse share the excitement of an ultrasound photograph of their baby.

Chapter Twenty

OBJECTIVES

- List indications for ultrasonic examination and the information that can be obtained from this procedure.
- Outline pertinent information to be discussed with the woman regarding her assessment of fetal activity.
- Identify criteria for the evaluation of fetal well-being by biophysical profile assessment.
- Discuss the nurse's role in teaching the woman the nipple stimulation contraction stress test and important factors to assess in evaluation of fetal heart rate response.
- Compare amniocentesis and chorionic villus sampling.
- Compare the procedures for the nonstress test and contraction stress test, including the indications, contraindications, and predictive value of each.

- Discuss implications of prenatal testing with regard to high-risk pregnancy management.

During the past two decades, increasing interest has been focused on the problems of the at-risk pregnant woman, her health management, and conditions that may affect her unborn child. It is now known that high-risk women and infants have a significantly greater chance of morbidity or mortality before or after delivery. Perinatal morbidity and mortality can be considerably reduced by early, skillful diagnosis and highly intensive antepartal care of the pregnant woman.

A variety of tests of fetal status are of value in monitoring the well-being of the fetus. These tests include ultrasound, computerized tomography, magnetic resonance imaging, fetoscopy, percutaneous umbilical blood sampling, chorionic villus sampling, measurements of specific hormones and enzymes in maternal blood and urine, amniocentesis, and fetal stress tests. Although the tests have been made as safe as possible, each procedure always involves some risk. Fetal morbidity, mortality, and status must be considered before suggesting the diagnostic procedures. In addition, the risk must be acceptable to the pregnant woman. Health care professionals may think the risk is minimal, but they are not the ones who will suffer the consequences of an untoward outcome.

Not all high-risk pregnancies require the same procedures. One must be certain that the advantages outweigh the potential risks and added expense. Each of these tests has its limitations in terms of screening, diagnostic accuracy, and applicability. No one test should be used to determine fetal status in the management of high-risk women. (For a summary of tests, see Table 20–1.)

● Nursing Process During Diagnostic Testing

Because many of the diagnostic tests are completed on an outpatient basis, the nurse has only brief contact with the woman and her support person. The nurse uses the nursing process to guide nursing care during these interactions.

Nursing Assessment

The nursing assessment begins with a history regarding the prenatal course and identification of possible indications for the particular diagnostic testing. The nurse assesses the information that the woman and her support person have regarding the test and the presence of any particular factors that may influence the teaching process.

Table 20–1   Summary of Screening and Diagnostic Tests

Goal	Test	When test may be done
To validate the pregnancy	Ultrasound for gestational sac volume	5 and 6 weeks after LMP
To determine how advanced the pregnancy is	Ultrasound: Crown-rump length Ultrasound: Biparietal diameter and femur length	7 to 10 weeks' gestation 13 to 40 weeks' gestation
To identify normal growth of the fetus	Ultrasound: Biparietal diameter Ultrasound: Head-abdomen ratio Ultrasound: Estimated fetal weight	Most useful from 20 to 30 weeks' gestation 13 to 40 weeks' gestation About 28 to 40 weeks' gestation
To detect congenital anomalies and problems	Ultrasound Chorionic villus sampling Fetoscopy Percutaneous blood sampling	18 to 40 weeks' gestation 8 to 12 weeks' gestation 18 weeks' gestation 2nd and 3rd trimesters
To localize the placenta	Ultrasound	Usually in 3rd trimester or before amniocentesis
To assess fetal status	Biophysical profile Maternal assessment of fetal activity Estriols Magnetic resonance imaging Nonstress test Contraction stress test	Approximately 28 weeks to delivery About 27 weeks to delivery During the 2nd and 3rd trimesters During the 2nd and 3rd trimesters Approximately 30 weeks to delivery Last few weeks of gestation
To diagnose cardiac problems	Fetal echocardiography	2nd and 3rd trimesters
To assess fetal lung maturity	Amniocentesis L/S ratio Phosphatidylglycerol Phosphatidylcholine Shake test	33 to 40 weeks 33 weeks to delivery 33 weeks to delivery 33 weeks to delivery 33 weeks to delivery
To obtain more information about breech presentation	Computerized tomography X ray	Just before labor is anticipated or during labor

During the test, the nurse completes needed assessments to monitor the status of the mother and her unborn child.

Analysis and Nursing Diagnosis

The primary nursing diagnoses are directed toward providing information regarding the diagnostic test and minimizing any risks to the mother and her unborn child. The woman may also be fearful of the outcome of the tests, and nurses can play an important role in providing support and counseling. Examples of nursing diagnoses that may be applicable include:

- Knowledge deficit related to insufficient information about the fetal assessment test, purpose, benefits, risks, and alternatives

- Fear related to unfavorable test results

Nursing Plan and Implementation

The nursing plan of care will be directed toward each specific nursing diagnosis. The nurse generally plays a vital role in providing information about the diagnostic test. The nurse assesses the woman's knowledge of the test and then provides information as needed. Some of the tests require written informed consent, and in these cases the physician is responsible for informing the woman about all aspects of the test. In this instance the nurse can reinforce information and clarify information that is not fully understood (see Box 20–1).

Contact with the expectant woman may be very brief. The nurse uses all her or his basic knowledge of communication, developmental psychology, cultural factors, and so forth to quickly establish a trusting relationship with the woman and her support person.

The nurse also functions as an advocate for the expectant woman by helping her clarify question areas and obtain needed information. The nurse frequently knows the areas for which most women have questions and can anticipate many of their fears. When the woman is not able to verbalize questions, the nurse can assist by bringing up questions that other women have had.

During the testing sessions, the nurse addresses the woman's fear by providing support and comfort measures. The presence of the nurse reassures the woman and helps her cope with the tests.

Evaluation

The expected outcomes for the woman who is having diagnostic testing are that she understands the reasons for the test and the test results and has had support during

Box 20–1   Sample Nursing Approaches to Pretest Teaching

Assess whether the woman knows the reason the screening or diagnostic test is being recommended.
Example:
"Has your doctor/nurse-midwife told you why this test is necessary?"
"Sometimes tests are done for many different reasons. Can you tell me why you are having this test?"
"What is your understanding about what the test will show?"

Provide an opportunity for questions.
Example:
"Do you have any questions about the test?"
"Is there anything that is not clear to you?"

Explain the test procedure paying particular attention to any preparation the woman needs to do prior to the test.

Example:
"The test that has been ordered for you is designed to . . ." (add specific information about the particular test. Give the explanation in simple language).

Validate the woman's understanding of the preparation.
Example:
"Tell me what you will have to do to get ready for this test."

Give permission for woman to continue to ask questions if needed.
Example:
"I'll be with you during the test. If you have any questions at any time, please don't hesitate to ask."

---

the test. In addition, the tests have been done without complication and the safety of the mother and her unborn child has been maintained.

● Indications for Diagnostic Testing

Women who are considered to be at risk and for whom the physician/nurse-midwife may order assessments of fetal well-being include women with:

- Chronic hypertension

- Pregnancy-induced hypertension

- Diabetes mellitus

- History of preterm labors or risk of preterm labor with this pregnancy

- Pregnancy beyond 41½ to 42 weeks

- Rh isoimmunization

- Previous unexplained stillborn or intrapartal fetal death

- Sickle cell hemoglobinopathies

- Suspected intrauterine growth retardation

- Maternal cyanotic heart disease

- Bleeding complications accompanying the pregnancy, such as abruptio placentae or placenta previa

- Hydramnios or oligohydramnios

Each of the listed complications may increase the risk to the expectant woman and her fetus. The list is not com-

plete; other preexisting medical diseases may place the woman at risk and necessitate diagnostic assessment of the fetus.

● Ultrasound

The introduction of ultrasound in the 1950s was a major advance in the practice of obstetrics. Although the first machines were crude compared to those in use today, they nevertheless permitted greater assessment of gestational age and placental localization for amniocentesis than was possible prior to their use. Newer machines with more capabilities have made ultrasound an integral part of age, health, and growth assessment of the fetus and have caused radical changes in the practice of perinatal medicine.

It is now possible to determine gestational age with much greater reliability than in previous years, diagnose fetal growth patterns, recognize fetal congenital anomalies, assess placental position and maturity, assess the effect of disease processes on the fetus, and ascertain fetal responses to its intrauterine environment. Ultrasound is also used to facilitate diagnostic and therapeutic measure such as amniocentesis, fetoscopy, chorionic villus sampling, intrauterine transfusion, and surveillance of ovarian follicle development.

Most ultrasound scanning is now performed using dynamic real-time imaging. Continuous, sequenced B-mode (brightness) images (in sequences of up to 40 images/second) are produced by transmission of sound waves via a transducer applied to the mother's abdomen. Echoes are reflected from tissues of varying densities back to the crystals in the transducer and converted to electrical signals, which are then amplified and displayed on the oscilloscope (similar to a television screen) (Figure 20–1). Real-time imaging gives the impression of motion because of the continuous rapid, fixed images produced and permits a visual image of the fetus as it functions in its environment. Such functions as fetal breathing, tone, movement, micturition, eye movement, and cardiac activity may all be assessed by means of imaging (Figure 20–2).

Ultrasound scanning is categorized as either level I or level II. A level I ultrasound scale may be performed by minimally trained individuals to assess gestational age, number of fetuses, fetal demise, and placental lakes (Jeanty & Romero 1984). A level II scan must be performed by a highly trained ultrasound clinician knowledgeable about assessment of specific congenital anomalies and abnormalities.

Although ultrasound testing can be beneficial, the NIH Consensus Development Conference on Ultrasound Imaging in Pregnancy recommends that it not be routinely used on all pregnant women because its long-term effects are not fully known (Kremkau 1984, Queenan 1984).

Diagnostic ultrasound has several advantages. It is painless, nonradiating to both the woman and fetus, and has no known harmful effects to either. Serial studies (several ultrasound tests done over a span of time) may be done for assessment and comparison. Soft tissue masses can be differentiated. The practitioner obtains results immediately. Finally, it is thought that ultrasound does not pose the same risk as other diagnostic or medical procedures, such as amniocentesis or intrauterine surgery, yet allows the clinician to "see" the fetus.

Safety of Ultrasound

Ultrasound images are created by the reflection of echoes that are produced when sound waves are dispersed to, and absorbed by, the tissue being scanned. Ultrasound scanning has been called both noninvasive and invasive. In the traditional sense, invasive procedures are those that pierce the skin or enter the body, as with an intravenous needle or nasogastric tube. Ultrasound is called noninvasive because it does not meet this criterion. However, since ultrasound does pass into the body, some sources call it an invasive procedure. Manning (1984) states that ultrasound scanning is invasive because it passes into the body and can affect tissue and individual cells. It is therefore a procedure that carries theoretical risks of tissue damage. Since it meets both definitions in some aspects, ultrasound scanning must be clearly explained when using the terms invasive or noninvasive.

The maximum safe level of ultrasound exposure has been defined as ≤ 100 milliwatts/cm^2 (mw/cm^2), and most ultrasound machines operate at ranges much lower than this, usually 10 to 20 mw/cm^2 (Manning 1984). There are

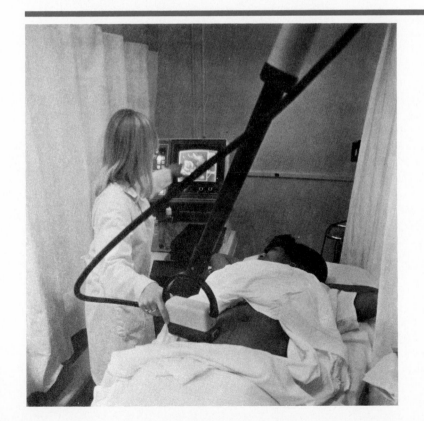

Figure 20–1   Ultrasound scanning permits visualization of the fetus in utero.

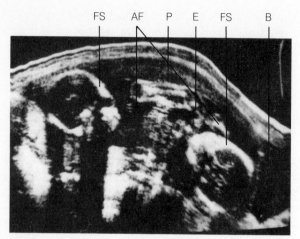

Figure 20–2　Ultrasound. Longitudinal scan demonstrating twin gestation, anterior placenta, fetal extremity. Both biparietal diameters (BPD) are at approximately 25 to 26 weeks' gestation. (AF = amniotic fluid; FS = fetal skull; E = extremity; B = woman's urinary bladder; P = placenta) (Courtesy Section of Diagnostic Ultrasound, Department of Diagnostic Radiology, Kansas University Medical Center.)

no reports to date of tissue damage using conventional diagnostic ultrasound imaging (Manning 1984). It is believed that ultrasound performed for indicated purposes carries no recognizable risk to mother or fetus and that it does provide information that can be of major benefit in pregnancy outcome.

In February 1984, the second and final public session of the Consensus Development Conference on Diagnostic Ultrasound Imaging in Pregnancy was convened by the National Institutes of Health (NIH). The 14-member panel reported that regarding fetal radiation, "For all practical purposes, fetal dose cannot be quantitated precisely" (Shearer 1984, p 26). The report further stated that in those situations for which ultrasound scanning is recommended (Box 20–2), no randomized controlled trials had yet shown improved management of pregnancy outcome.

Epidemiologic studies tend to support the safety of diagnostic ultrasound exposure in humans. Studies in animals using very high levels of ultrasound have caused effects such as a decrease in immune response, change in cell membrane function, and cell death. Because of the results of animal studies, routine ultrasound scanning is not recommended at this time (Shearer 1984).

Procedure

The woman is usually scanned with a full bladder except when ultrasound is used to localize the placenta prior to amniocentesis. When the bladder is full, the examiner can then assess other structures, especially the vagina and cervix, in relation to the bladder. This is partic-

Research Note

A lack of adequate human studies, and questions raised by animal studies about possible subtle, long-term or cumulative effects of ultrasound, prompted these researchers to investigate the use of ultrasound in their practice setting. Information collected retrospectively from 100 client charts included total number of ultrasounds performed, rationale for these, and delivery and outcome data.

One hundred twenty-nine ultrasounds were done on seventy-seven patients (from one to four per patient for 117 different reasons). Seventy percent of these reasons met the American College of Obstetricians and Gynecologists' guidelines for ultrasound use: Most often they were ordered to determine gestational age or to evaluate fetal growth.

The authors conclude that the well-established value of ultrasound warrants its continued use, but encourage providers to minimize the number and length of exposures and to provide for informed patient consent, including a discussion of the risks and benefits of the procedure. The authors also encourage nurses, physicians, and technicians to document the exposure dose and time for each type of ultrasound used during the antepartum and intrapartum period, including external fetal heart monitoring and doppler use.

Lewis C, Mocarski V: Obstetric ultrasound: Application in a clinic setting. J Obstet Gynecol Neonat Nurs 1987;16(January/February):56–60.

ularly important when vaginal bleeding is noted and placenta previa is the suspected cause. The woman is advised to drink 1 to 1½ quarts of water approximately 2 hours before the examination, and she is asked to refrain from emptying her bladder. If the bladder is not sufficiently filled, she is asked to drink three to four 8-oz glasses of water and is rescanned 30 to 45 minutes later.

Mineral oil or a transmission gel is generously spread over the woman's abdomen, and the sonographer slowly moves a transducer over the abdomen to obtain a picture of the contents of the uterus. Ultrasound testing takes 20 to 30 minutes. The woman may feel discomfort due to pressure applied over a full bladder. In addition, the woman lies on her back during the test; this position may cause shortness of breath, which may be relieved by elevating her upper body during the test.

Nursing Role

It is important for the nurse to ascertain whether the woman understands the reason the ultrasound is being sug-

Box 20–2   Ultrasound Can Be of Benefit in the Following Circumstances

Estimation of gestational age for patients (1) with uncertain clinical dates, (2) verification of dates of patients who are to undergo scheduled elective repeat cesarean delivery, induction of labor, or for other elective termination of pregnancy. Ultrasound confirmation of dating permits proper timing of cesarean delivery or labor induction to avoid premature delivery.

Evaluation of fetal growth (eg, when the patient has an identified etiology for uteroplacental insufficiency, such as severe preeclampsia, chronic hypertension, chronic renal disease, severe diabetes mellitus, or for other medical complications of pregnancy where fetal malnutrition, ie, IUGR or macrosomia, is suspected). Following fetal growth permits assessment of the impact of a complicating condition on the fetus and guides pregnancy management.

Vaginal bleeding of undetermined etiology in pregnancy. Ultrasound often allows determination of the source of bleeding and status of the fetus.

Determination of fetal presentation when the presenting part cannot be adequately determined in labor or the fetal presentation is variable in late pregnancy. Accurate knowledge of presentation guides management of delivery.

Suspected multiple gestation based upon detection of more than one fetal heartbeat pattern, or fundal height larger than expected for dates, and/or prior use of fertility drugs. Pregnancy management may be altered in multiple gestation.

Adjunct to amniocentesis. Ultrasound permits guidance of the needle to avoid the placenta and fetus, to increase the chance of obtaining amniotic fluid, and to decrease the chance of fetal loss.

Significant uterine size/clinical dates discrepancy. Ultrasound permits accurate dating and detection of such conditions as oligohydramnios and polyhydramnios, as well as multiple gestation, IUGR, and anomalies.

Pelvic mass detected clinically. Ultrasound can detect the location and nature of the mass and aid in diagnosis.

Suspected hydatidiform mole on the basis of clinical signs of hypertension, proteinuria, and/or the presence of ovarian cysts felt on pelvic examination or failure to detect fetal heart tones with a Doppler ultrasound device after 12 weeks. Ultrasound permits accurate diagnosis and differentiation of this malignancy from fetal death.

Adjunct to cervical cerclage placement. Ultrasound aids in timing and proper placement of the cerclage for patients with incompetent cervix.

Suspected ectopic pregnancy or when pregnancy occurs after tuboplasty or prior ectopic gestation. Ultrasound is a valuable diagnostic aid for this complication.

Adjunct to special procedures, such as fetoscopy, intrauterine transfusion, shunt placement, *in vitro* fertilization, embryo transfer, or chorionic villi sampling. Ultrasound aids instrument guidance that increases safety of these procedures.

Suspected fetal death. Rapid diagnosis enhances optimal management.

Suspected uterine abnormality (eg, clinically significant leiomyomata, or congenital structural abnormalities, such as bicornate uterus or uterus didelphys, etc). Serial surveillance of fetal growth and state enhances fetal outcome.

Intrauterine contraceptive device localization. Ultrasound guidance facilitates removal, reducing chances of IUD-related complications.

Ovarian follicle development surveillance. This facilitates treatment of infertility.

Biophysical evaluation for fetal well-being after 28 weeks of gestation. Assessment of amniotic fluid, fetal tone, body movements, breathing movements, and heart rate patterns assists in the management of high-risk pregnancies.

Observation of intrapartum events (eg, version/extraction of second twin, manual removal of placenta, etc). These procedures may be done more safely with the visualization provided by ultrasound.

Suspected hydramnios or oligohydramnios. Confirmation of the diagnosis is permitted, as well as identification of the cause of the condition in certain pregnancies.

Suspected abruptio placentae. Confirmation of diagnosis and extent assists in clinical management.

Adjunct to external version from breech to vertex presentation. The visualization provided by ultrasound facilitates performance of this procedure.

Estimation of fetal weight and/or presentation in premature rupture of membranes and/or premature labor. Information provided by ultrasound guides management decisions on timing and method of delivery.

(Box continues on following page.)

Box 20–2   Ultrasound Can Be of Benefit in the Following Circumstances (continued)

Abnormal serum alpha-fetoprotein value for clinical gestational age when drawn. Ultrasound provides an accurate assessment of gestational age for the AFP comparison standard and indicates several conditions (eg, twins, anencephaly) that may cause elevated AFP values.

Follow-up observation of identified fetal anomaly. Ultrasound assessment of progression or lack of change assists in clinical decision making.

History of previous congenital anomaly. Detection of recurrence may be permitted, or psychologic benefit to patients may result from reassurance of no recurrence.

Serial evaluation of fetal growth in multiple gestation. Ultrasound permits recognition of discordant growth, guiding client management, and timing of delivery.

Evaluation of fetal condition in late registrants for prenatal care. Accurate knowledge of gestational age assists in pregnancy management decisions of this group.

Source: Shearer MH: Revelations: A summary and analysis of the NIH consensus development conference on ultrasound imaging in pregnancy. *Birth* 1984;11(1):27.

---

gested. The nurse can provide an opportunity for the woman to ask questions and can act as an advocate if there are questions or concerns that need to be addressed prior to the ultrasound examination. The nurse explains the preparation needed and assures that adequate preparation is done. After the test is completed, the nurse can assist with clarifying or interpreting test results to the woman.

In some instances, with additional education, the nurse may actually perform the ultrasound exam. This is especially true in a birth setting with real-time ultrasound.

Clinical Application

Currently there are many uses for ultrasound in pregnancy (see Box 20–2). Some of the uses will be discussed in more detail.

EARLY PREGNANCY DETECTION

Pregnancy may be detected by diagnostic ultrasound as early as the fifth or sixth week following the LMP. A small collection of ringlike echoes may be seen within the uterus; this is called the gestational sac. Gestational sac

volume may be used to determine gestational age if performed before eight weeks. The error is less than one week (Manning 1985). Since most women do not seek prenatal care by this time, the practical application of this method is limited.

CLINICAL MEASUREMENTS

○   *MEASUREMENT OF CROWN–RUMP LENGTH*   During the first trimester, measurement of the crown–rump length (CRL) of the fetus is most useful for accurate dating of a pregnancy. The CRL is the longest length of the fetus (excluding the fetal limbs) and is the most accurate sonographic measurement used to establish gestational age (Figure 20–3). Because the curvature of the fetus becomes more pronounced after 12 weeks, CRL is not used after this time. Between 7 and 10 weeks CRL can predict gestational age within ±2.7 to ±4.7 days (Jeanty & Romero 1984). (Refer to Table 20–2 for CRL/gestational age measurements.)

○   *MEASUREMENT OF BIPARIETAL DIAMETER OF FETAL HEAD*   By far the most important and frequently used application of

Table 20–2   Normal CRL at Each Gestational Age

AGE	CRL	AGE	CRL	AGE	CRL	AGE	CRL	AGE	CRL	AGE	CRL
6+0	4	7+0	9	8+0	15	9+0	22	10+0	31	11+0	40
6+1	5	7+1	10	8+1	16	9+1	23	10+1	32	11+1	41
6+2	6	7+2	10	8+2	17	9+2	24	10+2	33	11+2	43
6+3	6	7+3	11	8+3	18	9+3	26	10+3	35	11+3	44
6+4	7	7+4	12	8+4	19	9+4	27	10+4	36	11+4	46
6+5	8	7+5	13	8+5	20	9+5	28	10+5	38	11+5	47
6+6	8	7+6	14	8+6	21	9+6	29	10+6	39	11+6	49

Note: CRL is expressed in millimeters. Age is expressed in weeks and days.

Source: Jeanty P, Romero R: *Obstetrical Ultrasound.* New York, McGraw-Hill, 1984, p 53.

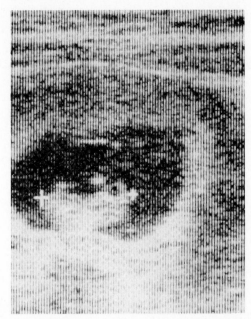

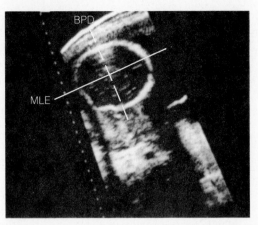

Figure 20–4 Transverse scan of 25 to 26 weeks' fetal skull. The BPD is measured perpendicular to midline echo (MLE). (Courtesy, Diagnostic Ultrasound Department, Section of Diagnostic Radiology, Kansas University Medical Center)

Figure 20–3 Measurement of crown–rump length. The CRL is measured from the top of the fetal head to the rump (excluding the legs). (From Jeanty P, Romero R: Obstetrical Ultrasound. New York, McGraw-Hill, 1984, p 53)

ultrasound is in the measurement of the biparietal diameter (BPD) of the fetal head. The BPD is the widest diameter of the fetal skull measured at the level of the thalamus and is perpendicular to the fetal midline echo (Figure 20–4). Measurement of the BPD provides the care giver with a useful tool for following fetal development.

Tables correlating the BPD with fetal gestation vary somewhat from one institution to the next, undoubtedly because of socioeconomic and geographic factors inherent in the populations for which the tables were derived (Table 20–3). Nevertheless, serial determinations on the same fetus using the same tables can be used as a gross measure

of the progress of fetal development. If growth of the fetal head follows a normal curve as gestation advances, one can be assured that the fetus is growing at a normal rate. However, if the curve begins to flatten, the physician must be on the alert for IUGR and must consider this a high-risk case. The fetus is evaluated by additional means, such as estriol determinations, nonstress tests, and possibly contraction stress tests.

The BPD measurements can be obtained beginning at 11 weeks of gestation but the BPD is too small for nomograms to be reliable until about 13 weeks. Detection of IUGR and an accurate prediction of fetal age can be most reliably achieved between 20 and 30 weeks of gestation, when the most rapid growth in the BPD occurs. After 40 weeks' gestation the BPD shows a growth of less than 1 mm/week; thus sonograms obtained at this point are of no value. The BPD measurement generally correlates closely with gestational age, especially if serial determinations were

Table 20–3 BPD vs. Weeks' Gestation

Week	BPD composite mean (cm)	Week	BPD composite mean (cm)
14	2.8	28	7.2
15	3.2	29	7.5
16	3.6	30	7.8
17	3.9	31	8.0
18	4.2	32	8.2
19	4.5	33	8.5
20	4.8	34	8.7
21	5.1	35	8.8
22	5.4	36	9.0
23	5.8	37	9.2
24	6.1	38	9.3
25	6.4	39	9.4
26	6.7	40	9.5
27	7.0		

Source: Queenan JT (ed): *Management of High-Risk Pregnancy,* ed 2. Oradell, NJ, Medical Economics Books, 1985, p 218.

obtained from early in the pregnancy. If only one determination is made late in pregnancy, the gestational age is less accurate and may vary by four weeks either way.

After 28 weeks the BPD alone should not be relied on to determine gestational age. The *cephalic index* (ratio of BPD to occipito-frontal (OF) diameter) should be evaluated to determine normality of the shape of the head. The cephalic index, which remains constant throughout pregnancy, is approximately 80 percent (mean 75 percent–85 percent) (Jeanty & Romero 1984) and is most useful in assessing the gestational age of the fetus in breech (fetal head crowded under maternal ribs) or vertex presentations (head descended into pelvis). If the cephalic index is abnormal, gestational age should be determined by other parameters, and abnormalities of the head should be considered and further assessed.

○ *MEASUREMENT OF FEMUR LENGTH* Measurement of femur length has been investigated by many as an alternative means of assessing gestational age and may even be considered a better indicator than the BPD because

> (1) it is considered less affected by growth disturbances, (2) it is easier to obtain, (3) the standard deviation for the femur measurement is smaller than for the BPD, and (4) the growth rate of the femur is greater than that of the BPD and therefore the late flattening of the curve is less pronounced (Jeanty & Romero 1984, p 60).

From 11 to about 13 weeks the nomograms are not reliable for BPD and femur length because the measurements are too small. Jeanty and Romero therefore recommend averaging the gestational age from both parameters. From 13 weeks until term, the BPD and/or femur are usually used to predict gestational age (Jeanty & Romero 1984).

To be truly accurate, femur growth rate charts should be developed by each institution with regard to the population served. Factors such as altitude and race would obviously have an effect on standards found in any given population.

○ *ABDOMINAL MEASUREMENTS* Measurement of the abdominal perimeter (measurement at the level of the fetal liver) provides data to aid in the detection of abnormal growth patterns. In IUGR, fetal abdominal girth ceases to increase due to the depletion of glycogen in the fetal liver and also to diminished accumulation of subcutaneous tissue overlying the fetal abdomen. Since different authors have reported differences in abdominal perimeter measurements, for optimum accuracy each institution should develop its own standards for its particular client population. Abdominal perimeter measurements alone are meaningless unless the gestational age of the fetus has been defined by CRL or serial BPDs. It appears to be most useful between 34 and 36 weeks' gestation in differentiating normal fetuses from those at risk for IUGR.

○ *HEAD-TO-ABDOMEN RATIO* The head perimeter (H) to abdomen perimeter (A) ratio is used to assess disproportion between the fetal head and body. Disproportion may be observed in asymmetrical IUGR and congenital anomalies such as microcephaly. The H:A ratio may also be used to evaluate head size in breeches that are being considered for vaginal delivery and fetal size in diabetic pregnancies (for possible shoulder dystocia). After 36 weeks the abdominal circumference will generally be larger than head circumference in a normal fetus (Hobbins et al 1983).

DETECTION OF CONGENITAL ANOMALIES

The role of ultrasound in the detection of structural and functional congenital anomalies is significant since these conditions contribute to 25 percent to 30 percent of all perinatal deaths and account for more than 65 percent of all deaths in high-risk gestations beyond 26 weeks (Manning 1985). Improvement in ultrasound resolution permits earlier and more accurate diagnosis of such conditions as hydrocephaly, anencephaly, meningomyelocele, encephalocele, and meningocele; thoracopulmonary, genitourinary, and musculoskeletal-cutaneous anomalies; and amniotic fluid, umbilical cord, and placental abnormalities. The use of the real-time ultrasound now permits detection of these types of anomalies and has had great impact on perinatal morbidity as a result of subsequent in utero therapy or early delivery and surgical correction of defects. Fetal anomalies are frequently associated with oligohydramnios or hydramnios, and the clinician should look for anomalies when these conditions are present.

FETAL GROWTH DETERMINATION

One of the most difficult problems facing the clinician is assessment of fetal growth. Ultrasound offers a valuable means of assessing intrauterine growth since the fetus can be measured serially.

Intrauterine growth retardation (IUGR) is classified as symmetrical (primary) or asymmetrical (secondary). In symmetrical IUGR, all organs are reduced in size with equal reduction in body weight and head size. At birth all measurements fall below the tenth percentile. This growth retardation is noted in the first half of the second trimester. It is associated with intrauterine viral infections, chromosomal disorders, major congenital malformations, and maternal malnutrition (Korones 1985).

In asymmetrical IUGR the head and brain are normal but there is a reduction in body size, apparently caused by a compromise in the uteroplacental blood flow. The decreased blood flow is associated with PIH, chronic hypertension, and chronic renal disease. This type of IUGR occurs in the majority of cases and is usually not evident prior to the third trimester. Fetuses with asymmetrical IUGR are particularly at risk for perinatal asphyxia, hypocalcemia, polycythemia, and hypoglycemia in the neo-natal period. Birth weight will be reduced to the 10th percentile, whereas cephalic size may be between the 25th and 30th percentile (Korones 1985).

Second to preterm delivery, IUGR is the greatest cause of perinatal mortality. Between 3 percent and 7 percent of all pregnancies are complicated by IUGR (Pernoll et al 1986).

The earlier the gestational age is accurately assessed, the more accurate the prediction of IUGR. If a growth-retarded fetus is suspected, serial ultrasounds should be done every two to three weeks.

On first examination, the estimated fetal weight (EFW) is figured as a percentile for that fetus. If the percentile is low, serial sonograms are warranted. If on repeat scan the fetus is at the same percentile, no abnormal growth has occurred. If the percentile increases, growth of the fetus has improved. If the fetus is at a lower percentile, fetal growth is slowing, and this fetus should be further assessed with other means of antenatal surveillance. Serial BPDs will closely assess the type of IUGR, and fetuses can be evaluated further with abdominal-chest measurements, nonstress and contraction stress tests, and biophysical profile. The additional assessments will help determine the optimal timing for delivery.

The question of when to deliver growth-retarded infants is still undecided. Some physicians, in light of pulmonary maturity, effect delivery of these infants by 37 to 38 weeks' gestation in hope of preventing long-term CNS deficits. Others choose to wait until other assessment parameters indicate fetal jeopardy (for example, a positive contraction stress test or an abnormal biophysical profile).

LOCALIZATION OF PLACENTA/AMNIOTIC FLUID POOL

Ultrasound is valuable in localizing the placenta for amniocentesis and in detecting placenta previa. Placentas appear to be located on the lower uterine segment in approximately 20 percent to 40 percent of pregnancies in the second trimester (Hibbard 1985). See Figure 20–5. By visualizing its location, the physician can avoid puncturing the placenta during amniocentesis. Ultrasound is used to locate a pool of amniotic fluid, thereby showing the physician exactly where and how deep to insert the needle for amniocentesis.

PLACENTAL GRADING

Grannum, Berkowitz, and Hobbins (1979) noted that throughout gestation the placenta undergoes maturational changes that may be visualized by ultrasound. These morphologic changes in the basal layer, chorionic plate, and intervening placental substance have been classified in

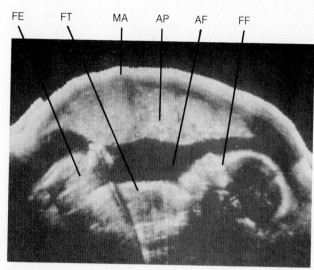

Figure 20–5   Ultrasound scan showing maternal abdomen (MA), anterior placenta (AP), profile of fetal face (FF), adequate amount of amniotic fluid (AF), fetal thorax (FT), and fetal extremities (FE). (From Hobbins JC, Winsberg F, Berkowitz RL: Ultrasonography in Obstetrics and Gynecology, ed 2. Baltimore, Williams & Wilkins, 1983, p 123)

terms of grades (0 to III), with increasing changes occurring from 12 weeks' gestation until term (Figure 20–6). The grade is described according to the presence of echogenic areas in the placental substance, basal layer, and chorionic plate. The reason for these changes is not clear (Spirit & Kagan 1980), but they seem to correlate with advancing placental maturity.

Any given placenta may contain more than one grade but the most mature grade should be used when total assessment is made. Grade I placentas may be noted at any time during gestation (after 12 weeks) and grade III placentas are rarely observed before the 36th week with the exception of women with hypertension or growth-retarded fetuses (Hobbins et al 1983).

Grannum, Berkowitz, and Hobbins (1979) noted in their original study that when correlating ultrasonic placental maturational changes with L/S ratios, the L/S ratio was 2:1 or greater in 100 percent of their cases with grade III placentas and in 88 percent with grade II placentas. Since that report, further studies have noted instances of false positive correlations with L/S ratios (Quinlan et al 1982). Consequently, it is felt that placental grading may be used to determine placental maturity but should not be used alone to predict fetal lung maturity.

Placental grading has been used with other assessments to estimate fetal maturity and determine timing of delivery. The Fetal Maturity Scoring System (Table 20–4) uses BPD, amniotic fluid volume (AFV), and placental grading to determine the timing of delivery (Queenan & Warsof 1985).

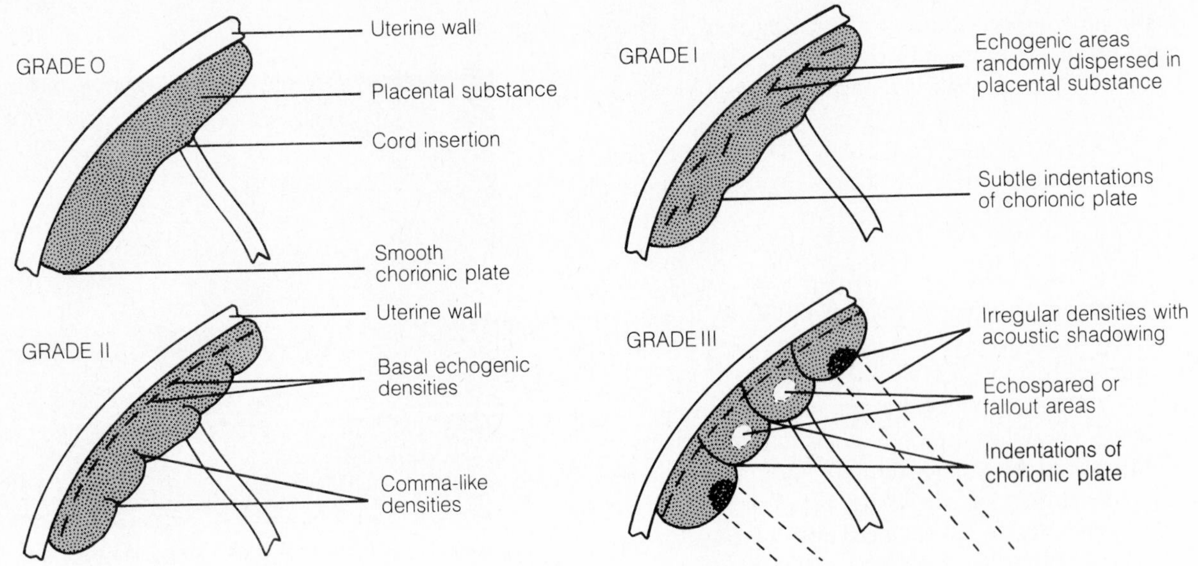

Figure 20–6 Diagrams showing the ultrasonic appearance of the placental grades. (From Grannum PAT, Berkowitz RL, Hobbins JC: The ultrasonic changes in the maturing placenta and their relation to fetal pulmonic maturity. *Am J Obstet Gynecol* 1979;133:916.)

BIOPHYSICAL PROFILE (BPP)

The biophysical profile (BPP), developed and reported in 1979 by Drs Frank Manning and Lawrence Platt, is an assessment of five biophysical variables: breathing movement, body movement, tone, amniotic fluid volume, and FHR reactivity. The BPP is used to assess the fetus at risk for intrauterine compromise. The first four variables are assessed by ultrasound scanning; FHR reactivity is assessed with the nonstress test. By combining these five assessments, the BPP helps to identify the compromised fetus and confirm the healthy fetus.

Specific criteria for normal and abnormal assessments are delineated in Table 20–5 with a score of 2 being assigned to each normal finding and 0 to each abnormal one for a maximum score of 10. The absence of a specific activity is difficult to interpret since it may be indicative of CNS depression or simply the resting state of a healthy fetus. Scores of 8 to 10 are considered normal (Platt et al 1985). Such scores seem to have the least chance of being associated with a compromised fetus unless a decrease in the amount of amniotic fluid is noted, in which case the infant should be delivered (Platt 1982). A prospective study of 1,184 high-risk women (Manning et al 1981) reported that perinatal mortality was reduced when this assessment profile was used for client management.

The advantages of the BPP are numerous. It is noninvasive, does not depend on accurate gestational age dating, requires a very short time to assess the different components, does not require the woman to have a full bladder, and can reduce the use of the contraction stress test (CST) in women who have nonreactive nonstress tests (NST). The test is not in wide use yet because not many physicians and nurses have been trained to perform the procedure and real-time ultrasound is not available in many birthing units.

Indications for BPP include those situations in which the NST and CST would be done. Assessment of these fetal biophysical activities is most useful in the evaluation of women who experience decreased fetal movement (who might subsequently have a nonreactive NST) and in the

Table 20–4 Fetal Maturity Scoring System

	Points*	BPD	Placental morphology	Amniotic fluid volume
Mature	3	Greater than 9.0 cm	Complete Grade II–Grade III	Crowding
Intermediate	2	8.8–9.0 cm	Grade I–incomplete Grade II	Normal
Nondiagnostic	0	Less than 8.8 cm	Grade 0	Generous

Points scored for each parameter. Seven points or more needed for delivery.

Source: Queenan JT (ed): *Management of High-Risk Pregnancy,* ed 2. Oradell, NJ, Medical Economics Books, 1985, p 225.

Table 20–5   Biophysical Profile Scoring: Technique and Interpretation*

Biophysical variable	Normal (score = 2)	Abnormal (score = 0)
1. Fetal breathing movements	≥1 episode of ≥30 sec in 30 min	Absent or no episode of ≥30 sec in 30 min
2. Gross body movements	≥3 discrete body/limb movements in 30 min (episodes of active continuous movement considered as single movement)	≤2 episodes of body/limb movements in 30 min
3. Fetal tone	≥1 episode of active extension with return to flexion of fetal limb(s) or trunk. Opening and closing of hand considered normal tone	Either slow extension with return to partial flexion or movement of limb in full extension or absent fetal movement
4. Reactive fetal heart rate	≥2 episodes of acceleration of ≥15 bpm and of ≥15 sec associated with fetal movement in 20 min	<2 episodes of acceleration of fetal heart rate or acceleration of <15 bpm in 20 min
5. Qualitative amniotic fluid volume	≥1 pocket of fluid measuring ≥1 cm in two perpendicular planes	Either no pockets or a pocket <1 cm in two perpendicular planes

Source: Manning FA, et al: Fetal assessment based on fetal biophysical profile scoring: Experience in 12,620 referred high-risk pregnancies. *Am J Obstet Gynecol* 1985;151(3):344.

management of IUGR, diabetic, and postterm pregnancies. The BPP differentiates the uncompromised fetus from the compromised one in postterm pregnancies (Johnson et al 1986) and, when used in the management of these pregnancies, can allow for a rational approach to client management when lack of cervical ripening does not suggest success with possible induction. Since perinatal mortality increases significantly for each week after 42 weeks of gestation, the BPP allows for continuation of the pregnancy until the cervix is ripe enough for induction or possible fetal jeopardy indicates immediate obstetric intervention.

A management protocol regarding BPP is outlined in Table 20–6 but to date there is no consensus of opinion regarding management based on abnormal BPP findings (Johnson et al 1986).

Other tests, such as the NST, will probably remain the primary tests for assessing the fetus at risk until more individuals are trained in the BPP procedure and more studies demonstrate its sensitivity, reliability, and prognostic value.

FETAL ECHOCARDIOGRAPHY AND FETAL BLOOD FLOW STUDIES

Ultrasound technology, in combination with Doppler devices, can be used to evaluate fetal cardiac structures and the functional status of fetal circulation. In fetal echocardiography, real-time ultrasound imaging is used to diagnose congenital cardiac disease. Blood velocity waveforms in umbilical vessels, which are an indicator of fetal well-

Table 20–6   Biophysical Profile Scoring: Management Protocol

Score	Interpretation	Recommended management
10	Normal infant, low risk for chronic asphyxia	Repeat testing at weekly intervals. Repeat twice weekly in diabetic patients and patients ≥42 wk
8	Normal infant, low risk for chronic asphyxia	Repeat testing at weekly intervals. Repeat twice weekly in diabetic patients and patients ≥42 wk. Indication for delivery = oligohydramnios
6	Suspected chronic asphyxia	Repeat testing within 24 hr. Indication for delivery = oligohydramnios or remaining ≤6
4	Suspected chronic asphyxia	≥36 score and favorable cervix. If <36 wk and lecithin/sphingomyelin ratio <2.0, repeat test in 24 hr. Indication for delivery = repeat score ≤6 or oligohydramnios
0–2	Strong suspicion of chronic asphyxia	Extend testing time to 120 min. Indication for delivery = persistent score ≤4, regardless of gestational age

Source: Manning FA, et al: Fetal assessment based on fetal biophysical profile scoring: Experience in 12,620 referred high-risk pregnancies. *Am J Obstet Gynecol* 1985;151(3):344.

being, are assessed by Doppler devices. These studies are particularly helpful in assessing fetuses who are at increased risk for development of cardiac anomalies. These include those fetuses with IUGR, dysrhythmias, and nonimmune hydrops and those whose mothers have cardiac disease, diabetes, collagen vascular disease, hydramnios, hypertension, a family history of congenital heart disease, metabolic disease, chromosome abnormalities, and certain intrauterine infections (Friedman 1985, Copel et al 1986).

Although only performed in selected perinatal centers throughout the world, these techniques provide valuable information regarding fetal status in potentially compromising situations. For example, through evaluation of fetal status via echocardiography, pharmacologic treatment of fetal arrhythmias has become possible prior to delivery. Many cases of congenital heart disease have been diagnosed prenatally and managed accordingly.

Echocardiography and Doppler blood flow studies are primarily recommended in those cases in which the fetus is suspected of having congenital anomalies, cardiac arrhythmias, or fetal distress such as that caused by congestive heart failure. Copel, Pilu, and Kleinman (1986) perform fetal echocardiography on all women found to have extracardiac anomalies by ultrasound. These procedures are also used to compare the quantity of fetal umbilical venous blood return to the estimated fetal weight to predict gestational age.

The advantage of obtaining this information prenatally is that parents as well as perinatal nursing and medical staff can be alerted for possible problems that may occur at the time of delivery or thereafter and thus plan accordingly. A fetus with a diagnosed problem may be serially evaluated and assessed more closely prior to delivery to permit optimum perinatal and neonatal management.

When fetal cardiac malformations are diagnosed by echocardiography, level II ultrasound scanning is performed to assess other fetal structures. Copel, Pilu, and Kleinman (1986) offer genetic amniocentesis to all clients with diagnosed fetal cardiac malformations since the risk of also having a fetal chromosome abnormality is 5 percent.

● Maternal Assessment of Fetal Activity

Assessment of fetal movement patterns has been used as a screening procedure in the evaluation of fetal status since 1971 when the clinical significance of various types of fetal activity was first described (Sadovsky 1985b). Clinicians now generally agree that vigorous fetal activity provides reassurance of fetal well-being and that marked decrease in activity or cessation of movement may indicate possible fetal compromise requiring immediate follow-up evaluation. Fetal movements are usually assessed by the woman but may also be evaluated by ultrasound and external fetal monitoring techniques.

Sadovsky (1985a) noted that although there is considerable variation among individuals, the average number of daily movements rises from about 200 at 20 weeks to a maximum of 575 at 32 weeks and gradually decreases to an average of 282 at term. In women with a multiple gestation, daily fetal movements are significantly higher. Although women report periods of markedly decreased fetal movement, this has been found to be associated with periods of fetal sleep, medications, smoking, and other factors. It has also been noted that some women are not as aware of fetal activity and that more fetal movements are usually noted on ultrasound assessment than by the woman herself. Although there are various types of fetal movements, women at high risk for fetal hypoxia have noted a reduction in or disappearance of fetal movements or changes in the type of fetal activity with a predominance of only weak movements prior to fetal death.

Because of the subjective nature of maternal assessment of fetal activity and the many factors that affect fetal reactivity (sound, drugs, smoking, fetal sleep states, blood glucose levels, and time of day), it is difficult to develop a protocol regarding this type of subjective assessment. The *movement alarm signal (MAS),* which is a reduction in fetal movement to three or fewer or cessation of movement for 12 hours, has been shown to be associated with fetal distress and indicates impending fetal death. This signal is associated with oligohydramnios, hydramnios, malformations, asymmetrical IUGR, Rh isoimmunization, and mothers with systemic lupus erythematosus (Sadovsky 1985b). Various studies have described different methods for counting and recording fetal activity, but there seems to be no significance to the number of daily movements unless the rate is very low.

One protocol is the *daily fetal movement response (DFMR) assessment,* a method described by Sadovsky. This protocol has been found to be practical and easy for maternal assessment (Figure 20–7). It involves having the woman count the number of times the fetus moves in 30 minutes (noting the strength of movements) three times a day. Four strong movements in 30 minutes on three occasions or at least 10 movements in 12 hours is considered reassuring. Because fetal demise has occurred 10 to 11 hours after cessation of fetal movement in diabetic women, these women should assess fetal movements in a 6 to 8 hour period. The presence of normal fetal movements is a reliable predictor of good fetal outcome in both high- and low-risk pregnancies. If the MAS is noted, further assessment of the fetus (NST, OCT, pulmonary maturity, and ultrasound to rule out malformations) must be done immediately to evaluate fetal status and determine management. A scoring system has been devised to identify a fetus at increased risk (Table 20–7). When the score is five or

Table 20–7   Scoring System to Use With MAS

Parameter	Definition		Score*
Contraction stress test (CST): *positive*	Three contractions followed by late decelerations (10-minute period)		2
Fetal movements acceleration (FMAC) test: *non-reactive*	Fewer than two accelerations associated with FM (20-minute period)		2
Daily fetal movements recording (DFMR): *pathologic*	Fewer than 10 movements (12-hour period) (DFM)		2
	Fewer than three or no movements (12-hour period) (MAS)		3
Fetal heart rate (FHR): *pathologic changes*	Base level: <100 bpm, >180 bpm	(3)	
	Repeated severe variable or late decelerations	(3)	
	Loss of long-term variability (amplitude <5, frequency <2)	(3)	3
	Constant sinusoidal pattern	(3)	
Lung maturity	L/S ratio ≥ 2		1

*If score is 5 or more, terminate pregnancy if fetus is viable.

Source: Sadovsky E: Fetal movements, in Queenan JT (ed): *Management of High-Risk Pregnancy,* ed. 2. Oradell, NJ, Medical Economics Books, 1985, p 190.

higher, it is suggested that pregnancy be terminated if the fetus is viable.

It is difficult to target a specific time that the expectant woman should begin assessing fetal movement. As soon as she begins to feel the movements of her baby, she should be counseled to note patterns of her own baby's activity and to report significant changes. Low-risk women should be counseled to count fetal movements daily beginning at about 27 weeks' gestation (Chez & Sadovsky 1984). It is recommended that they count the fetal movements twice daily for 20 to 30 minutes, or for up to an hour if necessary, early in the morning and in midafternoon or late evening. High-risk women should count movements three times a day. It is reassuring if 5 to 6 movements are noted during each counting period. If fewer than 10 movements are noted in a 12-hour period or 3 movements in 8 hours, or there is a significant change from strong and rolling movements to weak ones, the physician should be notified so that follow-up assessments can be made (Box 20–3).

It has been observed that sudden, strong, vigorous movements followed by cessation are characteristic signs of acute fetal distress and impending death, often caused by cord compression or sudden abruption (Sadovsky 1985a). Since DFMR would be of little use in such instances, women should immediately notify their physician if they note this type of fetal activity.

Although maternal assessment of fetal activity is a subjective means of evaluating fetal status, it has been found to be an excellent screening test for diagnosing chronic fetal distress. Furthermore, it is simple for the woman to perform, does not interfere with her normal routines, and costs nothing. Pregnant women need to understand that fetal movements are significant, that fetal activity changes during pregnancy, and that when movements weaken or cease they should contact their care giver for further evaluation.

Box 20–3   Assessing Fetal Activity: What to Tell Your Clients

Low risk

At 27 weeks count fetal movement twice daily for 20 to 30 minutes. Five or six movements during each counting period is a reassuring sign.

High risk

At 27 weeks count movements three times daily. If you note five to six movements in 30 minutes each time, stop counting. If you fail to note three movements in a half hour, continue counting for an hour or more.

All patients

If you note fewer than ten movements in a 12-hour period of counting, no movements in the morning, fewer than three movements in 8 hours, or become concerned for any reason, contact your obstetrician.

Source: Chez RA, Sadovsky E: Teaching patients how to record fetal movements. *Contemp OB/GYN* 1984;24:86.

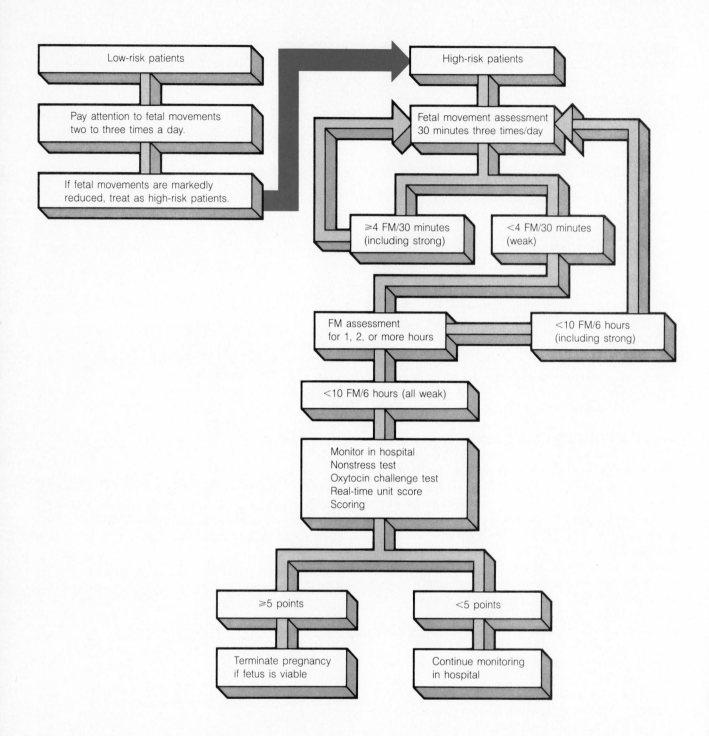

Figure 20–7 Protocol for daily fetal movement response (DFMR) assessment (From Sadovsky E: Monitoring fetal movement: a useful screening test. *Contemp OB/GYN* 1985;25:130)

As discussed in Chapter 16, women should be reassured that there are fetal rest-sleep states during which minimal or no movement may occur. Gross fetal movements may be absent for at least an hour as the fetus rests. Thus fetal movements may be a sign of fetal well-being, but episodic absence of movement is also characteristic of normal fetuses.

Nursing Role

The nurse assists in teaching the technique for DFMR. The nurse can also help the woman devise a daily record in which she can report fetal movements. The nurse is available for questions and to clarify areas of concern.

● Nonstress Test (NST)

The *nonstress test* (NST) has become a widely accepted method of evaluating fetal status. The test involves observation of acceleration of the fetal heart rate (FHR) with fetal movement. The test is based on the knowledge that the fetus is normally active throughout pregnancy and that good fetal activity will result in acceleration of the fetal heart rate when the normal fetus moves. Accelerations of the FHR imply an intact central and autonomic nervous system that is not being affected by intrauterine hypoxia.

The advantages of the NST are that it is relatively quick, inexpensive, and easy to interpret; it can be done in an outpatient setting; and there are no known side effects. The disadvantages are that it is sometimes difficult to obtain a suitable tracing, and the woman has to sit or lie relatively still for 20 to 30 minutes.

Interpretation of NST

The results of the NST are interpreted as follows:

● *Reactive test.* A reactive NST shows at least two accelerations of FHR with fetal movements, of 15 beats per minute, lasting 15 seconds or more, over 20 minutes (Figure 20–8).

● *Nonreactive test.* In a nonreactive test, the reactive criteria are not met. For example, the accelerations are not as much as 15 beats per minute, or do not last 15 seconds, and so on (Figure 20–9).

● *Unsatisfactory test.* An unsatisfactory NST has data that cannot be interpreted, or inadequate fetal activity.

Note that criteria for the NST appear to vary somewhat from one author to another. Some require two accelerations of FHR in 20 minutes; others require two in 10 minutes.

It is particularly important that anyone who performs the NST also understand the significance of any decelerations of the FHR during testing. If decelerations are noted, the physician/nurse-midwife should be notified for further evaluation of fetal status.

Procedure

The test may be done with the woman in a reclining chair or in bed in a semi-Fowler's or side-lying position. An electronic fetal monitor is applied (see discussion on p 616). The examiner applies two belts around the woman's waist. One belt holds a device that detects uterine or fetal movement. The other belt holds a device that detects the FHR.

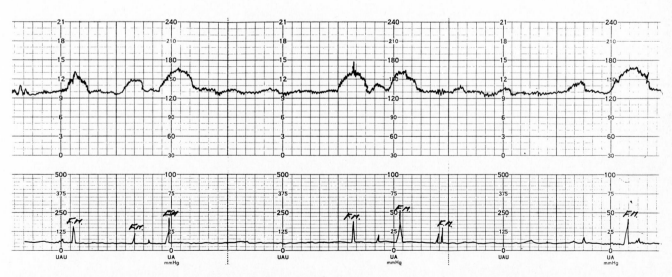

Figure 20–8   Example of a reactive nonstress test (NST). Accelerations of 15 beats/min, lasting 15 seconds with each fetal movement (FM). (Top of strip = fetal heart rate; bottom of strip = uterine activity tracing.)

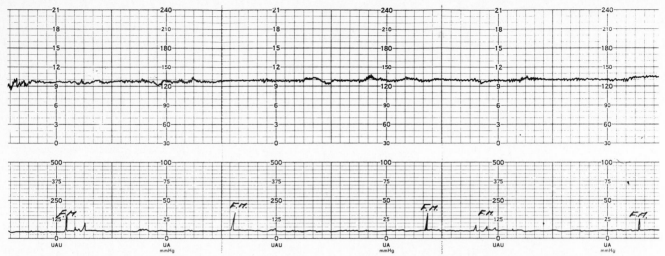

Figure 20–9 Example of a nonreactive NST. There are no accelerations of FHR with fetal movement (FM). Baseline FHR = 130 beats/min; tracing of uterine activity is on the bottom of the strip.

Recordings of the FHR are obtained for approximately 30 to 40 minutes (minimum of 20 minutes). The woman or nurse notes each fetal movement as it is recorded. If no fetal movements occur after 30 to 40 minutes of observation, the woman is given orange or other fruit juice or a light meal. Fetal movements often increase due to distention of the maternal stomach and elevation in blood glucose.

Prognostic Value

Bishop (1981) has reported that acceleration of FHR seems to be a function of advancing gestational age, fetal maturity, and fetal development. Bishop notes that there is a high occurrence of false positive results (that is, a nonreactive test) prior to 30 weeks' gestation. Since delivery is seldom indicated prior to this time, nonstress testing may not be justified before 30 weeks. The NST and the contraction stress test both have higher incidences of false positive rather than false negative results. Attainment of a reactive test appears to be indicative of fetal well-being, whereas nonreactive results do not necessarily indicate fetal jeopardy and therefore require further evaluation of fetal status by other parameters. The correlation between a reactive NST and a negative contraction stress test is high.

The high incidence of nonreactive NSTs appears to depend on many factors; therefore all nonreactive tests should be followed by additional testing. Some authors advocate rescheduling the NST again within the same 24 hours, while others suggest an immediate contraction stress test. When the NST is reactive, the test should be repeated in a week. Any change in maternal or fetal status (such as decreased fetal movement, falling estriols, vaginal bleeding, or deterioration of maternal condition) warrants more frequent testing. Many authors recommend testing twice a week for women with prolonged pregnancy, diabetes, or IUGR (Figure 20–10).

The NST has replaced the CST as the method of choice in antepartum surveillance in many facilities since the CST is time-consuming and poorly suited as a screening tool for significant numbers of women. Compared to the CST, the NST has many advantages. The NST is less expensive; no IV infusion is required; there are no contraindications; it may be performed away from a labor and delivery area; and the results are fairly easy to interpret. The NST can be used for surveillance of women with threatened preterm labor, previous classical cesarean section, and placenta previa and can be repeated often without side effects and with minimal inconvenience and expense to the woman.

Many physicians use the NST for all high-risk screening and reserve the CST for insulin-dependent women and those with IUGR, chronic hypertension, postterm pregnancies, or oligohydramnios. These clinicians believe that the CST may be a more sensitive indicator of impending fetal jeopardy in these specific situations. They believe that the CST is more sensitive to fetal oxygen reserves and that late decelerations will appear before there is a significant fall in pH, whereas accelerations disappear only after the fetus becomes acidotic and significantly hypoxic (Ward 1982).

Nursing Role

The nurse ascertains the woman's understanding of the NST and the possible results. The reasons for the NST and the procedure are reviewed prior to beginning the test. The nurse administers the NST, interprets the results, and reports the findings to the physician/nurse-midwife and the expectant woman.

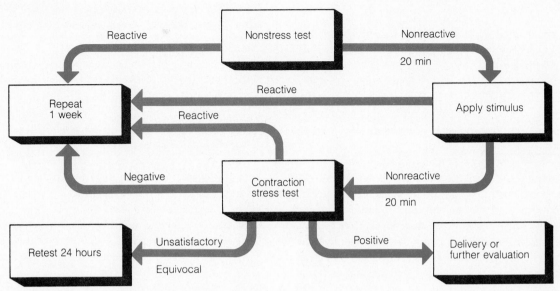

Figure 20–10 *Flow chart indicating recommended management of nonstress test* (From Evertson LR, et al: Antepartum fetal heart rate testing. 1. Evolution of the non-stress test. *Am J Obstet Gynecol* 1979;133(1):131)

Contraction Stress Test (CST)

The *contraction stress test (CST)* is a means of evaluating the respiratory function (oxygen and carbon dioxide exchange) of the placenta. It enables the health care team to identify the fetus at risk for intrauterine asphyxia by observing the response of the FHR to the stress of uterine contractions (spontaneous or induced). During contractions, intrauterine pressure increases. Blood flow to the intervillous space of the placenta is reduced momentarily, thereby decreasing oxygen transport to the fetus. A healthy fetus usually tolerates this reduction well. If the placental reserve is insufficient, fetal hypoxia, depression of the myocardium, and a decrease in FHR occur.

Indications and Contraindications

The CST is indicated for pregnancies at risk for placental insufficiency or fetal compromise because of the following:

- IUGR
- Diabetes mellitus
- Heart disease
- Chronic hypertension
- Preeclampsia-eclampsia
- Sickle cell disease
- Suspected postmaturity (42 weeks' gestation)
- History of previous unexplained stillborn or intrapartal loss

- Rh sensitization with meconium-stained amniotic fluid
- Abnormal estriol excretion
- Hyperthyroidism
- Renal disease
- Nonreactive NST
- Abnormal or suspicious biophysical profile

Contraindications for the CST are the following:

- Third trimester bleeding (placenta previa or marginal abruptio placentae)
- Previous cesarean delivery with classical uterine incision
- Instances in which the risk of possible preterm labor outweighs the advantage of the CST include:

  1. Premature rupture of the membranes

  2. Incompetent cervix or Shirodkar-Barter operation (cerclage—surgical procedure in which an incompetent cervix is encircled with suture to prevent it from dilating before term)

  3. Multiple gestation

General Procedure

A necessary component of the CST is the presence of uterine contractions that occur three times in ten minutes. The contractions may occur spontaneously, or they may be induced by oxytocin or nipple stimulation. The most common method of stimulating uterine contractions for a CST has been intravenous administration of oxytocin (Pitocin). This kind of CST is called the *oxytocin challenge test* (OCT). Many facilities now use the *nipple stimulation contraction stress test* (NSCST). The development of this method is based on the knowledge that endogenous oxytocin is produced in response to stimulation of the breasts or nipples.

The CST is performed on an outpatient basis by qualified obstetric nurses well acquainted with fetal monitoring and the interpretation of various FHR patterns. Most facilities require the tests be administered in or near the labor and delivery unit, in the event that adverse reactions to oxytocin stimulation occur. In many settings the physician/nurse-midwife must be present. The procedure, reasons for administering the test, equipment, and normal variations in monitoring that occur during the test should be clearly explained prior to the test to alleviate the woman's apprehension. A consent form may be signed. The woman should empty her bladder prior to beginning the CST, because she may be confined to bed for 1½ to 2 hours.

During the test, the woman assumes a semi-Fowler's or side-lying position to avoid supine hypotension. After the area of clearest fetoscopic heart tones is noted, the ultrasonic transducer (from the electronic fetal monitor) is placed on the woman's abdomen so that the FHR may be accurately recorded on the monitoring strip. (See Chapter 22 for further discussion of fetal monitoring.) To record uterine contractions, the tocodynamometer (pressure transducer) is placed over the area of the uterine fundus. For the first 15 minutes the nurse records baseline measurements, including blood pressure, fetal activity, variations of the FHR during fetal movement, and spontaneous contractions. In addition, pertinent medical and obstetric information may be obtained from the woman to aid in her further management.

After a 15-minute baseline recording, if three spontaneous contractions of good quality lasting 40 to 60 seconds have occurred in a 10-minute period, the results are evaluated and the test is concluded. If no contractions have occurred, or if they are insufficient for interpretation, nipple stimulation or intravenous oxytocin is used.

Nipple Stimulation Contraction Stress Test (NSCST)

In 1982 Garite and Freeman suggested manual stimulation of the mother's nipples to induce contractions sufficient for the CST. The test is also called breast self-stimulation test (BSST).

The exact mechanism by which nipple stimulation works and whether subsequent contractions are similar to those that occur in spontaneous labor or by the OCT have

---

Research Note

Nonstress tests (NSTs) and contraction stress tests (CSTs) have become common techniques to evaluate fetal well-being in pregnancies at risk. The traditional CST is obtained by intravenous infusion of oxytocin for one to three hours in order to stimulate three uterine contractions lasting 40 seconds in a ten-minute period. This technique is considered invasive, time-consuming, and expensive. Gantes and Kirchhoff proposed stimulating uterine contractions (UCs) via endogenous oxytocin released in response to breast massage.

The 30 subjects were instructed to massage alternate breasts with mineral oil for ten-minute periods for a maximum of 40 to 60 minutes. Fetal heart rate and uterine activity were electronically monitored. Of the 21 subjects who met the CST criteria of three uterine contractions in ten minutes, ninty-five percent did so within 40 minutes of initiating breast massage. Women who had uterine contractions prior to breast massage and were nearly at or at their due date were more likely to meet the CST criteria.

Overstimulation (uterine contractions longer than 120 seconds, three or more uterine contractions in five minutes, or five or more uterine contractions in ten minutes) occurred in three women, and two of them had fetal heart rate decelerations. For this reason Gantes and Kirchhoff caution practitioners to use monitoring with this procedure.

Gantes M, Kirchhoff KT, Work BA: Breast massage to obtain contraction stress test. Nurs Res 1985;34(November/December):338–341.

---

yet to be determined. With nipple stimulation, sensory nerve impulses are relayed to the neural cells of the hypothalamus where oxytocin is synthesized. These impulses cause the release of endogenous oxytocin from the neural cells, with subsequent transport to nerve terminals in the posterior pituitary gland into the bloodstream. The result is contractions similar to those caused by suckling stimulation during lactation.

Nipple stimulation has been found to be effective in inducing contractions sufficient for the CST. Most women have achieved satisfactory contractions within 15 to 30 minutes. Although the test seems simple to perform and no adverse fetal outcomes have been reported, the possibility of hyperstimulation and exaggerated uterine activity have been noted, occasionally with prolonged FHR decelerations (Figure 20–11). Hyperstimulation is defined as contractions lasting more than 90 seconds or occurring more frequently than every two minutes.

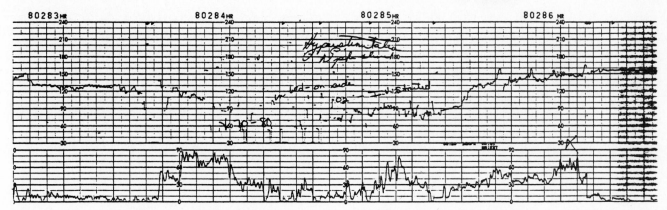

Figure 20–11   Hyperstimulation during nipple stimulation. The onset of contractions is shown two minutes following nipple stimulation. Panels 80284-80286 reveal hyperstimulation of more than 90 seconds and three contractions within an 8½-minute period with accompanying FHR deceleration to 70 to 80 beats per minute lasting 6½ minutes. (From McCluggage NA: Nipple stimulation contraction stress test. J Perinatol 1985;5(Summer):56)

Because pregnancies with compromised placental function are among those evaluated by the NSCST, exaggerated uterine activity and hyperstimulation could be potentially harmful to the fetus. It is suggested that this test be performed in or near a delivery unit where emergency fetal resuscitation, the administration of tocolytics, or immediate cesarean delivery can be performed if hyperstimulation and/or prolonged deceleration of the FHR occurs.

PROCEDURE

The nurse begins the NSCST by explaining the procedure to the woman. She is positioned in a sitting or side-lying position to maintain optimum uteroplacental circulation and to enhance the quality of the uterine contractions as they occur. When the woman lies on her side, uterine contractions seem to be less frequent but more intense than when she is in a semi-Fowler's position (Marshall 1986). The semi-Fowler's position is also more often associated with hyperstimulation (Marshall 1986). The woman's privacy should be protected, yet the nurse should stay with the woman during the whole procedure to remind her to cease stimulation at the appropriate time and to complete nursing assessments.

After the woman is comfortable, an electronic fetal monitor is applied, and a 15- to 20-minute strip is obtained to get a baseline and to determine uterine status. The FHR is evaluated for reactivity (NST). Nipple stimulation begins with the woman brushing her palm across one nipple through her shirt or gown for 2 to 3 minutes. Nipple stimulation should stop if a uterine contraction begins. The nipple stimulation continues after a 5-minute rest period. The process is continued until 40 minutes have elapsed or uterine contractions of at least 40 seconds in length occur at least three times in ten minutes (Marshall 1986). In some

settings, if no contractions occur after 15 to 20 minutes, the other nipple is stimulated in the same manner (Murray et al 1986). Bilateral stimulation should not be instituted unless unilateral stimulation fails to induce contractions; in these cases stimulation should be performed with caution to avoid hyperstimulation. The woman's blood pressure is assessed every 10 minutes throughout the procedure. The FHR is assessed for reactivity and the presence of decelerations. If a deceleration occurs, nipple stimulation is discontinued, the left lateral position is maintained, oxygen is begun per mask at 6 to 8 L/min, and the physician/nurse-midwife is notified (Marshall 1986). If contractions occur more frequently than every two minutes, and/or last more than 90 seconds, the nipple stimulation should be discontinued, the side-lying position maintained, the FHR carefully observed, and the physician/nurse-midwife notified (Marshall 1986). Oxygen may be administered. The woman's blood pressure and pulse should be assessed. In the presence of a hyperstimulation pattern the nurse should also be prepared to administer tocolytics or prepare for emergency delivery in the event of unresolved fetal distress.

The NSCST has been shown to be successful in terms of performance time and adequate contraction frequency. The same criteria that are used for the OCT are used for the NSCST. Embarrassment is rare if the procedure is thoroughly explained to the woman and is performed in a comfortable, relaxed, private environment. This test is commonly ordered twice weekly, like the OCT, since there is no guarantee that a negative test will be predictive of fetal well-being for one week as was previously thought (Ward 1982).

Since this test involves the induction of contractions by release of endogenous oxytocin, only knowledgeable nurses should be responsible for monitoring it.

The NSCST is equivalent to the administration of intravenous oxytocin but takes less time to perform, is less expensive, and causes less discomfort because no IV is used.

Oxytocin Challenge Test (OCT)

A CST can also be done by using intravenous oxytocin. This test is called an oxytocin challenge test (OCT). In this test an electrolyte solution such as lactated Ringer's solution is started as a primary infusion. A piggyback infusion of oxytocin in a similar solution is attached. An infusion pump is used so that the amount of oxytocin being infused can be measured accurately. The administration procedure is the same as for inducing labor through oxytocin administration. See Chapter 26 for further discussion. Oxytocin is administered until three uterine contractions lasting 40 to 60 seconds occur in a 10-minute period. If late decelerations are repetitive or occur more than three times, the oxytocin infusion should be discontinued and the physician notified immediately.

Prognostic Value

A CST is usually not done prior to 28 weeks' gestation primarily for two reasons:

1. In light of a positive test, delivery and extrauterine survival would be questionable at such an early gestational age.

2. Sufficient research has not been done to determine whether the same test results apply to a fetus of this gestation.

CSTs are usually begun at 32 to 34 weeks' gestation and are repeated once or twice a week until the woman delivers. Should the woman's condition deteriorate, the CST should be repeated as soon as possible.

A *negative CST* (Table 20–8 and Figure 20–12) has high prognostic value in that it implies that placental support is adequate. If that is the case, the physician can avoid premature intervention and gain approximately one additional week of intrauterine life for the fetus (Freeman 1975).

A woman who exhibits a *positive CST* (Table 20–8 and Figure 20–13) may have a fetus whose placental reserves are compromised. In many instances there is minimal baseline variability of the FHR (a condition that is usually not seen with healthy fetuses). Most frequently, acceleration of the FHR with fetal movement is absent or diminished, representing inadequate autonomic nervous system control of the fetal heart rate. Intravenous oxytocin-induced contractions may be stronger than would normally occur during labor as a result of hyperstimulation, which might not be detected with an external pressure transducer.

Women with positive test results may be managed differently according to their specific situation. Other parameters of fetal status must be taken into consideration, and on the basis of all available data, the pregnancy may be allowed to continue or labor may be induced.

If the CST is positive but the fetus demonstrates acceleration of FHR with fetal movement (reactive NST), the CST may have false positive results (about 50 percent of cases). Many of these women will tolerate trial induction of labor (Huddleston 1980).

If the CST is positive and there is no acceleration of FHR with fetal movement (nonreactive NST), the CST result appears ominous. It has been reported that loss of reactivity of the FHR is a late sign of fetal hypoxia, and this occurs later than appearance of late decelerations.

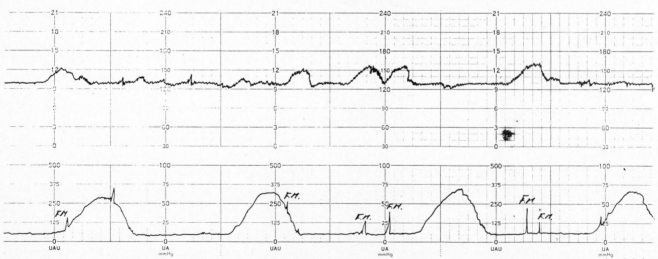

Figure 20–12   Example of a negative CST (and reactive NST). Baseline FHR = 130 with acceleration of FHR of at least 15 beats/min lasting 15 seconds with each fetal movement (FM). Uterine contractions recorded on bottom half of strip indicate three contractions in 8 minutes (with monitor paper speed at 3 cm/min).

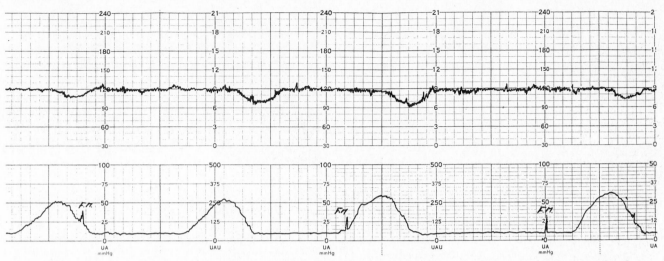

Figure 20–13 Example of a positive contraction stress test (CST). Repetitive late decelerations occur with each contraction. Note that there are no accelerations of FHR with three fetal movements (FM): Baseline FHR = 120 beats/min. Uterine contractions (bottom half of strip) occurred three times in 8 minutes.

Table 20–8 Interpretation of CST Results

CST	Findings	CST	Findings
Negative test	Three contractions of good quality in 10 min, lasting 40 or more sec, without late decelerations (Figure 20–12). Contraction of good quality lasting more than 90 sec; hyperstimulation without late deceleration. Usually associated with good variability of the FHR and acceleration of FHR with fetal movement.	Hyperstimulation	Contractions closer than every 2 min or lasting more than 90 sec with late decelerations; healthy fetus may show decelerations during a prolonged contraction. Repeat in 24 hr.
		Suspicious test	Nonrepetitive late decelerations occurring with less than 50% of contractions. Repeat in 24 hr.
Positive test	Occurrence of repetitive, persistent late decelerations with more than 50% of contractions; frequency of contractions need not be three in 10 min (Figure 20–13). Usually associated with decreased variability and lack of acceleration of the FHR with fetal movement.	Unsatisfactory test	Recording cannot be interpreted or contractions are inadequate, as a result of one or more of the following factors: 1. Obesity 2. Excessive maternal or fetal activity 3. Polyhydramnios 4. Fetal hiccups 5. Bowel sounds Repeat in 24 hr (may need to wait one week if unable to obtain contractions).

Kuschnick: "An Overview of Prenatal Screening and Genetic Counseling" *in* Human Prenatal Diagnosis, *Filliens and Russo, editors. Marcel Dekker, Inc., N.Y. 1985.*

Delivery is usually considered if it has been determined that the fetus's lungs are mature. Whether the woman with a positive CST should have a cesarean delivery depends on how rapidly the fetus must be delivered to avoid possible fetal distress, on the amount of dilatation, on the softness and effacement of the cervix ("ripeness") at the time, and on the woman's condition.

Although the NST is more commonly used for surveillance of fetal well-being in high-risk pregnancies, CST is still indicated for fetuses with IUGR, postmature fetuses, and pregnancies at particular risk for stillbirth. Because of the question of placental insufficiency in these situations, many authorities believe the CST is a better method of assessment than NST since it provides a test of stress to the fetus, who may have insufficient oxygen reserves. In addition this test may provide an earlier indication of impending uteroplacental insufficiency than lack of accelerations of the FHR.

Nursing Role

The nurse ascertains the woman's understanding of the CST and the possible results. The reasons for the CST and the procedure are reviewed before beginning the test. Written consent is required in some settings. In this case, the physician/nurse-midwife is responsible for fully informing the woman about the test. The nurse administers the CST, interprets the results, and reports the findings to the physician/nurse-midwife and the expectant woman. The nurse is available to clarify any further treatment ordered by the physician/nurse-midwife.

● Estriol Determinations

Estriol is a form of estrogen produced by the placenta. Its production depends on precursors from both the woman and fetus. For estrogen levels to be within normal limits, the mother, fetus, and placenta must be healthy, and all three must be functioning in harmony.

The amount of estriol in the maternal plasma or urine is an indication of the well-being of the maternal-fetal-placental unit. Estriol levels in both plasma and urine should increase as pregnancy advances, with significant amounts being produced in the third trimester. At term (40 weeks' gestation) the normal mean values of urine estriol are approximately 28 mg/24 hr and 14 ng/mL for plasma estriol (Kochenour 1982). Conditions that affect one of the parts of the maternal-fetal-placental unit can cause a decrease in the amount of estriol produced.

Determinations of estriol levels may be obtained by either a plasma (serum) or a urine test. Plasma tests are gradually replacing urine estriols because they are more quickly obtained and more accurate, although the woman must have a venopuncture each time. Urinary estriols require a 24-hour, accurate collection, which is often inconvenient for the pregnant woman but does not cause discomfort. Estriol level determinations are done serially (over time) in the management of high-risk women with hypertension, PIH, diabetes, renal disease, suspected placental insufficiency, IUGR, and postmaturity. Currently the role of estriol determinations is being questioned in light of other fetal assessment methods that are now available (Ray et al 1986).

Interpretation of Findings

The range of normal values is broad, and various patterns are seen in both plasma and urinary estriol levels. A single estriol measurement in the normal range does not necessarily indicate fetal well-being. Of more significance than any specific single value is the general trend in day-to-day or week-to-week values. Similar or gradually increasing estriol values are a sign of fetal well-being as long as the value stays above the critical level—12 ng/mL for plasma estriol and 12 mg/24 hrs for urinary estriol. A drop of 40 percent from the mean of the three previous highest consecutive values generally signifies fetal distress (Ray et al 1986).

● Amniocentesis

One of the most valuable studies available for the management of the pregnant woman is analysis of the amniotic fluid, which is obtained by a technique known as amniocentesis.

Determinations that can be made by amniocentesis early in the pregnancy include genetic studies. Later in the pregnancy, amniocentesis may be done for lung maturity studies such as L/S ratio and the presence of phosphatidylglycerol and phosphatidylcholine. This procedure is also used to determine the presence or absence of intrauterine infection with premature rupture of the membranes in preterm labor before tocolytic therapy is considered.

Amniotic fluid may be obtained by either transabdominal or suprapubic amniocentesis. Complications occur less than 1 percent of the time. The fetus, umbilical cord, or placenta may be punctured inadvertently, causing injuries ranging from minor scratches of fetal parts to intrauterine hemorrhage, leading to fetal distress and intrauterine fetal death. Placental perforation could result in hemorrhage from the fetal circulation, which could lead to fetal anemia or to increased sensitization of an Rh negative mother. Intraamniotic infection and induction of preterm labor are also hazards. Complications are rare, but the woman does need to be informed of them. A consent form is generally signed for this procedure.

Procedure

Amniocentesis may be done on an outpatient basis but needs to be performed near a delivery suite in case acute fetal distress is encountered. The woman should empty her bladder prior to the amniocentesis so that the bladder is not entered instead of the uterus. Amniotic fluid and urine may look similar, and if there is a possibility that urine was obtained during a suprapubic tap, the fluid should be checked for pH and protein content with a dipstick. Amniotic fluid has a high protein content, which is not a normal finding in urine unless the woman has been spilling protein in her urine as a result of preeclampsia or renal disease.

The abdomen is scanned by ultrasound to locate the placenta, fetus, and an adequate pocket of fluid. The amniocentesis, or "tap," is done immediately, before the fetus has the opportunity to move. The needle insertion site is of the utmost importance since the fetus, placenta, umbilical cord, bladder, and uterine arteries must all be avoided. The importance of locating the placenta cannot be stressed enough, especially in cases of Rh isoimmunization, in which trauma to the placenta increases fetal-ma-

ternal transfusion and worsens the immunization. In addition, if the placenta is anterior a suprapubic tap may be required to avoid puncturing the placenta. Except for very late in pregnancy, the fetal head can be displaced upward and the amniocentesis done suprapubically. If this is not feasible, it is usually done laterally (Figure 20–14). In the last few weeks of pregnancy, the fetus may occupy what appears to be all the available space in the uterus. There may be a decrease in the amount of available amniotic fluid. With the aid of ultrasound, fluid can usually be located, although in some cases it is impossible.

After the abdomen is scanned, the skin of the maternal abdomen is cleansed with povidone-iodine (Betadine). A 22-gauge spinal needle is inserted into the uterine cavity. Generally, fluid immediately flows into the needle. The first few drops are discarded, and then a syringe is attached to the needle and the fluid is aspirated (Figure 20–15). From 15 to 20 mL of amniotic fluid are withdrawn, placed in test tubes covered with tape (to shield the fluid from light to prevent breakdown of bilirubin and other pigments), and sent to the laboratory for analysis. The needle is withdrawn, and the FHR is assessed for ap-

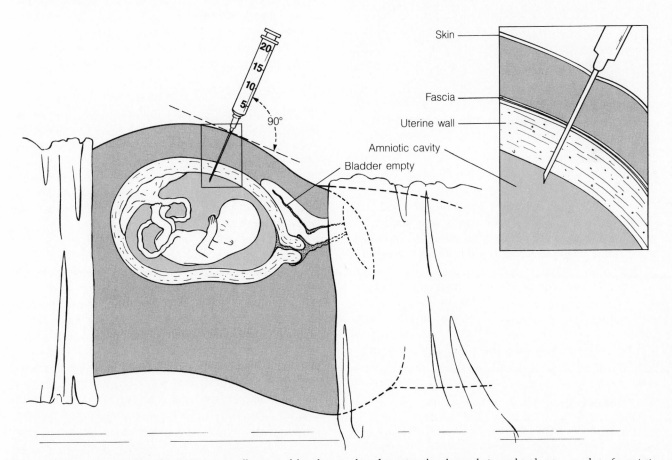

Figure 20–14 Amniocentesis. The woman is usually scanned by ultrasound to determine the placental site and to locate a pocket of amniotic fluid. As the needle is inserted, three levels of resistance are felt as the needle penetrates the skin, fascia, and uterine wall. When the needle is placed within the uterine cavity, amniotic fluid is withdrawn.

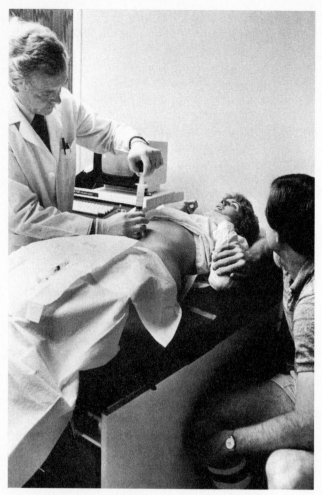

Figure 20–15 During the amniocentesis, amniotic fluid is aspirated into a syringe.

proximately 15 minutes. If the woman's vital signs and the FHR are normal, she is allowed to leave.

If the amniotic fluid becomes contaminated with blood, the fluid should be centrifuged immediately. The woman is observed closely for 30 to 40 minutes for alterations in the FHR. The blood should be tested to determine whether it is maternal or fetal.

Rh-negative women are given Rh-immune globulin after amniocentesis, provided that they are not already sensitized. If the amniotic fluid from these women is contaminated with blood, the sample should be tested to identify fetal cells. In this situation, a larger dose of immune globulin is required.

Nursing Role

The nurse assists the physician during the amniocentesis. Nursing responsiblities are listed in Procedure 20–1. In addition, the nurse supports the woman undergoing amniocentesis. Women are usually apprehensive about

what is about to happen as well as about the information that will be obtained by amniocentesis. The physician explains the procedure before the woman signs the consent form. As it is being performed, the woman may need additional emotional support. She may become anxious during the procedure. She may also become lightheaded, nauseated, and diaphoretic from lying on her back with a gravid uterus compressing the abdominal vessels. The nurse can provide support to the woman by further clarifying the physician's instructions or explanations, by relieving the woman's physical discomfort when possible, and by responding verbally and physically to the woman's need for reassurance.

Clinical Application

EVALUATION OF RH-SENSITIZED PREGNANCIES

The first studies of amniotic fluid were done in the early 1950s for the evaluation of bilirubin pigment in the amniotic fluid of Rh-sensitized mothers. The analyst could determine the degree to which the fetus was affected by looking at the optical density of the fluid.

Bevis (1956) reported that analysis of amniotic fluid of the Rh-sensitized mother could produce valuable information about the progress of her pregnancy. Liley (1961) produced a graph that is now universally used in determining the severity of hemolytic disease in the fetus (Figure 20–16).

If a sensitized Rh-negative woman produces an incompatible Rh-positive fetus, antibodies cross the placenta and cause hemolytic anemia in the fetus. Concentrations of bilirubin and other breakdown products from destroyed red blood cells can be detected in amniotic fluid by spectrophotometry. By plotting their concentration or optical density at 450 mu on a Liley curve, the physician can ascertain the degree to which the fetus is affected and the need for intervention or intrauterine transfusion.

Liley categorized the degree of hemolytic disease in three zones. If the optical density falls in zone I (low zone) at 28 to 31 weeks' gestation, the fetus will either be unaffected or have only mild hemolytic disease. Amniocentesis should be repeated in two or three weeks. When the optical density falls in zone II (midzone), amniocentesis is repeated frequently so that the trend can be determined. The age of the fetus and the trend in optical density indicate the necessity for intrauterine transfusion or premature delivery. Optical densities falling in zone III (high zone) indicate that the fetus is severely affected and death is a possibility. The decision concerning delivery or intrauterine transfusion depends on gestational age of the fetus. After about 32 or 33 weeks of gestation, early delivery and extrauterine treatment are probably preferred to performing intrauterine transfusion.

Procedure 20–1 Nursing Responsibilities During Amniocentesis

Objective	Nursing action	Rationale
Prepare woman.	Explain procedure. Reassure woman. Have woman sign consent form.	Information will decrease anxiety. Signing indicates woman's awareness of risks and consent to procedure.
	Have woman empty bladder.	Emptying bladder decreases risk of bladder perforation.
Prepare equipment.	Collect supplies: 22-gauge spinal needle with stylet 10 mL syringe 20 mL syringe Three 10 mL test tubes with tops (amber-colored or covered with tape)	Amniotic fluid must be shielded from light to prevent breakdown of bilirubin.
Monitor vital signs.	Obtain baseline data on maternal BP, pulse, respiration, and FHR. Monitor every 15 minutes.	Status of woman and fetus is assessed.
Locate fetus and placenta.	Provide assistance as physician palpates for fetal position. Assist with real-time ultrasound.	Real-time ultrasound is used to identify fetal parts and placenta and locate pockets of amniotic fluid. Amniocentesis is usually performed laterally in the area of fetal small parts where pockets of amniotic fluid are usually seen.
Cleanse abdomen.	Prep abdomen with Betadine or other cleansing agent.	Incidence of infection is decreased.
Collect specimen of amniotic fluid.	Obtain test tubes from physician; provide correct identification; send to lab with appropriate lab slips.	
Reassess vital signs.	Determine woman's BP, pulse, respirations, and FHR; palpate fundus to assess fetal and uterine activity; monitor woman with external fetal monitor for 20–30 minutes after amniocentesis. Have woman rest on left side	Fetus may have been inadvertently punctured. Uterine contractions may ensue following procedure; treatment course should be determined to counteract any supine hypotension and to increase venous return and cardiac output.
Complete client record.	Record type of procedure done, date, time, name of physician performing test, maternal-fetal response, and disposition of specimen.	Client records will be complete and current.
Educate woman.	Reassure woman; instruct her to report any of the following side effects: 1. Unusual fetal hyperactivity or lack of movement 2. Vaginal discharge—clear drainage or bleeding 3. Uterine contractions or abdominal pain 4. Fever or chills	Client will know how to recognize side effects or conditions that warrant further treatment.

EVALUATION OF FETAL MATURITY

In managing the woman and fetus at risk, the physician is constantly faced with the possibility of having to deliver an infant prior to term and before the onset of labor. There are many indications for early termination of pregnancy, including repeat cesarean delivery, premature rupture of the membranes, diabetes, hypertensive conditions in the pregnant woman, and placental insufficiency. Unfortunately, the most common cause of perinatal mortality is prematurity, especially in infants weighing 1500 g or less, and complications arising from pulmonary immaturity (Pernoll et al 1986); delivery of an infant with immature pulmonary function frequently results in RDS, also known as hyaline membrane disease (see Chapter 27).

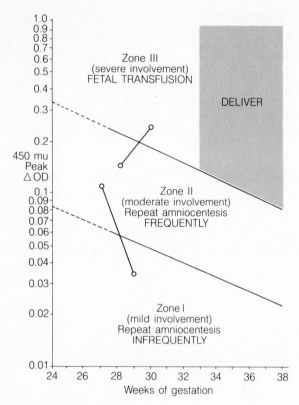

Figure 20–16   The density of amniotic fluid can be useful in determining the severity of erythroblastosis fetalis. There are three zones of optical density, which are correlated with the degree to which the fetus is affected by this condition. In this graph, management of the Rh-sensitized pregnacy is related to the condition of the fetus and gestational age. (Modified from Liley AW: Liquor amnii analysis in the management of the pregnancy complicated by rhesus sensitization. *Am J Obstet Gynecol* 1961;32:1359).

Because gestational age, birth weight, and the rate of development of organ systems do not necessarily correspond, it may be necessary to determine the lung maturation of the fetus by amniotic fluid analysis before elective delivery. Concentrations of certain substances in the amniotic fluid reflect the pulmonary condition of the fetus (see p. 557). In many cases, delivery of the infant can be delayed until the lungs show maturity.

L/S RATIO

The alveoli of the lungs are lined by a substance called *surfactant,* which is composed of phospholipids. Surfactant lowers the surface tension of the alveoli during extrauterine respiratory exhalation. By lowering the alveolar surface tension, surfactant stabilizes the alveoli, and a certain amount of air always remains in the alveoli during expiration. When a newborn with mature pulmonary function takes its first breath, a tremendously high pressure is needed to open the lungs. Upon breathing out, the lungs

do not collapse and about half the air in the alveoli is retained. An infant born too early in his or her development, when synthesis of surfactant is incomplete, is unable to maintain lung stability, resulting in underinflation of the lungs and development of RDS.

Fetal lung maturity can be assessed by determining the ratio of two components of surfactant—lecithin and sphingomyelin. Early in pregnancy the sphingomyelin concentration in amniotic fluid is more than that of lecithin, resulting in a low *lecithin/sphingomyelin* (L/S) *ratio.* At about 30 to 32 weeks' gestation, the amounts of the two substances become equal. The concentration of lecithin begins to exceed that of sphingomyelin, and at 35 weeks the L/S ratio is 2:1. Fetal lung maturity is assessed with 98 percent accuracy when the L/S ratio is 2:1 or greater; that is, when at least two times as much lecithin as sphingomyelin is found in the amniotic fluid (Figure 20–17). Infants of diabetic mothers are an exception to this and have a high incidence of false positive; the L/S ratio of 2:1 may not indicate lung maturity in these infants. Delayed maturation is often seen in infants of diabetic mothers because the high blood sugars interfere with biochemical development.

Some types of chronic intrauterine fetal stress cause an acceleration of lung maturation in the fetus. Prolonged rupture of membranes (over 24 hours) results in acceleration of lung maturation by approximately one week and therefore exerts a protective effect. Amnionitis and vaginal bleeding more than 24 hours before delivery also have a protective effect for the fetus (White et al 1986).

Although the L/S ratio has been one of the most universally used assays in evaluating pulmonary maturity,

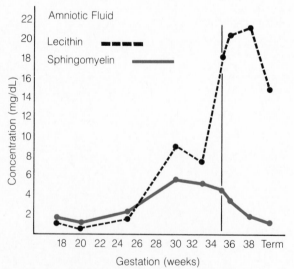

Figure 20–17   Mean concentrations in amniotic fluid of sphingomyelin and lecithin during gestation. The acute rise in lecithin at 35 weeks marks pulmonary maturity. (From Gluck L, et al: Diagnosis of the respiratory syndrome by amniocentesis. *Am J Obstet Gynecol* 1971;109:441.)

there are some associated limitations, including the following (Garite & Freeman 1986):

- It is time-consuming and expensive; it takes 4 to 5 hours to obtain if done in the same facility and more than 24 hours if it has to be sent away to a laboratory.

- Extensive training is required to perform the test.

- The presence of blood or other contaminants alters the results.

- There is a high rate of inaccuracy, that is, of predicting immaturity when the fetus is really mature.

Because of these problems, other tests have been developed and used to aid in assessing fetal lung maturity.

LUNG PROFILE

Some of the difficulties with the L/S ratio have been overcome by utilizing a lung profile of amniotic fluid to evaluate fetal lung maturity. The lung profile determines the presence of lecithin (phosphatidylcholine) and phosphatidylglycerol (PG), which are reported to be the major phospholipids of surfactant (Kogon et al 1986).

Lecithin accounts for approximately 80 percent of the total phospholipids in surfactant. Phosphatidylglycerol is the second most abundant phospholipid. Phosphatidylinositol (PI), increases in amniotic fluid after 26 to 30 weeks of gestation, peaks at 36 to 37 weeks, and then decreases gradually, whereas phosphatidylglycerol, appearing after 35 weeks, continues to increase until term. In instances of diabetes, complicated by premature rupture of the membranes, vascular disease, or severe preeclampsia-eclampsia, phosphatidylglycerol may be present before 35 weeks' gestation. It is helpful to know this fact, as early intervention in the event of lung maturation will lead to the best fetal outcome and prevention of RDS (Gabbe 1982).

The incidence of RDS in infants delivered of diabetic mothers with L/S ratios of 2:1 or greater is significant. Although it has been reported that in diabetic gestations a delay in the appearance of phosphatidylglycerol may occur, the presence of this phospholipid assists the physician in assessing the overall pulmonary status of the fetus in such pregnancies (Cunningham 1982).

Phosphatidylglycerol determination is also useful in blood-contaminated specimens. Since PG is not present in blood or vaginal fluids, its presence is reliable in predicting lung maturity (Creasy & Resnik 1984).

In recent years, lung maturity has been most frequently assessed by a combination of L/S ratio and PG. It appears that lung maturity can be confirmed in most pregnancies if PG is present in conjunction with an L/S ratio of 2:1.

Research on additional tests continues. Phosphatidylcholine phosphorus may be determined and its presence three to seven days before delivery is indicative of fetal lung maturity 94 percent of the time (Kogon et al 1986).

The fluorescence polarization test (also called microviscosimetry) is being used in some centers. Values of 0.320 are associated with fetal lung maturity (Garite & Freeman 1986).

SHAKE TEST (FOAM STABILITY TEST)

The shake test is a quick and inexpensive test for prediction of fetal lung maturity. It is based on the ability of surfactant in the amniotic fluid to form bubbles or foam in the presence of ethanol. The test requires 15 to 30 minutes. Exact amounts of 95 percent ethanol, isotonic saline, and amniotic fluid are shaken together for 15 seconds. The persistence of a complete ring of bubbles on the surface of the liquid after 15 minutes indicates a positive shake test, indicating lung maturity. There is a high false negative rate but a low false positive rate (Cruikshank 1982). Garite and Freeman (1986) have developed a fetal maturity cascade testing system for fetal maturity. The foam stability test is used first, and if it indicates maturity, no other test is done. If results are inconclusive or indicate immaturity, the next test is the fluorescence polarization test. If immaturity is again indicated, the L/S ratio is completed. More than half the time (63 percent), only a shake test is needed.

CREATININE LEVEL

Amniotic creatinine progressively increases as pregnancy advances. This may be due to excretion of fetal urine, which reflects fetal kidney function, or to muscle mass. The use of this value alone to assess maturity is not advisable since a high creatinine value may be a reflection of muscle mass in a particular fetus and not necessarily indicate kidney maturity. For example, the macrosomic fetus of a diabetic woman may have high creatinine levels due to increased muscle mass, or the small, growth-retarded infant of the hypertensive may demonstrate a low level of creatinine due to decreased muscle mass; in these cases creatinine values can be misleading if used without other data. Nevertheless, when fetal growth (muscle mass) and kidney maturity are at odds, the creatinine is still more indicative of fetal kidney maturity. Creatinine levels of 2 mg/dL of amniotic fluid seem to correlate closely with a pregnancy of 37 weeks or more (Creasy & Resnik 1984).

As long as the maternal serum creatinine is not elevated, measurement of creatinine level has a certain degree of reliability when used in conjunction with other maturity studies. An elevated maternal serum creatinine results in increased amniotic fluid levels. The woman's serum creatinine levels should be determined if the creatinine in the amniotic fluid is not what would normally be expected for a particular gestational age.

CYTOLOGIC EXAMINATION OF FETAL CELLS

One simple test of maturity, which can be done in the physician's office or at the bedside, is the staining of fetal fat cells in the amniotic fluid with Nile blue sulfate. The fetus sheds cells during its intrauterine life. In the last weeks of pregnancy the sebaceous glands gradually begin to function and cells are sloughed into the amniotic fluid. Sebaceous cells are different from other fetal cells in that they contain lipid globules. The number of these fat cells increases as the fetus matures, and the percentage of these cells present in the amniotic fluid gives an indication of gestational age. When the number of sebaceous cells (which stain orange with Nile blue sulfate) is 1 percent to 10 percent, the gestational age is between 34 and 38 weeks. Staining of 10 percent to 50 percent indicates 38 weeks' gestation or more (Creasy & Resnik 1984).

Identification of Meconium Staining

Any episode of hypoxia in utero may result in an increased fetal peristalsis, relaxation of the anal sphincter, and passage of meconium into the amniotic fluid. The amniotic fluid is normally clear, but the presence of meconium makes the fluid greenish.

Meconium staining may also be observed when amniocentesis is done. After the membranes have ruptured, meconium staining may be observed in the drainage from the vagina.

Once meconium staining is identified, more assessments must be made to determine if the fetus is suffering ongoing episodes of hypoxia.

Antenatal Genetic Screening

Antenatal intrauterine diagnosis by amniocentesis of many disorders that may result in a seriously deformed or mentally deficient child is a major advance in the field of perinatology. Indications for genetic amniocentesis and management are discussed in Chapter 9.

● ### Diagnostic Techniques of the Future
Chorionic Villus Sampling

Chorionic villus sampling (CVS), inaccurately referred to as chorionic biopsy, is performed in only a few medical centers throughout the world for first trimester prenatal diagnosis of genetic disorders. Although first proposed in 1968, it is still undergoing considerable research.

It is hoped that CVS will replace amniocentesis for prenatal diagnosis, except for diagnosis of neural tube defects (NTDs) (Ward 1985a). Because CVS makes possible earlier diagnosis of congenital defects, first trimester therapeutic abortion is possible if indicated and desired.

Villi in the chorion frondosum, present from 8 to 12 weeks, are believed to reflect fetal chromosome, enzyme, and DNA content, thereby permitting earlier diagnosis than can be obtained by amniocentesis. Various equipment has been used to aspirate chorionic villi from the placenta and three transcervical approaches have been used: "sampling by a flexible aspiration catheter under ultrasound guidance, by biopsy forceps under direct endoscopic vision, or by rigid biopsy forceps guided by ultrasound" (Brambati & Oldrini 1985, p 94).

After counseling regarding diagnosis and procedure technique, preliminary blood work is obtained. The morning of the procedure she is asked to fill her bladder, since displacement of an anteverted uterus may aid in positioning the uterus for catheter insertion. A high-resolution linear-array or sector ultrasound is used to determine uterine position, cervical position, size of the gestational sac, and CRL measurement and to identify the area of placental formation and cord insertion. The woman is then placed in lithotomy position; the vulva is cleansed with povidone-iodine solution (Betadine); and a sterile speculum is inserted into the vagina. The vaginal vault and cervix are cleansed with the same solution to decrease contamination from the vagina into the uterus. The anterior lip of the cervix is sometimes grasped with a tenacculum to aid in straightening anteflexion of the uterus. The catheter (or cannula) is slowly inserted under ultrasound guidance through the endocervix to the sampling site at the extraamniotic placental edge (outside the gestational sac) (Figure 20–18). The obturator is withdrawn from the catheter. A 30 mL syringe, containing 3 to 4 mL of Hank's solution with heparin, is attached and a sample of villi is aspirated by using a pressure of 5 to 10 mL (Brambati & Oldrini 1985). The contents of the syringe are flushed into a petri dish containing nutrient medium, and the villi are inspected microscopically and prepared for cell culture.

Complications of CVS include failure to obtain tissue, rupture of membranes or leakage of amniotic fluid, bleeding, intrauterine infection, spontaneous abortion, maternal tissue contamination of the specimen, and Rh isoimmunization. Rh negative women are given Rh_0 immune globulin to cover the risk of immunization from the procedure (Hogge et al 1986).

Fetal karyotype, diagnosis of hemoglobinopathies (eg, sickle cell anemia, alpha and some beta thalassemias), phenylketonuria, alpha antitrypsin deficiency, Down syndrome, Duchenne muscular dystrophy, and factor IX deficiency can be detected by this technique. Rapid sex determination can be made so that pregnancies with a male

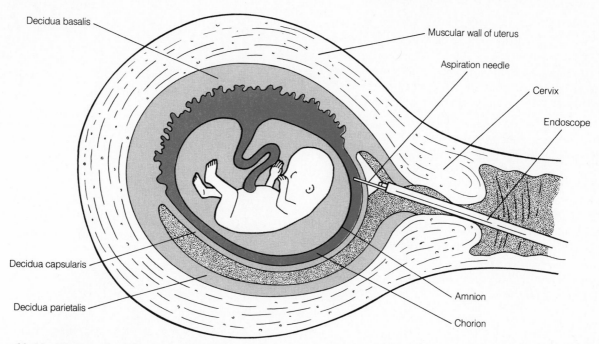

Figure 20–18 Diagram of eight-week pregnancy showing endoscopic needle aspiration of extraplacental villi. (From Rodeck CH, Morsman JM: First trimester chorion biopsy, in Ferguson-Smith MA (ed): *Early Prenatal Diagnosis.* New York, Churchill Livingstone, 1983, p 338.

fetus who would be affected in X-linked conditions can be identified early.

One of the greatest advantages to a mother undergoing this procedure is earlier diagnosis and decreased waiting time for results. Whereas amniocentesis is not done until at least 16 weeks' gestation, CVS is performed between 8 and 12 weeks. The CVS results are obtained in one to two weeks as compared to two to four weeks for amniocentesis. Earlier diagnosis may relieve many of the personal, social, and psychologic concerns of families.

Although the incidence of fetal loss is about 5 percent, deliveries that have occurred following this procedure have resulted in no neonatal malformations (Brambati & Oldrini 1985, Petrou et al 1983, Ward 1985b). Follow-up ultrasound and lab evaluation of each pregnancy must be done after performance of this procedure to evaluate fetal status; further neonatal follow-up studies are necessary to evaluate the long-term effects of this experimental technique.

NURSING ROLE

The nurse ascertains the woman's understanding of the CVS and the possible results. The reasons for the CVS and the procedure can be reviewed before the scheduled test. The nurse provides opportunities for questions and acts as an advocate when additional questions or concerns are raised. The nurse completes assessments following the procedure.

Fetoscopy

Fetoscopy, developed in 1972 but performed in only a few medical centers throughout the world, is a procedure for directly observing the fetus and obtaining a sample of blood or skin. It enables the physician to diagnose such conditions as fetal hemoglobinopathies, immunodeficient diseases, coagulation and metabolic disorders, chromosome abnormalities, Rh isoimmunization, and serious skin defects (Hobbins 1985). The associated risks include spontaneous abortion (5 percent), preterm delivery (9 percent) amniotic fluid leakage (1 percent) (Hobbins et al 1983), and intrauterine fetal death (Antsaklis et al 1985).

Prior to fetoscopy, women at risk for abnormalities are counseled by the genetic team. Indications, risks, and limitations of the procedure are thoroughly explained and a consent form is signed for the procedure, which is done at approximately 18 weeks' gestation. At this time vessels of the placental surface are of adequate size, and fetal parts are readily identifiable, yet therapeutic abortion would not be as hazardous at this time as if done at a later date.

Linear-array, real-time ultrasound is performed prior to and during fetoscopy to determine the gestational age, fetal position, placental location and thickness, location of umbilical cord insertion into the placenta, pockets of amniotic fluid, position of the part of the fetus or tissue to be viewed or sampled, and placement of the cannula (Antsaklis et al 1985). Following rapid intravenous sedation of the mother to decrease fetal activity, the abdomen is cleansed with povidone-iodine solution (Betadine), a local anesthetic solution may be injected into the maternal abdomen, and a 0.5 cm incision is made through the abdomen to the peritoneum.

A cannula, containing a trochar, is inserted through the incision into the uterus and the amniotic cavity to the site previously determined by ultrasound. The trochar is removed and amniotic fluid is withdrawn for genetic cell analysis and AFP level. A light source is connected to a 15 cm fiber-optic endoscope, which is about the diameter of a 16-gauge needle, and introduced through the cannula to visualize the fetus. The lens of the endoscope allows magnification up to 30 times, depending on the distance from the structure being visualized to the lens, and allows for a 55° field of vision (Rodeck & Nicolaides 1983).

If fetal blood sampling is to be performed, a 26- to 27-gauge needle is inserted through the side channel of the cannula and advanced until the vessel in the umbilical cord is pierced and a sample of blood is obtained (Figure 20–19).

The numerous indications for fetal blood sampling include suspicion of problems with hemoglobin or coagulation factors and need to assess for rubella, toxoplasmosis, and cytomegalovirus. In those facilities where percutaneous umbilical blood sampling (PUBS) is performed, fetoscopy is rarely performed for this purpose. During fetoscopy, blood samples can be taken from vessels in that portion of the cord that is a few centimeters from the placental insertion site. This is usually difficult, however, so a sample (approximately 0.5 mL) is collected from blood that leaks into the amniotic cavity after the needle is withdrawn from the vessel. Because blood aspirated by this method is mixed with amniotic fluid and diagnosis of various inherited diseases requires a pure fetal blood sample, in questionable situations blood is aspirated from a cord vessel at the placental insertion site.

Mother and fetus are monitored for several hours following the procedure for alterations in blood pressure and pulse, FHR abnormalities, uterine activity, vaginal bleeding, and loss of amniotic fluid. The woman is hospitalized until care givers are sure that no immediate complications have arisen. Rh negative mothers are given Rh_0 immune globulin unless the fetal blood is found to be Rh negative; antibiotics and tocolytics may or may not be given prophylactically. The following day, prior to discharge, a repeat ultrasound is performed to confirm the adequacy of amniotic fluid and fetal viability. Women are advised to avoid strenuous activity for one to two weeks following fetoscopy and to report any pain, bleeding, leakage of amniotic fluid, or fever.

Although amniocentesis permits the prenatal diagnosis of many sex-linked diseases, chromosome defects, and metabolic disturbances, the majority of fetal cells obtained by this procedure are not found to be viable, culture is difficult and lengthy, and many severe congenital abnormalities may only be diagnosed by direct visualization of the fetus or by analyzing fetal blood or skin tissue. Fe-

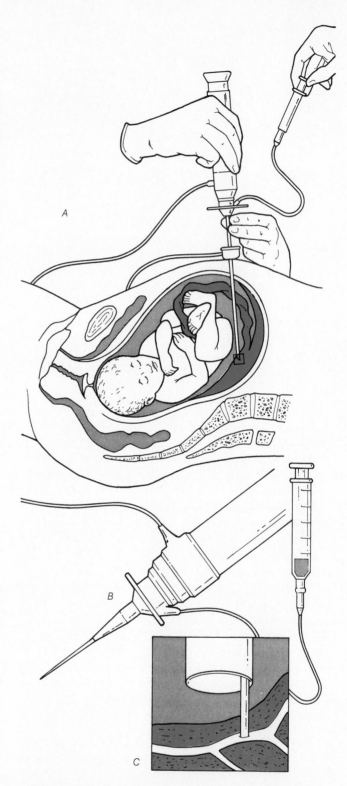

Figure 20–19 A Schematic diagram of fetoscopy for fetal blood sampling. B Detail of aspiration apparatus. C Detail of needle puncturing fetal blood vessel. (From McCormack MK: Amniocentesis for detection of sickle cell anemia and the thalassemia disorders using recombinant DNA methodologies, in Filkins K, Russo JF (eds): *Human Prenatal Diagnosis.* New York, Marcel Dekker, 1985, p 142)

toscopy has been used to view the extremities, spine, genitalia, and face in situations where the fetus is at risk for development of external abnormalities—such as limb and digital deformities, cleft lip and palate, and hereditary skin disorders—and genetic diseases affecting these structures.

As genetic amniocentesis, ultrasound, magnetic resonance imaging (MRI), chorionic villus sampling (CVS), and percutaneous umbilical blood sampling (PUBS) techniques become more sophisticated and conclusive of fetal conditions and more widely used, the need for fetoscopy will decrease except for unusual situations.

NURSING ROLE

The nurse clarifies the woman's understanding of fetoscopy, providing time for questions and acting as an advocate when additional areas of concern are raised. Following the test, the nurse completes assessments and continues to provide support.

Percutaneous Umbilical Blood Sampling (PUBS)

Since there is an approximately 5 percent risk of fetal loss associated with fetoscopy (Hobbins 1985), a new technique for obtaining pure fetal blood for prenatal diagnosis has been developed (Daffos et al 1985) and is beginning to replace fetoscopy in major centers. Although initially used at the time of therapeutic abortion to confirm diagnoses obtained by amniotic fluid analysis, this procedure has subsequently been used for diagnosis of hemophilias, hemoglobinopathies, congenital rubella, and toxoplasmosis and for fetal karyotyping. Percutaneous umbilical blood sampling (PUBS) is now being performed for second and third trimester prenatal diagnosis using fetoscopy only as a backup (Hobbins et al 1985).

The woman is scanned with a linear-array ultrasound transducer placed in a sterile glove, and a 25-gauge spinal needle is inserted into her abdomen through the skin alongside the transducer and into the fetal umbilical vein approximately 1 to 2 cm from the insertion of the cord into the placenta. The stylet is removed from the needle, and fetal blood is aspirated into a syringe containing an anticoagulant. Red blood cell size is determined to distinguish fetal from maternal cells. Premedication may be given to the woman if fetal movement is such that this becomes necessary.

No evidence of fetal bleeding during or following needle insertion was noted in one study (Hobbins et al 1985) and FHR monitoring following the procedure revealed no abnormal FHR patterns. Another report of over 400 cases (Daffos et al 1985) noted no fetal problems as a result of this procedure except for a transient fetal bradycardia in seven cases.

Although still undergoing considerable research, this new procedure appears to be a safe and simple way of obtaining fetal blood for prenatal diagnosis and therapy. It may replace fetoscopy because of the decreased risks, minimal expense, ease of performance, and the fact that it can be done on an outpatient basis.

NURSING ROLE

The nurse assesses the woman's understanding of the procedure and provides opportunities for additional questions. The nurse acts as an advocate when areas of concern are raised by helping the woman get additional information. The nurse completes needed assessments following the procedure.

Alpha-Fetoprotein (AFP) Screening

Alpha-fetoprotein (AFP) is a fetal serum protein produced in the yolk sac for the first six weeks and then by the fetal gastrointestinal tract and liver in the second trimester. The level of AFP in fetal plasma reaches a peak between 10 and 13 weeks and then declines until term, being excreted in fetal urine and subsequently into the amniotic fluid (Davis et al 1985). The AFP is found in the fetal circulation, amniotic fluid, and maternal serum. Elevated levels in amniotic fluid (AFAFP) or maternal serum (MSAFP) have been found to reflect open neural tube defects (NTD) such as spina bifida and anencephaly. Elevated levels have also been found in women with multiple gestation, incorrect gestational age, dead fetuses, and normal fetuses (Hobbins et al 1985).

The exact mechanism by which fetal AFP reaches the maternal circulation is unclear. Some authors state that it enters through the fetal kidneys and diffuses across the placenta to the maternal circulation (Jeanty & Romero 1984); others say it leaks through the meninges of the incomplete closure of the neural tube (spinal defect) (Hobbins et al 1985). Still others report that transfer cannot be explained on the basis of simple diffusion from the amniotic fluid to the maternal circulation, since they found no relationship between AFAFP and MSAFP levels (Barford et al 1985).

Maternal serum is assessed for AFP between 15 and 20 weeks' gestation. If the value is elevated, the results should be confirmed by a second sample. If the value is still elevated, a level II ultrasound is performed to rule out fetal abnormalities and an amniocentesis is performed to determine the AFAFP and acetylcholinesterase levels. The incidence of NTD has been found to be >95 percent when both these levels are elevated, and intestinal obstruction and ventral wall defects (gastroschisis and omphalocele) are likely if only AFP is elevated (Jeanty & Romero 1984).

How to Help Parents Make Informed Decisions Regarding Fetal Assessment Techniques

Diagnostic assessment and testing techniques increase in number and complexity with every passing year. Certainly the availability of these techniques has changed the outlook for pregnancies at risk or pregnancies with special problems. Using the new technology, the presence of the fetus can be confirmed and some congenital problems can be identified very early in the pregnancy. Indeed, fetal well-being can be assessed at various times throughout the pregnancy in order to identify problems and make treatment decisions. Because of these advantages, tests are used ever more frequently.

The childbearing couple needs to have as much information as possible in order to make informed decisions when faced with the array of new assessment technologies. Parents need to be clear about the purpose of the proposed test, the information that may be obtained, the risks and benefits for both the mother and the baby, and the alternatives that are available.

Although the majority of the diagnostic tests currently used are administered by physicians, nurses have an integral role in this arena as client educators and advocates. The nurse assesses the informational needs of the couple, provides the information, and ensures that the couple understands the diagnostic technique being used. The nurse does this in preparation for each test, even though the physician will still need to provide required information when obtaining a signed informed consent.

The provision of information and the securing of informed consent are essential, but occasionally problems can get in the way:

- To assure that the couple has a real choice about having the diagnostic test, the pertinent information needs to be provided ahead of time. It is difficult for parents to make other decisions or to refuse the test once they are in the actual test setting.
- It is often a challenge for nurses to obtain complete information regarding each new technique, and this may stand in the way of comprehensive and accurate teaching.
- Some nurses are unaware of the value they can bring to couples faced with diagnostic testing, and thus they ignore potential educational and advocacy roles.
- Often tests are done without any explanation to the couple. In some instances only the sketchiest information is provided. This makes it difficult for the couple to understand the situation and does not enable them to participate in their own care.
- Some physicians prefer that the couple not have much information, because this may cause them to worry unnecessarily. This approach can quickly lead to conflict when unanticipated problems arise and the couple feel they were not made aware of the potential risks.

In many areas of the country, measurement of MSAFP is presently being ordered routinely as a principal screening procedure for the detection of NTD. Because this method is sensitive but has low specificity, a level II ultrasound is usually performed prior to amniocentesis.

One research group (Hamilton et al 1985) noted an increased incidence of threatened and spontaneous abortion, antepartum hemorrhage, subsequent development of maternal hypertension, preterm labor, low birth weight, and other complications in pregnancies with normal fetuses when MSAFP levels were abnormally elevated. These authors suggest that in the absence of fetal abnormalities, women with elevated MSAFP levels should be closely followed and assessed during their pregnancy by biochemical and biophysical monitoring for fetal growth and the likelihood of preterm labor.

The incidence of NTD in the United States is 1 or 2:1000 (Queenan 1985). The number of false positive results depends on the cutoff level, but the higher the cutoff level, the greater the number of women who will be suspected of having an abnormal fetus requiring additional testing. Therefore, routine screening and cutoff level depend on the population area at high risk for NTD. There is controversy regarding the necessity for mass screening due to expense of testing, problems related to assay and interpretation of results, the number of false positive results, and the need for counseling. In any given population the cost-benefit ratio of this expensive screening test must be taken into consideration. Those women who may choose to be tested include those with a history of a child with a NTD, a strong family history of NTD, pregnant women with diabetes, and those residing in areas where NTD is prevalent (Queenan 1985).

Decreased levels of AFP in maternal serum have been found to be associated with fetal chromosome abnormalities (Merkatz et al 1984), and most recently with Down syndrome (trisomy 21), although the mechanism by which this occurs is not clear. Although reduced MSAFP levels have also been associated with trisomies 13 and 18, this cannot be explained by low levels of AFAFP (Davis et al 1985).

Specific cutoff values for any given set of maternal and gestational age groups are determined by the population being screened. Evaluation of any specific value is generally determined by the genetics department of the testing facility. Recommendations for follow-up assessment are then referred to the attending clinician responsible for the woman's prenatal course.

NURSING ROLE

The nurse ascertains the woman's understanding of the test and the possible results and clarifies any areas of questions.

Computerized Tomography (CT) Scanning

Computerized tomography (CT) is currently being performed in some regional perinatal centers throughout the country for assessment and management of women with breech presentations in labor (Gimovsky et al 1985). Minimal degrees of disproportion between the fetal head and maternal pelvis can greatly complicate the delivery of a fetus presenting as a breech. Pelvic diameters can be more accurately assessed by CT scanning than by previously used x-ray examination, and the exact degree of flexion and extension of the fetal head can be determined. This information assists the decision-making process regarding the safest delivery method for the fetus.

This method of evaluation is much superior to x-ray examination because of the significantly reduced dosage of radiation received. The International Commission on Radiologic Protection recommends that the fetus should not receive more than one rad during pregnancy. The fetus receives approximately 900 ± 100 millirad mean gonadal exposure via x ray; preliminary data suggest that the fetus receives only about 3 percent of this dose (approximately 20 millirad) via CT scan (Gimovsky et al 1985).

Magnetic Resonance Imaging (MRI)

The most recent advance in maternal-fetal assessment in the past few years has been magnetic resonance imaging (MRI). A major advantage of MRI is its ability to reveal previously inaccessible areas of the body without invasive techniques or risk of ionizing radiation. In addition, MRI can accurately distinguish between normal and impaired or diseased tissues and fetal and maternal anatomy. Although used in only a few selected regional perinatal centers and still undergoing considerable research, this new imaging technology is very promising as a complementary or alternative procedure to ultrasound imaging.

This type of imaging is similar to CT and ultrasound scanning. However, its advantages include the following:

- An image can be obtained in different planes.
- Fat and soft tissues can be differentiated easily.
- Assessment does not require the woman to have a distended bladder.
- The entire fetus can be imaged in one scan.

Disadvantages of MRI are its extreme expense to the woman, equipment expense, incapacity for real-time imaging, necessity of having a radiologist interpret findings, unavailability of imaging in the labor and delivery unit, longer performance time than ultrasound, difficulty in scanning when the fetus is moving a great deal, and occasional claustrophobia or intolerance by the woman of the confines of the magnetic unit for the extended periods of time required for scanning (45 to 60 minutes).

The woman is placed supine on a sliding table, which moves into a huge cylindrical unit. The outer layers of the cylinder contain coils of wires, which create a magnetic field when electricity is passed through them. The inner layers also contain coils of wires, which act like radio antennae, transmitting and receiving radio waves (energy) to and from the woman by creating a magnetic field and subsequently providing images of the part of the body being scanned (Johnson et al 1984).

Currently MRI can be used for confirmation of fetal abnormalities suggested by ultrasound examination, for pelvimetry, and for assessment of placental localization and size. In the future MRI may be used to assess fetal blood flow, nutritional status (IUGR), and intracranial anatomy.

No harmful effects have been reported in the literature, and clinical evidence to date indicates that MRI is safe. Even so, informed consent is required prior to performance of this procedure. The consent must include a statement such as, "There are no known or foreseeable hazards or risks associated with magnetic resonance imaging, although there may be risks to you or your baby at a future time which are currently unforeseeable" (Lowe et al 1985, p 629).

My first pregnancy was so tenuous that I didn't know from one moment to the next how it would end. I hoped for our baby's safety, but in the end the baby died. When I became pregnant the next time I was very nervous. Being able to see the baby on ultrasound helped me so much. I knew then that our baby was alive and growing.

KEY CONCEPTS

Diagnostic ultrasound is advantageous because it is noninvasive and painless, allows the physician to study

the gestation serially, is nonradiating to both the woman and her fetus, and to date has no known harmful effects.

The gestational sac may be detected as early as five or six weeks after the LMP.

During the first trimester, measurement of the CRL is most useful for accurate dating of a pregnancy.

The most important and frequently used ultrasound measurement is BPD.

Further ultrasound measurements that may be used include femur length, abdominal perimeter, and head-to-abdomen ratio.

Ultrasound offers a valuable means of assessing intrauterine fetal growth because the growth can be followed over a period of time.

A biophysical profile includes five variables (fetal breathing movement, body movement, tone, amniotic fluid volume, and FHR reactivity) to assess the fetus at risk for intrauterine compromise.

A new use of ultrasound is to examine fetal cardiac structures and functional status of the fetal circulation.

Maternal assessment of fetal activity can be used as a screening procedure in evaluation of fetal status.

A nonstress test (NST) is based on the knowledge that the heart rate normally increases in response to fetal activity. The desired result is a reactive test.

A contraction stress test (CST) provides a method for observing the response of the fetal heart rate to the stress of uterine contractions. The desired result is a negative test.

Amniocentesis can be used to obtain amniotic fluid for testing. A variety of tests are available to evaluate the presence of disease, genetic conditions, and fetal maturity.

The L/S ratio can be used to assess fetal lung maturity. The presence of PG may also provide information about fetal lung maturity.

Chorionic villus sampling is an experimental procedure that permits earlier diagnosis than is now available by amniocentesis.

Fetoscopy is a procedure for observing the fetus directly and obtaining a sample of blood or skin.

Percutaneous umbilical blood sampling (PUBS) is a new technique used in the second and third trimester for prenatal diagnosis.

Alpha-fetoprotein (AFP) screening of maternal serum provide information about the possibility of neural tube defects (NTDs) in the fetus.

Magnetic resonance imaging (MRI) can be used to assess previously inaccessible areas of the body via a noninvasive process without the risk of ionizing radiation. This procedure can accurately distinguish between normal and impaired or diseased tissues and fetal and maternal anatomy and pathology.

REFERENCES

Antsaklis AJ, **Benzie** RJ, **Hughes** RM: Fetoscopy: Fetal visualization and blood sampling in prenatal diagnosis, in **Filkins** K, **Russo** JF (eds): *Human Prenatal Diagnosis*. New York, Marcel Dekker, 1985, p 109.

Barford DA, **Dickerman** LH, **Johnson** WE: α-Fetoprotein: Relationship between maternal serum and alphafetoprotein levels. *Am J Obstet Gynecol* 1985;151(8):1038.

Bevis DCA: Blood pigments in haemolytic disease of the newborn. *J Obstet Gynecol* 1956;63:68.

Bishop EH: Fetal acceleration test. *Am J Obstet Gynecol* 1981;141:905.

Brambati B, **Oldrini** A: CVS for first-trimester fetal diagnosis. *Contemp OB/GYN* 1985;25:94.

Chez RA, **Sadovsky** E: Teaching patients how to record fetal movement. *Contemp OB/GYN* 1984;24(October):85.

Copel JA, **Pilu** G, **Kleinman** CS: Congenital heart disease and extracardiac anomalies: Associations and indications for fetal echocardiography. *Am J Obstet Gynecol* 1986;154(5):1121.

Copel JA, et al: Percutaneous umbilical blood sampling in the management of Kell isoimmunization. *Obstet Gynecol* 1986;67(2):288.

Creasy RK, **Resnik** R: *Maternal Fetal Medicine*. Philadelphia, Saunders, 1984.

Cruikshank DP: Amniocentesis for determination of fetal maturity. *Clin Obstet Gynecol* 1982;25:773.

Cunningham MD: Improved prediction of fetal lung maturity in diabetic pregnancies: A comparison of chromatographic methods. *Am J Obstet Gynecol* 1982;142:198.

Daffos F, **Capella-Pavlovsky** M, **Forestier** F: Fetal blood sampling during pregnancy with use of a needle guided by ultrasound: A study of 606 consecutive cases. *Am J Obstet Gynecol* 1985;153(6):655.

Davis RO, et al: Decreased levels of amniotic fluid α-fetoprotein associated with Down Syndrome. *Am J Obstet Gynecol* 1985;153(5):541.

Evertson LR, et al: Antepartum fetal heart rate testing. 1. Evolution of the nonstress test. *Am J Obstet Gynecol* 1979;133(1):131.

Freeman RK: The use of the oxytocin challenge test for antepartum clinical evaluation of uteroplacental respiratory function. *Am J Obstet Gynecol* 1975;121:487.

Friedman DM: Fetal echocardiography and doppler blood flow studies, in **Filkins** K, **Russo** JF (eds): *Human Prenatal Diagnosis.* New York, Marcel Dekker, 1985, vol 18, p 271.

Gabbe SG: Amniotic fluid indices of maturity, in **Queenan** JT, **Hobbins** JC (eds): *Protocols for High-Risk Pregnancies.* Oradell, NJ: Medical Economics Books.

Garite TJ, **Freeman** RK: EFM today: Nipple stimulation for antepartum testing. *Contemp OB/GYN* 1982;203:39.

Garite TJ, **Freeman** RK: Fetal maturity cascade: A rapid and cost effective method for fetal lung maturity testing. *Obstet Gynecol* 1986;67:619.

Gimovsky ML, et al: X-ray pelvimetry in a breech protocol: A comparison of digital radiography and conventional methods. *Am J Obstet Gynecol* 1985;153:887.

Gluck L, et al: Diagnosis of the respiratory distress syndrome by amniocentesis. *Am J Obstet Gynecol* 1971;109:441.

Grannum PAT, **Berkowitz** RL, **Hobbins** JC: The ultrasonic changes in the maturing placenta and their relation to fetal pulmonic maturity. *Am J Obstet Gynecol* 1979;133:915.

Hamilton PR, **Abdalla** HI, **Whitfield** CR: Significance of raised maternal serum α-fetoprotein in singleton pregnancies with normally formed fetuses. *Obstet Gynecol* 1985;65(4):465.

Hibbard LT: Placenta previa, in **Sciarri** JJ (ed): *Gynecology and Obstetrics.* Philadelphia, Harper & Row, 1985, vol 2, ch 49.

Hobbins JC: Fetoscopy, in **Queenan** JT (ed): *Management of High-Risk Pregnancy,* ed 2. Oradell, NJ, Medical Economics Books, 1985, p 231.

Hobbins JC, **Winsberg** F, **Berkowitz** RL: Normal and abnormal fetal anatomy, in *Ultrasonography in Obstetrics and Gynecology,* ed 2. Baltimore, Williams & Wilkins, 1983, p 113.

Hobbins JC, et al: Percutaneous umbilical blood sampling. *Am J Obstet Gynecol* 1985;152(1):1.

Hogge JS, **Hogge** WA, **Golbus** MS: Chorionic villus sampling. *J Obstet Gynecol Neonat Nurs* 1986;15:24.

Huddleston JF: Stress and non-stress testing, in **Sciarri** JJ (ed): *Gynecology and Obstetrics.* Phildelphia, Harper and Row, 1980, vol 3.

Jeanty P, **Romero** R: *Obstetrical Ultrasound.* New York, McGraw-Hill, 1984.

Johnson JM, et al: Biophysical profile scoring in the management of the postterm pregnancy: An analysis of 307 patients. *Am J Obstet Gynecol* 1986;154(2):269.

Johnson IR, et al: Imaging the pregnant human uterus with nuclear magnetic resonance. *Am J Obstet Gynecol* 1984;148(8):1136.

Kochenour NK: Estrogen assay during pregnancy. *Clin Obstet Gynecol* 1982;25(December):659.

Kogon DP, et al: Amniotic fluid phosphatidylglycerol and phosphatidylcholine phosphorus as predictors of fetal lung maturity. *Am J Obstet Gynecol* 1986;154(2):226.

Korones SB: The normal neonate, in **Sciarri** JJ (ed): *Gynecology and Obstetrics.* Philadelphia, Harper & Row, 1985, vol 2, ch 97.

Kremkau FW: Safety and long-term effects of ultrasound: What to tell your patients. *Clin Obstet Gynecol* 1984;27:269.

Leveno KJ, et al: Prolonged pregnancy. I. Observations concerning the causes of fetal distress. *Am J Obstet Gynecol* 1984;150(5):465.

Liley AW: Liquor amnii analysis in the management of the pregnancy complicated by rhesus sensitization. *Am J Obstet Gynecol* 1961;32:1359.

Lowe TW, et al: Magnetic resonance imaging in human pregnancy. *Obstet Gynecol* 1985;66(5):629.

Manning FA: Ultrasound in perinatal medicine, in **Creasy** RK, **Resnik** R (eds): *Maternal-Fetal Medicine.* Philadelphia, Saunders, 1984, pp 203.

Manning FA, et al: Fetal assessment based on fetal biophysical profile scoring: Experience in 12,620 referred high-risk pregnancies. *Am J Obstet Gynecol* 1985;151 (3):343.

Manning FA, et al: Fetal biophysical profile scoring: A prospective study in 1,184 high-risk patients. *Am J Obstet Gynecol* 1981;140:289.

Manning FA, **Platt** LD, **Sipos** L: Antepartum fetal evaluation: Development of a fetal biophysical profile. *Am J Obstet Gynecol* 1980;136(6):787.

Marshall C: The nipple stimulation contraction stress test. *J Obstet Gynecol Neonat Nurs* 1986;15:459.

McCluggage NA: Nipple stimulation contraction stress test. *J Perinatol* 1985;5(Summer):56.

McCormack MK: Amniocentesis for detection of sickle cell anemia and the thalessemia disorders using recombinant DNA methodologies, in **Filkins** K, **Russo** JF (eds): *Human Prenatal Diagnosis.* New York, Marcel Dekker, 1985.

Merkatz IR, et al: An association between low maternal serum α-fetoprotein and fetal chromosomal abnormalities. *Am J Obstet Gynecol* 1984;148:886.

Murray ML, **Canfield** S, **Harmon** J: Nipple stimulation-contraction stress test for the high-risk patient. *Am J Mat Child Nurs* 1986;11:331.

Patrick JE, et al: Human fetal breathing movements and gross fetal body movements at weeks 34–35 of gestation. *Am J Obstet Gynecol* 1978;130:693.

Pernoll ML, **Benda** GI, **Babson** SG: *Diagnosis and Management of the Fetus and Neonate at Risk.* St Louis: Mosby, 1986.

Petrou M, et al: Obstetric outcome in first trimester fetal diagnosis for the haemoglobinopathies. *Lancet* 1983;2: 1251.

Platt LD: A profile of fetal biophysical activities. *Contemp OB/GYN* 1982;19:225.

Platt LD, et al: A prospective trial of the fetal biophysical profile versus the nonstress test in the management of high-risk pregnancies. *Am J Obstet Gynecol* 1985;153(6):624.

Queenan JT: Maternal serum α-fetoprotein screening, in **Queenan** JT (ed): *Management of High-Risk Pregnancy,* ed 2. Oradell, NJ, Medical Economics Books, 1985, p 57.

Queenan JT: The NIH consensus report: A closer look. *Contemp OB/GYN* 1984;23(May):164.

Queenan JT, **Warsof** SL: Ultrasonography, in **Queenan** JT (ed): *Management of High-Risk Pregnancy,* ed 2. Oradell, NJ, Medical Economics Books, 1985, p 215.

Quinlan RW, et al: Changes in placental ultrasonic appearance. I. Incidence of Grade III changes in the placenta in correlation to fetal pulmonary maturity. *Am J Obstet Gynecol* 1982;144:468.

Ray DA, **Yeast** JD, **Freeman** RK: The current role of daily serum estriol monitoring in the insulin-dependent pregnant diabetic woman. *Am J Obstet Gynecol* 1986;154: 1257.

Rodeck CH, **Morsman** JM: First-trimester chorion biopsy, in **Ferguson-Smith** MA (ed): *Early Prenatal Diagnosis.* New York, Churchill Livingstone, 1983, p 338.

Rodeck CH, **Nicolaides** KH: Fetoscopy and fetal tissue sampling, in **Ferguson-Smith** MA (ed): *Early Prenatal Diagnosis.* New York, Churchill Livingstone, 1983, p 332.

Sadovsky E: Fetal movement, in **Queenan** JT (ed): *Management of High-Risk Pregnancy,* ed 2. Oradell, NJ, Medical Economics Books, 1985a, pp 183–193.

Sadovsky E: Monitoring fetal movement: A useful screening test. *Contemp OB/GYN* 1985b;25(April):123.

Schifrin BS, et al: Contraction stress test for antepartum fetal evaluation. *Am J Obstet Gynecol* 1975;45:436.

Shearer MH: Revelations: A summary and analysis of the NIH consensus development conference on ultrasound imaging in pregnancy. *Birth* 1984;11(1):23.

Spirit BA, **Kagan** EH: Sonography of the placenta, in **Raymond** HW, **Zwiebel** WJ (eds): *Seminars in Ultrasound.* New York: Grune & Stratton, 1980.

Spirit BA, **Kagan** EH, **Rozanski** RM: Abruptio placenta: Sonographic and pathologic correlation. *Am J Roentgenol Radium Ther Nucl Med* 1979;133:877.

Ward H: Chorionic villus sampling, in **Queenan** JT (ed): *Management of High-Risk Pregnancy,* ed 2. Oradell, NJ, Medical Economics Books, 1985, p 239.

Ward H: Symposium: Chorionic villus sampling: Something new in prenatal diagnosis. *Contemp OB/GYN* 1985;118.

Ward H: Symposium: NST or CST? What's best for spotting the high-risk fetus? *Contemp OB/GYN* 1985; 19(April):92.

White E, **Shy** KK, **Benedetti** TJ: Chronic fetal stress and the risk of infant respiratory distress syndrome. *Obstet Gynecol* 1986;67:57.

ADDITIONAL READINGS

Barss VA, **Frigoletto** FD, **Diamond** F: Stillbirth after nonstress testing. *Obstet Gynecol* 1985;65(4):541.

Boehm FH, et al: Improved outcome of twice weekly nonstress testing. *Obstet Gynecol* 1986;67(4):566.

Chervenal FA, **Isaacson** G: Sonographic detection of fetal neural axis anomalies. *Contemp OB/GYN* 1987;29(3):87.

Clark J, **Britton** K: Factors contributing to client nonuse of the Cardiff count-to-ten fetal activity chart. *J Nurse-Midwife* 1985;30(6):320.

Cohen FL: Neural tube defects: Epidemiology, detection, and prevention. *J Obstet Gynecol Neonat Nurs* 1987; 16(2):105.

Ernhart CB, et al: Intrauterine exposure to low levels of lead: The status of the neonate. *Arch Environ Health* 1986;41(5):287.

Fry ST: The ethical dimensions of policy for prenatal diagnosis technologies: The case of maternal serum alpha fetoprotein screening. *ANS* 1987;9(7):44.

Hogge JS, **Hogge** WA, **Golbus** MS: Chorionic villus sampling. *J Obstet Gynecol Neonat Nurs* 1986;15(January/February):24.

Huddleston JF, **Sutliff** G, **Robinson** D: Contraction stress test by intermittent nipple stimulation. *Obstet Gynecol* 1984;63(5):669.

Koren G, et al: Antenatal sonography of fetal malformations associated with drugs and chemicals. *Am J Obstet Gynecol* 1987:156(1):79.

Mayberry LJ, **Inturrisi-Levy** M: Use of breast stimulation for contraction stress tests. *J Obstet Gynecol Neonat Nurs* 1987;16(2):121.

McCluggage NA: Nipple stimulation contraction stress test. *J Perinatol* 1985;5(Summer):56.

Munsick RA: Similarities of Negro and Causasian fetal extremity lengths in the interval from 9–20 weeks pregnancy. *Am J Obstet Gynecol* 1987;156(1):183.

Sutliff JG, **Huddleston** JF: Antepartum bioelectric and biochemical fetal evaluation, in **Knuppel** RA, **Drukker** JE (eds): *High-Risk Pregnancy: A Team Approach.* Philadelphia, Saunders, 1986, p 38.

Thacker SB, **Berkelman** RL: Assessing the diagnostic accuracy and efficacy of selected antepartum fetal surveillance techniques. *OB/GYN Survey* 1986;41(3):121.

Thacker SB: The efficacy of intrapartum electronic fetal monitoring. *Am J Obstet Gynecol* 1987;156(1):24.

Williamson RA, et al: Abnormal pregnancy sonogram: selective indication for fetal karyotype. *Obstet Gynecol* 1987;69(1):15.

No matter how deeply we believe in the reasoning behind the decision to have an amniocentesis, the decision also offends our deepest wishes, dispersing a warm glow of inexpressible beauty with a grim, uncomforting light. (The New Yorker, "Talk of the Town")

Labor and Delivery

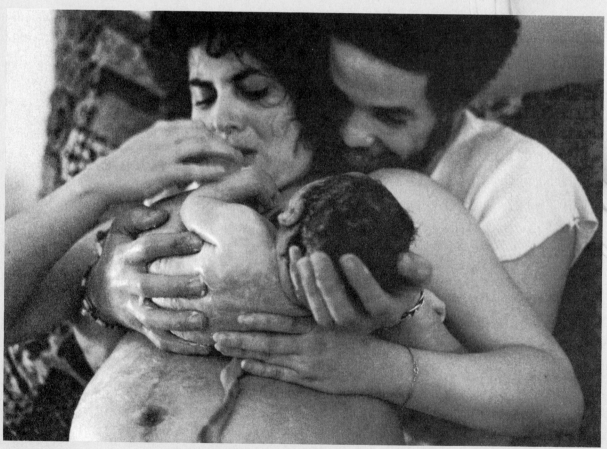

The nurse must respect and try to understand the particular style and needs
of each birthing couple.

Part Five

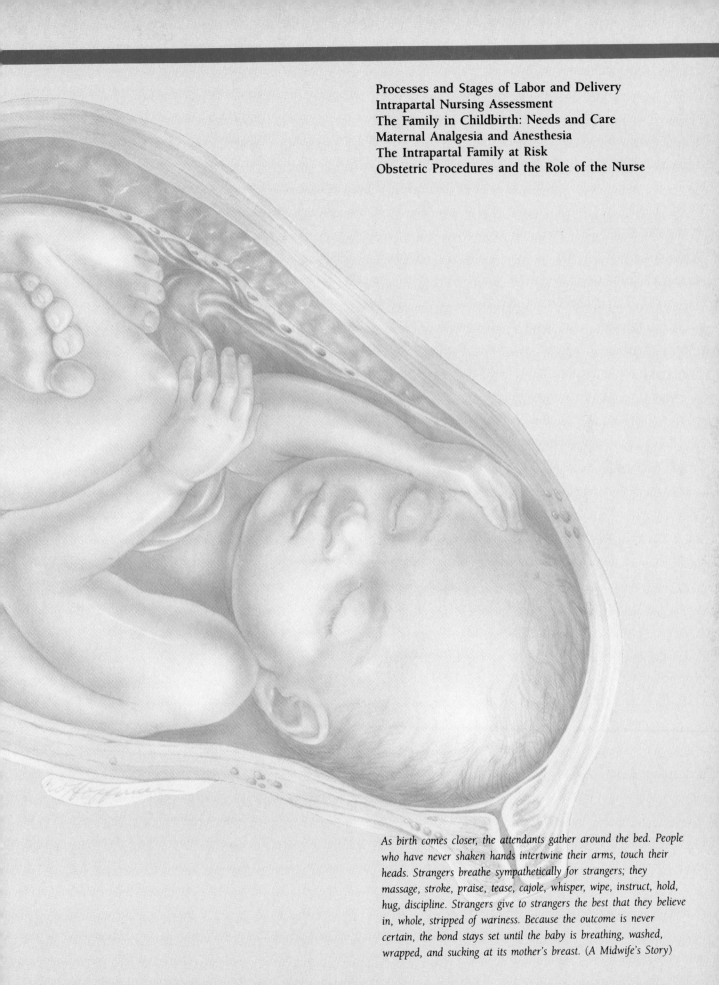

As birth comes closer, the attendants gather around the bed. People who have never shaken hands intertwine their arms, touch their heads. Strangers breathe sympathetically for strangers; they massage, stroke, praise, tease, cajole, whisper, wipe, instruct, hold, hug, discipline. Strangers give to strangers the best that they believe in, whole, stripped of wariness. Because the outcome is never certain, the bond stays set until the baby is breathing, washed, wrapped, and sucking at its mother's breast. (A Midwife's Story)

Processes and Stages of Labor and Delivery

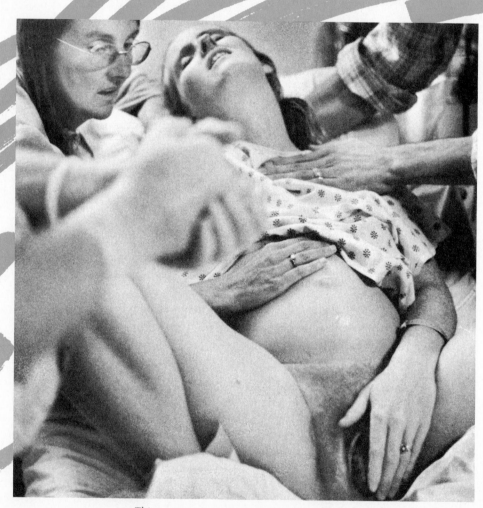

This nurse encourages a woman near the end of labor to rest between contractions and to feel her baby as the head begins to crown.

Chapter Twenty-One

OBJECTIVES

- **Relate the significance of each type of pelvis to the birth process.**
- **Examine the factors that influence labor and the physiology of the mechanisms of labor.**
- **Describe the fetal positional changes that constitute the mechanisms of labor.**
- **Explain the probable causes of labor onset and the premonitory signs of labor.**
- **Differentiate between false and true labor.**
- **Describe the physiologic and psychologic changes occurring in each of the stages of labor.**

T he process of labor and delivery signifies the end of the entire pregnancy cycle. During the months of gestation, the fetus and the pregnant woman have prepared to accom-

modate themselves to each other during the birth process. The fetus progresses through various stages of growth and development, preparing for the independence of extrauterine life. The pregnant woman undergoes various physiologic and psychologic adaptations during pregnancy that gradually prepare her for childbirth and mothering. For both the woman and her fetus the onset of labor marks a significant change in their relationship.

● Critical Factors in Labor

When examining the process of birth it is important to consider the birth canal, the baby, the uterine contractions, and the emotional state of the woman and her response to labor. It is sometimes helpful to remember these areas as the four Ps: passage (birth canal), passenger (fetus), powers (uterine contractions), and psyche (emotional state and response to labor). Each of the four Ps are further defined as follows:

1. Passage
   a. Size of the pelvis (diameters of the pelvic inlet, midpelvis, and outlet)
   b. Type of pelvis (gynecoid, anthropoid, platypelloid, or android)
   c. Ability of the cervix to dilate and efface and ability of the vaginal canal and introitus to distend

2. Passenger
   a. Fetal head (size and presence of molding)
   b. Fetal attitude (flexion or extension of the fetal body and extremities)
   c. Fetal lie
   d. Fetal presentation (the part of the fetal body entering the pelvis in a single or multiple pregnancy)
   e. Fetal position (relationship of the presenting part to the pelvis)

3. Powers
   a. The frequency, duration, and intensity of uterine contractions as the passenger is moved through the passage
   b. The duration of labor

4. Psyche

   a. Physical preparation for childbirth

   b. Sociocultural heritage

   c. Previous childbirth experience

   d. Support from significant others

   e. Emotional integrity

   f. Self-esteem

   g. Confidence

The progress of labor is critically dependent on the complementary relationship of these four factors. Abnormalities in the passage, the passenger, the powers, or the psyche can alter the outcome of labor and jeopardize both the pregnant woman and her fetus. Complications during labor and delivery are discussed in Chapter 25.

The Passage

In both males and females the pelvis provides support for the body weight and for the lower extremities. In the female, however, the pelvis must also adapt to the demands of childbearing (Pritchard et al 1985). Because the process of labor essentially involves the accommodation of the fetus to the bony pelvis through which it must descend, the size and shape of the maternal pelvis must be assessed by the health care team.

The true pelvis is divided into three sections: the inlet, the pelvic cavity (midpelvis), and the outlet. These are described in detail in Chapter 6, as are the pelvic measurements that influence the childbirth outcome. The techniques used to determine these measurements are described in Chapter 15.

TYPES OF PELVES

Familiarity with the types of pelves contributes to the understanding of the mechanism of labor and of the relationship of passage, passenger, and powers during the intrapartal period. The Caldwell-Moloy classification of the types of pelves is based on pertinent characteristics of both male and female pelves (Caldwell & Moloy 1933). Consideration is given to the size of the sacrosciatic notch, flaring of the pelvic brim, the shape of the inlet, and the relationship of the greatest anteroposterior diameter to the greatest transverse diameter.

The four classic types of pelves are *gynecoid, android, anthropoid,* and *platypelloid* (Figure 6–20). Mixed types of pelvic configurations occur more frequently than pure types. Each type of pelvis has specific implications for the process of labor and delivery (see Table 21–1).

○ *GYNECOID PELVIS*   Approximately 50 percent of female pelves are classified as gynecoid. The influence of a gynecoid pelvis on labor is favorable. Descent is facilitated because the fetal head usually engages in the transverse or oblique diameter with adequate flexion, and engagement occurs at midpelvis. The occipital anterior position at delivery is common (Oxorn 1986).

○ *ANDROID PELVIS*   Approximately 20 percent of female pelves are classified as android. The influence of an android pelvis on labor is not favorable. Descent into the pelvis is slow. The fetal head usually engages in the transverse or occipital posterior diameter in asynclitism with extreme

Table 21–1 Implications of Pelvic Type for Labor and Delivery

Pelvic type	Pertinent characteristics	Implications for birth
Gynecoid	Inlet rounded with all inlet diameters adequate Midpelvis adequate with parallel side walls Outlet adequate	Favorable
Android	Inlet heart shaped with short posterior sagittal diameter Midpelvis diameters reduced Outlet capacity reduced	Not favorable Descent into pelvis is slow Fetal head enters pelvis in transverse or posterior with arrest of labor frequent
Anthropoid	Inlet oval with long anteroposterior diameter Midpelvis diameters adequate Outlet adequate	Favorable
Platypelloid	Inlet oval with long transverse diameters Midpelvis diameters reduced Outlet capacity inadequate	Not favorable Fetal head engages in transverse Difficult descent through midpelvis Frequent delay of progress at outlet

Note: Description of pelvic shape is exaggerated for easier comprehension.

molding. Arrest of labor is frequent, requiring difficult forceps manipulation (rotation and extraction), and the deep, narrow pubic arch may lead to extensive perineal lacerations. Cesarean delivery may be required.

○ *ANTHROPOID PELVIS* Approximately 25 percent of female pelves are classified as anthropoid. The influence of the anthropoid pelvis on labor is favorable. Usually the fetal head engages in the anteroposterior or oblique diameter in the occipital-posterior position. Labor and delivery progress well.

○ *PLATYPELLOID PELVIS* Only 5 percent of the female pelves are classified as platypelloid. The influence of the platypelloid pelvis on labor is not favorable. The fetal head usually engages in the transverse diameter with marked asynclitism. If the infant can transverse the inlet, it rotates at or below the spines, and delivery is rapid through the wide arch. But frequently there is delay of progress at the inlet, requiring a cesarean delivery.

OTHER FACTORS

The passage is also affected by relaxin, a hormone released by the placenta. The presence of this hormone relaxes the pelvis and slightly increases the size of the pelvic diameters. During labor the pelvic diameters may be increased when the woman is in a squatting position or in a lateral Sims' position.

The Passenger

The unborn baby must accommodate itself to the maternal passage during labor. To pass through the relatively immobile pelvis, the fetus goes through a series of maneuvers to align its body with the maternal passage.

Movement of the fetus through the pelvis involves the articulation of the oval shapes of the fetus to the oval shapes presented by the maternal pelvis. The inlet of the more common gynecoid maternal pelvis presents a transverse oval (although the inlet is said to be rounded, the transverse diameters are slightly larger than the anteroposterior diameters). The outlet of the pelvis presents an oval passage that is anteroposterior or perpendicular to the ovoid of the inlet. The fetus brings to the laboring process two oval parts (head and shoulders) with a movable articulation at the neck. In a cephalic presentation (head first) the fetus enters the inlet with the first ovoid (the head), followed by the second ovoid (the shoulders) in a transverse direction. Herein lies the challenge of birth. The fetal head must enter the pelvic inlet in a transverse position and be rotated by the powers of labor to enter the midpelvis in an anteroposterior position. The shoulders of the fetus meanwhile must enter the inlet in a transverse position. As the head is lowered into the outlet, the shoulders

are compressed and rotated into the anteroposterior ovoid of the midpelvis (Oxorn 1986).

FETAL HEAD

The fetal head is composed of bony parts that can either hinder or enhance childbirth. Once the head (the least compressible and largest part of the fetus) has been delivered, there is rarely a delay in the birth of the rest of the body.

The fetal skull is composed of three major divisions: the face, the base of the skull, and the vault of the cranium (roof). The bones of the face and base are well fused and basically fixed. The base of the cranium is composed of the two temporal bones: the sphenoid and the ethmoid bones. The bones composing the vault are two frontal bones, two parietal bones, and the occipital bone (Figure 21–1). These bones are not fused, allowing this portion of the head to adjust in shape as the presenting part of the fetus passes through the narrow portions of the pelvis. This overlapping of the cranial bones under pressure of the powers of labor and the demands of the unyielding pelvis is called *molding*.

The *sutures* of the fetal skull are membranous spaces between the cranial bones. The intersections of the cranial sutures are called *fontanelles*. Presence of these sutures allows for molding of the fetal head and assists the examiner in identifying the position of the fetal head on vaginal examination. The important sutures of the cranial vault are as follows (see Figure 21–1):

● *Mitotic (frontal) suture:* Located between the two frontal bones; becomes the anterior continuation of the sagittal suture

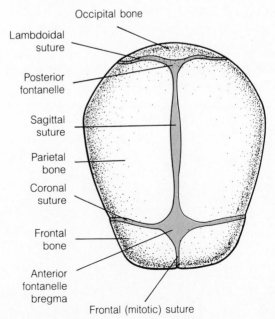

Figure 21–1   Superior view of the fetal skull

- *Sagittal suture:* Located between the parietal bones; divides the skull into left and right halves; runs anterioposterior, connecting the two fontanelles

- *Coronal sutures:* Located between the parietal and frontal lobes; extend transversely left and right from the anterior fontanelle

- *Lambdoidal suture:* Located between the two parietal bones and the occipital bone; extends transversely left and right from the posterior fontanelle

The anterior and posterior fontanelles are clinically useful in identifying the position of the fetal head in the maternal pelvis and in assessing the status of the newborn after birth. The anterior fontanelle is diamond-shaped and measures 2 × 3 cm; it facilitates growth of the brain by remaining unossified for as long as 18 months. The posterior fontanelle is much smaller and closes within 8 to 12 weeks after birth; it is shaped like a small triangle and marks the meeting point of the sagittal suture and the lambdoidal suture (Oxorn 1986).

Following are several important landmarks of the fetal skull (Figure 21–2):

- *Sinciput:* The anterior area known as the brow

- *Bregma:* The large diamond-shaped anterior fontanelle

- *Vertex:* The area between the anterior and posterior fontanelles

- *Posterior fontanelle:* The intersection between posterior cranial sutures

- *Occiput:* The area of the fetal skull occupied by the occipital bone, beneath the posterior fontanelle

- *Mentum:* The fetal chin

The diameters of the fetal skull vary considerably within normal limits. Some diameters shorten and others lengthen as the head is molded during labor. Fetal head diameters are measured between the various landmarks on the skull (Figure 21–3). The compound words used to designate the various diameters allow one to decipher which measurement is actually being reported. For example, the suboccipitobregmatic diameter notes the distance from the undersurface of the occiput to the center of the bregma, or anterior fontanelle. Fetal skull measurements are given in Figure 21–3.

Much can be learned from these diameters regarding the degree of extension or flexion of the fetal head. Extension of the head results in a larger diameter presenting than if the head is strongly flexed. Alterations in flexion of the fetal head can yield problems during the process of labor. The fetus endeavors to accommodate its most favorable head diameters to the limited measurements of the bony pelvis.

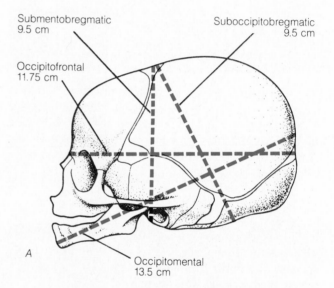

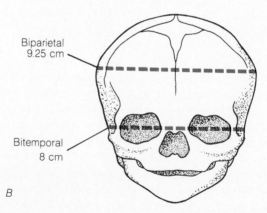

Figure 21–3 A Anteroposterior diameters of the fetal skull. When the vertex of the fetus presents and the fetal head is flexed with the chin on the chest, the smallest anteroposterior diameter (suboccipitobregmatic) enters the birth canal. B Transverse diameters of the fetal skull.

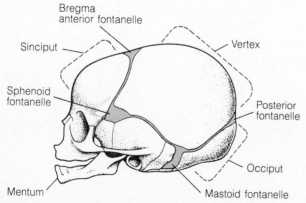

Figure 21–2 Lateral view of the fetal skull identifying the landmarks that have significance during birth

FETAL ATTITUDE

Fetal attitude, or habitus, refers to the relation of the fetal parts to one another. The normal attitude of the fetus, providing there is adequate amniotic fluid, is one of moderate flexion of the head and extremities on the abdomen and chest. This ovoid attitude has been called the *fetal position.* The back bows outward, the chin rests on the sternum, and the arms and thighs are flexed on the chest and abdomen. The fetus assumes various attitudes during the pregnancy, flexing and extending the arms, legs, and body. An extremely flexed and cramped attitude is maintained if the fetus has insufficient space in which to stretch, such as occurs in oligohydramnios (scant amniotic fluid).

Alterations in fetal attitude cause the fetus to present various diameters of the head to the maternal passage. With increased extension of the passenger's head, a larger diameter of the fetal skull must be accommodated by the pelvis. This alteration from a normal fetal attitude often contributes to a difficult labor. The fetus assumes a military attitude (chin up, shoulders back) when the head is moderately extended. Marked and excessive extension of the fetal head yield brow and face presentations.

FETAL LIE

Fetal lie refers to the relationship of the cephalocaudal axis of the fetus to the cephalocaudal axis of the pregnant woman. The fetus may assume either a transverse lie or a longitudinal lie. A *transverse lie* occurs when the long axis of the fetus is perpendicular to the woman's spine. The abdomen appears oval from left to right, with the buttocks of the fetus on one side and the head on the other. A *longitudinal lie* is assumed when the cephalocaudal axis of the fetus is parallel to the woman's spine. Depending on the fetal part entering the pelvis first, longitudinal lie may either be a cephalic (head) or breech (buttocks) presentation.

FETAL PRESENTATION

Fetal *presentation* is determined by the body part of the fetus that enters the pelvic passageway first. This portion of the fetus is referred to as *presenting part.* Depending on the attitude of the fetal extremities to its body and the fetal lie, the presentation is either cephalic, breech, or shoulder.

○ **CEPHALIC PRESENTATIONS** The fetal head presents itself to the passage in approximately 96 percent to 97 percent of term deliveries (Oxorn 1986). The cephalic presentations are classified according to the degree of flexion or extension of the fetal head. Thus the fetal attitude becomes critical in determining the type of cephalic presentation in each case.

There are four types of cephalic presentation. *Vertex presentation,* in which the head is completely flexed on the chest, is the most common cephalic presentation; the smallest diameter of the passenger's head (suboccipitobregmatic) enters the passage in this presentation (Figure 21–4A). *Military (median vertex) presentation* occurs when the fetal head is neither flexed nor extended and the occipitofrontal diameter is presented (Figure 21–4B). A *brow presentation* is assumed when the fetal head is partially extended and the occipitomental diameter, the largest anteroposterior diameter, is presented to the maternal pelvis (Figure 21–4C). The most extreme cephalic presentation is the *face presentation* in which the head is hyperextended (complete extension) and the submentobregmatic diameter presents to the maternal pelvis (Figure 21–4D).

○ **BREECH PRESENTATIONS** Breech or pelvic presentations occur in 3 percent of term births. These presentations are classified according to the attitude of the fetal hips and knees (see Figure 21–5 and Chapter 25, p 750). A *complete breech* occurs when the fetal knees and hips are both flexed, placing the thighs on the abdomen and the calves on the posterior aspect of the thighs. On vaginal examination both buttocks and feet can be palpated. Flexion of the hips and extension of the knees changes a complete breech to a *frank breech.* This presentation causes the fetal legs to extend onto the abdomen and chest, presenting the buttocks alone to the pelvis. The buttocks and genitals are palpable on vaginal examination when the fetus assumes a frank breech presentation. A *footling breech* presentation occurs when there is extension both at the knees and at the hips. A *single footling breech* presentation occurs if only one foot is presenting; a *double footling breech* occurs if both feet enter the pelvis first. In all variations of the breech presentation the sacrum is the landmark to be noted. See Chapter 25 for further discussion of the implications of the breech presentations for labor and delivery.

○ **SHOULDER PRESENTATION** A *shoulder presentation,* usually referred to as a *transverse lie,* is assumed by the fetus when its cephalocaudal axis lies perpendicular to the maternal spine (see Chapter 25, p 752). The fetus appears to lie crosswise in the uterus. Most frequently the shoulder is the presenting part in a transverse lie. In this case the acromion process of the scapula is the landmark to be noted. However, the fetal arm, back, abdomen, or side may present in a transverse lie. Unless the fetus rotates during labor to a longitudinal lie, the delivery must be accomplished by cesarean birth. See Chapter 25 for further discussion of the transverse lie and other malpresentations, and their effects on the labor and delivery processes.

The presentation of the fetus changes in the early part of the gestation. At 30 weeks' gestation there is a 75 percent chance that a malpositioned fetus will change to cephalic presentation. At 36 weeks' gestation, a malpositioned fetus will almost always maintain the malposition until delivery, and there is less than a 1 percent chance that a cephalic presentation will change to a malpresentation (Hughey 1985).

○ *FUNCTIONAL RELATIONSHIPS OF PRESENTING PART AND PASSAGE* *Engagement* of the presenting part takes place when the largest diameter of the presenting part reaches or passes through the pelvic inlet (Figure 21–6). The biparietal diameter is the largest dimension of the fetal skull to pass through the pelvis in a cephalic presentation. The intertrochanteric diameter is the largest to pass through the inlet in a breech presentation. Once the criteria for engagement have been met, the bony prominences of the presenting part are usually descending into the midpelvis and in most instances have reached the level of the ischial spines (Oxorn 1986).

A vaginal examination determines whether engagement has occurred. In primigravidas, engagement usually occurs two weeks before term. Multiparas, however, may experience engagement several weeks before the onset of labor or during the process of labor. If engagement has occurred, it means the adequacy of the pelvic inlet has been validated. Engagement does not suggest that the midpelvis and outlet are also adequate, however.

The presenting part is said to be *floating* (or ballottable) when it is freely movable above the inlet. When the presenting part begins to descend into the inlet, before engagement has truly occurred, it is said to be *dipping* into the pelvis.

Station refers to the relationship of the presenting part to an imaginary line drawn between the ischial spines of the maternal pelvis. In a normal pelvis, the ischial spines mark the narrowest diameter of the pelvis that the fetus must encounter. These spines are not sharp protrusions that harm the fetus but rather are blunted prominences at the midpelvis. The level of the ischial spines has been designated as zero station. Because in most instances the bony prominence of the presenting part has reached the level of the ischial spines, engagement is often said to occur at zero station. They are two distinct concepts, however (Figure 21–7). If the presenting part is higher than the ischial spines, a negative number is assigned, noting centimeters above zero station. Station −5 is at the inlet, and station +4 is at the outlet; the presenting part can be visualized

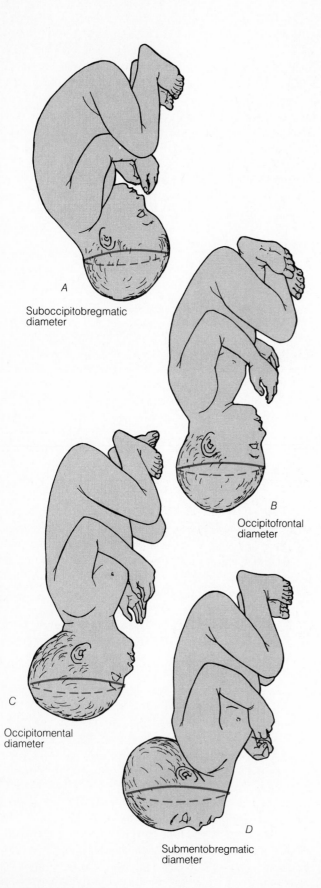

A
Suboccipitobregmatic diameter

B
Occipitofrontal diameter

C
Occipitomental diameter

D
Submentobregmatic diameter

Figure 21–4 Cephalic presentations. A Vertex presentation. Complete flexion of the head allows the suboccipitobregmatic diameter to present to the pelvis. B Military (median vertex) presentation, with no flexion or extension. The occipitofrontal diameter presents to the pelvis. C Brow presentation. The fetal head is in partial (halfway) extension. The occipitomental diameter, which is the largest diameter of the fetal head, presents to the pelvis. D Face presentation. The fetal head is in complete extension and the submentobregmatic diameter presents to the pelvis.

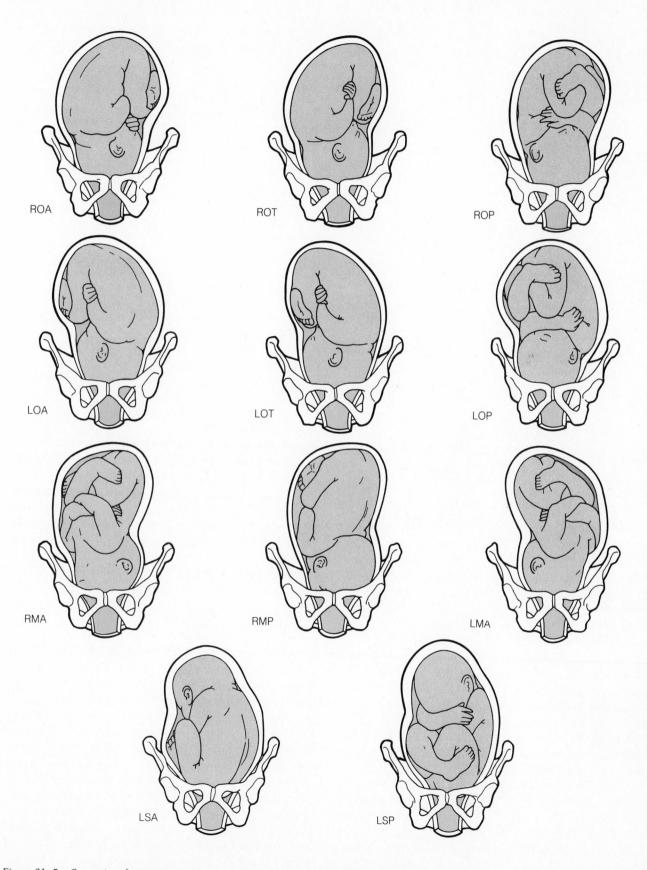

Figure 21–5 Categories of presentation (Courtesy Ross Laboratories, Columbus, Ohio)

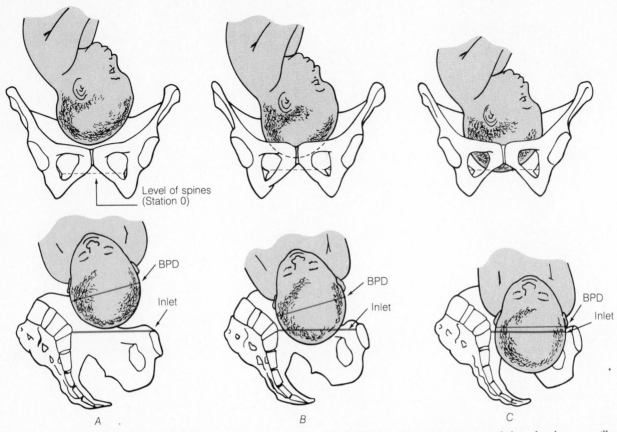

Figure 21–6   Process of engagement in cephalic presentation. A Floating: The fetal head is directed down toward the pelvis but can still easily move away from the inlet. B Dipping: The fetal head dips into the inlet but can be moved away by exerting pressure on the fetus. C Engaged: The biparietal diameter of the fetal head is in the inlet of the pelvis. In most instances the presenting part (occiput) will be at the level of the spines (zero station).

when viewing the woman's perineum—delivery is imminent. During the process of labor, the presenting part should move progressively from the negative stations to the midpelvis at zero station and into the positive stations. Failure of the presenting part to descend in the presence of strong contractions may be due to disproportion between the maternal pelvis and fetal presenting part, or a short and/or entangled umbilical cord.

When both pelvic and fetal planes are parallel, the relationship is said to be *synclitic.* Thus in a cephalic presentation, engagement occurs in synclitism when the biparietal diameter of the fetal head is parallel to the sacrum and the symphysis pubis. Engagement in synclitism takes place when the uterus is perpendicular to the inlet, not retroflexed or anteflexed. Synclitic engagement may also indicate that the pelvis is roomy.

Asynclitism indicates that the uterus is not perpendicular to the inlet and that the fetal head is not parallel to the planes of the pelvis. This usually occurs with small pelvic diameters or with weak abdominal musculature that allows the uterus to tilt anteriorly or posteriorly. When there is a large fetal head or small pelvic diameters, asynclitism facilitates engagement by allowing a smaller diam-

eter of the fetal head to enter the pelvis. Persistent asynclitism may cause difficulties, however, preventing normal rotation of the head in the pelvis (Oxorn 1986). See Table 21–2 for fetopelvic relationships.

FETAL POSITION

Fetal *position* refers to the relationship of the landmark on the presenting fetal part to the front, sides, or back of the maternal pelvis. The landmark on the fetal presenting part is related to four imaginary quadrants of the pelvis: left anterior, right anterior, left posterior, and right posterior. These quadrants assist in designating whether the presenting part is directed toward the front, back, left, or right of the passage. The landmark chosen for cephalic presentations is the occiput in vertex presentations and the mentum in face presentations. Breech presentations use the sacrum as the designated landmark, and the acromion process on the scapula is noted in shoulder presentations. If the landmark is directed toward the center of the side of the pelvis, it is designated as a *transverse position,* rather than anterior or posterior.

Three notations are used to describe the fetal position:

1. Right (R) or left (L) side of the maternal pelvis

2. The landmark of the fetal presenting part: occiput (O), mentum (M), sacrum (S), or acromion process (A)

3. Anterior (A), posterior (P), or transverse (T), depending on whether the landmark is in the front, back, or side of the pelvis

Abbreviations are formed from these notations to assist the health care team in communicating the fetal position. Hence, when the fetal occiput is directed toward the back and to the left of the passage, the abbreviation used in LOP (left-occiput-posterior). The term *dorsal* (D) is used when denoting the fetal position in a transverse lie; it refers to the fetal back. Thus the abbreviation RADA indicates that the acromion process of the scapula is directed toward the woman's right and the passenger's back is anterior.

Following is a list of the positions for various fetal presentations, some of which are illustrated in Figure 21–5.

Positions in vertex presentation:

ROA Right-occiput-anterior

ROT Right-occiput-transverse

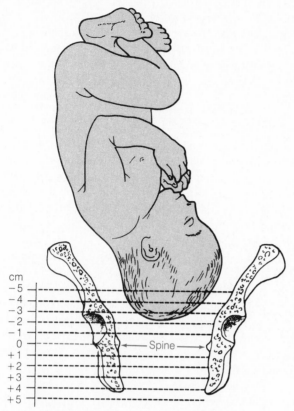

Figure 21–7 Measuring station of the fetal head while it is descending. In this view the station is − 2/ − 3.

Table 21–2 Fetopelvic Relationships

Presentation	Attitude	Presenting part	Landmark
Longitudinal lie (99.5%)			
Cephalic (96 to 97%)	Flexion	Vertex (posterior part)	Occiput (O)
	Military	Vertex (median part)	Occiput (O)
	Partial extension	Brow	Forehead (frontum) (Fr)
	Complete extension	Face	Chin (mentum) (M)
Breech (3 to 4%)			
Complete	Flexed hips and knees	Buttocks	Sacrum (S)
Frank	Flexed hips, extended knees	Buttocks	Sacrum (S)
Footling: single, double	Extended hips and knees	Feet	Sacrum (S)
Kneeling: single, double	Extended hips; flexed knees	Knees	Sacrum (S)
Transverse or oblique lie (0.5%)			
Shoulder	Variable	Shoulder, arm, trunk	Scapula (Sc or A)

Adapted from Oxorn H: *Human Labor and Birth,* 5 ed. Norwalk, Conn, Appleton-Century-Crofts, 1986, p 54.

ROP   Right-occiput-posterior

LOA   Left-occiput-anterior

LOT   Left-occiput-transverse

LOP   Left-occiput-posterior

Positions in face presentation:

RMA   Right-mentum-anterior

RMT   Right-mentum-transverse

RMP   Right-mentum-posterior

LMA   Left-mentum-anterior

LMT   Left-mentum-transverse

LMP   Left-mentum-posterior

Positions in breech presentation:

RSA   Right-sacrum-anterior

RST   Right-sacrum-transverse

RSP   Right-sacrum-posterior

LSA   Left-sacrum-anterior

LST   Left-sacrum-transverse

LSP   Left-sacrum-posterior

Positions in shoulder presentation:

RADA Right-acromion-dorsal-anterior

RADP Right-acromion-dorsal-posterior

LADA Left-acromion-dorsal-anterior

LADP Left-acromion-dorsal-posterior

The fetal position influences labor and delivery. For example, a posterior position causes a larger diameter of the fetal head to enter the pelvis than in an anterior position. With a posterior position, pressure on the sacral nerves is increased, causing the laboring woman backache and pelvic pressure and perhaps encouraging her to bear down or push earlier than normal. (See Chapter 25 for an in-depth discussion of malpositions and their management.)

Assessment techniques to determine fetal position include inspection and palpation of the maternal abdomen, and vaginal examination (see Chapter 22 for further discussion of assessment of fetal position).

The Powers

Primary and secondary powers work complementarily to deliver the fetus, the fetal membranes, and placenta from the uterus into the external environment. The primary power is uterine muscular contractions, which effect the changes of the first stage of labor—complete effacement and dilatation of the cervix. The second power is the use of abdominal and intercostal muscles in pushing during the second stage of labor. The pushing adds to the primary power after full dilatation has occurred.

UTERINE RESPONSE

In labor, *uterine contractions* are rhythmical but intermittent, which allows for a period of uterine relaxation between contractions. This period of relaxation allows uterine muscles to rest and provides respite for the laboring woman. It also restores uteroplacental circulation, which is important to fetal oxygenation and adequate circulation in the uterine blood vessels.

Each contraction has three phases: (a) *increment,* the "building up" of the contraction (the longest phase); (b) *acme* or the peak of the contraction; and (c) *decrement* or the "letting up" of the contraction. When describing uterine contractions during labor, the terms frequency, duration, and intensity are used. *Frequency* refers to the period of time between the beginning of one contraction to the beginning of the next contraction.

The *duration* of each contraction is measured from the beginning of the increment to the completion of decrement (Figure 21–8). In beginning labor, the duration is about 30 seconds. As labor continues duration lengthens to an average of 60 seconds with a range of 45 to 90 seconds (Varney 1980).

Intensity refers to the strength of the uterine contraction during acme. In most instances it is estimated by palpating the contraction but it may be measured directly through the use of an intrauterine catheter. When estimating intensity by palpation, the nurse determines whether it is mild, moderate, or strong by judging the amount of indentability of the uterine wall during the acme of a contraction. If the uterine wall can be indented easily, it is considered mild. Strong intensity would be achieved when the uterine wall cannot be indented. Moderate intensity falls between these two ranges. When intensity is measured by the use of an intrauterine catheter, the normal resting tonus (between contractions) averages 10 mm Hg of pressure. During acme the intensity ranges from 30 to 55 mm Hg of pressure (Cibils 1981). (See discussion on stages of labor, p. 595; and Chapter 22 for further discussion of assessment techniques.)

At the beginning of labor, the contractions are usually mild, of short duration, and relatively infrequent. As labor progresses, the duration lengthens, the intensity increases, and the frequency is every two to three minutes. It is important to remember the contractions are involuntary and the laboring woman cannot control their duration, frequency, or intensity.

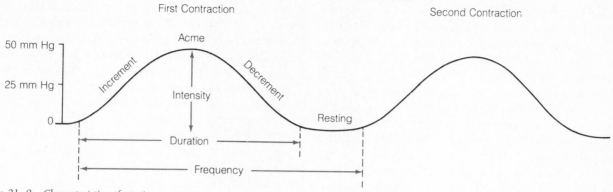

Figure 21–8   Characteristics of uterine contractions

The Psyche

Rubin (1984, p 52) notes that childbearing "requires an exchange of a known self in a known world for an unknown self in an unknown world. This is an act of courage. . . ." And no part of the childbearing period brings this more to light than labor. Every woman is uncertain about what her labor will be like: A woman anticipating her first labor faces a totally new experience, and even multiparas cannot be certain what each new labor will bring. The woman does not know whether she will live up to her expectations for herself in relation to her friends and relatives, whether she will be physically injured through laceration, episiotomy, or cesarean incision, or whether significant others will be as supportive as she hopes (Mercer 1981, Mercer 1985). The woman faces an irrevocable event—the birth of a new family member—and, consequently, disruption of life-style, relationships, and self-image. Finally, the woman must deal with concerns about her loss of control of bodily functions, emotional responses to an unfamiliar situation, and reactions to the pain associated with labor.

Various factors influence a woman's reaction to the physical and emotional crisis of labor (Table 21–3). Her accomplishment of the tasks of pregnancy, usual coping mechanisms in response to stressful life events, support system, and preparation for childbirth and cultural influences are all significant factors.

PREPARATION FOR LABOR

In her study of the psychosocial adaptations of pregnancy Lederman (1984) found that certain psychosocial factors of pregnancy were predictive of progress in labor. One such factor was related to a woman's psychological preparation for labor. Lederman found that expectant women prepared for labor through actions and through imaginary rehearsal. The actions frequently consisted of "nesting behavior" and a "psyching up" for the labor, which seemed to vary depending on the woman's sense of self-confidence, self-esteem, and previous experiences with stress. Specific actions to prepare for labor are usually focused on becoming better informed and prepared. Many women attended prenatal classes to learn about labor and to share the birth experience with their husbands. Others hoped that learning specific techniques of relaxation and breathing would allow them more control during labor so they could take a more active part. Additional information was gained through viewing films, reading books, and talking to other women.

An important developmental step for expectant women is to anticipate the labor in fantasy. Just as women "try on" the maternal role during pregnancy, fantasizing about labor seems to help the woman understand and become more prepared for labor. Her fantasies about the excitement of the baby's birth and the sharing of the experience involve her in constructive preparation even though she may still have some fears of labor. Women who have a great deal of apprehension about becoming a mother or a high fear of pain during labor are not able to fantasize the labor in positive ways and instead have many disturbing thoughts (Lederman 1984).

Positive fantasies seem to involve many areas. The woman thinks about the contractions and the work and pain that will be involved, and this seems to provide a

Table 21–3   Factors Associated With a Positive Birth Experience

Motivation for the pregnancy
Attendance at childbirth education classes
A sense of competence or mastery
Self-confidence and self-esteem
Positive relationship with mate
Maintaining control during labor
Support from mate or other person during labor
Not being left alone in labor
Trust in the medical/nursing staff

stimulus to becoming more prepared for labor. Lederman (1984) found that women who were able to visualize themselves as active participants in labor were usually well prepared and had positive self-images. Fantasy and thoughts about labor help the woman to have realistic ideas about the work, pain, and risks involved and to develop a sense of confidence in her ability to cope.

Many woman fear the pain of contractions. They not only see the pain as threatening but also associate it with a loss of control over their bodies and emotions. Our society seems to value control and cooperation with established routines in health care settings. When a woman is facing labor, especially for the first time, she may worry about her ability to withstand the pain of labor and maintain control over herself. Women are afraid of becoming fatigued and unable to relax because they may then act in a way that is undesirable or may induce bodily injury. In Lederman's study the women who were confident of their abilities usually had less fear than women who doubted their ability to maintain control of themselves.

COPING MECHANISMS

Westbrook (1979) suggests that "the ways in which a person copes with an event are dependent on how the event is experienced as well as the coping skills the person has acquired." Therefore, coping mechanisms related to pregnancy are expected to be consistent with those typical of the individual and influenced by perception of the experience. Westbrook looked at three groups of new mothers by socioeconomic level (working, middle, and upper-middle class) in relation to their perceptions of the positive and negative aspects of childbearing and their coping mechanisms. Positive aspects of childbearing include enhancement of the woman's femininity, feelings of well-being, sense of value as a person, and feelings of maturity.

Negative aspects of childbearing include rejection of the pregnancy and/or infant; anticipation of problems during labor (fear, poor performance, lack of support); fear of physical harm to self during labor; physical discomfort of pregnancy; problems of infant care and worries about conflicting advice; the family's coping abilities, and the well-being of the infant.

Perceptions of the pregnancy, labor, and delivery experience by women varied significantly by socioeconomic status because coping mechanisms vary from class to class. Some typical coping strategies are confrontation, avoidance, optimism, seeking interpersonal help, fatalism, and control. Working-class women expressed positive attitudes toward childbearing, experiencing it as a satisfying and enhancing experience. On the other hand, they had negative attitudes toward labor compared with the middle-class and upper-middle-class women. They complained of more physical discomfort and were, in general, more fearful of the physical processes of childbearing. These responses may reflect the perceptions of working-class women that they are less in control of events. It also suggests a greater use of fatalistic mechanisms and avoidance rather than confrontation (which is used more by middle-class and upper-middle-class women) in coping strategies. The working-class women also had the lowest attendance at childbirth classes despite adequate time, availability, and transportation, further indicating their reliance on avoidance of these activities related to perceived uncontrollable stresses (in this case, the childbirth classes were intended to help them to deal with physical control of labor).

SUPPORT SYSTEMS

The childbearing experience has traditionally been a group endeavor centered around the laboring woman. Long recognized as a major developmental transition or crisis, childbirth has brought with it numerous rites of passage (Chaney 1980). These rituals typically included both father and mother as well as significant members of the family and community. The role of the father has been often considered to have direct bearing on the outcome of the pregnancy (Heggenhougen 1980).

In most developed Western countries relatively little attention has been paid to the role of the father and support systems in childbirth. Changes in practice by the medical profession have not related to the needs of the family during childbirth. Instead the experience of the family has been forced to adapt to the needs of the caretakers. Only in the past decade has a significant thrust toward family-centered maternity care, and concern for the intrapartal needs of the family, been prevalent. As recently as the mid-1970s many hospitals continued to ban fathers from the labor rooms.

Current research and theory suggest that the support of the father or labor partner during birth positively affects the birth experience (Copstik 1986, Mishel & Braden 1987).

CHILDBIRTH PREPARATION CLASSES

Much attention has been focused on preparation during pregnancy as a way of increasing the woman's ability to cope during childbirth, decreasing her experienced stress, anxiety, and pain, and imparting satisfaction with the childbearing experience. Pain management has been viewed as the primary factor in providing a good childbirth experience (Humenick 1981, Mercer 1985), although current research does not support this concept. Doering and Entwisle (1975) point out that preparation for childbirth does not necessarily lead to a decrease in pain. Physical and psychologic awareness of the childbearing experience, that is, maternal awareness without spinal or general anesthesia or heavy analgesia, leads to increased experiences of satisfaction in childbearing. Humenick (1981) further sug-

Research Note

Lindell and Rossi observed whether women who received formal childbirth education and then delivered in a nondirective environment actually used the class instructions for positioning and breathing during second stage labor.

Independent witnesses observed 28 women who had attended classes for breathing and positioning. The nurse-midwives and nurses attending these births provided a nonprescriptive environment and refrained from directing positioning or expulsive efforts. Breathing methods observed included closed glottis (complete breath holding), open glottis (grunts, groans, and moans), and intermittent exhalation (both open and closed glottis in the same contraction). A variety of positions were used.

That data collected showed that 94 percent of the 17 women who were taught traditional pushing did not use breath holding and 59 percent did not maintain the position taught. The women who were instructed to use a variety of positions or to do what was most comfortable did comply. All of the women expressed high satisfaction with their ability to participate so fully. The length of second stage for these women was well within the accepted limits of normal, no forceps were used, and only 29 percent required episiotomy.

Nurses teaching childbirth classes may help clients feel more successful if they teach a variety of pushing techniques and positions. Labor and delivery nurses who provide a nondirective environment for women in second stage provide care that suits the individual needs of clients.

Lindell G, Rossi A: Compliance with childbirth education classes in second stage labor. Birth 1986;13(June):96–99.

gests that mastery, or control, of the childbearing experience is the key factor in perceived satisfaction. Humenick defines control as "continuing to be able to influence the decisions made, not surrendering all decisions and responsibilities to care providers, but rather maintaining a working alliance." In this respect childbirth education helps increase positive reactions to the birth experience because it provides the laboring woman and her support persons with greater opportunities to control, or master, her labor experience.

Factors relating to control, although complex, support the mastery model. Factors that have the potential to be supportive include knowledge of the labor and delivery process, acquisition of skills to be used in coping with labor, ability to influence decisions and obtain adequate and appropriate support from others, and adequate knowledge of alternatives. On the other hand, factors that may be potential stressors include fear and anxiety, excessive fatigue, low pain tolerance, a sense of helplessness, loss of dignity, feelings of being abandoned or alone, and threats to the life or health of the woman and fetus (Humenick 1981). Women who do not perceive themselves as controlling their lives or the stresses in their lives have greater anxieties regarding the actual birth experience (Lederman 1984). Women who attend childbirth preparation classes tend to need less medication during labor, are more aware, and perceive their experiences as more satisfying than women who do not attend.

In the mastery model, pain is included among the numerous stressors of both positive and negative aspects of pregnancy and childbearing. Childbirth preparation education provides the opportunity to increase control and accomplish the psychologic tasks women set for themselves in labor, thereby facilitating a more positive birth experience.

How the woman views the birth experience after the delivery may have implications for mothering behaviors. Mercer (1985) found a significant relationship between the birth experience and mothering behaviors. It appears that any activities—by the expectant woman or by maternal-child health care providers—that enhance the birth experience will be beneficial as the woman prepares for labor, experiences labor, and begins her new role as a mother.

● Physiology of Labor

Possible Causes of Labor Onset

For some reason, usually at the appropriate time for the uterus and the fetus, the process of labor begins. Although medical researchers have been conducting numerous studies to determine the exact cause, it still is not clearly understood. The relationship of some factors is presented in Figure 21–9. Some of the more widely accepted theories are discussed in the following sections.

OXYTOCIN STIMULATION THEORY

Throughout the course of pregnancy there is a slow increase in the amount of oxytocin in maternal circulating blood. The level increases more dramatically during labor and peaks in the second stage. The concentration of oxytocin receptors in the myometrium and decidua also increases and peaks during labor. Due to both of these factors, the uterus is increasingly sensitive to oxytocin as the pregnancy approaches term (38 to 40 weeks). However, there is no convincing evidence that maternal or fetal oxytocin initiates labor. Oxytocin does have an effect on the permeability of sodium in the myometrium and raises the intracellular calcium levels that are needed for muscle contraction (Hariharan et al 1986). Some researchers suggest

Factors that stimulate
uterine muscle contractions

Factors that act to
quiet the uterine muscles

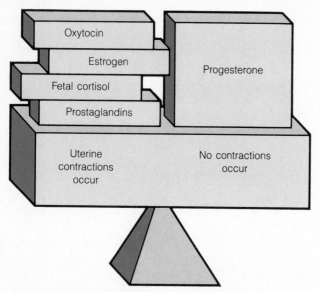

Figure 21–9   Factors affecting initiation of labor. The factors listed on the left have all been identified as providing stimulus to the beginning of labor. Progesterone exerts a relaxing effect, and a balance between all of the factors keeps the uterus quiet without contraction. When the relationship of factors changes, the balance is tipped and uterine labor begins.

that oxytocin has a dual action on two types of receptors in the uterus, with one leading to myometrial contractions and the other to stimulation of prostaglandin release (Hariharan et al 1986).

PROGESTERONE WITHDRAWAL THEORY

Progesterone has been reported to inhibit the estrogen effect of increased contractility by raising the resting membrane potential in the myometrial cells. It may stabilize the myometrial membrane-bound pools of calcium, thereby limiting uterine contractility (Hariharan et al 1986). Although some researchers feel there is insufficient evidence to show that progesterone levels in the maternal blood supply fall before labor, others report that progesterone metabolism in the fetal membranes is marked by decreases near term. The decrease in progesterone metabolism may be due to a progesterone-binding protein, which is present near term in the chorion and amnion. The decrease may facilitate prostaglandin synthesis in the chorioamnion, which increases uterine contractility. Although no general agreement exists regarding a decrease in progesterone metabolism, many researchers support the theory that a rising estrogen and decreasing progesterone ratio is important in raising levels of uterine contractility (Hariharan et al 1986).

ESTROGEN STIMULATION THEORY

Estrogen causes irritability of the myometrium, perhaps through an increase in concentrations of actin and myosin (contractile proteins) and adenosine triphosphate (ATP), which is the energy source for contractions. In addition, estrogen may promote prostaglandin synthesis in the decidua and fetal membranes. This enhances myometrial muscle contraction. Once the muscle cell is irritable and contracts, the presence of estrogen also enhances the propagation of impulses over the uterine muscle (Hariharan et al 1986).

FETAL CORTISOL THEORY

Liggins (1973) found that the removal of a fetal lamb's pituitary gland and adrenal cortex delays the onset of labor. Thus he has postulated that the fetus may play an important role in the initiation of labor. He also has reported premature labor in sheep that were infused with cortisol or ACTH. This phenomenon has not been confirmed in humans. However, a decrease in estrogen in both maternal and fetal plasma can be observed following maternal administration of corticosteroids. Research continues; there is a possibility that cortisol affects the biochemistry of the fetal membrane (Hariharan et al 1986).

FETAL MEMBRANE PHOSPHOLIPID–ARACHIDONIC ACID–PROSTAGLANDIN THEORY

According to the theory of fetal membrane phospholipid–arachidonic acid–prostaglandin interaction, estrogen promotes storage of esterified arachidonic acid in the fetal membranes. Withdrawal of progesterone activates phospholipase A_2, which is an enzymatic liberator. Phospholipase A_2 hydrolyzes phospholipids to liberate arachidonic acid in a nonesterified form. The arachidonic acid acts on PGE_2, $F_{2\alpha}$, or both in the decidual membranes. Prostaglandin stimulates the smooth muscle to contract, especially in the myometrium. Prostaglandin is present in increased quantities in the blood and amniotic fluid just prior to and during labor (Hariharan et al 1986). It has been suggested that the key to initiation of labor may be increased synthesis of PGE_2 in the amnion (Pritchard et al 1985).

Biochemical Interaction

The contraction wave of the uterus begins in the fundus, which contains the greatest concentration of myometrial cells, and moves downward throughout the entire myometrium. Because the contraction wave moves quickly, the myometrium appears to contract as a unit. Myometrial contraction efficiency depends on the presence of five factors:

1. Gap junctions must be present. Gap junctions of the myometrium are cell-to-cell contacts that promote synchronous contractions of smooth muscle cells and increase the effectiveness of the contractions. Gap junctions are prevalent at term and increase during labor in number and size. They begin to disappear within 24 hours after delivery. Gap junctions are present in premature labor. It is thought that estrogen, PGE_2, and $PGF_{2\alpha}$ promote formation of gap junctions and progesterone prevents them (Hariharan et al 1986, Pritchard et al 1985).

2. The contractile substances actin and myosin are essential for muscle contraction to occur.

3. A source of energy (ATP) must be available.

4. Cellular electrolyte exchange of calcium, sodium, and potassium is essential for muscle contraction.

5. The presence of an endocrine stimulus is necessary for conduction of the muscle contraction. During labor oxytocin, $PGF_{2\alpha}$, and acetylcholine are present.

All these factors work together to produce the uterine contractions of labor.

Myometrial Activity

Stretching of the cervix causes an increase in endogenous oxytocin, which increases myometrial activity. This is known as the *Ferguson reflex*. Pressures exerted by the contracting uterus vary from 20 to 60 mm Hg, with an average of 40 mm Hg.

In true labor the uterus divides into two portions. This division is known as the *physiologic retraction ring*. The upper portion, which is the contractile segment, becomes progressively thicker as labor advances. The lower portion, which includes the lower uterine segment and cervix, is passive. As labor continues, the lower uterine segment expands and thins out.

With each contraction the musculature of the upper uterine segment shortens and exerts a longitudinal traction on the cervix, causing effacement. *Effacement* is the taking up of the internal os and the cervical canal into the uterine side walls. The cervix changes progressively from a long, thick structure to a structure that is tissue-paper thin (Figure 21–10). In primigravidas, effacement usually precedes dilatation. This musculature remains shorter and thicker and does not return to its original length. This phenomenon is known as brachystasis. The space in the uterine cavity decreases as a result of brachystasis.

The uterus elongates with each contraction, decreasing the horizontal diameter. This elongation causes a straightening of the fetal body, pressing the upper pole against the fundus and thrusting the presenting part down toward the lower uterine segment and the cervix. The pres-

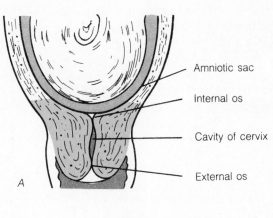

— Amniotic sac

— Internal os

— Cavity of cervix

— External os

A

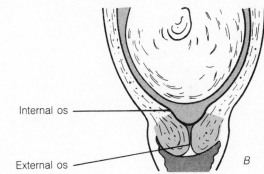

Internal os —

External os —

B

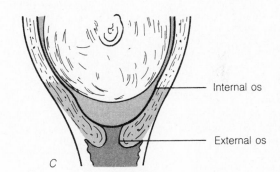

— Internal os

— External os

C

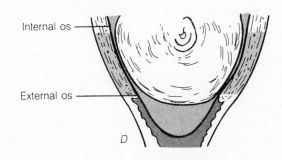

Internal os —

External os —

D

Figure 21–10 Effacement of the cervix in the primigravida. A At the beginning of labor there is no cervical effacement or dilatation. B Beginning cervical effacement. C Cervix is about one-half effaced and slightly dilated. D Complete effacement and dilatation.

sure exerted by the fetus is called the fetal axis pressure. As the uterus elongates, the longitudinal muscle fibers are pulled upward over the presenting part. This action, plus the hydrostatic pressure of the fetal membranes, causes *cervical dilatation*. The cervical os and cervical canal widen from less than a centimeter to approximately 10 cm, allowing delivery of the fetus. When the cervix is completely dilated and retracted up into the lower uterine segment, it can no longer be palpated.

The round ligament contracts with the uterus, pulling the fundus forward, thus aligning the fetus with the bony pelvis.

Intraabdominal Pressure

After the cervix is completely dilated, the maternal abdominal musculature contracts as the woman pushes. The pushing that the woman does aids in the expulsion of the infant and the placenta after delivery. If the cervix is not completely dilated, bearing down can cause cervical edema, which retards dilatation, and can cause maternal exhaustion as a result of straining. Tearing and bruising may also result from bearing down upon an incompletely dilated cervix.

Musculature Changes in the Pelvic Floor

The levator ani muscle and fascia of the pelvic floor draw the rectum and vagina upward and foward with each contraction, along the curve of the pelvic floor. As the fetal head descends to the pelvic floor, the pressure of the presenting part causes the perineal structure that was once 5 cm in thickness to change to a structure of less than a centimeter. Thus a normal physiologic anesthesia is produced as a result of the decreased blood supply to the area. The anus everts, exposing the interior rectal wall as the fetal head descends forward (Pritchard et al 1985).

● Maternal Systemic Response to Labor

Cardiovascular System

A strong contraction greatly diminishes or completely stops the blood flow in the branches of the uterine artery that supplies the intervillous space. This leads to a redistribution of the blood flow to the peripheral circulation and an increase in peripheral resistance, resulting in an increase of the systolic and diastolic blood pressure and a slowing of the pulse rate. The amount of change in maternal blood pressure and pulse is also dependent on the maternal position. Supine hypotension has an occurrence rate of 10 percent to 15 percent. When it occurs, it further taxes the cardiovascular system by decreasing venous return from the lower extremities (Albright et al 1986).

Cardiac output is increased by 10 percent to 15 percent during rest periods between contractions in early labor and by 30 percent to 50 percent in the second stage (Albright et al 1986). Additional increases and decreases in cardiac output mirror the changes in uterine pressure; that is, an increase in cardiac output as the contraction builds and peaks, and a slow return to precontraction cardiac output as the contraction diminishes.

There is an additional effect on hemodynamics during the bearing down efforts in the second stage. When the laboring woman holds her breath and pushes against a closed glottis (Valsalva maneuver), intrathoracic pressure rises. As intrathoracic pressure increases, the venous return is interrupted, which leads to a rise in the venous pressure. In addition, the blood in the lungs is forced into the left atrium, which leads to a transient increase in cardiac output, blood pressure, and pulse pressure and causes bradycardia. As venous return to the lungs continues to be diminished while the breath is held, a decrease in blood pressure, pulse pressure, and cardiac output occurs.

When the next breath is taken (Valsalva maneuver is interrupted), the intrathoracic pressure is decreased. Venous return increases, which leads to refilling of the pulmonary bed and results in recovery of the cardiac output and stroke volume. This process is repeated with each pushing effort.

Immediately after delivery, cardiac output peaks with an 80 percent increase over prelabor values, and then in the first 10 minutes decreases 20 percent to 25 percent. Cardiac output further decreases 20 percent to 25 percent in the first hour after delivery (Albright et al 1986).

Blood Pressure

As a result of increased cardiac output, systolic blood pressure rises during uterine contractions. In the immediate postpartal period the arterial pressure remains essentially normal even though the cardiac output increases due to peripheral vasodilation.

Supine hypotensive syndrome has been demonstrated radiographically in 90 percent of women at term. Although in clinical practice 10 percent to 15 percent of women demonstrate clinical symptoms (hypotension, tachycardia), some women may suffer supine hypotensive syndrome and remain asymptomatic due to compensatory mechanisms. These women are at risk because even though they are initially asymptomatic, placental perfusion is slowly compromised by arterial peripheral vasoconstriction (Albright et al 1986).

Women with the highest risk of developing supine hypotensive syndrome are nulliparas with strong abdominal muscles and tightly drawn abdominal skin, gravidas with hydramnios and/or multiple pregnancy, and obese women. Other predisposing factors include hypovolemia; dehydration; hemorrhage; metabolic acidosis; administration of narcotics, which results in vasodilation and inhibits compensatory mechanisms; and administration of regional anesthesia, which causes sympathetic blockade.

Fluid and Electrolyte Balance

Diaphoresis and hyperventilation occur during labor, which alters electrolyte and fluid balance from insensible loss. The muscle activity elevates the body temperature, which increases sweating and evaporation from the skin. The rise in the respiratory rate as the woman responds to the work of labor increases the evaporative water volume, because each breath of air must be warmed to the body temperature and humidified.

Gastrointestinal System

During labor, additional reduction of gastric motility and absorption of solid food occurs. The gastric emptying time is further prolonged. It is not uncommon for a laboring woman to vomit stomach contents of food that was ingested up to 12 hours previously.

Respiratory System

Oxygen consumption, which increased approximately 20 percent during pregnancy, is further increased during labor. During the early first stage oxygen consumption increases 40 percent, with a further increase of 100 percent during the second stage.

Minute ventilation increases to 20 to 25 L/min (normal 10 L/min), and in the unprepared and unmedicated woman it may reach 35 L/min or more. This hyperventilation results in a rise in the maternal pH in early labor, followed by a return to normal toward the end of the first stage. If the first stage is prolonged, the maternal pH may become acidotic (Albright et al 1986).

Hemopoietic System

Leukocyte levels may elevate to 25,000/mm³ or more during labor. Although the precise cause of the leukocytosis is unknown, it may be due to the strenuous exercise and stress response of labor (Pritchard et al 1985). It has been found that the longer a woman is in labor, the greater the elevation in leukocyte count (Acker et al 1985). In the absence of ruptured membranes or any signs of infection, this elevation seems to be a normal physiologic reaction.

Plasma fibrinogen increases, and blood coagulation time decreases. Blood glucose levels may decrease due to the increased activity of uterine and skeletal muscles (Varney 1980).

Marked changes in clotting factors VII, II, and X have occurred during pregnancy and continue through delivery. The most dramatic change occurs in factor VII. There is growing speculation that the increase is a phospholipid complex that is affected by trophoblastic tissue. By 40 weeks' gestation, the mean activity of factor VII is 248 percent above nonpregnant values, and the increase remains during delivery. There is a dramatic decrease during the first 30 minutes after delivery of the placenta. The decrease continues over the next few weeks of the postpartum period. Factor II increases to a mean activity factor of 136 percent. Factor X increases to 171 percent. These changes help protect against hemorrhage during delivery, but in addition, they place the woman at higher risk for thrombophlebitis (Dalaker 1986).

Renal System

The base of the bladder is pushed forward and upward when engagement occurs. The pressure from the presenting part may lead to edema of the tissues due to impaired drainage of blood and lymph from the base of the bladder (Pritchard et al 1985).

Approximately one-third to one-half of all laboring women have slight proteinuria (trace) as a result of muscle breakdown from exercise. An increase to 2+ or above is indicative of pathology (Varney 1980).

Response to Pain

THEORIES OF PAIN

Many theories of pain have evolved during the past century. The traditional theory of pain is known as the *specificity theory*. It proposes that a specific pain system carries messages from pain receptors in the body to a pain center in the brain. However, too many clinical facts are neglected in this model of a rigid, closed system. The amount and quality of pain experienced by an individual are modified by psychologic and environmental variables.

The simplest form of response to stimuli is a protective mechanism, the withdrawal reflex that occurs in the sensorimotor arc. For example, when the hand is placed on a hot object, pain nerve fibers transmit impulses to the dorsal root of the spinal cord. Each impulse is transmitted through synapses to the ventral root and returns to the local muscles as a motor impulse causing a jerking movement away from the hot object. This reaction occurs before the sensory information is processed by the brain; the hand is lifted before pain is perceived. Even this simple mechanism does not occur in isolation. The individual is thrown off balance by the reflex action, and immediately the entire body moves to restore equilibrium. This type of reflex action occurs during an intramuscular injection—the person flinches as the skin is penetrated.

The *pattern theory* of pain attempts to incorporate the psychologic aspects of pain ignored by the specificity theory. The pattern theory proposes that particular networks or patterns of nerve impulses are produced by the summation of sensory input at the dorsal horn cells. Pain results when the total output of these cells exceeds a critical level as a result of excessive stimulation of receptors or of pathologic conditions that enhance the summation of impulses. The patterns of impulses travel over multiple pathways and enter widespread regions of the brain.

When the mechanisms suggested by the specificity and pattern theories are examined, valuable complementary concepts come to light. The *gate-control theory* proposed by Melzack (1973) has attempted to integrate all aspects of pain into a comprehensive theory. According to this view, pain results from activity in several interacting specialized neural systems.

The gate-control theory proposes that a mechanism in the dorsal horn of the spinal column, probably the substantial gelatinosa, serves as a valve or gate that increases or decreases the flow of nerve impulses from the periphery to the central nervous system. The uterus-to-spinal cord pain pathway along a single sensory tract is illustrated in Figure 21–11. The gate mechanism is influenced by the size of the transmitting fibers and by the nerve impulses that descend from the brain. Psychologic processes such as past experiences, attention, and emotion may influence

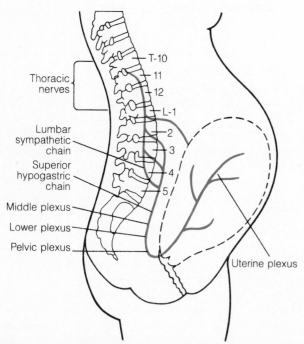

Figure 21–11   Pain pathway from uterus to spinal cord. Nerve impulses travel through the uterine plexus, pelvic plexus, inferior hypogastric plexus, middle and superior hypogastric, and the lumbar sympathetic chain and enter the spinal cord through the 12th, 11th, and 10th thoracic nerves. (Modified from Bonica JJ: Principles and Practice of Obstetric Analgesia and Anesthesia. Philadelphia, Davis, 1972, p 492)

pain perception and response by activating the gate mechanism. The gates may be opened or closed by central nervous system activities, such as anxiety or excitement, or through selective, localized activity (Melzack 1973). The gate-control theory has two important implications for obstetrics: Pain can be controlled by tactile stimulation; it can also be controlled by the use of distraction, suggestion, and imagery.

PAIN DURING LABOR

The pain associated with the first stage of labor is unique in that it accompanies a normal physiologic process. Even though perception of the pain of childbirth is greatly determined by cultural patterning, there is a physiologic basis for discomfort during labor. Pain during the first stage of labor arises from (a) dilatation of the cervix, (b) hypoxia of the uterine muscle cells during contraction, (c) stretching of the lower uterine segment, and (d) pressure on adjacent structures. The primary source of pain is dilatation or stretching of the cervix. Nerve impulses travel through the uterine plexus, inferior hypogastric (pelvic) plexus, middle hypogastric plexus, superior hypogastric plexus, and the lumbar sympathetic and lower thoracic chain and enter the spinal cord through the posterior roots of the 12th, 11th, and 10th thoracic and 1st lumbar nerves. As with other visceral pain, pain from the uterus is referred to the dermatomes supplied by the 12th, 11th, and 10th thoracic nerves. The areas of referred pain include the lower abdominal wall and the areas over the lower lumbar region and the upper sacrum (Figure 21–12).

During the second stage of labor, discomfort is due to (a) hypoxia of the contracting uterine muscle cells, (b) distention of the vagina and perineum, and (c) pressure on adjacent structures. The nerve impulses from the vagina and perineum are transmitted by way of the pudendal nerve plexus and enter the spinal cord through the posterior roots of the second, third, and fourth sacral nerves (Figure 21–13).

Pain during the third stage results from uterine contractions and cervical dilatation as the placenta is expelled (Figure 21–14). The mechanism for the transmission of nerve impulses is the same as for the first stage of labor. This stage of labor is short, and the primary need for anesthesia after this phase of the labor process is for repair of lacerations or an episiotomy if one has been done.

FACTORS AFFECTING RESPONSE TO PAIN

Because pain is a total psychosomatic experience, many factors affect the individual's perception of pain impulses. All human societies have developed patterns of behavior for the maternal role during childbirth. Some psychologic and environmental influences particularly appropriate to labor are discussed here.

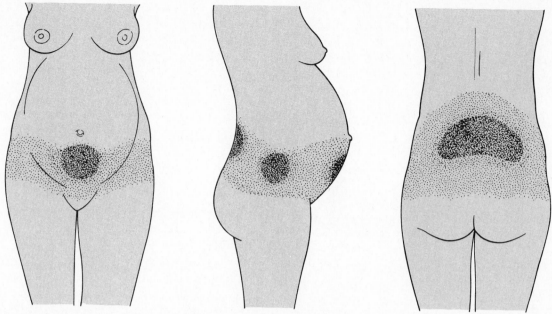

Figure 21–12   Area of reference of labor pain during the first stage. Density of stippling indicates intensity of pain. (From Bonica JJ: *Principles and Practice of Obstetric Analgesia and Anesthesia.* Philadelphia, Davis, 1972, p 108)

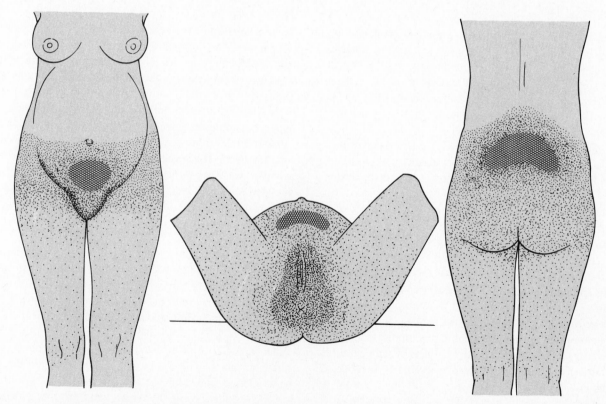

Figure 21–13   Distribution of labor pain during the later phase of the first stage and early phase of the second stage. Crosshatched areas indicate location of the most intense pain; dense stippling, moderate pain; and light stippling, mild pain. Note that the uterine contractions, which at this stage are very strong, produce intense pain. (From Bonica JJ: *Principles and Practice of Obstetric Analgesia and Anesthesia.* Philadelphia, Davis, 1972, p 109)

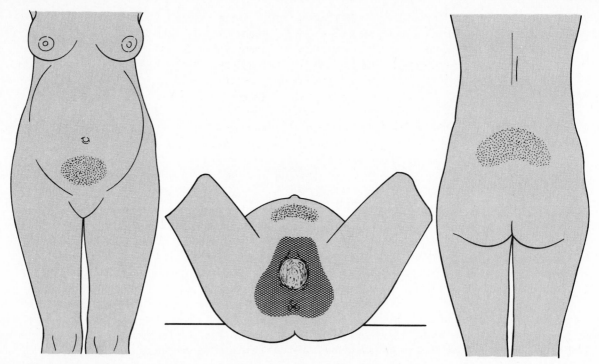

Figure 21-14   Distribution of labor pain during the later phase of the second stage and actual delivery. The perineal component is the primary cause of discomfort. Uterine contractions contribute much less. (From Bonica JJ: Principles and Practice of Obstetric Analgesia and Anesthesia. Philadelphia, Davis, 1972, p 109)

○   *EFFECT OF CHILDBIRTH EDUCATION* Preparation for childbirth has been shown to reduce the need for analgesia and the subjective experience of tension and stress that occurs during labor. A recent study (Delke et al 1985) demonstrated that Lamaze-prepared women had a decrease in fear, tension, and emotional stress.

○   *CULTURAL BACKGROUND* Medical and nursing professionals have their own health care culture expectations of the woman in labor. She is expected to use a breathing technique and relaxation methods. Value is placed on maintaining self-control and knowing what to expect during labor and birth. It is important to know that the health care professional will interpret pain according to the health care culture norms while various other cultures have other ways of responding to pain (Bates 1987). The absence of crying and moaning does not necessarily mean that pain is absent, nor does the presence of crying and moaning necessarily mean that pain relief is desired at that moment. Some cultures believe it is natural to communicate the pain experience, no matter how mild. Members of some cultures stoically accept pain out of fear or because it is expected of them.

Mexican women are taught to keep their mouths closed during labor and to avoid breathing in air that may cause the uterus to rise up (Kay 1982). Black women are expected to be stoic and not scream so that they will not cause others to think badly of the black race, and Navajo

women keep quiet to preserve the secrecy of the process (Kay 1982). The outward expression of the perceived pain may be difficult to interpret. Navajo women may be willing to receive pain medication but be hesitant to request it (Kay 1982).

The health care culture may use touching and the support of others to decrease pain during labor. Various other cultural groups may or may not value the same comfort measures. The traditional American Indian may want a female with her rather than her husband, and the Japanese woman may feel "ashamed" to be seen by her husband (Kay 1982). Hmong women usually prefer that their husbands remain with them in labor and be involved in comfort measures (Morrow 1986).

It is important, however, to avoid stereotyping women because of their ethnic backgrounds, since exposure to North American culture and expectations may modify the behavioral response to pain. Nurses who are providing support during labor must recognize that there are ways of reacting to pain that are different from their personal views of appropriate behavior. Nurses need to be familiar with the cultural beliefs of those they are likely to assist during labor and use this knowledge along with assessment skills to verify the type of support that is needed.

○   *FATIGUE AND SLEEP DEPRIVATION* Exhaustion may be so great that a laboring woman's attention wanders from the physical stimuli of childbirth, or it may have the opposite effect, lowering the powers of resistance and self-control to produce an exaggerated response. Fatigue from sleep deprivation affects an individual's response to pain in several ways. The fatigued person has less energy and a decreased ability to use such strategies as distraction or imagination as coping mechanisms in dealing with pain. The fatigued woman in labor may choose a less-demanding alternative, such as analgesia (McCaffery 1972). This is a particularly important factor in laboring clients because prolonged prodromal labor may interfere with sleep. A woman may begin the active phase of labor in an exhausted state and have difficulty coping with the discomfort of frequent contractions.

○ **PERSONAL SIGNIFICANCE OF PAIN** The significance of pain is closely related to the woman's self-concept as well as to cultural expectations. She may view labor as a fearful event, one she has dreaded throughout pregnancy, or she may view it as the happiest event of her life. Pain may be interpreted by some women as punishment for perceived sins, such as engaging in premarital intercourse or feeling ambivalent toward the pregnancy. Others who have had psychoprophylactic preparation for childbirth may consider the pain a test of their ability to cope with a challenging event. If such women do not handle the pain of labor according to their expectations, they tend to experience a sense of failure, which threatens not only their self-concept but also their ability to mother. Consequently, it is vital that childbirth instructors and nurses stress to each woman that the reaction to childbirth is varied and individual. A woman should not feel a sense of failure if she requires analgesia to assist her in coping. The primary goal of psychoprophylactic preparation is a childbirth experience that is satisfying to both father and mother.

○ **PREVIOUS EXPERIENCE** One's previous experience with pain affects one's ability to manage current and future pain. Particularly painful experiences can condition one to expect the same degree of pain in a similar situation. All persons, with very few exceptions, have experienced pain. It appears likely that those who have had more experience with pain are more sensitive to painful stimuli.

○ **ANXIETY** Anxiety related to pain must be approached on two levels, that associated with anticipation of pain and that associated with the presence of pain. While a moderate degree of anxiety about impending pain is necessary for the person to handle the pain experience, anxiety during the pain experience should be reduced as much as possible by nursing intervention. Anxiety during labor produces tension, which increases the intensity of the pain.

Anxieties unrelated to the pain can also intensify the pain experience. For many young women, admission for labor and delivery is their first hospitalization. Routine procedures, rules and regulations, equipment, and the general environment are unfamiliar and anxiety-provoking. For many women the spontaneous onset of labor has an element of surprise. Although the event is expected and even anticipated, few women are totally prepared for the actual onset of labor and hospitalization. Last-minute details must be completed. Arrangement for the care of other children have usually been made but now must actually be carried out. Having to leave young children for a few days is accompanied by varying degrees of anxiety for any mother.

○ **ATTENTION AND DISTRACTION** Both attention and distraction have an influence on the perception of pain. When pain sensation is the focus of attention, the perceived intensity is greater. The classic example is the football player who is unaware of an injury until the game is over and only then experiences painful sensations.

A sensory stimulus can serve as a distraction because the person's attention is focused on the stimulus rather than the pain, for example, providing a client with a back rub. Cutaneous sensations are carried by large-diameter afferent fibers, which can inhibit the pain sensation carried by small-diameter fibers. This is a component of the gate-control theory of pain discussed earlier. Cutaneous stimulation to relieve pain may also be explained by the theory of extinction or perceptual dominance. It is possible that sensory input may extinguish pain or raise its threshold.

● **Fetal Response to Labor**

In the presence of a normal fetus the mechanical and hemodynamic changes enforced by normal labor have no adverse fetal effect and in fact may have some positive effect on preparing the baby for extrauterine adaptation.

Heart Rate Changes

During labor, compression of the fetal head during contractions may lead to an early deceleration in fetal heart rate. In the second stage, decelerations may occur because of maternal bearing down efforts and from pressure on the umbilical cord as the fetus moves through the birth canal. (See Chapter 22 for further discussion of fetal heart rate patterns.)

Acid-Base Status in Labor

The first stage of labor is associated with a slow decrease in the fetal pH. As the second stage begins, there is a more rapid decrease due to an increase in uterine contractility and bearing down efforts of the laboring woman. There is also an increase in fetal base deficit and in P_{CO_2} and a drop in fetal oxygen saturation of about 10 percent (Creasy & Resnik 1984).

Fetal Movements

When the fetus is between 35 and 40 weeks, episodes of fetal breathing movements increase in the second and third hour following the mother's meals. There is also a marked increase during the night while the mother is asleep, which is thought to be part of a circadian rhythm in fetal breathing activity. In the healthy term fetus there are periods of apnea that last up to two hours. It has been noted that the incidence of fetal breathing movements slows markedly and may cease about three days before the onset of spontaneous labor (Creasy & Resnik 1984). It has been suggested that the absence of fetal breathing movements might be used to differentiate between true and false labor (Boylan et al 1985).

Gross fetal body movements occur at a rate of about 20 to 50 per hour in the term fetus. The number of movements do not normally increase prior to or during labor (Creasy & Resnik 1984).

Behavioral States

The behavioral states observed in the normal newborn may also be documented during the fetal state, and the pattern the fetus establishes seems to continue during labor even in the presence of uterine contractions. One study used ultrasound to observe fetal activity during labor (Griffin et al 1985). Two sleep states (quiet and active) were most prevalent, although quiet and active awake states were occasionally observed. A decrease in fetal heart rate variability accompanies the quiet sleep state, and there is also a decrease in fetal breathing movements and other general body activity. In all observed fetuses, the quiet sleep state lasted less than 40 minutes. The authors suggest that as long as other fetal heart rate parameters are within normal limits, a decrease in variability will usually indicate a normal behavioral sleep state.

Hemodynamic Changes

The adequate exchange of nutrients and gases to and from the fetal capillaries and the intervillous space depends on a number of factors, one of which is the fetal blood pressure. Fetal blood pressure serves as a protective mechanism for the normal fetus for the stresses of the anoxic period, which are enforced by the contracting uterus during labor. The fetal and placental reserve is enough to see the fetus through these anoxic periods without adversity.

Positional Changes

So that the fetus can make the transition from intrauterine life to extrauterine life, the fetal head and body must adjust to the passage by certain positional changes, often called *cardinal movements* or *mechanisms of labor*. These changes are described in the order in which they occur (Figure 21–15).

DESCENT

Descent is thought to occur because of four forces: (a) pressure of the amniotic fluid, (b) direct pressure of the fundus on the breech, (c) contraction of the abdominal muscles, and (d) extension and straightening of the fetal body. The head enters the inlet in the occiput transverse or oblique position because the pelvic inlet is widest from side to side. The sagittal suture is an equal distance from the maternal symphysis pubis and sacral promontory.

FLEXION

Flexion occurs as the fetal head descends and meets resistance from the soft tissues of the pelvis, the musculature of the pelvic floor, and the cervix.

INTERNAL ROTATION

The fetal head must rotate to fit the diameter of the pelvic cavity, which is widest in the anteroposterior diameter. As the occiput of the fetal head meets resistance from the levator ani muscles and their fascia, the occiput rotates from left to right and the sagittal suture aligns in the anteroposterior pelvic diameter.

EXTENSION

The resistance of the pelvic floor and the mechanical movement of the vulva opening anteriorly and forward assist with extension of the fetal head as it passes under the symphysis pubis. With this positional change, the occiput, then brow and face, emerge from the vagina.

RESTITUTION

The shoulders of the infant enter the pelvis obliquely and remain oblique when the head rotates to the anteroposterior diameter through internal rotation. Because of this rotation the neck becomes twisted. Once the head delivers and is free of pelvic resistance, the neck untwists, turning the head to one side (restitution), and aligns with the position of the back in the birth canal.

EXTERNAL ROTATION

As the shoulders rotate to the anteroposterior position in the pelvis, the head is turned farther to one side (external rotation).

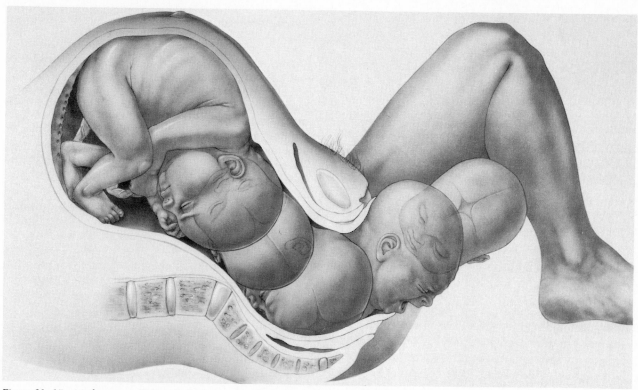

Figure 21–15 Mechanisms of labor. A, B Descent. C Internal rotation. D Extension. E External rotation.

EXPULSION

After the external rotation and through expulsive efforts of the laboring woman, the anterior shoulder meets the under surface of the symphysis pubis, slips under it, and as lateral flexion of the shoulder and head occurs, the anterior shoulder is born before the posterior shoulder. The body follows quickly (Oxorn 1986). The adaptations of the newborn to extrauterine life are discussed in Chapter 27.

● Premonitory Signs of Labor

Most primigravidas and many multiparas experience signs and symptoms of impending labor.

Lightening

The majority of primigravidas experience the phenomenon of *lightening* about two to three weeks before the onset of labor. This feeling occurs because the fetus begins to settle into the pelvic inlet. With its descent, engagement occurs, the uterus moves downward, and the fundus no longer presses on the diaphragm.

The woman can breathe more easily after lightening. With increased downward pressure of the presenting part, however, the woman may notice leg cramps or pains due to pressure on the nerves that course through the obturator foramen in the pelvis, increased pressure on urinary bladder, increased pelvic pressure, and increased venous stasis leading to dependent edema. Vaginal secretions increase due to congestion of the vaginal mucous membranes. In theory, primigravidas experience lightening because of increased intensity of Braxton Hicks contractions and the bracing action of abdominal muscles of good tone.

Braxton Hick Contractions

Prior to the onset of labor, *Braxton Hicks contractions,* the irregular, intermittent contractions that have been occurring throughout the pregnancy, may become uncomfortable. The pain seems to be in the abdomen and groin but may feel like the "drawing" sensations experienced by some with dysmenorrhea.

The contractions may occur for a few weeks, a few days, or just hours prior to the onset of true labor. False labor is uncomfortable and may be exhausting as the woman remains awake, wondering if "this is it." Since the contractions seem to be regular at times, she has no way of knowing if they are the beginning of true labor. She may come to the hospital for a vaginal examination to determine if cervical dilatation is occurring. Frequent episodes of false labor and trips back and forth to the physician's office or hospital may frustrate or embarrass the woman, who feels that she should know when she is really in labor. Reassurance by nursing personnel can ease embarrassment.

Cervical Changes

For some time the *"ripening"* (softening) of the cervix was thought to be caused by increasing intensity of Braxton Hicks contractions. Liggins (1978) suggests that softening of the cervix begins in the second half of pregnancy. A few days before the onset of labor, the cervix becomes even softer and begins to efface and dilate slightly. The mechanism for this ripening is biochemical and is the result of changes in the connective tissue of the cervix. A recent study (Ekman et al 1986) strongly suggested that the mechanism for this process rests with collagen as an important regulator of the cervical state and function in late pregnancy and term labor. In addition, PGE_2 was found to be important for cervical priming, initiation, and progress of term labor.

Bloody Show

With softening and effacement of the cervix, the mucous plug (accumulated cervical secretions that have closed off the opening of the uterine cavity) is often expelled, resulting in a small amount of blood loss from the exposed cervical capillaries. The resulting pink-tinged secretions are called *bloody show.*

Bloody show is considered a sign of imminent labor, which usually begins within 24 to 48 hours. Sometimes vaginal examination with manipulation of the cervix may also result in a blood-tinged discharge, which may be confused with bloody show.

Rupture of Membranes

In approximately 12 percent of women, the amniotic membranes rupture before the onset of labor. This is called rupture of membranes (ROM). Labor usually begins within 24 hours for 80 percent of these women. When the membranes rupture, the open pathway into the uterus causes danger of infection. If labor does not begin within 12 hours after rupture of the membranes, it is frequently induced if the pregnancy is near term (40 weeks). Opinion varies regarding how long to wait before inducing labor.

When the membranes rupture, the amniotic fluid may be expelled in large amounts. Danger of the umbilical cord washing out with the fluid (prolapse of umbilical cord) results if the presenting part does not fill the pelvis. Because of this threat and the possibility of infection, the woman is advised to notify her physician/nurse-midwife and proceed to the hospital. In some instances, the fluid is expelled in small amounts and may be confused with episodes of urinary incontinence associated with urinary urgency, coughing, or sneezing. The discharge may be checked to ascertain its source and to determine further action. After assessment the woman may feel embarrassed to find out she is having urinary incontinence. (See Chapter 22 for assessment techniques.)

I couldn't believe it—my membranes ruptured in church. One minute I was following the service and the next minute I felt a trickle of fluid running down my leg. Fortunately I made it out of the pew and into the ladies room before the big gush came. Once it passed I went back into the church and stood at the end of the pew, frantically beckoning to my husband. I was "sloshing" as we left church, but I had on black slacks and I don't think people could tell. It makes a great story now, but at the time it seemed like a wild way to start my first labor.

Sudden Burst of Energy

Some women report a sudden surge of energy 24 to 48 hours before labor. They may do their spring housecleaning or rearrange all the furniture (referred to as the "nesting instinct"). The nurse in prenatal teaching should warn prospective mothers not to overexert themselves at this time so that they will not be excessively tired at labor's onset. The cause of the energy spurt is unknown.

Other Signs

Additional premonitory signs may include a loss of 1 to 3 pounds resulting from fluid loss and electrolyte shifts produced by changes in estrogen and progesterone levels, and increased backache and sacroiliac pressure from the influence of relaxin hormone on the pelvic joints. Some women report diarrhea, indigestion, or nausea and vomiting just prior to the onset of labor. The causes are unknown.

Differences Between True and False Labor

The contractions of true labor produce progressive dilatation and effacement of the cervix. They occur regularly and increase in frequency, duration, and intensity. The discomfort of true labor contractions usually starts in the back and radiates around to the abdomen, and is not relieved by ambulation (in fact, it may intensify).

False labor contractions are called Braxton Hicks contractions, and they do not produce *progressive* cervical effacement and dilatation. Classically, they are irregular and do not increase in frequency, duration, and intensity. The contractions may be perceived as a hardening or "balling up" without discomfort, or discomfort may occur mainly in the lower abdomen and groin. The discomfort may be relieved by ambulation (Table 21–4).

It is helpful for the woman to know the characteristics of true labor contractions as well as the premonitory signs of ensuing labor. However, sometimes the only way to differentiate between true and false labor is by assess-

Table 21–4 Comparison of True and False Labor

True labor	False labor
Contractions are at regular intervals.	Contractions are usually irregular.
Intervals between contractions gradually shorten.	There is usually no change.
Contractions increase in duration and intensity.	There is usually no change.
Discomfort begins in back and radiates around to abdomen.	Discomfort is usually in abdomen.
Intensity usually increases with walking.	Walking has no effect or lessens contractions.
Progressive cervical dilatation and effacement occurs.	There is no change.

ment of dilatation. The woman must feel free to come in for accurate assessment of labor and should never be allowed to feel foolish if it is false labor. The nurse must reassure the woman that false labor is common and that it often cannot be distinguished from true labor except by vaginal examination.

● Stages of Labor and Delivery

There are three stages of labor. The *first stage* begins with the beginning of true labor and ends when the cervix is completely dilated at 10 cm. The *second stage* begins with complete dilatation and ends with the birth of the infant. The *third stage* begins with the expulsion of the infant and ends with the delivery of the placenta.

Some clinicians identify a *fourth stage* of labor. During this stage, which lasts 1 to 4 hours after delivery of the placenta, the uterus effectively contracts to control bleeding at the placental site (Pritchard et al 1985).

In this section we discuss the physiologic events and psychological changes that occur during labor and delivery. The care of the laboring woman is discussed in Chapter 23.

First Stage

The first stage of labor has traditionally been divided into the latent, active, and transitional phases. As a result of extensive study of labor patterns Friedman (1978) has suggested new titles to be used. He has further described and defined the active phase, according to cervical dilatation, as acceleration phase, phase of maximum slope, and deceleration phase. Friedman has also developed concepts based on the physiologic objectives of labor, calling them preparatory, dilational, and pelvic divisions. The preparatory division includes the latent and acceleration phase, the dilational division includes the phase of maximum slope,

and the pelvic division commences with the deceleration phase. Each phase of labor is characterized by physical and psychological changes (Figure 21–16 and Table 21–5).

Privacy, intimacy, calm, freedom to labor in any position, and the helpful presence of midwives are crucial to a spontaneous first stage of labor. (Michel Odent, quoted in *Pregnant Feelings*)

LATENT PHASE

The latent phase begins with the onset of regular contractions and is represented by a flat slope of cervical dilatation to 3 to 4 cm. As the cervix begins to dilate, it also effaces, although little or no fetal descent is evident. The latent phase averages 6.4 hours but should not exceed 20 hours for nulliparas, and averages 4.8 hours but should not exceed 14 hours in multiparas (Friedman 1978).

Uterine contractions become established during the latent phase and increase in frequency, duration, and intensity. They may start as mild contractions lasting 15 to 30 seconds with a frequqency of 15 to 30 minutes and progress to moderate ones lasting 30 to 40 seconds with a frequency of 5 to 7 minutes. They average 40 mm Hg during acme from a baseline tonus of 10 mm Hg.

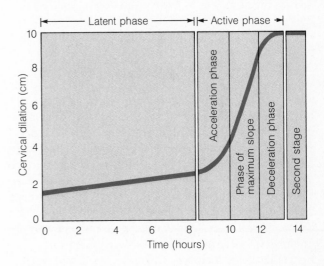

Figure 21–16 Composite of the average dilatation curve for nulliparous labor based on analysis of the data derived from the patterns traced by a large, nearly consecutive series of gravidas. The first stage is divided into a relatively flat latent phase and a rapidly progressive active phase. The active phase has three identifiable component parts: an acceleration phase, a linear phase of maximum slope, and a deceleration phase. (From Friedman EA: Labor: Clinical Evaluation and Management, ed 2. New York; Appleton-Century-Crofts, 1978, p 33)

Table 21–5   Characteristics of Labor in Nulliparas and Multiparas*

	Nulliparas	Multiparas
Duration of first stage		
Latent phase	6.4 (1.3–11.5 hours)	4.8 (0–9.7 hours)
Active phase	4.6 (1–8.2 hours)	2.4 (0.2–4.6 hours)
Total	11.0 (3.3–19.7 hours)	7.2 (0.1–14.3 hours)
Cervical dilation in active phase	1.2 cm/hr	1.5 cm/hr
Maximum rate of descent (cm/hr)	3.3 (1.0–5.6 cm/hr)	6.6 (2.6–10.6 cm/hr)
Duration of second stage (hr)	1.1 (0.3–1.9 hr)	0.39 (0.9–0.69 hr)

*All values given are ± 1 SD.

Adapted from Creasy RK, Resnik R: *Maternal-Fetal Medicine*. Philadelphia, Saunders, 1984, p 450.

In the early or latent phase of the first stage of labor, contractions are usually mild, and the woman feels able to cope. She may be relieved that labor has finally started and, while she may be anxious, is able to recognize and express those feelings of anxiety. She is often talkative and smiling and will be eager to talk about herself and answer questions. Excitement is high, and her mate or other support person is often just as elated.

ACTIVE PHASE

During the active phase, the cervix dilates from about 3 to 4 cm to 10 cm (complete dilatation), which marks the end of the first stage. Fetal descent is progressive.

The active period begins with the *acceleration phase* as cervical dilatation changes from a flat slope (as in the latent phase) to an upward curve. The *phase of maximum slope* covers the period of time when cervical dilatation progresses from approximately 3 to 4 cm to 8 cm. The cervical dilatation should be at least 1.2 cm/hr in nulliparas, and 1.5 cm/hr in multiparas (Friedman 1978).

The *deceleration phase* is the last part of the active phase. The cervical dilatation slows as it progresses from 8 to 10 cm and the rate of fetal descent increases. The average rate of descent is at least 1.0 cm/hr in nulliparas, and 2.0 cm/hr in multiparas. The deceleration phase should not be longer than three hours for nulliparas and one hour for multiparas (Friedman 1978). The deceleration phase may be referred to as *transition*.

During the active phase, contractions become more frequent, are longer in duration, and increase in intensity. By the end of the active phase, contraction frequency is usually every two to three minutes, with a duration averaging 60 seconds. The intensity is moderate to strong.

As the woman enters the early active phase, her anxiety tends to increase as she senses the fairly constant intensification of contractions and pain. She begins to fear a loss of control, and may exhibit coping mechanisms to maintain control. A decreased ability to cope may be noted along with a sense of helplessness. Women who have support persons available, particularly fathers, experience greater satisfaction and less anxiety throughout the birth process than those without these supports (Doering & Entwisle 1980).

The woman may demonstrate significant anxiety. She may become restless, frequently changing position. The most commonly expressed fear at this time is that of abandonment; it becomes crucial that the nurse be available as backup and relief for the support person. By the time the woman enters the active phase, she is inner focused and, often, tired. At the same time the support person may be feeling the need for a break, rest, or walk. The woman should be reassured that she will not be left alone and should always be told where her support persons are if they leave the room and where her nurse is should the woman need assistance.

She may also have fears about tearing open or splitting apart with the force of the contractions. Many women experience a sensation of pressure so great with the peak of a contraction that it seems to them that their abdomens will burst open with the force. She should be informed that this is a normal sensation and reassured that such bursting will not happen. By the time the woman reaches the deceleration phase (transition) she will most likely be withdrawn and inner focused. She may increasingly doubt her ability to cope with her labor. The deceleration or transition phase is associated with increasing apprehension and irritability. Not only does the woman not want to be left alone but also she may not want anyone to talk to or touch her. However, with the next contraction, she may ask for verbal and physical support. Other characteristics that may accompany this phase are hyperventilation as the woman increases her breathing rate, restlessness, difficulty understanding directions, a sense of bewilderment and anger at the contractions, statements that she "cannot take it anymore," requests for medication, hiccupping, belching, nausea, vomiting, beads of perspiration on upper lip, and increasing rectal pressure.

The woman in this phase is anxious to "get it over with" and is often terrified of being left alone. She may be amnesic and sleep between her now-frequent contractions. Her support persons may start to feel helpless and may turn to the nurse for increased participation as their efforts at alleviating the woman's discomfort seem less effective.

As dilatation approaches completion, increased rectal pressure and uncontrollable desire to bear down, increased amount of bloody show, and rupture of membranes may occur.

The exciting possibility exists today to rediscover our relationship with birth. To help us do so, we need to look for or create feminine images of birthing that can speak to us in our hours of birth. . . . British childbirth educator and anthropologist Sheila Kitzinger describes the vagina opening like a flower over the hard bud of the baby's head and tells of regions in India where an unopened flower is placed beside the laboring woman. Just as the flower opens during her labor, she knows that she too is opening. (Pregnant Feelings)

AMNIOTIC MEMBRANES

At the beginning of labor the amniotic membranes bulge through the cervix in the shape of a cone. As labor and dilatation progress, the membranes assume the shape of a large watch crystal. They may rupture before labor or any time during labor. If the chorion ruptures and the amnion remains intact, the infant may deliver with the amnion covering its head. The child is then said to be born with a *caul*. Rupture of membranes (ROM) generally occurs at the height of an intense contraction with a gush of the fluid out the introitus. If this occurs in transition, descent of the fetal head will follow.

Second Stage

The second stage of labor (also called the expulsive stage) begins with complete dilatation of the cervix (10 cm) and ends with delivery of the infant. It should be completed within an hour after the cervix becomes fully dilated for primigravidas (multiparas average 15 minutes). Contractions may be 60 to 90 seconds in duration, are strong in intensity, and have a frequency of two to three minutes. Descent of the fetal presenting part continues until it reaches the perineal floor (Figure 21–17).

As the fetal head descends, the woman develops the urge to push because of pressure of the fetal head on the sacral and obturator nerves. The urge to push may not occur immediately following complete dilatation. As she pushes, intraabdominal pressure is exerted from contraction of the maternal abdominal musculature. As the fetal head continues its descent, the perineum beings to bulge, flatten, and move anteriorly. There may be a further increase in the amount of bloody show. The labia begin to part with each contraction. Between contractions the fetal head appears to recede. With succeeding contractions and maternal pushing effort, the fetal head descends further, and crowning (encircling of the fetal head by the vaginal

opening) occurs, signifying that delivery is imminent (Figures 21–17 and 21–18).

The woman may feel a sense of relief that the delivery is near, and that she can now push. Some women feel a sense of control, which comes from being able to have active involvement. Others (particularly those without childbirth preparation) may become frightened, and tend to fight each contraction and any attempt of others to persuade them to push with contractions. Such behavior may be frightening and disconcerting to her support persons. The woman may feel she has lost control and become embarrassed and apologetic. She may demonstrate extreme irritability toward the staff or her supporters in an attempt to regain control over external forces against which she feels helpless. Some may feel acute and increasingly severe pain as the perineum distends. Usually, a psychoprophylactically prepared woman feels a sense of relief from the acute pain she felt during the transition phase.

I've been pregnant three times. Every time the childbirth educator, nurses, and doctors said that once I got past transition and could push the worst would be over and it wouldn't hurt so much. But that wasn't true for me. Pushing really hurt, too. Why didn't they tell me it would?

SPONTANEOUS DELIVERY (VERTEX PRESENTATION)

As the head distends the vulva with each contraction, the perineum becomes extremely thin and the anus stretches and protrudes. As extension occurs under the symphysis pubis, the head is born. After delivery of the head, restitution and external rotation of the head occurs. When the anterior shoulder meets the under side of the symphysis pubis, a gentle push by the mother aids in delivery of the shoulders. The body then follows.

Delivery of infants in other than vertex presentations is discussed in Chapter 25.

Third Stage

PLACENTAL SEPARATION

After the infant is delivered, the uterus firmly contracts, diminishing its capacity and the surface area of placental attachment. The placenta begins to separate because of this decrease in surface area. As this separation occurs, bleeding results in the formation of a hematoma between the placental tissue and the remaining decidua. This hematoma accelerates the separation process. The membranes are the last to separate. They are peeled off the uterine wall as the placenta extrudes into the vagina.

Signs of placental separation usually appear around one to five minutes after delivery of the infant (Pritchard et al 1985). These signs are (a) a globular-shaped uterus,

(b) a rise of the fundus in the abdomen, (c) a sudden gush or trickle of blood, and (d) further protrusion of the umbilical cord out of the introitus.

PLACENTAL DELIVERY

When the signs of placental separation appear, the woman may bear down to aid in placental expulsion. If this fails and the clinician has ascertained that the fundus is firm, gentle traction may be applied to the cord while pressure is exerted on the fundus. The weight of the placenta as it is guided into the placental pan aids in the

removal of the membranes from the uterine wall. A placenta is not considered to be retained until after 30 minutes have elapsed from completion of the second stage of labor.

If the placenta separates from the inside to the outer margins, it is delivered with the fetal or shiny side presenting (Figure 21–19). This is known as the *Schultze mechanism* of placental delivery, or more commonly *shiny Schultze*. If the placenta separates from the outer margins inward, it will roll up and present sideways with the maternal surface delivering first. This is known as the *Duncan method* of placental delivery, and is commonly called *dirty Duncan* because the placental surface is rough in appear-

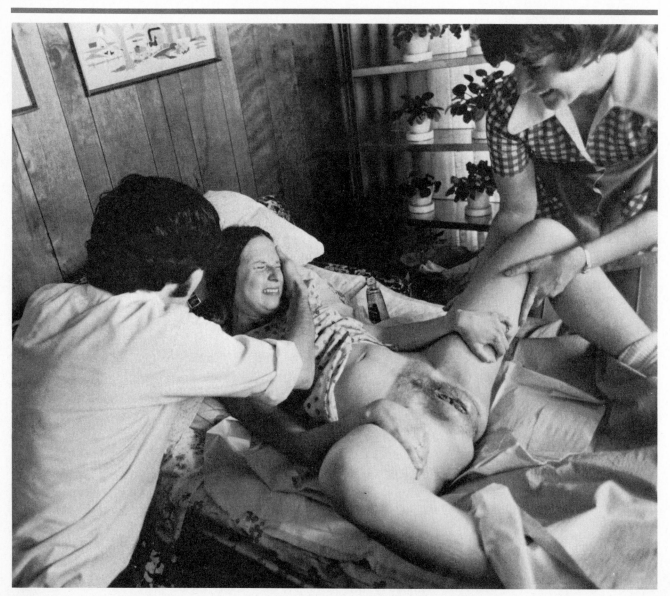

Figure 21–17   The birth sequence

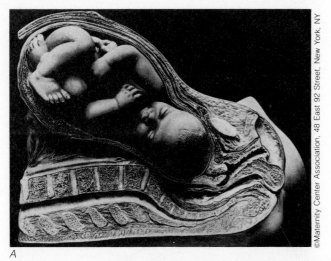

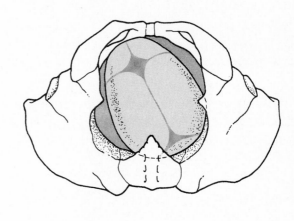

A

B

A, B. As labor begins, the fetal head settles down firmly on the cervix and engagement occurs. This view demonstrates an LOP position. The occiput is in the left posterior quadrant of the maternal pelvis. The cervix is long and thick with no dilatation.

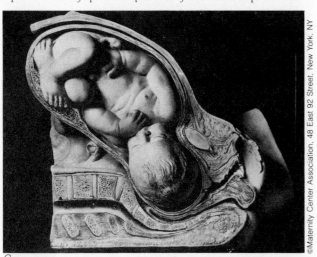

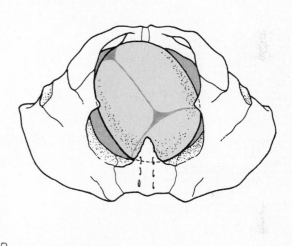

C

D

C, D. As the fetal head descends, flexion of the head occurs, and the occiput becomes the presenting part. Note the difference in the positions of the suture lines and anterior fontanelle (diamond shape) in views B and D. The cervix has begun to efface and dilate.

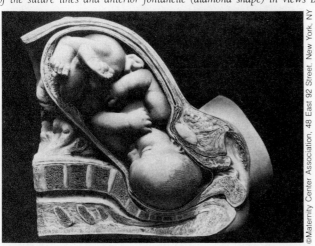

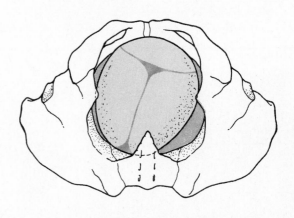

E

F

E, F. As the fetal head enters the bony pelvis, internal rotation takes place. In this view the fetal position is changing to occiput anterior. If the membranes are still intact, they precede the fetal head, the fluid acting as a cushion for the head during contractions. Note that the suture line in view F is almost vertical.

ance. This type is associated with increased blood loss and retention of placental fragments.

Nursing and medical interventions during the third stage of labor are discussed in detail in Chapter 23.

Fourth Stage

The period of time from 1 to 4 hours after delivery, in which physiologic readjustment of the mother's body begins, is sometimes designated the fourth stage of labor.

Hemodynamic changes occur with delivery. Blood loss at delivery may be up to 500 mL. With this blood loss, and the lifting of the weight of the gravid uterus from surrounding vessels, blood is redistributed into venous beds. This results in a moderate drop in both systolic and diastolic blood pressure, increased pulse pressure, and moderate tachycardia (Albright et al 1986).

The cerebrospinal fluid pressure, which increased during labor, now drops with the delivery of the neonate and rapidly recovers normal values (Albright et al 1986).

The uterus remains contracted and is in the midline of the abdomen. The fundus is usually midway between the symphysis pubis and umbilicus. Its contracted state provides for constriction of the vessels at the placental im-

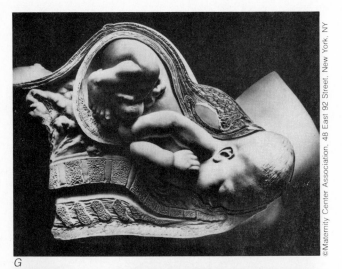

G

©Maternity Center Association, 48 East 92 Street, New York, NY

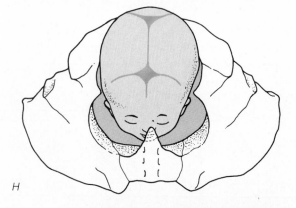

H

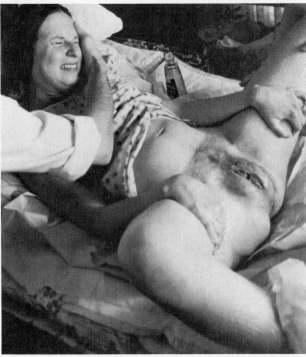

I

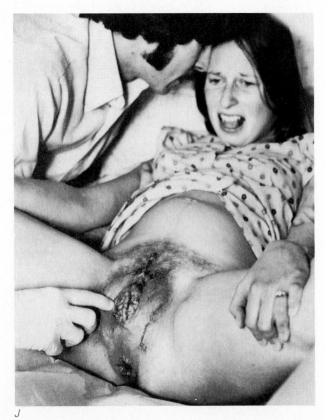

J

G, H, I, J. *Extension begins as the fetal head comes under the maternal symphysis pubis.*

plantation site. Immediately after delivery of the placenta, the cervix is patulous and thick.

Signs or symptoms of nausea and vomiting usually cease and the woman may be thirsty and hungry. She may experience a shaking chill, which is thought to be associated with the ending of the physical exertion of labor as well as change in intraabdominal pressure. It is not uncommon for the bladder to be hypotonic due to trauma during the second stage and/or the administration of anesthetics, which may decrease sensations. Hypotonic bladder leads to urinary retention. Management of this stage is discussed in Chapter 23.

KEY CONCEPTS

Four factors that continually interact during the process of labor and delivery are the birth canal (passage), the fetus (passenger), the uterine contractions and pushing efforts of the laboring woman (powers), and the emotional components the woman brings to the birth setting (psyche).

Four types of pelves have been identified and each has a different effect on labor. The gynecoid and anthropoid

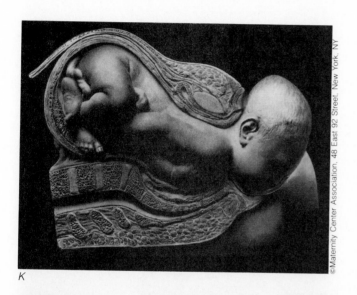

K

©Maternity Center Association, 48 East 92 Street, New York, NY

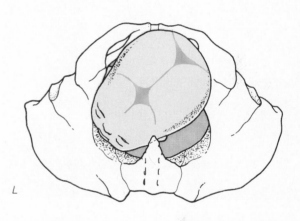

L

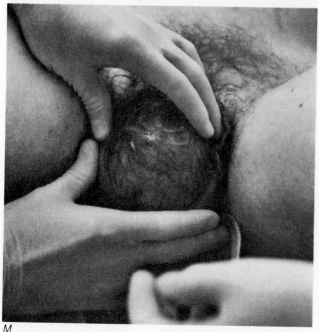

M

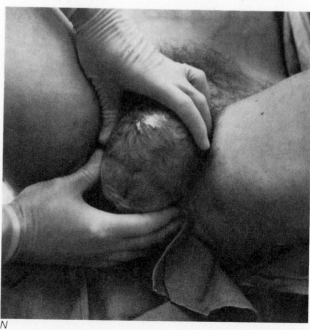

N

K, L, M, N. *In this view extension has occurred. The photos illustrate crowning, the birth of the head, and the beginning of external rotation.*

are favorable to labor and delivery. The android and platypelloid are associated with difficult labor because of diminished diameters.

Important parts of the maternal pelvis include the pelvic inlet, pelvic cavity, and pelvic outlet. The inclination of the symphysis pubis, shape of the side walls, and curvature of the coccyx are also important.

The fetus accommodates itself to the maternal pelvis in a series of movements called the cardinal movements of labor, which include descent, flexion, internal rotation, extension, and restitution.

The fetal head contains bones that are not fused. This allows for some overlapping and molding to facilitate birth.

Fetal *attitude* refers to the relation of the fetal parts to one another.

Fetal *lie* refers to the relationship of the cephalocaudal axis of the fetus to the maternal spine. The fetal lie is either longitudinal or transverse.

Fetal *presentation* is determined by the body part lying closest to the maternal pelvis. Fetal presentations are cephalic, breech, or shoulder.

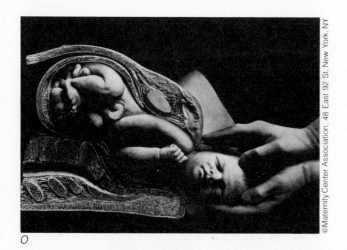

O

©Maternity Center Association, 48 East 92 St. New York, NY

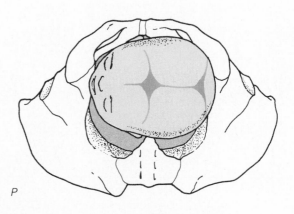

P

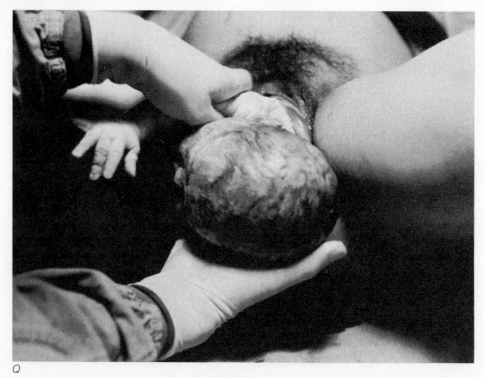

Q

O, P, Q. *External rotation is complete; the shoulders move into the widest part of the maternal pelvis.*

Fetal *position* is the relationship of the landmark on the presenting fetal part to the front, sides, or back of the maternal pelvis.

Engagement of the presenting part takes place when the largest diameter of the presenting part reaches or passes through the pelvic inlet.

Station refers to the relationship of the presenting part to an imaginary line drawn between the ischial spines of the maternal pelvis.

Each uterine contraction has an increment, acme, and decrement. Contraction frequency is the time from the beginning of one contraction to the beginning of the next contraction.

Duration of contractions refers to the period of time from the beginning to the end of one contraction.

Intensity of contractions refers to the strength of the contraction during acme. Intensity of contractions is termed as mild, moderate, or strong.

Possible causes of labor include oxytocin stimulation, progesterone withdrawal, estrogen stimulation, fetal

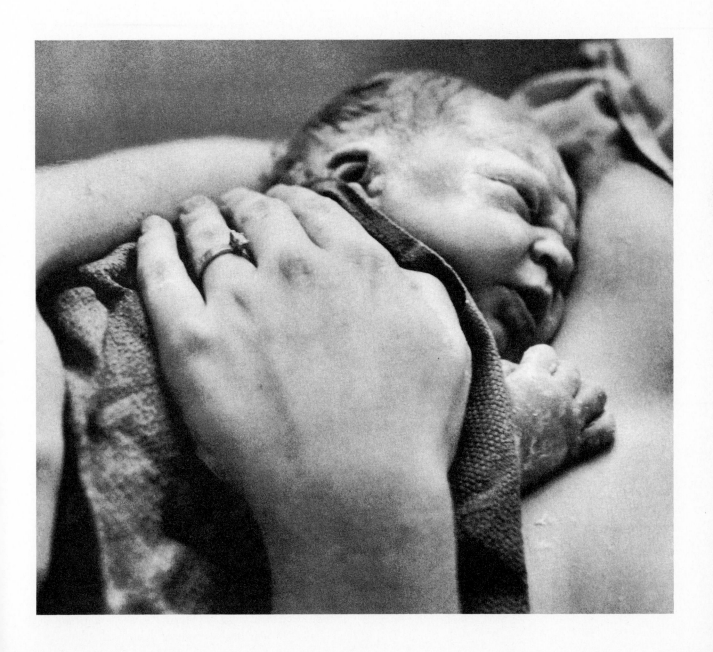

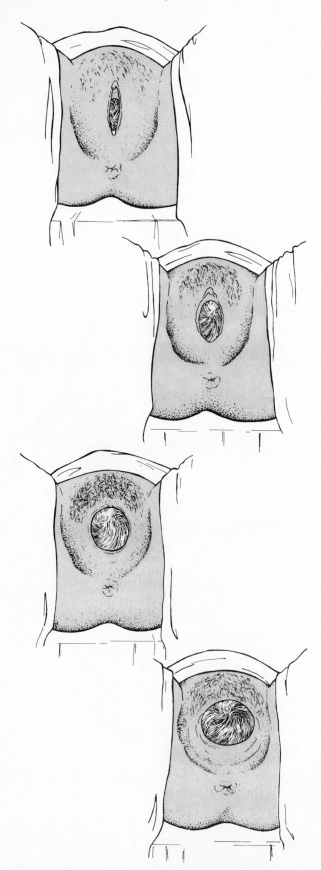

Figure 21–18 Progressive dilatation of the vaginal opening during the second stage of labor.

cortisol, and fetal membrane phospholipid–arachidonic acid–prostaglandin theory.

Labor stresses the coping skills of women. Women with prenatal education about childbrith usually report more positive responses to labor.

Factors that affect the response to labor pain include education, cultural beliefs, fatigue and sleep deprivation, personal significance of pain, previous experience, anxiety, and the availability of coping techniques.

Premonitory signs of labor include lightening, Braxton Hicks contractions, cervical softening and effacement, bloody show, sudden burst of energy, weight loss, and sometimes rupture of membranes.

There are four stages of labor and delivery. The first stage is from beginning of true labor to complete dilatation of the cervix. Second stage is from complete dilatation of the cervix to birth. Third stage is from birth to expulsion of the placenta. Fourth stage is from expulsion of the placenta to a period of one to four hours after.

Placental separation is indicated by lengthening of the umbilical cord, a small spurt of blood, change in uterine shape, and a rise of the fundus in the abdomen.

The placenta is delivered by Schultze or Duncan mechanism. This is determined by the way it separates from the uterine wall.

REFERENCES

Acker DB, et al: The leukocyte count in labor. *Am J Obstet Gynecol* 1985;153(7):737.

Aladjem S: *Obstetric Practice.* St Louis, Mosby, 1980.

Albright GA, et al: *Anesthesia in Obstetrics: Maternal, Fetal and Neonatal Aspects,* ed 2. Boston, Butterworths, 1986.

Bates MS: Ethnicity and pain: A biocultural model. *Soc Sci Med* 1987;24(1):47.

Bonica JJ: *Mechanisms and Pathways of Pain in Labor.* Chicago, Abbott Laboratories, 1960.

Bonica JJ: *Principles and Practice of Obstetric Analgesia and Anesthesia.* Philadelphia, Davis, 1972.

Boylan P, **O'Donovan** P, **Owens** OJ: Fetal breathing movements and the diagnosis of labor: A prospective analysis of 100 cases. *Obstet Gynecol* 1985;66(4):517.

Caldwell WE, **Maloy** HC: Anatomical variations in the female pelvis and their effect on labor with a suggested classification. *Am J Obstet Gynecol* 1933;26:479.

Calhoun MA: The Vietnamese woman: Health/illness attitudes and behaviors, in **Stern** PN: *Women, Health and Culture.* Washington, Hemisphere Publishing, 1986.

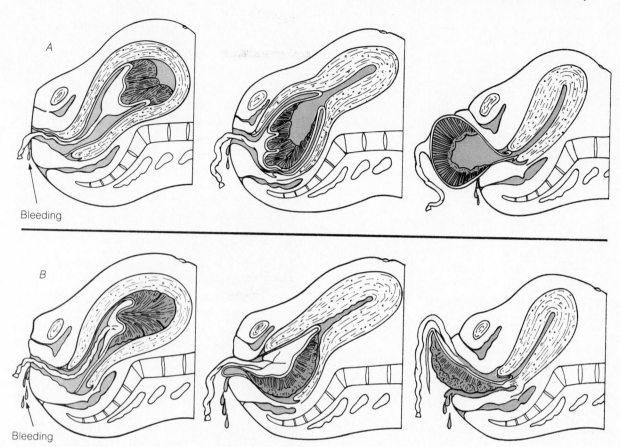

Figure 21–19   Placental separation and delivery. A Schultze mechanism. B Duncan mechanism

Challis JR, **Mitchell** BF: Hormonal control of preterm and term parturition. *Semin Perinatol* 1981;5(July):192.

Chaney JA: Birthing in early America. *J Nurs-Midwife* 1980;25(March/April):5.

Cibils LA: *Electronic Fetal-Neonatal Monitoring.* Boston, PSG, 1981.

Creasy RK, **Resnik**, R: *Maternal-Fetal Medicine.* Philadelphia, Saunders, 1984.

Copstik SM: Partner support and the use of coping techniques in labour. *J Psychosom Res* 1986;30(4):497.

Crandon AJ: Maternal anxiety and obstetric complications. *J Psychosom Res* 1978;23:109.

Dalaker K: Clotting factor VII during pregnancy, delivery and puerperium. *Br J Obstet Gynaecol* 1986;93:17.

Delke I, **Minkoff** H, **Grunebaum** A: Effect of Lamaze childbirth preparation on maternal plasma beta-endorphin immunoreactivity in active labor. *Am J Perinatol* 1985;2(4):317.

Doering SG, **Entwisle** DR: Preparation during pregnancy and ability to cope with labor and delivery. *Am J Orthopsych* 1975;45:825.

Ekman G, et al: Cervical collagen: An important regulator of cervical function in term labor. *Obstet Gynecol* 1986;67(5):633.

Friedman EA: *Labor: Clinical Evaluation and Management,* ed 2. New York, Appleton-Century-Crofts, 1978.

Griffin RL, **Caron** FJM, **van Geijn** HP: Behavioral states in the human fetus during labor *Am J Obstet Gynecol* 1985;152(7):828.

Hariharan S, **Takahashi** K, **Burd** L: Initiation of labor, in **Sciarri** JJ (ed): *Gynecology and Obstetrics.* Philadelphia, Saunders, 1986, chap 86.

Heggenhougen HK: Father and childbirth: An anthropological perspective. *J Nurse-Midwife* 1980;25(November/December):21.

Hughy MJ: Fetal position during pregnancy. *Am J Obstet Gynecol* 1985;153:885.

Humenick SS: Mastery: The key to childbirth satisfaction? A review. *Birth Fam J* 1981;8(Summer):79.

Huszar G: Biology and biochemistry of myometrial contractility and cervical maturation. *Semin Perinatol* 1981;5(July):216.

Kay MA: Anthropology of human birth. Philadelphia, Davis, 1982.

Lederman RP: *Psychosocial Adaptation in Pregnancy: Assessment of Seven Dimensions of Maternal Development.* Englewood Cliffs, NJ, Prentice-Hall, 1984.

Liggins GC: Fetal influences on myometrial contractility. *Clin Obstet Gynecol* 1973;16:148.

Liggins GC: Ripening of the cervix. *Semin Perinatol* 1978;2(July):261.

McCaffery M: *Nursing Management of the Patient With Pain.* Philadelphia, Lippincott, 1972.

Melzack R: *The Puzzle of Pain.* New York, Basic Books, 1973.

Mercer RA: A theoretical framework for studying factors that impact on the maternal role. *Nurs Res* 1981;30(March/April):73.

Mercer RT: Relationship of the birth experience to later mothering behaviors. *J Nurse-Midwife* 1985;30(July/August):204.

Mishel MH, **Braden** CJ: Uncertainty a mediator between support and adjustment. *West J Nurs Res* 1987;9(1):43.

Morrow K: Transcultural midwifery: Adapting to Hmong birthing customs in California. *J Nurse-Midwife* 1986;31(November/December):285.

Newton N: Some aspects of primitive childbirth. *JAMA* 1964;188(June):10.

Oxorn H: *Human Labor and Birth.* New York, Appleton-Century-Crofts, 1986.

Pritchard JA, **MacDonald** PC, **Gant** NF: *Williams Obstetrics,* ed 17. New York, Appleton-Century-Crofts, 1985.

Rubin R: *Maternal Identity and the Maternal Experience.* New York, Springer Publishing, 1984.

Varney H: *Nurse Midwifery.* Boston, Blackwell Scientific Publications, 1980.

Westbrook MT: Socioeconomic differences in coping with childbearing. *Am J Comm Psychol* 1979;7:397.

Berg G, **Andersson** RGG, **Ryden** G: Adrenergic receptors in human myometrium during pregnancy. *Am J Obstet Gynecol* 1986;154(3):601.

Chen SZ, et al: Effects of sitting position on uterine activity during labor. *Obstet Gynecol* 1987;69(January):67.

Dattel BJ, **Lan** F, **Roberts** JM: Failure to demonstrate decreased adrenergic receptor concentration or decreased agonist efficacy in term or preterm human parturition. *Am J Obstet Gynecol* 1986;154(2):450.

Giannopoulos G. et al: Prostaglandin E and F_2 receptors in human myometrium during the menstrual cycle and in pregnancy and labor. *Am J Obstet Gynecol* 1985;153(8):904.

Hahn DW, et al: Influence of ovarian steroids on prostaglandin- and leukotriene-induced uterine contractions. *Am J Obstet Gynecol* 1985;153(1):87.

McCosten JA, et al: Prostaglandin E_2 release on the fetal and maternal sides of the amnion and chorion decidua before and after term labor. *Am J Obstet Gynecol* 1987;156(January):173.

Orth-Gomer K, **Unden** AL: The measurement of social support in population surveys. *Soc Sci Med* 1987;24(1):83. Symposium: Managing pregnancy in patients over 35. *Contemp OB/GYN* 1987;29(May):180.

ADDITIONAL READINGS

Bell SE, **Whiteford** MB: Tai Dam health care practices: Asian refugee women in Iowa. *Soc Sci Med* 1987;24(4):317.

Birth usually feels like a steamy kitchen—similar to holiday preparations, except that the smells are different. The smell of sweat is more acrid, there are some fetid odors, there is the smell and steam rising from blood. The air is thick, pungent, fertile. It is hard not to be reminded of fresh straw and night stars. There is near and heady promise. (A Midwife's Story)

Intrapartal Nursing Assessment

Maternal Assessment
History
Intrapartal High-Risk Screening
Intrapartal Physical Assessment
Assessment of Pelvic Adequacy
Intrapartal Psychologic Assessment
Methods of Evaluating Labor Progress

Fetal Assessment
Determination of Fetal Position and Presentation
Evaluation of Fetal Status During Labor
Value of Electronic Fetal Monitoring
Psychologic Reactions to Electronic Monitoring
Nursing Care and Responsibilities
Additional Assessment Techniques

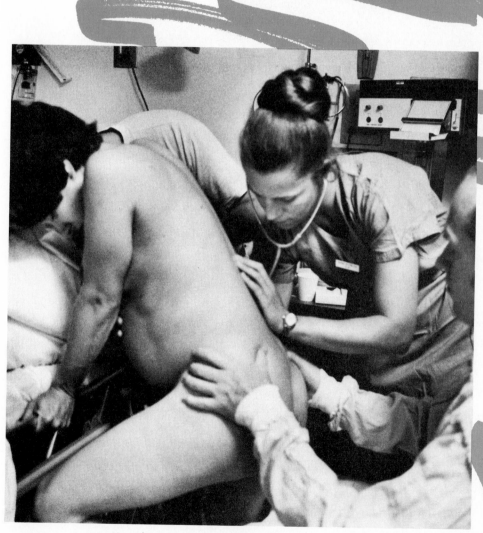

Here the nurse has encouraged her client to stand with one leg on a stool
to assist the baby in rotating from posterior to anterior position.

Chapter Twenty-Two

OBJECTIVES

- Summarize intrapartal physical and psychological assessments necessary for optimum maternal-fetal outcome.
- Define and identify the outer limits of normal progress of each of the phases and stages of labor.
- Compare the various methods of monitoring FHR and contractions, giving advantages and disadvantages of each.
- Differentiate between baseline and periodic changes in the FHR, and describe the criteria and significance of each.
- Outline the steps to be performed in the systematic evaluation of FHR tracings.
- Identify nonreassuring and ominous FHR patterns and the interventions that should be carried out in the management of each.
- Discuss the indications for fetal blood sampling and guidelines for management of labor for related pH values.
- Discuss information to be taught when EFM is used, and provide rationale for teaching.
- Discuss psychologic reactions to EFM and the role of the nurse.

The physiologic events that occur during labor call for many adaptations by the mother and fetus. Accurate and frequent assessment is crucial because the changes are rapid and involve two individuals, mother and child.

The nurse in the birth setting uses a wide variety of assessment skills to provide care to the mother and her child. The skills of observation, palpation, and auscultation are still important as the nurse watches for subtle clues that may indicate a problem is developing. The nurse's presence with the laboring woman provides an opportunity for ongoing assessment, even as the nurse quietly provides comfort measures and assists the coach in offering support. Experienced nurses seem to develop a sixth sense that enables them to anticipate the changes that may happen rapidly in the birth process.

In current practice, the "hands-on" techniques are enhanced by the use of ultrasound and electronic monitoring. These new techniques can be used to gather additional data and to validate the hands-on assessments. As with any new technological development, it is tempting to let the machine become an important focus of care. In the birth set-ting, where the contact between the couple and the nurse is so intense, "high-tech" assessments are easily meshed with "high-touch" assessments.

This chapter presents the assessments that are important in the birth setting.

● Maternal Assessment

History

The woman's history may be obtained in an abbreviated format when the woman is admitted to the labor and delivery area. Each agency has its own admission form but similar information is usually obtained. Relevant data include:

- Name and age
- Attending physician or certified nurse-midwife
- Personal data: blood type, Rh factor, results of serology testing, prepregnant and present weight, allergies to medications, foods, or substances
- History of previous illness, such as TB, heart disease, diabetes, convulsive disorders, thyroid disorders
- Problems in the prenatal course, for example, elevated blood pressure, bleeding problems, recurrent urinary tract infection
- Pregnancy data: gravida, para, abortions, term and preterm infants, number of living children, neonatal deaths
- The method chosen for infant feeding
- Type of prenatal education
- Requests regarding labor and birth (no enema, no analgesic or anesthetic, father and/or other support persons in attendance, and so on)

Intrapartal High-Risk Screening

As part of the history and assessment, the nurse should consider intrapartal factors that would increase the risk for the woman and her baby. Intrapartal high-risk factors are shown in Table 22–1. The table includes maternal and fetal or neonatal implications. The factors are presented prior to the intrapartal physical assessment guide so that they can be kept in mind during the assessment.

Intrapartal Physical Assessment

A physical examination is included as part of the admission procedure and as part of the ongoing care of the woman. The assessment becomes the basis for initiating nursing interventions.

Table 22–1 Intrapartal High-Risk Factors

Factor	Maternal implication	Fetal-neonatal implication
Abnormal presentation	↑ Risk of cesarean delivery ↑ Risk of prolonged labor ↑ Hypertension risk ↑ Nausea-vomiting	Prematurity ↑ Risk of congenital abnormality Neonatal physical trauma ↑ Risk of IUGR
Multiple gestation	↑ Uterine distention→ ↑ risk of postpartum hemorrhage ↑ Risk of cesarean delivery ↑ Risk of preterm labor	Low birth weight ↑ Risk of abortion Prematurity ↑ Risk of congenital anomalies Feto-fetal transfusion
Hydramnios	↑ Discomfort ↑ Dyspnea Edema of lower extremities	↑ Risk of esophageal or other high alimentary tract atresias ↑ Risk of CNS anomalies (myelocele)
Oligohydramnios	Maternal fear of "dry birth"	↑ Risk of congenital anomalies ↑ Risk of renal lesions ↑ Risk of IUGR ↑ Risk of fetal acidosis Postmaturity
Meconium staining of amniotic fluid	↑ Psychologic stress due to fear for fetus	↑ Risk of fetal asphyxia ↑ Risk of meconium aspiration ↑ Risk of pneumonia due to aspiration of meconium
Premature rupture of membranes	↑ Risk of infection (chorioamnionitis) ↑ Risk of preterm labor ↑ Anxiety Fear for the baby Prolonged hospitalization ↑ Risk of tocolytic therapy ↑ Infection risk	↑ Perinatal morbidity Prematurity ↓ Birth weight ↑ Risk of respiratory distress syndrome Prolonged hospitalization
Induction of labor	↑ Risk of hypercontractility of uterus ↑ Risk of uterine rupture ↑ Length of labor if cervix not ready ↑ Anxiety ↑ Pain in labor	Prematurity if gestational age not assessed correctly Hypoxia if hyperstimulation occurs
Abruptio placentae-placenta previa	Hemorrhage Uterine atony	Fetal hypoxia/acidosis Fetal exsanguination ↑ Perinatal mortality
Failure to progress in labor	Maternal exhaustion ↑ Risk of augmentation of labor ↑ Risk of cesarean delivery	Fetal hypoxia/acidosis Inracranial birth injury
Precipitous labor (<3 hours)	Perineal, vaginal, cervical lacerations ↑ Risk of PP hemorrhage	Tentorial tears Neonatal asphyxia
Prolapse of umbilical cord	↑ Fear of fetus Cesarean delivery	Acute fetal hypoxia/acidosis
Fetal heart aberrations	↑ Fear for fetus Cesarean delivery Continuous electronic monitoring and intervention in labor	Tachycardia, chronic asphyxic insult, bradycardia, acute asphyxic insult Chronic hypoxia Congenital heart block
Uterine rupture	Hemorrhage Cesarean delivery for hysterectomy Death	Fetal anoxia Fetal hemorrhage ↑ Neonatal morbidity and mortality
Postdates (>42 weeks)	↑ Anxiety ↑ Incidence of induction of labor ↑ Incidence of cesarean delivery ↑ Use of technology to monitor fetus	Postmaturity syndrome ↑ Risk of fetal-neonatal mortality ↑ Risk of antepartum fetal death

Intrapartal Physical Assessment Guide: First Stage of Labor

Assess/Normal findings	Alterations and possible causes of alterations*	Nursing responses to data base†
VITAL SIGNS		
Blood pressure: 90–140/60–90 or no more than 15–20 mm Hg rise over baseline BP during early pregnancy	High blood pressure (essential hypertension, preeclampsia, renal disease, apprehension or anxiety)	Evaluate history of preexisting disorders and check for presence of other signs of pre-eclampsia.
	Low blood pressure (supine hypotension)	Turn woman on her side and recheck blood pressure. Do not assess during contractions; implement measures to decrease anxiety and then reassess.
Pulse: 60–90 beats/min	Increased pulse rate (excitement or anxiety, cardiac disorders)	Evaluate cause, reassess to see if rate continues; report to physician.
Respirations: 16–24/min (or pulse rate divided by 4)	Marked tachypnea (respiratory disease)	Assess between contractions; if marked tachypnea continues, assess for signs of respiratory disease.
	Hyperventilation (anxiety)	Encourage slow breaths if woman is hyperventilating.
Temperature: 36.2–37.6C (98–99.6F)	Elevated temperature (infection, dehydration)	Assess for other signs of infection or dehydration.
WEIGHT		
15–30 lb greater than prepregnant weight	Weight gain >30 lb (fluid retention, obesity, large infant, hypertension of pregnancy)	Assess for signs of edema.
LUNGS		
Normal breath sounds (see irregular breath sounds)	Rales, rhonchi, friction rub (infection)	Reassess; refer to physician.
HEART		
Normal heart sounds; grade II/VI systolic ejection murmur is normally found in pregnant women due to extra blood volume passing through heart valves	Murmurs	Refer to physician.
FUNDUS		
At 40 weeks' gestation, located just below xyphoid process	Uterine size not compatible with estimated delivery time (SGA, hydramnios, multiple pregnancy)	Reevaluate history regarding pregnancy dating. Refer to physician for additional assessment.
EDEMA		
Slight amount of dependent edema	Pitting edema of face, legs, abdomen (preeclampsia)	Check deep tendon reflexes for hyperactivity, check for clonus; refer to physician.
HYDRATION		
Normal skin turgor	Poor skin turgor (dehydration)	Assess skin turgor; refer to physician for deviations.
PERINEUM		
Tissues smooth, pink color (see Prenatal Initial Physical Assessment Guide, Chapter 15)	Varicose veins of vulva	Exercise care while doing a perineal prep; note on client record need for follow-up in postpartal period; reassess after delivery.
Clear mucus	Profuse, purulent drainage	Suspect gonorrhea; report to physician; initiate care to newborn's eyes; notify neonatal nursing staff and pediatrician.

*Possible causes of alterations are placed in parentheses.
†This column provides guidelines for further assessment and initial nursing interventions.

Intrapartal Physical Assessment Guide: First Stage of Labor (continued)

Assess/Normal findings	Alterations and possible causes of alterations*	Nursing responses to data base†
Presence of small amount of bloody show that gradually increases with further cervical dilatation	Hemorrhage	Assess BP and pulse, pallor, diaphoresis; report any marked changes. (Note: Gaping of vagina and/or anus and bulging of perineum are suggestive signs of second stage of labor.)
ENERGY STATUS Sufficient energy to complete the work of labor	Exhaustion, acetone in urine (deficiency in metabolism of glucose and/or fat, decreasing uterine activity in long labor)	Provide ice chips or hard candy in early labor, IV with dextrose in late labor. Dipstick urine. Assess quality of contractions. Refer to physician.
LABOR STATUS Uterine contractions: Regular pattern	Failure to establish a regular pattern, prolonged latent phase Hypertonicity Hypotonicity	Evaluate whether woman is in true labor; ambulate if in early labor. Evaluate woman's status and contractile pattern.
Cervical dilatation: Progressive cervical dilatation from size of fingertip to 10 cm (Procedure 22–1, p 615)	Rigidity of cervix (frequent cervical infections, scar tissue, failure of presenting part to descend)	Evaluate contractions, fetal engagement, position, and cervical dilatation. Inform woman of progress
Cervical effacement: Progressive thinning of cervix (Procedure 22–1)	Failure to efface (rigidity of cervix, failure of presenting part to engage); cervical edema (pushing effort by woman before cervix is fully dilated and effaced, trapped cervix)	Evaluate contractions, fetal engagement, and position. Notify physician/nurse-midwife if cervix is becoming edematous; work with woman to prevent pushing until cervix is completely dilated.
Fetal descent: Progressive descent of fetal presenting part from station −5 to +4 (see Figure 22–1 on p 612)	Failure of descent (abnormal fetal position or presentation, macrosomic fetus, inadequate pelvic measurement)	Evaluate fetal position, presentation, and size. Evaluate maternal pelvic measurements.
Membranes: May rupture before or during labor	Rupture of membranes more than 12–24 hours before initiation of labor	Assess for ruptured membranes using Nitrazine test tape before doing vaginal exam. Instruct women with ruptured membranes to remain on bed rest if presenting part is not engaged. Keep vaginal exams to a minimum to prevent infection.

Findings on Nitrazine test tape:
Membranes probably intact
  yellow   pH 5.0
  olive   pH 5.5
  olive green   pH 6.0
 	
Membranes probably ruptured
  blue-green   pH 6.5
  blue-gray   pH 7.0
  deep blue   pH 7.5
	False-positive results possible if large amount of bloody show is present or if previous vaginal examination has been done using lubricant	Assess fluid for consistency, amount, odor; assess FHR frequently. Assess fluid at regular intervals for presence of meconium staining.

Amniotic fluid clear, no odor	Greenish amniotic fluid (fetal distress)	Assess FHR; do vaginal exam to evaluate for prolapsed cord; apply fetal monitor for continuous data; report to physician.
	Strong odor (amnionitis)	Take woman's temperature and report to physician.
FETAL STATUS FHR: 120–160 beats/min	< 120 or >160 beats/min (fetal distress); abnormal patterns on fetal monitor: decreased variability, late decelerations, variable decelerations (p 629)	Initiate interventions based on particular FHR pattern (p. 639)

Possible causes of alterations are placed in parentheses.
†This column provides guidelines for further assessment and initial nursing interventions.

Intrapartal Physical Assessment Guide: First Stage of Labor (continued)

Assess/Normal findings	Alterations and possible causes of alterations*	Nursing responses to data base†
Presentation: Cephalic, 97% Breech, 3%	Face or brow presentation	Report to physician; after presentation is confirmed as face or brow, woman may be prepared for cesarean delivery.
Position: LOA most common (Figures 22–2 and 22–3)	Persistent occipital-posterior position; transverse arrest	Carefully monitor maternal and fetal status.
Activity: Fetal movement	Hyperactivity (may precede fetal hypoxia)	Carefully evaluate FHR; may apply fetal monitor.
	Complete lack of movement (fetal distress or fetal demise)	Carefully evaluate FHR; may apply fetal monitor.
LABORATORY EVALUATION Hematologic tests Hemoglobin: 12–16 g/dL	< 12g (anemia, hemorrhage)	Evaluate woman for problems due to decreased oxygen-carrying capacity caused by lowered hemoglobin.
CBC Hematocrit: 38%–47% RBC: 4.2–5.4 million/μL WBC: 4,500–11,000/μL although leukocytosis to 20,000/μL is not unusual	Presence of infection or blood dyscrasias	Evaluate for other signs of infection or for petechia, bruising, or unusual bleeding.

*Possible causes of alterations are placed in parentheses.
†This column provides guidelines for further assessment and initial nursing interventions.

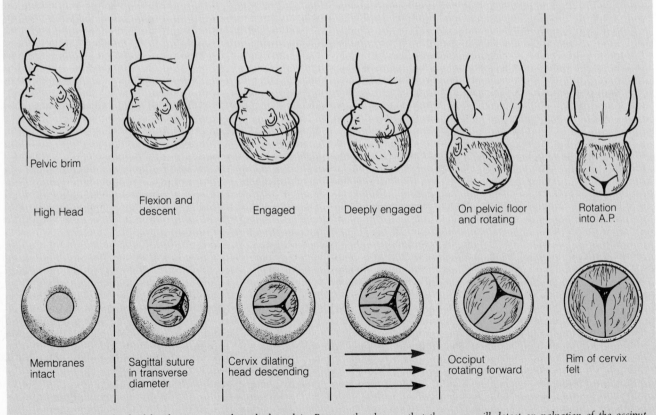

High Head	Flexion and descent	Engaged	Deeply engaged	On pelvic floor and rotating	Rotation into A.P.
Membranes intact	Sagittal suture in transverse diameter	Cervix dilating head descending		Occiput rotating forward	Rim of cervix felt

Figure 22–1 Top, the fetal head progressing through the pelvis. Bottom, the changes that the nurse will detect on palpation of the occiput through the cervix while doing a vaginal examination. (From Myles MF: Textbook for Midwives. Edinburgh, Scotland: Churchill Livingstone, 1975, p 246)

Intrapartal Physical Assessment Guide: First Stage of Labor (continued)

Assess/Normal findings	Alterations and possible causes of alterations*	Nursing responses to data base†
Serologic tests STS or VDRL test: Nonreactive	Positive reaction (see Chapter 15, Initial Prenatal Physical Assessment Guide)	For reactive test, notify newborn nursery and pediatrician.
Urinalysis Glucose: Negative	Glycosuria (low renal threshold for glucose, diabetes mellitus)	Assess blood glucose; test urine for ketones; ketonuria and glycosuria require further assessment of blood sugars.†
Ketone: Negative	Ketonuria (starvation ketosis)	
Proteins: Negative	Proteinuria (urine specimen contaminated with vaginal secretions, fever, kidney disease); proteinuria of 2+ or greater found in uncontaminated urine may be a sign of ensuing preeclampsia	Instruct woman in collection technique; incidence of contamination from vaginal discharge is common.
Red blood cells: Negative	Blood in urine (calculi, cystitis, glomerulonephritis, neoplasm)	Assess collection technique.
White blood cells: Negative	Presence of white blood cells (infection in genitourinary tract)	Assess for signs of urinary tract infection.
Casts: None	Presence of casts (nephrotic syndrome)	Inform clinician of finding.

†*Glycosuria should not be discounted. The presence of glycosuria necessitates follow-up.*

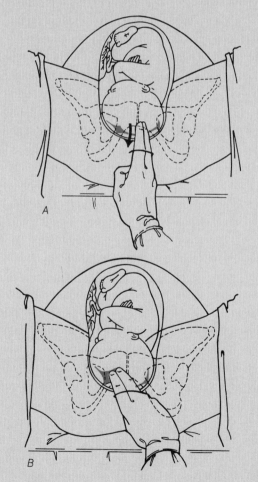

Figure 22-2   *Assessment of fetal position and station. A Palpate sagittal suture and assess station. B Identify anterior fontanelle.*

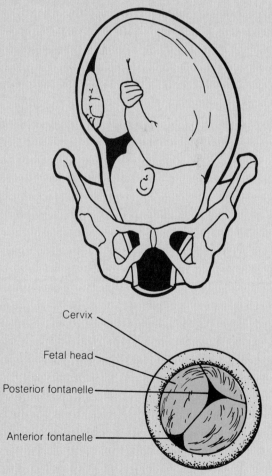

Figure 22-3   *Palpation of presenting part on LOA position. Posterior fontanelle is in upper right.*

The intrapartal physical assessment is not as complete and thorough as the initial prenatal physical examination (Chapter 15), but it does involve assessment of some body systems and of the actual labor process. The accompanying Intrapartal Physical Assessment Guide provides a framework for the maternity nurse's examination of the laboring woman.

The guide includes assessments performed immediately upon admission and continued as an ongoing assessment. Others may be assessed only once. Critical admission assessments include vital signs, labor status, fetal status, and laboratory and psychologic evaluation. These assessments will be continued throughout the labor process. Assessments that are done only once as part of the admission data, if time permits, include evaluation of weight, breasts, lungs, and heart (in many institutions assessments of breasts, lungs, and heart are omitted).

Assessment of Pelvic Adequacy

Clinical pelvimetry, which is a manual assessment of the pelvis, is usually performed in the prenatal period by the woman's primary care giver. Occasionally, however, a woman who is admitted to the birthing unit has had no prenatal care. Thus the nurse must perform an initial assessment of pelvic adequacy. When measurements are questionable, and/or labor is not progressing within normal limits, the diameters may be reassessed by x-ray or MRI examination at the discretion of the obstetrician.

Intrapartal Psychologic Assessment

Assessment of the laboring woman's psychologic status is an important part of the total assessment. The woman

Intrapartal Psychologic Assessment Guide

Assess/Normal findings	Alterations and possible causes of alterations*	Nursing responses to data base†
SUPPORT SYSTEM		
Physical intimacy of mother-father (or mother-support relationship): Caretaking activities such as soothing conversation, touching	Limited physical contact or continual clinging together (may reflect normal pattern for this couple or their attempt to cope with this situation)	Encourage caretaking activities that appear to comfort the woman; encourage support to the woman; if support is limited, the nurse may take a more active role.
Support person in close proximity	Maintaining a distance from woman for prolonged periods (may be normal pattern for this couple or may indicate strained relationship or anxiety due to labor)	Encourage support person to stay close (if this seems appropriate).
Relationship of mother-father (or support person): Involved interaction	Limited interaction (may reflect normal interaction pattern or strained relationship)	Support interactions; if interaction is limited, the nurse may provide more information and support.
ANXIETY		
Some anxiety and apprehension is within normal limits	Rapid breathing, nervous tremors, frowning, grimacing or clenching of teeth, thrashing movements, crying, increased pulse and blood pressure (anxiety, apprehension)	Provide support and encouragement.
PREPARATION FOR CHILDBIRTH		
The woman has some information regarding process of normal labor and delivery	Insufficient information	Add to present information base.
Woman has breathing and/or relaxation techniques to use during labor	No breathing or relaxation techniques (insufficient information)	Support breathing and relaxation techniques that the woman is using; provide information if needed.
RESPONSE TO LABOR		
Latent phase: relaxed, excited, anxious for labor to be well established	Inability to cope with contractions (fear, anxiety, lack of education)	Provide support and encouragement; establish trusting relationship.
Active phase: becomes more intense, begins to tire		
Transitional phase: feels tired, may feel unable to cope, needs frequent coaching to maintain breathing patterns		Provide support and coaching if needed.
Coping mechanisms: Ability to cope with labor through use of support system, breathing, relaxation techniques	Marked anxiety, apprehension (insufficient coping mechanisms)	Support coping mechanisms if they are working for the woman; provide information and support if she is exhibiting anxiety or needs additional alternatives to present coping methods.

*Possible causes of alterations are placed in parentheses.
†This column provides guidelines for further assessment and nursing interventions.

Procedure 22–1   Intrapartal Vaginal Examination

Objective	Nursing action	Rationale
Prepare woman.	Explain procedure, indications for carrying out procedure, and information being obtained.	Explanation of procedure decreases anxiety and increases relaxation.
	Position woman with thighs flexed and abducted; instruct her to put heels of feet together.	Prevents contamination of area during examination and allows for visualization of external signs of labor progress.
	Drape so that only the perineum is exposed. Encourage woman to relax her muscles and legs during procedure.	Provides as much privacy as possible.
Assemble and prepare equipment.	Have following equipment easily accessible: • Sterile disposable gloves • Lubricant • Nitrazine test tape prior to first examination	Examination is facilitated and can be done quickly.
Use aseptic technique during examination.	If leakage of fluid has been noted or if woman reports leakage of fluid, use Nitrazine test tape before doing vaginal exam.	Nitrazine test tape registers a change in pH if amniotic fluid is present (unless a lubricant has already been used).
	Put on both gloves; using thumb and forefinger of left hand, spread labia widely, insert well-lubricated second and index fingers of right hand into vagina until they touch the cervix.	Avoid contaminating hand by contact with anus; positioning of hand with wrist straight and elbow tilted downward allows fingertips to point toward umbilicus and find cervix.
Determine status of fetal membranes.	Palpate for movable bulging sac through the cervix; observe for expression of amniotic fluid during exam.	If intact, bag of waters feels like a bulge.
Determine status of labor progress during and after contractions.	Carry out vaginal examination during and between contractions.	Examination varies.
Identify degree of: 1. Cervical dilatation	Palpate for opening or what appears as a depression in the cervix.	Estimation of the diameter of the depression identifies degree of dilatation.
	Estimate diameter of cervical opening in centimeters (0–10 cm).	One finger represents approximately 1.5–2 cm cervical dilatation.
2. Cervical effacement	Palpate the thickness of the surrounding circular ridge of tissue; estimate degree of thinning in percentages (Figure 22–4).	Degree of thinning determines the amount of lower uterine segment that has been taken up into the fundal area.
Determine presentation and position of presenting part.	As cervix opens, palpate for presenting part and identify its relationship to the maternal pelvis.	Presenting part is easier to palpate through a dilated cervix and differentiation of landmarks is easier.
Determine station.	Locate lowest portion of presenting part.	Identification of station provides information as to degree of descent.
Inform woman about progress in labor.	Discuss findings of the vaginal examination and correlate them to woman's progress in labor.	Assists in identifying progress and reinforces need for frequency of procedure. Information is reassuring and supportive for woman and family.

brings to labor previous ideas, knowledge, and fears that can affect the labor and birth.

Assessment of psychologic parameters requires caring and skill. An atmosphere of rapport and support is essential for evaluating an area that is primarily subjective and allows great latitude in interpretation of responses and behavior. Information is gathered throughout all interactions with the laboring woman, and the observations and assessments are continuously analyzed and evaluated. For instance:

1. Do the woman's words and actions match?

Mrs Ames is admitted to the birthing unit. She appears unsure and hesitant during the admission process. With support and encouragement she begins to ask questions about the unit and is able to communicate her requests for the labor and delivery process. Although Mrs Ames was initially unsure and hesitant, her actions and words were congruent.

Mrs Martin is admitted in active labor. She smiles frequently and states through clenched teeth that she is "just fine." The nurse notes that her hands are tightly clenching

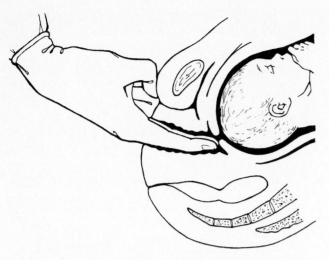

Figure 22–4 Vaginal palpation of cervical dilatation, effacement, amniotic membranes, and presenting part

the bed rails and her knuckles are white. Mrs Martin's words and actions are not congruent.

2. What coping behaviors are observed and are they effective?

3. What communication patterns are present and are they effective?

Assessment of the woman's psychologic status enables the nurse to meet her informational and support needs. The nurse can support the woman and her partner, or in the absence of a partner, the nurse may become the support person. See the accompanying Intrapartal Psychologic Assessment Guide.

Methods of Evaluating Labor Progress

CONTRACTION ASSESSMENT

Uterine contractions may be assessed by palpation and/or continuous electronic monitoring.

○ *PALPATION* Contractions are assessed for frequency, duration, and intensity by placing one hand on the uterine fundus. The hand is kept relatively still as excessive movement may stimulate contractions or may cause discomfort. To determine duration the time is noted when tensing of the fundus is first felt (begining of contraction) and again as relaxation occurs (end of contraction). During the acme of the contraction, intensity can be evaluated by estimating the indentability of the fundus. At least three successive contractions should be assessed to provide enough data to determine the contraction pattern. Since frequency is determined by noting the time from the beginning of one contraction to the beginning of the next, if contractions began at 7:00, 7:04, and 7:08, the frequency would be every four minutes.

○ *ELECTRONIC MONITORING* Electronic monitoring of the uterine contractions provides continuous data. In many agencies, it may be routinely done for all high-risk women and all women who are having oxytocin-induced labor.

○ *EXTERNAL MONITORING WITH TOCODYNAMOMETER* An indirect method for monitoring uterine activity is by use of the tocodynamometer, which contains a flexible disk that responds to pressure. This disk is strapped to the woman's abdomen directly over the fundus, which is the area of greatest contractility, and it records the external tension exerted by contractions (Figure 22–5). The pressure is amplified and recorded on graph paper. The advantages to this method are that (a) it may be used prior to rupture of membranes antepartally and intrapartally and (b) it provides a continuous recording of the duration and frequency of contractions. The major disadvantage is that this method does not record the magnitude or intensity of a contraction. Another disadvantage to this method is that sometimes the strap bothers the woman, because it must be snug to monitor uterine contractions accurately, and the straps require frequent readjustment as she changes position.

Internal monitoring of uterine pressure during labor is discussed on p 623.

Trying to figure out if I was in labor was quite a task. Here I was, a labor and delivery nurse, and I couldn't decide if my contractions were the real thing. I timed them, and about the time I decided this was It, they would slow down. How exasperating not to be able to really know! It was hard on me, because I felt surely a labor and delivery nurse should know for herself. But now I see that all women are in this spot. They want so much to be right, and we often treat them as if they *should* be able to know absolutely when it's the real thing. I'd like labor and delivery nurses to remember this.

CERVICAL ASSESSMENT

Cervical dilatation and effacement are evaluated directly by sterile vaginal examination (see Procedure 22–1, Intrapartal Vaginal Examination, p 615). The vaginal examination can also provide information regarding membrane status, fetal position, and station of the presenting part.

EVALUATION OF LABOR PROGRESS

○ *FRIEDMAN GRAPH* Evaluation of the intensity, frequency, and duration of contractions does not present the entire birthing picture. Nurses can document labor progress objectively by using the Friedman graph, which evaluates uterine activity, cervical dilatation, and fetal descent.

To use the Friedman graph, one needs a graph and

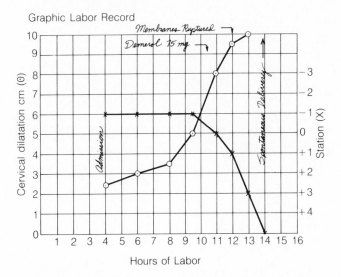

Graphic Labor Record

Figure 22–6 Example of charting labor progress on a Friedman graph (Modified from Friedman EA: An objective method of evaluating labor. *Hosp Pract* 1970;5(July):87)

skill in determining cervical dilatation and fetal descent. The numbers at the bottom of the graph in Figure 22–6 are hours of labor from 1 to 16. Vertically, at the left, cervical dilatation is measured from 0 to 10 cm. The vertical line on the right indicates fetal station in centimeters, from −5 to +5 (Friedman 1970). When one plots cervical dilatation and descent on the basic graph, a characteristic pattern emerges: an S curve represents dilatation and an inverse S curve represents descent.

When the laboring woman enters the hospital, she is asked at what time regular contractions began. A sterile vaginal examination determines cervical dilatation and the station of the presenting part of the fetus. This information is plotted on the graph. To determine the appropriate point to begin plotting data, the nurse must know how many hours the woman has been having regular contractions. In the example shown in Figure 22–6, on admission the cervix was dilated 2 to 3 cm after 4 hours of labor, and the station was −1. Later examinations are noted on the graph. When the woman was in the eleventh hour of labor, the graph indicates that cervical dilatation was 8 cm and the station was zero. At 14 hours of labor, the graph indicates spontaneous delivery.

When utilizing the Friedman graph, the following method may be used to calculate the progress in centimeters of cervical dilatation per hour (or maximum slope of active dilatation). Divide the difference between two consecutive observations by the intervening time interval to obtain the value for the slope in centimeters per hour. For example, in the case illustrated in Figure 22–6, at 9½ hours of labor, the cervix is dilated 5 cm. At 11 hours of labor, the cervix is dilated 8 cm. The difference between these two observations is 3 cm. Divide the difference by the intervening time interval, which is 1½ hours: 3 cm ÷ 1½ = 2 cm/hr.

Evaluation of the woman's labor progress through use of the Friedman graph will assist in identifying normal or abnormal labor patterns.

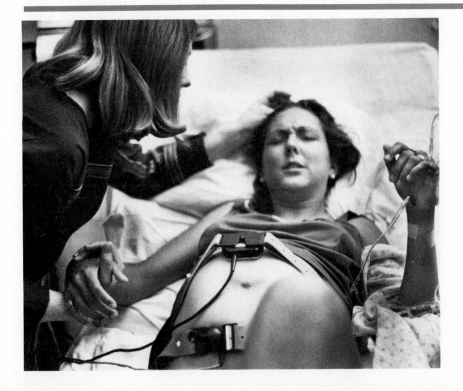

Figure 22–5 Woman in labor with external monitor applied

Fetal Assessment

Determination of Fetal Position and Presentation

Fetal position is determined by a combination of factors, using various senses and technology. Assessment of the maternal abdomen for fetal positon may be done by inspection, palpation, auscultation of fetal heart tones, determination of presenting part by vaginal examination, and utilization of ultrasound.

INSPECTION

The nurse should observe the woman's abdomen for size and shape. Attention should be given to the lie of the fetus by assessing whether the shape of the uterus projects up and down (longitudinal lie) or left and right, which indicates a transverse lie.

PALPATION

Use of Leopold's maneuvers provides a systematic evaluation of the maternal abdomen. Frequent practice with these maneuvers increases the proficiency of the examiner in determining fetal position by palpation. Difficulty may be encountered in performing these techniques on an obese woman or on a woman who has excessive amniotic fluid (hydramnios).

Leopold's maneuvers should be performed before listening to the fetal heart tones (FHT). Auscultation of the FHT is facilitated by locating the fetal back, because the sound of the heart tones is carried with more intensity through the fetal back and the uterine wall; it becomes diffused as it passes through the amniotic fluid.

Care should be taken to ensure the woman's comfort during Leopold's maneuvers. The woman should have recently emptied her bladder and should lie on her back with her abdomen uncovered. To aid in relaxation of the abdominal wall, the shoulders should be raised slightly on a pillow and the knees drawn up a little. The procedure should be completed between contractions. The examiner's hands should be warm (Figure 22–7).

Consideration should be given to several questions while inspecting and palpating the maternal abdomen:

- Is the fetal lie longitudinal or transverse?

- What is in the fundus? Am I feeling buttocks or head?

- Where is the fetal back?

- Where are the small parts or extremities?

- What is in the inlet? Does it confirm what I found in the fundus?

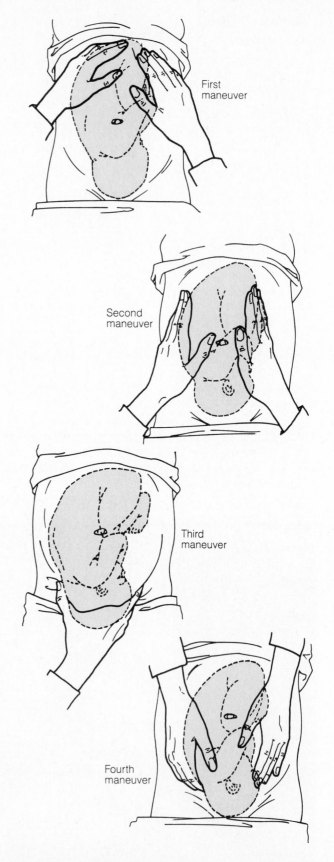

Figure 22–7 Leopold's maneuvers for determination of fetal position and presentation

- Is the presenting part engaged, floating, or dipping into the inlet?

- Is there fetal movement?

- How large is the fetus? (Appropriate for gestational age, excessively large?)

- Is there one fetus or more than one?

- Is fundal height proportionate to the estimated gestational age?

○ *FIRST MANEUVER* While facing the woman, the nurse palpates the upper abdomen with both hands (Figure 22–7). The nurse determines the shape, size, consistency, and mobility of the form that is found. The fetal head is firm, hard, and round and moves independently of the trunk. The breech feels softer and symmetrical and has small bony prominences; it moves with the trunk.

○ *SECOND MANEUVER* After ascertaining whether the head or the buttocks occupies the fundus, the nurse tries to determine the location of the fetal back and notes whether it is on the right or left side of the maternal abdomen. Still facing the woman, the nurse palpates the abdomen with deep but gentle pressure, using her palms (Figure 22–7). The right hand should be steady while the left hand explores the right side of the uterus. The maneuver is then repeated, probing with the right hand and steadying the uterus with the left hand. The fetal back should feel firm and smooth and should connect what was found in the fundus with a mass in the inlet. Once the back is located, the nurse validates the finding by palpating the fetal extremities (small irregularities and protrusions) on the opposite side of the abdomen.

○ *THIRD MANEUVER* Next the nurse should determine what fetal part is lying above the inlet by gently grasping the lower portion of the abdomen just above the symphysis pubis with the thumb and fingers of the right hand (Figure 22–7). This maneuver yields the opposite information from what was found in the fundus and validates the presenting part. If the head is presenting and is not engaged, it may be gently pushed back and forth.

○ *FOURTH MANEUVER* For this portion of the examination, the nurse faces the woman's feet and attempts to locate the cephalic prominence or brow. Location of this landmark assists in assessing the descent of the presenting part into the pelvis. The fingers of both hands are moved gently down the sides of the uterus toward the pubis (Figure 22–7). The cephalic prominence (brow) is located on the side where there is greatest resistance to the descent of the fingers toward the pubis. It is located on the opposite side from the fetal back if the head is well flexed. However, when the fetal head is extended, the occiput is the first cephalic prominence felt, and it is located on the same side as the back. Therefore, when completing the fourth maneuver, if the first cephalic prominence palpated is on the same side as the back, the head is not flexed. If the first prominence found is opposite the back, the head is well flexed (Oxorn 1986).

VAGINAL EXAMINATION

The vaginal examination reveals information regarding the fetus such as presentation, position, station, degree of flexion of the fetal head, and any swelling that might be present on the fetal scalp (caput succedaneum).

ULTRASOUND

Real-time ultrasound is frequently available in the birth setting and may be used to obtain specific information regarding the fetus. A real-time ultrasound may be done at this time to assess fetal lie, presentation, and position; obtain measurements of biparietal diameter to estimate gestational age; assess for anomalies when a vaginal examination reveals suspicious findings; and sometimes to confirm the presence of more than one fetus. (See Chapter 20 for further discussion of the use of ultrasound for fetal assessment.)

Evaluation of Fetal Status During Labor

AUSCULTATION OF FETAL HEART RATE

The fetoscope is essentially a special stethoscope that is used to listen to the fetal heart rate (FHR). The fetoscope has two major designs: One consists of a stethoscope attached to a metal band that goes over the nurse's head and conducts sound, enhancing the ability to hear the fetal heart; the other type is a stethoscope attached to a weighted bell approximately 3 inches in diameter, which is placed on the maternal abdomen (Figure 22–8).

Before listening to the FHR the first time, some nurses complete Leopold's maneuvers to assist in identifying the fetal presentation and position. The fetus is generally in a head-down (cephalic) presentation with its back to the mother's left side. Thus the nurse could anticipate that the fetal heart rate will be found in the lower quadrant of the maternal abdomen. As the presenting part descends and rotates through the pelvis during labor, the location of the FHR tends to descend and move toward the midline. The FHR can be heard most clearly at the fetal back (Figure 22–9).

After FHR is located, it is counted for 15 seconds and multiplied by 4 to obtain the number of beats per minute. The nurse should occasionally listen for a full minute through a contraction to detect any abnormal heart rate especially if tachycardia, bradycardia, or irregular beats are heard. If the FHR is irregular or has changed markedly from the last assessment, the nurse should listen for a full minute. The FHR should be auscultated every 30 to 60 minutes in early labor, every 15 minutes during active labor, and every 5 minutes during second stage of labor. It is especially important to listen during and after the contraction to detect any deceleration that might occur. It is also important to listen immediately after each contraction when the woman is pushing during second stage since fetal bradycardia frequently occurs as pressure is exerted on the fetal head during descent.

If decelerations (see p 629) are noted, the woman should be electronically monitored to rule out abnormalities in the FHR.

Only gross changes in FHR may be detected with the fetoscope. Subtle changes that occur in response to contractions may not be heard because it is difficult to hear the FHR during the peak of a contraction. Consequently, transient accelerations or decelerations in the FHR may be missed. In addition, occasional counting errors are inevitable. The auscultated FHR is an average measurement.

In current maternity care practice, a fetoscope may be used to assess the FHR during labor and delivery of the low-risk woman. In high-risk situations, an electronic fetal monitor will be used to provide continuous assessment of the FHR.

ELECTRONIC MONITORING

There are two methods of assessing FHR during labor: indirect (external) and direct (internal). The indirect method may be accomplished using a fetoscope, fetal electrocardiography, and Doppler ultrasound (intermittent or continuous). Direct monitoring provides continuous information about the FHR from a scalp electrode. Uterine contractions may be monitored externally with a tocodynamometer or internally with an intrauterine pressure catheter.

When the FHR is monitored electronically, the interval between two successive fetal heart beats is measured and the rate is displayed as if the beats occurred at the same interval for 60 seconds. For example, if the interval between two beats is 0.5 second, the rate for one full min-

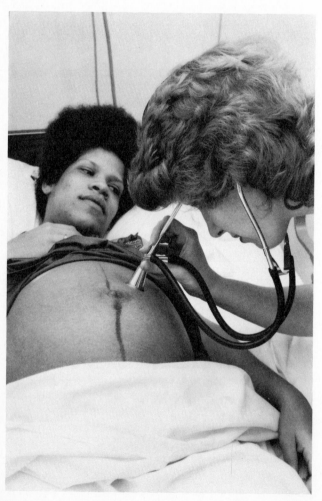
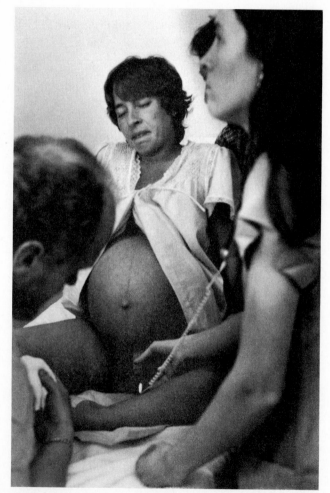

Figure 22–8 Two methods of assessing fetal heart rate. A Fetoscope. B Doppler

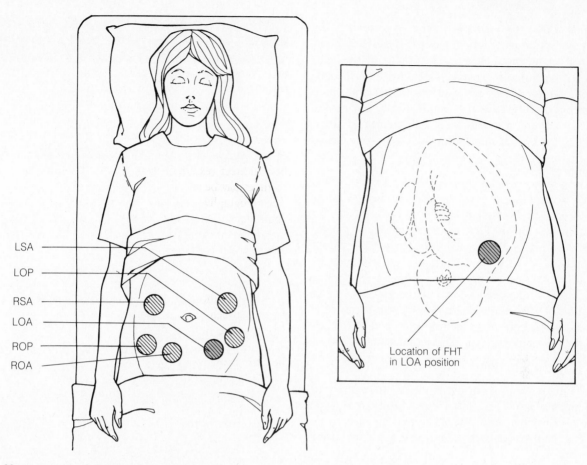

Figure 22–9 *Location of FHR in relation to the more commonly seen fetal positions*

ute would be 120 beats per minute. This measurement is called the instantaneous rate. The instantaneous rate provides documentation that the FHR varies from one moment to the next. Figure 22–10 compares instantaneous rates with those averaged by auscultation.

Electronic monitoring has major advantages over auscultation with the fetoscope. Electronic monitoring is a more reliable measure of fetal well-being. Fetal distress can be detected by observing the continuous FHR and the periodic changes that occur during and after uterine contractions. Interventions can be timely and thus more effective.

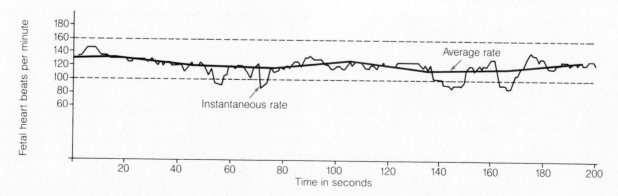

Figure 22–10 *Comparison of instantaneous and average FHR. The average FHR illustrates a more constant rate, while the instantaneous rate illustrates the normal variation of the FHR.* (From Hon E: *An Introduction to Fetal Heart Rate Monitoring*, ed 2. Los Angeles: University of Southern California School of Medicine, 1972, p 9)

○   *INDICATIONS FOR ELECTRONIC FETAL MONITORING* Any woman with previous history of medical or obstetric problems that might affect labor or the health of the fetus should be monitored by continuous electronic fetal monitoring. Some physicians advocate monitoring only those women considered to be at risk or at high risk, while many feel the procedure is mandatory for all women in labor. Specific indications for monitoring are listed in Box 22–1.

○   *EXTERNAL MONITORING* *External monitoring* of the fetus is usually accomplished by the use of ultrasound. A transducer, which emits continuous sound waves, is placed on the maternal abdomen. Prior to the placement of the ultrasonic transducer on the maternal abdomen, FHT should be auscultated to determine the area of clearest sounds for optimal clarity of the tracing. A water-soluble gel is applied to the crystals of the underside of the transducer to aid in conduction of fetal heart sounds. When placed correctly, the sound waves bounce off the fetal heart and are picked up by the electronic monitor. The actual moment-by-moment FHR is displayed simultaneously on a screen and on graph paper.

The transducer may inadvertently be directed toward a pulsating maternal vessel. In this case, the maternal signal will be noted rather than that of the fetal circulation. To avoid this, maternal pulse should be checked while using ultrasound.

Contractions can be monitored externally by use of a tocodynamometer (or "toco"), which is a pressure device (Figure 22–11). As the uterine muscles contract, pressure is exerted against a projection on the underside of the "toco," which has been applied to the maternal abdomen by means of an elastic belt. The pressure creates an electrical signal that is transmitted to the monitor and recorded on graph paper. Uterine contractions can be assessed for frequency but not for intensity. The intensity (which is displayed on the graph paper) is affected by how tightly the belt is applied around the maternal abdomen. When the belt is tight enough, one should be able to note the beginning of contractions on the monitor before or at the same time the woman begins to feel them. One of the most frequent complaints regarding the fetal monitor is the tightness of the belts, but if the reasons for monitoring are explained and the belts are frequently adjusted, most women are more understanding and do not object. Another problem with the external monitor is that some mothers may feel compelled to lie quietly to avoid the need to readjust the belts.

Some other disadvantages of external monitoring have been noted. In the case of a very obese woman, an active fetus, or hydramnios, the FHR may be difficult to monitor by external means. The recording may look "scratchy," and the data received will be incomprehensible.

Box 22–1   Indications for Electronic Monitoring

Fetal factors

  Decreased fetal movement
  Abnormal auscultory FHR
  Meconium passage
  Abnormal presentations/positions
  IUGR or SGA fetus
  Postdates (>42 weeks)
  Multiple gestation

Maternal factors

  Fever
  Infections
  Toxemia
  Disease conditions (eg, hypertension, diabetes)
  Anemia
  Rh isoimmunization
  Previous perinatal death
  Grandmultiparity
  Previous cesarean delivery
  Borderline/contracted pelvis

Uterine factors

  Dysfunctional labor
  Failure to progress in labor
  Oxytocin induction/augmentation
  Uterine anomalies

Complications of pregnancy

  Prolonged rupture of membranes
  Premature rupture of membranes
  Preterm labor
  Marginal abruptio placentae
  Partial placenta previa
  Occult/frank prolapse of cord
  Amnionitis

Regional anesthesia

Elective monitoring

The external monitor may react to extraneous noises, which are called artifacts, such as maternal bowel sounds, fetal movement, maternal movement, and noises emitted from the monitor and in the labor room. This may make it difficult to assess variability (moment-to-moment changes) in the FHR. Some of the new electronic fetal monitors are able to filter out any extraneous sounds and make the tracing look cleaner.

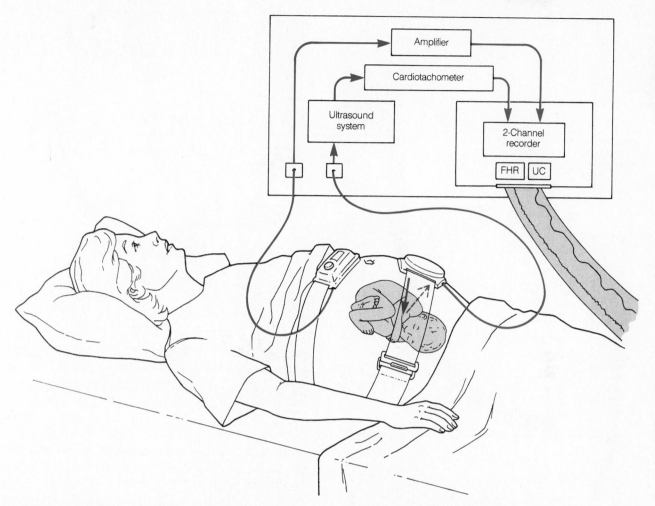

Figure 22–11   Tocodynamometer and ultrasonic technique to monitor maternal and fetal status during labor (From Hon E: *An Introduction to Fetal Heart Monitoring*. Los Angeles: University of California School of Medicine, 1972, p. 65)

○   *INTERNAL MONITORING*   Internal monitoring is accomplished through use of an internal spiral electrode, which is attached to the skin of the fetal head or buttocks, and an intrauterine pressure catheter (Figure 22–12). To insert the spiral electrode, the cervix must be dilated at least 2 cm, the presenting fetal part accessible by vaginal examination, and the membranes ruptured. Even though it is not possible to apply the electrode and catheter under strict sterile conditions, the procedure should be performed as aseptically as possible. The perineum should be cleaned with povidone-iodine solution (Betadine) or other cleansing agent. After determining fetal position by vaginal examination, the examiner (physician or nurse) inserts the electrode, which is encased in a plastic guide, to the level of the internal cervical os and attaches it to the presenting part, being careful not to apply it to the face, suture lines, scrotum, or fontanelles. The electrode is rotated clockwise until it is attached to the presenting part and is then dis-

engaged from the guide tube. The guide tube is removed, and the end wires are connected to a leg plate that is attached to the woman's thigh. The cable from the leg plate is connected to the monitor.

The spiral electrode provides an instantaneous and continuous recording of FHR that is more accurate than data provided by external monitoring.

Intensity of uterine contractions may be assessed by means of an intrauterine catheter (small polyethylene tubing), inserted directly into the uterine cavity. The guide tube encasing the catheter is advanced as far as the internal cervical os, and then the tubing is slowly threaded into the uterine cavity, usually in the area where fetal small parts are located. It is advanced only as far as the black marking indicated on the catheter, which should be visualized at the opening to the vaginal vault (Figure 22–13). The catheter and strain gauge are filled with sterile water (not saline as this will corrode the transducer). The gauge is then con-

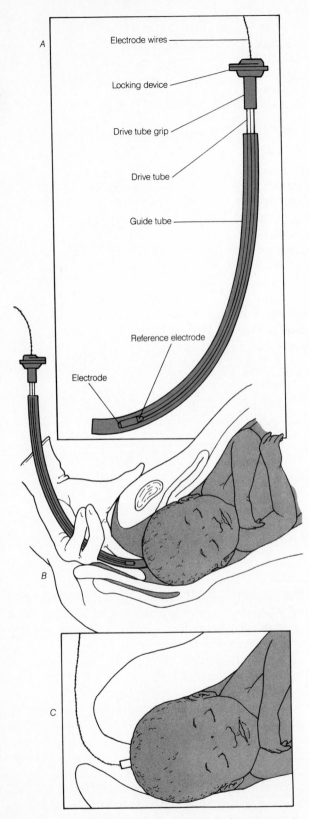

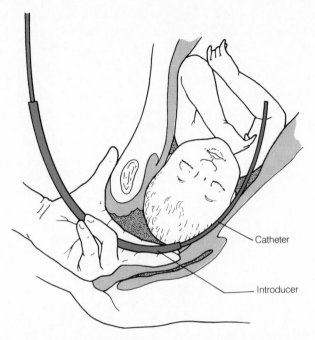

Figure 22–13   Technique of uterine catheter insertion. Note that the introducer (catheter guide) is inserted only about 1 cm inside the cervix. (From Perez RH: Fetal monitoring, in Protocols for Perinatal Nursing Practice. St Louis, Mosby, 1981, p 180)

nected to the monitor. For measurement of accurate baseline resting tone of the uterus, the strain gauge should be adjusted to the height of the maternal xiphoid process. With the woman in the supine position, this will approximate the level of the tip of the intrauterine catheter. By this means, a closed pressure system is maintained so that increases in intrauterine pressure with uterine contractions or hypertonus may be visualized.

The catheter is periodically flushed with sterile water to ensure patency and accurate resting tone. If the catheter becomes clogged with vernix or meconium, it will show an increase in baseline resting tone. If the woman changes position, the catheter should be flushed, the strain gauge readjusted, and the system recalibrated.

In many institutions the intrauterine catheter is used only during oxytocin augmentation, induction, or vaginal birth after cesarean. It is particularly important to quantitate the intensity and frequency of contractions to avoid hyperstimulation and possible uterine rupture due to overadministration of oxytocin. If the woman's labor is prolonged (per Friedman curve; see p 617), internal monitoring should be instituted to accurately assess the frequency and strength of contractions and resultant FHR pattern response. A slightly increased incidence of maternal infection (approximately 1 percent) may be noted following use of the intrauterine catheter, but this seems to depend on the duration of ruptured membranes and length of labor.

Figure 22–12   Technique for internal, direct fetal monitoring. A Spiral electrode. B Attaching spiral electrode to scalp. C Attached spiral electrode with guide tube removed. (Courtesy of Corometrics Medical Systems, Inc, Wallingford, Conn 06492. Operators Manual 112 Fetal Monitor)

It is of particular importance that the nurse evaluate the woman's labor status by means other than the fetal monitor. As with any type of technology, no machine is flawless, and the monitor cannot fill the role of the nurse. One should never rely solely on data recorded by a machine. Technology is only useful as an adjunct to good nursing assessment. All too often women are in active labor with adequate contractions that are regarded as "poor quality" because the monitor is not functioning properly. The nurse should routinely palpate the intensity of the contractions and compare the assessment with that of data recorded by the monitor.

The FHR tracing at the top of Figure 22–14 was obtained by internal monitoring, and the uterine contraction tracing at the bottom of the figure by external monitoring. Note the FHR is variable (the tracing moves up and down instead of in a straight line), and the tracing stays close to the line numbered 150. If the graph paper moves through the monitor at 3 cm per minute, each vertical dark line represents 1 minute. The frequency of the uterine contractions is every 2½ to 3 minutes. The duration of the contractions is 50 to 60 seconds.

○ *TELEMETRY* Fetal ECG and intrauterine pressure may be monitored through the use of telemetry. In telemetry a two-channel radio transmitter is placed into the vaginal vault, a pressure device is placed in the uterus, and a scalp electrode is applied to the presenting fetal part. Information derived from these sources is relayed to a cardiotachometer at a central nursing station where data may be evaluated. The advantage of telemetry is that it permits the woman to ambulate within a given distance from the monitor receiver. See Table 22–2 for comparison of various monitoring methods.

FETAL HEART RATE PATTERNS

Fetal heart rate is evaluated by assessing both baseline and periodic changes. Normal FHR ranges from 120 to 160 beats per minute. More important than FHR are the periodic changes that occur in response to the intermittent stress of uterine contractions and the baseline beat-to-beat variability of the fetal heart rate. A sick fetus may have a normal heart rate but demonstrate slight periodic changes and decreased variability indicative of intrauterine hypoxia.

○ *BASELINE RATE* The baseline refers to the range of FHR observed between contractions, during a ten-minute period of monitoring. The range does not include the rate present during decelerations.

○ *BASELINE CHANGES* Baseline changes in FHR are defined in terms of ten-minute periods of time. These changes are tachycardia, bradycardia, and beat-to-beat variability of the heart rate.

Tachycardia Tachycardia is defined as a rate of 160 beats per minute or more for a ten-minute segment of time.

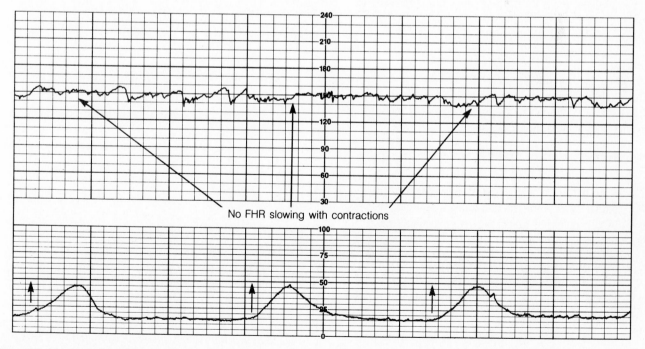

No FHR slowing with contractions

Figure 22–14 Normal FHR range is from 120 to 160. The FHR tracing in the upper portion of the graph indicates the FHR. The lower portion is a tracing of the uterine contraction.

Table 22–2 Advantages and Disadvantages of Various Monitoring Methods

Method	Advantages	Disadvantages
Fetoscope	Inexpensive Noninvasive Easy to use Easily transported	Intermittent information Gives no information regarding contractions Cannot assess variability or periodic changes in FHR unless severe Cannot hear FHT until 17–20 weeks' gestation
Doppler (pocket-sized ultrasound)	Inexpensive Noninvasive Easily transported Can hear FHT as early as 11–12 weeks	Gives no information regarding contractions Cannot assess variability Cannot assess periodic changes in FHR unless severe Intermittent information
External monitoring	Continuous information Noninvasive Uses: antepartal testing, and during labor Gives permanent record Can assess relative frequency of contractions Can assess decreased variability and periodic changes Useful for client teaching	Equipment is expensive Subject to artifact Cannot assess variability unless decreased and then must confirm with internal monitoring Cannot quantitate contractions Belts uncomfortable to some women Subject to double and half counting
Internal monitoring	Accurate, continuous information Monitors fetal ECG Not subject to artifact Client more mobile in bed, chair Can quantitate contractions Can assess short-term and long-term variability Accurate assessment of periodic changes Useful for client teaching	Will measure maternal heart rate if fetus is dead Equipment is expensive Need qualified and knowledgeable personnel to interpret Presenting part must be accessible, membranes must be ruptured, and cervix must be anterior and dilated enough for application of scalp electrode Requires knowledgeable personnel to apply equipment Client confined to bed or chair Slight increased risk of maternal or fetal infection Subject to double and half counting Invasive
Telemetry	Accurate, continuous information Client can be mobile (out of bed or in hall) Same advantages as internal monitoring	Equipment is expensive Invasive Not widely used at the present time Same disadvantages as internal monitoring

Moderate tachycardia has rates of 160 to 179 beats per minute. Severe tachycardia is defined as 180 beats per minute or more. Although tachycardia may occur without apparent reason, possible causes include:

- Extreme prematurity

- Maternal fever, which results in an increase in sympathetic nervous system stimulation and an increase in the maternal metabolic rate, thus increasing the fetal oxygen demand

- Mild or chronic fetal hypoxemia, which results in an effort by the fetus to compensate for the oxygen deficit with increased sympathetic nervous system stimulation

- Fetal infection, which results in a fetal stress reaction to pathogens

- Fetal anemia

- Beta sympathomimetic drugs given to the pregnant woman

- Maternal anxiety, which causes maternal epinephrine to cross the placenta

- Fetal tachyarrhythmias

- Maternal infection

- Thyrotoxicosis

- Maternal hyperthyroidism

- Maternal drugs that inhibit the transmission of vagal response to the S-A node (such as atropine, hydroxyzine, phenothiazine)

- Excessive fetal activity

Bradycardia Fetal bradycardia is defined as a rate of less than 120 beats per minute for a ten-minute segment of time. Mild bradycardia ranges from 100 to 119 beats per minute and is considered benign. Moderate bradycardia is a fetal heart rate less than 100 beats per minute. Severe bradycardia is an FHR less than 70 beats/min and is associated with a rapidly occurring fetal acidosis. Causes of fetal bradycardia include:

● Fetal hypoxia

● Fetal arrhythmias as seen with congenital heart block

● Drugs such as β-adrenergic (sympathetic) blocking agents (these include anesthetic agents used as paracervical and epidural blocks)

● Prolapse or prolonged compression of umbilical cord

● Hypothermia

● Initial response to acute asphyxia associated with maternal seizure, excessive uterine contractions, acute maternal hypotension, abruptio placentae, or fetal hemorrhage (due to rupture of anomalous fetal-placental vessel or torn vasa previa)

● End-stage bradycardia (due to continuous pressure on the fetal head during descent in the late second stage)

● Idiopathic sinus bradycardia

● Maternal systemic lupus erythematosus

Baseline Variability   One of the most important parameters of fetal well-being is noted in the variability of the FHR. The term *variability* refers to the irregularity of the FHR as noted on the graph paper. A healthy fetus normally demonstrates an irregular FHR baseline, which is caused by an interplay of the sympathetic and para-sympathetic nervous systems. Variability consists of two components—long-term and short-term variability—both of significance in evaluating fetal status.

● *Long-term variability* (LTV) refers to the larger rhythmic fluctuations of the FHR that occur from two to six times per minute with a normal range of six to ten beats per minute (Figure 22–15). Long-term variability is increased by fetal movement and decreased or absent when the fetus is in a sleep cycle. Long-term variability has been classified as follows (Hon 1976):

No variability   0–2 beats/min

Minimal variability   3–5 beats/min

Average variability   6–10 beats/min

Moderate variability   11–25 beats/min

Marked variability (saltatory) more than 25 beats/min

● *Short-term variability* (STV) refers to the differences between successive heart beats as measured by the

R–R wave interval of the QRS cardiac cycle and therefore represents actual beat-to-beat fluctuations in the FHR. These fluctuations average two to three beats/min. Short-term variability is classified as either present or absent.

Rather than counting specific beats, with practice one can usually become skillful in "eyeballing" the FHR variability. The LTV is noted as minimal (or none), average,

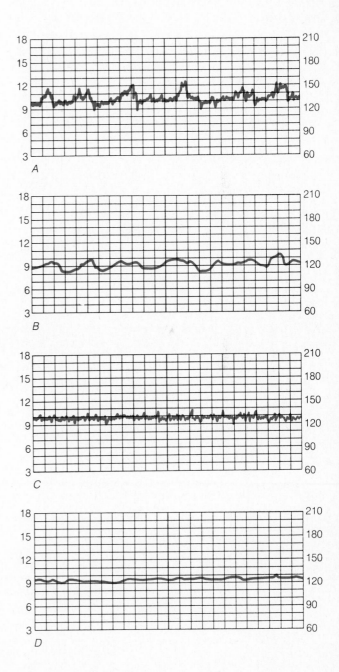

Figure 22–15   Long-term variability. A Moderate variability. B Average variability. C Minimal variability. D No variability.

or marked; the STV is noted as present or absent. Fluctuations are thought to be due to the interplay of the parasympathetic and sympathetic components of the autonomic nervous system, as mentioned earlier. When decreased LTV is noted, one must suspect some compromise of these mechanisms. Increased variability has not been as well defined, and the causes are unknown. The most important aspect of variability is that even in the presence of abnormal or questionable FHR patterns, if the variability is normal, the fetus is not suffering from cerebral asphyxia (Parer 1985b). During prolonged bradycardia or severe periodic changes (eg, late or severe variable decelerations, see

p 631), the fetus may decompensate and suffer cerebral and myocardial asphyxia and consequently demonstrate a decrease or loss of variability. If loss of variability accompanies tachycardia, fetal prognosis is usually poor (Boehm et al 1978), and immediate delivery of the fetus should be considered if fetal blood acid-base determination is not feasible.

The nurse needs to keep in mind that true STV can be evaluated only by internal monitoring. The external monitor may demonstrate "normal" variability, due to the presence of artifact, when in fact it is decreased. An appearance of decreased variability warrants application of an

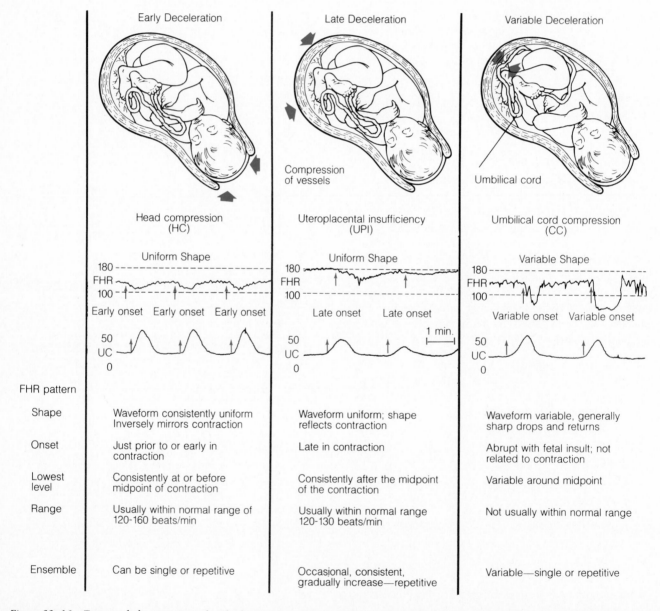

FHR pattern	Early Deceleration Head compression (HC)	Late Deceleration Uteroplacental insufficiency (UPI)	Variable Deceleration Umbilical cord compression (CC)
Shape	Waveform consistently uniform Inversely mirrors contraction	Waveform uniform; shape reflects contraction	Waveform variable, generally sharp drops and returns
Onset	Just prior to or early in contraction	Late in contraction	Abrupt with fetal insult; not related to contraction
Lowest level	Consistently at or before midpoint of contraction	Consistently after the midpoint of the contraction	Variable around midpoint
Range	Usually within normal range of 120-160 beats/min	Usually within normal range 120-130 beats/min	Not usually within normal range
Ensemble	Can be single or repetitive	Occasional, consistent, gradually increase—repetitive	Variable—single or repetitive

Figure 22–16 Types and characteristics of early, late, and variable decelerations (From Hon E: *An Introduction to Fetal Heart Rate Monitoring,* ed 2. Los Angeles: University of Southern California School of Medicine, 1976, p 29).

internal electrode. Decreased variability may be seen with the following conditions:

Administration of hypnotics, analgesics, and para-sympathetic blocking agents to the mother

Deep fetal sleep

Absence of fetal cortex (anencephaly)

Premature fetus (less than 28 weeks: variability present but less amplitude)

Fetal hypoxia and acidosis

Severe fetal tachycardia

Fetal anatomic brain damage

Stimuli such as maternal activity, abdominal palpation, fetal activity, and myometrial contractions may increase variability. Complete loss of variability may occur with complete heart block.

○ PERIODIC CHANGES *Periodic changes* are transient decelerations or accelerations of the FHR from the baseline that occur in response to contractions and fetal movement.

Accelerations are transient increases in the FHR normally caused by fetal movement. As the fetus moves in utero, the heart rate increases as it does in adults when they exercise. When the fetus quiets down the heart rate returns to normal. Acceleration often accompanies contractions, usually due to fetal movement in response to pressure of the contracting uterine musculature. Accelerations of this type are thought to be a sign of fetal well-being and adequate oxygen reserve. Accelerations may also be caused by partial occlusion of the umbilical cord. In this instance a transient period of decreased placental return and fetal hypotension are seen, resulting in a baroreceptor response that increases the FHR (Freeman & Garite 1981).

Accelerations may be periodic or sporadic and of uniform or variable shape (Krebs et al 1982). Periodic accelerations occur in conjunction with contractions; sporadic accelerations may occur with fetal movement.

Decelerations are periodic decreases in FHR from the normal baseline. Hon and Quilligan (1967) categorized them as early, late, and variable, according to when they occur in the contraction cycle and to their waveform (Figure 22–16).

Early Decelerations Early decelerations are due to pressure on the fetal head as it progresses down the birth canal. They have a uniform, smooth waveform that inversely mirrors that of the corresponding contraction. Beginning at the onset of the contraction and ending as the contraction ends, the nadir (lowest point) occurs at the peak of the contraction. The nadir is usually within the normal fetal heart rate range (Figure 22–17).

Early decelerations are generally benign and seen late in labor when the fetal head is on the perineum. Increased intracranial pressure results in local changes in cerebral blood flow, which in turn results in stimulation of vagal centers and produces a slowing of heart rate through the vagus nerve (Figure 22–18). If this pattern occurs early in labor, it may be due to head compression from cephalopelvic disproportion. A nurse must take great care in differentiating this type of deceleration from late decelerations: they look identical yet differ in time of onset.

Early decelerations are not associated with loss of variability, tachycardia, or other FHR changes nor are they associated with fetal hypoxia, acidosis, or low Apgar scores. Early decelerations are viewed as a reassuring FHR pattern unless seen in early labor or with lack of descent of the fetal head. In the latter instances, the nurse should assess the pelvis and fetal size for possible cephalopelvic disproportion.

Late Decelerations Late decelerations are due to uteroplacental insufficiency as the result of decreased blood flow and oxygen transfer to the fetus through the intervillous space during uterine contractions causing hypoxemia (Figure 22–19). They have a smooth, uniform shape that inversely mirrors the contraction (as do early decelerations) but are late in their onset and recovery. They begin at or within a few seconds after the peak of the contraction; the nadir is noted near the end of the contraction (Figure 22–20). They tend to occur with every contraction. When uteroplacental reserve is adequate, the fetus normally tolerates the transient stress of repetitive contractions. If fetal hypoxia occurs because of a decrease in uteroplacental blood flow (for example, from maternal hypotension or excessive uterine activity), late decelerations generally occur.

This pattern is always considered an ominous sign but does not necessarily require immediate delivery of the fetus. If late decelerations do not appear to be worsening and the variability of the FHR is normal, delivery may be delayed although the fetus warrants constant observation. Should decelerations worsen, tachycardia occur, or variability decrease, fetal blood sampling for pH determination is indicated to evaluate the acid-base status of the fetus.

Sometimes late decelerations are found to be due to supine position of the laboring woman. In this case decreased uterine blood flow to the fetus due to supine hypotension may be alleviated by raising the woman's upper trunk or turning her to the side to displace pressure of the gravid uterus on the inferior vena cava. If the woman remains flat on her back, the fetus will continue to have decelerations due to oxygen compromise.

Late decelerations normally occur within the normal heart rate range (120–160 beats/min) and may be quite obvious or very subtle and almost indistinguishable. Some fetuses at highest risk demonstrate a flat FHR baseline with late decelerations that are barely noticeable. It must be kept

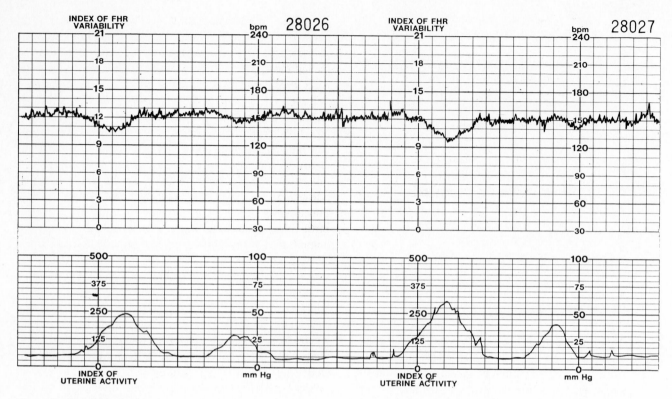

Figure 22–17 Early decelerations

in mind that the depth of the deceleration does not indicate the severity of the insult.

Chronic uteroplacental insufficiency during pregnancy results in intrauterine growth retardation and, if severe enough, antenatal death. When uteroplacental insufficiency is acute due to factors occurring during labor, fetal distress may ensue. If not properly treated intrapartal fetal death may occur.

Variable Decelerations Variable decelerations are appropriately named in that they vary in their onset, occurrence, and waveform. They are thought to be due to umbilical cord occlusion (which in essence cuts off the low-resistance fetal placental circulation) and the resulting increase in peripheral resistance in the fetal circulation, which causes fetal hypertension. The fetal hypertension results in stimulation of the baroreceptors in the aortic arch and carotid sinuses. This results in an outflow from the parasympathetic system, which causes a sudden slowing (bradycardia) of the fetal atrial pacemaker (Freeman & Garite 1981) (Figure 22–21). Either the fetus squeezes the cord or rolls over onto it, transient pressure is exerted on the cord from compression, or the cord is around the neck of the fetus. An occasional or isolated variable deceleration is usually benign. Variable decelerations that are repetitive and begin to worsen during the course of labor are of concern. Variable decelerations usually fall outside the normal FHR range and are classified as mild, moderate, and severe.

They are acute in onset, vary in duration and intensity, and abruptly disappear when the insult of cord compression is relieved (Figure 22–22).

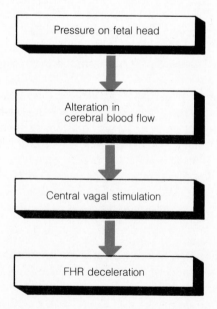

Figure 22–18 Mechanism of early deceleration (head compression) (Adapted from Freeman RK, Garite TJ: The physiologic basis of fetal monitoring, in *Fetal Heart Rate Monitoring.* Baltimore, Williams & Wilkins, 1981, ch 2, p 13)

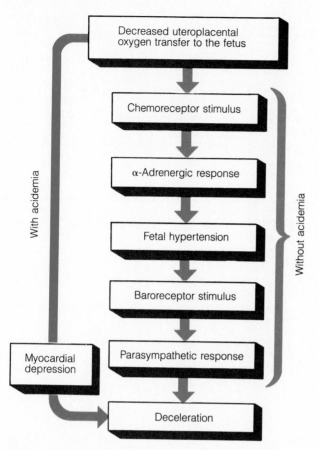

Figure 22–19 *Mechanism of late deceleration* (From Freeman RK, Garite TJ: The physiologic basis of fetal monitoring, in *Fetal Heart Rate Monitoring*. Baltimore, Williams & Wilkins, 1981, ch 2, p 15)

With repetitive decelerations, one should suspect a nuchal cord (umbilical cord around the neck) or occult prolapse of the cord. If this pattern becomes evident early in labor, variable decelerations may subsequently demonstrate a slow return to baseline (tailing) due to repetitive stress causing uteroplacental insufficiency. Acid-base status of the fetus should be assessed since cesarean delivery (or forceps delivery) might be indicated.

Decelerations that seem to deviate more from the baseline and widen are ominous and warrant further investigation. When they are prolonged and severe, a significant oxygen deficit develops from myocardial depression, resulting in hypoxemia and subsequent fetal metabolic acidosis (Freeman & Garite 1981). If hypoxia and acidosis are allowed to continue, fetal death may result.

With progressively worsening variable decelerations, an "overshoot" may occur. This is a blunt, smooth acceleration following the contraction and may be due to an attempt of the fetus to compensate for hypoxemia through sympathetic and adrenal mechanisms (Martin & Gingerich 1976).

Criteria for evaluation of variable decelerations vary from one author to another, and the very nature of these periodic changes can pose considerable anxiety regarding management. Dr. Robert Goodlin's "rule of the 60s" (in Parer 1984b, p 298) describes severe variable decelerations as having the following characteristics: variable decelerations below 60 beats per minute, 60 beats per minute below baseline FHR, or variable decelerations lasting more than 60 seconds in duration. These criteria seem to be the easiest to remember and perhaps the most practical.

Variable decelerations are frequently seen in labor when the membranes are ruptured. This decreases protection to the cord especially as the fetus descends down the birth canal. Variable decelerations usually do not warrant immediate delivery unless a rising baseline, loss of variability, and other ominous signs accompany them. Repositioning the woman often corrects this type of pattern.

Krebs, Petrie, and Dunn (1983) describe various "atypical variable decelerations," noting that variable decelerations are probably innocuous unless these features are present (Figure 22–23). They noted that the presence of these atypical decelerations should be regarded as signs of fetal hypoxia. The nurse should be cognizant of pattern interpretation and be able to recognize severe and "atypical" variables. A point to remember, however, is that in the presence of normal variability of the FHR, these variables have not been found to be associated with fetal acidosis and poor outcome.

Prolonged Decelerations Prolonged decelerations are those in which the FHR decreases from the baseline for two or more minutes (Figure 22–24). They may occur suddenly, and if the pattern is promptly corrected, FHR variability will remain good. Rebound tachycardia is an ominous sign implying that a state of hypoxia has occurred. Prolonged decelerations are frequently seen following paracervical or epidural block. These decelerations are thought to be due to fetal toxicity from fetal absorption of the drug through the uterine arteries or spasm of the uterine arteries resulting in decreased blood flow and hypoxia and reflex slowing of the FHR. Prolonged decelerations may often be seen with sudden occult or frank prolapse of the umbilical cord. When decelerations occur following administration of regional anesthesia, the woman should be turned on her side, evaluated for hypotension, and given a bolus of intravenous fluid (500 to 600 mL) to fill the dilated vascular space. This situation can usually be avoided by administering an IV bolus (800 to 900 mL) of lactated Ringer's or normal saline solution to the woman prior to administering regional anesthesia. Solutions containing dextrose should not be given since they may cause fetal hyperglycemia.

○ *SINUSOIDAL PATTERNS* An unusual pattern referred to as sinusoidal is occasionally seen. It is characterized by an undulant sinewave that is equally distributed above and

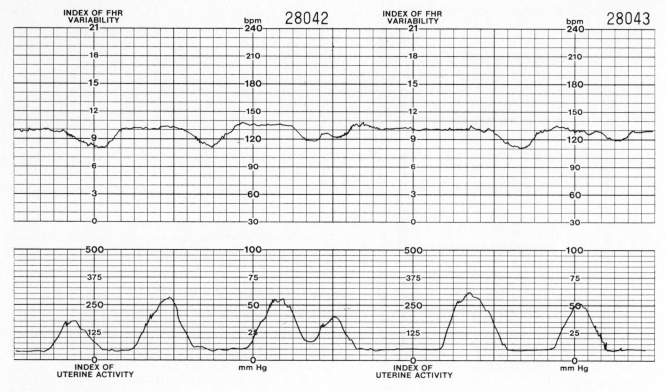

Figure 22–20   Late decelerations

below the baseline. The FHR usually ranges between 120 and 160 beats per minute. This wavelike baseline FHR usually has an amplitude of 5 to 15 beats per minute and

appears to oscillate in a regular, uniform pattern of 2 to 6 cycles per minute; there are differences of opinion about whether this is LTV. Fetal activity may be minimal or absent

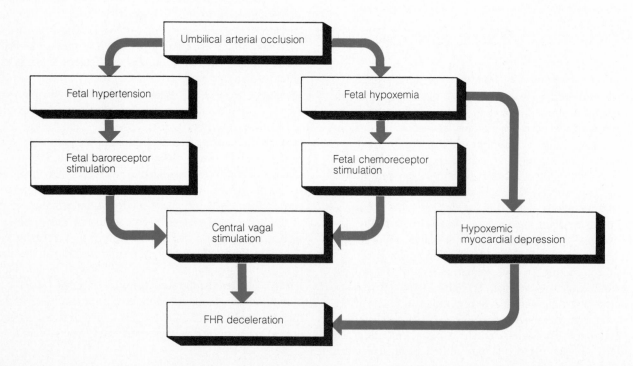

Figure 22–21   Mechanism of variable deceleration (Adapted from Freeman RK, Garite TJ: The physiologic basis of fetal monitoring, in *Fetal Heart Rate Monitoring.* Baltimore, Williams & Wilkins, 1981, ch 2, p 15)

and FHR accelerations are lacking. There is no beat-to-beat STV (Figure 22–25).

There is confusion regarding the definition and significance of the sinusoidal pattern, although the pattern seems to "imply severe fetal jeopardy and impending death" (Modanlou & Freeman 1982). In a review of the literature of 41 sinusoidal patterns, Modanlou and Freeman noted that true sinusoidal heart rate was seen most frequently in the severely affected Rh-sensitized fetus and neonate or in fetuses compromised by severe anemia of a different origin. It was also noted in fetuses and neonates with perinatal asphyxia and/or CNS insult. In addition, they found that the only cases in which true sinusoidal patterns were seen without significant morbidity were in fetuses whose mothers had received alphaprodine (Nisentil) analgesia during labor. They support the hypothesis that the cause of sinusoidal heart rate may be due to tissue hypoxia of the cardiac center.

The administration of nalbuphine hydrochloride (Nubain) has been associated with sinusoidal pattern (Feinstein et al 1986). Hatjis and Meiss (1986) noted in one study that the administration of intravenous butorphanol tartrate (Stadol) has also been noted to cause a sinusoidal pattern approximately 75 percent of the time it is given.

In the absence of analgesia-related occurrences, true sinusoidal FHR patterns noted intrapartally suggest fetal anemia or severe asphyxia. If noted by external monitoring,

internal fetal monitoring should be instituted, and cesarean delivery should be performed if the pattern is confirmed. Fetal blood sampling for determination of pH and hematocrit, ultrasound scan for signs of congestive heart failure and hydrops, and biophysical profile may aid in assessment, evaluation, and management of the fetus with this FHR pattern (Schneider & Tropper 1986).

○   *SALTATORY PATTERNS*   The saltatory pattern of marked or excessive variability is characterized by rapid variations in FHR that have a bizarre appearance. LTV occurs with a cycle frequency of three to six per minute, and the amplitude is greater than 25 beats per minute (Figure 22–26). The etiology of this pattern is uncertain. The fetus with this pattern may be moderately stressed, but no evidence to date indicates that fetal decompensation occurs with this pattern (Parer 1984b).

Value of Electronic Fetal Monitoring

In spite of several years of experience with fetal monitoring, the benefits in the normal labor are not yet conclusive. Certainly electronic monitoring has identified problems during labor that otherwise would have been undetected, and intervention has meant the survival of many infants who might otherwise have died during labor. In 1979 the Task Force of the National Institutes of Health recommended that electronic fetal monitors be considered

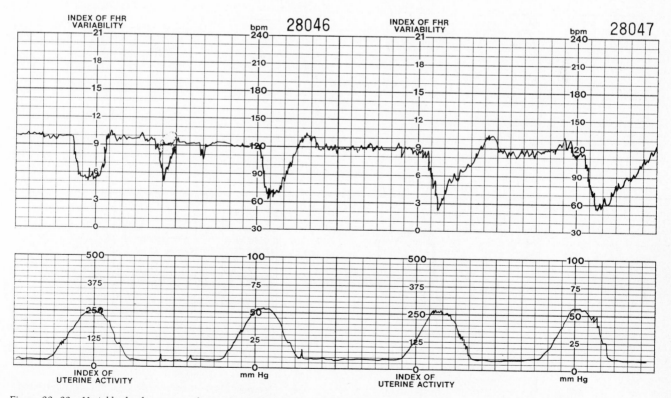

Figure 22–22 Variable decelerations with overshoot. The timing of the decelerations is variable and most have a sharp decline. An acceleration (overshoot) occurs after most of the decelerations.

in the management of high-risk clients "whenever the potential benefits of the technique exceed the known risks."

High-risk women, who account for approximately 25 percent of the obstetric population, account for only about one-half of the perinatal morbidity and mortality. The remainder of the perinatal casualties come from the low-risk group (75 percent of the obstetric population) (Wilson & Schifrin 1980). Obviously, classification of women according to risk prior to labor is not predictive of whether pregnancy outcome will be positive or not.

Only five randomized-controlled trial studies have compared auscultation to electronic fetal monitoring. Many clinicians believe these five studies are insufficient to support the monitoring of all laboring women. They conclude that in a well-screened population the value of electronic monitoring over careful auscultation is of little or no increased benefit. Others, however, prefer to use electronic fetal monitoring because it gives an indication of reassuring FHR patterns (normality) and an early indication of subtle FHR changes that might not be detected by auscultation by even the most experienced clinicians and nurses.

Parer (1984b) found evidence that monitoring decreases the intrapartal stillbirth rate by 1 to 2 per 1000 births and halves the neonatal death rate (saves 5 lives per 1000 births). According to this author, the benefit to the low-risk woman is one infant's life saved per 1000 births,

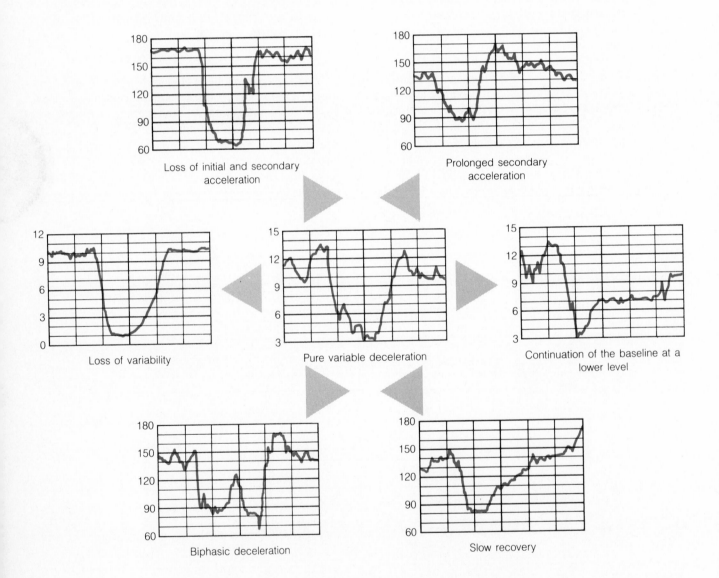

Figure 22–23 Atypical variable decelerations. The presence of any of these types of variable decelerations is very suggestive of fetal hypoxia, especially when variability is decreased. (From Krebs HB, Petrie RE, Dunn LJ: Atypical variable decelerations. *Am J Obstet Gynecol* 1983;145(3):298)

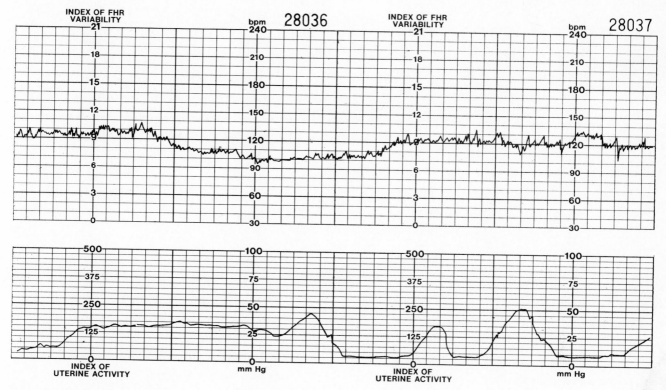

Figure 22–24 Prolonged deceleration

in addition to the permanent brain damage that might be avoided if women are monitored and managed accordingly. Unfortunately, electronic fetal monitoring is a better predictor of good outcome when patterns are reassuring than of poor fetal outcome when patterns are nonreassuring.

Psychologic Reactions to Electronic Monitoring

The nurse plays an important role in providing information about fetal monitoring. Many women have no knowledge of monitoring unless they have attended a prenatal class that dealt with this subject. Some women enter labor with preconceived negative ideas about this technology garnered from articles they have read in popular literature.

Studies regarding reactions of women to intrapartal electronic fetal monitoring reveal that most women react positively to the monitor; those with negative feelings seem to be in the minority. A study by Dulock and Herron (1976) noted that women had a more positive attitude after delivery than before delivery. Starkman (1976) stated that the most positive aspect of her study was that women with a previous history of intrapartal problems responded most favorably to the fetal monitor as a protector against disaster. Positive reactions expressed by women in documented studies include feelings that the fetal monitor offered reassurance as a protector (as an extension of the obstetri-

cian). It also acts as an aid in communication, an extension of the woman (as a provider of information to the physician), an extension of the fetus (confirmation that the baby is OK), and a facilitator of involvement of the woman's partner in the labor experience. The women appreciated the use of the monitor as a distraction or diversion during labor, and as an aid in mastery (for example, in Lamaze breathing).

Negative feelings about the monitor expressed by women included resentment (more attention paid to fetal monitor by partner and staff); physical discomfort; decreased mobility; and frustration due to mechanical difficulties with the monitor. The women who had negative reactions felt the monitor caused them anxiety (due to auditory information). They also experienced fear of injury to their baby (Molfese et al 1982).

Nurses should examine their own feelings about monitoring and give women the opportunity to talk about feelings regarding use of it. Nurses have influence in modifying attitudes and providing information. The nurse's attitudes influence the type of nursing care provided. If nurses express negativism or lack of confidence in the equipment they may not be able to incorporate this technology into their nursing assessment and therefore may give inadequate care and support to the woman.

The emphasis in maternity nursing is directed toward meeting the physical, emotional, and psychosocial needs of the woman with concern for the fetus. Use of the monitor enhances maternal and fetal surveillance, but the nurse

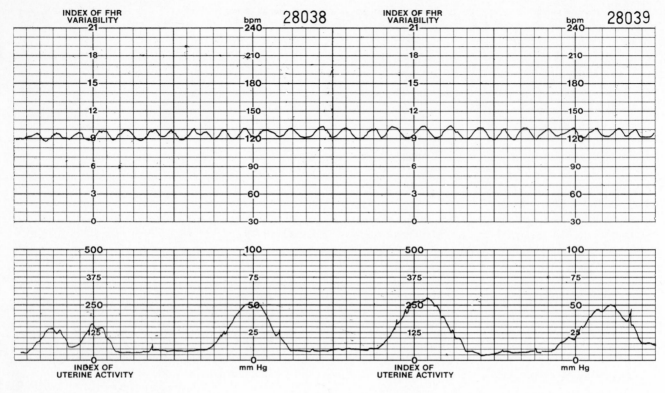

Figure 22–25 Sinusoidal pattern

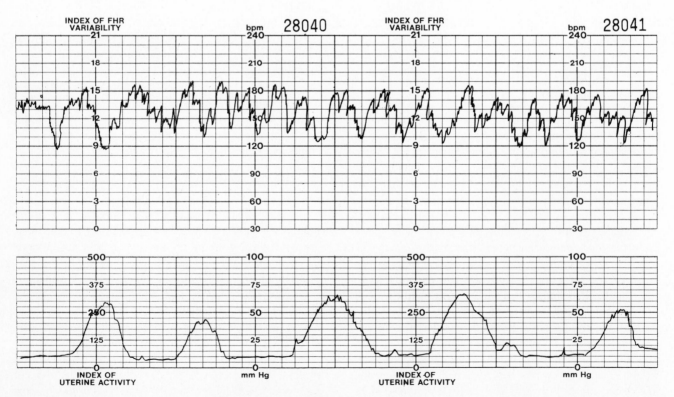

Figure 22–26 Saltatory pattern. Note pattern of marked variability.

must not lose sight of the woman's needs and overrely on the monitor. The monitor only provides information for the nurse's evaluation of the woman's status to provide the best care. Although technology should be appreciated for the additional information it offers, monitors do not care for women; nurses do.

Nursing Care and Responsibilities

Prior to application of the monitor, the nurse should fully explain to the woman the reason for it and the information that can be derived from its use. The nurse explains how the monitor can help identify the beginning of contractions and thus aid in breathing during the various phases of labor. An explanation alleviates apprehensions about equipment that may be totally unfamiliar to the woman. During labor it is advantageous to provide education regarding the use of the internal equipment as the care giver may quickly decide to convert to this method as a result of examination findings. Women who are informed about the possibility of internal monitoring are better prepared if a quick decision must be made to apply an electrode or catheter.

After the monitor is applied, basic information should be recorded on a label that is attached to the monitor strip. The data included are the date, time, woman's name, physician, hospital or agency number, age, gravida, para, estimated date of delivery, membrane status, maternal vital signs, and current medical problems. As the monitor strip continues to run and care is provided, it is important that documentation of occurrences during labor be recorded not only in the nurse's notes on the client's hospital record, but also on the fetal monitor tracing. The following information should be included on the tracing:

1. Vaginal examinations (dilatation, effacement, station, and position)

2. Amniotomy, spontaneous rupture of membranes, presence and consistency of meconium

3. Maternal vital signs

4. Maternal position changes

5. Application of spiral electrode and intrauterine pressure catheter

6. Medications, oxygen (route and flow rate), IV fluids, regional blocks

7. Maternal behaviors (emesis, coughing, hiccups)

8. Fetal blood sampling

9. Voiding or catheterization

This information is helpful in subsequent evaluation of maternal and fetal status. The tracing is considered to be a legal part of the medical record and is submissible in court. All pertinent information should be appropriately documented.

INTERPRETATION OF FHR TRACING

As in interpreting an ECG tracing, a systematic approach is required in evaluating FHR tracings to avoid misinterpretation of findings on the basis of inadequate or erroneous data. (See Box 22–2 for a method of systematic evaluation.) Developing a systematic approach to evaluation allows the nurse to make a more accurate and rapid assessment and to feel confident in communicating data to physicians and staff.

As a result of evaluation of the FHR tracing, the nurse makes decisions regarding care and the need for further assessment. The assumption is that labor and the response

---

Box 22–2   Evaluating FHR Tracings

Evaluation of the electronic monitor tracing begins by looking at the uterine contractions. Characteristics of the fetal heart rate are then evaluated.

Evaluate the uterine contraction pattern.

1. Determine the uterine resting tone.

2. Assess the contractions.

   What is the frequency?
   What is the duration?
   What is the intensity?

Evaluate the fetal heart rate tracing.

1. Determine the baseline.

   Is the baseline within normal range?
   Is there evidence of tachycardia?
   Is there evidence of bradycardia?

2. Determine FHR variability.

   Is short-term variability present or absent?
   Is long-term variability average? Minimal to absent? Moderate to marked?

3. Assess for periodic changes

   Are accelerations present?
   Do they meet the criteria for reactive NST?
   Are decelerations present?
   Are they uniform in shape? If so determine if they are early or late decelerations.
   Are they nonuniform in shape? If so determine if they are variable decelerations. Do they have a late component? Are they prolonged?

   Is a sinusoidal or saltatory pattern present?

of the fetus to uterine contractions will be within normal parameters. When possible problems are identified, the nurse responds with needed interventions (see Tables 22–3 and 22–4). The nurse also needs to be constantly aware of changes in the maternal-fetal condition and how the change might affect the FHR tracing. It is important to have a sound knowledge base regarding the cause of various FHR patterns so that appropriate assessments may be anticipated and completed.

All nurses who provide care to women in labor should be skilled in application of electronic monitoring equipment and assessment of baseline and periodic changes. A thorough understanding of the characteristics of "normal" FHR and FHR patterns is necessary to ensure immediate assistance and further evaluation if the FHR status is not normal (Table 22–5). A fetus who demonstrates a normal FHR pattern within 30 minutes prior to delivery will be vigorous at birth and have good Apgar scores about 98 percent of the time, providing: (1) delivery is accomplished within 30 minutes, (2) the fetus suffers no traumatic insult during delivery (eg, breech extraction or difficult forceps delivery), (3) the fetus has no serious congenital anomalies inconsistent with extrauterine life (Parer 1984b)

In the past nurses were told to refrain from "diagnosing" various FHR patterns. Since electronic fetal monitoring (EFM) has become a "standard" in hospital care (if only intermittently used) and the nomenclature for classification of periodic changes has been established, specific criteria have been delineated for classification of specific periodic changes. The nurse should know these criteria and use appropriate terminology in interpretation, documentation, and communication with other health team members. For example, if the FHR begins to decrease from the baseline at or after the peak of the contraction, inversely mirrors the contraction, has a uniform and smooth waveform, and returns to the baseline as the contraction wanes, the nurse can appropriately document and communicate to others that late decelerations are occurring. This is not a medical diagnosis but a recognition and documentation of an accepted standard of classification of FHR periodic change. Knowledge of EFM is necessary in order to attempt to correct nonreassuring patterns, document assessments correctly, communicate assessments to physicians, and provide follow-up management and evaluation to ensure optimum fetal outcome. (See Box 22–3).

Additional Assessment Techniques

MONITORING OF FETAL ACID-BASE STATUS

○   *FETAL SCALP SAMPLING*   When nonreassuring or confusing FHR patterns are noted, it becomes necessary to seek additional information regarding the acid-base status of the fetus. This is accomplished by means of fetal blood sampling, which is usually done from the fetal scalp, but may be performed on the fetus in the breech position.

When oxygen perfusion to the fetus is compromised, fetal hypoxia ensues and metabolism changes from aerobic to anaerobic, resulting in the production of lactic acid. This causes a state of acidosis and therefore a drop in the pH level. With fetal blood sampling, a higher correlation exists between low pH levels and low Apgar scores; with fetal monitoring, there is high correlation between normal FHR patterns and high Apgar scores. This may be due to the

Table 22–3   General Guidelines for Management of FHR Baseline Changes

FHR baseline	Nursing interventions
Normal	Evaluate maternal vital signs. Follow labor by means of vaginal examination at appropriate intervals. Assess and evaluate the quality of labor and FHR patterns. Document data and assessment of findings. Assure adequate hydration. Assist with maternal position changes. Maintain continual flow of communication.
Tachycardia	Report findings to physician/CNM. Assess maternal temperature. Assure adequate hydration. Reconfirm EDD. Monitor for changes in FHR pattern. Assist physician with fetal blood sampling if indicated (especially if decreased variability is present).
Bradycardia	Report findings to physician/CNM. Monitor for changes in FHR pattern (especially decreased variability). Assist physician with fetal blood sampling if indicated (especially with bradycardia on initial tracing).

Table 22–4   Guidelines for Management of Deceleration Patterns

Pattern	Nursing interventions
Early decelerations	Monitor for changes in FHR pattern. Evaluate for possible cephalopelvic disproportion if decelerations occur in early labor.

Variable decelerations
  Isolated or occasional
  Moderate
	Report findings to physician/CNM.
	Provide explanation to woman and partner.
	Monitor for changes in FHR pattern.
	Change maternal position to one in which FHR pattern is most improved.
	Discontinue oxytocin if it is being administered.
	Perform vaginal examination to assess for prolapsed cord or imminent delivery.
	Administer 100% oxygen by tight face mask at 6 to 8 L/min.
	Monitor FHR continuously to assess current status and for further changes in FHR pattern.

If variable decelerations are severe and uncorrectable and woman is in First stage	Report findings to physician/CNM. Provide explanation to woman and partner. Prepare for probable cesarean delivery.
Second stage labor	Prepare for vaginal delivery unless baseline variability is decreasing and/or FHR is progressively rising, then cesarean delivery if indicated. Assist physician with fetal scalp sampling. Prepare for cesarean delivery if scalp pH shows acidosis or downward trend.
Late decelerations occasional with average variability	Report findings to physician/CNM. Provide explanation to woman and partner. Monitor for further FHR changes. Maintain maternal position on left side. Maintain good hydration with IV fluids (normal saline or lactated Ringer's). Discontinue oxytocin if it is being administered. Administer oxygen by face mask at 6 to 8 L/min. Monitor maternal blood pressure and pulse for signs of hypotension; possibly increase flow rate of IV fluids to treat hypotension. Follow physician's orders for treatment for hypotension if present.
Late decelerations persistent with average variability	Report findings to physician/CNM. Provide explanation to woman and partner. Maintain maternal position on left side. Administer oxygen by face mask at 6 to 8 L/min. Discontinue oxytocin if it is being administered. Assess maternal blood pressure and pulse. Increase IV fluids to maintain volume and hydration (normal saline or lactated Ringer's). Assess labor progress (dilation and station). Assist physician with fetal blood sampling: If pH stays above 7.25, physician will continue monitoring and resample; if pH shows downward trend (between 7.25 and 7.20) or is below 7.20, prepare for delivery by most expeditious means.
Late decelerations with tachycardia and/or decreasing variability	Report findings to physician/CNM. Maintain maternal position on left side. Administer oxygen by face mask at 6 to 8 L/min. Discontinue oxytocin if it is being administered. Assess maternal blood pressure and pulse. Increase IV fluids (normal saline or lactated Ringer's). Assess labor progress (dilatation and station). Prepare for immediate cesarean delivery. Explain plan of treatment to woman and partner. Assist physician with fetal blood sampling.

fact that changes in fetal scalp blood pH occur only after significant anaerobic metabolism, whereas late decelerations may occur with early hypoxemia before the development of metabolic acidosis (Freeman & Garite 1981). Care givers must assess the risks of waiting against the risks

of intervention by cesarean delivery to achieve higher Apgar scores.

Parer (1984a) notes that fetal blood sampling may be of benefit in the following situations:

1. Absence of FHR variability on initial application of the monitor with no clear cause (eg, recent large maternal dose of centrally depressing drugs)

2. Absence of heart rate variability in a fetus with potential asphyxia, even in the presence of centrally depressing drugs (eg, in a gravida undergoing narcotic and magnesium sulfate treatment for preeclampsia)

3. A pattern of late decelerations with decreasing variability that cannot be abolished in a reasonable time (eg, 30 minutes)

4. A pattern of variable decelerations with decreasing variability that cannot be abolished in a reasonable time (eg, 30 minutes)

5. Puzzling or unusual, unexplained patterns, such as intermittent sinusoidal or regular "picket fence" pattern, which may simulate variability except for its repetitiousness

Fetal Blood Sampling Procedure Equipment needed for fetal blood sampling is available in sterile disposable trays. Items included are:

Three to six heparinized capillary tubes

A short capillary tube holder

A 2 mm blade on long handle

A conical beveled endoscope

Clay sealant

Silicone gel

Six to ten long sponge swabs

An extra light source is needed.

The woman's vulva and perineum should be thoroughly cleansed with povidone-iodine solution (Betadine) and sterile drapes arranged. A conical vaginal endoscope

Table 22–5 Characteristics of Normal Fetal Heart Rate Patterns

Baseline rate	120 to 160 beats/min
Baseline variability (amplitude range)	>6 beats/min
Periodic pattern	None or early decelerations or accelerations
Fetal outcome	Vigorous; Apgar score >7 at 5 min

Source: Parer JT: Fetal heart rate, in Creasy RK, Resnik R (eds): *Maternal-Fetal Medicine.* Philadelphia, Saunders, 1984, p 299.

Box 22–3 Reassuring and Nonreassuring FHR Patterns

FHR patterns need to be assessed for evidence that shows whether they are reassuring or nonreassuring. *Reassuring* patterns include (Freeman 1982):

1. No periodic changes

2. Early decelerations

3. Variable decelerations that do not exceed the following limits:

   a. Accelerations lasting less than 45 seconds

   b. Return to baseline is abrupt

   c. Baseline rate is not increasing

   d. Baseline variability is not decreasing

4. FHR accelerations

   a. With contractions

   b. With fetal movement

Nonreassuring patterns include (Freeman 1982):

1. Intermittent late deceleration with good FHR variability

2. Variable deceleration that exceeds the criteria (in reassuring patterns) with respect to duration and/or rate of return but still has good FHR variability and no rising baseline

3. Total loss of FHR variability with deceleration

4. Prolonged deceleration due to:

   a. Paracervical block

   b. Epidural block

   c. Supine hypotension

   d. Vaginal examination or manipulation

Ominous FHR patterns include (Freeman 1982):

1. Persistent, uncorrectable late decelerations with loss of FHR variability with or without fetal tachycardia

2. Variable decelerations accompanied by:

   a. Loss of FHR variability

   b. Fetal tachycardia

   c. Prolonged "overshoot"

   d. Blunted shapes

3. Sinusoidal FHR patterns

is inserted into the vagina and through the cervix to facilitate visualization of the fetal site to be sampled (Figure 22–27). Working through the endoscope, the physician cleanses the site to remove vernix, blood, and amniotic fluid. Silicone gel is then applied to the site to provide a surface for the formation of a globule of blood. The site is punctured with a 2 × 2 mm microscalpel. A small amount of blood is then collected in a long heparinized capillary tube and immediately assessed for pH value. Approximately 0.25 ml of blood is necessary for determination of fetal pH and base deficit. Two or three samples should be collected during each procedure to confirm reliability of pH.

The clotting mechanism is compromised when pH is lowered; therefore oozing at the site may occur for a period of time. Because loss of even minimal amounts of blood may be disastrous to the fetus, pressure is applied to the puncture site throughout two maternal contractions, then the site is observed throughout a third contraction. After the procedure the woman is observed for vaginal bleeding to assure that what may appear to be heavy bloody show is not a fetal hemorrhage from the puncture site. Results of pH determination should be readily available in 10 to 15 minutes for this procedure to be effective.

The major disadvantages of fetal blood sampling include the following (Freeman & Garite 1981):

1. The procedure is difficult.

2. The data are intermittent.

3. Scalp or buttocks data may not reflect data from the central circulation.

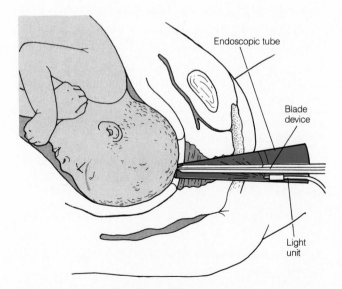

Figure 22–27 *Technique of obtaining fetal blood from scalp during labor* (From Creasy RK, Parer JT: Prenatal care and diagnosis, in Ruldolph AM (ed): *Pediatrics,* ed 16. Englewood Cliffs, NJ, Appleton-Century-Crofts, 1977)

4. There are risks of fetal bleeding and infection.

5. The data may be influenced by maternal acid-base status.

6. The data may be influenced by carbon dioxide retention.

Fetal Blood Sample Results   Normal pH values during labor are at or above 7.25 pH, with 7.20 to 7.24 pH considered preacidotic. Values below 7.20 pH indicate serious acidosis. Quilligan (1985) recommends sampling within 30 minutes to observe the trend if the pH is between 7.20 and 7.25, immediate resampling if it is less than 7.20, and immediate delivery by the most expeditious route (cesarean birth if necessary) if it remains below 7.20. Most clinicians consider a pH value of 7.25 or more as normal and resample only as indicated by FHR patterns and amount of variability. Values below 7.20 are considerd acidotic and warrant immediate delivery. Values between 7.20 and 7.25 are evaluated on the basis of several factors, including the relationship to maternal pH, the accuracy of the sampling and pH determination, the stage of labor, and the particular clinical situation (Parer 1984a). Fetal blood sampling may be repeated in 15 to 30 minutes depending on these factors.

Associated Factors   Some FHR patterns seem to be associated with abnormal fetal acid-base status. Short-term and long-term variability correlate better with fetal pH than deceleration patterns do. If STV and LTV are present, the pH will be in the normal range. If STV is present, the fetal pH is usually normal even in the presence of late decelerations. If STV is absent, however, the risk of acidosis increases. When STV is absent and variable decelerations are occurring, the pH will be in the preacidotic range. If late decelerations occur with no STV present, the pH will probably be in the acidotic range (Campbell et al 1986).

These findings are of particular significance when nonreassuring FHR patterns are observed and fetal acid-base determination is not feasible. One can be reassured that the fetus is not acidotic in almost 100 percent of cases if the variability remains normal (Boehm et al 1978, Krebs et al 1982, Parer 1984a). A pH above 7.25 predicts that the fetus will be vigorous in about 90 percent of cases; a pH less than 7.15 predicts a depressed fetus with only 80 percent reliability (Parer 1984a). Fetal blood sampling seems unnecessary when variability is normal since the fetus will be vigorous despite the pH value.

Although not clinically in use at present, it is possible to monitor fetal pH continuously by a pH electrode embedded in the fetal scalp tissue. This electrode does not measure fetal blood pH level per se but rather the subcutaneous tissue pH level. In hypoxia, an increase in alpha-adrenergic activity occurs initially with accompanying fetal hypertension, causing acidosis to occur in peripheral tissue more rapidly than in the central circulation. Conversely, as hypoxia is corrected, there may be a recovery lag of the pH value in the peripheral tissue (Freeman & Garite 1981).

Considerable skill is required for both continuous and intermittent fetal blood sampling. As yet, even intermittent sampling is not widely done due to the difficulty of the procedure and the scarcity of blood gas microanalyzers on or near the delivery unit to obtain immediate results.

○ *PERCUTANEOUS UMBILICAL BLOOD SAMPLING (PUBS)* In this new fetal assessment technique, fetal blood is obtained from the umbilical cord by means of a needle inserted in the maternal abdomen. The procedure can be performed at the bedside to assess fetal acid-base status during labor when FBS may not be feasible and FHR patterns are confusing or worrisome (Hobbins et al 1985). See Chapter 20 for a description of the procedure. The procedure is also most helpful in the management of women with idiopathic thrombocytopenic purpura. Early assessment of fetal platelet count by PUBS may allow these women to deliver vaginally rather than by cesarean when the fetus cannot be assessed by FBS due to inadequate dilatation of the cervix.

Although this technique is thought to be of low risk, and only minimal complications (transient bradycardia) have arisen, further study is required to assess the safety of the procedure.

SCALP STIMULATION TEST

Various stimuli have been used to arouse the fetus and cause acceleration of the FHR. This FHR characteristic has long been considered to be a reliable indicator of fetal well-being. One study suggested that a scalp stimulation test may be superior to measurement of fetal pH with regard to prediction of fetal well-being (Clark et al 1984). Methods used in the study were (1) 15 seconds of gentle digital pressure applied to the fetal scalp during vaginal examination and (2) application of an Allis clamp (closed to the first rachet) to the fetal scalp for 15 seconds. A positive response (accelerations of FHR of 15 beats/min for 15 sec) correlated in about 98 percent of cases with nonacidotic fetal status (pH >7.20). Furthermore, a greater percentage of fetuses responded to this biophysical test than to fetal scalp puncture during pH sampling. The scalp stimulation test may significantly reduce the necessity for fetal blood sampling and may be useful when nonreassuring FHR patterns are noted and fetal blood sampling is not feasible.

This procedure is certainly not without danger of trauma to the fetal scalp if a clamp is used, but is quite practical if only a digital exam is performed. It is a procedure that can be performed by any knowledgeable nurse caring for a woman in labor with a nonreassuring FHR pattern. Obviously this procedure would not be appropri-ate if the fetal head was not engaged and the membranes were intact because of the possibility of inadvertant rupture of the membranes and prolapse of the umbilical cord.

KEY CONCEPTS

Intrapartal assessment includes attention to both physical and psychological parameters of the laboring woman, assessment of the fetus, and ongoing assessment for conditions that place the woman and her fetus at increased risk.

A sterile vaginal examination determines status of fetal membranes; cervical dilatation and effacement; and fetal presentation, position, and station.

Uterine contractions may be assessed by palpation or by an electronic monitor. The electronic monitor may be used for external or internal monitoring.

Labor progress may be objectively evaluated using a Friedman graph, which plots cervical dilatation and fetal descent.

Leopold's maneuvers provide a systematic evaluation of fetal presentation and position.

Fetal presentation and position may also be assessed by vaginal examination, ultrasound, CT scan, and x ray.

The fetal heart rate may be assessed by auscultation (with a fetoscope) or electronic monitoring.

Electronic fetal monitoring is accomplished by indirect ultrasound or by direct methods that require the placement of a spiral electrode on the fetal presenting part.

Indications for electronic monitoring include fetal, maternal, and uterine factors; presence of pregnancy complications; regional anesthesia; and elective monitoring.

True variability of the FHR can only be assessed by direct electronic monitoring.

Baseline FHR refers to the range of FHR observed between contractions, during a ten-minute period of monitoring.

The normal range of FHR is 120 to 160 beats per minute.

Baseline changes of the FHR includes tachycardia, bradycardia, and variability.

Tachycardia is defined as a rate of 160 beats per minute or more for a ten-minute segment of time.

Bradycardia is defined as a rate of less than 120 beats per minute for a ten-minute segment of time.

Baseline variability is an important parameter of fetal well-being. It includes both long- and short-term variability.

Periodic changes are transient decelerations or accelerations of the FHR from the baseline. Accelerations are normally caused by fetal movement; decelerations may be termed early, late, variable, or sinusoidal.

Early decelerations are due to compression of the fetal head during contractions and are considered reassuring.

Late decelerations are associated with uteroplacental insufficiency and are considered ominous.

Variable decelerations are associated with compression of the umbilical cord.

Prolonged decelerations are those in which the FHR decreases from the baseline for two or more minutes.

Sinusoidal patterns are characterized by an undulant sinewave.

Saltatory patterns are characterized by marked or excessive variability and rapid variations in FHR that have a bizarre appearance.

Psychologic reactions to monitoring vary between feelings of relief and feelings of being tied down.

Labor and delivery nurses have responsibilities in recognizing and interpreting fetal monitoring patterns, notifying the physician/CNM of problems, and initiating corrective and supportive measures when needed.

Fetal acid-base status may be assessed by fetal scalp sampling or percutaneous umbilical blood sampling.

REFERENCES

Boehm FH, Graben AL, Hick MM: Coordinated metabolic and obstetric management of diabetic pregnancy. *South Med J* 1978;71:37.

Campbell WA, Vintzileos AM, Nochimson DJ: Intrauterine versus extrauterine management/resuscitation of the fetus/neonate. *Clin Obstet Gynecol* 1986;29(1):33.

Clark SL, Gimovsky ML, Miller FC: The scalp stimulation test: A clinical alternative to fetal scalp blood sampling. *Am J Obstet Gynecol* 1984;148(3):274.

Daffos F, Forestier F, Parlovsky MC: A new procedure for fetal blood sampling in utero: preliminary results of 53 cases. *Am J Obstet Gynecol* 1983;146(8):985.

Druzen M, et al: A possible mechanism for the increase in FHR variability following hypoxemia. Presented at the 26th Annual Meeting of the Society for Gynecological Investigation, San Diego, Calif, March 1979.

Dulock HL, Herron M: Women's responses to fetal monitoring. *J Obstet Gynecol Neonat Nurs* 1976;5(suppl):68s.

Feinstein SJ, et al: Sinusoidal fetal heart rate pattern after administration of nalbuphine hydrochloride: A case report. *Am J Obstet Gynecol* 1986;154(1):159.

Freeman RK: Fetal distress: Diagnosis and management. Presented at the Sixth International Symposium on Perinatal Medicine, Las Vegas, Nevada, 1982.

Freeman RK, Garite TJ: *Fetal Heart Rate Monitoring*. Baltimore, Williams & Wilkins, 1981.

Friedman EA: An objective method of evaluating labor. *Hosp Pract* 1970;5:82.

Gimovsky ML, et al: X-ray pelvimetry in a breech protocol: A comparison of digital radiography and conventional methods. *Am J Obstet Gynecol* 1983;153(4):887.

Hatjis CG, Meis PJ: Sinusoidal fetal heart rate pattern associated with butorphanol administration. *Obstet Gynecol* 1986;67(3):377.

Haverkamp AD, et al: A controlled trial of the differential effects of intrapartum fetal monitoring. *Am J Obstet Gynecol* 1979;134:399.

Hobbins JC, et al: Percutaneous umbilical blood sampling. *Am J Obstet Gynecol* 1985;152(1):1.

Hobel CJ, et al: Prenatal and intrapartum high risk screening. *Am J Obstet Gynecol* 1973;117:1.

Hon EH: *An Introduction to Fetal Heart Rate Monitoring*, ed 2. Los Angeles, USC School of Medicine, 1976.

Hon E, Quilligan EJ: The classification of fetal heart rate: II. A revised working classification. *Conn Med* 1967;31:779.

Krebs HB, Petrie RE, Dunn LJ: Atypical variable decelerations. *Am J Obstet Gynecol* 1983;145(3):297.

Krebs HB, et al: Intrapartum fetal heart rate monitoring. *Am J Obstet Gynecol* 1982;142:297.

Kubli EW, et al: Observations on heart rate and pH in the human fetus during labor. *Am J Obstet Gynecol* 1969;104:1190.

Martin CB, Gingerich B: Factors affecting the fetal heart rate: Genesis of FHR patterns. *J Obstet Gynecol Neonat Nurs* 1976;5(suppl):305.

Modanlou H, Freeman RK, Braly P: A simple method of fetal and neonatal heart rate beat-to-beat variability quantitation. *Am J Obstet Gynecol* 1977;127:861.

Modanlou HD, Freeman RK: Sinusoidal fetal heart rate pattern: Its definition and clinical significance. *Am J Obstet Gynecol* 1982;142:1033.

Molfese V, Sunshine P, Bennett A: Reactions of women to intrapartum fetal monitoring. *Obstet Gynecol* 1982;59:705.

Monheit A, Cousins L: When do you measure scalp and blood pH? *Contemp OB/GYN* 1981;18(August):55.

Myles MF: *Textbook for Midwives*. Edinburgh, Scotland, Churchill Livingston, 1975.

Neutra RR, Rienberg SE, Griedman EA: The effect of fetal monitoring on neonatal death rates. *N Engl J Med* 1978;299:324.

Oxorn H: *Human Labor and Birth*. New York, Appleton-Century-Crofts, 1986.

Parer JT: Fetal acid-base balance, in **Creasy** RK, **Resnik** R (eds): *Maternal-Fetal Medicine*. Philadelphia, Saunders, 1984a, pp 321–330.

Parer JT: Fetal heart rate, in **Creasy** RK, **Resnik** R (eds): *Maternal-Fetal Medicine*. Philadelphia, Saunders, 1984b, pp 285–319.

Paul RH, **Petrie** RH: Fetal intensive care: Current concepts. Los Angeles, USC School of Medicine, 1973.

Petrie R, **Pollack** KJ: Intrapartum fetal biochemical monitoring by fetal blood sampling. *J Obstet Gynecol Neonat Nurs* 1976;5(suppl):52s.

Quilligan EJ: Fetal bradycardia: watch or deliver? *Contemp OB/GYN* 1981;18(July):127.

Quilligan EJ: Identification of fetal distress, in **Queenan** JT (ed): *Management of High-Risk Pregnancy*, ed 2. Oradell, NJ, Medical Economics Books, 1985, p 135.

Schifrin BS, **Dame** L: Fetal heart rate pattern prediction of Apgar score. *JAMA* 1973;219:322.

Schneider EP, **Tropper** PJ: The variable deceleration, prolonged deceleration, and sinusoidal fetal heart rate. *Clin Obstet Gynecol* 1986;29(1):64.

Starkman MN: Psychological responses to the use of the fetal monitor during labor. *Psychosom Med* 1976;38:269.

Willson JR, **Carrington** E: *Obstetrics and Gynecology*, ed 6. St Louis, Mosby, 1979.

Wilson RW, **Schifrin** BS: Is any pregnancy low risk? *Obstet Gynecol* 1980;55:653.

Chen SZ, et al: Effects of sitting position on uterine activity during labor. *Obstet Gynecol* 1987;69(January):67.

Copstick SM, et al: Partner support and the use of coping techniques in labour. *J Psychosom Res* 1986;30(4):497.

Ganong LH, **Bzdek**, **Manderino** MA: Stereotyping by nurses and nursing students: A critical review of research. *Res Nurs Health* 1987;10:49.

Garite TJ, **Freeman** RK: Interpreting fetal heart tracings, in **Queenan** JT (ed): *Management of High-Risk Pregnancy*, ed 2. Oradell, NJ, Medical Economics Books, 1985, p 151.

Herbert W, et al: Clinical aspects of fetal heart auscultation. *Obstet Gynecol* 1987;69(April):574.

Hutson JM: Possible limitations of fetal monitoring. *Clin Obstet Gynecol* 1986;29(March):104.

Ingemarsson I, et al: Admission test: A screening test for fetal distress in labor. *Obstet Gynecol* 1986;68:800.

Kintz DL: Nursing support during labor. *J Obstet Gynecol Neonat Nurs* 1987;16(March/April):126.

Strickland OL: The occurrence of symptoms in expectant fathers. *Nurs Res* 1987;36(May/June):184.

Weishaar BB: A comparison of Lamaze and hypnosis in the management of labor *Am J Clin Hypn* 1986;28(April):214.

Young BK: Fetal stress and distress, in **Young** B (ed): *The Patient Within the Patient*. March of Dimes Birth Defects Foundation, Original Article Series, vol 21, no 5. Alan R Liss, 1985, p 155.

ADDITIONAL READINGS

Bargagliotti LA, **Trygstad** LN: Differences in stress and coping findings: A reflection of social realities of methodologies? *Nurs Res* 1987;36(May/June):170.

Bates MS: Ethnicity and pain: A biocultural model. *Soc Sci Med* 1987;24(1):47.

Bracero LA, et al: Fetal heart rate diagnosis that provides confidence in the diagnosis of fetal well-being. *Clin Obstet Gynecol* 1986;29(1):3.

There is a moment in the last few weeks of the first pregnancy that stands out beyond all others. At that moment the realization of how your baby is really going to be born hits you like a brick. Yes, all through the pregnancy you knew. But at this moment you know, without any way out, that this baby you feel kicking and turning—and surely weighing more than anyone expects—is going to come out your vagina. Let me tell you, that's quite a moment!

The Family in Childbirth: Needs and Care

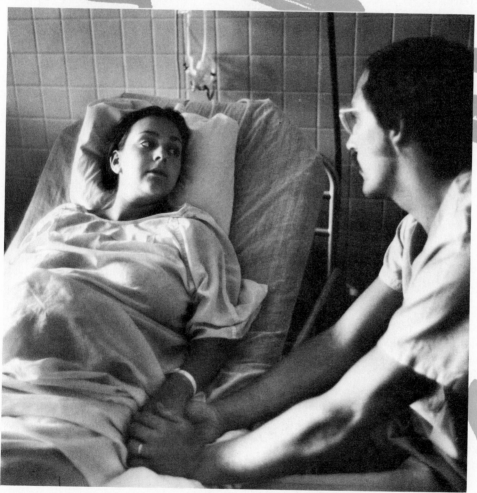

Nurses need to respect and encourage emotional support from the husband or partner of the woman in labor.

Chapter Twenty-Three

Care of the Family During the Second Stage of Labor
Nursing Goal: Assisting the Woman in Her Pushing Efforts
Nursing Goal: Preparation for Delivery
Nursing Goal: Assisting the Couple and Physican/Nurse-Midwife During Delivery
Physician/Nurse-Midwife Interventions
The Leboyer Method
Immediate Care of the Newborn
Apgar Scoring System
Care of the Umbilical Cord
Evaluation of the Newborn after Delivery
Newborn Identification Procedures
Care of the Family During the Third Stage
Nursing Goal: Initiation of Attachment
Physician/Nurse-Midwife Interventions
Care of the Family During the Fourth Stage
Nursing Goal: Preparation for the Recovery Period
Nursing Goal: Promotion of Maternal Physical Well-Being
Nursing Goal: Enhancing Attachment
Early Discharge
Case Study
Care of the Adolescent During Labor and Delivery
Nursing Goal: Promotion of Maternal and Fetal Well-Being
Nursing Goal: Support During Labor and Delivery
Care of the Woman and Newborn During Delivery in Less-Than-Ideal Circumstances
Precipitous Delivery
Out-of-Hospital Emergency Delivery

OBJECTIVES

- **Compare the advantages and disadvantages of alternative settings for labor and delivery.**
- **Identify options that women and their families have during the intrapartal period.**
- **Identify the data base to be obtained when a woman is admitted to a labor and delivery unit, and the associated nursing care.**
- **Discuss nursing interventions to meet the psychologic and physiologic needs of the woman during each stage of labor and delivery.**
- **Integrate knowledge of nursing care of the healthy woman and baby in the intrapartal period through use of the nursing process.**
- **Discuss immediate nursing care of the newborn following delivery.**
- **Describe early discharge programs and subsequent postpartal assessments.**

- **Discuss management of a delivery in less-than-optimal situations.**

I t is time for a child to be born. The waiting is over; labor has begun. The dreams and wishes of the past months fade as the expectant parents face the reality of the tasks of childbearing and childrearing that are ahead.

The couple is about to undergo one of the most meaningful and stressful events in their life together. The adequacy of their preparation for childbirth will now be tested. The coping mechanisms, communication, and support systems that they have established as a couple will be put to the test. In particular, the childbearing woman may feel that her psychologic and physical limits are about to be challenged.

Throughout the pregnancy, the couple has been involved in collecting information and making decisions about their childbearing experience. Many expectant parents are well-informed health care consumers who request alternatives to traditional maternity care. As a result, many hospitals now offer a variety of birthing experiences.

Maternity nurses have kept pace with the changing philosophy of childbirth and continue to bring personal caring and comfort to an increasingly high technology area (Tartasky 1985). Today's maternity nurse in the birth setting uses the full spectrum of nursing skills in working with childbearing families. Maternity nurses assess clients; gather information; provide information and teaching so that couples can make informed choices; function as a client advocate; collaborate with other health care professionals; ensure that they function within current nursing standards of care; and communicate with physicians and certified nurse-midwives. Maternity nurses have become an integral part of family-centered care as they provide support, encouragement, and safe, caring nursing care.

Providing nursing care to the childbearing couple is not only challenging but also tremendously rewarding. The nurse is participating in one of the most powerful emotional experiences in life.

Childbirth is usually joyous, but sometimes it is a time of grief and sadness. The needs of the childbearing couple in the event of crisis during or after labor and delivery are discussed in later chapters. This chapter describes the needs and nursing care of the family during normal labor and delivery.

● Using the Nursing Process During the Intrapartal Period

Maternity nurses will find that using the nursing process enhances their ability to provide individualized family-centered care during the intrapartal period. By applying the nursing process, nursing skills and theory, and their knowledge about childbirth, maternity nurses can function in a variety of birthing settings.

Nursing Assessment

When the laboring woman is admitted to the birthing unit, the first member of the health care team that she and her partner encounter is usually the nurse. The accuracy of the nurse's admission assessment of the woman's physical and psychological status is significant in determining the quality of the childbearing experience the couple will have. The nursing assessment is the basis for determining initial management of care by other members of the health care team.

The initial nursing assessment usually focuses on the imminence of delivery. Careful assessment of labor progress will help the nurse determine the priorities of care that must follow. After safety of the mother and fetus have been assured, the nursing assessment focuses on the woman's coping mechanisms and her support system. The nurse also determines the goals the couple have established for their birth experience.

During labor, the nurse continually reassesses maternal and fetal physical status and the couple's coping mechanisms in order to intervene appropriately.

Analysis and Nursing Diagnosis

Nursing diagnoses are based on physical and psychosocial assessments of the childbearing woman. Common nursing diagnoses in the intrapartal period include:

- Alteration in comfort: pain related to the birth process

- Potential ineffective individual coping related to ineffective labor coping strategies and/or unanticipated events

- Knowledge deficit related to breathing techniques and measures to increase comfort during labor and delivery

Nursing Plan and Implementation

Once nursing diagnoses are formulated, the nurse must determine which are most significant to the woman's well-being. Priorities of care differ for every woman admitted to the birthing unit. While physiological alterations usually form the basis for priorities of care when labor is progressing rapidly or high-risk factors are identified, this may not be the situation with a healthy woman admitted in early labor. After safety of the mother and fetus have

been assured, important factors that must be considered in developing the nursing plan of care include the woman's goals for her birth experience, her coping mechanisms, and the strength of her support systems. For example, the 16-year-old single nullipara who has had no prenatal care and comes to the hospital alone has different needs from the couple who planned the pregnancy and attended prepared childbirth classes. Nursing diagnoses and priorities for the plan of care will be quite different in these two situations. The nurse may be the 16-year-old girl's only support, but the couple may have only minimal need for the nurse's support.

A major challenge for the nurse is helping laboring women to achieve realistic goals for their birthing experience. Each woman is admitted to the birthing unit at a different phase in the laboring process and with a different level of wellness. The nurse may not have time to assess the choice of birthing options of a multipara whose delivery is imminent on admission or to support the goal of unmedicated labor in a primigravida who develops severe preeclampsia during her labor. Regardless of the individual factors each woman or couple brings to the labor, the nurse and the woman or couple work together to achieve a safe labor and birth.

To be effective, the nurse must use many types of interventions during labor and delivery. These include technical interventions; interventions that ensure that the birth setting is safe and comfortable for the woman and her baby; communication techniques for use with the laboring woman, her support person(s), and other members of the health team; and teaching techniques.

Evaluation

Evaluation of the effectiveness of nursing interventions is ongoing as the nurse continually reassesses the woman. Evaluation results in a constant cycle of nursing process application.

● Care of the Woman and Her Partner Upon Admission to the Birthing Unit

The woman is instructed during her prenatal visits to come to the birthing unit if any of the following occur:

- Rupture of the amniotic membranes

- Regular, frequent uterine contractions (nulliparas, 5 to 10 minutes apart for one hour; multiparas, 10 to 15 minutes apart for one hour)

- Any vaginal bleeding

Early admission means less discomfort for the laboring woman when traveling to the birth setting and more time to prepare for the birth. Sometimes the labor is advanced and birth is imminent, but usually the woman is in early labor at admission.

Special Nursing Considerations

INFORMED CONSENT

When the woman enters the health care facility, she may be facing a number of unfamiliar procedures that health care providers tend to take for granted as routine practice. It is important to remember that all women have the right to determine what happens to their bodies. *The client's informed consent should be obtained prior to any procedure that involves touching her body.* Informed consent requires that the woman be given information about the procedure or care, its reasons, potential benefits and risks, and possible alternatives. To give informed consent, whether verbal or signed, the woman should be considered a rational adult, and not under the influence of any medication that may affect her decision-making process. In most instances involving the nurse as the care giver, the informed consent may be verbal. Each nurse needs to be aware of the requirements of the state and the individual hospital (Trandel-Korenchuk 1982). (See Chapter 1 for additional discussion.)

ADMISSION ENVIRONMENT

The manner in which the woman and her partner are greeted by the maternity nurse influences the course of the woman's stay. It should be remembered that the sudden environment change and sometimes impersonal technical aspects of the admission procedures can produce additional sources of stress.

When I realized I was in labor, I cried for fear of hurting, fear of the unknown, fear of the end of my childhood. (Harriette Hartigan, *Women in Birth*)

If a woman is greeted in a brusque, harried manner, her anxiety usually increases, and she is less likely to look to the nurse for support. A calm, pleasant manner promotes calmness in the woman and indicates to her that what she has to say is important. It helps instill in the couple a sense of confidence in the staff's ability to provide quality care during this critical time.

ADMITTING A WOMAN WHO HAD PLANNED AN OUT-OF-HOSPITAL BIRTH

In most instances, out-of-hospital birth is a trouble-free, satisfying experience for the family. However, if a woman suddenly finds it necessary to seek hospital care, she is at risk both physiologically and psychologically. Either she, her fetus, or both are probably in distress if hospitalization is deemed necessary. Moreover, she is also vul-

nerable to disapproval, ridicule, and anger on the part of many hospital personnel. Her control over the birth process, which may have been a major factor in her decision to select out-of-hospital birth, is now almost totally gone. She must deal with her fears and concerns regarding the birth outcome, possible feelings of guilt and responsibility should the outcome be poor, and the unfamiliarity of her surroundings at this critical time. Other women who may find themselves in this position are those who cannot afford prenatal care and plan to enter the birth setting just before delivery (Curry & Howe 1985).

The nurse who has initial contact with the family must be careful to remain nonjudgmental in attitude or remarks. All care and procedures and the rationales for them should be carefully explained. No required procedure should be presented in a punitive way. The nurse can usually provide reassurance to the couple that their choice of birth location did not cause the current problem. Every effort should be made to give them any control and options possible in the new situation.

Initial Nursing Assessments

Following the initial greeting, the woman is taken into the labor or birthing room. Some couples prefer to remain together during the admission process, and others prefer to have the partner wait outside. As the nurse helps the woman undress and get into a hospital gown, or her own personal gown, the nurse can begin conversing with her to develop rapport and establish the nursing data base.

ASSESSMENT OF LABOR STATUS

The nurse immediately assesses the status of the woman's labor to develop nursing diagnoses and priorities of care in the admission process. Information that the nurse must obtain includes:

- Gravidity, parity
- Time of onset of true labor (generally defined as when contractions began to be five minutes apart)
- Frequency and duration of contractions on admission
- Status of membranes
- Presence of bloody show versus bleeding
- EDD
- Any significant prenatal history

  Present coping behaviors with contractions

See Table 23–1 for indicators of normal labor process.

On admission the woman and her support person are intensely focused on the changes occurring in her body, and are eager and relieved to share this information with

Table 23–1 Indicators of Normal Labor Process on Admission

Indicator	Normal characteristics
Uterine contractions	Frequency of not less than 2 minutes
	Duration of less than 75 seconds
	Uterine relaxation between contractions
	Discomfort in uterus occurs only with contractions
Fetal heart rate	Rate 120 to 160 with average variability
	Absence of variable or late decelerations
Maternal vital signs	B/P below 140/90 or less than $+30/+15$ above prepregnancy readings
	Pulse 60 to 100
	Temperature between 97.8 and 99.6F
If membranes ruptured	Fluid clear without odor

the nurse. They frequently share essential information about the status of the woman's labor before the nurse has an opportunity to ask specific questions about it. In many hospital settings the nursing staff has access to the woman's prenatal records and will know her gravidity, parity, EDD, and any significant prenatal history before she arrives on the unit. With the couple's cooperation, the nurse can collect a seemingly overwhelming amount of data very quickly without appearing rushed.

Maybe shock more than fear. All that preparation, but then you have to do it. This is not pretend. (Harriette Hartigan, *Women in Birth*)

ASSESSMENT OF FETAL AND MATERNAL VITAL SIGNS

After the laboring woman has changed into a gown, she is helped into bed for completion of the admission assessment. From the time the woman enters the birth setting, it is critical to remember that two people must be monitored; the laboring woman and the unborn baby. One of the vital signs to assess immediately after the laboring woman is in bed is the fetal heart rate. (Detailed information on monitoring the fetal heart rate is presented in Chapter 22.) If her membranes have ruptured prior to admission, a description of the color of the amniotic fluid is also important in determining the well-being of the fetus. Meconium-stained amniotic fluid is a possible sign of fetal distress when the fetus is in vertex presentation (Table 23-2).

Assessment of the fetus helps determine whether the rest of the admission process can proceed at a more leisurely pace or whether additional interventions have higher priority. For example, FHR of 110 beats per minute on auscultation or meconium-stained amniotic fluid are assessments indicating that a fetal monitor should be applied immediately to obtain additional data. The admission process will continue after these assessments are completed.

Throughout the admission it is important to have the woman indicate when a contraction is beginning; thus, contraction frequency, duration, and intensity are assessed as other data are gathered. The nurse needs to be aware that contractions may decrease in frequency with the trip to the birth unit. The contractions will resume when the woman is comfortable and relaxed again. The status of uterine contractions on admission helps the nurse determine the priorities of care. Contractions that are more than four minutes apart, with a duration of less than 40 seconds, are usually associated with early labor, and the admission process can usually progress in a leisurely manner. If the contractions are three minutes apart or less, with a duration of more than 45 seconds, and there have been previous labors, the admission needs to proceed more quickly.

Additional vital signs to assess are the woman's blood pressure, pulse, respiration, and oral temperature.

ASSESSMENT OF THE COUPLE'S PREPARATION FOR LABOR

Other necessary admission data require assessment of the woman's coping mechanisms, support system, and goals and expectations for her birthing experience. Examples of information collected from these assessments include:

- Attendance at childbirth education classes. If so, what kind (Lamaze, Bradley, etc)

- Name of support person

- Any expectations of her labor and delivery experience that she has discussed with her physician/CNM, such as no prep or enema, siblings in attendance, etc.

Some childbirth education classes and physicians/CNMs offer couples a checklist of options about their birthing experience. Couples who use the checklists are encouraged to share their choices with the nurse on admission (see Figure 18–2).

VAGINAL EXAMINATIONS

If the contraction pattern and behavioral response of the woman have not indicated rapid progress of labor, the vaginal exam can be delayed until this time. (If there are signs of excessive bleeding or if the woman has reported episodes of bleeding in the last trimester, a vaginal exam should not be done.) Before the sterile vaginal examination, the nurse informs the woman about the procedure and its purpose. Afterward the nurse tells the woman about the findings. Sterile vaginal exams should be kept at a minimum to reduce risks of infection whether membranes are ruptured or not.

Indications for vaginal exams during a normal labor are based on increased frequency, duration, and intensity of contractions. These changes in contractions are usually accompanied by some type of behavioral response in the laboring woman. Without these changes in the contraction pattern, it is unlikely that significant progress in cervical dilation and/or fetal descent has occurred.

Nursing Admission Interventions

After the nurse completes the admission assessment, her responsibilities focus on readying the laboring woman for delivery. Nursing actions include collecting a urine specimen, performing a prep and administering an enema if ordered, facilitating laboratory tests, and notifying the physician/nurse-midwife. In many hospitals the nursing admission interventions include requesting the woman to sign a delivery permit, fingerprinting the woman for the infant records, and fastening an identification bracelet to her wrist.

Table 23–2 Deviations from Normal Labor Process Requiring Immediate Intervention

Problem	Immediate action	Problem	Immediate action
Woman admitted with vaginal bleeding or history of painless vaginal bleeding	1. Do not perform vaginal examination. 2. Assess FHR. 3. Evaluate amount of blood loss. 4. Evaluate labor pattern. 5. Notify physician/ CNM immediately.	Prolapse of umbilical cord	1. Relieve pressure on cord manually. 2. Continuously monitor FHR; watch for changes in FHR pattern. 3. Notify physician/ CNM. 4. Assist woman into knee-chest position. 5. Administer oxygen.
Presence of greenish or brownish amniotic fluid	1. Continuously monitor FHR. 2. Evaluate dilatation status of cervix and determine whether umbilical cord is prolapsed. 3. Evaluate presentation (vertex or breech). 4. Maintain woman on complete bed rest on left side. 5. Notify physician/ CNM immediately.	Woman admitted in advanced labor; delivery imminent	1. Prepare for immediate delivery. 2. Obtain critical information: a. EDD b. History of bleeding problems c. Problems with this pregnancy d. FHR and maternal vital signs if possible e. Whether membranes are ruptured and how long since rupture f. Blood type and Rh 3. Direct another person to contact physician/CNM. Do not leave woman alone. 4. Provide support to couple. 5. Wash hands.
Absence of FHR and fetal movement	1. Notify physician/ CNM. 2. Provide truthful information and emotional support to laboring couple. 3. Remain with the couple.		

COLLECTION OF URINE SPECIMEN

After admission data are obtained, a clean voided midstream urine specimen is collected. The woman with intact membranes may walk to the bathroom. If the membranes are ruptured and the presenting part is not engaged, the woman is generally asked to remain in bed to avoid prolapse of the umbilical cord. The advisability of ambulation when membranes are ruptured depends on the woman's desires, physician/CNM requests, and agency policy.

The nurse can test the woman's urine for the presence of protein, ketones, and glucose by using a dipstick. This procedure is especially important if edema or elevated blood pressure is noted on admission. Proteinuria may be a sign of impending preeclampsia if it is 2+ or more, and the urine is not contaminated with blood or amniotic fluid. Ketonuria is a good index of starvation ketosis. Glycosuria is found frequently in pregnant women because of the increased glomerular filtration rate in the proximal tubules and the inability of these tubules to increase reabsorption of glucose. However, it may also be associated with latent diabetes and should not be discounted.

PREP AND ENEMA PROCEDURES

While the woman is collecting the urine specimen, the nurse can prepare the equipment for shaving the pubic area (the shaving is referred to as the *prep*) and for the enema if one is to be given. Prep orders vary, but many physicians/CNMs leave standing orders for prep measures. Complete preps, which involve the removal of all pubic, perineal, and rectal hair, were formerly done. A prep now is usually the removal of perineal hair below the vaginal orifice where an episiotomy or repair of a laceration would be done. The area can be shaved or clipped with a pair of sterile scissors. A miniprep is usually considered the removal of perineal hair from the labia parallel to the upper aspect of the vaginal orifice and downward to the rectum.

The use of preps is controversial. Some physicians/ CNMs believe that this form of skin preparation facilitates their work during the delivery, makes perineal repair easier, and prevents infection (Mahan & McKay 1983). Others believe a prep is unnecessary, since hair is minimal between the vagina and rectum, and that shaving may actually increase the risk of infection. Many women question the need for a prep and request that it be omitted. The nurse needs to ascertain the woman's wishes in this matter. Women who do not want a prep probably have already discussed it with the physician/CNM during the prenatal period. If the woman has not discussed her desire not to have a prep, the nurse acts as the woman's advocate in communicating the woman's wishes to the physician/CNM.

When a prep is to be done, the nurse explains the procedure to the woman. Most women feel embarrassed and vulnerable during this procedure, so the nurse needs to exercise great care to provide privacy and support.

The nurse performing a prep washes hands, dons disposable gloves, and positions the woman as for a vaginal examination. The nurse places a towel under the woman's buttocks and adjusts the lighting so that the perineal area can be well visualized. The woman is questioned about the presence of any moles or warts while the nurse is applying the soap solution with a gauze square or sponge provided in the prep set. The (right-handed) nurse holds the skin taut with the left hand and shaves in short strokes, holding the razor in the right hand and working downward to the vagina. When the perineum has been shaved, the woman is asked to turn to her left side and to assume the lateral Sims' position. The nurse pulls the upper buttock upward to expose the rectal area. After sudsing, the area around the rectum is shaved. The nurse must take care to prevent contaminants from the rectal area from entering the vaginal area.

Administration of an enema is also controversial. Proponents say the purposes of an enema are to (a) evacuate the lower bowel so that labor will not be impeded, (b) stimulate uterine contractions, (c) avoid embarrassment if bowel contents are expelled during pushing efforts, and (d) prevent contamination of the sterile field during delivery. Those who question the routine use of an enema on admission suggest that labor is impeded only by a severe bowel impaction, question whether labor is stimulated, and find that feces may still be expelled during pushing efforts. They also note that the enema is usually uncomfortable.

After determining the woman's wishes regarding an enema, the nurse notifies the physician/CNM. Some factors contraindicate the enema. They are vaginal bleeding, unengaged presenting part, rapid labor progress, and imminent delivery. These factors need to be identified. If an enema is to be given, the reasons and the procedure are explained to the woman. Then the enema is administered while she is on her left side.

If the membranes are intact and labor is not far advanced, the woman may expel the enema in the bathroom. Otherwise she is positioned on a bedpan in the bed. The side rails of the bed should be raised for safety.

Before leaving the labor area, the nurse must be sure that the woman knows how to operate the call system so that she can obtain help if she needs it. After the enema is expelled, the nurse monitors the FHR again to assess any changes. If the woman's partner has been out of the labor room, the couple is reunited as soon as possible.

LABORATORY TESTS

Laboratory tests may also be carried out during admission. Hemoglobin and hematocrit values help determine the oxygen-carrying capacity of the circulatory system and the ability of the woman to withstand blood loss at delivery.

Elevation of the hematocrit indicates hemoconcentration of blood, which occurs with edema, PIH, or dehydration. A low hemoglobin, in the absence of other evidence of bleeding, suggests anemia. Blood may be typed and cross-matched if the woman is in a high-risk category. A serology test for syphilis is obtained if one has not been done in the last three months or if an antepartal serology result was positive.

NOTIFICATION OF THE PHYSICIAN/NURSE MIDWIFE

Depending on how rapidly labor is progressing, the nurse notifies the physician/CNM before or after completing the admission procedures. The report should include the following information: cervical dilatation and effacement, station, presenting part, status of the membranes, contraction pattern, FHR, vital signs that are not in the normal range, gestational age, pregnancy complications, the woman's wishes, and her reaction to labor.

● Care of the Woman and Her Partner During the First Stage of Labor

Nursing care during the first stage of labor is influenced by the physical, psychologic, and cultural data obtained during admission. The primary goals of care are:

● To integrate the couple's cultural beliefs

● To promote maternal and fetal physical well-being

● To promote maternal comfort

Nursing Goal: Integration of Cultural Beliefs Influencing the Childbirth Experience

Knowledge of values, customs, and practices of different cultures is as important during labor as it is in the prenatal period. Without this knowledge, a nurse is less likely to understand a woman's behavior and may impose personal values and beliefs upon a woman. As cultural sensitivity increases, so does the likelihood of providing high-quality care.

MODESTY

In most cultures, modesty during childbirth is important. For example, Oriental, American Indian, and Mexican-American women view pregnancy as "female business" (Chung 1977). Some Oriental women are not accustomed to male physicians and attendants and may prefer female physicians and attendants. Modesty is of great concern to these women, and exposure of as little of the woman's body as possible is strongly recommended (Calhoun 1986). On the other hand, many American women have the desire to remove all clothing during birth if privacy is provided, and this should also be accepted.

PAIN EXPRESSION

The role of culture in determining attitudes toward and reactions to pain was first explored by Zborowski (1952). His study was conducted with four groups: Jewish, Italian, Irish, and "Old Americans." Old Americans were defined as whites whose grandparents were born in the United States. Italian and Jewish cultures tended to be more emotional in their responses to pain than the Irish and Old Americans, who exhibited little emotional complaining, but reported on their pain instead.

Differences in pain expression may also be seen among Orientals, blacks, and Mexican Americans. The laboring Oriental woman may not outwardly express pain for fear of shaming herself and her family (Hollingsworth et al 1980). Oriental women may be anxious about losing face by their behavior. Black women may also appear rather stoic in an effort to avoid showing weakness or calling undue attention to themselves (Kay 1982). Mexican-American women, on the other hand, may be more expressive during labor. One way they may express pain and suffering is through groaning and moaning (Murillo-Rohde 1979). Yet another behavior is for Mexican-American women in labor to keep their mouths closed for fear of making the uterus rise. They cry out only during exhalation (Kay 1978).

Understanding pain behavior helps lead to an accurate assessment of the woman's condition. Nonverbal communication becomes vital. In working with women of another culture, language is often a barrier; if possible, an interpreter should be used. It is also important to be aware of communication differences, so that a nurse does not inadvertently indicate hostility, rejection, or lack of interest to a woman.

In assessing a woman's pain, it is beneficial for the nurse to assess personal views of physical and psychologic distress. One study of nurses in six different cultures found that nurses' beliefs regarding suffering reflected their cultural backgrounds (Davitz et al 1976). For example, it was found that most Americans believe that Orientals feel less pain because their behavior does not appear to reflect pain. On the other hand, a nurse with a cultural background that dictates stoic behavior may have difficulty in understanding a woman who has learned to express pain freely. Awareness of one's own values leads to greater acceptance of another's behavior.

ROLE OF THE FATHER

In some cultures the husband or father attends the birth. In other groups the man is not present. In some

American Indian tribes, a midwife and female relatives traditionally assist the woman giving birth. In the traditional Navajo tribe, all family members view the birth process (Farris 1978). The Hmong father frequently remains with his wife during labor (Morrow 1986), but some Oriental and Vietnamese fathers do not participate in childbirth since it is considered "woman's work." An orthodox Jewish husband may not touch his wife during labor and delivery or postpartum because of her vaginal discharge. Historically, black women provided emotional support to a woman during childbirth. Today many black women prefer to have their mothers present instead of the newborn's father (Carrington 1978).

Who participates in the birth process is an important consideration for nurses. The participation of the father should not be assumed: His participation varies among cultures. A nurse's sensitivity to these different values alleviates stress for the family. Nurses should be aware that fathers often do perform definite functions even though they may not participate in the actual childbirth. In this case they are still viewed as active participants. They may adhere to certain taboos, perform certain rituals, experience couvade, or even simulate labor (Heggenhougen 1980).

CULTURAL BELIEFS: SOME EXAMPLES

A culture often assigns certain superstitions, taboos, and beliefs regarding spirits around significant events such as the delivery of a child. This activity is often a mechanism for dealing with anxiety. For example, in a rural Cambodian home, a laboring woman often lies on a bed with a fire beneath it to drive away evil spirits (Hollingsworth et al 1980). As soon as a baby is born to a Mexican-American woman, she places her legs together to prevent air from entering the womb (Kay 1978).

It is also common to prescribe certain activities for the relief of pain during childbirth. It is not uncommon for Southern white or black families to place a knife, razor, or ax under the bed to "cut the labor pains" (Murphee 1968). During labor, the Laguna Pueblo Indian woman often holds onto a belt that has been blessed (Farris 1978). In other tribes the medicine man may be called to give a special potion to the woman and to offer prayers for her. A badger claw is often given to a laboring Keresian Indian woman, since it is believed that badgers are good at "digging out" (Higgins & Wayland 1981).

In looking at specific practices on position, food, and drink during labor, obvious differences between cultures are apparent. In most non-European societies uninfluenced by Westernization, women assume an upright position in childbirth. For example, Hmong women who have emigrated from Laos to our country, report that squatting during childbirth is common in their culture (LaDu 1985). Some traditional American Indian women give birth in upright positions. For example, the Pueblo woman gives birth

on her knees, the Zuni woman kneels or squats while a midwife kneads her abdomen, and in some tribes teas made of juniper twigs may be given to relax the woman (Higgins & Wayland 1981). In some Southern black and white groups, three different teas are given "to keep the labor coming" and drinking of Coca Cola is encouraged (Murphee 1968). Some of these beliefs may be encountered by maternity nurses today.

Hmong women have special customs regarding childbirth. The beginning of labor signifies the beginning of a transition and entails certain dietary restrictions. The woman may want to be active and may be able to move about during labor. The husband is frequently present and actively involved in providing comfort. During labor the woman usually prefers only "hot" foods and warm water to drink. Traditionally, the woman prefers that the amniotic membranes are not ruptured until just before birth. It is thought that the escape of fluid at this time makes the birth easier. She may choose to kneel or squat for the birth of her baby. As soon as the baby is born, an egg needs to be soft-boiled and given to the mother to eat to restore her energy. During the postpartum period the mother prefers "warm" foods, such as chicken prepared with warm water and warm rice (Morrow 1986).

Vietnamese women also follow prescribed customs during pregnancy and birth (Calhoun 1986). While in labor, the woman usually maintains self-control and may smile throughout the labor. She may prefer to walk about during labor and to deliver in a squatting position. She may avoid drinking cold water and prefer fluids at room temperature. The newborn is protected from praise to prevent jealousy.

In working with women from another culture, an awareness of historical beliefs and practices helps the nurse understand their behavior. In many cases, certain old practices are retained either in part or in full. An awareness of cultural values is also necessary, since specific behavior is often dictated by these traditional views.

Nursing Goal: Promotion of Maternal and Fetal Physical Well-being

LATENT PHASE

After the admission process is completed, the nurse can help the laboring woman and her partner to become comfortable with the surroundings. The nurse can also assess their individual needs and plans for this experience. As long as there are no contraindications (such as vaginal bleeding or ROM with the fetus unengaged), the woman may be encouraged to ambulate (Figure 23–1). Many women feel much more at ease and comfortable if they can move around and do not have to remain in bed. In addition, ambulation may decrease the need for analgesics, shorten labor, and decrease the incidence of FHR abnormalities (Lupe & Gross 1986).

The nurse will need to assess the physical parameters of the woman and her fetus (Table 23–3). Maternal temperature is assessed every four hours unless the temperature is over 37.5C (99.6F), or the membranes are ruptured. In this case the temperature is taken every hour. Blood pressure, pulse, and respirations are assessed every hour. If the woman's blood pressure is over 140/90 or her pulse is more than 100, the physician or nurse-midwife must be notified. The blood pressure and pulse are then reassessed more frequently. Uterine contractions are assessed for frequency, intensity, and duration every 30 minutes. The FHR

is assessed every 30 minutes as long as it remains between 120 and 160 beats per minute with good long-term variability, short-term variability, and no variable or late decelerations.

The FHR should be assessed throughout one contraction and for about 15 seconds after the contraction to assure that there are no decelerations. If the FHR is not in the 120 to 160 range and/or decelerations are heard, continuous electronic monitoring is recommended. In some institutions, the external monitor is routinely attached for at least 15 minutes to assess fetal status. If no problems are noted, it is removed.

The laboring woman may be feeling some discomfort during contractions. The nurse can assist with diversions or by repositioning the woman. The woman may begin to use her breathing method during contractions (see the following discussion of management of pain).

If the laboring woman has not had childbirth education classes, the latent phase is a time when the nurse can do much teaching and anticipatory guidance. Most women are not too uncomfortable with contractions at this time and are responsive to teaching about breathing techniques they can use with contractions as labor progresses. In fact many women in the latent phase seek information about what to expect. The unprepared woman may hesitate to ask questions and thus can benefit even more from anticipatory guidance from the nurse. If the laboring woman's membranes are intact, a tour of the birthing facility can help decrease anxiety and distract her from her discomfort.

The nurse should offer fluids in the form of clear liquids and/or ice chips at frequent intervals. Because gastric-emptying time is prolonged during labor, solid foods are usually avoided.

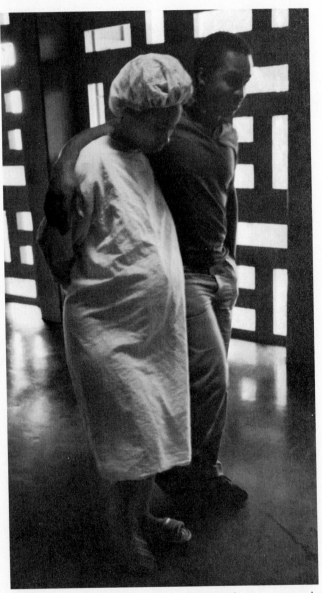

Figure 23–1   If there are no contraindications, the woman in early labor can be encouraged to walk around the birth facility.

ACTIVE PHASE

During this phase, the contractions have a frequency of 3 to 5 minutes, a duration of 30 to 60 seconds, and a moderate intensity. Contractions need to be assessed every 15 to 30 minutes. As the contractions become more frequent and intense, vaginal exams are done to assess cervical dilatation and effacement and fetal station and position. During the active phase, the cervix dilates from 4 to 7 cm, and vaginal discharge and bloody show increase. Maternal blood pressure, pulse, and respirations should be assessed every hour (unless elevated as previously noted). The FHR is assessed every 15 minutes.

During this phase, the laboring woman begins to withdraw from social interaction and focuses more on coping with her contractions; however, she does not want to be left alone. As she progresses into this phase, support in her breathing pattern with contractions becomes important (See Procedure 23–1).

Table 23–3 Nursing Assessments in the First Stage

Phase	Mother	Fetus
Latent	Blood pressure, pulse, respirations q 1 hr if in normal range Temperature q 4 hr unless over 37.5C (99.6F) or membranes ruptured, then q 1 hr Uterine contraction q 30 minutes	FHR q 30 min if normal characteristics present (average variability, baseline in the 120–160 BPM range, without late or variable decelerations). Note fetal activity. If electronic fetal monitor in place assess for reactive NST.
Active	Blood pressure, pulse, respirations q 1 hr if in normal range Uterine contractions q 30 min	FHR q 15 min if normal characteristics are present.
Transition	Blood pressure, pulse, respiration q 30 min	FHR q 15 minutes if normal characteristics are present.

A woman who has been ambulatory up to this point may now wish to sit in a chair or on a bed. If the woman wants to lie on the bed, she is encouraged to assume a side-lying position. The quality of contractions is often better in this position. A supine position should be avoided for another, more important reason: When the woman is supine, the weight of the uterus and fetus lie on the vena cava and obstruct venous return from the extremities. Reduction of blood volume results in fetal distress, which may initially be assessed only by observation of late decelerations on a fetal monitor strip. Severe fetal distress, which can be assessed by intermittent auscultation and the fetal monitor, may be accompanied by symptoms of shock in the mother. These symptoms can occur suddenly and include a drop in blood pressure, increased pulse, air hunger, pallor, and moist clammy skin. Turning the woman to a left lateral position and starting oxygen by face mask can relieve maternal and fetal symptoms rapidly.

It is important, therefore, for the nurse to assist the woman into a position of safety and comfort. When a lateral position is assumed, pillows can be placed between the woman's legs to support the joints. Pillows behind her back help support her body and remind her to remain in the lateral position. To increase comfort, the nurse can encourage the support person to give back rubs or effleurage or place a cool cloth on the woman's forehead or across her neck. If the laboring woman is alone, the nurse implements these comfort measures.

Because vaginal discharge increases, the nurse needs to change the absorbent pads (Chux) frequently. Washing the perineum with warm soap and water removes secretions and increases comfort.

Pharmacologic support may be administered at this time if the woman has a well-established contraction pattern and delivery is not expected within the next hour or two. If an analgesic is given, the woman must remain in bed to promote her safety. If no one can be at the bedside with her, the side rails should be up.

For the woman experiencing slow progress of labor, an intravenous electrolyte solution may be started to provide energy and prevent dehydration. If this occurs, it becomes even more important to encourage voiding every one or two hours to prevent bladder distention.

If the amniotic membranes have not ruptured previously, they may during this phase. When the membranes rupture, the nurse notes the color, amount, and odor of the amniotic fluid and the time of rupture and immediately auscultates the FHR. The fluid should be clear with no odor. Although the amount varies, the perineum usually remains damp with an almost constant spotting of fluid on the absorbent pad.

Fetal stress leads to intestinal and anal sphincter relaxation, and meconium may be released into the amniotic fluid. Meconium turns the fluid greenish-brown. Whenever the nurse notes meconium-stained fluid, an electronic monitor is applied to assess the FHR continuously.

The time of rupture is noted. Some clinicians suggest that delivery should occur within 24 hours of ROM. Others suggest that emphasis should be placed on assessment for signs of infection and that all invasive procedures (for example sterile vaginal exams) be kept to a minimum. An additional concern is prolapse of the umbilical cord, which may occur when membranes rupture before the fetus is engaged. The concern is that the amniotic fluid coming through the cervix will propel the umbilical cord downward into the pelvic cavity ahead of the presenting part. As the fetus descends, increased pressure against the umbilical cord would occur, cutting off the oxygen supply to the fetus. In the more extreme situation, the umbilical cord could prolapse through the cervix with the rupture of membranes. The FHR is auscultated immediately because a drop in the rate might indicate an undetected prolapsed

Procedure 23–1   Nursing Support of Breathing Techniques

Determine which breathing method the woman (couple) has learned.
Provide encouragement as needed in maintaining breathing pattern.
Provide support to the labor coach and assist as needed.

Lamaze breathing pattern cues

FIRST-LEVEL BREATHING

Pattern begins and ends with a cleansing breath (in through the nose and out through pursed lips as if cooling a spoonful of hot food). While inhaling through the nose and exhaling through pursed lips, slow breaths are taken moving only the chest. The rate should be approximately 6–9/minute or 2 breaths/15 seconds. The coach or nurse may assist by reminding the woman to take a cleansing breath and then the breaths could be counted out if needed to maintain pacing. The woman inhales as someone counts "one one thousand, two one thousand, three one thousand, four one thousand." Exhalation begins and continues through the same count.

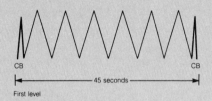

First-level breathing pattern for use during uterine contractions. The pattern begins and ends with a cleansing breath (CB).

SECOND-LEVEL BREATHING

Pattern begins and ends with a cleansing breath. Breaths are then taken in and out silently through the mouth at approximately 4 breaths/5 seconds. The jaw and entire body needs to be relaxed. The rate can be accelerated to 2–2½ breaths/second. The rhythm for the breaths can be counted out as "one and two and one and two and . . ." with the woman exhaling on the numbers and inhaling on *and*.

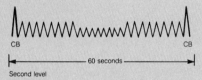

Second-level breathing pattern.

THIRD-LEVEL BREATHING

Pattern begins and ends with a cleansing breath. All breaths are rhythmical, in and out through the mouth. Exhalations are accompanied by a "Hee" or "Hoo" sound in a varying pattern, which begins as 3:1 (Hee Hee Hee Hoo) and can change to 2:1 (Hee Hee Hoo) or 1:1 (Hee Hoo) as the intensity of the contraction changes. The rate should not be more rapid than 2–2½/second. The rhythm of the breaths would match a "one and two and . . ." count.

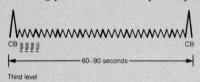

Third-level breathing pattern. Darkened "spike" represents Hoo.

Abdominal breathing pattern cues

The abdomen moves outward during inhalation and downward during exhalation. The rate remains slow with approximately 6–9 breaths/minute.

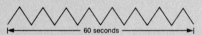

Breathing sequence for abdominal breathing.

Quick method

When the woman has not learned a particular method and is in active phase of labor, the nurse may teach her a combination of two patterns. Abdominal breathing may be used until labor is more advanced. Then a more rapid pattern can be used consisting of two short blows from the mouth followed by a longer blow. (This pattern is called "pant pant blow" even though all exhalations are a blowing motion.)

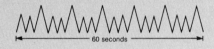

Pant-pant-blow breathing pattern.

---

cord. Immediate intervention is necessary to remove pressure on a prolapsed umbilical cord (see Chapter 19). See Table 22–2 for additional deviations from normal.

TRANSITION

During transition, the contraction frequency is every 2 to 3 minutes, duration is 45 to 90 seconds, and intensity is strong. Cervical dilatation increases from 8 to 10 cm, effacement is complete (100 percent), and there is usually

a heavy amount of bloody show. Contractions are assessed at least every 15 minutes. Sterile vaginal examinations are done more frequently because this stage of labor usually is accompanied by rapid change. Maternal blood pressure, pulse, and respirations are assessed at least every 30 minutes, and FHR is assessed every 15 minutes.

A common sign that a woman has entered transition is a decrease in coping mechanisms. A woman who has coped well with her labor through the active phase may now have difficulty in breathing effectively with contractions and may fear loss of control. This change is obviously a response to the change in contraction patterns. Even if she has not received an analgesic, the laboring woman in the transition phase often appears to doze between contractions. The woman who received an analgesic in the active phase will get better rest between contractions. The nurse can awaken the woman in either situation just before another contraction begins so she can begin her breathing pattern. Breathing the correct way with the woman during each contraction helps to guide her in maintaining effective coping mechanisms.

Comfort measures become very important in this phase of labor, but continual assessment is required to intervene appropriately. The woman may rapidly change from wanting a back rub and other "hands-on" care to wanting no one to touch her at all. The support person and the nurse need to follow her cues and change interventions as needed. Because the woman is breathing more rapidly, the nurse can increase her comfort by offering small spoons of ice chips to moisten her mouth or applying water-based jelly to dry lips.

Nausea and vomiting may appear suddenly. A readily available emesis basin decreases some anxiety for the laboring couple. A cool washcloth placed across the throat and a few slow deep breaths may decrease the feeling of nausea. If the woman vomits, comfort may be increased by cleansing her face with a cool cloth and swishing cool water in her mouth.

Diaphoresis increases, especially above the upper lip and on the forehead. Some women may even throw off their covers at this time. Leg tremors and hiccups are not uncommon in this phase.

As the fetal presenting part moves down the birth canal and complete dilatation approaches, the woman begins to feel increased rectal pressure. The woman indicates this by verbalizing the need to have a bowel movement or the urge to push, or by actually pushing by holding her breath with a contraction. A vaginal exam is done when any of these signs occur to determine if complete dilatation has been reached and effective pushing can begin. The nurse must discourage the woman from pushing until the cervix is completely dilated. Pushing during the first stage of labor does not facilitate progress of labor and is extremely tiring. It can actually prolong the first stage if cervical edema occurs. Excessive pressure from pushing before complete dilatation also increases the risk of cervical lacerations and fetal head trauma. To prevent pushing, the laboring woman must be encouraged to do rapid, shallow breathing (or panting) at the peak of the contraction when the urge to push is the greatest.

Nursing Goal: Promotion of Comfort

A labor and delivery nurse is in the unique position of assisting during one of the most profound experiences of human existence. This nurse has the privilege of sharing in each couple's personal miracle. But it is sometimes difficult for the nurse, who may be admitting a seventh woman toward the end of a busy shift, to share her enthusiasm and excitement. Nurses who care for women in labor face a challenge. They must integrate sophisticated technical skills with sensitivity and an awareness of the influence of the nurse's attitude and behavior on the laboring woman's perceptions. A warm and supportive nurse helps set the stage for a satisfying childbirth experience.

BEHAVIORAL RESPONSES TO LABOR

The woman's response to labor changes with each phase as labor progresses. This does not mean that each woman in labor responds in the same way. It does mean that regardless of a woman's coping mechanisms, her response to labor changes as contractions increase in frequency, duration, and intensity. In some women, the progress from the latent to the active phase may be more subtle than it is for others. Progress from the active phase to transition is usually more obvious. Awareness and sensitivity to even subtle changes are significant in assessing the progress of a normal labor. Identification of behavioral changes can reduce considerably the need for excessive vaginal examinations. Behavioral changes also signal the need for increased monitoring of indicators of maternal and fetal well-being, such as contraction patterns, FHR, and maternal blood pressure.

Although every woman's behavior changes as labor progresses, individual responses vary considerably due to many factors. In addition to uterine contractions, these factors include previous childbearing experiences, previous orientation to coping with pain, support systems, acceptance of pregnancy, childbirth education classes, physical variables, culture, the response of nurses and other members of the health team, level of wellness, and developmental level if the woman is an adolescent. Most of these factors cannot be changed by the nurse once the woman is admitted in labor. It is important, however, that the nurse recognize the significant influence of these factors and work with the woman to enhance her ability to cope with labor.

There are eight types of behavioral responses to pain (McCaffery 1979):

1. Physiologic manifestations

2. Body movement

3. Facial expression

4. Verbal statements

5. Vocal behavior

6. Physical contact

7. Response to environment

8. Patterns of handling pain

Many of these behaviors occur simultaneously. The most frequent physiologic manifestations are increased pulse and respiratory rates, dilated pupils, and increased blood pressure and muscle tension. In labor these reactions are transitory because the pain is intermittent. Increased muscle tension is most significant because it may impede the progress of labor. Women in labor frequently tighten skeletal muscles voluntarily during a contraction and remain motionless. Grimacing is also common. Verbal statements relating to pain and requests for intervention usually mean that the woman has reached her tolerance level. Vocalization may take many forms during the first stage of labor. A grunting sound typically accompanies the bearing-down effort during the second stage of labor.

Some women desire body contact during a contraction and may reach out to grasp the supporting person. As the intensity of the contraction increases with the progress of labor, the woman is less aware of the environment and may have difficulty hearing verbal instructions. The pattern of coping with labor contractions varies from the use of highly structured breathing techniques to loud vocalizations. Irritability and refusal of touch are common responses to the discomfort in the transition phase of the first stage of labor. The tense and frightened woman is more likely to lose control during any stage of labor.

COMFORT MEASURES

A decrease in the intensity of discomfort is one of the goals of nursing support during labor. Nursing measures used to decrease pain include:

- Ensuring general comfort

- Decreasing anxiety

- Providing information

- Using specific supportive relaxation techniques

- Incorporating the support person effectively

- Administering pharmacologic agents as ordered by the physician

○ *GENERAL COMFORT* General comfort measures are of utmost importance throughout labor. By relieving minor discomforts the nurse helps the woman use her coping mechanisms to deal with pain.

The woman should be encouraged to assume any position that she finds the most comfortable (Figure 23–2). A side-lying position on the left side is generally the most advantageous for the laboring woman, although frequent position changes seem to achieve more efficent contractions (Roberts et al 1983). Care should be taken that all the body parts are supported, with the joints slightly flexed. If the woman is more comfortable on her back, the head of the bed should be elevated to relieve the pressure of the uterus on the vena cava. Back rubs and frequent change of position contribute to comfort and relaxation.

Diaphoresis and the constant leaking of amniotic fluid can dampen the woman's gown and bed linen. Fresh, smooth, dry bed linen promotes comfort. To avoid having to change the bottom sheet following rupture of the membranes, the nurse may replace absorbent pads at frequent intervals. The perineal area should be kept as clean and dry as possible to promote comfort as well as to prevent infection. A full bladder adds to the discomfort during a contraction and may prolong labor by interfering with the descent of the fetus. The bladder should be kept as empty as possible by voiding every one to two hours. Even though the woman is voiding, urine may be retained because of the pressure of the fetal presenting part. A full bladder can be detected by palpation directly over the symphysis pubis. Some of the regional procedures for analgesia during labor contribute to the inability to void, and catheterization may be necessary.

The woman may experience dryness of the oral mucous membranes. Popsicles, ice chips, or a wet 4-by-4 sponge may relieve the discomfort. Some prepared childbirth programs advise the woman to bring suckers to help combat the dryness that occurs with some of the breathing patterns.

○ *HANDLING ANXIETY* The anxiety experienced by women entering labor is related to a combination of factors inherent to the process. A moderate amount of anxiety about the pain enhances the woman's ability to deal with the pain. An excessive degree of anxiety decreases her ability to cope with the pain and leads to increased tension, which causes increased pain and anxiety.

Anxiety not directly related to pain can be decreased in a number of ways. Anxiety is decreased as the nurse shares information, which eases fear of the unknown, and establishes rapport with the couple, which helps them preserve their personal integrity. In addition to being a good listener, the nurse must demonstrate genuine concern for the laboring woman. Remaining with the woman as much as possible conveys a caring attitude and dispels fears of abandonment. Praise for correct breathing, relaxation efforts, and pushing efforts not only encourages repetition of the behavior but also decreases anxiety about the ability to cope with labor (Stephany 1983).

A nurse's attitude of confidence in the woman's ability to handle the labor is very important. Even a frightened laboring woman seems to sense the nurse's confidence in her, and it gives her strength and courage to carry on.

○ *CLIENT TEACHING* Providing information about the nature of the discomfort that will occur during labor is

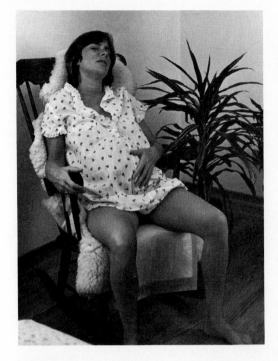

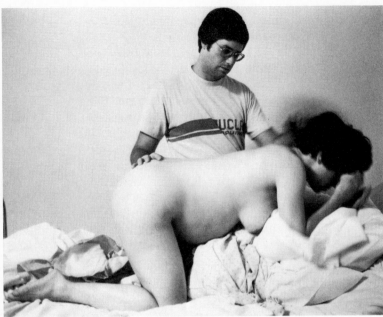

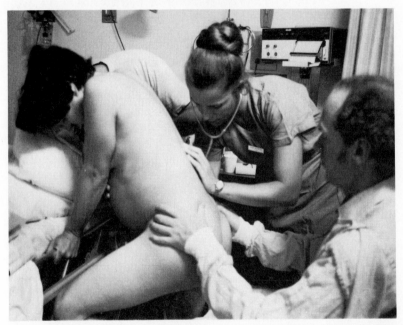

Figure 23–2 The laboring woman is encouraged to choose a position of comfort. The nurse modifies assessments and interventions as necessary.

important. Stressing the intermittent nature and maximum duration of the contractions can be most helpful. The woman can cope with pain better when she knows that a period of relief will follow. Describing the type of discomfort and specific sensations that will occur as labor progresses helps the woman recognize these sensations as normal and expected when she does experience them.

During the second stage, the woman may interpret rectal pressure as a need to move her bowels. The instinctive response is to tighten muscles rather than bear down

(push). A sensation of splitting apart also occurs in the latter part of the second stage, and the woman may be afraid to bear down. The woman who expects these sensations and understands that bearing down contributes to progress at this stage is more likely to do so.

Descriptions of sensations should be accompanied with information on specific comfort measures (Simkin 1982). Some women experience the urge to push during transition when the cervix is not fully dilated and effaced. This sensation can be controlled by panting, and instructions should be given prior to the time that panting is required.

A thorough explanation of surroundings, procedures, and equipment being used also decreases anxiety, thereby reducing pain (Frink & Chally 1984). Attachment to an electronic monitor can produce fear, because equipment of this type is associated with critically ill patients. The beeps, clicks, and other strange noises should be explained, and a simplified explanation of the monitor strip should be given. The nurse can emphasize that the use of the monitor provides a more accurate way to assess the well-being of the fetus during the course of labor. In addition, the nurse can show the woman and her coach how the monitor can help them use controlled breathing techniques to relieve pain. The monitor may indicate the beginning of a contraction just seconds before the woman feels it. The woman and coach can learn how to read the tracing to identify the beginning of the contraction. The disadvantages and possible risks also need to be discussed. The woman tends to lie more quietly to avoid disturbing the belts and transducers, and long-term fetal effects have been questioned.

○   ***SUPPORTIVE RELAXATION TECHNIQUES***   Tense muscles increase resistance to the descent of the fetus and contribute to maternal fatigue. This fatigue increases pain perception and decreases the woman's ability to cope with the pain. Comfort measures, massage, techniques for decreasing anxiety, and client teaching can contribute to relaxation. Other factors are adequate sleep and rest. The laboring woman needs to be encouraged to use the periods between contractions for rest and relaxation (Figure 23–3). A prolonged prodromal phase of labor may have prohibited sleeping. An aura of excitement naturally accompanies the onset of labor, making it difficult for the woman to sleep although the contractions are mild and infrequent.

Distraction is another method of increasing relaxation and coping with discomfort. During early labor, conversation or activities, such as light reading, cards, or other games, serve as distractions. Ambulation is an effective distraction and also helps stimulate labor. One technique that is effective for relieving moderate pain is to have the woman concentrate on a pleasant experience she has had in the past. This helps enhance relaxation between contractions and provides a focus point as she breathes with each contraction. As labor progresses the breathing pattern with contractions may be the main source of distraction. Another form of distraction is called visualization. With this technique the woman visualizes her body or her perineum relaxing (Morton 1983). It is probably most bene-

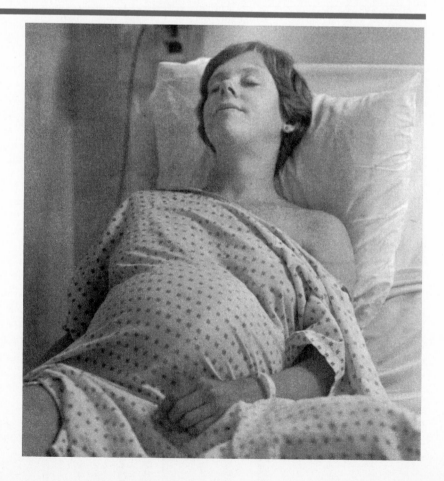

Figure 23–3   It is important for the laboring woman to conserve her energy and to reduce fatigue by relaxing between contractions.

ficial to begin practicing this technique early in pregnancy. However, even the woman in early labor can be taught this technique fairly quickly (see Box 23–1).

Touch is another type of distraction. Although some women regard touching as an invasion of privacy or threat to their independence, others want to touch and be touched during a painful experience.

The support person who has attended childbirth education classes is aware of various types of touch during labor, such as sacral pressure, a backrub, a light stroking of the arms, or hand holding. Those who have not attended can be taught about the importance of touch and shown what can be helpful. Most couples spontaneously use touch as part of their ongoing relationship. If the support person is not involved, and it appears that he wants to be, it is important for the nurse to encourage involvement. The nurse can model behaviors such as reaching out to touch the woman's hand or placing her hand at the woman's side within reach. The nurse can suggest the support person "take over" and perhaps sit beside the bed with one hand on the bed within reach. The woman who needs touch will reach out for contact. At other times the nurse can demonstrate how to do a back rub or provide sacral pressure.

Box 23–1 Simple Visualization Method

Direct a visualization by saying something like the following: "Think about a place you have been that has pleasant memories and feelings around it. A place that was relaxing, where all your stress disappeared. As you think about this place, take in a breath and remember the smells around it. If it was outside, feel the warmth of the sun or the way the breeze felt on your face. In your mind, sit in that place again. Let all your tension and tiredness leave your body as you feel the warmth and breezes."

Give the woman a few moments to think about her special place. Ask if she would like to share information about the setting. If the woman chooses to do this add the information to help her with the visualization (for example, "think about the mountain cabin and the warmth of the sun on your face as you sit in the rocking chair on the front porch," etc).

After the woman has a visualization set up, suggest thinking about it during contractions as a means of increasing relaxation and focusing concentration. You could say: "As each contraction begins, think about this special place for a moment and let your body relax. Keep a picture of your place in your mind as you breathe with the contraction. When the contraction is over, let your body stay relaxed. Feel the comfort of this room and support of those around you."

If no support person is present, the nurse provides this important comfort measure.

Effleurage, a light abdominal stroking, may be used at this time to maintain abdominal muscle relaxation. The technique is believed to work by providing stimulation to large-diameter fibers, which inhibits pain impulses carried by small-diameter fibers. Effleurage is effective for mild-to-moderate pain but is not very effective for intense pain (see Figure 18–4).

A shower or whirlpool bath may also be used as a comfort measure. The laboring woman may sit on a stool or chair in the shower with warm water directed onto her abdomen. In some birthing units the woman can sit in a whirlpool bath for prolonged periods, or she can recline in a bathtub of warm water. The nurse can continue her assessments but needs to be alert for the rupture of membranes, which may be more difficult to detect while the woman is in water.

Back pain associated with labor may be relieved by firm pressure on the lower back or sacral area. The nurse can show the support person how to place the palm of the hand in the small of the woman's back and provide slow and firm massage. Since much force is usually needed for sacral pressure to be effective, the nurse can offer to relieve the support person for short periods.

In addition to the measures just described, the nurse can enhance the woman's relaxation by providing encouragement and support for her controlled breathing techniques. The support person who has attended childbirth education classes with the woman is usually the most effective in helping the woman with her chosen breathing technique.

○   *CONTROLLED BREATHING*   Controlled breathing is helpful to the laboring woman. Used correctly, it increases the woman's pain threshold, permits relaxation, enhances the woman's ability to cope with the uterine contractions, and allows the uterus to function more efficiently.

Women usually learn Lamaze breathing in prenatal classes and practice it a number of weeks before delivery. If the woman has not learned Lamaze or another controlled breathing technique, teaching her may be difficult when she is admitted in active labor. In this instance, the nurse can teach slow, deep abdominal and pant-pant-blow breathing. In abdominal breathing, the woman moves the abdominal wall upward as she inhales and downward as she exhales. This method tends to lift the abdominal wall off the contracting uterus and thus may provide some pain relief. The breathing is deep and rhythmical. As transition approaches, the woman may feel the need to breathe more rapidly (see Procedure 23–1).

As the woman uses her breathing technique, the nurse can assess and support the interaction between the woman and her coach or support person. In the absence of a coach, the nurse assists the laboring woman by helping to identify the beginning of each contraction and encouraging her as she breathes through each contraction. Continued encouragement and support with each contraction throughout labor have immeasurable benefits (see Figure 23–4).

Hyperventilation is related to uneven breathing patterns, which occur most often with uncontrolled breathing during a contraction. Hyperventilation may also occur when a woman breathes very rapidly over a prolonged period of time. Hyperventilation is the result of an imbalance of oxygen and carbon dioxide (that is, too much carbon dioxide is exhaled, and too much oxygen remains in the body). The signs and symptoms of hyperventilation are tingling or numbness in the tip of the nose or the lips, fingers, or toes; dizziness; spots before the eyes; or spasms of the hands or feet (carpal-pedal spasms). If hyperventilation occurs, the woman should be encouraged to slow her breathing rate and to take shallow breaths. With instruction and encouragement, many women are able to change their breathing to correct the problem. Encouraging the woman to relax and counting out loud for her so she can pace her breathing during contractions are also helpful. If the signs and symptoms continue or become more severe (that is, if they progress from numbness to spasms), the woman can breath into a paper surgical mask, her hands cupped in front of her face, or a paper bag until symptoms abate. Breathing into a mask or bag causes rebreathing of carbon dioxide. The nurse should remain with the woman to reassure her.

In some instances, analgesics and/or regional anesthetic blocks may be used to enhance comfort and relaxation during labor. See Chapter 24 for a discussion of analgesia and anesthesia. Table 23–4 summarizes labor progress, possible responses of the laboring woman, and support measures.

● Care of the Family During the Second Stage of Labor

The second stage of labor begins when the cervix is completely dilated and is completed when the baby is delivered. During this stage, the primary nursing goals are:

- To assist the woman during pushing
- To prepare the couple and environment for delivery
- To assist the couple and clinician during delivery

Nursing Goal: Assisting the Woman in Her Pushing Efforts

During the second stage of labor, the cervix is completely dilated (10 cm). The uterine contractions continue as in the transition phase. Frequent sterile vaginal examinations are done to assess progress. Maternal pulse, blood pressure, and FHR are assessed every 5 to 15 minutes; some protocols recommend assessment after each contraction (Table 23–5). The woman usually feels an uncontrollable urge to push (bear down). The nurse can help by

Figure 23–4   The woman's partner provides support and encouragement during labor.

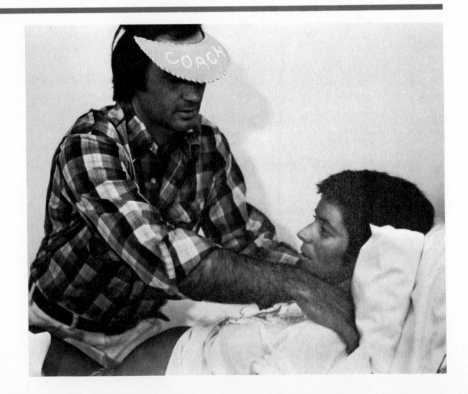

encouraging her and by assisting with positioning (see Figure 23–5). The woman can be propped up with pillows to a semireclining position.

I knew when I was completely dilated. I knew when to push and I did it without tearing. My body told me to listen. I knew what to do. (Harriette Hartigan, Women in Birth)

The nurse assists the woman in her pushing technique when the woman is ready. Exhale breathing is currently being advocated because it is effective yet avoids the adverse physiologic effects of the Valsalva maneuver. In exhale breathing the woman takes several deep breaths and then holds her breath for 5 to 6 seconds. Then, through slightly pursed lips, she exhales slowly every 5 to 6 seconds while continuing to hold her breath. The woman takes another breath and continues exhale breathing and pushing during the contraction (McKay 1981). She may also exhale in a continuous manner while pushing. In some facilities, the older Valsalva maneuver technique is used. Either technique seems to have the same effect on duration of the second stage (Knauth & Haloburdo 1986).

The woman is encouraged to rest between contractions. Although the laboring woman may appear exhausted at this time, most experience relief at being able to push with contractions. Perspiration increases with the pushing efforts, and a cool washcloth for forehead and face is most soothing.

When I began pushing, I felt in control because I could do something . . . I could push the baby out. I knew he was ready to be born. (Harriette Hartigan, Women in Birth)

Maternal positions such as standing, squatting while leaning back on a partner, lateral or Sims' position, and hands and knees may increase comfort and effectiveness of pushing. Some women feel that sitting on a toilet seat is a comfortable position that assists their pushing efforts. This position usually causes anxiety in the care givers, however, for fear that delivery may occur quickly in this most inopportune place.

Additional comfort measures may be used during this stage. Hot perineal, abdominal, and back compresses may be used to increase muscle relaxation. Perineal massage and stretching with a lubricant (Lubafax) may relieve the tearing and burning sensation as the perineal tissue distends. (At this time, perineal stretching is done by the CNM and not other nursing staff.)

Visualization techniques may be helpful. The woman can be encouraged to envision the infant descending the birth canal. Phrases such as "Open to your baby" and "Let the baby come; don't try to hold back" can be useful and calming (Sinquefield 1985, p 112).

I thought that the nurse . . . was really fantastic and was extremely helpful, and I always thought that I pushed better

when she was going through her whole thing of "take a breath in and breath out, and push, push, push!" . . . I felt like I was being trained for a track match or something . . . having that kind of support was really good. (RP Lederman, Psychosocial Adaptation in Pregnancy)

Nurses frequently have learned one way for assisting the woman during pushing efforts and may hesitate to encourage unique positions. It is important to support the woman's needs and to encourage a change in position if anticipated progress is not made.

Nursing Goal: Preparation for Delivery

A woman in labor for the first time (nullipara) is usually prepared for delivery when perineal bulging is noted. A multipara usually progresses much more quickly, so she may be prepared for delivery when the cervix is dilated 7 to 8 cm.

Research Note

The development and expansion of family-centered maternity services has made sibling-attended births increasingly common. While many studies have been done on the effect of the birth on the sibling, few, if any, previous studies have focused on the effect of sibling-attended birth on the mother and father.

Krutsky looked at why parents decide to have the children present and evaluated the effect of their presence on the parents. The study used an open-ended interview format for 16 couples with a total of 30 children ranging from 2 to 18 years old. All of the women had normal births in the birthing room of a small community hospital.

The parents in this study decided to have their children present at the birth because they thought the experience would be of benefit to the children's development and the shared experience would be of value to the family. In reviewing the experience, almost all the parents believed that their children's presence added to the feeling of family unity and as part of the positive experience of birth. All the parents said that they would include siblings at the next birth.

Nurses need to be informed about the various aspects of sibling-attended birth so that they can provide accurate information to interested parents during the prenatal period and can dispel myths about this emerging practice.

Krutsky CD: Siblings at birth: Impact on parents. *J Nurs Midwife* 1985;30(September/October):269.

Table 23–4 Normal Progress, Psychologic Characteristics, and Nursing Support During First and Second Stages of Labor

Phase	Cervical dilatation	Uterine contractions	Woman's response	Support measures
STAGE 1				
Latent phase (Friedman: latent phase)	1–4 cm	Every 15–30 min, 15–30 sec duration Mild intensity	Usually happy, talkative, and eager to be in labor Exhibits need for independence by taking care of own bodily needs and seeking information	Establish rapport on admission and continue to build during care. Assess information base and learning needs. Be available to consult regarding breathing technique if needed; teach breathing technique if needed and in early labor. Orient family to room, equipment, monitors, and procedures. Encourage woman and partner to participate in care as desired. Provide needed information. Assist woman into position of comfort; encourage frequent change of position; and encourage ambulation during early labor. Offer fluids/ice chips. Keep couple informed of progress. Encourage woman to void every one to two hours. Assess need for and interest in using visualization to enhance relaxation and teach if appropriate.
Active phase (Friedman: active phase-acceleration phase & phase of maximum slope)	4–7 cm	Every 3–5 min, 30–60 sec duration Moderate intensity	May experience feelings of helplessness; exhibits increased fatigue and may begin to feel restless and anxious as contractions become stronger; expresses fear of abandonment Becomes more dependent as she is less able to meet her needs	Encourage woman to maintain breathing patterns; provide quiet environment to reduce external stimuli. Provide reassurance, encouragement, support; keep couple informed of progress. Promote comfort by giving backrubs, sacral pressure, cool cloth on forehead, assistance with position changes, support with pillows, effleurage. Provide ice chips, ointment for dry mouth and lips. Encourage to void every one to two hours.
Transition (Friedman: active phase-deceleration phase)	8–10 cm	Every 2–3 min, 45–90 sec duration Strong intensity	Tires and may exhibit increased restlessness and irritability; may feel she cannot keep up with labor process and is out of control Physical discomforts Fear of being left alone May fear tearing open or splitting apart with contractions	Encourage woman to rest between contractions; if she sleeps between contractions, wake her at beginning of contraction so she can begin breathing pattern (increases feeling of control). Provide support, encouragement, and praise for efforts. Keep couple informed of progress; encourage continued participation of support persons. Promote comfort as listed above but recognize many women do not want to be touched when in transition. Provide privacy. Provide ice chips, ointment for lips. Encourage to void every one to two hours.

Table 23–4 Normal Progress, Psychologic Characteristics, and Nursing Support During First and Second Stages of Labor (cont)

Phase	Cervical dilatation	Uterine contractions	Woman's response	Support measures
STAGE 2	Complete		May feel out of control, helpless, panicky	Assist woman in pushing efforts. Encourage woman to assume position of comfort. Provide encouragement and praise for efforts. Keep couple informed of progress. Provide ice chips. Maintain privacy as woman desires.

PREPARATIONS IN THE BIRTHING ROOM

Couples often choose the birthing room for labor and delivery because of the more relaxed atmosphere maintained there. Not having to transfer a woman from the room where she has labored to a different room for delivery contributes tremendously to a relaxed atmosphere for both the woman and the nursing staff. It also avoids an uncomfortable transfer from one bed to another just before delivery. The needed equipment and supplies are brought to the birthing room when the birth is imminent (see Box 23–2).

Birthing rooms usually have birthing beds that can be adapted for delivery by removing a small section near the foot. Stirrups are available if needed or desired. In settings where birth is managed by nurse-midwives, an ordinary double bed is often found, which prevents the use of stirrups.

There are many other factors that facilitate the relaxed, nonmedical atmosphere in the birthing room. Other family members may be in attendance in addition to the support person. They are not usually required to change into scrub attire. Good handwashing technique is required of all staff, but they often do not wear caps and masks. Sterile gloves for the birth attendant and sterile equipment are still common, but the birth attendant does not usually put on a sterile gown, and the use of sterile drapes is kept to a minimum. Even medical interventions for a normal birth seem minimized in a birthing room in contrast to the delivery room setting.

PREPARATIONS IN THE DELIVERY ROOM

When it is time for the laboring woman to be moved to the delivery room, safety in transfer is a priority. Siderails must be used.

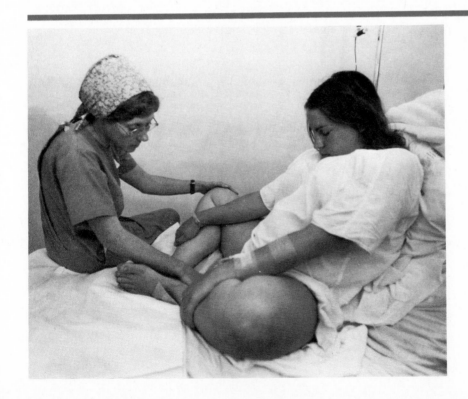

Figure 23–5 Nurse provides support during pushing efforts.

Table 23–5 Nursing Assessments in the Second Stage

Mother	Fetus
Blood pressure, pulse, respirations q 5–15 min. Just before delivery BP between each contraction. Uterine contraction palpated continuously.	FHR after each contraction.

Another priority is to provide privacy and preserve modesty for the laboring woman as she is pushed from her room to the delivery room. The woman is usually involved in her pushing efforts and may throw the covers off. Although she may be unaware of others at this time, after delivery she may be embarrassed that others were able to see her.

After being wheeled into the delivery room, the labor bed or transfer cart must be carefully supported against the birthing bed. This ensures the woman's safety during the transfer.

It is important that the woman move from one bed to another between contractions. If birth seems imminent, it is safer for the woman to deliver in her labor bed. Transfer to the delivery bed is then delayed until after the baby has been delivered and the cord has been clamped and cut.

During transfer and preparation of the woman for delivery, the woman's partner or support person is also preparing for delivery. In most facilities, the support person is required to don scrub suit, disposable boots, and perhaps cap and mask before entering the delivery room.

Since delivery is usually conducted under strict sterile precautions, all those who enter the delivery room wear scrub apparel and wash their hands. Caps and masks may be optional.

Nursing Goal: Assisting the Couple and Physician/Nurse-Midwife During Delivery

MATERNAL BIRTHING POSITIONS

The woman is usually positioned for delivery on a bed, birthing chair, or delivery table. The position that the woman assumes is determined not only by her individual wishes but also by the physician/nurse-midwife.

Stirrups, if used, are padded to alleviate pressure, and both legs should be lifted simultaneously to avoid strain on abdominal, back, and perineal muscles. The stirrups should be adjusted to fit the woman's legs. The feet are supported in the stirrup holders. The height and angle of the stirrups are adjusted so there is no pressure on the back of the knees or the calf, which might cause discomfort and postpartal vascular problems. The delivery table or bed

is elevated 30° to 60° to help the woman bear down, and handles are provided so she may pull back on them.

The upright posture for labor and delivery was considered normal in most societies until modern times. Squatting, kneeling, standing, and sitting were variously selected for birth by women. Only within the last two hundred years has the recumbent position become more usual in the Western world. Its use in this century has been reinforced because of the convenience it offers in applying new technology. The lithotomy position has thus become the conventional manner in which North American women give birth in hospitals. In searching for alternative positions, consumers and professionals alike are refocusing on

Box 23–2 Birthing Room Equipment and Supplies

Equipment for Delivery

Disposable pack containing drapes, towels, and gown
Instruments (scissors, clamps, etc)
Sterile gloves
Sterile, warmed baby blankets
Prep set for perineal scrub prior to delivery
Warmed sterile water

Equipment for the Newborn

Radiant-heated infant care unit
Bulb syringe
Device for assessing newborn's temperature
Oxygen
Suction equipment (DeLee suction trap)
Suction catheters (size 10, 12, and 14 French and sizes 8, 10, 12, and 14 French disposable plastic catheters with finger control)
Laryngoscope with a working light, Miller size 0 premature and size 1 blade
Endotracheal tubes size 2.5–4 mm or size 10, 12, and 14 and stylets for insertion if desired
Bag resuscitation set capable of delivering 100% oxygen

the comfort of the laboring woman rather than on the convenience of the birth attendant (see Figure 23–6 and Table 23–6).

○   *TRADITIONAL RECUMBENT POSITION*   The traditional lithotomy position for delivery enhances the maintenance of asepsis, assessment of FHR, and performance of episiotomy and repair. In contrast, when the comfort and well-being of the woman and fetus are considered, the following disadvantages have been noted:

1. There is a decrease of as much as 30 percent in the blood pressure of 10 percent of women.

2. Many women experience difficulty breathing because of pressure of the uterus on the diaphragm.

3. The uterine axis is directed toward the symphysis pubis instead of the pelvic inlet.

4. Aspiration of vomitus is more likely.

5. The woman may feel resentment at being forced to assume an "embarrassing" position.

6. Tightening of the vagina and perineum as the thighs are flexed may increase the need for an episiotomy.

7. The position may interfere with the frequency and intensity of contractions.

8. Stirrups cause excessive pressure on the legs.

9. The woman works against gravity.

These disadvantages may be lessened slightly if the woman is in a lithotomy position with her back elevated 30° to 40° (Fenwick 1984, McKay 1981).

○   *LEFT LATERAL SIMS'*   An alternative position favored by some women and birth attendants is the left lateral Sims'. In assuming this position for delivery, the woman lies on her left side with her left leg extended and her right knee drawn against her abdomen or flexed by her side or with both legs bent at the knees. Those who favor this position find it increases overall comfort, does not compromise venous return from the lower extremities, and diminishes the chances of aspiration should vomiting occur. Women also perceive the lateral Sims' as a more natural and comfortable position and less intrusive with no stirrups or overhead lights required. Birth attendants have found the position has a positive effect on the management of fetal shoulder dystocias. Fewer episiotomies are required in this position since the perineum tends to be more relaxed (Lehrman 1985). The disadvantages cited relate to the difficulty of cutting and repairing large episiotomies, and problems with difficult forceps deliveries (Lehrman 1985).

○   *SQUATTING*   The squatting position is favored by some women primarily for the positive use it makes of gravity. Squatting is thought to facilitate the entrance of the presenting part into the pelvic inlet, thus hastening engagement. A squatting bar may be used across a bed or on the floor to increase the woman's balance and provide some support (Figure 23–6D). During the second stage of labor, squatting increases the size of the pelvic outlet and helps in the woman's pushing efforts. Some birth attendants object to this position because the perineum is relatively inaccessible and it is difficult for them to control the birth process. Squatting also increases the difficulty of administering analgesia, using instruments, and monitoring fetal status.

○   *SEMI-FOWLER'S*   A semi-Fowler's position is advocated by some as an appropriate middle ground between the recumbent and upright positions. This position enhances the effectiveness of the abdominal muscle efforts while the woman is pushing and thereby shortens the second stage of labor. Raising and supporting the torso helps the woman view the birth process. At the same time, the birth attendant has access to the perineum. Many older delivery room tables are not capable of adjusting to a semi-Fowler's position. Supporting a woman in this position, however, is not difficult with most birthing beds.

○   *SITTING*   The sitting position is becoming an option for more women with the increased availability of birthing chairs. The use of delivery chairs can be traced back to ancient Egypt and was broadly used in ancient Greek, Roman, and Incan civilizations. In the wake of the nineteenth-century battle against puerperal fever, birthing chairs began to vanish on hygienic grounds. Birthing chairs are being used again during the second stage of labor and are perceived by some women who use them as a positive way to participate in the birth process. A supported sitting position may also be achieved in many of the newer birthing beds.

The upright sitting position offers advantages similar to squatting. It has been postulated that the weight of a term fetus is sufficient force in itself to supply much of what is needed to bring the newborn into the world. Proponents of the birthing chair state that it makes possible spontaneous deliveries in births that would have required operative assistance in the recumbent position. Women experiencing severe back pain have found use of the chair can diminish or eliminate the pain. The woman can curl forward and grasp her knees or ankles during pushing efforts. She can usually see the birth without aid of mirrors and following birth she can lift the baby up toward her face.

In a retrospective study, Shannahan and Cottrell (1985) found that duration of second stage and fetal outcome was not significantly affected by use of the birth chair. However, a potential for increased blood loss may exist.

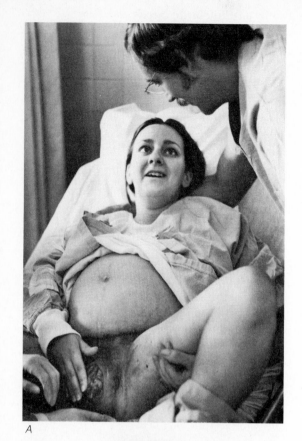

A

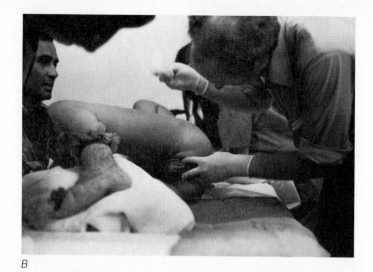

B

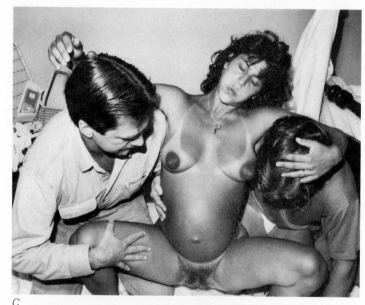

C

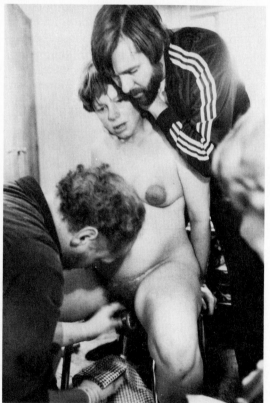

E

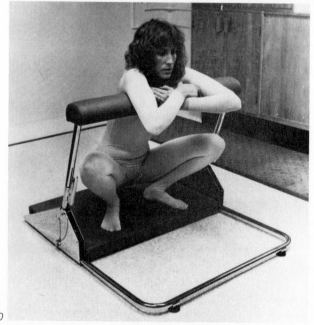

D

Table 23–6   Comparison of Birthing Positions

Position	Advantages	Disadvantages	Nursing implications
Sitting in birthing chair	Gravity aids descent and expulsion of infant. Does not compromise venous return from lower extremities. Chair can be tilted to various degrees. Woman can view birth process.	If woman is short, sitting with legs spread may increase tension on perineum, which may lead to lacerations. Position of body, legs, and feet cannot be altered. Potential for increased blood loss (Shannahan & Cottrell 1985)	Encourage woman to tilt the chair to increase her comfort. Assess for pressure points on legs.
Semi-Fowler's	Does not compromise venous return from lower extremities. Woman can view birth process.	If legs are positioned wide apart, relaxation of perineal tissues is decreased.	Assess that upper torso is evenly supported. Increase support of body by changing position of bed or using pillows as props.
Left lateral Sims'	Does not compromise venous return from lower extremities. Increased perineal relaxation and decreased need for episiotomy. Appears to prevent rapid descent.	It is difficult for the woman to see the birth if she desires.	Adjust position so that the upper leg lies on the bed (scissor fashion) or is supported by the partner or on pillows.
Squatting	Size of pelvic outlet is increased. Gravity aids descent and expulsion of newborn. Second stage may be shortened (McKay 1984).	May be difficult to maintain balance while squatting.	Help woman maintain balance. Use a squatting bar if available.
Sitting in birthing bed	Gravity aids descent and expulsion of the fetus. Does not compromise venous return from lower extremities. Woman can view the birth process. Leg position may be changed at will.		Assure that legs and feet have adequate support.

Figure 23–6   Birthing positions. Clockwise from upper left: A Lithotomy position with the woman's back elevated. B Side-lying delivery. Note that the woman's upper leg is supported by her partner. C Supported squatting position used in the second stage of labor. D Use of a bar to provide support when in the squatting position. E Birthing stool. (All photos by Suzanne Arms Wimberley except the one of the birthing bar, which is used with permission from Northwest Quality Innovations, Inc.)

CLEANSING THE PERINEUM

After being positioned for delivery, the woman's vulvar and perineal area is cleansed to increase her comfort and to remove the bloody discharge that is present prior to the actual birth. An aseptic technique such as the one that follows is recommmended.

After thoroughly washing her hands, the nurse opens the sterile prep tray, dons sterile gloves, and cleans the vulva and perineum with the cleansing solution (Figure 23–7). Some agency policy dictates the area be rinsed with sterile water. Beginning with the mons, the area is cleansed up to the lower abdomen. A second sponge is used to clean the inner groin and thigh of one leg, and a third is used to clean the other leg, moving outward to avoid carrying material from surrounding areas to the vaginal outlet. The last three sponges are used to clean the labia and vestibule with one downward sweep each. The used sponges are discarded.

SUPPORT OF THE COUPLE

The labor coach and/or support person is given a stool to sit on if desired. Both the woman and the coach are kept informed of procedures and progress and are supported throughout the delivery. In some birth settings, there is a mirror that can be adjusted so that the couple may watch the delivery. Hand mirrors are available in most birthing rooms.

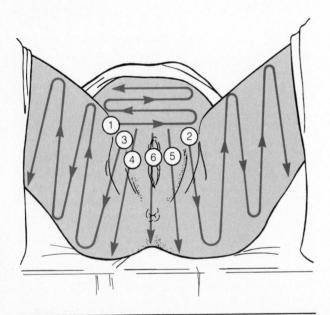

Figure 23–7 Cleansing the perineum prior to delivery. The nurse follows the numbered diagram, using a new sponge for each area. The woman in this drawing is in dorsal recumbent position to demonstrate the cleaning. The perineal scrub may be accomplished in any maternal position.

The woman's blood pressure and the FHR are monitored between contractions, and the contractions are palpated until delivery. The nurse and support person continue to assist the woman in her pushing efforts.

In addition to assisting the woman and her partner, the nurse also assists the physician or nurse-midwife in preparing for the delivery.

Physician/Nurse-Midwife Interventions

When the fetal head has distended the perineum about 5 cm, the clinician may perform certain hand maneuvers that are believed to prevent undue trauma to the fetal head and maternal soft tissues. With a towel draped over one hand, the clinician applies pressure on the chin of the fetus through the maternal perineum. The other hand exerts gentle pressure on the occiput. This is the modified Ritgen maneuver (Figure 23–8). This maneuver permits the head to be delivered slowly under the symphysis pubis, with the face sliding successfully over the perineum. The woman is encouraged to push with the contractions until the fetal chin clears the perineum. Then she is asked to blow to avoid too rapid a delivery of the fetal head. Some clinicians believe that Ritgen's maneuver causes a wider fetal head diameter to be presented on the perineum, which leads to an increased risk of perineal lacerations (Fenwick 1984).

After the infant's head is delivered, the clinician palpates the neck for the presence of a cord, which can be slipped over the fetal head if it is loose. If the cord is tight, it is double-clamped and cut.

Restitution and external rotation occur after the head is delivered. The only assistance needed during this time is support of the maternal perineum. While awaiting completion of external rotation, the clinician suctions the newborn's nose and mouth to remove mucus. When the newborn's shoulder appears at the symphysis pubis, the clinician may use both hands to grasp the newborn's head gently and pull downward for delivery of the anterior shoulder. Gentle upward traction facilitates delivery of the posterior shoulder.

Delivery of the newborn's body may be controlled by grasping the posterior shoulder with one hand, palm turned toward the perineum. The left hand may be used for this if the newborn is LOA. The right hand then follows along the infant's back, and the feet are grasped as they are delivered. The newborn's head is kept down and to the side as the newborn's feet, legs, and body are tucked under the clinician's left arm in a football hold. The clinician's right hand is then free for further care of the newborn and the newborn is securely held. The nose and mouth are suctioned with a bulb syringe, and respiratory passages are cleared.

There is considerable controversy about when to clamp and cut the cord. If the newborn is held at or below the vagina as cord clamping is delayed, as much as 50 to 100 mL of blood may be shifted from the placenta to the fetus. If the newborn is held 50 to 60 cm above the vagina, a negligible amount of blood is transferred to the newborn even after three minutes. The extra amount of blood added to the newborn's circulation may reduce the frequency of iron-deficiency anemia, which can occur later in infancy— or the circulatory overload may produce polycythemia and favor hyperbilirubinemia. Pritchard, MacDonald, and Gant (1985) advocate clamping the cord after clearing the newborn's airway, which takes about 30 seconds. The newborn is not elevated above the vagina.

The cord is clamped with two Kelly clamps and cut between them. The clamp on the placental side is placed on the mother's abdomen. A plastic cord clamp or umbilical tape may be applied on the newborn's cord about 2 cm from the newborn's abdomen, and then the Kelly clamp on the newborn's side may be removed.

Figure 23–9 on pp 672-673 depict the labor and delivery experience of one family.

The Leboyer Method

In 1975 Leboyer introduced a birthing technique directed toward easing the newborn's transition to extra-uterine life. In a conventional delivery the newborn is subjected to extreme changes in sensory input—bright lights, voices, suctioning, and being quickly dried and placed in blankets. Leboyer advocated a more soothing and tender approach to the handling of the newborn at delivery. The lights in the delivery room are dimmed, and the noise level, including talking, is kept to a minimum. As the newborn is delivered, the physician/nurse-midwife supports the infant by sliding a finger under each axilla, avoiding touching the head, to further reduce trauma. Suctioning is not done, and the newborn is placed on his or her stomach on the mother's bare abdomen. The mother is encouraged to gently stroke and touch the newborn in a massaging motion. Care is taken to keep the newborn's spine in a curved position similar to its position in utero.

Clamping of the umbilical cord is delayed until all pulsations have ceased out of respect for the innate rhythms of the new life. Leboyer (1976) believes that this delay helps the newborn's initial respiratory efforts as well as sheltering the newborn from anoxia at the time of birth.

After the umbilical cord is clamped, the newborn is gently and slowly placed in a water bath that has been warmed to 98 to 99F. The newborn remains in the bath until he or she is completely relaxed. The warm water recreates the intrauterine environment in temperature and weightlessness. Following the bath the infant is carefully and gently dried and wrapped in layers of warm blankets. The head and hands are always left to move and play. The newborn is then placed in a side-lying position to assure minimal stress on the spine and maximum freedom of movement. The infant is left alone to take in the new environment quietly.

Critics of the Leboyer method have expressed concerns about several of the techniques involved. They question the ability of the birth attendant to assess maternal and/or neonatal complications quickly or to calculate Apgar scores in an environment of dim light. Traditional practitioners are concerned about the potentially high neonatal bilirubin levels associated with delayed cord clamping. Other critics fear an increase in neonatal skin infections from the skin-to-skin contact between mother and newborn, as well as from immersion in the water bath. Hypothermia related to the bath is also cited as a risk of the Leboyer method. Although proponents suggest a beneficial long-term effect for the infant/child, there seems to be no evidence that gentle birth techniques such as the Leboyer method have an effect on temperment in infancy or a positive effect on child development (Maziade et al 1986). On the other hand, proponents and couples themselves cite the advantages of increased participation by the father in the birth process—particularly when he gives the bath— and the serenity of the birth experience (Crystle et al 1980).

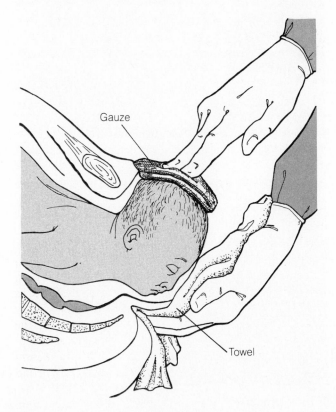

Gauze

Towel

Figure 23–8   Delivery by modified Ritgen maneuver

Once our little girls decided to be born, they didn't wait around. I thought surely Rebecca was going to pop out as I moved from the labor bed to the delivery table. The doctor didn't even get to sit down on the stool before she dropped into his hands. Hilary was born just seven minutes later, to much fanfare.

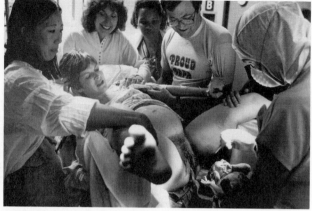

Delivery of the first twin. The nurse supports Pat's leg while Deborah, Steve, and the anesthesiologist provide encouragement.

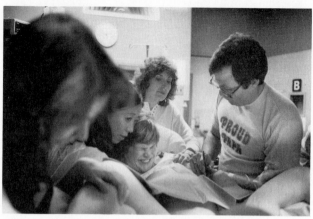

Pushing with the second baby. Everyone provides support.

The twins' birth was quite an exciting event for the hospital staff. It felt more like a party than a birth. Everyone urged me on, and they all cheered at each birth.

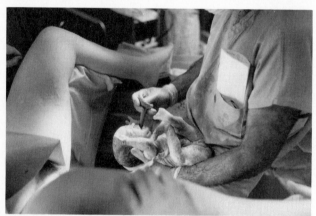

The baby's nose and mouth are suctioned.

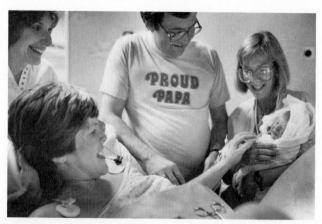

The nurse shows the first baby to Pat and Steve.

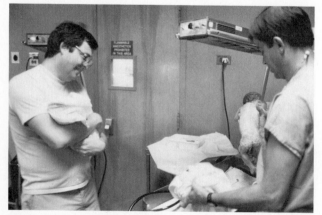

The pediatrician examines the second baby while Steve watches.

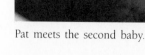

Pat meets the second baby.

Figure 23–9   A birth story

My favorite moment was when Steve, my husband, and Deborah, my friend, each held a baby up to my face and I nuzzled them. Later, in the recovery room, I got to hold them both for the first time.

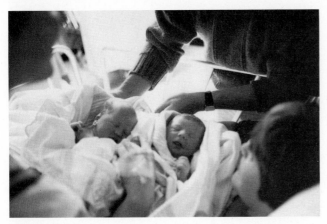

Hilary and Rebecca.

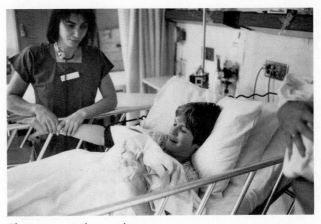

The nurse quietly completes assessments.

Rebecca has dark hair and is our quiet flower; Hilary is blond, outgoing, and into everything. I had pictured them that way when they were inside me, kicking me and each other. I had no trouble recognizing them when I saw them for the first time.

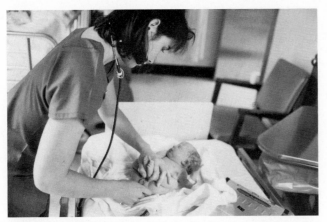

Assessments of the newborn include checking temperature.

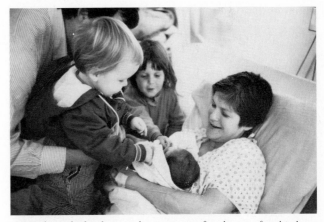

Amanda and Lloyd meet their sisters a few hours after birth.

Figure 23–9   A birth story (continued)

Immediate Care of the Newborn

Most immediate care of the newborn can be accomplished while the newborn is in the parent's arms or in the radiant-heated unit, which may be placed by the parents so they can see the baby. The physician/nurse-midwife places the newborn on the mother's abdomen or in the radiant-heated unit.

Since the first priority is to maintain respirations, the newborn is placed in a modified Trendelenburg position to aid drainage of mucus from the nasopharynx and tra-

chea. The newborn is also suctioned with a bulb syringe or DeLee mucus trap (see Procedure 23–2) as needed.

The second priority is to provide and maintain warmth, so the newborn is dried immediately. Warmth can be maintained by placing warmed blankets over the newborn or placing the newborn in skin-to-skin contact with the mother. If the newborn is in a radiant-heated unit, he or she is dried, placed on a dry blanket, and left uncovered under the radiant heat. Because radiant heat warms the outer surface of objects, a newborn wrapped in blankets will receive no benefit from radiant heat.

Procedure 23–2 DeLee Suction

Objective	Nursing action	Rationale
Clear secretions from newborn's nose and/or oropharynx if respirations are depressed and/or if amniotic fluid was meconium stained	Tighten the lid on the DeLee mucus trap collection bottle (Figure 23–10).	Avoids spillage of secretions and prevents air from leaking out of lid
	Place the whistle tip in your mouth; insert other end of tubing in newborn's nose or mouth 3 to 5 in; provide suction by sucking on whistle tip.	Provides suction Clears nasopharynx Gives gentle suction.
	Continue suction as tube is removed.	Avoids redepositing secretions in newborn's nasopharynx
	Continue reinserting tube and providing suction for as long as fluid is aspirated.	Facilitates removal of secretions
	Note: excessive DeLee suctioning can cause vagal stimulation, which causes decreased heart rate.	
	Occasionally the tube may be passed into the newborn's stomach to remove secretions or meconium that was swallowed before birth; if this is necessary, insert tube into newborn's mouth and then into the stomach. Provide suction and continue suction as tube is removed.	If meconium was present in amniotic fluid the baby may have swallowed some. Secretions and/or meconium aspirate may be removed from newborn's stomach to decrease incidence of aspiration of stomach contents.

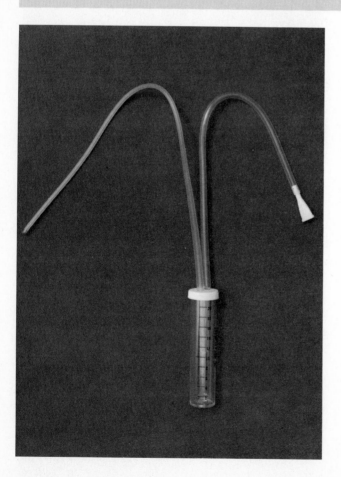

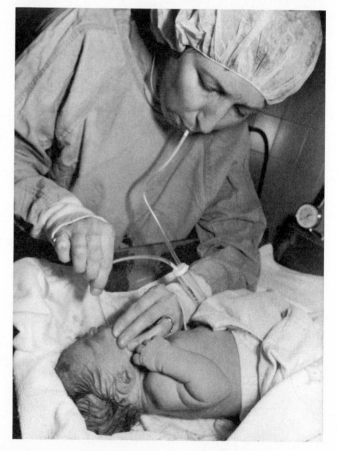

Figure 23–10   DeLee mucus trap

Apgar Scoring System

The Apgar scoring system (Table 23–7) was designed in 1952 by Dr. Virginia Apgar, an anesthesiologist. The purpose of the *Apgar score* is to evaluate the physical condition of the newborn at birth and the immediate need for resuscitation. The newborn is rated 1 minute after birth and again at 5 minutes and receives a total score ranging from 0 to 10 based on the following criteria:

1. The *heart rate* is auscultated or palpated at the junction of the umbilical cord and skin. This is the most important assessment. A newborn heart rate of less than 100 beats per minute indicates the need for immediate resuscitation.

2. The *respiratory effort* is the second most important Apgar assessment. Complete absence of respirations is termed *apnea*. A vigorous cry indicates good respirations.

3. The *muscle tone* is determined by evaluating the degree of flexion and resistance to straightening of the extremities. A normal newborn's elbows and hips are flexed, with the knees positioned up toward the abdomen.

4. The *reflex irritability* is evaluated by flicking the soles of the feet or by inserting a nasal catheter in the nose. A cry merits a full score of 2. A grimace is 1 point, and no response is 0.

5. The *skin color* is inspected for cyanosis and pallor. Newborns generally have blue extremities, and the rest of the body is pink, which merits a score of 1. This condition is termed *acrocyanosis* and is present in 85 percent of normal newborns at 1 minute after birth. A completely pink newborn scores a 2 and a totally cyanotic, pale infant is scored 0. Newborns with darker skin pigmentation will not be pink in color. Their skin color is assessed for pallor and acrocyanosis, and a score is selected based on the assessment.

A score of 8 to 10 indicates a newborn in good condition who requires only nasopharyngeal suctioning and perhaps some oxygen near the face. If the Apgar score is below 8, resuscitative measures may need to be instituted. See the discussion in Chapter 23.

Care of the Umbilical Cord

If the physician/CNM has not placed a cord clamp (Figures 23–11 and 23–12) on the newborn's umbilical cord, it is the responsibility of the nurse to do so. Before applying the cord clamp, the nurse examines the cut end for the presence of two arteries and one vein. The umbilical vein is the largest vessel, and the arteries are seen as smaller vessels. One artery in the umbilical cord is associated with genitourinary abnormalities. The number of vessels is recorded on the delivery room and newborn records. The cord is clamped approximately ½ to 1 inch from the abdomen to allow room between the abdomen and clamp as the cord dries. Abdominal skin must not be clamped, as this will cause necrosis of the tissue. The clamp is removed in the newborn nursery approximately 24 hours after the cord has dried.

Evaluation of the Newborn After Birth

As more newborns remain with their parents in the birth area, the initial evaluation of the newborn becomes even more important. Babies at risk must be identified at once so that stabilization or treatment is initiated quickly in the nursery. Although a full head-to-toe assessment is not necessary at this time, the evaluation must be thorough enough to determine that the newborn will not be compromised by remaining in the birth area. An initial newborn evaluation that identifies critical aspects is presented in Table 23–8.

Additional assessments focus on easily observed congenital anomalies. The head and face are observed for symmetry, and the mouth for an intact palate. The upper and lower extremities are inspected for the correct number of

Table 23–7 The Apgar Scoring System*

| Sign | Score | | |
	0	1	2
Heart rate	Absent	Slow—below 100	Above 100
Respiratory effort	Absent	Slow—irregular	Good crying
Muscle tone	Flaccid	Some flexion of extremities	Active motion
Reflex irritability	None	Grimace	Vigorous cry
Color	Pale blue	Body pink, blue extremities	Completely pink

*From Apgar V: The newborn (Apgar) scoring system: reflections and advice. *Pediatr Clin North Am* 1966;13(August):645.

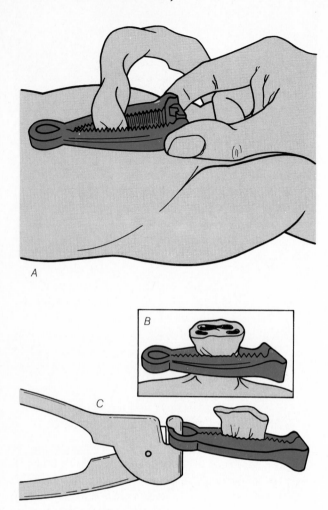

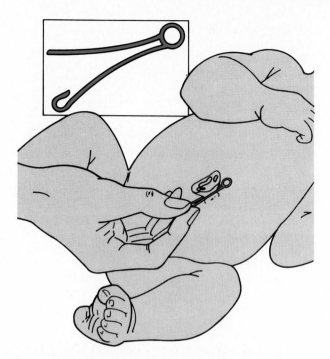

Figure 23–12 Hesseltine cord clamp. Two clamps are often used to reduce the possibility of hemorrhage should one inadvertently open. When the cord has dried, the clamp may be removed manually.

Figure 23–11 Hollister cord clamp. A Clamp is positioned ½ to 1 inch from the abdomen and then secured. B Cut cord. C Plastic device for removing clamp after cord has dried.

digits. The back is observed for any dimples, tufts of hair over the spine or lower back, and for any openings over the spinal column. At this time the anus may also be observed to determine if there is an opening.

This brief examination reveals any gross abnormalities and permits a quick determination of gestational age. Most of this examination is accomplished by visual assessment. Further neurologic assessment and an in-depth physical examination are performed in the newborn nursery (see Chapter 28).

The newborn may be weighed and measured in the delivery room/birthing room or in the newborn nursery.

Newborn Identification Procedures

To assure that the parents are given the correct newborn, the mother and baby are tagged with identical bands or bracelets before the newborn is separated from the mother. One bracelet is applied to the mother's wrist, and two bracelets are applied to the newborn—one on each wrist, one on a wrist and one on an ankle, or one on each ankle. The bands must be applied snugly to prevent loss.

Most hospitals footprint the newborn and fingerprint the mother for further identification purposes. When preparing to footprint the newborn, the nurse wipes the soles of both the newborn's feet to remove any vernix caseosa, which interferes with the placement of ink on the foot creases.

● Care of the Family During the Third Stage

The second stage of labor ends with delivery of the newborn and signals the beginning of the third stage. The placenta is expelled during the third stage.

Although care of the newborn is an immediate concern of the nurse, the nurse must keep in mind that physical changes are still occurring in the new mother. The tremendous reduction in uterine surface area causes the rapid process of detachment of the placenta from the uterine wall. The uterus continues to contract and relax rhythmically until the placenta is expelled, completing the third stage of labor. Although the maximum length of the third stage is considered to be 30 minutes, it usually lasts 5 to 10 minutes.

Table 23–8 Initial Newborn Evaluation

Assess	Normal findings
Respirations	Rate 30–60, irregular No retractions, no grunting
Apical pulse	Rate 120–160 and somewhat irregular
Temperature	Skin temp above 97.8F (36.5C)
Skin color	Body pink with bluish extremities
Umbilical cord	Two arteries and one vein
Gestational age	Should be 38–42 weeks to remain with parents for extended time
Sole creases	Sole creases that involve the heel

In general expect: scant amount of vernix on upper back, axilla, groin; lanugo only on upper back; ears with incurving of upper ⅔ of pinnae and thin cartilage that springs back from folding; male genitalia—testes palpated in upper or lower scrotum; female genitalia–labia majora larger; clitoris nearly covered

In the following situations, newborns should generally be stabilized rather than remaining with parents in the birth area for an extended period of time:

Apgar is less than 8 at one minute and less than 9 at five minutes, or a baby requires resuscitation measures (other than whiffs of oxygen).
Respirations are below 30 or above 60, with retractions and/or grunting.
Apical pulse is below 120 or above 160 with marked irregularities.
Skin temperature is below 97.8F (36.5C).
Skin color is pale blue, or there is circumoral pallor.
Baby is less than 38 or more than 42 weeks' gestation.
Baby is very small or very large for gestational age.
There are congenital anomalies involving open areas in the skin (meningomyelocele).

Nursing Goal: Initiation of Attachment

The beginning of the third stage is usually emotional for all involved. For the couple the birth of the healthy newborn is the culmination of the long months of pregnancy and the intense experience of labor. The expulsion of the newborn and the sound of the first cry creates an exhilarating and emotional moment for the new parents. The new mother may be exhausted but is elated and eager to see her new baby. The parents' concerns are usually about the well-being and gender of the baby. Given the alertness of newborns immediately after birth and the excitement and curiosity of the parents, it is an ideal time to initiate the attachment process. The baby may remain with the mother, and the nurse may help position the baby so that eye-to-eye contact is possible. The lights of the birthing room may be dimmed so that the baby's eyes open fully. The parents can be encouraged to explore and touch their baby.

I was hungry for the baby as he was born. I wanted to see, hold him. It was hours before I realized or even thought love in relation to him. (Harriette Hartigan, *Women in Birth*)

Physician/Nurse-Midwife Interventions

After the cord has been clamped and cut, the physician/nurse-midwife observes for the following signs of placental separation:

1. The uterus rises upward in the abdomen because the placenta settles downward into the lower uterine segment.

2. As the placenta proceeds downward, the umbilical cord lengthens.

3. A sudden trickle or spurt of blood appears.

4. The uterus changes from a discoid to a globular shape.

While waiting for these signs, the nurse or physician gently palpates the uterus to check for ballooning of the uterus caused by uterine relaxation and subsequent bleeding into the uterine cavity.

After the placenta has separated, it may be delivered by various techniques such as maternal effort, controlled cord traction, and fundal pressure. Maternal effort allows the placenta to deliver spontaneously and is best accomplished in an upright position. When the mother is in a dorsal recumbent or lithotomy positon, she or the nurse can help the process by splinting or supporting her abdominal muscles. The mother or nurse can place her palms over the lower abdomen, or the mother can flex her thighs over her abdomen. The mother then bears down to deliver the placenta.

Controlled cord traction may also be used to deliver the placenta. The physician/nurse-midwife first assures that separation has occurred and then places one hand above the symphysis with the palm against the anterior surface of the uterus. The uterus is displaced upward and backward as the mother is asked to relax her abdominal muscles and breathe through an open mouth. The elevation of the uterus straightens out the birth canal and facilitates delivery of the placenta, as well as protecting the uterus from inversion. Gentle traction is exerted on the umbilical cord. During this procedure the nurse encourages the mother to continue breathing through an open mouth and to relax her abdominal muscles.

Fundal pressure is not a method of choice because it is very uncomfortable for the mother and may damage uterine supports. If this method is needed, the mother is asked to relax her abdominal muscles and then the physician's/nurse-midwife's hand is placed behind the uterus with the fingers directed downward toward the maternal spine. With a quick "scooping" motion the contracted uterus is pressed downward in an arc. This motion is different from direct downward pressure, which folds the uterus over the lower segment and does not enhance movement of the placenta. During this procedure the nurse provides continued encouragement to maintain abdominal relaxation. This is very difficult due to the discomfort of the procedure (Long 1986).

After the delivery of the placenta, the physician/nurse-midwife inspects the placental membranes to make sure they are intact and that all cotyledons are present. This inspection is especially important with Duncan placentas. If there is a defect or a part missing from the placenta, a digital uterine examination is done. The vagina and cervix are inspected for lacerations, and any necessary repairs are made. The episiotomy may be repaired now if it has not been done previously. (See further discussion of episiotomy on pp 801–808.) The fundus of the uterus is palpated; normal position is at the midline and below the umbilicus. If the fundus is displaced, it may be because of a full bladder or a collection of blood in the uterus.

The time and mechanism (Schultze or Duncan) of delivery of the placenta are noted on the delivery record.

USE OF OXYTOCICS

Some physicians/CNMs advocate the use of oxytocic drugs (Pitocin, Syntocinon) to promote homeostasis by stimulating myometrial contractions after delivery and to reduce the incidence of third-stage hemorrhage (Long 1986).

The physician/CNM may request that 10 units of oxytocin be given intramuscularly at the time of delivery of the anterior shoulder of the infant; some believe that this facilitates delivery of the placenta (Long 1986). Others question whether this method increases the incidence of neonatal hyperviscosity because an additional bolus of blood may be infused into the fetus when the uterus contracts in response to the oxytocin. At other times, 10 units of oxytocin (Pitocin) may be administered IM, or by slow IV push at the time of placental delivery. It should be noted

that an IV bolus of oxytocin may cause profound hypotension and tachycardia (Marshall 1985). Some prefer to add 10 units of oxytocin to IV fluids administered over a period of hours. Additional information and associated nursing implications are presented in the Drug Guide–Oxytocin in Chapter 26.

Methylergonovine maleate (Methergine) may be given IM after delivery of the placenta to cause contraction of the uterus. Information regarding this drug and associated nursing implications are presented in the Drug Guide–Methergine in Chapter 34.

● Care of the Family During the Fourth Stage

The period immediately following delivery of the placenta is referred to as the fourth stage of labor and delivery. Actually the label is misleading since labor and delivery are completed with delivery of the placenta, and the next few hours are actually the immediate recovery phase. The fourth stage is usually defined as lasting one to four hours after delivery, or until vital signs are stable. Nursing care in this phase involves the basics of postpartum nursing care.

Since the fourth stage begins immediately after delivery of the placenta, repair of an episiotomy or vaginal lacerations is done at this time. The uterus is palpated at frequent intervals to ensure that it remains firmly contracted (medical interventions during this period are described on pp 679–681). If the mother has not held her baby yet, immediate newborn care can be completed at her side and within her reach so that she can touch her baby during this time. As soon as immediate care is completed, the new mother is usually eager to cuddle and explore her baby. If she plans to breast-feed her baby, and the baby is interested, she should be encouraged and helped to do so right after birth while the baby is awake and alert. Care should be taken not to try to force an uninterested baby to breast-feed as it will just lead to frustration for both mother and baby.

Behavioral characteristics of the newly delivered mother vary depending on such factors as the length of labor and the extent of interruption in normal sleep patterns. After the initial excitement of becoming acquainted with their new baby and notifying others of the birth, many new mothers are very tired and want to rest. Others are wide awake, eager to talk about their labor and satisfy basic body needs, such as hunger and thirst. Although labor is completed, the uterus is sensitive to touch and palpation of the uterus is not appreciated unless the woman understands the importance of the procedure.

The nursing goals of care for this stage are:

● To prepare the woman for the recovery period

- To promote maternal physical well-being

- To enchance attachment

Nursing Goal: Preparation for the Recovery Period

As soon as the physician/nurse-midwife completes her or his tasks, delivery drapes are removed. The nurse washes the perineum with gauze squares and sterile solution and dries the area with a sterile towel. If the woman is to remain in the birthing bed, the nurse helps her get clean and dry by placing clean absorbent pads beneath her and applying maternity pads. A clean gown is also provided

---

Research Note

Mercer examined the relationship between mothers' perceptions of their birth experiences and later mothering behaviors among specific age groups (15–19, 20–39, 30–42). The study included 242 mothers of healthy newborns, who described their perceptions by questionnaire and then were interviewed and rated on the Maternal Behavior Scale at 1, 4, 8, and 12 months postpartum.

The study data demonstrated a positive correlation between perceptions of the birth experience and maternal behavior at all interview dates in the teenage group, and in all but the eighth month date in the twenties group. The perception of the birth experience had little relationship with the maternal behaviors among the women who were 30 or older. Teens overall rated the experience less positively than the other age groups, and scored lower on mothering behaviors.

An increased feeling of control contributes to a feeling of mastery and therefore can result in a positive birth experience and positive mothering behavior. The teens more negative experience of childbirth may be due to their lack of knowledge and cognitive ability. The challenge for nurses is to make the experience as positive as possible for all women by increasing their understanding of events during labor and delivery and by encouraging participation in decision making. Teens in particular need early and repeated information about labor and delivery during the prenatal period, including simple and concrete information appropriate for their cognitive ability.

Mercer RT: Relationship of the birth experience to later mothering behaviors. *J Nurs-Midwife* 1985;30(July/August):204.

---

if necessary. Linen can be changed later when she first gets up to void.

If the woman delivered in the delivery room and stirrups were used, her perineum is cleaned and maternity pads applied before her legs are removed from the stirrups. In order to avoid muscle strain, both legs are removed from the stirrups at the same time. The legs may be "bicycled" to facilitate circulation return. The woman is transferred to a recovery room bed. If the mother has not had a chance to hold her infant, she may do so before she is transferred from the delivery room. The nurse ensures that the mother and father and newborn are given time to begin the attachment process.

Nursing Goal: Promotion of Maternal Physical Well-Being

The primary goal during the immediate recovery period is to ensure that the mother has minimal bleeding. The most significant source of bleeding is from the site where the placenta was implanted and where uterine vessels previously provided pooling of maternal blood to nourish the fetus. It is critical, therefore, that the fundus stay well-contracted in order to clamp off these uterine vessels and prevent hemorrhage. It is the nurse's responsibility to assess the mother's blood pressure, pulse, firmness and position of fundus, and amount and character of vaginal blood flow every 15 minutes for the first hour or two. Deviations from the normal ranges require more frequent checking (see Table 23–9). Blood pressure should return to the prelabor level, and pulse rate should be slightly lower than it was in labor. The return of the blood pressure is due to an increased volume of blood returning to the maternal circulation from the uteroplacental shunt. Baroreceptors cause a vagal response, which slows the pulse. The physiologic slowing may be offset by excitement, increased temperature, and/or dehydration. A rise in the blood pressure may be a response to oxytocic drugs or may be caused by preeclampsia. Blood loss may be reflected by a lowered blood pressure and a rising pulse rate.

The fundus should be firm at the umbilicus or lower and in the midline. The uterus should be palpated (Figure 23–13) but not massaged unless boggy (atonic). When a uterus becomes boggy, pooling of blood occurs within the uterus, resulting in the formation of clots. Anything left in the uterus prevents the uterus from contracting effectively. Thus, if it becomes boggy or appears to rise in the abdomen, the fundus should be massaged until firm; then with one hand supporting the uterus at the symphysis, the nurse should attempt to express retained clots.

A boggy uterus feels very soft instead of firm and hard. In some cases the uterus has relaxed so much that it cannot be found when the nurse attempts to palpate it. In this case, the nurse places her hand in the midline of the abdomen about at the level of the umbilicus and begins

Table 23–9 Maternal Adaptations Following Delivery

Characteristic	Normal finding
Blood pressure	Should return to prelabor level.
Pulse	Slightly lower than in labor.
Uterine fundus	In the midline at the umbilicus or 1–2 fingerbreadths below the umbilicus.
Lochia	Red (rubra), small to moderate amount (from spotting on pads to ¼–½ of pad covered in 15 minutes). Should not exceed saturation of one pad in first hour.
Bladder	Nonpalpable.
Perineum	Smooth, pink, without bruising or edema.
Emotional state	Wide variation, including excited, exhilarated, smiling, crying, fatigued, verbal, quiet, pensive, and sleepy.

to make kneading motions. This motion stimulates the uterine fundus to contract, and the nurse will feel the fundus tighten to a firm, hard object.

The nurse inspects the bloody vaginal discharge for amount and charts it as minimal, moderate, or heavy and should be bright red. A soaked perineal pad contains approximately 100 mL of blood. If the perineal pad becomes soaked in a 15-minute period, or if blood pools under the buttocks, continuous observation is necessary. As long as the woman remains in bed during the first hour, bleeding should not exceed saturation of one pad (Long 1986). Laceration of the vagina, cervix, or an unligated vessel in the episiotomy may be indicated by a continuous trickle of blood even though the fundus remains firm.

If the fundus rises and displaces to the right, the nurse palpates the bladder to determine whether it is distended. All measures should be taken to enable the mother to void. If she is unable to void, catheterization is necessary. Postpartal women have decreased sensations to void as a result of the decreased tone of the bladder due to the trauma imposed on the bladder and urethra during childbirth. The bladder fills rapidly as the body attempts to rid itself of the extra fluid volume returned from the uteroplacental circulation and of intravenous fluid that may have been received during labor and delivery. If the mother is unable to void, a warm towel placed across the lower abdomen or warm water poured over the perineum or spirits of peppermint poured into a bedpan may help the urinary sphincter relax and thus facilitate voiding. A distended bladder can cause uterine atony thus increasing postpartal bleeding.

The perineum is inspected for edema and hematoma formation. With episiotomies, an ice pack often reduces swelling and alleviates discomfort.

The following conditions should be reported to the physician/nurse-midwife: hypotension, tachycardia, uterine atony, excessive bleeding, or a temperature over 100F or 38C. The nurse should be aware that the blood pressure may not fall rapidly in the presence of dangerous bleeding in postpartal mothers because of the extra systemic volume.

However, an increasing pulse rate may be noted before a decrease in blood pressure is detected. A normal blood pressure with the mother in the Fowler's position is a good confirmation of a normotensive woman.

Women frequently have tremors in the immediate postpartal period. It has been proposed that this shivering response is caused by a difference in internal and external body temperatures (higher temperature inside the body

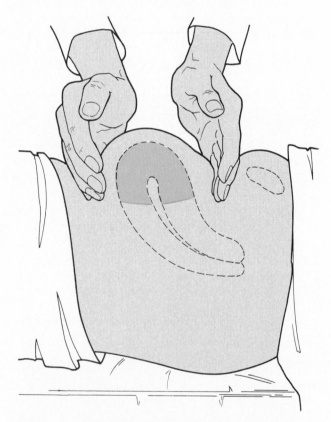

Figure 23–13 Suggested method of palpating the fundus of the uterus during the fourth stage. The left hand is placed just above the symphysis pubis, and gentle downward pressure is exerted. The right hand is cupped around the uterine fundus.

than on the outside). Another theory is that the woman is reacting to the fetal cells that have entered the maternal circulation at the placental site. A heated bath blanket placed next to the woman and, perhaps, a warm drink tend to alleviate the problem.

The couple may be tired, hungry, and thirsty. Some hospitals serve the couple a meal. The tired mother will probably drift off into a welcome sleep. The father should also be encouraged to rest, since his supporting role is physically and mentally tiring. The mother is usually transferred from the delivery unit to the postpartal unit after two hours or more depending on agency policy and if the following criteria are met:

- Stable vital signs
- No bleeding
- Nondistended bladder
- Firm fundus
- Sensations fully recovered from any anesthetic agent received during delivery

Nursing Goal: Enhancing Attachment

Evidence indicates that the first few hours and even minutes after birth are a sensitive period for attachment of mother and infant (Klaus & Kennell 1982). Separation during this critical period not only delays attachment but also may affect maternal and child behavior over a much longer period. At one month and one year after childbirth, mothers who were merely shown their infants after delivery and had them only briefly for 15- to 20-minute feeding periods demonstrated less eye contact and less soothing behavior during physical examination than did mothers who were allowed to hold their infants for an hour beginning one to two hours after delivery and for five hours on each of three succeeding days. The mothers with this extended contact asked twice as many questions about their children and used fewer commands at two years. The results of this and other research indicate that as soon as feasible the newborn needs to be united with his or her parents.

I feel different about my body now . . . feel proud of myself. I can do it again. I did such a great thing. (Harriette Hartigan, *Women in Birth*)

Klaus and Kennell (1982) believe the bonding experience can be enhanced by at least 30 to 60 minutes of early contact in privacy. If this period of contact can occur during the first hour after birth, the newborn will be in a quiet state and able to interact with parents by looking at them. Newborns also turn their heads in response to a spoken voice. (See Chapter 27 for further discussion of newborn states.)

The first parent–newborn contact may be brief (a few minutes) to be followed by a more extended contact after uncomfortable procedures (delivery of the placenta and suturing of the episiotomy) are completed. When the newborn is returned to the mother, she can be assisted to begin breast-feeding if she so desires. The nurse can help the mother to a more comfortable position for holding the infant and breast-feeding. Even if the newborn does not actively nurse, he or she can lick, taste, and smell the mother's skin. This activity by the newborn stimulates the maternal release of prolactin, which promotes the onset of lactation.

Darkening the delivery room by turning out most of the lights causes newborns to open their eyes and gaze around. This in turn enhances eye-to-eye contact with the parents. (*Note:* if the physician or nurse-midwife needs a light source, the spotlight can be left on.) Treatment of the newborn's eyes may also be delayed. Many parents who establish eye contact with the newborn are content to gaze quietly at their infant. Others may show more active involvement by touching and/or inspecting the newborn. Some mothers talk to their babies in a high-pitched voice, which seems to be soothing to newborns. Some couples verbally express amazement and pride when they see they have produced a beautiful, healthy baby. Their verbalization enhances feelings of accomplishment and ecstasy. Figure 35–4 shows a new parent establishing bonds with his newborn son.

Both parents need to be encouraged to do whatever they feel most comfortable doing. Some parents prefer limited contact with the newborn in the delivery room and private time together in a quieter environment, such as the recovery room or postpartal area. In spite of the current zeal for providing immediate attachment opportunities, nursing personnel need to be aware of parents' wishes. The desire to delay interaction with the newborn does not necessarily imply a decreased ability of the parents to bond to their newborn (see Chapter 35 for further discussion of parent–newborn attachment).

Early Discharge

More hospitals are offering new mothers—whether they deliver in a conventional labor and delivery setting, a birthing room, or an inhospital birth center—the option of discharge within a few hours after delivery. Most institutions have written policies and criteria about the mother and the newborn eligible for early discharge. Criteria for the mother may include any or all of the following:

- No antepartal or intrapartal complications
- A labor no longer than 30 hours for a primipara or 24 hours for a multipara

- An episiotomy or no greater than a third-degree laceration

- A spontaneous or low-forceps delivery

- Stable vital signs

- A firm uterine fundus

- Voiding without difficulty

- Ability to ambulate and provide care for herself and her newborn

- Help at home for one to three days

- Demonstrated understanding of home-care instructions

Early discharge criteria for the newborn may include:

- Stable vital signs

- Normal physical examination

- A hematocrit level of 45 percent to 65 percent and a Dextrostix result of greater than 45 percent

- At least one feeding

The desired practice is to follow up early discharges with home visits by labor and delivery, postpartum, or public health nurses. The early discharge option offers both financial benefits, by reducing the costs of obstetric care, and psychologic benefits, by reuniting families in their homes more quickly. The most frequent neonatal problem requiring readmission to the hospital is hyperbilirubinemia. Research suggests readmission may be due to the high percentage of breast-feeding mothers who are discharged early, the trend toward late cord clamping in the birth experience of this group, and the thorough assessment of nurses making home visits (Barton et al 1980).

Case Study

Allison and Scott Jones are expecting their first child. During the pregnancy, they attended prenatal classes and made special preparations in anticipation of using the birthing room at their local hospital. The pregnancy has proceeded without difficulty or problems.

When labor begins, they go to the hospital and are greeted by Marie Carlson, a nurse in the birthing unit. Ms Carlson helps Allison and Scott get settled and completes the admission process. Allison is having contractions every two to three minutes lasting 45 seconds, and cervical dilatation is 5 cm. She is breathing with each contraction and

focusing on a picture of their pet sheepdog, Max, as a focal point. Scott provides encouragement while he times contractions. He carefully unpacks their supply bag and they are quickly surrounded by extra pillows, knee socks for Allison, powder to use with effleurage, and suckers. They are both excited that the birth day is at hand.

Ms Carlson works to provide a comfortable, unhurried atmosphere. She is already acquainted with the Joneses because they have attended the prenatal classes that she teaches. She is familiar with their level of knowledge and will now work to support them as labor progresses. She notes that Allison and Scott are working well together in timing contractions and using relaxation techniques and breathing methods. She continues her assessments in a quiet manner and continues to offer support and encouragement to Allison and Scott. She assists Allison in position changes and helps arrange pillows to provide support. When Allison wants a backrub and effleurage, Ms Carlson takes over one of the activities as Scott does the other.

As Allison proceeds into transition, Ms Carlson notes that the Joneses need more encouragement and support, so she stays in constant attendance. She assesses maternal, fetal, and labor status and keeps the Joneses informed of their progress.

Dr Grey comes in to see the Joneses and stays close by because the labor is progressing rapidly. Toward the end of the transition, Ms Carlson prepares the equipment to be used during delivery. She assists Allison in her pushing efforts when the cervix has completely dilated. During the delivery, she assists Allison, Scott, and Dr Grey. The delivery is managed in the same unhurried manner. Ms Carlson assesses the physical parameters and offers continuing support as Allison delivers a baby girl of healthy appearance. Ms Carlson assesses the newborn quickly and then places her in her mother's arms.

The postdelivery recovery period is monitored closely so that any problems can be identified. Allison is recovering without problems and is eager to learn more about her new daughter. Ms Carlson talks to the Joneses to assess their level of knowledge and provides needed information. She does a physical assessment of the newborn and explains the findings to the Joneses. She assists Allison as she breast-feeds her baby for the first time. After the feeding, the nurse assists Scott in giving the baby her first bath. Ms Carlson has found that the bath time provides opportunities to talk and share information.

During the recovery period, Ms Carlson provides quiet time for the new family to be together and get acquainted.

A few hours after delivery, Ms Carlson assists the Joneses as they prepare for discharge. She will be making a visit to the Joneses' home the next morning to assess the mother and newborn and to provide information and continued support.

● Care of the Adolescent During Labor and Delivery

Each adolescent in labor is different. The nurse must assess what the adolescent brings to the experience by asking the following questions:

● Has the young woman received prenatal care?

● What are her attitudes and feelings about the pregnancy?

● Who will attend the birth and what is the person's relationship to her?

● What preparation has she had for the experience?

● What are her expectations and fears regarding labor and delivery?

● How has her culture influenced her?

● What are her usual coping mechanisms?

● Does she plan to keep the newborn?

The primary goals when caring for the adolescent during labor and delivery are:

● To promote maternal and fetal well-being

● To provide support to the adolescent

Nursing Goal: Promotion of Maternal and Fetal Well-Being

Any adolescent who has not had prenatal care requires close observation during labor. Fetal well-being is established by fetal monitoring. Adolescent women are at highest risk for pregnancy and labor complications and must be monitored intensively (Mercer 1979).

The nurse should be alert to any physiologic complications of labor in the adolescent. The young woman's prenatal record is carefully reviewed for risks. The adolescent is screened for PIH, CPD, anemia, drugs ingested during pregnancy, sexually transmitted disease, and size-date discrepancies.

Nursing Goal: Support During Labor and Delivery

One of the greatest fears of any laboring woman is being left alone. This fear is greater in the adolescent, whether or not she acknowledges it to those around her.

The support role of the nurse depends on the young woman's support system during labor. She may not be accompanied by someone who will stay with her during childbirth. Whether she has a support person or not, it is important for the nurse to establish a trusting relationship with the young woman. In this way, the nurse can help her maintain control and understand what is happening to her. Establishing rapport without recrimination for possible inappropriate behavior is essential. The adolescent who is given positive reinforcement for "work well done" will leave the experience with increased self-esteem, despite the emotional problems that may accompany her situation.

If a support person did accompany the adolescent, that person also needs the nurse's encouragement and support. Whether that person is the father of the baby, a parent, or a friend of the laboring adolescent, establishing rapport with the support person without recrimination is essential in gaining his or her cooperation. Without this sense of acceptance, the support person may isolate himself or herself from the laboring adolescent, thus increasing her anxiety. The nurse must explain changes in the young woman's behavior and show the support person ways to help the young woman cope. If the support person is also an adolescent, the nursing staff should reinforce the adolescent's feelings that he or she is wanted and important.

The adolescent who has taken childbirth education classes is generally better prepared than the adolescent who has had no preparation. The nurse must keep in mind, however, that the younger the adolescent, the less she may be able to participate actively in the process.

The very young adolescent (under age 14) has fewer coping mechanisms and less experience to draw on than her older counterparts have. Because her cognitive development is incomplete, the younger adolescent may have fewer problem-solving capabilities. Her ego integrity may be more threatened by the experience, and she may be more vulnerable to stress and discomfort.

The very young woman needs someone to rely on at all times during labor. She may be more childlike and dependent than older teens. The nurse must be sure that instructions and explanations are simple and concrete. During the transition phase, the young teenager may become withdrawn and unable to express her need to be nurtured. Touch, soothing encouragement, and measures to maintain her comfort help her maintain control and meet her needs for dependence. During the second stage of labor, the young adolescent may feel as if she is losing control and may reach out to those around her. By remaining calm and giving directions, the nurse helps her control feelings of helplessness.

The middle adolescent (age 14 to 16 years) often attempts to remain calm and unflinching during labor. If unable to break through the teenager's stoic barrier, the nurse needs to rise above frustration and realize that a caring attitude will still affect the young woman.

Many older adolescents feel that they "know it all," but they may be no more prepared for childbirth than their younger counterparts. The nurse's reinforcement and nonjudgmental manner will help them save face. If the adolescent has not taken classes, she may require preparation and explanations. The older teenager's response to the stresses of labor, however, is similar to that of the adult woman.

If the adolescent is planning to relinquish her newborn, she should be given the option of seeing and holding the infant. She may be reluctant to do this at first, but the grieving process is facilitated if the mother sees the infant. However, seeing or holding the newborn should be the young woman's choice. (See Chapter 34 for further discussion of the relinquishing mother and the adolescent parent.)

● Care of the Woman and Newborn During Delivery in Less-Than-Ideal Circumstances

Precipitous Delivery

Occasionally labor progresses so rapidly that the maternity nurse is faced with the task of delivering the baby. This is called a *precipitous delivery*. The attending maternity nurse has the primary responsibility for providing a physically and psychologically safe experience for the woman and her baby.

A woman whose physician or nurse-midwife is not present may feel disappointed, frightened, and abandoned, especially if she is not prepared through childbirth education. Fear is an inhibiting factor in childbirth; therefore, the nurse can support the woman by keeping her informed about the labor progress and assuring her that the nurse will stay with her. If delivery is imminent, the nurse must not leave the mother alone. Auxiliary personnel can be directed to contact the physician or nurse-midwife and to retrieve the emergency delivery pack ("precip pack"). An emergency delivery pack should be readily accessible to the labor rooms. A typical pack contains the following items:

1. A small drape that can be placed under the woman's buttocks to provide a sterile field

2. Several 4-by-4 gauze pads for wiping off the newborn's face and removing secretions from the mouth

3. A bulb syringe to clear mucus from the newborn's mouth

4. Two sterile clamps (Kelly or Rochester) to clamp the umbilical cord before applying a cord clamp

5. Sterile scissors to cut the umbilical cord

6. A sterile umbilical cord clamp, either Hesseltine or Hollister

7. A baby blanket to wrap the newborn in after delivery

8. A package of sterile gloves

As the materials are being gathered, the nurse must remain calm. The woman is reassured by the nurse's composure and feels that the nurse is competent.

The primary goal of nursing care is the safe delivery of the fetus whether it is in vertex or breech presentation.

NURSING GOAL: DELIVERY OF INFANT IN VERTEX PRESENTATION

The nurse who manages precipitous delivery in the hospital conducts it as follows. The woman is encouraged to assume a comfortable position. If time permits, the nurse scrubs her hands with soap and water and puts on sterile gloves. Sterile drapes are placed under the woman's buttocks.

At all times during the delivery, the nurse gives clear instructions to the woman, supports her efforts, and provides reassurance. The nurse needs to remain calm and proceed in a slow, confident manner.

When the infant's head crowns, the nurse instructs the woman to pant, which decreases her urge to push. The nurse checks whether the amniotic sac is intact. If it is, the nurse tears the sac with a clamp so the newborn will not breathe in amniotic fluid with the first breath.

The nurse may place an index finger inside the lower portion of the vagina and the thumb on the outer portion of the perineum and gently massage the area to aid in stretching of perineal tissues and to help prevent perineal lacerations. This is called "ironing the perineum."

With one hand, the nurse applies gentle pressure against the fetal head to maintain flexion and prevent it from popping out rapidly. *The nurse does not hold the head back forcibly.* Rapid delivery of the head may result in tears in the woman's perineal tissues. The rapid change in pressure within the fetal head may cause subdural or dural tears. The nurse supports the perineum with the other hand and allows the head to be delivered between contractions.

As the woman continues to pant, the nurse inserts one or two fingers along the back of the fetal head to check for the umbilical cord. If the cord is around the neck, the nurse bends her fingers like a fish hook, grasps the cord, and pulls it over the baby's head, loosens it, or slips it down over the shoulders. It is important to check that the cord is not wrapped around more than one time. If the cord is tightly looped and cannot be slipped over the baby's head, the nurse places two clamps on the cord, cuts the cord between the clamps, and unwinds the cord.

Immediately after delivery of the head, the mouth, throat, and nasal passages are suctioned. The nurse places one hand on each side of the head and instructs the woman to push gently so that the rest of the body can be delivered quickly. The newborn must be supported as it emerges.

The newborn is held at the level of the uterus to facilitate blood flow through the umbilical cord. The combination of amniotic fluid and vernix makes the newborn very slippery, so the nurse must be careful to avoid dropping the newborn. The nose and mouth of the newborn are suctioned again, using a bulb syringe. The nurse then dries the newborn quickly to prevent heat loss.

As soon as the nurse determines that the newborn's respirations are adequate, the infant can be placed on the mother's abdomen. The newborn's head should be slightly lower than the body to aid drainage of fluid and mucus. The weight of the newborn on the mother's abdomen stimulates uterine contractions, which aid in placental separation. The umbilical cord should not be pulled.

The nurse is alert for signs of placental separation (slight gush of dark blood from the vagina, lengthening of the cord, or a change in uterine shape from discoid to globular). When these signs are present, the mother is instructed to push so that the placenta can be delivered. In some instances the mother can squat, and this usually helps deliver the placenta. The nurse inspects the placenta to determine whether it is intact.

The nurse checks the firmness of the uterus. The fundus may be gently massaged to stimulate contractions and decrease bleeding. Putting the newborn to breast also stimulates uterine contractions through release of oxytocin from the pituitary gland.

The umbilical cord may now be cut. Two sterile clamps are placed approximately 2 to 4 inches from the newborn's abdomen. The cord is cut between them with sterile scissors. A sterile cord clamp (Hollister or Hesseltine) can be placed adjacent to the clamp on the newborn's cord, between the clamp and the newborn's abdomen. The clamp *must not* be placed snugly against the abdomen, because the cord will dry and shrink.

The area under the mother's buttocks is cleaned, and her perineum is inspected for lacerations. Bleeding from lacerations may be controlled by pressing a clean perineal pad against the perineum and instructing the woman to keep her thighs together.

If the physician's arrival is delayed or if the newborn is having respiratory distress, the newborn should be transported immediately to the nursery. *The newborn must be properly identified before he or she leaves the delivery area.*

○   *RECORD KEEPING*   The following information is noted and placed on a delivery record:

1. Position of fetus at delivery

2. Presence of cord around neck or shoulder (nuchal cord)

3. Time of delivery

4. Apgar scores at one and five minutes after birth

5. Gender of newborn

6. Time of delivery of placenta

7. Method of placental expulsion

8. Appearance and intactness of placenta

9. Mother's condition

10. Any medications that were given to mother or newborn (per agency protocol)

POSTDELIVERY   INTERVENTIONS   Postdelivery implications are the same as those on p 679.

NURSING GOAL: DELIVERY OF INFANT IN BREECH PRESENTATION

A significant factor in a breech delivery is that the smallest part of the fetus presents first; succeeding parts are progressively larger. The cervix is not as effectively dilated when the fetus is in breech presentation as it is when the fetus is in the vertex position. Therefore, descent is usually slow and may not occur until the cervix is fully dilated and the membranes rupture.

The emergency delivery of an infant in breech position is conducted similarly to that of an infant in vertex presentation. However, when the breech crowns, the nurse instructs the woman to blow so that the part is delivered between contractions. The nurse supports the breech in both hands. The infant's body is lifted slightly upward for delivery of the posterior shoulder and arm. The newborn may then be lowered, and the anterior shoulder and arm will pass under the symphysis.

Flexion of the head occurs as with other presentations. It is important to maintain the flexion. The nape of the neck pivots under the symphysis, and the rest of the head is borne over the perineum by a movement of flexion.

The remaining delivery and postdelivery interventions for breech birth are described in the preceding section on precipitous delivery of an infant in vertex presentation.

Out-of-Hospital Emergency Delivery

Every woman who is in labor should be transported to a care facility as soon as possible. However, this is not always possible. Emergency deliveries may be necessary in various locations, such as cars or out of doors. Home delivery is considered an emergency only if it is unexpected and unplanned.

If a hospital or birth center is not accessible and birth is imminent, the following are important considerations:

● Privacy for the delivering woman (or couple)

● A clean place to deliver

- Protection from infection

- Safeguard against hemorrhage

- Warmth for the baby

The nurse has three primary goals of care:

- To manage the delivery

- To promote neonatal well-being

- To facilitate parent–infant attachment

NURSING GOAL: MANAGEMENT OF DELIVERY

The woman who is laboring under such unusual circumstances will need a great deal of psychologic support. The beautiful experience that she had planned is now impossible, and she may react with hostility, bitterness, and resentment. In addition, she may be extremely frightened and alarmed by the lack of equipment and skilled personnel. An attitude of calm and confidence helps both the nurse and the woman maintain control.

The nurse must communicate to the woman in labor that her needs are understood. In addition, the nurse must reassure the woman that the nurse will work with the woman (and her support persons) to provide the best possible experience under the circumstances.

The mother should not be separated from her partner or other persons whom she wishes to be present. However, the expectant mother should be screened from curious strangers, both for privacy and asepsis. The less exposure the mother and newborn have to strangers, the less chance they have of contracting infections. If the woman is inside a shelter, folding chairs or carts draped with blankets or coats make an efficient screen, as do sleeping bags tied to low-hanging branches of trees if one is outdoors. A private room is desirable if available. Women in labor take precedence over any other individual or group when it comes to the use of space and transportation.

A clean surface should be provided for the woman. Unread newspapers, clean towels, blankets, garment bags turned inside out, the inside of a coat or even a shirt or pair of slacks turned inside out can be placed under the woman's hips to cover a floor, a carpet, or the ground.

If the room or car temperature can be regulated, a warm environment 26.7C to 28.9C (80F to 84F) degrees is preferred. Two roaring fires, one on each side of the woman, provide warmth if the delivery is outside.

The delivery can proceed as described for an in-hospital precipitous delivery. Substitutions may need to be made in equipment. Cord ties or new shoestrings may be used to tie the umbilical cord. The shoestrings should be boiled so that they shrink to prevent them from loosening and allowing blood to ooze from the cord. A clean soft cloth may be used to wipe off the newborn's face and the inside of the mouth. A new razor or scissors (clean or boiled) may be used to cut the cord. If necessary, the cord may be left intact and the placenta may be wrapped in a plastic bag and blanket. Care must be taken to keep the newborn and placenta close together so that no unnecessary traction is put on the umbilical cord, yet the newborn must be protected from heat loss as the placenta cools.

NURSING GOAL: PROMOTION OF WELL-BEING OF THE NEWBORN

The care of the newborn under out-of-hospital circumstances is directed toward the same goals as those born in a hospital or maternity center: protection from overstimulation, infection, and heat loss; adequate resuscitation; and facilitation of parent–infant attachment.

○ *PROTECTION FROM OVERSTIMULATION AND INFECTION* Loud music, very bright lights, and large numbers of extraneous personnel are usually not in evidence in hospitals, and they are contraindicated during any birth. Overstimulation can occur in the presence of a great deal of noise and activity. The chances of infection are increased by the number of people to whom the newborn is exposed.

At sites designated as shelters during natural disasters, such as schools or church basements, these forms of overstimulation are very much in evidence. Under these circumstances, the nurse attempts to provide the woman in labor a quiet, screened, and restricted area that has some soundproofing and indirect lighting. If this is not possible, the nurse should request that the noise level be lowered. If spotlights or lanterns are used, the newborn's eyes must be shielded, or the light should be adjusted so that it does not shine directly into the eyes. The number of people in the immediate area should be restricted to care givers, the expectant mother's family, and other support persons she chooses.

○ *PROTECTION FROM HEAT LOSS* Protecting the newborn from heat loss without a radiant warmer is a challenge to the nurse attending the family under emergency conditions. Any of several methods may be available. If the environment is unheated, that is, below 27.8C (82F), the nurse dries the newborn thoroughly, especially the hair. The nurse instructs the mother to roll onto her side (even if the placenta has not separated) and places the newborn on its side against the mother skin-to-skin, so they face each other. The mother and infant are then wrapped up together or covered with clothing, blankets, garment bags, layers of newspaper, or unused plastic food wrap.

When the mother and newborn are wrapped together, the nurse need not disturb their ambient environment to check the temperature. The mother can check the newborn's body temperature by feeling the infant's stomach with the back of her fingers.

Even if the environment is warmer than 27.8C (82F), it is necessary to dry thoroughly and protect the newborn.

○   *ENSURING ADEQUATE RESUSCITATION*   During an emergency situation outside of the hospital, resuscitation equipment may not be available. If there is mild respiratory depression of the newborn, he or she is:

1. Positioned on the side, with the head slightly lower than the trunk. This position facilitates drainage of mucus by gravity.

2. Cleared of mucus from the mouth with a soft rag or delivery person's finger.

3. Kept dry to avoid heat loss.

4. Stimulated by a back rub.

5. Given cardiopulmonary resuscitation if above measures are ineffective.

NURSING GOAL: FACILITATION OF PARENT– INFANT ATTACHMENT

The mother and father and newborn are encouraged to get to know each other. The nurse can point out the newborn's behavior and show the mother or couple how they can deal with this behavior. For example, if the newborn is looking at the mother's face, the nurse can encourage the mother to make eye-to-eye contact and to smile at the newborn. When the newborn puts fist or fingers in his or her mouth, the mother can offer to breast-feed. When the newborn no longer wants to nurse and shows signs of sleepiness, the mother can stroke the baby gently, hum, sing, or rock the newborn. Give-and-take behavior by the mother or couple helps alleviate much of their fear that the delivery under these unusual circumstances has adversely affected their ability to make bonds with or take care of their baby.

KEY CONCEPTS

Admission to the birth setting involves assessment of many physiological and psychological factors. The information gained helps the nurse establish priorities of care.

Before care is begun it is important to explain what will be done, the reasons, potential benefits and risks, and possible alternatives if appropriate. This helps the woman determine what happens to her body.

Behavioral responses to labor vary with the phase of labor; the preparation the woman has had; and her pre-vious experience, cultural beliefs, and developmental level.

The adolescent has special needs in the birth setting. Her developmental needs require specialized nursing care.

Each woman's cultural beliefs affect her needs for privacy, expression of discomfort, and expectations for the birth and the role she wishes the father to play in the birth event.

The laboring woman's comfort may be increased by general comfort measures, supportive relaxation techniques, methods of handling anxiety, controlled breathing, and support by a caring person.

The laboring woman fears being alone during labor. Even though there is a support person available, the woman's anxiety will be decreased when the nurse remains with her.

Maternal birthing positions include a wide variety of possibilities from side lying to sitting, squatting, and lying flat.

Immediate assessments of the newborn include evaluation of the Apgar score and an abbreviated physical assessment. These early assessments help determine the need for resuscitation and whether the newborn's adaptation to extrauterine life is progressing normally. The newborn who is not experiencing problems may remain with the parents for an extended period of time following birth.

Immediate care of the newborn following birth also includes maintenance of respirations, promotion of warmth, prevention of infection, and accurate identification.

The new parents and their baby are given time together as soon as possible after birth.

Nursing assessments continue after the birth and are important to assure that normal physiologic adaptations are happening after birth.

REFERENCES

Apgar V: The newborn (Apgar) scoring system: Reflections and advice. *Pediatr Clin North Am* 1966;13(August):645.
April IF: Mexican-American folk beliefs: How they affect health care. *Am J Mat Child Nurs* 1977;2(May/June):168.
Barton J, et al: Alternative birthing center: Experience in a teaching obstetric service. *Am J Obstet Gynecol* 1980; 137:377.

Brackbill Y, et al: Characteristics related to drug consumption of women choosing between nontraditional birth alternatives: A comparison. *J Nurs Midwife* 1984;29(May/June):177.

Burst HV: The influences of consumers on the birthing movement. *Top Clin Nurs,* October 1983, p 42.

Calhoun MA: The Vietnamese woman: Health/illness attitudes and behaviors, in **Stern** PN: *Women, Health and Culture.* Washington, Hemisphere, 1986.

Carr KC: Obstetric practices which protect against neonatal morbidity: Focus on maternal position in labor and birth. *Birth Fam J* 1980;7(Winter):249.

Carrington BW: The Afro American, in **Clark** AL (ed): *Culture, Childbearing, Health Professionals.* Philadelphia, Davis, 1978.

Chung JJ: Understanding the Oriental maternity patient. *Nurs Clin North Am* 1977;12(March):67.

Chute GE: Expectation and experience in alternative and conventional birth. *J Obstet Gynecol Neonat Nurs* 1985;14(January/February):61.

Crystle CD, et al: The Leboyer method of delivery: An assessment of risk. *J Reprod Med* 1980;25:267.

Curry MA, **Howe** CL: Nurses made a difference. *Am J Mat Child Nurs* 1985;10(July/August):225.

Daniels MB: The birth experience for the sibling: Description and evaluation of a program. *J Nurs Midwife* 1983;28(September/October):15.

Davitz LJ, et al: Suffering as viewed in six different cultures. *Am J Nurs* 1976;76:1296.

Farris L: The American Indian, in **Clark** AL (ed): *Culture, Childbearing, Health Professionals.* Philadelphia, Davis, 1978.

Fenwick L: Birthing: Techniques for managing the physiologic and psychosocial aspects of childbirth. *PN,* May/June 1984, p 51.

Frink BB, **Chally** P: Managing pain responses to cesarean childbirth. *Am J Mat Child Nurs* 1984;9(July/August):270.

Heggenhougen HK: Father and childbirth: An anthropological perspective. *J Nurs Midwife* 1980;25(November/December):21.

Higgins PG, **Wayland** JR: Labour and delivery in North America. *Nurs Times,* September 1981, midwifery suppl p 77.

Hollingsworth AO, et al: The refugees and childbearing: What to expect. *RN* 1980;43(November):45

Kaunitz AM, **Grines** DA: Childbirth without OB care: The bad old days revisited. *Contemp OB/GYN* 1985;26(July):165.

Kay MA: *Anthropology of Human Birth.* Philadelphia, Davis, 1982.

Kay MA: The Mexican American, in **Clark** AL (ed): *Culture, Childbearing, Health Professionals.* Philadelphia, Davis, 1978.

Klaus MH, **Kennell** JH: *Parent-Infant Bonding,* ed 2. St Louis, Mosby, 1982.

Knauth DG, **Haloburdo** EP: Effect of pushing techniques in birthing chair on length of second stage of labor. *Nurs Res* 1986;35(January/February):49.

Korones S. *High Risk Newborn Infants: The Basis for Intensive Nursing Care,* ed 3. St Louis, Mosby, 1981.

Kowba MD, **Schwirian** P: Direct sibling contact and bacterial colonization in newborns. *J Obstet Gynecol Neonat Nurs* 1985;14:412.

Krutsky CD: Siblings at birth: Impact on parents. *J Nurs Midwife* 1985;30(September/October):269.

LaDu EB: Childbirth care for Hmong families. *Am J Mat Child Nurs* 1985;10(November/December):382.

Leboyer F: *Birth Without Violence.* New York, Knopf, 1976.

Lehrman EJ: Birth in the left lateral position: An alternative to the traditional delivery position. *J Nurs Midwife* 1985;30(July/August):193.

Long PJ: Management of the third stage of labor: A review. *J Nurs Midwife* 1986;31(May/June):135.

Lupe PF, **Gross** TL: Maternal upright posture and mobility in labor: A review. *Obstet Gynecol* 1986;67(May):727.

MacLaughlin SM, **Johnston** KB: The preparation of young children for the birth of a sibling. *J Nurs Midwife* 1984;29(November/December):371.

Mahan CS, **McKay** S: Preps and enemas: Keep or discard? *Contemp OB/GYN* 1983;22(November):241.

Marshall C: The art of induction/augmentation of labor. *J Obstet Gynecol Neonat Nurs* 1985;14(January/February):22.

May KA, **Ditolla** K: In-hospital alternative birth centers: Where do we go from here? *Am J Mat Child Nurs* 1984;9(January/February):48.

Maziade M, et al: Influence of gentle birth delivery procedures and other perinatal circumstances on infant temperament: Development and social implications. *J Pediatr* 1986;108(January):134.

McCaffery M: *Nursing Management of the Patient with Pain,* ed 2. Philadelphia, Lippincott, 1979.

McKay SR: Maternal position during labor and birth: A reassessment. *J Obstet Gynecol Neonat Nurs* 1980;9:288.

McKay SR: Second stage labor: Has tradition replaced safety? *Am J Nurs* 1981;81:1061.

McKay SR: Squatting: An alternate position for the second stage of labor. *Am J Mat Child Nurs* 1984;8(May/June):181.

Mercer R: *Perspectives on Adolescent Health Care.* New York, Lippincott, 1979.

Morrow K: Transcultural midwifery: Adapting to Hmong birthing customs in California. *J Nurs Midwife* 1986;31(November/December):285.

Morton K: Beyond "choice" in childbirth. *Birth* 1983;10(Fall):179.

Murillo-Rohde I: Cultural sensitivity in the care of the Hispanic patient. *Wash State J Nurs* 1979(special suppl):25.

Murphee AH: A functional analysis of southern folk beliefs concerning birth. *Am J Obstet Gynecol* 1968;102(September):125.

Nobel E: Controversies in maternal effort during labor and delivery. *J Nurs Midwife* 1981;26(March/April):13.

Pritchard J, **MacDonald** PC, **Gant** NF: *Williams Obstetrics,* ed 17. New York, Appleton-Century-Crofts, 1985.

Roberts JE, **Mendez-Bauer** C, **Wodell** DA: The effects of maternal position on uterine contractility and efficiency. *Birth* 1983;10(Winter):243.

Shannahan MB, **Cottrell** BH: Effect of birth chair on duration of second stage labor, fetal outcome and maternal blood loss. *Nurs Res* 1985;34(March/April):89.

Simkin P: Preparing parents for second stage. *Birth* 1982;10(Winter):234.

Sinquefield G: Midwifery management of second stage of labor. *J Nurs Midwife* 1985;30(March/April):112.

Stephany T: Supporting the mother of a patient in labor. *J Obstet Gynecol Neonat Nurs* 1983;12(September/October):345.

Tartasky D: Human responses to high technology. *Am J Mat Child Nurs* 1985;10(July/August):242.

Trandel-Korenchuk DM: Informed consent: Client participation in childbirth decisions. *J Obstet Gynecol Neonat Nurs* 1982;11:379.

Wranesh BL: The effect of sibling visitation on bacterial colonization rate in neonates. *J Obstet Gynecol Neonat Nurs* 1982;11:211.

Young D: *Changing Childbirth: Family Birth in the Hospital.* Rochester, NY, Childbirth Graphics, 1982.

Zborowski M: Cultural components in responses to pain. *J Social Issues* 1952;8:16.

Zimmerman E: Home birth safety. *J Obstet Gynecol Neonat Nurs* 1980;9:191.

Bates MS: Ethnicity and pain: A biocultural model. *Soc Sci Med* 1987;24(1):47.

Bell SE, **Whiteford** MB: Tai Dam health care practices: Asian refugee women in Iowa. *Soc Sci Med* 1987;24(4):317.

Chen SZ, et al: Effects of sitting position on uterine activity during labor. *Obstet Gynecol* 1987;69(January):67.

Cohen WR: Steering patients through the second stage of labor. *Contemp OB/GYN* 1984;24(1):122.

Copstik SM, et al: Partner support and the use of coping techniques in labour. *J Psychosom Res* 1986;30(4):497.

Hutson JM: Possible limitations of fetal monitoring *Clin Obstet Gynecol* 1986;29(March):104.

Ingemarrson I, et al: Admission test: A screening test for fetal distress in labor. *Obstet Gynecol* 1986;68:800.

Kintz DL: Nursing support during labor. *J Obstet Gynecol Neonat Nurs* 1987;16(March/April):126.

Marecki M, et al: Early sibling attachment. *J Obstet Gynecol Neonat Nurs* 1985;14(September/October):412.

McKay S, **Roberts** J: Second stage labor: What is normal? *J Obstet Gynecol Neonat Nurs* 1985;14(March/April):101.

Romond JL, **Baker** IT: Squatting in childbirth: A new look at an old tradition. *J Obstet Gynecol Neonat Nurs* 1985; 14(5):406.

Symposium: Managing pregnancy in patients over 35. *Contemp OB/GYN* 1987;29(May):180.

Thacker SB: The efficacy of intrapartum electronic fetal monitoring. *Am J Ob Gyn* 1987;156(January):24.

Young BK: Fetal stress and distress, in **Young** B (ed): *The Patient Within the Patient.* March of Dimes Birth Defects Foundation, Original Article Series, vol 21, no 5. Alan R Liss, 1985, p 155.

ADDITIONAL READINGS

Arms S: *Immaculate Deception.* Boston, Houghton Mifflin, 1975.

Bargagliotti LA, **Trygstad** LN: Differences in stress and coping findings: A reflection of social realities or methodologies. *Nurs Res* 1987;36(May/June):170.

The sheer pleasure of the feeling of a born baby on one's thighs is like nothing on earth. (Margaret Drabble, in *Ever Since Eve*)

Maternal Analgesia and Anesthesia

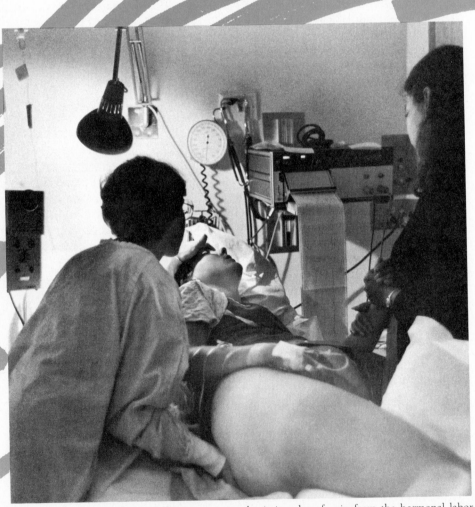

A nurse comforts a woman who is in a lot of pain from the hormonal labor
stimulant she is receiving.

Chapter Twenty-Four

OBJECTIVES

- Formulate a nursing care plan to meet the needs of a woman receiving systemic drugs for pain relief during labor.
- Differentiate between the major techniques of regional analgesia and anesthesia.
- Develop a nursing care plan to meet the specific needs of a woman receiving regional analgesia or anesthesia for pain relief during labor and/or delivery.
- Distinguish between the actions of inhalation and intravenous anesthetic agents used to provide general anesthesia for delivery and describe the nursing implications of both methods.
- Discuss the nursing role when complications of regional and general anesthesia occur.

The management of pain during childbirth is an important aspect of maternity health care. The discomfort associated with labor and delivery has been a subject of concern throughout history. A woman's attitude toward childbirth and pain reflects her culture. During the early Greek, Roman, and Egyptian civilizations, the art of assisting women in childbirth was highly developed. Unfortunately, the practices from these cultures were displaced during the Dark Ages by ignorance and superstition.

It was not until the nineteenth century that health care for mothers and babies began to improve. One significant clinical advance was the introduction of anesthetic agents into obstetrics. Ether and chloroform were first used for labor and delivery in Great Britain by Sir James Simpson of the University of Glasgow. An outraged clergy claimed that the pain of childbirth was decreed by God as punishment for the fall from grace in the Garden of Eden. They cited the Bible (Genesis 3:16) as proof that women must suffer: "Unto the woman He said, I will greatly multiply thy sorrow and thy conception; in sorrow thou shalt bring forth children. . . ." In his defense of the practice, Simpson also used the Bible (Genesis 2:21) to propose that God used anesthesia for the creation of Eve: "And the Lord God caused a deep sleep to fall upon Adam. . . ."

The use of chloroform by Queen Victoria for the birth of her eighth child was the event that finally ended the controversy and sanctioned the use of anesthetic agents for childbearing. Since that time, many agents and techniques have been introduced. The goal of pain relief in childbirth is alleviation of discomfort in the woman while ensuring the safety of both mother and fetus. To date, no method or agent has been discovered that can meet all these criteria. The search for a safe, effective method of pain relief during labor and delivery thus continues in the twentieth century.

Theories of pain and factors affecting maternal response to the pain of childbearing are discussed in Chapter 21.

• Methods of Pain Relief

Reduction or relief of pain during labor is achieved by several different methods, including psychoprophylactic methods (discussed in Chapters 18 and 23), systemic drugs, and regional nerve blocks.

The methods are not exclusive. The agents used for regional nerve blocks may enter general circulation and cause unwanted side effects. Systemic drugs such as meperidine (Demerol) may assist the tense psychoprophylactically prepared woman to regain control and progress to a satisfying childbirth experience. Regional nerve blocks with analgesic doses of anesthetic agents administered during the course of labor are compatible with the goals of prepared childbirth.

Although systemic analgesics and local anesthetic agents affect the fetus, so do the pain and stress experienced by the mother. Altered breathing techniques may lead to hypoventilation or hyperventilation, both of which cause a decrease of oxygen to the fetus (Oriel & Warfield 1984). During the pain and stress of labor there is an increase in maternal ventilation and oxygen consumption, which decreases the amount of oxygen available to the fetus. Hyperventilation leads to maternal metabolic acidosis and also shifts the maternal hemoglobin dissociative curve to the left, which may interfere with placental oxygen exchange.

Plasma epinephrine and norepinephrine levels are higher during labor than in the last trimester of pregnancy. The body's response to the pain and stress of labor causes a release of high levels of catecholamines, which also contribute to maternal metabolic acidosis (Albright et al 1986). A study of catecholamine levels in a small sample of women in labor before and after the administration of epidural anesthesia demonstrated a mean decrease of 56 percent in plasma epinephrine level and 19 percent in norepinephrine level (Snider et al 1983). Although it is not clear whether the decreases were due to alleviation of pain or denervation of the adrenal medulla, the researchers concluded that the reduction should result in increased uterine blood flow. When discussing medication alternatives with a prepared couple a positive approach should be taken to help them understand that maternal discomfort and anxiety may have as much adverse effect on the fetus as the administration of a small amount of an analgesic agent.

Many prepared couples approach childbirth confident that the psychoprophylactic techniques they have learned will enable them to cope with the discomforts of labor. There is a good deal of peer pressure on expectant parents to have the "ideal" birth experience. They may plan a natural childbirth with, perhaps, local infiltration anesthesia for episiotomy repair. The necessity for analgesia may elicit a sense of inadequacy and a feeling of guilt. The labor and delivery nurse has a very special role in assisting a woman and her partner to accept alterations in their original plan. Reassurance that accepting analgesia for discomfort is not a failure is important in maintaining the mother's self-esteem. The emphasis should be placed on the goal of a healthy, satisfying outcome for the family.

Systemic Drugs

The goal of pharmacologic pain relief during labor is to provide maximal analgesia with minimal risk for the mother and fetus. Three factors must be considered in the use of analgesic agents: (1) the effects on the mother, (2) the effects on the labor contractions, and (3) the effects on the fetus.

Maternal drug action is of primary importance because the well-being of the fetus depends on adequate functioning of the maternal cardiopulmonary system. Any alteration of function that disturbs the woman's homeostatic mechanism affects the fetal environment. Maintaining the maternal respiratory rate and blood pressure within normal range is thus of prime importance. The use of electronic fetal monitoring has provided a means of accurately assessing the effects of pharmacologic agents on uterine contractions. The Friedman labor curve provides a basis for determining the effects of drugs on the overall course of labor. (See Chapter 22 for discussion of the Friedman graph and electronic monitoring.)

All systemic drugs used for pain relief during labor cross the placental barrier by simple diffusion, with some agents crossing more readily than others. Drug action in the body depends on the rate at which the substance is metabolized by liver enzymes and excreted by the kidneys. The fetal liver enzymes and renal systems are inadequate to metabolize analgesic agents, so high doses remain active in fetal circulation for a prolonged period of time. The fetal

brain receives a greater amount of the cardiac output than the neonatal brain. The percentage of blood volume flowing to the brain is increased even further during intrauterine stress, so that the hypoxic fetus receives an even larger amount of a depressant drug. The blood-brain barrier is more permeable at the time of birth, a factor that also increases the amount of drug carried to the central nervous system. Premature fetuses are even more susceptible to the depressant effects and have higher blood concentrations because they have smaller blood and tissue volumes in which to distribute the drugs (Albright et al 1986).

ADMINISTRATION OF ANALGESIC AGENTS

The optimal time for administering analgesia is determined after making a complete assessment of many factors. In general, an analgesic agent is administered to nulliparas when the cervix has dilated to 5 or 6 cm, and to multiparas when the cervix has reached 3 or 4 cm dilatation. This is only a generalization, however; the character of the labor must be taken into account. Analgesia given too early may prolong labor, and analgesia given too late is of no value to the woman and may harm the fetus. In many institutions the nurse decides when to give the analgesic ordered by the physician/CNM. This decision is based on a complete assessment of the woman and the progress of labor.

Currently, a minimal amount of an analgesic agent is given during labor. Oral analgesics are not used because of poor absorption and prolonged gastric-emptying time. The intramuscular and intravenous routes are used instead. When the prescribed route is intramuscular, the needle must be of sufficient length to penetrate the muscle rather than only the subcutaneous fat. The intravenous route is preferred because it results in prompt, smooth, and more predictable action with a smaller total dose than the intramuscular route. When an agent is given intravenously it should be administered at a slow rate (see Table 24–1). It has been suggested that the intravenous injection be given with the onset of a contraction, when the blood flow to the uterus and the fetus is decreased. Whatever the route of administration, the power of suggestion on the part of the nurse greatly increases the effectiveness of the agent. The general principles for administering analgesic drugs are listed in Table 24–1.

NARCOTIC ANALGESICS

○   *MORPHINE*   Morphine is a pure agonist that exerts its analgesic action by attaching to opiate receptors in several brain structures. As an agonist, morphine has profound analgesic effects (Julien 1984). In addition, morphine, a CNS depressant, is thought to act on the corticothalamic pathways and the sensory areas of the brain. In

Table 24–1 General Nursing Principles for Administering Analgesic Drugs

1. The woman should be in an individual labor room.
2. The environment should be free from sensory stimuli, such as bright lights, noise, and irrelevant conversation, to allow the woman to focus on the drug action.
3. An explanation of the effects of the medication should be given, including how long the effects will last and how the drug will make the woman feel.
4. The woman should be encouraged to empty her bladder prior to administration of the drug.
5. The baseline FHR and maternal vital signs should be recorded prior to administration.
6. The physician's/CNM's written order should be checked, and the medication prepared and signed out on the narcotic or control sheet.
7. The woman should be asked again if she is allergic to any medication and her arm band should be checked for identification.
8. The drug should be administered by the route ordered, using correct technique.
9. The side rails should be pulled up for safety, and the reasons explained to the woman.
10. The medication, dosage, time, route, and site of administration should be charted on the nurse's notes and on the monitor strip.
11. The FHR should be monitored to assess the effects of the medication on the fetus, and the woman should be evaluated for the effectiveness of the analgesic agent.
12. The woman should not be left alone. If no support person is present and it is necessary for the nurse to leave, the woman should be given a short explanation and assurance that the nurse will return.
13. The woman's blood pressure, pulse, and respirations and the FHR should be rechecked after administration to identify untoward effects.

addition to raising the pain perception threshold, morphine alters the reaction to pain. It has selected action on the medulla, depressing the respiratory and cough centers and stimulating the vomiting center. Morphine also helps reduce increased cardiac output and does not depress the myocardium (Lavery 1985).

Morphine is not often used during labor. When it is used, the common dosage is 10 mg intramuscularly or 1 to 2 mg in incremental intravenous doses. The peak effect following intravenous administration occurs in approximately 20 minutes. After an intramuscular injection, the peak effect occurs in the second hour and analgesia lasts four to six hours. Adverse maternal effects include drowsiness, nausea and vomiting, itching, and light-headedness (Albright et al 1986). The maximum effect on the fetus is simultaneous with the maternal peak effect; fetal depression occurs and is most likely exhibited as decreased variability. Greater depression may occur with the morphine than with the use of meperidine because the fetal brain is more permeable to morphine (Albright et al 1986). Some clinicians feel that morphine sulfate and meperidine are associated with a similar incidence of neonatal respiratory depression at birth (Briggs et al 1986).

The woman who is receiving morphine for pain relief during labor requires frequent observation and electronic monitoring of the fetus. Maternal respiratory depression and orthostatic hypotension may occur, adding to the fetal depression caused by the agent. Vital signs must be taken frequently for early detection of any deviation from normal. The fetal heart rate, pattern, and variability are monitored continuously. The neonate's ability to sustain adequate respiration is observed closely following delivery. Oxygen, resuscitative equipment, and trained personnel must be available to manage untoward effects in the mother and baby. The opiate antagonists levallorphan (Lorfan) and naloxone (Narcan) must also be readily available.

○ *MEPERIDINE (DEMEROL)* Meperidine is a pure agonist and is the most frequently used agent for obstetric analgesia, especially where anesthesiologists are not available for continuous regional techniques. It is almost as effective as morphine but is thought to produce less respiratory depression in the mother and fetus. Meperidine is metabolized into the by-products of meperidinic acid, normeperidine, and normeperidinic acid, which are capable of depressing the neonatal respiratory center (McDonald 1985).

The intravenous route is preferred to intramuscular injection because it results in prompt, smooth, and more predictable action. In order to reduce the total drug dose necessary to achieve the desired analgesic effect, McDonald (1985) recommends titrated intravenous administration. Using this technique, the initial dose is 25 mg injected through a 25 gauge needle over a period of approximately one minute. Smaller intravenous doses are subsequently given as necessary to maintain analgesia. See Drug Guide–Meperidine Hydrochloride for further discussion and nursing implications.

○ *BUTORPHANOL TARTRATE (STADOL)* is a mixed agonist-antagonist agent. This type of agent can exert an analgesic effect when other more powerful agonists (such as morphine or meperidine) are not present in the body. In the presence of a more powerful agonist, the mixed agonist-antagonist reverses the analgesic effects. This action may precipitate withdrawal in drug-dependent adults.

The recommended dosage in labor is 2 mg intramuscularly or 1 mg intravenously every three to four hours. A titrated intravenous dose should begin with 0.5 mg. The onset is rapid, peaking at 5 minutes intravenously and 30 to 60 minutes intramuscularly, and the duration is two to four hours. It rapidly crosses the placental barrier.

As with the opiates, respiratory depression can occur. Additional adverse reactions include sedation, clamminess, nausea, dizziness, and a "floating feeling." Sedation is the most frequent side effect and occurs in 40 percent of those receiving the drug. Other side effects appear to occur at much lower rates than with the administration of meperidine (Maduska 1981).

Nursing Implications The respiratory depression and other effects are additive when administered with other central nervous system depressants such as sedatives, phenothiazides, and other tranquilizers, hypnotics, and general anesthetics. The respiratory and cardiac status of the mother should be evaluated by careful observation of vital signs. The maternal level of consciousness should also be checked frequently. Continuous electronic monitoring of the fetal heart rate, pattern, and variability is recommended. Respiratory depression can be reversed by naloxone (Narcan), which is a specific antagonist for this agent. This slightly depressed newborn is not likely to have prolonged drowsiness or sluggishness because the metabolites of butorphanol are inactive.

This agent should not be used for women with a known opiate dependency and should be used with caution if drug dependence is suspected.

Urinary retention following the administration of this drug is rare. The nurse should, however, be alert for bladder distention when a woman has received butorphanol for analgesia during labor, has intravenous fluids infusing, and receives regional anesthesia (epidural or subarachnoid block) for delivery. Butorphanol should be protected from light and stored at room temperature. This agent is not federally controlled and has been placed in the nonscheduled category. Hospitals vary in their own control of the drug.

○ *NALBUPHINE (NUBAIN)* Nalbuphine is a mixed agonist-antagonist, partial synthetic opiate that is structurally related to naloxone and oxymorphone but is pharmacologically similar to butorphanol and pentazocine. See the discussion of butorphanol for drug action and nursing implications. The recommended dosage by subcutaneous or intramuscular route is 10 to 20 mg, and the dose can be repeated in three to six hours. The initial dose for intravenous titration should be no greater than 5 mg. It is longer acting than butorphanol, but the respiratory depression apparently is not increased with cumulative doses (Am Soc Hosp Pharm 1985).

○ *OXYMORPHONE (NUMORPHAN)* Oxymorphone, a pure agonist, is a potent, semisynthetic substitute for morphine. See the discussion of morphine for drug action and nursing implications. The recommended dosage is 0.5 to 1.0 mg subcutaneously or intramuscularly, and it may be repeated every four to six hours as necessary. The initial intravenous dose is usually 0.5 mg.

○ *ALPHAPRODINE (NISENTIL)* Alphaprodine is a synthetic narcotic that is similar to morphine and meperidine. See morphine and meperidine for drug action and nursing implications. It has a rapid onset and a shorter duration (one to two hours) than meperidine. The recommended dose is 20 to 60 mg subcutaneously, or an initial 10 mg for intravenous titration (Drug Facts and Comparisons 1986). Alphaprodine should never be administered intramuscularly because the absorption rate is unpredictable with this route. This agent has been reported to cause a sinusoidal fetal heart rate pattern but Veren (1982) found no increase in fetal morbidity or mortality in infants exhibiting this pattern during the use of alphaprodine.

○ *PENTAZOCINE (TALWIN)* Pentazocine is a mixed agonist-antagonist synthetic analgesic. The agent causes less postural hypotension, nausea, vomiting, and dizziness than meperidine and crosses the placental barrier to a lesser extent (Albright et al 1986). It must be remembered that the drug's weak antagonistic properties may cause withdrawal symptoms in drug-dependent individuals. The recommended dose is 30 mg intramuscularly every two to three hours, or a smaller titrated intravenous dose (usually 20 mg) (Drug Facts and Comparisons 1986). Naloxone (Narcan) is a specific antagonist for respiratory depression.

Tissue damage can occur at the site of injection if multiple injections are given. Care should be taken that the agent is administered well into the muscle (avoid a short needle) and that the sites of injection are rotated if the drug is administered more than once. The nursing care of women receiving this agent is similar to nursing care with other analgesic agents.

OPIATE ANTAGONISTS

Opiate antagonists counteract the respiratory depressant effect of opiate-type narcotics by displacing the agonist from specific receptor sites in the central nervous system. In obstetrics, the administration of these agents is usually by the intravenous route for rapid effect.

○ *LEVALLORPHAN (LORFAN)* Levallorphan is a synthetic opiate antagonist that also has agonistic activity similar to morphine. If administered to a woman who has not received opiates recently, the agent causes respiratory depression, sedation, moderate bradycardia, and slight hypotension, as well as the unpleasant side effects of dysphoria and hallucinations. If given in the presence of large doses of morphine or morphinelike agents such as meperidine, alphaprodine, or pentazocine, levallorphan antagonizes most of the opiate-induced respiratory depression by increasing both depth and rate of respiration. If administered with other opiate drugs, it may even increase the chance of respiratory depression (Am Soc Hosp Pharm 1985).

The use of this agent has generally been replaced with naloxone. If naloxone is not available, levallorphan may be used in an initial maternal intravenous injection of 1 mg. The neonatal dose is 0.05 to 0.1 mg via umbilical cord vein. The neonatal dose may be repeated when it is certain that the asphyxia is opiate induced. Duration of action is two to five hours.

Nursing Implications If naloxone is unavailable and levallorphan is given, other resuscitative equipment and trained personnel must be available to care for the mother and infant. When the agent is administered to the mother five to ten minutes prior to delivery, the removal of the analgesic affect of the opiate may result in an uncomfortable, uncooperative woman who is suddenly in intense pain. The duration of levallorphan is shorter than that of opiates, so the nurse must be alert for a delayed return of opiate depression. An injection of levallorphan causes acute withdrawal symptoms in women who are physically dependent on opiates.

○ *NALOXONE (NARCAN)* Naloxone is a semisynthetic pure opiate antagonist devoid of agonistic (analgesic) properties. It exhibits little pharmacologic activity in the absence of opiates. Unlike levallorphan, naloxone can be used to reverse the mild respiratory depression following small doses of opiates. The drug is useful for respiratory depression caused by fentanyl, alpha-prodine, morphine, and meperidine as well as pentazocine and butorphanol (Am Soc Hosp Pharm 1985). *Naloxone is the drug of choice when the depressant is unknown because it will cause no further depression.* Although the agent may be given to the mother prior to delivery, many physicians feel it is preferable to wait and administer naloxone to the depressed infant. In this way the exact dose is known and the infant's response to the agent can be readily assessed. For neonatal dosage see Drug Guide–Narcan in Chapter 32.

Nursing Implications When naloxone is given, other resuscitative measures and trained personnel should be readily available. The duration of the drug is shorter than the analgesic drug it is acting as an antagonist for, so the nurse must be alert to the return of respiratory depression and the need for repeated doses. Naloxone should be given with caution in women with known or suspected opiate dependency because it may precipitate severe withdrawal symptoms in the newborn. For further discussion see Drug Guide–Narcan in Chapter 32.

ATARACTICS

Ataractic drugs do not relieve pain but decrease apprehension and anxiety, relieve nausea, and potentiate the effects of narcotics. Agents frequently used in labor include promethazine (Phenergan) and hydroxyzine (Vistaril). These agents may be given intramuscularly or intravenously. The peak action occurs within minutes when given intravenously and within 30 to 60 minutes when given intramuscularly.

Improved psychological preparation of the woman for labor and the use of the titrated technique for intravenous analgesia make the contribution of ataractics in labor questionable (McDonald 1985).

SEDATIVES

Sedatives formerly played an important role in the pharmacologic management of labor. However, barbiturates have the disadvantage of producing restlessness in the presence of moderate to severe pain, and they readily cross the placental barrier, causing respiratory depression in the newborn.

The principal use of barbiturates in current obstetric practice is in false labor or in the early stages of prodromal labor. An oral dose of 100 mg of secobarbital (Seconal) or pentobarbital (Nembutal) promotes relaxation and allows the woman to sleep a few hours. If the woman is in false labor, the contractions usually stop. Women in prodromal labor enter the active phase of labor in a more relaxed and rested state.

An increase in fetal depression has been reported when barbiturates are followed with opiate-type agents as labor progresses.

CONSIDERATIONS

There is no completely safe and satisfactory method of pain relief. When analgesia is used judiciously, however, it can be beneficial to the laboring woman and do little harm to the fetus. The woman who is free from fear and who has confidence in the medical and nursing personnel usually has a relatively comfortable first stage of labor and requires a minimum of medication. A positive attitude on the part of the professional nurse and the expectant parents is an essential part of pain relief.

Regional Analgesia and Anesthesia

Regional analgesia and anesthesia are achieved by injecting anesthetic agents (called *local anesthetics*) into an area that will bring the agent into direct contact with ner-

Drug Guide Meperidine Hydrochloride (Demerol)

Overview of Obstetrical Action

Meperidine hydrochloride is a narcotic analgesic that interferes with pain impulses at the subcortical level of the brain. In addition, it enhances analgesia by altering the physiologic response to pain, suppressing anxiety and apprehension, and creating a euphoric feeling. Meperidine hydrochloride is used during labor to provide analgesia. Peak analgesia occurs in 40 to 60 minutes with intramuscular and in 5 to 7 minutes with intravenous administration. Duration is 2 to 4 hours. Administration after labor has reached the active phase does not appear to delay labor or decrease uterine contraction frequency or duration. Meperidine HCl crosses the placental barrier and appears in the fetus 1 to 2 minutes after maternal intravenous injection (Briggs et al 1986).

Route, Dosage, Frequency
IM: 50 to 100 mg every 3 to 4 hours
IV: 25 to 50 mg by slow intravenous push every 3 to 4 hours

Maternal Contraindications
Hypersensitivity to meperidine, asthma

CNS depression

Respiratory depression

Fetal distress

Preterm labor if delivery is imminent

Hypotension

Respirations <12 per minute

Concurrent use with anticonvulsants may increase depressant effects

Maternal Side Effects
Respiratory depression

Nausea and vomiting, dry mouth

Drowsiness, dizziness, flushing

Transient hypotension

Tachycardia, palpitations

May precipitate or aggravate seizures in women prone to convulsive activity (Giacoia and Yaffee 1982)

Effect on Fetus/Neonate
Neonatal respiratory depression may occur if delivery occurs 60 minutes or longer after administration of the drug to the mother; incidence of respiratory depression peaks at 2 to 3 hours after administration (Briggs et al 1986)

Neonatal hypotonia, lethargy, interference of thermoregulatory response

Neurologic and behavioral alterations for up to 72 hours after delivery; presence of meperidine in neonatal urine up to 3 days following delivery (Briggs et al 1986)

May have depressed attention and social responsiveness for first 6 weeks of life (Briggs et al 1986)

Nursing Considerations

Assess the woman's history, labor and fetal status, maternal blood pressure and respirations to identify contraindications to administration

Intramuscular doses should be injected deeply to avoid irritation to subcutaneous tissue

Intravenous doses should be diluted and administered slowly

Provide for the woman's safety by instructing her to remain on bed rest, by keeping side rails up and placing call bell within reach

Evaluate effect of drug

Observe for maternal side effects

Observe newborn for respiratory depression, be prepared to initiate resuscitative measures and administer antagonist naloxone if needed

vous tissue. Local agents stabilize the cell membrane, which prevents initiation and transmission of nerve impulses and produces a temporary and reversible loss of sensation called a regional block. The regional blocks most commonly used in childbearing include peridural block (lumbar epidural), subarachnoid block (spinal for cesarean birth, low spinal or saddle block for vaginal delivery), pudendal block, and local infiltration. The regional blocks may be accomplished by a single injection or continuously by means of an indwelling plastic catheter. Before initiating any regional block, intravenous fluids should be infusing to provide hydration and direct access to the intravascular system in case of adverse effects. Regional blocks have gained widespread popularity in recent years and are particularly compatible with the goals of psychoprophylactic preparation for childbirth.

Essential prerequisites for the administration of regional analgesia and anesthesia are knowledge of the anatomy and physiology of pertinent structures, techniques for administration, the pharmacology of local anesthetics, and potential complications. With the exception of nurse anesthetists and nurse-midwives, who may perform procedures for which they have been trained, nurses in the United States may *not* legally administer anesthetic agents. However, the nurse must have an adequate knowledge of all aspects of regional anesthesia to provide support and give appropriate reinforcement of the administrator's explanation to the woman. The nurse who has a thorough understanding of the techniques and agents can also provide more efficient assistance to the administrator. The woman's safety is increased when the nurse recognizes complications and immediately initiates appropriate intervention.

The relief of pain associated with the first stage of labor can be accomplished by blocking the sensory nerves supplying the uterus with the techniques of paracervical, lumbar sympathetic, and peridural (epidural and caudal) blocks. The relief of pain associated with the second stage and delivery can be alleviated with pudendal, peridural, and subarachnoid (spinal, low spinal, and saddle) blocks (Figure 24–1).

ANESTHETIC AGENTS FOR REGIONAL BLOCKS

Local anesthetic agents block the conduction of nerve impulses from the periphery to the central nervous system by preventing the transmission of nerve impulses from the source of pain (Albright et al 1986). The types of nerve fibers are differentially sensitive to the various anesthetic agents. In general, the smaller the fiber, the more sensitive it is to local agents. It is possible to block the small C and A delta fibers, which transmit pain and temperature, without blocking the larger A alpha, A beta, and A gamma fibers, which continue to maintain a sense of pressure, muscle tone, position sense, and motor function.

Absorption of local anesthetics depends primarily on the vascularity of the area of injection. The agents also contribute to increased blood flow by causing vasomotor paralysis. Higher concentrations of drugs cause greater vasodilatation. Good maternal physical condition or a high metabolic rate aids absorption. Malnutrition, dehydration, electrolyte imbalance, and cardiovascular and pulmonary problems increase the potential for toxic effects. The pH of tissues affects the rate of absorption, which has implications for fetal complications such as acidosis. The addition of vasoconstrictors such as epinephrine delays absorption and prolongs the anesthetic effect. Recent studies have demonstrated that epinephrine decreases uteroplacen-

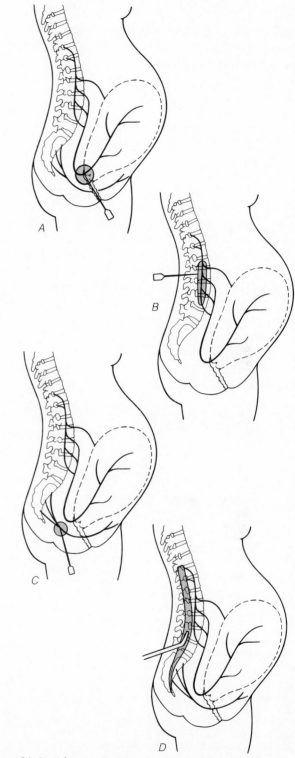

Figure 24–1   Schematic diagram showing pain pathways and sites of interruption. A Paracervical block: relief of uterine pain only. B Lumbar sympathetic block: relief of uterine pain only. C Pudendal block: relief of perineal pain. D Lumbar epidural block: dark area demonstrates peridural space and nerves affected, and the white tube represents continuous plastic catheter. (From Bonica JJ: Principles and Practice of Obstetric Analgesia and Anesthesia. Philadelphia, Davis, 1972, pp 492, 512, 521, 614)

tal blood flow, making it an undesirable additive in many situations. The breakdown of local anesthetics in the body is accomplished by the liver and plasma esterase, and the resulting substance is eliminated by the kidneys.

The weakest concentration and the smallest amount necessary to produce the desired results are advocated.

TYPES OF AGENTS

Three types of local anesthetic agents are currently available—the ester, amide, and opiate types. The ester type includes procaine hydrochloride (Novocain), chloroprocaine hydrochloride (Nesacaine), and tetracaine hydrochloride (Pontocaine). Esters are rapidly metabolized; therefore toxic maternal levels are not as likely to be reached, and placental transfer to the fetus is prevented. Amide types include lidocaine hydrochloride (Xylocaine), mepivacaine hydrochloride (Carbocaine), and bupivacaine hydrochloride (Marcaine). Amide types are more powerful and longer-acting agents. They readily cross the placenta, can be measured in the fetal circulation, and affect the fetus for a prolonged period. See Table 24–2.

The use of intrathecal and epidural routes for opiate-type agents is relatively new in obstetrical analgesia and anesthesia. Some of the agents being used include morphine, fentanyl, and meperidine. The mechanism of action seems to involve specific opiate receptors in the spinal cord (Albright et al 1986).

Advantages of these methods include (1) analgesia without the potential for toxic reaction, (2) long-lasting pain relief with little or no effect on voluntary muscle function or cardiovascular status, and (3) in small doses no effect on the fetus. The disadvantages identified so far include (1) pruritis, (2) nausea and vomiting, (3) urinary retention, (4) inadequate analgesia for perineal distention and delivery, and (5) respiratory depression.

A variety of agents and a wide range of doses have been used for epidural anesthesia with varying results. Dosages of meperidine have ranged from 25 mg to 100 mg, and achievement of acceptable analgesia has ranged from unacceptable to excellent (Hammonds et al 1982, Baraka et al 1982). All studies reported a high incidence of pruritis, nausea, and vomiting. The intrathecal route for morphine has provided good analgesia during labor with no

Table 24–2   Comparison of Local Anesthetic Agents (Esters and Amides)

	Procaine (Novocain)	Chloroprocaine (Nesacaine)	Tetracaine (Pontocaine)	Lidocaine (Xylocaine)	Mepivacaine (Carbocaine)	Bupivacaine (Marcaine)
Type	Ester	Ester	Ester	Amide	Amide	Amide
Potency	Low	Moderate	High	Moderate	Moderate	High
Onset	2–5 min	Rapid	Slow—up to 15 min	Rapid	7–15 min	4–17 min
Duration	Short—60 min	Short—40–60 min	Long—90–120 min	Intermed—70–90 min	Intermed—75–100 min	Long—90–180 min
Characteristics	Excellent for local infiltration. Unreliable for field blocks: poor permeability. Marked vasoconstriction occurs. Fetal effects negligible. Short shelf life; must be protected from light	Good spreading ability. Reliable, rapidly metabolized. Least likely to cause systemic drug reaction. Requires extreme care that subarachnoid space not penetrated. Drug of choice when fetal plasma levels are of concern	Excellent analgesia and relaxation. Not recommended for epidural due to spotty sensory and profound motor blockade. Fetal effects negligible. Available in crystalline form as Niphanoid (when mixed CSF cloudiness does occur)	Effective by all routes. Excellent spreading. Extremely stable. Causes little local vasodilation. Fetus can tolerate high concentrations provided acidosis and hypoxia are not present	Useful for all routes. Metabolized more slowly. Causes little vasodilation. Associated with fetal neurobehavioral changes. Not used for spinal anesthesia	Slow, unpredictable spread. Has weak motor block. Has the lowest degree of placenta transmission. The 0.75% solution is *not* to be used in obstetrics. *Not* approved for paracervical use. Associated with neonatal jaundice (Clark 1985) and late deceleration pattern (transient; no poor fetal outcome) (Abboud 1982)
		Addition of sodium bicarbonate may prevent neurological sequelae	Must be protected from light. Can be autoclaved only once	Can withstand repeated autoclaving	Can be autoclaved repeatedly. Spinal preparation cannot be autoclaved more than once	Noncardiotoxic. Can be autoclaved once for 15 min

Data sources: Drug Facts and Comparisons. St Louis, Lippincott, 1986. *Physician's Desk Reference.* Oradell, NJ, Medical Economics Books, 1986.

cardiorespiratory effect, but analgesia was inadequate for delivery (Baraka et al 1981, Justins et al 1982, Nybell-Lindahl et al 1981, McCaughey & Graham 1982, Bonnardot et al 1982). There was also a high incidence of nausea, vomiting, and pruritus in these groups. Brownridge (1983) reported only one incidence of delayed onset of depressed maternal respiration with 9000 doses of 50 mg of meperidine given epidurally to 2000 women following cesarean delivery.

ADVERSE MATERNAL REACTIONS TO ANESTHETIC AGENTS

Reactions to local anesthetic agents range from mild symptoms to cardiovascular collapse. Mild reactions include palpitations, vertigo, tinnitus, apprehension, confusion, headache, and a metallic taste in the mouth. Moderate reactions include more severe degrees of mild symptoms plus nausea and vomiting, hypotension, and muscle twitching, which may progress to convulsions and loss of consciousness. The severe reactions are sudden loss of consciousness, coma, severe hypotension, bradycardia, respiratory depression, and cardiac arrest. High concentrations of the agents may also cause local toxic effects on tissues. Anesthetic agents should not be used unless an intravenous line is in place.

Systemic toxic reactions most commonly occur with an excessive dose through too great a concentration or too large a volume. Accidental intravenous injection that suddenly increases the amount of the drug in maternal circulation results in depression of vasomotor, respiratory, and other medullary centers of the brain. It also depresses the heart and peripheral vascular bed. A massive intravascular dose can result in sudden circulatory collapse within one minute. Reactions to subcutaneous and extradural injection occur in 5 to 40 minutes. The short-acting agents can produce toxic reactions in 10 to 15 minutes (procaine), and the long-acting agents (mepivacaine), in 20 to 40 minutes. *It is imperative that the woman be under close supervision by knowledgeable personnel throughout the time that the agent is being used.*

If epinephrine has been added to the anesthetic agent to prolong the anesthesia, it is necessary to differentiate between reaction to the anesthetic agent and to the epinephrine. Reaction to epinephrine is characterized by pallor, perspiration, a greater increase in blood pressure and pulse than occurs with reactions to anesthetic agents, and dyspnea.

Psychogenic reactions can occur, with symptoms similar to systemic toxic reactions. This phenomenon may occur as the procedure is begun and prior to the injection of the anesthetic agent. Regardless of the cause, the symptoms must be treated.

Allergic reactions to anesthetic agents may also cocur. The manifestations of the antigen-antibody reaction include urticaria, laryngeal edema, joint pain, swelling of the tongue, and bronchospasm.

○ **INTERVENTIONS**

Treatment of Systemic Toxicity In the treatment of mild toxicity, the administration of oxygen and intravenous injection of a short-acting barbiturate to decrease anxiety is advocated. Preparation must be made to treat convulsions or cardiovascular collapse. Specific nursing interventions in the treatment of systemic toxicity are included in the nursing care plan for regional anesthesia.

Treatment of Convulsions The best treatment for convulsions is administration of oxygen, administration of 40 to 60 mg of succinylcholine, and intubation (Albright et al 1986). This method is quick, and succinylcholine can be given intramuscularly if necessary. It does not depress maternal myocardial and medullary centers, nor does it depress the fetus. This treatment has an advantage over treatment with short-acting barbiturates such as thiopental or pentobarbital, which depress maternal myocardial and medullary centers as well as the fetus. Overdosage is also more frequent with the short-acting barbiturates.

Treatment of Sudden Cardiovascular Collapse In sudden collapse, assisted ventilation with 100 percent oxygen through an endotracheal tube is indicated. The rate of intravenous fluids may be increased to support circulation. Vasopressors with inotropic (increases heart rate) action may be given, and in extreme cases, epinephrine and closed cardiac massage may be indicated.

PARACERVICAL BLOCK

The paracervical block is useful during the acceleration phase of the first stage of labor. It anesthetizes the inferior hypogastric plexus and ganglia to provide relief of pain from cervical dilatation but does not anesthetize the lower vagina or perineum. The woman should be in active labor and the cervix dilated 4 to 5 cm before initiation of the block. An indwelling catheter may be used for repeated injections and for the larger dose required for delivery. Agents commonly used for this procedure are lidocaine and chloroprocaine (Devore 1985).

This technique provides adequate anesthesia until the mother nears delivery, when another technique such as pudendal block becomes necessary.

○ **ADVANTAGES/DISADVANTAGES** The advantages of paracervical block include simplicity, and rapid onset of analgesia. The disadvantages include the following (Kyrc 1985):

- The vascularity of the area increases the possibility of rapid absorption of the agent with resulting systemic toxic reaction.

- Hematomas may occur as a result of uterine vessel damage.

- Fetal bradycardia frequently follows paracervical block with a reported incidence of 3 percent to 70 percent depending on the agent used and the presence of prior fetal distress.

o   *CONTRAINDICATIONS*   A paracervical block should not be used if there is evidence of placental insufficiency, fetal prematurity, or fetal distress (Albright et al 1986, p 212).

o   *TECHNIQUE*   A guide such as an Iowa trumpet or Kobak device is inserted into the lateral fornix of the vagina. A needle is inserted beyond the guide, and after aspirating to ensure that the needle is not in a blood vessel, between 5 and 10 mL of anesthetic solution is injected. The procedure is repeated on the opposite side (Figure 24–2).

o   *COMPLICATIONS*   The paracervical block was widely used in the 1960s and early 1970s but was almost abandoned as reports of intrauterine death appeared in the literature. Although the technique has been modified in the last decade and is used in Europe, it may become obsolete in the United States (Ueland 1986).

o   *NURSING ROLE*   Prior to the procedure, the maternal vital signs should be assessed to provide a baseline. The FHR is also assessed. An electronic fetal monitor is usually applied to provide a continuous assessment of the FHR. The procedure and expected results are explained to the woman, and any questions are answered. The nurse helps the woman into a dorsal recumbent position with her knees flexed so the agent can be administered. As the injection is given, the nurse provides support by maintaining communication, eye contact, or physical contact.

The FHR is continuously assessed. If bradycardia occurs, the woman is turned on her side and oxygen is administered. The bladder is assessed at frequent intervals because the woman may not be aware of the need to void. The amount of cervical dilatation is monitored because the paracervical block affects only the cervix and upper vagina. It is not sufficient for pain relief during delivery and episiotomy repair.

PERIDURAL BLOCK—EPIDURAL AND CAUDAL

Peridural anesthesia can provide pain relief throughout the course of labor. The peridural or *epidural space* is a potential space between the dura mater and the ligamentum flavum extending from the base of the skull to the end of the sacral canal (Figure 24–3). It contains areolar tissue, fat, lymphatics, and the internal vertebral venous plexus. Access to the space may be through the lumbar or caudal area. The technique is most frequently used as a continuous block to provide analgesia and anesthesia from active labor through episiotomy repair.

Disadvantages of peridural block are varied. Considerable skill is required for peridural techniques, and the incidence of success correlates highly with the skill and experience of the administrator. Pain relief is slower than with other methods, and a higher volume of anesthetic agent is required than for spinal anesthesia.

Fewer bony abnormalities occur in the lumbar vertebras than in the sacrum. The administrator must guard against accidental perforation of the dura mater, particularly with the lumbar epidural method, and against the

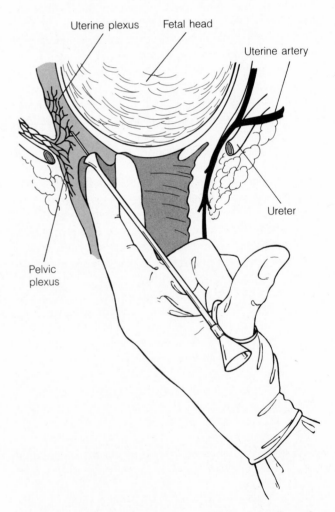

Figure 24–2 Technique for paracervical block with needle in place at appropriate distance beyond guide (From Bonica JJ: Principles and Practice of Obstetric Analgesia and Anesthesia. Philadelphia, Davis, 1972, p 515)

injection of an epidural dose into the spinal canal, with resultant high spinal anesthesia.

Peridural anesthesia is contradindicated when hemorrhage is present or likely to occur, if there is local infection at the site of injection (such as a pilonidal cyst), and in the presence of central nervous system disease or any condition in which a convulsive seizure or hypotension might have serious effects (cardiac or pulmonary disease).

The caudal block method for peridural anesthesia has been largely replaced by lumbar epidural block. The lumbar epidural method is technically easier to perform, less painful for the woman, and more reliable and requires a smaller amount of anesthetic agent.

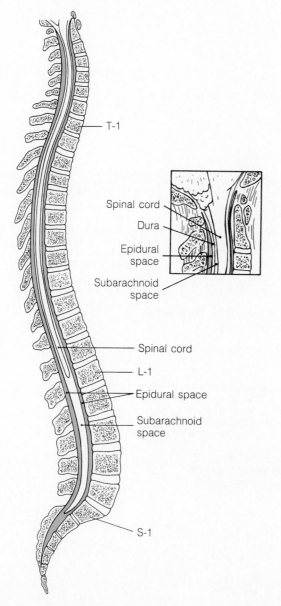

Figure 24–3 Epidural space

○   *LUMBAR EPIDURAL BLOCK* This method, particularly continuous lumbar epidural block, has become the obstetric analgesia and anesthesia of choice in many areas of the United States. It can be initiated as soon as active labor is established and is usually given when a nullipara is 5 to 6 cm dilated and a multipara is 3 to 4 cm dilated.

Advantages The lumbar epidural block produces good analgesia that alters maternal physiologic responses to pain and lowers maternal catecholamine levels (Joseppila 1984, Abboud et al 1984a). The mother is fully awake during labor and able to participate actively in delivery. This continuous technique allows different blocking for each stage of labor so that internal rotation can be accomplished and the reflex urge to bear down is preserved.

Disadvantages The disadvantages of the lumbar epidural block are that the onset of analgesia is delayed 10 to 20 minutes as compared to the pain relief provided by intravenous injections. Epidural block requires skilled personnel for administration and close observation of the mother and fetus. Variability of the fetal heart may decrease, which makes interpretation of the FHR tracing difficult. This technique is also thought to prolong labor and increase the rate of forceps delivery (Eggertsen & Steven 1984).

Contraindications The absolute contraindications for epidural block are client refusal, infection at the site of puncture, maternal problems with coagulation, allergy to the anesthetic agent, and chronic placental insufficiency. Relative contraindications include mild-to-moderate bleeding, moderate-to-severe fetal distress, prematurity, intrauterine growth retardation, postmaturity, and multiple fetuses.

The use of epidural (or spinal block) for cesarean delivery of a woman with herpetic lesions is very controversial. Some feel that the virus may be present on the skin and the skin puncture may allow for dissemination of the virus in the epidural or subarachnoid space. Ravindran (1982) reported no complications with epidural anesthesia in a sample of 30 women with herpetic lesions. Despite the fact that epidurals have been done without viral dissemination, Marx (1986) felt the risk to be too great unless there are significant contraindications to general anesthesia.

Technique for Lumbar Epidural Block The following steps must be taken in administering a lumbar epidural block:

1. The woman is placed on her left side, shoulders parallel, with her legs slightly flexed. *The spinal column is not kept convex, as it is for a spinal block, because that position reduces the peridural space to a greater degree and stretches the dura mater, making it more*

susceptible to puncture. (The epidural space is decreased during pregnancy because of venous engorgement. It is also smaller in obese and short individuals.)

2. The skin is prepared with an antiseptic agent.

3. A skin wheal is made to anesthetize the supraspinous and interspinous ligaments.

4. A short beveled 18-gauge needle with stylet is passed to the ligamentum flavum of the second, third, or fourth lumbar interspace (Figure 24–4). The ligamentum flavum is identified by its resistance to injection of saline or air. A rebound effect takes place.

5. Resistance disappears as the peridural space is entered.

6. Aspiration rules out penetration of a blood vessel.

7. A test dose of 2 to 3 mL of anesthetic agent is injected to make sure the dura mater has not been penetrated.

8. A test period of at least 5 minutes is allowed. During this time, vital signs and levels of anesthesia are checked to make sure that no untoward effects have occurred.

9. After checking again to make sure the dura mater has not been perforated, a single dose of 10 to 12 mL is injected to provide anesthesia for delivery.

Technique for Continuous Lumbar Epidural Block The procedure of a continuous lumbar epidural block is the same as for a lumbar epidural block through step 5, after which the following steps are taken:

6. A plastic catheter is threaded 3 to 5 cm beyond the tip of the needle. Hyperesthetic response in the leg, hip, or back is sometimes elicited if the soft catheter touches a nerve in the peridural space. The needle is removed. (The plastic catheter is *never* pulled back through the needle. Risk of shearing plastic catheters must be kept in mind.)

7. The catheter is taped in place.

8. A test dose of 2 to 3 mL of anesthetic agent is injected.

Table 24–3 Summary of Commonly Used Regional Blocks

Type of block	Area affected	Use during labor and birth	Nursing actions
Lumbar epidural	Vagina and perineum	Given in first stage and second stage of labor	Assess woman's knowledge regarding the block. Act as advocate to help her obtain further information if needed. Monitor maternal blood pressure to detect the major side effect, which is hypotension. Provide support and comfort. See Nursing Care Plan (p 706) for further nursing actions.
Pudendal	Perineum and lower vagina	Given in the second stage just prior to birth to provide anesthesia for episiotomy or for low forceps delivery	Assess woman's knowledge regarding the block. Act as advocate to help her obtain further information if needed.
Local infiltration	Perineum	Administered just before birth to provide anesthesia for episiotomy	Assess woman's knowledge regarding the block. Provide information as needed. Provide comfort and support. Observe perineum for bruising or other discoloration in the recovery period.

9. An analgesic dose of 5 to 6 mL is given for relief of uterine pain during the first stage of labor. Additional injections are made through the catheter as necessary.

10. An anesthetic dose of 10 to 12 mL is given just prior to delivery, with the woman sitting in an upright position.

Although other agents may be used for the epidural block, bupivacaine (Marcaine) is preferred because it produces analgesia of longer duration. Bupivacaine (Marcaine) and chloroprocaine (Nesacaine) produce good sensory analgesia with minimal motor blockade. A low concentration of the agent of choice is used to provide analgesia during labor, which avoids interference with fetal internal rotation due to paralysis of the perineal muscles. Reinforcing doses should be administered by the anesthesiologist before the anesthetic level has fallen considerably—otherwise tolerance to the agent and a reduction in the effectiveness of the block can occur. High concentrations are given for the "sitting dose" just prior to delivery to ensure good perineal relaxation.

A distressing maternal problem is inadequate block, unilateral block, or block failure. Epidural anesthesia has a higher failure rate than spinal anesthesia, because the catheter must be properly placed for adequate analgesia to occur. A one-sided block is fairly common and can be overcome by having the woman lie on the unanesthetized side and injecting more of the agent. A block may be effective except for a "spot" of pain in the inguinal or suprapubic area. Clark (1981) cites failure to block S_1 as the most likely cause. The insensitivity of the side of the foot to a pinprick demonstrates that S_1 is adequately blocked, since this area is innervated by that nerve.

Adverse Effects   The major side effect of epidural anesthesia is hypotension. This kind of anesthesia creates a sympathetic blockade, which causes a loss of peripheral resistance, a decrease in venous return to the heart, and a subsequent decrease in cardiac output resulting in lowered blood pressure. This problem can be minimized by placing a wedge under the right hip to displace uterine pressure on the vena cava and by overhydration prior to the procedure. From 500 to 1000 mL of fluid should be rapidly infused to increase blood volume and increase cardiac output. It is recommended that dextrose-free solutions be used because dextrose can cause fetal hyperglycemia with re-

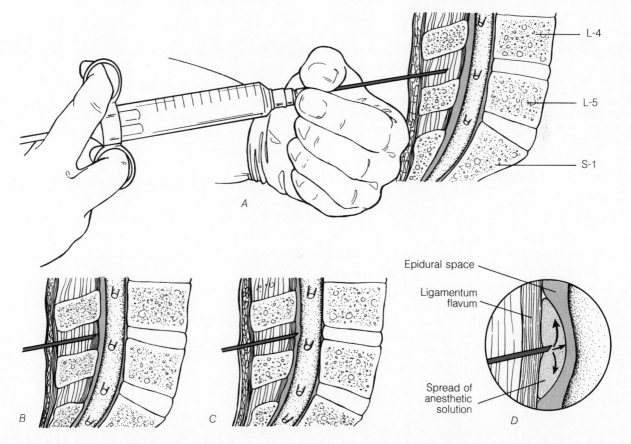

Figure 24–4   Technique of epidural block. A Proper position of insertion. B Needle in the ligamentum flavum. C Tip of needle in epidural space. D Force of injection pushing dura away from tip of needle. (From Bonica JJ: Principles and Practice of Obstetric Analgesia and Anesthesia. Philadelphia, Davis, 1972, p 631)

bound hypoglycemia the first few hours after birth (Kenepp et al 1982). Systolic pressure below 100 mm Hg or a fall in systolic pressure of greater than 30 percent of the baseline blood pressure requires treatment (Shnider et al 1983). The treatment of mild-to-moderate hypotension is to place the mother in a left lateral position, increase the rate of intravenous fluids, administer oxygen by mask to help decrease the nausea associated with a drop in blood pressure and increase fetal oxygenation, and provide reassurance to the mother. With severe or prolonged hypotension added treatment includes elevation of the mother's legs for two or three minutes to increase blood return from the extremities and administration of intravenous ephedrine. To avoid fetal compromise, it is essential to detect and treat hypotension as soon as it occurs. Maternal blood pressure and pulse must be taken every 1 to 2 minutes for 15 minutes after the injection and every 10 to 15 minutes thereafter. The regimen for initial surveillance should be repeated each time the epidural catheter is reinjected.

Other side effects include urinary retention, shivering, and headache. During epidural block the urge to void is diminished. The bladder must be checked carefully, and the woman should be encouraged to void at frequent intervals to avoid bladder distention. Catheterization may be necessary. Shivering may be caused by heat loss from increased peripheral blood flow or alteration of thermal input to the central nervous sytem when warm but not cold sensations have been suppressed. Reassurance for the mother and application of a warm blanket are the supportive therapies. Headache (of the type with spinal blocks) is not a side effect of epidural anesthesia, because the dura mater of the spinal canal has not been penetrated and there is no leakage of spinal fluid. Therefore, lying flat for a prescribed number of hours after delivery is not required. Both the mother and baby should be monitored for adverse reactions that develop long after the epidural is given (Fishburne 1984).

Complications One of the most serious complications of regional anesthesia, systemic toxic reaction, has been discussed in the section on adverse maternal reactions to anesthetic agents. Toxic reactions following a lumbar epidural may be caused by unintentional placement of the drug in the arachnoid or subarachnoid space, excessive amount of the drug in the epidural space (massive epidural), or accidental intravascular injection. Since large quantities of anesthetic agent are used for epidural block, the likelihood of toxic reactions is higher than with some of the other regional procedures. The incidence of drug reactions is relatively low but the possibility is always present. Neurologic sequelae have been reported with all anesthetic agents, but the unintentional injection of chloroprocaine (Nesacaine) into the subarachnoid space has been associated with prolonged neurological disorders (Shisky & Mallampati 1985). It has been suggested that prolonged

sensorimotor disturbances are due to a low pH and the sodium bisulfite additive in chloroprocaine (Gissen & Leith 1985, Wang et al 1984). The addition of sodium bicarbonate to the solution should decrease the possibility of nerve damage if accidental placement occurs.

Nursing Role The nurse assesses the maternal vital signs and the FHR for a baseline. The procedure and expected results are explained, and the woman's questions are answered. The woman is positioned on her left side with her shoulders parallel and her legs slightly flexed. After the block is given the woman will be returned to a supine position. The nurse takes the woman's blood pressure and pulse every 1 to 2 minutes during the first 15 minutes after the injection and every 10 to 15 minutes thereafter until they are stable.

If hypotension occurs, the nurse assists with corrective measures such as positioning the woman in a left side-lying position, increasing the flow rate of the intravenous infusion, and administering oxygen. The FHR should be assessed continuously during any hypotensive episode.

The bladder is assessed at frequent intervals because the epidural block lessens the urge to urinate. During the second stage of labor, the woman may also require more assistance with pushing, since she cannot feel her contractions and does not experience the urge to push.

Ambulation should be delayed until the anesthesia has worn off. This may take several hours, depending on the agent and the total dose. Motor control of the legs is weak but not totally absent after delivery. Return of complete sensation and the ability to control the legs are essential before ambulation is attempted. The woman must also be able to maintain blood pressure in a sitting or standing position.

Continuous Epidural Infusion Pumps The newest approach in epidural anesthesia is the use of a continuous infusion pump. Low concentrations of bupivacaine (Marcaine) were used in several studies (Kenepp et al 1982, Abboud et al 1984b). The advantages of this technique are considered to be (Morrison & Smedstad 1985):

- More stable level of analgesia, no return of painful contractions

- Lower blood concentrations of anesthetic agent

- Decreased total dose of local anesthetic

- Reduced risk if intravascular, intrathecal injection should occur

- Reduced incidence of hypotensive episodes due to decreased sympathetic block

- Minimal motor block for mother

- Ease of administration for unit personnel

Obviously, ease of administration does not indicate lack of need for close observation. Malfunctioning equipment with subsequent overdose is always a possibility. Checking the spread of analgesia and vital signs at frequent intervals is vital for the woman's safety since hypotension can still occur and immediate availability of resuscitative equipment and trained personnel must be assured. The main disadvantages are that hypotension can still occur, and the method has not been proven to be safer than intermittent injection.

The infusion pump used for injection of the local agent must have safety features such as accuracy, an adjustable flow rate that cannot be altered accidentally, and tubing that does not allow injection of other substances in error (Morrison & Smedstad 1985). Some infusion pumps are specifically designed for use in epidural anesthesia and have safety factors incorporated. At the present time, continuous epidural infusions should be administered with the same precautions used for intermittent injections.

SUBARACHNOID BLOCK (SPINAL, LOW SPINAL, OR SADDLE BLOCK)

In subarachnoid block, a local anesthetic agent is injected directly into the spinal fluid in the spinal canal to provide anesthesia for vaginal delivery and cesarean birth. For vaginal delivery, blockade to the T_{10} dermatome is usually effective, whereas cesarean delivery requires anesthesia to the T_8 dermatome (Figure 24–5). The term *saddle block* has been used to describe the subarachnoid block procedure used for vaginal delivery, but the term is incorrectly used in most cases because the area of the anesthesia is greater than the area anesthetized with a true saddle block (Pritchard et al 1985). However, *saddle block* is a more acceptable term to the general public than *low spinal block*.

The subarachnoid space is the fluid-filled area between the dura and the spinal cord. During pregnancy, the space decreases because of the distention of the epidural veins. Thus a specific dose of anesthetic produces a much higher level of anesthesia in the pregnant woman than in the nonpregnant woman. When a low spinal block is properly administered, failure rate is low.

○ *ADVANTAGES* The advantages are immediate onset of anesthesia, relative ease of administration, a smaller drug volume, and maternal compartmentalization of the drug.

○ *DISADVANTAGES* The primary disadvantage is intense blockade of sympathetic fibers resulting in a high incidence of hypotension. This leads to a greater potential for fetal hypoxia. In addition, uterine tone is maintained, which makes intrauterine manipulation difficult, and the level of spinal blockage is less predictable in laboring women.

○ *CONTRAINDICATIONS* Spinal anesthesia is contraindicated for women with severe hypovolemia, regardless of cause; central nervous system disease; infection over the site of puncture; maternal coagulation problems; and allergy to local anesthetic agents. Sepsis and active genital herpes may be considered relative rather than absolute contraindications. It is also contraindicated for women who do not wish to have spinal procedures (Albright et al 1986).

○ *TECHNIQUE* The following steps are followed in administering a subarachnoid block:

1. The woman is placed in a sitting position with feet supported on a stool. This may be uncomfortable because the block is not done until the fetal head begins to distend the perineum.

2. Intravenous infusion should be checked for patency.

3. The woman places her arms between her knees, bows her head, and arches her back to widen the intervertebral space.

4. Careful skin preparation is done, maintaining sterility.

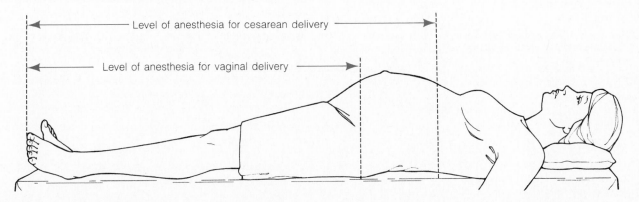

Figure 24–5 Levels of anesthesia for vaginal and cesarean deliveries (From *Regional Anesthesia in Obstetrics*. Clinical Education Aid No. 17, Columbus, Ohio, Ross Laboratories)

Nursing Care Plan: Regional Anesthesia—Lumbar Epidural

Pam Taylor is in labor with her first baby. Her contractions have been increasing in intensity, and she has been having difficulty remaining relaxed and continuing to breathe as she has been taught. She begins to ask for the regional anesthesia that she discussed with her obstetrician during the prenatal period. Although she has been planning to have a regional block, she is now not sure of the expected effects for herself and her baby. She begins to ask many questions. Mrs Taylor's vital signs are within normal limits, and the fetal status is normal.

Assessment

NURSING HISTORY

Maternal information
1. Allergies to drugs (especially anesthetic agents)
2. Psychological status
   a. What kind of anesthesia does Mrs Taylor want and what kind will she accept?
   b. Does she understand the procedure?
   c. What does she expect it to accomplish?
   d. Is she able to cope with the labor process, and can she follow directions?
3. Prenatal preparation and education
   a. Type of childbirth classes
   b. Degree of involvement in preparation classes
4. Presence of disease states
   a. Cardiovascular disorders
   b. Pulmonary disorders
   c. CNS disorders
   d. Metabolic problems
5. Course of current pregnancy
6. Support person available
Fetal information
1. Gestational age
   a. Calendar dates
   b. Ultrasound
2. Status of fetus
   a. Stability of FHR
   b. Result of assessments of fetal well-being

PHYSICAL EXAMINATION

1. Maternal vital signs and FHR to establish baselines
2. Estimation of pregnant uterus (Leopold's maneuver to determine fetal size, presentation, and position)
3. Quality of contractions
   a. Frequency
   b. Duration
   c. Intensity
4. Vaginal examination to determine
   a. Status of cervix
      (1) Dilatation
      (2) Effacement
   b. Maternal-fetal pelvic relationship
      (1) Presentation and position
      (2) Station of presenting part
   c. Rate of progress in labor
5. Determination whether site to be used for injection is free from infection

LABORATORY EXAMINATION

1. No specific tests required for mother
2. Fetal scalp blood samples if fetal distress occurs

ANALYSIS OF NURSING PRIORITIES

1. Maintaining a safe environment for the mother and fetus
2. Continuous monitoring of maternal status to detect and treat potential problems
3. Continuous monitoring of fetal status for same reason
4. Promoting thorough understanding of procedure through education of both parents

Nursing Diagnosis and Goals	Nursing Interventions	Rationale
NURSING DIAGNOSIS: Knowledge deficit related to regional analgesia and anesthesia. Anxiety related to procedures.	Provide thorough explanation of regional analgesia and anesthesia.	Regional anesthesia is frequently misunderstood and produces anxiety in clients.
SUPPORTING DATA: Mrs Taylor states she doesn't really understand what regional anesthesia means.	Thoroughly explain the regional procedure to be used.	Thorough explanation of procedure helps ensure client cooperation.
	Provide the opportunity for questions and discussions. Use charts and other teaching aids as necessary.	Misconceptions about procedure are frequent, and an accurate explanation can decrease anxiety.
Unfamiliarity with the specific procedures.	Evaluate emotional significance of regional anesthesia.	
GOALS: Mrs Taylor will be able to discuss the concept of regional anesthesia including the specific procedure planned for her, preparation, expected action, course, benefits, and risks.	Have legal permits signed.	Knowledge permits client to give informed consent.

Nursing Care Plan: Regional Anesthesia—Lumbar Epidural (continued)

Nursing Diagnosis and Goals	Nursing Interventions	Rationale
NURSING DIAGNOSIS: Potential for injury to mother and fetus related to anesthetic procedure.	Have Mrs Taylor empty her bladder.	Regional anesthesia interferes with the client's urge to void.
SUPPORTING DATA: Hypotension.	Assess maternal status and fetal status. Obtain baseline vital signs before procedure is initiated. Use fetal monitor to assess fetal heart rate, variability, and pattern.	Baseline vital signs verify status, provide basis for detecting deviation from normal. Abnormal fetal heart tracing indicates further investigation necessary before administering regional anesthesia.
GOALS: Mrs Taylor will not experience hypotension or other side effects.		
NURSING DIAGNOSIS: Potential for alteration in cardiac output due to decreased return of blood from extremities, resulting in decreased placental perfusion.	Initiate intravenous infusion.	Intravenous fluids maintain adequate hydration and provide systemic access in the event of maternal hypotension or other untoward events.
SUPPORTING DATA: Hypotension, presence of FHR deceleration, bradycardia and/or decreased variability.	Overhydrate the woman receiving an epidural block with 500–1000 mL fluid prior to procedure. Dextrose-free solution is recommended	Increased intravenous fluid intake increases blood volume and increases cardiac output to help minimize hypotension. Rapid infusion of fluids containing dextrose causes fetal hyperglycemia with rebound hypoglycemia in the first two hours after birth.
GOALS: Mrs Taylor will not experience hypotension or signs of fetal distress.		
NURSING DIAGNOSIS: Potential alteration in safe environment for mother and baby due to possible effects of anesthetic agents.	Assess Mrs Taylor's understanding of procedure and reinforce anesthesiologist's explanation. Include support person. Assist anesthesiologist with procedure.	Knowledge of procedure will increase woman's cooperation.
SUPPORTING DATA: Difficulty inserting needle. Numbness that extends beyond anticipated area. Altered sensorium.	Position Mrs Taylor correctly: 1. lateral position or upright position 2. back at edge of bed if in lateral position 3. back flexed enough to permit entry into interspinous space but not enough to cause tension on dura, which increases likelihood of accidental puncture of dura	Correct positioning of woman aids insertion of needle.
GOALS: Mrs Taylor will not experience an untoward reaction to the regional block.		

Nursing Care Plan: Regional Anesthesia—Lumbar Epidural (continued)

Nursing Diagnosis and Goals	Nursing Interventions	Rationale
NURSING DIAGNOSIS: Potential alterations in cardiac output due to sympathetic blockade.	Monitor uterus for onset of a contraction.	Uterine contraction during injection of anesthetic agent may increase upward spread to a higher level than desired.
	Converse with Mrs Taylor during test dose.	Altered sensorium may indicate a complication.
	Assist with injection and taping of catheter.	Catheter must be securely taped to prevent displacement.
	Take maternal blood pressure, pulse, and respiration every 5 minutes for 20–30 minutes.	Local anesthetic agent causes sympathetic blockade, may cause other complications. Regimen must also be followed after every reinjection.
SUPPORTING DATA: Hypotension. **GOAL:** Mrs Taylor will remain normotensive.		
NURSING DIAGNOSIS: Decreased gas exchange in fetus due to anesthetic agent.	Observe, record and report symptoms of hypotension: blood pressure <100 mm Hg or 25% fall in systolic pressure, nausea, and apprehension.	Maternal hypotension will decrease oxygenation of fetus. Early detection and immediate treatment decrease hypoxia in fetus.
SUPPORTING DATA: FHR: bradycardia, decelerations, decreased variability.	If hypotension occurs institute treatment measures: 1. Place Mrs Taylor with head flat and foot of bed elevated, left lateral position.	Gravity increases venous return to heart, increasing pulmonary blood volume; result is an increase in stroke volume and cardiac output with a rise in blood pressure.
	2. Increase IV fluid rate.	Blood volume increases and circulation improves.
	3. Administer O_2 by face mask at 8–10 L/min.	Increases oxygen content of circulating blood; mask is method of choice because woman in labor tends to breathe through her mouth.
	4. Administer vasopressor as ordered.	Vasoconstriction occurs; used only when blood pressure cannot be maintained by other means.
	Monitor blood pressure and pulse following delivery. Explain possible delayed effects of anesthetic agents on fetus.	Hypotension due to anesthetic agent may be delayed in onset. Anesthetic agents may produce neonatal neurobehavioral effects that could interfere with bonding.
	Assist Mrs Taylor to assume left lateral position.	Left lateral position prevents compression of vena cava assisting venous return from extremities.
	Monitor and record blood pressure and pulse every 15 to 20 minutes.	Early detection and treatment of hypotension can minimize effect on the fetus.
	Monitor fetal heart rate continuously.	Local anesthetic agents may cause loss of variability and late decelerations.

Nursing Care Plan: Regional Anesthesia—Lumbar Epidural (continued)

Nursing Diagnosis and Goals	Nursing Interventions	Rationale
	Observe, record, and report fetal bradycardia (FHR decrease of more than 20 beats), pattern of bradycardia, and decrease in variability. Institute measures to correct maternal hypotension if present.	Maternal hypotension causes decreased blood circulation to fetus and results in hypoxia. Anesthetic agents may cause decrease in variability, late decelerations (bupivacaine or sinusoidal pattern).
GOAL: FHR is 120–160 without decelerations.		
NURSING DIAGNOSIS: Potential for altered urinary elimination due to effects of epidural.	Assess bladder and encourage Mrs Taylor to void at frequent intervals.	Urinary retention frequently accompanies epidural block; client may be unaware of need to void.
SUPPORTING DATA: Mrs Taylor states she doesn't feel need to void. Bladder distention present. Mrs Taylor is unable to void.	Catheterize if necessary.	Client has been overhydrated and distention may (1) impede progress of labor, (2) increase chance of bladder trauma, and (3) cause lack of postpartum bladder tone. Anesthetic agents may decrease frequency of contractions. Return of uncomfortable contractions is an indication of need for reinjection of epidural catheter. Optimal time is prior to the return of painful contractions.
GOAL: Bladder distention is quickly identified and corrective actions taken.		
NURSING DIAGNOSIS: Potential for decreased frequency, duration, and intensity of contractions	Monitor contractions.	Woman does not have sensation of having contractions.
SUPPORTING DATA: Uterine contractions decrease in frequency and intensity.	Monitor contractions for return of sensation.	
GOAL: Normal uterine contraction pattern is maintained.		
NURSING DIAGNOSIS: Potential for maternal injury due to decreased motor control.	Assess progress of labor: increase in frequency and duration of contractions, observe for increase in show, perform vaginal examinations.	Woman who chooses epidural wants to experience and participate in labor and delivery.
SUPPORTING DATA: Mrs Taylor states she has little sensation and cannot control her legs.	Inform Mrs Taylor of progress in labor. Provide reassurance throughout labor. During second stage of labor coordinate Mrs Taylor's pushing effort with increased uterine pressure of contractions.	Loss of sensation may decrease awareness of the urge to "push" and the ability to push. Pushing without contraction will be ineffective and cause maternal exhaustion.

Nursing Care Plan: Regional Anesthesia—Lumbar Epidural (continued)

Nursing Diagnosis and Goals	Nursing Interventions	Rationale
SUPPORTING DATA: CON'T	Assist with "sitting dose" reinjection for delivery.	Additional anesthesia is necessary for perineal relaxation, delivery and episiotomy repair.
	Support extremities during movement. Position legs securely in stirrups (or on table for cesarean delivery).	Epidural block should not produce motor paralysis but the client may not have full control of extremities.
GOALS:	Ensure Mrs Taylor understands need for assistance with ambulation.	Motor control of the legs may be weak following epidural. Ambulation is delayed until complete sensation and ability to control legs has returned.
Mrs Taylors extremities are supported during movement. Mrs Taylor verbalizes need for assistance ambulating in the early postpartum period. Mrs Taylor asks for assistance in ambulation.		
NURSING DIAGNOSIS:		
Toxic systemic reaction.	Observe for and report symptoms of toxic reaction: excitement, disorientation, incoherent speech, muscle twitching, nausea and vomiting, and convulsions or severe reactions of sudden loss of consciousness, severe hypotension, bradycardia, respiratory depression, and cardiac arrest.	Larger volume of anesthetic agent used with epidural increases likelihood of toxic reaction.
	Small, more frequent doses of analgesic agent are recommended to avoid severe reactions.	
	Institute treatment immediately: 1. Support ventilation. 2. Increase IV fluids. 3. Administer muscle relaxant for convulsions as ordered. 4. Be prepared for respiratory and cardiac resuscitation.	Immediate treatment will lessen the effects of toxic systemic reactions on fetus.

Epilogue	
Mrs Taylor experienced no adverse effects from the regional block and had a normal labor and birth. She maintained comfort and a sense	of control throughout the whole experience. She asked for assistance to ambulate and was able to urinate shortly after the birth.

5. A skin wheal is made over L₃ or L₄.

6. The double-needle technique is advocated (Figure 24–6). A 20- or 21-gauge needle, with stylet used as an introducer, is passed through the wheal into the interspinous ligament, ligamentum flavum, and epidural space.

7. A 25- or 26-gauge needle is inserted into the larger needle and advanced through the dura into the subarachnoid space.

8. Upon removal of the stylet, a drop of fluid can be seen in the hub of the needle if the spinal canal has been entered.

9. The appropriate amount of anesthetic agent is injected slowly, and both needles are removed.

10. With hyperbaric solutions, the woman remains sitting up for 45 seconds.

11. The woman is placed on her back with a pillow

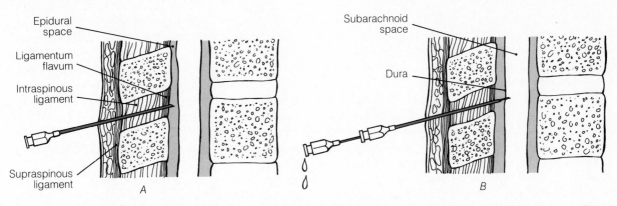

Figure 24–6   Double needle technique for spinal injection. A Large needle in epidural space. B 25–26 gauge needle in larger needle entering the spinal canal. (From Bonica JJ: Principles and Practice of Obstetric Analgesia and Anesthesia. Philadelphia, Davis, 1972, p 563)

under her head. Position changes can alter the dermatome level if done within three to five minutes. After ten minutes, a position change will not affect the level of anesthesia.

12. Blood pressure, pulse, and respiration must be monitored every one to two minutes for the first ten minutes then every five to ten minutes.

The sitting position is preferred for the administration of spinal (subarachnoid block) anesthesia. Since the procedure is not done until the presenting part is on the perineum, sitting on the edge of the delivery table may be very difficult for the laboring woman. The nurse helps the woman into a sitting position and provides encouragement and support during the procedure. The nurse informs the physician when a contraction is beginning so the anesthetic agent will not be injected at that time. After sitting upright for the prescribed number of minutes, the woman is placed in a recumbent position with her legs in stirrups.

In the absence of maternal hypotension or toxic reaction there is no direct effect on the fetus with subarachnoid block. The amount of anesthetic used is too small to reach fetal circulation in a quantity that might cause fetal depression. Spinal anesthesia was shown to be well tolerated by a healthy fetus when a maternal IV fluid load in excess of 1000 mL preceded the injection.

○   COMPLICATIONS   The complications of spinal anesthesia include hypotension, drug reaction, total spinal, neurological sequelae, and spinal headache. The side effects include nausea, shivering, and urinary retention as described in the section on lumbar epidural anesthesia. The hypotension that occurs with spinal anesthesia is more profound than with epidural anesthesia (Clark 1981). It is also important to note that hypotension following spinal anesthesia is the second most common cause of maternal death from anesthesia (Devore 1985). Hypotension can be min-

imized by hydration with 500 to 1000 mL of non-dextrose-containing fluids and displacing the uterus to the left. The practice of placing an already hypotensive woman in a sitting position following injection to prevent upward spread of hyperbaric solution is dangerous since it will cause venous pooling in the lower extremities, further decreasing the maternal blood pressure. The normal curve of the thoracic spine prevents cranial spread of an intrathecal agent. A pillow is placed under the mother's head to exaggerate the curve.

Treatment of hypotension is the same as with an epidural: positioning the women in a left lateral, head-down position and rapid infusion of intravenous fluids. The prevention of cardiovascular collapse requires early detection, supplemental oxygen, assisted ventilation, and measures to maintain the blood pressure. The extent to which the fetus is affected relates to the degree of maternal hypotension. When maternal hypotension has been reversed it is best to delay delivery for four to five minutes to allow the fetus to recover. Resuscitative equipment and trained personnel must be available to treat the mother and baby.

A total spinal occurs when there is paralysis of the respiratory muscles. It is a relatively rare but critical event. The symptoms are apnea, dilation of the pupils, loss of consciousness, and unobtainable blood pressure. The onset of symptoms usually occurs within minutes of the injection but can occur in a span of time ranging from 30 seconds to 45 minutes. Resuscitative treatment and support of blood pressure must begin immediately. If this complication occurs, it is important to remember that this woman is not asleep; although she may be paralyzed, she is aware of everything going on around her. She requires assurance that her respiration is being maintained and will continue to be maintained until she can breathe on her own.

Neurologic complications may occur coincidentally with spinal anesthesia such as with preexisting disease or faulty positioning of the woman. Genuine neurologic sequelae such as paralysis is extremely rare (Albright et al 1986).

Although much less serious than other complications, headache is an unpleasant aftermath of spinal anesthesia. It is the most frequent complication. Leakage of spinal fluid at the site of dural puncture is thought to be the cause. Several techniques have been suggested to decrease the possibility of headache. The use of a 25- or 26-gauge needle and entering the dura at a shallow angle rather than a right angle help reduce the incidence of leaking spinal fluid (Albright et al 1986). The incidence of spinal headache varies from about 70 percent after puncture with a 16-gauge needle to only about 2 percent with a 25-gauge spinal needle (Shnider & Levinson 1983). Hyperhydration and keeping the woman flat in bed for 6 to 12 hours after delivery have been recommended as preventive measures, but there is no evidence that these procedures are effective.

The postspinal block headache usually begins on the second postpartal day and lasts several days to a week. It may be of varying degrees of severity. The pain occurs or becomes worse when the woman sits or stands and decreases or ceases when she lies down or flexes and extends her head.

Treatment consists primarily of bed rest, increased fluids, and analgesics for the mild or moderate forms. Severe and incapacitating headache has been treated successfully by saline injection. In another technique, a "blood patch" is placed over the site of dural puncture. About 10 mL of blood is drawn from the woman and immediately injected into the epidural space over the site of the perforation; the clot applies pressure and seals off the leak. In many cases, this procedure has dramatically relieved symptoms. The success rate ranges from 89 percent to 100 percent.

○ *NURSING ROLE* Prior to the administration of a low spinal or saddle block for vaginal delivery, intravenous fluids should be infusing and the woman's knowledge about the procedure assessed. The woman should be able to verbalize what she thinks will happen and what is expected of her during the administration. Maternal vital signs and fetal heart rate are taken and recorded as a baseline for determining any deviation from normal during the procedure. The woman is then hydrated with 500 to 1000 mL of dextrose-free solution to maintain blood volume. Amount and time of increased infusion are noted and recorded.

The nurse positions the woman correctly on the delivery table, usually upright with her legs on a stool. The woman places her arms between her knees, bows her head (shoulders should be even with hips), and arches her back to widen the intervertebral spaces. The nurse supports the woman in this position and palpates the uterus to detect the beginning of a contraction. Intrathecal agents are not administered during a contraction because the increased pressure could cause a higher level of anesthesia than de-

sired. After the agent has been administered the woman is asked to sit upright for the length of time determined by the physician and is then assisted to the supine position with a wedge under her right hip to displace the uterus and a pillow is placed under her head. The nurse monitors blood pressure, pulse, and respirations every five minutes until delivery. Some physicians administer oxygen as a prophylactic measure. The mother should be kept informed of everything that is going on in the delivery room, particularly if she is receiving mask oxygen. Placing her legs in stirrups will facilitate venous return from the extremities. Both legs should be raised at the same time to avoid undue tension and possible injury to back muscles.

If hypotension should occur, the intravenous fluids should be increased and the uterus displaced manually to the left. Total spinal rarely occurs but the possibility must always be kept in mind. The woman should be observed for apnea, unconsciousness, pupil dilation, and unobtainable blood pressure. Prompt treatment may avert a catastrophe for the mother and/or baby. It is essential to establish an airway and give oxygen with positive pressure until the woman can be intubated and other emergency measures instituted.

Following delivery the legs should be lowered slowly and simultaneously. A sudden movement of the extremities when vasomotor paralysis is present can precipitate a hypotensive episode. Although the effectiveness of the supine position to avoid headache following a spinal is controversial, the physician's orders may include lying flat for six to eight hours.

The nursing interventions during administration of a spinal for cesarean delivery will be the same except for placing the legs in lithotomy position. It is even more important that the woman be kept informed about activities around her and reminded of the fact that she may have sensations but will not have pain. Reassurance and support of the mother are essential in helping her participate in the birth experience.

PUDENDAL BLOCK

The pudendal block technique provides perineal anesthesia for the second stage of labor, delivery, and episiotomy repair. An anesthetic agent is injected below the pudendal plexus, which arises from the anterior division of the second and third sacral nerves and the entire fourth sacral nerve. The pudendal nerve crosses the sacrosciatic notch and passes the tip of the ischial spine, where it divides into the perineal, dorsal, and inferior hemorrhoidal nerves. The perineal nerve, which is the largest branch of the pudendal plexus, supplies the skin of the vulvar area, the perineal muscles, and the urethral sphincter. The dorsal nerve supplies the clitoris, and the inferior hemorrhoidal nerve supplies the skin and muscles of the perianal region as well as the internal anal sphincter. Pudendal block provides relief of pain from perineal distention but does not relieve pain of uterine contractions.

Pudendal block is a relatively simple procedure but requires a thorough knowledge of pelvic anatomy to block the pudendal nerve adequately.

○ **ADVANTAGES/DISADVANTAGES** The advantages of pudendal block are ease of administration and absence of maternal hypotension. It also allows the use of low forceps for delivery. The disadvantages are that there is no relief from the pain of uterine contractions and it doesn't provide as good a block as the epidural or arachnoid techniques (Albright et al 1986).

A moderate dose of anesthetic agent (10 mL per side) has minimal effect on the woman and the course of labor. The urge to bear down during the second stage of labor may be eliminated, but the woman is able to do so with appropriate coaching. There is little effect on the uncompromised fetus unless overly rapid or intravascular injection occurs. The block may be done by a transvaginal or transperineal approach. Transvaginal injection is simpler, safer, and more direct, making it the procedure of choice.

○ **TECHNIQUE** A pudendal block is administered as follows:

1. The woman is placed in a lithotomy or dorsal recumbent position with her knees flexed.

2. A 12.7 to 15.24 cm, 22-gauge needle with guide is used to protect the vaginal wall and control needle depth.

3. The instrument is guided into the vagina until the ischial spine is reached (Figure 24–7).

4. The needle is advanced through the vaginal wall into the space where the pudendal nerve passes.

5. Following aspiration to make sure that the needle is not in a blood vessel, 3 to 5 mL of solution is injected.

6. The needle is advanced 1 cm more, aspiration is repeated, and another 3 to 5 mL of the agent is injected.

7. Injection of the agent into the pudendal nerve on the opposite side follows the same procedure.

Chloroprocaine (Nesacaine), which has a low toxicity, may be used if prompt but brief anesthesia is needed. Lidocaine (Xylocaine) has prompt effect and intermediate action. Other agents used are mepivacaine (Carbocaine) and bupivacaine (Marcaine).

The pudendal block is compatible with the goals of psychoprophylactic preparation for childbirth. The transvaginal technique must be done before the fetal head has

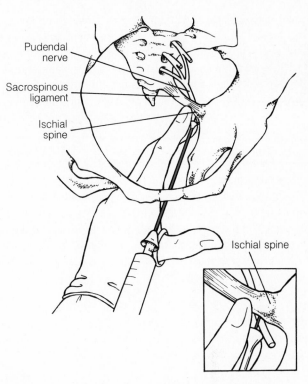

Figure 24–7 Technique for pudendal block. Inset shows needle extending beyond guide. (Modified from Bonica JJ: Principles and Practice of Obstetric Analgesia and Anesthesia. Philadelphia, Davis, 1972, p 495)

advanced too far in the birth canal. Demonstrable blood levels of anesthetic agents have been documented in the fetus but serious fetal complications are rare.

○ **COMPLICATIONS** Systemic toxic reaction can occur from accidental vascular injection. Other possible maternal complications specific to pudendal block include broad ligament hematoma, perforation of the rectum, and trauma to the sciatic nerve. Following delivery, neonatal bradycardia, hypoventilation or apnea, hypotonia, tonic seizures, and reduced responsiveness have been reported. These difficulties can usually be attributed to accidental injection of the fetal scalp.

○ **NURSING ROLE** The nurse explains the procedure and the expected effect and answers any questions. Pudendal block does not alter maternal vital signs or FHR, so additional assessments are not necessary.

LOCAL ANESTHESIA

Local anesthesia is accomplished by injection of an anesthetic agent into the intracutaneous, subcutaneous, and intramuscular areas of the perineum. It is generally used at the time of delivery for episiotomy repair and is especially useful for women delivering by psychoprophylactic methods of childbirth. The procedure is technically simple and is practically free from complications.

A disadvantage is that large amounts of solution must be used. Although any local anesthetic may be used, chloroprocaine (Nesacaine), lidocaine (Xylocaine), and mepivacaine (Carbocaine) are the agents of choice in local infiltration because of their capacity for diffusion.

○   *TECHNIQUE*   The technique of local anesthesia consists of injecting the agent with a long, beveled 22-gauge needle into the various fascial planes of the perineum (Figure 24–8). The procedure is deceptively simple; however, overdose may occur if the anesthetist does not wait for the anesthetic to take effect before injecting more solution. An excessive volume or concentration contributes to systemic toxic reactions and local toxic effects.

○   *NURSING ROLE*   The nurse explains the procedure and the expected effect and answers any questions. Local anesthetic agents have no effect on maternal vital signs or FHR, so additional assessments are unnecessary.

● General Anesthesia

The goal of obstetric anesthesia is to provide maximal pain relief with minimal side effects to the woman and her fetus. Anesthetic techniques and drugs should be selected to meet their needs. A general anesthesia may be needed for cesarean birth and surgical intervention with some obstetrical complications. The method used to achieve general anesthesia may be intravenous injection, inhalation of anesthetic agents, or a combination of both methods.

The leading cause of obstetric anesthetic death is regurgitation and aspiration of gastric contents. The physiologic changes in the gastrointestinal track during pregnancy include decreased gastric motility and delayed gastric emptying. The gastric contents are highly acid and produce chemical pneumonitis if aspirated. Every childbearing woman should be viewed as having a stomachful of hydrochloric acid. Prophylactic antacid therapy prior to general anesthesia has become common practice in the last decade.

Clear antacids such as sodium citrate, Bicitra (Gibbs & Banner 1984), and Alka Seltzer (Chen et al 1984) have recently been used one to three hours prior to scheduled cesarean delivery to decrease gastric pH. It is suggested that the woman be rotated from right to left and left to right to facilitate mixing of the antacids with gastric fluids when administered 15 to 20 minutes prior to surgery. There still remains a problem with gastric volume even when the pH has been decreased. Cimetidine (Tagamet) and ranitidine (Zantac) are being used to block production of gastric secretions thereby reducing gastric volume. These agents

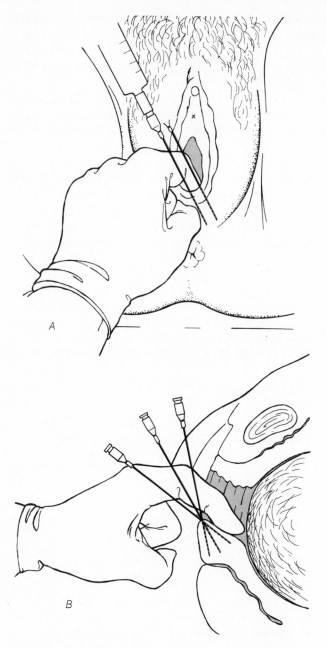

Figure 24–8 Local anesthesia. A Technique of local infiltration for episiotomy and repair. B Technique of local infiltration showing fan pattern for the fascial planes. (From Bonica JJ: Principles and Practice of Obstetric Analgesia and Anesthesia. Philadelphia, Davis, 1972, p 505)

were administered to over 10,000 women with no significant side effects in mother or infant (Moore et al 1984). Ranitidine, with a longer duration of action and lack of inhibition of hepatic drug metabolism, is the agent of choice (Moore et al 1984, Knodell 1982).

Metoclopramide (Reglan), which accelerates gastric emptying in labor, increases the lower esophageal sphincter tone, and decreases the incidence of vomiting, has also been used prior to general anesthesia. It is given intravenously about 30 minutes prior to surgery and is of value for the emergency cesarean delivery. A combination of cimetidine and metoclopramide has been used successfully (Capan et al 1983).

Because of the risk of aspiration the use of mask anesthesia without placement of an endotracheal tube can no longer be justified (Albright et al 1986, Devore 1985). In order to prevent possible regurgitation during intubation, the simplest and most effective method is to apply cricoid pressure. During the process of rapid induction of anesthesia, an assistant applies cricoid pressure as the woman loses consciousness. This is accomplished by depressing the cricoid cartilage 2 to 3 cm posteriorly so that the esophagus is occluded. Figure 24–9 shows the appropriate technique. Instead of using the other hand to support the neck, which helps avoid anatomical distortion, Crawford (1982) recommends that a firm foam rubber block be used. It is important to note that cricoid pressure is increased if active retching occurs and in any case should not be released until the cuffed endotracheal tube is in place.

Prior to induction of anesthesia, the mother should have a wedge placed under the right hip to displace the uterus and avoid vena caval compression in the supine position. She should also be preoxygenated with either three to five minutes of 100 percent oxygen or with four deep breaths of 100 percent oxygen in 15 seconds. Morris and Dewan (1985) found the latter to be as effective as breathing oxygen for three minutes. Of course intravenous fluids should be initiated so that access to the intravascular system is immediately available. The woman who has been in prolonged labor may also need to be hydrated if an infusion was not previously in place.

Many drugs have been used as obstetric anesthetic agents since chloroform was first used. Ether and nitrous oxide were first introduced in the eighteenth century for the relief of pain. Inhalation anesthetics depress the central nervous system in varying degrees, which correlate to the concentration of the agent in arterial blood entering cerebral circulation. By balancing the amount of a drug entering arterial circulation by way of the lung against the amount returning chemically intact to the lung by way of venous circulation, the anesthesiologist can control the concentration in the brain and keep the woman at the level of anesthesia desired. Inhalation anesthetics are considered to be safer than intravenously administered drugs because the circulating concentrations can be more quickly and better controlled. Once injected, intravenous agents cannot be retrieved and must be metabolized by the body for excretion.

Inhalation Anesthetics

Inhalation therapy should rarely, if ever, be used for an uncomplicated vaginal delivery (Albright et al 1986, Devore 1985).

NITROUS OXIDE

Nitrous oxide is the oldest analgesic and anesthetic gaseous agent. It provides rapid and pleasant induction; it is nonirritating, nonexplosive, and inexpensive; and it provides less disturbance in physiologic functioning than other agents. At a concentration of 40 percent, it produces excellent analgesia yet permits the laboring woman to cooperate. Little or no fetal depression occurs with this concentration. When used alone, there is no effect on the maternal respiratory center.

Nitrous oxide is generally used in combination with other agents for anesthesia. Although it is a good analgesic, nitrous oxide provides poor muscular relaxation. The main use of nitrous oxide is as an analgesic agent during the second stage of labor, as an induction agent or supplement to more potent inhalation anesthetics, and as a part of balanced anesthesia. In 1981 the FDA issued an advisory warning that chronic exposure to nitrous oxide may pose a risk of spontaneous abortion and congenital anomalies to the fetuses of health personnel.

HALOTHANE (FLUOTHANE)

Halothane, the vapor of a nonexplosive and nonflammable volatile liquid, is frequently used as a general anesthetic. Induction with this agent is smooth and rapid, safe and predictable. Halothane is nonirritating to the upper respiratory tract and causes little nausea or vomiting. It does cause depression of respiration and irritability of cardiac tissue. Only a moderate degree of muscle relaxation is produced. The agent increases blood flow to the uterus

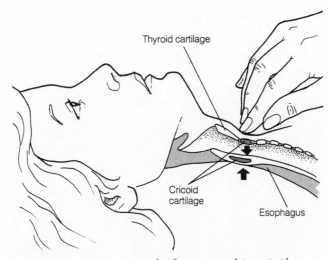

Figure 24–9 Proper position for fingers in applying cricoid pressure

and does not contribute to uterine relaxation when used in low doses.

ENFLURANE (ETHRANE)

Enflurane is considered by many to be the ideal inhalation agent since it provides cardiac stability, very good analgesia even at low levels, and a higher oxygen concentration than nitrous oxide. Effects are rapidly reversible, and the substance is rapidly eliminated by the fetus. Although seizure potential has been demonstrated on EEG, there has been no report of seizure activity (Albright et al 1986). The low solubility and rapid elimination may account for the lack of nephrotoxicity.

ISOFLURANE (FORANE)

Isoflurane is associated with low incidence of myocardial and ventilatory depression and does not cause seizure potential (Albright et al 1986). This agent is a good choice when uterine relaxation is essential. It provides relaxation while maintaining uterine blood flow and maternal blood pressure.

Intravenous Anesthetics

SODIUM THIOPENTAL (PENTOTHAL)

Sodium thiopental is an ultrashort-acting barbiturate that produces narcosis within 30 seconds after intravenous administration. Induction and emergence are smooth and pleasant, with little incidence of nausea and vomiting. The woman goes from the first stage of anesthesia to the first plane of the third stage so rapidly that the clinical signs of the levels in between are difficult to detect. Barbiturates are nonirritating to the respiratory tract and are nonexplosive. They differ from the inhalation anesthetics in two major ways: Little or no analgesia occurs, and the method of administration is less controllable.

Sodium thiopental is extremely irritating to tissues, and sloughing may result if infiltration occurs with high concentrations of the agent. Because of this effect, the integrity of the intravenous line must be checked prior to administration. The rapidity of action makes it valuable in convulsive states, particularly those that occur as side effects of local anesthetics. Maternal peak plasma concentration after injection may fall as much as 90 percent in 1 minute, so injection at the onset of a contraction prevents the fetus from receiving the transient high concentration of the agent. Hypotension, vasodilation, and laryngospasm may occur and muscle relaxation is inadequate.

Sodium thiopental is rarely used alone, because the dosage required for anesthesia produces profound central nervous system depression. It is most frequently used for induction.

KETAMINE HYDROCHLORIDE (KETALAR, KETAJECT)

The intravenous agent ketamine hydrochloride is a dissociative anesthetic with amnesic and analgesic properties. It is a useful alternative to sodium thiopental for induction of general anesthesia and is most frequently used as a single-dose induction of general anesthesia. Ketamine crosses the placental barrier within 60 to 90 seconds after injection, but causes little fetal depression with maternal doses of 0.5 to 1.0 mg/kg or less. Administration of higher doses is associated with neonatal respiratory depression and elevated bilirubin levels (Joyce et al 1986).

The advantages of ketamine are that induction is rapid and pleasant, and recovery from anesthesia is rapid. It is thought to produce less suppression of pharyngeal and laryngeal reflexes, thereby reducing risks of aspiration if vomiting should occur.

The disadvantages include a 10 percent to 20 percent increase in blood pressure and heart rate; increased oral secretions, which can be decreased by the administration of atropine; transitory apnea, which is usually associated with rapid intravenous injection, overdose, or prior medication with depressant drugs; skeletal muscle hypertonus, which is usually associated with excessive dosage and can be treated with intravenous succinylcholine; and unpleasant dreams. Use of ketamine may also induce amnesia about events surrounding delivery, which is unacceptable to many women.

Complications of General Anesthesia

The primary dangers of general anesthesia include fetal depression, uterine relaxation, and vomiting and aspiration.

FETAL DEPRESSION

Most general anesthetic agents reach the fetus in about two minutes. The depression in the fetus is directly proportional to the depth and duration of the anesthesia. The long-term significance of fetal depression in a normal delivery has not been determined. The poor fetal metabolism of general anesthetic agents is similar to that of analgesic agents administered during labor. General anesthesia is not advocated in cases in which the fetus is considered to be at high risk, particularly in premature delivery.

UTERINE RELAXATION

Most general anesthetic agents cause some degree of uterine relaxation as well as postpartal uterine atony. Following complicated vaginal delivery or cesarean delivery, the uterus must be carefully monitored for tone and vaginal flow must be observed frequently.

VOMITING AND ASPIRATION

Prevention of regurgitation has been discussed previously. If the recommended regime has not been used or has failed, the woman may aspirate gastric contents and develop a pneumonitis called Mendelson syndrome. The onset and severity of symptoms depend on whether the aspirate is solid food or liquid. Aspiration of solid food will cause coughing, bronchospasm, cyanosis, and shock. Immediate treatment is to place the delivery table in a 30° head-down position and quickly suction pharynx and larynx or remove the food with a gauze-wrapped finger. *Clearing the airway is the primary concern.* Intubation and 100 percent oxygen for pulmonary ventilation follow. A small volume pulmonary lavage may or may not be helpful.

If the aspirate is liquid, the onset and severity of symptoms are determined by the volume and pH of the fluid. The symptoms range from fine rales in the lungs, to tachypnea, tachycardia, and cyanosis, to pulmonary edema and circulatory failure. The right lung is usually affected because the right bronchus is larger than the left. Onset of symptoms ranges from immediately to six to eight hours later.

The pH of the aspirate determines subsequent treatment. Conservative management consists of oxygen (up to 100 percent) with or without positive pressure. If symptoms of infection are present, culture and sensitivity should be done and the organism treated appropriately. Chest percussion and postural drainage may be helpful in removing food particles or secretions.

Obviously the emergency interventions for aspiration just described constitute the recommended medical management of acute respiratory obstruction, but the *nursing* implications are very clear. Should aspiration occur, the labor and delivery room nurse should be prepared to act immediately by positioning the delivery table, turning the woman on her side, and initiating suction. During induction of and emergence from general anesthesia, the anesthesiologist must have an informed assistant able to provide help and give undivided attention if a crisis such as aspiration occurs.

● Neonatal Neurobehavioral Effects of Anesthesia and Analgesia

Recent studies have focused on the neonatal neurobehavioral effects of pharmacologic agents used during labor and delivery. The American Academy of Pediatrics has recommended the use of drugs that have been demonstrated to have the least effect during labor. While studies have shown that analgesic and anesthetic agents may alter the behavioral and adaptive functions of the neonate, the long-range importance of these findings has not been established.

There is a great deal of difficulty in interpreting study results. Few studies meet the criterion of solid scientific assessment of a clinical procedure. The majority are retrospective and uncontrolled. A survey of existing studies (Avard & Nimrod 1985) demonstrated that many studies had the following problems:

- Lack of a control group for comparison

- Sample size too small to achieve significance

- No blinding of observers, aware of therapeutic technique

- Lack of valid and reliable instruments for assessing neurobehavioral outcomes

- Confounding variables such as age, parity, gestational age not controlled for in the study design or analysis

- Lack of reliable and careful evaluation of neonatal drug concentration

- Too little detail for replication

One of the major problems is that studies do not distinguish between the effects of the drugs and the effects of the factors that caused the drugs to be necessary.

One study (Scanlon et al 1974) used the behavioral parameters first described by Brazelton to assess neonates' response to epidural anesthesia with lidocaine or mepivacaine and concluded that babies in these studies were "floppy but alert." In a later study (Scanlon et al 1976) bupivacaine was used as the epidural agent, and the infants did not show loss of muscle tone. This led the investigators to conclude that bupivacaine was the preferable agent. Numerous studies (Abboud et al 1982, 1983, 1984a, 1984b, 1985) tested the effect of lidocaine, chloroprocaine, and bupivacaine on the fetal, maternal, and neonatal response. They concluded there was no significant difference between the treatment groups and control groups. This finding is supported by two other researchers (Kileff et al 1984, Kuhnert et al 1984), who found only subtle changes but stated that other perinatal factors can influence neonatal behavior more than the agent used for anesthesia.

Hodgkinson and Hussain (1982) demonstrated dose-related depression and changes in neonatal EEG when meperidine was used during labor. Other researchers (Stefani et al 1982) compared nitrous oxide/oxygen and enflurane/oxygen as inhalation anesthesia with no anesthesia for vaginal delivery and found no differences in neonatal neurobehavioral response. While trying to determine the drug effect on the infant, it may be that other variables such as length of labor, parity, and drug dosage confound the issue.

Because of the methodological shortcomings in most studies, it is not possible to state whether there is a clearcut relationship between agents and outcomes. Neurobehavioral testing does not predict long-term outcome for the infant. Most of the agents are safe and effective when administered in the proper dosage, at the proper site, and with the proper precautions (Cooke & Spielman 1985).

● Analgesic and Anesthetic Considerations for the High-Risk Mother and Fetus

Up to this point the discussion of obstetric analgesia and anesthesia has dealt with the healthy mother and healthy fetus. Pain relief for high-risk women during labor and delivery requires skill in decision making, close observation, and awareness of potential threats to the mother and fetus. Safety for all involved necessitates the close cooperation of obstetrician, anesthesiologist, pediatrician, and labor and delivery nurse. The pathophysiologic changes that accompany maternal disorders have a direct influence on the choice of agent or technique. It is difficult to separate maternal and fetal complications, because whatever alters the mother's response will also affect the fetus. The effects on the woman cannot be considered without the potential effects on the fetus.

Preterm Labor

The preterm fetus has special risks and requirements. An immature fetus is more susceptible to depressant drugs because he or she has less protein available for binding; has a poorly developed blood-brain barrier, which increases the likelihood that pharmacologic agents will attain a higher concentration in the central nervous system; and has a decreased ability to metabolize and excrete drugs after birth. Analgesia during labor should be avoided whenever possible. If it becomes necessary, the smallest dose that will provide relief should be administered. Emotional support will be very valuable to the woman in this situation.

Pregnancy-Induced Hypertension

Pregnancies complicated by PIH are high-risk situations as indicated in Chapter 19. The potential for chronic placental insufficiency and/or preterm delivery are also present. The woman with mild PIH usually may have the analgesia or anesthesia of choice although the incidence of hypotension with epidural anesthesia is increased. This can usually be managed with judicial fluid increase and positioning.

The woman with severe PIH is a real challenge. Regional anesthesia seems to be the method of choice as long as hypotension can be avoided. Raising the central venous pressure by 3 to 4 cm H_2O with colloids or crystalloids helps avoid hypotension, but it must be remembered that this woman is already threatened with heart failure. The effect of fluid intake can be monitored with a CVP line or pulmonary catheter. It is important to monitor and record the fluid intake and output. Some physicians use vasopressors, while others avoid them because of the possible decrease in uterine blood flow to an already compromised fetus and the threat of a maternal cerebral vascular accident. McDonald (1985) feels that the dual catheter technique (used with caudal and epidural) is safe and effective for both the mother and fetus in PIH. Spinal anesthesia is rarely used because of the greater potential for hypotension.

With the use of general anesthesia, there is no threat of hypotension but there is a risk of aggravating maternal hypertension. The safest method for general anesthesia includes intubation, which may cause a hypertensive episode. Administration of nitroglycerine during this period will avoid the hypertensive episode (Hood et al 1985). The use of ketamine should be avoided in the induction procedure because of its potential to raise the blood pressure.

Diabetes Mellitus

Maternal diabetes mellitus requires careful surveillance throughout the childbearing period. The fetus may have compromised placental reserve, and hypotension during regional anesthesia can deplete this reserve even further. If labor can be managed without fetal distress, small doses of intravenous narcotics with pudendal block at delivery or the continuous epidural technique may be undertaken. If fetal distress occurs, surgical intervention is necessary. General anesthesia is frequently used, but McDonald (1985) has used the lumbar epidural technique with 3 percent chloroprocaine (Nesacaine) successfully for cesarean deliveries. All neonates in his study had one minute Apgar scores over 7 and good umbilical blood gases.

Cardiac Disease

Pregnancy imposes significant risk for the woman with cardiac disease. With mild mitral stenosis the anesthetic of choice is continual epidural anesthesia with low forceps delivery. This method avoids the cardiovascular changes associated with contractions and the Valsalva maneuver during bearing down in the second stage of labor. Hypotension can be avoided with carefully controlled intravenous fluids, and measuring CVP to avoid overload. A cesarean delivery may be done with epidural or general anesthesia. Ketamine should be avoided because it produces tachycardia.

Mitral valve prolapse is the most common congenital lesion seen during pregnancy. Most women will be asymptomatic but a few will experience palpitations, fatigue, anxiety, and chest pain. The anesthetic for the woman with this disorder may be general or regional, but hypovolemia and tachycardia must be avoided. Ketamine, atropine, meperidine, and ephedrine are contraindicated because of the possibility of inducing tachycardia.

The second most common valvular lesion is mitral regurgitation. Anesthetic agents that cause myocardial depression are hazards. The sympathetic blockade associated with regional anesthesia decreases peripheral resistance and improves left ventricle performance so lumbar epidural block is the preferred method of anesthesia.

Bleeding Complications

The most common causes of blood loss during the third trimester are placenta previa and abruptio placentae. With better techniques for diagnosing these conditions and determining the severity of maternal involvement and fetal maturity, the obstetrician can be more confident in the decision to manage the woman conservatively or aggressively.

The current trend is toward scheduled cesarean birth (McDonald et al 1985). When the maternal cardiovascular system is stable and there is no evidence of fetal distress, an epidural may be given for birth (Gibbs 1985). However, when either of these conditions results in active bleeding, the threat of hypovolemia must be treated immediately. Maternal hypovolemia and shock produce fetal hypoxia, acidosis, and possibly fetal demise.

Regional blocks are contraindicated during active bleeding because the sympathetic block causes vasodilatation and further reduction of the vascular volume. General anesthesia is recommended for these cases. While sodium thiopental may be used, it is a cardiac depressant and vasodilator and ketamine is a more appropriate choice for induction (Gibbs 1986). Following delivery of the infant and placenta, oxytocin should not be given as an intravenous bolus to contract the uterus because the vasodilatation produced causes a decrease in blood pressure and in total peripheral resistance. Oxytocin should be given as a dilute infusion to gain the oxytocic effect but avoid the incidence of cardiovascular changes (Gibbs 1985).

Obstetric Accidents

Prolapse of the cord is a serious emergency situation. In an otherwise uncomplicated labor, the cord may prolapse and be visible at the introitus or may be compressed in an occult manner. Fetal hypoxia with cerebral damage or death will occur unless immediate steps are taken to reduce compression of the cord. Manual elevation of the presenting part, steep Trendelenberg position, left pelvic tilt to avoid vena caval compression, and 65 percent to 70 percent maternal inspired oxygen will help maintain fetal circulation until cesarean delivery can be done. Rapid induction general anesthesia is the method of choice as long as the cord is pulsating.

The emergency cesarean delivery is a stressful situation for the obstetrical team and the mother. It is important during the flurry of activities not to lose sight of the woman's needs. Simple, concise explanations of the situation and what the woman might experience as a result of light anesthesia until delivery will help her cooperate. The support persons must also be kept fully informed. The optimal induction to delivery time is 10 to 12 minutes, but the interval between uterine incision and delivery has considerable influence on the infant's condition. With general anesthesia an interval of more than 90 seconds is associated with lower Apgar scores. An interval of three minutes produces fetal acidosis (Datta et 1981). Regardless of the situation, precautionary measures and the recommended procedure for induction of anesthesia should be followed so that maternal safety is not jeopardized.

KEY CONCEPTS

Pain relief during labor may be enhanced by psychoprophylactic methods and administration of analgesics and regional anesthesia blocks.

The goal of pharmacologic pain relief during labor is to provide maximal analgesia with minimal risk for the mother and fetus.

The optimal time for administering analgesia is determined after making a complete assessment of many factors. An analgesic agent is generally administered to nulliparas when the cervix has dilated 5 to 6 cm and to multiparas when the cervix has reached 3 to 4 cm dilatation.

Analgesic agents include meperidine, butorphanol, nalbuphine, oxymorphone, alphaprodine, and pentazocine.

Opiate antagonists counteract the respiratory depressant effect of the opiate narcotics by acting at specific receptor sites in the CNS. These drugs include levallorphan and naloxone.

Regional analgesia and anesthesia are achieved by injecting local anesthetic agents into an area that will bring the agent into direct contact with nerve tissue. Methods most commonly used in childbearing include peridural block (lumbar epidural), subarachnoid block (spinal, low spinal, or saddle block), pudendal block, and local infiltration.

Two types of local anesthetic agents used in regional blocks are amide and ester groups. The amides are absorbed quickly and can be found in maternal blood within minutes after administration, while the esters are metabolized more rapidly and have only limited placental transfer.

New agents in use for intrathecal and epidural routes include morphine, fentanyl, and meperidine.

Untoward reactions of the woman to local anesthetic agents ranges from mild symptoms, such as palpitations, to cardiovascular collapse.

The goal of general anesthesia is to provide maximal pain relief with minimal side effects to the woman and her fetus.

Complications of general anesthesia include fetal depression, uterine relaxation, vomiting, and aspiration.

The choice of analgesia and anesthesia for the high-risk woman and fetus requires careful evaluation.

REFERENCES

Abboud TK, et al: Continuous infusion epidural anesthesia in parturients receiving bupivacaine, chloroprocaine or lidocaine: Maternal, fetal and neonatal effects. *Anesth Analg* 1984a;63:421.

Abboud TK, et al: Effect of epidural analgesia during labor on fetal plasma catecholamine release. *Anesthesiology* 1984b;61(September):A413.

Abboud TK, et al: Lack of adverse neonatal neurobehavioral effects of lidocaine. *Anesth Analg* 1983;62:473.

Abboud TK, et al: Maternal, fetal and neonatal responses after epidural anesthesia with bupivacaine, chloroprocaine or lidocaine. *Anesth Analg* 1982;61:638.

Abboud TK, et al: The neonatal neurobehavioral effects of mepivacaine for epidural anesthesia during labor. *Anesthesiology* 1985;63(September):A449.

Albright GA, **Joyce** TH, **Stevenson** DK: *Anesthesia in Obstetrics,* ed 2. Boston, Butterworth, 1986.

American Academy of Pediatrics Committee on Drugs: Effect of medication during labor and delivery on infant outcome. *Pediatrics* 1978;62;402.

American Society of Hospital Pharmacists: Bupivacaine hydrochloride, in *Drug Information 85.* Bethesda, Md, 1985, p 1475.

Avard DM, **Nimrod** CM: Risks and benefits of obstetric epidural analgesia: A review. *Birth* 1985;12(Winter):215.

Baraka A, et al: Epidural meperidine-bupivacaine for obstetric analgesia. *Anesth Analg* 1982;61:652.

Baraka A, **Nouelhid** R, **Hajj** S: Intrathecal injection of morphine for obstetrical analgesia. *Anesthesia* 1981;54:136.

Biehl DR: Obstetrical anaesthesia update—1984. *Can Anaesth Soc J* 1984;31(3):523.

Bonica JJ: *Principles of Practice of Obstetric Analgesia and Anesthesia.* Philadelphia, Davis, 1972.

Bonnardot JP, et al: Maternal and fetal concentrations of morphine after intrathecal administration during labour. *Br J Anaesth* 1982;54:487,

Briggs GC, **Freeman** RK, **Yaffe** SJ: *Drugs in Pregnancy and Lactation,* ed 2. Baltimore, Williams & Wilkins, 1986.

Brownridge P: The management of headache following accidental dural puncture in obstetric patients. *Anaesth Intensive Care* 1983;11:4.

Brownridge P: A three-year survey of an obstetric epidural service with top-up doses administered by midwives. *Anaesth Intensive Care* 1982;10:298.

Bylsma-Howell M, et al: Placental transport of metoclopramide: Assessment of maternal and fetal effects. *Can Anaesth Soc J* 1983;30(5):487.

Capan LM, **Rosenberg** AD, **Carni** A: Effects of cimetidine-metoclopromide combination on gastric fluid volume and acidity. *Anesthesiology* 1983;59:A402.

Chambers WA, et al: Extradural morphine for relief of pain following cesarean section. *Br J Anaesth* 1983;55:1201.

Chandraratna PA, et al: Determination of cardiac output by transcutaneous continuous-wave ultrasonic Doppler computer. *Am J Cardiol* 1984;53:234.

Chen CT, et al: Evaluation of the efficacy of Alka Seltzer effervescent in gastric acid neutralizaion. *Anesth Analg* 1984;63:325.

Clark DA, et al: Bupivacaine alters red blood cell properties: A possible explanation for neonatal jaundice associated with maternal anesthesia. *Pediatr Res* 1985;19:341.

Clark RB: Conduction anesthesia: *Clin Obstet Gynecol* 1981;24:601.

Cohen SE, **Barrier** G: Does metoclopramide decrease gastric volume in cesarean section patients? *Anesthesiology* 1983;59:A403.

Cohen SE, **Woods** WA: The role of epidural morphine in the postcesarean patient: Efficacy and effects on bonding. *Anesthesiology* 1983;58:500.

Cooke BC, **Spielman** FJ: Problems associated with epidural anesthesia in obstetrics. *Obstet Gynecol* 1985;65(June):837.

Crawford JS: The "contracrecoid" cuboid aid to tracheal intubation, correspondence. *Anesthesia* 1982;37:345.

Crawford JS: Headache after lumbar puncture. *Lancet* 1981;2:418.

Datta S, et al: Epidural anesthesia for cesarean section in diabetic parturients: Maternal and neonatal acid base status, bupivacaine concentration. *Anesth Analg* 1981; 60(August):574.

Devore JS: Analgesia and anesthesia for delivery, in **Sciarra** JJ, **Dills** PV, **Gerbie** AB (eds): *Gynecology and Obstetrics.* Philadelphia, Harper & Row, 1985, vol 2.

Drug Facts and Comparisons. St Louis, Lippincott, 1986.

Eggertsen SC, **Steven** N: Epidural anesthesia and the course of labor and delivery. *J Fam Prac* 1984;18(2):309.

FDA Drug Bulletin. U.S. Dept. of Health and Human Services, Publication 11. Rockville, Md, 1981, p 21.

Ferguson JE II, et al: Maternal health complicatons, in **Albright** GA, et al: *Anesthesia in Obstetrics: Maternal, Fetal and Neonatal Aspects,* ed 2. Boston, Butterworth, 1986, chap 15.

Fishburne JI: Current concepts concerning the use of analgesia and anesthesia, in **Osofsky** HS (ed): *Advances in Clinical Obstetrics and Gynecology.* Baltimore, Williams & Wilkins, 1984.

Giacoia GP, **Yaffee** S: Perinatal pharmacology, in **Sciarra** JJ (ed): *Gynecology and Obstetrics.* Philadelphia, Harper & Row, 1982, vol 3.

Gibbs CP: Anesthetic management of the high risk mother, in **Sciarra** JJ, **Depp** R, **Eschenbach** DA (eds): *Gynecology and Obstetrics.* Philadelphia, Harper & Row, 1985, vol 3, chap 90.

Gibbs CP, **Banner** TC: Effectiveness of Bicitra as a preoperative antacid. *Anesthesiology* 1984;61:97.

Gibbs CP, et al: Epidural anesthesia: Leg wrapping prevents hypotension. *Anesthesiology* 1983;59:A405.

Gibbs CP, et al: Obstetric anesthesia: A national survey. *Anesthesiology* 1986;65(September):298.

Gissen D, **Leith** DE: Transient decreases in respiratory rate following epidural injections. *Anesthesiology* 1985; 62(June):822.

Hammonds W, et al: A comparison of epidural meperidine and bupivacaine for relief of labor pain. *Anesth Analg* 1982;61:187.

Hodgkins R, et al: Comparison of cimetidine (Tagamet) with antacid for safety and reducing gastric acidity before elective cesarean section. *Anesthesiology* 1983;59:86.

Hodgkinson R, **Husain** FJ: The duration of effect of maternally administered meperidine on neonatal behavior. *Anesthesiology* 1982;56:51.

Hood DD, et al: Use of nitroglycerine in preventing the hypertensive response to tracheal intubation in severe preeclampsia. *Anesthesiology* 1985;63(August):329.

James CF, **Caton** D, **Banner** T: Noninvasive determination of cardiac output during cesarean section. *Anesthesiology* 1984;61(September):413.

Johnson JR, et al: Use of cimetidine as an oral antacid in obstetric anesthesia. *Anesth Analg* 1983;62(August):720.

Joseppila R: Maternal and umbilical cord noradrenaline concentrations during labor with and without segmental extradural analgesia and during caesarean section. *B Jr Anaesth* 1984;56:251.

Joyce TH, **Albright** GA, **Longmire** S: Inhalation anesthetics and ketamine, in **Albright** GA, et al: *Anesthesia in Obstetrics: Maternal, Fetal and Neonatal Aspects,* ed 2. Boston, Butterworth, 1986, chap 8.

Julien RM: *Understanding Anesthesia.* Menlo Park, Calif, Addison-Wesley, 1984.

Justins DM, et al: A controlled trial of fentanyl in labor. *Br J Anaesth* 1982;54:409.

Kenepp NB, et al: Fetal and neonatal hazards of maternal hydration with 5 percent dextrose before cesarean section. *Lancet* 1982;1:1150.

Kileff ME, et al: Neonatal neurobehavioral responses after epidural anesthesia for cesarean section using lidocaine and bupivacaine. *Anesth Analg* 1984;63:413.

Kotelko DM, et al: Epidural morphine analgesia after cesarean delivery. *Obstet Gynecol* 1984;63(March):409.

Kuhnert BR, et al: Effect of maternal epidural anesthesia on neonatal behavior. *Anesth Analg* 1984;63:301.

Kyrc JJ: Local anesthetics in obstetrics, in **Sciarra** JJ, **Depp** R, **Eschenback** DA (eds): *Gynecology and Obstetrics.* Philadelphia, Harper & Row, 1985, vol 3.

Lavery JP: Morphine for obstetric analgesia. *Contemp OB/GYN,* 1985;(April):95.

Lester BM, **Heidelise** A, **Brazelton** TB: Regional obstetric anesthesia and newborn behavior: A reanalysis toward synergystic effects. *Child Dev* 1982;53:687.

Maduska AL: Butorphanol in obstetric anesthesia. *Anesth Dev* 1981;8:1417.

Marx G: Fundamental concerns, in **Albright** GA, et al (eds): *Anesthesia in Obstetrics,* ed 2. Boston, Butterworth, 1986, chap 10, p 251.

McCaughey W, **Graham** AL: The respiratory depression of epidural morphine. *Anaesthesia* 1982;37:990.

McDonald JS: Anesthesia and the high risk fetus, in **Sciarra** JJ, **Depp** R, **Eschenback** DA (eds): *Gynecology and Obstetrics.* Philadelphia, Harper & Row, 1985, chap 91.

McGuiness C, **Rosen** M: Enflurane as an analgesic in labor. *Anaesthesia* 1984;39:24.

Moore A, et al: Spinal fluid kinetics of morphine. *Clin Pharmacol Ther* 1984;35(January):40.

Moore DC, et al: Chloroprocaine neurotoxicity: Four additional cases. *Anesth Analg* 1982;61:155.

Moore TR, et al: Evaluation of continuous lumbar epidural anesthesia for hypotensive women in labor. *Am J Obstet Gynecol* 1985;152(4):404.

Morris MC, **Dewan** D: Pre-oxygenation for cesarean section: A comparison of two techniques. *Anesthesiology* 1985;62:827.

Morrison DH, **Smedstad** KG: Continuous epidurals for obstetric analgesia. *Can Anaesth Soc J* 1985;32(2):101.

Nybell-Lindahl G, et al: Maternal and fetal concentrations of morphine after fetal epidural administration during labor. *Am J Obstet Gynecol* 1981;139:20.

Oriel N, **Warfield** C: Pain relief during labor. *Hosp Prac* September 1984;30:151.

Oyama T, et al: Beta-endorphin in obstetrical analgesia. *Am J Obstet Gynecol* 1980;137:613.

Pedersen H, **Norishima** HO, **Finster** M: Anesthesia during pregnancy and parturition, in **Eskes** AB, **Finster** M (eds): *Drug Therapy During Pregnancy.* London, Butterworth, 1985.

Philipson EH, **Kuhnert** BR, **Syracuse** CD: Fetal acidosis, 2-chloroprocaine and epidural anesthesia. *Am J Obstet Gynecol* 1985;151(February):322.

Pritchard JA, **MacDonald** PC, **Gant** NF: *Williams Obstetrics,* ed 17. New York, Appleton-Century-Crofts, 1985.

Ravindran RS: Epidural analgesia in the presence of herpes simplex virus (type 2) infection. *Anesth Analg* 1982;61:714.

Remanathan S, et al: Maternal and fetal effects of prophylactic hydration with crystalloids or colloids before epidural anesthesia. *Anesth Analg* 1983;62:673.

Roberts WE, **Normal** PF, **Morrison** J: Pros and cons of meperidine for intrapartum analgesia. *Contemp OB/GYN,* 1984;(April):69.

Scanlon JW, et al: Neurobehavioral responses of newborn infants after maternal epidural anesthesia. *Anesthesiology* 1974;40(2):121.

Shisky MC, **Mallampati** SR: Prolonged neural blockade following caudal epidural block with chloroprocaine. *Reg Anesth* 1985;10:28.

Shnider SM, **Levinson** G. *Anesthesia for Obstetrics.* Baltimore, Williams & Wilkins, 1979.

Shnider SM, et al: Maternal catecholamines decrease during labor after lumbar epidural anesthesia. *Am J Obstet Gynecol* 1983;147(September):13.

Stefani SJ, et al: Neonatal neurobehavioral effects of inhalation analgesia for vaginal delivery. *Anesthesiology* 1982;56:351.

Stevenson DK, **Albright** CA, **Benitz** WE: Disorders of fetal growth and development, in **Albright** GA, et al: *Anesthesia in Obstetrics: Maternal, Fetal and Neonatal Aspects,* ed 2. Boston, Butterworth, 1986, chap 19.

Ueland K: Paracervical, pudendal, and field blocks, in **Albright** GA, et al: *Anesthesia in Obstetrics: Maternal, Fetal and Neonatal Aspects,* ed 2. Boston, Butterworth, 1986, chap 9.

Veren D, et al: The clinical significance of a sinusoidal FHR pattern associated with alphaprodine administration. *J Reprod Med* 1982;27(July):411.

Wang BC, et al: Effects of the anesthetic chloroprocaine on the anti-oxidant sodium bisulfate. *Anesth Analg* 1984;63(April):445.

Warren TM, et al: Comparison of maternal and neonatal effects of halothane, enflurane and isoflurane for cesarean delivery. *Anesth Analg* 1983;62(May):516.

ADDITIONAL READINGS

Albright GA, **Petree** BJ: Birthing, the obstetric nurse and psychoanalgesia, in **Albright** GA, et al: *Anesthesia in Obstetrics: Maternal, Fetal and Neonatal Aspects,* ed 2. Boston, Butterworth, 1986, chap 6.

Cohen SE: The aspiration syndrome. *Clin Obstet Gynecol* 1982;9:235.

Hollenbeck AR, et al: Labor and delivery medication influences parent-infant interaction in the first postpartum month. *Infant Behav Dev* 1984;7:201.

Jensen F, et al: Submucous paracervical blockade compared with intramuscular meperidine as analgesia during labor: A double blind study. *Obstet Gynecol* 1984; 64(November):724.

Poore M, **Foster** JC: Epidural and no epidural anesthesia: Differences between mothers and their experiences of birth. *Birth* 1985;12(Winter):205.

What we need is confidence in our bodies and our abilities to give birth. We need to reclaim the past by feeling our connection with all women who have given birth before us, and know that our bodies know and are equal to the task at hand. (Pregnant Feelings)

The Intrapartal Family at Risk

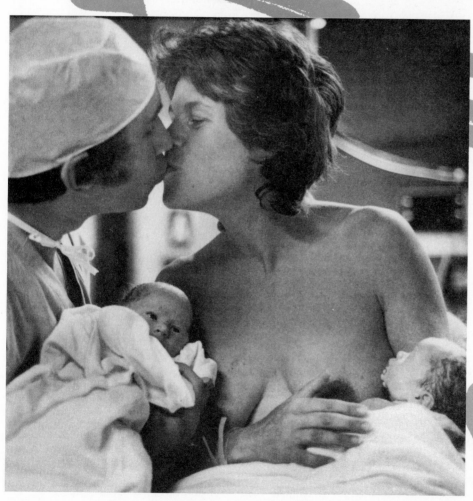

Despite the additional medical and nursing support required, the birth of twins can be an intimate and joyous event for the whole family.

Chapter Twenty-Five

Care of the Woman With Dysfunctional Labor
Hypertonic Labor Patterns
Hypotonic Labor Patterns
Prolonged Labor
Precipitous Labor

Care of the Woman With Premature Rupture of Membranes
Maternal Risks
Fetal-Neonatal Risks
Medical Therapy
Nursing Assessment
Nursing Diagnosis
Nursing Goal: Promotion of Maternal-Fetal Physical Well-Being
Nursing Goal: Client Education
Nursing Goal: Provision of Psychologic Support
Evaluative Outcome Criteria

Care of the Woman at Risk Due to Preterm Labor
Maternal Risks
Fetal-Neonatal Risks
Medical Therapy
Nursing Assessment
Nursing Diagnosis
Nursing Goal: Teaching Prevention Measures
Nursing Goal: Promotion of Maternal-Fetal Physical Well-Being During Labor
Nursing Goal: Provision of Emotional Support to the Family
Evaluative Outime Criteria

Care of the Woman With Postdate Pregnancy
Maternal Risks
Fetal-Neonatal Risks
Medical Therapy
Nursing Assessment
Nursing Diagnosis
Nursing Goal: Promotion of Fetal Well-Being
Nursing Goal: Promotion of Maternal Psychologic Support
Nursing Goal: Client Education
Evaluative Outcome Criteria

Care of the Woman With a Ruptured Uterus
Maternal Risks
Fetal-Neonatal Risks
Medical Therapy
Nursing Assessment
Nursing Diagnosis
Nursing Goal: Promotion of Maternal-Fetal Physical Well-Being
Nursing Goal: Provision of Emotional Support to the Woman and Family

Care of the Woman and Fetus at Risk Due to Fetal Malposition
Occiput-Posterior Position
Transverse Arrest

Care of the Woman and Fetus at Risk Due to Fetal Malpresentation
Brow Presentation
Face Presentation
Breech Presentation
Transverse Lie (Shoulder Presentation)
Compound Presentation

Care of the Woman and Fetus at Risk Due to Developmental Abnormalities
Macrosomia
Hydrocephalus
Other Fetal Malformations

Care of the Woman With a Multiple Pregnancy
Twin Pregnancy
Three or More Fetuses

Care of the Woman and Fetus in the Presence of Fetal Distress
Maternal Risks
Fetal-Neonatal Risks
Medical Therapy
Nursing Assessment
Nursing Diagnosis
Nursing Goal: Provision of Emotional Support to Family
Nursing Goal: Promotion of Maternal and Fetal Physical Well-Being

Care of the Family at Risk Due to Intrauterine Fetal Death
Maternal Risks
Medical Therapy
Nursing Assessment
Nursing Diagnosis
Nursing Goal: Provision of Emotional Support to the Family
Evaluative Outcome Criteria

Care of the Woman and Fetus at Risk Due to Placental Problems
Abruptio Placentae
Placenta Previa
Other Placental Problems

Care of the Woman With Disseminated Intravascular Coagulation
Medical Therapy
Nursing Assessment
Nursing Diagnosis
Nursing Goal: Promotion of Physical Well-Being
Nursing Goal: Provision of Emotional Support
Evaluative Outcome Criteria

Care of the Woman and Fetus at Risk Due to Problems Associated With the Umbilical Cord
Prolapsed Umbilical Cord
Umbilical Cord Abnormalities

OBJECTIVES

- Examine the psychologic factors that may contribute to complications during labor and delivery.
- Compare dysfunctional labor patterns.
- Relate various types of fetal malposition and malpresentation to possible associated problems.
- Describe abruptio placentae, placenta previa, and associated bleeding problems.
- Explain the nursing care that is indicated in the event of fetal distress.
- Discuss intrauterine fetal death including etiology, diagnosis, management, and the nurse's role in assisting the family.
- Distinguish variations that may occur in the umbilical cord and insertion into the placenta.
- Relate the implications of pelvic contractures to the labor and delivery process and outcome.
- Discuss complications of the third and fourth stages.

- Summarize the effects of childbirth complications on the family.

The successful completion of the 40-week gestational period requires the harmonious functioning of four components: the passenger, passage, powers, and psyche. (These components are described in depth in Chapter 21.) Briefly, the passenger includes all the products of conception: fetus, placenta, cord, membranes, and amniotic fluid. The passage comprises the vagina, introitus, and bony pelvis, and the powers are the myometrial forces of the contracting uterus. The psyche includes the intellectual and emotional processes of the pregnant woman as influenced by heredity and environment and her feelings about pregnancy and motherhood. Disruptions in any of the four components may affect the others and cause *dystocia* (abnormal or difficult labor).

● Using the Nursing Process With Families at Risk During the Intrapartal Period

The nursing process forms a basis for the provision of nursing care to the woman and her family when there are problems associated with the pregnancy.

Nursing Assessment

The nurse collects information regarding the woman's history and correlates it with known information regarding predisposing factors. The history helps the nurse identify pertinent assessments that need to be made.

Analysis and Nursing Diagnosis

The nurse looks for cues that may suggest the woman is at risk for problems during the intrapartal period. Sometimes subtle clues may be the only indication of a developing problem. The nurse operates on her or his knowledge of normal labor and delivery, and thus is able to identify problems quickly.

The nurse organizes the data and assessment information into nursing diagnoses that are appropriate for a woman at risk in the intrapartal period. Nursing diagnoses that may apply include:

- Knowledge deficit related to the possible implications and problems associated with intrapartal problems

● Potential for injury to the fetus related to decreased blood supply, secondary cord compression, problems during labor, or birth trauma

● Potential inadequate individual coping related to unanticipated problems in labor and/or birth

● Fear related to unknown outcome of the labor and birth

Nursing Implementation

After nursing diagnoses are identified, the nurse identifies nursing interventions to prevent or treat designated client problems. The nurse uses basic nursing skills and special intrapartal interventions to provide nursing care to the intrapartal family at risk.

Evaluation

Evaluation of the woman's response to care and the effectiveness of the nursing interventions is an ongoing process. As a result of evaluation, the nurse may redesign the plan of care or add other nursing interventions.

● Care of the Woman at Risk Due to Excessive Anxiety and Fear

Stress, anxiety, and fear have a profound effect on labor, particularly when complications occur that imply maternal or fetal jeopardy. A labor process that was initially viewed with confidence and happiness may now provoke anxiety and a variety of physiologic and psychologic responses.

Neural and endocrine changes are produced by stress and anxiety. The liver releases glucose to satisfy the body's increased energy needs. The bronchial tree dilates for increased oxygen intake. The anterior pituitary is stimulated, which results in an increase in production of glucocorticoids and mineralocorticoids by the adrenal cortex. These hormones promote the retention of sodium and the excretion of potassium and also stimulate the posterior pituitary to release antidiuretic hormone for the conservation of water. The loss of potassium is postulated to assist in the reduction of myometrial activity. The reduction of glucose stores from stress and anxiety decreases the availability of glucose used by a contracting uterus.

The sympathetic nervous system stimulates the adrenal medulla, resulting in the secretion of epinephrine, which increases the heart rate, cardiac output, and blood pressure. The sympathetic nervous system also stimulates the adrenals to release norepinephrine, which increases peripheral vasoconstriction and blood flow to the vital organs. This physiologic reaction can adversely affect the contracting uterus. The uterus responds to alpha-excitatory and beta-inhibitory effects of epinephrine. Through baroreceptor stimulation, epinephrine inhibits myometrial activity (beta-receptors), uterine contractility decreases, and labor is prolonged (Lederman 1984).

The anxiety, fear, and pain experienced by the laboring woman may produce a vicious cycle, resulting in increased fear and anxiety because of continued central pain perception. This leads to enhanced catecholamine release, which in turn increases physical distress and may result in myometrial dysfunction and ineffectual labor (Lederman et al 1985).

Nursing Assessment

Unless delivery is imminent or severe complications exist, the nurse begins the assessment by reviewing the woman's background. Factors such as age, parity, marital and socioeconomic status, culture, and knowledge and understanding of the labor process contribute to the woman's psychological response to labor.

As labor progresses, the nurse is alert for the woman's verbal and nonverbal behavioral responses to the pain and anxiety coexisting with labor. The woman who is agitated and noncompliant, or too quiet and compliant, may require further appraisal for anxiety. Verbal statements such as "Is everything okay?" "I'm really nervous," or "What's going on?" usually indicate some degree of anxiety and concern. Other women may be irritable, require frequent explanations, or repeat the same questions. The nurse further observes for nonverbal cues including a tense posture, clenched hands, or pain out of context to the stage of labor. Recognizing the impact of fatigue on pain and anxiety is another important nursing observation.

Nursing Diagnosis

Nursing diagnoses that may apply to the woman with excessive fear or anxiety include:

● Anxiety related to stress of the labor process

● Fear related to unknown outcome of labor

● Ineffective individual coping related to inability to use relaxation techniques during labor

Nursing Goal: Anticipatory Education During the Prenatal Period

Nursing research demonstrates that education is effective in minimizing the stress accompanying labor. Research findings generally indicate that women who participate in prenatal classes benefit by maintaining better control in labor, decreasing their use of ataractics and analgesics, manifesting more positive attitudes, and experiencing feelings of anticipation rather than fear (Genest 1981, Sasmor et al 1981).

Antepartal classes provide relevant information about the developmental and psychologic changes that can be expected during childbirth and teach relaxation strategies to reduce the anxiety and pain of labor. Couples learn coping mechanisms in the form of physical and emotional comfort measures, controlled breathing exercises, and relaxation techniques.

Nursing Goal: Provision of Support During Labor and Delivery

Prepared couples should be offered support and encouragement by the nurse as they employ the techniques they have learned. If the mother begins to lose control, the nurse can often assist the partner in helping the mother regain control. If anxiety is evident, the nurse should acknowledge and alleviate it, if possible, through comfort measures (see Chapter 23).

Unprepared couples can be taught many of these activities at the time of admission, especially if active labor has not begun. Clear but succinct information about the labor process, medical procedures, the environment, simple breathing exercises, and relaxation techniques can be given, thereby preventing or relieving some apprehension and fear. Even a woman in active labor who has had no prior preparation can achieve a great deal of relaxation from physical comfort measures, touch, constant attention, therapeutic interaction, and, possibly, analgesics.

The nurse's ability to help the woman and her partner cope with the stress of labor is directly related to the rapport established among them. By employing a calm, caring, confident, nonjudgmental approach, the nurse not only is able to acknowledge the anxiety, but also is often able to identify the source of the distress. Once the causative factors are known, the appropriate interventions, such as information, comfort measures, touch, or therapeutic communication, can be implemented.

Nursing Goal: Provision of Support During the Postpartal Period

If possible, the nurse should follow up with the mother after the labor and delivery to review the intrapartal process. Further explanations and reassurance may be offered as the woman's needs dictate. This is also an opportune time for the mother to share feelings about the labor.

Evaluative Outcome Criteria

Anticipated outcomes of nursing care include the following:

- The woman experiences a decrease in physiologic signs of stress and an increase in psychologic comfort.

- The woman is able to use effective coping mechanisms to manage her anxiety in labor.

- The woman's fear is decreased.

- The woman is able to verbalize feelings regarding her labor.

● Care of the Woman With Dysfunctional Labor

The myometrial forces of the contracting uterus depend on one or more contracting muscles stimulating the contraction of one or more adjacent muscles. The resulting wave of contractions then spreads for variable distances over the myometrium. The contractility of the uterus is affected by the following factors: (a) the energy source; (b) the ionic exchange of electrolytes; (c) the contractile proteins; and (d) the endocrine sources (Danforth & Scott 1986). See page 584 for further discussion. These four factors must interact for effective labor to occur. Any disruption in the interaction of these factors may result in ineffective, dysfunctional labor.

Dysfunctional labor that causes a delay in the delivery of the newborn is due to problems with the mechanisms of labor. Dysfunctional labor can have a profound effect on the woman as well as the fetus. Prolonged labor of over 24 hours' duration is associated with an increase in maternal and infant mortality, usually resulting from infection.

Fetal conditions associated with dysfunctional labor include fetal hypoxia and problems associated with cephalopelvic disproportion (CPD) between the maternal pelvis and fetus (such as bone fractures, internal hemorrhage, and neurologic changes resulting from compression).

Dysfunctional labor includes hypertonic and hypotonic labor patterns, prolonged labor, and precipitous labor. In hypertonic labor patterns, ineffectual contractions of poor quality occur in the latent phase of labor. In hypotonic labor patterns, early labor is well established with effective contractions, but the active phase of labor becomes prolonged or halts. Either type of dysfunctional labor may result in prolonged labor, which has potentially serious implications for the woman and fetus.

Hypertonic Labor Patterns

In *hypertonic* uterine motility, the resting tone of the myometrium rises more than 15 mm Hg and may rise as much as 50 to 85 mm Hg. The frequency of contractions is usually increased, whereas the intensity may be decreased (Figure 25–1B).

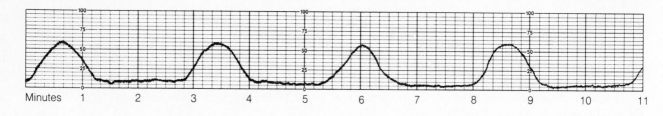

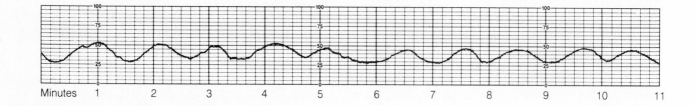

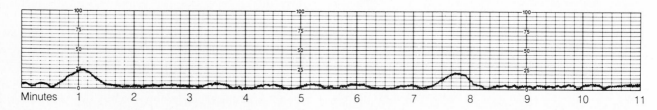

Figure 25–1 Comparison of labor patterns. A Normal uterine contraction pattern. Note contraction frequency is every 3 minutes, duration is 60 seconds. The baseline resting tone is below 10 mm Hg. B Hypertonic uterine pattern. Note in this example that the contraction frequency is every minute, duration is 50 seconds (which allows only a 10-second rest between contractions), intensity increases approximately 25 mm Hg during the contraction, and the resting tone of the uterus is increased. C Hypotonic uterine contraction pattern. Note in this example that the contraction frequency is every 7 minutes with some uterine activity between contractions, duration is 50 seconds, and intensity increases approximately 25 mm Hg during contractions.

The number of fibers in the myometrium that are not contracting and are free to receive new impulses from the pacemakers is diminished, which results in an increased resting tone due to premature interruption of the refractory period (Pritchard et al 1985).

Contractions are painful but ineffective in dilating and effacing the cervix, which may lead to a prolonged latent phase. Very anxious nulliparas at term or postterm are most commonly afflicted with hypertonic labor.

MATERNAL RISKS

Hypertonic labor patterns are extremely painful because of uterine muscle cell anoxia. There is an increase in uterine muscle tone but little cervical dilatation and effacement. Because hypertonic labor often occurs in the latent phase of labor, when dilatation may be no more than 2 or 3 cm, the woman may be accused of overreacting to her labor. She may be aware of the lack of progress and become anxious and discouraged. A woman who has prepared for her labor and delivery may feel frustrated as her coping mechanisms are severely tested.

FETAL-NEONATAL RISKS

Fetal distress occurs early, because contractions interfere with the uteroplacental exchange. If this distress goes unidentified, the fetus may be lost. In any situation in which pressure on the fetal head is prolonged, cephalhematoma, caput succedaneum, or excessive molding may occur (Figure 25–2).

MEDICAL THERAPY

As long as the membranes are intact and there are no indications of fetal distress, the goal of treatment is to arrest uterine activity and establish a more effective labor pattern. This is accomplished by promoting relaxation and reducing pain. Bed rest and sedation are common medical treatments. Oxytocin is not administered to a woman suffering from hypertonic uterine activity, because it is likely to accentuate the abnormal labor pattern (Pritchard et al 1985). If the hypertonic pattern continues and develops into a prolonged latent phase, the physician may use an oxytocin infusion and/or amniotomy as treatment methods. These methods are instituted only after CPD and fetal malpresentations have been ruled out. If signs of fetal distress become apparent, cesarean delivery may be necessary.

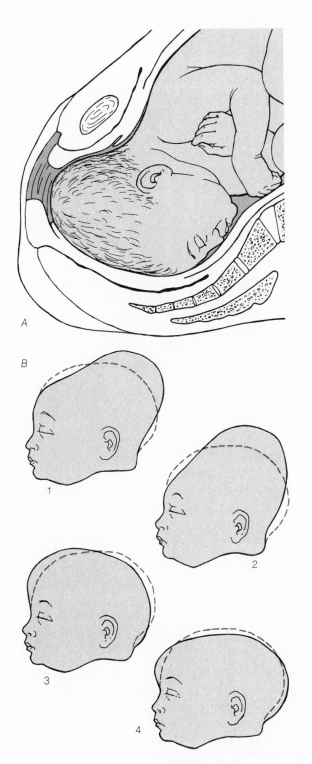

Figure 25–2 Effects of labor on fetal head. A Caput succedaneum formation. The presenting portion of the scalp is encircled by the cervix during labor, which causes swelling of the soft tissue. B Molding of fetal head in cephalic presentations: 1 occiput anterior, 2 occiput posterior, 3 brow, 4 face

NURSING ASSESSMENT

The relationship between the intensity of pain being experienced and the degree to which the cervix is dilating and effacing should be evaluated as a part of the labor assessment. Whether anxiety is having a deleterious effect on labor progress should also be noted, especially if the mother is a primigravida or is postterm. Evidence of increasing frustration and discouragement on the part of the mother and her partner may become apparent as labor ensues and their birth plan cannot be followed.

NURSING DIAGNOSIS

Nursing diagnoses that may apply to the woman in hypertonic labor include:

- Alteration in comfort: pain related to woman's inability to relax secondary to hypertonic uterine contractions

- Potential ineffective individual coping related to ineffectiveness of breathing techniques to relieve discomfort

- Anxiety related to slow labor progress

- Knowledge deficit related to lack of understanding regarding dysfunctional labor patterns

NURSING GOAL: PROVISION OF COMFORT AND SUPPORT TO THE LABORING WOMAN AND HER PARTNER

The woman experiencing a hypertonic labor pattern will probably be very uncomfortable because of the increased force of contractions. Her anxiety level and that of her partner may be high. The nurse attempts to reduce the woman's discomfort and promote a more effective labor pattern.

The nurse may wish to try a change of position for the woman; lateral position may correct the hypertonic pattern. Comfort measures include mouth care, effleurage, back rub, and change of linens. If sedation is ordered, the nurse ensures that the environment is conducive to relaxation. The labor coach may also need assistance in helping the woman cope. A calm understanding approach by the nurse offers the woman and her partner further support. Provision of information about the cause of the hypertonic labor pattern and assurances that the woman is not overreacting to the situation are also important nursing actions.

NURSING GOAL: PROMOTION OF MATERNAL-FETAL PHYSICAL WELL-BEING

Fluid balance must be maintained through adequate

hydration. Urine ketones should be monitored hourly. The couple should be informed of labor progress.

Nursing measures in the event of fetal-neonatal distress are given in the Nursing Care Plan on page 762.

NURSING GOAL: CLIENT EDUCATION

The laboring woman needs to have information about the dysfunctional labor pattern and the possible implications for herself and her baby. Information will help relieve anxiety and thereby increase relaxation and comfort. The nurse needs to explain treatment methods and offer opportunities for questions.

EVALUATIVE OUTCOME CRITERIA

Anticipated outcomes of nursing care include the following:

- The woman experiences a more effective labor pattern.

- The woman has increased comfort and decreased anxiety.

- The woman and her partner understand the hypertonic labor pattern.

Hypotonic Labor Patterns

In *hypotonic dysfunctional labor,* uterine activity in early labor has been within normal limits, but then a hypotonic pattern consisting of infrequent uterine contractions of mild to moderate intensity and a marked slowing or arrest of cervical dilatation and fetal descent occurs. In this pattern the myometrial resting tone is below 8 mm Hg. Fewer than two to three contractions occur in a ten-minute period (see Figure 25–1C) Hypotonic labor may occur when uterine fibers are overstretched from twins, large singletons, hydramnios, and grandmultiparity. Hypotonic uterine motility also occurs when sedation such as meperidine (Demerol) is given in the latent phase of labor or in the presence of various degrees of CPD. It may also occur with bladder and bowel distention. Clinically, hypotonic uterine motility may occur in the latent or active phase, but it is most often seen in the active phase. It is painless and responds to oxytocin if conditions permit its use.

MATERNAL RISKS

If labor is prolonged, intrauterine infection may result, along with maternal exhaustion and psychologic stress. Any woman with a dysfunctional labor pattern is a candidate for postpartal hemorrhage, but the woman with hypotonic labor is especially threatened. If the hypotonic pattern persists, the uterus may be less likely to contract efficiently after delivery, which can lead to postpartal hemorrhage.

FETAL-NEONATAL RISKS

Fetal and neonatal distress often accompany the intrauterine infection resulting from a prolonged hypotonic labor (Pritchard et al 1985). Antimicrobial therapy prescribed for the mother during labor appears to have little if any effect on preventing neonatal infection. Fetal tachycardia is observed on the electronic monitor or auscultated by the nurse. The newborn delivered of a mother with prolonged labor because of uterine hypotonia should be observed closely in the nursery for signs of sepsis.

MEDICAL THERAPY

Improving the quality of the uterine contractions while ensuring a safe outcome for the woman and her baby are the goals of therapy.

Prior to initiating treatment for hypotonic labor, the physician validates the adequacy of pelvic measurements and completes tests to establish gestational age if there is any question about fetal maturity. After CPD, fetal malpresentation, and fetal immaturity have been ruled out, oxytocin (Pitocin) may be given intravenously via an infusion pump to improve the quality of uterine contractions. Intravenous fluid is useful to maintain adequate hydration and prevent maternal exhaustion. Amniotomy may be done to stimulate the labor process.

An improvement in the quality of uterine contractions is demonstrated by noticeable progress in the labor process. If the labor pattern does not become effective, or if other complications develop, further interventions, including cesarean delivery, may be necessary.

NURSING ASSESSMENT

Assessing contractions (for frequency and intensity), maternal vital signs, and FHR provides the nurse with data to evaluate maternal-fetal status. The nurse is also alert for signs and symptoms of infection and dehydration. Because of the stress associated with a prolonged labor, observing the woman and her partner's degree of success with their coping mechanisms is also important.

NURSING DIAGNOSIS

Possible nursing diagnoses include:

- Alteration in comfort: pain related to inability to cope with uterine contractions secondary to dysfunctional labor

● Knowledge deficit related to lack of information regarding dysfunctional labor

NURSING GOAL: PROMOTION OF MATERNAL-FETAL PHYSICAL WELL-BEING

Nursing measures include frequent monitoring of contractions, maternal vital signs, and FHR. If meconium is present in the amniotic fluid, observing fetal status closely becomes more critical. Maintaining an intake and output record provides a way of determining maternal hydration or dehydration. The woman should be encouraged to void every two hours, and her bladder should be checked for distention. Because her labor may be prolonged, the woman must continue to be monitored for signs of infection (elevated temperature, chills, changes in characteristics of amniotic fluid). Vaginal examinations should be kept to a minimum. The nursing implications of oxytocin infusion are presented in Drug Guide–Oxytocin on page 802.

NURSING GOAL: PROVISION OF PSYCHOLOGIC SUPPORT

The nurse assists the woman and her partner to cope with the frustration of a lengthy labor process. A warm, caring approach coupled with techniques to reduce anxiety are very important strategies for the nurse to employ.

NURSING GOAL: CLIENT EDUCATION

The teaching plan must include information regarding the dysfunctional labor process and implications for the mother and baby. Disadvantages and alternatives of treatment also need to be discussed and understood.

EVALUATIVE OUTCOME CRITERIA

Nursing care is effective if:

● The woman understands the type of labor pattern that is occurring and the treatment plan.

● The woman and fetus have had the risk of infection reduced.

● The woman maintains comfort during labor.

Prolonged Labor

Labor lasting more than 24 hours is termed *prolonged labor*. In these cases usually the first stage is extended and the active and/or latent phase is prolonged. The cervix fails to dilate within a reasonable period of time. Early recognition and treatment are imperative to prevent maternal-fetal complications.

According to Oxorn (1986), the incidence of prolonged labor varies from 1 percent to 7 percent and is most common in the nullipara. The principal causes are CPD, malpresentations, malpositions, labor dysfunction, and cervical dystocia. Other influencing factors are excessive use of analgesics, anesthetics, and sedatives in the latent phase of labor; premature rupture of the membranes in the presence of an uneffaced, closed cervix; and reduced pain tolerance associated with high anxiety.

MATERNAL RISKS

Prolonged labor usually has a deleterious effect on the woman. Intense but unproductive pain from labor contractions in the latent phase or a prolonged active phase is likely to result in maternal exhaustion and moderate to severe stress. The woman also becomes a prime candidate for infection and hemorrhage from uterine atony, uterine rupture, or lacerations of the birth canal. An already stressful situation may be compounded by the necessity to deliver the fetus by forceps or cesarean birth.

FETAL-NEONATAL RISKS

Fetal distress may occur early or late in the labor depending on which phase of labor is prolonged. Utero-placental perfusion may be impeded by the length of the labor, resulting in fetal asphyxia. Premature rupture of the membranes (PROM) increases the risk of infection for both fetus and neonate. Prolapse of the cord may occur after rupture of the membranes if the presenting part fails to descend and engage. Continuing pressure on the head or a delivery by forceps may cause soft tissue edema and bruising, and in some instances, cerebral trauma (see Figure 25–2).

MEDICAL THERAPY

Management of prolonged labor begins with identification of any causal and complicating factors. Depending on these factors, the goal of treatment may be to stimulate labor through the administration of oxytocin or by performing an amniotomy.

Hydration is maintained with intravenous fluids, and anxiety is minimized with rest and sedation. In the event of serious maternal-fetal distress, delivery is likely to be by forceps or cesarean birth. Further discussion of the management of hypocontractility or hypercontractility patterns that may be precursors of prolonged labor is found on page 727.

NURSING ASSESSMENT

Monitoring maternal-fetal status is a primary nursing responsibility. The FHR patterns are assessed for signs of distress, including subtle tachycardia followed by brady-cardia, late decelerations, and decreasing variability. Amniotic fluid is observed for meconium staining and signs of infection. The nurse evaluates labor progress by considering the pattern of the contractions, the degree of cervical dilatation and effacement, and descent. Ongoing assessment of maternal hydration occurs throughout labor. If the woman is receiving oxytocin (Pitocin) therapy, the nurse watches maternal-fetal response to the treatment closely.

NURSING DIAGNOSIS

Possible nursing diagnoses include:

- Alteration in comfort: pain related to prolonged time in labor

- Potential ineffective individual coping related to ineffectiveness of breathing techniques to relieve discomfort and anxiety

- Potential for infection related to increased need for invasive assessments secondary to extended time in labor

NURSING GOAL: PROMOTION OF MATERNAL-FETAL PHYSICAL WELL-BEING

The nurse uses labor progress as an indicator of maternal-fetal status. If the fetus is in a vertex presentation, the nurse may evaluate the amount of pressure on the fetal head by the presence or absence of a caput succedaneum and/or molding. Calculating fluid intake and output and checking urine for presence of ketones provide the nurse with information about the maternal hydration state. If the woman is receiving oxytocin therapy, the nurse should implement appropriate nursing measures to ensure the safety of the woman and fetus. For further information on the administration of oxytocin, refer to Chapter 26 and Drug Guide—Oxytocin, page 802.

NURSING GOAL: PROVISION OF PSYCHOLOGIC SUPPORT

Following delivery the mother should be closely monitored for signs and symptoms of hemorrhage, shock, and infection. The newborn should be observed for signs and sepsis, cerebral trauma, and the appearance of cephalhematoma. Nursing actions for fetal distress are given on page 863.

Assisting the woman and her partner to deal with the anxiety and frustration of a prolonged labor is another important nursing responsibility. Support and encouragement become critical to assist the woman and her partner in coping with the numerous potential and actual problems

associated with prolonged labor. The nurse offers information as appropriate. Comfort measures such as a change in position, oral hygiene, skin care, and cool washcloths on the forehead may help the woman relax. Encouraging the involvement of her partner in care of the woman may further reduce anxiety.

EVALUATIVE OUTCOME CRITERIA

Nursing care is effective if:

- The woman and her partner are able to cope with the hypotonic pattern.

- The woman and fetus have had the risk of infection reduced.

- The woman maintains comfort during the labor.

Precipitous Labor

Precipitous labor is extremely rapid labor that lasts for less than three hours. The most common causes are low resistance in maternal tissues, which allows rapid cervical dilatation and fetal descent, and exceptionally strong uterine contractions, of which there are two types (Pritchard et al 1985). In the first type uterine contractility increases in intensity and frequency. Myometrial contractions exert pressures of 50 to 70 mm Hg, and the frequency of contractions is greater than five in a ten-minute period (Assali 1972). The second type is a myometrial tachysystole with only increased frequency.

Other contributing factors in precipitous labor are (a) multiparity, (b) large pelvis, (c) previous precipitous labor, and (d) a small fetus in a favorable position. One or more of these factors, plus strong contractions, result in a rapid transit of the infant through the birth canal (Pritchard et al 1985). Precipitous labor may also be caused by oxytocin overdose, which can occur during induction of labor. In this case, precipitous labor is caused by medical error.

Precipitous labor and precipitous delivery are not the same. A precipitous delivery is an unexpected, sudden, and often unattended birth. See page 685 for discussion of precipitous delivery.

MATERNAL RISKS

If the cervix is effaced and the maternal soft tissues are not resistant to stretching, maternal complications may be few. However, if the cervix is not ripe (soft) and the maternal soft tissues are resistant, lacerations of the cervix, vagina, perineum, and periurethral area may occur because the tissues do not stretch adequately. There is also a possibility of uterine rupture. When resistance is present, amniotic fluid embolism may occur (see page 783). The woman is also at risk for postpartal hemorrhage due to expanded uterine fibers and may lose control because of the rapidity of the labor process.

FETAL-NEONATAL RISKS

Decreased periods of uterine relaxation result in fetal hypoxia and hypercarbia. Clinically, an acidotic fetus demonstrates decreased beat-to-beat variability and eventually bradycardia. Vagal stimulation is elicited through hypoxic brain tissues, which causes the bradycardia. The same vagal stimulation causes an increase in intestinal motility, resulting in release of meconium in utero.

Rapid labor and delivery causes increased pressures on and in the fetal head and may cause cerebral trauma to the newborn. If the birth is unattended and unassisted, the newborn may suffer from lack of care in the first few minutes of life. Suffocation and aspiration are possible complications when resuscitation is not immediately available (Pritchard et al 1985).

MEDICAL THERAPY

Any woman with a history of precipitous labor requires close medical monitoring and preparation for an emergency delivery to facilitate a safe outcome for the mother and fetus. Drugs such as magnesium sulfate have been used in cases of precipitous labor. Tocolytic agents such as ritodrine may also prove effective (Pritchard et al 1985).

NURSING ASSESSMENT

Assessments of the woman with precipitous labor will reveal a contraction pattern that is accelerated beyond the normal labor pattern. As this more rapid pattern is identified, the need for more frequent assessments will be apparent. Frequent assessment of the fetal response to the rapid labor is important.

NURSING GOAL: MONITORING LABOR PROGRESS

If the woman is at risk for precipitous labor, the nurse is particularly attentive to the progress of labor and ensures that an emergency delivery pack is close at hand. The physician should be informed of any unusual findings on the Friedman graph (see Chapter 22). The nurse should be in constant attendance if at all possible.

To avoid hyperstimulation of the uterus and possible precipitous labor during oxytocin administration, the nurse should be alert to the danger of oxytocin overdosage (see Drug Guide—Oxytocin on page 802). If the woman receiving oxytocin develops an accelerated labor pattern, the oxytocin should be discontinued immediately, and the woman should be turned on her left side to improve uter-

ine perfusion. Oxygen may be started to increase the available oxygen in the maternal circulation; this increases the amount available for exchange at the placental site.

NURSING GOAL: PROMOTION OF PSYCHOLOGIC WELL-BEING

Comfort and rest may be promoted by assisting the woman to a comfortable position, providing a quiet environment, and administering sedatives as needed. Information and support are given before and after the delivery.

NURSING GOAL: ASSISTANCE DURING LABOR

An ensuing delivery may be slowed by having the woman pant or blow with each contraction. It is also helpful for the nurse to breathe with the woman during this time to help the woman pace her breathing. If delivery is imminent, the nurse can assist with the birth (Chapter 23). The nurse should never attempt to stop a delivery by holding the woman's legs together. This may cause trauma to the newborn's head and separation of the placenta.

EVALUATIVE OUTCOME CRITERIA

Nursing care is effective if:

- The woman and her baby are closely monitored during labor and a safe birth occurs.

- The woman feels support and enhanced comfort during labor and delivery.

● Care of the Woman With Premature Rupture of Membranes

Technically, premature rupture of the membranes (PROM) is defined as the spontaneous rupture of membranes prior to the onset of labor irrespective of the gestational age (Creasy & Resnik 1984). Premature rupture of the membranes may be further divided into the latent and interval periods. The latent period is the time from rupture of membranes to the onset of labor. The interval period is the time from rupture of membranes to delivery of the fetus (Creasy & Resnik 1984). Although rupture of the membranes long before term probably should be called *preterm rupture of the membranes* (Pritchard et al 1985), both terms are currently used in the clinical area.

Although the cause of PROM is unknown, a variety of contributing factors are correlated with its occurrence. An incompetent cervix may be the cause of second trimester PROM. Infection (UTI), hydramnios, trauma, multiple pregnancy, and maternal genital tract anomalies may also result in PROM.

The incidence of PROM is 3 percent at term and 18.5 percent with a preterm pregnancy (Creasy & Resnik 1984). In women with PROM at or near term, 70 percent are in labor within 12 hours, and only 5 percent are not in labor by 72 hours. As the gestational age decreases, the length of the latent period increases (Creasy & Resnik 1984). When the gestation is less than 37 completed weeks with PROM, the incidence of spontaneous labor within the first 24 hours is 50 percent; 70 percent of women have delivered within 72 hours (Creasy & Resnik 1984). In 10 percent of preterm labors the latent periods are greater than 14 days (Creasy & Resnik 1984).

Maternal Risks

The major maternal risks associated with PROM are ascending intrauterine infection and precipitation of preterm labor. Either event represents a major stressor for the woman.

Fetal-Neonatal Risks

A correlation exists among PROM, neonatal infection, and perinatal mortality. Infection, particularly of the respiratory tract, is the leading cause of fetal-neonatal death. The preterm fetus is further jeopardized by the associated increased risks of malpresentation (especially breech) and prolapse of the cord. An inverse relationship exists between preterm birth mortality and gestational age and the occurrence of RDS and neonatal sepsis.

Literature has suggested that a lengthier latent period following preterm rupture of the membranes may stimulate pulmonary maturity in the preterm infant and thereby reduce the rate of RDS (Creasy & Resnik 1984). The acceleration of the maturation of the lung is thought to occur because of the stress-producing situation. In contrast, other reports have provided only partial or no confirmation of the effect on the preterm newborn (Garite et al 1981, Simpson & Harbert 1984). Chapter 31 contains additional information on the preterm neonate.

Medical Therapy

The gestational age of the fetus and the presence or absence of infection determine the direction of medical treatment for PROM (Figure 25–3). If the fetus is preterm or infection is present, more drastic medical therapy is necessary to prevent complications that are potentially detrimental to the mother and her fetus-newborn.

After confirming with Nitrazine Paper and a microscopic examination (ferning test) that the membranes have ruptured, the gestational age of the fetus is calculated. Single or combination methods of calculation may be used, including Nägele's rule, fundal height, ultrasound to measure the fetal BPD, and amniocentesis to identify lung maturity. If maternal signs and symptoms of infection are evident, antibiotic therapy (usually by intravenous infusion) is initiated immediately, and the fetus is delivered vaginally or by cesarean birth regardless of the gestational age. Upon admission to the nursery the neonate is assessed for sepsis and placed on antibiotics. Chapter 32 provides further information about the neonate with sepsis.

Management of PROM in the absence of infection and gestation of less than 37 weeks is usually conservative. The woman is hospitalized on bed rest. An admission CBC and u/a are obtained. Continuous electronic fetal monitoring may be ordered at the beginning of treatment but usually is discontinued after a few hours, unless membranes are ruptured or the fetus is estimated to be very low birth weight (VLBW). Maternal B/P, pulse, and temperature and FHR are assessed every four hours. A WBC is ordered daily. Vaginal exams are avoided to decrease the chance of infection. As the gestation approaches 34 weeks, an amniocentesis may be done weekly to evaluate L/S and PG. After initial treatment and observation, some women may be followed at home. The woman is advised to continue bed rest (with bathroom privileges), monitor her temperature four times a day; avoid intercourse, douches, or tampons; and have a WBC every other day (Oxorn 1986, Danforth & Scott 1986). The woman is advised to contact her physician and return to the hospital if she has fever, uterine tenderness and/or contractions, increased leakage of fluid, or a foul vaginal discharge.

Opinions as to the efficacy of administering glucocorticoids (betamethasone or dexamethasone) prophylactically for PROM are sharply divided (Creasy & Resnik 1984, Avery et al 1986). When gestation is between 34 and 36 weeks, medical practice has been to delay delivery for 24 hours to allow natural elevation of maternal-fetal blood glucocorticoids, thereby contributing to fetal lung maturity. If gestation is between 28 and 32 weeks and labor can be delayed for 24 to 48 hours, betamethasone (Celestone) is frequently given. Glucocorticoids are not administered in the presence of uterine infection. (See Drug Guide—Betamethasone.) In research by Simpson and Harbert (1984), no difference was noted in the occurrence of respiratory distress syndrome (RDS) in the preterm neonate because of the administration glucocorticoids. Another study (Garite et al 1981) found no reduction in the incidence of RDS and also discovered an increased incidence of neonatal and maternal sepsis when glucocorticoids were given.

Some researchers suggest a short-term saline solution infusion into the amniotic cavity to treat variable or prolonged fetal heart decelerations once they appear (Nageotte et al 1985). When these researchers infused warmed (37°C), sterile normal saline through a uterine pressure catheter, they found a decreased incidence of variable decelerations and improvement of metabolic state at delivery.

Nursing Assessment

Determining the duration of the rupture of the membranes is a significant component of the intrapartal assessment. The nurse asks the woman when her membranes ruptured and when labor began, because the risk of infection may be directly related to the time involved. Gestational age is determined to prepare for the possibility of a preterm delivery. The nurse observes the mother for signs and symptoms of infection, especially by reviewing her WBC, temperature, and pulse rate and the character of her amniotic fluid. If the mother has a fever, hydration status should be checked. When a preterm or cesarean delivery

is anticipated, the nurse evaluates the coping abilities of the woman and her partner.

Nursing Diagnosis

Nursing diagnoses that may be used with PROM include:

● Potential for infection related to premature rupture of membranes

● Potential alteration in gas exchange in the fetus related to compression of the umbilical cord secondary to prolapse of the cord

● Potential ineffective individual coping related to unknown outcome of the pregnancy

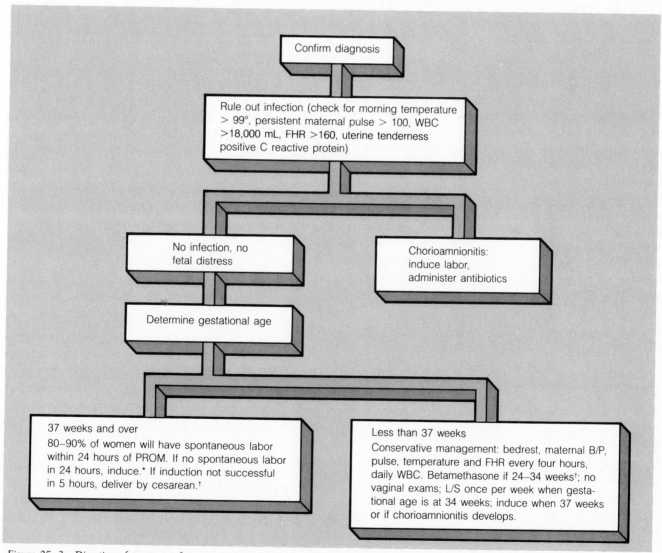

Figure 25–3 Direction of treatment for premature rupture of membranes. (From Oxorn H: *Human Labor and Birth,* ed 5. Norwalk, Conn, Appleton-Century-Crofts, 1986; Danforth DN: Other complications due to pregnancy, in Danforth DN, Scott JR (eds): *Obstetrics and Gynecology,* ed 5. Philadelphia, Lippincott, 1986)

Drug Guide Betamethasone (Celestone Solupan®)

Overview of Maternal-Fetal Action

"Betamethasone is a glucocorticoid which acts to accelerate fetal lung maturation and prevent hyaline membrane disease by inhibiting cell mitosis, increasing cell differentiation, promoting selected enzymatic actions, and participating in the storage and secretion of surfactant" (Bishop 1981). The best results are obtained when the fetus is between 30 and 32 weeks' gestation. It may be used as early as 26 weeks and as late as 34 weeks (Briggs et al 1986).

To obtain optimal results, delivery should be delayed for at least 24 hours after the end of treatment. If delivery does not occur, the effect of the drug disappears in about one week. A female fetus seems more likely than a male to obtain the most prophylactic effect (Briggs et al 1986).

Route, Dosage, Frequency
Prenatal maternal intramuscular administration of 12 mg of betamethasone is given once a day for 2 days. Repeated treatment will be needed on a weekly basis until 34 weeks of gestation (unless delivery occurs).

Contraindications
Inability to delay birth for 48 hours

Adequate L:S ratio

Presence of a condition that necessitates immediate delivery (eg, maternal bleeding)

Presence of maternal infection, diabetes mellitus, hypertension

Concomitant use of tocolytic agents, which may increase risk of maternal pulmonary edema (Bishop 1981)

Gestational age greater than 34 weeks

Maternal Side Effects
Bishop (1981) reports that suspected maternal risks include (a) initiation of lactation; (b) increased risk of infection; (c) augmentation of placental insufficiency in hypertensive women; (d) gastrointestinal bleeding; (e) inability to use estriol levels to assess fetal status; (f) pulmonary edema when used concurrently with tocolytics (such as ritodrine)

May cause Na^+ retention, K^+ loss, weight gain, edema, indigestion

Increased risk of infection if PROM present (Briggs et al 1986).

Effects on Fetus/Neonate
Lowered cortisol levels between 1 and 8 days following delivery (Giacoia & Yaffe 1982)

Possible suppression of aldosterone levels up to 2 weeks following delivery (Giacoia & Yaffe 1982)

Hypoglycemia

Increased risk of neonatal sepsis (Briggs et al 1986)

Animal studies have shown serious fetal side effects such as reduced head circumference, reduced weight of the fetal adrenal and thymus glands, and decreased placental weight (Briggs et al 1986). Human studies have not observed these effects however.

Nursing Considerations

Assess for presence of contraindications.

Provide education regarding possible side effects.

Administer deep into gluteal muscle, avoid injection into deltoid (high incidence of local atrophy).

Periodically evaluate BP, pulse, weight, and edema.

Assess lab data for electrolytes.

Nursing Goal: Promotion of Maternal-Fetal Physical Well-Being

Nursing actions should focus on the woman, her partner, and the fetus. The time her membranes ruptured and the time of labor onset are recorded. The nurse observes the woman for signs and symptoms of infection by frequently monitoring her vital signs (especially temperature and pulse), describing the character of the amniotic fluid, and reporting elevated WBC to the physician/nurse-midwife. Uterine activity and fetal response to the labor are evaluated, but vaginal exams are not done unless absolutely necessary. Comfort measures may help promote rest and relaxation. The nurse must also ensure that hydration is maintained, particularly if the woman's temperature is elevated.

Nursing Goal: Client Education

Provision of education is another important aspect of nursing care. The couple needs to understand the implications of PROM and all treatment methods. It is important to address side effects and alternative treatments. The couple needs to know that although the membranes are ruptured, fluid continues to be produced.

Nursing Goal: Provision of Psychologic Support

Providing psychologic support for the couple is critical. The nurse may reduce anxiety by listening empathetically, relaying accurate information, and providing explanations of procedures. Preparing the couple for a cesarean birth, a preterm neonate, and the possibility of fetal or neonatal demise may be necessary.

Evaluative Outcome Criteria

Nursing care is effective if:

- The woman's risk of infection and cord prolapse are decreased.

- The couple understands the implications of PROM and all treatments and alternative treatments.

- The pregnancy is maintained without trauma to the mother or her baby.

● Care of the Woman at Risk Due to Preterm Labor

Labor that occurs between 20 and 37 completed weeks of pregnancy is referred to as preterm labor (Creasy & Resnik 1984). The causes may be fetal, maternal, or placental factors. Premature rupture of the membranes occurs in 20 percent to 30 percent of the cases of preterm labor. In the other 70 percent to 80 percent of cases, no known cause has been identified (Danforth & Scott 1986). Maternal factors include cardiovascular or renal disease, diabetes, preeclampsia-eclampsia, abdominal surgery, a blow to the abdomen, uterine anomalies, cervical incompetence, and maternal infection (especially UTI). Uterine manipulation or displacement during abdominal surgery may contribute to the early onset of labor. Fetal factors include multiple pregnancy, hydramnios, and fetal infection.

Other cases reveal a strong correlation between preterm delivery and low socioeconomic status (education, income, occupation) and/or history of preterm births.

Risk-scoring tools help identify a large proportion of pregnant women who are at risk for preterm delivery. Table 15–1 presents one system for determining the risk of spontaneous preterm delivery. If this type of tool is used, it is important to reassess the risks and observe cervical changes as the pregnancy progresses.

CONTEMPORARY DILEMMA

How Small Is Too Small?

Advances in medical technology and obstetrical/perinatal care have influenced our perception of when a fetus is considered viable. In the past, many infants born prior to 28 weeks' gestation were considered nonviable. With aggressive perinatal management, the limits of birth weight have been progressively lowered. Now fetuses born weighing 750 to 1000 g (approximately 24 to 26 weeks' gestation) are surviving in increasing numbers. The greatest strides have been made with infants weighing over 1000 g, whose survival has doubled in the last 15 years. Many states now consider a live born fetus viable if it is at least 20 weeks' gestation or weighs 500 g or more. This change in the definition of viability raises many questions regarding obstetrical management of premature labor and delivery, decisions regarding initiation of resuscitation, provision of life support treatments and long-term care needs. The long-term physiologic and psychologic implications for these tiny infants and their families is not known.

This dilemma has produced many philosophical, ethical, legal, and economic questions. The questions include:

- What is a reasonable definition of viability?

- Is there a need for a consensus on the lower limits of birth weight at which efforts at resuscitation will not be made?

- Should the parameters used as a guide for critical decisions involving preterm viability be gestational age or birth weight?

- Who is to be involved in the decision regarding the course of action for "nonviable" fetuses, and when is the decision to be made?

- What are the legal, ethical, social, and economic implications of the current concept of fetal viability?

Maternal Risks

The major risks for the woman relate to psychologic stress factors related to her concern for her unborn child.

Fetal-Neonatal Risks

Mortality increases for neonates born before 37 weeks of gestation. Although the preterm infant is faced

Table 25–1 Criteria for Diagnosis of Preterm Labor

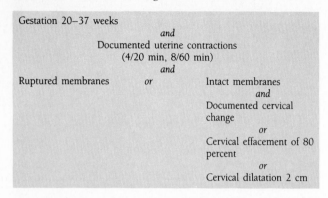

Gestation 20–37 weeks
and
Documented uterine contractions
(4/20 min, 8/60 min)
and
Ruptured membranes   *or*   Intact membranes
and
Documented cervical change
or
Cervical effacement of 80 percent
or
Cervical dilatation 2 cm

From Creasy RK, Resnik R: *Maternal Fetal Medicine.* Philadelphia, Saunders, 1984, p 424.

with many maturational deficiencies (fat storage, heat regulation, immaturity of organ systems), the most critical factor is the lack of development of the respiratory system—to the extent that life cannot be supported. In some instances, such as severe maternal diabetes or serious isoimmunization, continuation of the pregnancy may be more life-threatening to the fetus than the hazards of prematurity. See Chapter 31 for in-depth consideration of the preterm neonate.

Medical Therapy

The goal of medical therapy is to prevent preterm labor from advancing to a stage that no longer responds to medical treatment. If labor cannot be arrested, the priority becomes successful preterm delivery and its psychologic effect on the woman and her partner.

The mother who is at risk for preterm labor may benefit from participating in an early detection program. One such approach has resulted in increasing the proportion of preterm labor women who are eligible for tocolysis to over 80 percent with a concomitant 50 percent decrease in preterm deliveries (Herron et al 1982). The program itself uses an educational process to teach the woman to palpate for uterine contractions, to recognize the subtle symptoms of preterm labor, and to report these symptoms to her physician/nurse-midwife. If preterm labor occurs, prompt medical treatment is initiated.

Prior to considering tocolytic therapy, the physician/nurse-midwife must establish a diagnosis. Common criteria used for diagnosis are found in Table 25–1. Any medical condition that may contribute to preterm labor should also be treated, and maternal or fetal contraindications to inhibiting labor should be identified. Creasy and Resnik (1984) specify the following absolute and relative contraindications to interrupting labor:

Absolute contraindications

● Presence of severe PIH, which creates risk for the woman if the pregnancy continues

● Fetal complications (isoimmunization, gross anomalies)

● Ruptured membranes, which increases the risk of uterine infection (see exceptions, page 733)

● Hemorrhage

● Fetal death

● Severe renal disease

Relative contraindications

● Cervical dilatation of 5 cm or more

● Mild chronic hypertension

● Stable placenta previa

● Uncontrolled diabetes

● Maternal cardiac disease

Between 10 percent and 20 percent of women with preterm labor or PROM are candidates for long-term tocolytic treatment (Creasy & Resnik 1984). If the cervix is more than 3 to 4 cm dilated and more than 80 percent effaced, the effect of tocolytics on labor is reduced.

The drugs currently in use to arrest preterm labor are ritodrine (Yutopar), terbutaline sulfate (Brethine), and intravenous magnesium sulfate. Ritodrine, a β-mimetic agent, is currently FDA approved. See Drug Guide–Ritodrine on page 739.

Terbutaline sulfate (Brethine) a selective β receptor stimulator, may be used to arrest preterm labor. Although it is not FDA approved for this use, in some instances it is the drug of choice. It is given IV with an infusion pump. The side effects are similar to those of ritodrine (Bealle et al 1985).

Magnesium sulfate has long been used in treatment for PIH and has been gaining favor in the treatment of preterm labor because it is effective and has fewer side effects than β sympathomimetics. The usual recommended loading dose is 4 g IV over 20 minutes. The constant dose is then 1.5 g/hr. The dose may be increased by 0.5 g/hr every 30 minutes until contractions cease or a dose of 3.5 g/hr is reached. The therapy is maintained for 12 hours at the lowest rate to maintain cessation of contractions (Bealle et al 1985). The maternal serum level that is important for tocolysis seems to be 5–8 mg/dL or 4–7 mEq/L (Wilkins et al 1986). Side effects with the loading dose may include flushing, a feeling of warmth, headache, nausea, and dizziness. Other side effects include lethargy and sluggishness and a 2 percent risk of pulmonary edema if the woman has predisposing conditions such as multiple gestation or

Drug Guide   Ritodrine (Yutopar)

Overview of Obstetric Action

Ritodrine is a sympathomimetic β_2-adrenergic agonist. It exerts its effect on Type II beta receptors, which are found in uterine smooth muscle, bronchioles, and diaphragm. Stimulation of Type II receptors results in uterine relaxation, bronchodilation, vasodilation, and muscle glycogenolysis. As muscles in the vessel walls relax, hypotension is induced. The body compensates by increasing maternal heart rate and pulse pressure.

Ritodrine causes a potassium shift, which may cause hypokalemia. There may also be an increase in blood glucose and plasma insulin levels and stimulation of glycogen release from muscles and the liver (NAACOG 1984). Ritodrine is FDA-approved for use in treatment of preterm labor.

Route, Dosage, Frequency
Add 150 mg of ritodrine to 500 mL IV fluid and administer as a piggyback to a primary IV. The resulting dilution is 0.3 mg/mL. Note: Some authorities recommend a saline solution and others believe a dextrose solution reduces the incidence of pulmonary edema (Niebyl et al 1986). The initial dose is 0.1 mg/min (20 mL/hr on an adult infusion pump). The dose is increased 0.05 mg/min (10 mL/hr on an adult infusion pump) every 10 minutes until contractions cease. Maximum dosage is 0.35 mg/min (70 mL/hr on an adult infusion pump). When contractions cease, the infusion rate may be decreased by 0.5 mg/min (10 mL/hr on an adult infusion pump). The infusion may be maintained at a low rate for a period of hours to assure that contractions do not begin again. Before the intravenous infusion is discontinued, PO administration is begun (Shortridge 1983; Yutopar Drug Information 1984).

Gonik and Creasy (1986) recommend administration of oral ritodrine 30 minutes before ending IV ritodrine. The initial PO dose is 10–20 mg every 2 hours, and the time between doses may be increased to 3–4 hours based on uterine response and maternal pulse. The maternal pulse is maintained in the 90–100 BPM range.

This dosage can be administered safely to a maximum of 120 mg over 24 hours. The length of therapy varies.

Current research is directed toward the use of a single injection of ritodrine for other obstetric problems. Rapid relaxation of the uterus may be needed in the presence of tetanic contractions and cord prolapse (Ingemarsson et al 1985b). It has also been suggested for use with fetal bradycardia to improve the heart rate (Ingemarsson et al 1985a) and to inhibit labor in order to manage fetal distress (Caritis et al 1985).

Maternal Contraindications
Preterm labor accompanied by cervical dilatation greater than 4 cm, chorioamniotis, severe preeclampsia-eclampsia, severe bleeding, fetal death, significant IUGR contraindicate use of ritodrine, as do any of the following:

Hypovolemia, uncontrolled hypertension

Pulmonary hypertension

Cardiac disease, arrhythmias

Diabetes mellitus (use with caution)

Concurrent therapy with glucocorticoids (use with caution)

Gestation less than 20 weeks

Maternal Side Effects
Tachycardia, occasionally premature ventricular contractions (PVCs), increased stroke volume, slight increase in systolic and decrease in diastolic pressure, palpitations, tremors, nervousness, nausea and vomiting, headache, erythema, hypotension, shortness of breath (Bealle et al 1985)

Decreased peripheral vascular resistance, which lowers diastolic pressure → widening of pulse pressure

Hyperglycemia (usually peaks within 3 hours after initiation of therapy) (Hankins & Hauth 1985)

Metabolic acidosis

Hypokalemia (causes internal redistribution)

Pulmonary edema in women treated concurrently with glucocorticoids, and who have fluid overload (Benedetti 1983)

Increased concentration of lactate and free fatty acids

ST segment depression, T wave flattening, prolongation of QT interval (Hendricks et al 1986)

Increase in plasma volume as indicated by decreases in hemoglobin, hematocrit, and serum albumin levels (Philipsen 1981)

Possible neutropenia with long-term IV therapy (Wang & Davidson 1986)

Effects on Fetus/Neonate
Fetal tachycardia, cardiac dysrhythmias

Increased serum glucose concentration

Fetal acidosis

Fetal hypoxia

Neonatal hypoglycemia, hypocalcemia, ↑ WBC

Neonatal paralytic ileus, irritability, tremors

Neonatal hypotension at birth

May decrease incidence of neonatal respiratory distress syndrome (Lipshitz 1981)

(continued)

Drug Guide   Ritodrine (Yutopar) (continued)

Nursing Considerations

Position woman in left side-lying position to increase placental perfusion and decrease incidence of hypotension.

Complete a history and assessment to identify possible presence of infection and maternal-fetal contraindications to treatment.

Explain procedure, which will include electronic fetal monitor, IV, frequent assessments, possible use of cardiac monitor, blood samples, intake and output, and daily weight, and potential for development of side effects, especially increase in pulse and fetal heart rate.

Monitor uterine activity and fetal heart rate by electronic fetal monitor.

Assess maternal BP and pulse every 15 minutes while dosage is being increased and every 30 minutes while on maintenance IV (Shortridge 1983). As long as dosage is being increased, some agency protocols recommend taking maternal BP and pulse prior to dose increase. Notify physician if maternal pulse >120 bpm. (Note: Expect increase of 20–40 bpm. Maternal pulse may exceed 120 bpm for a brief period of time [NAACOG 1984]).

Assess respiratory rate and auscultate breath sounds with maternal vital signs. Note signs of pulmonary edema (rales and rhonchi). When oral therapy is begun, maternal BP, pulse, and respirations may be taken with each PO dose.

Monitor FHR with maternal assessments (Note: Expect increase of approximately 10 bpm. The rate should not exceed 180 bpm. Notify physician of rate >180 bpm).

Apply antiembolism stockings to prevent pooling of blood in extremities.

Encourage passive range of motion in legs every 1–2 hours.

Assess hydration status by evaluating intake/output, skin turgor, mucous membranes, and urine concentration.

Maintain intake and output records. Intake is usually limited to 2500 mL/day (Gonik & Creasy 1986) and 90–100 mL/hr (Shortridge 1983).

Assess output every hour until contractions cease, then every 4 hours (Shortridge 1983).

Weigh daily at same time after woman has emptied bladder, using same scales and same clothing.

Observe woman closely for problems associated with hypokalemia (muscle weakness, cardiac arrhythmia) and pulmonary edema (dyspnea, wheezing, coughing, rales or rhonchi, or tachypnea). Discontinue therapy if pulmonary edema or cardiac problems develop.

Assess lab data regarding electrolytes, glucose, and WBC.

Have β blocking agent available as antidote for betasympathomimetic therapy. Propranolol (Inderal) 0.25 mg IV is usually used (Shortridge 1983). It should be given by a physician and injected over at least 1 minute to reduce the potential for lowering the blood pressure and precipitating cardiac standstill. Cardiac monitoring should be continuous.

Provide psychosocial support. The threat of preterm labor produces anxiety. Provide information and counseling for the woman and partner, and encourage questions. Assist them in making life-style changes such as more frequent rest periods, cessation of employment, and possible changes in sexual activity. If woman is discharged on oral therapy, teach her to take medications on time to ensure optimum effect, to observe for signs of preterm labor, and to assess her pulse with each dose. The woman needs to report pulse above 120, palpitations, tremors, agitation, nervousness, chest pain, and any difficulty breathing.

If birth occurs when woman is on ritodrine therapy, assess newborn for presence of side effects (NAACOG 1984).

It is recommended to discontinue ritodrine in the presence of any of the following: Maternal heart rate above 140 bpm or fetal heart rate above 200 bpm, more than 6 maternal or fetal premature ventricular contractions/min, maternal systolic pressure above 180 mm Hg or diastolic below 40 mm Hg, chest pain, shortness of breath (Bealle et al 1985).

---

hydramnios (Wilkins et al 1986). See Drug Guide–Magnesium Sulfate on page 500 for other side effects. Fetal side effects may include hypotonia that persists for one or two days following birth (Wilkins et al 1986).

In comparison with IV ritodrine, magnesium sulfate has no recognizable effect on systolic or diastolic blood pressure (mean blood pressure is maintained and uteroplacental perfusion is maintained), no alteration of maternal heart rate (though it may cause a slight decrease in the fetal heart rate), no effect on cardiac output, and only a slight increase in placental blood flow (Thiagarajah et al 1985).

Long-term oral therapy may be accomplished with magnesium oxide, magnesium peroxide, or magnesium gluconate. The therapeutic dose is usually 250 to 450 mg every 3 hr. This dose maintains a maternal serum level of 2 to 2.5 mg, which is usually sufficient to prevent uterine contractions (Niebyl 1986).

Two new drugs may soon be used in the treatment of preterm labor. Hexaprenaline, another β mimetic drug, has less effect on maternal pulse and BP and FHR than ritodrine (Niebyl 1986). In some centers prostaglandin synthesis inhibitors (PSI) such as indomethacin (Indocin) are being investigated and used in selected instances. Early research indicates maternal side effects, such as oliguria and vasoconstriction, and potential fetal side effects, such as premature closure of ductus arteriosus, have been reported (Knight 1986).

Research is also being conducted on the use of calcium channel blockers such as nitrendipine and nifedipine to inhibit preterm labor (Sakamoto & Huszar, 1986, Veille et al 1986).

An additional treatment may be the administration of glucocorticoids (see discussion page 736).

Nursing Assessment

During the antepartal period, the nurse identifies the woman at risk for preterm labor by noting the presence of predisposing factors. During the intrapartal period, the nurse assesses the progress of labor and the physiologic impact of labor on the mother and fetus. The key nursing assessments during ritodrine therapy are listed in Box 25–1.

Nursing Diagnosis

Nursing diagnoses that may apply to the woman with preterm labor include:

- Knowledge deficit related to causes, identification, and treatment of preterm labor

- Fear related to early labor and delivery

- Potential for ineffective individual coping related to need for constant attention to pregnancy

Nursing Goal: Education for Self-Care

Once the woman at risk for preterm labor has been identified, she must be educated about the importance of preventing the onset of labor. Increasing the woman's awareness of the subtle symptoms of preterm labor is one of the most important teaching objectives of the nurse. The signs and symptoms of preterm labor include (Herron 1983):

- Uterine contractions that occur every ten minutes or less.

- Mild, menstrual-like cramps felt low in the abdomen.

- Feelings of pelvic pressure that may feel like the baby pressing down. The pressure may feel constant or intermittent.

- Low back ache, which may be constant or intermittent.

- A change in the vaginal discharge (an increase in amount or a change to more clear and watery or a pinkish tinge).

- Abdominal cramping with or without diarrhea.

The woman is also taught to evaluate contraction activity once or twice a day. She does so by lying down tilted to one side with a pillow behind her back for support. The woman places her fingertips on the fundus of the uterus, which is above the umbilicus (navel). She checks for contractions (hardening or tightening in the uterus) for about one hour. It is important for the pregnant woman to know that uterine contractions occur occasionally throughout the pregnancy. If they occur every ten minutes for one hour, however, the cervix could begin to dilate and labor could continue.

Box 25–1 Key Nursing Assessments During Ritodrine Therapy

Time interval	Assessment
During initial IV therapy and increases in infusion rate	
Every 10 or 15 minutes	FHR and maternal BP, pulse, and R. Auscultate lung sounds for rales and rhonchi. Be alert for complaints of dyspnea, chest tightness. Uterine activity.
Every hour	Assess output (should be over 30 cc/hr or match intake). Assess intake (should not exceed 90–100 mL/hr).
During maintenance IV therapy	
Every 30 minutes	Maternal BP, pulse, and R; FHR; lung sounds; uterine activity.
Every 4 hours	Intake and output.
During PO therapy	
Before each dose	Maternal BP, pulse, and R; FHR; lung sounds.
Every 4–8 hours	Intake and output.

Whenever lab work results are available, evaluate K^+ (for hypokalemia), hemoglobin, and hematocrit (for signs of hemodilution, which, together with hypokalemia, may be associated with pulmonary edema).

Box 25–2 Self-Care Measures to Prevent Preterm Labor

Rest two or three times a day lying on your left side.

Drink 2 to 3 quarts of water or fruit juice each day. Avoid caffeine drinks. Filling a quart container and drinking from it will eliminate the need to keep track of numerous glasses of fluid.

Empty your bladder at least every two hours during waking hours.

Avoid lifting heavy objects. If other small children are in the home, work out alternatives for picking them up, such as sitting on a chair and having them climb on your lap.

Avoid prenatal breast preparation such as nipple rolling or rubbing nipples with a towel. This is not meant to discourage breast feeding but to avoid the potential increase in uterine irritability.

Pace necessary activities to avoid overexertion.

Sexual activity may need to be curtailed or eliminated.

Find pleasurable ways to help compensate for limitations of activities and boost the spirits.

Try to focus on one day or one week at a time rather than longer periods of time.

If on bedrest, get dressed each day and rest on a couch rather than becoming isolated in the bedroom.

Prepared in consultation with Susan Bennett, RN, ACCE, Coordinator of the Prematurity Prevention Program.

The nurse ensures that the woman knows when to report signs and symptoms. If contractions occur every ten minutes (or less) for one hour, if any of the other signs and symptoms are present for one hour, or if clear fluid begins leaking from the vagina, she should telephone her physician/nurse-midwife, clinic, or hospital birthing unit and make arrangements to be checked for ongoing labor.

Care givers need to be aware that the woman is knowledgeable and attuned to changes in her body, and her call must be taken seriously. When a woman is at risk for preterm labor, she may have many episodes of contractions and other signs or symptoms. If she is treated positively, she will feel freer to report problems as they arise.

Other preventive measures the woman could follow are presented in Box 25–2.

Nursing Goal: Promotion of Maternal-Fetal Physical Well-Being During Labor

Provision of supportive nursing care to the woman in preterm labor is important during hospitalization. This care consists of promoting bed rest, monitoring vital signs (especially blood pressure and respirations), measuring intake and output, and continuous monitoring of FHR and uterine contractions. Placing the woman on her left side facilitates maternal-fetal circulation. Vaginal examinations are kept to a minimum. If tocolytic agents are being administered, the mother and fetus are monitored closely for any adverse effects.

Nursing Goal: Provision of Emotional Support to the Family

Whether preterm labor is arrested or proceeds, the woman and her partner experience intense psychologic stress. Decreasing the anxiety associated with the unknown and the risk of a preterm neonate is a primary aim of the nurse.

Providing emotional support for the woman and her partner during preterm labor and delivery is also important. Common behavioral responses include feelings of anxiety and guilt about the possibility that the pregnancy will terminate early. With empathetic communication, the nurse can facilitate the expression of these feelings, thereby helping the couple identify and implement coping mechanisms. The nurse also keeps the couple informed about the labor progress, the treatment regimen, and the status of the fetus so that their full cooperation can be elicited. In the event of imminent vaginal or cesarean delivery, the couple should be offered brief but ongoing explanations to prepare them for the actual birth process and the events following the birth.

EVALUATIVE OUTCOME CRITERIA

Nursing care is effective if:

- The woman understands the cause, identification, and treatment of preterm labor.
- The woman's fears about early labor and delivery are lessened.
- The woman feels comfortable in her ability to cope with her situation and has resources to call on.

- The woman understands self-care measures and can identify characteristics that need to be reported to her care giver.

- The woman and her baby have a safe labor and birth.

● Care of the Woman With Postdate Pregnancy

Postdate pregnancy has become recognized as an important problem. While many pregnancies extend beyond the anticipated due date, the true postdate pregnancy is associated with increased risk for asphyxia and trauma in the fetus.

Postdate pregnancy is one that extends more than 294 days or 42 weeks past the first day of the last menstrual period. Approximately 12 percent of women give birth after 294 days (41 full weeks), and only one third of these are truly postdate (Freeman 1986).

Maternal Risks

The postdate pregnancy does not pose any particular physiologic risks for the mother. Psychologic stress seems to increase as the due date is passed and the woman begins to worry about the termination of pregnancy and the welfare of her baby.

Fetal-Neonatal Risks

True postdate pregnancies are frequently associated with placental changes that cause a decrease in the uteroplacental–fetal circulation. This decreases the blood supply, oxygen, and nutrition for the fetus. In addition, oligohydramnios (decreased amount of amniotic fluid) is frequently present and may increase the risk of cord compression. Perinatal mortality increases significantly with a doubling of the mortality rate between 42 and 43 weeks. (See Chapter 31 for in-depth discussion of the postdate infant.)

Medical Therapy

Medical therapy is best begun in early pregnancy with accurate dating. It is difficult to establish the date of pregnancy accurately when it is far advanced.

Therapies that may be used when postdate pregnancy is suspected include weekly or twice weekly NST and/or CST, and fetal biophysical profile to provide information regarding fetal status.

Nursing Assessment

Assessment of the woman with postdate pregnancy usually occurs in the birth setting. The nurse needs to stay alert for evidence of variable decelerations of the FHR, which are associated with cord compression due to the oligohydramnios. Meconium may be present and would be evident when the amniotic membranes rupture. The woman's knowledge base regarding the condition, implications for her baby, risks, and possible interventions need to be assessed.

Nursing Diagnosis

Possible nursing diagnoses include:

- Knowledge deficit related to lack of information regarding postdate pregnancy

- Fear related to the unknown outcome for the baby

- Potential alteration in coping related to anxiety regarding the status of the baby

Nursing Goal: Promotion of Fetal Well-Being

The woman may be taught to assess fetal activity each day to become more familiar with fetal movement and to detect any decrease in movement. (See Chapter 20 for further discussion of fetal movement records.)

While in the birth setting, the fetal heart rate is monitored by continuous electronic monitoring. The FHR tracing is evaluated frequently for signs of distress.

Nursing Goal: Promotion of Maternal Psychologic Support

Women with pregnancies that extend past the due date frequently report that they would like more support from nursing personnel. In a recent study (Campbell 1986), women reported that they felt increased stress and anxiety and had more difficulty coping. Encouragement, support, and recognition of the woman's anxiety were all identified as helpful strategies by health personnel.

Nursing Goal: Client Education

The woman needs to have information regarding the postdate pregnancy. The implications and associated risks for the baby need to be addressed as well as possible treatment plans. The woman and her partner need opportunities to ask questions and clarify information.

Evaluative Outcome Criteria

Nursing care is effective if:

- The woman has knowledge regarding the postdate pregnancy.

- The woman and her partner feel supported and able to cope with the postdate pregnancy.

- Fetal status is maintained and any abnormalities are quickly identified and supportive measures are initiated.

Care of the Woman with a Ruptured Uterus

Unlike uterine perforation, a ruptured uterus involves the tearing of previously intact uterine musculature or an old uterine scar after the period of fetal viability. The rupture may be through the three muscular layers of the uterus (complete rupture) or through the endometrium and myometrium (incomplete rupture). The rupture can be caused by one or more of the following:

- A weakened cesarean scar, usually from a classic incision into the uterus (see Chapter 26)

- Obstetric trauma, such as may occur with any undue manipulation of the fetus at the time of delivery

- Mismanagement of oxytocin induction or stimulation during labor

- Obstructed labor

- Congenital or acquired defects

- External forces such as trauma

- Vaginal birth after cesarean

Maternal Risks

If a ruptured uterus remains untreated, irreversible shock and death may occur. When a rupture goes undetected for a period of time, peritonitis occasionally results.

Fetal-Neonatal Risks

In acute uterine rupture, the fetus extrudes into the abdominal cavity. The fetus, as it faces asphyxia, may become excessively active and exhibit bradycardia, which progresses to absence of heartbeat as it dies. All of this may take place within a few minutes.

Medical Therapy

In the presence of a threatened or actual rupture, emergency surgical intervention is performed to save the mother and her baby. Delivery is by cesarean birth. If the rupture (uterine tear) is small, the physician may be able to repair it. If the rupture is large, the physician may do a hysterectomy.

Nursing Assessment

The nurse should be alert for warning signs of impending uterine rupture, including the following:

1. Restlessness and anxiety from severe pain and strong uterine contractions may occur.

2. No indication of labor progress is found by vaginal examination in the presence of uterine contractions.

3. The lower uterine segment balloons out, simulating the appearance of a full bladder, and a pathologic retraction ring may be evident. This ring occurs when there is an abnormal division between the upper and lower uterine segments and is manifested by an indentation across the lower abdominal wall with acute tenderness above the symphysis.

4. On vaginal examination the cervix is found to stretch tautly around the presenting part, and a caput succedaneum may bulge out of the cervix in the vagina.

Nursing Diagnosis

Nursing diagnoses that may apply to the woman with a ruptured uterus include:

- Impaired gas exchange related to blood loss secondary to uterine hemorrhage

- Fear related to unknown outcome for herself and her baby

Nursing Goal: Promotion of Maternal-Fetal Physical Well-Being

The nurse may be the one to identify the warning signs of impending rupture or maternal hemorrhage if rupture has occurred. In acute rupture, the nurse quickly mobilizes the staff for emergency surgery. The nurse continues to assess the maternal-fetal status and initiates treatments to stabilize the woman during the hemorrhage.

Nursing Goal: Provision of Emotional Support to the Woman and Family

When the physiologic needs of the woman and the fetus are met, the nurse can focus on the emotional needs of the family. The family must have a clear understanding of the procedure and its implications for future childbearing. If fetal death has occurred, the mother and father should also be given an opportunity to grieve and to see their infant if they desire.

Evaluative Outcome Criteria

Nursing care is effective if:

- The woman's uterine rupture is quickly identified and supportive treatment is established

- The woman's fear is lessened

- The woman and her fetus have a safe delivery.

● Care of the Woman and Fetus at Risk Due to Fetal Malposition

Occiput-Posterior Position

Persistent occiput-posterior position of the fetus is probably one of the most common complications encountered in obstetrics. Although this position may be normal in some races because of a genetically small transverse diameter of the midpelvis, it is considered a malposition because of the maternal and fetal difficulties that may result. It should be remembered that the fetus generally tries to accommodate to the passage it has to travel through. For a fetus in an occiput-posterior position to rotate to an occiput-anterior position, it must rotate 135 degrees (ROP to ROT to ROA to OA), and most fetuses accomplish this. But some do not, and in those cases labor progress may cease or the fetus may be delivered in a posterior position.

MATERNAL RISKS

The woman may suffer a third or fourth degree perineal laceration or extension of a midline episiotomy during the second stage of labor.

FETAL-NEONATAL RISKS

There is no increased risk of fetal mortality due to the occiput-posterior position unless labor is protracted or an operative delivery is performed.

MEDICAL THERAPY

Medical treatment focuses on close monitoring of the maternal and fetal status and labor progress to determine whether vaginal or cesarean birth is the safer delivery method. According to Pritchard, MacDonald, and Gant (1985), vaginal delivery is possible as follows:

1. Await spontaneous delivery

2. Forceps delivery with the occiput directly posterior

3. Forceps rotation of the occiput to the anterior position and delivery (Scanzoni's maneuver; see Figure 25–4)

4. Manual rotation to the anterior position followed by forceps delivery

If the pelvis is roomy and the perineum is relaxed, as found in grandmultiparity, the fetus may have no particular problem delivering spontaneously in the occiput-posterior position. If, however, the perineum is rigid, the second stage of labor may be prolonged. A prolonged second stage is one that lasts over an hour in multiparas and two hours or more in nulliparas. One complication of the fetus delivering in the occiput-posterior position is the possibility of a third- or fourth-degree perineal laceration or extension of a midline episiotomy.

In the event of a prolonged second stage with arrest of descent due to occiput-posterior position, a midforceps or manual rotation may be done if no CPD is present. In cases of CPD, cesarean birth is the treatment of choice.

NURSING ASSESSMENT

Signs and symptoms of a persistent occiput-posterior position are a dysfunctional labor pattern, a prolonged active phase, secondary arrest of dilatation or arrest of descent, and complaints of intense back pain by the laboring woman. The back pain is caused by the fetal occiput compressing the sacral nerves. Further assessment may reveal a depression in the maternal abdomen above the symphysis. Fetal heart tones will be heard far laterally on the abdomen, and on vaginal examination one will find the wide diamond-shaped anterior fontanelle in the anterior portion of the pelvis. This fontanelle may be difficult to feel because of molding of the fetal head.

NURSING DIAGNOSIS

Nursing diagnoses that may apply to women with persistent occiput posterior include:

- Alteration in comfort related to unexpected back discomfort secondary to occiput posterior position

- Ineffective individual coping related to unanticipated discomfort and slow progress in labor

NURSING GOAL: FACILITATION OF FETAL POSITION CHANGE

Changing maternal posture has been used for many years to enhance rotation of OP or OT to OA. The woman may be placed on one side and then asked to move to the other side as the fetus begins to rotate. This side-lying position may promote rotation; it also enables the support

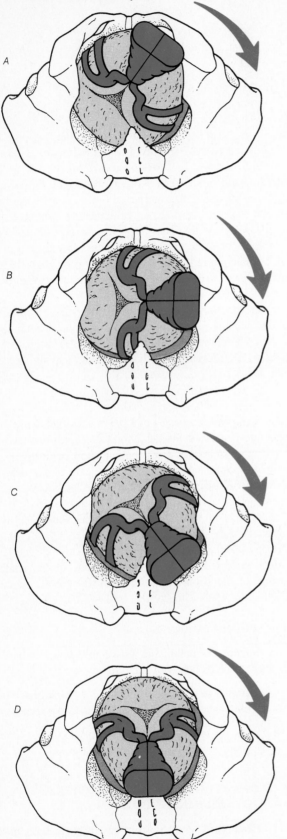

Figure 25-4 Scanzoni maneuver; anterior rotation. (From Oxorn H: *Human Labor and Birth,* ed 5. Norwalk, Conn, Appleton-Century-Crofts, 1986, p 401).

persons to apply counterpressure on the sacral area to decrease discomfort. A knee-chest position provides a downward slant to the vaginal canal, directing the fetal head downward on descent. Andrews and Andrews (1983) suggest that a hands and knees position is often effective in rotating the fetus. In addition to maintaining a hands and knees position on the bed, the woman may do pelvic rocking, and the support person may perform firm stroking motions on the abdomen. The stroking begins over the fetal back and swings around to the other side of the abdomen. After the fetus has rotated, the woman lies in a Sims' position on the side opposite the fetal back. Although Andrews and Andrews (1983) suggest that further research is warranted, these maternal position changes appear to be a safe, simple, and economical way to assist the change of fetal position.

EVALUATIVE OUTCOME CRITERIA

Nursing care is effective if:

- The woman's discomfort is decreased.

- The woman and her partner understand comfort measures and position changes that may assist her.

- The woman's coping abilities are strengthened.

- The woman and her partner feel supported and encouraged.

Transverse Arrest

In women with hypoactive labor or a diminished anteroposterior pelvic diameter (as seen with the platypelloid pelvis) or diminished tranverse diameter (in the android pelvis), an incomplete rotation may occur, resulting in a transverse arrest. This may also result in arrest of descent and a prolonged second stage of labor. In cases of severe molding and caput formation, the fetal scalp is visible at the vaginal opening even though the biparietal diameters have not entered the inlet. If labor is effective, spontaneous rotation may occur as labor continues.

MATERNAL RISKS

Manipulation during delivery can cause maternal soft tissue damage. Any prolonged pressure by the fetal head in one position may cause the woman later gynecologic problems, such as fistulas resulting from tissue anoxia. Postpartal hemorrhage may result from undetected lacerations or atony if the labor was hypoactive.

FETAL-NEONATAL RISKS

Unless a protraction or arrest disorder is present or an operative delivery is performed, fetal mortality is not increased with transverse position, because most fetuses do rotate spontaneously. Cerebral damage may be caused in cases of undetected CPD. The fetus should be closely observed in utero by the nurse, and at the time of delivery a pediatrician should be present if a midforceps delivery is anticipated.

MEDICAL THERAPY

The choice of medical treatment depends on the degree of fetal rotation. In the presence of a hypotonic labor pattern and no CPD, dilute oxytocin may be administered while closely monitoring the maternal-fetal response (Pritchard et al 1985). When rotation, uterine activity, and CPD are absent, delivery is often accomplished by midforceps, manual rotation, or vacuum extraction. If deep transverse arrest exists, forceps may be applied as long as excessive force is avoided. Cesarean birth is preferred, however.

NURSING ASSESSMENT

After identifying women who are candidates for transverse arrest, the nurse institutes ongoing review of the labor progress. If the labor becomes prolonged or a cesarean birth is necessary, the nurse assesses the coping abilities and knowledge level of the woman and her partner.

NURSING DIAGNOSIS

Nursing diagnoses that may apply to transverse arrest include:

- Ineffective coping related to unexpected problems in labor

- Knowledge deficit related to problems associated with transverse arrest

- Fear related to unknown labor outcome

NURSING GOAL: PROMOTION OF MATERNAL-FETAL PHYSICAL WELL-BEING

The nurse continues efforts to support and comfort the laboring woman. Continuous monitoring of contractions (character and frequency), amount of maternal discomfort, maternal vital signs, and fetal response to labor are important nursing interventions. The nurse notifies the physician/nurse-midwife in case of distress or dysfunctional labor.

The couple is prepared by the nurse for the extreme molding of the infant's head. The nurse remains alert for signs of postpartal hemorrhage.

EVALUATIVE OUTCOME CRITERIA

Nursing care is effective if:

- The mother and baby experience a safe labor and birth and any further complications are averted.

- The woman and her partner understand the associated problems of transverse arrest.

● Care of the Woman and Fetus at Risk Due to Fetal Malpresentation

Three vertex attitudes of the fetus are classified as abnormal presentations: the sinciput (military), brow, and face (Figure 25–5). The fetal body straightens out in these presentations from the classic fetal position to an S-shaped position. The sinciput presentation is probably the least difficult for the woman and fetus. In most cases, as soon as the head reaches the pelvic floor, flexion occurs and a vaginal delivery results.

In addition to the vertex malpresentation, the breech, shoulder (transverse lie), and compound presentations can cause significant difficulty during labor. These and the vertex presentations are discussed here.

Brow Presentation

The brow presentation occurs more often in the multipara than the nullipara and is thought to be due to lax abdominal and pelvic musculature. The largest diameter of the fetal head, the occipitomental, presents in this type of presentation. The nullipara whose fetus has a brow presentation commonly has a small infant. Upon descent into the inlet, the brow presentation frequently converts to an occiput position. Some brow presentations convert to face presentations.

MATERNAL RISKS

Delivery should be accomplished by cesarean birth in the presence of CPD or failure of a brow presentation to convert to an occiput or face presentation. With a vaginal birth, perineal lacerations are inevitable and may extend into the rectum or vaginal fornices.

FETAL-NEONATAL RISKS

Fetal mortality is increased due to injuries received during the delivery and/or infection because of prolonged labor. Trauma during the birth process can include tentorial tears, cerebral and neck compression, and damage to the trachea and larynx.

MEDICAL THERAPY

Active medical intervention is not necessary as long as cervical dilatation and fetal descent are occurring. In the presence of labor problems but no CPD, a manual conversion may be attempted. Some medical experts advocate midforceps delivery in the presence of complete dilatation and fetal station at +2. In the presence of failed conversions, CPD, or secondary arrest of labor, cesarean birth is the management of choice. Adequate resuscitation equipment and pediatric assistance should be available at the time of delivery.

NURSING ASSESSMENT

Leopold's maneuvers reveal a cephalic prominence on the same side as the fetal back. A brow presentation can be detected on vaginal examination by palpation of the diamond-shaped anterior fontanelle on one side and orbital ridges and root of the nose on the other side (Figure 25–6).

NURSING DIAGNOSIS

Nursing diagnoses that may apply to brow presentation include:

● Knowledge deficit related to the possible maternal-fetal effects of brow presentation

● Potential for injury to the fetus related to pressure on fetal structures secondary to brow presentation

NURSING GOAL: PROMOTION OF MATERNAL-FETAL PHYSICAL WELL-BEING

Nursing management of abnormal cephalic presentations include close observation of the woman for labor aberrations and of the fetus for signs of distress. The fetus should be observed closely during labor for signs of hypoxia as evidenced by late decelerations and bradycardia.

NURSING GOAL: PROVISION OF EMOTIONAL SUPPORT TO THE FAMILY

The nurse may need to explain the position to the laboring couple or to interpret what the physician/nurse-midwife has told them. The nurse should stay close at hand to reassure the couple, inform them of any changes, and assist them with labor-coping techniques.

In face and brow presentation, the appearance of the newborn may be affected. The couple may need help in beginning the attachment process because of the newborn's facial appearance. After the infant is inspected for gross abnormalities, the pediatrician and nurse can assure the

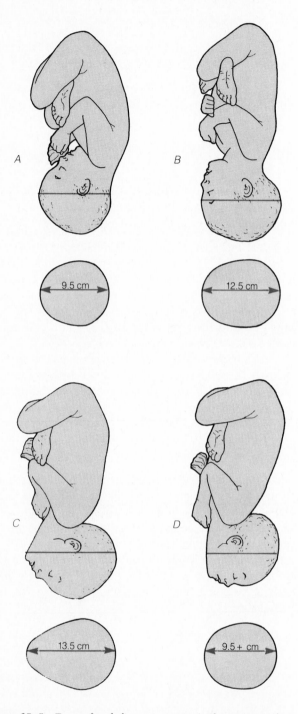

Figure 25–5 Types of cephalic presentation. A The occiput is the presenting part because the head is flexed and the fetal chin is against the chest. The largest AP diameter that presents and passes through the pelvis is approximately 9.5 cm. B Military presentation. The head is neither flexed nor extended. The presenting AP diameter is approximately 12.5 cm. C Brow presentation. The largest diameter of the fetal head (approximately 13.5 cm) presents in this situation. D Face presentation. The AP diameter is 9.5 cm. (From Danforth DN, Scott JR (eds): Obstetrics and Gynecology, ed 5. Philadelphia, Lippincott, 1986)

couple that the facial edema and excessive molding are only temporary and will subside in three or four days.

EVALUATIVE OUTCOME CRITERIA

Nursing care is effective if:

- The woman and her partner understand the implications and associated problems of brow presentation.

- The mother and her baby have a safe labor and delivery.

Face Presentation

Face presentation of the fetus occurs most frequently in multiparas, in preterm delivery, and in the presence of anencephaly. The head is hyperextended, and the chin is the presenting part.

MATERNAL RISKS

The risks of CPD and prolonged labor are increased with face presentation. As with any prolonged labor, the chance of infection is increased.

FETAL-NEONATAL RISKS

The fetus may develop caput succedaneum of the face during labor, and after delivery the edema gives the newborn a grotesque appearance. As with the brow presentation, the neck and internal structures may swell due to the trauma received during descent. Petechiae and ecchymoses are often seen in the superficial layers of the facial skin because of the birth trauma.

MEDICAL THERAPY

If no CPD is present, the chin (mentum) is anterior, and the labor pattern is effective, the objective of medical treatment is a vaginal delivery (Figure 25–7). Mentum posteriors can become wedged on the anterior surface of the

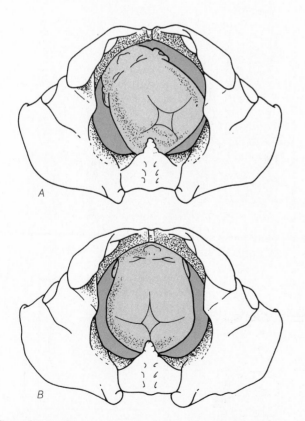

Figure 25–6 Brow presentation. A Descent. B Internal rotation. (From Oxorn H: *Human Labor and Birth*, ed 5. New York, Appleton-Century-Crofts, 1986, p 211)

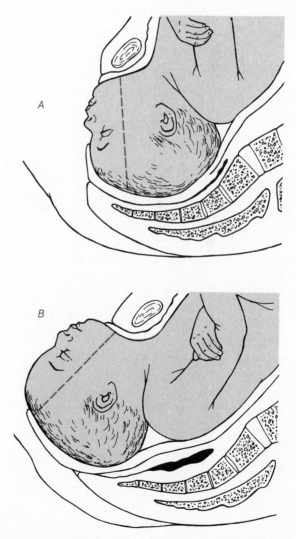

Figure 25–7 Mechanism of birth in mentoanterior position. A The submentobregmatic diameter at the outlet. B The fetal head is born by movement of flexion.

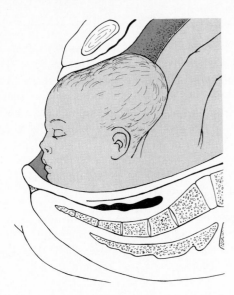

Figure 25–8   Face presentation. Mechanism of birth in mentoposterior position. Fetal head is unable to extend farther. The face becomes impacted.

sacrum (Figure 25–8). In this case as well as in the presence of CPD, cesarean birth is the management of choice.

NURSING ASSESSMENT

When performing Leopold's maneuvers, the nurse finds that the back of the fetus is difficult to outline, and a deep furrow can be palpated between the hard occiput and the fetal back (Figure 25–9). Fetal heart tones can be heard on the side where the fetal feet are palpated. It may be difficult to determine by vaginal examination whether a breech or face is presenting, especially if facial edema is already present. During the vaginal examination, palpation of the saddle of the nose and the gums should be attempted. When assessing engagement, the nurse must remember that the face has to be deep within the pelvis before the biparietal diameters have entered the inlet.

NURSING DIAGNOSIS

Nursing diagnoses that may apply to the woman with a fetus in face presentation include:

- Fear related to unknown outcome of the labor

- Potential for injury to the newborn's face related to edema secondary to the birth process

NURSING GOAL: PROMOTION OF MATERNAL-FETAL WELL-BEING

Nursing interventions are the same as for the brow presentation.

EVALUATIVE OUTCOME CRITERIA

Nursing care is effective if:

- The woman and her partner understand the implications and associated problems of face presentation.

- The mother and her baby have a safe labor and birth.

Breech Presentations

The exact cause of breech presentation (Figure 25–10) is unknown. This malpresentation occurs in 3 percent to 4 percent of all pregnancies and has a threefold to tenfold increase in perinatal morbidity and mortality in comparison to cephalic presentation (Mazor et al 1985). Breech presentation is frequently associated with preterm birth, placenta previa, hydramnios, multiple gestation, and grandmultiparity. The fetus in breech presentation is three times more likely to have congenital anomalies than a fetus in cephalic presentation (Mazor et al 1985). Because of the

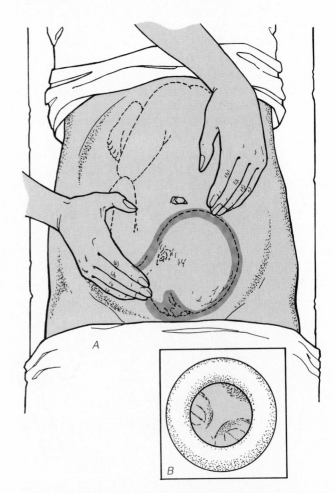

Figure 25–9   Face presentation. A Palpation of the maternal abdomen with the fetus in RMP. B Vaginal examination may permit palpation of facial features of the fetus.

increased incidence of congenital anomalies, an ultrasound may be done late in pregnancy to identify fetal problems or the presence of placenta previa (Mazor et al 1985).

MATERNAL RISKS

Breech presentation may prolong labor because the breech does not exert as much pressure on the cervix as the fetal head. This increases the mother's risk of infection.

Prior to the mid-1970s more than 90 percent of breeches were born vaginally. Since then, approximately 90 percent of breeches have been born by cesarean delivery (Bodmer et al 1986). Cesarean delivery involves more risk for the mother than vaginal delivery.

FETAL-NEONATAL RISKS

The fetus is at increased risk for prolapsed cord once the membranes rupture because there is more space around the body as it rests against the cervix.

The most critical problem with a breech presentation is that the largest part of the infant (the head) delivers last. In the presence of unrecognized cephalopelvic disproportion, the fetal head may not fit through the maternal pelvis (head entrapment), and the baby may die before any other action can be taken.

The increased incidence of perinatal mortality and

morbidity may also be associated with any of the following (Avery & Taeusch 1984):

- Increased risk of intracranial hemorrhage from traumatic delivery of the head

- Spinal cord injuries caused by stretching and manipulating of the infant's body and hyperextension of the fetal head

- Hemorrhage into the fetal abdominal viscera because of rupture of internal organs especially the kidneys, spleen, and liver due to manipulation

- Brachial plexus palsy

- Fracture of the long bones

- Fetal/neonatal asphyxia

- Aspiration

- Bruising with secondary jaundice

MEDICAL THERAPY

For the mother, a vaginal birth has less risk than a cesarean. Therefore, an increasing number of physicians are performing external version to convert a breech to cephalic presentation so that vaginal birth is possible. If a version is not done or is unsuccessful, birth will most likely be by

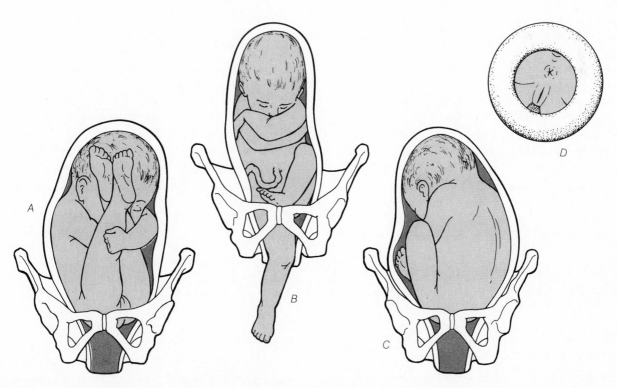

Figure 25–10 Breech presentation. A Frank breech. B Incomplete (footling) breech. C Complete breech in LSA position. D On vaginal examination, the nurse may feel the anal sphincter. The tissue of the fetal buttocks feels soft.

cesarean. The childbearing woman needs to know the implications of breech presentation and understand the rationale behind the delivery method chosen.

To minimize infant mortality and morbidity, medical management includes searching for any evidence of any actual or potential complications that justify cesarean birth as the delivery of choice. Pritchard, MacDonald, and Gant (1985) list the following criteria for vaginal delivery: (1) The pelvis is determined to be adequate when examined by x-ray pelvimetry, (2) the fetus presents as a frank breech with a fetal weight less than 3500 grams as estimated by a sonogram or two or more experienced clinicians, (3) spontaneous labor as demonstrated by progressive dilation and effacement of the cervix and fetal descent, (4) clinicians skilled in breech delivery and infant resuscitation.

NURSING ASSESSMENT

Frequently it is the nurse who first recognizes a breech presentation. On palpation the hard vertex is felt in the fundus and ballottement of the head can be done independently of the fetal body. The wider sacrum is palpated in the lower part of the abdomen. If the sacrum has not descended, on ballottement the entire fetal body will move. Furthermore, FHTs are usually auscultated above the umbilicus. Passage of meconium from compression of the infant's intestinal tract on descent is common.

The nurse is particularly alert for a prolapsed umbilical cord, espcially in incomplete breeches, because space is available between the cervix and presenting part through which the cord can slip. If the infant is small and the membranes rupture, the danger is even greater. This is one reason why any woman admitted to the labor and delivery suite with a history of ruptured membranes should not be ambulated until a full assessment, including vaginal examination, is performed.

NURSING DIAGNOSIS

Nursing diagnoses that may apply to breech presentation include:

- Potential for impaired gas exchange in the fetus related to interruption in umbilical blood flow secondary to compression of the cord

- Knowledge deficit related to the implications and associated complications of breech presentation on the mother and fetus

NURSING GOAL: PROMOTION OF MATERNAL-FETAL WELL-BEING

During labor it is important for the nurse to continue to make frequent assessments to evaluate fetal and maternal status. The nurse needs to be aware of the associated problems and look for subtle clues of beginning problems. The nurse provides teaching and information regarding the breech presentation and the nursing care needed.

NURSING GOAL: ASSISTANCE DURING VAGINAL DELIVERY

Although many infants in breech presentations are delivered by cesarean birth, a few are born vaginally. The nurse should include Piper forceps as a part of the delivery table setup. During the delivery process, the nurse may have to assist in the support of the infant's body if the physician elects to use forceps. The circulating nurse should monitor the FHR closely during the delivery.

If the family and physician elect a cesarean birth, the nurse intervenes as with any cesarean birth.

EVALUATIVE OUTCOME CRITERIA

Nursing care is effective if:

- The woman and her partner understand the implications and associated problems with breech presentation.

- The mother and baby have a safe labor and delivery.

- Major complications are recognized early and corrective measures are instituted.

Transverse Lie (Shoulder Presentation)

A transverse lie occurs in approximately 1 of every 300 to 400 deliveries (Seeds & Cefalo 1982). The infant's long axis lies across the woman's abdomen, and on inspection the contour of the maternal abdomen appears widest from side to side (Figure 25–11).

Maternal conditions associated with a transverse lie are grandmultiparity with lax uterine musculature; obstructions such as bony dystocia, placenta previa, neoplasms, and fetal anomalies; hydramnios; and preterm labor. It is not uncommon in multiple gestations for one or more of the fetuses to be in a transverse lie. Careless vaginal examinations before engagement may convert a dipping fetal head or breech presentation into a transverse lie. Premature amniotomy may also assist a fetus who has not firmly entered the inlet to assume this position.

MATERNAL RISKS

Labor can be dysfunctional in the presence of a transverse lie. Uterine rupture can occur. As in any case of prolonged labor, the woman is more prone to infection.

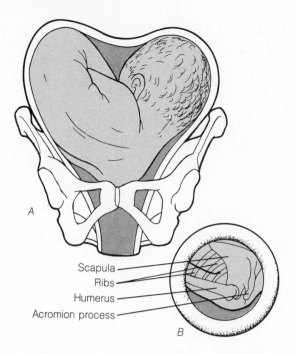

Scapula
Ribs
Humerus
Acromion process

A

B

Figure 25–11 A Transverse lie (shoulder presentation). B On vaginal examination the nurse may feel the acromion process as the fetal presenting part.

FETAL-NEONATAL RISKS

One danger of transverse lie is a prolapsed umbilical cord, because there is nothing in the pelvic inlet to serve as a blocking agent. Prolapse of a fetal arm may also occur. If the woman is allowed to labor in the presence of a transverse lie, the fetus may succumb from asphyxia and trauma.

MEDICAL THERAPY

With a viable fetus at term in the transverse lie, the medical goal is delivery by cesarean birth. External version for vaginal delivery may be attempted if the following criteria are met:

- There is no indication for rapid termination of labor.

- The fetus is highly movable.

- Contractions are not strong and frequent.

- There is no cephalopelvic disproportion.

- The membranes are intact.

- There is an adequate amount of amniotic fluid.

- Placenta previa has been ruled out.

When the required critieria are met, attempts at external version are appropriate prior to the onset of labor or in early labor. (See discussion in Chapter 26.)

NURSING ASSESSMENT

The nurse can identify a transverse lie by inspection and palpation of the abdomen, by auscultation of FHTs in the midline of the abdomen (not conclusive), and by vaginal examination.

On palpation no fetal part is felt in the fundal portion of the uterus or above the symphysis. The head may be palpated on one side and the breech on the other. Fetal heart tones are usually auscultated just below the midline of the umbilicus. On vaginal examination, if a presenting part is palpated, it is the ridged thorax or possibly an arm that is compressed against the chest.

NURSING DIAGNOSIS

Nursing diagnoses that may apply when transverse lie is present include:

- Knowledge deficit related to possible implications and problems associated with transverse lie

- Potential impaired gas exchange in the fetus related to decrease in blood flow secondary to cord compression associated with prolapsed cord

- Fear related to unknown outcome of birth

NURSING GOAL: PROMOTION OF MATERNAL-FETAL WELL-BEING

The primary nursing actions are to assist in the interpretation of the fetal presentation and to provide information and support to the couple. The nurse assesses maternal and fetal status frequently and prepares the woman for an operative birth. The nurse explains to the parents the need for cesarean and the assessments and care surrounding a cesarean. (See Chapter 26 for further information regarding teaching with cesarean birth.)

EVALUATIVE OUTCOME CRITERIA

Nursing care is effective if:

- The transverse lie is recognized promptly and crucial assessments are completed.

- The mother and baby have a safe delivery.

- The couple understands the implications and associated problems of transverse lie.

Compound Presentation

A compound presentation is one in which there are two presenting parts. It can occur when the pelvic inlet is not totally occluded by the primary presenting part. If the prolapsed part is a hand, the delivery is generally not difficult. Sometimes the hand slips back and occasionally it is delivered alongside the head; however, this may increase the chance of laceration (Pritchard et al 1985).

A compound presentation becomes a medical emergency when one of the presenting parts is the umbilical cord (see the discussion on prolapse of the umbilical cord on page 780).

● Care of the Woman and Fetus at Risk Due to Developmental Abnormalities

Macrosomia

Fetal macrosomia occurs when a neonate weighs more than 4000 g at birth. This condition is more common among offspring of large parents and diabetic women and in cases of grandmultiparity and postmaturity.

MATERNAL RISKS

The pelvis that is adequate for an average-sized fetus may be disproportionately small for an oversized fetus. Distention of the uterus causes overstretching of the myometrial fibers, which may lead to dysfunctional labor and an increased incidence of postpartal hemorrhage. If the oversized fetus acts as an obstruction, the chance of uterine rupture during labor increases.

FETAL-NEONATAL RISKS

Fetal prognosis is guarded. If a macrosomic fetus is unsuspected and labor is allowed to continue in the presence of disproportion, the fetus can receive cerebral trauma from intermittent forceful contact with the maternal bony pelvis. During difficult operative procedures performed at the time of vaginal delivery, the fetus may become asphyxiated or receive neurologic damage from pressure exerted on its head.

Shoulder dystocia can occur if the shoulders become wedged between the sacrum and the pubic bone. During manual attempts to facilitate delivery, there is a danger of overstretching the fetal neck. If the cord has also been brought down into the bony pelvis and delivery is delayed, asphyxia from cord compression can occur.

MEDICAL THERAPY

The occurrence of the maternal and fetal problems associated with excessively large infants may be somewhat lessened by identifying macrosomia prior to the onset of labor. If a large fetus is suspected, the maternal pelvis should be evaluated carefully. An estimation of fetal size can be made by palpating the crown-rump length of the fetus in utero, but the greatest errors in estimation occur

on both ends of the spectrum—the macrosomic fetus and the very small fetus. Fundal height can give some clue. Ultrasound or x-ray pelvimetry may give further information about fetal size. Whenever the uterus appears excessively large, hydramnios, an oversized fetus, or multiple pregnancies must be considered as possible causes.

When fetal weight is estimated to be 4500+ g and there is any abnormality of the labor pattern, a cesarean should be considered (Acker et al 1985, O'Leary 1986).

Unfortunately, in some situations a diagnosis of an oversized fetus is not made until numerous attempts to deliver the newborn have not been successful. If shoulder dystocia occurs and delivery cannot be completed by various maneuvers, the physician may find it necessary to fracture the clavicles to save the neonate's life. Appropriate pediatric and anesthesia support must be available to reduce the sequelae of the traumatic delivery.

NURSING ASSESSMENT

The nurse assists in identifying women who are at risk for a large fetus or those who exhibit signs of macrosomia. Because these women are prime candidates for dystocia and its complications, the nurse frequently assesses the FHR for indications of fetal distress and evaluates the rate of cervical dilatation and fetal descent.

The presence of a protraction and/or arrest disorder may be associated with an increased incidence of shoulder dystocia (Acker et al 1986).

NURSING DIAGNOSIS

Nursing diagnoses that may apply to the woman with a macrosomic fetus include:

● Potential for injury to the fetus related to trauma during the birth process

● Potential for infection related to traumatized tissue secondary to maternal tissue damage during birth

● Knowledge deficit related to the implications and possible problems associated wtih birth of a macrosomic baby

NURSING GOAL: PROMOTION OF MATERNAL-FETAL PHYSICAL WELL-BEING

The nurse should use the Friedman graph to monitor these labors closely for dysfunction. The fetal monitor is applied for continuous fetal evaluation. Early decelerations could mean disproportion at the bony inlet. Any sign of labor dysfunction or fetal distress should be reported to the physician.

The nurse inspects these neonates after delivery for skull fractures, cephalhematoma, and Erb palsy and informs the nursery of any problems. If the nursery staff is aware of a difficult delivery, the newborn will be observed more closely for cerebral and neurologic damage.

Postpartally, the nurse checks the uterus for potential atony and the maternal vital signs for deviations suggesting shock.

NURSING GOAL: PROVIDING EMOTIONAL SUPPORT

The nurse provides support for the laboring woman and her partner and information regarding the implications and possible associated problems. During the birth, the nurse continues to provide support and encouragement to the couple.

EVALUATIVE OUTCOME CRITERIA

Nursing care is effective if:

- The woman and her partner understand the implications and some of the possible associated problems.

- The mother and baby have a safe labor and birth.

Hydrocephalus

In hydrocephalus, 500 to 1500 mL of cerebrospinal fluid accumulates in the ventricles of the brain. The rate of occurrence, 1 in 2000 fetuses, represents about 12 percent of the severe malformations found at birth (Pritchard et al 1985). When this condition exists before birth, severe CPD results because of the enlarged cranium of the fetus.

MATERNAL RISKS

Obstruction of labor can occur, and if the uterus is allowed to continue contracting without medical interference, uterine rupture can result.

FETAL-NEONATAL RISKS

Outlook for the fetus is poor. Frequently, other congenital malformations accompany this condition, such as spina bifida and myelomeningocele. The neonate may be severely brain damaged and often succumbs during delivery or afterward in the nursery because of malformations and the presence of infection.

MEDICAL THERAPY

Medical intervention is directed toward delivering the fetus by the least traumatic means. It is important to know the degree of hydrocephalus and whether other anomalies or abnormalities are present that would make it very un-

likely that the baby could live after the birth. When anomalies that are incompatible with life are present, the decision regarding the method of birth needs to be discussed between the physician and the parents. A cesarean birth may give the newborn the best chance, but if the predicted chance of survival is very small, or if the fetus is already dead, a cesarean birth unnecessarily increases the risk to the mother. The decisions regarding method of delivery are not easy; they are best made by the physician and parents together.

NURSING ASSESSMENT

The nurse performing abdominal palpation discovers the presence of a hard mass just above the symphysis; this is the unengaged head. If the presentation is breech, it is difficult on external palpation to distinguish between the breech and an enlarged head. An ultrasound is indicated in the presence of breech presentations to evaluate the cranium. Vaginal examination with a vertex presentation reveals wide suture lines and a globular cranium.

Additional nursing assessments focus on the information needs of the woman and her partner. It is also important to assess their emotional state in order to provide support.

NURSING DIAGNOSIS

Nursing diagnoses that may apply include:

- Grief related to knowledge of the baby's anomalies

- Knowledge deficit related to the implications of hydrocephalus

NURSING GOAL: PROVISION OF EMOTIONAL SUPPORT TO THE FAMILY

The nurse helps the couple cope with the crisis and to deal with their grief (see discussion on page 789).

NURSING GOAL: PROMOTION OF MATERNAL-FETAL PHYSICAL WELL-BEING

The nurse assists with diagnostic procedures and interprets the findings if the couple has questions after conversations with the physician. The type of assistance at delivery will depend on the method chosen.

EVALUATIVE OUTCOME CRITERIA

Nursing care is effective if:

- The parents receive accurate information regarding their child and have their questions answered in a caring manner.

- The parents have support in beginning the grief process and have resources available in the days ahead.

- The parents are able to participate in the selection of the method of birth.

- The parents have their wishes respected in handling the labor and birth and in decisions regarding their baby.

Other Fetal Malformations

Enlargement of various fetal parts could result in dystocia. These fetal problems include enlargement of fetal organs, such as the liver or bladder, and incomplete twinning, in which a partially developed twin is attached to the fetus. It is not uncommon for malpresentations and malpositions to accompany this type of gestation. Hydramnios often accompanies the pregnancy that has a neurologically damaged fetus with defective swallowing (see page 784).

Identification of an enlarged fetal part that may cause dystocia often does not take place until delivery attempts have been fruitless. Careful examination of sonograms may lead to earlier diagnosis.

Cesarean birth is recommended to avoid a difficult vaginal delivery if a developmental problem is diagnosed early.

Nursing tasks fall in the realm of physical and emotional support of the laboring couple. Physical support includes physiologic maintenance of the woman's body functions during labor and assistance with comfort measures. Emotional support includes helping the couple with the grief process if the baby dies (see further discussion on p 761).

● Care of the Woman With a Multiple Pregnancy

Twin Pregnancy

The incidence of twin pregnancy in the United States is approximately 1 in 85 to 90 births (Polin & Frangipane 1986). Twins may be either monozygotic or dizygotic. When two fetuses develop from the fertilization of one ovum, the twins are categorized as *monozygotic*. The twins are further classified as diamniotic, dichorionic, or monochorionic, depending on the period in which the division of the ovum occurs (Figure 13–21). Monozygotic twins are identical and thus the same sex.

Dizygotic twins result from the fertilization of two separate ova. They are diamniotic, dichorionic, and fraternal. They may or may not be the same sex and are not identical.

According to Pritchard, MacDonald, and Gant (1985), the incidence of monozygotic twins is independent of race, heredity, age, parity, and fertility therapy. However,

the incidence of dizygotic twinning is highly influenced by these factors. The specific factors associated with dizygotic twinning are: increased maternal age; increased parity; a family history of twins; increased maternal nutrition; increased frequency of coitus, as in the first three months of marriage; pregnancies that occur within one month of stopping birth control pills; and race (black) (Polin & Frangipane 1986).

The perinatal morbidity and mortality rates for twins are increased as compared to single pregnancies, and the mortality rate for monozygotic twins is three times the rate for fraternal twins. The incidence of preterm delivery is 12 times that of single births and only 5 percent of twins reach 40 weeks of gestation (Polin & Frangipane 1986).

MATERNAL RISKS

In addition to the normal physiological changes in pregnancy, the woman with twins has further changes in the cardiovascular system. The blood volume is increased an additional 500 mL. The heart does not enlarge but cardiac output is increased in the second and third trimesters. The change in cardiac output is accomplished by an increase in heart rate and contractility. These changes probably reduce cardiac reserve so maternal activity and exercise should be tailored to take these physiological changes into consideration (Veille et al 1985).

A multiple pregnancy is associated with numerous problems for the childbearing woman:

- Spontaneous abortions are more common, possibly because of genetic defects or poor placental implantation or development.

- Maternal anemia occurs because the maternal system is nurturing more than one fetus.

- The increased incidence of PIH is thought to result from an oversized uterus and increased amounts of placental hormones.

- Third trimester bleeding from placenta previa and abruptio placenta occurs more frequently.

- Hydramnios may be due to increased renal perfusion from cross-vessel anastomosis of monozygotic twins.

Complications during labor include (a) uterine dysfunction due to an overstretched myometrium, (b) abnormal fetal presentations, and (c) preterm labor. With rupture of membranes and hydramnios, abruptio placentae can occur. Danger of placental abruption after the delivery of the first twin also exists because of a decrease in the surface area of the uterus to which the placenta is still attached.

The woman pregnant with twins may experience more physical discomfort during her pregnancy, such as shortness of breath, dyspnea on exertion, backaches, and pedal edema, because of the oversized uterus.

Occasionally multiple pregnancies are not diagnosed until the time of delivery; this occurs most often in cases of preterm labor. If the family has physically, psychologically, and financially prepared for one baby, problems can arise when they are suddenly confronted with more than one child. Infants of multiple pregnancies frequently require intensive care, and this may cause financial and emotional stress.

FETAL-NEONATAL RISKS

Fetal problems in the presence of twin pregnancy are numerous. Congenital anomalies are twice as common (Polin & Frangipane 1986). Labor is usually preterm, which has the potential to cause problems for the newborns.

Twins with monochorionic placentas may develop artery-to-artery anastomosis, which comprises fetoplacental circulation. One twin is overperfused and is born with polycythemia and hypervolemia and may have hypertension with an enlarged heart. This twin's amniotic sac exhibits hydramnios because of the increased renal perfusion and excessive voiding. The other twin has hypovolemia and exhibits IUGR. In the newborn period the neonate with increased perfusion has an increased chance of hyperbilirubinemia as the system tries to rid itself of the extra red blood cells. The other twin is anemic, with all the problems that SGA infants exhibit.

Twins that share the same amniotic sac have some special problems. They have an increased chance of becoming entangled in each others umbilical cords and this problem is responsible for a stillborn rate of over 50 percent. They are also more likely to have vasa previa, and developmental problems after birth. Their intelligence quotients are slightly lower than normal, and there is an increased incidence of learning disabilities (Polin & Frangipane 1986).

Conjoined or Siamese twins occur when the division of the embryonic disk is incomplete. The incidence is 1 in 50,000 births and 1 in 400 pairs of monozygotic twins. The stillborn rate is 40 percent (Sakala 1986).

MEDICAL THERAPY

The goals of medical care are the promotion of normal fetal development for both fetuses, preventing the delivery of preterm fetuses, and diminishing fetal trauma during labor.

Once the presence of twins has been detected, preventing and treating problems that infringe on the development and delivery of normal fetuses is a significant medical activity. Prenatal care is comprehensive. The woman's visits are more frequent than those of the woman with one fetus. The childbearing woman needs to understand nutritional implications, assessment of fetal activity, signs of preterm labor, and danger signs.

Since there are no factors that predispose the childbearing women to conjoined twins, all pregnancies with twins should be examined by ultrasound to rule out this problem. Ultrasound exams later in gestation are more likely to provide evidence of conjoining than early ones. Diagnostic clues include continuous external skin contour and identical body parts on the same level (Sakala 1986). Once diagnosed it is important to identify the extent of the conjoining and evaluate the twins' postnatal viability. This helps the physician determine what type of birth to recommend.

Serial ultrasounds are done to assess the growth of each fetus and to provide early recognition of IUGR. A program of bed rest is usually advised beginning in the 26th week. Some physicians believe that bed rest in the lateral position enhances uterine–placental–fetal blood flow and decreases the risk of preterm labor. Others question the value of bed rest, especially for the prevention of uterine contractions, which seem to precede preterm labor (Newman et al 1986).

Testing usually begins at 30 to 34 weeks' gestation and may include NST, fetal biopysical profile, and in some instances CST. A reactive NST is associated with good fetal outcome if delivery occurs within one week of the testing. The NST is done every three to seven days until delivery or results become nonreactive (Polin & Frangipane 1986). If the NST is nonreactive, some physicians recommend a CST, while others avoid this test because of the associated risk of stimulating preterm labor (Lodeiro et al 1986). The fetal biophysical profile is also accurate in assessing fetal status with twin pregnancies. Some researchers have found that a fetal biophysical score of 8 is associated with a reactive NST and suggest that both of these tests do not need to be done at the same time (Lodeiro et al 1986).

Intrapartal management and assessment require careful attention to maternal and fetal status. The mother should have an IV in place with a large bore needle. Anesthesia and cross-matched blood should be readily available. The twins are monitored by electronic fetal monitoring. The labor may progress very slowly or very quickly.

The decision regarding method of delivery may not be made until labor occurs, and the method depends on a variety of factors. The presence of maternal complications such as placenta previa, abruptio placentae, or severe PIH usually indicate the need for cesarean birth. Fetal factors such as severe IUGR, preterm birth, fetal anomalies, fetal distress, or unfavorable fetal position or presentation also require cesarean delivery.

Any combination of presentations and positions can occur with twins (Figure 25–12). Approximately 50 percent of twins are delivered by cesarean, which is chosen in the hope of reducing complications for the twins, especially birth asphyxia (Bell et al 1986).

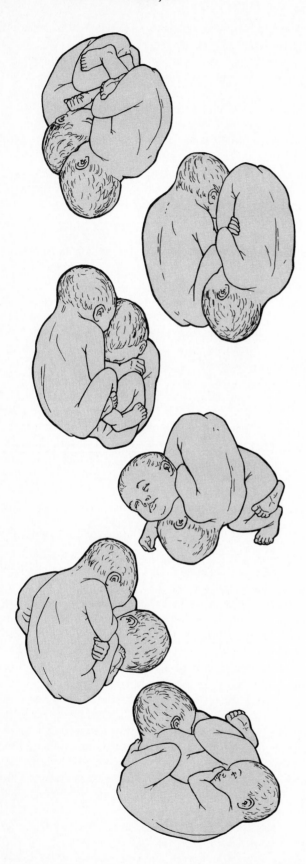

Figure 25-12   Types of twin presentations

Vaginal delivery is planned when the following factors are present (Polin & Frangipane 1986):

● Gestation is greater than 32 weeks and estimated fetal size is greater than 2000 g each.

● Twin A (the fetus closest to the cervix) is the largest twin.

● Twin A is vertex. Some authorities (Olofsson & Rydhstrom 1985) include frank breech as long as x-ray pelvimetry indicates no CPD.

● Twin B is vertex, breech, or transverse and smaller than twin A.

● There is no evidence of fetal distress.

● There is no CPD.

Since most breech presentations are delivered by cesarean, many physicians choose cesarean birth if either of the twins is breech.

An anesthesiologist should be present during the vaginal delivery in case a cesarean delivery needs to be done. One additional obstetrician is usually available to assist in the event that complications occur. The presence of two pediatricians, two nurses to care for the babies, and two labor and delivery nurses is usually recommended.

Since labor is frequently preterm and the labor progress difficult to predict, the mother is usually not given analgesics. An epidural may be used for the last part of labor and delivery or local anesthesia may be given at the time of delivery.

The twins are continually monitored by electronic fetal monitoring. After the birth of twin A, twin B is observed by ultrasound to assess position and descent into the pelvis. If twin B is in a transverse lie, the obstetrician converts it to a double footling breech by internal podalic version. The anesthesiologist administers general anesthesia such as halothane to effect good uterine relaxation during this procedure.

In some instances the second twin may need to be born by cesarean. Complications that would require this include profound fetal distress when vaginal delivery is not imminent; prolapse of the cord; and contractions of the uterus that trap the second twin (Polin & Frangipane 1986).

Delivery in the presence of dysfunctional labor due to overstretched uterine fibers can be managed with cesarean birth or infusion of diluted oxytocin. There is little agreement on the benefits and dangers of the two methods or on the most beneficial type of analgesia and anesthesia to employ for labor and delivery. In the presence of an unstable maternal circulatory system, as found with PIH, regional anesthetic agents such as epidurals or caudals can cause hypovolemic shock due to the blocking of the sympathetic nervous system. Large and continuous doses of narcotics can cause neonatal respiratory depression, especially if these infants are premature, as twins frequently are. Paracervical blocks have been known to cause transient fetal bradycardia. Pritchard, MacDonald, and Gant (1985) advocate the use of the pudendal block at the time of a vaginal delivery.

The placentas are examined after delivery. If the twins are of the same sex, the placentas are sent to the pathology laboratory for examination to determine whether they are monozygotic or dizygotic twins.

NURSING ASSESSMENT

When obtaining a maternal history, it is important to identify a family history of twinning. Equally important is a history of medication taken to enhance fertility. These facts should be noted on the antepartal record.

At each antepartal clinic visit, the nurse should measure the fundal height. Any growth, fetal movement, or heart tone auscultation out of proportion to gestational age by dates is indicative of twins. During palpation, many small parts on all sides of the abdomen may be felt. If twins are suspected, the nurse should attempt to auscultate two separate heartbeats in different quadrants of the maternal abdomen. Use of the Doppler device may be helpful. Conclusive evidence of twins is found on sonography.

During the prenatal visits, the nurse should determine the family's level of preparation for integrating more than one new member.

During labor it is important to monitor both twins. An external electronic monitor can be applied to both twins, or if conditions permit, the internal monitor can be applied to twin A and the external monitor to twin B. The heart rates may be auscultated on different quadrants of the maternal abdomen, but continuous monitoring is more beneficial. Signs of distress should be reported to the obstetrician.

After multiple deliveries, mothers are closely monitored for postpartal hemorrhage.

NURSING DIAGNOSIS

Nursing diagnoses that may apply to a woman with a twin pregnancy include:

- Fear related to unknown outcome of the birth process

- Ineffective individual coping related to uncertainty about the labor and birth plan

- Knowledge deficit related to implications and problems associated with twin pregnancy

- Potential for impaired gas exchange in the twins related to decreased oxygenation secondary to cord compression

NURSING GOAL: PRENATAL EDUCATION FOR SELF-CARE

Antepartally, the woman may need counseling about diet and daily activities. The nurse can help her plan meals to meet her increased needs. An increase of 300 calories or more over the recommended daily dietary allowance established by the Food and Nutrition Board of the National Research Council is advised for uncomplicated pregnancy (see Table 17–1). The daily intake of protein should be increased as much as 1.5 g/kg of body weight. Daily iron supplements of 60 to 80 mg and an additional 1 mg of folic acid are recommended.

Occasionally in multiple pregnancies women exhibit nausea and vomiting past the first trimester. A diet consisting of dry, nongreasy foods may be helpful. Antiemetics may be necessary to provide relief. The woman is more prone to have a feeling of fullness after eating, but this may be alleviated by eating small but frequent meals.

Maternal hypertension is treated with bed rest in the lateral position to increase uterine and kidney perfusion. The nurse can help the woman schedule frequent periods of rest during the day. Family members or friends may be willing to care for the woman's other children periodically to allow her time to get rest. Back discomfort can be alleviated by pelvic rocking, good posture, and good body mechanics.

Teaching regarding prevention and recognition of preterm labor is very important. For further discussion see page 741.

NURSING GOAL: PREPARATION FOR DELIVERY

The nurse must prepare to receive two neonates instead of one. This means a duplication of everything, including resuscitation equipment, radiant warmers, and newborn identification papers and bracelets. Two staff members should be available for newborn resuscitation.

If twins are discovered at the time of delivery, the nurse must move quickly to prepare for the second newborn. The pediatric team may need to be notified at this time. While one nurse is monitoring the second twin in utero, the other nurse is caring for the already delivered newborn and preparing to ensure correct identification of the neonates. Special precautions should be observed to ensure correct identification of the neonates. The first born is usually tagged Baby A and the second, Baby B.

NURSING GOAL: PROVISION OF SUPPORT TO THE FAMILY

The nurse determines the woman's or family's need for referral to social welfare agencies or public health clinics for follow-up care. The family may be unprepared financially and psychologically for the arrival of twins and thus at risk for further difficulties.

EVALUATIVE OUTCOME CRITERIA

Nursing care is effective if:

- The woman gains knowledge regarding the implications and problems associated with twin pregnancy.
- The woman feels she is able to cope with the pregnancy and birth.
- The woman understands the treatment plan and how to gain further information.
- The mother and her babies have a safe prenatal course, labor, and birth.

Three or More Fetuses

When three or more fetuses are present, maternal and fetal problems are potentiated. The more fetuses conceived, the smaller they tend to be at the time of delivery. Delivery of three or more fetuses is best accomplished by cesarean birth because of the risk of fetal insult due to decreased placental perfusion and hemorrhage from the separating placenta during the intrapartal period (Pritchard et al 1985). Complicated obstetric maneuvers such as breech extraction and podalic version, the risk of prolapse of the cord, and an increase in fetal collision provide additional reasons for cesarean birth.

● Care of the Woman and Fetus in the Presence of Fetal Distress

When the oxygen supply is insufficient to meet the physiological demands of the fetus, fetal distress results. The condition may be acute, or chronic, or a combination of both. A variety of factors may contribute to fetal distress. The most common are related to cord compression and uteroplacental insufficiency associated with placental abnormalities and preexisting maternal disease. If the resultant hypoxia persists and metabolic acidosis follows, the situation is potentially life threatening to the fetus.

The most common initial signs of fetal distress are meconium-stained amniotic fluid (in a vertex presentation) and changes in the FHR. The presence of ominous FHR patterns, such as late or severe variable decelerations, decrease or lack of variability, and progressive acceleration in the FHR baseline, are indicative of hypoxia. Fetal scalp blood samples demonstrating a pH value of 7.20 or less provide a more sophisticated indication of fetal problems

and are generally obtained when questions about fetal status arise. (For further discussion, see page 638.)

MATERNAL RISKS

Indications of fetal distress greatly increase the psychologic stress a laboring woman must face.

FETAL-NEONATAL RISKS

Prolonged fetal hypoxia may lead to mental retardation or cerebral palsy and ultimately to fetal demise.

MEDICAL THERAPY

When there is evidence of possible fetal distress, treatment is centered on relieving the hypoxia and minimizing the effects of anoxia on the fetus. Initial interventions include changing the mother's position and administering oxygen by mask at 6 to 10 L per minute. If electronic fetal monitoring has not yet been used, it is usually instituted at this time. If oxytocin is in use, it should be discontinued. Fetal scalp blood samples are taken.

NURSING ASSESSMENT

The nurse reviews the woman's prenatal history to anticipate the possibility of fetal distress. When the membranes rupture, it is important to assess FHR and to observe for meconium staining. As labor progresses, the nurse is particularly alert for even subtle changes in the FHR pattern and the fetal scalp pH, if available. Reports by the mother of increased or greatly decreased fetal activity may also be associated with fetal distress. For further discussion of FHR patterns and characteristics, see page 625.

NURSING DIAGNOSIS

Nursing diagnoses that may apply are presented in the nursing care plan on page 762.

NURSING GOAL: PROVISION OF EMOTIONAL SUPPORT TO THE FAMILY

The professional staff may become so involved in assessing fetal status and initiating corrective measures that they fail to give explanations and emotional support to the woman and her partner. It is imperative to provide both full explanations of the problem and comfort to the couple. In many instances, if delivery is not imminent, the woman must undergo cesarean delivery. This operation may be a source of fear and frustration for the couple, especially if they were committed to a shared, prepared birth experience.

NURSING GOAL: PROMOTION OF MATERNAL AND FETAL PHYSICAL WELL-BEING

The nurse stays alert for clues of fetal distress, initiates corrective measures, and answers any questions the couple have. Additional information regarding nursing interventions are presented in the Nursing Care Plan on page 762.

EVALUATIVE OUTCOME CRITERIA

Nursing care is effective if:

- The woman and her family feel supported and able to cope with their situation.

- The fetal distress is identified quickly, and corrective, supportive measures are instituted.

- The fetal heart rate remains in normal range or supportive measures maintain the FHR as normal as possible.

● Care of the Family at Risk Due to Intrauterine Fetal Death

Fetal death, often referred to as fetal demise, accounts for one-half of the perinatal mortality after 20 weeks' gestation. Intrauterine fetal death (IUFD) results from unknown causes or a number of physiologic maladaptions including preeclampsia-eclampsia, abruptio placentae, placenta previa, diabetes, infection, congenital anomalies, and isoimmune disease.

. . . She was smooth-skinned, as if very finely made. I was riveted by the look of peace on her face. And profoundly confused by the umbilical cord knotted so tightly about her neck. . . . It was the absence of life. . . . . Usually I felt as if I was helping give life, but here I was unneeded; death had managed for itself. . . . I wrapped the baby in old soft flannel. I covered her and carried her to her parents. (A Midwife's Story)

MATERNAL RISKS

Prolonged retention of the fetus may lead to the development of disseminated intravascular coagulation (DIC) (also referred to as consumption coagulopathy). After the release of thromboplastin from the degenerating fetal tissues into the maternal bloodstream, the extrinsic clotting system is activated, triggering the formation of multiple tiny blood clots. Fibrinogin and factors V and VII are subsequently depleted, and the woman begins to display symptoms of DIC. Fibrinogen levels begin a linear descent three to four weeks after the death of the fetus and continue

to decrease without appropriate medical intervention. An in-depth discussion of DIC is found on p 778.

MEDICAL THERAPY

Abdominal x-ray examination may reveal Spalding's sign, an overriding of the fetal cranial bones. In addition, maternal estriol levels fall. Diagnosis of IUFD is confirmed by absence of heart action on real-time ultrasonography.

The goals of therapy are to deliver the fetus within two weeks of fetal death and to assist the family with the grieving process. In 75 percent of these circumstances, spontaneous labor begins within two weeks of the fetal death (Quilligan 1980). Artificial rupture of the membranes is avoided because of the risk of introducing infection. If labor does not begin, oxytocin or prostaglandins may be administered to induce labor.

Nursing Assessment

Cessation of fetal movement reported by the mother to the nurse is frequently the first indication of fetal death. It is followed by a gradual decrease in the signs and symptoms of pregnancy. Fetal heart tones are absent, and fetal movement is no longer palpable. Once fetal demise is established, the nurse assesses the family's ability to adapt to their loss. Open communication among the mother, her partner, and the health team members contributes to a more realistic understanding of the medical condition and its associated treatments. The nurse may discuss prior experiences the family has had with stress and what they feel were their coping abilities at that time. Determining what social supports and resources the family has is also important.

Birth and death together. It's confusing and frightening enough for adults, but how are young children to understand it? For them the baby never really existed, or lived only briefly. What does this mean for them? Why are the parents so distraught? Too often, children's feelings about these issues are ignored or misunderstood. When parents are struggling to deal with their own feelings, they find it even harder to respond to the emotional needs of their other children. (When Pregnancy Fails)

Nursing Diagnosis

Nursing diagnoses that may apply include:

- Grieving related to an actual loss

- Alteration in family process related to loss of a family member

- Ineffective individual coping related to depression in response to loss of child

(Text continues on page 764.)

Nursing Care Plan: Potential for Fetal Distress

Kim Smith is admitted to the birthing room accompanied by her husband Ken. This is their first baby, and they are excited about the labor process. During the admission exam the nurse notes the presence of meconium in the amniotic fluid, the cervix is dilated 3 cm with 50 percent effacement, and the fetal station is − 3/− 4. FHR is 140. The nurse assists Mrs Smith into bed and helps position her on her left side. The nurse asks about fetal movement and discovers that Mrs Smith has been assessing fetal movement daily for the past month and the "baby has been real consistent in movements each day." While they are talking, Mrs Smith asks what the "funny-colored fluid" is.

Since the initial assessment of the fetus indicates normal status, the nurse sits with Mrs Smith and explains the implication of meconium-stained fluid and gives some introductory information about the birthing room.

The nurse begins her care, knowing that additional assessments must be made because the station and dilatation place Mrs Smith at increased risk for cord prolapse. In addition meconium is present in the amniotic fluid. The nurse knows that this may or may not be associated with fetal distress.

Assessment

NURSING HISTORY

Presence of predisposing factors
- Preexisting maternal disease
- Maternal hypotension, bleeding
- Placental abnormalities

Course of pregnancy
Estimated gestational age
Support person available
Educational preparation
Changes in fetal movement patterns

PHYSICAL EXAMINATION

1. Examine the pregnant uterus to determine fetal size and position.
2. Determine gestational age.
3. Evaluate contractions.
4. Determine whether membranes are intact or ruptured.
5. Check for signs of fetal distress:
   - FHR decelerations, decreased variability, tachycardia followed by bradycardia
   - Presence of meconium in the amniotic fluid
   - Fetal scalp blood pH determination ≤ 7.20

LABORATORY EVALUATION

Material hemoglobin and hematocrit
Urinalysis
Fetal scalp blood pH

Analysis of Nursing Priorities

1. Evaluate maternal and fetal status for variations requiring immediate intervention.
2. Identify and correct interferences with transplacental gas exchange.
3. Identify and report FHR decelerations and lack of baseline variability.
4. In presence of severe fetal asphyxia, prepare woman for immediate delivery (either vaginally or by cesarean).
5. Provide opportunities to explain treatments, discuss problems, questions, and concerns of the woman and her family.

Nursing Diagnosis and Goals	Nursing Interventions	Rationale
NURSING DIAGNOSIS: Potential impaired gas exchange in the fetus related to change in uteroplacental blood flow: interruption of blood flow (cord compression) or decreased blood flow (uteroplacental insufficiency)	Apply electronic fetal monitor.	Presence of meconium may be indicative of fetal distress. Continuous FHR monitoring will provide more data on fetal status.
SUPPORTING DATA: Presence of meconium in amniotic fluid Fetal presenting part at − 3/− 4 with 3 cm cervical dilatation.	Maintain Mrs Smith in side-lying position.	Side-lying position promotes optimum uteroplacental–fetal perfusion.
	Evaluate fetal monitor tracing. If variable decelerations are present, change maternal position. Also change maternal position in the presence of: Decreasing or loss of variability	Presence of variable decelerations is indicative of cord compression. Maternal position change may relieve compression on the cord and improve blood flow. These are additional signs of fetal distress.
	Rising baseline	
	Falling baseline	
	Tachycardia	
	Bradycardia	
	Late decelerations	
	Observe for further meconium staining of amniotic fluid	Fetal hypoxic episode leads to increased intestinal peristalsis and anal sphincter relaxation, resulting in meconium release.

Nursing Care Plan: Potential for Fetal Distress (continued)

Nursing Diagnosis and Goals	Nursing Interventions	Rationale
	Assess maternal BP and pulse. If hypotensive, start IV fluids or increase rate of IV fluids already being administered. Note amniotic fluid on a frequent basis for amount of fluid and increasing amounts of meconium. Explain the need for continued bed rest.	Maternal hypotension affects placental–fetal perfusion. Correction of hypotension may relieve or lessen fetal distress. Characteristics of the amniotic fluid may indicate fetal distress. Amount of dilatation and fetal station increase the risk of cord prolapse especially when the woman is in an upright position.
GOAL: FHR will remain in normal range (120–160) with good variability and no variable or late decelerations.		
NURSING DIAGNOSIS: Knowledge deficit related to potential problems associated with meconium staining		
SUPPORTING DATA: Mrs Smith asks questions regarding the amniotic fluid.	Provide information regarding implications of meconium staining. For example: It may indicate fetal distress now or in recent past, the fetus needs to be carefully assessed, at delivery the baby's nose and mouth will be carefully suctioned to remove all meconium fluid from nose and mouth before the baby breathes.	Providing information helps decrease anxiety and enables woman to be an active participant in her care. The presence of meconium may be associated with problems in labor or at the birth of the baby.
GOAL: Mr and Mrs Smith understand the potential problems associated with meconium-stained fluid and the recommended treatment.		
NURSING DIAGNOSIS: Fear related to chance of problems occurring with the baby.		
SUPPORTING DATA: Mrs Smith frequently asks how the baby is doing. She looks at the fetal monitor tracing frequently. Mr Smith waits anxiously each time an assessment is done.	Provide information regarding the electronic fetal monitor. Explain how the machine works, what to expect, and what may indicate a problem. Explain the assessments that need to be made, the reasons for them, and the findings as assessments are completed. Stay with the couple.	Information regarding the monitor and procedures decreases fear by increasing knowledge base. It also increases the control the couple feels. Ongoing reports of findings and progress help decrease fear. The nurse's presence helps provide support and decreases anxiety and fear.
GOAL: Mr and Mrs Smith will gain more information that will decrease their fears for the baby.		

A few hours later, the nurse notes severe decelerations and decreased variability on the fetal monitoring strip. The nurse recognizes that these are signs of cord compression. As she begins immediate interventions, the nurse explains what is needed to Mr and Mrs Smith. The nurse asks a colleague to notify the obstetrician.

Nursing Care Plan: Potential for Fetal Distress (continued)

Nursing Diagnosis and Goals	Nursing Interventions	Rationale
NURSING DIAGNOSIS: Impaired gas exchange in the fetus related to interruption of blood flow due to cord compression	Administer O_2 per face mask at 6–10 L/min.	Administration of O_2 may increase amount of oxygen available for transport to fetus. Tight face mask is used because laboring woman tends to breathe through her mouth. Administration of at least 6 L/min is needed to clear the face mask of CO_2.
SUPPORTING DATA: Presence of severe decelerations Decreased variability	Change maternal position and assess FHR for improvement. If no improvement, change position again. Perform vaginal exam to assess cervical dilation, effacement, fetal station, and especially for prolapse of cord. Assess maternal BP and pulse. If hypotensive, start IV fluids or increase rate of IV fluids already being administered. Continue to monitor FHR.	Change of position may relieve pressure on the cord and improve placental–fetal blood exchange. Dilatation status may indicate amount of time from delivery and helps determine type of delivery. If cord is prolapsed, the pressure is relieved manually. Maternal hypotension affects placental–fetal perfusion. Correction of hypotension may relieve or lessen fetal distress. FHR provides information regarding fetal status.
GOAL: The fetus will have the compression on the umbilical cord relieved. The variable decelerations will cease and the variability will improve.		
NURSING DIAGNOSIS: Fear related to fetal status	Keep parents informed of fetal status. Provide honest information. Stay with parents at all times.	Truthful information relieves anxiety and helps parents cope with situation. The nurse's presence is reassuring.
GOAL: Mr and Mrs Smith receive information and support		
Epilogue		
Mrs Smith was prepared for emergency cesarean birth. Mr Smith was able to accompany her, and his presence helped provide support.		Their baby had minimal difficulty after birth, and after initial stabilization the Smiths were able to hold their new son.

- Ineffective family coping related to death of a child

- Anxiety related to death of a child

A friend asked if we had named our stillborn baby. After telling her the name, we both began referring to the baby by her name, Sarah. It felt so good to call her a name. (*When Pregnancy Fails*)

Nursing Goal: Provision of Emotional Support to the Family

The parents of a stillborn infant suffer a devastating experience, precipitating an intense emotional trauma. During the pregnancy, the couple has already begun the attachment process, which now must be terminated through the grieving process. The behaviors that couples exhibit while mourning may be associated with the five stages of grieving described by Elizabeth Kübler-Ross (1969). Often the first stage is *denial* of the death of the fetus. Even when the initial health care provider suspects fetal demise, the couple is hoping that a second opinion will be different. Some couples may not be convinced of the death until they view and hold the stillborn infant. The second stage is *anger,* resulting from the feelings of loss, loneliness, and perhaps guilt. The anger may be projected at significant others and health team members, or it may be omitted when the death of the fetus is sudden and unexpected. *Bargaining,* the third stage, may or may not be present depending on the couple's preparation for the death of the fetus. If the death is unanticipated, the couple may have no time for bargaining. In the fourth stage, *depression* is evidenced by preoccupation, weeping, and withdrawal. Physiologic postpartal depression appearing 24 to 48 hours after delivery may compound the depression of grief. The final stage is *acceptance,* which involves the process of resolution. This is a highly individualized process that may take months to complete.

In some facilities, a checklist is used to make sure important aspects of working with the parents are addressed. The checklist becomes a communication tool between staff members to share information particular to this couple (Beckey et al 1985; Carr and Knupp 1985). Such a checklist might include the following items:

- When the fetal death is known before admission, inform the admission department and nursing staff so that inappropriate remarks are not made.

- Allow the woman and her partner to remain together as much as they wish. Provide privacy by assigning them to a private room.

- Stay with the couple and do not leave them alone and isolated.

- As much as possible, have the same nurse provide care to increase the support for the couple. Develop a care plan to provide for continuity of care.

- Have the most experienced labor and delivery nurse auscultate for fetal heart tones. This avoids the searching that a more inexperienced nurse might feel compelled to do. Avoid the temptation to listen again "to make sure" (Whitaker 1986).

- Listen to the couple; do not offer explanations. They require solace without minimizing the situation.

- Facilitate the woman and her partner's participation in the labor and delivery process. When possible, allow them to make decisions about who will be present and what ritual will occur during the birth process. Allow the woman to make the decision regarding whether to have sedation during labor and delivery. Provide a quiet supportive environment; ideally the labor and delivery should occur in a labor room or possibly a birthing room rather than the delivery room.

- Give parents accurate information regarding plans for labor and birth.

- Provide ongoing opportunities for the couple to ask questions.

- Arrange for the woman to be assigned to a room that is away from new mothers and babies. Let the woman decide if she wants to be on another unit. If early discharge is an option, allow the family to make that selection.

- Encourage the couple to experience the grief that they feel. Accept the weeping and depression. A couple may have intense feelings that they are unable to share with each other. Encourage them to talk together and allow emotions to show freely.

- Give the couple an opportunity to see and hold the stillborn infant in a private quiet location. (Advocates of seeing the stillborn believe that viewing assists in dispelling denial and enables the couple to progress to the next step in the grieving process.) If they choose to see their stillborn infant, prepare the couple for what they will see by saying "the baby is cold," "the baby is blue," "the baby is bruised," or other appropriate statements.

- Some families may elect to bathe or dress their stillborn; support them in their choice.

- Take a photograph of the infant, and let the family know it is available if they want it now or some time in the future.

- Offer a card with footprints, crib card, ID band, and possibly a lock of hair to the parents. These items may be kept with the photo if the parents do not want them at this time (Beckey et al 1985).

- Prepare the couple for returning home. If there are siblings, each will progress through age-appropriate grieving. Provide the parents with information about normal mourning reactions, both psychologic and physiologic.

- Furnish the mother with educational materials that discuss the changes she will experience in returning to the nonpregnant state.

- Provide information about community support groups including group name, contact person if possible, and phone number. Use materials such as the book *When Hello Means Goodbye* by Schwiebert & Kirk (1985).

- Remember it is not so important to "say the right words." The caring support and human contact that a couple receives is important and can be conveyed through silence and your presence.

The nurse experiences many of the same grief reactions as the parents of a stillborn infant. It is important to have support persons and colleagues available for counseling and support.

Evaluative Outcome Criteria

Nursing care is effective if:

- The family members express their feelings about the death of their baby.

- The family participates in decisions regarding whether to see their baby and in other decisions regarding the baby.

- The family has resources available for continued support.

- The family knows the community resources available and has names and phone numbers to use if they choose.

- The family is moving into and through the grieving process.

I knew something was wrong just by the way everyone was scurrying around in the delivery room and by that terrible silence. Then we knew the baby was dead. The doctor's only comment was, "It must be congenital," as if to say it certainly must be my fault, not his. Then a nurse said: "It would be worse if you had a five-year-old that died." I suppose she was right, but it certainly didn't make me feel any better. Later, the doctor said, "You're young, you'll have lots more kids." I was appalled—I was thirty-three already. Where do they learn all these stupid comments? (*When Pregnancy Fails*)

● Care of the Woman and Fetus at Risk Due to Placental Problems

Maintenance of placental function is paramount to assure fetal well-being and continuance of the pregnancy. Because the placenta is so vascular, problems that develop are usually associated with maternal and possible fetal hemorrhage. Causes and sources of hemorrhage are reviewed in Table 25–3.

Abruptio Placentae

Abruptio placentae is the premature separation of a normally implanted placenta from the uterine wall. Premature separation is considered a catastrophic event because of the severity of the hemorrhage that occurs. The incidence varies according to the population studied and the diagnostic criteria used, which accounts for rates of 1 in 86 to 1 in 750 (Pritchard et al 1985). Whether the incidence has stabilized or declined over the last two to three decades is not readily apparent. It is clear, however, that the risk of recurrence in subsequent pregnancies is as

Table 25–3 Causes and Sources of Hemorrhage

Causes and sources	Signs and symptoms
ANTEPARTAL PERIOD	
Abortion	Vaginal bleeding Intermittent uterine contractions Rupture of membranes
Placenta previa	Painless vaginal bleeding after seventh month
Abruptio placentae	
Partial	Vaginal bleeding; no increase in uterine pain
Severe	No vaginal bleeding Extreme tenderness of abdominal area Rigid, boardlike abdomen Increase in size of abdomen
INTRAPARTAL PERIOD	
Placenta previa	Bright red vaginal bleeding
Abruptio placentae	Same signs and symptoms as listed above
Uterine atony in stage III	Bright red vaginal bleeding Ineffectual contractility
POSTPARTAL PERIOD	
Uterine atony	Boggy uterus Dark vaginal bleeding Presence of clots
Retained placental fragments	Boggy uterus Dark vaginal bleeding Presence of clots
Lacerations of cervix or vagina	Firm uterus Bright red blood

much as 30 times the risk in the general population (Green 1984).

The cause of abruptio placentae is largely unknown. Theories have been proposed relating its occurrence to decreased blood flow to the placenta through the sinuses during the last trimester. Excessive intrauterine pressure caused by hydramnios or multiple pregnancy, maternal hypertension, cigarette smoking, alcohol ingestion, increased maternal age and parity, trauma, and sudden changes in intrauterine pressure (as with amniotomy) have been suggested as contributing factors.

PATHOPHYSIOLOGY

Premature separation of the placenta may be divided into three types (Figure 25–13):

1. *Marginal.* The blood passes between the fetal membranes and the uterine wall and escapes vaginally. Separation begins at the periphery of the placenta; this marginal sinus rupture may or may not become more severe.

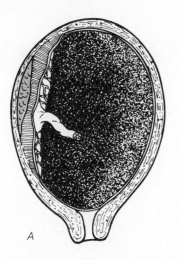
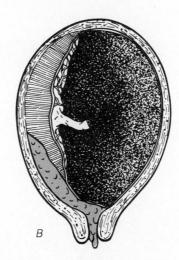
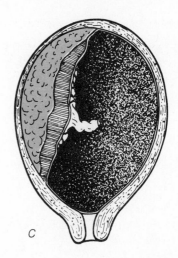

Figure 25–13   Abruptio placentae. A Central abruption with concealed hemorrhage. B Marginal abruption with external hemorrhage. C Complete separation. (From Abnormalities of the Placenta, Clinical Educational Aid No. 12, Ross Laboratories, Columbus, Ohio)

2. *Central.* The placenta separates centrally, and the blood is trapped between the placenta and the uterine wall. Entrapment of the blood results in concealed bleeding.

3. *Complete.* Massive vaginal bleeding is seen in the presence of almost total separation.

The signs and symptoms of these three types of placental abruption are given in Table 25–4. In severe cases of central abruptio placentae, a blood clot forms behind the placenta. With no place to escape, the blood invades the myometrial tissues between the muscle fibers. This occurrence accounts for the uterine irritability that is a significant sign of premature separation of the placenta. If hemorrhage continues, eventually the uterus turns entirely blue in color. After delivery of the neonate, the uterus contracts only with difficulty. This syndrome is known as a *Couvelaire uterus* and frequently necessitates hysterectomy.

As a result of the damage to the uterine wall and the retroplacental clotting with covert abruption, large amounts of thromboplastin are released into the maternal blood supply, which in turn triggers the development of disseminated intravascular coagulation (DIC) and the resultant hypofibrinogenemia. Fibrinogen levels, which are ordinarily elevated in pregnancy, may drop to incoagulable amounts within a matter of minutes as a result of rapidly developing premature separation of the placenta. Further information on DIC is found on p 778.

MATERNAL RISKS

Maternal mortality is approximately 6 percent. Problems following delivery depend in large part on the severity of the intrapartal bleeding, coagulation defects (DIC), hypofibrinogenemia, and length of time bewteen separation and delivery. Moderate to severe hemorrhage results in hemorrhagic shock, which ultimately may prove fatal to the mother if not reversed. In the postpartal period, mothers who have suffered this disorder are at risk for hemorrhage and renal failure due to shock, vascular spasm, intravascular clotting, or a combination of the three. Another cause of renal failure is incompatible emergency blood transfusion. Failure is directly proportional to the number of units transfused.

FETAL-NEONATAL RISKS

Perinatal mortality associated with premature separation of the placenta is about 15 percent. In severe cases in which separation is almost complete, infant mortality is 100 percent. In less severe separation, fetal outcome depends on the level of maturity. The most serious complications in the neonate arise from preterm labor, anemia, and hypoxia. If fetal hypoxia progresses unchecked, irreversible brain damage or fetal demise may result. With thorough assessment and prompt action on the part of the health team, fetal and maternal outcome can be optimized.

MEDICAL THERAPY

Because of the risk of DIC, evaluating the results of coagulation tests is imperative. In DIC, fibrinogen levels and platelet counts are usually decreased; prothrombin times and partial thromboplastin times are normal to prolonged. If the values are not markedly abnormal, serial testing may be helpful in establishing an abnormal trend that is indicative of coagulopathy. Another very sensitive test

Table 25-4 Differential Diagnosis

	Placenta previa	Abruptio placentae
Onset	Quiet and sneaky	Sudden and stormy
Bleeding	External	External and concealed
Color of blood	Bright red	Dark venous
Anemia	= Blood loss	> Apparent blood loss
Shock	= Blood loss	> Apparent blood loss
Toxemia	Absent	May be present
Pain	Only labor	Severe and steady
Uterine tenderness	Absent	Present
Uterine tone	Soft and relaxed	Firm to stony hard
Uterine contour	Normal	May enlarge and change shape
Fetal heart tones	Usually present	Present or absent
Engagement	Absent	May be present
Presentation	May be abnormal	No relationship

From Oxorn H: *Human Labor and Birth,* ed 5. Norwalk, Conn, Appleton-Century-Crofts, 1986, p 507.

determines fibrin degradation products levels; these values rise with DIC.

After establishing the diagnosis, emphasis is placed on maintaining the cardiovascular status of the mother and developing a plan for effecting the delivery of the fetus. Which birth method is selected depends on the condition of the woman and fetus; in many circumstances, cesarean birth may be the safest option.

If the separation is mild and gestation is near term, labor may be induced and the fetus delivered vaginally with as little trauma as possible. If the induction of labor by rupture of membranes and oxytocin infusion by pump does not initiate labor within eight hours, a cesarean birth is usually done. A longer delay would increase the risk of increased hemorrhage, with resulting hypofibrinogenemia. Supportive treatment to decrease risk of DIC includes typing and cross-matching for blood transfusions (at least three units), clotting mechanism evaluation, and intravenous fluids.

In cases of moderate to severe placental separation, a cesarean delivery is done after hypofibrinogenemia has been treated by intravenous infusion of cryoprecipitate or plasma. Vaginal delivery is impossible in the event of a Couvelaire uterus, because it would not contract properly in labor. Cesarean birth is necessary in the face of severe hemorrhage to allow an immediate hysterectomy to save both woman and fetus.

The hypovolemia that accompanies severe abruptio placentae is life threatening and must be combated with whole blood. If the fetus is alive but in distress, emergency cesarean birth is the method of choice. With a stillborn fetus, vaginal birth is preferable unless shock from hemorrhage is uncontrollable. Intravenous fluids of a balanced salt solution such as lactated Ringer's are given through a 16- or 18-gauge cannula (Pritchard et al 1985). Central venous pressure (CVP) monitoring may be needed to evaluate intravenous fluid replacement. A normal CVP of 10 cm H_2O is the goal (Berkowitz 1983). The CVP is evaluated hourly, and results are communicated to the physician. Elevations of CVP may indicate fluid overload and pulmonary edema. The hematocrit is maintained at 30 percent through the administration of packed red cells and/or whole blood (Berkowitz 1983).

Laboratory testing is ordered to provide ongoing data regarding hemoglobin, hematocrit, and coagulation status. A clot observation test may be done at the bedside to evaluate coagulation status. A glass tube containing 5 mL of maternal blood is inverted four to five times. If a clot fails to form in six minutes, a fibrinogen level of less than 150 mg/dL is suspected. If a clot is not formed in 30 minutes, the fibrinogen level may well be less than 100 mg/dL. A clot observation test may be completed by a physician or a nurse.

Measures are taken to stimulate labor to prevent DIC. An amniotomy may be performed and oxytocin stimulation is given to hasten delivery. Progressive dilatation and effacement usually occur (Pritchard et al 1985).

Electronic monitoring of the uterine contractions and resting tone between contractions provides information regarding the labor pattern and effectiveness of the oxytocin induction. Since uterine resting tone is frequently increased with abruptio placentae, it must be evaluated frequently for further increase. Abdominal girth measurements may be ordered hourly and are obtained by placing a tape measure around the maternal abdomen at the level of the umbilicus. Another method of evaluating uterine size, which increases as more bleeding occurs at the site of abruption, is to place a mark at the top of the uterine fundus. The distance from the symphysis pubis to the mark may be evaluated hourly.

NURSING DIAGNOSIS

Nursing diagnoses that may apply to the woman with abruptio placentae are presented in the Nursing Care Plan on page 770.

NURSING GOAL: PROVISION OF EMOTIONAL SUPPORT TO THE FAMILY

The psychologic aspects of nursing care are very important. Maternal apprehension increases as the clinical picture changes. Factual reassurance and an explanation of the procedures and what is happening are essential for the emotional well-being of the expectant couple. The nurse can reinforce positive aspects of the woman's condition, such as normal FHR, normal vital signs, and decreased evidence of bleeding.

Other nursing care measures are addressed in the Nursing Care Plan on page 770.

EVALUATIVE OUTCOME CRITERIA

Nursing care is effective if:

● Any signs of fetal distress are recognized promptly and corrective measures are begun.

● The woman and her baby have a safe labor and birth without further complications for the mother or child.

● The hemorrhage ceases and any hypovolemia is corrected as indicated by normal blood studies and normal vital signs.

Placenta Previa

In placenta previa, the placenta is improperly implanted in the lower uterine segment. This implantation may be on a portion of the lower segment or over the internal os (Figure 25–14). As the lower uterine segment contracts and dilates in the later weeks of pregnancy, the placental villi are torn from the uterine wall, thus exposing the uterine sinuses at the placental site. Bleeding begins, but because its amount depends on the number of sinuses exposed, it may initially be either scanty or profuse.

The cause of placenta previa is unknown. Statistically it occurs in about 1 of every 167 deliveries, with 20 percent of the cases being complete, and is more common in multiparas (Pritchard et al 1985). Women with a previous history of placenta previa, as well as those who have undergone a low cervical cesarean delivery, appear to be at greater risk for its occurrence. Other factors associated with placenta previa are increased incidences of IUGR, placenta accreta, breech, and transverse lie (Danforth & Scott 1986).

MEDICAL THERAPY

The goal of medical care is to identify the cause of bleeding and to provide treatment that will ensure delivery of a mature newborn. Indirect diagnosis is made by localizing the placenta through tests that require no vaginal examination. The most commonly employed diagnostic test is the ultrasound scan (Figure 25–15). If placenta previa is ruled out, a vaginal examination can be performed with

(Text continues on page 774.)

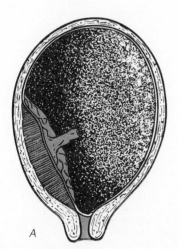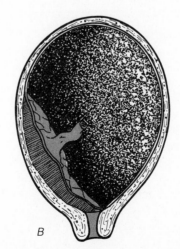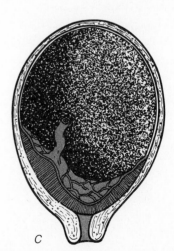

Figure 25–14   *Placenta previa. A Low placental implantation. B Partial placenta previa. C Complete placenta previa.* (From *Abnormalities of the Placenta,* Clinical Educational Aid No. 12, Ross Laboratories, Columbus, Ohio)

Nursing Care Plan: Hemorrhage

Karen Clark is admitted to the birthing room accompanied by her husband Mike. Mrs Clark tells the nurse that she has been having some dark vaginal bleeding. This is her second child. Her EDD is one week away. Mrs Clark has uterine contractions every 5 minutes lasting 45 seconds. Her vital signs are 120/80, P 80, R 18, FHR 140 with STV of 10 BPM, and no periodic changes. The nurse defers a vaginal exam because of the presence of bleeding. An ultrasound exam is done to try to establish the presence of placental problems. While waiting for the obstetrician and the results of the ultrasound the nurse begins care.

Assessment

NURSING HISTORY

Identify factors predisposing to hemorrhage:
1. Presence of preeclampsia-eclampsia
2. Overdistention of the uterus
   a. Multiple pregnancy
   b. Hydramnios
3. Grandmultiparity
4. Advanced age
5. Uterine contractile problems
   a. Hypotonicity
   b. Hypertonicity
6. Painless vaginal bleeding after seventh month
7. Presence of hypertension
8. Presence of diabetes
9. History of previous hemorrhage or bleeding problems, blood co-agulation defects, abortions
10. Retained placental fragments
11. Lacerations

Determine:
Religious preference to establish whether the woman will permit a blood transfusion
Course of present pregnancy
Education for childbirth
Support person available

Analysis of Nursing Priorities

1. If IV is not present, start one in large vein with large-bore plastic cannula.
2. Evaluate blood loss (if possible, measure or weigh blood-soaked pads to facilitate adequate replacement).
3. Monitor vital signs, particularly pulse and BP.
4. Measure urine output.
5. Administer oxygen as necessary.
6. Evaluate fetal status.
7. Maintain fetal life-support mechanisms.
8. Do not perform vaginal or rectal exam until placenta previa has been ruled out.
9. Provide information regarding the cause of the hemorrhage.
10. Discuss the assessment techniques and treatment associated with the hemorrhage.
11. Provide opportunities for questions and individual concerns of the woman and her family.

PHYSICAL EXAMINATION

Severe abdominal pain
Painless vaginal hemorrhage
Shock symptoms (decreased blood pressure, increased pulse, pallor)
Uterine tetany or uterine atony
Portwine amniotic fluid with abruptio placentae
Changes in FHR

LABORATORY EVALUATION

Hemoglobin and hematocrit
Type and cross-match
Fibrinogen levels
PTT
Platelet count

Nursing Diagnosis and Goals	Nursing Interventions	Rationale
NURSING DIAGNOSIS: Potential fluid volume deficit related to blood loss	Observe, record, and report blood loss.	Hypovolemia causes decreased venous return to the heart and subsequent decrease in cardiac output. Decreased cardiac output initiates sympathoadrenal response, which leads to increased peripheral resistance and tachycardia in an effort to maintain adequate tissue perfusion. Decreased blood flow to kidneys causes stimulation of juxtaglomerular apparatus to release hormones; this leads to retention of sodium ions and water (mechanism to increase blood volume) and increased reabsorption of water by distal tubules, which increases intravascular volume. Cells do not receive sufficient O_2 or nutrients because of vasoconstriction of venules and arterioles (caused by increased catecholamines).

Nursing Care Plan   Hemorrhage (continued)

Nursing Diagnosis and Goals	Nursing Interventions	Rationale
SUPPORTING DATA: Presence of dark vaginal bleeding	Complete assessments associated with decreased blood volume.	Release of catecholamines and cortisol during shock also stimulates release of fatty acids for energy production. As fatty acids are metabolized, ketones increase. Ketones are normally oxidized in the liver, but the hypoperfused liver cannot do this adequately, resulting in increase in metabolic acidosis.
	1. Monitor rate and quality of respirations frequently.	Initially respiratory rate increases as a result of sympathoadrenal stimulation, resulting in increased metabolic rate; pain and anxiety may cause hyperventilation.
	2. Monitor pulse rate frequently.	Increased pulse rate is an effect of increased epinephrine.
	3. Assess pulse quality by direct palpation. Determine pulse deficit by comparing apical-radial rates.	Pulse quality reflects circulatory status.
	4. Compare present BP with Mrs Clark's baseline BP; note pulse pressure.	Thready pulse indicates vasoconstriction and reflects decreased cardiac output; peripheral pulses may be absent if vasoconstriction is intense. Bounding pulse may indicate overload. Hypotension indicates loss of large amount of circulatory fluid or lack of compensation in circulatory system. As cardiac output decreases, there is usually a fall in pulse pressure. Peripheral vasoconstriction may make accurate readings difficult.
	5. Monitor urine output (decrease to less than 30 mL/hr is sign of shock): a. Insert Foley catheter. b. Measure output hourly. c. Measure specific gravity to determine concentration of urine.	Vasoconstrictor effect of norepinephrine decreases blood flow to kidneys, which decreases glomerular filtration rate and the output of urine. Inability to concentrate urine may indicate renal damage from vasoconstriction and decreased blood perfusion.
	6. Assess skin for presence of following: a. Pallor and cyanosis: *Pallor* in brown-skinned persons appears yellowish-brown; black-skinned individuals appear ashen gray; generally pallor may be observed in mucous membranes, lips, and nail beds. *Cyanosis* is assessed by inspecting lips, nail beds, conjunctiva, palms, and soles of feet at regular intervals; evaluate capillary refilling by pressing on nail bed and observing return of color; compare by testing your own nail bed. b. Coldness c. Clamminess	Skin reflects amount of vasoconstriction. Pallor is determined by intensity of vasoconstriction. Cyanosis occurs when the amount of unoxygenated hemoglobin in the blood is ≤5 g/dL blood. Produced by slow blood flow. Caused by sympathetic stimulation of sweat glands.
	Assess state of consciousness frequently.	
	If Mrs Clark's condition deteriorates a subclavian catheter may be inserted to obtain CVP readings.	Diminished cerebral blood flow causes restlessness and anxiety; as shock progresses, state of consciousness decreases.

Nursing Care Plan: Hemorrhage (continued)

Nursing Diagnosis and Goals	Nursing Interventions	Rationale
	Measure CVP: Insert catheter into superior vena cava; intravenous fluid should run freely through catheter before measuring, and baseline zero mark should be marked on woman's chest; normal CVP is 5–10 cm H_2O.	Provides estimation of volume of blood returning to heart and ability of both chambers in right heart to propel blood. Low CVP indicates a decrease in the circulating volume of blood (hypovolemia).
	Assess amount of blood loss: 1. Count pads. 2. Weigh pads and chux (1 g = 1 mL blood approximately). 3. Record amount of flow in a specific amount of time (for example, 50 mL bright red blood on pad in 20 min).	In childbearing women, blood is replaced according to estimates of actual blood loss, rather than using parameters of increased and decreased BP.
	Observe for signs and symptoms of hemorrhage.	Bleeding often stops as shock develops but resumes as circulation is restored.
	If partial abruptio placentae is diagnosed, nurse will: 1. Evaluate blood loss. 2. Assess uterine contractile pattern and tenderness. 3. Monitor maternal vital signs. 4. Assess fetal status. 5. Assess cervical dilatation and effacement.	
	If severe abruptio placentae is diagnosed: 1. Perform same assessments as for partial abruptio placentae. 2. Measure CVP. 3. Assess blood loss. 4. Observe for signs and symptoms of disseminated intravascular coagulation (DIC).	
GOALS: Mrs Clark's blood loss will be minimized, and her vital signs will remain stable.		

Mrs Clark's labor progresses, and she begins to have increased amounts of dark blood and bright red bleeding. Lab work is ordered and the results indicate a fall in the hemoglobin and hematocrit. Mrs Clark appears anxious and is very fatigued. Her BP decreases and pulse rate increases. An indwelling bladder catheter is inserted to assess urine output.

NURSING DIAGNOSIS: Impaired gas exchange related to reduction of hemoglobin	Position Mrs Clark in a side-lying or supine position with a rolled blanket under her right hip.	Either position keeps more blood volume available to vital centers and avoids pressure on vena cava.
	Avoid Trendelenburg position.	Trendelenburg position shifts heavy uterus against diaphragm and may compromise respiratory function.
SUPPORTING DATA: Decreased hemoglobin	Administer whole blood.	Corrects reduced oxygen-carrying capacity.
Anxiety	Administer O_2 by face mask at 6–10 L/min.	Woman in labor is mouth breather; using face mask assures better oxygen delivery.
Fatigue	Monitor fetal status.	Decreased blood volume and resulting hypotension affects the uteroplacental–fetal blood flow.

Nursing Care Plan: Hemorrhage (continued)

Nursing Diagnosis and Goals	Nursing Interventions	Rationale
GOAL: Mrs Clark's hemoglobin will be within normal limits.		
NURSING DIAGNOSIS: Decreased cardiac output related to hypovolemia	Relieve decreased blood pressure by administration of whole blood.	Hypotension results from decreased blood volume.
	While waiting for whole blood to be available, infuse isotonic fluids, plasma, plasma expanders, or serum albumin.	Degree of hypovolemia may be assessed by CVP, hemoglobin, and hematocrit.
SUPPORTING DATA: Hypotension Tachycardia		
GOAL: Mrs Clark's status will stabilize as indicated by normal BP and pulse.		
NURSING DIAGNOSIS: Potential alteration in tissue perfusion related to fluctuations of blood supply to vital organs.	Monitor urine output hourly: 1. 50 mL/hr or more indicates safe renal perfusion. 2. Less than 30 mL/hr indicates inadequate renal perfusion (tubular ischemia and necrosis can result).	This provides excellent measure of organ perfusion.
	Monitor adequacy of fluid volume by evaluating CVP.	
SUPPORTING DATA: Urine output of less than 30 mL/hr.		
GOAL: Mrs Clark's urine output will be monitored and a rate of at least 30 mL/hr will be maintained.		
NURSING DIAGNOSIS: Potential impaired fetal gas exchange related to decreased blood volume and hypotension	Assess and monitor fetal heart rate (range 120–160 beats/min).	Hemorrhage from woman disrupts blood flow pattern to fetus, possibly compromising fetal status.
	Observe for meconium in amniotic fluid.	Hypoxia causes increased motility of fetal intestines and relaxation of abdominal muscles, with release of meconium into amniotic fluid.
	Assist in obtaining fetal blood sample (pH <7.2 indicates severe jeopardy).	
SUPPORTING DATA: FHR patterns that indicate decreased variability, tachycardia or bradycardia, late decelerations		
GOAL: The FHR will remain within normal limits without signs of stress or distress.		

Nursing Care Plan: Hemorrhage (continued)

Nursing Diagnosis and Goals	Nursing Interventions	Rationale
NURSING DIAGNOSIS: Fear related to an unknown outcome and potential maternal/fetal jeopardy	Explain all procedures to decrease anxiety. Answer questions.	Knowledge increases confidence and ability to cope.
SUPPORTING DATA: Anxiety Apprehension		
GOAL: Mrs Clark will have questions answered and will feel less anxious.		
NURSING DIAGNOSIS: Potential alteration in tissue perfusion to vital organs related to depletion of fibrinogen and increased thromboplastin	Evaluate blood levels; at term, normal fibrinogen level is 375–700 mg/dL; critical level required to clot blood is 100 mg/dL. Observe for signs and symptoms of DIC. Determine whether fetal demise is cause of fibrinogen depletion; conduct coagulation studies and measure fibrinogen levels; induce labor if patient is at risk.	Fibrinogen and fibrin are lost because of their accumulation in a retroplacental clot; further fibrinogen loss and additional coagulation failure may result from intravascular clotting and fibrinolysis. Dead fetus releases thromboplastin, which interferes with the clotting mechanism and lowers fibrinogen level.
SUPPORTING DATA: Decreased fibrinogen levels, platelet count Elevated PTT	Monitor the administration of blood components as necessary (whole blood, platelets, cryoprecipitate, plasma). Presence of hemorrhage: Note previous interventions and rationale. Minimize anxiety with an empathetic approach and explanations.	Maintain the hematocrit value at 30% and above; elevate the platelet count and the fibrinogen levels. Increase Mrs Clark's feelings of security.
GOAL: Mrs Clark's clotting status will return to normal as indicated by normal lab work.		

Epilogue
Mrs Clark's condition was stabilized and an emergency cesarean delivery was done. Her husband was able to accompany her into the operating room for the cesarean delivery and provided support by talking with her and holding her hand as she went to sleep. Their baby had Apgars of 8 and 9 and Mr Clark was able to hold the baby soon after birth. When Mrs Clark recovered from the general anesthesia, Mr Clark brought their baby girl into the recovery room so they all could get acquainted.

a speculum to determine the cause of bleeding (such as cervical lesions).

Direct diagnosis of placenta previa can only be made by feeling the placenta inside the cervical os. However, such an examination may cause profuse bleeding due to tearing of tissue in the cotyledons of the placenta. Because of the danger of bleeding, a vaginal examination should be performed only if ultrasound is not available, the pregnancy is near term, and there is profuse vaginal bleeding. The examination may be done using a double setup procedure. In this situation, it must be determined whether the cause of the bleeding is placenta previa or advanced labor with copious bloody show (which is normal). *Double setup* means that the delivery room is set up for the vaginal examination and normal vaginal birth and for a cesarean birth should placenta previa be present and the examination precipitates brisk bleeding. Adequate personnel must be present to respond to treatment decisions.

The differential diagnosis of placental or cervical bleeding takes careful consideration. Partial separation of the placenta may also present with painless bleeding, and a true placenta previa may not demonstrate overt bleeding until labor begins, thus confusing the diagnosis. Another important fact to note is that the causes of slight-to-moderate antepartal bleeding episodes in 20 percent to 25 percent of women are never accurately diagnosed.

Care of the women with painless late gestational bleeding depends on (a) the week of gestation during which the first bleeding episode occurs and (b) the amount of bleeding (Figure 25–16). If the pregnancy is less than 37 weeks' gestation, expectant management is employed to delay delivery until about 37 weeks' gestation to allow the fetus to mature. Expectant management involves stringent regulation of the following:

1. Bed rest with bathroom privileges only as long as the woman is not bleeding

2. No rectal or vaginal exams

3. Monitoring of blood loss, pain, and uterine contractility

4. Evaluating FHTs with external monitor

5. Monitoring of vital signs

6. Complete laboratory evaluation: hemoglobin, hematocrit, Rh factor, and urinalysis

7. Intravenous fluid (lactated Ringer's) with drip rate monitored

8. Two units of cross-matched blood available for transfusion

If frequent, recurrent, or profuse bleeding persists, or if fetal well-being appears threatened, a cesarean birth may be performed before 37 weeks.

NURSING ASSESSMENT

Assessment of the woman with placenta previa must be ongoing to prevent or treat complications that are po-

tentially lethal to the mother and fetus. Painless, bright red vaginal bleeding is the best diagnostic sign of placenta previa. If this sign should develop during the last three months of a pregnancy, placenta previa should always be considered until ruled out by examination. The first bleeding episode is generally scanty. If no rectal or vaginal examinations are performed, it often subsides spontaneously. However, each subsequent hemorrhage is more profuse.

The uterus remains soft, and if labor begins, it relaxes fully between contractions. The FHR usually remains stable unless profuse hemorrhage and maternal shock occur. As a result of the placement of the placenta, the fetal presenting part is often unengaged, and transverse lie is common.

Blood loss, pain, and uterine contractility are appraised by the nurse from both subjective and objective perspectives. Maternal vital signs and the results of blood and urine tests provide the nurse with additional data about the woman's condition. FHR is evaluated with an external fetal monitor. Another pressing nursing responsibility is observing and verifying the family's ability to cope with the anxiety associated with an unknown outcome.

NURSING DIAGNOSIS

Nursing diagnoses that may apply are presented in the Nursing Care Plan on page 770.

NURSING GOAL: PREPARATION FOR DOUBLE SETUP PROCEDURE

Before a double setup procedure is performed, the laboring couple should be physiologically and psycho-

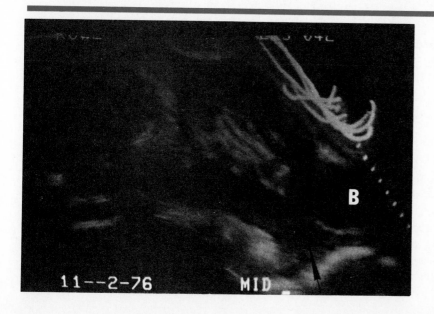

Figure 25–15 Ultrasound of placenta previa

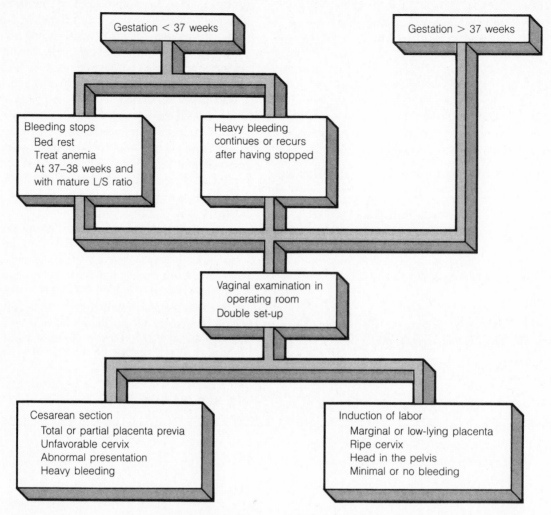

Figure 25–16 Management of placenta previa (From Oxorn H: *Human Labor and Birth.* Norwalk, Conn, Appleton-Century-Crofts, 1986, p 510)

logically prepared for possible surgery (Chapter 26). A whole-blood setup should be readied for intravenous infusion and a patent intravenous line established before any intrusive procedures are undertaken. The maternal vital signs should be monitored every 15 minutes in the absence of hemorrhage and every 5 minutes with active hemorrhage. The external tocodynamometer should be connected to the maternal abdomen to monitor uterine activity continuously.

NURSING GOAL: PROMOTION OF PHYSICAL WELL-BEING

The nurse continues to monitor the woman and her fetus to determine the status of the bleeding and to determine the mother's and baby's responses. Vital signs, intake and output, and other pertinent assessments must be made frequently. The nurse evaluates the electronic monitor tracing to evaluate the fetal status.

NURSING GOAL: PROVISION OF EMOTIONAL SUPPORT TO THE FAMILY DURING EXPECTANT MANAGEMENT

Emotional support for the family is an important nursing care goal. When active bleeding is occurring, the assessments and management must be directed toward physical support. However, emotional aspects need to be addressed simultaneously. The nurse can explain the assessments being completed and the treatment measures that need to be done. Time can be provided for questions, and the nurse can act as an advocate in obtaining information for the family. Emotional support can also be offered by staying with the family and the use of touch.

NURSING GOAL: PROMOTION OF NEONATAL PHYSIOLOGIC ADAPTATION

The newborn's hemoglobin, cell volume, and erythrocyte count should be checked immediately and then monitored closely. The newborn may require oxygen and administration of blood.

NURSING GOAL: PROVISION OF CARE TO THE WOMAN WITH BLEEDING

Additional information regarding nursing care is addressed in the Nursing Care Plan on page 770.

EVALUATIVE OUTCOME CRITERIA

Nursing care is effective if:

- The cause of hemorrhage is recognized promptly and corrective measures are taken.

- The woman's vital signs remain in the normal range.

- The woman and her baby have a safe labor and birth.

- Any other complications are recognized and treated early.

- The family understands what has happened and the implications and associated problems of placenta previa.

Other Placental Problems

Other problems of the placenta can be divided into those that are developmental and those that are degenerative. Developmental problems of the placenta include placental lesions, placental succenturiata, circumvallate placenta, and battledore placenta (Figure 25–17). Degenerative changes include infarcts and placental calcification.

PLACENTAL LESIONS

Angiomatous tumors, metastatic tumors, and cysts are classified as placental lesions. About one-third of placental tumors are associated with maternal hydramnios. Maternal complications can result from hydramnios (see page 784). Perinatal mortality is high because of the high rate of prematurity.

SUCCENTURIATE PLACENTA

In succenturiate placenta, one or more accessory lobes of fetal villi have developed on the placenta, with vascular connections of fetal origin (Figure 25–17A). Vessels from the major to the minor lobe(s) are supported only

by the membranes, thus increasing the risk of the minor lobe being retained during the third stage of labor.

The gravest maternal danger is postpartal hemorrhage if this minor lobe is severed from the placenta and remains in the uterus. All placentas should be examined closely for intactness. If vessels appear to be severed at the margin of the placenta, the uterus should be explored for retained placental tissue. This condition is not usually diagnosed until after the delivery of the placenta (Pritchard et al 1985). If the vascular connections rupture between the lobes, life-threatening fetal hemorrhage can result. At birth the infant should be inspected for pallor, cyanosis, retractions, tachypnea, tachycardia, and feeble pulse. The infant's cry will be weak and the muscle tone flaccid.

CIRCUMVALLATE PLACENTA

In circumvallate placenta, the fetal surface of the placenta is exposed through a ring opening around the umbilical cord (Figure 25–17B). The vessels descend from the cord and end at the margin of the ring instead of coursing through the entire surface area of the placenta. The ring is composed of a double fold of amnion and chorion with some degenerative decidua and fibrin between. The cause of this condition is unknown. Maternal-fetal problems include an increased incidence of late abortion or fetal death,

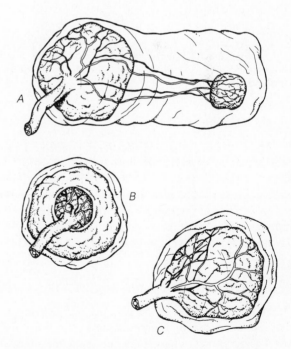

Figure 25–17 Placental variations. A Succenturiate placenta. B Circumvallate placenta. C Battledore placenta. (From Abnormalities of the Placenta, Clinical Educational Aid No. 12, Ross Laboratories, Columbus, Ohio)

DIC Coagulation Process

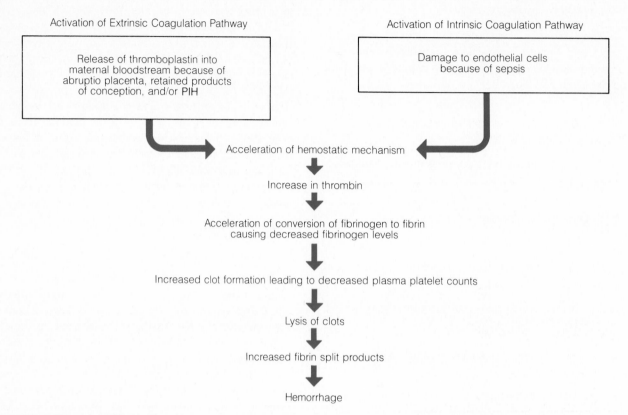

Figure 25–18   DIC coagulation process

antepartal hemorrhage, prematurity, and abnormal maternal bleeding during or following the third stage of labor, resulting from improper placental separation or shearing of membranes from the placenta.

BATTLEDORE PLACENTA

In the case of battledore placenta, the umbilical cord is inserted at or near the placental margin (Figure 25–17C). As a result, all fetal vessels transverse the placental surface in the same direction. The chances of preterm labor are high because of interference with fetal circulation and nutrition. Fetal distress or bleeding during labor is also likely because of cord compression or vessel rupture.

PLACENTAL INFARCTS AND CALCIFICATIONS

In the aging process the placenta may develop infarcts and calcifications. They become significant if they cover a large enough area to interfere with the uterine–placental–fetal exchange. Altered exchange can also occur with certain maternal disease processes, such as hypertension. Infarcts are most often seen in cases of severe pregnancy-induced hypertension and in women who smoke.

● Care of the Woman With Disseminated Intravascular Coagulation

Disseminated intravascular coagulation is an abnormal overstimulation of the coagulation process, secondary to an underlying disease. The coagulation process remains essentially the same, but certain medical conditions hasten and intensify the response to the point that hemorrhage may be life-threatening as coagulation factors are overconsumed (Figure 25–18).

Sepsis in the childbearing woman may activate the intrinsic coagulation pathway because of damage to the endothelial cells. The extrinsic pathway is activated by the release of thromboplastin from damaged tissues in such conditions as abruptio placentae, PIH, chorioamnionitis, and retained products of conception. The normally high levels of tissue thromboplastin in the placenta and decidua of the uterus may contribute to the occurrence of DIC. Amniotic fluid released into the bloodstream from amniotic fluid emboli and intraamniotic saline infusions activates both pathways. With the initiation of the coagulation process, massive numbers of clots form rapidly. Fibrinogen becomes depleted as it is converted to fibrin. Platelets are entrapped in the clots, leading to a decrease in the number of platelets. The coagulation process also activates plasminogen conversion to plasmin, which can lyse fibrinogen (dissolve clots), and as the fibrin clots are destroyed, fibrin split products having an anticoagulant effect are released. Because of the elevated fibrin split products level, the decrease in the number of platelets, and the reduced fibrinogen level, the outcome is generalized bleeding. Ischemia of the organs follows from the vascular occlusion of the numerous fibrin thrombi. The multisite hemorrhages result in shock and potentially death.

The clinical manifestations of DIC begin subtly and become more overt with severity of the disease. The signs and symptoms are indicators of the degree of bleeding, which ranges from generalized hemorrhage to minor generalized bleeding to localized bleeding in the form of purpura and petechiae.

Medical Therapy

The goals of therapy are early diagnosis and supportive treatment of the woman with DIC. Confirmation of DIC is made with several blood tests. The prothrombin time (PT) test evaluates the extrinsic pathway in clotting. The PT is prolonged in DIC. The intrinsic pathway is evaluated by testing the partial thromboplastin time, which is also prolonged in DIC. Both platelets and fibrinogen levels decrease. Platelet counts below $50,000/\mu L$ result in spontaneous bleeding. Fibrinogen levels may be within normal ranges but will be lower than the initial level. The number of fibrin split products is elevated. The frequency of testing depends on the severity of the disease (Berkowitz 1983).

Cases of DIC can frequently be resolved by correcting the underlying cause. In the childbearing woman, terminating the pregnancy removes the causative factor. Until delivery can be accomplished, supportive therapy is critical to maintain maternal-fetal status.

Initial treatment includes evaluation of vital signs; assessment of vaginal bleeding, uterine contractility, and resting tone; continuous FHR monitoring; and fetal blood studies. Intravenous infusions of lactated Ringer's are given through a 16- or 18-gauge cannula. An indwelling bladder catheter is used to allow better evaluation of urinary output, which should be maintained at 30 mL per hour to assure adequate renal perfusion. Anemia (hematocrit less than 30 percent) is treated by giving packed red cells. Each unit generally increases the hematocrit by 3 points and the hemoglobin by 1 to 1.5 g. Fresh frozen plasma may also be used to replace fibrinogen, factors V and VII, and antithrombin III. If fibrinogen levels are very low, cryoprecipitate is used. Each unit of cryoprecipitate provides 250 mg of fibrinogen and raises the fibrinogen level by approximately 5 mg/dL (Berkowitz 1983).

The administration of heparin is a controversial issue. Heparin is used to decrease thrombin generation and activity. When the causative factor cannot be removed, as with infection or in self-limiting cases in childbearing women, heparin is not used routinely. In some instances, the use of heparin may even increase the hemorrhage (Berkowitz 1983).

Vaginal delivery without an episiotomy is the preferred birthing method as it avoids the surgical incision of numerous tissues and further stress on the hemostatic system (Berkowitz 1983). Conduction anesthesia should be avoided because of the chance of bleeding from injection puncture sites and the formation of hematomas.

Nursing Assessment

The nurse should carefully observe for signs and symptoms of DIC in women who are candidates for this complication. Bleeding from injection sites, epistaxis, bleeding gums, and the presence of purpura and petechiae on the skin may be signs of developing DIC.

Clinical evidence may also be apparent in the results of laboratory blood tests specific to DIC. As appropriate, the nurse continues to assess maternal-fetal status by checking vital signs, uterine activity, FHR, and urinary output.

The nurse documents and reports signs and symptoms of DIC to the physician as well as any changes in the FHR, maternal vital signs, and uterine activity.

Nursing Diagnosis

Nursing diagnoses that may apply to the woman with DIC include:

- Fear related to unknown outcome of the labor and birth

- Potential impaired gas exchange related to impaired oxygen-carrying ability of blood secondary to hemorrhage

- Potential for infection related to decreased hemoglobin

Nursing Goal: Promotion of Physical Well-Being

In the event of a major blood loss, nursing measures are directed toward assessment of maternal-fetal status and corrective or supportive treatment measures. The nurse is also responsible for monitoring administration of blood products.

Protecting the woman from further bleeding involves interventions such as padding the side rails, avoiding IM injections, assessing IV insertion sites, and placing the blood pressure cuff carefully to prevent bruising.

Nursing Goal: Provision of Emotional Support

Meeting the woman's psychologic needs is another nursing priority. Accurate, informative explanations should be offered frequently. The nurse who listens and projects warmth and understanding is most likely to help the woman cope with her anxiety and frustration.

Evaluative Outcome Criteria

Nursing care is effective if:

- The woman's circulatory status is restored to normal and blood loss is replaced.

- The mother and baby have a safe labor and delivery and further complications are quickly identified and treated.

- The parents understand the complication that occurred and are able to participate in decision making as much as possible.

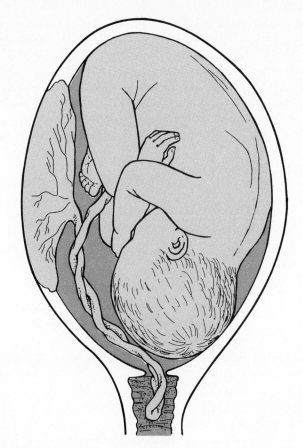

Figure 25–19 Prolapse of the cord

● Care of the Woman and Fetus at Risk Due to Problems Associated With the Umbilical Cord

Prolapsed Umbilical Cord

Conditions associated with a prolapsed cord include breech presentation, transverse lies, contracted inlets, small fetus, extra long cord, low-lying placenta, hydramnios, and twin gestations. Any time the inlet is not occluded and the membranes rupture, the cord can be washed down (Figure 25–19) into the birth canal in front of the presenting part.

MATERNAL RISKS

When predisposing factors to cord prolapse exist, the woman should be considered high risk and should be monitored closely. If prolapse occurs prior to complete cervical dilatation, cesarean delivery is the treatment of choice.

FETAL-NEONATAL RISKS

Because with each contraction the umbilical cord becomes compressed between the maternal pelvis and the presenting part, fetal distress is common. If the cord ceases to pulsate, it is generally indicative of fetal demise.

MEDICAL THERAPY

Preventing the occurrence of prolapse of the cord is the preferred medical approach. If the prolapse does happen, relieving the compression on the cord is critical to fetal outcome. The medical and nursing team must work together to facilitate delivery.

Bed rest is indicated for all laboring women with a history of ruptured membranes, until engagement with no cord prolapse has been documented. Furthermore, at the time of spontaneous rupture of membranes or amniotomy, the FHR should be auscultated for at least a full minute and again at the end of a contraction and after a few contractions. If fetal bradycardia is detected on the auscultation, the woman should be examined to rule out a cord prolapse. In the presence of cord prolapse, electronic monitor tracings show severe, moderate, or prolonged variable decelerations with baseline bradycardia. If these patterns are found, the woman is examined vaginally.

If a loop of cord is discovered, the gloved fingers are left in the vagina, and attempts are made to lift the fetal head off the cord to relieve compression until the physician arrives. This is a life-saving measure. Oxygen is begun, and FHR is monitored to see if the cord compression is adequately relieved.

The force of gravity can be employed to relieve the compression. The woman assumes the knee-chest position or the bed is adjusted to the Trendelenburg position and the woman should be transported to the delivery or operating room in this position. The nurse must remember that the cord may be occultly prolapsed with an actual loop extending into the vagina or lying alongside the presenting part. It may be pulsating strongly or so weakly that it is difficult to determine on palpation of the cord whether the fetus is alive.

Occasionally a cord prolapses out the vagina. If this condition is identified in a home situation, some of the previously discussed life-saving actions can be implemented by the nurse. The lateral Sims' position may be more feasible for the woman if the position is to be assumed for any extended period of time. The pelvis should be elevated on pillows. Compression on the cord can be relieved in the vagina as in the hospital situation, and wet dressings soaked in a mild salt solution should be wrapped around the protruding cord. The woman should be transported to the hospital immediately. If the cord is pale, limp, and obviously not pulsating, no action is necessary other than transport. At no time should attempts be made to replace the cord into the uterus, because this could cause devastating trauma to the cord and could greatly increase the possibility of intrauterine infection. Vaginal delivery (with or without forceps) is possible if the following criteria are met:

- The cervix is completely dilated.

- A vertex is presenting at least at zero station.

- The membranes are ruptured.

- Pelvic measurements are adequate.

If these conditions are not present, cesarean delivery is the method of choice. The woman is taken to the delivery room while the nurse vaginally relieves the pressure on the cord until the infant has been delivered. The medical and nursing team must work together quickly to facilitate delivery in this obstetric emergency.

NURSING ASSESSMENT

By reviewing the nursing history, the nurse ascertains whether the woman is at risk for prolapse of the cord. Particularly when the presenting part is not engaged and spontaneous or artificial rupture of the membranes occurs, the nurse observes the perineum and evaluates the FHR for changes that may signify a prolapsed cord. During labor, bradycardia accompanied by variable decelerations may also indicate prolapse.

NURSING DIAGNOSIS

Nursing diagnoses that may apply to the woman with a prolapsed cord include:

- Potential impaired gas exchange in the fetus related to decreased blood flow secondary to compression of the umbilical cord

- Fear related to unknown outcome.

NURSING GOAL: PROMOTION OF FETAL WELL-BEING

In addition to monitoring the woman closely for the occurrence of this complication, the nurse must be prepared to intervene instantaneously if the cord prolapses. Relieving the compression of the cord alleviates fetal distress and increases the likelihood of delivering a healthy live newborn.

NURSING GOAL: PROVISION OF EMOTIONAL SUPPORT TO THE FAMILY

In the event of fetal death, assisting the family to deal with their loss becomes a priority. See discussion on p 761.

EVALUATIVE OUTCOME CRITERIA

Nursing care is effective if:

- The FHR remains in normal range with supportive measures.

- The fetus is born safely.

- The woman and her partner feel supported.

- The woman and her partner understand the problem and the corrective measures that are undertaken.

Umbilical Cord Abnormalities

Umbilical cord abnormalities include congenital absence of an umbilical artery, insertion variations, cord length variations, and knots and loops of the cord. Insertion variations include velamentous insertion and vasa previa, and cord length problems include long and short cords.

CONGENITAL ABSENCE OF UMBILICAL ARTERY

Absence of an umbilical artery may have serious fetal implications. The incidence of all types of fetal anomalies is 25 percent with a "two-vessel" cord.

Immediately after the umbilical cord is cut, it should be inspected to determine whether the correct number of vessels is present. If an artery is absent, the nurse should examine the newborn more closely for anomalies and gestational age problems.

INSERTION VARIATIONS

In a *velamentous insertion* condition, the vessels of the umbilical cord divide some distance from the placenta in the placental membranes (Figure 25–20). Velamentous insertions occur more frequently in multiple gestations than in singletons. Other placental anomalies often accompany this condition, such as succenturiate placenta. The velamentous insertion is more easily compressed or kinked during pregnancy or labor because of the lack of Wharton's jelly to protect it. If the vessels become torn during labor, fetal hemorrhage can occur and is signaled by FHR abnormalities accompanied by vaginal bleeding.

When the vessels of a velamentous insertion transverse the internal os and appear in front of the fetus, a *vasa previa* has occurred. Fetal hemorrhage with asphyxia is likely to result because the hemorrhage will probably be diagnosed as maternal.

CORD LENGTH VARIATIONS

The average length of the umbilical cord is 55 cm. Although short cords rarely cause complications directly, they have been associated with umbilical hernias in the fetus, abruptio placentae, and cord rupture. Long cords tend to twist and tangle around the fetus, causing transient variable decelerations. A long cord rarely causes fetal death, however, because it is generally not pulled tight until descent at the time of delivery. With a long cord and an active fetus, one or more true knots can result. Again, these knots usually are not pulled tight enough to cause fetal distress until the infant has been delivered, and the cord can then be clamped and cut.

MEDICAL THERAPY

Preventing serious fetal complications and examining the newborn for anomalies that coexist with umbilical cord abnormalities are the goals of medical treatment.

In the presence of any vaginal bleeding during labor, continuous monitoring of the fetus is imperative. Monitoring is best done with the aid of the external electronic monitor. Any signs of fetal distress should be reported immediately. In the presence of bleeding, laboratory tests may be used to differentiate fetal from maternal red blood cells. Fetal hemorrhage is resolved by termination of the pregnancy vaginally or through cesarean delivery and by correction of neonatal anemia. Expediting the delivery, whether vaginally or surgically, is paramount when severe fetal distress is apparent. Following the birth, the pediatric

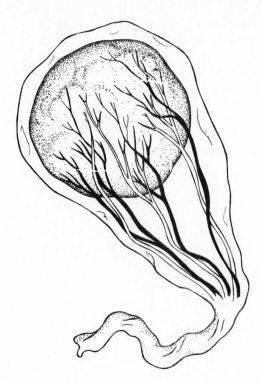

Figure 25–20 Placenta with a velamentous umbilical cord insertion

team rules out or treats the complications or anomalies that may occur.

NURSING ASSESSMENT

The presence of umbilical abnormalities may not become evident until the birth of the fetus. During labor, the nurse should observe for signs of fetal distress and vaginal bleeding that may signify a problem with the cord.

NURSING DIAGNOSIS

Nursing diagnoses that may apply include:

- Potential alteration of gas exchange in the fetus related to decreased blood flow secondary to placental abnormalities

- Knowledge deficit related to lack of information regarding implications and associated problems with placental abnormalities

NURSING GOAL: PROMOTION OF MATERNAL WELL-BEING

The nurse is alert for unusual bleeding during the labor and birth. Following the delivery, the placenta is inspected for abnormalities.

NURSING GOAL: PROMOTION OF FETAL WELL-BEING

Often any mild or moderate variable deceleration can be successfully managed by the nurse. Repositioning of the mother often alleviates pressure on the cord if this is the reason for the deceleration.

EVALUATIVE OUTCOME CRITERIA

Nursing care is effective if:

● The mother and baby have a safe labor and birth.

● The mother's bleeding is assessed quickly and corrective measures are taken.

● Care of the Woman and Fetus at Risk Due to Amniotic Fluid-Related Complications

Amniotic Fluid Embolism

Amniotic fluid embolism can occur naturally after a tumultuous labor or from oxytocin induction with hypertonic uterine contractions. In the presence of a small tear in the amnion or chorion high in the uterus, the fluid may leak into the chorionic plate and enter the maternal circulation through the gaping venous system. The fluid can also enter at areas of placental separation or cervical tears. Under pressure from the contracting uterus, the fluid is driven into the maternal system. Amniotic fluid embolus occurs more often in multiparas. The incidence is 1 in 15,000 to 20,000 pregnancies with a mortality rate of 80 percent (Clark et al 1986).

MATERNAL RISKS

This condition frequently occurs during or after the delivery when the woman has had a difficult, rapid labor. Suddenly she experiences respiratory distress, circulatory collapse, acute hemorrhage, and cor pulmonale, as the embolism blocks the vessels of the lungs. The more debris in the amniotic fluid (such as meconium), the greater the maternal problems. The acute hemorrhage is a result of DIC (page 778), which is caused by the thromboplastinlike material found in amniotic fluid, in which factor VII is not essential. It has been demonstrated in vitro and in vivo that mucus, which is also found in amniotic fluid, induces coagulation by activation of factor X.

Maternal mortality is extremely high. In suspected cases in which the women survive, it is difficult to determine whether an amniotic fluid embolism actually occurred.

FETAL-NEONATAL RISKS

Delivery must be facilitated immediately to obtain a live birth. In many cases the delivery has already occurred or the fetus can be delivered vaginally with forceps. If labor has been tumultuous, the fetus may suffer problems associated with dysfunctional labor.

MEDICAL THERAPY

The goals of medical therapy are to maintain oxygenation, support the cardiovascular system and blood pressure, and assess coagulopathy (Clark 1986).

Any woman exhibiting chest pain, dyspnea, cyanosis, frothy sputum, tachycardia, hypotension, and massive hemorrhage needs the cooperation of every member of the health team if her life is to be saved. Medical and nursing interventions are supportive. Recovery is contingent upon the return of the mother's cardiovascular and respiratory stability. If necessary the delivery is assisted to enhance the health of the newborn.

NURSING ASSESSMENT

The nurse must be especially observant for manifestations of amniotic fluid embolism when the labor has been short and difficult. Signs and symptoms of respiratory and circulatory collapse are sudden, acute, and severe and require immediate medical intervention.

NURSING DIAGNOSIS

Nursing diagnoses that may apply include:

● Potential alteration of gas exchange related to anxiety, restlessness, and dyspnea secondary to amniotic fluid embolism

● Fear related to unknown outcome of the complication

NURSING GOAL: MAINTENANCE OF OXYGENATION

Every delivery room should be equipped with a working oxygen unit. In the absence of the physician, the nurse administers oxygen under positive pressure until medical help arrives. An intravenous line is quickly established. If respiratory and cardiac arrest occurs, cardiopulmonary resuscitation (CPR) is initiated immediately.

NURSING GOAL: PROVISION OF CARDIOVASCULAR SUPPORT

The nurse readies the equipment necessary for blood transfusion and for the insertion of the CVP line. As the blood volume is replaced, using fresh blood to provide clotting factors, the CVP is monitored frequently. In the presence of cor pulmonale, fluid overload could easily occur.

When DIC is controlled with fibrinogen replacement, the nurse is responsible for obtaining fibrinogen and other medications needed. Intravenous heparin may be life saving.

NURSING GOAL: PROMOTION OF FETAL-NEONATAL WELL-BEING

As one nurse helps the physician maintain maternal homeostasis, another nurse intervenes as necessary to maintain the well-being of the fetus in utero and the newborn after delivery.

EVALUATIVE OUTCOME CRITERIA

Nursing care is effective if:

- The mother's signs and symptoms are recognized and corrective measures taken quickly.

- Fetal distress is recognized and corrective measures taken early.

- The mother and her baby are stabilized and no further complications develop.

Hydramnios

Hydramnios occurs when there is over 2000 mL of amniotic fluid. The exact cause of hydramnios is unknown; however, it often occurs in cases of major congenital anomalies. It is postulated that a major source of amniotic fluid is found in special amnion cells that lie over the placenta (Danforth & Scott 1986). During the second half of the pregnancy, the fetus begins to swallow and inspire amniotic fluid and to urinate, which contributes to the amount present. In cases of hydramnios, no pathology has been found in the amniotic epithelium. However, hydramnios is associated with fetal malformations that affect the fetal swallowing mechanism and neurologic disorders in which the fetal meninges are exposed in the amniotic cavity. This condition is also found in cases of anencephaly in which the fetus is thought to urinate excessively due to overstimulation of the cerebrospinal centers. When a monozygotic twin manifests hydramnios, it is possible that the twin with the increased blood volume urinates excessively. The weight of the placenta has been found to be increased in some cases of hydramnios, indicating that increased functioning of the placental tissue may be contributory.

There are two types of hydramnios: chronic and acute. In the chronic type, the fluid volume gradually increases. Most cases are of this variety. In acute cases, the volume increases rapidly over a period of a few days.

MATERNAL RISKS

When the amount of amniotic fluid is over 3000 mL, the woman experiences shortness of breath and edema in the lower extremities from compression of the vena cava. If hydramnios is severe enough, she can experience intense pain. The acute form of hydramnios tends to be more severe. Milder forms of hydramnios occur more frequently and are associated with minimal symptoms. Hydramnios is associated with such maternal disorders as diabetes and Rh sensitization.

Antepartally, if the amniotic fluid is removed too rapidly, abruptio placentae can result from a decreased attachment area. Because of these overstretched fibers, uterine dysfunction can occur intrapartally, and there is increased incidence of postpartal hemorrhage.

FETAL-NEONATAL RISKS

Fetal malformations and premature delivery are common with hydramnios; thus perinatal mortality is high. Prolapsed cord can occur when the membranes rupture, which adds a further complication for the fetus. The incidence of malpresentations is also increased.

MEDICAL THERAPY

Hydramnios is managed with supportive treatment unless the intensity of the woman's distress and symptoms dictate otherwise.

If the accumulation of amniotic fluid is severe enough to cause maternal dyspnea and pain, hospitalization and removal of the excessive fluid are required. This can be done vaginally or by amniocentesis. The dangers of performing the technique vaginally are prolapsed cord and the inability to remove the fluid slowly. If amniocentesis is performed, it should be done with the aid of sonography to prevent inadvertent damage to the fetus and placenta. The fluid should be removed slowly to prevent abruption (Pritchard et al 1985).

When performing amniocentesis it is vital to maintain sterile technique. The nurse can offer support to the couple by explaining the procedure to them. The nurse assists the clinician in interpreting sonographic findings.

NURSING ASSESSMENT

Hydramnios should be suspected when the fundal height increases out of proportion to the gestational age. As the amount of fluid increases, the nurse may have difficulty palpating the fetus and auscultating the FHR. In more severe cases, the maternal abdomen appears extremely tense and tight on inspection. On sonography, large spaces can be identified between the fetus and the uterine wall. An anencephalic infant or a dilated fetal stomach resulting from esophageal atresia may also be identified, and multiple gestations may be confirmed. An x-ray fetogram will also show a radiolucent area of space and any fetal skeletal defects.

NURSING DIAGNOSIS

Nursing diagnoses that may apply include:

- Potential alteration in gas exchange related to pressure on the diaphragm secondary to hydramnios
- Fear related to unknown outcome of the pregnancy

NURSING GOAL: ASSISTANCE DURING AMNIOCENTESIS

When amniocentesis is performed, it is vital to maintain sterile technique to prevent infection. The nurse can offer support to the couple by explaining the procedure to them. The nurse assists the clinician in interpreting sonographic findings.

NURSING GOAL: PROVISION OF EMOTIONAL SUPPORT TO THE FAMILY

If the fetus has been diagnosed with a congenital defect in utero or is born with the defect, psychologic support is needed to assist the family. Often the nurse collaborates with social services to offer the family this additional help.

EVALUATIVE OUTCOME CRITERIA

Nursing care is effective if:

- The woman and her partner understand the procedure, implications, risks, and characteristics that need to be reported to the care giver.

Oligohydramnios

Oligohydramnios, in which the amount of amniotic fluid is severely reduced and concentrated, is a rare maternal finding. The exact cause of this condition is unknown. It is found in cases of postmaturity, with IUGR secondary to placental insufficiency, and in fetal conditions associated with renal and urinary malfunction. If oligohydramnios occurs in the first part of pregnancy, there is a danger of fetal adhesions (one part of the fetus may adhere to another part). Pulmonary hypoplasia has been found, theoretically due to lack of fluid inhaled in the terminal air sacs (Pritchard et al 1985). An increased incidence of major anomalies involving major organ systems

and low 5-minute Apgar scores has also been found (Bastide et al 1986). The perinatal mortality rate was more than doubled.

MATERNAL RISKS

Labor can be dysfunctional and can begin before term. It is usually extremely painful for the woman, and progress is protracted.

FETAL-NEONATAL RISKS

Fetal hypoxia may occur due to umbilical cord compression. At birth these infants appear wrinkled and leathery, and serious skeletal deformities are often found (Pritchard et al 1985).

In some research centers, a new technique is being explored as a supportive therapy for oligohydramnios. Sterile normal saline is infused slowly into the amniotic cavity. This treatment seems to decrease the incidence of variable decelerations in the FHR because the increase in fluid volume helps relieve pressure on the umbilical cord.

● Care of the Woman With Cephalopelvic Disproportion

The birth passage includes the maternal bony pelvis, beginning at the pelvic inlet and ending at the pelvic outlet, and the maternal soft tissues within these anatomic areas. A contracture in any of the described areas can result in cephalopelvic disproportion (CPD). Abnormal fetal presentations and positions occur in CPD as the fetus attempts to accommodate to its passage.

The gynecoid and anthropod pelvic types are usually adequate for vertex delivery, but the android and platypelloid types predispose to CPD. Certain combinations of types also can result in pelvic diameters inadequate for vertex delivery. (See Chapter 15 for a description of the types of pelves and their implications for childbirth.) Clues that may lead to suspicion of contractures of the maternal pelvis are presented in Box 25–3.

Types of Contractures

CONTRACTURES OF THE INLET

The pelvic inlet is contracted if the shortest anterior-posterior diameter is less than 10 cm or the greatest transverse diameter is less than 12 cm. The anterior-posterior diameter may be approximated by measuring the diagonal conjugate, which in the contracted inlet is less than 11.5 cm. Clinical and x-ray pelvimetry are used to determine the smallest anterior-posterior diameter through which the fetal head must pass. Sonography then can be used to

Box 25–3   Clues to Contractures of Maternal Pelvis

- Diagonal conjugate <11.5 cm (contracture of inlet), outlet <8 cm (contracture of outlet)
- Unengaged fetal head in early labor in primigravidas (consider contracture of inlet, malpresentation, or malposition)
- Hypotonic uterine contraction pattern (consider contracted pelvis)
- Deflexion of fetal head (fetal head not flexed on fetal chest; may be associated with occiput posterior)
- Uncontrollable pushing prior to complete dilatation of cervix (may be associated with occiput posterior)
- Failure of fetal descent (consider contracture of inlet, midpelvis, or outlet)
- Edema of anterior portion (lip) of cervix (consider obstructed labor at the inlet)

measure the biparietal diameter of the fetal head, which averages 9.5–9.8 cm.

When both diameters are contracted, the incidence of difficult deliveries increases. The risks associated with inlet contractures are numerous. The course of labor tends to be prolonged with unsatisfactory dilatation of the cervix. Because the entire force of the labor contractions is exerted on the membranes, PROM may occur. The lack of fetal descent in the nullipara before the onset of labor may potentiate the risk of prolapse of the cord. In these cases, vertex presentations assume other presentations, such as face and shoulder. Pathologic retraction rings and uterine rupture may also develop. Perinatal mortality increases for the fetus. Excessive molding and skull fractures may lead to fetal intracranial hemorrhage. A large caput succedaneum may also form.

The management of inlet contractures begins with assessment of the size and presentation of the fetus, the pelvic configuration, uterine activity, cervical dilatation, and any problems during previous labors and deliveries. Based on these findings, the decision is made to proceed with a trial labor or a cesarean delivery.

CONTRACTURES OF THE MIDPELVIS

Contractures of the midpelvis are more common than inlet contractures. The plane of the midpelvis is formed from the margin of the symphysis pubis through the ischial spines and touches the sacrum near the fourth or fifth vertebra. Although a satisfactory method of measuring the midpelvis manually does not exist, prominent spines, converging pelvic walls, or a narrow sacrosciatic notch can be ascertained on vaginal examination. Midpelvis contractures

cause transverse arrest of the head, leading to potentially difficult midforceps delivery.

The treatment goal is to allow the natural forces of labor to push the biparietal diameter of the fetal head beyond the potential interspinous obstruction. Although forceps may be used, they cause difficulty because pulling on the head destroys flexion and the space is further diminished. A bulging perineum and crowning indicate that the obstruction has been passed.

CONTRACTURES OF THE OUTLET

An interischial tuberous diameter of less than 8 cm constitutes an outlet contracture. Outlet and midpelvic contractures frequently occur simultaneously. Whether vaginal delivery can occur depends on the woman's interischial tuberous diameters and the fetal posterosagittal diameter.

Implications of Pelvic Contractures

MATERNAL RISKS

Labor is prolonged and protracted in the presence of CPD, and PROM can result from the force of the unequally distributed contractions being exerted on the fetal membranes. In obstructed labor, uterine rupture can also occur. With protracted descent, necrosis of maternal soft tissues can result from pressure exerted by the fetal head. Eventually necrosis can cause fistulas from the vagina to other nearby structures. Difficult forceps deliveries can also result in damage to maternal soft tissue.

FETAL-NEONATAL RISKS

If the membranes rupture and the fetal head has not entered the inlet, there is a grave danger of cord prolapse. Extreme molding of the fetal head can result in skull fracture or intracranial hemorrhage. Traumatic forceps deliveries can cause damage to the fetal skull and CNS.

MEDICAL THERAPY

The goal of medical treatment is to assess the maternal pelvis accurately and determine whether CPD is present.

Fetopelvic relationships can be appraised by x-ray pelvimetry when the pregnancy is at term or in early labor. The x-ray pelvimetry provides measurements for the maternal pelvic inlet, midpelvis, outlet, degree of fetal descent, and selected diameters of the fetal head (Figures 25–21, 25–22).

When pelvimetry is used in combination with ultrasonography, the mechanisms of labor are even more predictable.

In addition to x-ray pelvimetry, assessment techniques such as careful manual examination of the pelvis and the new technique of magnetic resonance imaging (MRI) are used to identify inadequate diameters and determine the treatment plan (Silbar 1986).

When the pelvic diameters are borderline or questionable, a trial of labor (TOL) may be advised. In this process, the woman continues to labor and careful, frequent assessments of cervical dilatation and fetal descent are made by the physician and nurse. As long as there is continued progress, the TOL continues. If progress ceases, the decision for a cesarean birth is made.

NURSING ASSESSMENT

The adequacy of the maternal pelvis for a vaginal delivery should be assessed intrapartally as well as ante-

partally. During the intrapartal assessment, the size of the fetus and its presentation, position, and lie must also be considered. (See Chapter 22 for intrapartal assessment techniques.)

The nurse should suspect CPD when labor is prolonged, cervical dilatation and effacement are slow, and engagement of the presenting part is delayed.

NURSING DIAGNOSIS

Nursing diagnoses that may apply include:

- Knowledge deficit related to lack of information regarding implications and associated complications of CPD

- Fear related to unknown outcome of labor

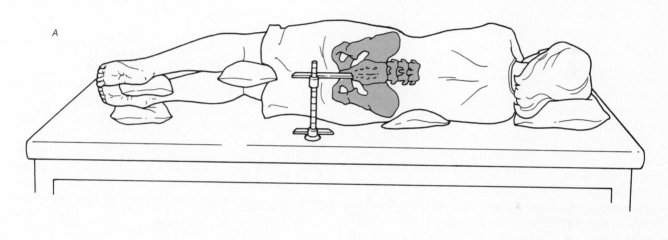

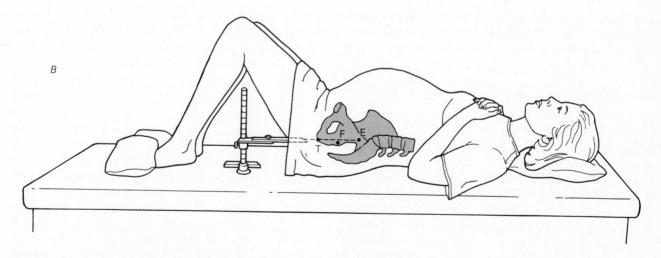

Figure 25–21   Colcher-Sussman method for x-ray pelvimetry. X-ray pelvimetry is obtained by placing a ruler at the level of points to be measured. The markings on the ruler are projected onto the x-ray film and become the known length with which to compare the other measurements. The measurements are recorded on a special chart for interpretation: E = inlet, F = midpelvis, T = outlet. (From Matthies HJ: X-ray pelvimetry, in Sciarri JJ (ed): Gynecology and Obstetrics. Philadelphia, Harper & Row, 1986, vol 2, chap 63, pp 2, 3)

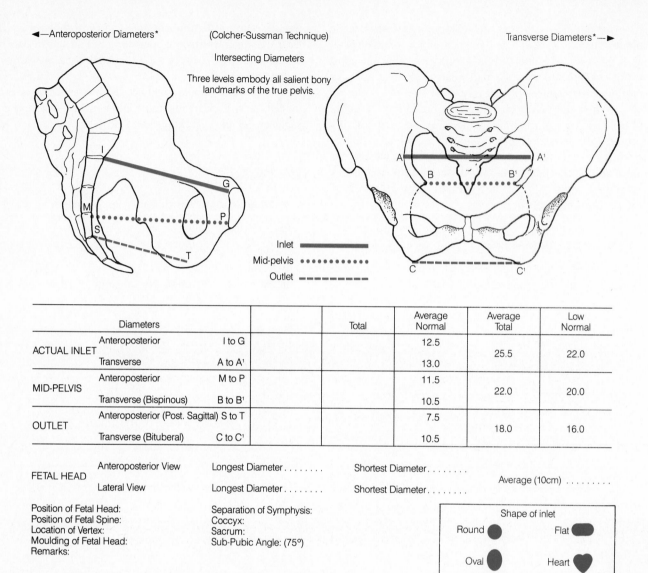

	Diameters			Total	Average Normal	Average Total	Low Normal
ACTUAL INLET	Anteroposterior	I to G			12.5		
	Transverse	A to A¹			13.0	25.5	22.0
MID-PELVIS	Anteroposterior	M to P			11.5		
	Transverse (Bispinous)	B to B¹			10.5	22.0	20.0
OUTLET	Anteroposterior (Post. Sagittal) S to T				7.5		
	Transverse (Bituberal)	C to C¹			10.5	18.0	16.0

FETAL HEAD	Anteroposterior View	Longest Diameter........	Shortest Diameter........	Average (10cm) ....
	Lateral View	Longest Diameter........	Shortest Diameter........	

Position of Fetal Head:
Position of Fetal Spine:
Location of Vertex:
Moulding of Fetal Head:
Remarks:

Separation of Symphysis:
Coccyx:
Sacrum:
Sub-Pubic Angle: (75°)

Shape of inlet
Round   Flat
Oval   Heart

Figure 25–22   X-ray pelvimetry chart. The assessed diameters are recorded on the chart. Average normals are identified for the inlet, midpelvis, and outlet. The chart also identifies low normal measurements.

NURSING GOAL: PROMOTION OF MATERNAL AND FETAL WELL-BEING

Nursing actions during the TOL are similar to care during any labor with the exception that the assessments of cervical dilatation and fetal descent are more frequent. Contractions should be monitored continuously, and the labor progress may be charted on the Friedman graph. The fetus should also be monitored continuously. Any signs of fetal distress are reported to the physician immediately.

NURSING GOAL: POSITION CHANGES TO INCREASE PELVIC DIAMETERS

The mother may be positioned in a variety of ways to increase the pelvic diameters. Sitting or squatting in-

creases the outlet diameters and may be effective in instances where there is failure of or slow fetal descent. Changing from one side to the other, and/or maintaining a hands and knees position may assist the fetus in occiput posterior position to change to an occiput anterior. The mother may instinctively want to assume one of these positions. If not, the nurse may encourage a change of position.

NURSING GOAL: PROVISION OF EMOTIONAL SUPPORT

A couple may need support in coping with the stresses of complicated labor. The nurse should keep the couple informed of what is happening and explain the procedures that are being used. This knowledge can reassure the couple that measures are being taken to resolve the problem.

EVALUATIVE OUTCOME CRITERIA

Nursing care is effective if:

- The woman's fear is lessened.

- The woman has additional knowledge regarding the problems, implications, and treatment plans.

● Care of the Woman at Risk Due to Complications of Third and Fourth Stages

Lacerations

Lacerations of the cervix or vagina may be indicated when bright red vaginal bleeding persists in the presence of a well-contracted uterus. The incidence of lacerations is higher when the childbearing woman is young or a nullipara, has an epidural, has forceps delivery and an episiotomy (Bromberg 1986), and has not done perineal massage or preparation during pregnancy (Avery & Burket 1986). Vaginal and perineal lacerations are often categorized as first, second, third, or fourth degree:

- First degree laceration is limited to the fourchet, perineal skin, and vaginal mucous membrane.

- Second degree laceration involves the perineal skin, vaginal mucous membrane, underlying fascia, and muscles of the perineal body; it may extend upward on one or both sides of the vagina.

- Third degree laceration extends through the perineal skin, vaginal mucous membranes, and perineal body and involves the anal sphincter; it may extend up the anterior wall of the rectum.

- Fourth degree laceration is the same as the third degree but extends through the rectal mucosa to the lumen of the rectum; it may be called a third degree laceration with a rectal wall extension.

Placenta Accreta

The chorionic villi attach directly to the myometrium of the uterus in *placenta accreta*. Two other types of placental adherence are *placenta increta,* in which the myometrium is invaded, and *placenta percreta,* in which the myometrium is penetrated. The adherence itself may be total, partial, or focal, depending on the amount of placental involvement.

The primary complication with placenta accreta is maternal hemorrhage. An abdominal hysterectomy may be

the necessary treatment, depending on the amount and depth of involvement.

For further discussion of hemorrhage following delivery see Chapter 36.

Inversion of Uterus

Uterine inversion occurs when the uterus turns inside out during the third stage of labor. This rare occurrence can be caused by a lax uterine wall coupled with undue tension on an umbilical cord when the placenta has not separated. Forceful pressure on the fundus with a dilated cervix and sudden emptying of the uterine contents may be contributing factors. Maternal bleeding with shock is rapid and profound. The fundus is absent from the abdominal cavity on palpation.

Restoration of the uterus to its normal position manually or by surgical intervention is the goal of medical treatment. The uterus is replaced manually by grasping the vaginal mass, spreading the cervical ring with the fingers and thumb, and steadily forcing the fundus upward. The woman is often placed under deep anesthesia for this procedure.

Relaxation of the uterus may be accomplished by administering 2 g magnesium sulfate intravenously (Grossman 1981). Oxytocin is given only after the restored uterus returns to its normal configuration.

● Complicated Childbirth: Effects on the Family and the Role of the Nurse

A complicated pregnancy and difficult labor and delivery are crisis situations that can test the coping mechanisms of every individual involved. The family may respond to the crisis in relatively typical ways or may respond dysfunctionally.

During the antepartal period of a normal, low-risk pregnancy, resolution of any ambivalence about the pregnancy usually occurs when fetal movement is felt. With a complicated pregnancy, feelings of ambivalence may continue as the family experiences fear and anxiety about the woman's health and the health and welfare of the fetus. Hostile behaviors and feelings of guilt may be displayed as a woman questions her ability to bear healthy children, a father blames himself for the pregnancy, or the family accuses the health care team of poor management.

If a pregnancy is going well, the parents begin to develop a desire to nurture and love their child as they prepare for their parenting role. With a complicated pregnancy, the uncertainty about the outcome for the fetus inhibits the parents' ability to adapt to the pregnancy and hinders the evolvement of feelings of adequacy as parents.

When an infant is stillborn or dies following delivery, the couple must mourn and deal with the pain of detaching themselves. As the parents respond to their loss, they experience the anger, guilt, pain, and sadness associated with the grieving process.

Parents of an ill or deformed infant must not only resolve their feelings of guilt and grief, but they must also prepare themselves to care for that child. This couple may be unable to face the possibility that their infant may not survive. They may doubt their ability to care properly for the child. The great costs of caring for the high-risk child may create financial difficulties for the family. The emotional toll of caring for such a child may also be extreme.

The birth of an ill, abnormal, or stillborn infant presents the couple with the reality that they may have been fearing throughout the pregnancy. It is imperative that the medical and nursing staff respond in supportive and sympathetic ways. Typically, however, health care personnel minimize eye contact and avoid communication with the woman or family. Sympathies expressed to the couple commonly include such statements as "The poor thing is better off," "It was God's will," or "You can try again." Such expressions seem insensitive, are often very painful, and may result in the couple being reluctant to share their loss with anyone close to them. The couple may feel alone and isolated, even from each other.

When a malformed infant is born, powerful reactions are not unusual even among care givers. Such a child is frequently the focus of a great deal of staff attention in the nursery. After they have seen the newborn, they feel shock and sadness similar to that experienced by the parents. This reaction is especially common for those who have had little experience with congenital anomalies. In an effort to deal with their reactions, they have a tendency to avoid the parents. In such instances it is frequently helpful to provide the staff with occasions to talk through their feelings so that they can be more supportive of the family's grief. In some centers with intensive care nurseries, this practice has been formalized through regular staff meetings and has been of great benefit to staff and, indirectly, to families.

Providing emotional support to the family is a vital nursing role. When a labor is complicated or when the fetus dies, the woman should have consistent support and not be left alone. The partner should be encouraged to remain, and the nurse should be present to observe the woman or couple and to provide support. By attending and responding with empathy, the nurse helps the couple acknowledge their loss and begin their grieving process. Using comfort measures to meet basic needs also demonstrates a caring attitude.

When a malformed infant is born, the couple must deal with their mourning and with the future needs of their child. Attachment may be facilitated by keeping parents and their newborn together as much as possible. The newborn can frequently be returned to the parents after a brief physical assessment in the nursery. The contact between the parents and infant may ultimately be a source of great satisfaction to the parents.

KEY CONCEPTS

Stress, anxiety, and fear have a profound effect on labor, particularly when complications occur that imply maternal or fetal jeopardy.

A hypertonic labor pattern is characterized by painful contractions that are not effective in effacing and dilating the cervix. It usually leads to a prolonged latent phase.

Hypotonic labor patterns begin normally and then progress to infrequent, less intense contractions. If there are no contraindications, IV oxytocin is used as treatment.

Prolonged labor lasts more than 24 hours.

Precipitous labor is extremely rapid labor that lasts for less than three hours. It is associated with an increased risk to the mother and newborn infant.

Spontaneous rupture of the membranes prior to labor is called premature rupture of the membranes. Associated problems include amnionitis and prolapse of the umbilical cord.

Preterm labor occurs between 20 and 37 weeks of completed pregnancy. The major problems are associated with the extrauterine adaptation of the preterm infant due to lack of development and immaturity of major organ systems.

The occiput posterior position of the fetus during labor prolongs the labor process, causes severe back discomfort in the laboring woman, and predisposes her to vaginal and perineal trauma and lacerations during birth.

The types of fetal malpresentations include face, brow, breech, and shoulder.

A fetus/newborn weighing more than 4000 g is termed *macrosomic*. Problems may occur during labor, delivery, and in the early neonatal period.

Preventing and treating problems that infringe on the development and delivery of normal fetuses are significant medical-nursing activities once the presence of twins has been detected.

Intrauterine fetal death poses a major nursing challenge to provide support and caring for the parents.

Major bleeding problems in the intrapartal period are abruptio placentae and placenta previa.

Prolapse of the umbilical cord may occur quickly, and the major goal of therapy is the immediate relief of pressure on the umbilical cord.

Contractures of the maternal pelvis predispose to CPD.

REFERENCES

Acker DB, **Sachs** BP, **Friedman** EA: Risk factors for shoulder dystocia. *Obstet Gynecol* 1985;66:762.

Acker DB, **Sachs** BP, **Friedman** EA: Risk factors for shoulder dystocia in the average-weight infant. *Obstet Gynecol* 1986;67:614.

Andrews CM, **Andrews** EC: Nursing, maternal postures, and fetal positions. *Nurs Res* 1983;32:6.

Assali NS: *Pathophysiology of Gestation: Maternal Disorders.* New York: Academic Press, 1972.

Avery MD, **Burket** BA: Effect of perineal massage on the incidence of episiotomy and perineal laceration in a nurse-midwifery service. *J Nurs-Midwife* 1986;31(May/June):128.

Avery ME, **Taeusch** HW: *Schaffer's Diseases of the Newborn.* Philadelphia, Saunders, 1984.

Avery ME, et al: Update on prenatal steroid for prevention of respiratory distress. *Am J Obstet Gynecol* 1986;155:2.

Bealle MH, et al: A comparison of ritodrine, terbutaline, and magnesium sulfate for the suppression of preterm labor. *Am J Obstet Gynecol* 1985;153:854.

Beckey RD, et al: Development of a perinatal grief checklist. *J Obstet Gynecol Neonat Nurs* 1985;14(May/June):194.

Bell D, et al: Birth asphyxia, trauma, and mortality in twins: Has Cesarean section improved outcome? *Am J Obstet Gynecol* 1986;154:235.

Benedetti TJ: Maternal complications of parenteral B-sympathomimetic therapy for premature labor. *Am J Obstet Gynecol* 1983;145:1.

Berkowitz RL: *Critical Care of the Obstetric Patient.* New York, Churchill Livingstone, 1983.

Bishop EH: Acceleration of fetal pulmonary maturity. *Obstet Gynecol* 1981;58(suppl):48.

Bodmer B, et al: Has use of cesarean section reduced the risks of delivery in the preterm breech presentation? *Am J Obstet Gynecol* 1986;154:244.

Briggs GC, **Freeman** RK, **Yaffe** SJ: *Drugs in Pregnancy and Lactation,* ed 2. Baltimore, Williams & Wilkins, 1986.

Bromberg MH: Presumptive maternal benefits of routine episiotomy: A literature review. *J Nurs-Midwife* 1986; 31(May/June):121.

Butane P, et al: Mothers' perceptions of their labor experiences. *Am J Mat Child Nurs* 1980;9:73.

Campbell B: Overdue delivery: Its impact on mothers-to-be. *Am J Mat Child Nurs* 1986;11(May/June):170.

Caritis SN, **Lin** LS, **Wong** LK: Evaluation of the pharmacodynamics and pharmacokinetics of ritodrine when ad-

ministered as a loading dose. *Am J Obstet Gynecol* 1985; 152:1026.

Carr D, **Knupp** SF: Grief and perinatal loss: A community hospital approach to support. *J Obstet Gynecol Neonat Nurs* 1985;14(March/April):130.

Clark SL, et al: Squamous cells in the maternal pulmonary circulation *Am J Obstet Gynecol* 1986;154(January):104.

Cohen W, **Friedman** EA (eds): *Management of Labor.* Baltimore, University Park Press, 1983.

Creasy RK: Prevention of preterm birth. *Birth Defects* 1983;19(5):97.

Creasy RK, **Resnik** R: *Maternal Fetal Medicine: Principles and Practice.* Philadelphia: Saunders, 1984.

Creasy RK, et al: A system for predicting spontaneous preterm birth. *Obstet Gynecol* 1980;55:692.

Danforth DN, **Scott** JR: *Obstetrics and Gynecology,* ed 5. Philadelphia, Lippincott, 1986.

Freeman RK: Problems of postdate pregnancy. *Contemp OB/GYN* 1986;28(October):73.

Friedman EA: *Labor: Clinical Evaluation and Management.* New York, Appleton-Century-Crofts, 1978.

Garite TJ, et al: Prospective randomized study of corticosteroids in the management of premature rupture of the membranes and premature gestation. *Am J Obstet Gynecol* 1981;141:508.

Genest M: Preparation for childbirth—Evidence for efficacy: A review. *J Obstet Gynecol Neonat Nurs* 1981;10:82.

Giacoia GP, **Yaffe** S: Perinatal pharmacology, in **Sciarri** JJ (ed): *Gynecology and Obstetrics.* Philadephpia, Harper & Row, 1982, vol 3, chap 100.

Gimoisky MC, **Paul** RF: Singleton breech presentation in labor. *Am J Obstet Gynecol* 1982;143:733.

Gonik B, **Creasy** RK: Preterm labor: Its diagnosis and management. *Am J Obstet Gynecol* 1986;154:3.

Green JR: Placental abnormalities: Placenta previa and abruptio placentae, in **Creasy** RK, **Resnik** R (eds): *Maternal Fetal Medicine: Principles and Practice.* Philadelphia, Saunders, 1984.

Grossman RA: Magnesium sulfate for uterine inversion. *J Reprod Med* 1981;26:261.

Hankins GD, **Hauth** JC: A comparison of the relative toxicities of beta-sympathomimetic tocolytic agents. *Am J Perinatol* 1985;2(October):338.

Hendricks SK, **Keroes** J, **Katz** M: Electrocardiographic changes associated with ritodrine-induced maternal tachycardia and hypokalemia. *Am J Obstet Gynecol* 1986; 154:921.

Herron M: *Recognizing Premature Labor May Prevent Premature Birth.* San Francisco, University of California, 1983.

Herron M, et al: Evaluation of a preterm birth prevention program preliminary report. *Obstet Gynecol* 1982;59:452.

Hicks EC: Obstetrical emergencies: A systematic approach for nursing intervention. *Nurs Clin North Am* 1983;17:1.

Ingemarsson I, **Arulkumaran** S, **Ratnam** SS: Single injection of terbutaline in term labor: I. Effect on fetal pH in cases with prolonged bradycardia. *Am J Obstet Gynecol* 1985a;153:859.

Ingemarsson I, **Arulkumaran** S, **Ratnam** SS: Single injection of terbutaline in term labor: II. Effect on uterine activity. *Am J Obstet Gynecol* 1985b;153:865.

Knight A: PSIs—tocolytics of last resort? *Contemp OB/GYN* 1986;27(January):191.

Kübler-Ross E: *On Death and Dying.* New York, Macmillan, 1969.

Lederman RP, **Lederman** E, **Work** B: Anxiety and epinephrine in multiparous women in labor: Relationship to duration of labor and fetal heart rate pattern. *Obstet Gynecol* 1985;153:870.

Lederman RP: *Psycho-Social Adaptation in Pregnancy.* Englewood Cliffs, New Jersey, 1984.

Lipshitz J: Beta-adrenergic agonists. *Semin Perinatol* 1981;5(July):252.

Lipshitz J, **Schneider** JM: Inhibition of labor, in **Sciarri** JJ (ed): *Gynecology and Obstetrics.* Philadelphia, Harper & Row 1980, vol 3, chap 87.

Lodeiro JG, et al: Fetal biophysical profile in twin gestations. *Obstet Gynecol* 1986;67:824.

Mazor M, **Hagay** ZJ, **Biale** Y: Fetal malformations associated with breech delivery. *J Reprod Med* 1985;30:884.

Miller JM, et al: A comparison of magnesium sulfate and terbutaline for the arrest of premature labor. *J Reprod Med* 1982;27:348.

NAACOG: Preterm labor and tocolytics. *OGN Nurs Practice Resource* 1984;10(September).

Nageotte MP, et al: Prophylactic intrapartum amnioinfusion in patients with preterm premature rupture of membranes. *Am J Obstet Gynecol* 1985;153:557.

Newman RB, et al: Uterine activity during pregnancy in ambulatory patients: Comparison of singleton and twin gestations. *Am J Obstet Gynecol* 1986;154(3):530.

Niebyl J (moderator): Symposium: Tocolytics: When and how to use them. *Contemp OB/GYN* 1986;27(June):146.

O'Driscoll K, **Foley** M: Correlation of decrease in perinatal mortality and increase in cesarean section rates. *Obstet Gynecol* 1983;61:1.

O'Driscoll K, et al: Active management of labor as an alternative to high cesarean section rate for dystocia. *Obstet Gynecol* 1984;63:485.

O'Leary JA: Shoulder dystocia: An ounce of prevention. *Contemp OB/GYN* 1986;27(4):78.

Olofsson P, **Rydhstrom** H: Twin delivery: How should the second twin be delivered? *Am J Obstet Gynecol* 1985;153:479.

Oxorn H: *Human Labor and Birth,* ed 5. New York, Appleton-Century-Crofts, 1986.

Penticuff JH: Psychologic implications in high-risk pregnancy. *Nurs Clin North Am* 1982;17:1.

Petrie RH: Tocolysis using magnesium sulfate. *Semin Perinatol* 1981;5:266.

Philipsen T, et al: Pulmonary edema following ritodrine-saline infusion in premature labor. *Obstet Gynecol* 1981;58:304.

Polin JI, **Frangipane** WL: Current concepts in management of obstetric problems for pediatricians: II. Modern concepts in the management of multiple gestation. *Ped Clin North Am* 1986;33(3):649.

Pritchard JA, **MacDonald** PC, **Gant** NF: *Williams Obstetrics,* ed 17. Norwalk, Conn, Appleton-Century-Crofts, 1985.

Quilligan EJ: *Current Therapy in Obstetrics and Gynecology.* Philadelphia, Saunders, 1980.

Sakala EP: Obstetric management of conjoined twins. *Obstet Gynecol* 1986;67:21S.

Sakamoto H, **Huszar** G: Pharmacologic levels of nitrendipine do not affect actin-myosin interaction in the human uterus and placenta. *Am J Obstet Gynecol* 1986;154:402.

Sasmor JL, et al: Childbirth education in 1980. *J Obstet Gynecol Neonat Nurs* 1981;10:155.

Schwiebert P, **Kirk** P: *When Hello Means Goodbye.* Oregon Health Sciences University, 1985.

Seeds JW, **Cefalo** RC: Malpresentations. *Clin Obstet Gynecol* 1982;25:145.

Shortridge LA: Using ritodrine hydrochloride to inhibit preterm labor. *Am J Mat Child Nurs* 1983;8(January/February):58.

Silbar EL: Factors related to the increasing cesarean section rates for cephalopelvic disproportion. *Am J Obstet Gynecol* 1986;154(May):1095.

Simpson GF, **Harbert** GM Jr: Use of betamethasone in management of preterm gestation with rupture of membranes. *Am J Obstet Gynecol* 1984;66(August):168.

Thiagarajah S, **Harbert** GM, **Bourgeois** FJ: Magnesium sulfate and ritodrine hydrochloride: Systemic and uterine hemodynamic effects. *Am J Obstet Gynecol* 1985;153(November):666.

Veille JC, **Morton** MJ, **Burry** KJ: Maternal cardiovascular adaptations to twin pregnancy. *Am J Obstet Gynecol* 1985;153:261.

Veille JC, et al: The effect of a calcium channel blocker (nifedipine) in uterine blood flow in the pregnant goat. *Am J Obstet Gynecol* 1986;154:1160.

Wang R, **Davidson** BJ: Ritodrine-induced neutropenia. *Am J Obstet Gynecol* 1986;154:924.

Wilkins IA, et al: Long-term use of magnesium sulfate as a tocolytic agent. *Obstet Gynecol* 1986;67:38S.

Work BA: Caring for genital tract birth trauma. *Contemp OB/GYN* 1982;20(November):82.

Young DC, et al: Potassium and glucose concentrations without treatment during ritodrine tocolysis. *Am J Obstet Gynecol* 1983;145:105.

Yutopar Drug Information Insert. Astra Pharmaceutical Products, Westborough, Mass, 1984.

Zacharias JF: Childbirth education classes: Effects on attitudes toward childbirth in high-risk indigent women. *J Obstet Gynecol Neonat Nurs* 1981;10:265.

ADDITIONAL READINGS

Areskog B, **Uddenberg** N, **Kjessler:** Postnatal emotional balance in women with and without antenatal fear of childbirth. *J Psychosomatic Res* 1984;28(3):213.

Borg S, **Lasker** J: *When Pregnancy Fails: Families Coping with Miscarriage, Stillbirth and Infant Death.* Boston, Beacon Press, 1981.

Cefalo RC: Managing missed abortion and antepartum fetal death. *Contemp OB/GYN* 1983;22(August):17.

Cronenwett L, **Brickman** P: Models of helping and coping in childbirth. *Nurs Res* 1983;32:2.

Druzin ML, **Toth** M, **Ledger** WJ: Nonintervention in premature rupture of the amniotic membranes. *J Reprod Med* 1986;163(July):5.

Geden E, et al: Identifying procedure components for analogue research of labor pain. *Nurs Res* 1983;32:2.

Gustaitis R, **Young** EWD: *A Time to Be Born, A Time to Die.* Reading, Mass, Addison-Wesley, 1986.

Halfar MM: Frequency of labor dysfunction in nulliparas over the age of thirty. *J Nurs-Midwife* 1985;30(November/December):333.

Howe CL: Physiologic and psychosocial assessment in labor. *Nurs Clin North Am* 1982;17:1.

Larsen JF, et al: Ritodrine in the treatment of preterm labor: Second Danish multicenter study. *Obstet Gynecol* 1986;67:607.

Manderino MM, **Bzdek** VM: Effects of modeling and information on reactions to pain: A childbirth preparation analogue. *Nurs Res* 1984;33:1.

Mercer RT, et al: Relationship of psychosocial and perinatal variables to perception of childbirth. *Nurs Res* 1983;32:4.

Sinquefield G: Midwifery management of prodromal labor. *J Nurs-Midwife* 1985;30(November/December):342.

Vintzileos AM, et al: Fetal biophysical profile and the effect of premature rupture of the membranes. *Obstet Gynecol* 1986;67:818.

Vintzileos AM, et al: Fetal breathing as a predictor of infection in premature rupture of the membranes. *Obstet Gynecol* 1986;67:813.

When I found I was pregnant the first time, I was amazed. When I found I was pregnant the second time, I thought "How can that be? We don't 'do it' that often." (Having a child can really affect your sex life.) When I found out I was pregnant the third time, and that we were expecting twins, I just felt tired.

Obstetric Procedures and the Role of the Nurse

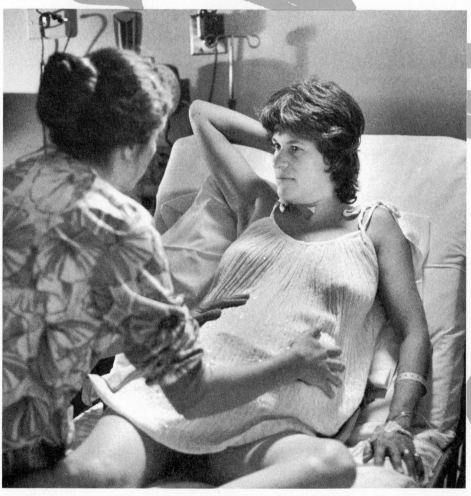

When explaining possible procedures, it's important for the nurse to be sensitive to the laboring woman's fears and anxieties.

Chapter Twenty-Six

OBJECTIVES

- Examine the method of external version and the related nursing interventions.
- Discuss the use of amniotomy in current maternity care.
- Compare methods for inducing labor, explaining their advantages and disadvantages.
- Describe the types of episiotomies performed, the rationale for each, and the associated nursing intervention.
- Describe the indications for forceps delivery and types of forceps that may be used.
- Discuss the use of vacuum extraction, including indications, procedure, complications, and related nursing interventions.
- Determine the indications for cesarean birth, the impact on the family unit, preparation and teaching needs, and associated nursing interventions.
- Discuss vaginal birth after cesarean (VBAC).
- Describe the prerequisites for a trial of labor (TOL) after previous cesarean delivery and associated nursing care.

Most births occur without the need for operative obstetric intervention. In some instances, however, obstetric procedures are necessary to maintain the safety of the mother and her baby. The use of obstetric procedures, especially cesarean delivery, has increased in recent years due in part to better diagnostic techniques and a philosophy of more rapid intervention in labor.

Some women are prepared for the possible use of operative procedures such as the need for cesarean delivery in the presence of CPD. Many women know that episiotomies are also commonly used. However, most women expect to have a "natural" labor and birth and do not anticipate the need for any medical interventions. This presents a challenge to maternity nurses. Information may be included in prenatal classes so that expectant women know the types of procedures that may be needed and the situations that would necessitate intervention. When the woman is in labor it is important to provide information regarding any procedure to make sure the woman and her partner understand what is proposed, the anticipated benefits and possible risks, and any possible alternative treatments. Some obstetric procedures require written informed consent and others do not. Even if written consent is not required, it is important to provide accurate, comprehensive, easily understood information so the woman will be better able to participate in her care.

● Care of the Woman During Version

Version is the alteration of fetal position by abdominal or intrauterine manipulation to accomplish a more favorable fetal presentation for delivery. Alteration of the breech or shoulder presentation is attempted by external (or cephalic) version, that is, external manipulation of the maternal abdomen. Internal (or podalic) version is attempted by introduction of the obstetrician's entire hand into the uterine cavity. Internal version is attempted only under certain conditions in multiple gestations for delivery of the second twin.

External Version

If breech or shoulder presentation (transverse lie) is detected in the later weeks of pregnancy an external version may be attempted. The procedure is done after 37 weeks' gestation because most fetuses still in breech presentation at this time will not spontaneously convert to a vertex presentation (Figure 26–1).

The prerequisites for cephalic version are (Pritchard et al 1985, Danforth & Scott 1986):

1. The presenting part must not be engaged.

2. The abdominal wall must be thin enough to permit accurate palpation.

3. The uterine wall must not be irritable.

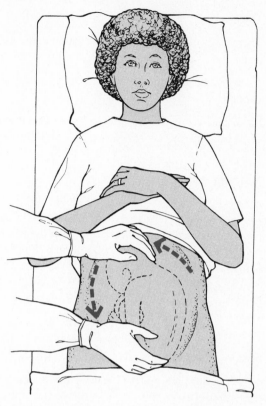

Figure 26–1   External (or cephalic) version of fetus. A new technique involves pressure on the fetal head and buttocks so that the fetus completes a "backward flip" or "forward roll."

4. There must be a sufficient quantity of amniotic fluid in the uterus, and the membranes must be intact. Oligohydramnios or rupture of the membranes makes the amniotic fluid inadequate for unrestricted turning of the fetus.

5. There must be a reactive NST.

The contraindications to external version are (Hansen 1984, Danforth & Scott 1986):

1. Fetopelvic disproportion that would prevent a vaginal birth

2. Multiple gestation

3. Oligohydramnios

4. Nonreactive NST

5. Gross fetal abnormality

6. Suspected IUGR

7. History of premature labor

8. Placenta previa

9. Uterine scar

One study showed a version success rate of 77 percent, and there were no spontaneous reversions from vertex to breech (Dyson et al 1986). There were also no significant maternal or fetal problems. Some researchers have reported an overall ratio of successful external cephalic version to spontaneous version of 3:1. There seems to be a variation in success rates in differing ethnic groups with a significantly lower success rate in white nulliparas. This may be explained by the known tendency of the presenting part to engage in white nulliparous women several weeks prior to labor whereas in black women the presenting part frequently does not engage until labor begins (Hofmeyr et al 1986).

Nursing Assessment

As the woman is admitted, the nurse begins her assessment by validating that no contraindications to the version are present. Maternal vital signs and FHR are assessed and the NST is done to ascertain reactivity of the FHR. Maternal vital signs are assessed prior to the version and every 5 minutes throughout the procedure and for 30 minutes following it. The fetus is monitored continuously with ongoing evaluation of the FHR.

Version Procedure

The version is accomplished in a birthing unit rather than an outpatient setting in case further intervention is necessary. The obstetrician evaluates the results of laboratory studies, which usually include a hemoglobin, hematocrit, blood type, and Rh. An ultrasound exam is completed just prior to the version to validate fetal presentation and locate the placenta. The fetus is monitored electronically and a nonstress test is done. After these initial assessments intravenous ritodrine or terbutaline is given to achieve uterine relaxation. The obstetrician does the version by rotating the fetus in a backward or forward flip and holds it in the new position as the intravenous infusion is discontinued. The version is discontinued immediately in the presence of severe maternal discomfort or significant fetal bradycardia (less than 90 bpm for more than 60 seconds) or if the attempt is unsuccessful after a maximum of 15 minutes (Dyson et al 1986).

Nursing Role

The nurse completes the assessments previously discussed. Assessments of the maternal-fetal response to the β-mimetic are also done (see Drug Guide p 739). The nurse also provides information for the woman and her partner. The admission period and time when the initial NST is performed are excellent opportunities for educating the woman. The woman should be encouraged to express her understanding and expectations of the procedure, verbalize her fears, and ask questions. The possibility of failure of the procedure and operative intervention if the fetus becomes distressed should be discussed. Explaining what will occur in either of these circumstances will better prepare the woman if intervention becomes necessary.

● **Care of the Woman During an Amniotomy**

Amniotomy is the artificial rupture of the amniotic membranes (AROM). It is probably the most common operative procedure in obstetrics. It is usually performed in the late active or transition phase of labor or in the second stage just prior to delivery, but it may be done earlier as a means of inducing (beginning) labor. Amniotomy may also be done to allow access to the fetus for scalp blood sampling, to apply an internal fetal heart monitoring electrode, or to insert an intrauterine pressure catheter.

Opinion varies regarding the advisability of AROM. When AROM is not done, 66 percent of membranes will remain intact until the end of the first stage (Marshall 1985).

Amniotomy seems to be a successful method of induction. When there is a favorable cervix (some cervical dilatation and effacement), 40 percent of women are delivered within 4 hours of the AROM and 85 percent within 12 hours (Marshall 1985).

The advantages of amniotomy as a method of labor induction are:

1. The contractions elicited are similar to those of spontaneous labor.

2. There is usually no risk of hypertonus or rupture of the uterus.

3. The woman does not require close surveillance as with oxytocin infusion.

4. Fetal monitoring is facilitated because amniotomy does not interfere with the following:

   a. Scalp blood sampling for pH determinations

   b. Scalp electrode application

   c. Intrauterine catheter placement

5. The color and composition of amniotic fluid can be evaluated.

The disadvantages of amniotomy are:

1. Once an amniotomy is done, delivery must occur regardless of subsequent findings that suggest delaying birth.

2. The danger of a prolapsed cord is increased.

3. There is a risk of infection from ascending organisms.

4. Compression and molding of the fetal head are increased.

5. Labor may not be successfully induced, necessitating cesarean delivery.

Nursing Assessment

Before an amniotomy is performed, the fetus is assessed for presentation, position, and station. The nurse has already completed these assessments, but the obstetrician will also assess these factors before doing the AROM. Unless the head is well engaged in the pelvis, most obstetricians do not advocate an amniotomy because of the danger of a prolapsed cord. Other risks are abruptio placentae, infection, and amniotic fluid embolus.

AROM Procedure

While performing a sterile vaginal examination, the physician introduces an amnihook (or other rupturing device) into the vagina. A small tear is made in the amniotic membrane. Following rupture of the membranes, amniotic fluid is allowed to escape. Opinion varies regarding how much fluid should escape. Proponents of slow escape suggest that slow escape of the amniotic fluid decreases the chance of prolapse of the umbilical cord or abruptio placentae that may occur with sudden reduction in uterine volume (Niswander 1985). They stress that the amniotomy should be done between contractions if the presenting part is at a station of +1 or above. Those favoring escape of a large amount of fluid believe it reduces uterine volume, which results in contraction of the myometrium, which produces more effective contractions (Niswander 1985).

Nursing Role

The laboring woman needs to understand the AROM procedure, and its purpose, anticipated benefits, and risks. The nurse is frequently the person who provides this information. Prior to AROM it is helpful to explain the sensations the laboring woman will feel in order to decrease anxiety. The laboring woman can expect to feel the draining of amniotic fluid onto her perineum but usually she will not feel discomfort.

It is imperative that the FHR be auscultated before and immediately after the procedure so that any changes from the previous FHR pattern can be noted. If changes are marked, the nurse should check for prolapse of the cord. The amniotic fluid should be inspected for amount, color, odor, and presence of meconium or blood. The findings are documented in the chart and on the fetal monitoring strip.

The perineal area is cleaned and dried after the procedure. There is now an open pathway for organisms to ascend into the uterus, so strict sterile precautions must be taken when doing vaginal examinations, the number of vaginal exams must be kept to a minimum, and the woman's temperature should be monitored every hour.

Care of the Woman During Induction of Labor

The American College of Obstetricians and Gynecologists defines *induction of labor* as the initiation of uterine contractions before the onset of labor by medical and/or surgical means for the purpose of accomplishing birth (ACOG 1987). The procedure may be either elective or medically indicated because of the presence of a maternal and/or fetal problem.

Elective induction is defined by the Food and Drug Administration as "the initiation of labor for the convenience of an individual with a term pregnancy who is free of medical indications." The FDA prohibits oxytocin use for elective induction of labor in the absence of medical indications (Dept HEW 1978). The practice of elective induction is questionable in some centers because of the associated maternal risks and the possibility of delivering a preterm infant. The woman should be carefully evaluated for the presence of a medical condition that would contraindicate the procedure. Accurate gestational dating is essential. Elective induction may be indicated for a woman who has had previous precipitous labors (lasting less than three hours) to avoid an unexpected out-of-the-hospital delivery.

Indicated induction may be considered in the presence of a preexisting maternal disease such as diabetes mellitus, chronic hypertensive vascular disease, and renal disease. Since these diseases are associated with possible placental insufficiency, fetoplacental function tests should be done to assist the physician in determining the need for and the timing of an induction. Additional tests for fetal maturity are necessary to determine the neonate's capacity for extrauterine survival.

Additional indications for medically indicated induction include severe preeclampsia-eclampsia, abruptio placentae, premature rupture of membranes, postterm pregnancy, severe fetal hemolytic disease, intrauterine growth retardation, and intrauterine fetal death (Niswander 1985).

The most frequently used methods of induction are amniotomy, intravenous oxytocin (Pitocin) infusion, or both. The use of PGE_2 to induce labor is currently being investigated.

Oxytocin infusion and prostaglandin administration are discussed later in this section. See p 798 for a discussion of amniotomy.

Contraindications

All contraindications to spontaneous labor and vaginal delivery are contraindications to the induction of labor (Niswander 1985, Pritchard et al 1985).

Maternal contraindications are:

- Client refusal
- Previous uterine incision (cesarean birth, hysterotomy, myomectomy)
- Obstructions of the birth canal from soft tissue masses (myomas, fibroids, large cysts)
- Invasive carcinoma of the cervix
- Presence of herpesvirus type 2
- Cephalopelvic disproportion
- Placenta previa centrally located
- Grand multiparity (five or more pregnancies)
- Overt uterine overdistention (hydramnios, multiple fetuses)

Fetal contraindications are:

- Severe fetal distress or abnormal results of contraction stress test

Table 26–1   Prelabor Status Evaluation Scoring System*

Factor	Assigned value			
	0	1	2	3
Cervical dilatation	Closed	1–2 cm	3–4 cm	5 cm or more
Cervical effacement	0%–30%	40%–50%	60%–70%	80% or more
Fetal station	−3	−2	−1, 0	+1, or lower
Cervical consistency	Firm	Moderate	Soft	
Cervical position	Posterior	Midposition	Anterior	

*Modified from Bishop EH: Pelvic scoring for elective induction. *Obstet Gynecol* 1964;24:266.

- Low-birth-weight or preterm fetus
- Abnormal fetal presentation (transverse, or possibly breech)

Before induction is attempted, appropriate assessment must indicate that both the woman and fetus are ready for the onset of labor. This includes evaluation of fetal maturity and cervical readiness.

Labor Readiness

FETAL MATURITY

Early diagnosis of pregnancy with adequate recorded data during the early months of pregnancy, including serial sonograms, is helpful in determining the expected date of delivery. External abdominal examination of the growing uterus and amniotic fluid studies are also beneficial in assessing fetal maturity.

CERVICAL READINESS

The findings on vaginal examination will help determine whether cervical changes favorable for induction have occurred. Bishop (1964) developed a prelabor scoring system that has proved helpful in predicting the inducibility of women (Table 26–1). Components evaluated are cervical dilatation, effacement, consistency, and position, as well as the station of the fetal presenting part. A score of 0, 1, 2, or 3 is given to each assessed characteristic. The higher the total score for all the criteria, the more likely it is that labor will ensue. The lower the total score, the higher the failure rate. A favorable cervix is the most important criterion for a successful induction.

The presence of a cervix that is anterior, soft, more than 50 percent effaced, and dilated at least 3 cm, with the fetal head at + 1 station or lower is favorable for successful induction (Danforth & Scott 1986).

A "ripe" cervix is so widely accepted an indicator for success that several methods (including laminaria, catheters, and PG gel) to enhance ripening are being investigated (Marshall 1985). In a recent study (Salmon et al 1986), which investigated cervical ripening by breast stimulation, women began gentle unilateral breast stimulation of alternate breasts for 1½ hours under monitoring in the hospital. Then the stimulation was continued for three hours daily for the next three days at home. There were no maternal or fetal problems and there was a significant change in the Bishop score.

Oxytocin Infusion

Intravenous administration of oxytocin is an effective method of initiating uterine contractions (inducing labor).

During administration, the goal is to achieve two to three uterine contractions with a duration of 40 to 60 seconds in ten minutes with good uterine relaxation and return to the baseline tone between contractions (Niswander 1985).

MEDICAL THERAPY

Ten units of oxytocin (Pitocin) are added to 1 L of intravenous fluid (usually 5 percent dextrose in balanced salt solution—for example, 5 percent dextrose in lactated Ringer's). The resulting mixture will contain 10 mU of oxytocin per milliliter (1 mU/min = 6 mL/hr) and the prescribed dose can be calculated easily. Other dosage concentrations are presented in the Drug Guide on p 802.

A second bottle of intravenous fluid is prepared and used to start and maintain the infusion. This avoids infusing a large dose of oxytocin as the line is begun and provides additional fluids while the oxytocin solution is being kept at a low infusion rate. After the infusion is started, the oxytocin solution is piggybacked into the primary tubing port closest to the catheter insertion. This allows only a small amount of oxytocin to backflow into the tubing and assures greater dosage accuracy. The FDA recommends an initial dosage of 1 to 2 mU/min and further states the dosage "may be gradually increased in increments of no more than 1 to 2 mU/min until the patient experiences a contraction pattern similar to normal labor."

Depending on the rate of infusion, maximum effect is reached in approximately 20 to 60 minutes; therefore it has been considered advisable to increase the infusion rate at intervals of no less than every 30 minutes to a maximum rate of 20 mU/min with increases based on an evaluation of uterine, fetal, and maternal response to present dose (Danforth 1982; ACOG 1987).

If the desired effects are not achieved with a dose of 20 mU/min, it is unlikely that higher doses will be successful, and they may increase the hazards to the woman and fetus (Danforth & Scott 1986; Pritchard et al 1985). Currently the rate of infusion (dosage of oxytocin) and suggested frequency of advancing the rate are in question.

There is a triphasic response of the uterus to oxytocin. During the incremental phase, there is an even increase in uterine activity. The next phase, the stable phase, is reached when the uterine activity remains constant in spite of increased oxytocin doses. After the stable phase has been established further increases in rate will result in the third phase, which is characterized by increased frequency of contractions, a fall in mean uterine pressure, and increased uterine baseline tone. The increased frequency may develop into tachysystole, polysystole, or prolonged tetanic contractions (Marshall 1985).

Oxytocin induction is not without some associated risks. Rapid progression of infusion rates or continuance of a particular rate without adequate assessment of the uterine contractions may lead to hyperstimulation of the uterus, compromise of the fetus due to decreased placental perfusion, a rapid labor and delivery with the danger of cervical or perineal lacerations, or uterine rupture. Whenever 20 mU/min or more of oxytocin is infused, the antidiuretic effect of oxytocin results in a marked decrease in the free water clearance by the kidney, and urinary output decreases significantly. Water intoxication may result (Niswander 1985).

NURSING ASSESSMENT

Close observation and accurate assessments are mandatory to provide safe, optimal care for both woman and fetus. Baseline data (maternal temperature, pulse, respiration, blood pressure, and FHR) should be obtained before beginning the infusion. A fetal monitor is used to provide continuous data. Many institutions recommend obtaining a 15-minute recording and NST before the infusion is started to obtain baseline data on uterine contractions and FHR.

Before each advancement of the infusion rate, assessments of the following should be made: (a) maternal blood pressure and pulse; (b) rate and reactivity of the FHR tracing (any bradycardia or decelerations are noted); and (c) contraction status, frequency, intensity, duration, and resting tone between contractions. During the induction, urinary output is assessed to identify any problems with retention, fluid deficit, and possible development of water intoxication.

As contractions are established, vaginal examinations are done to evaluate cervical dilatation, effacement, and station. The frequency of vaginal examinations primarily depends on the number of pregnancies and on characteristics of contractions. For example, a nullipara with contractions every five to seven minutes, each lasting 30 seconds, who does not perceive her contractions does not usually require a vaginal examination, but when her contractions are every two to three minutes, lasting 50 to 60 seconds with good intensity, a vaginal examination will be needed to evaluate her status.

When evaluating the need for analgesia, a vaginal examination should be performed to avoid giving the medication too early and increasing the risk of prolonging labor and to identify advanced dilatation and imminent delivery. The administration of analgesia within two to four hours before delivery may result in respiratory difficulties for the newborn.

NURSING DIAGNOSIS

The nursing diagnoses that may be appropriate for labor induction are presented in the Nursing Care Plan on p 804.

NURSING GOAL: PROMOTION OF MATERNAL-FETAL PHYSICAL WELL-BEING

Pritchard, MacDonald, and Gant (1985) recommend that the woman not be left alone during oxytocin infusion. Niswander (1985) recommends constant attendance during the first 20 to 30 minutes of infusion and for 20 to 30 minutes after each increase in dose. During this time assessment is directed to the maternal and fetal response to the infusion.

For additional information on nursing interventions, see Drug Guide–Oxytocin on page 802, and Nursing Care Plan: Induction of Labor on page 804.

Intravenous oxytocin may be given for augmentation of labor; see Drug Guide–Oxytocin for further discussion.

Prostaglandin Administration

Prostaglandin E_2 vaginal suppositories are used extensively in the management of intrauterine fetal demise in the second trimester of pregnancy. However, approval for their use the third trimester is pending evaluation of safety and efficacy.

The use of prostaglandin $F_{2\alpha}$ ($PGF_{2\alpha}$) and prostaglandin E_2 (PGE_2) for induction is fairly routine in England, and is currently being studied for use in the United States and Canada (Neal 1984).

Macer, Buchanan, and Yonekurs (1984) conducted a study using a 3 mg prostaglandin E_2 vaginal suppository with intravenous oxytocin for the induction of labor. They found the E_2 suppository was successful in ripening the cervix and in inducing labor. More than half the women had a successful induction with only the E_2 suppository; the remaining women also required IV oxytocin.

● Care of the Woman During an Episiotomy

An episiotomy is a surgical incision of the perineal body that extends downward from the vaginal orifice. It is done with sharp scissors with rounded points. The episiotomy is done to minimize stretching of the perineal tissues and subsequent symptomatic relaxation of the perineum, to decrease the incidence of perineal lacerations, to decrease the length of the second stage, and to decrease trauma to the fetal head during delivery (Varner 1986, Bromberg 1986).

The routine use of episiotomies is becoming an increasingly controversial issue. Various authors have found no evidence to support the listed reasons for episiotomies (Banta & Thacker 1982, Thacker & Banta 1983, Buekens et al 1985, Varner 1986). To date there is no significant data to substantiate the claim that an episiotomy prevents perineal stretching and subsequent relaxation of the peri-

Drug Guide–Oxytocin (Pitocin)

Overview of Obstetric Action

Oxytocin (Pitocin) exerts a selective stimulatory effect on the smooth muscle of the uterus and blood vessels. Oxytocin affects the myometrial cells of the uterus by increasing the excitability of the muscle cell, increasing the strength of the muscle contraction, and supporting propagation of the contraction (movement of the contraction from one myometrial cell to the next). Its effect on the uterine contraction depends on the dosage used and on the excitability of the myometrial cells. During the first half of gestation, little excitability of the myometrium occurs and the uterus is fairly resistant to the effects of oxytocin. However, from midgestation on, the uterus responds increasingly to exogenous intravenous oxytocin. When at term, cautious use of diluted oxytocin, administered intravenously, results in a slow rise of uterine activity.

The circulatory half-life of oxytocin is 3–4 minutes, but the uterine effects last 20–30 minutes.

The effects of oxytocin on the cardiovascular system can be pronounced. There may be an initial decrease in the blood pressure, but with prolonged administration, a 30 percent increase in the baseline blood pressure may be noted. Cardiac output and stroke volume are increased. With doses of 20 mU/min or above, the antidiuretic effect of oxytocin results in a decrease of free water exchange in the kidney and a marked decrease in urine output (Marshall 1985).

Oxytocin is used to induce labor at term and to augment uterine contractions in the first and second stages of labor. Oxytocin may also be used immediately after delivery to stimulate uterine contraction and thereby control uterine atony.

Oxytocin is not thought to cross the placenta because of its molecular weight and the presence of oxytocinase in the placenta (Giacoia & Yaffe 1982). Oxytocin has an antidiuretic effect.

Route, Dosage, Frequency

For induction of labor: Add 10 units Pitocin (1 mL) to 1000 mL of intravenous solution. (The resulting concentration is 10 mU oxytocin per 1 mL of intravenous fluid.) Using an infusion pump, administer IV, starting at 0.5 mU/min and increasing the rate stepwise at no less than every 30–60 minutes until good contractions (every 2–3 minutes, each lasting 40–60 seconds) are achieved. The maximum rate is 20 mU/min (Cibils 1981). Decrease oxytocin by similar increments once labor has progressed to 5–6 cm dilatation (ACOG 1987).

0.5 mU/min =	3 mL/hr	8 mU/min =	48 mL/hr
1.0 mU/min =	6 mL/hr	10 mU/min =	60 mL/hr
1.5 mU/min =	9 mL/hr	12 mU/min =	72 mL/hr
2 mU/min =	12 mL/hr	15 mU/min =	90 mL/hr
4 mU/min =	24 mL/hr	18 mU/min =	108 mL/hr
6 mU/min =	36 mL/hr	20 mU/min =	120 mL/hr

Protocols may vary from one agency to another.

For augmentation of labor: Prepare and administer IV Pitocin as for labor induction. Increase rate until labor contractions are of good quality. The flow rate is gradually increased at no less than every 30 minutes to a maximum of 10 mU/min (Pritchard et al 1985).

In some settings, or in a situation when limited fluids may be administered, a more-concentrated solution may be used. When 10 U Pitocin is added to 500 mL IV solution the resulting concentration is 1 mU/min = 3 mL/hr. If 10 U Pitocin is added to 250 mL IV solution the concentration is 1 mU/min = 1.5 mL/hr.

For administration after delivery of placenta: One dose of 10 units Pitocin (1 mL) is given intramuscularly or by slow intravenous push or added to IV fluids for continuous infusion.

Maternal Contraindications

Severe preeclampsia-eclampsia

Predisposition to uterine rupture (in nullipara over 35 years of age, paragravida 4 or more, overdistention of the uterus, previous major surgery of the cervix or uterus)

Cephalopelvic disproportion

Malpresentation or malposition of the fetus, cord prolapse

Preterm infant

Rigid, unripe cervix; total placenta previa

Presence of fetal distress

Maternal Side Effects

Hyperstimulation of the uterus results in hypercontractility, which in turn may cause the following:

Abruptio placentae

Impaired uterine blood flow → fetal hypoxia

Rapid labor → cervical lacerations

Rapid labor and delivery → lacerations of cervix, vagina, perineum, uterine atony, fetal trauma

Uterine rupture

Water intoxication (nausea, vomiting, hypotension, tachycardia, cardiac arrhythmia) if oxytocin is given in electrolyte-free solution or at a rate exceeding 20 mU/min.

Hypotension with rapid IV bolus administration postpartum.

(continued)

Drug Guide—Oxytocin (Pitocin) (continued)

Effect on Fetus/Neonate
Fetal effects are primarily associated with the presence of hypercontractility of the maternal uterus. Hypercontractility causes a decrease in the oxygen supply to the fetus, which is reflected by irregularities and/or decrease in FHR. Hyperbilirubinemia.

Nursing Considerations

Explain induction of augmentation procedure to client.

Apply fetal monitor and obtain 15-minute tracing and NST to assess FHR before starting IV oxytocin.

For induction or augmentation of labor, start with primary IV and piggy-back secondary IV with oxytocin.

Assure continuous fetal and uterine contraction monitoring.

Assess FHR, maternal blood pressure, pulse, and uterine contraction frequency, duration, and resting tone before each increase in oxytocin infusion rate.

Record all assessments and IV rate on monitor strip and on client's chart.

Record all client activities (such as change of position, vomiting), procedures done (amniotomy, sterile vaginal examination), and administration of analgesics on monitor strip to allow for interpretation and evaluation of tracing.

Assess cervical dilatation as needed.

Apply nursing comfort measures.

Discontinue IV oxytocin infusion and infuse primary solution when (a) fetal distress is noted (bradycardia, late or variable decelerations, meconium staining); (b) uterine contractions are more frequent than every 2 minutes; (c) duration of contractions exceeds more than 60 seconds (Pritchard et al 1985); or (d) insufficient relaxation of the uterus between contractions or a steady increase in resting tone are noted; in addition to discontinuing IV oxytocin infusion, turn client to side, and if fetal distress is present, administer oxygen by tight face mask at 6–10 L/min; notify physician.

---

neal tissues (Varner 1986). A slightly higher incidence of tears has been found when the woman has a mediolateral episiotomy (Buekens et al 1985). There is no significant data to support the need to do an episiotomy to decrease the pressure on the full-term infant's head (Varner 1986).

Even those who question the routine use of episiotomies would not hesitate to agree that an episiotomy is necessary for a forceps delivery, large fetus and anticipated difficult delivery, breech presentation, or use of a vacuum extractor.

The associated complications are laceration, excessive blood loss, infection, and pain that may continue for weeks or months following delivery. Thacker and Banta (1983) estimate that 10 percent of women have an additional 300 cc blood loss from the episiotomy alone.

Episiotomy Procedure

The episiotomy is performed just before delivery, when the presenting part has begun to distend the perineum and the fetus will be delivered with the next three or four contractions (Varner 1986). There are two types in current practice: midline and mediolateral (Figure 26–2). A midline episiotomy is performed along the median raphe of the perineum. It extends down from the vaginal orifice to the fibers of the rectal sphincter. This type of episiotomy avoids muscle fibers and major blood vessels because it divides the insertions of the superficial perineal muscles. A midline episiotomy is preferred if the perineum is of adequate length and no difficulty is anticipated during delivery, because the blood loss is less and the incision is easy to repair and heals with less discomfort for the mother. The major disadvantage is that a tear of the midline incision may extend through the anal sphincter and rectum.

In the presence of a short perineum or an anticipated difficult delivery, a mediolateral episiotomy provides more room and decreases the possibility of a traumatic extension into the rectum. The mediolateral episiotomy begins in the midline of the posterior fourchette (in order to avoid incision into the Bartholin's gland) and extends at a 45° angle downward to the right or left (the direction depending on the handedness of the clinician). The mediolateral episiotomy may be complicated by greater blood loss, a longer healing period, and more postpartal discomfort for the mother.

The episiotomy is usually performed with regional or local anesthesia but may be performed without anesthesia in emergency situations. It is generally proposed that as crowning occurs, the distention of the tissues causes numbing. Adequate anesthesia must be given for the repair.

Repair of the episiotomy (episiorrhaphy) and any lacerations are accomplished either during the period between delivery of the neonate and before delivery of the placenta or after the delivery of the placenta.

Nursing Care Plan: Induction of Labor

Mrs Brookens is at 40 weeks' gestation and is admitted to the birthing unit for induction of labor. Her husband RJ is with her. They both seem excited about this first labor and birth and hopeful that delivery will occur today. They have attended prenatal classes and have practiced the techniques together for many weeks. They ask many questions about how the induction works and what the labor will be like.

Assessment

HISTORY

Previous pregnancies
Present pregnancy course
Childbirth preparation
Estimated gestational age

PHYSICAL EXAMINATION

1. Examination of pregnant uterus (Leopold's maneuvers to determine fetal size and position)
2. Vaginal examination to evaluate cervical readiness
   a. Ripe cervix: feels soft to the examining finger, is located in a medial to anterior position, is more than 50% effaced, and is 2–3 cm dilated
   b. Unripe cervix: feels firm to the examining finger, is long and thick, perhaps in a posterior position, with little or no dilatation
3. Presence of contractions
4. Membranes intact or ruptured
5. Fetal size (Leopold's maneuvers, ultrasound)
6. Fetal readiness
7. CPD evaluation
8. Maternal vital signs and FHR before beginning induction

LABORATORY EVALUATION

Fetal maturity tests (L/S ratio, creatinine concentrations, ultrasonography)
Maternal blood studies (CBC, hemoglobin, hematocrit, blood type, Rh factor)
Urinalysis

ANALYSIS OF NURSING PRIORITIES

1. Monitor and evaluate status of mother and fetus continuously throughout the induction.
2. Provide continuous physical and emotional support.
3. Evaluate and monitor uterine response to induction.
4. Evaluate and monitor fetal response to induction.
5. Continuously evaluate client for complications associated with induction (abruptio placentae, fetal distress, any rise or decrease in maternal BP, hemorrhage, shock, uterine rupture, tetanic contractions).

CLIENT/FAMILY EDUCATIONAL FOCUS

1. Provide information about the induction procedure, including action and side effects of medications and expected action.
2. Provide information about the fetal monitor, how it works, and the information that can be obtained from it.
3. Provide opportunities for questions and individual concerns of the client and family.

Nursing Diagnosis and Goals	Nursing Interventions	Rationale
NURSING DIAGNOSIS: Knowledge deficit related to induction procedure	Assess their feelings regarding induction. They may ask, "Will this work?" "How long will it take?" "Will it hurt more?"	Mrs Brookens may be apprehensive about what will happen, or feel a sense of failure that she cannot "go into labor by herself."
SUPPORTING DATA: Mrs Brookens asks questions about the induction.	Assess knowledge base regarding the induction process Provide needed information (for example, when the cervix is ripe, contractions should begin in 30–60 minutes); length of labor depends on a number of factors Assess knowledge of breathing techniques; if she does not have a method to use, teach breathing techniques before starting oxytocin infusion	After assessing knowledge base, appropriate information can be given to allay apprehension. Use of breathing techniques during contractions will help relaxation; although a woman may be apprehensive about induction, teaching a new breathing method will be easier before contractions are present.
GOAL: Mr and Mrs Brookens can discuss the induction procedure, the benefits, and potential risks.		

Nursing Care Plan: Induction of Labor (continued)

Nursing Diagnosis and Goals	Nursing Interventions	Rationale
NURSING DIAGNOSIS: Potential alteration in cardiac output related to positional changes and the weight of the uterus on the vena cava	Position Mrs Brookens on her side; encourage her to avoid supine position. Monitor maternal BP and pulse and FHR every 15–20 minutes. If she becomes hypotensive: 1. Keep her on her side, may change to other side. 2. Discontinue oxytocin infusion 3. Increase rate of primary IV 4. Monitor FHR 5. Notify physician 6. Assess for cause of hypotension	Side-lying position maintains optimal blood flow to uterus and placenta. Mrs Brookens is frequently on her back at beginning of induction while monitors are attached and IV is started; vena cava is obstructed, causing maternal hypotension, which may lead to fetal bradycardia; initial hypotension is secondary to peripheral vasodilatation induced by oxytocin, which causes diminished blood supply to placenta and resultant decrease in O$_2$ supply to fetus. Actions are directed toward improving blood flow and oxygenation of tissues.
SUPPORTING DATA: Decrease in BP and increase in pulse rate Breathlessness Cool, moist skin		
GOAL: Mrs Brookens will maintain vital signs within normal range with no significant increase or decrease.		
NURSING DIAGNOSIS: Potential alteration in tissue perfusion (placenta) related to hypertonic contraction pattern	Apply monitor to obtain 15 minutes of tracing prior to starting induction.	Establishes baseline data.
	Administer oxytocin in electrolyte solution.	Oxytocin has slight antidiuretic effect, especially when administered in electrolyte-free solutions.
	Assess and record fluid intake and output. Monitor for nausea, vomiting, hypotension, tachycardia, cardiac arrhythmias.	Provides information on hydration status. These are signs and symptoms of water intoxication; they must be differentiated from other problems.
	Assess FHR by continuous electronic fetal monitoring. Obtain 15-minute tracing prior to beginning induction to evaluate fetal status; *do not* start infusion or advance rate (if induction has already begun) if FHR is not in range of 120–160 beats/min, if decelerations are present, or if variability decreases.	Will provide continuous data regarding fetal response to induction.
	Assess maternal BP and pulse before beginning induction and then before each increase in infusion rate; do not advance infusion rate in presence of maternal hypertension or hypotension or radical changes in pulse rate.	To establish baseline data and to assess client response to induction; client status may change rapidly.
	Assess contraction frequency, duration, and intensity prior to each increase in infusion rate.	Evaluates uterine response to induction.
	Do not increase rate of infusion if contractions are every 2–3 minutes, lasting 40–60 seconds, with moderate intensity.	Desired effect has been obtained.

Nursing Care Plan: Induction of Labor (continued)

Nursing Diagnosis and Goals	Nursing Interventions	Rationale
	Discontinue oxytocin infusion if: 1. Contractions are more frequent than every 2 minutes 2. Contraction duration exceeds 90 seconds 3. Uterus has elevated resting tone (NAACOG 1988)	Uterus is being overstimulated and serious complications may develop for woman and fetus.
	Increase oxytocin IV infusion rate every 30–60 minutes until adequate contractions are achieved; do *not* exceed an infusion rate of 20 mU/min (ACOG 1987)	Uterine response to oxytocin may be individualized.
	Check infusion pump to assure oxytocin is infusing; check whether pump is on, chamber refills and empties, level of fluid in IV bottle becomes lower; if problem is found, correct it, and restart infusion at beginning dose. Check piggy-back connection to primary tubing to assure solution is not leaking	Oxytocin may not be infusing due to pump, mechanical, or human error.
	Evaluate cervical dilatation by vaginal examination with each oxytocin dosage increase after labor is established.	When cervix responds by stretching or pulling, *do not* increase oxytocin dosage; overdosage may occur, causing rapid labor with possible cervical lacerations and fetal damage; when there is no change in the cervix, additional oxytocin is needed.
	Observe contraction frequency and duration. In presence of contractions lasting over 90 seconds: 1. Discontinue oxytocin infusion 2. Assess maternal status 3. Assess fetal status	Contractions lasting over 90 seconds with decreased resting tone may result in fetal hypoxia. Ruptured uterus or abruptio placentae can result from drug-induced tumultuous labor.
	Monitor FHR continuously (normal range is 120–160/min). In episodes of bradycardia (<120 beats/min) lasting for more than 30 sec, administer O_2 by face mask at 4–7 L/min. Stop oxytocin infusion. Position woman on left side if quick recovery of FHR does not occur.	O_2 deficiency may occur over a long period of time; in cases of placental insufficiency or cord compression, compensated tachycardia may be evoked.
	Carefully evaluate fetal tachycardia (>160 beats/min). Sustained tachycardia may necessitate discontinuation of oxytocin infusion. Assess for presence of meconium staining.	Persistent fetal tachycardia causes more prominent O_2 deficiency (hypoxia) and CO_2 increase in fetal blood. Vasoconstriction occurs, with increased fetal blood flow through coronary arteries, brain, and placenta; this increased demand on myocardial performance leads to cardiac decompensation if oxygen exchange is impaired and hypoxia continues. Fetal hypoxia may also cause central vasomotor center to release adrenal catecholamines; at term, this enhances depolarization of cardiac pacemaker cells, which will result in direct bradycardia. Bradycardia or subsequent reflex tachycardia temporarily remedies the O_2 deficiency.

SUPPORTING DATA:
Uterine contraction frequency every 2 minutes and/or duration greater than 75–90 seconds with strong intensity.

GOAL:
Uterine contraction pattern will be approximately every 2½ to 3 min with duration of about 60 seconds.

Nursing Care Plan: Induction of Labor (continued)

Nursing Diagnosis and Goals	Nursing Interventions	Rationale
NURSING DIAGNOSIS: Alteration in comfort related to uterine contractions	Provide support to client as she uses breathing techniques. Encourage use of effluerage, back rub, and other supportive measures. Assess need for analgesia or anesthesia.	Contractions may build up more quickly with oxytocin induction. Techniques help maintain relaxation and thereby decrease pain sensation. After labor is well established, analgesia or epidural anesthesia may be given without delaying progress.
SUPPORTING DATA: Mrs Brookens winces when the contractions occur and has difficulty keeping her body relaxed. **GOAL:** Mrs Brookens will be able to maintain her breathing pattern and other comfort measures will be able to relax her body during contractions.		

Epilogue

Mrs Brookens' labor progressed at a normal rate for a first labor and she gave birth to a 6 pound, 12½ ounce girl. There were no complications associated with the labor or birth. Mr and Mrs Brookens and their new daughter were able to leave the birthing unit after 24 hours as they had planned.

Nursing Role

The woman needs to be supported during the repair as she may feel some pressure sensations. In the absence of adequate anesthesia, she may feel pain. Placing a hand on her shoulder, and talking with her can provide comfort and distraction from the repair process. If the woman is having more discomfort than she can comfortably handle, the nurse needs to act as an advocate in communicating the woman's needs to the physician/nurse-midwife. At all times the woman needs to be the one who decides whether the amount of discomfort is tolerable, and she should never be told "This doesn't hurt." She is the person experiencing the discomfort, and her evaluation must be respected. If there are just a few (three to five) stitches left, she may choose to forego more local anesthesia, but she should be given the choice.

The type of episiotomy and type of suture used (usually chromic catgut 00 or 000) are recorded on the delivery record. This information should also be included in a report to the recovery room, so that adequate assessments can be made and relief measures can be instituted if necessary.

Pain relief measures may begin immediately after delivery with application of an ice pack to the perineum. For optimal effect the ice pack should be applied for 20 to 30 minutes and removed for at least 20 minutes before being reapplied. The perineal tissues should be assessed frequently to prevent injury from the ice pack. After the fourth stage is completed, warm sitz baths (101°F to 105°F) are recommended to increase circulation to the area and promote healing. The use of cool sitz baths is currently being investigated, with some women reporting increased pain relief from using a lukewarm sitz bath to which ice chips have been added (Varner 1986; Ramler and Roberts 1986). The episiotomy site should be inspected every 15 minutes during the first hour after delivery and thereafter daily for redness, swelling, tenderness, and hematomas. Mild analgesic sprays and oral analgesics are ordered as needed. The mother will need instruction in perineal hygiene care and may need instructions about use of the analgesic spray. (See Chapter 34 for additional discussion of relief measures.)

● Care of the Woman During Forceps Delivery

Forceps are designed to provide two functions: traction and rotation of the fetus. There are two types of forceps deliveries: low or outlet, forceps and midforceps (see Figure 26–3). The delivery is termed *outlet forceps delivery* when the fetal head is visible on the perineum without spreading the labia. *Midforceps delivery* occurs when the head is engaged but the head is not visible on the perineum. Midforceps may also be used for rotation of the fetal head to an occiput-anterior position. The use of outlet forceps delivery has increased slightly, and the use of mid-

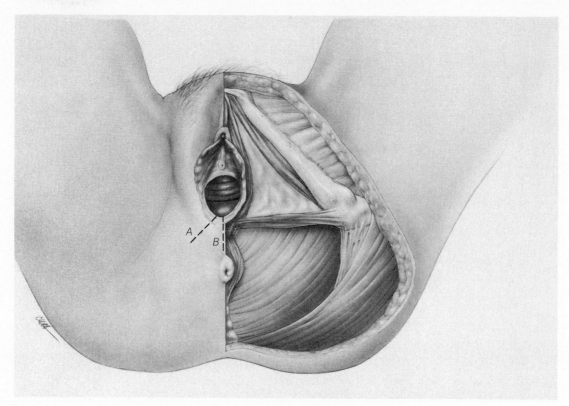

Figure 26–2   The two most common types of episiotomies are midline and mediolateral.

forceps delivery has decreased significantly over the past few years (Laufe 1985, Laube 1986). Types of forceps used are shown in Figure 26–4.

Indications

Indications for the use of forceps include any condition that threatens the life of the woman or fetus. Maternal conditions include heart disease, acute pulmonary edema, intrapartal infection, exhaustion, or the administration of epidural or spinal anesthesia. Fetal conditions include prolapsed cord, premature placental separation, and fetal distress. Forceps may be used electively to shorten the second stage of labor and spare the woman pushing effort, or when regional or general anesthesia has affected the woman's motor innervation and she cannot push effectively. Forceps are advocated in preterm infant delivery (Pritchard et al 1985).

Complications

Perinatal morbidity and mortality appear to be increased with midforceps deliveries. One research group (Friedman et al 1977) found a lower IQ score in children three to four years old who were delivered by midforceps, compared with those delivered by low forceps or sponta-

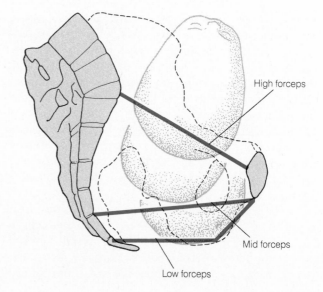

Figure 26–3   Classification of forceps deliveries. With low (outlet) forceps the fetal head is on the perineum. The fetal head is engaged and at the level of the spines with midforceps. When the fetal head is not engaged, a forceps application is called high forceps. High forceps are no longer used.

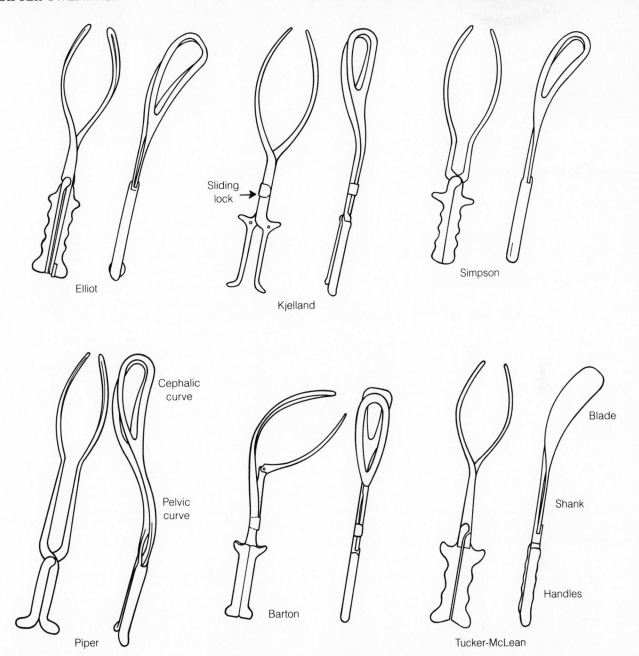

Figure 26–4   Forceps are composed of a blade, shank, and handle and may have a cephalic and pelvic curve. (Note labels on Piper and Tucker-McLean forceps). The blades may be fenestrated (open) or solid. The front and lateral views of these forceps illustrate differences in blades, open and closed shank, and cephalic and pelvic curves. Elliot, Simpson, and Tucker-McLean forceps are used as outlet forceps. Kjelland and Barton forceps are used for midforceps rotations. Piper forceps are used to provide traction and flexion of the aftercoming head of a fetus in breech presentation.

neously. Another group (Dierker et al 1985) found that 46 percent of the women had third-degree perineal lacerations, and 22 percent had a blood loss of more than 500 mL. In light of questions about the method that provides the best outcome for the fetus and the current medicolegal climate, a cesarean delivery is frequently chosen over midforceps (Laube 1986).

Prerequisites for Forceps Application

Use of forceps requires complete dilatation of the cervix and knowledge of the exact position and station of the fetal head. The membranes must be ruptured to allow a firm grasp on the fetal head. The presentation must be vertex or face with the chin anterior, and the head must be engaged, preferably on the perineum. *Under no circumstances should there be any CPD* (Pritchard et al 1985).

Trial or Failed Forceps Delivery

In a trial forceps procedure, the physician attempts to use forceps with the knowledge that there is a degree of CPD. A complete setup for immediate cesarean delivery needs to be available before the forceps are applied. If a good application cannot be obtained or if no descent occurs with the application, cesarean delivery is the method of choice. A failed forceps procedure is an attempt to deliver with forceps without success (Pritchard et al 1985).

Nursing Assessment

The obstetrician completes assessments to determine if the prerequisites for forceps application are present. The nurse continues the second stage assessments and carefully notes uterine contractions in order for the obstetrician to time the application of the forceps. The nurse auscultates FHR before, during, and after the forceps application. Early decelerations may occur due to the head compression from the forceps.

Nursing Role

The nurse can explain the procedure briefly to the woman. With adequate regional anesthesia, the woman should feel some pressure but no pain. The nurse encourages her to maintain breathing techniques to prevent her from pushing during application of the forceps (Figure 26–5). The nurse monitors contractions and with each contraction the physician will provide traction as the woman pushes. The FHR should be monitored continuously by the circulating nurse until the delivery. It is not uncommon to observe bradycardia as traction is being applied to the forceps. This bradycardia results from head compression and is transient in nature. With midforceps rotations, pediatric assistance may be needed immediately after delivery. Adequate resuscitation equipment should be readied.

Occasionally the neonate will have a forceps bruise from the application. The parents should be informed about the presence of a bruise and told that it will disappear in a few days. The neonate should be inspected for cerebral trauma and Erb's palsy if there was a difficult forceps extraction.

The mother should be assessed for perineal bruising, swelling, hematoma, hemorrhage, and postpartum infection.

● Care of the Woman During Vacuum Extraction

Vacuum extraction is an obstetric procedure with widespread use throughout the world, although it has not gained as much popularity in the United States (Greis et al 1981). The vacuum extractor is composed of a suction cup attached to a suction bottle (pump) by tubing. The suction cup, which comes in various sizes, is placed against the fetal occiput. Care must be taken to ensure that the cervix or vaginal tissue is not trapped under the cup. The pump is used to create negative pressure (suction) and an artificial caput ("chignon") is formed. The physician then applies traction in coordination with uterine contractions and the fetal head is delivered (Figure 26–6).

The most common indication for use of the vacuum extractor is prolonged second stage labor. The vacuum extractor is preferred to forceps in cases of borderline CPD, when successful passage of the fetal head requires the availability of all potential space inside the vaginal canal. Other indications for its use include (a) fetal distress, (b) malpositions such as OP or OT, and (c) such maternal complications as cardiopulmonary disease, shock, PIH, and abruptio placentae (Greis et al 1981). Contraindications for use of the vacuum extractor include the presence of CPD, face, or breech presentation.

The theoretical advantages of the vacuum extractor are a great reduction in intracranial pressure during traction and no impingement on maternal soft tissue (Pritchard et al 1985). Risks of vacuum extraction may include abrasion of the fetal scalp and cephalohematoma (Fall et al 1986).

Nursing Role

During the procedure, the woman should be informed about what is happening. If adequate regional anesthesia has been administered, the woman feels only pressure during the procedure. The fetus should be auscultated at least every five minutes, and proper infant resuscitation equipment should be readied if fetal problems are anticipated. The parents need to be informed that the caput (chignon) on the baby's head will disappear in a few hours.

Assessment of the newborn should include inspection and continued observation for cerebral trauma.

● Care of the Family During Cesarean Birth

Cesarean birth is the delivery of the infant through an abdominal and uterine incision. The word *cesarean* is derived from the Latin word *caedere*, meaning "to cut." Ce-

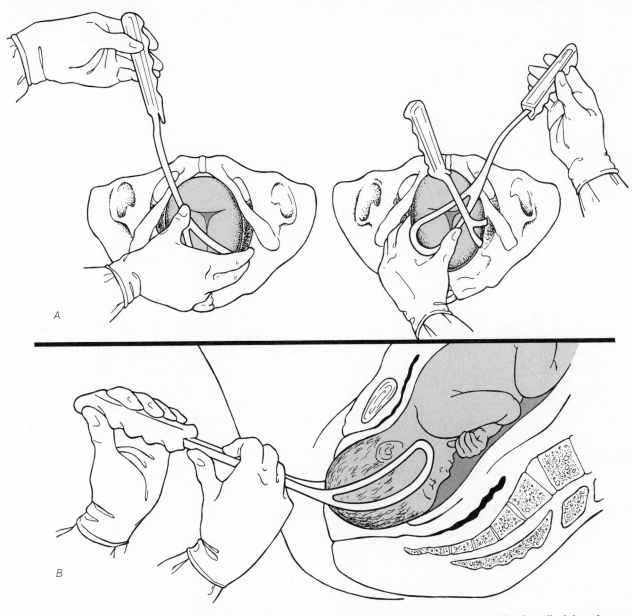

Figure 26–5 Application of forceps in occiput anterior (OA) position. A The left blade is inserted along the left side wall of the pelvis, over the parietal bone. B The right blade is inserted along the right side wall of the pelvis over the parietal bone. C With correct placement of the blades, the handles lock easily. During contractions, traction is applied to the forceps in a downward and outward direction to follow the birth canal.

sarean birth is one of the oldest surgical procedures known to modern man. Until the twentieth century, cesarean delivery was primarily equated with an attempt to salvage the fetus of a dying woman. Today cesarean birth has become a common occurrence, with approximately one out of every five neonates being delivered by this method.

As a result of a nearly threefold increase in the incidence of cesarean births, a National Institutes of Health (NIH) Consensus Development Conference was held in September 1980 to address issues concerning cesarean childbirth (NIH 1980). Findings of the NIH Cesarean Birth Task Force will be discussed throughout this section.

Indications

Cesarean births are performed in cases of breech presentation, preterm infant, fetal distress, dysfunctional labor, and uteroplacental insufficiency associated with maternal

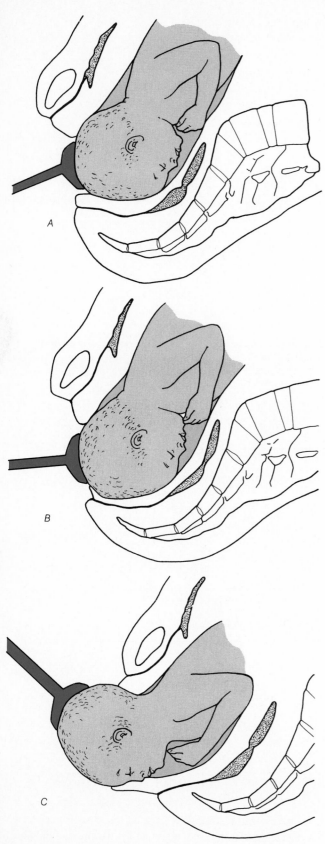

Figure 26–6　Vacuum extractor traction. A Traction outward and posteriorly. B Traction outward and horizontally. C Traction outward and anteriorly

disease conditions (Iams & Reiss 1985, Westgren & Paul 1985). The most common indication for cesarean delivery is dystocia caused by CPD. Other indications for the procedure include prolapsed cord, placenta previa, abruptio placentae, IUGR, prolonged rupture of the membranes, genital herpes, prematurity, fetal distress, and, occasionally, tumors blocking the vagina. Primary cesarean deliveries are increasingly done for breech presentations in nulliparas.

In the United States the incidence of cesarean birth has increased from 5.5 percent in 1970 to 16 percent in 1980 and 21.1 percent in 1984 (Eckholm 1986). This trend is also evident in Canada, Ireland, Great Britain, and the Netherlands. Factors that are thought to contribute to this increased rate are technologic advancements, social changes, changes in childbearing practices, increasing capability for infant survival, advances or changes in medical care, obstetric attitudes and practices, and the increasing percentage of complicated births.

Four diagnostic categories have had the greatest influence on the increased incidence of cesarean birth. Dystocia (abnormal or difficult labor, CPD) accounted for 30 percent of the increase followed by repeat cesarean (25 to 30 percent), breech presentation (10 to 15 percent), and fetal distress (10 to 15 percent) (NIH 1980).

Technologic and medical advancements have altered the attitude toward cesarean birth from a "procedure of last resort" to an "alternative birth method." Technologic advancements include:

1. Refinements in surgical techniques for entry and closure of the uterus

2. Monitoring of maternal and fetal physiology to identify pairs at risk from the forces of labor and vaginal delivery

3. Developments in anesthesia enhancing maternal participation and comfort during delivery, as well as reducing depressant effects on the fetus

4. Pharmacology and parenteral fluid therapy, which decrease hazards of maternal hemorrhage and infection

Social changes are also associated with increasing numbers of cesarean deliveries. In conjunction with initiation of federal programs in the 1960s to promote maternal and child health, the socioeconomic disparity of women having cesarean births has decreased. A trend toward women receiving care from an obstetrician and delivering in larger hospitals is also evident. The increasing rate of cesareans in larger hospitals (greater than 1000 deliveries per year) has been higher than in smaller hospitals. Although there is no reliable data to support the claims, some speculate that the trend toward third-party reimbursement and defensive obstetrics to avoid malpractice lawsuits might also be contributing factors (NIH 1980, Philipson & Rosen

1985) One study (Silbar 1986) suggested that the increased cesarean delivery rate was due to more frequent diagnosis of CPD and increased size of the fetus (by 100 g) and paralleled a decline in forceps-assisted deliveries.

Changes in childbearing practices are also related to the increasing rate of cesarean deliveries. Because the decreasing size of American families, the percentage of primigravida deliveries has increased. The incidence of cesarean births is nine times greater for primigravidas than for multigravidas (Stichler & Affonso 1980). An increasing number of women are choosing to have their children later in life. Age is associated with a higher incidence of uterine inertia or dystocia, common conditions necessitating cesarean delivery (Boehm et al 1981).

Although in 90 percent of all the primary cesarean births, the neonate weighs more than 2500 g, increasing numbers of cesareans are being done for low-birth-weight or preterm neonates (NIH 1980). Some contend that this mode of delivery is more advantageous than subjecting the vulnerable preterm neonate to the stresses of a vaginal birth. It is difficult to assess the true effect of operative deliveries on neonatal mortality. Improved neonatal survival rates are also attributed to higher numbers of neonatal intensive care units, improvement in the specialty areas of maternal-fetal and neonatal medicine, and improved technology.

Changes in obstetric management have also resulted in the higher number of cesarean births. Improved antepartal monitoring, and electronic monitoring during labor for fetal distress are considered contributing factors. Standard management of breech presentation and difficult forceps deliveries has changed from vaginal delivery toward cesarean birth.

Although the rationale for cesarean delivery is to improve pregnancy outcome, insufficient data exist regarding morbidity risk to the mother and neonate to support this claim. The NIH (1980) summarized the following data for cesarean birth outcomes:

Dystocia: No evidence that the infant greater than 2500 g had survival advantage.

Repeat cesarean: No mortality/morbidity data relative to risks or benefits to client or infant.

Breech: Insufficient data in terms of preferred method for all fetuses regardless of weight.

Fetal distress: No evidence relative to mortality risks associated with the method of delivery.

Whether pregnancy outcome is improved with cesarean birth remains an unanswered and controversial issue.

Electronic fetal monitoring to assess fetal distress has often been blamed for the increased cesarean birth rate. Some contend that fetal distress is diagnosed more often than it actually exists, resulting in unnecessary cesarean births. Yet controlled studies have shown that in *experienced* hands a liberal use of fetal monitoring in low-risk and high-risk clients does not cause a rise in the overall incidence of cesarean deliveries (Boehm et al 1981). Electronic fetal monitoring does not necessarily raise the incidence of diagnosed fetal distress in a given population unless the population itself changes. The liberal attitude toward cesarean delivery for breech and other high-risk conditions has contributed more to its increased incidence than electronic fetal monitoring has.

Management of breech presentation has accounted for about 15 percent of the rise in the cesarean rate during the last 10 years. This trend was based on the increased incidence of neonatal morbidity and mortality thought to be secondary to vaginal delivery of breech presentations.

A cesarean delivery is avoided if possible when the fetus is dead or too small to survive outside the uterus. The abdominal route increases maternal morbidity and mortality risks without any advantage for the fetus.

Maternal Mortality and Morbidity

Cesarean births have two to four times the maternal mortality of vaginal deliveries (Petitti 1985). Mortality, although low (less than 0.02 percent), is most often due to anesthesia accidents and/or underlying medical conditions such as cardiac disease, renal disease, diabetes, or severe PIH.

Morbidity varies widely and depends on the population assessed and the circumstances necessitating abdominal delivery. Major complications resulting from surgery include hemorrhage, blood clots, injury to the bladder or intestines and, most frequently, infection. The incidence of endometritis is 6 percent to 10 percent, and urinary tract and wound infection occur at a lower rate (Petitti 1985). Overall the risk is five to ten times greater after cesarean delivery (Gibbs 1985).

Factors associated with increased risk for endometritis include onset and length of labor, rupture of the amniotic membranes prior to delivery, number of vaginal examinations, internal fetal monitoring, duration of operation, and anemia.

Surgical Techniques

SKIN INCISIONS

The skin incision for a cesarean delivery is either transverse (Pfannenstiel) or vertical and is not indicative of the type of incision made into the uterus. The transverse incision is made across the lowest and narrowest part of the abdomen. Since the incision is made just below the pubic hair line, it is almost invisible after healing. The limitations of this type of skin incision are that it does not allow for extension of the incision if needed. Since it usually requires more time, this incision is used when time is not of the essence (eg, with CPD or failure to progress and no fetal or maternal distress). The vertical incision is made between the navel and the symphysis pubis. This type of incision is quicker and is therefore preferred in cases of fetal distress and preterm, or macrosomic infants. A variation of the vertical incision is the paramedian (just off center). This incision allows for stronger scar formation and is recommended for obese women (Morrison & Wiser 1986). The type of skin incision is determined by time factor, client preference, or physician preference.

UTERINE INCISIONS

The type of uterine incision is contingent on the need for the cesarean. The choice of incision affects the woman's opportunity for a subsequent vaginal delivery and her risks of a ruptured uterine scar with a subsequent pregnancy.

The two major types of uterine incisions are in the lower uterine segment or in the upper segment of the uterine corpus.

The lower uterine segment incision most commonly used is a transverse incision, although a vertical incision may also be used (Figure 26–7). The transverse incision is preferred for the following reasons (Morrison & Wiser 1986, Danforth & Scott 1986, Pritchard et al 1985):

1. The lower segment is the thinnest portion of the uterus and involves less blood loss.

2. It requires only moderate dissection of bladder from underlying myometrium.

3. It is easier to repair.

4. The site is less likely to rupture during subsequent pregnancies.

5. There is a decreased chance of adherence of bowel or omentum to the incision line.

The disadvantages are:

1. It takes longer to make and repair this incision.

2. It is limited in size because of the presence of major blood vessels on either side of the uterus.

3. It has a greater tendency to extend laterally into the uterine vessels.

4. The incision may stretch and become a thin window, but it usually does not create problems clinically until a subsequent labor ensues.

The lower uterine segment vertical incision is preferred for multiple gestation, abnormal presentation, placenta previa, fetal distress, and preterm and macrosomic fetuses. Disadvantages of this incision include:

1. The incision may extend downward into the cervix.

2. More extensive dissection of the bladder is needed to keep the incision in the lower uterine segment.

3. If it extends upward into the upper segment, hemostasis and closure is more difficult.

4. The chance of rupture with subsequent labor is increased (Morrison & Wiser 1986, Danforth & Scott 1986; Pritchard et al 1985).

One other incision, the classic incision, was the method of choice for many years but is used infrequently now. This vertical incision was made into the upper uterine segment. There was more blood loss, and it was more difficult to repair. Most important, there was an increased risk of uterine rupture with subsequent pregnancy, labor, and delivery because the upper uterine segment is the most contractile portion of the uterus.

Nursing Role

PREPARATION FOR CESAREAN BIRTH

Cesarean birth is an alternative method of delivery. Since one out of every five deliveries is a cesarean, preparation for this possibility should be an integral part of every childbirth education curriculum. The attitude of the instructor in conveying factual information will affect the woman's reaction to an unplanned cesarean birth. The instructor can emphasize the similarities between cesarean and vaginal births to minimize undertones of "normal" versus "abnormal" delivery (Affonso 1981, Cox & Smith 1982). This will diminish feelings of anger, loss, and grief. Discussion about the couple's childbirth expectations may identify potential problem areas and further informational needs (Frink & Chally 1984).

All couples should be encouraged to discuss with their obstetrician what the approach would be in the event of a cesarean. They can also discuss their needs and desires as a couple under those circumstances. Their preferences may include the following:

• Participating in the choice of anesthetic

• Father (or significant other) being present during the procedures and/or delivery

• Father (or significant other) being present in the recovery or postpartum room

• Audio recording and/or taking pictures of the birth

• Delayed instillation of eye drops to promote eye contact between parent and infant in the first hours after delivery

• Physical contact or holding the newborn while on the delivery table and/or in the recovery room (if the mother cannot hold the newborn the father can hold the baby for her)

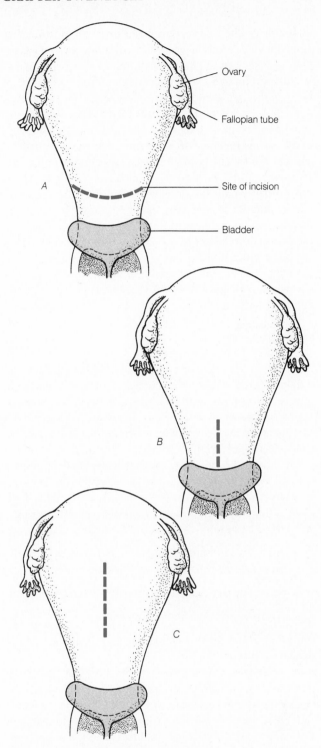

Figure 26–7 Incisions in lower uterine segment A *Transverse (Kerr incision).* B *Vertical (Sellheim incision).* C *Classic*

- Breast-feeding on the delivery table and/or in the recovery room.

Information that couples need about cesarean delivery includes:

- Events in the preparatory phase

- Description or viewing of the delivery room

- Types of anesthesia for delivery and analgesia available postpartum

- Sensations that may be experienced

- Roles of significant others

- Interaction with neonate

- Immediate recovery phase

- Postpartal phase

The context in which this information is given should be "birth-oriented" rather than surgery-oriented.

PREPARATION FOR REPEAT CESAREAN BIRTH

When a couple is anticipating a cesarean birth, they have time to analyze and synthesize the information and to prepare for some of the specifics. Many hospitals or local groups (such as C-Sec Inc) provide preparation classes for cesarean birth. The instructor should impart a feeling of normalcy and factual information, which will allow a couple to make choices and participate in their birth experience. Couples who have had previous negative experiences need an opportunity to describe what they felt contributed to these events. They should be encouraged to identify what they would like to have altered and to list interventions that would make the experience more positive. Those who have had positive experiences need reassurance that their needs and desires will be met in the same manner. In addition, an opportunity should be given to discuss any fears or anxieties.

A specific concern of the woman facing a repeat cesarean is "anticipation of the pain experience." She needs reassurance that subsequent cesareans are often less painful than the first. She will not experience the extreme fatigue that followed the primary cesarean if it was preceded by a long and/or strenuous labor. Giving this information will enable her to cope more effectively with stressful stimuli, including pain. The nurse can remind the woman that she has already had experience with how to prevent, cope with, and alleviate painful stimuli.

PREPARATION FOR EMERGENCY CESAREAN DELIVERY

Usually a couple is prepared for an emergency cesarean by either the "last minute" or the "mutual decision" approach. All too frequently childbirth attendants wait until the last minute to inform the woman of the need for a cesarean delivery under the guise of "sparing the couple undue anxiety." Ironically, the woman's reaction to this delayed approach is not only excessive anxiety but also anger, shock, and resentment resulting in a state of crisis or panic

Research Note

Previous studies done on middle class women belonging to the "natural childbirth culture" demonstrate that for these women cesarean birth is seen as a devastating interference with nature. Sandelowski and Bustamunte studied the response of a low-income population to cesarean birth. They interviewed 50 primarily black, indigent women during their hospital recovery period following a cesarean birth. Of these women 22 were available for a brief follow-up telephone interview one month later.

The researchers found that these women used "distancing" prenatally and postdelivery to protect themselves from the threatening and undesirable event. Prenatally, most of the women denied that cesarean birth was something that could happen to them. This "not-me" theme was evident not only in 28 women who did not expect a cesarean section, but also in 2 who suspected that they might have one, and in 1 of 14 who knew that they would have one. After delivery 42 of the women coped by separating themselves from or minimizing their association with the event and by attributing the need for the cesarean to factors removed from their own person. Most of the women also focused on the outcome of the birth to evaluate the experience rather than perceiving the experience as an end to be evaluated in itself. The women who had previous vaginal births compared the two different birth experiences in terms of physical rather than affective or cognitive components of birth. For the most part, women in this study had few expectations of childbirth and were neither depressed nor happy, but simply "OK," suggesting a model of cesarean childbirth experience different from the previously reported middle class model.

Sandelowski M, Bustamunte R: Cesarean birth outside the natural childbirth culture. Res Nurs Health 1986;9(June):81–88.

(Cox & Smith 1982). In contrast, the mutual decision approach between the birth attendants and the woman keeps the family fully informed as developments occur. The physician/nurse-midwife presents all the facts, suggests alternatives, and describes likely outcomes of nonintervention, allowing the expectant parents to participate in the decision making. The opportunity to make choices and have control over their birthing experience is the major factor influencing a couple's positive perception of the event (Cox & Smith 1982).

The period preceding surgery must be used to its greatest advantage. The couple needs some time for privacy to assimilate the information given to them and to gather strength to face this new crisis. It is imperative that care givers use their most effective communication skills. Silence is often interpreted by the woman as indicating danger for her and her fetus and/or care giver anger resulting from her failure to perform (Affonso 1981). The woman may experience panic and/or fear. She may be confused and numb to instructions. It is essential for the attendant to address the salient points regarding what the couple may anticipate during the next few hours. Ask "What questions do you have about the decision?" This gives the couple an opportunity for further clarification. Prepare the woman in increments, giving her information and the rationale for each procedure before commencing. In brief, before carrying out a procedure tell her (a) what you are going to do; (b) why you are going to do it; and (c) what sensations she may experience. This allows the woman to be informed and to consent to the procedure. The woman experiences a sense of control, and therefore less helplessness and powerlessness.

Often the phenomenon of memory lapse is more pronounced during crisis or panic states. "Missing pieces" are unremembered events or segments of time. Although not unique to cesarean birth this phenomenon contributes to a sense of loss or missing out for the woman. Her inability to remember may contribute to feelings of depression or anger. It is important for the delivery nurse to visit the client during the postpartal period to fill in the "missing pieces." Women, whether awake or asleep for the delivery, have confirmed the value of having the event relived for them minute-by-minute and event-by-event. This process is valuable because

- It allows for reality orientation and correction of the woman's misperceptions or misinformation.

- It aids in psychologic integration of the birth event.

- It fosters the attachment process.

Preparation of the woman for surgery involves more than the procedures of establishing intravenous lines and urinary catheter, or doing an abdominal prep. As discussed previously, good communication skills are very influential in helping the woman stay in control. Therapeutic touch and eye contact do much to maintain reality orientation and control. These measures reduce anxiety for the client during the stressful preparatory period. All women will experience some degree of anxiety and apprehension: behavioral manifestations of anxiety include withdrawal, crying, apologies, or inappropriate laughter. Increased heart rate, blood pressure, body temperature, dilated pupils, pallor, and/or dry mouth are physiologic signs of anxiety. Anxiety also affects senses such as sight, hearing, and cognitive grasp. Severe anxiety often results in distortion of reality. The nurse should continually assess how the woman is perceiving the event and coping with her apprehension.

If the cesarean delivery is scheduled and not an emergency, the nurse has ample time for preoperative teaching. The woman needs to practice her turning, coughing, and deep breathing. It is helpful if she is taught to splint her abdominal muscles when she coughs.

To prepare the woman for the surgery, she is given nothing by mouth. To reduce the likelihood of serious pulmonary damage should aspiration of gastric contents occur, antacids may be administered within 30 minutes of surgery. If epidural anesthesia is used, the nurse may assist with the procedure, monitor the woman's blood pressure and response, and continue EFM if it is used. An abdominal and perineal prep is done (from below breasts to the pubic region), and an indwelling catheter is inserted to prevent bladder distention and obstructed delivery. The woman must sign an operative permit. At least two units of whole blood are readied for administration. An intravenous line is started, with a needle of adequate size to permit blood administration, and preoperative medication is ordered. The pediatrician should be notified and adequate preparation made to receive the infant. The nurse should make sure that the infant warmer is functional, and that appropriate resuscitation equipment is available. The circulating nurse assists in positioning the woman on the operating table. Fetal heart rate should be ascertained before surgery and during preparation, since fetal hypoxia can result from aortocaval compression. The operating table may be adjusted so it slants slightly to one side, or a wedge (folded blanket or towels) may be placed under the right hip. The uterus should be displaced about 15° from the midline (Bassell 1985). This helps relieve the pressure of the heavy uterus on the vena cava and lessens the incidence of vena caval compression and supine maternal hypotension. The suction should be in working order, and the urine collection bag should be positioned under the operating table to ensure proper urinary drainage. A last-minute check is done to ensure that the fetal scalp electrode has been removed if the woman was internally monitored.

Delivery

Every effort should made made to include the father in the birth experience. Hospital routines can be established to provide for the father's presence in the operating room.

The NIH Task Force on Cesarean Birth (1980), after considering this issue, concluded that "in spite of the widespread fears of adverse effects . . . there is no evidence of harm from fathers' participation." The American College of Obstetrics and Gynecology position statement states that they "cannot perceive strong medical indications or contraindications of the presence of fathers in the operating suite" (Affonso 1981). In fact it has been found that the father's presence during the cesarean procedure leads to a more positive evaluaton of the birth experience later by both the mother and father (Affonso 1981). When the father was present for the delivery, the mother required less postpartal medication for pain, experienced less loneliness, and was less anxious about the baby's health.

When the father attends the cesarean birth, he must scrub and wear a surgical gown and mask as do others in the operating suite. A stool can be placed beside the woman's head. The father can sit nearby to provide physical touch, visual contact, and verbal reassurance to his partner.

Other measures can be taken to promote the participation of the father who chooses not to be in the delivery room. They are:

1. Allowing the father to be near the delivery room where he can hear the newborn's first cry

2. Encouraging the father to carry or accompany the infant to the nursery for the initial assessment

3. Involving the father in postpartal care in the recovery room

In addition to meeting the emotional and informational needs of the expectant parents, other nursing functions are carried out to assure physiologic support and safety of the woman and neonate. The nurse should stand by to connect the suction when the operating team is ready and should record the actual time the incision is made and the infant is delivered. An oxytocin preparation is administered intravenously just as the infant is born.

After delivery, the nurse assesses the Apgar score and completes the initial assessment and identification procedures as after a vaginal birth. Every effort must be made to assist the parents in bonding with the infant. At least one of the mother's arms should be freed to enable her to touch and stroke the infant. The baby can be given to the father to hold until she or he must be taken to the nursery.

Repeat administration of oxytocin during surgery may be necessary to control uterine bleeding. The circulating nurse assists with the application of the dressing to the incision and, with the aid of other staff, helps the woman back into bed.

Analgesia and Anesthesia

There is no perfect anesthesia for cesarean delivery. Each has its advantages, disadvantages, possible risks, and side effects. Goals for analgesia and anesthesia administration include safety, comfort, and emotional satisfaction for the client. Effects of analgesia and anesthesia on the neonate vary. Different pharmacologic agents cross the placenta at different rates into the fetal bloodstream and are metabolized at varying rates. Other factors associated with the effects of drugs on the neonate include (a) dosage, (b) route of administration, (c) maternal metabolism, (d) health of fetus, and (e) length of time between administration of drug and delivery of the neonate. There are two classifications of anesthesia for cesarean delivery: general and conduction (spinal and epidural). See Chapter 24 for further discussion.

Immediate Postpartal Recovery Period

The postpartal recovery room must be equipped with suction and oxygen to ensure a patent airway and avoid respiratory obstruction resulting from secretions. The nurse caring for the postpartal woman should check the mother's vital signs every 5 minutes until they are stable, then every 15 minutes for an hour, then every 30 minutes until she is discharged to the postpartal floor. The nurse should remain with the woman until she is stable.

The dressing and perineal pad must be checked every 15 minutes for at least an hour, and the fundus should be gently palpated to determine whether it is remaining firm. The fundus may be palpated by placing a hand to support the incision. Intravenous oxytocin is usually administered to promote the contractility of the uterine musculature. If the woman has been under general anesthesia, she should be positioned on her side to facilitate drainage of secretions, turned, and assisted with coughing and deep breathing every 2 hours for at least 24 hours. If she has received a spinal or epidural anesthetic, the level of anesthesia should be checked every 15 minutes until sensation has fully returned. It is important to monitor intake and output and to observe the urine for bloody tinge, which could mean surgical trauma to the bladder. The physician prescribes medication to relieve the mother's pain and nausea, and this should be administered as needed. Some physicians use a single dose of epidural morphine (5 to 7.5 mg) for postsurgical pain relief. Facilitation of parent-infant interaction following birth and postpartal care is discussed in Chapter 35.

Vaginal Birth After Cesarean (VBAC)

The trend is increasing to have a trial of labor and vaginal delivery after a primary cesarean in cases of nonrecurring indications (for example, cord accident, placenta previa, fetal distress). This trend has been influenced by consumer demand and a growing body of evidence suggesting that a properly conducted vaginal delivery after a cesarean poses less risk for maternal and neonatal mortality and morbidity than does a repeat cesarean (Lavin et al 1982, Cohen and Estner 1983, Porreco 1985). A review of the literature (Lavin et al 1982) revealed that of those women allowed a trial of labor, 66.7 percent were successful in deliverying vaginally. Successful vaginal delivery occurred in 74.2 percent of women with a nonrecurrent indication for their previous cesarean and in 33.3 percent of those whose indication for previous cesarean was CPD. Women who had a prior vaginal delivery were more likely to deliver vaginally than those who did not (Lavin et al

1982). Wilf and Franklin (1984) found similar results with a VBAC success rate of 78.6 percent. Although a classic uterine scar increases the probability of uterine rupture, the precise increased risk cannot be accurately determined. Following an extensive review of the literature Flamm (1985) concluded that "Spontaneous or traumatic rupture of an unscarred uterus is often complete and catastrophic. In contrast, 'rupture' of a prior low transverse uterine incision is most often incomplete and inconsequential" (p 736).

As the philosophy turns more to VBAC, some areas are still controversial, such as the use of oxytocin induction/augmentation, type of anesthesia, use with postdate pregnancy, and the number of previous cesareans. In a review of over 600 cases Flamm (1985) found no increase in maternal or fetal mortality with oxytocin induction/augmentation. Regional anesthesia has been in question because of fear that it will mask the pain of uterine rupture. In a study of over 600 cases in the last four years, there were two uterine ruptures and one was masked. This does not support significantly increased risk to the mother and her fetus (Flamm 1985). Postdate pregnancies have posed management problems that are more complicated with a history of previous cesarean birth. One study (MacKenzie et al 1984) reported a 76 percent VBAC success rate in women with postdate pregnancy. The question of acceptable number of previous cesareans remains unanswered.

Although there is no clear argument on guidelines for VBAC, the general principles are the following (ACOG 1982, Flamm 1985, Porreco 1985):

1. Early in the pregnancy the woman and physician discuss the options for a trial of labor and VBAC to allow for questions, planning, and increased opportunity for shared decision making.

2. Contraindications for vaginal delivery (such as CPD, placenta previa, abruptio placentae, and medical/obstetrical complications) are ruled out.

3. Previous medical records are available to substantiate a low segment uterine incision and whether previous problems occurred. A classic uterine incision would preclude a VBAC.

4. The VBAC is conducted in a fully equipped facility with emergency equipment and personnel readily available.

5. Blood products are readily available.

6. Oxytocin is used judiciously.

7. Regional anesthesia is considered, and if it is used, the woman is carefully assessed.

8. Continuous electronic monitoring equipment is available for monitoring the contractile pattern and the fetal heart rate.

Nursing Care Plan: Cesarean Birth

Mr and Mrs Chavez are attending prenatal classes for cesarean birth at the birthing center. They are anticipating the birth of their first child.

Assessment

HISTORY

Present pregnancy course
Estimated gestational age
Childbirth preparation
Sensitivity to medications and anesthetic agents
Past bleeding problems

PHYSICAL EXAMINATION

1. Fetal size, fetal status (FHR), and fetal maturity
2. Lung and cardiac status
3. Complete physical examination prior to administration of anesthetic

LABORATORY EVALUATION

CBC
Hemoglobin and hematocrit
Type and cross-match for two units whole blood
Rh
Prothrombin time
VDRL
Urinalysis

Analysis of Nursing Priorities

1. Provide couple with factual information and support in preparation for their cesarean birth to enable them to make choices, feel in control, and minimize feelings of anxiety, loss, guilt, and helplessness.
2. Support the couple's desires to participate in their birth experience within the constraints or options of the situation.
3. Encourage couple to participate in the decision-making process for the cesarean birth experience and care during the preparatory, recovery, and postpartal periods.

Nursing Diagnosis and Goals	Nursing Interventions	Rationale
NURSING DIAGNOSIS: Knowledge deficit related to the cesarean birth	Integrate cesarean birth information into childbirth preparation classes. Emphasize the similarities between vaginal and cesarean delivery. Minimize perceptions of "normal" versus "abnormal" birth.	Couples may deny the possibility of an unplanned cesarean birth. Preparatory needs are basically the same for all couples anticipating childbirth. A good knowledge base will allow for adaptive coping responses should they deliver in either manner.
SUPPORTING DATA: Mr and Mrs Chavez ask many questions about the cesarean.	Provide factual information.	Information enables couples to make choices and participate in their birth experience.
	Encourage couple to discuss with obstetrician the approach and birth preferences in the event of a vaginal or cesarean birth.	Opportunity to discuss needs and desires minimizes unrealistic expectations, disappointment and/or feelings of loss; promotes understanding of options, beliefs of birth attendant, and hospital policies; and allows couple to do anticipatory problem solving and develop effective coping behaviors.
	Encourage expression of feelings.	Enable couple to work through fears, ambivalent or unresolved feelings, and grief associated with loss of vaginal birth.
	Assess reaction to and interpretation of past cesarean birth experiences.	Identify need for information and opportunity to work through fears or unresolved feelings.
	Encourage the development of mutual support by couples sharing their experiences and common concerns.	Decrease sense of being "different" or "alone" by realizing that their fears and concerns are not unique and feelings of anger or guilt are normal.

Nursing Care Plan: Cesarean Birth (continued)

Nursing Diagnosis and Goals	Nursing Interventions	Rationale
	Create a safe, nonthreatening environment for couples to work through unresolved negative feelings.	Negative feelings may contribute to distortion of information, impede learning, and affect expectations of upcoming birth experience.
	Encourage couples to identify events that would make this birth experience more positive.	Allow for anticipatory problem solving, and enhance ability to meet goals and expectations for birth event.
	Cover most salient points of what to anticipate: 1. What is going to happen to the woman's body and how it will feel 2. What and why specific procedures will be done 3. How to handle discomfort associated with procedures	Knowing what to expect increases coping capability.
	Provide couple with brief period of privacy.	They need an opportunity to pool their coping strengths to deal with the anxiety of the situation.
	Inquire if couple has any questions about the decision.	Give opportunity for further clarification.
	Prepare Mrs Chavez in increments, giving information and rationale for each procedure.	Crisis-altered cognitive grasp leads to information not being heard or misinterpreted.
	Avoid silence.	Silence is often interpreted by the client as frightening and/or negative.
	Employ eye contact and therapeutic touch.	Convey a feeling of caring and reality orientation.
GOAL: Mr and Mrs Chavez will understand the procedure associated with the cesarean and have a chance to ask questions and raise their concerns.		
Mrs Chavez is admitted for a cesarean and because of the prenatal classes she is able to anticipate most aspects of the preparation. Mr Chavez stays with her and is able to provide support. He is planning to be present during the cesarean.		
NURSING DIAGNOSIS: Potential alteration in respiratory function due to decreased air exchange secondary to shallow breathing with incisional pain and ineffective cough.	Teach deep breathing and coughing. Teach abdominal splinting while deep breathing and coughing. Assess lung sounds.	Promotes good air exchange. Provides support and decreases pain. Provides data on respiratory status.
SUPPORTING DATA: Shallow respirations Productive cough	Explain that she will be turned every two hours.	Provides aeration of lungs and assists in preventing pulmonary complications.
GOAL: Mrs Chavez will deep breath and cough at regular intervals to maintain effective respiratory function.		

Nursing Care Plan: Cesarean Birth (continued)

Nursing Diagnosis and Goals	Nursing Interventions	Rationale
NURSING DIAGNOSIS: Alteration of comfort related to incisional pain and uterine involution	Administer analgesic medications. Change position and support body parts with pillows. Provide quiet environment to enhance rest.	Provides relief of pain. Promotes comfort. Promotes comfort.
SUPPORTING DATA: Mrs Chavez groans when moving and requests pain medication frequently.		
GOAL: Mrs Chavez will have pain relieved.		
NURSING DIAGNOSIS: Potential alteration in tissue perfusion related to excessive blood loss secondary to inadequate contraction of the uterus after delivery		
SUPPORTING DATA: Heavy vaginal bleeding (lochia rubra) Uterine fundus not firm and possibly out of the midline and above the umbilicus	Evaluate firmness and position of fundus. Palpate fundus after pain medication is administered to promote patient comfort. Fundus may be palpated from side of abdomen to avoid discomfort. Evaluate lochia.	Monitor involution. Palpation of fundus causes discomfort to the woman and is frequently neglected and therefore becomes increasingly important. Avoid tenderness at incisional site. Lochia progresses from rubra to serosa to alba. Increase in flow indicates inefficient contraction of uterus and/or subinvolution.
GOAL: Mrs Chavez will maintain normal tissue perfusion. Blood pressure and pulse will remain within normal limits. Fundus is firm, in midline, and below the umbilicus.		
NURSING DIAGNOSIS: Potential alterations in parenting	Provide information about the baby as soon as possible.	Interaction may be impaired because of recovery from anesthesia and discomfort in first few hours after delivery.
SUPPORTING DATA: Due to anesthesia for cesarean delivery and discomfort associated with the incision, Mrs Chavez is not able to interact with the newborn as much as she had wanted. The newborn is not able to remain with the parents for an extended period of time immediately following birth.	Provide opportunities for the parents to be with the baby as soon as possible. Provide opportunities for Mrs Chavez to discuss her feelings about the cesarean birth and her self-image as a mother.	Feelings of failure associated with birthing experience can be generalized to ability to assume mothering role.
GOAL: Mr and Mrs Chavez will have opportunities to interact with their baby and will move into a positive attachment.		

Epilogue

Mrs Chavez had a successful cesarean delivery, and her husband was able to accompany her. They were able to hold their new son moments after his birth. Mrs Chavez's immediate recovery period was without complications although she experienced a lot of pain. Careful positioning and administration of analgesia was helpful in increasing her comfort.

NURSING ROLE

Staffing is a prime consideration when a woman is having a VBAC because of the need to provide continuous care. Close observation is essential throughout the labor and delivery process. Along with routine labwork, the woman's blood should be typed and cross-matched for two units of whole blood. Continuous EFM is usually ordered. Support measures during labor include those used with any laboring woman although this woman may need additional support and encouragement. Fear of the process and possible outcome is not only a patient problem. Labor and delivery staff have long believed that a woman with a previous cesarean who begins labor is in an emergency situation because of the danger of uterine rupture. It is difficult for them now to consider this a normal happening and be fully supportive. But the nurse's support and encouragement is essential.

KEY CONCEPTS

An external (or cephalic) version may be done after 37 weeks' gestation to change a breech presentation to a cephalic. The benefits of the version are that a lower-risk vaginal delivery may be anticipated. The version is accomplished with the use of tocolytics to relax the uterus. An internal podalic version is used only when needed during the vaginal birth of a second twin.

Amniotomy (AROM) is probably the most common procedure in obstetrics. The risks are prolapse of the umbilical cord and infection.

Indicated induction of labor is done for many reasons. The methods include amniotomy, prostaglandins, and oxytocin infusion.

Nursing responsibilities are heightened during an induced labor.

An episiotomy may be done just prior to delivery of the fetus. Although in this country it is very prevalent, it is becoming more controversial.

Forceps deliveries can be low outlet or midforceps. Low outlet forceps are the most common and are associated with few maternal-fetal complications. Midforceps are associated with more complications but when needed are an important aid to delivery.

A vacuum extractor is a soft pliable cup attached to suction that can be applied to the fetal head and used in much the same way as forceps.

At least one in five births is now accomplished by cesarean delivery. The increase in the cesarean delivery rate has been influenced by many factors. The nurse has a vital role in providing information, support, and encouragement to the couple participating in a cesarean birth.

Vaginal birth after cesarean (VBAC) is becoming more popular and the success rate is more than 60 percent. Overcoming the old fears of uterine rupture is a high priority for both the parents and the medical community.

REFERENCES

ACOG Guidelines for vaginal birth after cesarean childbirth, Committee Statement, January 7, 1982.

ACOG: *Induction and Augmentation of Labor,* Technical Bulletin No. 110, November 1987.

ACOG: *Induction of Labor,* Technical Bulletin No. 49, May 1978.

Affonso DD: *Impact of Cesarean Childbirth.* Philadelphia, Davis, 1981.

Banta D, **Thacker** SB: The risks and benefits of episiotomy: A review. *Birth* 1982;9(Spring):25.

Bassell GM: Anesthesia for cesarean section. *Clin Obstet Gynecol* 1985;28(December):722.

Bishop EH: Pelvic scoring for elective inductions. *Obstet Gynecol* 1964;24:266.

Boehm FH, et al: The effect of electronic fetal monitoring on the incidence of cesarean section. *Am J Obstet Gynecol* 1981;140(June):295.

Bromberg MH: Presumptive maternal benefits of routine episiotomy: A literature review. *J Nurs-Midwife* 1986; 31(May/June):121.

Buekens P, et al: Episiotomy and third degree tears. *Br J Obstet Gynaecol* 1985;92:820.

Cibils LA: *Electronic Fetal-Maternal Monitoring.* Boston, PSG Publishing, 1981.

Cohen NW, **Estner** LJ: Silent knife: Cesarean section in the United States. *Society,* November/December 1983, p 95.

Cox BE, **Smith** EC: The mother's self-esteem after a cesarean delivery. *Am J Mat Child Nurs* 1982;7(September/October):309.

Danforth DN: *Obstetrics and Gynecology,* ed 4. Philadelphia, Harper & Row, 1982.

Danforth DN, **Scott** JR: *Obstetrics and Gynecology,* ed 5. Philadelphia, Harper & Row, 1986.

Department of Health, Education, and Welfare: New restrictions on oxytocin use, Food and Drug Administration Bulletin, Vol 8, October/November 1978.

Dierker LJ, et al: The midforceps: Maternal and neonatal outcomes. *Am J Obstet Gynecol* 1985;152:176.

Dyson DC, **Ferguson** JE, **Hensleigh** P: Antepartum external cephalic version under tocolysis. *Obstet Gynecol* 1986;67(January):63.

Eckholm E: Curbs sought in caesarean deliveries. *New York Times,* August 11, 1986, p A10.

Fall O, et al: Forceps or vacuum extraction? A comparison of effects on the newborn. *Acta Obstet Gynaecol Scand* 1986;65:75.

Flamm BL: Vaginal birth after cesarean section: Controversies old and new. *Clin Obstet Gynecol* 1985;28 (December):735.

Friedman E, et al: Dysfunctional labor. XII. Long-term effects on infant. *Am J Obstet Gynecol* 1977;127:779.

Frink BB, **Chally** P: Managing pain responses to cesarean childbirth. *Am J Mat Child Nurs* 1984;9(July/August):270.

Giacoia GP, **Yaffe** S: Perinatal pharmacology, in **Sciarri** JJ (ed): *Gynecology and Obstetrics*. Philadelphia, Harper & Row, 1982, vol 3, chap 100.

Gibbs CE: Planned vaginal delivery following cesarean section. *Clin Obstet Gynecol* 1985;23(June):507.

Greis JB, et al: Comparison of maternal fetal effects of vacuum extraction with forceps or cesarean deliveries. *Obstet Gynecol* 1981;57(May):571.

Hansen GF: Version of the fetus, in **Iffy** L, **Charles** D (eds): *Operative Perinatology*. New York, Macmillan, 1984.

Hofmeyr GJ, **Myer** IG, **Simko** G: External cephalic version and spontaneous version rates: Ethnic and other determinants. *Br J Obstet Gynaecol* 1986;93(January):13.

Iams JD, **Reiss** R: When should labor be interrupted by cesarean delivery. *Clin Obstet Gynecol* 1985;28 (December):745.

Laube DW: Forceps delivery. *Clin Obstet Gynecol* 1986;29(June):286.

Laufe LE: Obstetric forceps, in **Sciarri** JJ (ed): *Gynecology and Obstetrics*. Hagerstown, Md, Harper & Row, 1985, vol 2, chap 72.

Lavin JP, et al: Vaginal delivery in patients with prior cesarean section. *Obstet Gynecol* 1982;59(February):135.

Macer J, **Buchanan** D, **Yonekurs** ML: Induction of labor with prostaglandin E$_2$ vaginal suppositories. *Obstet Gynecol* 1984;64:664.

Mackenzie I, **Bradley** S, **Embrey** M: Vaginal prostaglandins and labour induction for patients previously delivered by caesarean section. *Br J Obstet Gynaecol* 1984;91:7.

Marshall C: The art of induction/augmentation of labor. *J Obstet Gynecol Neonat Nurs* 1985;14(January/February):22.

Morrison JC, **Wiser** WL: Cesarean birth: Surgical techniques, in **Sciarri** JJ (ed): *Gynecology and Obstetrics*. Hagerstown, Md, Harper & Row, 1986, vol 2, chap 83.

NAACOG: *The Nurse's Role in the Induction/Augmentation of Labor,* January 1988.

Neal R: Induction of labor with vaginally administered prostaglandin E$_2$. *Can Med Assoc J* 1984;131:907.

NIH Cesarean Birth Task Force. National Institute of Child Development statement on cesarean childbirth, 1980. USDHHS, Building HHH, Rm 447F8, Washington, DC 20201.

Niswander KR: Induction of labor, in **Sciarri** JJ (ed): *Gynecology and Obstetrics*. Hagerstown, Md, Harper & Row, 1985, vol 2, chap 71.

Petitti DB: Maternal mortality and morbidity with cesarean section. *Clin Obstet Gynecol* 1985;28(December):763.

Philipson EH, **Rosen** MG: Trends in the frequency of cesarean births. *Clin Obstet Gynecol* 1985;28(December):691.

Porreco RP: High cesarean section rate: A new perspective. *Obstet Gynecol* 1985;65:307.

Pritchard JA, **MacDonald** PC, **Gant** NF: *Williams Obstetrics,* ed 17. New York, Appleton-Century-Crofts, 1985.

Ramler D, **Roberts** J: A comparison of cold and warm sitz baths for relief of postpartum perineal pain. *J Obstet Gynecol Neonat Nurs* 1986;15(November/December):471.

Salmon YM, et al: Cervical ripening by breast stimulation. *Obstet Gynecol* 1986;67(January):21.

Silbar EL: Factors related to the increasing cesarean section rates for cephalopelvic disproportion. *Am J Obstet Gynecol* 1986;154:1095.

Stichler JF, **Affonso** DD: Cesarean birth. *Am J Nurs* 1980;80(March):466.

Thacker SB, **Banta** HB: Benefits and risks of episiotomy: An interpretive review of the English language literature, 1860–1980. *Obstet Gynecol Surv* 1983;38:322.

Varner MW: Episiotomy: Techniques and indications. *Clin Obstet Gynecol* 1986;29(June):309.

Westgren M, **Paul** RH: Delivery of the low birth weight infant by cesarean section. *Clin Obstet Gynecol* 1985;28(December):752.

Wilf RT, **Franklin** JB: Six years' experience with vaginal births after cesareans at Booth Maternity Center in Philadelphia. *Birth* 1984;11(Spring):1.

ADDITIONAL READINGS

Heritage CK, **Cunningham** MD: Association of elective repeat delivery and persistent pulmonary hypertension of the newborn. *Am J Obstet Gynecol* 1985;152:627.

Kitzinger S: Episiotomy. *ICEA Review* 1985;9(2):1.

Leveno KJ, **Cunningham** FG, **Pritchard** JA: Cesarean section: An answer to the House of Horne. *Am J Obstet Gynecol* 1985;153:838.

Prins RP, et al: Preinduction cervical ripening with sequential use of prostaglandin E$_2$ gel. *Am J Obstet Gynecol* 1986;154:1275.

Savona-Ventura C: The role of external cephalic version in modern obstetrics. *Obstet Gynecol* 1986;41:393.

Trofatter KF, et al: Preinduction cervical ripening with prostaglandin E$_2$ (Prepidil) gel. *Am J Obstet Gynecol* 1985;153:268.

Wyman AC: Cesarean birth: What to expect. *Lamaze Parents Magazine,* 1986, p 50.

As women in childbirth we bring our complete selves to the experience: body, mind, emotions, habits, past experiences, lessons to be learned . . . a woman births as she lives, expressing this continuity of birth within the rest of a woman's life. (Birthing Normally: A Personal Growth Approach to Childbirth)

The Newborn

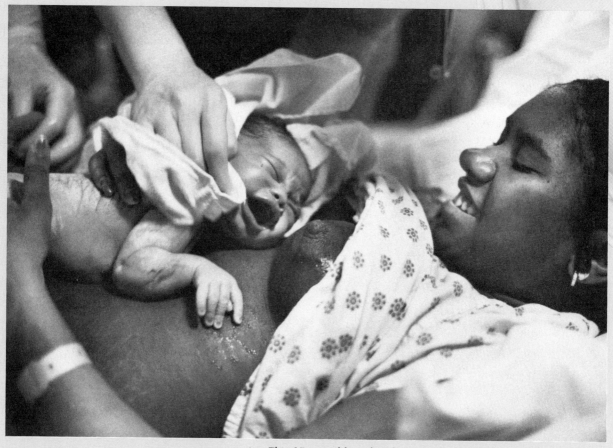

This 15-year-old mother, having just given birth without any medical intervention, takes great pride and joy in her still wet infant.

Part Six

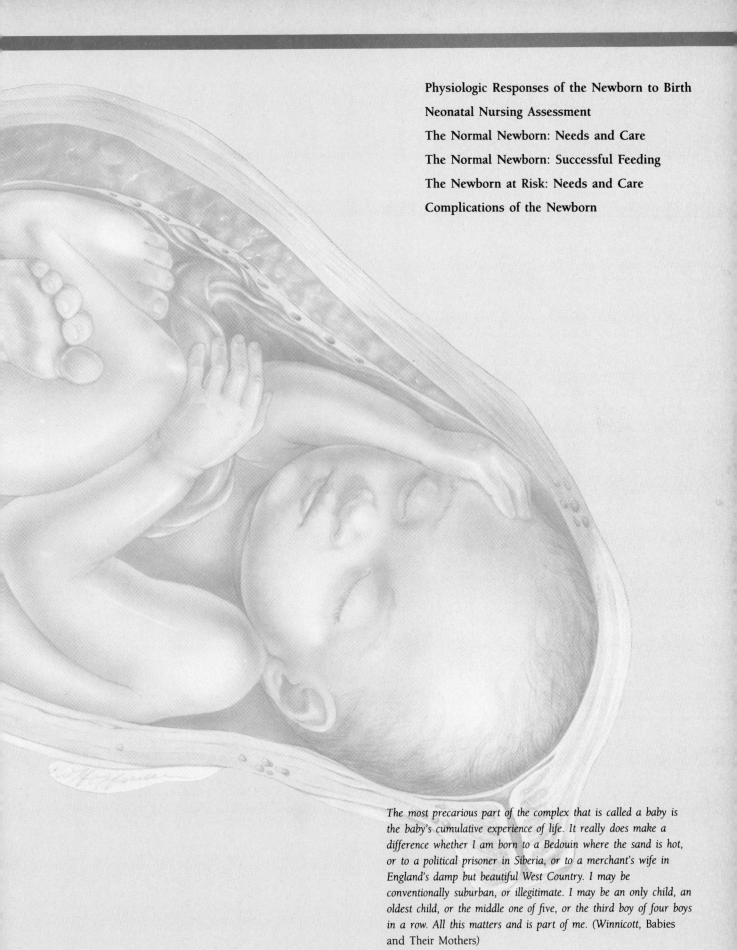

The most precarious part of the complex that is called a baby is the baby's cumulative experience of life. It really does make a difference whether I am born to a Bedouin where the sand is hot, or to a political prisoner in Siberia, or to a merchant's wife in England's damp but beautiful West Country. I may be conventionally suburban, or illegitimate. I may be an only child, an oldest child, or the middle one of five, or the third boy of four boys in a row. All this matters and is part of me. (Winnicott, Babies and Their Mothers)

Physiologic Responses of the Newborn to Birth

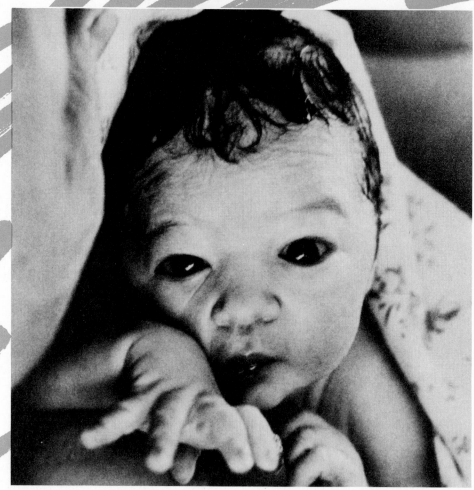

Chapter Twenty-Seven

This half-hour-old baby, nuzzling at her mother's breast, suddenly lifts her head and looks directly into her mother's eyes.

Gastrointestinal Adaptations
Fetal-Neonatal Transitional Physiology
Digestive Function
Urinary Adaptations
Kidney Development and Function
Characteristics of Neonatal Urinary Function
Immunologic Adaptations
Neurologic and Sensory/Perceptual Adaptations
Intrauterine Factors Influencing Newborn Behavior
Characteristics of Neonatal Neurologic Function
Behavioral States of the Newborn
Sensory Capacities

OBJECTIVES

- Summarize the cardiovascular and respiratory changes that occur during the transition to extrauterine life.
- Summarize the major mechanisms of heat loss in the newborn and how the newborn produces heat.
- Describe the functional abilities of the newborn's gastrointestinal tract and liver.
- Explain the steps involved in conjugation and excretion of bilirubin in the newborn.
- Examine the reasons why the newborn develops jaundice.
- Identify three reasons why the newborn's kidneys have difficulty in maintaining fluid and electrolyte balance.
- List the immunologic responses available to the newborn.
- Describe how various factors affect the newborn's blood values.
- Describe the normal sensory/perceptual abilities seen in the newborn period.

The newborn period includes the time from birth through the first 28 days of life. During this period, the newborn adjusts from intrauterine to extrauterine life. The nurse must be knowledgeable about a newborn's normal biopsychosocial adaptations to recognize deviations from it.

To begin life as an independent being, the baby must immediately establish pulmonary ventilation in conjunction with marked circulatory changes. These radical and rapid changes are crucial to the maintenance of life. All other neonatal body systems change their functions or establish themselves over a longer period of time.

● Respiratory Adaptations

The following must occur to establish respiratory function:

1. Extrauterine respiratory movements begin.

2. Air entry overcomes opposing forces so that the lungs expand.

3. Some air remains in the alveoli during expiration, thus preventing lung collapse. (The amount of air remaining is called the functional residual capacity.)

4. Pulmonary blood flow increases, and cardiac output is redistributed.

Although the previous events occur at birth, certain intrauterine factors also enhance the newborn's ability to breathe.

Intrauterine Factors Supporting Respiratory Function

FETAL LUNG DEVELOPMENT

The respiratory system is in a continuous state of development during fetal life, and the development continues into the neonatal period. During the first 20 weeks of gestation, development is limited to the differentiation of pulmonary, vascular, and lymphatic structures.

At 20 to 24 weeks alveolar ducts begin to appear, followed by primitive alveoli at 24 to 28 weeks. During this time, the alveolar epithelial cells begin to differentiate into type I cells (structures necessary for gas exchange) and type II cells (structures that provide for the synthesis and storage of surfactant). *Surfactant* is composed of a group of surface-active phospholipids, of which one component, lecithin, is the most critical for alveolar stability.

At 28 to 32 weeks the number of type II cells increases further, and surfactant is produced by a choline pathway within the type II cells. Surfactant production by this pathway peaks at about 35 weeks and remains high until term, parallelling late fetal lung development. At this time, the lungs are structurally developed enough to permit maintenance of good lung expansion and adequate exchange of gases (Avery 1987).

Clinically, the peak production of surfactant by the choline pathway corresponds closely with the marked decrease in incidence of idiopathic respiratory distress syndrome after 35 weeks' gestation. Production of sphingomyelin remains constant throughout gestation. The neonate delivered before the L/S ratio is 2:1 will have varying degrees of respiratory distress. (See discussion of L/S ratio in Chapter 32.)

FETAL BREATHING MOVEMENTS

The ability of the neonate to breathe air immediately upon exposure to extrauterine life appears to be the consequence of weeks of intrauterine practice. In this respect, breathing can be perceived as a continuation of an intrauterine process as the lungs convert from a fluid to a gas medium. Fetal breathing movements (FBM) occur as early as 11 weeks' gestation (see Chapter 20 for discussion). Goldstein and Reid (1980) propose that FBMs are essential for development of chest wall muscles (including the diaphragm) and to a lesser extent for regulating lung fluid volume and, therefore, lung growth.

Initiation of Breathing

To maintain life, the lungs must function immediately after birth. Two radical changes must take place for the lungs to function:

1. Pulmonary ventilation must be established through lung expansion following birth.

2. A marked increase in the pulmonary circulation must occur.

The first breath of life—the gasp in response to chemical, tactile, thermal, and mechanical changes associated with birth—initiates the serial opening of the alveoli. Thus begins the transition from a fluid-filled environment to an air-breathing, independent, extrauterine life.

MECHANICAL EVENTS

During the latter half of gestation, the fetal lungs produce fluid continuously. This secretion fills the lungs almost completely, expanding the air spaces. Some of the lung fluid drains out of the lungs into the amniotic fluid and is then swallowed by the fetus.

Secretion of lung fluid diminishes 48 hours before onset of labor. However, approximately 80 to 110 mL of fluid remains in the respiratory passages of a normal term fetus at the time of delivery. This fluid must be removed from the lungs to permit adequate movement of air.

The primary mechanical event involved in initiation of breathing and the removal of fluid from the lungs is the compression of the thorax as the fetal body passes through the birth canal. As the fetal chest is compressed, thus increasing intrathoracic pressure, approximately one-third of the fluid is squeezed out of the lungs. After the birth of the newborn's trunk, the chest wall recoils. This chest recoil is thought to produce a small, passive inspiration of air (negative intrathoracic pressure sucks air in), which is drawn into the lungs to replace the fluid that was squeezed out. After this first inspiration, the newborn exhales, with crying, against a partially closed glottis, creating a positive intrathoracic pressure. The high positive pressure distributes the inspired air through the alveoli and begins the establishment of functional residual capacity. On expiration, the diaphragm descends, creating greater pressure within the alveoli than outside. Fluid flows from the alveoli across the alveolar membranes into the pulmonary interstitial tissue.

With each succeeding breath, the lungs expand, stretching the alveolar walls and enlarging the alveolar pores. The expansion of the pores facilitates movement of the remaining lung fluid into the interstitial tissue. Since the protein concentration is higher in the pulmonary capillaries, the interstitial fluid passes by osmosis into the capillaries and lymphatics. As pulmonary vascular resistance decreases, pulmonary blood flow increases, and more fluid is absorbed into the bloodstream. In the normal term newborn, movement of lung fluid to the interstitial tissue is rapid, but movement into lymph and blood vessels may take several hours (Korones 1986).

Some of the inspired air is also forced into the proximal airways. An air–liquid interface (the surface boundary between these two components) is established in the smaller airways and alveoli. About 70 percent of the alveoli fluid is reabsorbed within 2 hours after birth, and it is completely absorbed within 12 to 24 hours after birth (Korones 1986). Figure 27–1 summarizes the initiation of respiration.

Although the initial expiration should clear the airways of accumulated fluid and permit further inspiration, some clinicians feel it is wise to suction mucus and fluid from the newborn's mouth and oropharynx. They use a

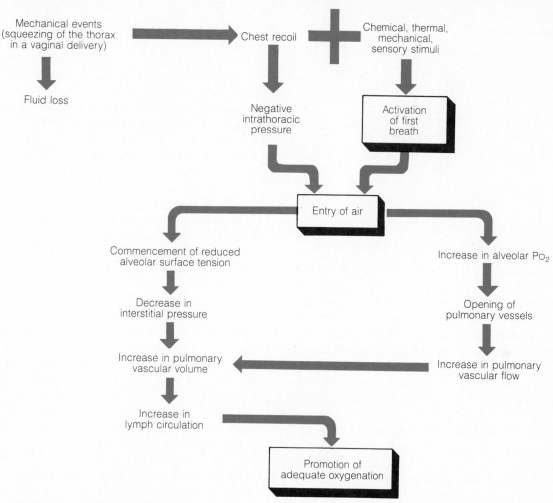

Figure 27–1 Initiation of respiration in the neonate

DeLee or bulb syringe as soon as the newborn's head and shoulders are delivered and again as the newborn adapts to extrauterine life and stabilizes (see Procedure 23–2 and Chapter 23).

Problems associated with lung clearance and/or initiation of respiratory activity may be caused by a variety of factors. The lymphatics may be underdeveloped, thus decreasing the rate at which the fluid is absorbed from the lungs. Complications that occur antenatally or during labor and delivery can interfere with adequate lung expansion, resulting in increased pulmonary vascular resistance, and decreased blood flow. These complications include inadequate compression of the chest wall in a very small neonate, the absence of chest wall compression in the neonate delivered by cesarean birth, or severe asphyxia at birth.

CHEMICAL STIMULI

An important chemical stimulator that contributes to the onset of breathing is transitory asphyxia of the fetus and newborn. Elevation in PCO_2 and decrease in pH and

PO_2 are the natural outcome of normal vaginal delivery with cessation of placental gas exhange and umbilical cord pulsation and cutting. These changes, which are present in all newborns to some degree, stimulate the aortic and carotid chemoreceptors, initiating impulses that trigger the medulla's respiratory center. Although brief periods of asphyxia are a significant stimulator, prolonged asphyxia is abnormal and acts as a central nervous system depressant.

THERMAL STIMULI

A significant decrease in ambient temperature after delivery [(from 37C (98.6F) to 21C–23.9C (70F–75F)] is enough thermal stimulus for initiation of breathing. As skin nerve endings are stimulated to transmit impulses to the medullary respiratory control center, the newborn responds with rhythmic respirations. Excessive cooling may result in profound depression and evidence of cold stress (see p 1033), but the normal temperature changes that occur at birth are apparently within acceptable physiologic limits.

SENSORY STIMULI

As the fetus is delivered from an environment characterized by sensory deprivation to one of sensory overstimulation, a number of sensory influences help initiate respiration. They include the numerous tactile, auditory, and visual stimuli of birth. Historically, vigorous stimulation was provided by slapping the buttocks or heels of the newborn, but today greater emphasis is placed on gentle physical contact. Thoroughly drying the infant provides stimulation in a far more comforting way and also decreases heat loss.

FACTORS OPPOSING THE FIRST BREATH

Three major factors may oppose the initiation of respiratory activity: (1) alveolar surface tension, (2) viscosity of lung fluid within the respiratory tract, and (3) degree of lung compliance.

Because of surface tension within the alveoli, there is a constant tendency for surfaces to contract. The small airways and alveoli would collapse between each inspiration were it not for the presence of surfactant, which reduces the cohesive force between the moist surfaces of the alveoli. Surfactant promotes lung expansion by preventing the alveoli from completely collapsing with each expiration and increases lung *compliance* (the ability of the lung to fill with air easily). When surfactant is decreased, compliance is also decreased and the pressure needed to expand the lungs with air increases. Resistive forces of the fluid-filled (presence of viscous lung fluid) lung in conjunction with the small radii of the respiratory airways require the generation of pressures of 40 to 80 cm of water for the initial inflation of the lung. The first breath generally establishes a functional residual capacity (FRC) that is 30 percent to 40 percent of the fully expanded lung volume. The FRC allows alveolar sacs to remain partially expanded on expiration. This residual air in the lungs after expiration alleviates the need for continuous high pressure for successive breaths. Subsequent breaths require only 6 to 8 cm H_2O pressure to open alveoli during inspiration. Indeed, the first breath of life is usually the most difficult.

Cardiopulmonary Physiology

With the onset of respiration, the functions of the cardiovascular and respiratory systems become interrelated; hence the term *cardiopulmonary adaptation*. As air enters the lungs, PO_2 rises in the alveoli, which stimulates the relaxation of the pulmonary arteries and triggers a decrease in the pulmonary vascular resistance. At the same time, the lowered surface tension decreases interstitial pressure. As pulmonary vascular resistance decreases, the vascular flow in the lung increases by 20 percent, followed by an increase of 85 percent at 7 hours of life and 100 percent at 24

hours of life. This greater blood volume to the lungs contributes to the conversion from fetal circulation to newborn circulation.

After pulmonary circulation is established, blood is distributed throughout the lung, although the alveoli may or may not be fully open. For adequate oxygenation to occur, sufficient blood must be delivered by the heart to the lungs. It is important to remember that shunting of blood is common in the early newborn period. This bidirectional blood flow, or right-to-left shunting through the ductus arteriosus, may divert a significant amount of blood away from the lungs depending on the pressure changes of respiration, crying, and the cardiac cycle. This shunting in the newborn period is also responsible for the unstable transitional period to neonatal respiratory functions.

OXYGEN TRANSPORT

The transportation of oxygen to the peripheral tissues depends on the type of hemoglobin in the red blood cell. In the fetus and neonate, a variety of hemoglobins exist, the most significant being fetal hemoglobin (Hb F) and adult hemoglobin (Hb A). Approximately 70 percent to 90 percent of hemoglobin in the fetus and neonate is of the fetal variety. The greatest difference between Hb F and Hb A is related to the transport of oxygen.

In the newborn, the greater affinity of Hb F for oxygen causes the shift to the left in the oxygen dissociation curve (Figure 27–2). More oxygen is bound to Hb F, which makes oxygen saturation in the newborn relatively greater than in the adult, but less oxygen is available to the tissues. This is beneficial for the fetus, who must maintain adequate oxygen uptake in the presence of very low oxygen tension (umbilical venous PO_2 cannot exceed the uterine venous PO_2). Because of this phenomenon, hypoxia in the neonate is particularly difficult to recognize because of the high concentration of oxygen in the blood. Clinical manifestations of cyanosis are lacking until low blood levels of oxygen are present. Shifts to the left in the curve may also be caused by alkalosis (increased pH) and hypothermia. Acidosis, hypercarbia, and hyperthermia may cause the oxygen dissociation curve to shift to the right.

Other factors that regulate oxygen supply to the tissues are blood oxygen capacity and cardiac output (Glader 1984). Oxygen capacity is the maximum amount of hemoglobin and oxygen that can be bound together and is directly affected by hemoglobin concentration. One gram of hemoglobin is able to combine with 1.34 mL of oxygen. The actual amount of oxygen-bound hemoglobin divided by the oxygen capacity gives a percentage signifying *oxygen saturation*. Oxygen saturation, which is controlled by arterial oxygen tension (PaO_2) and hemoglobin-oxygen affinity usually has values between 96 percent and 98 percent. A significant reduction in the oxygen capacity results in an

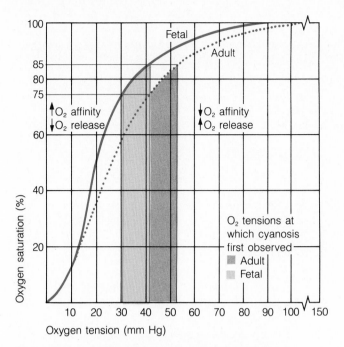

Figure 27-2 Fetal oxygen dissociation curve (Modified from Klaus M, Fanaroff AA: *Care of the High Risk Infant.* Philadelphia, Saunders, 1986, p 234)

increased cardiac output to compensate for the decreased oxygen concentration of the hemoglobin.

Maintaining Respiratory Function

The ability of the lung to maintain oxygen (oxygenation) and carbon dioxide exchange (ventilation) is influenced by such factors as lung compliance and airway resistance. Lung compliance is influenced by the elastic recoil of the lung tissue and by anatomic variation. Anatomic differences between the neonate and the adult influence lung compliance. The infant has a relatively large heart and mediastinal structures that reduce available lung space. The large abdomen further encroaches on the high diaphragm to decrease lung space. Anatomically, the neonatal chest is equipped with weak intercostal muscles, a rigid rib cage with horizontal ribs, and a high diaphragm that restricts the space available for lung expansion. Ventilation is also limited by airway resistance, which depends on the radii, length, and number of airways.

Characteristics of Neonatal Respiration

The normal neonatal respiratory rate is 30 to 50 breaths per minute. Initial respirations may be largely diaphragmatic, with shallow and irregular depth and rhythm. They are primarily abdominal and synchronous with the chest movement. Short periods of apnea are to be expected. When the breathing pattern is characterized by apnea last-

ing 5 to 15 seconds, *periodic breathing* is occurring. Periodic respiration is rarely associated with differences in skin color or heart rate changes, and it has no prognostic significance. Tactile or other sensory stimulation increases the inspired oxygen and converts periodic breathing patterns to normal breathing patterns. Neonatal sleep states in particular influence respiratory patterns. The pattern is reasonably regular in deep sleep. Periodic breathing occurs with rapid-eye-movement (REM) sleep, and grossly irregular breathing is evident with motor activity, sucking, and crying.

The neonate is an obligatory nose breather, and any obstruction will cause respiratory distress, so it is important to keep the throat and nose clear. If respirations drop below 30 or exceed 60 per minute when the infant is at rest, or if dyspnea or cyanosis occurs, the physician should be notified. Immediately after birth and for the first two hours after birth, respiratory rates of 60 to 70 breaths per minute are normal. Some initial dyspnea or cyanosis may also be normal. Any increased use of the intercostal muscle (retracting) may indicate respiratory distress.

● Cardiovascular Adaptations

As described on p 828, blood flow to the lungs increases with the first respirations of the normal newborn. This greater blood volume contributes to the conversion from fetal circulation to neonatal circulation.

Fetal-Neonatal Transitional Anatomy and Physiology

The lungs of the fetus do not function in utero; therefore, it is necessary to have a special circulatory system that will bypass most of the blood supply to the lungs. (See Chapter 13 for a discussion of fetal circulation and Figure 13–13 for a pictorial presentation.) During fetal life, blood with higher oxygen content is diverted to the heart and brain. Blood in the descending aorta is less oxygenated and supplies the kidneys and intestinal tract. Limited amounts of blood, pumped from the right ventricle toward the lungs, enters the pulmonary vessels. In the fetus, increased pulmonary resistance forces most of the blood through the ductus arteriosus into the descending aorta (Table 27–1).

Marked changes occur in the cardiovascular system at birth. Expansion of the lungs with the first breath decreases the pulmonary vascular resistance and left atrial pressure. This physiologic mechanism marks the beginning of newborn circulation and cardiopulmonary adaptations (Figure 27–3). As the newborn adapts to extrauterine life, there are five major areas of change in circulatory function:

1. *Increased aortic pressure and decreased venous pressure.* With severing of the cord, the placental vascular bed is eliminated and the intravascular space is reduced.

Table 27–1 Fetal and Neonatal Circulation

System	Fetal	Neonatal
Pulmonary blood vessels	Constricted with very little blood flow; lungs not expanded	Vasodilation and increased blood flow; lungs expanded; increased oxygen stimulates vasodilation.
Systemic blood vessels	Dilated with low resistance; blood mostly in placenta	Arterial pressure rises due to loss of placenta; increased systemic blood volume and resistance.
Ductus arteriosus	Large with no tone; blood flow from pulmonary artery to aorta	1. Reversal of blood flow. Now from aorta to pulmonary artery due to increased left atrial pressure. 2. Ductus is sensitive to increased oxygen and body chemicals and begins to constrict.
Foramen ovale	Patent with large blood flow from right atrium to left atrium	Increased pressure in left atrium attempts to reverse blood flow and shuts one-way valve.

Consequently, aortic (systemic) blood pressure is increased. At the same time, separation from the placenta results in decreased blood return via the inferior vena cava, and in a small decrease in pressure within the venous circulation.

2. *Increased systemic pressure and decreased pulmonary artery pressure.* With the loss of the low-resistance placenta, pressure increases in the systemic circulation, resulting in greater systemic resistance. At the same time, lung expansion promotes increased pulmonary blood flow, and the increased blood PO_2 associated with initiation of respirations produces vasodilatation of pulmonary blood vessels. The combination of increased pulmonary blood flow and vasodilatation results in decreased pulmonary artery resistance. As a result of opening the vascular beds, the systemic vascular pressure decreases, causing perfusion of the other body systems.

3. *Closure of the foramen ovale.* Closure of the foramen ovale is a function of atrial pressures. In utero, pressure is greater in the right atrium, and the foramen ovale is open. Decreased pulmonary resistance and increased pulmonary blood flow result in increased pulmonary venous return into the left atrium, thereby increasing left atrial pressure slightly. The decreased pulmonary vascular resistance also causes a decrease in right atrial pressure. The pressure gradients are now reversed, left atrial pressure is greater, and the foramen ovale is functionally closed. Although the foramen ovale closes one to two hours after birth, a slight right-to-left shunting may occur in the early neonatal period. Any increase in pulmonary resistance may result in reopening of the foramen ovale, causing a right-to-left shunt. Permanent closure occurs within several months.

4. *Closure of the ductus arteriosus.* Initial elevation of the systemic vascular pressure above the pulmonary vascular pressure increases pulmonary blood flow by causing a reversal of the flow through the ductus arteriosus. Blood now flows from the aorta into the pulmonary artery. Furthermore, although the presence of oxygen causes the pulmonary arterioles to dilate, an increase in blood PO_2 triggers the opposite response in the ductus arteriosus—active constriction. In utero, the placenta provides prostaglandin E_2, which causes ductus vasodilation. With the loss of the placenta and increased pulmonary blood flow, prostaglandin E_2 levels drop, leaving the active constriction by PO_2 unopposed. If the lungs fail to expand or if PO_2 levels drop, the ductus remains patent. Fibrosis of the ductus occurs within 3 weeks after birth, but functional closure is accomplished within 15 hours after birth.

5. *Closure of the ductus venosus.* Although the mechanism of initiating closure of the ductus venosus is not known, it appears to be related to mechanical pressure changes after severing of the cord, redistribution of blood, and cardiac output. Closure of the bypass forces perfusion of the liver. Fibrotic closure occurs within three to seven days (Korones 1986) (Figure 27–4).

Characteristics of Neonatal Cardiovascular Function

HEART RATE

Shortly after the first cry and the advent of cardiopulmonary circulation, the newborn heart rate accelerates to 175 to 180 beats per minute. Thereafter the rate follows a fairly uniform course, decelerating to 115 beats per minute at 4 to 6 hours of life, then rising and leveling off at

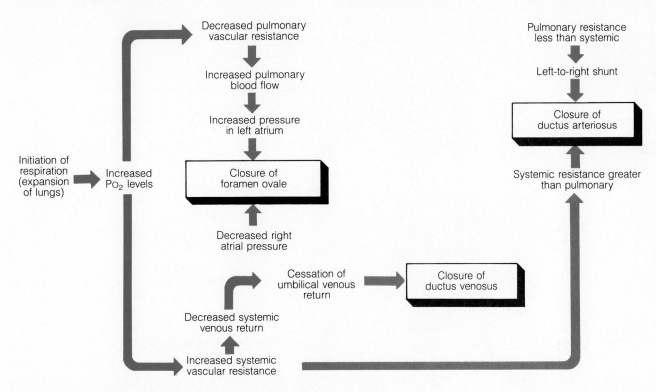

Figure 27–3   Transitional circulation: conversion from fetal to neonatal circulation

approximately 120 beats per minute at 12 to 24 hours of life (Smith & Nelson 1976). The range of the heart rate in the full-term neonate is 100 beats per minute while asleep and 120 to 150 while awake. Resting heart rates are as low as 70 to 90 beats per minute, and rates as high as 180 while crying have been reported as normal. Apical pulse rates should be obtained by auscultation for a full minute, preferably when the neonate is asleep. Peripheral pulses should also be evaluated to detect any lags or unusual characteristics.

BLOOD PRESSURE

During the newborn period, the blood pressure tends to be highest immediately after birth and then descends to its lowest level about three hours of age. By four to six days of life, the blood pressure rises and plateaus at a level approximately the same as the initial level (Smith & Nelson 1976). Blood pressure is particularly sensitive to the changes in blood volume that occur in the transition to neonatal circulation. Figure 27–5 diagrams this response.

Blood pressure values during the first 12 hours of life vary with the birth weight. In the full-term resting neonate, the average blood pressure is 74/47 mm Hg and 64/39 mm Hg for the preterm newborn. Crying may cause an elevation of 20 mm Hg in both the systolic and diastolic blood pressure, thus accuracy is more likely in the quiet newborn.

The measurement of blood pressure is best accomplished by using the Doppler technique or a 1 to 2 inch cuff and a stethoscope over the brachial artery.

HEART MURMURS

Murmurs are usually produced by turbulent blood flow. Murmurs may be heard when blood flows across an abnormal valve or across a stenosed valve, when there is an atrial septal or ventricular septal defect, or when there is increased flow across a normal valve.

In newborns, 90 percent of all murmurs are transient and not associated with anomalies. They usually involve incomplete closure of the ductus arteriosus or foramen ovale. Soft murmurs may be heard as the pulmonary branch arteries increase their blood flow from 7 percent to 50 percent of combined ventricular output during transition, causing physiologic peripheral pulmonary stenosis. With early discharge, murmurs associated with ventricular septal defect and patent ductus arteriosus are not being picked up until the first well-baby checkup at four to six weeks of age. It should also be noted that murmurs are sometimes absent in seriously malformed hearts.

Murmurs can be related to persistent fetal circulation or fluid overload. Significant murmurs will occasionally be heard, including the murmur of a persistent patent ductus arteriosus, aortic or pulmonic stenosis, or a small ventric-

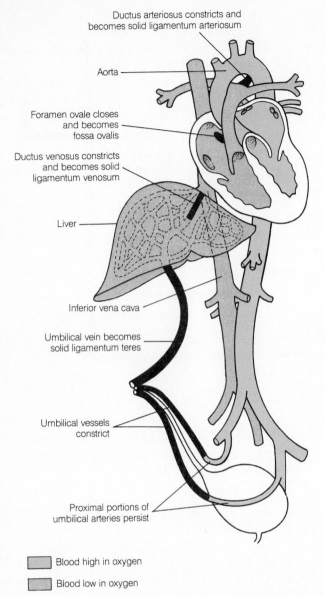

Ductus arteriosus constricts and becomes solid ligamentum arteriosum

Aorta

Foramen ovale closes and becomes fossa ovalis

Ductus venosus constricts and becomes solid ligamentum venosum

Liver

Inferior vena cava

Umbilical vein becomes solid ligamentum teres

Umbilical vessels constrict

Proximal portions of umbilical arteries persist

☐ Blood high in oxygen

☐ Blood low in oxygen

Figure 27–4 Major changes that occur in the newborn's circulatory system (From Hole JW: Human Anatomy and Physiology, ed 2. Dubuque, Iowa, William C. Brown, 1981, p 757. All rights reserved. Reprinted by permission.)

ular septal defect. Presence of a split S_2 may be reassuring, whereas a gallop may be an ominous finding. See Chapter 32 for discussion of congenital heart defects.

CARDIAC OUTPUT

In the first two hours after birth when the ductus arteriosus remains mostly patent, about one-third of the ventricular output is returned to the pulmonary circulation. Minimal amounts of blood may also shunt from left to right through the foramen ovale. As a result, the left ventricle has a significantly greater volume load than the right ven-

tricle. In the adult, right and left ventricular outputs are equal; in the neonate, right ventricular output equals systemic blood flow, and left ventricular output equals pulmonary blood flow. Systemic blood volume and pulmonary blood volume are *not* equal in the neonate. The newborn's combined cardiac output (left and right ventricular) is greater per unit of body weight than in later childhood.

CARDIAC WORKLOAD

Prior to birth, the right ventricle does approximately two-thirds of the cardiac work. This workload is seen in the increased size and thickness of the right ventricle at birth and may explain why left-sided heart defects are less tolerable than right-sided lesions after birth. After birth the left ventricle must assume a larger share of the cardiac workload, and it increases in size and thickness (Avery & Taeusch 1984).

● Hematologic Adaptations

In the fetus, the hemoglobin and erythrocyte counts are high because of the nature of fetal circulation. Fetal blood (umbilical vein) in-utero is 50 percent oxygen saturated; this relative hypoxia causes increased amounts of erythropoietin to be secreted, resulting in active erythropoiesis (an increase in nucleated red blood cells and reticulocytes). After birth (8 to 12 weeks postnatally), erythropoietin is again produced by the kidney. In the first days of life, hemoglobin concentration may rise by 1 to 2 g/dL above fetal levels as a result of placental transfusion, low oral fluid intake, and diminished extracellular fluid volume. By one week postnatally, peripheral hemoglobin decreases and is back to fetal blood levels. The hemoglobin level

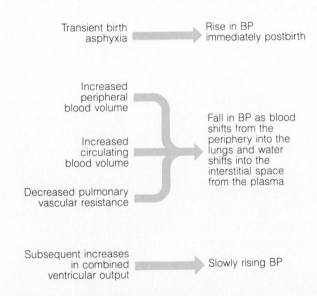

Transient birth asphyxia ⟹ Rise in BP immediately postbirth

Increased peripheral blood volume

Increased circulating blood volume

Decreased pulmonary vascular resistance

⟹ Fall in BP as blood shifts from the periphery into the lungs and water shifts into the interstitial space from the plasma

Subsequent increases in combined ventricular output ⟹ Slowly rising BP

Figure 27–5 Response of BP to neonatal changes in blood volume

declines progressively thereafter during the first three months after birth, then begins to increase slowly as the infant grows to adulthood. The initial decline in hemoglobin creates a phenomenon known as *physiologic anemia of infancy* (Hatch & Sumner 1981). A factor that influences the degree of physiologic anemia is the nutritional status of the neonate. Supplies of vitamin E, folic acid, and iron may be inadequate given the amount of growth in the later part of the first year of life. Hemoglobin values fall, mainly from a decrease in red cell mass rather than from the dilutional effect of increasing plasma volume. Other contributing factors are that red cell survival is lower in neonates than in adults, and red cell production is less. Neonatal red blood cells have a life span of 80 to 100 days, which is approximately two-thirds of an adult's red blood cell life span.

Leukocytosis is a normal finding because the trauma of birth stimulates increased production of neutrophils during the first week of life. Neutrophils then decrease to 35 percent of the total leukocyte count by two weeks of age.

The thymus provides lymphoblasts to the lymph nodes and other lymphoid tissue, which then play a role in antibody formation. Lymphocytes attain two-thirds of the adult's value by 20 weeks' gestation and gradually continue to increase until term. Megakaryocytes appear in the liver and spleen as platelets at about 11 weeks' gestation and approach adult values by 30 weeks. Lymphocytes eventually become the predominant type of leukocyte, and the total white blood count falls.

Blood volume of the term infant is estimated to be 80 to 85 mL/kg of body weight. The true amount of blood volume varies based on the amount of placental transfusion received. The concentration of serum electrolytes in the blood indicates the fluid and electrolyte status of the baby. See Table 27–2 for normal term newborn electrolyte and blood values. Hematologic values in the newborn are affected by several factors, including:

The site of the blood sample. Hemoglobin and hematocrit levels taken simultaneously are significantly higher in capillary blood than in venous blood. Sluggish peripheral blood flow creates red blood cell stasis, thereby increasing their concentration in the capillaries. Because of this, blood samples taken from venous blood sites are more accurate.

Delayed cord clamping and the normal shift of plasma to the extravascular spaces. Neonatal hemoglobin and hematocrit values are higher when a placental transfusion occurs postnatally. Placental vessels contain about 100 mL of blood at term, most of which can be transfused into the newborn by holding the newborn below the level of the placenta and by late clamping of the cord (Figure 27–6). Blood volume increases by 40 percent to 60 percent with late cord clamping (Korones 1986). The increase is reflected by a rise in hemoglobin level and an increase in the hematocrit to 65 percent about 48 hours after birth (compared with 48 percent when the cord is clamped immediately). For greatest accuracy, the initial hemoglobin and hematocrit levels should be measured in the cord blood, although this is not a routine practice.

Gestational age. There appears to be a positive association between increasing gestational age, higher red blood cell numbers, and greater hemoglobin concentration. This means that the gestational age of the newborn influences the values.

Prenatal and/or perinatal hemorrhage. Occurrence of significant prenatal or perinatal bleeding decreases the hematocrit level and causes hypovolemia.

● Temperature Regulation

Temperature regulation is the maintenance of thermal balance of the loss of heat to the environment at a rate equal to the production of heat. Newborns are *homeothermic;* they attempt to stabilize their internal (core) body temperatures within a narrow range in spite of significant temperature variations in their environment.

Thermoregulation in the newborn is closely related to the rate of metabolism and oxygen consumption. Within a specific environmental range called the *thermal neutral zone* (TNZ), the rates of oxygen consumption and metabolism are minimal, and internal body temperature is maintained because of thermal balance. For an unclothed full-

Table 27–2   Normal Term Newborn Blood Values

Laboratory data	Normal range
Hemoglobin	15–20 g/dL
Hematocrit	43%–61%
WBC	10,000–30,000/mm³
Neutrophils	40%–80%
Immature WBC	3%–10%
Platelets	100,000–280,000/mm³
Reticulocytes	3%–6%
Blood volume	82.3 mL/kg (third day after early cord clamping) 92.6 mL/kg (third day after delayed cord clamping)
Sodium mmol/L	124–156
Potassium mmol/L	5.3–7.3
Chloride mmol/L	90–111
Calcium mg/dL	7.3–9.2
Glucose mg/dL	40–97

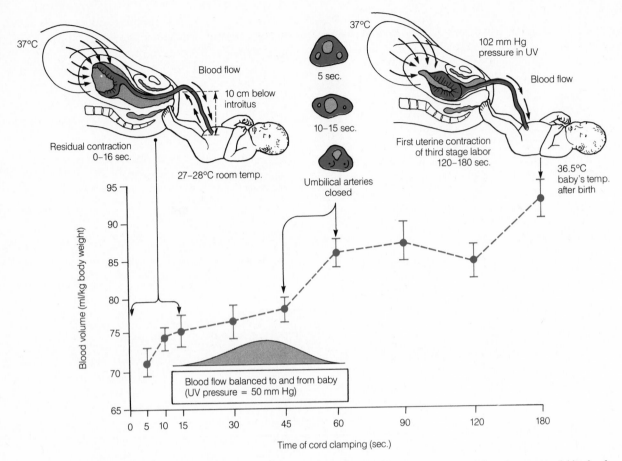

Figure 27–6 *Schematic illustration of the mechanisms in placental transfusion (normal term deliveries). The mean neonatal blood volume at 30 minutes is plotted against time of cord clamping after birth (mean + SE, data from 114 full-term infants). Note episodic, stepwise increments in blood volume at 10, 60, and 180 seconds (From Yao AC, Lind J: Placental Transfusion: A Clinical and Physiological Study. Springfield, Ill, Charles C. Thomas, 1982)*

term newborn, the TNZ range is an ambient temperature of 32 to 34C (89.6–93.2F). The limits for an adult are 26 to 28C (78.8–82.4F). Thus, the normal newborn requires higher environmental temperatures to maintain a thermoneutral environment than does the adult. See Table 27–3 for suggested TNZ ranges based on gestational weight and postnatal age.

Several newborn characteristics affect the establishment of a TNZ. The newborn has decreased subcutaneous fat and a thin epidermis, with blood vessels closer to the skin than those of an adult. Therefore, the circulating blood is influenced by changes in environmental temperature, and in turn influences the hypothalmic temperature-regulating center.

The flexed posture of the term infant decreases the surface area exposed to the environment, thereby reducing heat loss. Other neonatal characteristics such as size and age may also affect the establishing of a TNZ. Preterm SGA neonates require higher environmental temperatures to achieve a thermoneutral environment while a larger, well-insulated newborn may be able to cope with lower environmental temperature. If the environmental temperature falls below the lower limits of the TNZ, the newborn responds with increased oxygen consumption and raised metabolism, which results in greater heat production. Prolonged exposure to the cold may result in depleted glycogen stores and acidosis. Oxygen consumption also increases if the environmental temperature is above the TNZ.

To accomplish thermal regulation, the neonate must possess a system of surface sensors to perceive temperature differences, a central control system (the hypothalamus), and a means to adjust heat production and heat loss (vasomotor control) (Avery 1987). Vasomotor control aids the retention of heat through vasoconstriction and permits heat loss through vasodilatation.

Heat Loss

A newborn is at a distinct disadvantage in maintaining a normal temperature because of its larger body surface in relation to mass and a limited amount of insulating subcutaneous fat. With a body weight approximately 5 percent of the adult's and a body surface nearly 15 percent of the adult's, the full-term newborn loses about four times as

Table 27–3   Neutral Thermal Environmental Temperatures*

Age and weight	Range of temperature (°C)†	Age and weight	Range of temperature (°C)†
0–6 HOURS		**72–96 HOURS**	
Under 1200 g	34.0–35.4	Under 1200 g	34.0–35.0
1200–1500 g	33.9–34.4	1200–1500 g	33.0–34.0
1501–2500 g	32.8–33.8	1501–2500 g	31.1–33.2
Over 2500 (and >36 weeks)	32.0–33.8	Over 2500 (and >36 weeks)	29.8–32.8
6–12 HOURS		**4–12 DAYS**	
Under 1200 g	34.0–35.4	Under 1500 g	33.0–34.0
1200–1500 g	33.5–34.4	1501–2500 g	31.0–33.2
1501–2500 g	32.2–33.8	Over 2500 (and >36 weeks)	
Over 2500 (and >36 weeks)	31.4–33.8	4–5 days	29.5–32.6
		5–6 days	29.4–32.3
12–24 HOURS		6–8 days	29.0–32.2
Under 1200 g	34.0–35.4	8–10 days	29.0–31.8
1200–1500 g	33.3–34.3	10–12 days	29.0–31.4
1501–2500 g	31.8–33.8		
Over 2500 (and >36 weeks)	31.0–33.7	**12–14 DAYS**	
		Under 1500 g	32.6–34.0
24–36 HOURS		1500–2500 g	31.0–33.2
Under 1200 g	34.0–35.0	Over 2500 (and >36 weeks)	29.0–30.8
1200–1500 g	33.1–34.2		
1501–2500 g	31.6–33.6	**2–3 WEEKS**	
Over 2500 (and >36 weeks)	30.7–33.5	Under 1500 g	32.2–34.0
		1500–2500 g	30.5–33.0
36–48 HOURS			
Under 1200 g	34.0–35.0	**3–4 WEEKS**	
1200–1500 g	33.0–34.1	Under 1500 g	31.6–33.6
1501–2500 g	31.4–33.5	1500–2500 g	30.0–32.7
Over 2500 (and >36 weeks)	30.5–33.3		
		4–5 WEEKS	
48–72 HOURS		Under 1500 g	31.2–33.0
Under 1200 g	34.0–35.0	1500–2500 g	29.5–32.2
1200–1500 g	33.0–34.0		
1501–2500 g	31.2–33.4	**5–6 WEEKS**	
Over 2500 g (and >36 weeks)	30.1–33.2	Under 1500 g	30.6–32.3
		1500–2500 g	29.0–31.8

*Adapted from Scopes and Ahmed (1966). For his table, Scopes had the walls of the incubator 1–2 degrees warmer than the ambient air temperatures.
†Generally speaking, the smaller infants in each weight group will require a temperature in the higher portion of the temperature range. Within each time range, the younger the infant, the higher the temperature required.

From Klaus MH, Fanaroff AA: *Care of the High-Risk Neonate,* ed 3. Philadelphia, Saunders, 1986, p 103.

much heat as an adult (Danforth & Scott 1986). The neonate's poor thermal stability is primarily due to excessive heat loss rather than to impaired heat production. Because of the risk of hypothermia, minimizing heat loss in the newborn after delivery is essential (see Chapters 23 and 29 for nursing measures).

Two major routes of heat loss are from the internal core of the body to the body surface, and from the external surface to the environment. Usually the core temperature is 0.5C higher than the skin temperature, providing for the continuous transfer or conduction of heat to the surface. The greater the difference in temperatures between core and skin, the more rapid the transfer. Heat loss from the body surface to the environment takes place by four avenues—convection, radiation, evaporation, and conduction.

- *Convection* is the loss of heat from the warm body surface to the cooler air currents. Air-conditioned rooms, oxygen by mask, and removal from an incubator for procedures done without an overhead warmer increase convective heat loss of the neonate.

- *Radiation* losses occur when heat transfers from the heated body surface to cooler surfaces and objects not in direct contact with the body. The walls of a room or of an incubator are potential causes of heat loss by radiation, even if the ambient temperature of the isolette is within the thermal neutral range for that infant.

- *Evaporation* is the loss of heat incurred when water is converted to a vapor. The newborn is particularly prone to lose heat by evaporation immediately after delivery, when the infant is wet with amniotic fluid, and during baths.

Conduction is the loss of heat to a cooler surface by direct skin contact. Chilled hands, cool scales, cold examination tables, and cold stethoscopes can cause loss of heat by conduction.

After birth, the highest losses of heat generally result from radiation and convection because of the newborn's large body surface compared with weight, and from thermal conduction because of the marked difference between core temperature and skin temperature. The newborn can respond to the cooler environmental temperature with adequate peripheral vasoconstriction, but this mechanism is less effective because of the minimal amount of fat insulation present, the large body surface, and ongoing thermal conduction. Because of these factors, minimizing the baby's heat loss and preventing hypothermia are imperative. Nursing measures for preventing hypothermia can be found in Chapter 29.

Heat Production (Thermogenesis)

Upon being exposed to a cool environment, the neonate requires additional heat. Several sources of heat production, or *thermogenesis,* are available, including increased basal metabolic rate, muscular activity, and chemical thermogenesis (also referred to as *nonshivering thermogenesis*) mediated through the release of catecholamines (Avery & Taeusch 1984).

Nonshivering thermogenesis is unique to the newborn and uses the newborn's stores of brown adipose tissue. *Brown adipose tissue* (BAT), or brown fat, is the primary source of heat in the cold-stressed newborn. It first appears in the fetus at 26 to 30 weeks' gestation and continues to increase in supply until 2 to 5 weeks after the birth of a full-term neonate, unless it is depleted by cold stress. Brown fat is deposited in the midscapular area, around the neck, and in the axillas, with deeper placement around the trachea, esophagus, abdominal aorta, kidneys, and adrenal glands (Figure 27–7). It constitutes 2 percent to 6 percent of the newborn's total body weight. Brown fat receives its name from its dark color, which is due to its enriched blood supply, dense cellular content, and abundant nerve endings.

The structures of brown and white fat cells differ, as do their functions. In brown fat, the large numbers of fat cells facilitate the speed with which triglycerides can be metabolized to produce heat. Energy is provided by the presence of glycogen and large numbers of mitochondria releasing adenosine triphosphate (ATP) for rapid metabolic turnover and production of heat. In addition, brown fat possesses a rich blood supply to enhance distribution of heat throughout the body, and a nerve supply for initiation

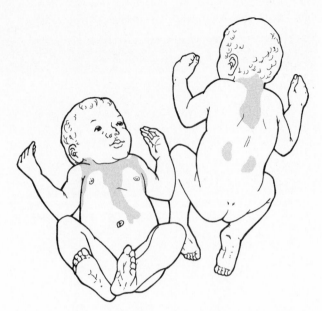

Figure 27–7   The distribution of brown adipose tissue (brown fat) in the neonate (Adapted from Davis V: Structure and function of brown adipose tissue in the neonate. *J Obstet Gynecol Neonat Nurs* 1980;9(November/December):364)

of metabolic activity. This type of metabolism is specific to the newborn. The brown fat is metabolized and used within several weeks after birth (Korones 1986).

Chemical thermogenesis occurs when skin receptors perceive environmental temperature changes and transmit sensations to the CNS, which in turn stimulates the sympathetic nervous system. Release of norepinephrine by the adrenal gland and at local nerve endings in the brown fat causes the metabolism of the triglycerides to fatty acids, thereby releasing heat to be distributed to the body. Brown fat is a major producer of heat for the cold-stressed neonate because of its greater heat production capacity.

Shivering, a form of muscular activity common in the cold adult, is rarely seen in the newborn, although it has been observed at ambient temperatures of 15C (59F) or less. If shivering does appear, it means the infant's metabolic rate has already doubled and the extra muscular activity does little to produce needed heat.

After being exposed to cold, thermographic studies of newborns show an increase in the skin heat over the brown fat deposits in the neonate between 1 and 14 days of age. If the brown fat supply has been depleted, the metabolic response to cold will be limited or lacking. An increase in basal metabolism as a result of hypothermia results in an increase in oxygen consumption. A decrease in the environmental temperature of 2C (36F) is a drop sufficient to double the oxygen consumption of a term neonate (Avery & Taeusch 1984).

The normal term neonate is usually able to cope with the increase, but the preterm neonate may be unable to increase ventilation to the necessary level of oxygen consumption. As a consequence, providing the newborn with an optimal thermal environment is absolutely necessary to prevent neonatal cold stress and the resulting metabolic physiologic responses. (See Chapter 32 for discussion of cold stress.)

Hypoxia and the effect of certain drugs (such as Demerol) may also prevent metabolism of brown fat. Demerol given to the laboring woman leads to a greater fall in the newborn's body temperature during the neonatal period. It is important to remember that neonatal hypothermia prolongs as well as potentiates the effects of many analgesic and anesthetic drugs in the neonate.

Response to Heat

Sweating is the usual initial response of the newborn to hyperthermia. The neonate has six times as many sweat glands as the adult, but the newborn's activity level is one-third that of the adult. The glands have limited function until after the fourth week of extrauterine life. Dissipation of heat is accomplished by peripheral vasodilation and evaporation of insensible water loss. Oxygen consumption and metabolic rate also increase in response to hyperthermia. Severe hyperthermia can lead to death or gross brain damage if the baby survives (Korones 1986).

● Hepatic Adaptations

In the newborn, the liver is frequently palpable 2 to 3 cm below the right costal margin. It is relatively large and occupies about 40 percent of the abdominal cavity. The neonatal liver plays a significant role in iron storage, carbohydrate metabolism, conjugation of bilirubin, and coagulation.

Iron Storage

As red blood cells are destroyed after birth, the iron is stored in the liver until needed for new red blood cell production. Neonatal iron stores are proportional to total body hemoglobin content and length of gestation. The term newborn has about 270 mg of iron at birth, and about 140 to 170 mg of this amount is in the hemoglobin (Avery & Taeusch 1984). If the mother's iron intake has been adequate, enough iron will be stored to last until the fifth month of neonatal life. At this time, foods containing iron or iron supplements must be given to prevent anemia in the infant.

Carbohydrate Metabolism

At term, the newborn's cord blood glucose is 70 percent to 80 percent of the maternal blood. Neonatal carbohydrate reserves are relatively low. One-third of this reserve is in the form of liver glycogen. Neonatal glycogen stores are twice that of the adult. Blood glucose levels are influenced by a balance between liver glucose output and peripheral uptake, body temperature, insulin concentration, and muscular activity. The newborn enters an energy crunch at the time of birth with the removal of the maternal glucose supply and the increased energy expenditure associated with the birth process and extrauterine life. Fuel sources are consumed at a faster rate because of the work of breathing, loss of heat when exposed to cold, activity, and activation of muscle tone. Glucose is the main source of energy in the first few (four to six) hours after delivery. The blood glucose level falls rapidly and then stabilizes at values of 50 to 60 mg/dL for several days; by the third day postnatally the mean values increase to 60 to 70 mg/dL. If the fetus or neonate experiences hypoxia, the glycogen stores are used and may be depleted to meet metabolic requirements. As stores of liver and muscle glycogen and blood glucose decrease, the neonate compensates by changing from a predominantly carbohydrate metabolism to fat metabolism. Energy is derived from fat and protein as well as from carbohydrates. The amount and availability of each of these "fuel substrates" depends on constraints imposed by immature metabolic pathways (lack of specific enzymes or hormones) in the first few days of life.

Conjugation of Bilirubin

Unconjugated (indirect) bilirubin is a breakdown product derived from hemoglobin that is released from lysed red blood cells and heme pigments found in cell elements (nonerythrocyte bilirubin). Unconjugated bilirubin is not in excretable form and is a potential toxin. Total serum bilirubin is the sum of direct and indirect bilirubin.

The fetus does not conjugate bilirubin, which allows it to cross the placenta. Fetal unconjugated bilirubin is normally excreted by the placenta in utero, so total bilirubin at birth is usually less than 3 mg/dL unless an abnormal hemolytic process has been present. Postnatally, the infant must conjugate bilirubin (convert a lipid-soluble pigment into a water-soluble pigment) in the liver, producing a rise in serum bilirubin in the first few days of life.

Unconjugated albumin-bound bilirubin is taken up by the liver cells. Since albumin does not transfer into the liver cells, the bilirubin must be transferred to two other intracellular binding proteins labeled Y and Z. These determine the amount of bilirubin held in a liver cell for processing and consequently the potential amount of bilirubin uptake into the liver. The clearance and conjugation of bilirubin depend on the glucuronyl transferase enzyme. Activity of this enzyme results in the attachment of unconjugated bilirubin to glucuronic acid (product of liver glycogen) producing conjugated, direct bilirubin. It is excreted into the tiny bile ducts, then into the common duct and duodenum. The conjugated bilirubin then progresses down the intestines, where bacteria transform it into urobilinogen. This product is not reabsorbed but is excreted as a yellow-brown pigment in the stools.

The newborn liver has relatively less glucuronyl transferase activity at birth and in the first few weeks of life than an adult. This reduction in activity predisposes to decreased conjugation of bilirubin and increased susceptibility to jaundice.

Even after the bilirubin has been conjugated and bound, it can be converted back to unconjugated bilirubin by enterohepatic circulation. In the intestines β-glucuronidase enzyme acts to split off (deconjugate) the bilirubin from glucuronic acid if it has not first been reduced by gut bacteria to urobilinogen; the free bilirubin is reabsorbed though the intestinal wall and brought back to the liver via portal vein circulation. This recycling of the bilirubin and decreased ability to clear bilirubin from the system are prevalent in babies who have very high β-glucuronidase activity levels as well as delayed bacterial colonization of the gut.

PHYSIOLOGIC JAUNDICE (ICTERUS NEONATORUM)

The fetal liver begins to metabolize bilirubin at 12 weeks of gestation, but this ability disappears by 36 weeks. The fetus does not conjugate bilirubin so that it can cross the placenta to be excreted. Physiologic jaundice, caused by accelerated lysis of fetal red blood cells, impaired conjugation of bilirubin, and increased bilirubin reabsorption from the intestinal tract does *not* have a pathologic basis but is a normal biologic response of the newborn.

Oski (1984) describes six factors whose interactions may give rise to physiologic jaundice:

1. *Greater bilirubin loads to the liver.* In the neonate, the combination of an increased blood volume, largely due to delayed cord clamping, and accelerated lysis of the fetal red blood cell contributes to an increased bilirubin level in the blood. The neonate has a shorter erythrocyte (RBC) life span (80 to 100 days instead of 120) and a proportionately larger amount of nonerythrocyte bilirubin formed than the adult. Therefore, newborns have two to three times greater production or breakdown of bilirubin.

2. *Defective uptake of bilirubin from the plasma.* If the newborn does not ingest adequate calories, the formation of hepatic binding proteins diminishes, resulting in higher bilirubin levels.

3. *Defective conjugation of the bilirubin.* Decreased glucuronyl-transferase activity results in greater bilirubin values. The presence of the enzyme $3\alpha 20\beta$ propregnandiol in breast milk is thought to further impede the conjugation of bilirubin.

4. *Defect in bilirubin excretion.* A congenital infection may cause impaired excretion. Delay in introduction of bacterial flora and decreased intestinal mobility can also delay excretion.

5. *Inadequate hepatic circulation.* Decreased oxygen supplies to the liver associated with neonatal hypoxia or congenital heart disease lead to a rise in the bilirubin level.

6. *Increased reabsorption of bilirubin from the intestine.* Reduced bowel motility, intestinal obstruction, or delayed passage of meconium increases the circulation of bilirubin in the enterohepatic pathway, thereby resulting in higher bilirubin values.

About 50 percent of full-term neonates and 80 percent of preterm neonates exhibit physiologic jaundice on about the second or third day after birth. The characteristic icteric (yellow) color results from increased levels of unconjugated bilirubin. These are a normal product of red blood cell hemolysis and reflect a temporary inability of the body to eliminate bilirubin. The manifestations of physiologic jaundice appear *after* the first 24 hours postnatally. This differentiates physiologic jaundice from pathologic jaundice (Chapter 32), which is clinically evident at birth or within the first 24 hours of postnatal life. Serum levels of bilirubin are about 4 to 6 mg/dL before yellow coloration of the skin and sclera appears.

During the first week, unconjugated bilirubin levels in physiologic jaundice should not exceed 12 to 12.5 mg/dL in the full-term or preterm newborn (Sills & Coen 1984). Peak bilirubin levels are reached between days 3 and 5 in the full-term infant and between days 5 and 6 in the preterm infant. These values are established for European and American newborns. Chinese, Japanese, Korean, and American Indian neonates have considerably higher bilirubin levels that persist for longer periods with no apparent ill effects (Oski 1984).

Nursery environment, including lighting, hinders the early detection of the degree and type of jaundice. Pink walls and artificial lights mask the beginning of jaundice in newborns. Daylight assists the observer in early recognition by eliminating distortions caused by artificial light.

The following nursery procedures are designed to decrease the probability of high bilirubin levels:

● The infant's body temperature is maintained at 36.4C (97.6F) or above, since chilling results in acidosis. This condition in turn decreases available serum albumin–binding sites, weakens albumin-binding powers, and causes elevated unconjugated bilirubin levels.

● Stool is monitored for amount and characteristics. Bilirubin is eliminated in the feces; inadequate stooling may result in reabsorption and recycling of bilirubin. Early breast-feeding is encouraged because the laxative effect of colostrum increases excretion of stool.

- Early feedings are also encouraged to promote intestinal elimination and bacterial colonization, and to provide caloric intake necessary for formation of hepatic binding proteins.

If jaundice is suspected, the nurse can quickly assess the neonate's coloring by pressing his or her skin with a finger. As the blanching occurs, the nurse can observe the icterus (yellow coloring). If jaundice becomes apparent, nursing care is directed toward keeping the neonate well hydrated and promoting intestinal elimination. For specific nursing management and therapies, see the Nursing Care Plan on p 1048.

Physiologic jaundice may be very upsetting to parents; they require emotional support and thorough explanation of the condition. Necessary hospitalization of the newborn for a few additional days may also be disturbing to parents. They should be encouraged to provide for the emotional needs of their newborn by continuing to feed, hold, and caress the infant. If the mother is discharged, the parents should be encouraged to return for feedings and feel free to telephone or visit whenever possible. In many instances, the mother, especially if she is breast-feeding, may elect to remain hospitalized with her infant; this decision should be supported. As an alternative to extended hospitalization, some newborns are treated in home phototherapy programs (Jaundiced babies . . .1984).

BREAST-FEEDING JAUNDICE

Breast-feeding is implicated in prolonged jaundice in some newborns. According to Korones (1986) 1 percent to 5 percent of newborns being breast-fed will develop breast-feeding jaundice. The breast-fed jaundiced newborn's bilirubin level begins to rise about the fourth day after the mother's milk has come in. The level peaks at two to three weeks of age and may reach 20 to 25 mg/dL without intervention (Oski 1984).

It is theorized that some women's breast milk may contain several times the normal concentration of certain free fatty acids. These free fatty acids may inhibit the conjugation of bilirubin or increase lipase activity, which disrupts the red blood cell membrane. Increased lipase activity enhances absorption of bile across the GI tract membrane, thereby increasing the enterohepatic circulation of bilirubin. In the past it was thought that the breast milk of women whose newborns have breast-feeding jaundice contained an enzyme that inhibited glucuronyl transferase.

Newborns with breast milk jaundice appear well, and at present there is an absence of documented kernicterus with this type of jaundice. Even so it is suggested that traditional guidelines should be followed (Neville & Neifert

1983). Interruption of nursing may be advised if bilirubin reaches presumed toxic levels of approximately 20 mg/dL or if the interruption is necessary to establish the cause of the hyperbilirubinemia (Oski 1984). Within 24 to 36 hours after discontinuing breast-feeding, the newborn's serum bilirubin levels begin to fall dramatically, returning to normal levels in four to eight days.

Many physicians believe that breast-feeding may be resumed once other causes of jaundice have been ruled out, although the bilirubin concentration may rise 1 to 3 mg/dL with a subsequent decline (Oski 1984). Nursing mothers need encouragement and support in their desire to nurse their infants, assistance and instruction regarding pumping and expressing milk during the interrupted nursing period, and reassurance that nothing is wrong with their milk or mothering abilities.

Coagulation

The liver plays an important part in blood coagulation during fetal life and continues this function to some degree during the first few months following birth. Coagulation factors II, VII, IX, X (synthesized in the liver), and prothrombin are activated under the influence of vitamin K and therefore are considered vitamin K-dependent. The absence of normal flora needed to synthesize vitamin K in the newborn gut results in low levels of vitamin K and creates a transient blood coagulation deficiency between the second and fifth day of life. From a low point at about 2 to 3 days after birth, these coagulation factors rise slowly, but reach adult levels at nine months of age or later.

Vitamin K dependent coagulation factors increase in response to dietary intake and bacterial colonization of the intestines. An injection of vitamin K (AquaMEPHYTON) is given prophylactically on the day of birth to combat potential clinical bleeding problems. (Hemorrhagic disease of the newborn is discussed in more depth in Chapter 32.) Breast milk contains one-quarter the amount of vitamin K per deciliter in cow's milk, so milk intake restores prothrombin time faster than breast-feeding (Korones 1986) if there is a bleeding problem. Other coagulation factors with low cord blood levels are XI, XII, and XIII. Fibrinogen and factors V and VII are near adult ranges (Oski & Naiman 1982).

Platelet counts at birth are in the same range as for adults, but newborns may manifest mild transient platelet aggregation functioning defect. This platelet defect is accentuated by phototherapy (Hatch & Sumner 1981).

Prenatal maternal therapy with phenytoin sodium (Dilantin) or phenobarbital also causes abnormal clotting studies and neonatal bleeding in the first 24 hours after birth. Infants born to mothers receiving coumarin (warfarin) compounds may bleed because these agents cross the placenta and accentuate existing vitamin K-dependent factor deficiencies.

● Gastrointestinal Adaptations

Fetal-Neonatal Transitional Physiology

Full maturity of the gastrointestinal tract is achieved by 36 to 38 weeks' gestation with the presence of enzymatic activity and the ability to transport nutrients. The intestines are about 240 to 300 cm in length at term, or about three to four times the crown-to-heel length of the newborn. Differentiation and maturation of the structures necessary for digestion progress from the proximal to the distal parts of the sytem. Development of the secretory and absorbing surfaces is greater than that of the supporting musculature. All glandular elements found in the adult mucosa are present at birth, but the fetal structures are shallower and less functional.

By birth, the neonate has experienced swallowing, gastric emptying, and intestinal propulsion. In utero, swallowing is accompanied by gastric emptying and peristalsis of the fetal intestinal tract. By the end of gestation, peristalsis becomes much more active in preparation for extrauterine life. Fetal peristalsis is also stimulated by anoxia, causing the expulsion of meconium into the amniotic fluid.

Air enters the stomach immediately after birth. The small intestine is filled within 2 to 12 hours and the large bowel within 24 hours. The salivary glands are immature at birth and little saliva is manufactured until the infant is about three months old. The newborn's stomach has a capacity of 50 to 60 mL. It empties intermittently, starting within a few minutes of the beginning of a feeding and ending between two and four hours after feeding.

The cardiac sphincter is immature, as is nervous control of the stomach, so some regurgitation may be noted in the neonatal period. Regurgitation of the first few feedings during the first day or two of life can usually be lessened by avoiding overfeeding and by burping the newborn well during and after the feeding.

When no other signs and symptoms are evident, vomiting is limited and ceases within the first few days of life. Continuous vomiting or regurgitation should be observed closely. If the newborn has swallowed bloody or purulent amniotic fluid, lavage may be indicated to relieve the problem.

Normal term newborns pass meconium within 12 to 48 hours of birth (Avery & Taeusch, 1984). Meconium is formed in utero from the amniotic fluid and its constituents, together with intestinal secretions and shed mucosal cells. It is recognized by its thick, tarry, dark green appearance. Transitional (thin brown to green) stools consisting of part meconium and part fecal material are passed for the next day or two, after which the stools become entirely fecal. Generally, the stools of a breast-fed newborn are pale yellow (but may be pasty green); they are more liquid and more frequent than those of formula-fed neonates, whose are paler in color. Bowel movement is individualized but ranges from one every two to three days to as many as ten daily.

Digestive Function

The term neonate has adequate intestinal and pancreatic enzymes to digest most simple carbohydrates, proteins, and fats. The newborn's gastric acidity is equal to an adult's but becomes less acidic in about a week and remains lower than that of adults for two to three months. The stomach secretes pepsinogen, which is necessary for protein digestion and production of hydrochloric acid. Both pepsinogen and hydrochloric acid are necessary for the digestion of milk prior to its entrance into the small bowel. Digestion and absorption of nutrients are primarily functions of the small bowel, where pancreatic secretions digest starches and proteins. Bile secretions from the gallbladder through the bile duct aid in fat absorption, and duodenal secretions complete this complex process.

DIGESTION OF CARBOHYDRATES

The carbohydrates requiring digestion in the newborn are usually disaccharides (lactose, maltose, sucrose), which are split into monosaccharides (galactose, fructose, and glucose) by the enzymes of the intestinal mucosa. Lactose is the primary carbohydrate in the breast-feeding newborn and is generally easily digested and well absorbed. The only enzyme lacking at birth is pancreatic amylase, which remains relatively deficient during the first few months of life. Therefore, newborns have trouble digesting starches (changing more complex carbohydrates into maltose).

DIGESTION OF PROTEINS

Although proteins require more digestion than carbohydrates, they are well digested and absorbed from the neonatal intestine. Protein digestive enzymes have been present in the fetus from about midgestation. The proteolytic enzymes of the intestinal mucosa facilitate hydrolysis of protein while enterocytes transfer resultant amino acids to the blood.

DIGESTION OF FATS

Fats are digested and absorbed less efficiently by the newborn than by the child because of the minimal activity of the pancreatic enzyme lipase in the newborn. The neonate excretes 10 percent to 20 percent of the dietary fat intake, compared with 10 percent for the adult. The fat in breast milk is absorbed more completely by the newborn than is the fat in straight cow's milk because it consists of more medium-chain triglycerides and contains lipase. (See Chapter 30 for a more detailed discussion of infant nutrition.)

Adequate digestion and absorption are essential for neonatal growth and development. If optimal nutritional support is available, postnatal growth ideally should parallel intrauterine growth; that is, after 30 weeks of gestation, the fetus gains 30 g per day and adds 1.2 cm to body length daily. Caloric intake is often insufficient for weight gain until the newborn is five to ten days old. During this time there may be a weight loss of 5 percent to 10 percent. Shift of intracellular water to extracellular space and insensible water loss account for the expected 5 percent to 10 percent weight loss. Failure to lose this weight when caloric intake is inadequate may indicate fluid retention.

● Urinary Adaptations

Kidney Development and Function

Certain physiologic features of the newborn's kidneys are important to consider when looking at the newborn's ability to manage body fluids and excretional function:

1. The term newborn's kidneys have a full complement of functioning nephrons.

2. The glomerular filtration rate of the newborn's kidney is low in comparison with the adult rate. Because of this physiologic inefficiency, the newborn's kidney is unable to dispose of water rapidly when necessary.

3. The juxtamedullary portion of the nephron has limited capacity to reabsorb Na^+ and H^+ and concentrate urine. The limitation of tubular reabsorption can lead to inappropriate loss of substances present in the glomerular filtrate, such as amino acids and bicarbonate.

Full-term newborns are less able than adults to concentrate urine (reabsorb water back into the serum) because the tubules are short and narrow. There is a greater capacity for glomerular filtration than for tubular reabsorption-secretion. Although feeding practices may affect the osmolarity of the urine, the maximum concentrating ability of the newborn is a specific gravity of 1.025. The inability to concentrate urine is due to the limited excretion of solutes (principally sodium, potassium, chloride, bicarbonate, urea, and phosphate) in the growing newborn. The ability to concentrate urine fully is attained by three months of age.

Since the newborn has difficulty concentrating urine, the effect of excessive insensible water loss or restricted fluid intake is unpredictable. The newborn kidney is also limited in its dilutional capabilities. Maximal dilution ability is specific gravity of 1.001. Concentrating and dilutional limitations of renal function are important considerations in monitoring fluid therapy to avoid dehydration and overhydration.

Characteristics of Newborn Urinary Function

Many newborns void in the delivery room and it goes unnoticed. Among normal newborns, 92 percent void by 24 hours after birth and 99 percent void by 48 hours (Fanaroff & Martin 1983). A newborn who has not voided by 72 hours should be assessed for adequacy of fluid intake, bladder distention, restlessness, and symptoms of pain. Appropriate clinical personnel should be notified if indicated.

The initial bladder volume is 6 to 44 mL of urine. Unless edema is present, normal urinary output is often limited, and the voidings are scanty until fluid intake increases. (The fluid of edema is eliminated by the kidneys, so infants with edema have a much higher urinary output.) The first two days postnatally, the newborn voids two to six times daily, with a urine output of 30 to 60 mL per day. The newborn subsequently voids 5 to 25 times every 24 hours, with a volume of 30 to 50 mL/kg per day.

Following the first voiding, the newborn's urine frequently appears cloudy (due to mucus content) and has a high specific gravity, which decreases as fluid intake increases. Occasionally pink stains ("brick dust spots") appear on the diaper. These are caused by urates and are innocuous. Blood may occasionally be observed on the diapers of female infants. This *pseudomenstruation* is related to the withdrawal of maternal hormones. Males may have bloody spotting from a circumcision. In the absence of apparent causes for bleeding, the clinician should be notified. Normal urine during early infancy is straw-colored and almost odorless, although odor occurs when certain drugs are given or when infection is present. Box 27–1 contains urinalysis values of the normal newborn.

● Immunologic Adaptations

The cells that constitute the immune system appear early in fetal life, but usually are not *fully* activated until sometime after birth. The newborn possesses varying de-

Box 27–1   Newborn Urinalysis Values
Protein <5–10 mg/dL
WBC <2–3
RBC 0
Casts 0
Bacteria 0

grees of nonspecific and specific immunity. The nonspecific mechanism of opsonization—the process of coating invasive bacteria to ready them for ingestion by phagocytic cells—is impaired. Immunoglobulins (specific immunity) are a type of antibody secreted by the lymphocytes and plasma cells into the body fluids. Fetal albumin, globulin, and other immunoglobulins are present throughout the last trimester of gestation.

The three major types of immunoglobulins—IgG, IgA, and IgM—are primarily involved in immunity. Of these three, only IgG crosses the placenta. When IgG antibodies are transferred to the fetus in utero, *passive acquired immunity* results, because the fetus does not produce the antibodies itself. Because a transfer of maternal immunoglobulin occurs primarily during the third trimester, preterm infants (especially those born prior to 34 weeks) may be more susceptible to infection.

The fetus receives immunity in utero (if mother has specific antibodies) to tetanus, diphtheria, smallpox, measles, mumps, poliomyelitis, and a variety of other bacterial and viral diseases. IgG is very active against bacteria. The IgG level in newborns is 700 to 1300 mg/dL (Danforth & Scott 1986). The period of resistance varies: Immunity against common viral infections such as measles may last four to eight months, whereas immunity to certain bacteria may disappear within four to eight weeks.

IgM immunoglobulins in the expectant mother are primarily antibodies to blood group antigens, gram negative enteric organisms, and some viruses. Because IgM does not normally cross the placenta, most or all IgM immunoglobulins are produced by the fetus/newborn as part of the initial antigen-antibody response to practically all infectious agents. IgM levels in the newborn range from 0 to 20 mg/dL (Korones 1986). Elevated levels of IgM at birth (greater than 20 mg/dL) may indicate placental leaks or, more commonly, antigenic stimulation in utero. Consequently, elevations suggest that the infant was exposed to an intrauterine infection such as rubella, syphilis, toxoplasmosis, herpesvirus, or cytomegalovirus. The lack of available maternal IgM in the newborn also accounts for the infant's increased susceptibility to gram negative enteric organisms such as *E. coli.*

The functions of IgA immunoglobulins are not fully understood, although they appear to provide protection mainly on secreting surfaces such as the respiratory tract, gastrointestinal tract, and eyes. Serum IgA does not cross the placenta and is not normally produced by the fetus in utero. Unlike the other immunoglobulins, IgA has a secretory form that is not affected by gastric action. Colostrum, the forerunner of breast milk, is very high in secretory form of IgA. Consequently, it provides some passive immunity to the baby of a breast-feeding mother. Newborns begin to produce secretory IgA in their intestinal mucosa at about four weeks after birth.

The incredible attributes of the newborn have a major purpose. They prepare the baby for interaction with the family and for life in the world. (*The Amazing Newborn*)

● Neurologic and Sensory/Perceptual Adaptations

The newborn's brain is about one-quarter the size of an adult's, and myelination of nerve fibers is incomplete. Unlike the cardiovascular or respiratory systems, which undergo tremendous changes at birth, the nervous system is minimally influenced by the actual birth process.

Because many biochemical and histologic changes have yet to occur in the newborn's brain, the postnatal period is considered a time of risk to the development of the brain and nervous system. For neurologic development—including development of intellect—to proceed, the brain and other nervous system structures must mature in an orderly, unhampered fashion.

Intrauterine Factors Influencing Newborn Behavior

The newborn responds to and interacts with the environment in a predictable pattern of behavior that is somewhat shaped by his or her intrauterine experience. This intrauterine experience is affected by intrinsic factors such as maternal nutrition and external factors such as the mother's physical environment. Depending on the newborn's intrauterine experience, neonatal behavioral responses to various stresses vary from dealing quietly with the stimulation, to becoming overreactive and tense, to a combination of the two.

Brazelton (1975, 1977) found a positive association between newborn behavior and nutritional status of the pregnant woman. Newborns with higher birth weight attended and responded to visual and auditory cues and exhibited more mature motor activity than low-birth-weight newborns.

Factors such as exposure to intense auditory stimuli in utero can eventually be manifested in the behavior of the newborn. For example, the fetal heart rate initially increases when the pregnant woman is exposed to an auditory stimuli, but repetition of the stimuli leads to decreased FHR. Thus the newborn who was exposed to intense noise during fetal life is significantly less reactive to loud sounds postnatally.

Characteristics of Newborn Neurologic Function

Partially flexed extremities with the legs near the abdomen is the usual position of the normal newborn. When awake, the newborn may exhibit purposeless, uncoordinated bilateral movements of the extremities. The organization and intensity of the newborn's motor activity are influenced by a number of factors including the following (Brazelton 1984): (a) sleep-wake states; (b) presence of environmental stimuli such as heat, light, cold, and noise; (c) conditions causing a chemical imbalance, such as hypoglycemia; (d) hydration status; (e) state of health; and (f) recovery from the stress of labor and delivery. If movements are absent, minimal, or obviously asymmetrical, neurologic dysfunction should be suspected.

Eye movements are observable during the first few days of life. An alert neonate is able to fixate on faces and brightly colored objects. If a bright light shines in the newborn's eyes, the blinking response is elicited.

The cry of the newborn should be lusty and vigorous. High-pitched cries, weak cries, or no cries are all causes for concern.

Growth of the newborn's body progresses in a cephalocaudal (head-to-toe), proximal-distal fashion. The newborn is somewhat hypertonic; that is, there is resistance to extending the elbow and knee joints. Muscle tone should be symmetrical. Diminished muscle tone and flaccidity may indicate neurologic dysfunction.

Specific symmetrical deep tendon reflexes can be elicited in the newborn. The knee jerk is brisk; a normal ankle clonus may involve three or four beats. Plantar flexion is present. Other reflexes, including the Moro, grasping, rooting, and sucking reflexes are characteristic of neurologic integrity.

Performance of complex behavioral patterns reflects the newborn's neurological maturation and integration. The newborn who can bring a hand to his mouth is demonstrating motor coordination as well as a self-quieting technique, thus increasing the complexity of the behavioral response. Neonates also possess complex organized defensive motor patterns as exhibited by the ability to approach and remove an obstruction, such as a cloth across the face.

Behavioral States of the Newborn

The behavior of the newborn can be divided into two categories, the sleep state and the alert state (Prechtl & Beintema 1964, Brazelton 1984). These postnatal behavioral states are similar to those that have been identified during pregnancy (Nijhuis et al 1982, Tuck 1986). Subcategories are identified under each major category.

SLEEP STATES

The following sleep states have been identified in the newborn:

1. *Deep or quiet sleep.* Deep sleep is characterized by closed eyes with no eye movements, regular even breathing, and jerky motion or startles at regular intervals. Behavioral responses to external stimuli are likely to be delayed. Startles are rapidly suppressed, and changes in state are not likely to occur.

2. *Active REM.* Irregular respirations, eyes closed with REM, irregular sucking motions, minimal activity, and irregular but smooth movement of the extremities can be observed in active REM sleep. Environmental and internal stimuli initiate a startle reaction and a change of state.

These sleep cycles are defined based on length of the time cycle. The length of the cycle is contingent upon the age of the newborn. At term, REM active sleep and quiet sleep occur in intervals of 45 to 50 minutes. Rapid eye movement is also present in both the first half and second half of quiet sleep. When viewed in percentages, about 45 percent to 50 percent of the total sleep of the neonate is active sleep, 35 percent to 45 percent is quiet (deep) sleep, and 10 percent of sleep is transitional between these two periods. It is hypothesized that REM sleep stimulates the growth of the neural system. Over a period of time, the neonate's sleep-wake patterns become diurnal; that is, the infant sleeps at night and stays awake during the day. (See Chapter 28 for in-depth discussion of assessment of neonatal states.)

ALERT STATES

In the first 30 to 60 minutes after birth, many neonates display a quiet alert state, characteristic of the first period of reactivity (Saigal et al 1981) (Figure 27–8). About 12 to 18 hours after birth, the infant is again alert when the second period of reactivity occurs. (A further description of these two periods of reactivity is found on p 897.) These periods of alertness tend to be short the first two days after birth to allow the baby to recover from the birth process. Subsequently, alert states are of choice or of necessity (Brazelton 1984). Increasing choice of wakefulness by the newborn indicates a maturing capacity to achieve and maintain consciousness. Heat, cold, and hunger are but a few of the stimuli that can cause wakefulness by necessity. Once the disturbing stimuli are removed, sleep tends to recur.

The following are subcategories of the alert state (Brazelton 1984):

1. *Drowsy or semidozing.* The behaviors common to the drowsy state are open or closed eyes, fluttering eyelids, semidozing appearance, and slow, regular movements of the extremities. Mild startles may be noted from time to time. Although the reaction to a sensory stimulus is delayed, a change of state often results.

2. *Wide awake.* In the wide awake state, the neonate is alert and follows and fixates on attractive objects, faces, or auditory stimuli. Motor activity is minimal, and the response to external stimuli is delayed.

3. *Active awake.* The eyes are open and motor activity is quite intense with thrusting movements of the extremities in the active awake state. Environmental stimuli increase startles or motor activity, but discrete reactions are difficult to distinguish because of generalized high activity level.

4. *Crying.* Intense crying is accompanied by jerky motor movements. Crying serves several purposes for the newborn. It may be used as a distraction from disturbing stimuli such as hunger and pain. Fussiness often allows the neonate to discharge energy and reorganize behavior. Most important, crying elicits an appropriate response of help from the parents.

Sensory Capacities

The newborn is able to process and respond to complex visual stimulation. For example, when a bright light is flashed into the neonate's eyes, the initial response is blinking, constriction of the pupil, and perhaps a slight startle reaction. However, with repeated stimulation, the newborn's response repertoire gradually diminishes and

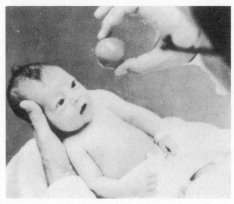

Figure 27–9   Following a red ball (From Avery ME, Taeusch HW (eds): *Schaffer's Diseases of the Newborn.* Philadelphia, Saunders, 1984, p 71)

disappears; this is known as *habituation.* The capacity to ignore repetitive disturbing stimuli is a neonatal defense mechanism readily apparent in the noisy well-lighted nursery.

In addition to being able to disregard specific stimuli, the newborn has the ability to be alert to, to follow, and to fixate on complex visual stimuli that have a particular appeal and attractiveness to the neonate. The newborn prefers the human face and eyes and bright shiny objects. As the face or object is brought into the line of vision, the neonate responds with bright, wide eyes, still limbs, fixed

Figure 27–8   Mother and baby gaze at each other. This quiet, alert state is the optimal state for interaction between baby and parents.

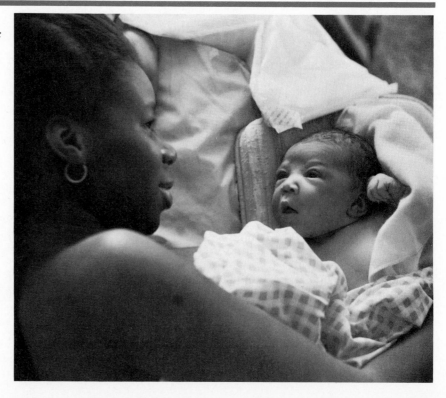

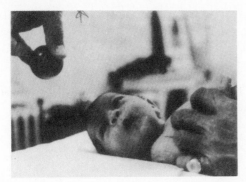

Figure 27–10   Head turning to follow (From Avery ME, Taeusch HW (eds): *Schaffer's Diseases of the Newborn*. Philadelphia, Saunders, 1984, p 71)

staring. This intense visual involvement may last several minutes, during which time the neonate is able to follow the stimulus from side to side. Figures 27–9 and 27–10 illustrate these responses. The newborn uses this sensory capacity to become familiar with family, friends, and surroundings.

AUDITORY CAPACITY

The newborn responds to auditory stimulation with a definite, organized behavior repertoire. The stimulus used to assess auditory response should be selected to match the state of the newborn. A rattle is appropriate for light sleep, a voice for an awake state, and a clap for deep sleep. As the neonate hears the sound, the cardiac rate rises, and a minimal startle reflex may be observed. If the sound is appealing, the newborn will become alert and search for the site of the auditory stimulus.

OLFACTORY CAPACITY

Neonates are able to distinguish their mother's breast pads from those of other mothers by one week postnatally (Brazelton 1984). Apparently this phenomenon is related to the ability of the neonate to select by smell.

TASTE

The newborn responds differently to varying tastes. Sugar, for example, increases sucking. Sucking pattern variations also exist in newborns fed cow's milk or human breast milk (Brazelton 1984). When breast-feeding, the neonate sucks in bursts with frequent regular pauses. The bottle-fed newborn tends to suck at a regular rate with infrequent pauses. The pauses in feeding may be used to interject social communication between the mother and neonate, whether at regular or irregular intervals.

TACTILE CAPACITY

The neonate is very sensitive to being touched, cuddled, and held. Often a mother's first response to an upset or crying newborn is touching or holding. Swaddling, a hand on the abdomen, or holding the arms to prevent a startle reflex are other methods that may soothe the newborn. The settled neonate is then able to attend to and interact with the environment.

SUCKING

When awake and hungry, the neonate displays rapid searching motions in response to the rooting reflex. Once feeding begins, the newborn establishes a sucking pattern according to the method of feeding. Finger sucking is present not only postnatally but also in utero. The neonate frequently uses sucking as a self-quieting activity, which assists in the development of self-regulation.

KEY CONCEPTS

Establishing pulmonary ventilation and the resulting cardiovascular changes are essential for extrauterine survival.

The production of surfactant is crucial to keeping the lungs expanded during expiration by reducing alveolar surface tension.

Neonatal respiration is initiated primarily by chemical and mechancial events in association with thermal and sensory stimulation.

The characteristics of newborn respirations differ from adult respirations because the newborn is an obligatory nose breather. Respirations move from being primarily shallow, irregular, and diaphragmatic to synchronous abdominal and chest breathing.

Periodic breathing is normal, and newborn sleep states affect breathing patterns.

The status of the cardiopulmonary system may be measured by evaluating the heart rate, blood pressure, cardiac output, and presence or absence of murmurs.

Oxygen transport in the newborn is significantly affected by the presence of greater amounts of HbF (fetal hemoglobin) than HbA (adult hemoglobin), which holds oxygen easier but releases it to the body tissues only at low PO$_2$ levels.

Blood values in the newborn are modified by several factors such as site of the blood sample, gestational age,

prenatal and/or perinatal hemorrhage, and the timing of the clamping of the umbilical cord.

Blood glucose level should reach 60 to 70 mg/dL by the third postnatal day.

The newborn is considered to have established thermoregulation when oxygen consumption and metabolic activity are minimal.

Excessive heat loss occurs from radiation and convection because of the newborn's larger surface area when compared to weight; and from thermal conduction because of the marked difference between core temperature and skin temperature.

The newborn generates additional heat primarily by chemical, or nonshivering, thermogenesis.

The primary source of heat in the cold-stressed newborn is brown adipose fat.

The normal newborn possesses the ability to digest and absorb nutrients necessary for neonatal growth and development.

The newborn's liver plays a crucial role in iron storage, carbohydrate metabolism, conjugation of bilirubin, and coagulation.

The newborn's stools change from meconium (thick, tarry, dark green) to transitional stools (thin, brown-to-green) and then to the distinct forms for either breast-fed newborns (yellow-gold, soft, or mushy) or bottle-fed newborns (pale yellow, formed, and pasty).

Controversy continues to exist about the relationship of breast-feeding and the development of prolonged jaundice.

The neonatal kidney is characterized by a decreased rate of glomerular flow, limited tubular reabsorption, limited excretion of solutes, and limited ability to concentrate urine. Most newborns void by between 24 and 48 hours of extrauterine life.

The immune system in the newborn is not fully activated until sometime after birth, but the newborn does possess some specific and nonspecific immunologic abilities.

Neurologic and sensory/perceptual functioning in the newborn is evident from the newborn's interaction with the environment, presence of synchronized motor activity, and well-developed sensory capacities.

Intactness of the nervous system is indicated by the state of alertness, resting posture, cry, and quality of muscle tone and motor activity.

The behavioral states in the neonate can be divided into sleep states and alert states.

REFERENCES

Avery GB: *Neonatology: Pathophysiology and Management of the Newborn.* Philadelphia, Lippincott, 1987.

Avery ME, **Taeusch** H.W. (eds). *Schaffer's Diseases of the Newborn.* Philadelphia, Saunders, 1984.

Brazelton TB, et al: The behavior of nutritionally deprived Guatemalan neonates. *Dev Med Child Neurol* 1977;19:364.

Brazelton TB, et al: Biomedical variables and neonatal performance of Guatemalan infants. Presented to American Academy of Cerebral Palsy, New Orleans, 1975.

Brazelton TB: Neonatal behavior and its significance, in **Avery** ME, **Taeusch** HW (eds): *Schaffer's Diseases of the Newborn.* Philadelphia, Saunders, 1984.

Danforth DH and **Scott** R, (eds): *Obstetrics and Gynecology,* ed 5. Philadelphia, Harper & Row, 1986.

Fanaroff AA, **Martin** RJ: *Behrman's Neonatal-Perinatal Medicine,* ed 3. St Louis, Mosby, 1983.

Glader BE: Erythrocyte disorders in infancy, in **Avery** ME, **Taeusch** HW (eds): *Schaffer's Diseases of the Newborn.* Philadelphia, Saunders, 1984.

Goldstein JD, **Reid** LM: Pulmonary hypoplasia resulting from phrenic nerve agenesis and diaphragmatic amyoplasia. *J Pediat* 1980.97:282.

Hatch DJ, **Sumner** E: *Neonatal Anaesthesia.* Chicago, Year Book Medical Publishers, 1981.

Jaundiced babies bloom with home phototherapy. *Am J Nurs* 1984; 84(7):871.

Korones SB: *High Risk Newborn Infants: The Basis for Intensive Care Nursing,* ed 4. St. Louis, Mosby, 1986.

Neville MC, **Neifert** MR: *Lactation: Physiology, Nutrition, and Breastfeeding.* New York, Plenum Press, 1983.

Nijhuis JG, et al: Are there behavioral states in the human fetus? *Early Human Dev* 1982;6:177.

Oski FA: Physiologic jaundice, in **Avery** ME, **Taeusch** HW (eds): *Schaffer's Diseases of the Newborn.* Philadelphia, Saunders, 1984.

Oski FA, JL **Naiman**: *Hematologic Problems in the Newborn,* ed 3. Philadelphia, Saunders, 1982.

Prechtl HFR, **Beintema** DL: *The Neurological Examination of the Full-Term Newborn Infant.* London, William Heinemann, 1964.

Saigal S, et al: Observations on the behavioral state of newborn infants during the first hour of life. *Am J Obstet Gynecol* 1981;139(March 15):716.

Scopes J and **Ahbmed** I: Range of critical temperatures in sick and premature newborn babies. *Arch Dis Child* 1966;41:417.

Sills JA, **Coen** RW: The neonate, in **Creasy** RK, **Resnik** R (eds): *Maternal Fetal Medicine.* Philadelphia, Saunders, 1984.

Smith CA, **Nelson** NM: *The Physiology of the Newborn Infant,* ed 4. Springfield, Ill, Charles C Thomas, 1976.

Tuck SM: Ultrasound monitoring of fetal behavior. *Ultrasound Med Biol* 1986;12(April):307.

ADDITIONAL READINGS

Avery ME, **Fletcher** BD, **Williams** RG: *The Lung and Its Disorders in the Newborn Infant,* ed 4. Philadelphia, Saunders, 1981.

Bernhardt J: Sensory capabilities of the fetus. *Am J Mat Child Nurs* 1987;12(1):44.

Chess S, **Thomas** A: Temperamental differences: A critical concept in child health care. *Pediatric Nurs* 1985;11(May/June):167.

Choi EC, **Hamilton** RK: The effects of culture on mother-infant interaction. *J Obstet Gynecol Neonat Nurs* 1986;15(3):256.

Creasy RK, **Resnik** R: *Maternal Fetal Medicine.* Philadelphia, Saunders, 1984.

Daze AM, **Scanlon** JW: *Neonatal Nursing.* Baltimore, University Park Press, 1985.

Dierker LJ, **Rosen** MG: Studying life before birth: The human brain develops. *P/N* 1986;10(4):10.

Dodman N: Newborn temperature control. *Neonatal Netw* 1987;5(6):19.

Guyton A: *Textbook of Medical Physiology.* Philadelphia, Saunders, 1985.

Heck LJ, et al: Serum glucose levels in term neonates, during the first 48 hours of life. *J Pediatr* 1987;110 (January):119.

Koldvsky O: Perinatal adaptation of gastrointestinal tract functions in man. *P/N* 1987;11(1):31.

Martin RG: Drug disposition in the neonate. *Neonatal Netw* 1986;4(4):14.

Ruchala P: The effect of wearing head coverings on the axillary temperatures of infants. *Am J Mat Child Nurs* 1985;10(July/August):240.

Saul K, **Warburton** D: Increased incidence of early onset hyperbilirubinemia in breast-fed versus bottle-fed infants. *J Perinatol* 1984;4(3):36.

Tan KL: Blood pressure in full term healthy neonates. *Clin Pediatr* 1987;26(January):21.

When the nurse took my first child and put him to my breast his tiny mouth opened and reached for me as if he had known forever what to do. (Leslie Kenton, All I Ever Wanted Was a Baby)

Neonatal Nursing Assessment

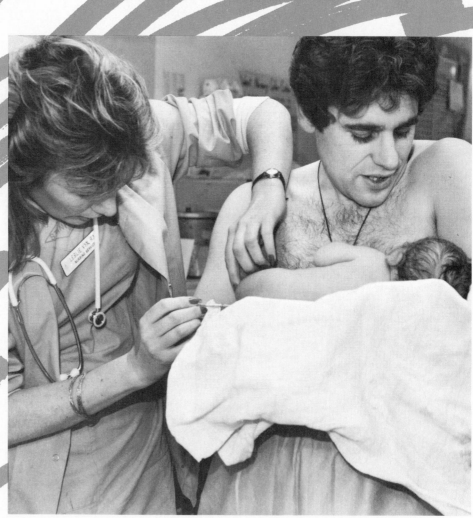

This nurse is taking the temperature of a half-hour-old baby, born by cesarean, while his father holds him skin to skin.

Chapter Twenty-Eight

OBJECTIVES

- **Describe the normal physical and behavioral characteristics of the newborn.**
- **Summarize the components of a complete newborn assessment.**
- **Explain the various components of the gestational age assessment.**
- **Describe the neurologic and/or neuromuscular characteristics of the newborn and the reflexes that may be present at birth.**
- **Describe the categories of the neonatal behavioral assessment.**

Unlike adults, newborns communicate needs primarily by behavior. Because nurses are the most consistent observers of the newborn, they must be able to interpret this behavior into information about the neonate's condition and to respond with appropriate nursing interventions. This chapter focuses on the assessment of the neonate and interpretation of findings.

Assessment of the newborn is a continuous process used to evaluate development and adjustments to extrauterine life. In the delivery room, Apgar scoring and careful observation of the newborn form the basis of the assessment and are correlated with information such as:

- Maternal history
- Duration of labor
- Maternal analgesia and anesthesia
- Complications of labor or delivery
- Treatment instituted in the delivery room, in conjunction with determination of clinical gestational age

- Identification of the newborn's classification by weight and gestational age and related potential neonatal mortality risk
- Physical examination of the newborn

The nurse incorporates data from these sources with the assessment findings during the first one to four hours after birth to formulate a plan for nursing intervention.

Timing of Newborn Assessments

The first 24 hours of life are significant because during this period the newborn makes the critical transition from intrauterine to extrauterine life. The risk of mortality and morbidity is statistically high during this period. Assessment of the infant is essential to ensure that the transition is proceeding successfully.

There are three major assessments of newborns while they are in the birth facility. The first assessment is done immediately after birth in the delivery room to determine the need for resuscitation or other interventions. The newborn who is stable can stay with the parents after delivery to initiate early attachment. The newborn who has complications is taken to the nursery for further evaluation and intervention.

A second evaluation is done in the first one to four hours after birth as part of the routine admission procedures. During this assessment, the nurse carries out a brief physical examination to evaluate the newborn's adaptation to extrauterine life and to estimate gestational age. Any problems that place the newborn at risk are assessed further during this time.

Prior to discharge, a physician or nurse-practitioner does a complete physical examination for legal purposes. A behavioral assessment is also done at this time.

This chapter presents the procedures for estimating gestational age and performing the complete physical examination and behavioral assessment. Chapter 23 discusses the immediate postdelivery assessment. Chapter 29 describes the brief assessment performed during the first four hours of life.

Parental Involvement

The various neonatal assessments and the data obtained from them are only as effective as the degree to which the findings are shared with the parents and incorporated into the interaction between parents and infant. Parents must be included in the assessment process from the moment of their child's birth. The Apgar score and its meaning should be explained immediately to the parents. As soon as possible, the parents should be a part of the physical and behavioral assessments. The examiner should emphasize the uniqueness of their infant.

The nurse can encourage the parents to identify the unique behavioral characteristics of their infant and to learn nurturing activities. Attachment is promoted when parents are allowed to explore their infant in private, identifying individual physical and behavioral characteristics. The nurse's supportive responses to the parents' questions and observations are essential throughout the assessment process. With the nurse's help, attachment and the beginning of interactions between family members are established.

Something very special occurs within the first hour after birth. If the environment is quiet, the birthing without complications, the lights lowered, the handling diminished, newborn infants— aside from all the physiological adaptations they must make— begin in a uniquely human way to adapt to the new experience of being in the world. (*The Amazing Newborn*)

● Estimation of Gestational Age

The nurse must establish the newborn's gestational age in the first four hours after birth so that careful attention can be given to age-related problems. Traditionally, the gestational age of a neonate was determined from the date of the pregnant woman's last menstrual period. This method was accurate only 75 percent to 85 percent of the time. Because of the problems that develop with the newborn who is preterm or whose weight is inappropriate for gestational age, a more accurate system was developed to evaluate the newborn. Once learned, the procedure can be done in a few minutes.

Clinical *gestational age assessment tools* have two components: external physical characteristics and neurologic and/or neuromuscular development evaluations. Physical characteristics generally include sole creases, amount of breast tissue, amount of lanugo, cartilagenous development of the ear, testicular descent, and scrotal rugae or labial development. These objective clinical criteria are not influenced by labor and delivery and do not change significantly within the first 24 hours after birth.

During the first 24 hours of life, the newborn's nervous system is unstable; thus, neurologic evaluation findings based on reflexes or assessments dependent on the higher brain centers may not be reliable. If the neurologic findings drastically deviate from the gestational age derived by evaluation of the external characteristics, a second assessment is done in 24 hours.

The neurologic components (excluding reflexes) can aid in assessing neonates of less than 34 weeks' gestation.

Between 26 and 34 weeks, neurologic changes are significant, whereas significant physical changes are less evident. The important neurologic changes consist of replacement of extensor tone by flexor tone in a caudocephalad progression. Neurologic examination facilitates assessment of functional or physiologic maturation in addition to physical development.

Of the current gestational assessment aids, Dubowitz and Dubowitz's tool is the most thoroughly documented and validated way to assess intrauterine growth alterations and preterm neonates (Robertson 1979). This assessment tool lists physical characteristics and neuromuscular tone components to be assessed on admission to the nursery.

Ballard's *estimation of gestational age* by maturity rating is a simplified version of the Dubowitz tool. The Ballard tool omits some of the neuromuscular tone assessments, such as head lag, ventral suspension (which is difficult to assess in very ill newborns or those on respirators), and leg recoil. The scoring method of Ballard's tool is much like that of the Dubowitz tool; each physical and neuromuscular finding is given a value, and the total score is matched to a gestational age (Figure 28–1). The maximum score on the Ballard's tool is 50, which corresponds to a gestational age of 44 weeks.

For example, upon completing a gestational assessment of a one-hour-old newborn, the nurse gives a score of 3 to all the physical characteristics, for a total of 18, and gives a score of 3 to all the neuromuscular assessments, for a total neurologic score of 18. The physical characteristics score of 18 is added to the neurologic score of 18 for a total score of 36, which correlates with 38+ weeks' gestation. Since all newborns vary slightly in the development of physical characteristics and maturation of neurologic function, the scores will vary instead of all being 3, as in the example.

The Dubowitz and Ballard tools are less accurate for neonates of less than 28 weeks' or more than 43 weeks' gestation. Some nurseries use the physical characteristics component of Brazie and Lubchenco's "Estimation of Gestational Age Chart" (Appendix G) as the initial assessment for all neonates admitted to the nursery.

In carrying out gestational age assessments, the nurse should keep in mind that some maternal conditions such as PIH and diabetes may affect certain gestational assessment components and warrant further study. Maternal diabetes, although it appears to accelerate fetal physical growth, seems to retard neurologic maturation. Maternal hypertensive states, which retard growth, seem to speed neurologic maturation. Newborns of preeclamptic-eclamptic women suffer a poor correlation with the criteria involving active muscle tone and edema. Babies with respiratory distress syndrome tend to be flaccid and edematous and to assume a "frogleg" posture. These characteristics affect the scoring of the neuromuscular components of the assessment tool.

Estimation of Gestational Age
by Maturity Rating
Symbols: X=First exam   O=Second exam

Neuromuscular Maturity

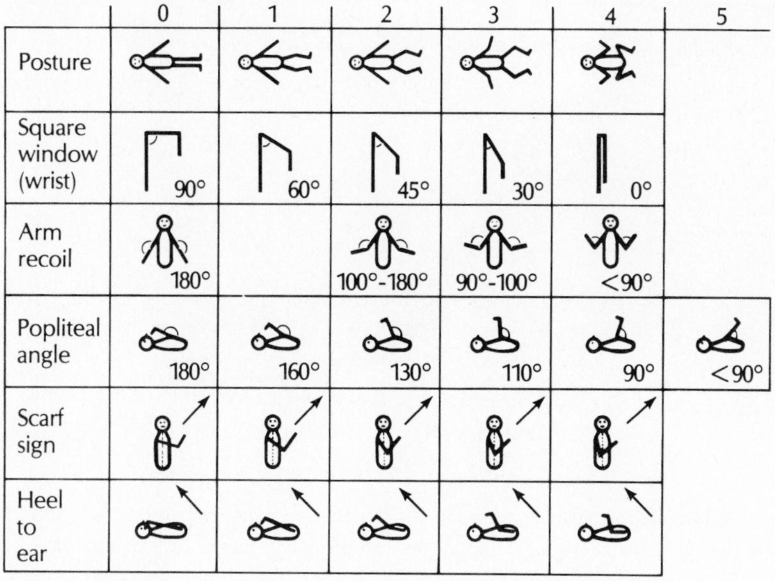

Gestation by dates _____ wks.

Birth date _____ Hour _____ am/pm

APGAR _____ 1 min _____ 5 min

Score	Wks
5	26
10	28
15	30
20	32
25	34
30	36
35	38
40	40
45	42
50	44

Physical Maturity

	0	1	2	3	4	5
Skin	gelatinous red, transparent	smooth pink, visible veins	superficial peeling and/or rash, few veins	cracking pale area, rare veins,	parchment, deep cracking, no vessels	leathery, cracked, wrinkled
Lanugo	none	abundant	thinning	bald areas	mostly bald	
Plantar creases	no crease	faint red marks	anterior transverse crease only	creases anter. 2/3	creases cover entire sole	
Breast	barely percept.	flat areola, no bud	stippled areola, 1-2 mm bud	raised areola, 3-4 mm bud	full areola, 5-10 mm bud	
Ear	binna flat, stays folded	sl. curved pinna, soft with slow recoil	well-curv. pinna, soft but ready recoil	formed and firm with instant recoil	thick cartilage, ear stiff	
Genitals (male)	scrotum empty, no rugae		testes decending, few rugae	testes down, good rugae	testes pendulous, deep rugae	
Genitals (female)	prominent clitoris and labia minora		majora and minora equally prominent	majora large, minora small	clitoris and minora completely covered	

Figure 28–1 Newborn maturity rating and classification (From Ballard JL, et al: A simplified assessment of gestational age. Classification of the low-birth-weight infant, in Klaus MH, *Pediatr Res* 1977;11:374. Figure adapted from Sweet AY: Fanaroff AA: *Care of the High-Risk Infant.* Philadelphia, Saunders, 1977, p 47).

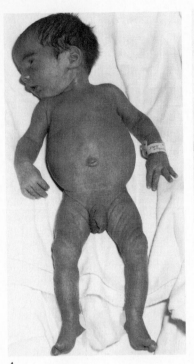
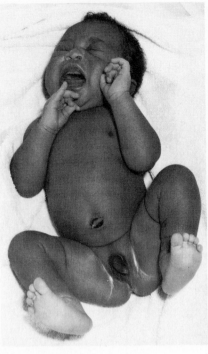
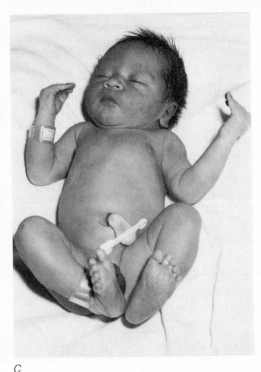

A   B   C

Figure 28–2   Resting posture. A Infant exhibits beginning of flexion of the thigh. The gestational age is approximately 31 weeks. Note the extension of the upper extremities. B Infant exhibits stronger flexion of the arms, hips, and thighs. The gestational age is appoximately 35 weeks. C The full-term infant exhibits hypertonic flexion of all extremities. (From Dubowitz L, Dubowitz V: Gestational Age of the Newborn. Menlo Park, Calif, Addison-Wesley, 1977)

Assessment of Physical Characteristics

The nurse first evaluates observable characteristics without disturbing the baby. Selected physical characteristics common to both gestational assessment tools are presented here in the order in which they might be evaluated most effectively:

1. *Resting posture,* although a neuromuscular component, it should be assessed as the baby lies undisturbed on a flat surface (Figure 28–2).

2. *Skin* in the preterm neonate appears thin and transparent, with veins prominent over the abdomen early in gestation. As term approaches, the skin appears opaque because of increased subcutaneous tissue. Disappearance of the protective vernix caseosa promotes skin desquamation.

3. *Lanugo,* a fine hair covering, decreases as gestational age increases. The amount of lanugo is greatest at 28 to 30 weeks and then disappears, first from the face, then from the trunk and extremities.

4. *Sole (plantar) creases* are reliable indicators of gestational age in the first 12 hours of life. After this, the skin of the foot begins drying, and superficial creases appear. Development of sole creases begins

at the top (anterior) portion of the sole and, as gestation progresses, proceeds to the heel (Figure 28–3). Peeling may also occur. Plantar creases vary with race. Black newborns' sole creases may be less developed at term.

5. The *areola* is inspected and the *breast bud tissue* is gently palpated by application of the forefinger and middle finger to the breast area and is measured in centimeters or millimeters (Figure 28–4). At term gestation, the tissue will measure between 0.5 and 1 cm (5 to 10 mm). During the assessment the nipple should not be grasped because skin and subcutaneous tissue will prevent accurate estimation of size. The nurse may also cause trauma to the breast tissue if this procedure is not done gently.

As gestation progresses, the breast tissue mass and areola enlarge. However, a large breast tissue mass can occur as a result of conditions other than advanced gestational age. The infant of a diabetic mother tends to be large for gestational age (LGA) and the accelerated development of breast tissue is a reflection of subcutaneous fat deposits. Small for gestational age (SGA) term or postterm newborns may have used subcutaneous fat (which would have been deposited as breast tissue) to survive in utero;

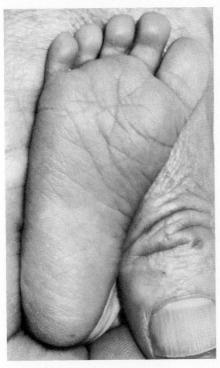
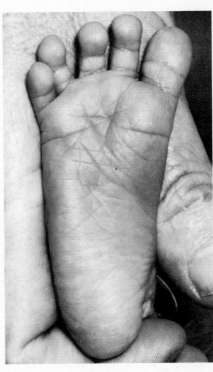
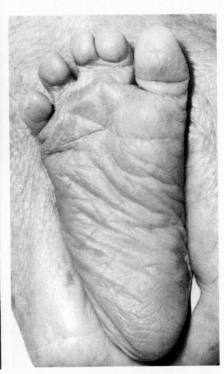

A   B   C

Figure 28–3   Sole creases. A Infant has a few sole creases on the anterior portion of the foot. Note the slick heel. The gestational age is approximately 35 weeks. B Infant has a deeper network of sole creases on the anterior two-thirds of the sole. Note the slick heel. The gestational age is approximately 37 weeks. C The full-term infant has deep sole creases down to and including the heel as the skin loses fluid and dries after birth; sole (plantar) creases can be seen even in preterm newborns. (From Dubowitz L, Dubowitz V: Gestational Age of the Newborn. Menlo Park, Calif, Addison-Wesley, 1977)

as a result, their lack of breast tissue may indicate a gestational age of 34 to 35 weeks, even though other factors indicate a *term* or *postterm* neonate.

6. *Ear form and cartilage distribution* develop with gestational age. The cartilage gives the ear its shape and substance (Figure 28–5). In a newborn of less than 34 weeks' gestation the ear is relatively shapeless and flat; it has little cartilage, so the ear folds over on itself and remains folded. By approximately 36 weeks' gestation, some cartilage and slight incurving of upper pinna are present, and the pinna springs back slowly when folded. (This response is tested by holding the top and bottom of the pinna together with the forefinger and thumb and then releasing it, or by folding the pinna of the ear forward against the side of the head and releasing it, and observing the response.) By term, the newborn's pinna is firm, stands away from the head, and springs back quickly from the folding.

7. *Male genitals* are evaluated for size of the scrotal sac, the presence of rugae, and descent of the testes (Figure 28–6). Prior to 36 weeks, the small scrotum has few rugae, and the testes are palpable in the inguinal canal. By 36 to 38 weeks, the testes are in the upper scrotum, and rugae have developed over the anterior portion of the scrotum. By term, the testes are generally in the lower scrotum, which is pendulous and covered with rugae.

8. The appearance of the *female genitals* depends in part on subcutaneous fat deposition and therefore relates to fetal nutritional status (Figure 28–7). The clitoris varies in size and occasionally is so large that it is difficult to identify the sex of the infant. This may be caused by adrenogenital syndrome, which causes the adrenals to secrete excessive amounts of androgen and other hormones. At 30 to 32 weeks' gestation, the clitoris is prominent, and the labia majora are small and widely separated. As gestational age increases, the labia majora increase in size. At 36 to 40 weeks, they nearly cover the clitoris. At 40 weeks and beyond, the labia majora cover the labia minora and clitoris.

In the full-term female newborn, some tissue may protrude from the floor of the vagina. This tissue, the hymenal tag, is a normal segment of the hymen and disappears in several weeks (Korones 1986).

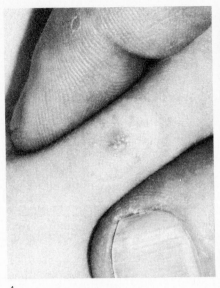
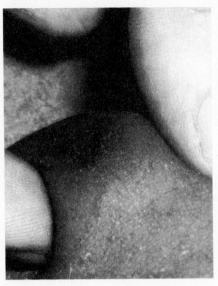
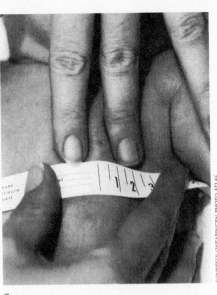

A   *B*   *C*

Figure 28–4   Breast tissue. A Newborn has a visible raised area. On palpation the area is 4 mm. The gestational age is 38 weeks. B Newborn has 10 mm breast tissue area. The gestational age is 40 to 44 weeks. C Gently compress the tissue between middle and index finger and measure the tissue in centimeters or millimeters. Absence of or decreased breast tissue often indicates premature or SGA newborn. (From Dubowitz L, Dubowitz V: Gestational Age of the Newborn. Menlo Park, Calif, Addison-Wesley, 1977; Swearingen PL: The Addison-Wesley Photo-Atlas of Nursing Procedures. Menlo Park, Calif, Addison-Wesley, 1984)

Other physical characteristics assessed by some gestational age scoring tools include the following:

1. *Vernix* covers the preterm newborn. The postterm newborn has no vernix. After noting vernix distribution, the delivery room nurse dries the newborn to prevent evaporative heat loss, thus disturbing the vernix. The delivery room nurse must communicate to the neonatal nurse the amount of vernix and the areas of vernix coverage.

2. *Hair* of the preterm newborn has the consistency of matted wool or fur and lies in bunches rather than in the silky, single strands of the term neonate's hair.

3. *Skull firmness* increases as the newborn matures. In a term neonate the bones are hard, and the sutures are not easily displaced. The clinician should not attempt to displace the sutures forcibly.

4. *Nails* appear and cover the nail bed at about 20 weeks' gestation. Nails extending beyond the fingertips may indicate a postterm neonate.

Assessment of Neurologic Status

The central nervous system of the human fetus matures at a fairly constant rate. Specific neurologic parameters have been correlated with gestational age. Tests have been designed to evaluate neurologic status as manifested by neuromuscular tone. In the fetus, neuromuscular tone

develops from the lower to the upper extremities. The neurologic evaluation requires more manipulation and disturbances than the physical evaluation of the neonate.

The neuromuscular evaluation (see Figure 28–1) is best performed when the infant has stabilized. The following characteristics are evaluated:

1. *Ankle dorsiflexion* is determined by flexing the ankle on the shin. The examiner uses a thumb to push on the sole of the newborn's foot while the fingers support the back of the leg. Then the angle formed by the foot and the interior leg is measured (Figure 28–8). This sign can be influenced by intrauterine position and congenital deformities.

2. The *square window sign* is elicited by flexing the baby's hand toward the ventral forearm. The angle formed at the wrist is measured (Figure 28–9).

3. *Recoil* is a test of flexion development. Because flexion first develops in the lower extremities, recoil is first tested in the legs. The neonate is placed on his or her back on a flat surface. With a hand on the newborn's knees and while manipulating the hip joint, the nurse places the baby's legs in flexion, then extends them parallel to each other and flat on the surface. The response to this maneuver is recoil of the neonate's legs. According to gestational age, they may not move or they may return slowly or quickly to the flexed position.

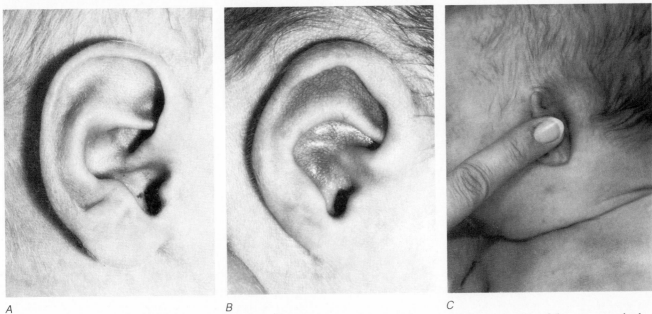

A   *B*   *C*

Figure 28–5 Ear form and cartilage. A The ear of the infant at approximately 36 weeks' gestation shows incurving of the upper two-thirds of the pinna. B Infant at term shows well-defined incurving of the entire pinna. C If the auricle stays in the position in which it is pressed, or returns slowly to its original position, it usually means the gestational age is less than 38 weeks. (From Dubowitz L, Dubowitz V: Gestational Age of the Newborn. Menlo Park, Calif, Addison-Wesley 1977; Swearingen PL: The Addison-Wesley Photo-Atlas of Nursing Procedures. Menlo Park, Calif, Addison-Wesley, 1984)

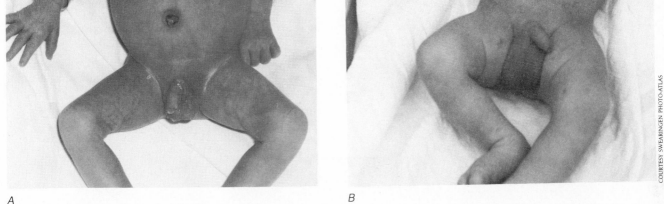

A   *B*

Figure 28–6 Male genitals. A A preterm infant's testes are not within the scrotum. The scrotal surface has few rugae. B Term infant's testes are generally fully descended. The entire surface of the scrotum is covered by rugae. (From Dubowitz L, Dubowitz V: Gestational Age of the Newborn. Menlo Park, Calif, Addison-Wesley, 1977; Swearingen PL: The Addison-Wesley Photo-Atlas of Nursing Procedures. Menlo Park, Calif, Addison-Wesley, 1984)

Recoil in the upper extremities is tested by flexion at the elbow and extension of the arms at the newborn's side. While the baby is in the supine position, the nurse completely flexes both elbows, holds them in this position for five seconds, extends the arms at the baby's side, and releases them. Upon release, the elbows of a full-term newborn form an angle of less than 90° and rapidly recoil back to flexed position. The elbows of preterm newborns have slower recoil time and form a less-than-90° angle. Arm recoil is also slower in healthy but fatigued newborns after birth; therefore arm recoil is best elicited after the first hour of birth when the baby has had time to recover from the stress of delivery.

4. The *popliteal angle* (degree of knee flexion) is determined with the newborn supine and flat. The thigh is flexed on the abdomen/chest, and the nurse places the index finger of the other hand behind the newborn's ankle to extend the lower leg until resistance is met. The angle formed is then measured. Results vary from no resistance in the very immature infant to an 80° angle in the term infant.

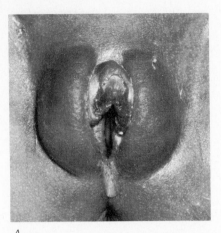
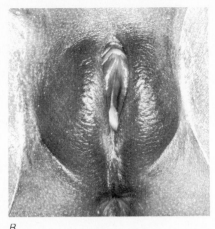
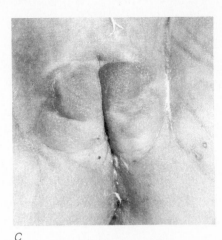

A   B   C

Figure 28-7 Female genitals. A Infant has a prominent clitoris. The labia majora are widely separated, and the labia minora, viewed laterally, would protrude beyond the labia majora. The gestational age is 30 to 36 weeks. B The clitoris is still visible; the labia minora are now covered by the larger labia majora. The gestational age is 36 to 40 weeks. C The term infant has well-developed, large labia majora that cover both the clitoris and labia minora. (From Dubowitz L, Dubowitz V: Gestational Age of the Newborn. Menlo Park, Calif, Addison-Wesley, 1977)

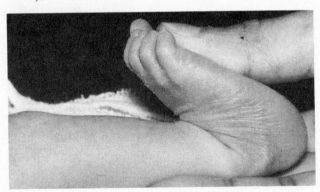
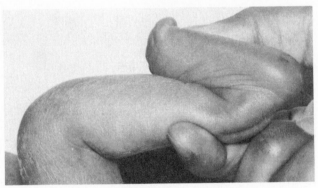

A   B

Figure 28-8 Ankle dorsiflexion. A A 45° angle is indicative of 32 to 36 weeks' gestation. A 20° angle is indicative of 36 to 40 weeks' gestation. B An angle of 0° is common at gestational age of 40 weeks or more. (From Dubowitz L, Dubowitz V: Gestational Age of the Newborn. Menlo Park, Calif, Addison-Wesley, 1977)

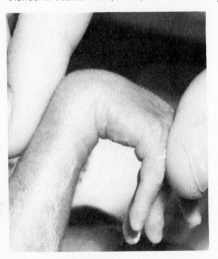
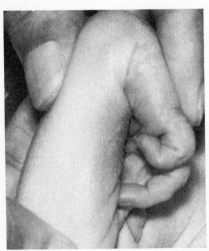
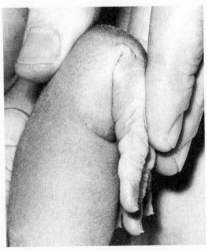

A   B   C

Figure 28-9 Square window sign. A This angle is 90° and suggests an immature newborn of 28 to 32 weeks' gestation. B A 30° angle is commonly found from 38 to 40 weeks' gestation. C A 0° angle occurs from 40 to 42 weeks. (From Dubowitz L, Dubowitz V: Gestational Age of the Newborn. Menlo Park, Calif, Addison-Wesley, 1977)

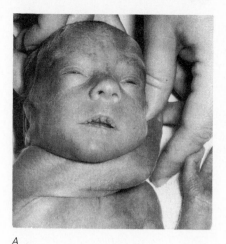
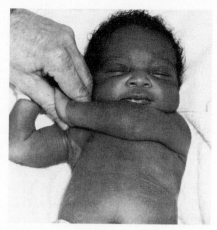
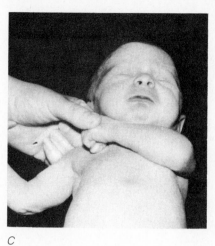

A   *B*   *C*

Figure 28–10 Scarf sign. A No resistance is noted until after 30 weeks' gestation. The elbow can be readily moved past the midline. B The elbow is at midline at 36 to 40 weeks' gestation. C Beyond 40 weeks' gestation, the elbow will not reach the midline. (From Dubowitz L, Dubowitz V: Gestational Age of the Newborn. Menlo Park, Calif, Addison-Wesley, 1977)

5. The *heel-to-ear maneuver* is performed by placing the baby in a supine position and, while stabilizing the hip on the bed, gently drawing the foot toward the ear on the same side until resistance is felt. Both the popliteal angle and the proximity of the foot to the ear are assessed. In a very preterm newborn, the leg will remain straight and the foot will go to the ear or beyond. Maneuvers involving the lower extremities of newborns who had frank breech presentation should be delayed to allow for resolution of leg positioning (Ballard et al 1979).

6. The *scarf sign* is elicited by placing the neonate supine and drawing an arm across the chest toward the infant's opposite shoulder until resistance is met. The location of the elbow is then noted in relation to the midline of the chest (Figure 28–10).

7. *Head lag (neck flexors)* is measured by pulling the baby to a sitting position and noting the degree of head lag. Total lag is common in infants up to 34 weeks' gestation, whereas the postmature newborn (42 + weeks) will hold the head in front of the body line.

8. *Ventral suspension (horizontal position)* is evaluated by holding the newborn prone on the examiner's hand. The position of head and back and degree of flexion in the arms and legs are then noted. Some flexion of arms and legs indicates 36 to 38 weeks' gestation; fully flexed extremities, with head and back even, are characteristic of a term neonate.

9. *Major reflexes* such as sucking, rooting, grasping, Moro, tonic neck, and others are evaluated and scored.

An interesting supplementary method for estimating gestational age is to view the vascular network of the cornea with an ophthalmoscope. The amount of vascularity present over the surface of the lens correlates with gestational age. In babies of less than 27 weeks' gestation, the cornea is cloudy and the vascular network is not visible; after 34 weeks' gestation, the vascular network has generally disappeared completely.

Determination of gestational age and correlation with birth weight (Figure 28–11) enables the nurse to assess the infant more accurately and to anticipate possible physiologic problems. This information is then used in conjunction with a complete physical examination to determine priorities and to establish a plan of care appropriate to the individual infant.

● **Physical Assessment**

After the initial determination of gestational age and related potential problems, a more extensive physical assessment is done. (The nursing student is expected to be able to do most of the assessments, although she or he may not be required to know all the alterations and possible causes.) The nurse should choose a warm, well-lighted area that is free of drafts. Completing the physical assessment in the presence of the parents provides an opportunity to acquaint them with their unique newborn. The examination is performed in a systematic, head-to-toe manner, and all findings are recorded. When assessing the physical and neurologic status of the newborn, the nurse should first consider general appearance and then proceed to specific areas.

A guide for systematically assessing the newborn appears on pages 874–885. Normal findings, alterations, and related causes are presented and correlated with suggested

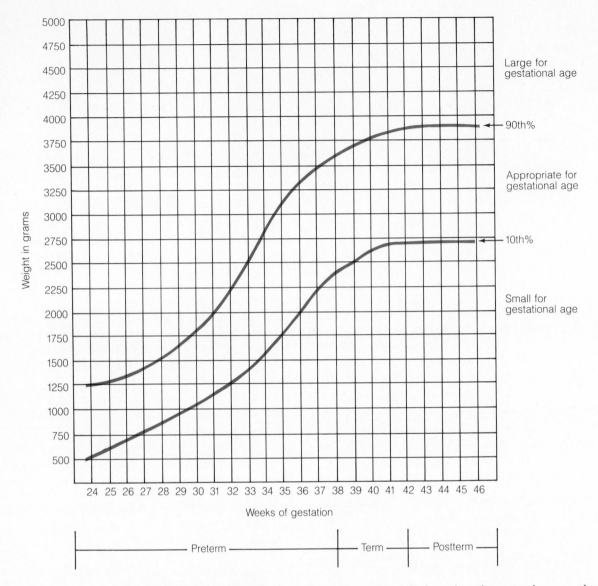

Figure 28–11   Classification of newborns by birth weight and gestational age. The newborn's birth weight and gestational age are plotted on the graph. The newborn is then classified as large for gestational age, appropriate for gestational age, or small for gestational age. (From Battaglia FC, Lubchenco LO: A practical classification of newborn infants by weight and gestational age. J Pediatr 1967;71:161)

nursing responses. The findings are typical for a full-term newborn.

General Appearance

The newborn's head is disproportionately large for the body. The center of the baby's body is the umbilicus rather than the symphysis pubis, as in the adult. The body appears long and the extremities short. The flexed position that the neonate maintains contributes to the short appearance of the extremities. The hands are tightly clenched. The neck looks short because the chin rests on the chest.

Newborns have a prominent abdomen, sloping shoulders, narrow hips, and rounded chests. They tend to stay in a flexed position similar to the one maintained in utero and will offer resistance when the extremities are straightened. After a breech delivery, the feet are usually dorsiflexed, and it may take several weeks for the newborn to assume typical newborn posture.

Weight and Measurements

The normal full-term Caucasian newborn has an average birth weight of 3405 g (7 lb, 8 oz), whereas black,

Oriental, and American Indian newborns are usually somewhat smaller. Other factors that influence weight are age and size of parents, health of mother, and interval between pregnancies. After the first week and for the first six months, the neonate's weight will increase about 198 g (7 oz) weekly.

Approximately 70 percent to 75 percent of the neonate's body weight is water. During the initial newborn period (the first three or four days), there is a physiologic weight loss of 5 percent to 10 percent for term newborns because of fluid shifts. This weight loss may reach 15 percent for preterm newborns. Large babies may tend to lose more weight because of greater fluid loss in proportion to birth weight. If weight loss is greater than expected, clinical reappraisal is indicated. Factors contributing to weight loss include small fluid intake resulting from delayed breastfeeding or a slow adjustment to the formula, increased volume of meconium excreted, respiration, and urination. Weight loss may be marked in the presence of temperature elevation because of associated dehydration.

The length of the normal newborn is difficult to measure because the legs are flexed and tensed. To measure length, the nurse should place infants flat on their backs with legs extended as much as possible (Figure 28–12). The average length is 49.4 cm (19.5 in), with the normal range being 45.8 to 52.3 cm (18 to 20.5 in). The newborn will grow approximately an inch a month for the next six months. This is the period of most rapid growth.

At birth, the newborn's head is one-third the size of an adult's head. The circumference of the newborn's head is 33 to 35 cm (13 to 14 in). For accurate measurement, the tape is placed over the most prominent part of the occiput and brought to just above the eyebrows (Figure 28–13A). The circumference of the newborn's head is approximately 2 cm greater than the circumference of its chest at birth and will remain in this proportion for the next few months. (Factors that alter this measurement are discussed on page 876.)

The average circumference of the chest at birth is 32 cm (12.5 in). Chest measurements should be taken with the tape measure at the lower edge of the scapulas and brought around anteriorly directly over the nipple line (Figure 28–13B). The abdominal circumference or girth may also be measured at this time by placing the tape around the newborn's abdomen at the level of the umbilicus, with the bottom edge of the tape at the top edge of the umbilicus.

Temperature

Initial assessment of the newborn's temperature is critical. In utero, the temperature of the fetus is about the same as or slightly higher than the expectant mother's. When the baby enters the outside world, his or her temperature can suddenly drop as a result of exposure to drafts and the skin's heat-loss mechanisms. If no heat conservation measures are instituted, the normal term newborn's deep body temperature falls 0.1C (0.2F) per minute; skin temperature lowers 0.3C (0.5F) per minute. Marked decrease in skin temperature occurs within ten minutes after exposure to room air (Korones 1986). The temperature should stabilize within 8 to 12 hours. Temperature should be monitored at least every hour until stable, then every 4 hours for 24 hours (AAP 1983). Many institutions use a continuous probe, or measurements are obtained every 15 to 30 minutes for the first hour, then each hour for four hours. (See Chapter 27 for a discussion of the physiology of temperature regulation.)

Body temperature can be assessed either by the rectum, axilla, or skin. Rectal temperature is assumed to be the closest approximation to core temperature, but this depends on the depth of the thermometer insertion. Normal rectal temperature is 36.6C to 37.2C (97.8 to 99F). The rectal route is not recommended as a routine method as it may predispose to rectal mucosal irritation and increase chances of perforation (AAP 1983). If the temperature is taken rectally, the nurse holds the thermometer in the rectum for five minutes (Figure 28–14A). Rectal temperatures were previously advocated to detect imperforate anus, but nurses can make this assessment by observing the newborn's stools.

Axillary temperature reflects body temperature and the body's compensatory response to the thermal environment. Axillary temperatures are recommended as an alternative to rectal temperatures. Axillary temperatures are reliable as a close estimation of the rectal temperature (Korones 1986). In preterm and term newborns, there is less than 0.10C (0.20F) difference between the two sites. If the axillary method is used, the thermometer must remain in place at least three minutes unless an electronic thermometer is used (Figure 28–14B). Normal axillary temperature ranges from 36.5C to 37C (97.7F to 98.6F). Axillary temperatures can be misleading because the friction caused by apposition of the inner arm skin and upper chest wall and the nearness of brown fat to the probe may elevate the temperature.

The best measure of skin temperature is by means of continuous skin probe rather than axillary temperature, especially for small newborns or newborns maintained in incubators or under radiant warmers. Normal skin temperature is 36C to 36.5C (96.8F to 97.7F). Skin temperature assessment allows time for initiation of interventions prior to a more serious fall in core temperatures.

Temperature instability, a deviation of more than 1C (2F) from one reading to the next, or a subnormal temperature may indicate an infection. In contrast with an elevated temperature in older children, an increased temperature in a newborn may indicate reactions to too much covering, too hot a room, or dehydration. Dehydration, which tends to increase body temperature, occurs in newborns whose feedings have been delayed for any reason. Newborns respond to overheating (temperature greater than 37.5C or 99.5F) by increased restlessness and eventually by perspiration. The perspiration is initially seen on the head and face, then on the chest.

Skin

The skin of the newborn should be pink tinged or ruddy in color and warm to the touch. The ruddy color results from increased concentration of red blood cells in the blood vessels and from limited subcutaneous fat deposits.

ACROCYANOSIS

Acrocyanosis (bluish discoloration of the hands and feet) may be present in the first two to six hours after birth. This condition is due to poor peripheral circulation, which results in vasomotor instability and capillary stasis, especially when the baby is exposed to cold. If the central circulation is adequate, the blood supply should return quickly to the extremity after the skin is blanched with a finger.

Mottling (lacy pattern of dilated blood vessels under the skin) occurs as a result of general circulation fluctuations. It may last several hours to several weeks or may come and go periodically.

HARLEQUIN SIGN

Harlequin (clown) color change is occasionally noted: A deep red color develops over one side of the newborn's body while the other side remains pale, so that the skin resembles a clown's suit. This color change results from a vasomotor disturbance in which blood vessels on one side dilate while the vessels on the other side constrict. It usually lasts from 1 to 20 minutes. Affected neonates may have single or multiple episodes.

JAUNDICE

Jaundice is first detectable on the face (where skin overlies cartilage) and the mucous membranes of the mouth. It is evaluated by blanching the tip of the nose, the forehead, or the gum line. This procedure must be carried out in appropriate lighting. If jaundice is present, the area will appear yellowish immediately after blanching. Another area to assess for jaundice is the sclera. Evaluation and determination of the cause of jaundice must be initiated immediately to prevent possibly serious sequelae. The jaundice may be related to breast-feeding (small incidence), hematomas, immature liver function, or bruises from for-

ceps, or it may be caused by blood incompatibility, pitocin augmentation or induction, or severe hemolytic process. For detailed discussion of causes and assessment of jaundice see Chapter 32.

ERYTHEMA NEONATORUM TOXICUM

Erythema toxicum is a perifollicular eruption of lesions that are firm, vary in size from 1 to 3 mm, and consist of a white or pale yellow papule or pustule with an erythematous base. The rash may appear suddenly, usually over the trunk and diaper area, and is frequently widespread. The lesions do not appear on the palms of the hands or the soles of the feet. The peak incidence is at 24 to 48 hours of life. The cause is unknown and no treatment is necessary. The lesions disappear in a few hours or days. If a maculopapular rash appears and there is a question whether it is erythema toxicum, a smear of the aspirated papule will show numerous eosinophils on staining and no bacteria will be cultured.

SKIN TURGOR

Skin turgor is assessed to determine hydration status, the need to initiate early feedings, and the presence of any infectious processes. The usual place to assess skin turgor is over the abdomen. Skin should be elastic (return to original shape).

VERNIX CASEOSA

Vernix caseosa, a whitish cheeselike substance, covers the fetus while in utero and lubricates the skin of the newborn. The skin of the term or postterm newborn has less vernix and is frequently dry and peeling, especially on the hands and feet. *Milia,* which are plugged sebaceous glands, appear as raised white spots on the face, especially across the nose.

MONGOLIAN SPOTS

Mongolian spots are macular areas of bluish-black pigmentation found on the lumbar dorsal area and the buttocks. They are common in Oriental and black infants and newborns of other dark-skinned races (Color Plate VII). They gradually fade during the first or second year of life.

FORCEPS MARKS

Forceps marks may be present after a difficult forceps delivery. The newborn may have reddened areas over the cheeks and jaws. It is important to reassure the parents that these will disappear, usually within one or two days.

Transient facial paralysis resulting from the forceps pressure is a rare complication.

TELANGIECTATIC NEVI

Telangiectatic nevi, or *"stork bites,"* appear as pale pink or red flat, dilated capillaries and are fequently found on the eyelids, nose, lower occipital bone, and nape of the neck. These lesions are common in light complexioned neonates and are more noticeable during periods of crying. These areas blanch easily, have no clinical significance, and fade during infancy, usually disappearing by the second birthday. In many children, they reappear during crying episodes.

NEVUS FLAMMEUS

Nevus flammeus, or port-wine stain, is a capillary angioma directly below the epidermis. It is a nonelevated, sharply demarcated, red-to-purple dense area of capillaries (Color Plate X). The size and shape are variable, but it commonly appears on the face. It does not grow in size, does not fade with time, and does not blanch as a rule. In the black infant, the nevus flammeus appears jet black in color. The birthmark may be concealed by using an opaque cosmetic cream. If convulsions, contralateral hemiplegia, or intracortical calcifications accompany the nevus flammeus, it is suggestive of Sturge-Weber syndrome with involvement of the fifth cranial nerve.

NEVUS VASCULOSUS

Nevus vasculosus, or "strawberry mark," is a capillary hemangioma. It consists of newly formed and enlarged capillaries in the dermal and subdermal layers. It is a raised, clearly delineated, dark red, rough-surfaced birthmark commonly found in the head region. Such marks usually grow (often rapidly) for several months and become fixed in size by eight months. They then begin to shrink and start to resolve spontaneously several weeks to months after peak growth is reached. Except in rare cases, they are completely gone by the time the child is 7 years old. Parents can be told that resolution is heralded by a pale purple or gray spot on the surface of the hemangioma. The best cosmetic effect is achieved when the lesions are allowed to resolve spontaneously.

Birthmarks are frequently a cause of concern for the parents. Guilt feelings are common in the presence of misconceptions about the cause. Birthmarks should be identified and explained to the parents. By providing appropriate information about the cause and course of birthmarks, the nurse frequently relieves the fears and anxieties of the family.

Head

GENERAL APPEARANCE

The newborn's head is large (approximately one-fourth of the body size), with soft, pliable skull bones. The head may appear asymmetrical in the newborn of a vertex delivery. This asymmetry, called *molding,* is caused by over-riding of the cranial bones during labor and delivery (Figure 28–15). The degree of molding varies with the amount and length of pressure exerted on the head. Within a few days after delivery, the overriding usually diminishes and the suture lines become palpable. Because head measurements are affected by molding, a second measurement is indicated a few days after delivery. The heads of breech-born newborns and those delivered by cesarean birth are characteristically round and well shaped since pressure was not exerted on them during birth. Any extreme differences in head size may indicate microcephaly or hydrocephalus. Variations in the shape, size, or appearance of the head measurements may be due to *craniostenosis* (premature closure of the cranial sutures) and *plagiocephaly* (asymmetry caused by pressure on the fetal head during gestation).

Two *fontanelles* ("soft spots") may be palpated on the infant's head. Fontanelles, which are openings at the juncture of the cranial bones, can be measured with the fingers. Accurate measurement necessitates that the examiner's finger be measured in centimeters. The diamond-shaped *anterior fontanelle* is 3 to 4 cm long by 2 to 3 cm wide. It is located at the juncture of the frontal and parietal bones. The *posterior fontanelle,* smaller and triangular, is formed by the parietal bones and the occipital bone. The fontanelles will be smaller immediately after birth than several days later because of molding. The anterior fontanelle closes within 18 months, whereas the posterior fontanelle closes within 8–12 weeks.

The fontanelles are a useful indicator of the newborn's condition. The anterior fontanelle may swell when the newborn cries or may pulsate with the heartbeat, which is normal at rest. A bulging fontanelle usually signifies increased intracranial pressure, and a depressed fontanelle indicates dehydration. The sutures between the cranial bones should be palpated for amount of overlapping.

In addition to being inspected for degree of molding and size, the head should be evaluated for soft tissue edema and bruising.

CEPHALHEMATOMA

Cephalhematoma is a collection of blood resulting from ruptured blood vessels between the surface of a cranial bone and the periosteal membrane (Figure 28–16). The scalp in these areas feels loose and slightly edematous. These areas emerge as defined hematomas between the first

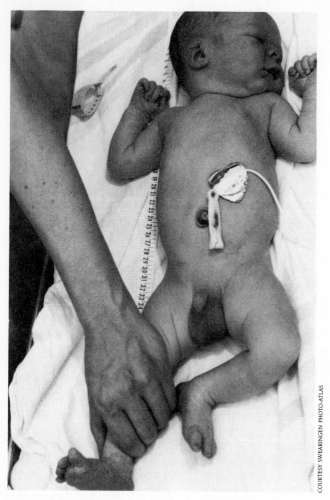

Figure 28–12 Measuring the length of a newborn (From Swearingen PL: *The Addison-Wesley Photo-Atlas of Nursing Procedures.* Menlo Park, Calif, Addison-Wesley, 1984)

COURTESY SWEARINGEN PHOTO-ATLAS

and second day. Although external pressure may cause the mass to fluctuate, it does not increase in size when the infant cries. Cephalhematomas may be unilateral or bilateral and do not cross suture lines. They are relatively common in vertex deliveries and may disappear slowly over a few weeks.

CAPUT SUCCEDANEUM

Caput succedaneum is a localized, easily identifiable soft area of the scalp, generally resulting from a long and difficult labor or vacuum extraction. The sustained pressure of the presenting part against the cervix results in compression of local blood vessels, and venous return is slowed. This causes an increase in tissue fluids, an edematous swelling, and occasional bleeding under the periosteum. The caput may vary from a small area to a severely elongated head. The fluid in the caput is reabsorbed within 12 hours or a few days after birth. Caputs resulting from vacuum extractors are sharply outlined, circular areas up to 2 cm thick. They disappear more slowly than naturally occurring edema. It is possible to distinguish between a cephalhematoma and a caput because the caput overrides suture lines (Figure 28–17), whereas the cephalhematoma, because of its location, never crosses a suture line.

Face

The newborn's face is well designed to help the infant suckle. Sucking (fat) pads are located in the cheeks, and labial tubercles (sucking calluses) are frequently found in the center of the upper lip. The chin is recessed, and the nose is flattened. The lips are sensitive to touch, and the sucking reflex is easily initiated.

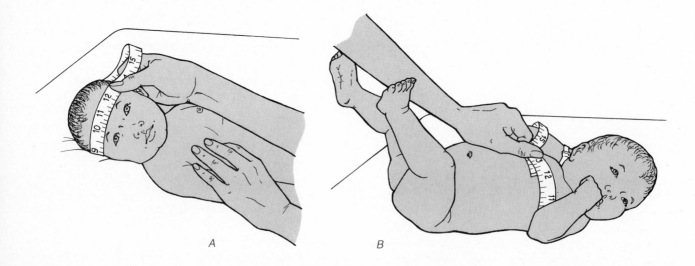

A

B

Figure 28–13 A Measuring the head circumference of the newborn. B Measuring the chest circumference of the newborn.

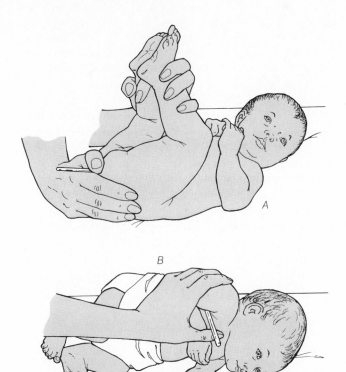

Figure 28–14   A The rectal thermometer must be held in place for 5 minutes and the legs supported. B The axillary temperature should be taken for 3 minutes. The newborn's arm should be tightly but gently pressed against the thermometer and the newborn's side as illustrated.

Symmetry of the eyes, nose, and ears is evaluated. See the Neonatal Physical Assessment Guide on p 876 for deviations in symmetry and variations in size, shape, and spacing of facial features. Facial movement symmetry should be assessed to determine the presence of facial palsy.

Facial paralysis appears when the neonate cries; the affected side is immobile and the palpebral (eyelid) fissure widens (Figure 28–18). Paralysis may result from forceps delivery or pressure on the facial nerve from the maternal pelvis during birth. Facial paralysis usually disappears within a few days to three weeks.

EYES

The eyes of the Caucasian neonate are a blue or slate blue gray. Scleral color tends to be bluish because of its relative thinness. The infant's eye color is usually established at approximately three months, although it may change any time up to one year. Dark-skinned neonates tend to have dark eyes at birth.

The eyes should be checked for size, equality of pupil

size, reaction of pupils to light, blink reflex to light, and edema and inflammation of the eyelids. The eyelids are usually edematous during the first few days of life because of the delivery and manipulation of the eyelids during administration of eye prophylaxis. The instillation of silver nitrate drops in the newborn's eyes increases the incidence of chemical conjunctivitis. This conjunctivitis appears in a few hours after instillation but disappears without treatment in one to two days. If infectious conjunctivitis exists, the newborn has the same purulent (greenish-yellow) discharge as in chemical conjunctivitis. But it is caused by staphylococci or a variety of Gram-negative bacteria and requires treatment with ophthalmic antibiotics. Onset is usually after the second day. Edema of the orbits or eyelids may persist for several days until the neonate's kidneys can evacuate the fluid.

Small subconjunctival hemorrhages appear in about 10 percent of newborns and are commonly found on the inner aspect of the sclera. These are caused by the changes in vascular tension during birth. They will remain for a few weeks and are of no pathologic significance. Parents need reassurance that the infant is not bleeding from within the eye and that vision will not be impaired.

The neonate may demonstrate transient strabismus caused by poor neuromuscular control of eye muscles (Figure 28–19). It gradually regresses in three to four months. The "doll's eye" phenomenon is also present for about ten days after birth. As the newborn's head position is changed to the left and then to the right, the eyes move

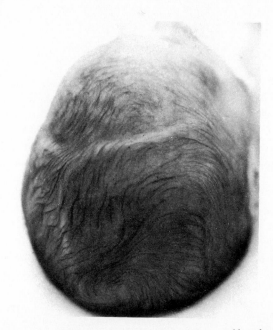

Figure 28–15   Overlapped cranial bones produce a visible ridge in a small, premature infant. Easily visible overlapping does not often occur in term infants. (From Korones SB: High-Risk Newborn Infants, ed 4. St Louis, Mosby, 1986)

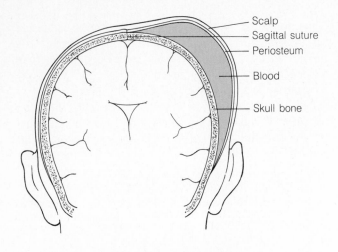

A

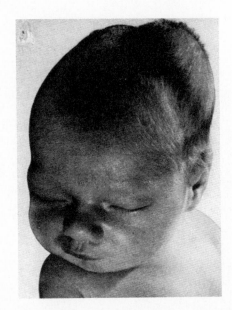

B

Figure 28–16 Cephalhematoma is a collection of blood between the surface of a cranial bone and the periosteal membrane. This is a cephalhematoma over the left parietal bone. (Photo reproduced with permission from Potter EL, Craig JM: Pathology of the Fetus and Infant, *ed 3. Copyright 1975 by Year Book Medical Publishers, Chicago.)*

to the opposite direction. This results from underdeveloped integration of head-eye coordination.

The nurse should observe the neonate's pupils for opacities or whiteness and for the absence of a normal red reflex. Red reflex is a red-orange flash of color observed when an ophthalmoscope light reflects off the retina. In dark-colored newborns, the retina may appear more greyish. Absence of red reflex occurs with cataracts. Congenital cataracts should be suspected in infants of mothers with a history of rubella, cytomegalic inclusion disease, or syphilis.

The cry of the newborn is commonly tearless because the lacrimal structures are immature at birth and are not usually fully functional until the second month of life. Some newborns may produce tears during the neonatal period. Poor oculomotor coordination and absence of accommodation limit visual abilities, but the newborn does have peripheral vision and can fixate on near objects (9–12 in) for short periods (Ludington-Hoe 1983). The newborn can perceive faces, shapes, and colors and begins to show visual preferences early. The neonate blinks in response to bright lights, to a tap on the bridge of the nose (glabellar reflex), or to a light touch on the eyelids. Pupillary light reflex is also present. Examination of the eye is best accomplished by rocking the newborn from an upright position to the horizontal a few times or by other methods that will elicit an opened-eye response.

NOSE

The newborn's nose is small and narrow. Infants are characteristically nose breathers for the first few months of

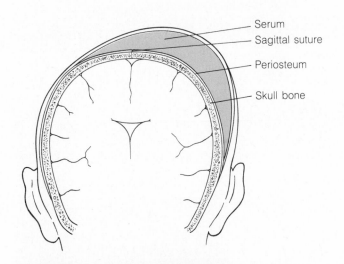

A

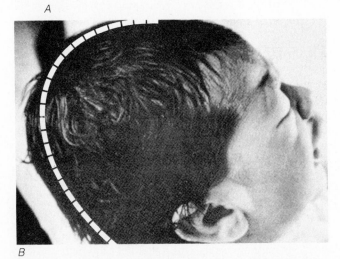

B

Figure 28–17 Caput succedaneum is a collection of fluid (serum) under the scalp. (Photo courtesy Mead Johnson Laboratories, Evansville, Ind)

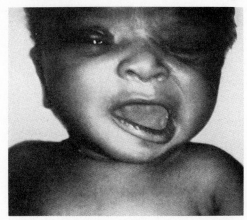

Figure 28–18   Facial paralysis. Paralysis of the right side of the face from injury to right facial nerve. (Courtesy of Dr. Ralph Platow, in Potter EL, Craig JM: *Pathology of the Fetus and Infant,* ed 3. Copyright 1975 by Year Book Medical Publishers, Chicago)

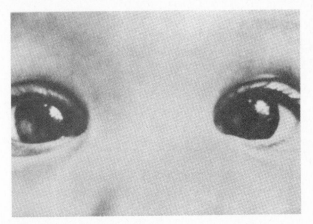

Figure 28–19   Transient strabismus may be present in the newborn due to poor neuromuscular control. (Courtesy Mead Johnson Laboratories, Evansville, Ind)

life. The newborn generally removes obstructions by sneezing. Nasal patency is assured if the baby breathes easily with mouth closed. If respiratory difficulty occurs, the nurse checks for choanal atresia (see page 878).

The newborn has the ability to smell after the nasal passages are cleared of amniotic fluid and mucus. This ability is demonstrated by the search for milk. Infants will turn their heads toward the milk source, whether bottle or breast.

MOUTH

The lips of the newborn should be pink, and a touch on the lips should produce sucking motions. Saliva is normally scant. The taste buds are developed prior to birth, and the newborn can easily discriminate between sweet and bitter.

The easiest way to examine the mouth completely is to stimulate infants gently to cry by depressing their tongue, thereby causing them to open the mouth fully. It is extremely important to observe the entire mouth to look for a cleft palate, which can be present even in the absence of a cleft lip. The examiner places a clean index finger along the hard and soft palate to feel for any openings (Figure 28–20).

Occasionally, an examination of the gums will reveal *precocious teeth* on the lower central incisor. If they appear loose, they should be removed to prevent aspiration. Gray-white lesions (*inclusion cysts*) on the gums may be confused with teeth. On the hard palate and gum margins, *Epstein's pearls,* small glistening white specks (keratin-containing cysts) that feel hard to the touch are often present. These usually disappear in a few weeks and are of no significance. Thrush may appear as white patches that look like milk curds adhering to the mucous membranes and that cause

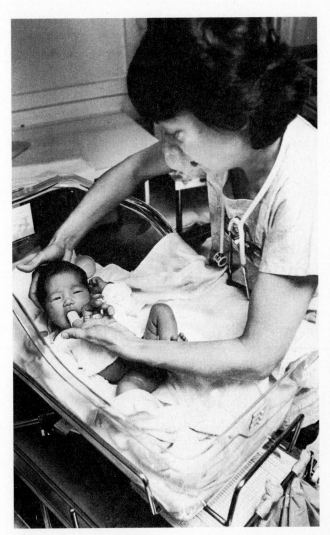

Figure 28–20   The nurse inserts the index finger into the newborn's mouth and feels for any openings along the hard and soft palates.

bleeding when removed. Thrush is caused by *Candida albicans,* often acquired from an infected vaginal tract during birth, and is treated with a preparation of nystatin (Mycostatin).

A *tongue-tied* neonate has a ridge of frenulum tissue attached to the underside of the tongue at varying lengths from its base, causing a heart shape at the tip of the tongue. "Clipping the tongue," or cutting the ridge of tissue, is not recommended. This ridge does not affect speech or eating, but cutting does create an entry for infection.

Transient nerve paralysis resulting from birth trauma may be manifested by asymmetrical mouth movements when the neonate cries or by difficulty with sucking and feeding.

EARS

The ears of the newborn may be crumpled or flattened against the skull and should have well-formed cartilage (appropriate for gestational age). In the normal newborn, the top of the ear should be parallel to the outer and inner canthus of the eye. The ears should be inspected for shape, size, and position. *Low-set ears* are characteristic of many syndromes and may indicate chromosomal abnormalities (especially trisomies 13 and 18), mental retardation, and/or internal organ abnormalities, especially bilateral renal agenesis as a result of embryologic developmental deviations (Figure 28–21). A preauricular skin tag and dermal sinus may be present just in front of the ear. Preauricular tags are ligated at the base and allowed to slough off.

Visualization of the tympanic membranes is not usually done soon after birth since blood and vernix obliterate the ear canal.

Following the first cry, the newborn's hearing improves. Hearing becomes acute as mucus from the middle ear is absorbed and the eustachian tube is aerated. Risk factors (Duara et al 1986) associated with potential hearing loss include:

- The presence of hearing loss in any family member prior to the age of 50 years
- Serum bilirubin level greter than 20 mg/dL for the full-term newborn
- Suspected maternal rubella infection during pregnancy, resulting in congenital rubella syndrome
- Congenital defects of the ear, nose, or throat
- Small neonatal size, particularly less than 1500 g at birth
- Perinatal asphyxia

The newborn's hearing is evaluated by response to loud or moderately loud noises unaccompanied by vibra-

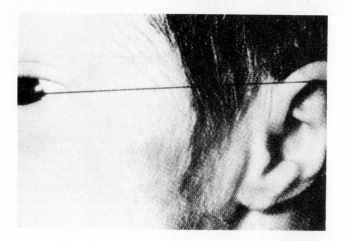

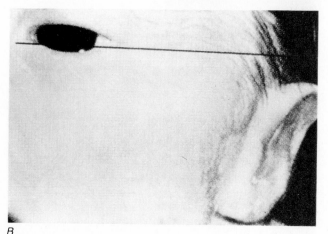

B
Figure 28–21   The position of the external ear may be assessed by drawing a line across the inner and outer canthus of the eye to the insertion of the ear. A Normal position. B True low-set. (Courtesy Mead Johnson Laboratories, Evansville, Ind)

tions. The sleeping neonate should stir or awaken in response to the nearby sounds.

Neck

A short neck, creased with skin folds, is characteristic of the normal newborn. Because muscle tone is not well developed, the neck cannot support the full weight of the head, which rotates freely. The head lags considerably when the neonate is pulled from a supine to a sitting position, but the prone newborn is able to raise the head slightly. The neck is palpated for masses and presence of lymph nodes and is inspected for webbing. Adequacy of range of motion and neck muscle function is determined by fully extending the head in all direction. Injury to the sternocleidomastoid muscle (congenital torticollis) must be considered in the presence of neck rigidity.

The clavicles are evaluated for evidence of fractures, which occasionally occur during difficult deliveries or in neonates with broad shoulders. The normal clavicle is straight. If fractured, a lump and a grating sensation during movements may be palpated along the course of the side of the break. The Moro reflex (p 885) is also elicited to evaluate bilateral equal movement of the arms. If the clavicle is fractured, the response will be demonstrated only on the unaffected side.

Chest

The thorax is cylindrical at birth, and the ribs are flexible. The general appearance of the chest should be assessed. A protrusion at the lower end of the sternum, called the *xiphoid cartilage,* is frequently seen. It is under the skin and will become less apparent after several weeks as the infant accumulates adipose tissue.

Engorged breasts occur frequently in both male and female newborns. This condition, which occurs by the third day, is a result of maternal hormonal influences and may last up to two weeks (Figure 28–22). The infant's breast should not be massaged or squeezed, because this practice may cause a breast abscess. Extra or *supernumerary nipples* are occasionally noted below and medial to the true nipples (Figure 28–23). These harmless pink spots vary in size and do not contain glandular tissue (Korones 1986). Accessory nipples can be differentiated from a pigmented nevi (mole) by placing the fingertips alongside the accessory nipple and pulling the adjacent tissue laterally. The accessory nipple will appear dimpled. At puberty the accessory nipple may darken.

Cry

The newborn's cry should be strong, lusty, and of medium pitch. A high-pitched, shrill cry is abnormal and

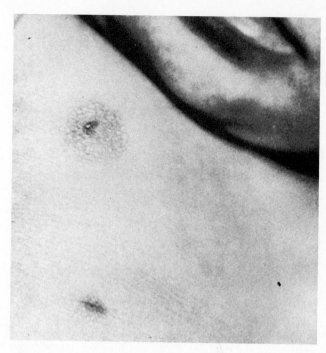

Figure 28–23   Extra or supernumerary nipples may appear below and medial to the true nipples. (Courtesy Mead Johnson Laboratories, Evansville, Ind)

may indicate neurologic disorders or hypoglycemia. Cries usually vary in length after consoling measures are used. The baby's cry is an important method of communication and alerts caretakers to changes in his or her condition and needs.

Respiration

Normal breathing for a term newborn is predominantly diaphragmatic, with associated rising and falling of the abdomen during inspiration and expiration. The normal range is 30 to 60 respirations per minute. Any signs of respiratory distress, nasal flaring, intercostal or xiphoid retractions, or tachypnea (sustained or greater than 60 respirations per minute) should be noted. Hyperextension (chest appears high) or hypoextension (chest appears low) of the anteroposterior diameter of the chest should also be noted. Both the anterior and posterior chest are auscultated. Some breath sounds are heard better when the neonate is crying, but localization and identification of breath sounds are difficult in the newborn. Upper airway noises and bowel sounds may also be heard over the chest wall and make auscultation difficult. Since sounds may be transmitted from the unaffected lung to the affected lung, the absence of breath sounds cannot be diagnosed. Air entry may be noisy in the first couple of hours until lung fluid resolves, especially in cesarean births.

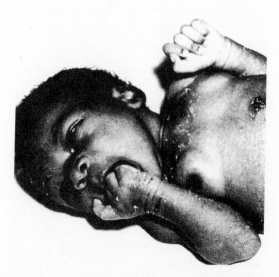

Figure 28–22   Breast hypertrophy (From Korones SB: *High-Risk Newborn Infants,* ed 4. St Louis, Mosby, 1986)

Heart

Heart rates can be as rapid as 180 beats per minute in newborns and fluctuate a great deal. Normal range is 120 to 150 beats per minute. Auscultation provides the nurse with valuable assessment data. The heart is examined for rate and rhythm, position of apical impulse, and heart sound intensity.

The pulse rate is variable and follows the trend of respirations in the neonatal period. The pulse rate is influenced by physical activity, crying, state of wakefulness, and body temperature. Auscultation is performed over the entire precordium, below the left axilla, and below the scapula. Apical pulse rates are obtained by auscultation for a full minute, preferably when the neonate is asleep.

The placement of the heart in the chest should be determined when the neonate is in a quiet state. The heart is relatively large at birth and is located high in the chest, with its apex somewhere between the fourth and fifth intercostal space.

A shift in the mediastinum to either side may indicate pneumothorax, dextrocardia (heart placement on the right side of the chest), or a diaphragmatic hernia. The experienced nurse can diagnose these and many other problems early with a stethoscope. Normally, the heart beat has a "toc tic" sound. A slur or slushing sound (usually after the first sound) may indicate a *murmur*. Although 90 percent of all murmurs are transient and are considered normal (Korones 1986), they should be observed closely by a physician.

A low-pitched, musical murmur heard just to the right of the apex of the heart is fairly common in newborns. Occasionally, significant murmurs will be heard, including the murmur of a patent ductus arteriosus, aortic or pulmonary stenosis, or small ventricular septal defect. However, some significant murmurs may not appear immediately after birth. See Chapter 32 for a discussion of congenital heart defects.

Peripheral pulses (brachial, femoral, pedal) are also evaluated to detect any lags or unusual characteristics. Brachial pulses are palpated bilaterally for equality and compared with the femoral pulses. Femoral pulses are palpated by applying gentle pressure with the middle finger over the femoral canal (Figure 28–24). Decreased or absent femoral pulses indicate coarctation of the aorta and require additional investigation. A wide difference in blood pressure between the upper and lower extremities also indicates coarctation. The measurement of blood pressure is best accomplished by using the Doppler technique or a 1 to 2 inch cuff and a stethoscope over the brachial artery.

Blood pressures are not routinely measured on newborns unless they are having distress, are premature, or are suspected of having some anomaly. Blood pressure is usually 80–60/45–40 mm Hg at birth, and by the tenth day of life it rises to 100/50 mm Hg. It may be difficult to obtain the diastolic pressure or to hear the blood pressure with a standard sphygmomanometer.

Abdomen

The nurse can learn a great deal about the newborn's abdomen without disturbing the infant. It should be cylindrical and protrude slightly. A certain amount of laxness of the abdominal muscles is normal. A scaphoid appearance suggests the absence of abdominal contents. No cyanosis should be present, and few if any blood vessels should be apparent to the eye. There should be no gross distention or bulging. The more distended the abdomen, the tighter the skin becomes, with engorged vessels appearing. Distention is the first sign of many of the abnormalities found in the gastrointestinal tract.

Prior to palpation of the abdomen, the presence or absence of bowel sounds should be auscultated for in all four quadrants. Palpation can cause a transient decrease in intensity of the bowel sounds.

Abdominal palpation should be done systematically. The nurse palpates each of the four abdominal quadrants and moves in a clockwise direction until all four quadrants have been palpated for softness, tenderness, and the presence of masses.

When palpating the abdomen, the nurse should feel for the liver and both kidneys. The newborn's liver is large in proportion to the rest of the body and can usually be felt between 1 and 2 cm below the right costal margin. Kidneys are more difficult to feel, but examination is facilitated if done within four to six hours after birth, before the intestines become distended with air and feedings are initiated. By placing a finger at the posterior flank and pushing upward while pressing downward with the opposite hand, each kidney may be palpated as a firm oval mass between the examiner's finger and hand. The lower pole of the kidney is usually found 1 to 2 cm above the umbilicus. The spleen tip may be palpated in the lateral aspect of the left upper quadrant in the normal newborn.

Umbilical Cord

Initially the umbilical cord is white and gelatinous in appearance, with the two umbilical arteries and one umbilical vein readily apparent. Because a single umbilical artery is frequently associated with congenital anomalies, the vessels should be counted as part of the newborn assessment. The cord begins drying with one or two hours after delivery and is shriveled and blackened by the second or third day. Within seven to ten days, it sloughs off, although a granulating area may remain for a few days longer.

Cord bleeding is abnormal and may result because the cord was inadvertently pulled or because the cord

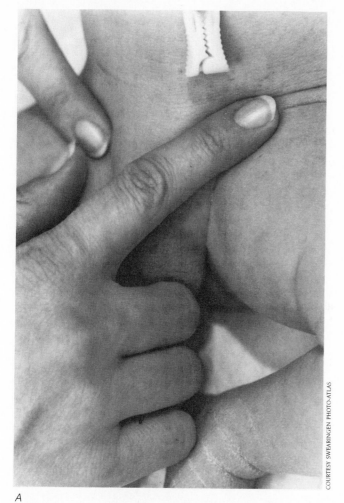

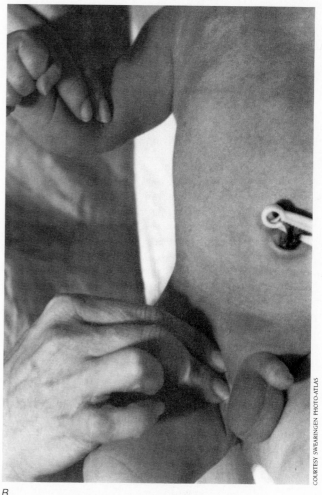

A

B

Figure 28–24   A *Bilaterally palpate the femoral arteries for rate and intensity of the pulses. Press fingertip gently at the groin as shown.* B *Compare the femoral pulses to the brachial pulses by palpating the pulses simultaneously for comparison of rate and intensity.* (From Swearingen PL: *The Addison-Wesley Photo-Atlas of Nursing Procedures.* Menlo Park, Calif, Addison-Wesley, 1984)

clamp was loosened. Foul-smelling drainage is also abnormal and is generally caused by infection. Such infection requires immediate treatment to prevent the development of septicemia. If the neonate has a patent urachus (abnormal connection between the umbilicus and bladder), moistness or draining urine may be apparent at the base of the cord.

Genitals

FEMALE INFANTS

The labia majora, labia minora, and clitoris are examined, and the nurse notes the size of each as appropriate for gestational age. A vaginal tag or hymenal tag is often evident and will usually disappear in a few weeks. During the first week of life, the neonate may have a vaginal discharge composed of thick whitish mucus. This discharge, which can become tinged with blood, is referred to as *pseu-domenstruation* and is caused by the withdrawal of maternal hormones. Smegma, a white cheeselike substance, is often present under the labia.

MALE INFANTS

The penis is inspected to determine whether the urinary orifice is correctly positioned. *Hypospadias* occurs when the urinary meatus is located on the ventral surface of the penis. It occurs most commonly in white infants in the United States. *Phimosis* is a condition commonly occurring in newborn males in which the opening of the prepuce is narrowed and the foreskin cannot be retracted over the glans. This condition may interfere with urination, so the adequacy of the urinary stream should be evaluated.

The scrotum is inspected for size and symmetry and should be palpated to verify the presence of both testes. The testes are palpated separately between the thumb and forefinger, with the thumb and forefinger of the other hand placed together over the inguinal canal. Scrotal edema and discoloration are common in breech deliveries. *Hydrocele* (collection of fluid surrounding the testes in the scrotum) is common in newborns and should be identified.

Anus

The anal area is inspected to verify that it is patent and has no fissure. Imperforate anus and rectal atresia may be ruled out by a digital examination. The passage of the first meconium stool is also noted. Atresia of the gastrointestinal tract or meconium ileus with resultant obstruction must be considered if the newborn does not pass meconium in the first 24 hours of life.

Extremities

Extremities are examined for gross deformities, extra digits or webbing, clubfoot, and range of motion. The normal neonate's extremities appear short, are generally flexible, and move symmetrically.

ARMS AND HANDS

Nails extend beyond the fingertips in term infants. Fingers and toes should be counted. *Polydactyly* is the presence of extra digits on either the hands or feet. Polydactyly is more common in black infants. If the infant has polydactyly and the parents do not, a dominant genetic disorder can be ruled out. *Syndactyly* refers to fusion (webbing) of fingers or toes. Hands should be inspected for normal palmar creases. A single palmar crease, called *simian line* (see Figure 9–23) is frequently present in children with Down syndrome. (See Chapter 9 for further discussion.)

Brachial palsy, which is partial or complete paralysis of portions of the arm, results from trauma to the brachial plexus during a difficult delivery. It occurs most commonly when strong traction is exerted on the head of the neonate in an attempt to deliver a shoulder lodged behind the symphysis pubis in the presence of shoulder dystocia. Brachial palsy may also occur during a breech delivery if an arm becomes trapped over the head and traction is exerted.

The portion of the arm affected is determined by the nerves damaged. *Erb-Duchenne paralysis* involves damage to the upper arm (fifth and sixth cervical nerves) and is the most common type. Injury to the eighth cervical and first thoracic nerve roots and the lower portion of the plexus produces the relatively rare *lower arm injury.* The *whole arm type* results from damage to the entire plexus.

With Erb-Duchenne paralysis (Erb's palsy) the newborn's arm lies limply at the side (Figure 28–25). The elbow is held in extension, with the forearm pronated. The

newborn is unable to elevate the arm, and therefore the Moro reflex cannot be elicited on the affected side. When lower arm injury occurs, paralysis of the hand and wrist results; complete paralysis of the limb occurs with the whole arm type.

Treatment involves passive range-of-motion exercises to prevent muscle contractures and to restore function. The nurse should carefully instruct the parents in the correct method of performing the exercises and supervise practice sessions. In more severe cases, splinting of the arm is indicated until the edema decreases. The arm is held in a position of abduction and external rotation with the elbow flexed 90°. The "Statue of Liberty" splint is commonly used, although similar results are obtained by attaching a strip of muslin to the head of the crib and tying the other end around the wrist, thereby holding the arm up.

Prognosis is related to the degree of nerve damage resulting from trauma and hemorrhage within the nerve sheath. Complete recovery occurs within a few months with minimal trauma. Moderate trauma may result in some partial paralysis. Recovery is unlikely with severe trauma, and muscle wasting may develop.

LEGS AND FEET

The legs of the newborn should be of equal length, with symmetrical skin folds. *Ortolani's maneuver* is per-

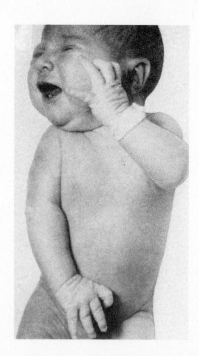

Figure 28–25 Erb's palsy resulting from injury to the fifth and sixth cervical roots of brachial plexus (Photo reproduced with permission from Potter EL, Craig JM: Pathology of the Fetus and Infant, ed 3. Copyright 1975 by Year Book Medical Publishers, Chicago)

formed to rule out the possibility of congenital hip dysplasia. With the baby supine, the nurse places thumbs on
the inner thighs and fingers on the outer aspect of the
neonate's leg from the knee to the head of the femur. The
legs are flexed, abducted, and pressed downward. If a click
is felt under the index finger and there is resistance to
abduction, a dislocation exists (Figure 28–26).

The feet are then examined for evidence of a talipes
deformity (clubfoot). Intrauterine position frequently
causes the feet to appear to turn inward (Figure 28–27);
this is termed a "positional" clubfoot. If the feet can easily
be returned to midline by manipulation, no treatment is
indicated. Further investigation is indicated when the foot
will not turn to a midline position or align readily and is
considered a "true" clubfoot.

Back

With the baby prone, the nurse examines the back.
The spine should appear straight and flat, since the lumbar
and sacral curves do not develop until the infant begins to
sit. The base of the spine is then examined for a dermal

sinus. The nevus pilosus ("hairy nevus") is only occasionally found at the base of the spine in newborns, but it is
significant because it is frequently associated with spina
bifida.

Neurologic Status

The neurologic examination assesses the intactness of
the neonatal nervous system. It should begin with a period
of observation, noting the general physical characteristics
and behavior of the newborn. Important behaviors to assess
are the state of alertness, resting posture, cry, and quality
of muscle tone and motor activity.

Partially flexed extremities with the legs abducted to
the abdomen is the usual position of the neonate. When
awake, the newborn may exhibit purposeless, uncoordinated bilateral movements of the extremities. If these movements are absent, minimal, or obviously asymmetrical, neurologic dysfunction should be suspected. Eye movements
are observable during the first few days of life. An alert
neonate is able to fixate on faces and brightly colored objects. If a bright light shines in the newborn's eyes, the

(Text continues on page 886.)

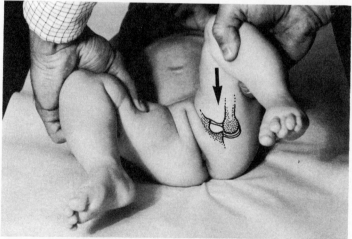
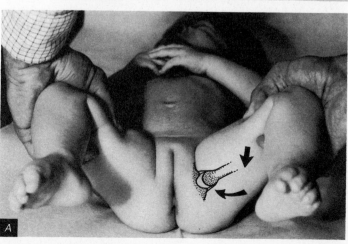
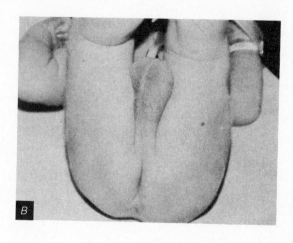

Figure 28–26 Congenital dislocation of the right hip. A
Ortolani's maneuver puts downward pressure on the hip and
then inward rotation. If the hip is dislocated, this will force the
femoral head over the acetabular rim with a noticeable "clunk."
B Dislocated right hip in a young infant as seen on gross
inspection. (From Smith DW: Recognizable Patterns of
Human Deformation. Philadelphia, Saunders, 1981)

Neonatal Physical Assessment Guide

Assessment and normal findings	Alterations and possible causes*	Nursing responses to data base†
VITAL SIGNS		
Blood pressure		
At birth: 80–60/45–40 mm Hg Day 10: 100/50 mm Hg (may be unable to measure diastolic pressure with standard sphygmomanometer)	Low BP (hypovolemia, shock)	Monitor BP in all cases of distress, prematurity, or suspected anomaly. Low BP; refer to physician immediately so measures to improve circulation are begun.
Pulse: 120–150 beats/min (if asleep 100/min; if crying, up to 180/min)	Weak pulse (decreased cardiac output) Bradycardia (severe asphyxia)	Assess skin perfusion by blanching (capillary refill test). Correlate finding with BP assessments; refer to physician.
	Tachycardia (over 160 beats/min at rest) (infection, CNS problems)	Carry out neurologic and thermoregulation assessments.
Respirations		
30–50 breaths/min Synchronization of chest and abdominal movements Diaphragmatic and abdominal breathing	Tachypnea (pneumonia, RDS) Rapid, shallow breathing (hypermagnesemia due to large doses given to mothers with PIH)	Identify sleep-wake state; correlate with respiratory pattern.
Transient tachypnea	Expiratory grunting, subcostal and substernal retractions; flaring of nares (respiratory distress); apnea (cold stress, respiratory disorder) Respirations below 30 breaths/min (maternal anesthesia or analgesia)	Evaluate for all signs of respiratory distress; report findings to physician.
Crying		
Strong and lusty Moderate tone and pitch Alternate periods of excitability and quietness Cries varying in length 3–7 min after consoling measures are used	High-pitched, shrill (neurologic disorder, hypoglycemia) Weak or absent (CNS disorder, laryngeal problem)	Discuss neonate's use of cry for communication. Assess and record abnormal cries.
Temperature		
Axilla 36.5–37C (97.7–98.6F) Rectal 36.6–37.2C (97.8–99F); 36.8C (98.8F) desired Heavier neonates tend to have higher body temperatures	Elevated temperature (room too warm, too much clothing or covers, dehydration, sepsis, brain damage) Subnormal temperature (brain stem involvement, cold) Swings of more than 2F from one reading to next or subnormal temperature (infection)	Notify physician of elevation or drop. Counsel parents on possible causes of elevated or low temperatures, appropriate home care measures, when to call physician. Teach parents how to take rectal and/or axillary temperature; assess parents' information regarding use of thermometer; provide teaching as needed.
Weight		
2950–3515 g (6.5–7.75 lb)	<2748 g (<6 lb) = SGA or preterm infant >4050 g (>9 lb) = LGA (infants of diabetic mothers)	Plot weight and gestational age to identify high-risk infants. Ascertain body build of parents. Counsel parents regarding appropriate caloric intake.
Within first 3 to 4 days, normal weight loss of 5%–10% Large babies tend to lose more due to greater fluid loss in proportion to birth weight except IDMs	Loss greater than 15% (small fluid intake, loss of meconium and urine, feeding difficulties)	Notify physician of net losses or gains. Calculate fluid intake and losses from all sources (insensible water loss, radiant warmers, and phototherapy lights).
Length		
45 cm (18 in) to 52.3 cm (20.5 in) Grows 10 cm (4 in) during first 3 months	Less than 45 cm (congenital dwarf) Short/long bones proximally (achondroplasia) Short/long bones distally (Ellis-Van Creveld syndrome)	Assess for other signs of dwarfism. Determine other signs of skeletal system adequacy. Plot progress at subsequent well-baby visits.

*Possible causes of alterations are placed in parentheses.
†This column provides guidelines for further assessment and initial nursing interventions.

Neonatal Physical Assessment Guide (continued)

Assessment and normal findings	Alterations and possible causes*	Nursing responses to data base†
POSTURE		
Body usually flexed, hands tightly clenched, neck appears short as chin rests on chest In breech deliveries, feet are usually dorsi-flexed	Only extension noted, inability to move from midline (trauma, hypoxia, immaturity) Constant motion	Record spontaneity of motor activity and symmetry of movements. If parents express concern about neonate's movement patterns, reassure and evaluate further if appropriate.
SKIN		
Color		
Color consistent with racial background	Pallor of face, conjunctiva (anemia, hypothermia, anoxia)	Discuss with parents common skin color variations to allay fears.
Pink-tinged or ruddy color over face, trunk, extremities	Beefy red (hypoglycemia, immature vasomotor reflexes, polycythemia)	Document extent and time of occurrence of color change.
Common variations: acrocyanosis, circumoral cyanosis, or harlequin color change	Meconium staining (fetal distress) Icterus (hemolytic reaction from blood incompatibility, sepsis)	Obtain Hb and hematocrit values. Assess for respiratory difficulty. Differentiate between physiologic or pathologic jaundice.
Mottled when undressed	Cyanosis (choanal atresia, CNS damage or trauma, respiratory or cardiac problem, cold stress)	Assess degree of (central or peripheral) cyanosis and possible causes; refer to physician.
Minor bruising over buttocks in breech presentation and over eyes and forehead in facial presentations		Discuss with parents cause and course of minor bruising related to labor and delivery.
Texture		
Smooth, soft, flexible; may have dry, peeling hands and feet	Generalized cracked or peeling skin (SGA or postterm; blood incompatibility; metabolic, kidney dysfunction)	Report to physician.
	Seborrhea-dermatitis (cradle cap) Absence of vernix (postmature) Yellow vernix (bilirubin staining)	Instruct parents to shampoo the scalp and anterior fontanelle area daily with soap; rinse well; avoid use of oil.
Elastic, returns to normal shape after pinching	Maintains tent shape (dehydration)	Assess for other signs and symptoms of dehydration.
Pigmentation		
Clear; milia across bridge of nose or forehead will disappear within a few weeks		Advise parents not to pinch or prick these pimplelike areas.
Café-au-lait spots (one or two)	Six or more (neurologic disorder such as Van Recklinghausen disease, cutaneous neurofibromatosis)	
Mongolian spots common in dark-skinned infants over lumbar dorsal area and buttock		Assure parents of normalcy of this pigmentation; it will fade in first year or two.
	Xanthoma (benign or may be associated with abnormal metabolism of lipids)	Reassure parents that xanthoma plaques will disappear in a few weeks.
Erythema toxicum	Impetigo (group A β-hemolytic streptococcus or *Staphylococcus aureus* infection)	If impetigo occurs, instruct parents about hand-washing and linen precautions during home care.
Telangiectatic nevi birthmarks	Hemangiomas: Nevus flammeus (port-wine stain) Nevus vascularis (strawberry hemangioma) Cavernous hemangiomas	Collaborate with physician. Counsel parents about birthmark's progression to allay misconceptions. Record size and shape of hemangiomas. Refer for follow-up at well-baby clinic.
Rashes	Rashes (infection)	Assess location and type of rash (macular, papular, vesicular). Obtain history of onset, prenatal history, and related signs and symptoms.
Petechiae of head or neck (breech presentation, cord around neck)	Generalized petechiae (clotting abnormalities)	Determine cause; advise parents if further health care is needed.

*Possible causes of alterations are placed in parentheses.
†This column provides guidelines for further assessment and initial nursing interventions.

Neonatal Physical Assessment Guide (continued)

Assessment and normal findings	Alterations and possible causes*	Nursing responses to data base†
HEAD		
General appearance, size, movement		
Round, symmetrical, and moves easily from left to right and up and down; soft and pliable	Asymmetrical, flattened occiput on either side of head (plagiocephaly) Head held at angle (torticollis)	Instruct parents to change infant's sleeping positions frequently.
	Unable to move head side-to-side (neurologic trauma)	Determine adequacy of all neurologic signs.
Circumference: 33–35 cm (13–14 in); 2 cm greater than chest circumference	Extreme differences in size may be microencephaly (Cornelia de Lange syndrome, CID, rubella, toxoplasmosis, chromosome abnormalities), hydrocephalus (meningomyelocele achondroplasia), anencephaly (neural tube defect) Head 3 cm or more larger than chest circumference (preterm, hydrocephalus)	Measure circumference from occiput to frontal area using metal or paper tape. Measure chest circumference using metal or paper tape and compare to head circumference. Record measurements on growth chart. Reevaluate at well-baby visits.
One-fourth of body size		Record measurements on growth chart.
Size increases 2 in. during first 4 months of life		Reevaluate at well-baby visits.
Common variations:		
Molding—overriding cranial bones Breech and cesarean newborns' heads are round and well shaped	Cephalhematoma (trauma during delivery; persists up to 3 weeks) Caput succedaneum (long labor and delivery; disappears in 1 week)	Reassure parents regarding common manifestations due to birth process and when they should disappear.
Fontanelles		
Palpation of juncture of cranial bones		
Anterior fontanelle; 3–4 cm long by 2–3 cm wide, diamond-shaped	Overlapping of anterior fontanelle (malnourished or preterm infant)	Discuss normal closure times with parents and care of "soft spots" to allay misconceptions.
Posterior fontanelle; 1–2 cm at birth, triangle-shaped	Premature closure of sutures (craniostenosis) Late closure (hydrocephalus)	Refer to physician. Observe for signs and symptoms of hydrocephalus.
Slight pulsation	Moderate to severe pulsation (vascular problems)	Refer to physician.
Moderate bulging noted with crying or pulsations with heartbeat	Bulging (increased intracranial pressure, meningitis)	
	Sunken (dehydration)	Evaluate hydration status.
HAIR		
Texture		
Smooth with fine texture variations (Note: variations dependent on ethnic background)	Coarse, brittle, dry hair (hypothyroidism) White forelock (Waardenburg syndrome)	Instruct parents regarding routine care of hair and scalp.
Distribution		
Scalp hair high over eyebrows (Spanish-Mexican hairline begins mid-forehead and extends down back of neck)	Low forehead and posterior hairlines may indicate chromosomal disorders	Assess for other signs of chromosomal aberrations. Refer to physician.
FACE		
Symmetrical movement of all facial features, normal hairline, eyebrows, and eyelashes present		Assess and record symmetry of all parts, shape, regularity of features, sameness or differences in features.
Spacing of features		
Eyes at same level; nostrils equal size, cheeks full, and sucking pads present	Eyes wide apart—ocular hypertelorism (Apert syndrome, cri-du-chat, Turner syndrome)	Observe for other signs and symptoms indicative of disease states or chromosomal aberrations.
Lips equal on both sides of midline	Abnormal face (Down syndrome, cretinism, gargoylism)	

*Possible causes of alterations are placed in parentheses.
†This column provides guidelines for further assessment and initial nursing interventions.

Neonatal Physical Assessment Guide (continued)

Assessment and normal findings	Alterations and possible causes*	Nursing responses to data base†
Spacing of features (continued)		
Chin recedes when compared to other bones of face	Abnormally small jaw—micrognathia (Pierre Robin syndrome, Treacher Collins syndrome)	Maintain airway. Initiate surgical consultation and referral.
Movement		
Makes facial grimaces	Inability to suck, grimace, and close eyelids (cranial nerve injury)	Initiate neurologic assessment and consultation.
Symmetrical when resting and crying	Asymmetry (paralysis of facial cranial nerve)	Assess and record symmetry of all parts, shape, regularity of features, sameness or differences in features.
Frontal and maxillary sinuses	Frontal—absent at birth Maxillary—nontender	
EYES		
General placement and appearance		
Bright and clear, even placement; slight nystagmus	Gross nystagmus (damage to third, fourth, and sixth cranial nerves)	
Concomitant strabismus	Constant and fixed strabismus	Reassure parents that strabismus is considered normal up to 6 months.
Move in all directions		
Blue or slate blue gray (permanent color established by 3 months of age)	Lack of pigmentation (albinism) Brushfield spots (may indicate Down syndrome)	Discuss with parents any necessary eye precautions. Assess for other signs of Down syndrome.
Brown color at birth in dark-skinned infants		Discuss with parents that permanent eye color is usually established by 3 months of age.
Eyelids		
Position: above pupils but within iris, no dropping	Elevation or retraction of upper lid (hyperthyroidism) "Setting sun" (hydrocephalus), ptosis (congenital or paralysis of oculomotor muscle)	Assess for signs of hydrocephalus and hyperthyroidism. Evaluate interference with vision in subsequent well-baby visits.
Eyes on parallel plane Epicanthal folds in Oriental and 20% of Caucasian newborns	Upward slant in non-Orientals (Down syndrome) Epicanthal folds (Down syndrome, cri-du-chat syndrome)	Assess for other signs of Down syndrome.
Movement		
Blink reflex in response to light stimulus		
Inspection		
Edematous for first few days of life, resulting from delivery and instillation of silver nitrate (chemical conjunctivitis); palpation; no lumps or redness	Purulent drainage (infection); infectious conjunctivitis (staphylococcus or Gram-negative organisms) Marginal blepharitis (lid edges red, crusted, scaly)	Initiate good hand-washing. Refer to physician. Evaluate infant for seborrheic dermatitis; scales can be removed easily.
Cornea and retina		
Clear Corneal reflex present Circular red reflex	Ulceration (herpes infection); large cornea or corneas of unequal size (congenital glaucoma) Clouding, opacity of lens (cataract)	Refer to ophthalmologist. Assess for other manifestations of congenital herpes; institute nursing care measures.
Sclera		
May appear bluish in newborn, then white; slightly brownish color frequent in blacks	True blue sclera (osteogenesis imperfecta)	Refer to physician.
Pupils		
Pupils are equal in size, round, and react to light by accommodation	Anisocoria—unequal pupils (CNS damage) Dilatation or constriction (intracranial damage, retinoblastoma, glaucoma) Pupils nonreactive to light or accommodation (brain injury)	Refer for neurologic examination.

*Possible causes of alterations are placed in parentheses.
†This column provides guidelines for further assessment and initial nursing interventions.

Neonatal Physical Assessment Guide (continued)

Assessment and normal findings	Alterations and possible causes*	Nursing responses to data base†
Pupils (contined)		
Slight nystagmus in infant who has not learned to focus	Nystagmus (labyrinthine disturbance, CNS disorder)	
Pupil light reflex demonstrated at birth or by 3 weeks of age		
Conjunctiva		
Chemical conjunctivitis	Pale color (anemia)	Obtain hematocrit and hemoglobin.
Subconjunctival hemorrhage		Reassure parents that chemical conjunctivitis will subside in 1–2 days and subconjunctival hemorrhage disappears in a few weeks.
Palpebral conjunctiva (red but not hyperemic)	Inflammation or edema (infection, blocked tear duct)	
Vision		
20/150	Cataracts (congenital infection)	Record any questions about visual acuity and initiate follow-up evaluation at first well-baby checkup.
Tracks moving object to midline		
Fixed focus on objects at a distance of about 7 in; may be difficult to evaluate in newborn		
Prefers faces, geometric designs, and black and white to colors		
Lashes and lacrimal glands		
Presence of lashes (lashes may be absent in preterm infants)	No lashes on inner two-thirds of lid (Treacher Collins syndrome); bushy lashes (Hurler syndrome); long lashes (Cornelia de Lange syndrome)	
Cry commonly tearless	Excessive tearing (plugged lacrimal duct, natal narcotic abstinence syndrome)	Demonstrate to parents how to milk blocked tear duct.
		Refer to ophthalmologist if tearing is excessive before third month of life.
NOSE		
Appearance		
External nasal aspects		
May appear flattened as a result of delivery process	Continued flat or broad bridge of nose (Down syndrome)	Arrange consultation with specialist.
Small and narrow in midline; even placement in relationship to eyes and mouth	Low bridge of nose; beaklike nose (Apert syndrome, Treacher Collins syndrome)	Initiate evaluation of chromosomal abnormalities.
	Upturned (Cornelia de Lange syndrome)	
Patent nares bilaterally (nose breathers)	Blockage of nares (mucus and/or secretions)	Inspect for obstruction of nares.
Sneezing common to clear nasal passages	Flaring nares (respiratory distress)	
	Choanal atresia	
Internal nasal aspects		
Pink and firm mucous membranes		
Septum midline and without polyps or tumors	Deviated or perforated septum; tumors or polyps of septum	Collaborate with physician.
No swelling or nasal discharge	Swelling and erythema (infection)	Note and record characteristics of nasal discharge.
Smelling abilities		
Identifies odors; appears to smell breast milk	No response to stimulating odors	Inspect for obstructions of nares.

*Possible causes of alterations are placed in parentheses.
†This column provides guidelines for further assessment and initial nursing interventions.

Neonatal Physical Assessment Guide (continued)

Assessment and normal findings	Alterations and possible causes*	Nursing responses to data base†
MOUTH		
Function of facial, hypoglossal, glossopharyngeal, and vagus nerves		
Symmetry of movement and strength	Mouth draws to one side (transient seventh cranial nerve paralysis due to pressure in utero or trauma during delivery, congenital paralysis) Fishlike shape (Treacher Collins syndrome)	Initiate neurologic consultation. Administer eye care if eye on affected side is unable to close.
Presence of gag, swallowing, and sucking reflexes Adequate salivation	Suppressed or absent reflexes	Evaluate other neurologic functions of these nerves.
Palate (soft and hard)		
Hard palate dome-shaped Uvula midline with symmetrical movement of soft palate	High-steepled palate (Treacher Collins syndrome)	
Palate intact, sucks well when stimulated	Clefts in either hard or soft palate (polygenic disorder)	Initiate a surgical consultation referral.
Epithelial (Epstein's) pearls appear on mucosa		Assure parents that these are normal in newborn and will disappear at 2 or 3 months of age.
Esophagus patent; some drooling common in newborn	Excessive drooling or bubbling (esophageal atresia)	Test for patency of esophagus.
Tongue		
Free-moving in all directions, midline	Lack of movement or asymmetrical movement Tongue-tied	Further assess neurologic functions. Test reflex elevation of tongue when depressed with tongue blade.
	Deviations from midline (cranial nerve damage)	Check for signs of weakness or deviation.
Pink color, smooth to rough texture, non-coated	White cheesy coating (thrush) Tongue has deep ridges	Differentiate between thrush and milk curds. Reassure parents that tongue pattern may change from day to day.
Tongue proportional to mouth	Large tongue with short frenulum (cretinism, Down and other syndromes)	Evaluate in well-baby clinic to assess development delays. Initiate referrals.
EARS		
External ear		
Without lesions, cysts, or nodules	Nodules, cysts, or sinus tracts in front of ear. Adherent earlobes	Evaluate characteristics of lesions. Counsel parents to clean external ear with washcloth only; discourage use of cotton-tip applicators.
	Preauricular skin tags	Refer to physician for ligation.
Inner canal		
Bony landmarks present (may not be visible)	Bulging (infection) Discharge, disagreeable odor (infection)	Assess for other signs of infections.
Tympanic membrane light color, pearly gray Translucent, intact	Ruptured tympanic membrane	Remove wax and vernix debris with wire loop or curette under constant visualization.
Hearing		
With first cry, eustachian tubes are cleared		
Absence of all risk factors	Presence of one or more risk factors	Assess history of risk factors for hearing loss.
Attends to sounds; sudden or loud noise elicits Moro reflex	No response to sound stimuli (deafness)	Test for Moro reflex.

*Possible causes of alterations are placed in parentheses.
†This column provides guidelines for further assessment and initial nursing interventions.

Neonatal Physical Assessment Guide (continued)

Assessment and normal findings	Alterations and possible causes*	Nursing responses to data base†
NECK		
Appearance		
Short, straight, creased with skin folds	Abnormally short neck (Turner syndrome) Arching or inability to flex neck (meningitis, congenital anomaly)	Report findings to physician.
Posterior neck lacks loose extra folds of skin	Webbing of neck (Turner syndrome, Down syndrome, trisomy 18)	Assess for other signs of the syndromes.
Head moves freely from side to side	Neck rigidity (congenital torticollis, eleventh cranial nerve damage)	
Sternocleidomastoid muscle should be symmetrical on both sides If infant is held upright and body tilted, head returns to upright position		
Trachea (palpate from top to bottom with thumb and index fingers) Slightly right of midline	Deviated left or right (pneumothorax, tumor of chest or neck)	
Thyroid		
Thyroid not usually palpable in newborn No masses	Palpate for lymph nodes and masses	
Clavicles		
Straight and intact	Knot or lump on clavicle (fracture during difficult delivery)	Obtain detailed labor and delivery history; apply figure 8 bandage.
Moro reflex elicitable	Unilateral Moro reflex response on unaffected side (fracture of clavicle, brachial palsy, Erb-Duchenne paralysis)	Collaborate with physician.
Symmetrical movement of shoulders	Hypoplasia	
CHEST		
Appearance and size		
Circumference: 32.5 cm, 1–2 cm less than head Wider than it is long		Measure at level of nipples after exhalation.
Normal shape without depressed or prominent sternum	Funnel chest (congenital or associated with Marfan syndrome)	Determine adequacy of other respiratory and circulatory signs.
Lower end of sternum (xiphoid cartilage) may be protruding; is less apparent after several weeks	Continued protrusion of xiphoid cartilage (Marfan syndrome, "pigeon chest")	Assess for other signs and symptoms of various syndromes.
Sternum 8 cm long	Barrel chest	
Expansion and retraction		
Bilateral expansion	Unequal chest expansion (pneumonia, pneumothorax, respiratory distress)	Assess respiratory effort regularity, flaring of nares, difficulty on both inspiration and expiration.
No intercostal, subcostal, or suprasternal retractions	Retractions (respiratory distress)	Record and consult physician.
Auscultation		
Breath sounds are louder in infants Heard bilaterally	Decreased breath sounds (decreased respiratory activity, atelectasis, pneumothorax)	Perform assessment and report to physician any positive findings.
Chest and axilla clear on crying	Increased breath sounds (resolving pneumonia or in cesarean births)	

*Possible causes of alterations are placed in parentheses.
†This column provides guidelines for further assessment and initial nursing interventions.

Neonatal Physical Assessment Guide (continued)

Assessment and normal findings	Alterations and possible causes*	Nursing responses to data base†
Bronchial breath sounds (heard where trachea and bronchi closest to chest wall, above sternum and between scapulae)		
Bronchial sounds bilaterally Air entry clear Rales may indicate normal newborn atelectasis Cough reflex absent at birth appears in 2 or more days	Adventitious or abnormal sounds (respiratory disease or distress)	
Breasts		
Flat with symmetrical nipples Breast tissue diameter 5 cm or more at term Distance between nipples 8 cm	Lack of breast tissue (preterm or SGA)	
Breast engorgement occurs on third day of life; liquid discharge may be expressed in term infants	Breast abscesses	Reassure parents of normalcy of breast engorgement.
Nipples	Supernumerary nipples Dark-colored nipples	
HEART		
Auscultation		
Location: lies horizontally, with left border extending to left of midclavicle		
Regular rhythm and rate	Arrhythmia (anoxia), tachycardia, bradycardia	Refer all arrhythmia and gallop rhythms.
Determination of point of maximal impulse (PMI)	Malpositioning (enlargement, abnormal placement, pneumothorax, dextrocardia, diaphragmatic hernia)	Initiate cardiac evaluation.
Usually lateral to midclavicular line at third or fourth intercostal space		
Functional murmurs No thrills	Location of murmurs (possible congenital cardiac anomaly)	Evaluate murmur: location, timing, and duration; observe for accompanying cardiac pathology symptoms; ascertain family history.
Horizontal groove at diaphragm shows flaring of rib cage to mild degree	Marked rib flaring (vitamin D deficiency) Inadequacy of respiratory movement	Initiate cardiopulmonary evaluation; assess pulses and blood pressures in all four extremities for equality and quality.
ABDOMEN		
Appearance		
Cylindrical with some protrusion; appears large in relation to pelvis; some laxness of abdominal muscles No cyanosis, few vessels seen Diastasis recti—common in black infants	Distention, shiny abdomen with engorged vessels (gastrointestinal abnormalities, infection, congenital megacolon) Scaphoid abdominal appearance (diaphragmatic hernia) Increased or decreased peristalsis (duodenal stenosis, small bowel obstruction)	Examine abdomen thoroughly for mass or organomegaly. Measure abdominal girth. Report deviations of abdominal size. Assess other signs and symptoms of obstruction.
	Localized flank bulging (enlarged kidneys, ascites, or absent abdominal muscles)	Refer to physician.
Palpation		
Nontender	Tense abdomen with marked rigidity or resistance to pressure (infection)	Take temperature and assess other signs and symptoms.
No palpable masses	Solid masses (Wilm's tumor)	Avoid deep palpation of abdomen; initiate referral.
Liver		
Liver 1–2 cm below right costal margin	Enlarged liver (sepsis, erythroblastosis)	Report and record size, consistency, and tenderness.

*Possible causes of alterations are placed in parentheses.
†This column provides guidelines for further assessment and initial nursing interventions.

Neonatal Physical Assessment Guide (continued)

Assessment and normal findings	Alterations and possible causes*	Nursing responses to data base†
Spleen		
Tip under left costal margin	Enlarged spleen (trauma)	
Kidney		
Posterior flank firm, oval mass, not enlarged, less commonly palpable	Displaced kidney (Wilm's tumor, neuroblastoma, polycystic kidney, agenesis)	Initiate nephrologic consultation.
Umbilicus		
No protrusion of umbilicus Protrusion of umbilicus common in black infants Bluish white color Cutis navel (umbilical cord projects); granulation tissue in navel	Umbilical hernia Patent urachus (congenital malformation) Omphalocele Gastroschisis Redness or exudate around cord (infection) Yellow discoloration (hemolytic disease, meconium staining)	Measure umbilical hernia by palpating the opening and record it; it should close by 1 year of age; if not, refer to physician. Instruct parents on cord care and hygiene.
Two arteries and one vein apparent Begins drying 1–2 hours after birth No bleeding	Single umbilical artery (congenital anomalies)	
Auscultation and percussion		
Soft bowel sounds heard shortly after birth; heard every 10–30 sec	Bowel sounds in chest (diaphragmatic hernia) Absence of bowel sounds	Collaborate with physician.
	Hyperperistalsis (intestinal obstruction)	Assess for other signs of dehydration and/or infection.
Femoral pulses		
Palpable, equal, bilateral	Absent or diminished femoral pulses (coarctation of aorta)	Monitor blood pressure in upper and lower extremities.
Inguinal area		
No bulges along inguinal area No inguinal lymph nodes felt	Inguinal hernia	Initate referral. Continue follow-up in well-baby clinic.
Bladder		
Percusses 1–4 cm above symphysis Emptied about 3 hours after birth; if not, at time of birth Urine—inoffensive, mild odor	Failure to void within 24–48 hours after birth Exposure of bladder mucosa (exstrophy of bladder) Foul odor (infection)	Check if baby voided at birth. Consult with clinician; obtain urine specimen if infection is suspected.
GENITALS		
Gender clearly delineated	Ambiguous genitals	Refer for genetic consultation.
MALE		
Penis		
Slender in appearance, 2.5 cm long, 1 cm wide at birth Normal urinary orifice, urethral meatus at tip of penis	Micropenis (congenital anomaly) Meatal atresia	Observe and record first voiding.
	Hypospadias, epispadias	Collaborate with physician in presence of abnormality.
Noninflamed urethral opening	Urethritis (infection)	Palpate for enlarged inguinal lymph nodes and record painful urination.
Foreskin adheres to glans; prepuce can be retracted beyond urethral opening	Ulceration of meatal opening (infection, inflammation)	Evaluate whether ulcer is due to diaper rash; counsel regarding care.
Uncircumcised foreskin tight for 2–3 months	Phimosis—if still tight after 3 months	Instruct parents to retract foreskin gently for cleaning at monthly intervals after 4 months of age.
Circumcised Erectile tissue present		Teach parents how to care for circumcision.

*Possible causes of alterations are placed in parentheses.
†This column provides guidelines for further assessment and initial nursing interventions.

Neonatal Physical Assessment Guide (continued)

Assessment and normal findings	Alterations and possible causes*	Nursing responses to data base†
Scrotum		
Skin loose and hanging or tight and small; extensive rugae and normal size	Large scrotum containing fluid (hydrocele)	Shine a light through scrotum (transilluminate) to verify diagnosis.
Normal skin color	Red, shiny scrotal skin (orchitis)	
Scrotal discoloration common in breech		
Testes		
Descended by birth; not consistently found in scrotum	Undescended testes (cryptorchidism)	If testes cannot be felt in scrotum, gently palpate femoral, inguinal, perineal, and abdominal areas for presence.
Testes size 1.5–2 cm at birth	Enlarged testes (tumor) Small testes (Klinefelter syndrome or adrenal hyperplasia)	Refer and collaborate with physician for further diagnostic studies.
FEMALE		
Mons		
Normal skin color; area pigmented in dark-skinned infants		
Labia majora cover labia minora; symmetrical size appropriate for gestational age	Hematoma, lesions	Evaluate for recent trauma.
Clitoris		
Normally large in newborn Edema and bruising in breech delivery	Hypertrophy (hermaphroditism)	
Vagina		
Urinary meatus and vaginal orifice visible (0.5 cm circumference)	Inflammation; erythema and discharge (urethritis)	Collect urine specimen for laboratory examination.
Vaginal tag or hymenal tag disappears in a few weeks	Congenital absence of vagina	Refer to physician.
Discharge; smegma under labia	Foul smelling discharge (infection)	Collect data and further evaluate reason for discharge.
Bloody or mucoid discharge	Excessive vaginal bleeding (blood coagulation defect)	
BUTTOCKS AND ANUS		
Buttocks symmetrical	Pilonidal dimple	Examine for possible sinus. Instruct parents about cleaning this area.
Anus patent and passage of meconium within 24–48 hours after birth	Imperforate anus, rectal atresia (congenital gastrointestinal defect)	Evaluate extent of problems. Initiate surgical consultation. Perform digital examination to ascertain patency.
No fissures, tears, or skin tags	Fissures	
EXTREMITIES AND TRUNK		
Short and generally flexed; extremities move symmetrically through range of motion but lack full extension	Unilateral or absence of movement (spinal cord involvement) Fetal position continued or limp (anoxia, CNS problems, hypoglycemia)	Review birth record to assess possible cause.
All joints move spontaneously; good muscle tone, of flexor type, birth to 2 months	Spasticity when infant begins using extensors (cerebral palsy, lack of muscle tone, "floppy baby" syndrome)	Collaborate with physician.
Arms		
Equal in length Bilateral movement Flexed when quiet	Brachial palsy (difficult delivery) Erb-Duchenne paralysis Muscle weakness, fractured clavicle Absence of limb or change of size (phocomelia, amelia)	Report to clinician.

*Possible causes of alterations are placed in parentheses.
†This column provides guidelines for further assessment and initial nursing interventions.

Neonatal Physical Assessment Guide (continued)

Assessment and normal findings	Alterations and possible causes*	Nursing responses to data base†
Hands		
Normal number of fingers	Polydactyly (Ellis-Van Creveld syndrome) Syndactyly—one limb (developmental anomaly) Syndactyly—both limbs (genetic component)	Report to physician.
Normal palmar crease	Simian line on palm (Down syndrome)	
Normal size hands	Short fingers and broad hand (Hurler syndrome)	
Nails present and extend beyond fingertips in term infant	Cyanosis and clubbing (cardiac anomalies) Nails long (postterm)	
Spine		
C-shaped spine Flat and straight when prone Slight lumbar lordosis Easily flexed and intact when palpated At least half of back devoid of lanugo Full-term infant in ventral suspension should hold head at 45° angle, back straight	Spina bifida occulta (nevus pilosus) Dermal sinus Myelomeningocele Head lag, limp, floppy trunk (neurologic problems)	Evaluate extent of neurologic damage; initiate care of spinal opening.
Hips		
No sign of instability	Sensation of abnormal movements, jerk, or snap of hip dislocation	Examine all newborn infants for dislocated hip prior to discharge from hospital.
Hips abduct to more than 60° Iliac crests are equal		If this suspected, refer to orthopedist for further evaluation. Reassess at well-baby visits.
Inguinal and buttock skin creases		
Symmetrical inguinal and buttock creases	Asymmetry (dislocated hips)	Refer to orthopedist for evaluation, counsel parents regarding symptoms of concern and therapy.
Legs		
Legs equal in length Legs shorter than arms at birth Legs one-third overall length of body when infant supine with legs flexed at knees	Shortened leg (dislocated hips) Lack of leg movement (fractures, spinal defects)	Refer to orthopedist for evaluation. Counsel parents regarding symptoms of concern and discuss therapy.
Feet		
Foot is in straight line Positional clubfoot—based on position in utero Fat pads and creases on soles of feet	Talipes equinovarus (true clubfoot)	Discuss differences between positional and true clubfoot with parents. Teach parents passive manipulation of foot. Refer to orthopedist if not corrected by 3 months of age.
Talipes planus (flat feet) normal under 3 years of age		Reassure parents that flat feet are normal in infant.
NEUROMUSCULAR		
Motor function		
Symmetrical movement and stength in all extremities	Limp, flaccid, or hypertonic (CNS disorders, infection, dehydration, fracture)	Appraise newborn's posture and motor functions by observing activities and motor characteristics.
May be jerky or have brief twitchings	Tremors (hypoglycemia, hypocalcemia, infection, neurologic damage)	Evaluate electrolyte imbalance and neurologic functioning.
Head lag not over 45°	Delayed or abnormal development (preterm, neurologic involvement)	
Neck control adequate to maintain head erect briefly	Asymmetry of tone or strength	

*Possible causes of alterations are placed in parentheses.
†This column provides guidelines for further assessment and initial nursing interventions.

Neonatal Physical Assessment Guide (continued)

Assessment and normal findings	Alterations and possible causes*	Nursing responses to data base†
Reflexes		
Moro		
Response to sudden movement or loud noise should be one of symmetrical extension and abduction of arms with fingers extended; then return to normal relaxed flexion Fingers form a C Present at birth, disappears at 1–4 months of age	Asymmetry of body response (fractured clavicle, injury to brachial plexus) Consistent absence (brain damage)	Discuss normality of this reflex in response to loud noises and/or sudden movements.
Rooting and sucking		
Turns in direction of stimulus to cheek or mouth; opens mouth and begins to suck; difficult to elicit after feeding; disappears by 7 months of age Sucking is adequate for nutritional intake and meeting oral stimulation needs; disappears by 12 months	Poor sucking or easily fatiguable (preterm, breast-fed infants of barbiturate-addicted mothers) Absence of response (preterm, neurologic involvement, depressed infants)	Evaluate strength and coordination of sucking. Observe neonate during feeding and counsel parents about mutuality of feeding experience and neonate's responses.
Palmar grasp		
Fingers grasp adult finger when palm is stimulated and hold momentarily; lessens at 3–4 months of age	Asymmetry of response (neurologic problems)	Evaluate other reflexes and general neurologic functioning.
Plantar grasp		
Toes curl downward when sole of foot is stimulated; lessens by 8 months	Absent (defects of lower spinal column)	
Stepping		
When held upright and one foot touching a flat surface, will step alternately; disappears at 4–5 months of age	Asymmetry of stepping (neurologic abnormality)	Evaluate muscle tone and function on each side of body. Refer to specialist.
Babinski		
Hyperextension of all toes when one side of sole is stroked from heel upward across ball of foot	Absence of response (low spinal cord defects)	Refer for further neurologic evaluation.
Tonic neck		
Fencer position—when head is turned to one side, extremities on same side extend and on opposite side flex; this reflex may not be evident during early neonatal period; disappears at 3–4 months of age Response often more dominant in leg than in arm	Absent after 1 month of age or persistent asymmetry (cerebral lesion)	
Prone crawl		
While on abdomen, neonate pushes up and tries to crawl	Absence or variance of response (preterm, weak or depressed infants)	Evaluate motor functioning. Refer to specialist.
Trunk incurvation		
In prone position, stroking of spine causes pelvis to turn to stimulated side	Failure to rotate to stimulated side (neurologic damage)	

*Possible causes of alterations are placed in parentheses.
†This column provides guidelines for further assessment and initial nursing interventions.

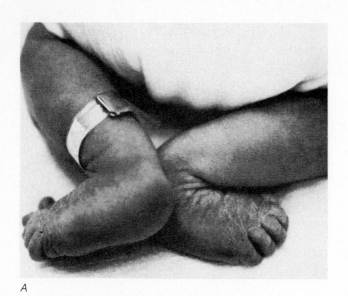

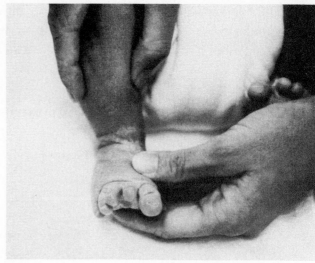

A   B

Figure 28–27   A Bilateral talipes equinovarus seen with infant in supine position. B To determine the presence of clubfoot, the nurse moves the foot to the midline. Resistance indicates true clubfoot.

blinking response is elicited. The cry of the newborn should be lusty and vigorous. High-pitched cries, weak cries, or no cries are all causes for concern.

Muscle tone is evaluated with the head of the neonate in a neutral position as various parts of the body are passively moved. The newborn is somewhat hypertonic; that is, extention of the elbow and knee joints is resisted. Muscle tone should be symmetrical. Diminished muscle tone and flaccidity require further evaluation.

Neonatal tremors are common in the full-term newborn and must be evaluated to differentiate them from a convulsion. A fine jumping of the muscle is likely to be a central nervous system disorder and requires further evaluation. Tremors may also be related to hypoglycemia or hypocalcemia. Neonatal seizures may consist of no more than chewing or swallowing movements, deviations of the eyes, rigidity, or flaccidity, because of central nervous system immaturity.

Specific deep tendon reflexes can be elicited in the neonate but have limited value unless they are obviously asymmetrical. The knee jerk is brisk; a normal ankle clonus may involve three or four beats. Plantar flexion is present.

The central nervous system of the newborn is immature and characterized by a variety of reflexes. Because the newborn's movements are uncoordinated, methods of communication are limited, and control of bodily functions is drastically limited, the reflexes serve a variety of purposes. Some are protective (blink, gag, sneeze), some aid in feeding (rooting, sucking), and some stimulate human interaction (grasping). Neonatal reflexes and general neurologic activity should be carefully assessed.

The most common reflexes found in the normal neonate are the following:

- The *tonic neck reflex (fencer position)* is elicited when the neonate is supine and the head is turned to one side. In response, the extremities on the same side straighten, whereas on the opposite side they flex (Figure 28–28). This reflex may not be seen during the early neonatal period, but once it appears it persists until about the third month.

- The *grasp reflex* is elicited by stimulating the palm with a finger or object. The neonate will grasp and hold the object or finger firmly enough to be lifted momentarily from the crib (Figure 28–29).

- The *Moro reflex* is elicited when the neonate is startled by a loud noise or is lifted slightly above the crib and then suddenly lowered. In response, the newborn straightens arms and hands outward while the knees flex. Slowly the arms return to the chest, as in an embrace. The fingers spread, forming a C, and the infant may cry (Figure 28–30).

- The *rooting reflex* is elicited when the side of the neonate's mouth or cheek is touched. In response, the newborn turns toward that side and opens the lips to suck (Figure 28–31).

- When an object is placed in the neonate's mouth, the *sucking reflex* is elicited.

● The *Babinski reflex*, or hyperextension of all toes, occurs when the lateral aspect of the sole is stroked from the heel upward and across the ball of the foot.

● When the newborn is prone, stroking the spine causes the pelvis to turn to the stimulated side. This is called *trunk incurvation*.

In addition to these reflexes, the newborn can blink, yawn, cough, sneeze, and draw back from pain (protective reflexes). Neonates can even move a little on their own. When placed on their stomachs, they push up and try to crawl (*prone crawl*). When he or she is held upright with one foot touching a flat surface, the neonate puts one foot in front of the other and walks (*stepping reflex*) (Figure 28–32). This reflex is most pronounced at birth and is lost at about 4–5 months of age.

Table 28–1 summarizes the evoking stimulus and response of the common newborn reflexes.

Brazelton (1984) recommends the following steps as a means of assessing central nervous system integration:

1. Insert a clean finger into the newborn's mouth to elicit a sucking reflex.

2. As soon as the neonate is sucking vigorously, assess hearing and vision responses by noting sucking changes in the presence of a light, rattle, and a voice.

3. The neonate should respond with a brief cessation of sucking followed by continuous sucking with repeated stimulation.

This examination demonstrates auditory and visual integrity as well as the ability for complex behavioral interactions.

One of the newborn's first responses is to move into a quiet but alert state of consciousness. The baby is still; his body molds to yours; his hands touch your skin; his eyes open wide and are bright and shiny. He looks directly at you.

This special alert state, this innate ability to communicate, may be the initial preparation for becoming attached to other human beings. One feels awed by the intensity and appealing power of this little bud of humanity meeting the world for the first time. (*The Amazing Newborn*)

● **Behavioral Assessment**

Two conflicting forces influence parents' perceptions of their infant. One is the parents' preconceptions, based on hopes and fears, of what their newborn will be like. The other is their initial reaction to their baby's temperament, behaviors, and physical appearance. Nurses can assist parents in identifying their baby's specific behaviors.

Brazelton (1973) developed a tool that has revolutionized our understanding and perception of the newborn's capabilities and responses, permitting us to recognize each infant's individuality. *Brazelton's neonatal behavioral assessment* tool provides valuable guidelines for assessing the newborn's state changes, temperament, and individual behavior patterns. It provides a means by which the health care provider, in conjunction with the parents

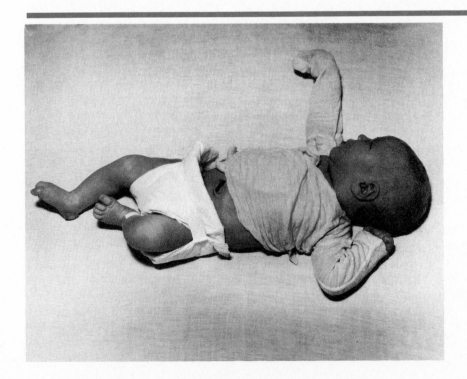

Figure 28–28 Tonic neck reflex

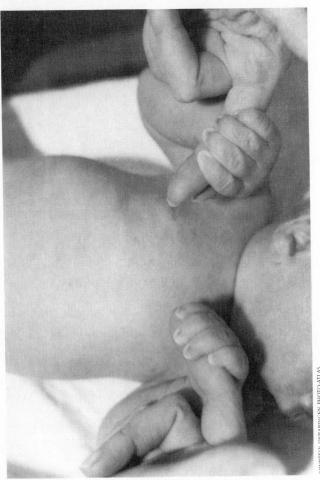

COURTESY SWEARINGEN PHOTO-ATLAS

Figure 28–29 Grasping reflex (From Swearingen PL: *The Addison-Wesley Photo-Atlas of Nursing Procedures*. Menlo Park, Calif, Addison-Wesley, 1984)

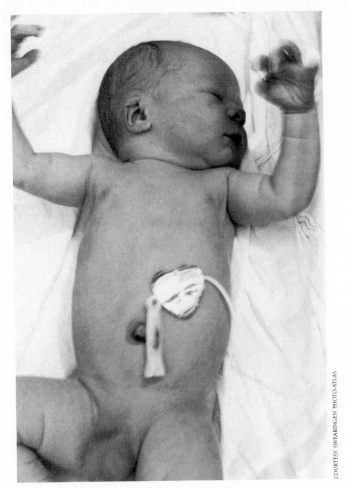

COURTESY SWEARINGEN PHOTO-ATLAS

Figure 28–30 Moro reflex (From Swearingen PL: *The Addison-Wesley Photo-Atlas of Nursing Procedures*. Menlo Park, Calif, Addison-Wesley, 1984)

(primary caregivers), can identify and understand the individual newborn's states. Parents learn which responses, interventions, or activities best meet the special needs of their infant, and this understanding fosters positive attachment experiences.

The assessment tool attempts to identify the newborn's repertoire of behavioral responses to the environment and also documents the newborn's neurologic adequacy and capabilities. The examination usually takes 20 to 30 minutes and involves about 30 tests. It should be noted that to administer the complete assessment tool accurately and ensure reliability, the nurse must have completed a training course. The scale includes 27 behavioral items, which are scored on a nine-point scale, and 20 elicited reflexes, which are scored on a three-point scale. Some items are scored according to the newborn's response to specific stimuli. Others, such as consolability and alertness, are scored as a result of continuous behavioral observations throughout the assessment.

Generally the tool is set up so that the midpoint is the norm for most items. The Brazelton assessment tool differs from most in that the newborn's score is determined not on the average performance but on the best. Since the first few days after birth are a period of behavioral disorganization, the complete assessment should be done on the third day after delivery. Every effort should be made to elicit the best response. This may be accomplished by repeating tests at different times or by testing during situations that facilitate the best possible response, such as when parents are alerting their baby by holding, cuddling, rocking, and singing to them.

The assessment of the newborn should be carried out initially in a quiet, dimly or softly lit room, if possible. The newborn's state of consciousness should be determined, because scoring and introduction of the test items are correlated with the sleep or awake state. The newborn's state depends on physiologic variables, such as the amount of time from the last feeding, positioning, environmental tem-

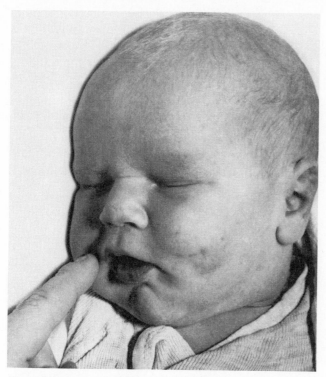

Figure 28-31   Rooting reflex

Habituation   The infant's ability to diminish or shut down innate responses to specific repeated stimuli, such as a rattle, bell, light, or pinprick to heel, is assessed.

Orientation to inanimate and animate visual and auditory assessment stimuli   How often and where the newborn attends to auditory and visual stimuli are observed. The infant's orientation to the environment is determined by an ability to respond to clues given by others and by a natural ability to fix on and to follow a visual object horizontally and vertically. This capacity and parental appreciation of it are important for positive communication between infant and parents; the parents' visual (*en face*) and auditory (soft, continuous voice) presence stimulates their infant to orient to them. Inability or lack of response may indicate visual or auditory problems. It is important for parents to know that their infant can turn to voices by 3 days of age and can become alert at different times with a varying degree of intensity in response to sounds.

Motor activity   Several components are evaluated. Motor tone of the newborn is assessed in the most

perature, and health status; presence of such external stimuli as noises and bright lights; and the wake-sleep cycle of the infant. An important characteristic of the neonatal period is the *pattern of states,* as well as the transitions from one state to another. The pattern of states is a predictor of the infant's receptivity and ability to respond to stimuli in a cognitive manner. Babies learn best in a quiet, alert state and in an environment that is supportive and protective and that provides appropriate stimuli.

The nurse should observe the newborn's sleep-wake patterns (as discussed in Chapter 27) and the rapidity with which the newborn moves from one state to another, ability to be consoled, and ability to diminish the impact of disturbing stimuli. The following questions may provide the nurse with a framework for assessment:

- Does the newborn's response style and ability to adapt to stimuli indicate a need for parental interventions that will alert the newborn to the environment so that he or she can grow socially and cognitively?

- Are parental interventions necessary to lessen the outside stimuli, as in the case of the baby who responds to sensory input with intensity?

- Can the baby control the amount of sensory input that he or she must deal with?

The behaviors and the sleep-wake states in which they are assessed are categorized as follows:

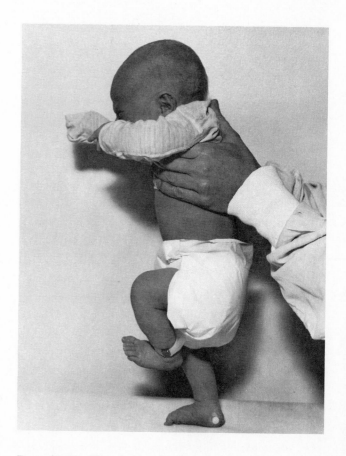

Figure 28-32   The stepping reflex disappears after about one month.

Table 28–1 Common Reflexes of the Neonate

Reflex name	Evoking stimulus	Response
Blinking reflex	Light flash	Eyelids close.
Pupillary reflex	Light flash	Pupil constricts.
Rooting reflex	Light touch of finger on cheek close to mouth	Head rotates toward stimulation; mouth opens and attempts to suck finger. Disappears by about 4 months of age.
Sucking reflex	Finger (or nipple) inserted into mouth	Rhythmic sucking.
Moro reflex	Infant lying on back: slightly raised head suddenly released; infant held horizontally, lowered quickly about 6 in, and stopped abruptly	Arms are extended, head is thrown back, fingers are spread wide; arms are then brought back to center convulsively with hands clenched; spine and lower extremities are extended. Disappears by about 6 months of age.
Startle reflex	Loud noise	Similar to Moro reflex flexion in arms; fists are clenched.
Grasping reflex	Finger placed in palm of hand	Infant's fingers close around and grasp object.
Tonic neck reflex	Head turned to one side while infant lies on back	Arm and leg are extended on the side the infant faces. Opposite arm and leg are flexed.
Abdominal reflex	Tactile stimulation or tickling	Abdominal muscles contract.
Withdrawal reflex	Slight pinprick to the sole of the infant's foot	Leg flexes.
Walking reflex	Infant supported in an upright position with feet lightly touching a flat surface	Rhythmic stepping movement. Disappears at about 4 months of age.
Babinski reflex	Gentle stroking on the sole of the foot	Fanning and extension of the toes (adults respond to this stimulation with flexion of toes).
Plantar, or toe-grasping, reflex	Pressure applied with the finger against the balls of the infant's feet	A plantar flexion of all toes. Disappears by the end of the first year of life.

Adapted from Mott SR, Frazekas NF, James SR: *Nursing Care of Children and Families: A Holistic Approach.* Menlo Park, Calif, Addison-Wesley, 1985.

characteristic state of responsiveness. This summary assessment includes overall use of tone as the neonate responds to being handled—whether during spontaneous activity, prone placement, or horizontal holding—and overall assessment of body tone as the neonate reacts to all stimuli.

Variations Frequency of alert states, state changes, color changes (throughout all states as examination progresses), activity, and peaks of excitement are assessed.

Self-quieting activity Assessment is based on how often, how quickly, and how effectively newborns can use their resources to quiet and console themselves when upset or distressed. Considered in this assessment are such self-consolatory activities as putting hand to mouth, sucking on a fist or the tongue, and attuning to an object or sound. The infant's need for outside consolation must also be considered, for example, seeing a face; being rocked, held, or dressed; using a pacifier; and having extremities restrained.

Cuddliness or social behaviors This area encompasses the infant's need for and response to being held. Also considered is how often the newborn smiles. These behaviors influence the parents' self-esteem and feel-ings of acceptance or rejection. Cuddling also appears to be an indicator of personality. Cuddlers appear to enjoy, accept, and seek physical contact; are easier to placate; sleep more; and form earlier and more intense attachments. Noncuddlers are active, restless, have accelerated motor development, and are intolerant of physical restraint. Smiling, even as a grimace reflex, greatly influences parent-infant feedback. Parents identify this response as positive.

KEY CONCEPTS

A perinatal history, determination of gestational age, physical examination, and behavior assessment forms the basis for complete newborn assessment.

The common physical characteristics included in the gestational age assessment are: skin, lanugo, sole (plantar) creases, breast tissue and size, ear form and cartilage, and genitalia.

The neuromuscular components of gestational age scoring tools are usually posture, square window sign, popliteal angle, arm recoil, heel to ear, and scarf sign.

By assessing the physical and neuromuscular components of a gestational age tool, the nurse can determine the gestational age of the newborn.

After determining the gestational age of the baby, the nurse can assess how the newborn will make the transition to extrauterine life and anticipate potential physiologic problems.

In-depth knowledge of normal newborn physical characteristics and common variations is essential for the newborn nurse.

Normal ranges for vital signs assessed in the newborn are: Heart rate—120–150 beats/min; respirations—30–60 respirations/min; axillary temperature—36.5C–37C (97.7F–98.6F), or skin temperature—36C–36.5C (96.8F–97.7F), or rectal temperature—36.6C–37.2C (97.8F–99F); and blood pressure at birth of 80–60/45–40 mm Hg.

Normal newborn measurements include: Weight range 2950–3515 g (6lb, 8oz–7lb, 12 oz), with weight dependent on maternal size and age; length range 45.8–52.3 cm (18–20.5 in); and head circumference range of 33–35 cm (13–14 in)—approximately 2 cm larger than the chest circumference.

The newborn nursery nurse performs the physical examination by completing the less-disturbing components first and then proceeding in a head-to-toe approach.

Commonly elicited newborn reflexes are tonic neck, Moro, grasp, rooting, sucking, and blink.

An important role of the nurse during the physical and behavioral assessments of the newborn is to teach parents about their newborn and involve them in their baby's care. This facilitates the parents' identification of their newborn's uniqueness and allays their concerns.

REFERENCES

AAP Committee on Fetus and Newborn & ACOG Committee on Obstetrics: *Guidelines for Perinatal Care.* Evanston, Ill, American Academy of Pediatrics, 1983.

Avery GB (ed): *Neonatology,* ed 3. Philadelphia, Lippincott, 1987.

Ballard JL, et al: A simplified score for assessment of fetal maturation of newly born infants. *J Pediatr* 1979; 95(November):769.

Brazelton T: *The Neonatal Behavioral Assessment Scale.* Philadelphia, Lippincott, 1973.

Brazelton T: Neonatal behavior and its significance, in **Avery** ME, **Taeusch** HW (eds): *Schaffer's Diseases of the Newborn.* Philadelphia: Saunders, 1984.

Duara S, et al: Neonatal screening with auditory brainstem responses: Results of a follow-up audiometry and risk factor evaluation. *J Pediatr* 1986;108(2):276.

Korones SB: *High-Risk Newborn Infants,* ed 4. St Louis, Mosby, 1986.

Ludington-Hoe SM: What can newborns really see? *Am J Nurs* 1983; 83:1286.

Robertson A: Commentary: Gestational age. *J Pediatr* 1979; 95(November):732.

ADDITIONAL READINGS

Budreau G: Postnatal cranial molding and infant attractiveness: Implications for nursing. *Neonatal Netw* 1987;5(April):13.

Haddock B, **Vincent** P, **Merow** D: Axillary and rectal temperatures of full-term neonates: Are they different? *Neonatal Netw* 1986;5(1):36.

Judd JM: Assessing the newborn from head to toe. *Nurs* 1985;15:12.

Klaus M, **Klaus** PH: *The Amazing Newborn.* Reading, Mass, Addison-Wesley, 1985.

Korones SB: The normal neonate: Assessment of early physical findings, in **Sciarra** JJ, et al (eds): *Gynecology and Obstetrics.* Hagerstown, Md, Harper & Row, 1985, vol 2.

Lascari AD: "Early" breast-feeding jaundice: Clinical significance. *J Pediatr* 1986;108(January):156.

Powell ML: *Assessment and Management of Developmental Changes and Problems in Children,* ed 2. St Louis, Mosby, 1982.

Scanlon JW, et al: *A System of Newborn Physical Examination.* Baltimore, University Park Press, 1979.

Sendak MJ, **Harris** AP: Neonatal pulse oximetry in the delivery room: Review of recent investigations. *P/N* 1987;11(1):8.

Stephen SB, **Sexton** PR: Neonatal axillary temperatures: Increases in readings over time. *Neonatal Netw* 1987; 5(6):25.

White PL, et al: Comparative accuracy of recent abbreviated methods of gestational age determination. *Clin Pediatr* 1980;19(5):319.

Zachman RD, et al: Neonatal blood pressure at birth by the Doppler method. *Am Heart J* 1986;111(January):189.

She was not red nor even wrinkled, but palely soft, each feature delicately reposed in its right place, and she was not bald but adorned with a thick, startling crop of black hair. (Margaret Drabble, The Millstone)

The Normal Newborn: Needs and Care

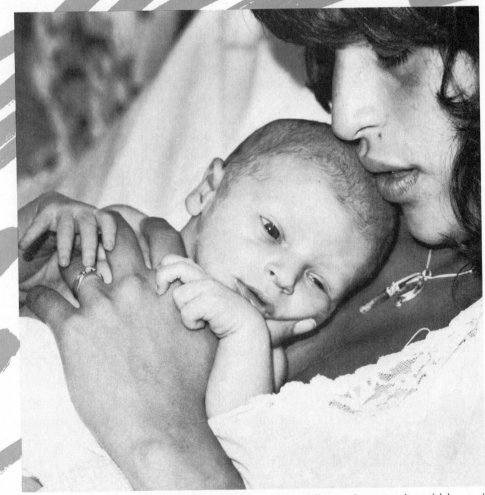

A young Italian-American mother rests following her unmedicated labor and delivery, her 8-hour-old baby still in her arms, awake and alert.

Chapter Twenty-Nine

OBJECTIVES

- **Summarize the essential areas of information to be obtained about a newborn's birth experience and immediate postnatal period.**

- **Explain the physiological and behavioral responses of newborns during periods of reactivity and possible interventions needed.**

- **Discuss the major nursing considerations and activities to be carried out during the first four hours after birth (admission and transitional period) and subsequent daily care.**

- **Identify the assessments and activities that should be included in a daily care plan for a normal newborn.**

- **Determine common parental concerns regarding their newborns.**

- **Describe the topics and related content to be included in parent education classes on newborn/infant care**

At the moment of birth, numerous physiologic adaptations begin to take place in the newborn's body. Because of these dramatic changes, the newborn requires close observation to determine how smoothly she or he is making the transition to extrauterine life. The newborn also requires care that enhances her or his chances of making the transition successfully.

The two broad goals of nursing care during this period are to promote the physical well-being of the newborn and to promote the establishment of a well-functioning family unit. The first goal is met by providing comprehensive care to the newborn while he or she is in the nursery. The second goal is met by teaching parents how to care for their new baby and by supporting their parenting efforts so that they feel confident and competent.

● Using the Nursing Process During the Normal Newborn Period

Nursing Assessment

Assessment during the neonatal period gives the nurse an opportunity to identify any actual or potential physical problems facing the newborn. Careful assessment of the general characteristics, variations, and responses of the newborn helps the nurse differentiate between normal physiologic adaptations and abnormal findings that require further evaluation. Individual temperament and behavior patterns are also assessed.

During the newborn assessment, the nurse determines the presence of any psychosocial factors that may affect the family's ability to integrate its newest member. The nurse's assessment should reveal the extent of the family's need for information, support, and instruction about child care. Identifying the family's strengths is just as important as identifying problems because these strengths can be incorporated in the care plan. To perform an accurate family assessment, the nurse must be knowledgeable about the characteristics of the expanding family.

An accurate assessment is essential during this period, since the plan of care is based on the findings of the assessment. If the assessment is inadequate, the plan of care will most likely be ineffective as well. The newborn's successful transition to extrauterine life may ultimately depend on the nurse's ability to identify physiologic needs correctly. The family's ability to meet the physical and psychological needs of the newborn may be affected by the nurse's accuracy in identifying their strengths and weaknesses.

Assessment is performed on a daily basis while the newborn is present on the birthing unit. The daily assessment period is an opportune time for parent education. The nurse can explain the newborn's physiological and behavioral changes and responses as the assessment proceeds.

Analysis and Nursing Diagnosis

Nursing diagnoses are based on an analysis of findings of the assessment. Physiologic alterations of the newborn form the basis of many nursing diagnoses. Nursing diagnoses that may apply are:

- Ineffective airway clearance related to mucus obstruction

- Potential alteration in urinary elimination related to circumcision

- Potential alteration in nutrition: less than body requirements related to limited nutritional/fluid intake

- Alteration in comfort: acute pain related to heel sticks for blood glucose and hematocrit

- Potential for alteration in tissue perfusion related to cold stress

Nursing diagnoses that may apply to family functioning are:

- Knowledge deficit related to lack of experience in infant care

- Knowledge deficit related to decision about male circumcision

- Alterations in parenting related to the need to integrate the newborn into the family unit

Identification, prioritization, and documentation of the nursing diagnoses are essential for developing a thoughtful, systematic plan of care.

Nursing Plan and Implementation

Even though most newborns are healthy, every newborn has physiological needs that must be met. The family also has needs, which are usually psychologic and educational. To meet these needs in an organized fashion, the neonatal nurse must develop a plan of care based on the assessment findings and nursing diagnoses.

A nursing care plan is important to ensure consistent and comprehensive care. Even though most newborns and their mothers remain in the birthing unit for a brief period, they may have several nurses administering care during their stay. When there is one care plan implemented by all personnel caring for the family, the goals of care are more likely to be achieved. Redundancy or missed interventions are less likely, and parent education can proceed at a steady pace, even though different nurses are teaching.

Evaluation

Through ongoing observations nurses evaluate whether the newborn's body systems are successfully maturing and adapting to extrauterine life. This evaluation is based on knowledge of the expected cardiovascular, pulmonary, renal, and neurologic changes that occur in the days immediately following birth.

To evaluate the daily nursing care given to the newborn, the nurse notes whether complications have developed in the baby. The success of parent education can be evaluated by how well the parents perform baby care measures and how comfortable they feel in caring for their baby.

This moment of meeting seemed to be a birthtime for both of us; her first and my second life. Nothing, I knew, could ever be the same again. (Laurie Lee, Two Women)

● Care of the Newborn in the First Four Hours of Life

After delivery, the baby is formally admitted to the health care facility. The admission procedures include an assessment to ensure that the newborn's adaptation to extrauterine life is proceeding normally and several interventions to promote successful adaptation.

If the initial assessment indicates that the newborn is not at risk physiologically, many of the routine admission procedures are performed in the presence of the parents in the maternal recovery area. The care measures indicated by the assessment findings may be performed by the nurse or by the parents under the supervision of the nurse in an effort to educate and support the parents. Other interventions may be delayed until the infant has been transferred to an observational nursery.

Nursing Assessment

As discussed in Chapter 27, the newborn's physiologic adaptations to extrauterine life occur rapidly. All the body systems are affected. Thus the newborn requires close monitoring during the first few hours of life so that any deviation from normal can be identified immediately.

During the assessment in the first four hours after birth, the nurse focuses on the newborn's physiologic adaptations. A complete physical examination is done later by the physician or nurse practitioner, usually within the first 24 hours of life or just prior to discharge (see Chapter 28 and Box 29–1).

If the newborn is transferred to an observational nursery for the first four-hour assessment, the nurse receiving the infant first checks and confirms the newborn's identification. The delivery nurse who carries the baby to the nursery communicates via a concise verbal report all significant information regarding the newborn. The essential data to be reported and recorded as part of the newborn's chart include the following:

1. *Condition of the newborn.* Pertinent information includes the newborn's Apgar scores at one and five minutes, resuscitative measures required in the delivery room, vital signs, voidings, and passing of meconium. Complications to be noted are excessive mucus, delayed spontaneous respirations or responsiveness, abnormal number of cord vessels, and obvious physical abnormalities.

2. *Labor and delivery record.* A copy of the labor and delivery record should be placed in the newborn's chart. The record contains all the significant data about the birth, for example, duration, course, and status of mother and fetus throughout labor and delivery and any analgesia or anesthesia administered to the mother. Particular care is taken to note any variation or difficulties such as prolonged rupture of membranes, abnormal fetal position, meconium-stained amniotic fluid, signs of fetal distress during labor, nuchal cord (cord around the newborn's neck at delivery), precipitous delivery, and use of forceps.

3. *Antepartal history.* Any maternal problems that may have compromised the fetus in utero, such as pre-eclampsia, spotting, illness, recent infections, or a history of maternal substance abuse, are of immediate concern in the assessment of the newborn. Information about maternal age, EDD, previous pregnancies, and existing siblings is also included.

4. *Parent-infant interaction information.* Parental interactions with their newborn and their desires regarding care, such as rooming-in, circumcision, and type of feeding, are noted. Information about other children in the home, available support systems, and interactional patterns within each family unit assists in providing comprehensive care.

In the absence of any newborn distress, the nurse continues with the admission assessment by taking the newborn's vital signs. The initial temperature should be taken by the axillary method, which is safer than the rectal method and correlates closely with rectal temperature in the newborn (Mayfield et al 1984). Normal axillary temperature is 36.5C to 37C (97.7F–98.6F). Some hospitals still choose to use a rectal thermometer for the initial temperature, theorizing that rectal patency can be assessed simultaneously. Equally successful alternative methods for assessing anal patency are digital examination or use of a sterile, flexible rubber catheter. Patency can also be assessed by observing the newborn having a bowel movement.

Once the initial temperature assessment is made, the core temperature is monitored either by obtaining an axillary temperature at intervals or by placing a skin sensor on the newborn for continuous reading. The usual skin sensor placement site is on the newborn's abdomen (Figure 29–1), but placement on the upper thigh or arm gives a reading more closely correlated with the mean body temperature (Avery & Taeusch 1984). The axillary temperature should be monitored every hour for the first 4 hours and then once every 4 hours for the first 24 hours.

The apical pulse and respirations are assessed every 15 to 30 minutes for one hour and then every one to two hours until stable. The apical pulse is best assessed while the newborn is at rest. The newborn's respirations may be irregular and still be normal. The normal pulse range is 120 to 150 beats per minute, and the normal respiratory range is 30 to 60 respirations per minute.

Blood pressure is assessed by auscultation, palpation, or by Doppler or Dinemapp instrument (Figure 29–2). If a Dinemapp or Doppler device is used, the newborn's extremities must be immobilized during the assessment, and the cuff should cover two-thirds of the upper arm or upper leg. Movement, crying, and inappropriate cuff size can give inaccurate measurements of the blood pressure.

The newborn is weighed in grams and pounds. Most parents understand pound measurement (Figure 29–3). The scales are covered each time an infant is weighed to

Box 29–1 Timing and Types of Newborn Assessments

1. Evaluation immediately after delivery by nurse to determine need for resuscitation or if newborn is stable and can remain with parents to initiate attachment.

2. Assessment within first one to four hours after birth:
   - Evaluate adaptation to extrauterine life.
   - Determine gestational age.
   - Evaluate for high-risk problems.

3. Assessment within first 24 hours or prior to discharge:
   - Perform complete physical examination. (Depending on agency protocol, the nurse may complete some components on her own, with a physician or nurse practitioner completing the exam prior to discharge.)
   - Evaluate behavior.

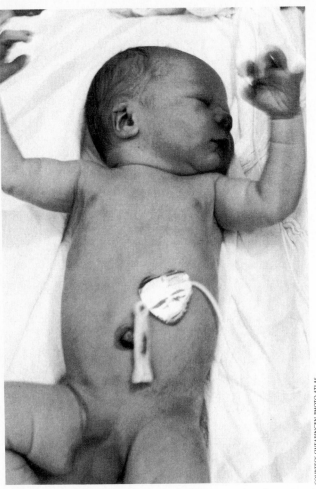

Figure 29–1 *A skin thermal sensor is placed on the newborn's abdomen, upper thigh, or arm and secured with porous tape or a foil-covered foam pad. (From Swearingen P:* The Addison-Wesley Photo-Atlas of Nursing Procedures. *Menlo Park, Calif, Addison-Wesley, 1984)*

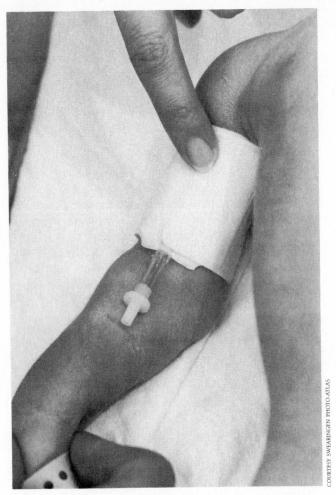

Figure 29–2 *The Dinemapp and Doppler devices use ultrasound to measure the systemic blood pressure. The cuff can be applied to either the neonate's upper arm or thigh. (From Swearingen P:* The Addison-Wesley Photo-Atlas of Nursing Procedures. *Menlo Park, Calif, Addison-Wesley, 1984)*

prevent cross-infection and heat loss from conduction. The newborn is measured; the measurements are recorded in both centimeters and inches. Three routine measurements are (a) length, (b) circumference of the head, and (c) circumference of the chest (Figures 28–12, 28–13). In some facilities, abdominal girth may also be determined. The nurse rapidly appraises the baby's color, muscle tone, alertness, and general state. Gestational age is estimated and the physical examination is completed (for further discussion, see Chapter 28). A hematocrit and blood glucose evaluation is routinely done on all newborns in many institutions (see Procedure 32–2).

The assessment during the first four hours after birth provides a basis for establishing nursing diagnoses regarding the infant and setting priorities for care and family education needs (Haun et al 1984). In many settings, the father accompanies the newborn to the nursery. This is an excellent opportunity for him to get to know his child

while the nurse systematically examines and explains the newborn's responses and characteristics. It is also an excellent opportunity for the astute nurse to take note of the father's bonding process and comfort level with the newborn. The nurse must recognize that the father may be overwhelmed by the unfamiliar nursery setting. However, he will benefit from observing and interacting with the nurse who cares for his baby.

The nurse must also be able to assess the newborn's physiological adaptation and behavior during the transitional periods (see Box 29–2). The baby usually shows a predictable pattern of behavior during the first several hours after birth.

PERIODS OF REACTIVITY

○　*FIRST PERIOD OF REACTIVITY*　This phase lasts approximately 30 minutes after birth. During this phase the newborn is awake and active and may appear hungry and have a strong sucking reflex. This is a natural opportunity to initiate breast-feeding if this is the mother's choice. Bursts of random, diffuse movements may alternate with relative immobility. Respirations are rapid, as high as 80 breaths per minute, and there may be chest retractions, transient flaring of the nares, and grunting. The heart rate is rapid and irregular. Bowel sounds are absent.

○ *SLEEP PHASE* The newborn's activity gradually diminishes, and the heart rate and respirations decrease as the baby enters the sleep phase. First sleep usually occurs an average of three hours after birth, and may last from a few minutes to two to four hours. During this period, the newborn will be difficult to awaken and will show no interest in sucking. Bowel sounds become audible, and cardiac and respiratory rates return to baseline values.

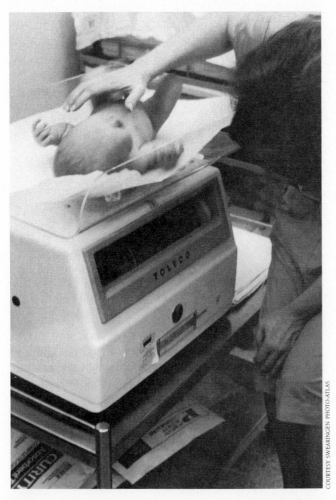

Figure 29–3 The scale is balanced before each weight, with the protective pad in place. The caretaker's hand is poised above the infant as a safety measure. (From Swearingen P: The Addison-Wesley Photo-Atlas of Nursing Procedures. Menlo Park, Calif, Addison-Wesley, 1984)

> ### Box 29–2 Key Signs of Newborn Transition
>
> Pulse: 120–150 beats/min.
>   During sleep as low as 100 beats/min; if crying, up to 180 beats/min.
> Respirations: 30–60 respirations/min.
>   Predominantly diaphragmatic but synchronous with abdominal movements.
> Temperature: Axillary: 36:5C–37C (97.7F–98.6F)
>   Skin: 36C–36.5C (96.8F–97.7F)
> Dextrostix: greater than 45 mg %
> Hematocrit: less than 65 percent–70 percent central venous sample
> Blood pressure: 90–60/45–40 mm Hg

○ *SECOND PERIOD OF REACTIVITY* The newborn is again awake and alert. This phase lasts four to six hours in the normal newborn. Physiologic responses are variable during this stage. The heart and respiratory rates increase; however, the nurse must be alert for apneic periods, which may cause a drop in the heart rate. The newborn must be stimulated to continue breathing during such times. The newborn may develop rapid color changes, becoming mildly cyanotic or mottled during these fluctuations. Production of respiratory and gastric mucus increases, and the baby responds by gagging, choking, and regurgitating. Continued close observation and interventions may be necessary to maintain a clear airway during this period of reactivity. The gastrointestinal tract becomes more active. The first meconium stool is frequently passed during this second active stage, and the initial voiding may also occur at this time. The newborn will indicate readiness for feeding by such behaviors as sucking, rooting, and swallowing. If feeding was not initiated in the first period of reactivity, it is done at this time. See p 900 for further discussion of this first feeding.

Nursing Admission Interventions

In addition to the continuous observations and assessment of the newborn during the admission period, the nurse's primary care goals are as follows:

- To maintain a clear airway
- To maintain a neutral thermal environment
- To prevent complications, such as hemorrhage and infection
- To facilitate parent-newborn attachment
- To initiate oral feedings

The nurse evaluates the newborn's need to remain under observation by assessing the newborn's ability to maintain a clear airway, maintain body temperature, maintain stable vital signs, demonstrate normal neurologic status and no observable complications, and tolerate the first feeding. If these criteria are met, it indicates a successful beginning adaptation to extrauterine life. The baby is moved to a regular nursery or to rooming-in. This transfer usually takes place between 6 and 12 hours after birth.

If 24 hours have passed and the first voiding and passage of stool has not occurred, the nurse continues the normal observation routine while also assessing for abdominal distention, status of bowel sounds, hydration, fluid intake, and temperature stability.

Nursing Goal: Maintenance of a Clear Airway

The nurse positions the newborn on his or her side. If necessary, a bulb syringe (Figure 29–10) or DeLee suction (Procedure 23–2, and Figure 23–10) is used to remove mucus from the nasal passages and oral cavity. Another routine but controversial practice in some institutions is use of the DeLee catheter to remove mucus from the stomach to help prevent possible aspiration. This practice can cause vagal nerve stimulation, which can result in bradycardia and apnea in the unstabilized neonate.

Nursing Goal: Maintenance of a Neutral Thermal Environment

A neutral thermal environment is essential to minimize the newborn's need to expend calories to maintain body heat in the optimal range of 36.5C to 37.0C (97.7F–98.6F). If the newborn becomes hypothermic, the physiologic response can lead to metabolic acidosis, hypoxia, and shock (Kemp et al 1982).

A neutral thermal environment is best achieved by performing the assessment and interventions with the newborn unclothed and under a radiant warmer. The thermostat of the radiant warmer is controlled by the thermal skin sensor taped to the newborn's abdomen, upper thigh, or arm. The sensor indicates when the newborn's temperature exceeds or falls below the acceptable temperature range. The nurse should be aware that leaning over the newborn may block the radiant heat waves from reaching the newborn.

It is common practice in some institutions to cover the neonate's head with a stockinette or knit cap to prevent further heat loss in addition to placing the baby under a radiant warmer. A recent study (Ruchala 1985) comparing axillary temperatures of neonates whose heads were covered and those remaining uncovered failed to demonstrate a significant difference two hours after birth. However, the neonates whose heads were uncovered had a slightly lower temperature on admission to the newborn nursery and, once under the radiant warmer, a slightly greater temperature increase than those whose heads were covered. More definitive studies are necessary. However, these limited results lead to the question whether heat can more effectively be conserved by using a head covering while the newborn is outside the radiant warmer but not when the newborn is under the radiant warmer (to avoid a barrier effect).

When the newborn's temperature is normal and vital signs are stable (about two to four hours after birth), the baby may be given a sponge bath. However, this admission bath may be postponed for some hours if the newborn's condition dictates or the parents desire it. The admission sponge bath and shampoo are done quickly to minimize heat loss. The bath takes place while the baby is either under the radiant warmer or in the bassinet in the parents' room. The temperature is rechecked after the bath and if it is stable, the newborn is dressed, wrapped, and placed in an open crib at room temperature. If the baby is unable to maintain his or her axillary temperature at 36.5C (97.7F) or more, the newborn is returned to the radiant warmer. The nurse implements measures to prevent neonatal heat loss, such as using heat shields, keeping the infant dry and covered, and avoiding cool surfaces or use of cold instruments. The infant is also protected from drafts, open windows or doors, or air conditioners. Blankets and clothing are stored in a warm place. (See discussion on nonshivering thermogenesis and the mechanism of heat loss in Chapter 27.)

Nursing Goal: Prevention of Complications

A prophylactic injection of vitamin K is given to prevent hemorrhage, which can occur due to low prothrombin levels in the first few days of life (see the accompanying Drug Guide–Vitamin K_1 phytonadione). The potential for hemorrhage is considered to result from the absence of gut bacterial flora, which influences the production of vitamin K in the newborn (see Chapter 32 for further discussion). Controversy exists over whether the administration of vitamin K may predispose the newborn to significant hyperbilirubinemia. However, Pritchard, MacDonald, and Gant (1985) indicate there is no evidence to support this concern as long as a standard dose of 1 mg is given. Recently some people have questioned whether research supports giving vitamin K to newborns who have had a nontraumatic delivery.

The vitamin K injection is given intramuscularly in the middle one third of the vastus lateralis muscle located in the lateral aspect of the thigh (Figure 29–4). An alternate site is the rectus femoris muscle in the anterior aspect of the thigh. However, this site is near the sciatic nerve and femoral artery and should be used with caution (Figure 29–5).

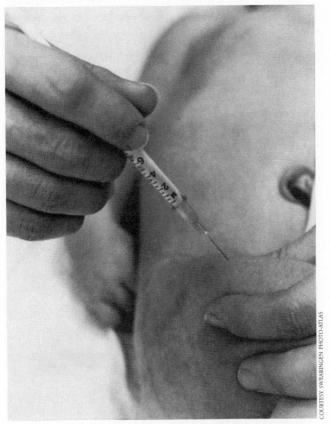

COURTESY SWEARINGEN PHOTO-ATLAS

Figure 29–4   Bunch the tissue of the upper thigh (vastus lateralis muscle) and quickly insert the needle at a 90° angle to the thigh. Aspirate, then slowly inject the solution to distribute the medication evenly and minimize the baby's discomfort. Remove the needle and massage the site with an alcohol swab. (From Swearingen P: The Addison-Wesley Photo-Atlas of Nursing Procedures. *Menlo Park, Calif, Addison-Wesley, 1984)*

The nurse is also responsible for giving the legally required prophylactic eye treatment for *Neisseria gonorrhoeae,* which may have infected the newborn during the birth process. The traditional drug of choice is 1 percent silver nitrate solution. Other antibiotic ophthalmic ointments used instead of silver nitrate include erythromycin (Ilotycin, see the accompanying Drug Guide–Erythromycin), tetracycline, or penicillin.

To instill silver nitrate, the nurse punctures the wax container of 1 percent silver nitrate with a sterile needle, pulls down the infant's lower eyelid, and administers one or two drops into the lower conjunctival sac (Figure 29–6). After instillation, the eye is closed to spread the medication. The other eye is treated in the same manner. Controversy exists as to the value of flushing the eye with sterile water following the instillation of the silver nitrate. The American Academy of Pediatrics, however, recommends that the eyes not be flushed after instillation of silver nitrate. The skin around the newborn's eye should be wiped

to prevent staining of the skin. Silver nitrate and the other medications can cause chemical conjunctivitis, and silver nitrate has a higher incidence of this effect. Chemical conjunctivitis causes the newborn some discomfort and may interfere with the baby's ability to focus on the parents' faces. The resulting edema, inflammation, and discharge may cause concern if the parents have not been given information that the side effects will clear in 24 to 48 hours and that this prophylactic eye treatment is necessary for the newborn's well-being.

During the first 24 hours of life, the nurse is constantly alert for signs of distress. If the newborn is with his or her parents during this period, extra care must be taken to teach them how to maintain their newborn's temperature, recognize the hallmarks of physiologic distress, and respond immediately to signs of respiratory problems. Their repertoire of responses should include nasal and oral suctioning, vigorous fingertip stroking of the newborn's spine to stimulate respiratory activity, positioning, and resuscitative measures if necessary. The nurse also must be available immediately should the baby develop distress (see Box 29–3).

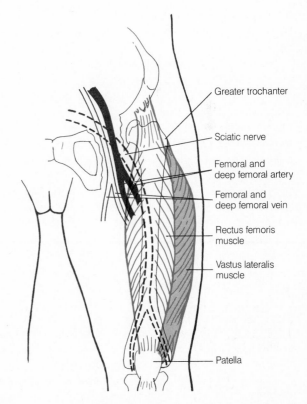

Greater trochanter

Sciatic nerve

Femoral and deep femoral artery

Femoral and deep femoral vein

Rectus femoris muscle

Vastus lateralis muscle

Patella

Figure 29–5   The middle third of the vastus lateralis muscle is the preferred site for intramuscular injection in the newborn. The middle third of the rectus femoris is an alternate site, but its proximity to major vessels and the sciatic nerve necessitates caution in using this site.

Drug Guide   Vitamin K₁ phytonadione (AquaMEPHYTON)

Overview of Neonatal Action

Phytonadione is used in prophylaxis and treatment of hemorrhagic disease of the newborn. It promotes liver formation of the clotting factors II, VII, IX, and X. At birth the neonate does not have the bacteria in the colon that is necessary for synthesizing fat-soluble vitamin K₁, therefore the newborn may have decreased levels of prothrombin during the first 5–8 days of life reflected by a prolongation of prothrombin time.

Route, Dosage, Frequency
Intramuscular injection is given in the lateral thigh muscle. A one-time only prophylactic dose of 0.5–1.0 mg is given in the delivery room or upon admission to the newborn nursery. May need to repeat 6–8 hours later especially if mother received anticoagulants during pregnancy.

Neonatal Side Effects
Pain and edema may occur at injection site. Possible allergic reactions such as rash and urticaria.

Nursing Considerations

Observe for bleeding (usually occurs on second or third day). Bleeding may be seen as generalized ecchymoses or bleeding from umbilical cord, circumcision site, nose, or gastrointestinal tract. Results of serial PT and PTT should be assessed.

Observe for jaundice and kernicterus especially in preterm infants.

Observe for signs of local inflammation.

Nursing Goal: Initiation of First Feeding

The timing of the first feeding varies depending on whether the newborn is to be breast-fed or bottle-fed. Mothers who choose to breast-feed their newborns may seek to put their baby to the breast while in the delivery room or recovery area. This practice should be encouraged since successful, long-term breast-feeding during infancy appears to be related to beginning breast-feedings in the first few hours of life (Beske & Garvis 1982). Bottle-fed babies usually begin the first feedings by 5 hours of age, during the second period of reactivity, when they awaken and appear hungry.

Signs indicating newborn readiness for the first feeding are: active bowel sounds, absence of abdominal distention, and a lusty cry that quiets with rooting and sucking behaviors when a stimulus is placed near the lips (see p 921).

Nursing Goal: Facilitation of Attachment

Eye-to-eye contact between the parents and baby is extremely important during the early hours after birth, when the newborn is in the first period of reactivity. The newborn is alert during this time, the eyes are wide open, and often direct eye contact is made with human faces within optimal range for visual acuity (7 to 8 inches). It is theorized that this eye contact is an important foundation in establishing attachment in human relationships (Klaus & Klaus 1985). Consequently the prophylactic eye medi-

cation is often delayed to provide an opportunity for this period of eye contact between parents and their newborn, thus facilitating the attachment process.

A Mayan Indian saying tells us: "In the baby lies the future of the world. The mother must hold him close so he will know the world is his. The father must take him to the highest hill so he can see what his world is like." (*The Amazing Newborn*)

Box 29–3   Key Signs of Newborn Distress

- Increased rate (more than 60/min) or difficult respirations
- Sternal retractions
- Excessive mucus
- Facial grimacing
- Cyanosis (generalized)
- Abdominal distention or mass
- Lack of meconium elimination within 24 hours after birth
- Inadequate urine elimination
- Vomiting of bile-stained material
- Jaundice of the skin

Drug Guide Erythromycin (Ilotycin) ophthalmic ointment

Overview of Neonatal Action

Erythromycin (Ilotycin) is used as prophylactic treatment of ophthalmia neonatorum, which is caused by the bacteria *Neisseria gonorrhoeae*. Preventive treatment of gonorrhea in the newborn is required by law. Erythromycin is also effective against ophthalmic chlamydial infections. It is either bacteriostatic or bactericidal depending on the organisms involved and the concentration of drug.

Route, Dosage, Frequency
Ophthalmic ointment is instilled as a narrow ribbon or strand, ¼-inch long, along the lower conjunctival surface of each eye, starting at the inner canthus. It is instilled only once in each eye. Administration may be done in the delivery room or later in the nursery so that eye contact is facilitated and the bonding process is not interrupted.

Neonatal Side Effects
Sensitivity reaction; may interfere with ability to focus and may cause edema and inflammation. Side effects usually disappear in 24–48 hours.

Nursing Considerations

Wash hands immediately prior to instillation to prevent introduction of bacteria

Do not irrigate the eyes after instillation

Observe for hypersensitivity

● Daily Newborn Care

The nurse is responsible for the daily assessment of the health of the newborn and routine daily care. While performing assessment and care tasks, the nurse can encourage the parents to participate, thus strengthening the family unit and enhancing the parents' confidence in their ability to care for their baby. Due to today's changing family structures and lack of extended family, many new parents have had no opportunities to learn about babies. They often look to the nurse for guidance and information. The nurse must have a complete understanding of newborn needs to be able to anticipate and answer questions.

Nursing Assessment

Routine daily assessments vary among birthing facilities. However, the following should be assessed daily while the newborn baby is in the birthing setting.

- *Vital signs.* These are taken once a shift or more, depending on the newborn's status.
- *Weight.* The baby should be weighed at the same time each day for accurate comparisons. A weight loss of up to 10 percent for term infants is expected during the first week of life. This is the result of limited intake, loss of excess extracellular fluid, and passage of meconium. Parents should be told about the expected weight loss, the reason for it, and the expectations for regaining the birth weight.
- *Skin color.* Changes in skin color may indicate the need for closer assessment of temperature, cardiopulmonary status, hematocrit, and bilirubin levels.
- *Intake/output.* Fluid intake and voiding and stooling patterns are recorded.
- *Umbilical cord.* The cord is assessed for signs of hemorrhage or infection, such as oozing and foul smell
- *Circumcision.* The circumcision is assessed for signs of hemorrhage and infection. The first voiding after a circumcision is also a significant assessment in order to evaluate for possible urinary obstruction due to trauma and edema.
- *Newborn nutrition.* Caloric and fluid intake are recorded. The nurse is also responsible for assessing the mother's skill and education needs regarding breast-feeding or bottle-feeding.
- *Parent education.* The nurse assesses the parent's knowledge of newborn and infant care. The nurse also assesses whether the parent's learning needs can be met in a group setting or require individual teaching.
- *Attachment.* Ongoing attachment between newborn and parents is assessed. Some indications of possible difficulties in attachment are verbalizations indicating disappointment with the newborn and lack of eye contact and physical comforting behaviors. Attachment is promoted by encouraging all family members to be involved with the new member of the family.

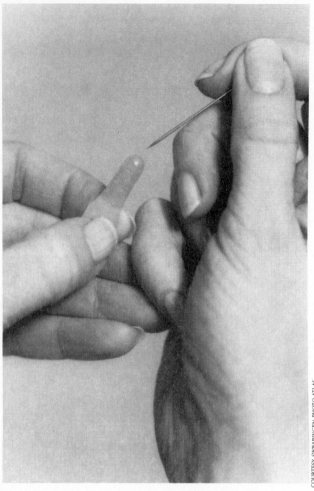
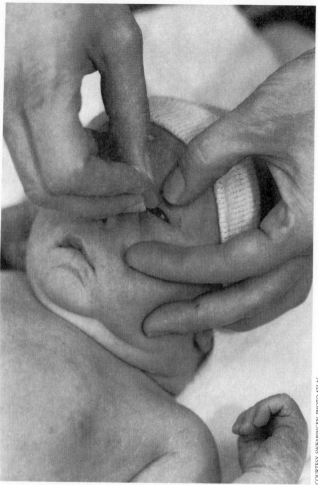

Figure 29–6   Silver nitrate instillation. A Wax container is punctured with a needle. B One or two drops of 1 percent silver nitrate solution are instilled in each lower conjunctival sac. (From Swearingen P: The Addison-Wesley Photo-Atlas of Nursing Procedures. Menlo Park, Calif, Addison-Wesley, 1984)

The goals for daily care of the newborn are similar to those upon admission to the nursery:

- To maintain cardiorespiratory function

- To maintain a neutral thermal environment

- To promote adequate hydration and nutrition

- To prevent complications

- To promote safety

- To foster family-newborn attachment

- To enhance parent knowledge of newborn care

Nursing Goal: Maintenance of Cardiopulmonary Function

The newborn should always be placed in a prone or propped, side-lying position when left unattended to pre-

vent aspiration and facilitate drainage of mucus. A bulb syringe is kept within easy reach should the baby need oral-nasal suctioning. If the newborn has respiratory difficulty, the airway is cleared. Vigorous fingertip stroking of the baby's spine will frequently stimulate respiratory activity. A cardiorespiratory monitor can be used on newborns who are not being observed at all times and are at risk for decreased respiratory or cardiac function. Indicators of risk are pallor, cyanosis, a ruddy color, apnea, or other signs of instability.

Nursing Goal: Maintenance of Neutral Thermal Environment

Every effort is made to maintain the newborn's temperature within the normal range. The nurse must make certain the newborn is undressed and exposed to the air as little as possible. A stockinette or knit head covering should be used for the small newborn who has less subcutaneous fat to act as insulation in maintaining body heat. The ambient temperature of the room where the newborn is kept should be monitored routinely and kept at approximately 37.8C (70F). Parents should be advised to dress the newborn in one more layer of clothing than is necessary for an adult to maintain thermal comfort. A newborn whose temperature falls below optimal levels will use calories to maintain body heat rather than for growth. Chilling also decreases the affinity of serum albumin for bilirubin, thereby increasing the likelihood of newborn jaundice.

A newborn who is overheated will increase activity and respiratory rate in an attempt to cool the body. Both measures deplete caloric reserves. In addition the increased respiratory rate leads to increased insensible fluid loss.

Nursing Goal: Promotion of Adequate Hydration and Nutrition

Nutrition is addressed in depth in Chapter 30. Adequate hydration is enhanced by maintaining a neutral thermal environment and by offering early and frequent feedings. Early feedings promote gastric emptying and increase peristalsis, thereby decreasing the potential for hyperbilirubinemia by decreasing the amount of time fecal material is in contact with beta glucuronidase in the small intestine. This enzyme is capable of freeing the bilirubin from the feces, allowing bilirubin to be reabsorbed into the vascular system.

Excessive handling of the newborn can cause an increase in the newborn's metabolic rate and caloric use. The nurse should be alert to the baby's subtle cues of fatigue. These include turning the head away from eye contact, decrease in muscle tension and activity in the extremities and neck, and loss of eye contact, which may be manifested by fluttering or closure of the eyelids. The nurse quickly ceases stimulation when signs of fatigue emerge. The nurse's care should demonstrate to the parents the need for awareness of newborn cues and the use of periods of alertness in the baby for contact and stimulation.

Nursing Goal: Prevention of Complications

Pallor may be an early sign of hemorrhage and must be reported to the physician. The newborn is placed on a cardiorespiratory monitor to permit continuous assessment. If cyanosis develops and is unrelieved by administration of oxygen, it is likely the newborn is in hypovolemic shock, which necessitates emergency interventions and Trendelenburg positioning. All newborns are at risk from hemorrhage, but this is especially true following a circumcision procedure (see p 911).

Infection in the nursery is best prevented by requiring that all personnel having direct contact with newborns follow a three-minute scrub procedure at the beginning of each shift. The hands must also be washed well before and after contact with every newborn or after touching any soiled surface such as the floor or one's hair or face. Parents are often instructed to use an antiseptic hand cleaner before touching the baby as well. Anyone with an infection should refrain from working with newborns until the infection has cleared. Some agencies ask fathers, siblings, and grandparents to wear a gown over their street clothes and to wash their hands before handling the newborn.

Research Note

Research has demonstrated the importance of contact between mother and newborn in the first hours and days of life in establishing an optimal relationship. Despite the benefits of rooming-in, many babies still spend large amounts of time in a nursery for various reasons. Karraker's study was done to explore the social environment of infants in a normal newborn nursery.

The 67 infants in the study were observed in six sessions, one week apart, to note the adult-infant interchanges that took place and to explore the influence of individual infant differences on interactions.

The collected data showed that infants received adult attention an average of 5.5 percent of the time they were in the nursery. The most common attention activities included changing and rearranging infant clothing, changing diapers, or moving a bassinet. Infrequent adult behaviors included feeding, smiling, rocking, and sitting and holding (infants were usually fed by the mothers). The infants who received the most attention were those who cried more, those who were older, and those who the nursery attendants rated low on a physical attractiveness scale.

Nurses need to look carefully at the quality of the time newborns spend in the nursery. Early infancy is a time for humans to learn contingent relationships. In this study observers noted a lag time of greater than eight minutes between infant crying and adult response. Nurses need both to encourage mothers to room-in and to provide a nursery experience that will optimize infant development by setting expected contact times for these newborns.

Karraker KH: Adult attention to infants in a newborn nursery. Nurs Res 1986;35(November/December):358–363.

Nursing Goal: Promotion of Safety

It is essential to verify the identity of the newborn, by comparing the numbers and names on the identification bracelets of mother and newborn before giving a baby to a parent. Other safety issues are specifically covered later in the sections on circumcision, positioning and handling, bathing, nail care, and safety considerations.

Nursing Goal: Fostering Newborn and Parent Attachment

Attachment is promoted by encouraging all family members to be involved with the new member of the family. Specific interventions are examined in depth in Chapter 35.

Nursing Goal: Enhancement of Parent Knowledge of Infant Care

To meet parent needs for information, the nurse who is responsible for the daily care of the mother and newborn should assume the primary responsibility for education. Nearly every contact with the parents presents an opportunity for sharing information that can facilitate the parents' sense of competence in newborn care. The nurse also needs to recognize and respect the fact that there are many good ways to provide safe baby care. The parents' methods of giving care should be reinforced rather than contradicted, unless their care methods are harmful to the newborn.

The information in the following section is provided to increase the nurse's knowledge of infant care and can also be used to meet parents' needs for information.

● Parent Education

Parents may be familiar with handling and caring for infants, or this may be their first time to interact with a newborn. If they are new parents, the sensitive nurse gently teaches them by example and instructions geared to their needs and previous knowledge about the various aspects of newborn care.

The nurse observes how parents interact with their infant during feeding and caregiving activities. Rooming-in, even for a short time, offers opportunities for the nurse to provide information and evaluate whether the parents are comfortable with changing diapers and wrapping, handling, and feeding their newborn. Do both parents get involved in the infant's care? Is the mother depending on someone else to help her at home? Does the mother give excuses for not wanting to be involved in her baby's care? ("I am too tired," "My stitches hurt," or "I will learn later.") All these considerations need to be taken into account when evaluating the educational needs of the parents.

Several methods may be used to teach parents about newborn care. Daily child care classes are a nonthreatening way to convey general information. Individual instruction is helpful to answer specific questions or to clarify an item that may have been confusing in class (Figure 29–7). Discharge planning is essential to verify the mother's knowledge when she leaves the hospital. Follow-up calls or visits after discharge lend added support by providing another opportunity for parents to have their questions answered. The essential areas to be covered by a nurse in educating parents before discharge are described in the following sections.

With the new life come new rhythms. Or perhaps I should say no rhythms. The day is divided into phone calls, meals eaten

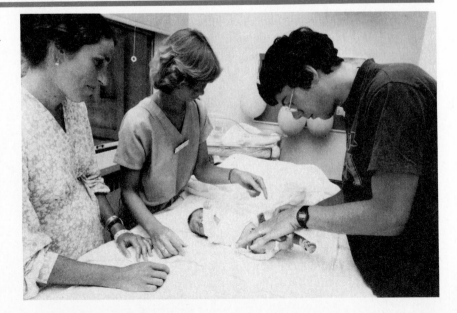

Figure 29–7 Individualizing parent education. Father returns demonstration of diapering his daughter.

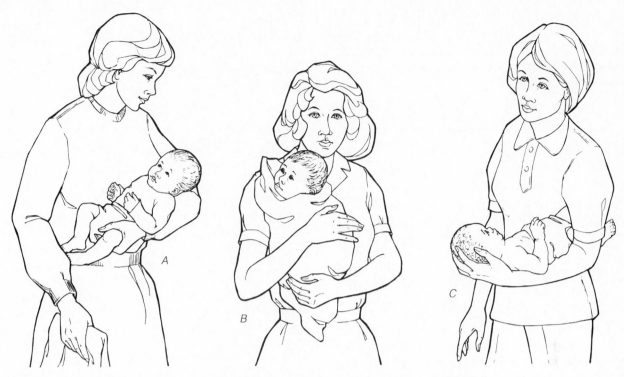

Figure 29–8   Various positions for holding an infant. A Cradle hold. B Upright position. C Football hold

on the run, visitors who've come to see the baby, trips from hospital to home to walk the dog.

The new life brings new thoughts, new perceptions of the world.

Why don't men take paternity leaves? Why is time off, if any, basically reserved for women? Why don't we take a month off. In those first few chaotic days, filled with ecstasy and fear, the family needs to be together. Being together in times of joy and sadness is what a family is. A month's distance from the office grind, from the bottom line could not help but create a healthier world. (Dennis Donziger, *Daddy*)

Positioning and Handling

Methods of positioning and handling the newborn are demonstrated to parents if needed. As the parents provide care, the nurse can enhance parental confidence by giving them positive feedback. If the parents encounter problems, the nurse can express confidence in their abilities to master the new skill or information, suggest alternatives, and serve as a role model.

How to pick up a newborn is one of the first concerns of anyone who has not handled many babies. When the infant is the in side-lying position, he or she is easily picked up by sliding one hand under the baby's neck and shoulders and the other hand under the buttocks or between the legs, then gently lifting the newborn from the crib. This technique provides security and support for the head (which the baby is unable to support until the age of 3 or 4 months).

After the baby is out of the crib, one of three holds may be used (Figure 29–8). The *cradle hold* is frequently used during feeding. It provides a sense of warmth and closeness, permits eye contact, frees one of the nurse's or parent's hands, and provides security because the cradling protects the newborn's body. Extra security is provided by gripping the thigh with the hand while the arm supports the infant's body. The *upright position* provides security and a sense of closeness and is a good position for burping the infant.

One hand should support the neck and shoulders, while the other hand holds the buttocks or is placed between the newborn's legs. The *football hold* frees one of the caregiver's hands and permits eye contact. This hold is ideal for shampooing, carrying, or breast-feeding. It frees the mother to talk on the telephone or answer the door at home or do the myriad of tasks that await her attention.

The newborn infant is most frequently positioned on the side with a rolled blanket or diaper behind the back for support (Figure 29–9). This position aids drainage of mucus and allows air to circulate around the cord. It is also more comfortable for the newly circumcised male. After feeding, the newborn is placed on the right side to prevent aspiration and to aid digestion; this position makes it easier to expel air bubbles from the stomach.

Once the cord is healed, many newborns prefer to lie on their stomachs. Newborns have enough head control to turn their heads from side to side to prevent suffocation. The baby's position should be changed periodically during the early months of life, because neonatal skull bones are soft, and flattened areas may develop if the newborn consistently lies in one position. The newborn should not be left in a supine position when unattended due to the danger of aspiration.

Nasal and Oral Suctioning

Most babies are obligatory nose breathers for the first months of life. They generally maintain air passage patency by coughing or sneezing. During the first few days of life, however, the newborn has increased mucus, and gentle suctioning with a bulb syringe may be indicated. The nurse can demonstrate the use of the bulb syringe in the nose and mouth and have the parents do a return demonstration. The parents should repeat this demonstration before discharge so they will feel more confident and comfortable with the procedure.

To suction the newborn, the bulb syringe is compressed, then the tip is placed in the nostril, and the bulb is permitted to reexpand slowly as the nurse or parent releases the compression on the bulb (Figure 29–10). The drainage is then compressed out of the bulb onto a tissue. The bulb syringe may also be used in the mouth if the newborn is spitting up and unable to handle the excess secretions. The bulb is compressed; the tip of the bulb syringe is placed about 1 inch in one side of the infant's mouth; and compression is released. This draws up the excess secretions. The procedure is repeated on the other side of the mouth. The center of the baby's mouth is avoided because suction in this area might stimulate the gag reflex. The bulb syringe should be washed in warm, soapy water and rinsed in warm water after each use. A bulb syringe should always be kept near the newborn.

Parents have a great fear that their baby will choke and may be relieved if they know how to take action if such an event occurs. They should be advised to turn the newborn's head to the side as soon as there is any indication of gagging or vomiting.

Bathing

An actual bath demonstration is the best way for the nurse to provide information to parents. Because excess bathing and use of soap will dry out the baby's sensitive skin, bathing should be done every other day or twice a week. Sponge baths are recommended for the first two weeks or until the umbilical cord completely falls off and has healed.

Supplies (see Box 29–4) can be kept in a plastic bag or some type of container to avoid hunting for them each time. The mother may want to use a small plastic tub, a clean kitchen or bathroom sink, or a large bowl. Expensive baby tubs are not necessary, but some parents may prefer to purchase them.

Before starting, if no one else is at home, the parent may want to take the phone off the hook and put a sign on the door to prevent being disturbed or decide just to ignore these intrusions. Having someone home during the first few baths will be helpful because that person can get forgotten items and provide moral support. The room should be warm and free of drafts.

SPONGE BATH

After the supplies are gathered, the tub (or any of the containers mentioned above) is filled with water that is warm to the touch. The water temperature is tested with

Figure 29–9 The most common sleeping position of the newborn is on the side. The little girl shown here does not need the additional support provided by a rolled blanket.

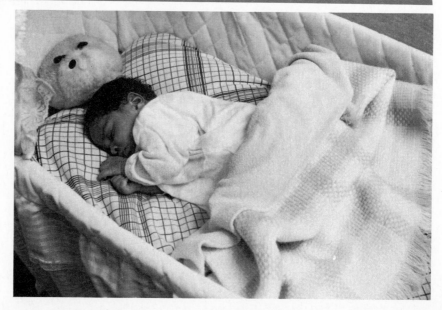

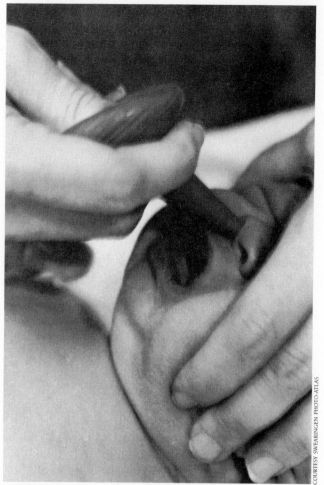

Figure 29-10 Nasal and pharyngeal suctioning. The bulb is compressed, then the tip is placed either in the nostril or mouth; the bulb is allowed to reexpand as the compression of the bulb is released. (From Swearingen P: The Addison-Wesley Photo-Atlas of Nursing Procedures. Menlo Park, Calif, Addison-Wesley, 1984)

an elbow or forearm. Parents may also choose to purchase a thermometer to help them determine when the bath water is at approximately 37.8C (100F) and safe to use. Soap should not be added to the water. The infant should be wrapped in a blanket, with a T-shirt and diaper on. This helps keep the newborn warm and secure.

To start the bath, a washcloth is wrapped around the index finger once. Each eye is gently wiped from inner to outer corner. This direction is the way eyes naturally drain, and wiping in this direction prevents irritation of the eyes. A different portion of the washcloth is used for each eye to prevent cross-contamination. Cotton balls can also be used for this purpose, using a new one for each eye. Some swelling and drainage may be common the first few days after birth.

The ears are washed next by wrapping the washcloth once around an index finger and gently cleaning the external ear and behind the ear. Cotton swabs are never used

in the ear canal because it is possible to put the swab too far into the ear and damage the ear drum. In addition, the swab may pack any discharge farther down into the ear canal.

The remainder of the baby's face is then wiped with the soap-free washcloth. Many babies start to cry at this point. The face should be washed every day and the mouth and chin wiped off after each feeding.

The neck is washed carefully but thoroughly with the washcloth. Soap may now be used. Formula or breast milk and lint collect in the skin folds of the neck, so it may be helpful to sit the baby up, supporting the neck and shoulders with one hand while washing the neck with the other hand.

The baby's T-shirt is now removed and the blanket unwrapped. The chest, back, and arms are wet with the washcloth. The parent may then lather the hands with soap and wash the baby's chest, back, and arms. Wetting the cord is avoided, if possible, because it delays drying. Soap is rinsed off with the wet washcloth, and the upper part of the body is dried with a towel or blanket. The baby's upper body is then wrapped with a dry clean blanket to prevent a chill.

Next the infant's legs are unwrapped, wet with the washcloth, lathered, rinsed, and well dried. If the infant has dry skin, a *small* amount of unperfumed lotion or ointment (petroleum jelly or A and D ointment) may be used. Ointments are better than lotions for dry cracked feet and hands. Baby oil is not recommended because it clogs skin pores. Powders aggravate dry skin and are also avoided.

Both baby oil and baby powder can cause serious respiratory problems if inhaled. Parents should be warned of this danger and advised to take measures to prevent these substances from being aspirated by the baby. If parents want to use powder, advise them to select one that is talc free. The powder should be shaken into the parent's hand and then placed on the infant rather than shaking the powder directly over the baby.

The genital area is cleaned daily with soap and water and with water after each wet or dirty diaper. Girls are

---

Box 29-4 Bath Supplies

Washcloths
Towels
Blanket
Unperfumed mild soap (eg, Ivory, Neutragena)
Shampoo
Petroleum jelly or A and D ointment
Rubbing alcohol
Cotton balls
Diapers
Clean clothes

washed from the *front* of the genital area toward the rectum to avoid fecal contamination of the urethra and thus to the bladder. Newborn girls often have a thick, white mucous discharge or a slight bloody discharge from the vagina. This discharge is normal for the first one to two weeks and should be wiped off gently with a damp cloth at diaper changes.

Parents of uncircumcised newborn boys should clean the penis daily. Periodically the parents can gently check for retraction. If the foreskin does not retract with minimal pressure, there is no need to attempt to wash under it. Normal cleaning of the small exposed area of the glans is sufficient. Newborn boys who have been circumcised also need daily gentle cleaning. A very wet washcloth is rubbed over a bar of soap. The washcloth is squeezed above the baby's penis, letting the soapy water run over the circumcision site. The area is rinsed off with plain warm water and lightly patted dry. A small amount of petroleum jelly, A and D ointment, or bactericidal ointment may be put on the circumcised area, but excessive amounts may block the meatus and should be avoided.

Baby powder (or cornstarch) is not recommended for diaper rash. Baby powder may cake with urine and irritate the infant's perineal area. Cornstarch may promote fungal infection. Ointments that provide a barrier, such as zinc oxide, A and D ointment, or petroleum jelly are more effective for diaper rash. If the ointment does not help the rash, parents using disposable diapers should try another brand of diaper. If cloth diapers are used, a different detergent or fabric softener may alleviate the problem. If the rash persists, parents should discuss the problem with a nurse practitioner or physician because it may be a yeast or fungal infection.

The umbilical cord should be kept clean and dry. The close proximity of the umbilical vessels makes the cord a common portal for infection. Various preparations such as triple dye, alcohol, hexachlorophene, Betadine, and Bacitracin are used for cord care in newborn nurseries to promote drying and provide a bactericidal effect. Triple dye may be used and seems to be a highly effective antistaphylococcal agent (Andrich & Golden 1984). At discharge, most parents are advised to clean the area around the cord with a cotton ball and alcohol two to three times a day until the cord is completely gone and the stump is healed. The cord stump generally falls off in 7 to 14 days. The diaper should be folded down to allow air to circulate around the cord. The care provider should be consulted if bright red bleeding or puslike drainage occurs or if the area remains unhealed two to three days after the cord stump has sloughed off.

The last step in bathing is washing the infant's hair (some suggest doing this step first). The newborn is swaddled in a dry blanket, leaving only the head exposed and held in the football hold with the head tilted slightly down-

ward to prevent water running in the eyes. Water should be brought to the head by a cupped hand. The hair is moistened and lathered with a small amount of shampoo. A *very* soft brush may be used to massage the shampoo over the entire head. The brush may be used over the soft spots. The hair is then rinsed and toweled dry. Oils or lotions are not used on the newborn's head unless there is evidence of cradle cap. Moistening the scaly area with lotion a half an hour or more before shampooing softens the crusts or scales and makes it easier to remove them. To assist in preventing cradle cap, the infant's hair should be brushed every day and the hair washed during baths.

TUB BATHS

The infant may be put in a tub after the cord has fallen off and the circumcision site is healed (approximately two weeks) (Figure 29–11). Infants usually enjoy a tub

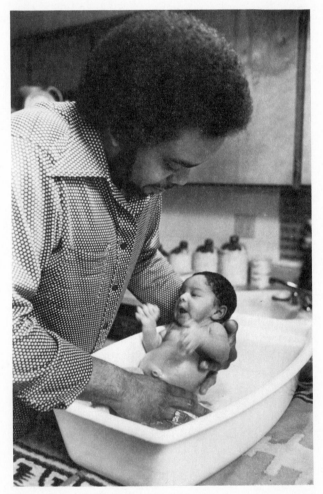

Figure 29–11　When bathing the infant, it is important to support the head. Note that the cord site has healed on this 2-week-old baby.

bath more than a sponge bath, although some newborns cry during either type.

Only 3 or 4 inches of water are needed in the tub. To prevent slipping, a washcloth is placed in the bottom of the tub or sink, or the baby can be brought into a tub with the parent.

The face is washed in the same manner as for a sponge bath. The parent then places the newborn in the tub using the cradle hold and grasping the distal thigh. The neck is supported by the parent's elbow in the cradle position. An alternative hold is to support the newborn's head and neck with the parent's forearm while grasping the distal shoulder and arm.

Because wet infants are slippery, some parents have found that pulling a cotton sock (with the holes cut out for the fingers) over the arm will prevent the baby from slipping.

The body may be washed with a soapy washcloth or hand. To wash the baby's back, the parent places his or her noncradling hand on the infant's chest with the thumb under the infant's arm closest to the parent. Gently tipping the baby forward onto the supporting hand frees the cradling arm to wash the back of the baby. After the bath the baby is lifted out of the tub in the cradle position, dried well, and wrapped in a dry blanket. The hair can then be washed in the same way as for a sponge bath.

Nail Care

The nails of the newborn are seldom cut in the hospital. During the first days of life, the nails may adhere to the skin of the fingers, and cutting is contraindicated. Within a week the nails separate from the skin and frequently break off. If the nails are long or if infants are scratching themselves, the nails may be trimmed. This is most easily done while babies sleep. Nails should be cut straight across using adult cuticle scissors or blunt-ended infant cuticle scissors.

Wrapping the Newborn

Wrapping helps the newborn maintain body temperature and provides a feeling of closeness and security. When wrapping, a blanket is placed on the crib (or secure surface) in the shape of a diamond. The top corner of the blanket is folded down slightly, and the baby's body is placed with the head at the upper edge of the blanket. The right corner of the blanket is wrapped around the infant and tucked under the left side (not too tightly—newborns need a little room to move). The bottom corner is then pulled up to the chest, and the left corner is wrapped around the baby's right side (Figure 29–12). This wrapping technique can be shared with a new mother so she will feel more skilled in handling her baby.

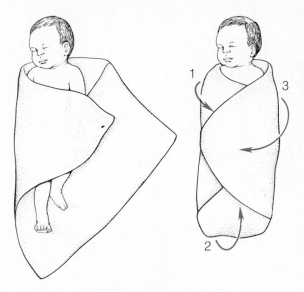

Figure 29–12 Steps used for wrapping a baby

Dressing the Newborn

Newborns need to wear a T-shirt, diaper (plastic pants if using cloth diapers), and a sleeper. On a fairly cool day, they should also be wrapped in a light blanket while being fed.

A good rule of thumb is for the parent to add one more light layer of clothing than the parent is wearing. An infant may be covered with a blanket in air-conditioned buildings. The blanket should be unwrapped or removed when inside a warm building.

At home the amount of clothing the infant wears is determined by the temperature. Families who maintain the home at 60F to 65F should dress the infant more warmly than those who maintain the temperature at 70F to 75F.

Infants should wear head coverings outdoors to protect their sensitive ears from drafts. Parents must also be advised of the ease with which a baby's skin can burn when exposed to the sun. To prevent sunburn the baby should remain shaded, wear a light layer of clothing, or be protected with a sunscreen product.

Diaper shapes vary and are subject to personal preference (Figure 29–13). Prefolded and disposable diapers are usually rectangular. Diapers may also be triangular or kite-folded. Extra material is placed in front for boys and toward the back for girls to aid in absorbency.

Baby clothing should be laundered separately using a mild soap or detergent. Diapers may be presoaked before washing. All clothing should be rinsed twice to remove soap and residue and to decrease the possibility of rash. Some babies may not tolerate clothing treated with fabric softeners; in this case softeners should be avoided.

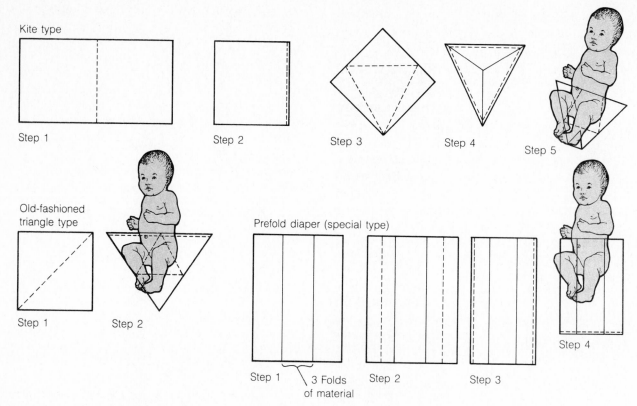

Kite type

Step 1   Step 2   Step 3   Step 4   Step 5

Old-fashioned triangle type

Step 1   Step 2

Prefold diaper (special type)

Step 1   3 Folds of material   Step 2   Step 3   Step 4

Figure 29–13   Three basic diaper shapes. Dotted lines indicate folds.

Temperature Assessment

The nurse must demonstrate how to take rectal and axillary temperatures for parents. A return demonstration is the only way to evaluate their understanding. The nurse shows them how to shake down a thermometer before inserting it.

When parents take a rectal temperature, the infant should be supine with the legs held up in one hand, exposing the rectum. The end of the rectal thermometer is lubricated with petroleum jelly, and the thermometer is inserted just until the silver bulb is covered, approximately half an inch. The thermometer is held in place five minutes. A baby is never left alone with a thermometer in place and the adult must maintain a hold on the thermometer at all times. Some pediatricians feel that rectal temperatures are more accurate and prefer that parents take temperatures this way. Parents may be more receptive to taking axillary temperatures and should make their preferences known to the caregiver.

To take an axillary temperature, the thermometer is placed under one of the infant's arms, making sure that the bulb of the thermometer is underneath the armpit. It is held in place three to four minutes (Figure 28–14).

A parent needs to take the newborn's temperature only when the signs of illness are present. Parents are advised to call their physician or pediatric nurse practitioner immediately if any of the signs listed in Box 29–5 occur.

Parents should also check with their clinician for advice about over-the-counter medications they should have in the medicine cabinet. All parents should be advised to avoid giving any form of aspirin to their infants for any illness that may be viral. Use of aspirin in viral illnesses has been linked to Reye syndrome in children under 19 years of age. Flu, colds, teething, constipation, diarrhea, and other common ailments and their management should be discussed with the clinician before they occur.

Box 29–5   When Parents Should Call Their Health Care Provider

If any of the following signs are present parents need to call their health care provider.

- Temperature above 38.4C (101F) or below 36.1C (97F).

- More than one episode of projectile vomiting

- Refusal of two feedings in a row

- Lethargy (listlessness)

- Cyanosis with or without a feeding

- Absence of breathing longer than 15 seconds

Stools and Urine

The appearance and frequency of the newborn's stools can cause concern for parents. The nurse prepares parents by discussing and showing pictures of meconium stools, transitional stools, and the difference between breast-milk and formula stools.

Although each baby develops his or her own stooling patterns, parents can be given an idea of what to expect. Parents should be told that breast-fed babies may have six to ten small, loose yellow stools per day or only one stool every few days. Bottle-fed infants may have only one or two stools a day. The stools are more formed and will be yellow or yellow-brown in color. The parents may also be shown pictures of a constipated stool (small, pelletlike) and diarrhea (loose, green, or perhaps blood-tinged). Parents should understand that a green color is common in transitional stools so that transitional stools are not confused with diarrhea the first week of a newborn's life.

Constipation may be an indication that the baby needs additional fluid intake or that excessive solids have been introduced to the diet. The parent might try discontinuing or decreasing the intake of solids, offering additional water, or adding fruit to the diet in an attempt to reverse the constipation (Chow et al 1984).

Babies normally void six to ten times per day. Fewer than six wet diapers a day may indicate the newborn needs more fluids.

Sleep and Activity

Perhaps nothing is more individual to each baby than the sleep-activity cycle. It is important for the nurse to recognize the individual variations of each newborn and to assist parents as they develop sensitivity to their infant's communication signals and rhythms of activity and sleep.

The newborn demonstrates several different sleep-wake states (see Chapter 27) after the initial periods of reactivity described earlier. It is not uncommon for a baby to sleep almost continuously for the first two to three days following birth, awakening only for feedings every three or four hours. Some newborns bypass this stage of deep sleep and may require only 12 to 16 hours of sleep. The parents need to know that this is normal.

Quiet sleep is characterized by regular breathing and no movement except for sudden body jerks. During this sleep state, normal household noise will not awaken the infant. In the *active sleep state,* the newborn has irregular breathing and fine muscular twitching. The newborn may cry out during sleep, but this does not mean he or she is uncomfortable or awake. Unusual household noise may awaken the infant more easily in this state; however, the newborn will quickly go back to sleep.

Wide awake is a state in which newborns are quietly involved with the environment. They watch a moving mo-
bile, smile, and, as they become older, discover and play with their hands and feet. When infants become uncomfortable due to wet diapers, hunger, or cold, they enter the *active awake and crying state.* In this state, the cause of the crying should be identified and eliminated. Sometimes parents are frustrated as they try to identify the external or internal stimuli that are causing the angry, hurt crying. Parents need to be told that the baby's state may be changed from crying to quiet alert by moving the baby toward an upright position where scanning and exploration is possible (Klaus & Klaus 1985).

CRYING

For the newborn, crying is the only means of expressing needs vocally. Parents and caregivers learn to distinguish different tones and qualities of the neonate's cry. The amount of crying is highly individual. Some will cry as little as 15 to 30 minutes in 24 hours or as long as 2 hours every 24 hours. When crying continues after causes such as discomfort or hunger are eliminated, the newborn may be comforted by swaddling or by rocking and other reassuring activities. There is some indication that infants who are held more tend to be calmer and cry less when not being held. Excessive crying should be noted and assessed, taking other factors into consideration. After the first two or three days, newborns settle into individual patterns.

● Circumcision

Circumcision is a surgical procedure in which the prepuce, an epithelial layer covering the penis, is separated from the glans penis and is excised. This permits exposure of the glans for easier cleaning.

The parents make the decision about circumcision for their newborn male child. In most cases the choice is based on cultural, social, and family tradition. To guarantee informed consent, parents should be informed about possible long-term medical effects of circumcision and noncircumcision during the prenatal period.

In the past, this procedure was recommended for all newborn males. In recent years, however, the American Academy of Pediatrics Committee on Fetus and Newborn (1975) has stated that there are no valid medical reasons for routine newborn circumcision. In fact the procedure should not be performed if the newborn is premature or compromised, has a known bleeding problem, or is born with a genitourinary defect such as hypospadias or epispadias, which may necessitate the use of the foreskin in future surgical repairs (Pritchard et al 1985).

Circumcision was originally a rite of the Jewish religion. The practice gained widespread cultural acceptance in the United States but is done infrequently in many European countries. Many parents choose circumcision because they want the infant to have a similar physical appearance to the father or the majority of other children, or they may feel that it is expected by society (Harris 1986).

Another frequently cited reason for circumcising newborn males is to prevent the need for anesthesia, hospitalization, pain, and trauma should the procedure be needed later in life. Pritchard, MacDonald, and Gant (1985) note that only 5 percent to 10 percent of males are estimated to be in this category.

Parents must be informed about potential risks and outcomes of circumcision. Hemorrhage, infection, difficulty in voiding, separation of the edges of the circumcision, discomfort, and restlessness are early potential problems. Later there is the risk that the glans and urethral meatus can become irritated and inflamed from contact with ammonia from urine. Ulcerations and progressive stenosis may develop. Adhesions, entrapment of the penis, and damage to the urethra are all potential complications that could require surgical correction (Gibbons 1984).

Parents who are doubtful about their ability to use good hygienic practices in caring for their uncircumcised male infant and child require information from the nurse. They should be told that the foreskin and glans are two similar layers of cells that separate from each other. The separation process begins prenatally and is normally completed at between 3 and 6 years of age. In the process of separation, sterile sloughed cells build up between the layers. This buildup looks similar to the smegma secreted after puberty, but it is harmless. Occasionally during the daily bath, the parents can gently test for retraction. If retraction has occurred, daily gentle washing of the glans with soap and water is sufficient to maintain adequate cleanliness (Gibbons 1984). The child should be taught to incorporate this practice into his daily self-care activities.

If circumcision is to be done, the procedure is not usually done until the day before discharge when the newborn is well stabilized and there is less chance of cold stress. The parents may also choose to have the circumcision done after discharge. However, they need to be advised that if the baby is older than 1 month, he will probably be hospitalized, and the procedure will be done in surgery under general anesthesia.

The nurse's responsibilities during a circumcision are to determine if the parents have any further questions about the procedure and to ensure that the circumcision permit is signed. The nurse gathers the equipment and prepares the newborn by removing the diaper and placing him on a circumcision board or some other type of restraint (Figure 29–14). In the Jewish ceremonies, the infant is held by the parent and given wine before the procedure.

There are a variety of techniques for circumcision (Figures 29–15, 29–16), and all produce minimal bleeding. During the procedure, the nurse assesses the newborn's response. One consideration is pain experienced by the newborn. Some physicians use local anesthesia for this procedure. Successful pain relief has been achieved with the use of lidocaine to block the penile dorsal nerve (Kirya & Werthmann 1978).

The nurse can provide comfort measures such as lightly stroking the baby's head and talking to him. Following the circumcision he should be held and comforted by a parent (Lubchenco 1980) or the nurse. The nurse must be alert to any cues that these measures are overstimulating the newborn instead of comforting him. Such cues are turning away of the head, increased generalized body movement, skin color changes, hyperalertness, and hiccoughing (D'Apolito 1984).

After the circumcision a small petroleum jelly gauze strip is applied to help control bleeding and to keep the diaper from adhering to the site in all procedures except the Plastibell. The petroleum jelly gauze is left in place for one to two days. It need not be changed unless it becomes contaminated with stool. A and D ointment may be used instead of petroleum jelly. A large amount is placed on the penis at each diaper change or at least four to five times a day for at least 48 hours.

The baby's voiding is assessed for amount, adequacy of stream, and presence of blood. If bleeding does occur, light pressure is applied intermittently to the site with a sterile gauze pad, and the physician is notified. The newborn may cry when he voids. He should be positioned on his side with the diaper fastened loosely to prevent undue pressure. He may remain fussy for several hours and be less interested in feedings.

Before discharge, the parents should be instructed to observe the penis for bleeding or possible signs of infection. A whitish yellow exudate around the glans is granulation tissue. It is normal and not indicative of an infection. The exudate may be noted for about two or three days, and should not be removed.

The parents should be instructed to squeeze water gently over the penis and pat it dry after each diaper change. The diaper is loosely fastened for two to three days, because the glans remains tender for this length of time.

If the Plastibell is used, parents are informed that it will remain in place for three or four days and then fall off. If it is still in place after eight days, it may require manual removal by the clinician (Gibbons 1984).

● Discharge Planning

The nurse can do much to assist parents in feeling comfortable with newborn care. By discussing with parents how to meet their newborn's needs and ensure his or her safety, the nurse can get the new family off to a good start. The nurse also plays a vital role in fostering parent-infant attachment.

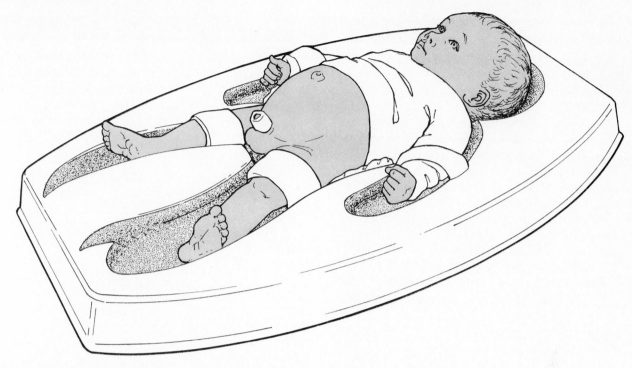

Figure 29–14 *Proper positioning of the infant on a circumcision restraining board*

In addition to the information the nurse provides to parents during their stay in the birthing site, the nurse should provide information about safety, the newborn screening program, and follow-up care before the mother and baby are discharged.

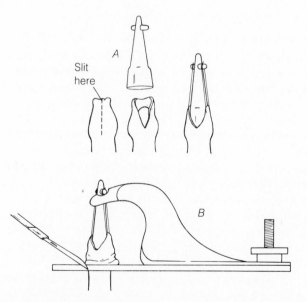

Figure 29–15 *When the Yellen or Gomco clamp is used for circumcision, the prepuce is drawn over the cone (A), and the clamp is applied (B). Pressure is maintained for three to five minutes, and then the excess prepuce is cut away.*

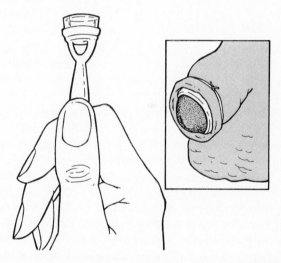

Figure 29–16 *When the Plastibell is used for circumcision, the bell is fitted over the glans. A suture is tied around the bell's rim and the excess prepuce is cut away. The plastic rim remains in place for three to four days until healing takes place. The bell may be allowed to fall off or removed if still in place after eight days.*

Safety Considerations

The nurses can be an excellent role model for parents in the area of safety. Newborns should always be positioned on the stomach or side with a blanket rolled up behind them. Correct use of the bulb syringe must be demonstrated. The baby should never be left alone anywhere but

To Circumcise or Not to Circumcise?

Circumcision is the most frequently performed surgical procedure in the United States. Circumcisions are carried out on anywhere from 30 percent of males born in alternative birth settings to 80 percent to 90 percent of those born in traditional hospital settings. This surgical procedure continues in spite of the American Academy of Pediatrics 1975 statement that "there is no absolute medical indication for routine circumcision of the newborn . . . circumcision of the male neonate cannot be considered an essential component of adequate total health care" (American Academy of Pediatrics 1975, p 10).

What then motivates parents to have their male newborns circumcised? Various reasons have been given for the circumcision, including: traditional practice (It's always been done—why question it?); wanting the child to have a similar appearance to the father; rites of passage into manhood (religious and cultural rites); desire to conform to the dominant culture; sexual adequacy and cosmetic appearance; and hygiene. Opponents provide equally strong rationale

and cultural data for not carrying out this procedure. It is important for nurses to identify and acknowledge the sociocultural motivating factors involved in the decision to circumcise or not to circumcise.

The current controversy over the continuation of the practice of circumcision raises important issues and concerns of parents.

- When is the optimal time for providing parents information about the circumcision procedure?

- What information should be provided to facilitate an informed choice?

- How do sociocultural factors influence the continued practice of circumcision?

- How does the health professional's ethnocentrism affect the information provided parents?

- Does a child have a right to an intact body? Or to avoid exposure to potential harm?

in the crib. The mother is reminded that while she and the newborn are together in the hospital, she should never leave the baby alone because newborns spit up frequently the first day or two after birth.

Accidents are the number one cause of death in children, with car accidents causing the most deaths, followed by poisonings. Half the children killed or injured in automobile accidents could have been protected by the use a federally approved car seat. Newborns should go home from the hospital in a car seat (not an infant carrier seat). The seat should be positioned to face the rear of the car until the baby is a year old or weighs 20 pounds. At this time the bone structure is adequately mineralized and better able to withstand a forward impact in a five-point harness restraint belt. Children should always ride in a car seat until they are 4 years old (depending on size of the child), no matter how short the trip. In many states, the use of car seats for children up to the age of 4 is mandatory.

All medications must be locked up. Newborns quickly grow into toddlers who can climb to medicine cabinets. Medications look like candy to a toddler. Whenever medication is given, children should be told they are taking medicine instead of calling it candy. Plants should be put above a toddler's reach; many are poisonous. All cleaning supplies must be moved to high, out-of-the-way cupboards. Parents are told to cover electrical outlets and keep electrical cords out of sight. Newborns do not need pillows or stuffed animals in the crib while they sleep; these items

could cause suffocation. Mattresses should fit snugly in a crib to prevent entrapment and suffocation, and the crib should be inspected regularly to determine whether it is in safe working order.

Newborn Screening Program

Before the newborn and mother are discharged from the hospital, parents are informed about the normal screening tests for newborns and should be told when to return to the hospital or clinic to have the tests completed. *Newborn screening tests* detect disorders that cause mental retardation, physical handicaps, or death if left undiscovered. Inborn errors of metabolism can usually be detected within one to two weeks after birth and important treatment begun before any damage has occurred. The disorders that can be identified from a drop of blood obtained by a heel stick on the second or third day are galactosemia, homocystinuria, hypothyroidism, maple syrup urine disease, phenylketonuria (PKU), and sickle cell anemia. Parents should be instructed that a second blood specimen will be required after 7 to 14 days when the newborn's defects are clearly apparent. However, it must be clarified that an abnormal test result is not diagnostic. More definitive tests must be performed to verify the results (Avery & Taeusch 1984). If additional tests are positive, treatment is initiated. These conditions may be treated by dietary means or by administration of the missing hormones. The inborn conditions cannot be cured, but they can be treated. Although they are not contagious, they may be inherited (Chapter 9).

Follow-Up Care

Each newborn will have variations in normal physiologic responses. Parents need to learn how to interpret these changes in their child. To assist parents in caring for their newborn at home, some physicians encourage pediatric prenatal visits so that this contact is established before the birth (Sprunger & Preece 1981). Public health nurses have long been involved in newborn care and parent education (Lauri 1981). Hospitals are now expanding their primary care functions to the new family to include one home visit by the primary nurse who cared for the family in the hospital. The hospital nursery staff may also make themselves available as a 24-hour telephone resource for the new mother who needs additional support and consultation during the first few days at home with her newborn.

Routine well-baby visits should be scheduled with the clinic, pediatric nurse practitioner, or physician.

Parents should be taught all necessary care-giving methods before discharge. A checklist may be helpful to see if the teaching has been completed. The nurse needs to review all areas for understanding or questions with the mother, without rushing, taking time to answer all queries. The mother should have the physician's phone number, address, and any specific instructions. Having the birthing unit or nursery phone number is also reassuring to a new mother. The parents are encouraged to call with questions.

Documentation

The final step of discharge planning is documentation. Any concerns of the parents or nurse are noted. The nurse records which demonstrations and/or classes the mother and/or father attended and their expressed understanding of the instructions given to them.

KEY CONCEPTS

The overall goal of newborn nursing care is to provide comprehensive care while promoting the establishment of a well-functioning family unit.

The period immediately following birth, during which adaptation to extrauterine life occurs, requires close monitoring to identify any deviations from normal.

Nursing goals during the first four hours after birth (admission period) are to: maintain a clear airway,

maintain a neutral thermal environment, prevent hemorrhage and infection, and initiate bathing and oral feedings.

The first period of reactivity lasts for 30 minutes after birth. The newborn is alert and hungry at this time, making this a natural opportunity to promote attachment.

The second period of reactivity requires close monitoring by the nurse as apnea, decreased heart rate, gagging, choking, and regurgitation are likely to occur and require nursing intervention.

The newborn is routinely given prophylactic vitamin K to prevent possible hemorrhagic disease of the newborn.

Prophylactic eye treatment for *Neisseria gonorrhoeae* is legally required on all newborns.

Essential daily care includes assessments of the vital signs, weight, overall color, intake/output, umbilical cord and circumcision, newborn nutrition, parent education, and attachment.

The physician should be notified if there is evidence of bright red bleeding or puslike drainage near the cord stump or if the umbilicus remains unhealed.

Following a circumcision the newborn must be observed closely for signs of bleeding, inability to void, and signs of infection.

Signs of illness in newborns include: temperature above 38.4C (101F) or below 36.1C (97F), more than one episode of projectile vomiting, refusal of two feedings in a row, lethargy, cyanosis, and absence of breathing for longer than 15 seconds.

Newborn screening for galactosemia, homocystinuria, hypothyroidism, maple syrup urine disease, phenylketonuria, and sickle cell anemia is done on all newborns in the first 1 to 3 days, with a second blood specimen drawn after 7 to 14 days.

REFERENCES

American Academy of Pediatrics, Committee on Fetus and Newborn: Report of the Ad Hoc Task Force on Circumcision. *Pediatrics* 1975;56(October):10.

Andrich M, Golden S: Umbilical cord care. *Clin Pediatr* 1984;23:342.

Avery M, Taeusch Jr H: *Schaffer's Diseases of the Newborn*, ed 5. Philadelphia, Saunders, 1984.

Benitz W, Tatro D: *The Pediatric Drug Handbook*. Chicago, Year Book Medical Publishers, 1981.

Beske E, Garvis M: Important factors in breast feeding success. *Am J Mat Child Nurs* 1982;7(May/June):174.

Chow M, et al: *Handbook of Pediatric Primary Care,* ed 2. New York, Wiley, 1984.

D'Apolito K: The neonate's response to pain. *Am J Mat Child Nurs* 1984;9(July/August)256.

Gibbons M: Circumcision: The controversy continues. *Pediatr Nurs* 1984;10(March/April):103.

Harris CC: Cultural values and the decision to circumcise. *IMAGE* 1986;18(Fall):98.

Haun N, Porter E, Chance G: Care of the normal neonate. *Can Nurs* 1984;80(October):37.

Kemp C, Silver H, O'Brien D: *Current Pediatric Diagnosis and Treatment,* ed 7. Los Altos, Calif, Lange Medical Publications, 1982.

Kirya C, Werthmann M: Neonatal circumcision and penile dorsal nerve block: A painless procedure. *J Pediatr* 1978;92:998.

Klaus M, Klaus P: *The Amazing Newborn.* Menlo Park, Calif, Addison-Wesley, 1985.

Lauri S: The public health nurse as a guide in infant child care and education. *J Adv Nurs* 1981;6:297.

Lubchenco L: Routine neonatal circumcision: A surgical anachronism. *Clin Obstet Gynecol* 1980;23:1135.

Mayfield S, et al: Temperature measurement in term and preterm neonates. *J Pediatr* 1984;104(February):271.

Pritchard J, MacDonald P, Gant N: *Williams Obstetrics,* ed 17. East Norwalk, Conn, Appleton-Century-Crofts, 1985.

Ruchala P: The effect of wearing head coverings on the axillary temperatures of infants. *Am J Mat Child Nurs* 1985;10(July/August):240.

Sprunger LW, Preece EW: Use of pediatric prenatal visits by family physicians. *J Fam Pract* 1981;13:1007.

Evans M, Hansen B: *A Clinical Guide to Pediatric Nursing,* ed 2. Norwalk, Conn, Appleton-Century-Crofts, 1985.

Hayden GF, et al: Providing free samples of baby items to newly delivered parents. An unintentional endorsement? *Clin Pediatr* 1987;26(March):14.

Klaus M, Kennell J: *Parent-Infant Attachment,* ed 2. St Louis, Mosby, 1982.

Lincoln GA: Neonatal circumcision: Is it needed? *J Obstet Gynecol Neonat Nurs* 1986;15(November/December):463.

Marcus D: Child car seats: A must for safety. *Pediatr Nurs* 1981;7(May/June):13.

Osborn LM, et al: Hygiene care in uncircumcised infants. *Pediatrics* March 1981;67:365.

Panwar S: Introducing family-centered care for mothers and newborns. *Nursing Management* 1986;17(November):45.

Pelosi MA, Apuzzio J: Making circumcision safe and painless. *Contemp OB/GYN* 1984;24:42.

Sandstrom I: Ophthalmia neonatorum with special reference to chlamydia trachomatis: Diagnosis and treatment. *Acta Paediatr Scand* 1986;330(suppl):4.

Tedder JI: Newborn circumcision. *J Obstet Gynecol Neonat Nurs* 1987;16(January/February):42.

Tomlinson PS: Father involvement with first-born infants: Interpersonal and situational factors. *Pediatr Nurs* 1987;13(March/April):101.

Wagner T, Hindi-Alexander M: Hazards of baby powder. *Pediatr Nurs* 1984;10(March/April):124.

Wieser M, Castiglia P: Assessing early father-infant attachment. *Am J Mat Child Nurs* 1984;9(March/April):104.

ADDITIONAL READINGS

Chess S, Thomas A: Temperamental differences: A critical concept in child health care. *Pediatr Nurs* 1985;11(May/June):167.

Choi ES, Hamilton RK: The effects of culture on mother-infant interaction. *J Obstet Gynecol Neonat Nurs* 1986;15(May/June):256.

Cunningham N, et al: Infant carrying, breastfeeding, and mother-infant relations, letter. *Lancet* 1987;1(February):379.

Dunn DM, White DG: Interactions of mothers with their newborns in the first half-hour of life. *J Adv Nurs* 1981;6:271.

When our daughter was laid in my arms right after birth she was so delicate. I had not dared to hope that we would be blessed with a girl because there were so few girls in my husband's family. Our two-year-old niece was the first girl in 107 years, so I had pretty much decided that another boy would be just fine. But here she was, right here in my arms.

I think mothers wish for daughters. There is a oneness between women that is unique and not easily explained. That special feeling has persisted, even though she is so grown up now. I still feel very lucky to have a daughter.

The Normal Newborn: Successful Feeding

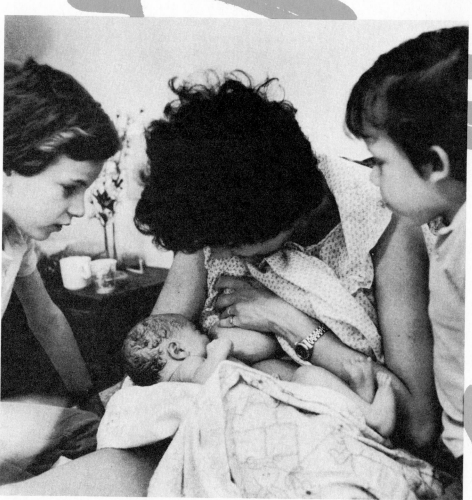

With her 4- and 6-year-old sons looking on, a nurse who has just given birth in an alternative birthing environment puts her hour-old baby to her breast.

Chapter Thirty

OBJECTIVES

- Compare the nutritional value and composition of breast milk and formula preparations.
- Identify the benefits of breast-feeding for both mother and infant.
- Develop guidelines for helping both breast-feeding and bottle-feeding mothers to feed their infants successfully.
- Delineate nursing responsibilities for client education about problems the breast-feeding mother may encounter at home.
- Describe an appropriate process for weaning an infant from breast-feeding.
- Discuss the use of supplemental foods in the diet of infants under 1 year old.

Feeding their newborn is an exciting, satisfying, and often worrisome task for parents. Meeting this essential need of their new child helps parents strengthen their attachment to their child and fosters their self-images as nurturers and providers. Whether a woman chooses to breast-feed or bottle-feed, she can be reassured that she can adequately meet her infant's needs. Questions may arise, however, and the nurse works with the woman to help her develop skill in her chosen method. The nurse provides information, assists the parent, and answers questions as necessary. In every interaction it is the nurse's responsibility to do and say things that increase rather than decrease the family's sense of confidence.

This chapter considers various aspects of infant nutrition. The first part of the chapter focuses on the nutritional needs of infants and compares breast milk and formula. The next portion of the chapter describes feeding techniques for both breast-feeding and bottle-feeding. The final portion of the chapter focuses on nutritional assessment of the infant and addresses such concerns as supplemental feeding.

● Nutritional Needs of the Newborn

The newborn's diet must supply nutrients to meet the rapid rate of physical growth and development. A neonatal diet should provide adequate calories and include protein, carbohydrate, fat, water, vitamins, and minerals. The recommendations in Table 30–1 are based on limited research data but give generalizations about requirements for optimal nutrition for the first year of life.

The calories (120 cal/kg/day) in the newborn's diet are divided among protein, carbohydrate, and fat and should be adjusted according to the infant's weight. Protein is needed for rapid cellular growth and maintenance. Carbohydrates provide energy. The fat portion of the diet provides calories, regulates fluid and electrolyte balance, and is necessary for the development of the neonatal brain and neurologic system.

Water requirements are high (140–160 mL/kg/day) because of the newborn's inability to concentrate urine. Fluid needs are further increased in illness or hot weather.

The iron intake of the infant will be affected by accumulation of iron stores during the fetal life, and the mother's iron and other food intake if she is breast-feeding. Ingestion of ascorbic acid (usually in the form of fruit juices) and meat, poultry, and fish are known to enhance absorption of iron in the mother just as it does later in the infant. Adequate minerals and vitamins are needed by the newborn to prevent deficiency states such as scurvy, cheilosis, and pellagra (Eckstein 1980).

Breast Milk

Three types of milk are produced during the establishment of lactation: (a) colostrum, (b) transitional milk, and (c) mature milk. *Colostrum* is a yellowish or creamy-appearing fluid that is thicker than later milk and contains more protein, fat-soluble vitamins, and minerals. It also contains high levels of immunoglobulins, which may be a source of immunity for the newborn. Colostrum produc-

Table 30–1 Nutritional Needs of the Normal Newborn

	At birth	At 1 year
Calories	120/kg/day	100/kg/day
Protein	1.9 g/100 kcal*	1.7 g/100 kcal*
Fat	30%–55% of total calories	30%–50% of total calories
Carbohydrate	35%–55% of total calories	35%–55% of total calories
Water	330 mL†	700 mL
Calcium	388 mg	299 mg
Phosphate	132 mg	110 mg
Magnesium	16 mg	13.5 mg
Iron	7 mg	7 mg
Copper	Not established	Not established
Zinc	Not established	Not established
Vitamins		
A	100–200 IU*	100–200 IU*
D	0.4 mg/dL*	0.4 mg/dL*
E	0.4 mg/dL*	0.4 mg/dL*
K	75 mg/day*	75 mg/day*
C	10 mg/day*	10 mg/day*
Thiamine	0.2 mg/100 kcal*	0.2 mg/100 kcal*

*Estimated to be approximately equivalent to levels in breast milk.
†Approximately.

Adapted from information contained in Eckstein EF: *Food, People, and Nutrition.* Westport, Conn, AV Publishing, 1980.

tion begins early in pregnancy and may last for several days after delivery. However, in most cases colostrum is replaced by transitional milk within two to four days after delivery. *Transitional milk* is produced from the end of colostrum production until approximately two weeks postpartum. This milk contains elevated levels of fat, lactose, water-soluble vitamins, and more calories than colostrum.

The final milk produced, *mature milk,* has a high percentage of water. Although it appears similar to skim milk and may cause mothers to question whether their milk is "rich enough," mature breast milk provides 20 kcal/ounce, as do most prepared formulas. However, the percentage of calories derived from protein is lower in breast milk than in formulas, with a greater proportion of calories being derived from carbohydrates in the form of lactose (Pipes 1985). The nitrogen wastes of protein metabolism are, thereby, lessened in the breast-fed newborn, which has a positive effect on the immature renal system.

The American Academy of Pediatrics (1981) recommends breast milk as the optimal food for the first four to six months of life. The advantages that breast-feeding provides to newborns and infants are generally immunological, nutritional, and psychosocial.

Immunologic advantages identified by Pipes (1985), Gulick (1986), and Anholm (1986) include varying degrees of protection from respiratory and gastrointestinal infections, otitis media, meningitis, sepsis, and allergies. This protection has a positive impact on the health of the breast-fed baby into the infant and toddler period (Gulick 1986). Secretory IgA, which is present in colostrum and breast milk, has antiviral, antibacterial, and antigenic-inhibiting properties. It is theorized that the immature intestine allows antigenic macromolecules, such as those found in cow's milk, to cross the mucosa of the small intestine. Secretory IgA plays a role in decreasing the permeability of the intestine to these macromolecules. Other properties in colostrum and breast milk that act to inhibit the growth of bacteria and/or viruses are *Lactobacillus bifidus,* lysozymes, lactoperoxidase, lactoferrin, transferrin, and various immunoglobulins or antibodies. Immunoglobulins to the poliomyelitis virus are also present in the breast milk of immune mothers. Due to the fact that this may inhibit the desired intestinal infection and immune response of the infant, some clinics suggest that breast-feedings be withheld for 30 to 60 minutes following the administration of the Sabin oral polio vaccine. Table 30–2 identifies the factors in breast milk with specific antibacterial and antiviral actions.

In addition to its immunologic properties, breast milk is known to be nonallergenic and is not affected by unsafe water or insect-carried disease (Joseph 1981).

Breast milk is composed of lactose, lipids, polyunsaturated fatty acids, and amino acids, especially taurine, and has a whey to casein protein ratio that facilitates the digestion, absorption, and full use of breast milk compared to formulas (Gulick 1986). Some researchers feel the high concentration of cholesterol and the balance of amino acids in breast milk make it the best food for myelination and neurologic development. It is also suggested that high cholesterol levels in breast milk may stimulate the production of enzymes that lead to more efficient metabolism of cholesterol, thereby reducing its long-term harmful effects on the cardiovascular system (Kemp et al 1982, Anholm 1986).

Table 30–2   Antibacterial and Antiviral Factors in Breast Milk

Factor	Shown in vitro to be active against
ANTIBACTERIAL FACTORS	
L. bifidus growth factor	Enterobacteriaceae, enteric pathogens
Secretory IgA	E. coli, E. coli enterotoxin, C. tetani, C. diphtheriae, D. pneumoniae, Salmonella, Shigella
C1-C9	Effect not known
Lactoferrin	E. coli, C. albicans
Lactoperoxidase	Streptococcus, Pseudomonas, E. coli, S. typhimurium
Lysozyme	E. coli, Salmonella, M. lysodeikticus
Lipid (unsaturated fatty acid)	S. aureus
Milk cells	By phagocytosis: E. coli, C. albicans
	By sensitized lymphocytes: E. coli
ANTIVIRAL FACTORS	
Secretory IgA	Polio types 1,2,3; Coxsackie types A9, B3, B5; ECHO types 6, 9; Semliki Forest virus; Ross River virus; rotavirus
Lipid (unsaturated fatty acids and monoglycerides)	Herpes simplex; Semliki Forest virus, influenza, dengue, Ross River virus, Murine leukemia virus, Japanese B encephalitis virus
Nonimmunoglobulin macromolecules	Herpes simplex; vesicular stomatitis virus
Milk cells	Rotavirus; induced interferon active against Sendai virus; sensitized lymphocytes? phagocytosis

From Pipes P: *Nutrition in Infancy and Childhood.* St Louis, Times Mirror/Mosby, 1985.

Breast milk provides newborns with minerals in more acceptable doses than those provided by formulas (Riordan & Countryman 1980). The iron found in breast milk, even though much lower in concentration than that of prepared formulas, is much more readily and fully absorbed and appears sufficient to meet the infant's iron needs for the first four to six months of age (Picciano & Deering 1980). The American Academy of Pediatrics states that there is generally no need to give supplemental iron to breast-fed newborns before the age of 6 months. Supplemental iron may be detrimental to the ability of breast milk to protect the newborn by interfering with lactoferrin, an iron-binding protein that enhances the absorption of iron and has anti-infective properties.

Another advantage of breast milk is that all its components are delivered to the infant in an unchanged form, and vitamins are not lost through processing and heating. If the breast-feeding mother is taking daily multivitamins and her diet is adequate, the only supplements necessary are vitamin D and fluoride until the infant is 6 months old (American Academy of Pediatrics 1981). If the mother's diet or vitamin intake is inadequate or questionable, care givers may choose to prescribe additional vitamins for the infant.

The psychosocial advantages of breast-feeding are primarily those associated with attachment. Breast-feeding enhances attachment by providing the opportunity for frequent, direct skin contact between the newborn and the mother. The newborn's sense of touch is highly developed at birth and is a primary means of communication. The tactile stimulation associated with breast-feeding can communicate warmth, closeness, and comfort. The increased closeness provides both newborn and mother with the opportunity to learn each other's behavioral cues and needs. The mother's sense of accomplishment in being able to satisfy her baby's needs for nourishment and comfort is enhanced when the newborn sucks vigorously, and is satiated and calmed by the breast-feeding. Some mothers prefer breast-feeding as a means of extending the close, unique, nourishing relationship between mother and baby that existed prior to delivery. In the event of a twin birth, breast-feeding not only is possible but also enhances the mother's individualization and attachment to each newborn. The fantasized single baby is replaced more readily with the reality of two individual babies when the mother has close and frequent contact with each (Gromada 1981). Other studies have been cited that associate breast-feeding with improved language and cognitive development as well as scholastic ability (Anholm 1986).

One disadvantage of breast-feeding is that most drugs taken by the mother are transmitted through breast milk and may cause harm to the infant (see Appendix J for specific drugs and their possible effect on the neonate). Jaundice caused by breast milk may be another reason to interrupt breast-feeding. Breast-feeding can normally be resumed after 48 hours without resulting in further hyperbilirubinemia.

A mother's poor nutritional, physical, or mental health or a personal aversion to breast-feeding may be contraindications to nursing. Difficulty in maintaining milk supply, concern over the adequacy of the breast milk to meet the newborn's needs, sore nipples, resumption of a heavy work schedule, and constant demands on her time are other reasons mothers discontinue breast-feeding. Lack of support and encouragement from health care providers or family may also contribute to a woman's decision to stop breast-feeding.

Opinion varies as to the advisability of continuing breast-feeding in the event of another pregnancy. Some feel the nutritional demands on the pregnant mother are too great and advocate gradual weaning. Others suggest that with adequate rest, a proper diet, and strong emotional support, continued breast-feeding during pregnancy is a valid choice. The practice of nursing one infant throughout

Research Note

Morgan explored the concerns of 78 primiparous breast-feeding mothers who all had normal deliveries and healthy term babies. The mothers were observed and interviewed six times from the initial postpartum period to six months postpartum.

The data from this research showed that the biggest decline in breast-feeding occurred between two and four months postpartum, most commonly due to a perception of inadequate milk or a return to work.

At the two-week and one-, two-, and four-month home visits, the most common concern of the mother was a perception of insufficient milk or a perception that the milk looked too thin. Other concerns included nipple and breast discomfort (at two weeks), fatigue, and feeding technique. At six months, of the 65 percent of mothers who were still nursing only a few had questions about technique.

The results of this study emphasize the importance of adequate teaching about breast-feeding during pregnancy and the postpartum period, particularly including information about the characteristics of breast milk and about evaluating the amount of milk. In addition, the repetitiveness of the concerns despite repeated advice indicates a need for support and education throughout the breast-feeding period, which could be provided by the pediatric nurse or by a support group such as La Leche League.

Morgan J: A study of mothers' breastfeeding concerns. Birth 1986;13(June):104–108.

pregnancy and then breast-feeding both infants after delivery is called *tandem nursing* (Lawrence 1980). When pregnancy occurs, the decision is best made on an individual basis after considering maternal health and motivation and the age of the first child.

Even though many mothers obtain information about breast-feeding from written sources, family and friends, and La Leche League, the nurse needs to be a ready source of information, encouragement, and support as well. The nurse can be helpful during the time when parents are deciding whether to breast-feed, after the birth process when breast-feedings are just being established, and after the family returns home.

Formula

Numerous types of commercially prepared lactose formulas adequately meet the nutritional needs of the infant. These milk formulas contain different amounts of amino acids: tyrosine and phenylalanine are more prevalent in formula milk; the taurine present in breast milk is absent in cow's milk formula. Bottle-fed babies do gain weight faster than breast-fed babies because of the higher protein in commercially prepared formula than in human milk.

Bottle-fed infants up to 6 months of age may gain as much as 1 ounce per day and tend to regain their birth weight by ten days after birth (Pipes 1985). Healthy breast-fed babies, however, gain approximately ½ ounce per day in the first six months of life (Stahl & Guida 1984) and tend to regain their birth weight about 14 days postpartum. Formula-fed infants generally double their weight within 3½ to 4 months, whereas nursing infants double their weight at about 5 months of age.

Formulas contain mostly saturated fatty acids, whereas breast milk is higher in unsaturated fatty acids. Calcium, sodium, and chloride, which occur in higher concentrations in some commercially made formulas, may be detrimental to the newborn's kidneys. Their immature state may not be ready to handle such high loads of solutes. This high solute load may also lead to thirst in the formula-fed infant, causing overfeeding and possibly obesity (Evans & Glass 1979).

Another potential problem with formulas is an allergic reaction in the newborn. The small intestine of the infant is permeable to macromolecules such as those found in cow's milk and milk-based formulas. The introduction of foreign proteins in formula may cause an allergy.

Clinicians recommend the use of iron-fortified formulas or supplements to mothers who are bottle-feeding as iron deficiency anemia is still very prevalent. The recommended iron dosage is 7 mg per day. However, the nurse must be aware that too much iron in the form of extra iron-fortified cereal or a too high formula iron content may interfere with the infant's natural ability to defend against disease (Picciano & Deering 1980). Parents also need to be informed about the constipation that sometimes results from iron-enriched formula and about various methods of alleviating the constipation. Opinion varies about the use of vitamin supplements for newborns, but it is generally agreed that commercially prepared formulas adequately meet the needs of the healthy newborn and infant.

Many companies make an enriched formula that is similar to breast milk. These formulas all have sufficient levels of carbohydrate, protein, fat, vitamins, and minerals to meet the newborn's nutritional needs.

The American Academy of Pediatrics recommends that infants be given breast milk or formula rather than whole milk until 1 year of age. However, the American Academy of Pediatrics Committee on Nutrition (1983) has more recently noted that no research studies to date have identified any conclusive evidence of harm to the infant who is given whole cow's milk along with adequate supplementary feedings after age 6 months. Table 30–3 compares the components of breast milk, unmodified cow's milk, and a commercially standardized formula. Table 30–4 describes some of the commonly prescribed formulas for healthy newborns, infants with milk allergies, and infants with certain metabolic disorders.

Neither unmodified cow's milk nor skim milk is an acceptable alternative for newborn feeding. The protein content in cow's milk is too high (50 percent to 75 percent more than human milk), is poorly digested, and may cause bleeding of the gastrointestinal tract. Unmodified cow's milk is also inadequate in vitamins. Skim milk lacks adequate calories, fat content, and essential fatty acids necessary for proper development of the neonate's neurological system. It provides excessive protein and also causes problems as a result of altered osmolarity. Nutritionists advise against use of unmodified cow's milk, cow's milk with decreased fat content, or skim milk for children under 2 years of age.

● Newborn Feeding

Initial Feeding

The time when the first feeding is given should be determined by the physiological and behavioral cues of the newborn. The nurse should assess for active bowel sounds, absence of abdominal distention, and a lusty cry, which quiets and is replaced with rooting and sucking behaviors when a stimulus is placed near the lips (Kemp et al 1982). These signs are indicators that the newborn is hungry and physically ready to tolerate the feeding. Assessment of the newborn's physiologic status is of primary and ongoing concern to the nurse throughout the first feeding.

The initial feeding provides an opportunity to assess the newborn for symptoms of tracheoesophageal fistula or esophageal atresia (see Chapter 32 for further discussion).

Table 30-3   Composition of Mature Breast Milk, Unmodified Cow's Milk, and a Routine Infant Formula

Composition/dL	Mature breast milk	Cow's milk	Routine formula (20 cal) with iron
Calories	75.0	69.0	67.0
Protein, g	1.1	3.5	1.5
Lactalbumin %	80	18	60
Casein %	20	82	40
Water, ml	87.1	87.3	90
Fat, g	4.5	3.5	3.8
Carbohydrate, g	7.1	4.9	7.0
Ash, g	0.21	0.72	0.34
Minerals			
Na, mg	16.0	50.0	21.0
K, mg	51.0	144.0	69.0
Ca, mg	33.0	118.0	46.0
P, mg	14.0	93.0	32.0
Mg, mg	4.0	13.0	5.3
Fe, mg	0.05	Tr.	1.3
Zn, mg	0.15	0.4	0.42
Vitamins			
A, IU	182.0	140.0	210.0
C, mg	5.0	1.0	5.3
D, IU	2.2	4.2	42.3
E, IU	0.18	0.04	0.83
Thiamin, mg	0.01	0.03	0.04
Riboflavin, mg	0.04	0.17	0.06
Niacin, mg	0.2	0.1	0.7
Curd size	Soft	Firm	Mod. firm
	Flocculent	Large	Mod. large
pH	Alkaline	Acid	Acid
Anti-infective properties	+	±	−
Bacterial content	Sterile	Nonsterile	Sterile
Emptying time	More rapid		

From Avery GB: *Neonatology,* ed. 3 Philadelphia, Lippincott, 1987, p 1192.

In cases of esophageal atresia, the feeding is taken well initially, but as the esophageal pouch fills, the feeding is quickly regurgitated unchanged by stomach contents. If a fistula is present, the infant gags, chokes, regurgitates mucus, and may become cyanotic as fluid passes through the fistula into the lungs.

It is the practice in most institutions to offer the newborn an initial feeding of a few milliliters of plain sterile water one to six hours after birth. Parents of breast-fed infants need to be informed of the rationale for using sterile water for the first feeding and of the fact that it will not significantly hinder the newborn's intake of breast milk. If aspiration should occur, as is often the case with a tracheoesophageal fistula, the water is readily absorbed by the lung tissue. Glucose water should not be used, since it will damage the newborn's lung tissue if aspirated (Avery 1987). The sterile water feeding provides an opportunity for the nurse to assess the effectiveness of the newborn's suck, swallow, and gag reflexes. A softer nipple made for preterm infants may be used if the newborn appears to tire easily. Extreme fatigue coupled with rapid respiration, circumoral cyanosis, and diaphoresis of the head and face may indicate cardiovascular complications and should be assessed further.

Some mothers who plan to breast-feed will ask to nurse their newborns immediately following birth. This practice provides stimulation for milk production, aids in maternal-newborn attachment, and enhances the probability that the mother will be successful in her efforts to breast-feed. If the newborn appears to have difficulty nursing, the sterile water feeding by the nurse allows an opportunity for assessment. If the water feeding is taken without difficulty and retained, the mother may resume breast-feeding.

Some institutions substitute glucose water for the sterile water after the newborn has successfully taken between 5 and 15 mL without any signs of distress. Early glucose water substitution provides sugar needed to prevent hypoglycemia. Other institutions use sterile water for the first two feedings to rule out the danger of aspiration.

The newborn will usually take 15 to 30 mL at this first feeding. For the breast-fed newborn this means that there are signs of being satisfied after 3 to 5 minutes of strong sucking at the breast.

It is not unusual for the neonate to regurgitate some mucus and water following a feeding even if it was taken without difficulty. Consequently, the newborn is observed closely and positioned on the right side after a feeding to

Table 30–4 Pediatric Formulas

Formula (Company)	Carbohydrate	Protein	Fat	Stool characteristics	Explanation
Enfamil (Mead Johnson)	Lactose	Nonfat milk	Soy, coconut oils	Formed, greenish-brown with very little free water around stool	Can be used with infants with fat intolerance. Appropriate formula for normal infants who have no special nutritional requirements
Similac (Ross)	Lactose	Nonfat milk	Soy, coconut, corn oils	Formed, greenish-brown with very little free water around stool	Iron may be added to any of these formulas to supply a dependable daily intake; for premature infants; for offspring of anemic mothers; for infants of multiple births; for infants with low birth weights and those who grew rapidly; for infants who have lost blood
SMA (Wyeth)	Lactose	Electrolyzed whey, nonfat milk	Coconut, safflower, soybean oils	Similar to breast milk stools: small volume, pasty yellow, some free water	
Isomil (Ross)	Sucrose, cornstarch, corn syrup solids	Soy protein isolates	Soy, coconut, corn oils	Mushy, yellow-green with more free water than cow's milk stools	Used for children with milk allergies
Neomulsoy (Syntex)	Sucrose	Soy protein isolates	Soy oil		
Nursoy (Wyeth)	Sucrose, corn syrup	Soy protein isolates	Coconut, oleic, safflower, soybean oils, and soy oil		
Prosobee (Mead Johnson)	Sucrose, corn syrup	Soy protein isolates	Soy oil		Metabolic defects, eg. galactosemia
Lofenalac (Mead Johnson)	Corn syrup solids, tapioca starch	Hydrolyzed casein (most of phenylalanine removed)	Corn oil	Similar to cow's milk formula: formed, greenish-brown with very little free water around stool	Used in children with phenylketonuria in whom a low phenylalanine diet is needed

From Mott S, Fazekas N, James S: *Nursing Care of Children and Families.* Menlo Park, Calif, Addison-Wesley, 1985 p 214.

aid drainage and facilitate gastric emptying. To decrease this mucus, some nurseries routinely aspirate the stomach contents and do gastric lavage when the neonate is admitted from labor and delivery. This practice has the potential for causing bradycardia and apnea. Inability to pass the gastric tube suggests the possiblity of atresia. If this occurs, the procedure should be stopped and the newborn assessed further.

Establishing a Feeding Pattern

Following the initial feeding, some hospitals establish artificial three- or four-hour time frames for feedings. This scheduling may present difficulties for the new mother trying to establish lactation just as it fails to recognize and respond to the individual needs of the newborn infant. Breast milk is rapidly digested by the newborn, who may desire to nurse every 1½ to 3 hours initially, with one or two feedings during the night.

Rooming-in permits the mother to feed the infant as needed. When rooming-in is not available, a supportive nursing staff and flexible nursery policies will allow the mother to feed on demand when the infant is hungry. Nothing is more frustrating to a new mother than attempting to nurse a newborn who is sound asleep because he or she is either not hungry or exhausted from crying. Once lactation is established and the family is home, a feeding pattern agreeable to both mother and child is usually established.

Formula-fed newborns may awaken for feedings every two to five hours but are frequently satisfied with feedings every three to four hours. Because formula is digested more slowly, the bottle-fed infant may go longer between feedings and may begin skipping the night feeding

Table 30–5 Infant Feeding Behaviors

Age	Hunger behavior	Feeding behavior	Satiety behavior
Birth to 13 weeks (0–3 months)	Cries; hands fisted; body tense	Rooting reflex; medial lip closure; strong suck reflex; suck-swallow pattern; tongue thrust and retraction; palmomental reflex, gags easily, needs burping	Withdraws head from nipple; falls asleep; hands relaxed; relief of body tension
14–24 weeks (4–6 months)	Eagerly anticipates; grasps and draws bottle to mouth; reaches with open mouth	Aware of hands; generalized reaching; intentional hand to mouth; tongue elevation; lips purse at corners—pucker; shifts food in mouth—prechewing; tongue protrudes in anticipation of nipple; tongue holds nipple firm; tongue projection strong; suck strength increases; coughs and chokes easily; preference for tastes	Tosses head back; fusses or cries; covers mouth with hands; ejects food; distracted by surroundings
28–36 weeks (7–9 months)	Reacts to food preparation sounds; vocalizes hunger; reaches out	Biting (first teeth); turns palm toward face; draws lower lip with food; thumb-finger grasp and palmar grasp; increased dexterity of hands; lateral tongue movement; mature swallow; chewing begins—vertical jaw protrusion; sucking decreases; holds bottle; handles cup awkwardly	Changes posture; closes mouth; shakes head "no"; plays with and throws utensils
40–52 weeks (10–12 months)	Vocalizes; grasps utensils	Tongue licks food from lower lip; holds and transfers to mouth; drinks from cup with spillage; lateral chewing movements; sticks out tongue; demands to feed self	Shakes head "no"; sputters

From Mott S, Fazekas N, James S: *Nursing Care of Children and Families.* Menlo Park, Calif, Addison-Wesley, 1985 p 216.

within about six weeks. This is very individualized depending on the size and development of the infant.

Both breast-fed and bottle-fed infants experience growth spurts at certain times and require increased feeding. The mother of a breast-fed infant may meet these increased demands by nursing more frequently to increase her milk supply; however, it will take about 24 hours for the milk supply to increase adequately to meet the new demand (Kemp et al 1982). A slight increase in feedings will meet the needs of the formula-fed infant.

Providing nourishment for her newborn is a major concern of the new mother. Her feelings of success or failure may influence her self-concept as she assumes her maternal role. With proper instruction, support, and encouragement from health care providers, feeding becomes a source of pleasure and satisfaction to both parents and infant. Table 30–5 can be used to assist parents in identifying their baby's cues indicating hunger and satiation.

● Promotion of Successful Infant Feeding

Feeding their baby is the task that parents may see as the center of the relationship between themselves and the new family member. Whether the mother has chosen to bottle-feed or breast-feed, the nurse can help the mother have a successful experience while in the hospital and during the early days at home. Feeding and caring for newborns may be routine tasks for the nurse, but the success or nonsuccess that a mother achieves the first few times may determine her feelings about herself as an adequate mother.

As an expression of personality, the response of the newborn to caring is important. A parent may interpret the newborn's behavior as rejection, which may alter the progress of parent-child relationships. A parent may also interpret the sleepy infant's refusal to suck or inability to retain formula as evidence of his or her incompetence as a parent. Likewise, the breast-feeding mother may deduce that the newborn does not like her if he or she fails to take her nipple readily. Conversely, infants pick up messages from the muscular tension of those holding them.

A nurse who is sensitive to the needs of the mother can form a relationship with her that permits sharing of knowledge about techniques and emotions connected with the feeding experience. Breast-feeding women frequently express disappointment in the help given to them by hospital nurses, saying they would like more encouragement, support, and practical information about feeding their newborn (Beske & Garvis 1982). This desire and need also applies to nonnursing mothers. Consistency in teaching by nursing personnel is paramount. A new mother becomes very frustrated if she is shown a number of different methods of feeding her newborn.

The decision by the mother about whether to breast-feed or bottle-feed is usually made by the sixth month of pregnancy and often even before conception. The decision is frequently based on the influences of relatives, especially the father and maternal grandmother (Beske & Garvis 1982), friends, and social customs rather than on knowledge about the nutritional and psychologic needs of herself and her newborn. With the technologic advances in formula production and the availability of knowledge about breast-feeding techniques, the mother should be confident that the choice she makes will promote normal growth and development of her newborn.

If the mother makes the decision to breast-feed at the time of delivery without prenatal preparation or support from her partner or other members of her family, she may encounter difficulty. It is necessary for the nurse to

Research Note

Aberman and Kirchhoff looked at the process by which mothers make infant feeding decisions. The 51 primarily black, single, low-income primiparas and multiparas in the study responded to a questionnaire designed to find out when final infant feeding decisions were made, who or what influenced the decision, and whether nurses gave mothers information about infant feeding.

Of the women in the study 62 percent said that they had made their decision by the end of the first trimester of pregnancy, and 82 percent said they had done so before the third trimester. Their decisions were most often influenced by books, mothers, or sisters. No respondent identified a nurse or doctor as an influence. Mothers chose to breast-feed because it was better for the baby's health. Mothers chose to bottle-feed because of convenience, because of previous experience with the method, or because they needed to return to work or school. Half the mothers said that a nurse never discussed feeding with them either during pregnancy or the postpartum. Of the 20 percent who attended childbirth classes, half said that they were influenced by class discussions.

Nurses need to reevaluate the timing of their teaching about infant feeding. Advantages and disadvantages of methods need to be presented early in pregnancy to help women make well-informed decisions. The lack of influence of health care professionals on choice of feeding method found in this study should be of concern to nurses.

Aberman S, Kirchhoff T: Infant feeding practices: Mothers' decision making. J Obstet Neonat Nurs 1985;14(September/October):394–398

find out before delivery whether the woman really wants to breast-feed or has made the decision based on social or family influences (Mullett 1982).

The nurse's primary responsibility is to support the feeding method decision and to help the family achieve a positive result. No woman should be made to feel inadequate or superior because of her choice in feeding. There are advantages and disadvantages to breast- and bottle-feeding, but positive bonds in parent-child relationships may be developed with either method.

Immediately before feeding, the mother should be made as comfortable as possible. Preparations may include voiding, washing her hands, and assuming a position of comfort.

The cesarean birth mother needs support so that the infant does not rest on her abdomen for long periods of time. If she is breast-feeding, she may be more comfortable lying on her side with a pillow behind her back and one between her legs. The nurse can position the newborn next to the woman's breast and place a rolled towel or small pillow behind the infant for support. The mother will initially need assistance turning from side to side and burping the newborn. She may prefer to breast-feed sitting up with a pillow on her lap and the infant resting on the pillow rather than directly on her abdomen. It may be helpful to place a rolled pillow under the arm supporting the infant's head. Bottle-feeding cesarean birth mothers frequently use the sitting position, too. If incisional pain makes this position difficult, the bottle-feeding mother may also assume the side-lying position. The infant can be positioned in a semi-sitting position against a pillow close to the mother, who can hold the bottle in her upper hand.

Depending on the newborn's level of hunger, the parents may want to use the time before feeding to get acquainted with their infant. The presence of the nurse during part of this time to answer questions and provide reinforcement of parenting skills will be helpful for the family.

For the sleepy baby, a period of playful activity—such as gently rubbing the feet and hands or adjusting clothing and loosening coverings to expose the infant to room air may increase alertness so that, when the feeding is initiated, the infant is ready and sucks eagerly. It may allow the active newborn an opportunity to calm down so that he or she can find and grasp the nipple effectively. After the feeding, when the infant is satisfied and asleep, parents may explore the characteristics unique to their newborn. Hospital routines must be flexible enough to allow this time for the family. Rooming-in offers spontaneous, frequent encounters for the family and provides opportunities to practice handling skills, thereby increasing confidence in care after discharge. It may also allow for demand rather than scheduled feeding times, and this should be encouraged.

Cultural Considerations in Infant Feeding

Breast-feeding has been the traditional feeding method for most cultures. However, bottle-feeding has become extremely popular much to the chagrin of some older members of a culture. Navajo elders, for instance, believe that breast-feeding ensures respect and obedience because the child remains close to the mother, while the bottle-fed infant will be more disobedient (Clark 1981).

Western practices encourage the new mother to breast-feed as soon as possible, but in many cultures (for example, Mexican American, Navajo, Filipino, and Vietnamese) colostrum is not offered to the newborn. Breast-feeding begins only after the milk flow is established. Interestingly, when a group of Vietnamese mothers who delayed breast-feeding until the third day after delivery was studied, it was found they had no difficulty breast-feeding (Ward et al 1981).

In many Oriental cultures the newborn is given boiled water until the mother's milk flows. The newborn is fed on demand and cries are responded to immediately. If the crying continues, evil spirits may be blamed and a priest's blessing may be necessary. Although many of the Hmong women of Laos combine breast-feeding with some bottle-feeding, they find it unacceptable to express their milk or pump their breasts. Thus other methods of providing relief should be suggested if breast engorgement develops (LaDu 1985).

In the black American culture there is much emphasis on feeding. Solid foods are introduced early and may even be added to the infant's formula. For the traditional Mexican American, a fat baby is considered a healthy baby and infants are fed on demand. "Spoiling" is encouraged and a colicky baby may be given mint or olive oil for relief.

Bottle-Feeding: Education for Self-Care

The mother who has chosen to bottle-feed her infant should be encouraged to assume a comfortable position with adequate arm support so she can easily hold her infant. Most women cradle their infants in the crook of the arm close to the body, which provides the intimacy and cuddling so essential to an infant. With the great emphasis placed on successful breast-feeding, the teaching needs of the bottle-feeding new mother may be overlooked. If she has had only limited experience in feeding infants, she may need some guidelines to feed her newborn successfully. The following important principles should be included in the teaching provided:

1. Bottles should always be held, not propped. Positional otitis media may develop when the infant is fed horizontally, because milk and nasal mucus may occlude the eustachian tube. Holding the infant provides a rest for the feeder, social and close physical contact for the baby, and an opportunity for parent-child interaction and bonding. Once feeding is initiated, the child should be held securely to provide physical closeness and facilitate eye contact (Figure 30–1).

2. The nipple should have a hole big enough to allow milk to flow in drops when the bottle is inverted. Too large an opening may cause overfeeding or regurgitation because of rapid feeding. If feeding is too fast, the nipple should be changed and the infant should be helped to eat more slowly by stopping the feeding frequently for burping and cuddling.

3. The nipple should be pointed directly into the mouth, not toward the palate or tongue, and should be on top of the tongue. The nipple should be full of liquid at all times to avoid ingestion of extra

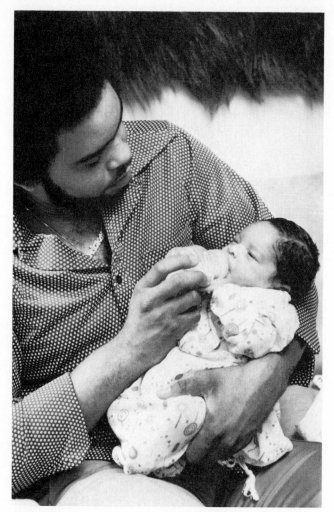

Figure 30–1   An infant is supported comfortably during bottle-feeding.

amounts of air, which decreases the amount of feeding and increases discomfort.

4. The infant should be burped at intervals, preferably at the middle and end of the feeding. The infant who seems to swallow a great deal of air while sucking may need more frequent burping. In addition, if the infant has cried before being fed, air may have been swallowed, and the infant should be burped before beginning to feed or after taking just enough to calm down. Burping is done by holding the infant upright on the shoulder or by holding the infant in a sitting position on the feeder's lap with chin and chest supported on one hand. The back is then gently patted or stroked with the other hand. Too-frequent burping may confuse a newborn who is attempting to coordinate sucking, swallowing, and breathing simultaneously.

5. Newborns frequently regurgitate small amounts of feedings. This may look like a large amount to the inexperienced parent, however, and she or he may require reassurance that this is normal. Initially it may be due to excessive mucus and gastric irritation from foreign substances in the stomach from birth. Later, regurgitation may result when the infant feeds too rapidly and swallows air. It may also occur when the infant is overfed and the cardiac sphincter allows the excess to be regurgitated. Because this is such a common occurrence, experienced parents and nurses generally keep a "burp cloth" available. Although regurgitation is normal, vomiting or a forceful expulsion of fluid is not. When forceful expulsion occurs, further evaluation may be indicated, especially if other symptoms are present.

6. A fat baby is not necessarily a healthy one. Parents should be encouraged to avoid overfeeding or feeding infants every time they cry. Infants should be encouraged but not forced to feed and should be allowed to set their own pace once feedings are established. Parents sometimes set artificial goals— "The baby must take all five ounces"—and tend to keep feeding the child until those goals are met, even though the infant may not be hungry. Overfeeding results in infant obesity. During early feedings, however, the infant may need simple tactile stimulation—such as gently rubbing feet and hands, adjusting clothing, and loosening coverings—to maintain adequate sucking for a sufficient time to complete a full feeding.

Formula preparation and sterilization techniques are always important to discuss with families. Cleanliness remains an essential component but sterilization is necessary only if the water source is questionable. (Procedure 30–1 describes methods of sterilization.) Bottles may be effectively prepared in dishwashers (nipples may be weakened by the temperature of dishwashers and therefore should be washed thoroughly by hand with soap and water and rinsed well) or washed thoroughly in warm soapy water and rinsed well. Tap water, if from an uncontaminated source, may be used for mixing powdered formulas, which are less expensive than the concentrated or ready-to-use prepared formulas. Whole or evaporated milk may be diluted with water and sweetened with a sugar source such as corn syrup, depending on the age of the infant and caloric requirements.

Bottles may be prepared individually or up to one day's supply of formula may be prepared at one time. Extra bottles are stored in the refrigerator and should be warmed slightly before feeding. Ready-to-use disposable bottles of formula are very convenient, but are also expensive.

Breast-Feeding

LACTATION

The female breast is divided into 15 to 24 lobes separated from one another by fat and connective tissue. These lobes are subdivided into lobules, composed of small units called *alveoli* where milk is synthesized by the alveolar secretory epithelium. The lobules have a system of lactiferous ductiles that join larger ducts and eventually open onto the nipple surface. During pregnancy increased levels of estrogen stimulate breast duct proliferation and development, and elevated progesterone levels promote the development of lobules and alveoli in preparation for lactation.

Delivery results in a rapid drop in estrogen and progesterone with a concomitant increase in the secretion of *prolactin* by the anterior pituitary. This hormone promotes milk production by stimulating the alveolar cells of the breasts. When the newborn sucks on the mother's nipple, *oxytocin* is released from the posterior pituitary. This hormone increases the contractility of the myoepithelial cells lining the walls of the mammary ducts, and a flow of milk results. This is called the *letdown reflex*. Mothers have described the letdown reflex as a prickling or tingling sensation during which they feel the milk coming down. It is not unusual for the breasts to leak some milk prior to feeding.

The letdown reflex can be stimulated by the newborn's sucking, presence, or cry, or even by maternal thoughts about her baby. It may also occur during sexual orgasm because oxytocin is released. Conversely, the mother's lack of self-confidence, fear of, embarrassment about, or pain connected with breast-feeding may prevent the milk from being ejected into the duct system. Milk production is decreased with repeated inhibition of the letdown reflex. Failure to empty the breasts frequently and completely also decreases production, because as milk accumulates and is not withdrawn, the buildup of pressure in the alveoli suppresses secretion.

Once lactation is well established, prolactin production decreases. Oxytocin and sucking continue to be the facilitators of milk production. The release of oxytocin in response to the infant's suckling is beneficial to the new mother. Oxytocin stimulates uterine contraction and thus promotes rapid involution.

EDUCATION FOR SELF-CARE

The nurse caring for the breast-feeding mother should help the woman achieve independence and success in her feeding efforts (Figure 30–2). Prepared with a knowledge of the anatomy and physiology of the breast and lactation, the components and positive effects of breast milk, and techniques of breast-feeding, the nurse can help

Procedure 30–1   Methods of Bottle Sterilization

Terminal sterilization

ADVANTAGES

1. Safest, most efficient method
2. More easily learned

DISADVANTAGES

1. Prolonged cooling period (1–2 hr)
2. Not suitable for disposable bottles

PROCEDURE

1. Assemble equipment and wash hands.
2. Thoroughly wash bottles, caps, and nipples in warm soapy water; squeeze some water through holes to rid them of accumulated milk; rinse well.
3. Wash the lid of the formula can (if using a liquid) and prepare formula according to directions.
4. Fill the bottles with the desired amount of formula and loosely apply the nipples and caps; one or two bottles of water may be prepared at the same time.
5. Place the prepared bottles in a large kettle or bottle sterilizer and add the appropriate amount of water (as specified on the sterilizer or 2–3 in. if a kettle is used).
6. Cover the sterilizer, bring the water to a gentle boil and boil for 25 min.
7. Remove from heat but let the bottles remain in the sterilizer with the lid on until the sides of the pan are cool to the touch.
8. Remove the bottles, tighten the lids, and refrigerate until needed.

Aseptic method of sterilization

ADVANTAGES

1. May be modified for use with disposable bottles

DISADVANTAGES

1. Difficult to learn, contamination more likely

PROCEDURE

1. Same as steps 1 and 2 of terminal method.
2. Place all equipment needed (bottles, nipples, caps, can opener, tongs, measuring pitcher, and spoon) in a large kettle or sterilizer; cover with water and boil for 5 min.
3. In another pan boil the amount of water necessary to make the formula (boil for 5 min).
4. Drain the water from the sterilizer pan and let the equipment cool for a few minutes.
5. Remove the measuring pitcher, being certain to touch only the handle.
6. Use the sterilized can opener to open a can of formula after first washing the lid with soapy water and rinsing well; pour the formula into the prepared measuring pitcher and add the correct amount of boiled water, mix with the prepared spoon.
7. Use tongs to remove the bottles from the sterilizer and fill them with the desired amount of formula; (one or two bottles of water may also be prepared by boiling enough additional water).
8. Use the tongs to set the nipples on the bottles; and then apply the caps, touching only the edges.
9. Refrigerate until needed.

To modify for disposable bottles:
Complete all steps as directed except *do not boil the bottles* with the other equipment and allow the water to cool for 15–20 min before preparing the formula (the plastic bag may melt if the formula is too hot).

---

the woman and her family use their own resources to achieve a successful experience. The objectives involved in breast-feeding are (a) to provide adequate nutrition, (b) to establish an adequate milk supply, and (c) to prevent trauma to the nipples. All instructions are aimed toward these goals.

The newborn who is breast-feeding should be put to breast as soon as possible, depending on the situation of birth. Some infants are not interested so soon, but for those who are, early breast-feeding affords a soothing experience and has considerable physiologic and psychologic benefit

for the mother. Colostrum has sufficient nutrients to satisfy the infant until milk is established in two to four days. Establishment of lactation depends on the strength of the infant's suck and the frequency of nursing.

Positioning of the baby at the breast is a critical factor. The entire body of the infant should be turned toward the mother's breast, with the mouth adjacent to the nipple. The mother should not have to lift her shoulder or breast to direct the nipple into the infant's mouth. The nipple should be directed straight into the mouth, not toward the palate or tongue, and as much of the areola as possible

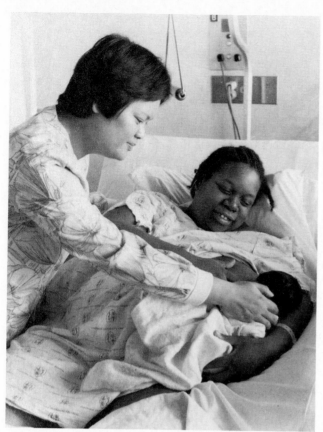

Figure 30–2 For many mothers, the nurse's support and knowledge are instrumental in establishing successful breast-feeding.

feeding (five minutes, then seven minutes, etc) is not helpful in preventing nipple soreness as was previously believed (Slaven & Harvey 1981, deCarvalho et al 1984, L'Esperance & Frantz 1985). Furthermore, since letdown may take up to three minutes to occur, in the first few days at least, artificial time limits may actually interfere with successful feeding. In working to avoid undue nipple trauma it is important, then, to be certain that the nipple is properly positioned and that the infant's mouth covers a large portion of the areola.

The mother is encouraged to alternate the breast she offers to the infant first at each feeding. A convenient way for the mother to remember which breast to begin with is to fasten a small safety pin to the bra cup on that side. Generally the infant will empty the breasts during a feeding.

If a full breast appears to be occluding the infant's nares, the mother should either lift the breast slightly or gently press the breast away from the nares. Pressure must be gentle to avoid inadvertently pulling the breast from the infant's mouth.

The mother is instructed in techniques for breaking suction prior to removing the infant from the breast. By inserting a finger into the infant's mouth beside the nipple, she can break the suction, and the nipple may be removed without trauma. Burping between feedings on each breast

should be included so that, as the baby sucks, the jaws compress the ducts that are directly beneath the areola (Figure 30–3). To do this, the mother holds her breast with her thumb placed on the upper portion of the breast and the remainder of her fingers cupped under her breast. She then lightly brushes the infant's lips with the nipple. Through the rooting reflex, the infant can locate the nipple. The mother should avoid stimulating both cheeks, which only confuses the hungry infant.

If the mother does not have a prominent or everted nipple, she may try rolling the nipple between her thumb and forefinger or stretching the nipple by pressing in and outward around the nipple prior to the feeding. Nurses should avoid the temptation to substitute a regular nipple shield to correct nipple positions. The shield tends to confuse the baby, as the artificial nipples on the shields are softer and easier to feed from, and the baby may refuse the human nipple when it is reoffered. This problem, termed "nipple confusion," may also be avoided if sterile water or dextrose and water feedings are not routinely given to breast-feeding infants. Following feedings, the nipples should be assessed for trauma so that corrections may be made in position and technique for the next feeding. Current literature suggests that imposing time limits for breast-

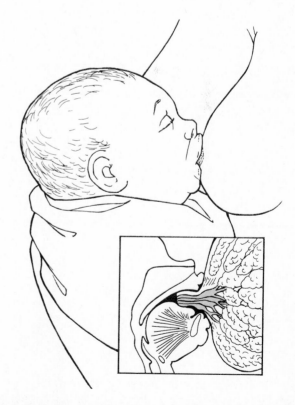

Figure 30–3 To nurse effectively, it is important that the infant's mouth cover the majority of the areola to compress the ducts below. (Courtesy Ross Laboratories, Columbus, Ohio)

and at the end of the feeding continues to be necessary. If the infant has been crying, it is also advisable to burp before beginning feeding.

Initially more milk is produced than is required by the infant. Later the amount of milk will be produced to meet nutritional need, manifested through sucking. Milk may tend to leak until supply meets demand. The mother should expect this and use breast pads in her bra to absorb the secretions. She should be cautioned to remove wet pads frequently to avoid irritation to the nipples or infection. The mother may also be taught to apply direct pressure to the breast with her hand or forearm. This will often stop the leaking.

The use of supplementary feedings for the breast-feeding infant may weaken or confuse the sucking reflex and may interfere with successful outcome. Often parents are concerned because they have no visual assurance regarding the amount consumed. The mother may be reassured about adequacy of intake if she listens for sounds of swallowing while the baby is nursing. In addition, if the infant gains weight and has six or more wet diapers a day, he or she is receiving adequate amounts of milk. Activity levels and intervals between feedings may also indicate how satisfied the infant is. Parents should know that, because breast milk is more easily digested than formulas, the breast-fed infant becomes hungry sooner. Thus the frequency of breast-feedings may be greater, particularly after discharge, when fatigue or excitement may decrease milk supply temporarily. Increasing the frequency of feedings alleviates problems during these periods. The parents may also expect the infant to demand more frequent nursing during periods when growth spurts are expected, such as 10 days to 2 weeks, 5 to 6 weeks, 2½ to 3 months, and 4½ to 6 months (Riordan 1983).

The mother may be taught to express her milk manually and freeze it for bottle-feeding if she will be absent for a scheduled feeding. Breast milk should be frozen in plastic bottles; if glass bottles are used, the antibodies will adhere to the sides of the bottle and their benefits will be lost. Manual expression to relieve maternal discomfort and to maintain the milk supply is advisable if the mother must go several hours without feeding. The mother's milk supply will decrease unless the breasts are emptied regularly.

Milk may be expressed by hand or by using a breast pump. Expression of milk is used to collect milk for supplemental feedings. It is also used to relieve breast fullness or engorgement and to help build the woman's milk supply. To express her milk manually, the woman first washes her hands, and then massages her breast to stimulate letdown. To massage her breast, the woman grasps the breast with both hands at the base of the breast near the chest wall. Using the palms of her hands she then firmly slides her hands toward her nipple. She repeats this process several times. Then she is ready to begin hand expression. The woman generally uses her left hand for her right breast and right hand for her left breast. However, some women find it preferable to use the hand on the same side as the breast (right hand for right breast). The nurse should encourage the woman to use the method she finds most effective. She grasps the areola with her thumb on the top and her first two fingers on the lower portion (Figure 30–4). Without allowing her fingers to slide on her skin, she

Figure 30–4 Hand position for manual expression of milk.

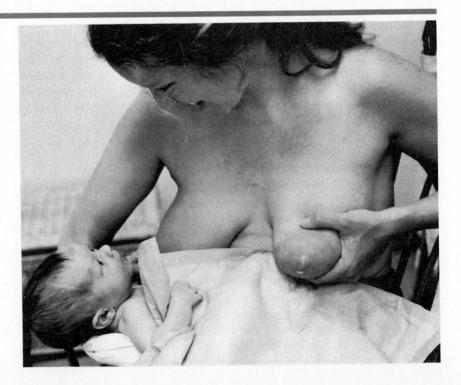

pushes inward toward the chest and then squeezes her fingers together while pulling foward on the areola (Figure 30–5). She can use a container to catch any fluid that is squeezed out. She then repositions her hand by rotating it slightly so that she can repeat the process. She continues to reposition her hand and repeat the process to empty all the milk sinuses.

Hand or electric breast pumps are useful for building and maintaining a milk supply when the infant is not able to nurse (premature infant, ill infant, infant with breast milk jaundice, mother on medications that are excreted in the breast milk) or for the working mother who regularly misses certain feedings (Figure 30–6). Hand pumps are more portable, can be purchased by the mother, and are less expensive. Electric pumps are more efficient but are bulky and expensive. They may be rented in many areas. Breast pumps work by suction to express the milk. Some have collection systems for easy milk saving. Many agencies have a variety of pumps available and provide instruction on correct methods of pumping the breasts. Videotapes or photographs are also useful in demonstrating the process to new mothers.

La Leche League is an organized group of volunteers who work to provide education about breast-feeding and assistance to women who are breast-feeding infants. They sponsor activities, have printed material available, offer one-to-one counseling to mothers with questions or problems, and provide group support to breast-feeding mothers.

Numerous books and pamphlets are also available to help the breast-feeding mother. The mother needs the support of all family members, her physician/nurse-midwife, pediatrician or pediatric nurse practitioner, and all nursing personnel because it is often the attitudes of these people that ultimately lead the woman to success or failure.

MEDICATIONS AND BREAST-FEEDING

It has long been recognized that certain medications taken by the mother may have an effect on her infant. A drug may affect the newborn in one of three ways (Platzer et al 1980):

1. Lactation may be inhibited, thereby decreasing the supply of breast milk.

2. The newborn's physiologic processes may be directly affected by the drug if it crosses into the breast milk.

3. The mother's physical or emotional ability to care for her newborn may be altered.

Certain characteristics of a drug influence whether it passes into the breast milk, including its degree of protein binding. In general, unbound drugs enter the breast milk. Other factors are (a) the degree of ionization (drugs tend to cross in un-ionized form); (b) molecular weight (drugs with a molecular weight greater than 200 will not cross into the breast milk); (c) mechanism of transport (drugs enter breast milk by active transport, simple diffusion, or carrier-mediated diffusion); and (d) solubility of the drug (the alveolar epithelium presents a lipid barrier that tends to be more permeable when colostrum is present). The effects of the drug are also influenced by the infant's ability to absorb the drug from the gastrointestinal tract and by

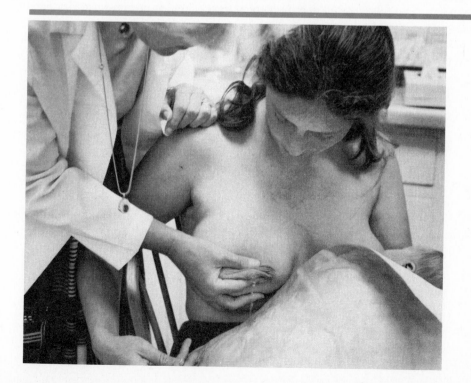

Figure 30–5 Manual expression of milk

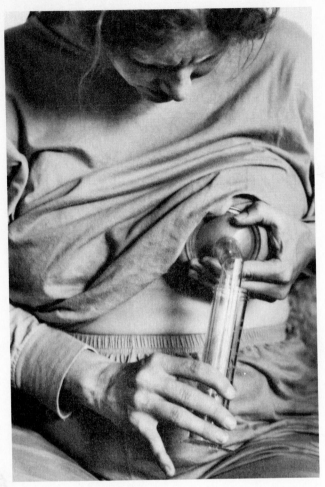

Figure 30–6   Hand-held breast pump

his or her ability to detoxify the drug and excrete it (Lawrence 1980).

Four adjustments should be made to decrease the effects on her infant when administering drugs to a nursing mother (Lawrence 1980):

1. The use of long-acting drug forms, which are usually detoxified in the liver, should be avoided. The infant may have difficulty excreting them and accumulation may be a problem.

2. Absorption rates and peak blood levels should be considered in scheduling the administration of the drugs. Less of the drug crosses into the milk if the medication is given immediately after the woman has nursed her baby.

3. The infant should be closely observed for any signs of drug reaction including rash, fussiness, lethargy, or changes in sleeping habits or feeding pattern.

4. Using an appropriate table, whenever possible a drug should be selected that shows the least tendency to pass into breast milk.

The mother should be given information of the potential of most drugs to cross into breast milk. She should also be advised to tell any physician who may prescribe medications for her that she is breast-feeding. Clinicians who do not routinely care for obstetric or pediatric clients may not be familiar with the effects on breast milk of the drugs they prescribe and may need to consult the obstetrician. The positive and negative effects of the medication on the woman and her infant must be considered carefully.

POTENTIAL PROBLEMS IN BREAST-FEEDING

Many women stop nursing because the problems encountered seem to have no solutions. Anticipatory guidance about remedies and solutions to the problems is the nurse's role. This allows the mother to provide her infant with the nutritional and emotional experience that she has planned for during the pregnancy. Box 30–1 summarizes self-care measures the nurse can suggest to a woman with a breast-feeding problem.

○   *ABNORMAL NIPPLES*   As discussed in Chapter 16, nipple inversion can be helped during the antepartal period by doing Hoffman's exercises and/or wearing special breast shields (see Figures 16–5, 16–6). For the breast-feeding woman with problems because of nipple inversion, several measures can be suggested. She can manually shape the nipple as the newborn begins to nurse. Application of ice may cause nipple erection. Wearing a breast shield will also cause the nipple to become erect, thus allowing the infant to nurse.

○   *INADEQUATE LETDOWN*   To ensure adequate letdown, the mother is advised to massage her breasts prior to nursing. Application of warm compresses or a warm shower may also help. The mother may find it beneficial, at least initially, to nurse in a quiet place, free of distractions and interruptions. She should try to relax (relaxation techniques may be useful) and focus on her infant and her milk flow. Many women find that having a drink of water or juice before and during the feeding promotes adequate letdown. If letdown difficulties persist, the physician can prescribe a synthetic oxytocin nasal spray. This spray is used for only a day or so to condition the letdown reflex.

Overfatigue can inhibit letdown. The new mother should be encouraged to rest when the baby naps. Many women find it helpful to nurse while lying down, especially at night. The new mother will also benefit from some quiet time alone or a change of activity such as a walk, a meal out with a friend, or time for a favorite activity.

○   *NIPPLE SORENESS*   The mother should be told that some soreness often occurs initially with breast-feeding and that the problem will clear as soon as the letdown reflex is established. The infant should not be switched to bottle-

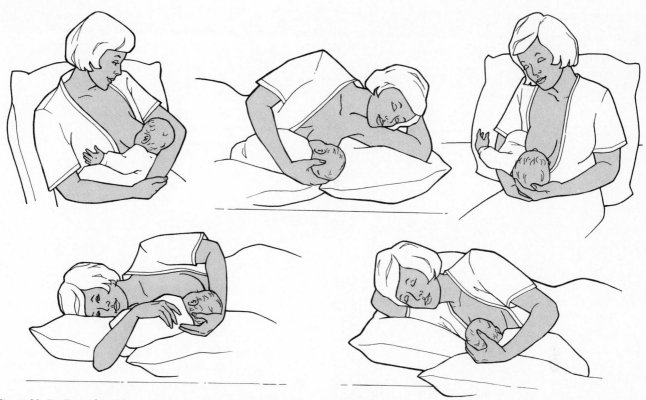

Figure 30–7   Examples of breast-feeding position changes to facilitate thorough breast emptying and prevent nipple soreness.

feeding or have feedings delayed as this will only cause engorgement and more soreness.

Because the area of greatest stress to the nipple is in line with the newborn's chin and nose, nipple soreness may be decreased by encouraging the mother to rotate positions when feeding the infant. Figure 30–7 illustrates the cradle hold, football hold, and maternal side-lying positions. Changing positions alters the focus of greatest stress and promotes more complete breast emptying.

Nipple soreness may also develop if the infant develops faulty sucking habits. An infant may retract the tongue rather than positioning it correctly under the breast. Consequently the tongue does not act as a cushion and the infant's jaw may bruise the nipple. Soreness may also develop if the infant falls asleep with the breast in his or her mouth. This leads to problems because of continuous negative pressure on the nipple (L'Esperance & Frantz 1985).

Occasionally the infant grasps only the nipple in his or her mouth. Vigorous sucking produces little milk because the milk sinuses under the areola are not compressed. This results in a frustrated infant and marked soreness for the mother. The problem is overcome by positioning the infant with as much areola as possible in his or her mouth.

Nipple soreness is especially pronounced during the first few minutes of the feeding. If the mother is not expecting this, she may become discouraged and quickly

stop. The letdown reflex may take a few minutes to activate, and it may not occur if the mother stops nursing too quickly. The problem is compounded if the infant does not empty the mammary ducts; the infant is unsatisfied, and the possibility of breast engorgement increases.

Because nipple soreness can also result from an overeager infant, the mother may find it helpful to nurse more frequently. This helps ease the vigorous sucking of a ravenous infant. The woman can also apply ice to her nipples and areola for a few minutes prior to feeding. This promotes nipple erectness and numbs the tissue to ease the initial discomfort. To prevent excoriation and skin breakdown, the nipples and areola should be washed with water and then allowed to dry thoroughly. Drying may be accomplished by leaving the bra flaps down for several minutes after feeding or by exposing the nipples to sunlight or ultraviolet light, for 30 seconds at first and gradually increasing to 3 minutes. Drying the nipples with a hair dryer on low heat setting also facilitates drying and promotes healing.

If the woman finds that her bra or clothing rub against her nipples and add to her discomfort, she may insert shields into her bra to prevent this. Both Medela Shells and Woolrich Shields, for example, relieve friction and promote air circulation.

The mother may use substances such as lanolin, Massé Breast Cream, Eucerin cream, or A and D ointment on the nipples between feedings. These should be lightly

Box 30–1   Self-Care Measures for the Woman with Breast-Feeding Problems

Abnormal Nipples

Use Hoffman's exercises antepartally to increase pro-tractility (see Chapter 16).

Use special breast shields such as Woolrich or Esch-mann.

Use hand to shape nipple when beginning to nurse.

Apply ice for a few minutes prior to feeding to im-prove nipple erection.

If all else fails, use nipple shield for a few minutes until nipple becomes erect, then switch to reg-ular nursing.

Inadequate Letdown

Massage breasts prior to nursing.

Feed in a quiet, private place, away from distraction.

Take a warm shower before nursing to relax and stim-ulate letdown.

Apply warm pack for 20 minutes before nursing.

Use relaxation techniques and focus on letdown.

Drink water, juice, or noncaffeinated beverages before and during feeding.

Avoid overfatigue by resting when the baby sleeps, feeding while lying down, and having quiet time alone.

Develop a conditioned response by establishing a routine for starting feedings.

Allow the baby sufficient time (at least 10 to 15 min-utes per side) to trigger the letdown reflex.

If all else fails obtain a prescription for oxytocin nasal spray from the health care provider.

Nipple Soreness

Ensure that infant is correctly positioned at breast.

Rotate breast-feeding positions.

Use finger to break suction before removing infant from the breast.

Hold baby close when feeding to avoid undue pulling on nipple.

Don't allow baby to sleep with nipple in mouth.

Nurse more frequently.

Begin nursing on less sore breast.

Apply ice to nipples and areola for a few minutes prior to feeding.

Protect nipples to prevent skin breakdown:

—Clean milk gently from nipple with warm water.

—Allow nipples to air dry, or dry nipples with hair dryer set to low heat, or expose nipples to sunlight.

If clothing rubs nipples, use ventilated shields to keep clothing away from skin.

Lightly apply protective substance such as lanolin, Massé Breast Cream, Eucerin cream, or A and D ointment between feedings.

Apply tea bags soaked in warm water.

Change breast pads frequently.

Nurse long enough to empty breasts completely.

Cracked Nipples

Use interventions discussed under sore nipples.

Inspect nipples carefully for cracks or fissures.

Use a nipple shield if it is helpful; some women find it contributes to their discomfort.

Temporarily stop nursing on the affected breast and hand express milk for a day or two until cracks heal.

Maintain healthy diet. Protein and vitamin C are es-sential for healing.

Use a mild analgesic such as acetaminophen for dis-comfort.

Consult health care providers if signs of infection de-velop (see Chapter 36).

Breast Engorgement

Nurse frequently (every 1½ to 3 hours).

Wear a well-fitting supportive bra at all times.

Take a warm shower or apply warm compresses to trigger letdown.

Massage breasts and then hand express some milk to soften the breast so the infant can "latch on."

Breast-feed long enough to empty breast.

Alternate starting breast.

Take a mild analgesic 20 minutes before feeding if discomfort is pronounced.

Plugged Ducts (Caked Breasts)

Nurse frequently and for long enough to empty the breasts completely.

Rotate feeding position.

Massage breasts prior to feeding, in a warm shower when possible.

Maintain good nutrition and adequate fluid intake.

applied after the nipples have dried thoroughly to avoid trapping moisture on the skin. A *light* coat of the substance is applied to the areola and nipple with care to avoid the end of the nipple where the duct openings are located. In most cases the lubricant will be absorbed prior to the next feeding. If the infant objects to the taste of the substance, however, it may be washed off with warm water (no soap) before beginning the next feeding.

A woman may use breast pads inside her bra to prevent leaking of milk onto her clothes. These pads should be changed frequently so that the nipples remain dry. Breast pads with plastic liners interfere with air circulation; The plastic should be removed before using them.

Older remedies for nipple soreness are receiving renewed acceptance. For instance, tea bags may be moistened in warm water and applied to the nipples. The tannic acid seems to help toughen the nipples, and the warmth is soothing and promotes healing.

If the nipple soreness has a sudden onset, it may be caused by a thrush infection transmitted from the infant to the mother. White patches or streaks in the infant's mouth indicate a need for treatment of the mouth and nipple infection. If the problem is treated, the mother can usually continue breast-feeding.

○   *CRACKED NIPPLES*   Nipple soreness is frequently coupled with cracked nipples. Whenever a breast-feeding mother complains of soreness, the nipples must be carefully examined for fissures or cracks, and the mother should be observed during breast-feeding to see whether the infant is correctly positioned at the breast. If the positioning is correct and cracks exist, interventions are necessary. The mother's first reaction may be to cease nursing on the sore breast, but this may aggravate the problem if engorgement and plugged ducts result. All the interventions described for sore nipples may be used. It may also help the mother to begin nursing on the less sore breast. This allows the letdown reflex to occur in the affected breast, and the infant does more vigorous sucking on the less tender breast, which decreases trauma to the cracked nipple.

With severe cases, the temporary use of a nipple shield for nursing may be necessary. For the mother's comfort, analgesics may be taken after nursing.

○   *BREAST ENGORGEMENT*   About the time their milk initially comes in, many women complain of feelings of engorgement. Their breasts are hard, painful, and warm and appear taut and shiny. At first this fullness is caused by venous congestion due to the increased vascularity in the breasts. Later the problem may be compounded by the pressure of accumulating milk.

The mother should be encouraged to wear a well-fitting nursing bra 24 hours a day. The bra supports the breasts and prevents further discomfort from tension and pulling on the Cooper's ligament. Frequent nursing is also helpful in preventing or decreasing engorgement. Breast-feeding every 1½ to 3 hours initially keeps the breasts emptied, increases the circulation in the breast, and helps remove the fluid that might lead to engorgement.

Because the breast is quite hard, nursing may be difficult for the infant and painful for the mother. Manual expression of milk or the use of a nontraumatic breast pump to initiate the flow may be helpful, as is the judicious use of analgesics. Warmth is often soothing, and the mother who has problems with engorgement may find a warm shower comforting. It is also useful in stimulating the letdown reflex. The mother may find it helpful to stand in the shower and manually express some milk before feeding. To prevent discomfort, it is advisable to avoid having the spray beat directly on the nipples and breasts. Warm, moist cloths may also be used for relief. Additional relief measures include the use of ice packs between feedings, with hot packs applied 20 minutes prior to a feeding. The engorgement is generally relieved within 12 to 24 hours.

○   *PLUGGED DUCTS*   Some mothers experience plugging of one or more ducts, especially in conjunction with or following engorgement. This is often referred to as caked breasts. Manifested as an area of tenderness or "lumpiness" in an otherwise well woman, plugging may be relieved by the use of heat and massage. The mother can be encouraged to massage her breasts from her chest wall forward to the nipple while standing in a warm shower or following the application of hot packs to the breast (Riordan 1983). She should then nurse her infant, starting on the unaffected breast if the plugged breast is tender. Frequent nursing will help prevent the problem and fatigue as well. In cases of repeatedly plugged ducts or caked breasts, it may be necessary for the mother to limit her fat intake to polyunsaturated fats and to add lecithin to her diet (Lawrence 1980).

BREAST-FEEDING AND THE WORKING MOTHER

Often a mother returning to work elects to continue breast-feeding her infant. This decision requires planning on her part and family encouragement and assistance. She will find this easier to accomplish if she has six to eight weeks at home to establish lactation before returning to work. She should use this time to accustom her infant to taking supplemental feedings from a bottle. This permits others to care for the baby while the mother works. A few days before returning to work she can begin manually expressing and freezing her milk for her infant's use while she is gone. At work it will be necessary for her to pump her breasts during lunch or coffee breaks to avoid the discomfort of full breasts. Because milk production follows the principle of supply and demand, if breasts are not pumped, the milk supply will decrease.

Sometimes a mother has a flexible schedule and can return home to nurse at lunch time or have the baby brought to her. If this is not possible, the infant may be fed expressed milk or a supplemental bottle of formula. If the mother is expressing milk at work for use the next day, she must be certain to keep it refrigerated and use it within 48 hours. Breast milk can be frozen in plastic bottles or bags and stored for up to six months.

To maintain an adequate milk supply the working mother must pay special attention to her fluid intake. She can ensure an adequate intake by drinking extra fluid at each break and whenever possible during the day. In addition, it is helpful to nurse more on weekends, to nurse during the night, to eat a nutritionally sound diet, and to continue manual expression or pumping when not nursing (Reifsnider & Myers 1985).

Night nursing presents a dilemma in that it may help a working mother maintain her milk supply but may also contribute to fatigue. Some women choose to have the infant sleep with them so that breast-feeding is more easily accomplished. Other women find it difficult to sleep soundly when the infant is in the same bed. For the mother who works long hours or has a rigid work schedule, the best alternative may be to limit breast-feeding to morning and evening feedings with supplemental feedings at other times. This choice allows her to maintain a close relationship with the infant and provides some of the unique benefits of breast milk.

WEANING

The decision to wean the baby from the breast may be made for a variety of reasons including family or cultural pressures, changes in the home situation, pressure from the woman's partner, or a personal opinion about when weaning should occur. For the woman who is comfortable with breast-feeding and well-informed about the process, the appropriate time to wean her infant will become evident if she is sensitive to the child's cues. Often weaning falls between periods of great developmental activity for the child. Thus weaning commonly occurs at 8 to 9 months, 12 to 14 months, 18 months, 2 years, and 3 years of age. Within our society, however, weaning commonly occurs before the child is 9 months old, although it may occur any time from soon after birth to 4 years of age (Lauwers & Woessner 1983).

If weaning is timed to respond to the child's cues, and if the mother is comfortable with the timing, it can be accomplished with less difficulty than if the process is begun before both mother and child are ready emotionally. Nevertheless, weaning is a time of emotional separation for mother and baby; it may be difficult for them to give up the closeness of their nursing sessions. The nurse who is understanding about this possibility can help the mother see that her infant is growing up and plan other comforting, consoling, and play activities to replace breast-feeding. A gradual approach is the easiest and most comforting way to wean the child from breast-feedings. Other activities can enhance the parent-infant attachment process.

During weaning, the mother should substitute one cup-feeding or bottle-feeding for one breast-feeding session over several days to a week so that her breasts gradually produce less milk. Eliminating the breast-feedings associated with meals first facilitates the mother's ability to wean the infant as satiation with food lessens the desire for milk (Bishop 1985). Over a period of several weeks she should substitute more cup-feedings or bottle-feedings for breast-feedings. Many mothers continue to nurse once a day in the early morning or late evening for several months until the milk supply is gone. The slow method of weaning prevents breast engorgement and allows infants to alter their eating methods at their own rates.

Supplemental Foods

Opinions vary widely about when to add new foods and what kinds of supplemental foods to add to the infant's diet. Health care professionals need to help mothers plan their children's diet. If reasons are offered for giving or withholding specific foods, more parental cooperation can be expected (Broussard 1984).

The proper time to add foods to the infant's diet should be determined by the physiologic ability to accept foods other than milk. Before 4 to 6 months of age, the infant's tongue pushes upward and forward in the oral cavity in a sucking, thrusting motion. If solids are offered, the tongue reflexively pushes them forward. After this age the tongue is able to move solids toward the pharynx in a movement synchronized with swallowing. During this same age the infant learns to grasp objects and bring them toward the mouth. These are early physiologic indicators that the infant's neurologic development is adequate to begin supplemental foods. Immunologically, it appears that the tendency to develop food allergies secondary to the absorption of macromolecules may be lessened if solids are introduced after 6 months of age, when the infant's intestinal mucosa is producing IgA (American Academy of Pediatrics 1981).

Because breast milk or formula meets all the requirements of growth for the normal infant until 6 months of age, only after 6 months does the child need extra iron, water, carbohydrate, and vitamin C. Foods should be introduced in small amounts, one new food every three to seven days, in order to identify any food allergy, but the sequence of foods given is not critical. Rice cereal is usually the first solid food offered, primarily because it is iron-fortified and believed to be the least allergenic of the cereals. Strained fruits and vegetables are usually the next foods offered and can be given in whatever order the parent chooses. Most commercially prepared baby foods are now available without added salt or sugar. Mothers should be cautioned against adding extra salt or sugar to the infant's food; their long-term effects on the infant's future growth and blood pressure and the need for salt are currently under study. Some clinicians also advocate withholding cow's milk, eggs, and wheat until the infant is six to nine months old. These are known to be allergenic substances for many persons.

Many mothers choose to prepare solid foods by blenderizing the foods normally eaten by the family. Infant-sized portions can be frozen in an ice cube tray and then stored in separate freezer bags. Mothers need to be warned that the excessive salt and sugar content often found in canned foods is inappropriate for the infant. Frozen vegetables and fresh fruits are generally free of these additives. Meats blenderized for the infant should also be prepared without seasoning.

For the infant who is on a total vegetarian diet, it is important to offer a broad mixture of cereals, vegetables, fruits, and legumes. The infant should also receive either breast milk or soy formula and supplemental vitamin D in order to assure an adequate intake of essential nutrients (Rudy 1984).

Solids are offered to an infant by various means. Some parents add the solids to the bottle of formula or use an infant feeder with a nipple adapter. These methods delay development of the infant's eating skills by prolonging the time when nourishment is obtained by sucking. To foster appropriate development, parents should be encouraged to offer solids by spoon or allow the infant to use the fingers in a hand-to-mouth motion.

Parents need to be advised that putting an infant to bed with a bottle of formula or juice or allowing the infant to breast-feed intermittently while sleeping beside the mother through the night may foster tooth decay and ear infections. Cavities are prevented by the saliva bathing the teeth and washing away the cariogenic materials. The flow of saliva diminishes rapidly once the infant has fallen asleep, and the milk or juice is left in contact with the teeth. The subsequent decay is referred to as bottle mouth syndrome. It is believed ear infections are more likely to occur when the infant feeds in a horizontal position allowing the milk to pool near the pharyngeal opening to the eustachian tube. To avoid both of these conditions, parents should be encouraged to hold the infant during feedings, spend quiet time comforting and consoling the infant, and then place the drowsy infant in the crib without a bottle.

Parents need to be advised that the infant needs extra water between meals when solid food is added because the solute load on the infant's kidneys will be increased. Juices, however, add extra calories to the diet and often are delayed until the infant is 9 to 12 months old and can drink from a cup.

● Nutritional Assessment of the Infant

During the early months of life, the food offered to and consumed by infants will be instrumental in their proper growth and development. At each well-baby visit the nurse assesses the nutritional status of the newborn. Assessment should include four components:

- Nutritional history from the parent
- Weight gain since the last visit
- Growth chart percentiles
- Physical examination

The nutritional history reports the type, amount, and frequency of milk and supplemental foods being given to the infant on a daily basis. The healthy formula-fed infant should generally gain 1 ounce per day for the first six months of life and 0.5 ounce per day for the second six months. Healthy breast-fed babies may fall within these weight gain parameters but may also be normal while gaining 0.5 ounce per day for the first six months (Stahl & Guida 1984). Individual charts show the infant's growth with respect to height, weight, and head circumference. The important consideration is that infants continue to grow at their own individual rates.

For the breast-feeding mother who is concerned about whether her infant is getting adequate nutrition, the nurse can recommend looking for an appearance of weight gain and counting the number of wet diapers in a 24-hour period. Six wet diapers or more in a day indicates adequate nutrition is being attained in the totally breast-fed infant. If additional water is ingested, this count is low. The presence of urine can most accurately be assessed when the diaper is free of feces. This is most likely prior to feedings. The gastrocolic reflex often stimulates stooling following a feeding. For the anxious parent, another means of reassurance of adequate intake and output is to keep a record of the frequency and duration of feedings and the exact number of wet and/or soiled diapers. Keeping a record tends to give the worried parent a sense of control and a tangible indication on which to rule out or base concern (Humphrey 1985).

The physical examination will assist in identifying any nutritional disorders. Edema, dermatitis, cheilosis, or bleeding gums may be caused by excess protein intake, or riboflavin, niacin, or vitamin C deficiency, respectively. Iron deficiency should be suspected in a pale, diaphoretic, irritable infant who is obese and consumes more than 35 to 40 ounces of formula per day (Driggers 1980).

By calculating the nutritional needs of infants, the nurse can recommend a diet that supplies appropriate nutrition for infant growth and development. The assessment is especially helpful in counseling mothers of infants under 6 months of age in view of the tendency to add too many supplemental foods or offer too much formula to infants of this age. Clinicians generally advise that an infant should not be given more than 32 ounces of formula in one day. If additional calories are needed, supplemental foods should be added to the diet. Conversely, if the caloric intake is adequate or excessive, formula alone gives the infant enough calories and introduction of solid foods can be delayed until later.

When an infant's caloric intake and weight gain is found to be excessive, clinicians do not advise putting the infant on a weight reduction diet because tissue growth is rapid during this period and must be supported. The appropriate advice is to provide a maintenance caloric intake as a means of allowing the infant to maintain weight while growing in length and age.

Identification of appropriate nutritional intake can be done by comparing the infant's dietary intake with the desired caloric intake, weight, age, and the number of calories needed by the infant. Most commercial formulas prescribed for the normal healthy newborn contain 20 calories per ounce. If the infant is eating solids, the caloric value of those foods must be determined and included in the calculation of nutritional intake. With knowledge of the amount of calories needed by the infant according to weight and the advised maximum ounces of formula per day (Tables 30–6, 30–7), the nurse can counsel the parents about how many ounces per day the child needs to meet caloric requirements. The following case studies show the effectiveness of these assessments.

Case Study: Age 1 Week

Jamie, age 1 week, is visited at home by the nurse associated with a health maintenance organization (HMO). Jamie is Mrs Adam's first child, and Mrs Adams is concerned about whether Jamie is getting adequate nourishment. Jamie weighed 7 pounds at birth and has regained her birth weight after an 11-ounce (10 percent) loss. Mrs Adams reports that Jamie takes 3 ounces of formula at each of seven feedings during a 24-hour period, does not spit up any formula, and has eight to ten wet diapers a day.

NURSING ASSESSMENT

Using Table 30–6, the nurse calculates 1-week-old Jamie's dietary needs as follows:

Jamie's weight = 7 lb
24 hr caloric need = 385
Needed formula for 24 hr = 19 oz
Jamie's 24-hr intake = 21 ounces (20 cal/ounce) = 420 calories

NURSING DIAGNOSIS

● Alteration in nutrition: more than body requirement related to formula intake that is greater than necessary to meet Jamie's growth needs

PLAN

Encourage Mrs Adams to offer Jamie 2¾ ounces of formula at each of the seven feedings a day.

Use Table 30–5 to advise Mrs Adams of cues that indicate hunger and satiation.

Table 30–6 Approximate Number of Ounces of 20 Calorie/Ounce Formula Needed to Meet Infant Caloric Needs

Weight of infant	Caloric need (24 hr)	Ounces infant formula (24 hr)
Birth to 3 months		
6 lb	330	16.5
7 lb	385	19
8 lb	440	22
9 lb	495	25
10 lb	550	27.5
11 lb	605	30
12 lb	660	33
13 lb	715	36
14 lb	770	38.5
3–6 months		
10 lb	520	26
11 lb	572	28.5
12 lb	624	31
13 lb	676	34
14 lb	728	36.5
15 lb	780	39
16 lb	832	41.2
17 lb	884	44
18 lb	936	47
19 lb	988	49.5
20 lb	1040	52
21 lb	1092	54.5
22 lb	1144	57

Reprinted with permission from Markesberry B: Watching baby's diet: A professional and parent guide. *Am J Nurs* 1979;4:180

Table 30–7 Average Recommended Levels of Caloric Intake*

Birth to 3 months	55 calories/lb
3–6 months	52 calories/lb
6–9 months	50 calories/lb
9–12 months	47 calories/lb

*Caloric needs may vary up to 10 percent for individual infants on a day-to-day basis. This would amount to only a 2 to 3 ounce variation in amount of formula per day.

From *Recommended Dietary Allowances,* ed 8, Washington, DC, National Academy of Sciences, 1980

Explore alternative methods for providing comfort to a newborn.

Case Study: Age 1 Month

Mrs Baker has brought 1-month-old Daniel into the pediatric nurse practitioner's office for a well-child visit. Daniel weighed 8 pounds and was 21 inches in length at birth. At this visit Daniel weighs 10 pounds and is 22 inches in length. Using standardized growth grids to plot the weight and length, the nurse notes that Daniel's weight has been on or just above the fiftieth percentile since birth, and the length has remained at the seventy-fifth percentile.

Daniel is presently taking between 4 and 5 ounces of formula six times a day. Mrs Baker has not begun supplementing Daniel's diet with solid foods but reports that her mother has advised her to add 1 to 2 tablespoons of rice cereal to the bedtime bottle in order to get Daniel to sleep through the night.

The nurse uses Table 30–6 to assess Daniel's intake and to demonstrate to Mrs Baker whether Daniel needs the additional calories that would be provided by the cereal.

NURSING ASSESSMENT

Daniel's intake = 24 to 30 ounces of formula (20 calories/ounce) = 480 to 600 calories
Daniel's needs at 10 pounds = 550 calories and 27.5 ounces/24 hr

NURSING DIAGNOSIS

- Knowledge deficit related to the correct time to introduce solid foods into Daniel's diet

PLAN

Reassure Mrs Baker that Daniel's intake is adequate.

Advise Mrs Baker that although many infants begin to sleep through the night at 6 weeks of age, others take longer to accomplish this.

Advise Mrs Baker that solid food supplements would add unnecessary calories to Daniel's diet and encourage excessive weight gain.

Use Table 30–5 to advise Mrs Baker of cues indicating hunger and satiation.

KEY CONCEPTS

Breast milk is the optimal food for the first four to six months of life.

The newborn needs 110 to 120 cal/kg/day and 140 to 160 ml of water/kg/day.

Mature breast milk and commercially prepared formulas (unless otherwise noted) provide 20 cal/ounce.

Breast-fed infants need supplements of vitamin D and fluoride. However, there is no need to give supplemental iron to breast-fed infants before 6 months of age.

A disadvantage of breast-feeding is that most drugs taken by the mother are transmitted through breast milk.

Formula-fed infants regain their birth weight by 10 days of age and gain 1 ounce/day for the first six months and 0.5 ounce/day for the second six months; birthweight is doubled at 3.5 to 4 months of age. Healthy breast-fed babies gain approximately 0.5 ounce/day in the first six months of life, regain their birth weight by about 14 days of age, and double their birth weight at approximately 5 months of age.

Formula-fed infants need no vitamin or mineral supplements other than iron, if it is not already in the formula, and fluoride if it is not obtained in the water system.

Signs indicating newborn readiness for the first feeding are: active bowel sounds, absence of abdominal distention, and a lusty cry that quiets, with rooting and sucking behaviors when a stimulus is placed near the lips.

The first newborn feeding should be of sterile water to assess the ability to ingest fluids and to minimize lung danger if aspiration occurs.

The bottle-feeding mother may require assistance with feeding and burping her infant. She will also benefit from information about feeding schedules, types of formula, and the like.

Breast-feeding mothers should be encouraged to ensure that the infant is correctly positioned at breast, with a large portion of the areola in his or her mouth. The mother is advised to rotate position to ensure that all ducts are emptied.

To prevent sore nipples the nurse can encourage the breast-feeding mother to allow her breasts to air dry after feeding.

The breast-feeding mother needs to increase her caloric intake by about 200 calories. It is also essential that she consume adequate amounts of liquid to promote milk production.

Infants should receive formula or breast milk until 1 year of age.

The use of skim milk, cow's milk with lowered fat content, or unmodified cow's milk is not recommended for children under 2 years old.

Nutritional assessment of the infant includes: nutritional history from parent, weight gain, growth chart percentiles, and physical examination.

Breast-fed infants are probably getting adequate nutrition if they are gaining weight and have at least six wet diapers a day when not receiving additional water supplements.

Formula intake should not exceed 32 ounces in 24 hours. If additional calories are needed, supplemental foods should be added to the diet.

After six months supplemental foods should be added to the diet starting with small amounts and adding one new food every three to seven days.

REFERENCES

American Academy of Pediatrics, Committee on Nutrition: The use of whole cow's milk in infancy. *Pediatrics* 1983;72:253.

American Academy of Pediatrics, Committee on Nutrition: Nutrition and lactation. *Pediatrics* 1981;68:435.

Anholm P: Breast feeding: A preventive approach to health care in infancy. *Issues Comp Pediatr Nurs* 1986;9:1.

Avery G: *Neonatology*, ed 3. Philadelphia, Lippincott, 1987.

Beske JE, **Garvis** M: Important factors in breastfeeding success. *Am J Mat Child Nurs* 1982;7:(May/June):174.

Bishop W: Weaning the breastfed toddler or preschooler. *Pediatr Nurs* 1985;11(May/June):211.

Broussard A: Anticipatory guidance: Adding solids to the infant's diet. *J Obstet Gynecol Neonat Nurs* 1984;13(July/August):239.

Clark AL (ed): *Culture, Childbearing, Health Professionals.* Philadelphia, Davis, 1978.

Clark AL: *Culture and Childrearing.* Philadelphia, Davis, 1981.

deCarvalho M, et al: Does the duration and frequency of early breastfeeding affect nipple pain? *Birth* 1984;11 (Summer):81.

Driggers D: Infant nutrition made simple. *Am Fam Physician* 1980;22:113.

Eckstein E: *Food, People and Nutrition.* Westport, Conn, AV Publishing, 1980.

Evans H, **Glass** L: Breastfeeding: Advantages and potential problems. *Pediatr Ann* 1979;8:110.

Gromada K: Maternal-infant attachment: The first step toward individualizing twins. *Am J Mat Child Nurs* 1981; 6(March/April):129.

Gulick E: Infant health and breastfeeding. *Pediatr Nurs* 1986;12(January/February):51.

Hanson LA, et al: Protective factors in milk and the development of the immune system. *Pediatrics* 1985; 75(suppl):172

Humphrey N: Common questions about breastfeeding. *Children's Nurse* 1985;3(February):1.

Joseph S: Anatomy of the infant formula controversy. *Am J Dis Child* 1981;135:889.

Kemp C, et al: *Current Pediatric Diagnosis and Treatment,* ed 7. Los Altos, Calif, Lange Medical Publications, 1982.

LaDu EB: Childbirth care for Hmong families. *Am J Mat Child Nurs* 1985;10(November/December):382.

Lauwers J, **Woessner** C: *Counseling the Nursing Mother.* Wayne, NJ, Avery Publishing, 1983.

Lawrence RA: *Breastfeeding: A Guide for the Medical Profession.* St Louis, Mosby, 1980.

L'Esperance C, **Frantz** K: Time limitation for early breastfeeding. *J Obstet Gynecol Neonat Nurs* 1985;14(March/April):114.

Mullett SE: Helping mothers breast-feed. *Am J Mat Child Nurs* 1982;7:178.

Picciano M, **Deering** R: The influence of feeding regimens on iron status during infancy. *Am J Clin Nutr* 1980;33:746.

Pipes P: *Nutrition in Infancy and Childhood,* ed 3. St Louis, Mosby, 1985.

Pritchard JA, **MacDonald** PC, **Gant** N. *Williams Obstetrics,* ed 17. New York, Appleton-Century-Crofts, 1985.

Platzer AC, et al: Drug administration via breast milk. *Hosp Pract* 1980;15(September):111.

Reifsnider E, **Myers** ST: Employed mothers can breastfeed, too! *Am J Mat Child Nurs* 1985;10(July/August):256.

Riordan J: *A Practical Guide to Breastfeeding.* St Louis, Mosby, 1983.

Riordan J, **Countryman** B: Basics of breastfeeding. Part III: The biological specificity of breast milk. *J Obstet Gynecol Neonat Nurs* 1980;9(September/October):273.

Rudy C: Vegetarian diets for children. *Pediatr Nurs* 1984;10(September/October):329.

Slaven S, **Harvey** D: Unlimited suckling time improves breastfeeding. *Lancet* 1981;1:392

Stahl M, **Guida** D: Slow weight gain in the breast-fed infant: Management options. *Pediatr Nurs* 1984;10(March/April):117.

Ward BG, et al: Vietnamese refugees in Adelaide: An obstetric analysis. *Med J Aust* 1981;1:72.

ADDITIONAL READINGS

Balkam JAJ: Guidelines for drug therapy during lactation. *J Obstet Gynecol Neonat Nurs* 1986;15:(January/February): 65.

Beall MH: Breastfeeding: Some drug admonitions. *Contemp OB/GYN* 1987;29(February):49.

Boyer DB: Serum indirect bilirubin levels and meconium passage in early fed normal newborns. *Nurs Res* 1987;36(May/June):174.

Hot milk in cool bottles . . . microwave oven. *Emerg Med* 1987;19(January 30):109.

Janas LM, et al: Quantities of amino acids ingested by human milk-fed infants. *J Pediatrics* 1986;109(November): 802.

Jones D: Breast-feeding practices. *Nurs Times* 1987;83 (January 21–27):56.

Jordan PL; Breastfeeding as a risk factor for fathers. *J Obstet Gynecol Neonat Nurs* 1986;15(March/April):94.

Meier P, **Anderson** GC: Responses of small preterm infants to bottle- and breast-feeding. *Am J Mat Child Nurs* 1987;12(March/April):97.

Morse JM, et al: Minimal breastfeeding. *J Obstet Gynecol Neonat Nurs* 1986;15(July/August):333.

Niebyl JR: Making the breastfeeding decision. *Contemp OB/GYN* 1986;28(September):43.

Position of the American Dietetic Association: Promotion of breastfeeding. *J Am Diet Assoc* 1986;86(November):1580.

Raihu NCR: Why LBW infants thrive on human milk. *Contemp OB/GYN* 1985;25(June):112.

Riordan J, **Riordan** M: Drugs in breast milk. *Am J Nurs* 1984;84(March):328.

Scrimshaw SCM, et al: Factors affecting breastfeeding among women of Mexican origin or descent in Los Angeles. *Am J Pub Health* 1987;77(April):467.

Simic BS: Childhood obesity as a risk factor in adulthood and its prevention. *Prev Med* 1983;12(January):47.

I had been told that most babies ate every three or four hours and slept the rest of the time. Not mine! She wanted to nurse every two hours, and sometimes more often than that. Sometimes she would sleep for an hour, sometimes for fifteen minutes. I loved her, but I also felt consumed by her needs. It was hard to adjust to the fact that I couldn't get anything finished, whether it was an article I was reading or folding the laundry. At the end of the day I would realize I hadn't accomplished anything. Once I accepted the fact that I was not going to function at my old efficient rate (at least for a while) and stopped feeling guilty about what I wasn't getting done, I felt freer to enjoy the time I was spending with my baby. (The New Our Bodies, Ourselves)

The Newborn at Risk: Needs and Care

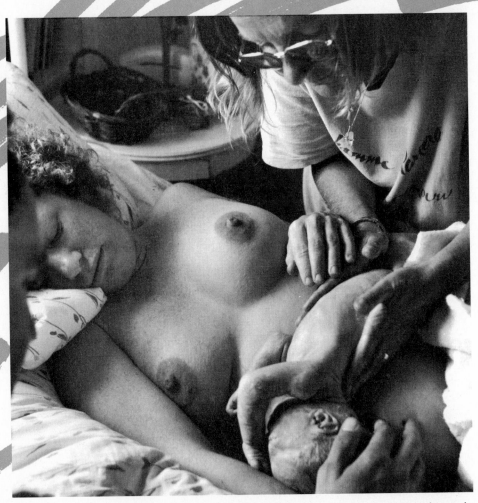

Rather than putting this premature infant immediately into an incubator, the nurse-midwife places the newborn on the mother's abdomen, with its head lowered to assist mucus drainage, and strokes its back to stimulate the central nervous system. The mother and father can then also comfort and warm the infant with their hands while the nurse-midwife carefully monitors its progress.

Chapter Thirty-One

OBJECTIVES

- **Discuss the physiologic characteristics of the preterm newborn that predispose each body system to various complications of prematurity.**

- **Compare the underlying etiologies of the similar physiologic complications of preterm appropriate-for-gestational-age (AGA) and small-for-gestational-age (SGA) newborns.**

- **Use supporting data to identify nursing diagnoses required to plan interventions for the care of the AGA preterm newborn.**

- **Compare the characteristics and potential complications of the postterm newborn and the infant with postmaturity syndrome.**

- **Explain the effects of selected maternal health problems on the fetus.**

- **Discuss interventions to facilitate parent-infant attachment with the high-risk newborn.**

- **Identify nursing actions necessary to support family members dealing with the crisis of preterm birth.**

Within the last 20 years, the field of neonatology has expanded greatly. Many levels of nursery care have evolved in response to increasing knowledge about the neonate: special care; transitional care; and low-, medium-, and high-risk care. The nurse is an important care giver in all these nurseries. As a member of the multidisciplinary health care team, the nurse has contributed to the high level of perinatal care available today.

In addition to the availability of high-level neonatal care other factors influence the outcome for these at-risk infants. These factors include:

- Birth weight

- Gestational age

- Type and length of neonatal illness

- Environmental and maternal factors

● Identification of At-Risk Newborns

An at-risk infant is one who is susceptible to illness (morbidity) or even death (mortality) because of dysmaturity, immaturity, physical disorders, or complications of birth. In most cases, the infant is the product of a pregnancy involving one or more predictable risk factors, including:

- Low socioeconomic level of the mother

- Exposure to environmental dangers such as toxic chemicals

- Preexisting maternal conditions such as heart disease and diabetes

- Obstetric factors such as age or parity

- Medical conditions related to pregnancy such as prenatal maternal infection

- Obstetric complications such as abruptio placentae

Various risk factors and their specific effects on the pregnancy outcome are listed in Table 15–2.

Because these factors and the perinatal risks associated with them are known, the birth of many at-risk newborns can often be anticipated and prepared for through adequate prenatal care. The pregnancy can be closely monitored, treatment can be instituted as necessary, and arrangements can be made for delivery to occur at a facility with appropriate equipment and personnel to care for both mother and child.

Identification of at-risk infants cannot always be made before labor, since the course of labor and delivery or how the infant will withstand the stress of labor is not known prior to the actual process. Thus during labor, fetal heart monitoring has played a significant role in detecting fetuses in distress.

Immediately after birth the Apgar score is a valuable tool in identifying the at-risk neonate. The lower the Apgar score at 5 minutes after birth, the higher the percentage of neurologic abnormalities (such as cerebral palsy) seen after 1 year. The percentage also increases significantly as birth weight decreases (Korones 1986).

The newborn classification and neonatal mortality risk chart is another useful tool in identifying newborns at risk (Figure 31–1). Before this classification tool was developed, birth weight of less than 2500 g was the sole criterion for determination of immaturity. It was eventually recognized that an infant could weigh more than 2500 g but still be immature. Conversely, an infant less than 2500 g might be functionally at term or beyond. Thus birth weight and gestational age together became the criteria used to assess neonatal maturity and mortality risk.

According to the newborn classification and neonatal mortality risk chart, *gestation* is divided as follows:

- Preterm = 0–37 (completed) weeks

- Term = 38–41 (completed) weeks

- Postterm = 42+ weeks

As shown in Figure 31–1, large-for-gestational-age (LGA) infants are those above the curved line labeled 90 percent. Appropriate-for-gestational-age (AGA) infants are those between the lines labeled 10th percentile and 90th percentile. Small-for-gestational-age (SGA) infants are those below the curved line labeled 10th percentile. A newborn is assigned to a category depending on birth weight and gestational age. For example, a newborn classified as Pr SGA is preterm and small for gestational age. The full-term newborn whose weight is appropriate for gestational age is classified F AGA.

Neonatal mortality risk is the chance of death within the neonatal period, that is, within the first 28 days of life. As indicated in Figure 31–1, the neonatal mortality risk decreases as both gestational age and birth weight increase. Infants who are preterm and small for gestational age have the highest neonatal mortality risk. The mortality for LGA infants has decreased at most perinatal centers because of improved management of diabetes in pregnancy and increased recognition of potential problems with LGA infants.

Neonatal morbidity can be anticipated based on birth weight and gestational age. In Figure 31–2 the infant's birth weight is located in the vertical column, and the gestational age in weeks is found horizontally. The area where the two meet on the graph identifies commonly occurring problems. This tool assists in determining the needs of particular infants for special observation and care. For example, an infant of 2000 g at 40 weeks' gestation should be carefully assessed for evidence of fetal distress, hypoglycemia, congenital anomalies, congenital infection, and polycythemia.

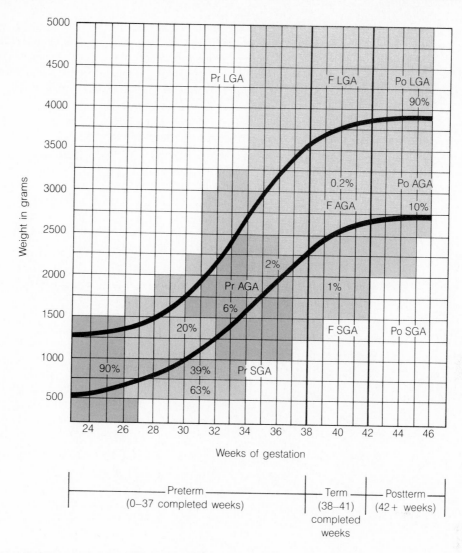

Figure 31–1 Newborn classification and neonatal mortality risk chart. (From Koops BL, Morgan LP, Battaglia FC: Neonatal mortality risk in relationship to birth weight and gestational age. *J Pediatr* 1982;101(6):969)

● Using the Nursing Process for At-Risk Newborns

Nursing Assessment

Assessment of the at-risk newborn is an ongoing nursing process. It begins with the history of the newborn, which includes family and maternal history and other factors that may influence in utero development.

In the delivery room the nurse correlates the Apgar scores and careful observation with information about the duration of labor, maternal analgesia and anesthesia, and complications of the labor and delivery process. Assessment continues when the newborn is admitted to the nursery. All previous assessments, Apgar scores, and treatments immediately after birth are evaluated in conjunction with the physical assessment of the newborn. As discussed in Chapter 28, the physical examination includes all of the following:

● Complete head-to-toe assessment, observing for cardiorespiratory function, temperature, and congenital anomalies

● Clinical determination of gestational age

● Classification of the baby as AGA, SGA, or LGA and correlation with the morbidity risk for the specific classification (Figure 31–2).

Analysis and Nursing Diagnosis

Many of the nursing diagnoses for the at-risk newborn are based on careful analysis of the assessment data and are centered around alteration in physiologic process, and the newborn's response to procedures or stimuli. Nursing diagnoses may include:

● Impaired gas exchange related to respiratory distress secondary to fluid aspiration or surfactant deficiency

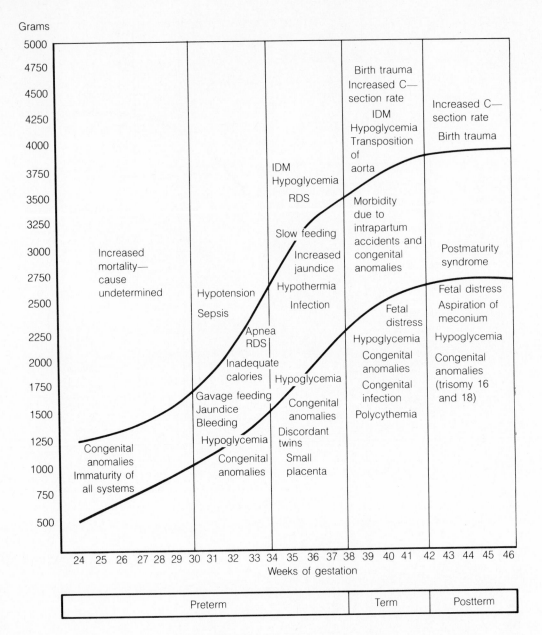

Figure 31–2 *Neonatal morbidity by birth weight and gestational age* (From Lubchenco LO: *The High Risk Infant.* Philadelphia, Saunders, 1976, p 122)

- Alteration in nutrition: less than body requirements related to inadequate fluid intake

- Alteration in thermoregulation related to hypothermia secondary to inadequate subcutaneous tissue.

The psychosocial needs of these newborns and their parents may be addressed in such nursing diagnoses as:

- Ineffective family coping related to birth of potentially ill newborn

- Knowledge deficit related to potential long-term de-

velopmental outcomes secondary to at-risk newborn complications

Nursing Plan and Implementation

When all the data are gathered and analyzed, the care plan is developed. Nursing care of the at-risk newborn depends on minute-to-minute observations of the changes in the neonate's physiologic status. It is essential to a baby's survival that the neonatal nurse understand the basic physiologic principles that guide nursing management of the at-risk neonate. The organization of nursing care must be directed toward:

- Decreasing physiologically stressful situations
- Constantly observing for subtle signs of change in clinical condition
- Interpreting laboratory data and coordinating interventions
- Conserving the infant's energy, especially in frail, debilitated newborns
- Providing for developmental stimulation and sleep cycle
- Assisting the family in attachment behaviors

Nursing Evaluation

The success of the care plan is confirmed by continuous assessments of the neonate's behavior, communication with family and health team members, and use of diagnostic measures.

The at-risk newborn is the newest member of a family, so it is imperative to incorporate the parents into the plan of care. They must be kept informed of their newborn's condition and progress, involved in care, and given frequent opportunities to interact with their newborn and voice their fears and concerns. They should also be assisted in learning about their baby and how to care for their baby. The nurse should make every effort to evaluate on an ongoing basis how the family is being incorporated into the care of their newborn and how they are adjusting to this new member of the family.

● Care of the Preterm (Premature) Newborn

A preterm newborn is any infant born before 38 weeks' gestation. The length of gestation and thus the level of maturity vary even in the "premature" population. Figure 31–3 shows a preterm newborn.

The incidence of preterm births in the United States ranges from 7 percent of white newborns to 14 percent to 15 percent of nonwhites. The causes of preterm labor are poorly understood, but more and more of the variables that influence preterm labor and delivery are being identified (see Chapter 25 for a discussion of preterm labor and delivery).

With the help of modern technology, some babies under 500 g and between 23 and 26 weeks' gestation are surviving. But the mortality rates are the highest among these newborns.

The major problem of the preterm newborn is variable immaturity of all systems. The degree of immaturity depends on the length of gestation. For example, newborns of 32 weeks' gestation can be expected to exhibit more immaturity than newborns of 36 weeks' gestation. The degree of immaturity also presents problems of management. Maintenance of the preterm newborn falls within narrow physiologic parameters. "Catch-up care" is usually not possible if ground is lost in initial management. Improper physiologic management (or lack of management) adds

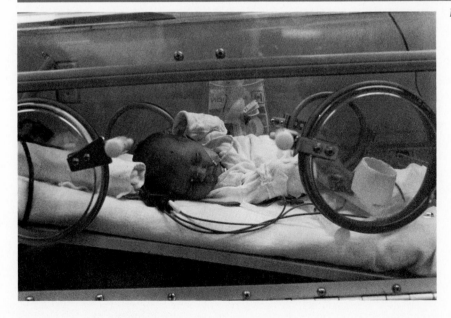

Figure 31–3   Preterm infant

stress and feeds the vicious cycle of physiologic deterioration.

The preterm newborn must traverse the same complex, interconnected pathways from intrauterine to extrauterine life as the term newborn. Because of immaturity, the preterm neonate is ill-equipped to make this transition smoothly.

Physiologic Characteristics and Risks of the Preterm Newborn

RESPIRATORY PHYSIOLOGY AND CONSIDERATIONS

The preterm newborn is at risk for respiratory problems because the lungs are not fully mature and ready to take over the process of oxygen and carbon dioxide exchange until 37 to 38 weeks' gestation. The length of time needed varies; some infants who are born before 37 to 38 weeks do not develop respiratory distress, and some infants born at 37 weeks experience severe respiratory distress. The most critical influencing factor in the development of respiratory distress is the preterm baby's ability to produce adequate amounts of surfactant. Surfactant prevents alveolar collapse when the baby exhales and increases lung compliance (ability of the lung to fill with air easily). When surfactant is decreased, compliance is also lessened, and the inspiratory pressure needed to expand the lungs with air increases (see Chapter 27 for discussion of respiratory adaptation and development).

Besides adequate surfactant production, alveolar sacs must be present in sufficient number to provide the surface area needed to accomplish oxygen and carbon dioxide exchange. The term infant has about 24 million alveoli, while the adult has 200 million to 600 million (Korones 1986).

Lung development begins at around 24 days of fetal life, when the primitive lung bud appears (Figure 31–4). The primitive lung bud branches at about 26 to 28 days to form the major right and left bronchi. Throughout gestation, growth and branching continue, forming terminal bronchioles to respiratory bronchioles, from which arise alveolar ducts. The alveolar ducts are differentiated by approximately 24 weeks' gestation and give rise to thin-walled terminal air sacs. From 24 weeks until birth, growth and development of these terminal air sacs or premature alveoli are continuous. At about 24 to 26 weeks' gestation, the surface area available for gas exchange is very limited (because of inadequate number and size of alveoli) and inadequate surfactant is produced, making survival at this time unlikely.

By 27 to 28 weeks, more alveolar sacs have developed, and more capillaries are in contact with the alveolar membrane. This allows some exchange of oxygen and car-

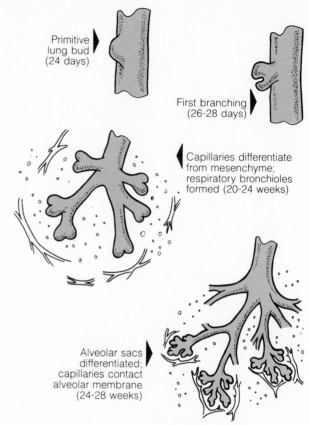

Figure 31–4 Development of primitive lung bud and subsequent branching into surrounding mesenchyme. (From Korones SB: High Risk Newborn Infants, ed 4. St Louis, Mosby, 1986)

bon dioxide from the alveoli to the capillaries, and from the capillaries to the alveoli. Surfactant production at this time is unstable and inadequate, but with respiratory assistance, survival is possible. The newborn is at risk, however, for many complications, such as RDS, hypoxemia, acidemia, intraventricular hemorrhage, cold stress, and metabolic imbalances, any one of which may compromise ultimate survival.

Between 29 and 30 weeks, additional differentiation of the alveolar sacs occurs and additional surfactant is released. After 30 weeks' gestation, growth of new primitive alveoli is rapid, and by 34 to 36 weeks, mature alveoli are present (Korones 1986). Also by this time surfactant production increases rapidly as the second pathway of surfactant production begins optimal functioning. If the fetus is unstressed and without iatrogenic complications, adequate amounts of surfactant should be produced for lung expansion and gas exchange at this time. In the presence of asphyxia, hypoxemia, acidemia, or cold stress, surfactant production is impaired, resulting in increased chances of respiratory distress. The more immature the infant, the more devastating the physiologic complications.

CARDIOVASCULAR PHYSIOLOGY AND CONSIDERATIONS

In the preterm infant, the muscular coat of the pulmonary arterioles is incompletely developed. This muscular development occurs late in gestation; therefore the more premature the infant, the less muscular the pulmonary arterioles (Avery 1987). With decreased pulmonary ateriole musculature, vasoconstriction is not as significant in response to decreased oxygen levels. Therefore, the healthy preterm infant has a lower pulmonary vascular resistance than a full-term infant. This factor leads to increased left-to-right shunting through the ductus arteriosus, which steps up the blood flow back into the lungs. On the other hand, the preterm infant who develops respiratory distress and its complications (acidemia and hypoxemia) is at greater risk for increasing pulmonary vascular resistance (decreased PO_2 triggers vasoconstriction), which decreases blood flow through the lungs, causing additional hypoxemia and acidemia. The ductus arteriosus responds to rising oxygen levels by vasoconstriction; in the preterm infant, who is more susceptible to hypoxia, the ductus may remain open. A patent ductus increases the blood volume to the lungs, causing pulmonary congestion, increased respiratory effort, and higher oxygen consumption.

THERMOREGULATION

Maintaining a normal body temperature in the preterm baby presents a nursing challenge. Heat production is a factor over which the nurse has little control, yet heat loss is a major problem that the nurse can do much to prevent.

Heat production in the preterm infant is primarily a result of normal metabolic functions. Heat is produced by the oxidation of glucose and free fatty acids and also by the metabolism of brown fat. Two limiting factors in heat production, however, are the availability of glycogen in the liver (glycogen stores are primarily laid down during the third trimester) and the amount of brown fat available for metabolism (the preterm newborn does not have a full complement of brown fat). If the baby is chilled after birth, both glycogen and brown fat stores are metabolized rapidly for heat production, leaving the newborn with no reserves in the event of future stress. Since the muscle mass is small in preterm infants, and muscular activity is diminished (they are unable to shiver), little heat is produced.

One of the greatest threats to the preterm baby is heat loss. Heat loss occurs as a result of several physiologic and anatomic factors:

1. The preterm baby has a much larger ratio of body surface to body weight. This means that the baby's ability to produce heat (body weight) is much less than the potential for losing heat (surface area). The loss of heat in a preterm newborn weighing 1500 g is five times greater per unit of body weight than in an adult (Korones 1986). Without an adequate thermal environment, the preterm baby is at risk for excessive heat loss.

2. The preterm baby has very little subcutaneous fat, which is the human body's insulation. Without adequate insulation, heat is easily conducted from the core of the body (warmer temperature) to the surface of the body (cooler temperature). Heat is lost from the body as the blood vessels transport blood from the body core to the subcutaneous tissues. The preterm baby's blood vessels lie close to the skin surface, and without adequate insulation (fat), more heat is given off as the blood circulates throughout the body.

3. The posture of the preterm baby is another important factor influencing heat loss. Flexion of the extremities decreases the amount of surface area exposed to the environment; extension increases the surface area exposed to the environment and thus increases heat loss. The gestational age of the newborn influences the amount of flexion, from completely hypotonic and extended at 28 weeks to strong flexion displayed by 36 weeks (Figure 28–2).

In summary, the more preterm an infant the less capable he or she is of maintaining heat balance because of disproportionate body surface area, decreased subcutaneous fat, and increased heat loss due to body posture. Prevention of heat loss by providing a neutral thermal environment is one of the most important considerations in nursing management of the preterm newborn. Cold stress, with its accompanying severe complications, can be prevented (see Chapter 32).

DIGESTIVE PHYSIOLOGY AND CONSIDERATIONS

The basic structure of the gastrointestinal (GI) tract is formed early in gestation, so even the very preterm newborn is able to take in some nourishment. Maturation of the digestive and absorptive processes is more variable, however, and occurs later in gestation. In addition, many of the problems that compromise adequate nutrition are a result of immaturity of systems other than the GI tract. The renal system is unable to concentrate urine. The respiratory system may be so immature that the newborn's cough is weak or absent. Poor suck and swallow reflexes are a result of immaturity of the neurologic system. Severe illness of the newborn may also prevent intake of adequate nutrients.

The quality as well as the quantity of protein ingested is important to small preterm infants. These babies lack the enzymes necessary to convert certain essential amino acids into other nonessential amino acids (American Academy of Pediatrics 1985). Amino acids that are known to be essential for preterm infants but are not essential for term infants include histidine, tyrosine, and cystine.

Another factor in protein composition is the whey-to-casein ratio. Because of immaturity of the kidneys, the preterm infant is unable to handle the increased solute load (increased osmolarity) of a protein that is high in casein. The baby requires a protein high in whey. Preterm babies fed cow's milk protein with a whey/casein ratio of 18:82 have been shown to have more complications such as azotemia and hyperammonemia than those fed a formula (or human milk) with a ratio of 60:40 (American Academy of Pediatrics 1985).

Absorption of saturated fat, another difficulty for the preterm infant, is presumed to be a result of decreased concentration of bile salt and deficiency of pancreatic lipase. Polyunsaturated fatty acids or medium-chain triglycerides (MCTs) are well absorbed since they do not require lipase for digestion or bile salts for absorption. These fatty acids and MCTs may be added to the formula to provide additional calories for growth. But there is evidence that the use of MCTs may increase the frequency of abdominal distention, loose stools, and vomiting, which might limit the gain achieved by the improved absorption; therefore, addition of MCTs to the formula is controversial (Okamoto et al 1982).

Most simple sugars are well absorbed by the preterm infant and do not present a problem in digestion. Some evidence suggests that lactose digestion may not be fully functional during the first few days of life. Polycose (glucose supplement derived from corn starch) may be added to preterm infant formulas to provide adequate calories without increasing osmolarity, which may lead to an increased incidence of necrotizing enterocolitis. When carbohydrate malabsorption does occur one should suspect necrotizing enterocolitis (see Chapter 32), and the baby's stools should be watched carefully for reducing substances (Clinitest-positive results that indicate sugar in stools), which suggest possible carbohydrate malabsorption.

Because of the factors just discussed and the preterm newborn's general immaturity, certain problems inherent in the feeding process include the following:

- Marked danger of aspiration and its associated complications because of the infant's poorly developed gag reflex, incompetent esophageal cardiac sphincter, and poor sucking and swallowing reflexes

- Small stomach capacity, which limits the amount of fluid that can be introduced to meet high caloric requirements

- Decreased absorption of essential nutrients because of immaturity, malabsorption, and nutritional loss associated with vomiting and diarrhea

- Fatigue associated with sucking, which may lead to increased basal metabolic rate, increased oxygen requirements, and its sequelae of complications

- Feeding intolerance and necrotizing enterocolitis due to diminished blood flow to the intestinal tract because of shock or prolonged hypoxia at birth

RENAL PHYSIOLOGY AND CONSIDERATIONS

The kidneys of the preterm infant are immature in comparison with those of the full-term infant, which poses clinical problems in the management of fluid and electrolyte balance. Specific characteristics of the preterm infant include the following:

- The glomerular filtration rate (GFR) is lower due to decreased renal blood flow. Since the GFR is directly related to lower gestational age, the more preterm the infant the less the GFR, and the closer to term the greater the GFR. The GFR is also decreased in the presence of diseases or conditions that decrease the renal blood flow and/or oxygen content, such as severe respiratory distress, perinatal asphyxia, and congestive heart failure. Anuria and/or oliguria may be observed in the preterm infant after severe asphyxial insult with associated hypotension.

- The preterm infant's kidneys are limited in their ability to concentrate urine or to excrete excess amounts of fluid. This means that if excess fluid is administered, the infant is at risk for fluid retention and overhydration. If too little is administered, the infant will become dehydrated, because of the inability to retain adequate fluid.

- The kidneys of the preterm infant begin excreting glucose (glycosuria) at a lower serum glucose level than adult kidneys. Therefore, glycosuria with hyperglycemia is common (Oh 1981).

- The buffering capacity of the kidney is less, predisposing the infant to metabolic acidosis. Bicarbonate is excreted at a lower serum level, and excretion of acid is accomplished more slowly. Therefore, after periods of hypoxia or insult, the kidneys require a longer time to excrete the lactic acid that accumulates. Sodium bicarbonate is frequently required to treat the metabolic acidosis.

- The immaturity of the renal system also affects the infant's ability to excrete drugs. Because excretion time is longer, many drugs are given over longer intervals in the preterm infant (for example, every 12 hours instead of every 8 hours). Urine output must be carefully monitored when the infant is receiving nephrotoxic drugs such as gentamicin, nafcillin, and others. In the event of poor urine output, drugs can become toxic in the infant much more quickly than in the adult.

HEPATIC PHYSIOLOGY AND CONSIDERATIONS

Immaturity of the preterm newborn's liver predisposes the infant to several problems. First, glycogen is stored in the liver throughout gestation, reaching approximately 5 percent of the weight of the liver by term (Klaus & Fanaroff 1986). After birth, the glycogen stores are rapidly used for energy. Glycogen deposits are affected by asphyxia in utero, and after birth by both asphyxia and cold stress. The baby born preterm has decreased glycogen stores at birth because of low gestational age and frequently experiences stress, which uses up the glycogen rapidly. Therefore the preterm newborn is at high risk for hypoglycemia and its sequelae.

Iron is also stored in the liver and the amount greatly increases during the last trimester of pregnancy. Therefore, the preterm newborn is born with low iron stores. If subject to hemorrhage, rapid growth, and excess blood sampling, the preterm newborn is likely to become iron depleted more quickly than the term newborn. Many preterm babies require transfusions of packed cells to replace the blood withdrawn by frequent blood sampling.

Conjugation of bilirubin in the liver is also impaired in the preterm infant until approximately 37 weeks' gestation. Thus, bilirubin levels increase more rapidly and to a higher level than in the full-term infant (Avery 1987). Early clinical assessment of jaundice at nontoxic bilirubin levels is more difficult in preterm newborns, because they lack subcutaneous fat.

IMMUNOLOGIC PHYSIOLOGY AND CONSIDERATIONS

The preterm infant is at a much greater risk for infection than the term infant. This increased susceptibility is partially attributable to low gestational age but may also be the result of an infection acquired in utero, which precipitates preterm labor and delivery.

In utero, the fetus receives passive immunity against a variety of infections from maternal IgG immunoglobulins, which cross the placenta (see Chapter 27). Because most of this immunity is acquired in the last trimester of pregnancy, the preterm infant has few antibodies at birth, which provide less protection and become depleted earlier than in a full-term infant. This may be a contributing factor in the higher incidence of recurrent infection during the first year of life as well as in the immediate neonatal period (Korones 1986).

The other immunoglobulin significant for the preterm infant is secretory IgA, which does not cross the placenta but is found in breast milk in significant concentrations. Breast-milk's secretory IgA provides immunity to the mucosal surfaces of the GI tract, providing protection from enteric infections such as those caused by E. coli and Shigella. Ill preterm infants may be unable to have breast milk and thus are at risk for enteric infections. In addition, the incidence of necrotizing enterocolitis affects more formula-fed than breast-fed infants (Avery 1987).

Another altered defense against infection in the preterm infant is the skin surface. In very small infants the skin is easily excoriated, and this factor, coupled with many invasive procedures, places the infant at great risk for nosocomial infections. It is vital to use good hand-washing techniques in the care of these infants to prevent unnecessary infection.

HEMATOLOGIC PHYSIOLOGY AND CONSIDERATIONS

The normal cord hemoglobin in an infant of 34 weeks' gestation is approximately 16.8 g/dL and total blood volume ranges from 89 mL/kg to 105 mL/kg (Avery 1987). Because of the small total blood volume, any blood loss is highly significant to the preterm infant. For this reason, all blood taken for sampling must be recorded. Blood is generally replaced when the infant has lost 10 percent of total blood volume.

CENTRAL NERVOUS SYSTEM PHYSIOLOGY AND CONSIDERATIONS

Because the period of most rapid brain growth and development occurs during the third trimester of pregnancy, the closer to term an infant is delivered, the better the neurologic prognosis. The degree of immaturity of the preterm infant's neurologic functioning depends on the length of gestation. Polysynaptic connections are found only in the early stages of fetal development, and myelination of nerve cells is incomplete.

Lining the ventricles is an ependymal layer or membrane, and the germinal matrix, a structure present only until term. This germinal matrix is a highly vascular area, with very thin and fragile capillary walls. The matrix provides little supportive tissue for the fragile blood vessels. Before 32 weeks' gestation, an infant is much more susceptible to hemorrhage of these tiny vessels, because they are vulnerable to hypoxic events that damage vessel walls and cause them to rupture. Most often, hemorrhage occurs in the germinal matrix, through the ependymal wall and into the ventricles of the brain to circulate within the cerebral spinal fluid (Korones 1986).

REACTIVITY PERIODS AND BEHAVIORAL STATES

The newborn infant's response to extrauterine life is characterized by two periods of reactivity, as discussed in Chapter 27. Because of the immaturity of all systems in comparison to those of the full-term neonate, the preterm infant's periods of reactivity are delayed. If the infant is very ill, these periods of reactivity may not be observed at all, as the infant may be hypotonic and unreactive for several days after birth.

At the preterm newborn grows and the condition stabilizes, it becomes increasingly possible to identify behavioral states and traits unique to each infant. This is a very important part of nursing management of the high-risk infant, because it facilitates parental knowledge of their infant's cues for interaction.

In general, stable preterm infants do not demonstrate the same behavioral states as term infants. Preterm infants are more disorganized in their sleep-wake cycles and are unable to attend as well to the human face and objects in the environment. Neurologically, their responses are weaker (sucking, muscle tone, states of arousal) than full-term infants' responses (Gorski et al 1979).

By observing each infant's patterns of behavior and responses, especially the sleep-wake states, the nurse can teach parents optimal times for interacting with their infant. The parents and nurse can plan nursing care around the times when the infant is alert and best able to attend. In addition, the more knowledge parents have about the meaning of their infant's responses and behaviors, the better prepared they will be to meet their newborn's needs and to form a positive attachment with their child.

Management of Nutrition and Fluid Requirements

Providing adequate nutrition and fluids for the preterm infant is a major concern of the health care team. It is now recognized that early feedings are extremely valuable in maintaining normal metabolism and lowering the possibility of such complications as hypoglycemia, hyperbili-

rubinemia, hyperkalemia, and azotemia. However, the preterm newborn is at risk for complications that may develop because of immaturity of the digestive system.

The composition of the "best-suited formula" for the preterm infant is a subject of much discussion and research. Over the past decade many formulas have been tried and revised in an attempt to meet the unique nutritional needs of the preterm infant. Breast milk as the primary source of nutrition for the preterm infant has also been a topic of recent debate and research.

NUTRITIONAL REQUIREMENTS

Enteral caloric intake necessary for growth in an uncompromised healthy preterm infant is 120 to 150 kcal/kg/day. In addition to these relatively high caloric needs, the preterm infant requires more protein (3 to 4 g/kg/day, as opposed to 2.0 to 2.5 g/kg/day for the full-term infant). To meet these needs, a number of higher-calorie, higher-protein formulas are available that meet the preterm infant's nutritional demands yet do not overtax the concentration abilities of the immature kidneys.

In addition to a higher calorie and protein formula, it is recommended that preterm infants receive supplemental multivitamins and vitamin E. The requirement for vitamin E is increased by a diet high in polyunsaturated fats (those tolerated best by preterm infants). Preterm infants fed iron-fortified formulas have higher red cell hemolysis and lower vitamin E concentrations, and thus require additional vitamin E. Vitamin E supplements decrease susceptibility to hemolytic anemia (American Academy of Pediatrics 1985).

Since two-thirds of the calcium and phosphorus in the newborn's body is deposited in the last trimester of gestation, the preterm infant is deficient in these minerals. Rickets and significant bone demineralization have been

Table 31–1 Oral Feeding Schedule for the Low-Birth-Weight Infant

Time and substance*	Less than 1000 g		1001–1500 g		1501–2000 g		More than 2000 g	
	Amount	Frequency	Amount	Frequency	Amount	Frequency	Amount	Frequency
First "drink": sterile H₂O, 5% glucose	1–2 mL	1 hr	3–4 mL	2 hr	4–5 mL	2–3 hr	10 mL	3 hr
Formula: Subsequent feedings, 12–72 hr	Increase 1 mL every other feeding to maximum 5 mL	1 hr	Increase 1 mL every other feeding to maximum 10 mL	2 hr	Increase 2 mL every other feeding to maximum 15 mL	2–3 hr	Increase 5 mL every other feeding to maximum 20 mL	3 hr
Formula: Final feeding schedule, 150 mL/kg	10–15 mL	2 hr	20–28 mL	2–3 hr	28–37 mL	3 hr	37–50 mL	3–4 hr

Supplemental IV fluids should be given to fulfill fluid requirements of 140–160 mL/kg or to give urine specific gravities of 1.008–1.010 and caloric requirements of 90–130 cal/kg.

Modified from Avery GB (ed): *Neonatology*, ed 3. Philadelphia, Lippincott, 1987, p 1196.

Table 31–2 Commonly Used Preterm Formulas

	Contents per dL (usual dilution)								
		CARBOHYDRATE			PROTEIN			FAT	OSMOLALITY
Formula	Caloric content	g/dL	Type	g/dL	Whey/casein ratio	g/dL	Type		mOsm/kg H₂O
Enfamil 24 Premature Formula	81	8.9	60% polycose 40% lactose	2.4	60/40	4.1	40% MCT 40% corn		300
SMA "Preemie"	81	8.6	50% lactose 50% maltodextrins	2.0	60/40	4.4	27% coconut 25% oleic		268
Similac Special Care Infant Formula	81	8.6	50% lactose 50% polycose	2.2	60/40	4.4	50% MCT 30% corn		300
Similac 24 w/Iron	81	8.5	lactose	2.2	18/82	4.3	60% coconut		360
Similac PM 60/40	68	7.6	lactose	1.6	60/40	3.5	60% coconut		260
SMA 24	81	4.2	lactose	1.8	60/40	4.2	oleo, soy, coconut		364

Modified from Avery ME, Taeusch HW (eds): *Schaffer's Diseases of the Newborn,* ed 5. Philadelphia, Saunders 1984, p 974.

documented in very low-birth-weight infants and otherwise healthy preterm infants. One research group (Ziegler et al 1983) recommends 210 mg of elemental calcium/kg/day for a 1000 g premature infant. For larger premature infants, 150 to 180 mg/kg/day may be sufficient.

Special formulas currently available for preterm infants have increased calcium and phosphorus supplementation. These may lead to mineral acquisition similar to that acquired in utero if the infant can tolerate a minimum of 150 mL/kg/day (Greer et al 1982) If other formulas are used, enteral supplements are recommended. In addition to calcium and phosphorus supplementation, vitamin D intake should be at least 500 IU/day to facilitate retention of calcium and increase bone densities (American Academy of Pediatrics 1985).

SCHEDULE OF FEEDINGS

Sterile water is the fluid of choice for the first few feedings, since lung tissue reactions are less severe should aspiration occur. Feeding regimens are then established based on the weight and estimated stomach capacity of the infant (Table 31–1). In many instances it is necessary to supplement the oral feedings with parenteral fluids to maintain adequate hydration and caloric intake.

FORMULAS FOR PRETERM NEWBORNS

The formula of choice for feeding the preterm infant varies somewhat among institutions and areas of the country. However, most of the formulas contain protein with a whey/casein ratio of 60:40, a similar proportion to that found in breast milk, and a caloric value of 24 calories per ounce (Table 31–2). Initial feedings may be diluted to 12 calories per ounce and gradually increased, as the infant tolerates them, to 24-calorie formulas. Breast milk is widely used to feed preterm infants. Besides its many benefits for the infants, it allows the mother to contribute to the infant's well-being (Figure 31–5). It is a nursing responsibility to inform mothers of their option to breast-feed if they choose to do so. The nurse should be aware of the advantages and possible disadvantages of breast-feeding, such as decreased growth rate, hyponatremia, lactose intolerance, and rickets if breast milk is the sole source of food.

METHODS OF FEEDING

Various feeding methods are used for the preterm infant, depending on the infant's gestational age, health and physical condition, and neurologic status. The methods, criteria for selection, description, and nursing responsibilities associated with each method are summarized in the following sections.

○ **NIPPLE FEEDING** Nipple feeding is used in infants who are 34 weeks' gestation and have a coordinated suck and swallow reflex. Infants who are showing consistent weight gain (20 to 30 g per day) are also nipple fed, since they have the extra strength that sucking requires.

Method The infant feeds from a bottle. The feeding should take no longer than 15 to 20 minutes. A premature

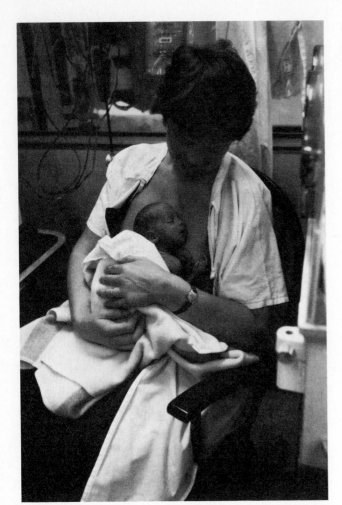

Figure 31–5   A mother visits the intensive care unit to breast-feed her preterm infant.

infant nipple or a regular-sized nipple may be used, depending on the infant's strength and ability (nippling requires more energy than other methods). The infant is fed in a semisitting position and burped gently after each half ounce or ounce.

Nursing Responsibilities   The infant's ability to suck is assessed. Sucking may be affected by age, asphyxia, sepsis, intraventricular hemorrhage or other neurologic insult. Before initiating nipple feeding, the infant is observed for any signs of stress, such as tachypnea (more than 60 respirations/min), respiratory distress, or hypothermia, which may increase the risk of aspiration. During the feeding, the infant should be observed for signs of difficulty with feeding (tachypnea, cyanosis, bradycardia, lethargy, and uncoordinated suck and swallow). After the feeding, the infant is gently burped and positioned on the right side or abdomen.

○   *GAVAGE FEEDING*   The gavage feeding method is used with preterm infants (less than 34 weeks' gestation) who lack or have a poorly coordinated suck and swallow reflex or are ill.

Gavage feeding may be used as an adjunct to nipple feeding if the infant tires easily or as an alternative if an infant is losing weight because of the energy expenditure required for nippling. It is also used when term or preterm infants are unable to nipple feed due to neurologic insult, such as asphyxia or CNS depression.

Method   An orogastric tube is passed into the infant's stomach. Correct placement of the tube is verified, and formula is passed through the tube into the infant's stomach (see Procedure 31–1 for description).

Nursing Responsibilities   See Procedure 31–1.

○   *TRANSPYLORIC, NASOJEJUNAL, OR NASODUODENAL TUBE FEEDING*   Transpyloric, nasojejunal, or nasoduodenal feeding by tube is used with very small preterm infants who are ventilator dependent or tachypneic, have chronic lung disease, recurrent aspiration, or repeated residuals with other methods of feeding.

Method   Transpyloric, nasojejunal, or nasoduodenal feeding involves a continuous infusion of formula into the duodenum or jejunum of the baby to prevent vomiting. An indwelling feeding tube is passed through the nostril, into the stomach, past the pylorus, and into the small intestine. Tube placement is confirmed by x-ray examination. A constant infusion pump is used to administer small amounts of formula continuously. The tube is left in place and changed every three days.

Potential Risks   Although this feeding method has advantages (for example, decreased risk of aspiration), it poses risks of stomach or intestinal perforation and accidental bolus infusion by the pump. In addition, formula bypasses the digestive activity of the stomach. The transpyloric method is never used in some centers, where the risks are believed to outweigh the benefits (Pereira & Lemons 1981).

Nursing Responsibilities   The nurse assists with the passing of the tube, observing the infant's vital signs and watching for any intolerance of the procedure. After feedings have begun, the nurse:

● Measures abdominal girth every two to three hours and prior to each feeding to check for distention

● Checks gastric residual every two to three hours (by oral tube inserted into stomach along with the feeding tube)

Procedure 31–1   Gavage Feeding

Objective	Nursing Action	Rationale
Ensure smooth accomplishment of the procedure.	Gather necessary equipment including: 1. No. 5 or No. 8 Fr. feeding tube 2. 10–30 mL syringe 3. ¼-in. paper tape 4. Stethoscope 5. Appropriate formula 6. Small cup of sterile water Explain procedure to parents.	Considerations in choosing size of catheter include size of the infant, area of insertion (oral or nasal), and rate of flow desired. The very small infant (less than 1600 g) requires a 5 Fr. feeding tube; an infant greater than 1600 g may tolerate a larger tube. Orogastric insertion is preferred over nasogastric insertion as most infants are obligatory nose breathers. If nasogastric insertion is used, a No. 5 catheter should be used to minimize airway obstruction. The size of the catheter will influence the rate of flow. The syringe is used to aspirate stomach contents prior to feeding, to inject air into the stomach for testing tube placement, and for holding measured amount of formula during feeding. Tape is used to mark tube for insertion depth as well as for securing tube during feeding. Stethoscope is needed to auscultate rush of air into stomach when testing tube placement. Sterile water may be used to lubricate feeding tube when inserted nasally. With oral insertion, there are enough secretions in the mouth to lubricate the tube adequately. The cup of sterile water may also be used to test for placement by placing the end of the tube into the water to check for air bubbles from the lungs. However, this test may not be accurate as air may also be present in the stomach (Avery 1987).

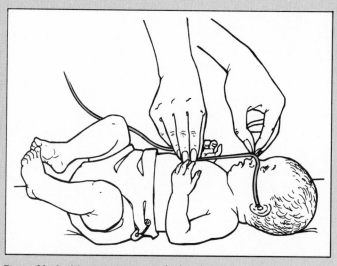

Figure 31–6   Measuring gavage tube length

Insert tube accurately into stomach.	Position infant on back or side with head of bed elevated.	This position allows easy passage of the tube.
	Take tube from package and measure the distance from the tip of the ear to the nose to the xiphoid process, and mark the point with a small piece of paper tape (Figure 31–6).	This measuring technique ensures enough tubing to enter stomach.
	If inserting tube nasally, lubricate tip in cup of sterile water. Shake excess drops to prevent aspiration.	Water should be used, as opposed to an oil-based lubricant, in case the tube is inadvertently passed into a lung.

Procedure 31-1 Gavage Feeding (continued)

Objective	Nursing Action	Rationale
	Stabilize infant's head with one hand, and pass the tube via the mouth (or nose) into the stomach, to the point previously marked. If the infant begins coughing or choking or becomes cyanotic or aphonic, remove the tube immediately.	Any signs of respiratory distress signal likelihood that tube has entered trachea. Orogastric insertion is less likely to result in passage into the trachea than nasogastric insertion.
	If no respiratory distress is apparent, lightly tape tube in position, draw up 0.5–1.0 mL of air in syringe, and connect it to tubing. Place stethoscope over the epigastrium and briskly inject the air (Figure 31–7).	Nurse should hear a sudden rush of air as it enters stomach.

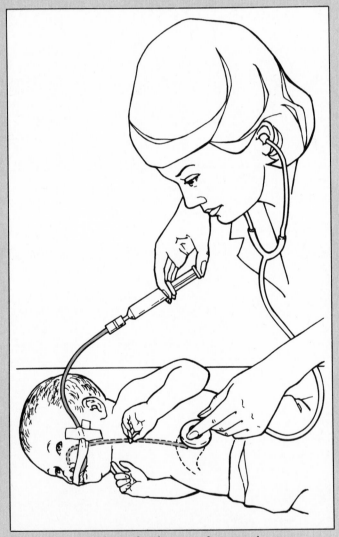

Figure 31–7 Auscultation for placement of gavage tube

Procedure 31–1 Gavage Feeding (continued)

Objective	Nursing Action	Rationale
	Aspirate stomach contents with syringe, and note amount, color, and consistency. Return residual to stomach unless otherwise ordered to discard it.	Residual formula should be evaluated as part of the assessment of infant's tolerance of gavage feedings. It is not discarded, unless particularly large in volume or mucoid in nature, because of the potential for causing an electrolyte imbalance.
	If only a clear fluid or mucus is found upon aspiration and if any question exists as to whether the tube is in the stomach, the aspirate can be tested for pH.	Stomach aspirate tests in the 1–3 range for pH.
Introduce formula into stomach without complication.	Hold infant for feeding or position on right side if infant cannot be held.	Positioning on side decreases the risk of aspiration in case of emesis during feeding.
	Separate syringe from tube, remove plunger from barrel, reconnect barrel to tube, and pour formula into syringe.	Feeding should be allowed to flow in by gravity. It should not be pushed in under pressure with a syringe.
	Elevate syringe 6–8 in. over infant's head. Allow formula to flow at slow, even rate.	Raising column of fluid increases force of gravity. Nurse may need to initiate flow of formula by inserting plunger of syringe into barrel just until formula is seen to enter feeding tube. Rate should be regulated to prevent sudden stomach distention, with possibility of vomiting and aspiration.
	Continue adding formula to syringe until desired volume has been absorbed. Then rinse tubing with 2–3 mL sterile water.	Rinsing tube ensures that infant receives all of formula. It is especially important to rinse tube if it is going to be left in place, because this decreases risk of clogging and bacterial growth in tube.
	Remove tube by loosening tape, folding the tube over on itself, and quickly withdrawing it in one smooth motion. If tube is to be left in, position it so that infant is unable to remove it.	Folding tube over on itself minimizes potential for aspiration of fluid, which would otherwise flow from tubing as it passes epiglottis. A tube left in place should be replaced at least every 24 hours.
Maximize feeding pleasure of infant.	Whenever possible hold infant during gavage feeding. If it is too awkward to hold infant during feeding, be sure to take time for holding afterward.	Feeding time is important to infant's tactile sensory input.
	Offer a pacifier to infant during feeding.	Infants fed for long periods by gavage can lose their sucking reflex. Sucking during feeding comforts and relaxes infant, making formula flow more easily. One study showed that infants allowed to suck during feedings were able to nipple sooner and were discharged earlier than a control group of infants who did not suck during tube feedings.

- Observes and records rate of infusion hourly to make sure the correct amount is infusing

- Changes infusion setup every eight hours to decrease chances of bacterial growth in the formula

- Ensures that no more than three hours' worth of formula is hung at one time to prevent "dumping" of excess formula

- Checks all stools for blood and glucose (signs of necrotizing enterocolitis)

○ *TOTAL PARENTERAL NUTRITION* Total parenteral nutrition (TPN) is used in situations that contraindicate feeding the infant through the GI tract. Contraindications include GI anomalies requiring surgical intervention, necrotizing enterocolitis, intolerance of feedings, and extreme prematurity.

Method The TPN method provides complete nutrition to the infant intravenously. Hyperalimentation gives calories, vitamins, minerals, protein, and glucose. Intralipids must also be administered to provide essential fatty acids. Hyperalimentation may be infused through either a central or a peripheral line. Intralipids may only be infused peripherally, and if added as a piggyback to the hyperalimentation, they must be piggybacked as close to the infusion site as possible and not through the filter.

Nursing Responsibilities The nurse needs to monitor serum glucose levels carefully during TPN. Urine is checked for protein, sugar, and specific gravity at least every eight hours. The intravenous rate is monitored hourly to maintain accurate intake (do not "catch up" if behind). The intravenous site should be observed hourly for signs of infiltration (hyperalimentation is extremely caustic and causes severe tissue destruction if it infiltrates). Fluid intake and output are carefully monitored (hyperglycemia causing an osmotic diuresis can lead to dehydration). The nurse observes for signs of reaction to intralipids, for example, dyspnea, vomiting, elevated temperature, or cyanosis.

Whichever method of feeding is selected for an infant, the nurse should carefully watch for any signs and symptoms of feeding intolerance, including:

- Increasing gastric residuals (more than 2 mL)

- Abdominal distention (measured routinely before feedings)

- Guaiac-positive stools (occult blood in stools)

- Presence of glucose in the stools

- Vomiting

- Diarrhea

FLUID REQUIREMENTS

Calculation of fluid requirements takes into account the infant's weight and postnatal age. Fluid is normally lost through urine, sweat, feces, and insensible water loss (lungs and skin). The preterm infant loses more fluid through the skin than the term infant because of decreased insulating fat and blood vessels close the surface. Higher environmental temperature, phototherapy, and radiant warmers may increase fluid loss an additional 50 percent.

Recommendations for fluid therapy in the preterm newborn are approximately 80 to 100 mL/kg/day for the first day of life; 100 to 120 mL/kg/day for day 2; and 120 to 150 mL/kg/day by day 3 of life. These amounts may be increased up to 200 mL/kg/day if the baby is very small, receiving phototherapy, or under a radiant warmer. The baby may need less fluid if a heat shield is used, the environment is more humid, or humidified oxygen is being provided.

Parameters that indicate adequate fluid and nutritional intake in the preterm newborn include:

1. Urine

   a. Volume at 1–3 mL/kg/hr
   b. Specific gravity at 1.006–1.013
   c. Absence of glycosuria when checked by Dipstix or Clinitest

2. Normoglycemic state

   a. Absence of hypoglycemia (Dextrostix value below 45 mg/dL) or clinical symptoms
   b. Absence of hyperglycemia (Dextrostix value above 130 mg/dL). Hyperglycemia may occur with glucose infusion greater than 10 percent or formula greater than 50 percent carbohydrate.

Research Note

Meier and Pugh's intensive study of the breast- and bottle-feeding behavior of three less-than-1500 g infants questioned the common assumption that breast-feeding is too strenuous for preterm infants and needs to be postponed until a certain weight is achieved. The infants in this study were 35 or more weeks' gestation. The researchers collected data by examining infant medical records, conducting unstructured interviews, and videotaping alternating breast- and bottle-feeding sessions.

The researchers found that while breast-feeding sessions took longer than bottle-feeding sessions (45 vs 15 minutes), the infants independently paced the feedings by alternating bursts of nutritive sucking with nonnutritive sucking and lengthy interactional periods. The infants showed no signs of distress during these feedings but did have increased incidents of gagging and burping during bottle-feedings. One baby had a longer period of bottle-feeding before initiation of breast-feeding and had much more difficulty adapting to the human breast.

Nurses working in NICUs need to be sensitive to the needs of these babies and of mothers who wish to breast-feed. The babies need a flexible feeding schedule so that they can nurse during an alert state when they can most effectively coordinate sucking and swallowing, and flexible feeding times to allow the baby to "self-pace." Breast-feeding should begin as soon as the baby can coordinate sucking and swallowing and can control body temperature outside of an Isolette regardless of weight.

Meier P, Pugh E: Breastfeeding behavior of small preterm infants. Am J Mat Child Nurs 1985;10(November/December):396–401.

3. Continued weight gain of 20 to 30 g per day (initially, no gain may be noted for several days, but total weight loss should not exceed 15 percent of the total body weight or more than 1 percent to 2 percent per day).

4. Normal blood pH 7.35 to 7.45

5. Some institutions add the criteria of head circumference growth and increase in body length of 1 cm/week, once the infant is stable.

Common Complications of Preterm Newborns and Their Medical Management

The goals of medical therapy are to meet the growth and development needs of the preterm newborn and to anticipate and manage the complications associated with prematurity. Complications associated with prematurity that require medical intervention are respiratory distress syndrome (RDS), patent ductus arteriosus (PDA), apnea, and intraventricular hemorrhage (IVH). Long-term problems include retinopathy of prematurity (ROP) and bronchopulmonary dysplasia (BPD).

An in-depth discussion of RDS and BPD, including pathophysiology, medical management, and nursing care, is contained in Chapter 32. Patent ductus arteriosus, apnea, intraventricular hemorrhage, retinopathy of prematurity, and other complications are discussed in this section.

PATENT DUCTUS ARTERIOSUS

Spontaneous closure of the connection between the aorta and pulmonary artery is often delayed in preterm newborns. It is more frequently seen in the larger (>1500 g), less severely ill newborns. The overall incidence of patent ductus arteriosus (PDA) is 20 percent with a 12 percent incidence of significant shunting of blood (Dooley 1984).

Emergence of a hemodynamically significant PDA is often evident around the third day of life when the premature infant is recovering from RDS. Initially, when the preterm neonate is hypoxic secondary to RDS, the pulmonary vascular resistance (PVR) may exceed the systemic resistance and right-to-left shunting through the ductus will occur. However, as the RDS improves and adequate oxygenation is maintained, the PVR will fall and the shunt will reverse to left-to-right flow. This significantly increases the pulmonary blood flow and leads to left ventricular volume overload, pulmonary edema, and congestive failure. Oxygenation is again compromised and ventilator requirements will increase, leading to the possibility of long-term pulmonary sequelae.

Ductal patency with left-to-right shunting is manifested as congestive heart failure with a continuous or systolic murmur, active precordium (visible heart pulsation), bounding pulses (increased pulse pressure), tachycardia, tachypnea, hepatomegaly, and pulmonary edema, which lead to signs of respiratory distress and continued oxygen and ventilator requirements. Chest radiographs reveal cardiomegaly with increased pulmonary vascularity.

Patency of the ductus arteriosus can be demonstrated by aortic contrast echocardiography. This technique visualizes microbubbles that result when saline is injected into an umbilical artery catheter as they pass left-to-right through the patent ductus. Since the left atrium and aorta are usually the same size, regular echocardiography can also demonstrate a patent ductus by determining an increase in left atrial size compared to the aortic root dimension.

The goal of medical therapeutic intervention is to achieve ductal closure. Early identification of symptomatic infants and prompt intervention will minimize long-term sequelae. Three methods are currently used, separately or in combination, to effect closure:

1. *Medical therapy.* Fluid is restricted and diuretics are used to reduce the effects of volume overload on the cardiovascular system. Digoxin was formerly used as part of medical therapy, but recent data suggests that it has little to offer the preterm infant with PDA and may have significant side effects (Dooley 1984).

2. *Pharmacologic therapy.* Administration of prostaglandin synthetase inhibitors such as indomethacin impairs synthesis of the E series prostaglandins responsible for dilatation of the ductus and can effect ductal closure. Indomethacin is effective, but it is not without side effects and must be used cautiously. Since it is protein bound it will compete with bilirubin for binding sites. In addition to impairing synthesis of E prostaglandins, indomethacin impairs synthesis of thromboxane A_2, which is responsible for platelet aggregation. Prolonged bleeding times after the initial dose persist until 48 hours after completion of a three-dose administration. However, clinical bleeding appeared to be limited to occult hematuria rather than to major hemorrhagic complications (Corrazza et al 1984).

Indomethacin administration is also associated with transient renal dysfunction, which is dose-related and reversible. Combined use of indomethacin and aminoglycosides leads to increased trough and peak levels of gentamicin if dose adjustment is not undertaken when renal dysfunction occurs (Zarfin et al 1985).

3. *Surgical therapy.* The ductus may be surgically ligated. A national collaborative study compared all

three therapies alone or in combination and followed the infants until one year of age (Gersony et al 1983, Peckham et al 1984). Results show the preferable mode of therapy in infants with hemodynamically significant PDA is a trial of medical therapy alone at the time of diagnosis followed by intravenous administration of indomethacin as backup therapy if indicated. Medical therapy alone was effective in approximately one-third of the cases. About 45 percent of the cases required indomethacin following a trial of medical therapy, and the remainder required surgical ligation. No significant differences in outcome (at one year of age) were identified with any of the therapies.

Patent ductus arteriosus will often prolong the course of illness in a preterm newborn and lead to chronic pulmonary dysfunction. Early identification is essential for prompt treatment to minimize the complications that may have long-term sequelae.

APNEA

Apnea (cessation of breathing for more than 20 seconds) is a common problem in the preterm infant (of less than 36 weeks' gestation) and is thought to be primarily a result of neuronal immaturity, a factor that contributes to the preterm infant's irregular breathing patterns. The immaturity of the preterm's CNS increases the baby's vulnerability to any adverse factors affecting nerve cell metabolism. Impaired nerve cell metabolism in turn can impair respiratory neurons in the brain stem. Factors that adversely affect brain nerve cells include hypoxia, acidosis, edema, intracranial bleeding, hyperbilirubinemia, hypoglycemia, hypocalcemia, and sepsis.

○ *NURSING RESPONSIBILITIES* Apneic onset is often insidious; cardiorespiratory monitoring allows for early recognition and intervention, thus decreasing the need for resuscitative efforts. The nurse checks during each shift to make sure alarms are set and working properly. Apnea may occur during feeding, suctioning, or while stooling. On the other hand, there may be no observable activity related to apnea. All episodes of apnea are documented. The documentation includes activity at the time of apnea, length of episode, and treatment required to bring the baby out of the apneic spell. This data is useful in determining etiology and possible treatment.

The nurse must make careful observations and quickly assess the need for intervention. The intervention required depends on the severity of the apneic episode and the baby's response. If an apneic episode occurs the nurse may:

1. Observe the infant briefly to see if treatment is necessary or if the infant will begin breathing spontaneously.

2. Begin stimulation by gently rubbing the soles of the feet, the ankles, and the infant's back. Rubbing bony prominences is uncomfortable to the infant and therefore more stimulating than rubbing other areas of the body.

3. Suction nasopharynx and oropharynx, provide additional oxygen, and prepare for bag and mask ventilation if the infant is dusky, cyanotic, or bradycardic. Obstruction of the airway by mucus or formula may result in apnea and bradycardia. Clearing the airway while providing increased oxygen concentration and stimulation may resolve apneic episode. If the infant does not respond, bag and mask ventilation may be required to relieve cyanosis and return heart rate to normal.

4. Prepare for intubation and use of the respirator for ventilation if the infant has frequent apneic episodes that require bag and mask ventilation. Ventilatory assistance may be necessary to prevent possible sequelae of frequent apneic spells with resulting hypoxemia.

5. Prepare for septic workup if the infant is not already on antibiotics.

6. Administer oxygen and warm humidified air per physician order to control dyspnea and cyanosis. Increased oxygen may alleviate episodes of apnea and bradycardia. Monitor and record the oxygen concentration every two hours.

7. Report and assess variations in blood gases and laboratory reports. Apnea is associated with elevated PCO_2, decreased PO_2, and other electrolyte imbalances.

8. Maintain thermal neutrality. Temperature instability may precipitate apnea.

Drug management includes administration of theophylline per physician order for intractable neonatal apnea. Theophylline acts as a CNS stimulant that increases respiratory drive and alveolar ventilation.

The care given an apneic baby should include gentle handling to prevent unnecessary stress on the baby. Keeping the airway clear is very important, but nasopharyngeal suctioning should be done gently and only as necessary, since it can cause apnea. Use of indwelling orogastric or nasogastric tubes is preferred to intermitent passage of feeding tubes. The nurse provides IV fluids as ordered to maintain adequate fluid and electrolyte balance. Severe apnea may preclude oral feeding for a time, and the infant may require nutritional maintenance with intravenous therapy. Adequate nutrition prevents catabolism of body tissues, as well as biochemical aberrations such as hypoglycemia, hyperglycemia, acidosis, or electrolyte imbalance. Following feedings, the baby should be positioned prone or supported on its right side with the head of the bed elevated.

INTRAVENTRICULAR HEMORRHAGE

Intraventricular hemorrhage (IVH) is the most common type of intracranial hemorrhage in the small preterm infant. Those most susceptible to IVH are infants weighing less than 1500 g or of less than 34 weeks' gestation. The incidence of intracranial hemorrhage in these newborns is approximately 50 percent (Kauffman 1986).

An IVH frequently occurs after an insult to the infant that results in hypoxia but may also be related to venous pressure changes and increases in osmolality in the bloodstream. Events leading to hypoxia include respiratory distress, birth trauma, and birth asphyxia, with the more immature infants being at higher risk for both of these complications. Hypoxia can cause abnormalities in autoregulation of cerebral blood flow that permit transmission of increased arterial pressure to the fragile cerebral arterioles. Autoregulation is the ability of the arterioles to maintain a stable cerebral blood flow by dilation in response to decreases in blood pressure and constriction in response to increases in blood pressure. Hypercapnia, a common complication of respiratory distress, causes vasodilation of the cerebral blood vessels, which increases the tendency to rupture. Volume expanders are sometimes required to reverse hypotension, which is not uncommon in the preterm infant, and leads to increased central venous pressure. Administration of sodium bicarbonate to relieve acidosis causes an increase in osmolarity, which also contributes to rupture of the tiny blood vessels within the brain.

The most common site of hemorrhage is in the periventricular subependymal germinal matrix where there is a rich blood supply and the capillary walls are thin and fragile (see p 951). In 85 percent of these cases, lumbar puncture will generally produce bloody spinal fluid with elevated protein and low glucose levels. Computerized axial tomography (CAT) or ultrasound scanning can be used to identify both the site and the extent of hemorrhage.

The clinical signs observed in an infant with IVH are variable. The infant may suddenly "crash" (characterized by pallor and shocklike appearance) and die or may show very subtle signs or no signs at all. The most common manifestations are neurological signs (hypotonia, lethargy, temperature instability, nystagmus, bulging fontanelle, falling hematocrit, apnea, bradycardia, hypotension, and a worsening in the respiratory condition (increasing hypoxia) with

metabolic acidosis. Seizures may occur, and decerebrate posturing may be observed.

Although the thrust of current research seems to be focused on preventive measures (Kauffman 1986), at present there are no proven methods to meet this goal. Therapeutic efforts include supportive care of the infant with an IVH and prevention or early recognition of posthemorrhagic hydrocephalus. Acute treatment of the infant with IVH depends to a large extent on the severity of the presenting symptoms. Hypoxemia, acidemia, and apnea should be corrected by adequate oxygenation, ventilation, and bicarbonate administration. Phenobarbital is administered to control seizures. Blood is administered as needed to normalize the hematocrit. Serial lumbar punctures or ventricular reservoirs have been used to relieve increased intracranial pressure and decrease CSF protein level. These techniques, however, have not been proved to prevent hydrocephalus. Many hemorrhages resolve spontaneously. However, placement of a ventriculoperitoneal shunt is required if progressive ventricular dilatation is documented.

The outcome for the infant depends on the size of the bleed and the gestational age of the infant. The most severe hemorrhages may cause motor deficits, hydrocephalus, hearing loss, and blindness. Less severe bleeds may have no observable sequelae (Hellmann & Vannucci 1982).

○   *NURSING RESPONSIBILITIES*   Nursing care of a newborn with IVH is mainly observational and supportive. All related parameters should be monitored closely (vital signs, fontanelle tenseness, seizure activity, hematocrit, blood pressure, and changes in muscle tone or activity). The nurse should prepare the infant and assist with lumbar puncture for spinal fluid analysis. While administering replacement whole blood or albumin, the nurse should monitor blood pressure. Thermal neutrality must be maintained. After a suspected bleed, the occipital frontal circumference should be checked closely as hydrocephalus may occur. The nurse also monitors for signs of increased intracranial pressure (apnea, bradycardia, hypotension). Serial head ultrasounds may be done.

In caring for the infant with an IVH, the nurse provides support for the parents by identifying their level of understanding and facilitating interdisciplinary communication with them. When infants suffer massive intraventricular hemorrhage, the option of no treatment may be considered, and the parents must be involved in this decision (Carey 1983). As a member of the interdisciplinary team, the nurse can identify the parents' needs and provide continuing supportive care.

RETINOPATHY OF PREMATURITY

Premature neonates are particularly susceptible to characteristic retinal changes known as retinopathy of prematurity (ROP). This disease has previously been referred to as retrolental fibroplasia (RLF), but the new term is gaining acceptance because it describes the phases of the condition more accurately.

Until recently ROP was thought to be exclusively the result of excessive use of oxygen in the treatment of premature infants. However, many authors have reported that ROP also occurs in premature infants who never received oxygen, in full-term infants with cyanotic congenital heart disease, and in certain other congenital anomalies. The disease is now viewed as multifactorial in origin.

Increased survival of VLBW infants may be the most important factor in the increased incidence of ROP. Infants weighing less than 1500 g, particularly those infants of less than 1000 g, are at greatest risk for increased incidence and severity of ROP. Recent data indicate an occurrence rate of about 7 percent in infants with birth weights in the 1000 to 1500 g range. In those with birth weights below 1000 g, the incidence can be as high as 42 percent. The susceptibility of these infants is thought to be due to many factors, including immaturity, a wide range of medical problems, and associated therapies (Lucey & Dangman 1984).

A new international classification of ROP has been developed to describe the disease and the extent of retinal changes (Committee for the Classification of Retinopathy of Prematurity 1984). International use of this classification will allow the collaborative clinical trials needed for further documentation of the disease and collection of data in current therapies.

The fetal retina is unique in that its vascularization does not begin until the fourth month of gestation, with the temporal peripheral area of retinal vasculature lagging in development. Vascularization is not completed until term. Consequently, the immature vascular system is susceptible to damage in the preterm neonate and occasionally in the term neonate. In the early, acute stages of ROP, immature retinal vessels constrict. If the vasoconstriction is sustained, vascular closure follows and irreversible capillary endothelial damage occurs. This disintegration of vessels is called vaso-obliteration. New vessels will eventually emerge from the point of vaso-obliteration, but they will lack normal structural integrity. In the later stages of ROP, vasoproliferation occurs as the new vessels erupt through the retina to proliferate into the vitreous body. The fragile vessels often rupture to produce retinal and vitreous hemorrhage. Scar tissue forms and traction may occur, leading to retinal detachment and subsequent blindness.

The goal of therapy is early identification and selective intervention. In the absence of therapeutic intervention, detection will at least enable early counseling and support of the parents when visual defects are suspected. Progressive vasoproliferation can be documented by serial ophthalmoscopic examinations. An initial fundal examination with an indirect ophthalmoscope should be performed between 4 and 8 weeks of age (Avery & Taeusch 1984). In 1974 the American Academy of Pediatrics recommended eye examinations for all infants of less than 36 weeks' gestation or all infants who weighed less than 2000 g and received oxygen therapy. Frequency of repeat examinations will depend on the rapidity of progression or the severity of the disease.

Preventive care is based on maintaining the small premature infant in as stable a physiologic condition as possible. Treatment of the acute stages of ROP with laser or cryotherapy is still experimental. Reports of effectiveness and side effects are varied. The treatment obliterates the neovascularization (new vessel formation) and reduces the traction that causes retinal detachment. Since most acute cases of ROP regress spontaneously with no long-term visual impairment, the possibility of regression must be weighed against the hazards of unproven treatment. Based on the new international classification of ROP, a multicenter study is currently being undertaken to test the effectiveness of cryotherapy when at least 50 percent risk for retinal detachment is suspected (Palmer & Phelps 1986).

When infants have suffered bilateral traction and retinal detachment, surgical vitrectomy and scleral buckling have been used experimentally. These surgeries are technically difficult due to the small size of the infant's eye. Since they are experimental, further follow-up is required for evaluation.

○   *NURSING RESPONSIBILITIES*   Nursing care for the visually impaired infant must concentrate on parental support and education. When the crisis of premature birth is quickly followed by the devastating news of suspected visual impairment or blindness, the parents will need extensive support by all members of the management team. The parents again experience overwhelming anxiety and uncertainty about their infant's future abilities.

Premature infants with blindness due to ROP may be at increased risk of cognitive and emotional problems. The evidence suggests that this increased risk may be due to environmental factors rather than to inherent intellectual or neurologic factors. Isolation, overprotectiveness, understimulation, and parental despair or emotional withdrawal may have accentuated the problems of blindness (Teplin 1983). Figure 31–8 demonstrates the "vicious cycle" leading to emotional and developmental problems that may arise when the problems of parental attachment to a premature infant are compounded by the news of visual impairment.

Nurses can prevent the development of this cycle by helping parents develop appropriate attachment behaviors. Parents can be assured that their infant will be able to recognize them by voice and touch. They must also be told that visually impaired infants may not show recognition or feeling by changes in facial expressions. They will need to

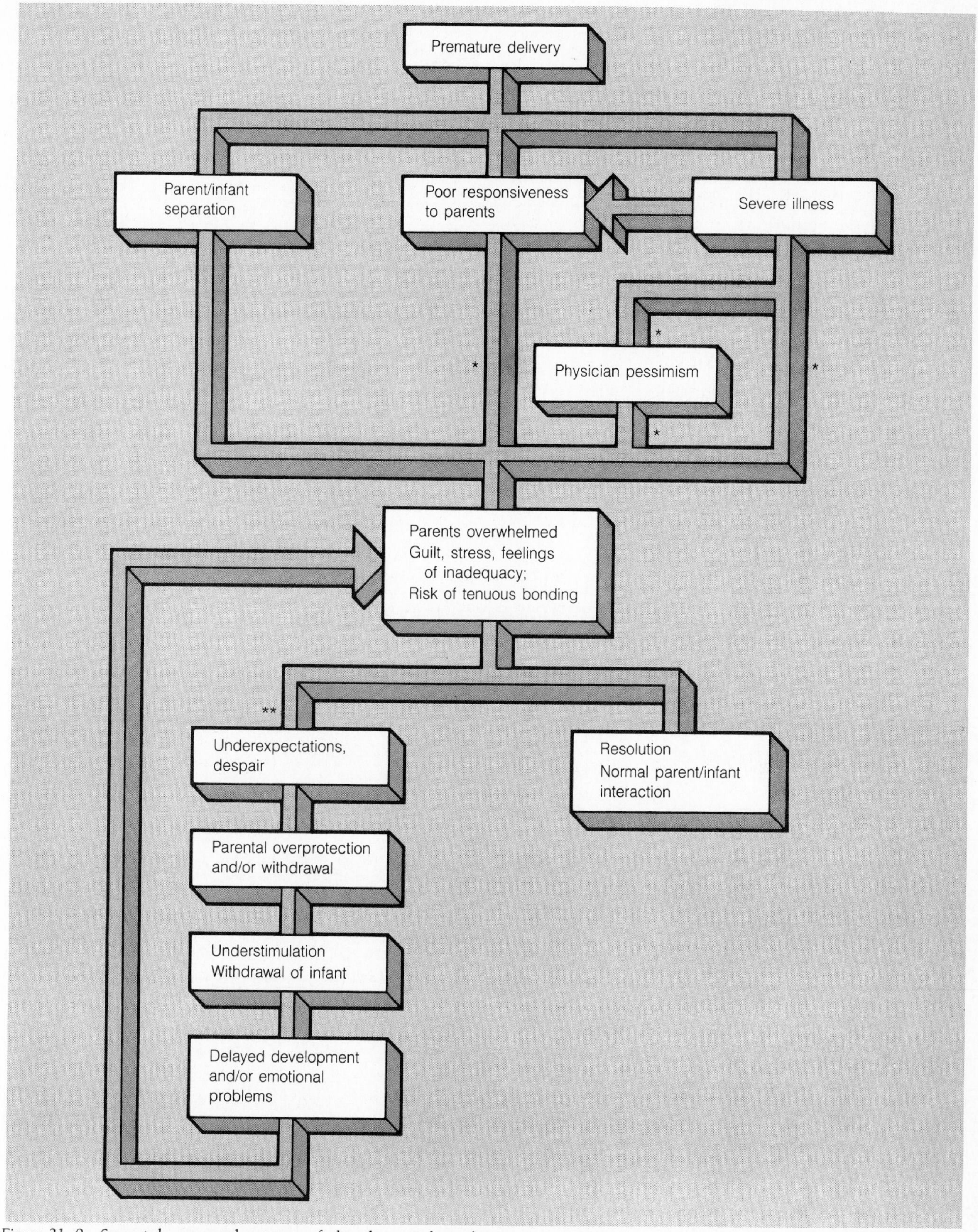

Figure 31–8 *Suggested causes and outcomes of altered parental attachment to premature infants with blindness due to ROP. A single asterisk indicates factors affecting attachment in all premature babies that are exacerbated by discovery of blindness. A double asterisk indicates onset of "vicious cycle" leading to emotional/developmental problems (pseudoretardation). (From Teplin SW: Development of blind infants and children with retrolental fibroplasia: Implications for physicians.* Pediatrics *1983;71:6)*

look for other cues or body language that their infant uses for self-expression.

In caring for the infant, the nurse can model specific developmental intervention activities and give the parents information on normal developmental milestones. Since the visually impaired chlid uses the other senses for exploration, parents can be taught specific activities to enhance their child's learning. Developmental goals and sample activities are listed in Table 31–3.

Prior to discharge, the management team should provide detailed information about and contacts with available community services and resource groups. Community agencies can provide support and direction for the parents as their child grows and new problems are encountered.

SENSORINEURAL HEARING LOSS

It is estimated that 1 in 50 preterm infants suffers a loss of hearing. Those at increased risk include infants with congenital viral infections, hyperbilirubinemia, perinatal asphyxia, and birth trauma. Damage from ototoxic drugs

such as gentamicin and furosemide (Lasix) is variable and related to multiple factors, including renal function, age, duration of treatment, and concomitant administration of other ototoxic agents (Eviator 1984).

SPEECH DEFECTS

The most frequently observed speech defects involve delayed development of receptive and expressive ability that may persist into the school-age years.

NEUROLOGIC DEFECTS

The most common neurologic defects include cerebral palsy, hydrocephalus, seizure disorders, lower IQ scores, and learning disabilities. However, the socioeconomic climate and family support systems have been shown to be important factors influencing the child's ultimate school performance in the absence of major neurologic defects (Vohr & Coll 1985).

When evaluating the infant's abilities and disabilities, it is important for parents to understand that the devel-

Table 31–3 Developmental Goals and Sample Activities for Blind Infants and Children (Partial Listing)

Goal	Sample activities toward goal
INFANTS (0–2 YR)	
Parent-infant emotional attachment	Early positive parent-infant contact during newborn-infant hospitalization Promotion of maximal holding, carrying, and talking to infant Social/emotional support of parents by family, professionals, parent groups
Active exploration of environment; improving tactile/auditory discrimination	Strengthening neck and trunk by encouraging prone position; discouraging prolonged supine lying Repetitive games to encourage reaching for sound cues Liberal exposure to new textures, sounds, smells, and sights (to encourage residual vision) Encouraging hands together in midline
Increasing independence and mobility	Encouraging self-feeding (despite mess) Encouraging tactile search for dropped toys Expecting/tolerating minor bumps, bruises
Language development	Parents' contingent "talking" to infant vocalizations Consistent and repetitive use of labels for objects, activities, body parts Prevention of prolonged exposure to noncontingent sound (eg, TV, radio)
PRESCHOOL-AGED (2–5 YR)	
Social interaction	Encouraging interaction with peers, including nonhandicapped (eg, nursery school) Setting behavioral limits
Self-help skills	Teaching specific techniques for toileting, dressing, bathing, etc
Mobility and orientation	Games that teach directional concepts (eg, up, down, under) Concrete techniques for safely walking in a room
Concepts/"real world" experiences	Frequent exposures to sounds/textures of everyday environments (eg, yard, grocery store, gas station)
EARLY SCHOOL-AGED (6–10 YR)	
Reading	Determination of optimal mode(s), ie, Braille, large-print, use of optical aids, recorded books
Improved orientation and mobility	Individualized orientation and mobility training

Source: Teplin SW: Development of blind infants and children with retrolental fibroplasia: Implications for physicians. *Pediatrics* 1983;71:10.

opmental level cannot be evaluated based on chronological age. Developmental progress must be evaluated from the expected date of birth, not from the actual date of birth. In addition, the parents need the consistent support of health care professionals in the long-term management of their infant. Many new and ongoing concerns arise as the high-risk infant grows and develops; the goal is to promote the highest quality of life possible.

LONG-TERM NEEDS AND OUTCOME

The care of the preterm infant and the family is not complete upon discharge from the nursery. Follow-up care is extremely important because many developmental problems are not noted until the infant is older and begins to demonstrate motor delays or sensory disability.

Within the first year of life, low-birth-weight preterm infants face higher mortality than term infants. Causes of death include sudden infant death syndrome (SIDS), which occurs about five times more frequently in the low-birth-weight infant, and respiratory infections and neurologic defects. Morbidity is also much higher among preterm infants, with those weighing less than 1500 g at highest risk for long-term complications.

Nursing Assessment

Accurate assessment of the physical characteristics and gestational age of the preterm newborn is imperative to anticipate the special needs and problems of this baby. Physical characteristics vary greatly depending on the gestational age, but the following characteristics are frequently present:

- Color—usually pink or ruddy but may be acrocyanotic; observe for cyanosis, jaundice, pallor, or plethora

- Skin—reddened, translucent, blood vessels readily apparent, lack of subcutaneous fat

- Lanugo—plentiful, widely distributed

- Head size—appears large in relation to body

- Skull—bones pliable, fontanelle smooth and flat

- Ears—minimal cartilage, pliable, folded over

- Nails—soft, short

- Genitals—small; testes may not be descended

- Resting position—flaccid, froglike

- Cry—weak, feeble

- Reflexes—poor sucking, swallowing, and gag

- Activity—jerky, generalized movements (seizure activity is abnormal)

Determination of gestational age in preterm newborns requires knowledge and experience in administering gestational assessment tools. The tool used should be specific, reliable, and valid. For a discussion of gestational age assessment tools, see Chapter 28.

Nursing Diagnosis

Nursing diagnoses that may apply to the preterm newborn include:

- Potential impairment of gas exchange related to newborn respiratory distress secondary to immature pulmonary vasculature

- Ineffective breathing patterns: apnea related to immature central nervous system

- Alteration in metabolic processes related to cold stress

- Alteration in cardiac output: decreased output secondary to activity intolerance

- Alteration in nutrition: less than body requirements related to weak suck and swallow reflexes

- Fluid volume deficit related to dehydration secondary to high insensible water losses

- Ineffective parental coping related to anger/guilt at having delivered a premature baby

Nursing Goal: Maintenance of Respiratory Function

There is increased danger of respiratory obstruction in preterm newborns because their bronchi and trachea are so narrow that mucus can obstruct the airway. The nurse must maintain patency through judicious suctioning.

Positioning of the newborn can also affect respiratory function. The nurse should slightly elevate the infant's head to maintain the airway. Because the newborn has weak neck muscles and cannot control head movement, the nurse should ensure that this head position is maintained. The nurse should avoid placing the infant in the supine position because the newborn has difficulty raising the chest due to weak chest and abdominal muscles. The prone position is best for facilitating chest expansion. Weak or absent cough or gag reflexes increase the chance of aspiration in the premature newborn. The nurse should ensure that the infant's position facilitates drainage of mucus or regurgitated formula.

The nurse monitors heart and respiratory rates with cardiorespiratory monitors and observes the newborn to identify alterations in cardiopulmonary status. Nursery nurses must be alert to signs of respiratory distress, including:

- Cyanosis—serious sign when generalized

- Tachypnea—sustained respiratory rate greater than 60/min after first four hours of life

- Retractions

- Expiratory grunting

- Flaring nostrils

- Apneic episodes

- Presence of rales or rhonchi on auscultation

- Inadequate breath sounds

The nurse who observes any of these alterations records and reports them for further evaluation. If respiratory distress occurs, the nurse administers oxygen per physician order to relieve hypoxemia. If hypoxemia is not treated immediately, it may result in patent ductus arteriosus or metabolic acidosis. If oxygen is administered to the newborn, the nurse monitors the oxygen concentration with devices such as the transcutaneous oxygen monitor (tcPO$_2$) or the pulseoximeter. Monitoring of oxygen concentration in the baby's blood is essential since hyperoxemia can lead to blindness (ROP, p 962).

The nurse must also consider respiratory function during feeding. To prevent aspiration and increased energy expenditure and oxygen consumption, the nurse must ensure that the infant's gag and suck reflexes are intact before initiating oral feedings. To minimize oxygen consumption, the body temperature must be maintained around 36.5C±0.2C (97.7F±0.5F).

Nursing Goal: Maintenance of Neutral Thermal Environment

Provision of a neutral thermal environment minimizes the oxygen consumption expended to maintain a normal core temperature; it also prevents cold stress and facilitates growth by decreasing the calories needed to maintain body temperature. The preterm infant's immature central nervous system provides poor temperature control, and stores of brown fat are decreased. A small infant (<1200 g) can lose 80 cal/kg/day through radiation of body heat.

The nurse can minimize heat loss and temperature instability effects by taking the following measures:

1. Warm and humidify oxygen without blowing it over the face to avoid increasing oxygen consumption.

2. Place the baby in a double-walled Isolette, and use a heat shield over small preterm infants.

3. Avoid placing the baby on cold surfaces such as metal treatment tables and cold x-ray plates; pad cold surfaces with diapers and use radiant warmers during procedures; and warm hands before handling the baby to prevent heat transfer via convection/conduction.

4. Warm the blood before exchange transfusions.

5. Keep the skin dry and place a cap on the baby's head to prevent heat loss via evaporation. (The head makes up 25 percent of the total body size.)

6. Keep Isolettes, radiant warmers, and cribs away from windows and cold external walls and out of drafts to prevent heat loss by radiation.

7. Use a skin probe to monitor the baby's skin temperature. The temperature should be 36C to 37C (96.8F to 97.7F). Temperature fluctuations indicate hypothermia or hyperthermia.

Nursing Goal: Maintenance of Fluid and Electrolyte Status

Maintenance of hydration is accomplished by providing adequate intake based on the neonate's weight, gestational age, chronological age, and volume of sensible and insensible water losses. Adequate fluid intake should provide sufficient water to compensate for increased insensible losses and to provide the amount needed for renal excretion of metabolic products. Insensible water losses can be minimized by providing a high ambient humidity, humidifying oxygen, using heat shields, covering the skin with plastic wrap, and placing the infant in a double-walled Isolette.

The nurse evaluates the hydration status of the baby by assessing and recording signs of dehydration. Signs of dehydration include sunken fontanelle, loss of weight, poor skin turgor (skin returns to position slowly), dry oral mucous membranes, decreased urine output, and increased specific gravity (>1.013). The nurse must also identify signs of overhydration by observing the newborn for edema or excessive weight gain and by comparing urine output with fluid intake.

The preterm infant should be weighed at least once daily at the same time each day. Weight change is one of the most sensitive indicators of fluid balance.

Intake and output is measured accurately. A comparison of intake and output measurements over an 8-hour or 24-hour period provides important information about renal function and fluid balance. Assessment of patterns and whether they show a net gain or loss over several days is also essential to fluid management. Blood serum levels and pH should be monitored to evaluate for electrolyte imbalances.

Accurate hourly intake calculations should be maintained when administering intravenous fluids. Since the preterm infant is unable to excrete excess fluid, it is important to maintain the correct amount of intravenous fluid to prevent fluid overload. This can be accomplished by using neonatal or pediatric infusion pumps. To prevent electrolyte imbalance and dehydration, care must be taken to give the correct IV solutions and volumes and concentrations of formulas. Urine specific gravity and pH are obtained periodically. Urine osmolality provides an indication of hydration, although this factor must be correlated with other assessments (for example, serum sodium). Hydration is considered adequate when the urine output is 1 to 3 cc/kg/hr.

Nursing Goal: Prevention of Infection

The nurse is responsible for minimizing the preterm newborn's exposure to pathogenic organisms. The preterm newborn is susceptible to infection because of an immature immune system and thin and permeable skin. Invasive procedures, techniques such as umbilical catheterization and mechanical ventilation, and prolonged hospitalization place the infant at greater risk for infection.

Strict hand washing, reverse isolation, and use of equipment for only one infant help minimize exposure of the preterm newborn to infectious agents. Many intensive care nurseries require a two- to three-minute scrub using iodined antibacterial solutions, which decrease growth of Gram-positive cocci and Gram-negative rod organisms. Other specific nursing interventions include limiting visitors; requiring visitors to wash their hands; and maintaining strict aseptic practices when changing intravenous tubing and solutions (IV solutions and tubing should be changed very 24 hours), administering parenteral fluids, and assisting with sterile procedures. Isolettes and radiant warmers should be changed weekly. There should be minimal use or avoidance of chemical skin preps and tape, which may cause skin trauma.

If infection (sepsis) occurs in the preterm newborn, the nurse may be the first to identify the subtle clinical signs associated with infection. The nurse informs the clinician of the findings immediately and implements the treatment plan per clinician orders in the presence of infection. For specific nursing care required for the newborn with an infection, see Chapter 32.

Nursing Goal: Provision of Adequate Nutrition and Prevention of Fatigue During Feeding

The first feeding may be sterile water in small amounts given every two to three hours. These small amounts are increased slowly by one to two mL. Formula or breast milk (with or without fortifiers to increase caloric content) is incorporated into the feedings slowly, initially may be at a quarter strength, then half strength, and so on. This is done to avoid overtaxing the digestive capacity of the preterm newborn.

Special formulas (eg, Similac Special Care, Preemie Enfamil) are used to meet the caloric needs of the preterm newborn. These special formulas are concentrated to supply more calories in less volume. Small, frequent feedings of high-calorie formula are used because the newborn has limited gastric capacity and decreased gastric emptying.

The feeding method depends on the feeding abilities and health status of the preterm newborn; see the discussion of various feeding methods on p 953. Both nipple and gavage methods are initially supplemented with intravenous therapy until oral intake is sufficient to support growth. Growth usually occurs when 120 to 150 cal/kg/day are provided, and this prevents metabolic catabolism and hypoglycemia. Growth is evaluated by an increase in weight, length, and body measurements.

The nurse must be watchful for any signs of respiratory distress or fatigue during feedings. Prior to each feeding, the nurse measures abdominal girth and auscultates the abdomen to determine the presence and quality of bowel sounds. Such assessments promote early detection of abdominal distention and decreased peristaltic activity, which may indicate necrotizing enterocolitis (NEC) or paralytic ileus. The nurse also checks for residual formula in the stomach prior to feeding. This is done when the newborn is fed by gavage or transpyloric method or in the presence of abdominal distention in a nipple-fed newborn. The presence of residual formula is an indication of intolerance to the type or amount of feeding or the increase in amount of feeding. Residual formula is usually readministered because digestive processes have already been initiated.

Preterm newborns who are ill or fatigue easily with nipple feedings are usually fed by gavage or transpyloric feeding. The infant is essentially passive with these methods, thus conserving energy and calories. As the baby matures, gavage feedings are replaced with nipple feedings to assist in strenthening the sucking reflex and meeting oral and emotional needs. The nurse establishes a nipple-feeding program that is begun and progresses slowly, such as one nipple feeding per day, then one nipple feeding per shift, and then a nipple feeding every other feeding. Daily weights are monitored because often there is a small weight loss when nipple feedings are started. After feedings, the baby is placed on the right side (with support to maintain this position) or on the abdomen. These positions enhance gastric emptying and decrease the chance of aspiration if regurgitation occurs. Gastroesophageal reflux is not uncommon in preterm newborns.

The nurse involves the parents in feeding their preterm baby. This is essential to the development of attachment between parents and infant. In addition, such involvement increases parental knowledge about the care of their infant and helps them cope with the situation.

Nursing Goal: Promotion of Parent-Infant Attachment

Preterm newborns are generally separated from their parents for prolonged periods. Illness or complications may be detected in the first few hours or days following birth. The resultant interruption in parent-newborn bonding necessitates intervention to ensure successful attachment of parent and child.

Nurses should take measures to promote positive parental feelings toward the newborn. Photographs of the baby are given to parents to have at home or to the mother if she is in a different hospital. The infant's name is placed on the Isolette as soon as it is known to help the parents feel that their infant is a unique and special person. The telephone number of the nursery and/or intensive care unit and names of staff members are given to parents so that they have access to information about their baby at any time of day or night. Equipment and therapies are explained to parents, and the explanations are repeated as often as necessary to familiarize them with the treatment and decrease their anxiety.

Parents are included in determining the baby's plan of care. Early involvement in the care and decisions regarding their baby provide parents with realistic expectation for their baby. Their daily participation (if possible) is encouraged, as are early and frequent visits. The nurse provides opportunities for parents to touch, hold, talk to, and care for the baby. Parents are started with simple tasks, based on the nurse's assessment of the parent's skill and coping abilities. Early success in performing simple tasks builds parents' confidence in their care-taking abilities.

The rhythmic tides of her sleeping and feeding spaciously measured her days and nights. Her frail absorption was a commanding presence, her helplessness strong as a rock. (Laurie Lee, *Two Women*)

Nursing Goal: Promotion of Sensory Stimulation

Within the past 20 years, increased attention has been given to the infant's need for sensory stimulation. Evidence suggests that the infant who receives tactile, kinesthetic, and auditory stimulation has fewer apneic spells, decreased stooling, improved weight gain, and advanced CNS functioning (Klaus & Kennell 1982).

With prolonged separation and the NICU environment, individualized baby sensory stimulation programs are necessary. The nurse plays a key role in determining the appropriate type and amount of sensory (visual, tactile, and auditory) stimulation.

New research into the unique behavioral characteristics of the preterm infant highlight many responses that reflect disorganization of the autonomic system. This work suggests that some preterm infants are not developmentally able to deal with more than one sensory input at a time. The Assessment of Preterm Infant Behavior (APIB) scale (Als et al 1982) identifies the individual preterm newborn behaviors according to five areas of development. The preterm baby's behavioral reactions to stimulation are observed, and developmental interventions are then based on reducing stress and optimizing the newborn's behavioral organization (Cole & Frappier 1985). Parents are ideally equipped to meet the baby's need for stimulation. Stroking, rocking, cuddling, singing, and talking can all be an integral part of the baby's care. Visual stimulation in the form of mobiles and en face interaction with the caregiver are also important. Teaching the parents to read behavioral cues will help them move at their infant's own pace when providing stimulation.

Nursing Goal: Preparation for Discharge

Parents of preterm babies should receive the same postpartal teaching as any parent taking a new infant home. In preparing for discharge, parents are encouraged to spend time just before discharge caring directly for their baby. This familiarizes the parents with their baby's behavior patterns and helps them establish realistic expectations about the infant.

Discharge instruction includes breast- and bottle-feeding techniques, formula preparation (including bottle sterilization), and vitamin administration. Mothers of preterm babies desiring to breast-feed are taught to pump their breasts to keep the milk flowing and provide milk even before discharge. This activity (pumping) allows breast-feeding after discharge from the hospital. Information on bathing, diapering, hygiene, and normal elimination patterns is given. Parents should be told to expect changes in the color of the baby's stool, number of bowel movements, and timing of elimination when the infant is switched from bottle to breast-feeding. This information can prevent unnecessary concern by the parents. Normal growth and development patterns, reflexes, and activity for preterm infants are discussed. Care of the preterm infant with complications, prevention of infections, and the need for continued medical follow-up are emphasized.

Families with preterm infants usually do not need to be referred to community agencies, such as visiting nurse assistance. Referral may be necessary if the infant has severe congenital abnormalities, feeding problems, or complications with infections or respiratory problems, or if the parents seem unable to cope with an at-risk baby. Parents of preterm infants can benefit from meeting with others in a similar situation to share common experiences and concerns. Nurses can refer parents to support groups sponsored by the hospital or by others in the community.

Evaluative Outcome Criteria

Nursing care is effective if:

- The preterm newborn is free of respiratory distress and establishes effective respiratory function.

- The preterm newborn gains weight and shows no signs of fatigue and/or aspiration during feedings.

- The parents are able to verbalize their anger and guilt feelings about the birth of a preterm baby and show attachment behavior such as frequent visits and growing confidence in their participatory care activities.

● Care of the Postterm Newborn

The postterm newborn is any newborn delivered after 42 weeks' gestation (product of a prolonged pregnancy). In the past, the terms *postterm* and *postmature* were used interchangeably. The term *postmature* is now used only when the infant is delivered after 42 weeks of gestation and also demonstrates characteristics of the *postmaturity syndrome* (Hendriksen 1985).

Prolonged pregnancy occurs in approximately 3.5 percent to 10 percent of all pregnancies (Hobart & Depp 1982). The cause of postterm pregnancy is not completely understood, but several factors are known to be associated with it, including primiparity, high multiparity (more than four), and a history of prolonged pregnancies (Affonso & Harris 1980). Many pregnancies classified as prolonged are thought to be due only to inaccurate obstetrical dates.

Most babies born as a result of prolonged pregnancy are of normal size and health; some keep on growing and are over 4000 g, which supports the premise that the postterm fetus can remain well nourished. Intrapartal problems for these healthy but large fetuses are CPD and shoulder dystocia. At birth about 5 percent of postterm newborns show signs of postmaturity syndrome (Oxorn 1986). The major portion of the following discussion will address the fetus who is not tolerating the prolonged pregnancy, is suffering from uteroplacental compromise to blood flow and resultant hypoxia, and is considered to have postmaturity syndrome.

Common Complications of the Postmature Syndrome Newborn

The truly postmature newborn is at high risk for morbidity and has a mortality rate two to three times greater than term infants. The majority of deaths occur during labor, since by that time the fetus has used up necessary reserves. Because of decreased placental function, oxygenation and nutrition transport are impaired, leaving the fetus prone to hypoglycemia and asphyxia when the stresses of labor begin. The problems in surviving postmature babies are caused by inadequate placental function, decreased oxygen and glucose reserves, and the stress of labor. The most common disorders of the postmature newborn are:

- Hypoglycemia, from nutritional deprivation and resultant depleted glycogen stores.

- Meconium aspiration in response to in utero hypoxia. In the presence of oligohydramnios the meconium cannot be diluted and the danger of aspirating thick meconium is increased. Severe meconium aspiration syndrome increases the baby's chance of developing persistent fetal circulation and pneumothorax (see Chapter 32).

- Polycythemia due to increased production of RBCs in response to hypoxia.

- Congenital anomalies of unknown cause.

- Seizure activity because of hypoxic insult.

- Cold stress because of loss or poor development of subcutaneous fat.

The long-term effects of postmaturity syndrome are unclear. At present studies do not agree on the effect of postmaturity syndrome on weight gain and IQ scores.

Medical Therapy

The goal of medical therapy is identification and management of the postmature newborn's potential problems.

Antenatal management is directed at differentiating the fetus who has postmaturity syndrome from the fetus who at birth is large, well-nourished, and equally alert and has experienced an equally long gestation. Table 31–4 depicts a system that attempts to distinguish in utero the fetus who may have postmaturity syndrome and requires intervention from the healthy fetus who is tolerating the prolonged (postterm) pregnancy.

Antenatal tests that can be done to evaluate fetal status and determine obstetrical management include fetal ultrasound, and the NST and CST. These tests and their use in postterm pregnancy are discussed in more depth in Chapters 20 and 25.

If the amniotic fluid is meconium stained, the baby's airway should be suctioned by the clinician prior to deliv-

Table 31-4   Evaluation of Fetal Status in True Prolonged Pregnancy

Clinical parameters	Positive	Guarded	Negative
Uterine size	Increasing	No increase	Decreasing
Amniotic fluid volume	Appropriate	Diminished	Oligohydramnios
Fetal activity	Unchanged	Diminished	Absent
Maternal weight	Increasing	Decreasing	
Estriol levels	Stable/increasing	Chronically low	Decrease ≥35%
Ultrasound (growth-adjusted sonographic age)	Maintenance of growth percentile	Decrease in growth percentile	Cessation of growth
Nonstress test	Reactive	Nonreactive: spontaneous variables	Spontaneous late deceleration
Oxytocin challenge test	Negative	Ambiguous: variable decelerations	Positive
Intrapartum monitoring	Baseline 100–140 beats/min, normal pattern, variability of 6–15 beats/min	Baseline <150 beats/min, decreased variability, variable decelerations	Baseline <150 beats/min, absent variability, repetitive late decelerations

From Hobart JM, Depp R: Prolonged pregnancy, in Sciarra JJ (ed): *Gynecology and Obstetrics*. Philadelphia, Harper & Row, 1982, p 5.

ery of the chest and trunk and before the baby takes its first breath to minimize the chance of meconium aspiration syndrome. For detailed discussion of medical management and nursing assessments and care, see Chapter 32.

Hypoglycemia is monitored by serial glucose determinations. The baby may be placed on glucose infusions or given early feedings if respiratory distress is not present. Postmature newborns are often voracious eaters.

Peripheral and central hematocrits are tested to assess the presence of polycythemia. Oxygen is provided for respiratory distress. A partial exchange transfusion may be necessary to prevent adverse sequelae such as hyperviscosity.

Nursing Assessment

The newborn with postmaturity syndrome appears alert. This wide-eyed, alert appearance is not necessarily a positive sign as it may indicate chronic intrauterine hypoxia.

The infant has dry, cracking, parchmentlike skin without vernix or lanugo (Figure 31–9). Fingernails are long, and scalp hair is profuse. The infant's body appears long and thin. The wasting involves depletion of previously stored subcutaneous tissue causing the skin to be loose. Fat layers are almost nonexistent.

Postmature newborns frequently have meconium staining, which colors the nails, skin, and umbilical cord. The varying shades (yellow to green) of meconium staining can give some clue about whether the expulsion of meconium was a recent or chronic, long-standing event.

Prolonged pregnancy itself is not responsible for the postmaturity syndrome. The previously described characteristics of the postmature newborn are primarily caused by a combination of advanced gestational age, placental

insufficiency, and continued exposure to amniotic fluid (Clifford 1957).

Nursing Diagnosis

Nursing diagnoses that may apply to the postmature newborn include:

- Potential for cellular injury related to hypothermia secondary to decreased liver glycogen and brown fat stores
- Alteration in nutrition: less than body requirements related to increased use of glucose secondary to in utero stress
- Alteration in exchange of oxygen and carbon dioxide in the lungs and at the cellular level related to airway

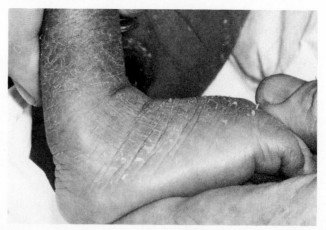

Figure 31–9   The postterm infant has deep cracking and peeling of skin.

obstruction from potential meconium aspiration in utero

Nursing Goal: Promotion of Physical Well-Being

Nursing interventions are primarily supportive measures.

They include the following:

- Observation of cardiopulmonary status, since the stresses of labor are poorly tolerated and severe asphyxia can ensue at birth

- Provision of warmth to counterbalance poor response to cold stress and decreased liver glycogen and brown fat stores

- Frequent monitoring of blood glucose and initiation of early feeding (at 1 or 2 hours of age) or intravenous glucose per physician order

- Observation for the common disorders identified earlier and institution of nursing care and medical management as ordered

Nursing Goal: Provision of Emotional Support to the Parents

The nurse encourages parents to express their feelings and fears regarding the newborn's condition and potential long-term problems. For further discussion, see p 990.

Evaluative Outcome Criteria

Nursing care is effective if:

- The postterm newborn establishes effective respiratory function.

- The postmature baby is free of metabolic alterations (hypoglycemia) and maintains a stable temperature.

● Care of the Small-for-Gestational-Age (SGA) Newborn

A small-for-gestational-age (SGA) newborn is any newborn who at birth is at or below the tenth percentile (intrauterine growth curves) on the newborn classification chart (Figure 31–1). It should be noted that intrauterine growth charts are influenced by altitude and ethnicity. When assigning SGA classification to a newborn, birth weight charts should be based on the local population into which the newborn is born (Guidelines for Perinatal Care 1983). An SGA newborn may be preterm, term, or postterm. Other terms used to designate a growth-retarded

newborn include *intrauterine growth retarded* (IUGR), *small for dates* (SFD), and *dysmature*. For this discussion, SGA and IUGR will be used interchangeably.

Between 3 percent and 7 percent of all pregnancies are complicated by IUGR. Growth-retarded infants have a fivefold greater incidence of perinatal asphyxia and an eightfold higher perinatal mortality than normal infants (Hobbins 1982).

Causes of Growth Retardation

The causes of IUGR may be maternal, placental, or fetal factors and may not be apparent antenatally. Intrauterine growth is linear in the normal pregnancy from approximately 28 to 38 weeks' gestation. After 38 weeks, growth is variable, depending on the growth potential of the fetus and placental function. The most common causes of growth retardation are:

- *Malnutrition.* Maternal nutrition has not been found to influence the birth weight of the newborn significantly unless starvation occurs during the last trimester of pregnancy. Before the third trimester, the nutritional supply far exceeds the needs of the fetus. By the third trimester the nutritional supply becomes a limiting factor to fetal growth.

- *Vascular complications.* Complications associated with PIH (preeclampsia and eclampsia), chronic hypertensive vascular disease, and advanced diabetes mellitus cause diminished blood flow to the uterus.

- *Maternal disease.* Maternal heart disease, substance abuse (drugs and alcohol), sickle cell anemia, phenylketonuria, and asymptomatic pyelonephritis are associated with SGA.

- *Maternal factors.* Factors such as small stature, primiparity, grand multiparity, smoking, lack of prenatal care, age (<16 or >40), and low socioeconomic class (which can result in poor health care), poor education, and poor living conditions are associated with SGA.

- *Environmental factors.* Such factors include high altitude, x rays, and maternal use of drugs, such as antimetabolics, anticonvulsants, and trimethadione, which have teratogenic effects.

- *Placental factors.* Placental conditions such as infarcted areas, abnormal cord insertions, single umbilical artery, placenta previa, or thrombosis may affect circulation to the fetus, which becomes more deficient with increasing gestational age.

- *Fetal factors.* Congenital infections (rubella, toxoplasmosis, syphilis, cytomegalic inclusion disease) or malformations, multiple pregnancy (twins or triplets), discordant twins, chromosomal syndromes, and inborn errors of metabolism can predispose a fetus to IUGR.

Antenatal identification of fetuses with IUGR is the first step in the detection of common disorders of the SGA newborn. The perinatal history of maternal conditions and examination of the placenta and newborn are also important in identifying this at-risk newborn.

Patterns of Intrauterine Growth Retardation (IUGR)

Growth occurs in two ways: increase in cell number and increase in cell size. If the insult occurs early, during the critical period of organ development in the fetus, fewer new cells are formed, organs are small, and organ weight is subnormal. In contrast, growth failure that begins later in pregnancy affects not the total number of cells but only their size. The organs are normal, but their size is diminished.

There are two clinical pictures of SGA newborns. These clinical presentations are classified as either symmetric (proportional) IUGR or asymmetric (disproportional) IUGR.

Symmetric IUGR is caused by long-term maternal conditions (such as chronic hypertension, severe malnutrition, chronic intrauterine infection, substance abuse, and anemia) or fetal genetic abnormalities (Bree & Mariona 1980). Symmetric IUGR can be noted by ultrasound in the first half of the second trimester with its onset prior to 32 weeks' gestation. In symmetric IUGR there is chronic prolonged retardation of growth in size of organs, weight, length, and, in severe cases, head circumference.

Asymmetric IUGR is associated with an acute compromise of uteroplacental blood flow. Some associated causes are placental infarcts, PIH, and poor weight gain in pregnancy. The growth retardation is usually not evident before the third trimester. Asymmetric IUGR can be detected on ultrasound after 36 weeks, when the size of the head of a normal fetus becomes smaller than the abdominal circumference. In asymmetric IUGR, the head circumference remains larger than the abdominal circumference. Thus measuring only the biparietal diameter on ultrasound will cause a failure to detect asymmetric IUGR (Oxorn 1986).

Birth weight is reduced below the 10th percentile, whereas cephalic size may be between the 15th and 90th percentile. Asymmetric SGA neonates are particularly at risk for perinatal asphyxia, pulmonary hemorrhage, hypocalcemia, and hypoglycemia in the neonatal period (Bree & Mariona 1980).

Despite growth retardation, physiologic maturity develops according to gestational age. Therefore, the SGA newborn may be more physiologically mature than the pre-term AGA newborn and less predisposed to complications of prematurity such as respiratory distress syndrome and hyperbilirubinemia. The SGA newborn's chances for survival are better because of organ maturity, although this newborn still faces many other potential difficulties in the newborn period and long-term problems.

Common Complications of the SGA Newborn

The problems occurring most frequently in the SGA newborn include:

- *Perinatal asphyxia.* The SGA infant suffers chronic hypoxia in utero, which leaves little reserve to withstand the demands of normal labor and delivery. Thus intrauterine asphyxia occurs with its potential systemic problems.

- *Aspiration syndrome.* In utero hypoxia can cause the fetus to gasp during delivery, resulting in aspiration of amniotic fluid into the lower airways. Hypoxia can also lead to relaxation of the anal sphincter and passage of meconium. This can result in aspiration of the meconium from the oropharynx with the first few breaths after birth.

- *Heat loss.* Diminished subcutaneous fat (used for survival in utero), depletion of brown fat in utero, and a large surface area decrease the IUGR newborn's ability to conserve heat. The effect of surface area is diminished somewhat because of the flexed position assumed by the term SGA newborn.

- *Hypoglycemia.* The high metabolic rate (secondary to heat loss and poor hepatic glycogen stores) of the SGA infant causes hypoglycemia. In addition, the infant is compromised by inadequate supplies of enzymes to activate gluconeogenesis (conversion of nonglucogen sources such as fatty acids and proteins to glucose).

- *Hypocalcemia.* Decreased calcium levels occur secondary to birth asphyxia and preterm birth.

- *Polycythemia.* The number of red blood cells is increased in the SGA newborn. This finding is considered a physiologic response to in utero chronic hypoxic stress

Infants who have significant IUGR tend to have a poor prognosis, especially when born before 37 weeks' gestation. Factors contributing to poor outcome for these infants are as follows:

- *Congenital malformations.* Congenital malformations occur 10 to 20 times more frequently in SGA infants than in AGA infants. The more severe the IUGR, the greater the chance for malformation as a result of impaired mitotic activity and cellular hypoplasia.

- *Intrauterine infections.* When infants are exposed to intrauterine infections such as rubella and cytomegalovirus, they are profoundly affected by direct invasion of the brain and other vital organs by the offending virus.

- *Continued growth difficulties.* It is generally agreed that SGA newborns tend to be shorter than newborns of the same gestational age but will have appropriate size growth. Miller (1985) reports that asymmetrical IUGR infants can be expected to catch up in weight to normal growth infants by 3 to 6 months of age. Symmetric SGA infants reportedly have varied growth potential but tend not to catch up to their peers. It is important to remember that the rate of growth during the newborn's first year of life remains the best predictor of later growth potential (Avery & Taeusch 1984).

- *Learning difficulties.* Often SGA newborns exhibit poor brain development and subsequent failure to catch up, and minimal cerebral dysfunction is not uncommon. Dysfunction is characterized by hyperactivity, short attention span, and poor fine motor coordination (reading, writing, and drawing). Poor scholastic performance is also a common problem (Parkinson et al 1981). Some hearing loss and speech defects also occur.

Korones (1986) reported that SGA newborns born into families of high socioeconomic levels do as well as their peers at age 10 to 12 years while, at the same age, SGA neonates from families of low socioeconomic levels function below their peers. This finding suggests that the environment of the symmetrical SGA neonate can play a vital role in long-term outcome.

Medical Therapy

The goal of medical therapy is early recognition and implementation of medical management of the potential problems associated with SGA babies.

Nursing Assessment

The nurse is responsible for assessing gestational age and identifying signs of potential complications associated with SGA infants.

All body parts of the symmetric IUGR infant are in proportion, but they are below normal size for the baby's gestational age. Therefore the head does not appear overly large or the length excessive in relation to the other body parts. These newborns are generally vigorous (Korones 1986).

The asymmetric IUGR infant appears long, thin, and emaciated, with loss of subcutaneous fat tissue and muscle mass. The baby has loose skin folds; dry, desquamating skin; and a thin and often meconium-stained cord. The head appears relatively large (although it approaches normal size) because the chest size and abdominal girth are decreased. The baby may have a vigorous cry and appear deceptively alert (Figure 31–10).

Nursing Diagnosis

Nursing diagnoses that may apply are included in the Nursing Care Plan beginning on p 974.

Nursing Goal: Promotion of Physical Well-Being

Hypoglycemia, the most common metabolic complication of IUGR, produces such sequelae as CNS abnormalities and mental retardation. In addition to hypoglycemia, conditions such as asphyxia, hyperviscosity, and cold stress may also affect the baby's outcome. Meticulous attention to physiologic parameters is essential for immediate nursing management and reduction of long-term disorders (see the Nursing Care Plan, p 975).

Nursing Goal: Provision of Follow-Up Care

The long-term needs of the SGA newborn include scrupulous follow-up evaluation of patterns of growth and possible disabilities that may later interfere with learning or motor functioning. Long-term follow-up care is especially necessary for those infants with congenital malformations, congenital infections, and obvious sequelae from physiologic problems. In addition, the parents of the IUGR neonate need support, because a positive atmosphere can

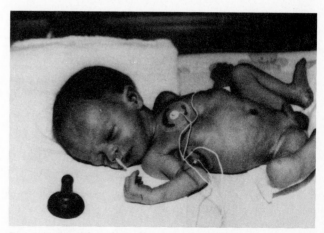

Figure 31–10 The infant with symmetric IUGR appears long, thin, and emaciated. The gestational age of the infant shown here is 41 weeks. He weighed approximately 1560 g at birth.

Nursing Care Plan: SGA Newborn

Julie Adams was born at 40 weeks' gestation by maternal dates and confirmed by gestation age assessment. Her asymmetric IUGR was evidenced by a weight of 1800 g, length of 49 cm, and head circumference of 34 cm (of these only the weight falls below the tenth percentile for this gestational age). Julie's mother is a 24-year-old G1 P1 and was diagnosed as having PIH at 37 weeks' gestation. She is a smoker and had a marginal placenta previa. Amniotic fluid was meconium stained and Apgars were 5 at 1 minute and 7 at 5 minutes.

Assessment

NURSING HISTORY	LABORATORY EVALUATION
Identification of predisposing factors include: a. PIH b. Smoking c. Low socioeconomic class d. Placental previa	a. Dextrostix less than 35 mg/dL b. Venous hematocrit of 68%
PHYSICAL EXAMINATION	ANALYSIS AND NURSING PRIORITIES
a. Large-appearing head in proportion to chest and abdomen b. Loose dry skin c. Long, thin, emaciated appearance, scarcity of subcutaneous fat d. Sparse scalp hair e. Vigorous cry and very alert appearance	a. Support effective breathing. b. Provide a neutral thermal environment. c. Provide for adequate nutrition and fluid needs. d. Protect from infection. e. Observe for signs of meconium aspiration, hypoglycemia, polycythemia, and metabolic alteration resulting from cold stress. f. Support emotional well-being of Julie's parents, facilitate parent-newborn bonding, and provide sensory stimulation for Julie.

Nursing Diagnosis and Goals	Nursing Interventions	Rationale
NURSING DIAGNOSIS: Impaired gas exchange related to meconium aspiration	Maintain airway patency through judicious suctioning.	Respiratory distress in SGA newborns is due to in utero hypoxia and aspiration of meconium.
SUPPORTING DATA: Julie has had a sustained respiratory rate above 60 resp/min, intermittent cyanosis, sternal retractions, expiratory grunting, and nasal flaring.	Maintain adequate body temperature (36C±0.2C (97.7F±0.5F)) to avoid increased oxygen consumption. Observe for worsening signs of respiratory distress such as generalized cyanosis; worsening retractions, grunting, and nasal flaring, as evidenced by Silverman respiratory index; sustained tachypnea; apnea episodes; inequality of breath sounds; presence of rales and rhonchi. Administer oxygen per order for relief of respiratory distress signs (see Chapter 32 for nursing care and treatment of meconium aspiration, infant resuscitation). Implement treatment plan for respiratory distress. Monitor glucose levels.	Respiratory distress increases consumption of glucose.
GOAL: Julie's respirations will be 30–50/min with no periods of apnea or evidence of worsening distress.		
NURSING DIAGNOSIS: Potential for injury related to impaired thermoregulatory mechanisms and cold stress secondary to decreased subcutaneous fat	Provide NTZ range for Julie based on her postnatal weight.	Neutral thermal environment charts used for preterm infant are not reliable for weight of SGA infant.
SUPPORTING DATA: Provision of appropriate neutral thermal environment since birth has assisted Julie in maintaining her temperature.	Use a skin probe to maintain Julie's skin temperature at 36C–36.5C.	A neutral thermal environment requires minimal oxygen consumption to maintain a normal core temperature.

Nursing Care Plan: SGA Newborn (continued)

Nursing Diagnosis and Goals	Nursing Interventions	Rationale
	Obtain axillary temps and compare to registered skin probe temp. If discrepancy exists evaluate potential cause.	Discrepancies between axillary and skin probe monitor temp may be due to mechanical causes or the burning of brown fat.
	Adjust and monitor incubator or radiant warmer to maintain skin temperature.	
	Minimize heat losses and prevent cold stress by: 1. Warming and humidifying oxygen without blowing over face in order to avoid increasing oxygen consumption 2. Keeping skin dry 3. Keeping isolettes, radiant warmers, and cribs away from windows and cold external walls and out of drafts 4. Avoiding placing infant on cold surfaces such as metal treatment tables, cold x-ray plates 5. Padding cold surfaces with diapers and using radiant warmers during procedures 6. Warming blood for exchange transfusions	
	Observe for signs and symptoms of cold stress: decreased temperature, lethargy, pallor (for further discussion see p 1033)	Physical principles of heat loss effects include: 1. Evaporation—lungs and skin when cooling occurs as a result of water evaporation 2. Convection—air currents 3. Conduction—skin contact with cooler object 4. Radiation—loss of warmth to cooler surrounding objects
		Hypothermia is a potential problem for SGA infant because: 1. SGA infant has decreased stores of brown fat available for thermogenesis, because SGA infant has used these stores in utero for survival. 2. SGA infant has poor insulation due to use of subcutaneous tissue in utero for survival.
GOAL: Julie's temperature will be stable and maintained within normal limits.		
NURSING DIAGNOSIS: Potential for injury related to glycogen stores and impaired gluconeogenesis	Monitor Dextrostix per SGA protocol and report values <45 mg/dL.	Combined with depletion of glycogen stores, impaired gluconeogenesis predisposes SGA infants to profound hypoglycemia within first 2 days of life.
	Observe, record, and report signs of hypoglycemia: cyanosis, lethargy, jitteriness, seizure activity, and apnea.	Hypoglycemia in SGA infant is indicated by whole blood sugar less than 20 mg/dL.
SUPPORTING DATA: Julie's initial Dextrostix was less than 45 mg/dL and a blood glucose is subsequently drawn. Results are normoglycemia (greater than 20 mg/dL of blood glucose)	Initiate feeding schedule for SGA newborns per agency protocol.	Frequent monitoring of Dextrostix assists in identifying decreasing glucose levels.
	Provide glucose intake either through early enteral feeding (before 4 hrs) or by IV per physician's order. See further discussion of hypoglycemia in Chapter 32.	Provision of glucose through early feedings (begin before 4 hrs of age) assists in maintaining glucose levels.
GOAL: Julie will have a normal blood glucose level		

Nursing Care Plan: SGA Newborn (continued)

Nursing Diagnosis and Goals	Nursing Interventions	Rationale
NURSING DIAGNOSIS: Alteration in nutrition: less than body requirements related to SGA's increased metabolic rate	Initiate test water feeding at 1 hr of age, then proceed to 5% glucose/water. Move early to formula feeding q2–3 hrs.	Sterile water is desirable for first feedings because it causes fewer pulmonary complications in the presence of gastrointestinal tract abnormalities and/or aspiration of feeding.
SUPPORTING DATA: Julie has lost more weight than 2% per day. She tires easily when given formula by nipple.		SGA newborns require more calories/kg for growth than AGA newborns because of increased metabolic activity and oxygen consumption secondary to increased percentage of body weight made up by visceral organs.
	Supplement oral feedings with intravenous intake per orders. Use concentrated formulas that supply more calories in less volume, such as Similac 24.	Small, frequent feedings of high caloric formula are used because of limited gastric capacity and decreased gastric emptying.
	Promote growth by providing caloric intake of 120–150 cal/kg/day in small amounts.	Growth is evaluated by increase in weight, length, and body measurements.
		Decrease in exhaustion is an important consideration in feeding SGA infant.
	Observe, record, and report signs of respiratory distress or fatigue occurring during feedings.	Adequate nutritional intake promotes growth and prevents such complications as metabolic catabolism and hypoglycemia.
	Supplement gavage or nipple feedings with intravenous therapy per physician order until oral intake is sufficient to support growth.	Gavage feedings require less energy expenditure on the part of the newborn.
	Establish a nipple feeding program that is begun slowly and progresses slowly, such as nipple feed once per day, nipple feed once per shift, and then nipple feed every other feeding. Monitor daily weight with anticipation of small amount of weight loss when nipple feedings start.	Nipple feeding, an active rather than passive intake of nutrition, requires energy expenditure and burning of calories by infant.
GOAL: Julie will gain weight and tolerate nipple feedings without tiring.		
NURSING DIAGNOSIS: Alteration in tissue perfusion related to increased blood viscosity		
SUPPORTING DATA: Venous hemoglobin >22 g/dL Venous hematocrit >65% Respiratory distress Cyanosis Tachycardia	Initiate screening of hematocrit on admission to nursery.	Polycythemia may occur in half of all SGA infants. Exact etiology of polycythemia in SGA is not known but is thought to be a physiologic response to chronic hypoxia with increased erythropoietin production.
	Observe, record, and report symptoms, including: 1. Decrease in peripheral pulses, discoloration of extremity, alteration in activity or neurologic depression, renal vein thrombosis with decreased urine output, hematuria, or proteinuria in thromboembolic conditions. 2. Tachycardia or congestive heart failure. 3. Respiratory distress syndrome, cyanosis, tachypnea, increased oxygen need, labored respirations, or hemorrhage in respiratory system.	Polycythemia is defined as a central venous hematocrit above 65%–70% in the first week of life. Hyperviscosity is resultant "thickness" of red-cell rich blood so that its ability to perfuse the tissues is disturbed due to thickness and decrease in deformability of cells. Symptoms are caused by poor perfusion of tissues.

Nursing Care Plan: SGA Newborn (continued)

Nursing Diagnosis and Goals	Nursing Interventions	Rationale
	Watch for other signs of increased hematocrit such as hyperbilirubinemia. Implement therapy per physician's order to reduce central venous hematocrit to 60% or less by using partial exchange of plasma rather than phlebotomy without volume replacement.	As the increase in red blood cells begins to break down, hyperbilirubinemia may present.
GOAL: Julie will have a normal hemoglobin level.		

See further discussion of polycythemia in Chapter 32.

Nursing Diagnosis and Goals	Nursing Interventions	Rationale
NURSING DIAGNOSIS: Potential for infection related to decreased immunologic response	Initiate a plan of care to prevent exposure to infection such as handwashing, reverse isolation, and individual equipment.	Newborns born to hypertensive mothers tend to be neutropenic and leukopenic.
SUPPORTING DATA: Julie is a SGA newborn and has had feeding difficulties, which required intravenous line insertion.	Observe, and report other signs of sepsis such as: lethargy/irritability, temperature instability, respiratory distress, and hypotension.	
GOAL: Julie will be free of infection or infection will be controlled.	Implement treatment per orders in presence of infection (refer to section on sepsis neonatorum, p 1060, for review of nursing care).	
NURSING DIAGNOSIS: Potential alteration in parenting related to prolonged separation of Julie and her parents secondary to illness	Support emotionally the psychologic well-being of family, including positive parent-infant bonding and sensory stimulation of infant. Include parents in determining infant's plan of care and encourage their participation. Encourage parents to visit frequently. Provide opportunities for parents to touch, hold, talk to, and care for infant. Determine the type and amount of appropriate sensory stimulation and implement sensory stimulation program.	Parent-infant bonding begins in first few hours or days following birth of an infant. Preterm infants experience prolonged periods of separation from their parents, which necessitates intervention to ensure parent-infant bonding.
SUPPORTING DATA: Julie is hospitalized for 3 weeks because of feeding problems and possible sepsis. Her parents are only able to visit once a day because they live 50 miles from the hospital.		
GOAL: Julie's parents will bond with her and have realistic expectations about her.		

Nursing Care Plan: SGA Newborn (continued)

Nursing Diagnosis and Goals	Nursing Interventions	Rationale
NURSING DIAGNOSIS: Parental knowledge deficit concerning care of newborn at home	Prepare for discharge by instructing parents in such areas as feeding techniques, formula preparation (including bottle sterilization), and breast-feeding; bathing, diapering, and hygiene; rectal temperature monitoring; administration of vitamins; sibling rivalry; care of complications and preventing exposure to infections; normal elimination patterns, normal reflexes and activity, and how to promote normal growth and development without being overprotective; returning for continued medical care; and availability of community resources if indicated.	Parents should receive the same postpartum teaching as any parent taking a new infant home. Parents need to understand the changes to expect in color of the infant's stool and number of bowel movements plus odor from bottle or breast-feeding in order to avoid unnecessary concern. Preterm infants usually do not require referral to community agencies such as visiting nurse associations unless there is a specific problem requiring assistance. Infants with congenital abnormalities, feeding problems, or resolving complications with infections or mothers unable to cope with defective infants are examples of conditions requiring referral to community resources.
SUPPORTING DATA: Julie's parents ask about taking care of her at home. "She's so small and sick and doesn't eat very well. Will she really be OK? What if I make a mistake?"		
GOAL: Julie's parents are comfortable taking her home. They are able to demonstrate normal infant care and assessments of possible complications, and know when to return for follow-up.		

Epilogue	
Julie is going home with her parents 3 weeks to the day after her birth. She is now gaining weight (20 g/day) and taking 2 ounces of formula every 3 hours by nipple without respiratory distress or fatigue. Her parents are eager to take Julie home. They have just completed	parent classes on infant care and CPR. As they wait for the discharge papers, they talk to and smile at Julie, and she watches them and smiles.

enhance the baby's growth potential and the child's ultimate outcome.

● Care of the Large-for-Gestational-Age (LGA) Newborn

A large-for-gestational-age (LGA) neonate is one whose birth weight is at or above the 90th percentile on the intrauterine growth curve (at any week of gestation). The majority of LGA newborns have been incorrectly categorized because of miscalculation of dates due to postconceptual bleeding (Korones 1986). Careful gestational age assessment is essential to identify the potential needs and problems of such infants.

The best-known condition associated with excessive fetal growth is maternal diabetes (Classes A–C); however, only a minority of large newborns are born to diabetic mothers. The cause of the majority of cases of LGA new-

borns is unclear, but certain factors or situations have been found to correlate with their birth.

● Genetic predisposition is correlated proportionally to the prepregnancy weight and to weight gain during pregnancy. Large parents tend to have large infants.

● Multiparous women have three times the number of LGA infants as primigravidas.

● Male infants are traditionally larger than female infants.

● Infants with erythroblastosis fetalis, Beckwith-Wiedemann syndrome, or transposition of the great vessels are usually large.

The increase in the LGA infant's body size is characteristically proportional, although head circumference and body length are in the upper limits of intrauterine growth. The exception to this rule is the infant of the diabetic mother, whose body weight increases only in proportion to length.

Common Complications of the LGA Newborn

Common disorders of the LGA infant include:

- *Birth trauma because of cephalopelvic disproportion.* Often these infants have a biparietal diameter greater than 10 cm or a fundal height measurement greater than 42 cm without the presence of hydramnios. Because of their excessive size, there are more breech presentations and shoulder dystocias. These complications may result in asphyxia, fractured clavicles, brachial palsy, facial paralysis, phrenic nerve palsy, depressed skull fractures, and intracranial bleeding.

- *Increased incidence of cesarean deliveries due to fetal size.* These births are accompanied by all the risk factors associated with cesarean deliveries.

- *Hypoglycemia, polycythemia, and hyperviscosity.* These disorders are most often seen with erythroblastosis fetalis and Beckwith-Wiedemann syndrome and in infants of diabetic mothers.

NURSING RESPONSIBILITIES

The perinatal history, in conjunction with ultrasonic measurement of fetal skull and gestational age testing, is important in identifying an at-risk LGA newborn. Nursing management is directed toward early identification and immediate treatment of the common disorders. Essential components of the nursing assessment are monitoring vital signs and screening for hypoglycemia and polycythemia. The nursing care involved in the complications associated with LGA newborns applies to the care needed by the infant of a diabetic mother and will be discussed in the next section.

● Care of the Infant of a Diabetic Mother (IDM)

Infants of diabetic mothers (IDMs) are considered at risk and require close observation the first few hours to the first few days of life. Mothers with severe diabetes or diabetes of long duration (type 1, or White's classes D–F, associated with vascular complications) may give birth to SGA infants. The typical IDM (type 1, or White's classes B and C), however, is LGA. He or she is fat, macrosomic, and plethoric (Figure 31–11). The cord and placenta are also large.

The infant is not edematous since IDMs have decreased total body water, particularly in the extracellular spaces. Their excessive weight is due to increased weight of the visceral organs, cardiomegaly, and increased body fat. The only organ not affected is the brain.

The excessive fetal growth of the IDM is caused by exposure to high levels of maternal glucose, which readily crosses the placenta. The fetus responds to these high glucose levels with increased insulin production and hyperplasia of the pancreatic beta cells. The main action of the insulin is to facilitate the entry of glucose into muscle and fat cells in a function similar to a cellular growth hormone. Once in the cells, glucose is converted to glycogen and stored. Insulin also inhibits the breakdown of fat to free fatty acids, thereby maintaining lipid synthesis, increasing the uptake of amino acids and promoting protein synthesis. Insulin is an important regulator of fetal growth and metabolism.

Common Complications of the IDM

Although IDMs are usually large, they are immature in physiologic functions and exhibit many of the problems of the preterm infant. The complications most often seen in an IDM are:

- *Hypoglycemia.* After birth the most common problem of an IDM is hypoglycemia. Even though the high maternal blood supply is lost, this newborn continues to produce high levels of insulin, which deplete the blood glucose within hours after birth. IDMs also have less ability to release glucagon and catecholamines, which normally stimulate glucagon breakdown and glucose release. The incidence of hypoglycemia in IDMs varies from 2 percent to 75 percent. The wide range in incidence of hypoglycemia in IDMs is thought to be due to the degree of success in controlling the maternal diabetes, differences in

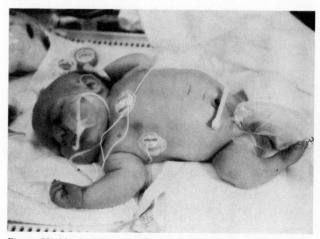

Figure 31–11   Macrosomic infant of diabetic mother. X-ray examination of this infant revealed caudal regression of the spine.

maternal blood sugars at the time of delivery, length of labor, the class of maternal diabetes, and early versus late feedings of the newborn.

- *Hypocalcemia.* Tremors are the obvious clinical sign of hypocalcemia. This complication may be due to the increased incidence of prematurity among IDMs and to the stresses of difficult pregnancy, labor, and delivery, which predispose any infant to hypocalcemia. Diabetic women tend to have higher calcium levels at term, which may cause secondary hypoparathyroidism in their infants (Korones 1986). Other factors may include vitamin D antagonism secondary to elevated cortisol and hyperphosphatemia from tissue catabolism.

- *Hyperbilirubinemia.* This condition may be seen at 48 to 72 hours after birth. It may be caused by slightly decreased extracellular fluid volume, which increases the hematocrit level. Enclosed hemorrhages resulting from complicated vaginal delivery may also cause hyperbilirubinemia. There may also be an increase in rate of bilirubin production in the presence of polycythemia.

- *Birth trauma.* Since most IDMs are LGA, trauma may occur during labor and delivery (see p 979).

- *Polycythemia.* This condition may be caused by the decreased extracellular volume in IDMs. Current research centers on the fact that hemoglobin A_{lc} binds oxygen, which decreases the oxygen available to the fetal tissues. This tissue hypoxia stimulates increased erythropoietin production, which increases the hematocrit level (Shannon et al 1986).

- *Respiratory distress.* This complication occurs especially in newborns of White's classes A–C diabetic mothers. Increasing evidence suggests that IDMs may have normal levels of the phospholipids that make up surfactant, which leads others to theorize that the composition of the lipids themselves are altered in the lungs of IDMs (Avery & Taeusch 1984). Other researchers (Duara et al 1985) report radiographic findings of segmental reticulogranular disease, especially in lung bases, in a small number of IDMs. They theorize that fetal hyperinsulinemia may block normal maturation of basal lung areas, which results in a disease clinically and radiographically distinct from RDS. RDS does not appear to be a problem for infants born of diabetic mothers in White's classes D–F; instead the stresses of poor uterine blood supply may lead to increased production of steroids, which accelerates lung maturation.

- *Congenital birth defects,* such as transposition of the great vessels, ventricular septal defect, patent ductus,

small left colon syndrome, and caudal regression syndrome.

Medical Therapy

The goal of medical therapy is the early detection of and intervention in the problems associated with being born an IDM. Key prenatal management is directed toward control of maternal hyperglycemia, which minimizes the common complications of IDMs: pulmonary problems, macrosomia, polycythemia, and hypoglycemia.

Because the onset of hypoglycemia occurs at 2 hours of age in IDMs (with a spontaneous rise to normal levels by 4 to 6 hours), blood glucose determinations should be done on cord blood and at 1, 2, 4, 6, 12, and 24 hours of age (Korones 1986).

IDMs who are symptomatic should be given 10 percent to 15 percent glucose intravenously immediately after birth at the volume of fluids necessary for the hydration of the infant. The rate of 4 to 6 mg/kg/min usually maintains normoglycemia in the IDM (Avery 1987). Once the blood glucose has been stable for 24 hours, the solution is then decreased in concentration with careful attention to the neonate's blood glucose level. Dextrose (25 percent to 50 percent) as a rapid infusion is contraindicated because it may lead to severe rebound hypoglycemia following an initial brief increase in glucose level.

Nursing Diagnosis

Nursing diagnoses that may apply to IDMs include:

- Alteration in nutrition: less than body requirements related to increased glucose metabolism secondary to hyperinsulinemia

- Impaired gas exchange related to respiratory distress secondary to impaired production of surfactant

- Ineffective family coping related to the illness of the baby

Nursing Goal: Promotion of Physical Well-Being

Nursing care of the IDM is directed toward early detection and ongoing monitoring of hypoglycemia (by doing glucose tests) and polycythemia (by obtaining central hematocrits). For specific nursing interventions for hypoglycemia and polycythemia, see Chapter 32. In caring for the IDM baby, the nurse assesses for signs of respiratory distress, hyperbilirubinemia, birth trauma, and congenital anomalies. Close and ongoing nursing assessments and care are essential in decreasing the potential harmful effects of the problems associated with being an IDM.

Nursing Goal: Promotion of Family Adaptation

Education of parents is directed toward prevention of macrosomia and resultant fetal/neonatal problems by better diabetic control for future pregnancies. Parents are advised that with prompt care, most IDMs' neonatal problems have no significant sequelae.

Evaluative Outcome Criteria

Nursing care is effective if:

● The IDM is free of respiratory distress and metabolic alterations.

● The parents understand the cause of the IDM baby and preventive steps they can initiate to decrease the impact of maternal diabetes on subsequent fetuses.

● The parents verbalize their concerns surrounding their baby's health problems and understand the rationale behind management of their newborn.

● Care of the Newborn of a Substance-Abusing Mother

The newborn of an alcoholic or drug-addicted woman will also be alcohol- or drug-dependent. After birth, when an infant's connection with the maternal blood supply is severed, the baby suffers withdrawal. In addition, the drugs ingested by the mother may be teratogenic, resulting in congenital anomalies.

Alcohol Dependency

The fetal alcohol syndrome (FAS) includes a series of malformations frequently found in infants born to women who have been chronic severe alcoholics (Jones et al 1973). It has been estimated that the complete FAS syndrome occurs in 1 or 2 live births per 1000. The syndrome occurs partially in 3 to 5 live births per 1000 (Abel 1985).

Controversy surrounds the exact cause of FAS. Although it is known that ethanol freely crosses the placenta to the fetus, it is still not known whether the alcohol alone or the break-down products of alcohol cause the damage. It is possible that alcohol itself may not harm the fetus but rather that the break-down product acetaldehyde, which is cytotoxic and teratogenic, is the culprit (Tanmer 1985). Pregnant women with inherited acquired defects of mitochondrial aldehyde dehydrogenase may have acetaldehyde levels well over the danger limit (35 mol/L) for their fetus, even after modest alcohol intake (Dunn et al 1979). This may explain why "social drinking" can sometimes cause adverse fetal effects, while heavy drinking may have no effect at all on the fetus.

Some studies have shown ethanol-induced uterine vessel vasoconstriction, which exposes the fetus to hypoxia (Altura et al 1982).

Other factors in conjunction with alcohol may contribute to the teratogenic effects. The factors include drugs (diazepam, nicotine, and caffeine), in addition to poor diet and low socioeconomic status (Iosub et al 1981). Cavdar (1984) theorizes that severe zinc deficiency produced by overconsumption of alcohol may be the major factor leading to dysmorphogenesis. This might also account for the association of immune deficiency with FAS, since zinc plays a crucial role in cell-mediated immune functions.

LONG-TERM COMPLICATIONS

The long-term prognosis for the FAS neonate is less than favorable. Most infants with FAS are growth-deficient at birth, and few infants have demonstrated postnatal catch-up growth. In fact most FAS infants are evaluated for failure to thrive. It has been found that decreased adipose tissue is a constant feature of persons with FAS.

Feeding problems are frequently present during infancy and preschool years. These infants have a delay in the normal progression of oral feeding development but have a normal progression of oral motor function. Many FAS infants nurse poorly and have persistent vomiting until 6 to 7 months of age. They have difficulty adjusting to solid foods and show little spontaneous interest in food (Streissguth & LaDue 1985). They continue to have feeding problems into adolescence, including eustachian tube dysfunction and malocclusion, which may result from midface malformation in utero (Streissguth & LaDue 1985).

Central nervous system dysfunctions are the most common and serious problem associated wth FAS. Most children exhibiting FAS are mildly to severely mentally retarded. The more dysmorphic the features, the lower the IQ scores. Providing a better environment for infants with FAS has been found to have no remarkable influence on IQ (Iosub et al 1981), which indicates that the brain damage occurred prenatally. These children are often hyperactive and show a high incidence of speech and language abnormalities indicative of CNS disorders. The brain is the organ most sensitive to damage from alcohol in the fetus.

MEDICAL THERAPY

Prevention of alcohol-induced complications is the foremost goal of medical therapy. This can be accomplished by educating the pregnant woman about the risks of alcohol ingestion and having the woman eliminate, or at least significantly reduce, her alcohol intake (Rosett et al 1983,

Larsson et al 1985). It has been found that reducing alcohol intake during midpregnancy can prevent growth retardation, although malformations will still occur.

The medical goal during the neonatal period is the management of CNS dysfunction and withdrawal. Seizures are treated with phenobarbital or diazepam.

NURSING ASSESSMENT

Newborns with FAS show the following characteristics:

- *Abnormal structural development and CNS dysfunction,* including mental retardation, microcephaly, and hyperactivity.

- *Growth deficiencies.* Infants with FAS are often IUGR with weight, length, and head circumference being affected. These infants continue to show a persistent postnatal growth deficiency with weight being more affected than linear growth.

- *Distinctive facial abnormalities.* These include short palpebral fissures, midfacial and maxillary hypoplasia, micrognathia, hypoplastic upper lip, and diminished or absent philtrum.

- *Associated anomalies.* Abnormalities affecting cardiac (primarily septal), ocular, renal, and skeletal (especially involving joints such as congenital dislocated hips) systems are often noted.

Withdrawal symptoms of the alcohol-dependent neonate have been documented in children with normal facial features as well as in those with the typical features of FAS (Coles et al 1984). These symptoms include tremors, seizures, sleeplessness, unconsolable crying, abnormal reflexes, activeness with little ability to maintain alertness and attentiveness to environment, abdominal distention, and exaggerated mouthing behaviors such as hyperactive rooting and increased nonnutritive sucking (Clarren et al 1985).

Signs and symptoms of withdrawal often appear within 6 to 12 hours and at least within the first three days of life. Seizures after the neonatal period are rare. Alcohol dependence in the infant is physiologic, not psychologic.

NURSING DIAGNOSIS

Nursing diagnoses that may apply to the FAS newborn include:

- Alteration in nutrition: less than body requirements related to decreased food intake and hyperirritability

- Potential for injury related to seizure activity secondary to CNS dysfunction or chemical dependence

- Ineffective family coping related to potential developmental delay and/or guilt over the diagnosis

NURSING GOAL: PROMOTION OF PHYSICAL WELL-BEING

The nurse's awareness of the signs and symptoms of fetal alcohol effects is important in structuring and guiding nursing care. Nursing care of the FAS newborn is aimed at avoiding heat loss, protecting the infant from injury during seizures, administering medications such as phenobarbital or diazepam to limit convulsions, monitoring intravenous fluid therapy, and reducing environmental stimuli. The FAS baby is most comfortable in a quiet, dimly lit environment. Because of their feeding problems, these infants require extra time and patience during feedings.

Mothers should be informed that breast-feeding is not contraindicated but that excessive alcohol consumption may intoxicate the newborn and inhibit the letdown reflex. The nurse must monitor the newborn's vital signs closely and observe for evidence of seizure activity and respiratory distress.

NURSING GOAL: PROMOTION OF FAMILY ADAPTATION

Infants affected by maternal alcohol abuse are also at risk psychologically. Restlessness, sleeplessness, agitation, resistance to cuddling or holding, and frequent crying can be frustrating to parents as their efforts to relieve the distress are unrewarded. Feeding dysfunction can also result in frustrations for the care giver and digestive upsets for the infant. Frustration may cause the parents to punish the baby or result in the unconscious desire to "stay away from the infant." Either outcome may create an unstable family environment, and result in the infant's failure to thrive.

The nurse should focus on providing support for the parents and reinforcing positive parenting activity. Prior to discharge, parents are provided with opportunities to provide baby care so that they can feel confident in their interpretations of their baby's cues and ability to meet the baby's needs. Referring the family to social services and visiting nurse or public health nurse associations is essential for the well-being of the infant. Follow-up care and teaching can strengthen the parents' skills and coping abilities and help them create a stable, healthy environment for their family.

EVALUATIVE OUTCOME CRITERIA

Nursing care is effective if:

- The FAS newborn is able to tolerate feedings and gain weight.

- The FAS infant's hyperirritability and/or seizures are controlled and the baby has suffered no physical injuries.

- The parents are able to identify the special needs of their newborn and accept outside assistance as needed.

Drug Dependency

Almost all drugs ingested by a pregnant woman cross the placenta and enter the fetal circulation. Thus the fetus can develop drug-associated problems in utero or soon after birth.

During the antenatal period, the greatest risk to the fetus is intrauterine asphyxia. This is often a direct result of fetal withdrawal, secondary to maternal withdrawal. Fetal withdrawal is accompanied by hyperactivity with increased oxygen consumption, which, if not adequately compensated, can lead to fetal asphyxia. Moreover, narcotic-addicted women tend to have a higher incidence of PIH, abruptio placentae, and placenta previa, which lead to placental insufficiency and fetal asphyxia.

The birth weight of newborns of narcotic-addicted women may depend on the type of drug the mother uses. Women using predominantly heroin have SGA newborns. Women maintained on methadone have higher birth weight newborns, some of whom are LGA (Merker et al 1985).

Addicted newborns often have low Apgar scores at birth. Low scores may be related to the intrauterine asphyxia or the medication the woman received during labor. The use of a narcotic antagonist (naloxone or levallorphan) to reverse respiratory depression in the newborn is contraindicated. These drugs may precipitate acute withdrawal in the baby.

COMMON COMPLICATIONS OF THE DRUG-ADDICTED NEWBORN

The newborn of a woman who abused drugs during her pregnancy is predisposed to the following problems:

- *Respiratory distress.* The addicted newborn frequently suffers respiratory stress, mainly meconium-aspiration pneumonia and transient tachypnea. Meconium aspiration is usually secondary to increased oxygen consumption and activity experienced by the fetus during intrauterine withdrawal. Transient tachypnea may develop secondary to the inhibitory effects of narcotics on the reflex responsible for clearing the lungs. Respiratory distress syndrome occurs less in heroin-addicted newborns even in the presence of prematurity because they have tissue-oxygen unloading capabilities comparable to those of a 6-week-old term infant. In addition, heroin stimulates production of glucocorticoids via the anterior pituitary gland.

- *Jaundice.* Newborns of methadone-addicted women may develop jaundice due to prematurity. Heroin contributes to early maturity of the liver, leading to a lower incidence of hyperbilirubinemia for these babies.

- *Congenital anomalies.* The incidence of anomalies of the genitourinary and cardiovascular systems is slightly increased in infants of drug-addicted mothers.

- *Behavioral abnormalities.* Babies exposed to cocaine have poor state organization and decreased interactive behaviors when tested with the Brazelton Neonatal Behavioral Assessment Scale (Chasnoff 1985).

- *Withdrawal.* The most significant postnatal problem of the drug-addicted newborn is that of narcotic withdrawal (usually from heroin or methadone). The onset of the withdrawal manifestations usually occurs within the first 72 hours after birth. For heroin-addicted newborns a majority of withdrawal symptoms are seen within the first 24 to 48 hours. For newborns exposed to barbiturates, symptoms may be delayed for several days. Withdrawal for cocaine-addicted infants may occur four to five days after birth. For methadone-addicted infants, withdrawal may be delayed two to three weeks but can occur earlier. In most cases, the withdrawal manifestations peak in the newborn about the third day and subside by the fifth to seventh day. One study reported an increased frequency of withdrawal in infants born to women maintained on more than 50 mg of methadone, but no relationship was observed between the severity of withdrawal and the maternal dose (Stimmell et al 1983).

LONG-TERM COMPLICATIONS

The physical and mental development of infants of drug-addicted mothers falls within normal limits up to two years of age. Although these infants demonstrate higher incidence of gastrointestinal and respiratory illnesses, it is believed these are related not to narcotic addiction but to lack of education regarding proper infant care, feeding, and hygiene. Another important problem is the high incidence (5 percent) of sudden infant death syndrome (SIDS) among these newborns (Lemons 1983). The occurrence of SIDS may be even higher in those infants who have had moderate-to-severe postnatal withdrawal.

MEDICAL THERAPY

The goal of medical therapy is prevention through prenatal management of the addicted women (see Chapter 19) and pharmacologic management of neonatal narcotic withdrawal. For optimal fetal and neonatal outcome, the narcotic-addicted woman should receive complete prenatal care as soon as possible. She should be started on a methadone program with a reduction in dosage to 20 mg or less, if possible. The aim of methadone maintenance during pregnancy is the prevention of heroin use. Thus the dose of methadone used for maintenance should be sufficient to ensure this goal even if the dose is greater than 20 mg (Stimmel et al 1983). It is not recommended that the woman be withdrawn completely from narcotics while pregnant since this induces fetal withdrawal with poor newborn outcomes.

About 50 percent of newborns of addicted mothers experience withdrawal symptoms severe enough to require treatment. Drugs used to control withdrawal symptoms are phenobarbital or paregoric. Attention to nutritional support is important in light of the increase in energy expenditure that withdrawal may entail. The American Academy of Pediatrics (1983) recommends use of a formula that supplies 24 calories per ounce to provide 150 to 250 cal/kg/day.

NURSING ASSESSMENT

Early identification of the newborn needing medical or pharmacologic interventions decreases the incidence of mortality and morbidity. During the newborn period, nursing assessment focuses on:

- Discovering the mother's last drug intake and dosage level. This is accomplished through the perinatal history and laboratory tests.

- Assessing the complications related to intrauterine withdrawal such as SGA, intrauterine asphyxia, and prematurity. (For nursing care of SGA newborns, see p 972; for nursing care of premature newborns, see p 960; for nursing care of the infant who suffered intrauterine asphyxia, see Chapter 32.)

- Identifying the signs and symptoms of newborn withdrawal. The signs and symptoms of newborn withdrawal can be classified in five groups:

1. Central nervous system signs

   a. Hyperactivity
   b. Hyperirritability (persistent high-pitched cry)
   c. Increased muscle tone
   d. Exaggerated reflexes
   e. Tremors, seizures
   f. Sneezing, hiccups, yawning

   g. Short, unquiet sleep
   h. Fever

2. Respiratory signs

   a. Tachypnea
   b. Excessive secretions

3. Gastrointestinal signs

   a. Disorganized, vigorous suck
   b. Vomiting
   c. Drooling
   d. Sensitive gag reflex
   e. Hyperphagia
   f. Diarrhea
   g. Abdominal cramping

4. Vasomotor signs

   a. Stuffy nose, yawning, sneezing
   b. Flushing
   c. Sweating
   d. Sudden, circumoral pallor

5. Cutaneous signs

   a. Excoriated buttocks
   b. Facial scratches
   c. Pressure point abrasions

Although many of the signs and symptoms of narcotic withdrawal are similar to those seen with hypoglycemia and hypocalcemia, glucose and calcium values are reported to be within normal limits for this group of infants (Harper et al 1977).

NURSING DIAGNOSIS

Nursing diagnoses that may apply to drug-dependent newborns include:

- Alteration in nutritional and fluid requirements: less than body requirements related to vomiting and diarrhea, uncoordinated suck and swallow reflex, hypertonia secondary to withdrawal

- Alteration in comfort related to skin excoriation over bony prominences secondary to constant activity

- Alteration in parenting related to hyperirritable behavior

NURSING GOAL: PROMOTION OF PHYSICAL WELL-BEING

Care of the drug-dependent newborn is based on reducing withdrawal symptoms and promoting adequate respiration, temperature, and nutrition. Specific nursery care measures include:

- Temperature regulation.

- Careful monitoring of pulse and respirations every 15 minutes until stable; stimulation if apnea occurs.

- Small frequent feedings, especially in the presence of vomiting, regurgitation, and diarrhea.

- Intravenous therapy as needed.

- Medications as ordered, such as phenobarbital, paregoric, diazepam (Valium), or chlorpromazine hydrochloride (Thorazine). Methadone should not be given because of possible neonatal addiction to it.

- Proper positioning on the right side to avoid possible aspiration of vomitus or secretions.

- Observation for problems of SGA or LGA newborns.

- Swaddling to minimize injury.

NURSING GOAL: PROMOTION OF FAMILY ADAPTATION

Parents should be prepared for what they can expect for the first few months at home. At the time of discharge the mother should be instructed to anticipate mild jitteriness and irritability in the newborn, which may persist from 8 to 16 weeks, depending on the initial severity of the withdrawal. The nurse should help the mother learn feeding techniques and comforting measures. Parents are to be counseled regarding available resources, such as support groups, and signs and symptoms that require further care. Ongoing evaluation is necessary because of the potential for long-term problems.

EVALUATIVE OUTCOME CRITERIA

Nursing care is effective if:

- The newborn tolerates feedings, gains weight, and has a decreased number of stools.

- The parents learn ways to comfort their newborn.

- The parents are able to cope with their frustrations and begin to use outside resources as needed.

Care of the Newborn With AIDS

An increasing number of newborns are being born with or acquiring AIDS in the newborn period or early infancy. Perinatal and neonatal modes of transmission have been identified as transplacental, breast-feeding, and/or contaminated blood. For discussion of fetal/neonatal AIDS characteristics and nursing care of the newborn with AIDS, see chapter 19.

Care of the Family of the At-Risk Newborn

The Effects of Maternal-Infant Separation on Attachment

Studies of maternal-infant interactions in most human cultures have found that mother and infant remain together, usually for three to seven days after birth, without prolonged periods of separation. Only in the high-risk and preterm nurseries of the Western world are mothers and infants separated after birth.

This separation has a historical basis. In the early 1900s, it was discovered that newborn survival rates were improved if strict isolation procedures and visitor restrictions were enforced for all newborns. Of course, infection-preventing practices have rendered such isolation practices relatively obsolete for the normal newborn. The health of infants at risk, however, is extremely fragile, and separation from parents is necessary to allow treatment of complications.

The question that arises is whether interruptions in maternal contact and care giving can disrupt the process of maternal-infant attachment. The evidence seems to indicate that such interruptions may have a negative effect on bonding. It has been found, for example, that a disproportionately high number of battered or neglected children were born prematurely and stayed in an intensive care nursery for prolonged periods following birth.

What exactly in the attachment process is being interrupted by early maternal-infant separation? The period immediately after birth has been described as the *maternal sensitive period*. During this period certain behaviors have been identified as specific for development of attachment, bonding, and effective mothering. These behaviors include seeing and touching the newborn. Immediate performance of these behaviors is often impossible if the infant is preterm or has a congenital anomaly.

Animal studies demonstrate that interruption of maternal behavior patterns results in rejection of the offspring, inability to recognize the offspring, and indiscriminate feeding of other young. Research with humans also suggests that interference with maternal behavior patterns during the early postpartal period can disturb the developing relationship between the mother and child. Early maternal anxieties about the infant may also have long-lasting effects on the mother-baby relationship (Klaus & Kennell 1982).

Parental Adjustments to the At-Risk Newborn

The events of premature labor and delivery abruptly terminate the normal adaptive processes to pregnancy. Taylor and Hall (1979) have devised a schematic representation interrelating the initiation-to-end course of the main psychologic processes that occur during pregnancy (Figure 31–12). Because pregnancy can be viewed as a developmental crisis, the pregnant woman spends much energy reworking unresolved conflicts she may have with her mother. In addition, as the pregnancy progresses to term, the mother-to-be begins voicing a desire to have the pregnancy end; these feelings usually coincide with a fetal gestation age that is maximal for extrauterine survival. It is believed that the mother's desire either to retain the pregnancy or "let it go" might affect her attitude toward delivery and her infant. When an infant is delivered prior to term, the mother may not have had sufficient time to rework conflicts or be prepared to let the pregnancy go. As a result, the mother harbors feelings not only of anxious concern over the labor and delivery and survival of the infant, but also of separation, helplessness, failure, and loss of control over the ability to produce the desired outcome.

Feelings of guilt and failure also often plague the mothers of preterm newborns. They may ask themselves "Why did labor start? What did I do (or not do)?" A woman may have guilt fantasies, and wonder "Was it because I had sexual intercourse with my husband (a week, three days, a day) ago?" "Was it because I carried three loads of wash up from the basement?" "Am I being punished for something done in the past—even in childhood?"

The birth of the newborn with congenital abnormalities also engenders feelings of guilt and failure. As in the birth of a preterm infant, the woman may entertain ideas of personal guilt: "What did I do (or not do) to cause this?" "Am I being punished for something?"

Parental reactions and steps of attachment are altered by the birth of a preterm infant or one with a congenital anomaly. A variety of new feelings, reactions, and stresses must be recognized and dealt with before the family can work toward the establishment of a healthy parent-infant relationship.

Kaplan and Mason (1974) view maternal reactions to preterm births as an acute emotional disorder. They have identified four psychologic tasks as essential for coping with the stress and for providing a basis for the maternal-infant relationship:

1. Anticipatory grief as a psychologic preparation for possible loss of the child, while still hoping for his or her survival.

2. Acknowledgment of maternal failure to produce a term infant, expressed as anticipatory grief and de-

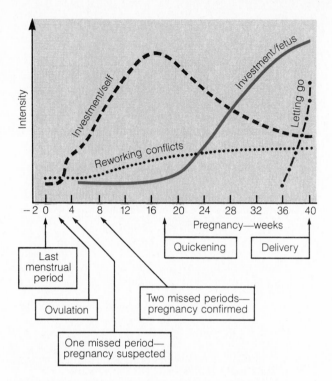

Figure 31–12   Relationship between basic psychologic processes and milestones of pregnancy. General agreement exists about the sequence and time courses of the processes of investment in self, investment in fetus, and letting go as represented here. The process of reworking unresolved conflicts with the woman's own mother is represented only tentatively. (From Taylor PM, Hall BL: Parent-infant bonding problems and opportunities in a perinatal center. Semin Perinatol 1979;3:375)

pression and lasting until the chances of survival seem secure.

3. Resumption of the process of relating to the infant, which was interrupted by the threat of nonsurvival. This task may be impaired by continuous threat of death or abnormality, and the mother may be slow in her response of hope for the infant's survival.

4. Understanding of the special needs and growth patterns of the preterm infant, which are temporary and yield to normal patterns.

Klaus and Kennell (1982), on the other hand, feel that with extra, sustained support and early contact with her infant a mother need not necessarily become involved in anticipatory preparation for her child's possible death.

Most authorities agree that the birth of a preterm infant or a less-than-perfect infant does require major adjustments as the parents are forced to surrender the image they had nurtured for so long of their ideal child.

Solnit and Stark (1961) postulate that grief and mourning of the loss of the loved object—the idealized child—mark parental reactions to a child with abnormalities. The parents must grieve the loss of the valued object—their wished-for perfect child. Simultaneously, they must adopt the imperfect child as the new love object. Parental responses to a child with health problems may also be viewed as a five-staged process (Klaus & Kennell 1982):

1. *Shock* is felt at the reality of the birth of this child. This stage may be characterized by forgetfulness, amnesia of the situation, and a feeling of desperation.

2. There is disbelief (*denial*) of the reality of the situation, characterized by a refusal to believe the child is defective. This stage is exemplified by assertions that "It didn't really happen!" "There has been a mistake; it's someone else's baby."

3. *Depression* over the reality of the situation and a corresponding grief reaction follows acceptance of the situation. This stage is characterized by much crying and sadness. Anger about the reality of the situation may also occur at this stage. A projection of blame on others or on self and feelings of "not me" are characteristic of this stage.

4. Equilibrium and *acceptance* are characteristic of a decrease in the emotional reactions of the parents. This stage is variable and may be prolonged because of a prolongation of the threat to the infant's survival. Some parents experience chronic sorrow in relation to their child.

5. *Reorganization* of the family is necessary to deal with the child's problems. Mutual support of the parents facilitates this process, but the crisis of the situation may precipitate alienation between the parental partners.

These stages of parental adjustment are similar to the stages of dying and of grieving. Indeed, reorganization is necessary to deal with a crisis concerning a child at risk.

In the birth of either a child with an anomaly or a preterm infant, the process of mourning is necessary for attachment to the less-than-perfect child. *Grief work*, the emotional reaction to a significant loss, must occur before adequate attachment to the actual child is possible. Parental detachment precedes parental attachment.

It is essential that the mother be reunited with her infant as soon as possible after birth so that:

1. She knows that her infant is alive.

2. She knows what the infant's real problems are. Fantasies of the infant's problems may be more devastating than the reality of the problem. Early acquaintance between mother and infant allows a realistic perspective of the baby's condition.

3. She can begin the grief work over the loss of the idealized child and begin the process of attachment to the actual child.

4. She can share the experience of the infant's problems with the father, who may have already seen and touched the infant.

The nurse should guard against indiscriminate admission of normal newborns to the intensive care unit because of prior high-risk conditions, such as cesarean birth, fetal bradycardia, or short periods of rapid breathing after birth. It has been found that while these unjustified short-term admissions to special care nurseries cause no long-term maternal-infant attachment problems, they do cause unnecessary anxiety and unhappiness for the parents.

Nursing Assessment

Development of a nurse-family relationship facilitates information gathering in areas of concern. A concurrent illness of the mother or other family members or other concurrent stress (lack of hospitalization insurance, loss of job, age of parents) may alter the family response to the baby. Feelings of apprehension, guilt, failure, and grief that are verbally or nonverbally expressed are important aspects of the nursing history. These observations enable all professionals to be aware of the parental state, coping behaviors, and readiness for attachment, bonding, and caretaking. Appropriate nursing observations during interviewing and relating to the family include:

1. *Level of understanding.* Observations concerning the ability to assimilate information given and to ask appropriate questions; the need for constant repetition of "the same" information.

2. *Behavioral responses.* Appropriateness of behavior in relation to information given; lack of response; "flat" affect.

3. *Difficulties with communication.* Deafness (reads lips only); blindness; dysphagia; understanding only of foreign language.

4. *Paternal and maternal education level.* Parents unable to read or write; only eighth grade completed; mother an MD, RN, or PhD; and so on.

Documentation of such information, obtained by the nurse through continuing contact and development of a therapeutic family relationship, enables all professionals to understand and use the nursing history in providing continuous individual care.

Visiting and care-giving patterns give an indication of the level or lack of parental attachment. A record of visits, caretaking procedures, affect (in relating to the newborn), and telephone calls is essential. Serial observations must be obtained, rather than just isolated instances of concern. Grant (1978) has developed a conceptual framework depicting adaptive and maladaptive responses to parenting of a preterm or less-than-perfect infant (Figure 31–13).

If a pattern of distancing behaviors evolves, appropriate intervention should be instituted. Follow-up studies have found that a statistically significant number of preterm, sick, and congenitally defective infants suffer from failure to thrive, battering, or other disorders of mothering. Early detection and intervention will prevent these aber-

rations in mothering behaviors from leading to irreparable damage or death.

Nursing Diagnosis

Nursing diagnoses that may apply to the family of a newborn at risk include:

- Grief related to loss of idealized newborn

- Fear related to emotional involvement with an at-risk newborn

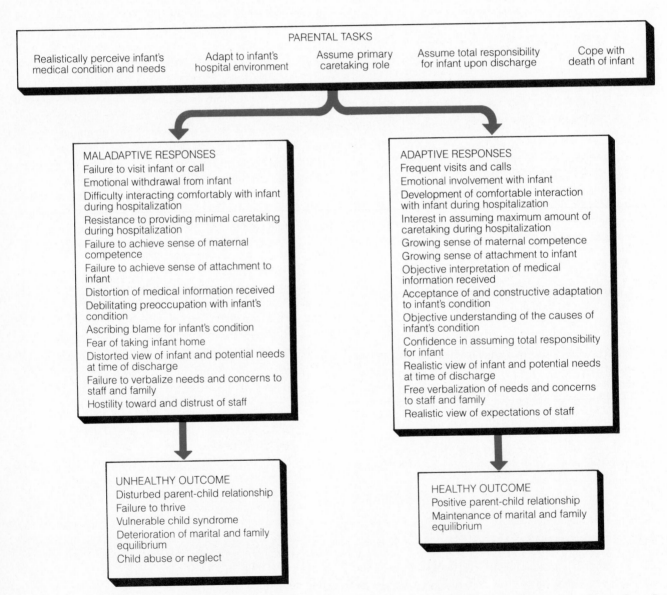

Figure 31–13 Maladaptive and adaptive parental responses during crisis period showing unhealthy and healthy outcomes (From Grant P: Psychosocial needs of families of high-risk infants. *Fam Comm Health* 1978;11:93, by permission of Aspen Systems Corporation)

● Alteration in parenting related to impaired bonding secondary to feelings of inadequacy about caretaking activities

Nursing Goal: Preparation of Parents for Initial Viewing of Newborn

Before parents see their child, the nurse must prepare them for the viewing. It is important that a positive, realistic attitude regarding the infant be presented to the parents rather than a pessimistic one. An overly negative, fatalistic attitude further alienates the parents from their infant and retards attachment behaviors. Instead of allowing attachment and bonding to develop, the mother will begin the process of anticipatory grieving, and once started, this process is difficult to reverse.

In preparing parents for the first view of their infant, it is important for a professional to have looked at the baby. The parents should be prepared to see both the deviations and the normal aspects of their infant. All infants exhibit strengths as well as deficiencies. The nurse may say, "Your baby is small, about the length of my two hands. She weighs 2 lb, 3 oz but is very active and cries when we disturb her. She is having some difficulty breathing but is breathing without assistance and in only 35 percent oxygen."

The equipment being used for the at-risk newborn and its purpose should be described before the parents enter the intensive care unit. Many intensive care units have booklets for parents to read before entering the unit. Through explanations and pictures, the parents can be better prepared to deal with the feelings they may experience when they see their infant for the first time.

Nursing Goal: Support of Parents During Their Initial Viewing of the Newborn

Upon entering the unit, parents may be overwhelmed by the sounds of monitors, alarms, and respirators, as well as by the unfamiliar language and "foreign" atmosphere. It is more reassuring when parents are prepared and accompanied to the unit by the same person(s). The primary physician and primary nurse caring for the newborn should be with the parents when they first visit their baby. Parental reactions are varied, but there is usually an element of initial shock. Provision of chairs and time to regain composure will assist the parents. Slow, complete, and simple explanations—first about the infant and then about the equipment—allay fear and anxiety.

As parents attempt to deal with the initial stages of shock and grief at the birth of a premature or less-than-perfect baby, they may fail to assimilate new information. They may require constant repetition by the nurse to accept the reality of the situation, procedures, equipment, and the infant's condition on subsequent visits.

Misconceptions about equipment and its placement on the infant and about its potential harm are common. Such statements as "Does the fluid go into the brain?" "Does the white wire on the abdomen go into the stomach?" and "Does the monitor make the baby's heart beat?" imply much fear for the infant's safety and misconception about the machines. These worries are easily overcome by simple explanations of all equipment being used.

Concern about the infant's physical appearance is common, yet may remain unvoiced. Parents may express such concerns as "He looks so small and red—like a drowned rat." "Why do her genitals look so abnormal?" "Will that awful looking mouth [cleft lip and palate] ever be normal?" Such questions need to be anticipated by the nurse and addressed. Use of pictures, such as of an infant after cleft lip repair, may be reassuring to doubting parents. Knowledge of the development of a "normal" preterm infant will allow the nurse to make reassuring statements such as "The baby's labia may look very abnormal to you, but they are normal for her maturity. As she grows, the outer lips of the labia will become larger and the clitoris will be covered and the genitals will then look as you expect them to. She is normal for her level of maturity."

The tone of the neonatal intensive care unit is set by the nursing staff. Development of a safe, trusting environment depends on viewing the parents as essential care givers and not as "visitors" or "nuisances" in the unit. Pleasant, relaxed physical surroundings convey the sense of hospitality and encourage parents to "be at home." Provision of chairs, privacy when needed, and easy access to staff and facilities are all important in developing an open, comfortable environment. An uncrowded and welcoming atmosphere lets parents know "You are welcome here." However, even in crowded physical surroundings, an attitude of openness and trust can be conveyed by the nursing staff.

A trusting relationship is essential for collaborative efforts in caring for the infant. Nurses must therapeutically use their own responses to relate on a one-to-one basis with the parents. Each individual has different needs, different ways of adapting to crisis, and different means of support. Professionals must use techniques that are real and spontaneous to them and avoid adopting words or actions that are foreign to them. Nurses must also gauge their interventions to match the parents' pace and needs.

Nursing Goal: Facilitation of Attachment If Neonatal Transport Occurs

Smaller hospitals may be unable to care for sick infants. Transport to a regional referral center may be necessary. These centers may be as far as 500 miles from the parents' community; it is therefore essential that the mother see and touch her infant before he or she is transported. Facilitation of this important contact may be the responsibility of the referring hospital staff as well as the transport team. Bringing the mother to the nursery or taking the infant in a warmed transport incubator to the mother's bedside will allow her to see the infant before transportation to the center.

Once the infant has reached the referral center, parents also appreciate a telephone call relaying the infant's condition during the transport, safe arrival at the center, and present condition. A member of the transport team is often the best person to make the call, as the team has already begun a trusting relationship with the parents and are most knowledgeable about the infant.

Support of parents, with explanations from the professional staff, is crucial. Occasionally the mother may be unable to see the infant before transport, for example, if she is still under general anesthesia or experiencing complications such as shock, hemorrhage, or seizures. In these cases, before the infant is transported a photograph of the infant should be taken to be given to the mother, along with an explanation of the infant's condition, problems, and a detailed description of the infant's characteristics, to facilitate the attachment process until the mother can visit. An additional photograph is also helpful for the father to share with siblings and/or the extended family. With the increased attention to improved fetal outcome, maternal transports, rather than neonatal transports, are occurring more frequently. This practice gives the mother of a high-risk infant the opportunity to visit and care for her infant during the early postpartal period.

Nursing Goal: Promotion of Touching

Mothers visiting a small or sick infant may need several visits to become comfortable and confident in their abilities to touch the infant without injuring him or her. Barriers such as incubators, incisions, monitor electrodes, and tubes may delay the mother's confidence. Knowledge of this "normal" delay in touching behavior will enable the nurse to understand parental behavior.

Klaus and Kennell (1982) have demonstrated a significant difference in the amount of eye contact and touching behavior of mothers of preterm infants. Whereas mothers of normal newborns progress within minutes to palm contact of the infant's trunk, the mother of a preterm infant is slower in her progression from fingertip to palm contact and from the extremities to the trunk. The progression to palm contact with the infant's trunk may take several visits, as illustrated in Figure 31–14.

Through support, reassurance, and encouragement, the nurse can facilitate the mother's positive feelings about her ability and her importance to her infant. Touching facilitates "getting to know" the infant and thus establishes a bond with the infant. Touching as well as seeing the infant helps the mother to realize the "normals" and potentials of her baby.

Nursing Goal: Facilitation of Parental Care-Taking

Bonding can be facilitated by encouraging parents to visit and become involved in their baby's care (Figure 31–15). When visiting is impossible, the parents should feel free to phone whenever they wish to receive information about their baby. A warm, receptive attitude is very supportive. Nurses can also facilitate parenting by personalizing a baby to the parents, by referring to the infant by name, or by relating personal behavioral characteristics to the parents. Remarks such as "Jenny loves her pacifier" help make the infant more individual and unique.

Caretaking may be delayed for the mother of a preterm, defective or sick infant. The variety of equipment needed for life support is hardly conducive to anxiety-free caretaking by the parents. However, even the sickest infant may be cared for, if even in a small way, by the parents. As a facilitator of parental caretaking, it is the responsibility of the nurse to promote the parents' success. Demonstration and explanation, followed by support of the parents in initial caretaking behaviors, positively reinforce this behavior. Changing the infant's diaper, giving their infant skin care or oral care, or helping the nurse turn the infant may at first be anxiety-provoking for the parents, but they will become more comfortable and confident in caretaking and receive satisfaction from the baby's reactions and their ability "to do something." Complimenting the parents' competence in caretaking also increases their self-esteem, which has received recent "blows" of guilt and failure. It is vitally important that the parents never be given a task if there is any possibility that they will not be able to accomplish it.

Often mothers have ambivalent feelings toward the nurse, in the face of their own inability to provide the sophisticated care needed by the infant. As the mother watches the nurse competently perform the caretaking tasks, she feels both grateful to the nurse for the skill and expertise and jealous of the nurse's ability to care for her infant. These feelings may be acted out in criticism of the care being received by her infant, in manipulation of staff, or in personal guilt about such feelings. Instead of fostering (by silence) these inferiority feelings within mothers, nurses are in a special position to recognize these feelings and to intervene appropriately to facilitate mother-infant attachment.

Nurses who are understanding and secure will be able to support the parents' egos instead of collecting rewards for themselves. To reinforce positive parenting behaviors, professionals must first believe in the importance of the parents. The nurse could hardly convince a doubting

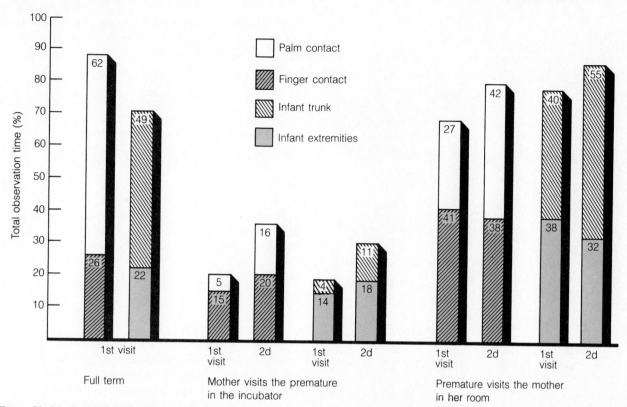

Figure 31–14 Fingertip and palm contact on the trunk or extremities of a newborn in three groups of mothers: (1) 12 mothers of full-term infants at their first visit; (2) 9 mothers who visited their preterm infants in incubators in the intensive care unit; and (3) 14 mothers whose preterm infants were brought to their maternity rooms and placed in their beds (From Klaus MH, Kennell JH: Parent-Infant Bonding, ed 2. St Louis, Mosby, 1982)

parent of her or his importance to the infant unless the nurse really believes it. The attitude of the professionals communicates acceptance or rejection to the parents, regardless of what is said. During this crisis period, it is essential that attitudes *and* words say: "You are a good mother/father. You are a good person. You have an important contribution to make to the care of your infant." Unless as much care is taken in facilitating parental attachment as in providing physiologic care, the outcome will not be a healthy family.

Verbalizations by the nurse that improve parental self-esteem are essential and easily shared. Breast-feeding is possible and in many centers this is recommended for preterm or sick infants for nutrition as well as for defense against the development of necrotizing enterocolitis. In addition to physiologic use, breast milk is important because of the emotional investment of the mother. Pumping, storing, labeling, and delivering quantities of breast milk is time-consuming and a "labor of love" for mothers. Positive remarks regarding breast milk reinforce the maternal behavior of caretaking and providing for her infant: "Breast milk is something that only you can give your baby" or "You really have brought a lot of milk today" or "Look how rich this breast milk is" or "Even small amounts of milk are important, and look how rich it is."

If the infant begins to gain weight while being fed breast milk, it is important to point this out to the mother. Parents should also be advised that initial weight loss with beginning nipple feedings is common because of the increased energy expended when the infant begins active rather than passive nutritional intake.

Provision of care by the parents is appropriate even for very sick or defective infants who are likely to die. It has been found that detachment is easier after attachment, because the parents are comforted by the knowledge that they did all they could for their child while he or she was alive.

Nursing Goal: Provision of Continuity in Information Giving

During crisis, maintenance of interpersonal relationships is difficult. Yet in a newborn intensive care area, the parents are expected to relate to many different care providers. It is important that parents have as few professionals as possible relaying information to them. A primary nurse should coordinate and provide continuity in information giving to parents. Care providers are individuals and thus will use different terms, inflections, and attitudes. These subtle differences are monumental to parents and only con-

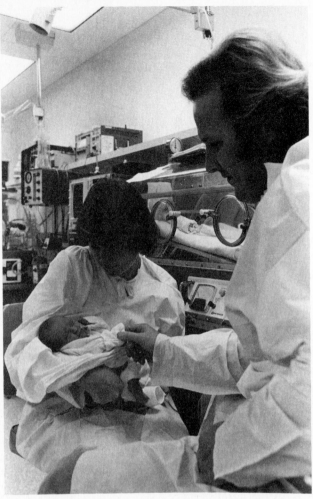

Figure 31–15 It is important that the parents of high-risk infants be given the opportunity to get acquainted with their children. Physical contact is extremely important in the bonding process and should be encouraged whenever possible.

fuse, confound, and produce anxiety. Several relationships with trusted professionals minimize unnecessary anxiety and concern and facilitate open communication. The nurse not only functions as a liaison between the parents and the wide variety of professionals interacting with the infant and parents but also offers clarification, explanation, interpretation of information, and support to the parents.

Nursing Goal: Use of Family's Support System

The parents should be encouraged to deal with the crisis with help from their support system. The support system attempts to meet the emotional needs and provide support for the family members in crisis and stress situations. Biologic kinship is not the only valid criterion for a support system; an emotional kinship is the most important factor. In our mobile society of isolated nuclear families, the support system may be a next-door neighbor, a best friend, or perhaps a school chum.

The nurse must search out the significant others in the lives of the parents and help them understand the problems so that they can be a constant parental support.

Nursing Goal: Facilitation of Family Adjustment

The impact of the crisis on the family is individual and varied. In constructing a conceptual framework for family crisis Hill (1974) has formulated an equation to show the relationship of all elements:

A (the event) → interacting with B (the family's crisis-meeting resources) → interacting with C (the definitions the family makes of the events) → produces X (the crisis).

The stressful event (A), a situation for which the family has little or no preparation, may be classified according to the source of trouble: *extra-family events,* which may solidify the family, and *intra-family events,* which may reflect negatively on the adequacy of the family.

Marked changes in the configuration, such as addition of a new member (normal or preterm infant, infant with congenital anomaly) may also be a stressful occasion for the family members. The ability of the family to adapt to changing situations is the basis of the crisis-meeting resource (B). This adaptability to events depends on the definition (C) ascribed to each event by the family. Thus, an interplay of an event, the crisis-meeting resources, and the family definition of the event produces the crisis situation.

Information about the ability of the family to adapt to the situation is obtained through the nurse-family relationship. The event itself (normal newborn, preterm infant, infant with congenital anomaly) can then be viewed as it is defined by the family, and appropriate intervention can be instituted.

Because the family is a unit composed of individuals who must deal with the situation, it is important to encourage open intrafamily communication. Secret-keeping should not be encouraged, especially between spouses, because secrets undermine the trust of their relationship. Well-meaning rationales such as "I want to protect her," "I don't want him to worry about it," and so on can be destructive to open communication and to the basic element of a relationship—trust.

The nurse should be particularly sensitive to open communication when the mother is in an institution separate from the infant. The father is the first to visit the infant and relays information regarding the infant's care and condition to the mother. In this situation, the mother has had minimal contact, if any, with her infant. Because of her anxiety and isolation, she may mistrust all those who provide information (the father, nurse, physician, or extended family) until she can see for herself. This alone can put tremendous stress on the relationship between the spouses. The parents (and family) should be given information together. This practice helps overcome misunderstandings and misinterpretations and helps to promote "working through" together.

The entire family—siblings as well as relatives—should be encouraged to visit and receive information about the baby. Methods of intervention in assisting the family to cope with the situation include providing support, confronting the crisis, and understanding the reality. Support, explanations, and the helping role must extend to the kin network, as well as to the nuclear family, in an attempt to aid them in communication and support ties with the nuclear family.

It is also essential to meet the needs of the individuals involved. Desires and needs of the individuals must be respected and facilitated; differences are tolerable and able to exist side by side. Eliciting the parents' feelings is easily accomplished with the question: "How are you doing?" The emphasis is on *you,* and the interest must be sincere.

Families with children in the newborn intensive care unit become friends and support one another. To encourage the development of these friendships and to provide support, many units have established parent groups. The core of the groups consists of parents who previously have had an infant in the intensive care unit. Most groups make contact with families within a day or two of the infant's admission to the unit, either through phone calls or visits to the hospital. Early one-on-one parent contacts help families work through their feelings better than discussion groups. This personalized method gives the grieving parents an opportunity to express personal feelings about the pregnancy, labor, and delivery and their "different than expected" infant with others who have experienced the same feelings and with whom they can identify (Elsas 1981).

Nursing Goal: Provision of Predischarge Teaching

Predischarge planning begins once the infant's condition becomes stable and indications suggest the newborn will survive. Through adequate predischarge teaching, the parents are able to transform their feelings of inadequacy and competition with the nurse into feelings of self-assurance and attachment. From the beginning the parents should be included in the infant's care and taught about the infant's special needs and growth patterns. This teaching and involvement is best facilitated by a nurse who is familiar with the infant and his or her family over a period of time and who has developed a comfortable and supportive relationship with them.

The nurse's responsibility is to provide instructions in an optimal environment for parental learning. Learning should take place over time, to avoid the necessity of bombarding the parents with instructions in the day or hour before discharge.

Routine well-baby care, such as bathing, temperature taking, formula preparation, and breast-feeding are learned by the parents. Parents are also trained in the special procedures specific for their newborn. These procedures may include gavage or gastrostomy feedings, tracheostomy or enterostomy care, administration of medications, and CPR. Before discharge, the parents should be as comfortable as possible with these tasks and should demonstrate independence. Written tools and instructions are useful for parents to refer to once they are home with the infant, but these should not replace actual participation in the infant's care.

Teaching and learning methods are used in assessment of parental readiness to learn. Parents often enjoy doing minimal caretaking tasks with gradual expansion of their role. Many intensive care units provide facilities for parents to room-in with their infants for a few days before discharge. This allows parents a degree of independence in the care of their infant with the security of nursing help nearby. This practice is particularly helpful for anxious parents, parents who have not had the opportunity to spend extended time with their infant, or parents who will be giving a high level of physical care at home, such as tracheostomy care.

Referrals to community health services are done before discharge. The visiting nurses' association, public health nurses, or social services can assist the parents in the stressful transition from hospital to home by providing the necessary home teaching and support. Some intensive care nurseries have their own parent support groups to help bridge the gap between hospital and home care. Parents can also find support from a variety of community support organizations, such as mother of twins groups, or trisomy 13 clubs, March of Dimes Birth Defects Foundation, handicapped children services, and teen mother and child programs. Each community has numerous agencies capable of assisting the family in adapting emotionally, physically, and financially to the chronically ill infant. The nurse should be familiar with community resources and help the parents identify which agencies may benefit them.

The nurse helps parents recognize the growth and development needs of their infant. A development program begun in the hospital can be continued at home, or parents may be referred to an infant development program in the community.

Arrangements are made for medical follow-up care before discharge. The infant may need to be followed up by a family pediatrician, a well-baby clinic, or a specialty clinic. The first appointment should be made before the infant is discharged from the hospital.

The nurse evaluates the need for special equipment for infant care (such as a respirator, oxygen, apnea monitor) in the home. Any extra equipment or supplies should be placed in the home before the infant's discharge. The nurse can be instrumental in helping the parents assess the newborn's needs and coordinate services.

Evaluative Outcome Criteria

Nursing care is effective if:

- The parents are able to verbalize their feelings of grief and loss.

- The parents verbalize their concerns about their baby's health problems, care needs, and potential outcome.

- The parents are able to participate in their infant's care and show attachment behaviors.

● Considerations for the Nurse Who Works With At-Risk Newborns

Support cannot be given unless it can be received. Working in an emotional environment of "lots of living and lots of dying" takes its toll on staff. The emotional needs and feelings of the staff must be recognized and dealt with in order to enable them to support the parents. An environment of openness to feelings and support in dealing with their own human needs and emotions is essential for staff. Such techniques as group meetings, individual support, and primary care nursing may assist in maintaining staff mental health.

The staff NICU nurses may never see the long-term results of the specialized, sensitive care they give to parents and their newborns. Their immediate evidence of effective care may be only the beginning of resolution of parental grief, discharge of a recovered thriving infant to the care of happy parents, and reintegration of family life.

KEY CONCEPTS

Early identification of potential high-risk fetuses through assessment of prepregnant, prenatal, and intrapartal factors facilitates strategically timed nursing observations and interventions.

High-risk neonates, whether they are premature, SGA, LGA, postterm, or infant of a diabetic or substance-addicted mother, have many similar problems—although their problems are based on different physiologic processes.

The common problems of the preterm newborn are a result of the baby's immature body systems. Potential problem areas include respiratory distress (respiratory distress syndrome), patent ductus arteriosus, hypothermia and cold stress, feeding difficulties and necrotizing enterocolitis, marked insensible water loss and loss of buffering agents through the kidneys, infection, anemia of prematurity, apnea and intraventricular hemorrhage, retinopathy of prematurity, and behavioral state disorganization. Long-term needs and problems include bronchopulmonary dysplasia, speech defects, sensorineural hearing loss, and neurologic defects.

Postterm newborns frequently encounter the following intrapartal problems: CPD (shoulder dystocia) and birth traumas, hypoglycemia, polycythemia, meconium aspiration, cold stress, and possible seizure activity. Long-term complications may involve poor weight gain and low IQ scores.

Small-for-gestational-age newborns are associated with perinatal asphyxia and resulting aspiration syndrome, hypothermia, hypoglycemia, hypocalcemia, polycythemia, congenital anomalies, and intrauterine infections. Long-term problems include continued growth and learning difficulties.

Large-for-gestational-age newborns are at risk for birth trauma as a result of cephalopelvic disproportion, hypoglycemia, polycythemia, and hyperviscosity.

Infants of diabetic mothers are at risk for hypoglycemia, hypocalcemia, hyperbilirubinemia, polycythemia, and respiratory distress due to delayed maturation of their lungs.

Newborns of alcohol dependent mothers are at risk for physical characteristic alterations and the long-term complications of feeding problems; CNS dysfunction, including lower IQ, hyperactivity, and language abnormalities; and congenital anomalies.

Newborns born to drug-dependent mothers experience drug withdrawal as well as respiratory distress, jaundice, congenital anomalies, and behavioral abnormalities.

With early recognition and intervention, the potential long-term physiologic and emotional consequences of these difficulties can be avoided or at least lessened in severity.

Parents of at-risk newborns need support from nurses and health care providers to understand the special needs of their baby and to feel comfortable in an overwhelmingly strange environment.

REFERENCES

Abel EL: Prenatal effects of alcohol on growth: A brief overview. *Fed Proc* 1985;44:2318.

Affonso DD, **Harris** TR: Postterm pregnancy: Implications for mother and infant, challenge for the nurse. *J. Obstet Gynecol Neonat Nurs* 1980;9:139.

Als H, et al: Assessment of preterm infant behavior (APIB), in **Fitzgerald** HE, **Lester** BM, **Yogman** MW (eds): *Theory and Research in Behavioral Pediatrics.* New York, Plenum, 1982, vol 1.

Altura BM, et al: Alcohol produces spasms of human umbilical blood vessels: Relationship of fetal alcohol syndrome (FAS). *Eur J Pharmacol* 1982;86:311.

American Academy of Pediatrics Committee on Nutrition: Nutritional needs of low-birthweight infants. *Pediatrics* 1985;75(5):976.

American Academy of Pediatrics: Report: Neonatal drug withdrawal. *Pediatrics* 1983;72:895.

Avery GB (ed): *Neonatology.* ed 3. Philadelphia, Lippincott, 1987.

Avery ME, **Taeusch** HW (eds): *Schaffer's Diseases of the Newborn.* Philadelphia, Saunders, 1984.

Bree RL, **Mariona** FG: The role of ultrasound in the evaluation of normal and abnormal fetal growth, in **Raymond** HW, **Zwiebel** WJ (eds): *Seminars in Ultrasound.* New York, Grune & Stratton, 1980.

Carey BE: Intraventricular hemorrhage in the preterm infant. *J Obstet Gynecol Neonat Nurs* 1983;12(suppl):60s.

Cavdar AO: Fetal alcohol syndrome, malignancies, and zinc deficiency. *J Pediatr* 1984;105(2):335.

Chasnoff IJ, et al: Cocaine use in pregnancy. *N Engl J Med* 1985;313(September):666.

Clarren SK, **Bowden** DM, **Astley** S: The brain in the fetal alcohol syndrome. *Alcohol Health Res World,* Fall 1985, p 20.

Clifford S: Postmaturity. *Adv Pediatr* 1957;9:13.

Cloherty JP, **Stark** AR (eds): *Manual of Neonatal Care,* ed 2. Boston, Little, Brown, 1985.

Cole JG, **Frappier** PA: Infant stimulation reassessed: A new approach to providing care for the preterm infant. *J Obstet Gynecol Neonat Nurs* 1985;14(6):471.

Coles CD, et al: Neonatal ethanol withdrawal: Characteristics in clinically normal, nondysmorphic neonates. *J Pediatr* 1984;105(3):445.

The Committee for the Classification of Retinopathy of Prematurity: An international classification of retinopathy of prematurity. *Arch Ophthalmol* 1984;102:1130.

Corrazza MS, et al: Prolonged bleeding time in preterm infants receiving indomethacin for patent ductus arteriosus. *J Pediatr* 1984;105:292.

Dooley KJ: Management of the premature infant with a patent ductus arteriosus. *Pediatr Clin N Am* 1984;31:1159.

Duara S, et al: A newly recognized profile in neonatal lung disease with maternal diabetes. *Am J Radiol* 1985;144:637.

Dunn PM, et al: Metronidazole and the fetal alcohol syndrome. *Lancet* 1979;2(July):144.

Elsas TL: Family mental health care in the neonatal intensive care unit. *J Obstet Gynecol Neonat Nurs* 1981;10(May/June):204.

Eviator L: Evaluation of hearing in the high-risk infant. *Clin Perinatol* 1984;11(1):153.

Gersony WM, et al: Effects of indomethacin in premature infants with patent ductus arteriosus: results of a national collaborative study. *J Pediatr* 1983;102:895.

Gorski PA, et al: Stages of behavioral organization in the high-risk neonate: Theoretical and clinical considerations. *Semin Perinatol* 1979;3:61.

Grant P: Psychosocial needs of families of high-risk infants. *Fam Com Health* 1978;1(November):91.

Greer FR, et al: Effects of increased calcium, phosphorus, and vitamin D intake on bone mineralization in very low-birth-weight infants fed formulas with Polycose and medium-chain triglycerides. *J Pediatr* 1982;100(6):951.

Guidelines for Perinatal Care. Chicago, American Academy of Pediatrics and American College of Obstetricians and Gynecologists, 1983.

Harper RG, et al: Maternal ingested methadone, body fluid methadone, and the neonatal withdrawal syndrome. *Am J Obstet Gynecol* 1977;129(4):417.

Hellmann J, **Vannucci** RC: Intraventricular hemorrhage in premature infants. *Semin Perinatol* 1982;6:42.

Hendriksen A: Prolonged pregnancy: A literature review. *J Nurs-Midwife* 1985;39(1):33.

Hill R: Generic features of families under stress, in **Parad** HJ (ed): *Crisis Interventions.* New York, Family Services Association of America, 1974.

Hobart JM, **Depp** R: Prolonged pregnancy, in **Sciarra** JJ (ed): *Gynecology and Obstetrics.* Philadelphia, Harper & Row, 1982, vol 3.

Hobbins JC: Fetoscopy, in **Queenan** JT, **Hobbins** JC (eds): *Protocols for High Risk Pregnancies.* Oradell, NJ, Medical Economics Co, 1982.

Iosub S, et al: Fetal alcohol syndrome revisited. *Pediatrics* 1981;68(October):475.

Jones KL, et al: Pattern of malformation in offspring of chronic alcoholic mothers. *Lancet* 1973;1(June):1267.

Kaplan DM, **Mason** EA: Maternal reactions to premature birth viewed as an acute emotional disorder, in **Parad** HJ (ed): *Crisis Interventions*. New York, Family Services Association of America, 1974.

Kauffman RE: Therapeutic intervention to prevent intracerebral hemorrhage in preterm infants. *J Pediatr* 1986;108:323.

Klaus MH, **Fanaroff** AA: *Care of the High-Risk Neonate*. Philadelphia, Saunders, 1986.

Klaus MH, **Kennell** JH: *Maternal-Infant Bonding,* ed 2. St Louis, Mosby, 1982.

Korones SB: *High-Risk Newborn Infants: The Basis for Intensive Care Nursing,* ed 4. St Louis, Mosby, 1986.

Larsson G, **Bohlin** AB, **Tunell** R: Prospective study of children exposed to variable amounts of alcohol in utero. *Arch Dis Child* 1985;60:316.

Lemons PK: Victims of addiction. *Crit Care Update* 1983;10(5):12.

Lucey JF, **Dangman** B: A reexamination of the role of oxygen in retrolental fibroplasia. *Pediatrics* 1984;73(1):82.

Merker L, **Higgins** P, **Kinnard** E: Assessing narcotic addiction in neonates. *Pediatr Nurs* 1985;(May/June), p 177.

Miller HC: Prenatal factors affecting intrauterine growth retardation. *Clin Perinatol* 1985;12(June):307.

Oh W: Renal functions and clinical disorders in the neonate. *Clin Perinatol* 1981;4:321.

Okamoto E, et al: Use of medium-chain triglycerides in feeding the low-birth-weight infant. *Am J Dis Child* 1982;136(5):428.

Oxorn H: *Human Labor and Birth,* ed 5. Norwalk, Conn, Appleton-Century-Crofts, 1986.

Palmer EA, **Phelps** D: Multicenter trial of cryotherapy for retinopathy of prematurity. *Pediatrics* 1986;77:428.

Parkinson CE, **Wallis** S, **Harvey** D: School achievement and behavior of children who were small-for-dates at birth. *Dev Med Child Neurol* 1981;23:41.

Peckham GJ, et al: Clinical course to 1 year of age in premature infants with patent ductus arteriosus: Results of a multicenter randomized trial of indomethacin. *J Pediatr* 1984;105:285.

Pereira GR, **Lemons** JA: Controlled study of transpyloric and intermittent gavage feeding in the small pre-term infant. *Pediatrics* 1981;67:68.

Rosett HL, et al: Patterns of alcohol consumption and fetal development. *Obstet Gynecol* 1983;61:539.

Shannon K, et al: Erythropoiesis in infants of diabetic mothers. *Ped Res* 1986;20(2):161.

Solnit A, **Stark** M: Mourning and the birth of a defective child. *Psychoanal Study Child* 1961;16:505.

Stimmel B, et al: Fetal outcome in narcotic-dependent women: The importance of the type of maternal narcotic used. *Am J Drug Alcohol Abuse* 1983;9(4):383.

Streissguth AP, **La Due** RA: Psychological and behavioral effects in children prenatally exposed to alcohol. *Alcohol Health & Res World* 1985;10(Fall):6.

Tanmer JE: Disposition of ethanol in maternal venous blood and the amniotic fluid. *J Obstet Gynecol Neonat Nurs* 1985;14(6):484.

Taylor PM, **Hall** BL: Parent-infant bonding: Problems and opportunities in perinatal center *Semin Perinatol* 1979;3(1):75.

Teplin SW: Development of blind infants and children with retrolental fibrolasia: Implications for physicians. *Pediatrics* 1983;71:6.

Vohr BR, **Coll** CT: Neurodevelopmental and school performance of very low-birth-weight infants: A seven-year longitudinal study. *Pediatrics* 1985;76(3):345.

Zarfin Y, et al: Possible indomethacin-aminoglycoside interaction in preterm infants. *J Pediatr* 1985;106:511.

Ziegler EE, **Bega** RL, **Fomon** SJ: Nutritional requirements of the premature infant, in **Suskind** RM (ed): *Symposium on Pediatric Nutrition*. New York, Raven Press, 1983.

ADDITIONAL READINGS

Adamkin DH: Use of intravenous fat emulsions. Part 2. *Perinatal/Neonatal* 1986;10(July/August):48.

Anderson GC, **Marks** EA, **Wahlberg** V: Kangaroo care for premature infants. *Am J Nurs* 1986;July:807.

Armentrout D: Attitudes/beliefs/feelings held by neonatal nurses toward the care and management of fetal-infants. *Neonatal Network* 1986;4(February):21.

Boyes SM: AIDS virus in breast milk: A new threat to neonates and donor milk banks. *Neonatal Network* 1987;5(April):37.

Budreau G: Postnatal cranial molding and infant attractiveness: Implications for nursing. *Neonatal Network* 1987;5(April):13.

Cagle CS: Access to prenatal care and prevention of low birth weight. *Am J Mat Child Nurs* 1987;12(July/August):235.

Eden RD, et al: Perinatal characteristics of uncomplicated postdate pregnancies. *Obstet Gynecol* 1987;69(March):296.

Gates E: Obstetrical decision making in the delivery of the extremely premature infant. *Neonatal Network* 1986;4(February):7.

Inglis AD: AIDS and the neonatal ICU. *Neonatal Network* 1986;5(December):39.

Linton PT: Behavioral development of the premature infant. *Perinatal/Neonatal* 1986;10(July/August):27.

McCormick A: Special considerations in the nursing care of the very-low-birth-weight infant. *J Obstet Gynecol Neonat Nurs* 1984;13(6):357.

Meirer P, **Anderson** GC: Responses of small preterm infants to bottle- and breast-feeding. *Am J Mat Child Nurs* 1987;12(March/April):97.

Nelson D, **Heitman** R, **Jennings** C: Effects of tactile stimulation on premature infant weight gain. *J Obstet Gynecol Neonat Nurs* 1986;15(May/June):262.

Salitros PH: Transitional infant care: A bridge to home for high risk infants. *Neonatal Network* 1986;4(February):35.

Sherwen LN: The nursing role in helping the high-risk mother in crisis master maternal tasks. *J Perinatol* 1986;6:75.

Smith SM: Primary care in the NICU: A parent's perspective. *Neonatal Network* 1987;5(February):25.

Sterk MB: Understanding parenteral nutrition: A basis for neonatal nursing care. *J Obstet Gynecol Neonat Nurs* 1983;12(suppl):45s.

Trotter CW, et al: Perinatal factors and the developmental outcome of preterm infants. *J Obstet Gynecol Neonat Nurs* 1982;11:83.

Trouy MB, **Ward-Larson** C: Sibling grief. *Neonatal Network* 1987;5(February):35.

Wagner P, **Segall** ML: The NICU graduate: A multidisciplinary approach to complex home care. *Perinatal/Neonatal.* 1987;11(July/August):12.

When we chose the name Jonathan before the birth of our son, I thought I wouldn't use the shorter versions of the name. However, in the hospital, people referred to him by nicknames. They always talked about Jonny, or asked me how Jon was. I was pleased to hear these names. He sounded like a real person even though he had so many problems and was dying.(When Pregnancy Fails)

Complications of the Newborn

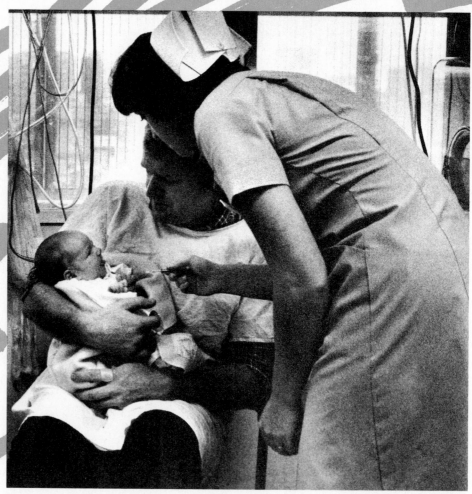

A neonatal nurse in Melbourne, Australia, gives an injection to an ill 3-day-old baby girl, held by her visiting father.

Chapter Thirty-Two

OBJECTIVES

- Based on the labor record, Apgar score, and observable physiologic indicators, identify infants in need of resuscitation and describe the appropriate method of resuscitation.

- Differentiate the various types of respiratory distress patterns.

- Use the nursing process to make nursing diagnoses and plan the care for an infant with respiratory distress syndrome.

- Differentiate between physiologic and pathologic jaundice based on onset, etiology, severity, and duration of disease.

- Use nursing assessment and diagnosis to identify nursing responsibilities in caring for the neonate receiving phototherapy or an exchange transfusion.
- Explain the relationship between the disease process and the clinical manifestations of an infant with persistent pulmonary hypertension of the newborn.
- Describe key indicators for nursing assessment of the infant at risk for necrotizing enterocolitis.
- Describe the nursing assessment of clinical manifestations that would lead the nurse to suspect neonatal sepsis.
- Relate the consequences of maternal syphilis, gonorrhea, or herpesvirus to the management of the infant in the neonatal period.
- Discuss selected metabolic abnormalities (including cold stress, hypoglycemia, and hypocalcemia), their effects on the neonate, and the nursing implications.
- Discuss selected hematologic problems such as anemia and the nursing implications for each problem.
- Discuss the nurse's role in the care of an infant with hemolytic disease.
- Correlate the clinical manifestations of bronchopulmonary dysplasia with the underlying disease process.
- Discuss nursing assessments and care of selected congenital anomalies.
- Discuss the clinical manifestations and nursing care of newborns with cardiac defect.

Marked homeostatic changes occur during the transition from fetal to neonatal life. The most rapid anatomic and physiologic changes of this period occur in the cardiopulmonary system. Thus the major problems of the newborn are usually related to this system. These problems include asphyxia, respiratory distress, patent ductus arteriosus, jaundice, hemolytic disease, and anemia. Ideally, problems are anticipated and identified prenatally, and appropriate intervention measures are begun at that time.

- ## Care of the Newborn At Risk Due to Asphyxia

Neonatal asphyxia results from circulatory, respiratory, and biochemical factors. Circulatory patterns that accompany asphyxia represent an inability to make the transition to extrauterine circulation—in effect a return to fetal-like circulatory patterns. Failure of lung expansion and establishment of respiration rapidly produces hypoxia (decreased PaO_2), acidosis (decreased pH), and hypercarbia (increased PCO_2). These biochemical changes result in pulmonary vasoconstriction, with retention of high pulmonary vascular resistance, hypoperfusion of the lungs, and a large right-to-left shunt through the ductus arteriosus. The foramen ovale opens (as right atrial pressure exceeds left atrial pressure), and blood flows from right to left.

Biochemical changes that occur in asphyxia contribute to these circulatory changes. The most profound biochemical aberration is a change from aerobic to anaerobic metabolism in the presence of hypoxia. This results in the accumulation of lactate and the development of metabolic acidosis. A concomitant respiratory acidosis may also occur due to a rapid increase in PCO_2 during asphyxia. In response to hypoxia and anaerobic metabolism, the amounts of free fatty acids (FFA) and glycerol in the blood increase. Glycogen stores are also mobilized to provide a continuous glucose source for the brain. Hepatic and cardiac stores of glycogen may be consumed rapidly during an asphyxial attack.

The neonate is supplied with protective mechanisms against hypoxial insults. These defenses include a relatively immature brain and a resting metaoblic rate less than that observed in the adult, an ability to mobilize substances within the body for anaerobic metabolism and use the energy more efficiently; and an intact circulatory system able to redistribute lactate and hydrogen ion in tissues still being perfused (Klaus & Fanaroff 1986). Unfortunately, severe prolonged hypoxia will overcome these protective mechanisms, resulting in brain damage or death of the neonate.

The newborn who is apneic on delivery requires immediate resuscitative efforts. The need for resuscitation can be anticipated if specific risk factors are present during the pregnancy or labor and delivery period.

Risk Factors Predisposing to Asphyxia

Need for resuscitation may be anticipated in antepartal, intrapartal, or neonatal situations.

ANTEPARTAL RISK FACTORS FOR RESUSCITATION

1. Previous obstetric history of fetal or neonatal death; premature or growth retarded infant; infant weighing 10 lb or more

2. Maternal conditions that affect the placenta or fetus—preeclampsia-eclampsia, postterm (more than 42 weeks), preexisting hypertension, diabetes, infection, chronic renal disease, maternal obesity, and cardiac disease

3. Maternal age—younger than 15 or over 35 years

4. Isoimmunization

5. Abruptio placentae or placenta previa

6. Multiple gestation

7. Abnormal presentation

8. Preterm infant

9. Prolonged rupture of the membranes

10. Hydramnios or oligohydramnios

11. Abnormal estriol levels

12. Less-than-mature L/S ratio

13. Maternal drug usage (narcotic, barbiturate, tranquilizer, or alcohol)

14. Anemia (hemoglobin less than 10 mg/dL)

INTRAPARTAL RISK FACTORS FOR RESUSCITATION

1. Abnormal labor pattern—dystocia, precipitous delivery

2. Meconium-stained amniotic fluid

3. Fetal heart rate patterns—tachycardia (greater than 160/min without maternal temperature elevation); bradycardia (less than 120/min, particularly associated with smooth baseline, an ominous sign); irregular rate; lack of baseline variability of FHR (smooth or fixed); lack of significant variability with fetal movement; ominous patterns (moderate to severe variable deceleration and late deceleration of any magnitude)

4. Abnormal fetal presentation—breech, transverse lie, shoulder

5. Prolapsed cord

6. Abruptio placentae or placenta previa

7. Indications for cesarean delivery

NEONATAL RISK RACTORS FOR RESUSCITATION

1. Difficult delivery

2. Fetal blood loss

3. Apneic episode unresponsive to tactile stimulation

4. Cardiac arrest

5. Inadequate ventilation

Medical Therapy

The initial goal of medical management is to identify the fetus at risk for asphyxia, so that resuscitative efforts can begin at delivery. Particular attention must be paid to at-risk pregnancies during the intrapartal period. Labor and delivery are asphyxiating processes and often the at-risk fetus has less tolerance to the stress of labor and delivery.

Fetal biophysical assessment and monitoring (fetal and maternal pH and blood gases) during the intrapartal period may help identify fetal distress. If fetal distress is present, appropriate measures can be taken to deliver the fetus immediately, before major damage occurs, and to treat the asphyxiated newborn.

The fetal biophysical profile includes tests for heart rate accelerations associated with fetal movement, sustained fetal breathing movements, fetal limb or trunk movements, extension and flexion movements, and measurement of amniotic fluid volume. Use of this testing procedure improves the ability to predict an abnormal perinatal outcome (Baskett et al 1984). Fetal scalp blood sampling (p 638), a valuable assessment tool, may indicate asphyxic insult and related degree of fetal acidosis if considered in relation to stage of labor, uterine contractions, and ominous FHR patterns. Normal fetal pH ranges from 7.3 to 7.35. The pH falls gradually during the first stage of labor. During the second stage and delivery, it decreases more drastically. The stress of labor causes an intermittent decrease in exchange of gases in the placental intervillous space, which causes a fall in pH and fetal acidosis. The acidosis is primarily metabolic rather than respiratory, because exchange of CO_2 is more rapid than exchange of hydrogen ions in the placenta.

During labor, a fetal pH of 7.25 or higher is considered normal. A pH value of 7.21–7.24 is considered as "preacidosis." A pH value of 7.20 or less is considered an ominous sign of fetal asphyxia. However, low fetal pH without associated hypoxia can be caused by maternal acidosis secondary to prolonged labor, dehydration, and maternal lactate production. One research group (Bowen et al 1986) found that only 50 percent to 70 percent of newborns were depressed when severe acidosis (pH 7.20) was present. Concurrent testing of maternal venous pH and fetal pH may help to rule out contributing maternal acidosis or to identify maternal alkalosis, which might result in a false normal fetal pH finding in the presence of fetal compromise.

The treatment of asphyxia is resuscitation. The goal of resuscitation is to provide an adequate airway with expansion of the lungs, to decrease the PCO_2 and increase the PO_2, to support adequate cardiac output, and to minimize oxygen consumption by reducing heat loss (Avery & Taeusch 1984).

Initial resuscitative management of the neonate is extremely important. The infant should be kept in a head-down position prior to the first gasp to avoid aspiration of the oropharyngeal secretions. The oropharynx and naso-pharynx must be suctioned immediately. By clearing the nasal and oral passages of fluid that may obstruct the air-way, a patent airway is established. Suction is always per-formed before resuscitation so that mucus, blood, meconium, or formula is not aspirated into the lungs.

After the first few breaths, the infant is kept in a flat position under a radiant heat source and is dried quickly to maintain skin temperature at about 36.5C (97.7F). Drying is also a good stimulation to breathing. Heat loss through evaporation is tremendous during the first few minutes of life. The temperature of a wet 1500 g baby in a 16C (62F) delivery room drops 1C every 3 minutes. Hypothermia increases oxygen consumption and in an asphyxiated infant increases the hypoxic insult and may lead to severe acidosis and development of respiratory distress.

Appraisal of the infant's need for resuscitation begins at the time of birth. The time of the first gasp, first cry, and onset of sustained respirations should be noted in order of occurrence. The Apgar score (p 675) is important in determining the severity of neonatal depression and the immediate course of necessary action (Table 32–1).

Breathing is established by employing the simplest form of resuscitative measures initially, with progression to more complicated methods as required.

1. Simple stimulation is provided by rubbing the back.

2. If respirations have not been initiated or are inadequate (gasping or occasional respirations), the lungs must be inflated with positive pressure. The mask is positioned securely on face (over nose and mouth; avoiding the eyes) with head in "sniffing" or neutral position (Figure 32–1). Hyperextension of the infant's neck will obstruct the trachea. An airtight connection is made between the infant's face and the mask (thus allowing the bag to inflate). The lungs are inflated rhythmically by squeezing the bag. Oxygen can be delivered at 100 percent with an anesthesia or Laerdal bag and adequate liter flow, whereas an Ambu or Hope bag delivers only 40 percent oxygen, unless it has been adapted. In addition, it may not be possible to maintain adequate inspiratory pressure with Ambu or Hope bags. In a crisis situation it is crucial that 100 percent O_2 be delivered with adequate pressure.

3. The rise and fall of the chest is observed for proper ventilation. Air entry and heart rate are checked by auscultation. Manual resuscitation is coordinated with any voluntary efforts. The rate of ventilation should be between 30 and 50 breaths per minute. Pressure should be less than 30 cm of H_2O. If ventilation is adequate, the chest moves with each inspiration, bilateral breath sounds are audible, and the lips and mucous membranes become pink. If

color and heart rate fail to respond to ventilatory efforts, poor or improper placement of an endotracheal tube may be the cause; if the neonate is intubated properly, pneumothorax, diaphragmatic hernia, or hypoplastic lungs (Potter's syndrome) may exist. Distention of the stomach is controlled by inserting a nasogastric tube for decompression.

4. Intubation (Figure 32–2, Procedure 32–1) is rarely needed. Most newborns can be resuscitated by bag and mask ventilation.

Once breathing has been established, the heart rate should increase to over 100 beats/min. If the heart rate is less than 60 beats/min, external cardiac massage is begun. (Cardiac massage is commenced immediately if there is no detectable heart beat.)

1. The infant is positioned *properly* on a firm surface.

2. The resuscitator uses two fingers (Figure 32–3), or may stand at the foot of the infant and place both thumbs at the junction of the middle and lower third of the sternum, with the fingers wrapped around and supporting the back.

3. The sternum is depressed approximately two-thirds of the distance to the vertebral column (1.0–1.5 cm), at a rate of 80 to 100 beats per minute.

4. A 3:1 ratio of heartbeat to assisted ventilation is used.

Drugs that should be available in the delivery room include those needed in the treatment of shock, cardiac arrest, and narcosis. Oxygen, because of its effective use in ventilation, is the drug most often used.

If by 5 minutes after delivery, the neonate has not responded to the resuscitation with spontaneous respira-

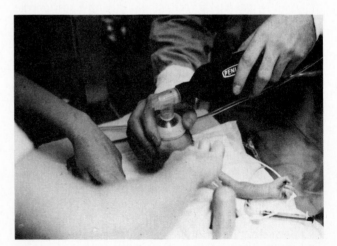

Figure 32–1 Resuscitation of infant with bag and mask. Note that the mask covers the nose and mouth and the head is in a neutral position.

Table 32–1 Guidelines for Resuscitation of the Neonate

Apgar score	Heart rate	Arterial blood pH*	Appearance	Resuscitative measures
9 or 10	>100	7.30–7.40 (normal)	Regular respirations; flexed extremities; cries in response to flicking of soles of feet; may be dusky or show acro-cyanosis	Place under radiant heat source and dry immediately; gently suction airway.
7 or 8	60–100	7.20–7.29 (slight acidosis)	Decreased tone, cyanotic, or dusky and dyspneic; respirations may be shallow, irregular, or gasping; heart rate is normal; fair response to flicking of sole	Dry and place under warmer; give oxygen near face.
5 or 6	60–100	7.10–7.19 (moderate acidosis)	Same as for Apgar 7 or 8	Dry and place under warmer; clear airway and stimulate through drying process. If still not improved, place in "sniff" position and begin ventilation (100% O_2) with bag and mask, using pressure of 30 cm H_2O at rate of 30–50 per min. If difficulty persists, reevaluate maternal history of drug administration, especially if heart rate responds to ventilation but there is no spontaneous respiration. Give narcotic antagonist (Narcan) if indicated. Mildly depressed newborns will usually develop regular spontaneous respirations within 5 minutes. If tracheal aspiration reveals blood or meconium, directly visualize with laryngoscope and suction as needed before administering positive pressure.
3 or 4	<60	7.00–7.09 (marked acidosis)	White and limp, little or no respiratory effort; Jaw is slack during suctioning	For Apgar 3–4: Dry under warmer; clear airway; consider immediate intubation. Hold O_2 near face during intubation. Ventilate after direct visualization with laryngoscope and appropriate suctioning. Check breath sounds. If heart rate remains low (0–<60), immediately institute external cardiac massage. Correction of hypotension is usually via umbilical vein. Obtain blood gas values (pH, PCO_2, PO_2) and BP.
0 to 2	<60	<7.00 (severe acidosis)	Same as for Apgar 3 or 4	

*Correlations of Apgar score and arterial blood pH adapted from Saling E: Technical and theoretical problems in electronic monitoring of the human fetal heart. *Int J Gynecol Obstet* 1972;10:211, and from Korones S: *High-Risk Newborn Infants: The Basis for Intensive Nursing Care*, ed 3. St Louis, Mosby, 1986.

tions and a heart rate above 100 beats per minute, it may be necessary to correct the acidosis and provide the myocardium with glucose. The most accessible route for administering medications is the umbilical vein. In a severely asphyxiated neonate, sodium bicarbonate (2 to 4 mEq/kg) is given to correct metabolic acidosis. If bradycardia is profound, epinephrine (0.01 mL/kg of a 1:10,000 solution) is given through the umbilical vein catheter, the peripheral

IV, or the endotracheal tube (in the absence of venous access). Bradycardia can also be treated with atropine (0.03 mg/kg intravenously). Calcium gluconate (1 or 2 mL/kg of a 10 percent solution) intravenously is used for arrhythmias, poor cardiac output despite adequate ventilation, and severe hypocalcemia or hyperkalemia. Dextrose can be given to correct hypoglycemia. Usually a 10 percent dextrose in water intravenous solution is sufficient to prevent

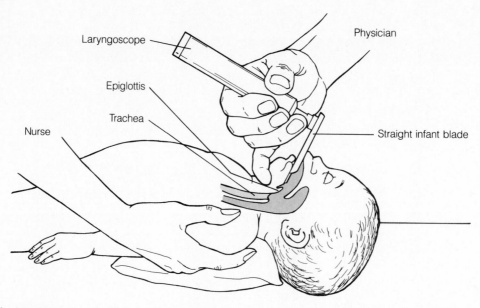

Figure 32–2   Endotracheal intubation is accomplished with the infant's head in the sniff position. The clinician places the fifth finger under the chin to hold the tongue forward.

or treat hypoglycemia in the delivery room. Naloxone hydrochloride (0.02 mg/mL neonatal solution intravenously or intramuscularly), a narcotic antagonist, is used to reverse narcotic depression. See Drug Guides–Sodium Bicarbonate and Naloxone.

In the advent of shock (low blood pressure or poor peripheral perfusion) the neonate should be given a volume expander. Fresh frozen plasma, plasminate, packed red blood cells, and whole blood can also be used for volume expansion and treatment of shock.

Nursing Assessment

Communication between the obstetric office or clinic and the labor and delivery nurse facilitates the identification of potential newborns in need of resuscitation. Upon arrival of the woman in the birthing area, the nurse should have the antepartal record and should note any contributory perinatal history factors and assess present fetal status. As labor progresses, nursing assessments include ongoing monitoring of fetal heartbeat and its response to contractions, assisting with fetal scalp blood sampling, and observing for expulsion of meconium, thereby identifying fetal asphyxia and hypoxia. In addition, the nurse should alert the resuscitation team and the practitioner responsible for care of the neonate of any potential high-risk patients in the labor and delivery area.

Nursing Diagnosis

Nursing diagnoses that may apply to the newborn with asphyxia include:

- Ineffective breathing pattern related to lack of spontaneous respirations at birth secondary to in utero asphyxia

- Decreased cardiac output related to impaired oxygenation

- Ineffective parental coping related to baby's lack of spontaneous respirations at birth and fear of losing their newborn

Nursing Goal: Preparation of Resuscitation Equipment

Following identification of possible high-risk situations, the next step in effective resuscitation is assembling

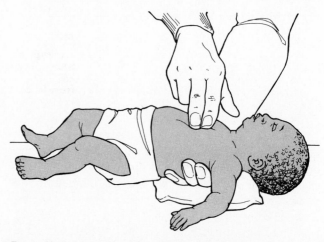

Figure 32–3   External cardiac massage. The midsternum is compressed with two fingertips at a rate of 80–100 beats/min.

Procedure 32–1   Tracheal Intubation

Objective	Nursing Action	Rationale
Facilitate atraumatic insertion of endotracheal tube in support of adequate tissue oxygenation	Gather necessary equipment, ensuring that all possible variations are available: 1. Laryngoscope handle with extra batteries and bulbs	Intubation is usually performed as an emergency measure. It is potentially hazardous to the newborn. If prolonged, iatrogenic effects include local orotracheal tissue damage and/or generalized hypoxia. Necessary equipment should be available on unit emergency cart.
	2. Detachable blades of curved and straight variety—infant and small child lengths	Curved blades are used when unusual tongue and jaw formations make straight blades inadequate. Smallest internal diameter endotracheal tube (2.5 mm) is used in very small neonates, with sizes increasing according to weight and length.
	3. Variety of uncuffed endotracheal tubes 4. Adapters for oxygen hookup between endotracheal tube and ventilator or resuscitation bag 5. Infant and pediatric masks and resuscitation bags 6. Oxygen tubing and flow meter with wall outlet adapter 7. Suction equipment (Procedure 32–3, p 1031) 8. Benzoin and 1-in. adhesive tape	In infants, uncuffed tubes can provide adequate seal.
	Immediately set up oxygen supply system and suction equipment. Suction and preoxygenate infant by mask and bag.	Infant should be as well oxygenated as possible before intubation begins to delay onset of hypoxemia. Oropharyngeal suctioning prior to intubation can facilitate visualization of epiglottis.
	Position and immobilize infant during laryngoscopy and tube insertion (Figure 32–2).	Most frequently used position is supine with very slight extension of head. Hold oxygen near neonate's face while he or she is being intubated.
	In the event of an unsuccessful intubation attempt, reoxygenate prior to next attempt	
	After appropriate placement of the tube has been determined (usually by portable x-ray), secure tube in that position. 1. Apply tincture of benzoin to clean and dry upper lip and cheeks of the infant. Allow it to dry. 2. Apply overlapping split 1-in. adhesive tape around tube and onto lips and cheeks.	Tube is inserted to a point just above the carina, which ensures effective ventilation of both lungs. With poor handling techniques, it is possible to dislodge tube, causing intubation of mainstem bronchus (usually on right) with no ventilation of other lung or causing complete extubation. Taping tube minimizes possibility of dislodgement. Some practitioners suture tube to tape.
	Measure length of tube from oral exit point to its connection point every 4 hr. Assess bilateral breath sounds and chest excursion symmetry for equality every hour.	Frequent monitoring of tube length and respiratory status are measurable criteria for evaluation of tube placement.

Precautions

Only skilled practitioners should attempt to intubate newborns in an emergency situation. Intubation of unanesthetized infants is usually carried out only in a profoundly obtunded patient. Insertion and suctioning of endotracheal tubes call for use of aseptic technique to minimize pulmonary infection. Assessment for signs and symptoms of tube obstruction and/or pneumothorax (especially with mechanical ventilation) should be of utmost priority for the nurse caring for an intubated infant.

Drug Guide   Sodium Bicarbonate

Overview of Neonatal Action

Sodium bicarbonate is an alkalizing agent. It buffers hydrogen ions caused by accumulation of lactic acid from anaerobic metabolism occurring during hypoxemia. Sodium bicarbonate thereby raises the blood pH, reversing the metabolic acidosis. Sodium bicarbonate should *only* be used to correct severe metabolic acidosis in asphyxiated newborns once adequate ventilation has been established (Avery 1987).

Note: Sodium bicarbonate dissociates in solution into sodium ion and carbonic acid, which can split into water and carbon dioxide. The carbon dioxide must be eliminated via the respiratory tract.

Route, Dosage, Frequency

For resuscitation and severe asphyxiation: intravenous push via umbilical vein catheter for quick infusion. Dosage is 2 mEq/K: 4 mL of 0.5 mEq/mL (4.2 percent) or 2 mL of mEq/mL (8.4 percent). 8.4 percent solution diluted at least 1:1 with sterile water to decrease the osmolarity; infuse at rate no faster than 1 mEq/kg/min (Avery 1987). Can repeat every 15 minutes if needed for total of 4 doses. For marked metabolic acidosis: a pH of less than 7.05 and a base deficit of 15 mEq/L or more should be corrected using a 0.5 mEq/mL solution of sodium bicarbonate at a rate of 1 mEq/kg/min or slower. Calculate total dosage by the following formula:

$$mEq = 0.3 \times weight\ (kg) \times base\ deficit\ in\ mEq/L$$

Neonatal Contraindications

Inadequate respiratory ventilation that causes a rise in PCO_2 and a decrease in pH

Presence of edema; metabolic or respiratory alkalosis; and hypocalcemia, anuria, or oliguria

Neonatal Side Effects

Hypernatremia, hyperosmolarity, fluid overload

Intracranial hemorrhage (rapid infusion of bicarbonate increases serum osmolarity, causing a shift of interstitial fluid into the blood and capillary rupture)

Nursing Considerations

Assess for any contraindications.

Monitor intake and output rates.

Assess adequacy of ventilation by monitoring respiratory status, rate, and depth; ventilate as necessary.

Dilute bicarbonate prior to administration into umbilical vein catheter (for resuscitation) or peripheral IV to prevent sloughing of tissue.

Evaluate effectiveness of drug by monitoring arterial blood gases for PCO_2, bicarbonate concentration, and pH determination.

Incompatible with acidic solutions.

Administration with calcium creates precipitates.

---

the necessary equipment and ensuring proper functioning (See Box 32–1). It is desirable to provide for pH and blood gas determination as well. Necessary equipment includes a radiant warmer, a device that should be in every delivery room. This equipment provides an overhead radiant heat source that is servocontrolled (a thermostatic mechanism that is taped to the infant's abdomen triggers the radiant warmer to turn on or off in order to maintain a level of thermoneutrality) and an open bed for easy access to the newborn. It is essential that the nurse keep the infant warm. The infant is dried quickly to prevent evaporative heat loss and is placed under the radiant warmer.

Resuscitative equipment in the delivery room must be sterilized after each use. In the high-risk nursery the need for resuscitation may occur at any time. Therefore, every newborn should have his or her own bag and mask available at the bedside. This equipment must be sterilized before use on another infant.

Equipment reliability must be maintained before an emergency arises. Inspect all equipment—bag and mask, oxygen and flow meter, laryngoscope, suction machines—for damaged or nonfunctioning parts before a delivery or assembly at the infant's bedside. A systematic check of the emergency cart and equipment should be a routine responsibility of each shift.

Nursing Goal: Provision and Documentation of Resuscitation

Training and knowledge about resuscitation are vital to personnel in the delivery setting for both normal and high-risk births. Since resuscitation is at least a two-person effort, the nurse should call for assistance so that there is adequate staff available. The resuscitative efforts should be recorded on the newborn's chart so that all members of the health care team will have access to this information.

Drug Guide   Naloxone Hydrochloride (Narcan)

Overview of Neonatal Action

Naloxone hydrochloride (Narcan) is used to reverse respiratory depression due to acute narcotic toxicity. It displaces morphinelike drugs from receptor sites on the neurons; therefore, the narcotics can no longer exert their depressive effects. Naloxone reverses narcotic-induced respiratory depression, analgesia, sedation; hypotension, and pupillary constriction (Berkowitz et al 1981).

Route, Dosage, Frequency
Intravenous dose is 0.01 mg/kg, usually through umbilical vein, although naloxone can be given intramuscularly. Neonatal dose is supplied as 0.02 mg/mL solution (0.5–1.0 mL for preterms and 2 mL for full-terms). Reversal of drug depression occurs within 1 to 2 minutes. The duration of action is variable (minutes to hours) and depends on amount of drug present and rate of excretion. Dose may be repeated in 5 minutes. If no improvement after two or three doses, naloxone administration should be discontinued. If initial reversal occurs, repeat dose as needed.

Neonatal Contraindications
Must be used with caution in infants of narcotic-addicted mothers as it may precipitate acute withdrawal syndrome. Respiratory depression resulting from nonmorphine drugs such as sedatives, hypnotics, anesthetics, or other nonnarcotic CNS depressants.

Neonatal Side Effects
Excessive doses may result in irritability and increased crying, and possibly prolongation of PTT
Tachycardia

Nursing Considerations

Monitor respirations closely—rate and depth.

Assess for return of respiratory depression when naloxone effects wear off and effects of longer-acting narcotic reappear.

Have resuscitative equipment, O_2, and ventilatory equipment available.

Monitor bleeding studies.

Incompatible with alkaline solutions.

Nursing Goal: Parent Education

Delivery room resuscitation is particularly distressing for the parents. If the need for resuscitation is anticipated, the parents should be assured that a team will be present at the delivery to care specifically for their infant. As soon as stabilization is accomplished, a member of the interdisciplinary team should discuss the infant's condition with the parents. The parents may have many fears about the need for resuscitation and the condition of their infant following the resuscitation.

Evaluative Outcome Criteria

Nursing care is effective if:

● The risk of asphyxia is promptly identified, and intervention is started early.

● The newborn's metabolic and physiologic processes are stabilized, and recovery is proceeding without sequelae.

● The parents can verbalize the reason for resuscitation and what was done to resuscitate their newborn.

● The parents can verbalize their fears about the re-

suscitation process and potential implications for their baby's future.

● ### Care of the Newborn With Respiratory Distress

One of the severest conditions to which the newborn may fall victim is respiratory distress—an inappropriate respiratory adaptation to extrauterine life. The nursing care of a baby with respiratory distress requires understanding of the normal pulmonary and circulatory physiology (Chapter 27), the pathophysiology of the disease process, clinical manifestations, and supportive and corrective therapies. Only with this knowledge can the nurse make appropriate observations concerning responses to therapy and development of complications. Unlike the verbalizing adult client, the newborn communicates needs only by behavior. The neonatal nurse interprets this behavior as clues about the individual baby's condition.

Idiopathic Respiratory Distress Syndrome (Hyaline Membrane Disease)

Respiratory distress syndrome (RDS), also referred to as *hyaline membrane disease* (HMD), is a complex disease

Box 32-1 Newborn Resuscitation Equipment

1. Radiant warmer

2. Stethoscope

3. Bag (that can deliver 100 percent oxygen)

4. Mask (two mask sizes: one preterm and one newborn)

5. Tubing and pressure gauges for bag

6. Oxygen, flow meter, and provision for warmth and humidification

7. Suction equipment
   a. DeLee trap
   b. Bulb syringe
   c. Mechanical suction apparatus
   d. Suction catheters (No. 5, 6, and 8 Fr)

8. Intubation equipment
   a. Magill forceps
   b. Endotracheal tubes—sizes 2.5, 3.0, 3.5, 4.0 mm (fitted with adapter)
   c. Wire stylets for tubes
   d. Laryngoscope handle with two blades—size 0 (premature), size 1 (newborn)
   e. Four extra batteries
   f. Two extra bulbs

9. Nasogastric tube (for decompression of stomach)

10. Infant plastic airway

11. K-Y lubricating jelly

12. Benzoin

13. Cotton applicators

14. Adhesive tape

15. Scissors

16. Safety pins (for attachments)

17. Syringes (tuberculin, 3, 5, and 10 mL)

18. Umbilical artery catheter tray (No. 3.5 and 5 Fr catheters)

19. IV solution and tubing

20. Drugs (solutions)
    a. Sodium bicarbonate (0.5 mEq/mL)
    b. Epinephrine (0.01 mL/kg of 1:10,000 solution)
    c. Dextrose (10 percent D/W for IV for hypoglycemia)
    d. Calcium gluconate (10 percent solution)
    e. Narcan (0.02 mg/mL neonatal solution)
    f. Volume expanders (plasma or human plasma protein fraction [plasminate])
    g. Normal saline (for suctioning)
    h. Atropine (0.4 mg/0.5 mL)

21. Blood pressure cuff and gauge or pressure transducer

22. Doppler (to measure blood pressure)

23. ECG electrodes and heart rate monitor

affecting primarily preterm infants and accounts for approximately 7000 deaths per year in the United States alone. The syndrome occurs more frequently in premature white infants than in black infants and almost twice as often in males as in females.

The factors precipitating the pathologic changes of RDS have not been determined, but two main factors are associated with its development:

1. *Prematurity.* All preterm newborns—whether AGA, SGA, or LGA—and especially IDMs are at risk for RDS. The incidence of RDS increases with the degree of prematurity, with most deaths occurring in newborns weighing less than 1500 g. The maternal and fetal factors resulting in preterm labor and delivery, complications of pregnancy, cesarean birth (indications for), and familial tendency are all associated with RDS.

2. *Asphyxia.* Asphyxia, with a corresponding decrease in pulmonary blood flow, may interfere with surfactant production

Development of RDS indicates a failure to synthesize lecithin at the rate required to maintain alveolar stability. Upon expiration this instability increases atelectasis, which causes hypoxia and acidosis. These inhibit surfactant production and cause pulmonary vasoconstriction. Thus the central pathophysiologic defect, lung instability due to this abnormality in the surfactant system, precipitates the biochemical aberrations of hypoxemia (decreased PO_2), hypercarbia (increased PCO_2), and acidemia (decreased pH), which further increases pulmonary vasoconstriction and hypoperfusion. The cycle of events of RDS leading to eventual respiratory failure is diagrammed in Figure 32-4.

Because of these pathophysiologic conditions, the neonate must expend increasing amounts of energy to reopen the collapsed alveoli with every breath, so that each breath becomes as difficult as the first. The progressive expiratory atelectasis upsets the physiologic homeostasis of the pul-

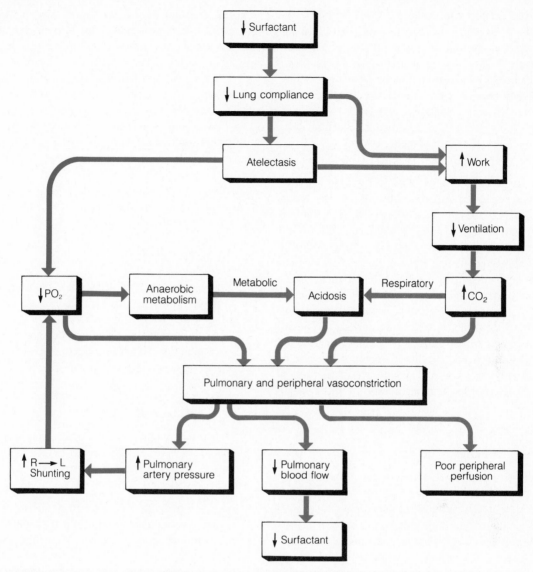

Figure 32–4   Cycle of events of RDS leading to eventual respiratory failure (Modified from Gluck L, Kulovich MV: Fetal lung development. *Pediatr Clin North Am* 1973;20:375)

monary and cardiovascular systems and prevents adequate gaseous exchange. Lung compliance decreases, and stiff lungs, which account for the difficulty of inflation, labored respirations, and the increased work of breathing, are the result.

The physiologic alterations of RDS produce the following complications:

1. *Hypoxia.* Hypoxia produces physiologic complications and consequences that increase the hypoxia and decrease pulmonary perfusion. As a result of hypoxia, the pulmonary vasculature constricts, pulmonary vascular resistance increases, and pulmonary blood flow is reduced. Increased pulmonary vascular resistance may precipitate a return to fetal circulation

as the ductus opens and blood flow is shunted around the lungs. Hypoxia also causes impairment or absence of metabolic response to cold, reversion to anaerobic metabolism resulting in lactate accumulation (acidosis), and impaired cardiac output, which decreases perfusion to vital organs.

2. *Respiratory acidosis.* Increased PCO_2 and decreased pH are results of alveolar hypoventilation. Carbon dioxide retention and resultant respiratory acidosis are the measure of ventilatory inadequacy, so that persistently rising PCO_2 and decrease in pH are poor prognostic signs of pulmonary function and adequacy.

3. *Metabolic acidosis.* Decreased pH and decreased bicarbonate levels may be results of impaired delivery of oxygen at the cellular level. Because of the lack of oxygen, the neonate begins an anaerobic pathway of metabolism, with an increase in lactate levels and a resultant base deficit. As the lactate levels increase, the pH becomes acidotic (decreased pH), and the buffer base decreases in an attempt to compensate and maintain acid-base homeostasis.

The classic radiologic picture of RDS is diffuse reticulogranular density (bilaterally), with portions of the air-filled tracheobronchial tree outlined by the opaque lungs (air-bronchogram). Opacification of the lung fields or "white-out" may be due to massive atelectasis, diffuse alveolar infiltrate, or pulmonary edema. The progression of radiologic findings parallels the pattern of resolution (four to seven days in uncomplicated, mild, or moderate RDS) and the time of surfactant reappearance.

The gross pathologic picture at autopsy reveals lungs that are dark red-purple, airless, and liverlike in consistency. Atelectasis is widespread, and the lungs are difficult to inflate. The presence of hyaline membranes in overdistended terminal bronchioles and alveoli reveals destruction and damage to the basement membrane of the alveolar cells.

MEDICAL THERAPY

The primary goal of prenatal management is the prevention of preterm delivery through aggressive treatment of premature labor and possible administration of glucocorticoids to enhance fetal lung development (see p 734). The goals of postnatal therapy are maintenance of adequate oxygenation and ventilation, correction of acid-base abnormalities, and provision of the supportive care required to maintain homeostasis.

Supportive medical management consists of ventilatory therapy, transcutaneous oxygen and carbon dioxide monitoring, correction of acid-base imbalance, environmental temperature regulation, adequate nutrition, and protection from infection. Ventilatory therapy is directed toward prevention of hypoventilation and hypoxia. Mild cases of RDS may require only increased humidified oxygen concentrations. Use of continuous positive airway pressure (CPAP) may be required in moderately afflicted infants. Severe cases of RDS require mechanical ventilatory assistance, with positive end-expiratory pressure (PEEP) (Figure 32–5).

NURSING ASSESSMENT

Increasing cyanosis, tachypnea, grunting respirations, nasal flaring, and significant retractions are characteristics of the disease. Table 32–2 reviews clinical findings associated with respiratory distress. The Silverman-Andersen index (Figure 32–6) may be helpful in evaluating the signs of respiratory distress.

NURSING DIAGNOSIS

Nursing diagnoses that may apply are included in the Nursing Care Plan: Respiratory Distress Syndrome, p 1016.

NURSING GOAL: PROMOTION OF PHYSICAL WELL-BEING

Based on clinical parameters the neonatal nurse implements therapeutic approaches to maintain physiologic

Figure 32–5 Infant on a respirator

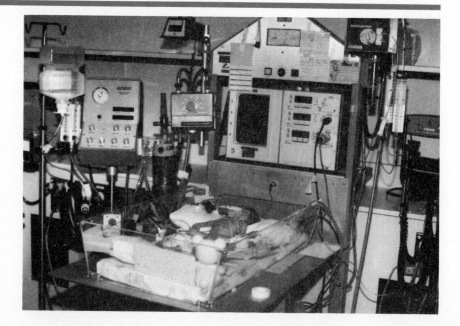

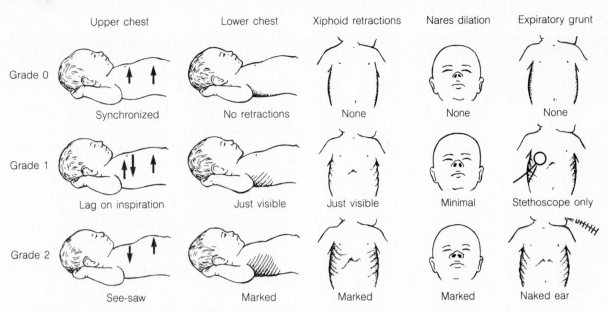

	Upper chest	Lower chest	Xiphoid retractions	Nares dilation	Expiratory grunt
Grade 0	Synchronized	No retractions	None	None	None
Grade 1	Lag on inspiration	Just visible	Just visible	Minimal	Stethoscope only
Grade 2	See-saw	Marked	Marked	Marked	Naked ear

Figure 32–6 Evaluation of respiratory status using the Silverman-Andersen index (From Ross Laboratories, Nursing Inservice Aid no. 2, Columbus, Ohio; and Silverman WA, Andersen DH: *Pediatrics* 1956;17:1, copyright © 1956, American Academy of Pediatrics)

homeostasis and provides supportive care to the newborn with RDS (see Nursing Care Plan: Respiratory Distress Syndrome, p 1016).

NURSING GOAL: PROVISION OF MECHANICAL VENTILATORY ASSISTANCE

Nursing interventions and criteria for instituting mechanical ventilatory assistance are included in Table 32–3. Methods of transcutaneous monitoring and nursing interventions are included in Table 32–4 on p 1028. Ventilatory assistance with high-frequency jet ventilations (Carlo et al 1984) and intratracheal administration of surfactant (Hallman et al 1985) are two new experimental therapeutic interventions that show positive preliminary results for treatment of infants with RDS.

Transient Tachypnea of the Newborn (Type II Respiratory Distress Syndrome)

Some newborns, primarily AGA and near-term infants, develop progressive respiratory distress that resembles classic RDS. These infants have usually had some intrauterine or intrapartal asphyxia due to maternal oversedation, cesarean birth, maternal bleeding, prolapsed cord, breech delivery, or maternal diabetes. The result is failure by the newborn to clear the airway of lung fluid, mucus, and other debris or an excess of fluid in the lungs due to aspiration of amniotic or tracheal fluid.

Usually little or no difficulty is experienced at the onset of breathing. However, shortly after admission to the nursery, expiratory grunting, flaring of the nares, and mild cyanosis may be noted in room air. Tachypnea is usually present by 6 hours of age, with respiratory rates as high as 100 to 140 breaths per minute.

MEDICAL THERAPY

The goal of medical management is to identify the type of respiratory distress and to institute treatment.

X-ray examination is performed. Initial x-ray findings may be identical to those showing RDS within the first three hours. However, radiographs of infants with transient tachypnea usually reveal a generalized overexpansion of the lungs (hyperaeration of alveoli), which is identifiable principally by flattened contours of the diaphragm. Dense streaks (increased vascularity) radiate from the hilar region. These perihilar streaks may represent engorgement of the lymphatics, which participate in clearance of alveolar fluid upon initiation of air breathing. Occasionally one or more dense patches indicates areas of collapse and/or large fluid accumulations.

Ambient oxygen concentrations as high as 70 percent may be required to correct the cyanosis initially. Thereafter, oxygen requirements usually decrease over the first 48 hours unlike those infants with RDS, which increase during this time.

The infants should be improving by 24 to 48 hours, except for modest O_2 dependence (less than 30 percent). The duration of the clinical course of transient tachypnea is approximately four days (96 hours). Early acidosis, both respiratory and metabolic (with moderate elevations of PCO_2), is easily corrected. Ventilatory assistance is rarely needed, and most of these infants survive.

Table 32–2   Clinical Findings Associated With Respiratory Distress

Clinical picture	Significance
SKIN	
Color	
Pallor or mottling	Represents poor peripheral circulation due to systemic hypotension and vasoconstriction and pooling of independent areas (usually in conjunction with severe hypoxia).
Cyanosis (bluish tint)	Depends on hemoglobin concentration, peripheral circulation, intensity and quality of viewing light, and acuity of observer's color vision; frankly visible in advanced hypoxia; central cyanosis is most easily detected by examination of mucous membranes and tongue.
Jaundice (yellow discoloration of skin and mucous membranes due to presence of unconjugated (indirect) bilirubin)	Metabolic aberrations (acidosis, hypercarbia, asphyxia) of respiratory distress predispose to dissociation of bilirubin from albumin-binding sites and deposition in the skin and central nervous system.
Edema (presents as slick, shiny skin)	Characteristic of preterm infant because of low total protein concentration with decrease in colloidal osmotic pressure and transudation of fluid; edema of hands and feet frequently seen within first 24 hours and resolved by fifth day in infant with severe RDS.
RESPIRATORY SYSTEM	
Tachypnea (normal respiratory rate 30–50/min; elevated respiratory rate 60+/min)	Increased respiratory rate is the most frequent and easily detectable sign of respiratory distress after birth; a compensatory mechanism that attempts to increase respiratory dead space to maintain alveolar ventilation and gaseous exchange in the face of an increase in mechanical resistance. As a decompensatory mechanism it increases work load and energy output (by increasing respiratory rate), which causes increased metabolic demand for oxygen and thus increase in alveolar ventilation (of already over-stressed system). During shallow, rapid respirations, there is increase in dead space ventilation, thus decreasing alveolar ventilation.
Apnea (episode of nonbreathing of more than 20 sec in duration; periodic breathing, a common "normal" occurrence in preterm infants, is defined as apnea of 5–10 sec alternating with 10–15 sec periods of ventilation)	Poor prognostic sign; indicative of cardiorespiratory disease, CNS disease, metabolic alterations, intracranial hemorrhage, sepsis, or immaturity; physiologic alterations include decreased oxygen saturation, respiratory acidosis, and bradycardia.
Chest	Inspection of thoracic cage includes shape, size, and symmetry of movement. Respiratory movements should be symmetrical and diaphragmatic; asymmetry reflects pathology (pneumothorax, diaphragmatic hernia). Increased anteroposterior diameter indicative of air-trapping (meconium aspiration syndrome).
Labored respirations (Silverman-Andersen chart in Figure 32–6 indicates severity of retractions, grunting, and flaring, which are signs of labored respirations)	Indicative of marked increase in work of breathing.
Retractions (inward pulling of soft parts of chest cage—suprasternal, substernal, intercostal, subcostal—at inspiration)	Reflect significant increase in negative intrathoracic pressure necessary to inflate stiff, noncompliant lung; infants attempt to increase lung compliance by using accessory muscles; markedly decreases lung expansion; seesaw respirations are seen when chest flattens with inspiration and abdomen bulges; retractions increase work and O_2 need of breathing, so that assisted ventilation may be necessary due to exhaustion.
Flaring nares (inspiratory dilation of nostrils)	Compensatory mechanism that attempts to lessen resistance of narrow nasal passage.
Expiratory grunt (Valsalva maneuver in which infant exhales against closed glottis, thus producing audible moan)	Produces increase in transpulmonary pressure, which decreases or prevents atelectasis, thus improving oxygenation and alveolar ventilation; intubation should not be attempted unless infant's condition is rapidly deteriorating, because it prevents this maneuver and allows aveoli to collapse.
Rhythmic movement of body with labored respirations (chin tug, head bobbing, retractions of anal area)	Result of use of abdominal and other respiratory accessory muscles during prolonged forced respirations.
Auscultation of chest reveals decreased air exchange with harsh breath sounds or fine inspiratory rales, rhonchi may be present.	Decrease in breath sounds and distant quality may indicate interstitial or intrapleural air or fluid.

Table 32–2 Clinical Findings Associated With Respiratory Distress (continued)

Clinical picture	Significance
CARDIOVASCULAR SYSTEM	
Continuous systolic murmur may be audible	Patent ductus arteriosus is common occurrence with hypoxia, pulmonary vasoconstriction, right-to-left shunting, and congestive heart failure.
Heart rate usually within normal limits (fixed heart rate may occur with a rate of 110–120/min)	Fixed heart rate indicates decrease in vagal control.
Point of maximal impulse usually located at fourth to fifth intercostal space, left sternal border.	Displacement may reflect dextrocardia, pneumothorax, or diaphragmatic hernia.
HYPOTHERMIA	Inadequate functioning of metabolic processes that require oxygen to produce necessary body heat.
MUSCLE TONE	
Flaccid, hypotonic, unresponsive to stimuli	May indicate deterioration in neonate's condition and possible CNS damage, due to hypoxia, acidemia, or hemorrhage.
Hypertonia and/or seizure activity	

Radiographs are usually normal within a week and the infant is well within two to five days. If progressive deterioration occurs to the extent that assisted ventilation is required, a diagnosis of superimposed sepsis must be considered and treatment measures initiated. For nursing actions, see the Nursing Care Plan: Respiratory Distress Syndrome, p 1016.

Meconium Aspiration Syndrome

The presence of meconium in amniotic fluid indicates an asphyxial insult to the fetus. The physiologic response to asphyxia is increased intestinal peristalsis, relaxation of the anal sphincter, and passage of meconium into the amniotic fluid.

Approximately 10 percent of all pregnancies will have meconium-stained fluid. This fluid may be aspirated into the tracheobronchial tree in utero or during the first few breaths taken by the newborn. Prolonged labor is associated with meconium aspiration syndrome (MAS). This syndrome primarily affects term, SGA, and postterm newborns.

Presence of meconium in the lungs produces a ball-valve action (air is allowed in but not exhaled), so that alveoli overdistend; rupture with pneumomediastinum or pneumothorax is a common occurrence. The meconium also initiates a chemical pneumonitis in the lung with oxygen and carbon dioxide trapping and hyperinflation. Secondary bacterial pneumonias are common. Clinical manifestations of MAS include: (a) fetal hypoxia in utero a few days or a few minutes prior to delivery indicated by a sudden increase in fetal activity followed by diminished activity, slowing of fetal heart rate or weak and irregular heartbeat, and meconium staining of amniotic fluid; and (b) presence of signs of distress at delivery, such as pallor, cyanosis, apnea, slow heartbeat, and low Apgar scores (be-

low 6) at one and five minutes. As the victims of intrauterine asphyxia, meconium-stained neonates or newborns who have aspirated meconium are often depressed at birth and require resuscitative efforts to establish adequate respiratory effort.

After the initial resuscitation, the severity of clinical symptoms correlates with the extent of aspiration. Mechanical ventilation is frequently required from birth due to immediate signs of distress (generalized cyanosis, tachypnea, and severe retractions). An overdistended, barrel-shaped chest with increased anteroposterior diameter is common. Auscultation reveals diminished air movement with prominent rales and rhonchi. Abdominal palpation may reveal a displaced liver due to diaphragmatic depression secondary to the overexpansion of the lungs (Nugent 1983). Yellowish staining of the skin, nails, and umbilical cord is usually present.

The chest x-ray film reveals nonuniform, coarse, patchy densities and hyperinflation (9- to 11-rib expansion). The densities are associated with focal areas of irregular aeration, some of which appear atelectatic or consolidated, while others appear emphysemic. Evidence of pulmonary air leak is frequently present. These infants have massive biochemical aberrations, which include: (a) extreme metabolic acidosis resulting from the cardiopulmonary shunting and hypoperfusion; (b) extreme respiratory acidosis due to shunting and alveolar hypoventilation; and (c) extreme hypoxia, even in 100 percent O_2 concentrations and with ventilatory assistance. The extreme hypoxia is also caused by the cardiopulmonary shunting and resultant failure to oxygenate.

MEDICAL THERAPY

The combined efforts of the obstetrician and pediatrician are needed to prevent MAS. The most effective form of preventive management is outlined as follows:

Table 32–3 Assisted Ventilatory Methods

Types	Functions and rationale	Nursing interventions
Continuous positive airway pressure (CPAP)	Application of gas with greater than atmospheric pressure to airway during spontaneous respiratory effort. Infant must have spontaneous respirations, because apnea is absolute criterion for assisted ventilation; persistently low PaO_2 (below 50 while breathing 50%–60% O_2)(Avery 1987), and repeated apneic episodes are criteria for CPAP application (usually via endotracheal tube or nasal prongs; when high distending pressures are used abdominal distention may occur).*	Maintain CPAP system through knowledge of elements of system and function of each. Monitor oxygen concentration as ordered; place an orogastric tube and leave open for decompression; monitor manometer reading and document distending pressure; make adjustments when baby is quiet; humidify and warm oxygen; suction as needed for patency; clean nasal prongs, assess nares for irritation, and give mouth care every two hours. Evaluate response of infant to CPAP application or adjustment by arterial blood gases and by clinical condition (same as for evaluation under oxygen therapy). As a general rule, first decrease concentrations of oxygen, then slowly reduce pressure until neonate is able to maintain adequate arterial oxygenation with CPAP system at 3 cm H_2O.
Assisted ventilation ventilators Pressure-cycled respirators (operate by cessation of inspiratory phase when preset pressure has been reached)	Tidal volume and compliance of thorax and lungs is smaller in infants than in adults; tidal volume is variable for newborn (7–10 mL/kg)	Understand and maintain type of ventilatory support; check and record patency of system and respirator parameters (at least every hour), rate, volume, pressure, oxygen concentrations, mean airway pressure, flow, and gas temperature. Perform chest physiotherapy and suction when indicated; humidify and warm gas; reposition baby every 2 hours and inspect skin for breakdown; monitor for signs of extubation (sudden deterioration, decreased breath sounds, bradycardia, audible crying); maintain alarms on at all times.
Volume-cycled respirators (deliver predetermined volume of air with each respiratory cycle; pressure is developed within system so that delivery of a known volume to a stiff lung increases pressure within system)	Certain conditions decrease lung compliance and resistance, such as atelectasis, respiratory distress syndrome; with use of increased pressures, there is increased incidence of complications (see p 1009)	
Time-cycled respirators (used by adjustment of inspiratory and expiratory phases of respiration)	Indications for use of mechanical ventilation are* 1. Apnea—absolute indication. 2. Hypoxia—evidenced by PaO_2 less than 50 mm Hg (torr) 3. Hypercarbia—evidenced by $PaCO_2$ greater than 60 mm Hg (torr) or rapidly rising respiratory acidosis (pH less than 7.20)	Keep bag and mask at bedside in the event of mechanical failure of ventilator or accidental or necessary extubation; if mechanical failure occurs, support neonate with bag and mask until corrections are made (an indispensable member of team is respiratory therapist). For reintubation, keep proper size of tracheal tube at bedside. Evaluate response of infant to assisted ventilation or adjustments within system by arterial blood gas determinations and by clinical condition (same as for evaluations under oxygen therapy).

*The criteria for instituting CPAP or controlled ventilation are somewhat arbitrary and vary from institution to institution. Clinical assessments of severity of respiratory distress, transcutaneous monitoring of PO_2, rate of rise of PCO_2, oxygen requirements, and frequency or duration of apneic episodes are essential.

1. After the head of the neonate is delivered and the shoulders and chest are still in the birth canal, the nasopharynx and oropharynx are suctioned with a DeLee catheter. (The same procedure is followed with a cesarean delivery.)

2. Immediately after delivery of the neonate, intubation and direct suctioning of the trachea through an endotracheal tube is performed.

   a. The resuscitator places his or her mouth over the endotracheal tube and sucks on the tube as it is withdrawn from the trachea (a paper mask is placed over the tube to present inhalation of meconium by the resuscitator).

b. If meconium is suctioned from the trachea, the neonate is reintubated and suctioned until the airway is cleared.

c. It is recommended that the neonate not be lavaged with normal saline once intubated, as this procedure forces the meconium into the small airways.

If the newborn is not adequately suctioned on the perineum, respiratory or resuscitative efforts will push meconium into the airway and into the lungs. Stimulation of the neonate is avoided to minimize respiratory movements. Further resuscitative efforts as indicated follow the same principles mentioned earlier in this chapter, p 1002. Resuscitated neonates should be immediately transferred to the nursery for closer observation. An umbilical arterial line may be used for direct monitoring of arterial blood pressures; blood sampling for pH, and blood gases; and infusion of intravenous fluids, blood, or medications.

Treatment usually involves high ambient oxygenation and controlled ventilation. Low positive end-expiratory pressures (PEEP) are desired to avoid air leaks. Unfortunately, high pressures may be needed to cause sufficient expiratory expansion of obstructed terminal airways or stabilize airways that are weakened by inflammation so that the most distal atelectatic alveoli are ventilated. Systemic blood pressure and pulmonary blood flow must be maintained. Intravenous tolazoline (Priscoline) or isoproterenol (Isuprel) may be used to increase the pulmonary blood flow by overcoming the arterioles' vasoconstriction and pulmonary vasospasm, which has created a right-to-left cardiopulmonary shunt. Tolazoline must be used with extreme caution as dramatic falls in blood pressure can occur.

Treatment also includes chest physiotherapy (chest percussion, vibration, and drainage) to remove the debris. Prophylactic antibiotics are frequently given. Bicarbonate may be necessary for several days for severely ill newborns. Mortality in term or postterm infants is very high, because they are so difficult to oxygenate.

NURSING ASSESSMENT

During the intrapartal period, the nurse should observe for signs of fetal hypoxia and meconium staining of amniotic fluid. At delivery, the nurse assesses the newborn for signs of distress. During the ongoing assessment of the newborn, the nurse carefully observes for complications such as pulmonary air leaks; anoxic cerebral injury manifested by cerebral edema and/or convulsions; anoxic myocardial injury evidenced by congestive heart failure or cardiomegaly; DIC resulting from hypoxic hepatic damage with depression of liver-dependent clotting factors; anoxic renal damage demonstrated by hematuria, oliguria or an-

uria; fluid overload; sepsis secondary to bacterial pneumonia; and any signs of intestinal necrosis from ischemia, including gastrointestinal obstruction or hemorrhage.

NURSING DIAGNOSIS

Nursing diagnoses that may apply to the newborn with meconium aspiration syndrome include:

- Ineffective gas exchange related to presence of respiratory distress secondary to aspiration of meconium and amniotic fluid during delivery

- Alteration in nutrition: less than body requirements related to respiratory distress and increased energy requirements

- Ineffective parental coping related to life-threatening illness in term newborn

NURSING GOAL: PREVENTION OF MECONIUM ASPIRATION

Initial interventions are primarily aimed at prevention of the aspiration by assisting with the removal of the meconium from the infant's naso- and oropharynx prior to the first extrauterine breath.

NURSING GOAL: PROMOTION OF PHYSICAL WELL-BEING

When significant aspiration occurs, therapy is supportive with the primary goals of maintaining appropriate gas exchange and minimizing sequelae. Nursing interventions after resuscitation should include: maintenance of adequate oxygenation and ventilation, temperature regulation, glucose strip test at 2 hours of age to check for hypoglycemia, observation of intravenous fluids, calculation of necessary fluids (which may be restricted in first 48–72 hours due to cerebral edema), and provision of caloric requirements.

EVALUATIVE OUTCOME CRITERIA

Nursing care is effective if:

- The risk of MAS is promptly identified and early intervention is initiated.

- The newborn is free of respiratory distress and metabolic alterations.

- The parents verbalize their concerns about their baby's health problem/survival and understand the rationale behind management of their newborn.

Nursing Care Plan: Respiratory Distress Syndrome

Joey Roberts was born at 1290 g, 31 weeks AGA to a 19-year-old, G 1, P 0, AB 0, A positive mother. Pregnancy was complicated by partial abruption requiring cesarean delivery. Joey required bag and mask resuscitation in the delivery room. Apgars were 3 at one minute and 6 at five minutes. On admission to the intensive care nursery, he exhibited severe respiratory distress with cyanosis, nasal flaring, audible grunting, severe intracostal and substernal retractions, and a res-

piratory rate of 68. Auscultation revealed coarse breath sounds with audible rales. He was placed in a 40% oxygen hood. Initial chest X ray revealed a diffuse reticulogranular pattern with visible air bronchograms. Arterial blood gases showed a pH of 7.20 with $PaCO_2$ of 60 and PaO_2 of 49 mm Hg. He was started on an IV of 10% glucose at 80 mL/kg/day.

Assessment

NURSING HISTORY

Identification of predisposing factors including:
a. 31 weeks preterm AGA
b. 19-year-old mother
c. Hx of partial placenta abruption
d. Apgar 3 at one minute and 6 at five minutes
e. Required bag and mask resuscitation in DR

PHYSICAL EXAMINATION

Tachypnea (over 60 respirations/min), expiratory grunting (audible), substernal/intercostal retractions.
Followed by flaring of nares on inspiration, cyanosis and pallor, rhythmic movement of body and labored respirations, chin tug.
Auscultation: There is decreased air exchange with coarse breath sounds and, upon deep inspiration, rales.
Increasing oxygen concentration requirements to maintain adequate Po_2 levels.

LABORATORY EVALUATION

Arterial blood gases (indicating respiratory failure): PaO_2 49 mm Hg and PCO_2 60 mm Hg, pH 7.20
X ray: Diffuse reticulogranular density bilaterally, with (air-filled tracheobronchial tube outlined by opaque lungs) air bronchogram; hypoexpansion
Dextrostix: 40 mg/dL

ANALYSIS OF NURSING PRIORITIES

1. Assure adequate oxygenation.
2. Provide for assisted ventilatory exchange.
3. Determine and correct acid-base imbalances.
4. Take supportive measures to maintain homeostasis—maintain neutral thermal environment, provide for adequate fluid and electrolyte and caloric requirements, prevent infection.
5. Provide for the emotional needs of the infant with respiratory distress without overstimulation and meet the needs of the family.
6. Observe possible complications of therapy and institute appropriate nursing interventions.

Nursing Diagnosis and Goals	Nursing Interventions and Actions	Rationale
NURSING DIAGNOSIS: Impaired gas exchange related to inadequate lung surfactant	Initial observation of respiratory effort, ventilatory adequacy—observation of chest wall movement, skin, mucous membranes, color; estimation of degree and equality of air entry by auscultation, arterial blood gases, and pH determination.	Alveoli of normal infant remain stable during expiration due to presence of surfactant. Alveoli of infant with RDS lack surfactant and collapse with expiration.
SUPPORTING DATA: Cyanosis Increased respiratory effort Expiratory grunting Retractions Hypoxemia—PaO_2 49 Hypercarbia—$PaCO_2$ 60 Acidemia—pH 7.20 Respiratory failure Altered level of infant activity Lethargy	Maintain on respiratory and cardiac monitors—note rates every 30–60 min or more often as indicated by the severity of infant's distress. Check and calibrate all monitoring and measuring devices every 8 hr. Calibrate oxygen devices to 21% and 100% O_2 concentrations. Control and monitor oxygen concentrations at least every hour.	Alveolar atelectasis and intrapulmonary shunting results in poor gas exchange, hypoxemia, hypercarbia, and acid-base derangements. Grunting, a compensatory mechanism, increases transpulmonary pressure, overcomes high surface tension, forces and prevents atelectasis, and thus enables improved oxygenation and a rise in PaO_2.
	Administer oxygen by oxygen hood—a small transparent head hood that contains an inlet and carbon dioxide outlet (Figure 32–7).	Provides a constant oxygen environment. Incubators are not recommended for long-term oxygen delivery since the concentration is difficult to regulate and fluctuates when portholes are opened for care giving.
	Maintain Joey in stable oxygen concentration by increasing or decreasing oxygen by 5%–10% increments and then obtain arterial blood gases.	Stable concentration of oxygen is necessary to maintain PaO_2 within normal limits (50–70 mm Hg). Sudden increase or decrease in O_2 concentration may result in disproportionate increase or decrease in PaO_2 due to vasoconstriction in response to hypoxemia.

Nursing Care Plan: Respiratory Distress Syndrome (continued)

Nursing Diagnosis and Goals	Nursing Interventions and Actions	Rationale
	Joey's response to therapy is evaluated by arterial blood gases, transcutaneous oxygen monitoring, and clinical assessment.	
	Observe for: 1. Pink color, cyanosis (central or acrocyanosis), duskiness, pallor 2. Respiratory effort (evaluation at rest), rate of respirations, patterns (apnea, periodic breathing), quality (easy, unlabored; abdominal, labored), auscultation (site of breath sounds—overall or part of lung fields—describe quality of breath sounds every 1–2 hr), accompanying sounds with respiratory effort (change from previous observations) 3. Activity—less active, flaccid, lethargic, unresponsive; increased activity, restless, irritable; inability to tolerate exertion, crying, sucking, or nursing care activity 4. Circulatory response (evaluate at rest); rate, regularity, and rhythm of heart rate; periods of bradycardia; alterations of blood pressure	
	Observations of clinical condition are taken serially for comparison and changes.	
	Observations should be taken while infant is receiving oxygen and with any oxygen adjustment.	
	Return O_2 concentration to previous levels if there is deterioration in neonate's condition or drop below desired transcutaneous oxygen monitor (TCM) levels. Repeat arterial blood gases (keep PaO_2 50–70 mm Hg). Gases should be done within 15–20 min after any change in ambient O_2 concentration or after inspiratory or expiratory pressure changes.	Any deterioration of clinical condition with oxygen adjustments (usually a decrease in ambient oxygen concentration) indicates inability of neonate to compensate for hypoxia.

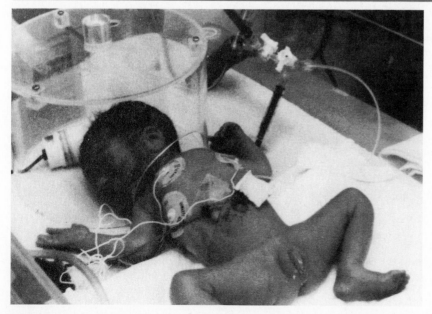

Figure 32–7 Infant in oxygen hood

Nursing Care Plan: Respiratory Distress Syndrome (continued)

Nursing Diagnosis and Goals	Nursing Interventions and Actions	Rationale
	Record and report clinical observations and action taken.	
	Maintain stable environment prior to collection of artierial blood gas sample:	Values used to determine adequate oxygenation—normal PaO_2 50–70 mm Hg. Adequate ventilation—normal $PaCO_2$ 35–45 mm Hg. Acid-base balance—normal pH 7.35–7.45.
	1. Maintain constant O_2 concentration at least 15–20 min before sample	Accurate arterial blood determinations are essential in management of any infant receiving oxygen, because presence or absence of cyanosis is unreliable.
	2. Avoid any disturbances of infant 15 min before gases are drawn.	Crying or struggling may cause hyperventilation or breath holding and may increase shunting of blood.
	Do not suction; if suction is absolutely necessary, delay blood sample.	
	Maintain temperature of sample (pH should be measured at body temperature).	
	Provide arterial blood gas setup (a 3 mL syringe with heparinized solution and a heparinized tuberculin syringe) to obtain blood sample.	Use of temporal, radial, or brachial arteries takes skill, is time-consuming, and may have serious consequences; therefore, most common technique for sampling is through umbilical artery catheter (Procedure 32–2, p 1024).
	After blood sample is taken, recheck flow through line to assure patency and prevent establishment of clot.	
	Replace blood used to clear line.	Total blood volume of infant is small; blood removed to clear catheter must be returned to prevent hypovolemia, anemia.
	Use heparinized flush solution before restarting IV solution to prevent clots in the line.	
GOALS: Respirations will be 30–50/min, regular without episodes of apnea. Oxygen therapy will be discontinued without evidence of complications. Complications of oxygen or ventilator therapy will be absent or minimized.		

Joey is now 28 hours old and has progressive respiratory distress. His PaO_2 is now 40 mm Hg, and his $PaCO_2$ is 65 in 75% oxygen. His respiratory effort is increased, he is now hypotensive, and has had 2 episodes of bradycardia. The decision is made to intubate Joey and place him on assisted ventilation. Joey is also placed on ampicillin and gentamicin because of the catheter insertion, intubation, and temperature instability.

	Nursing Interventions and Actions	Rationale
	Assess need for assisted ventilatory measures. Criteria for assisted ventilation: 1. Apnea 2. Hypoxia (PaO_2 <50 mm Hg) 3. Hypercarbia ($PaCO_2$ >60 mm Hg) 4. Respiratory acidosis (pH <7.20)	
	Set up CPAP or PEEP (see Table 32–3). Position infant in "sniffing" position. See Figure 32–2 for intubation.	Application of CPAP or PEEP produces same stabilization force on alveoli as grunting does and produces same effect—improved oxygenation and rise in Pao_2.
	Set up for endo/nasotracheal intubation and assist (see Procedure 32–1).	Delivery of CPAP or PEEP can only be done by use of nasal prongs, nasopharyngeal tube, or oral intubation.

Nursing Care Plan: Respiratory Distress Syndrome (continued)

Nursing Diagnosis and Goals	Nursing Interventions and Actions	Rationale
	Attempts at intubation should not exceed 30 sec and should be terminated with evidence of hypoxia and bradycardia.	
	Determine proper placement of tube by presence and quality of breath sounds. If breath sounds are better on one side, tube may be in right main stem bronchus; slowly withdraw tube and auscultate chest for equal bilateral breath sounds.	
	Extubate if breath sounds are heard over stomach. Reoxygenate prior to another intubation attempt.	Tube is in esophagus.
	Tube is properly placed if chest moves symmetrically, infant cannot cry, color and muscle tone improve with effective oxygenation.	
	Heart rate and rhythm improve with effective oxygenation.	
	Confirm placement by chest x ray. Secure and maintain with tape a properly positioned tube.	
	Observe nasal passage for position and deformity. Keep tube in neutral position without pulling on alae nasi. Observe for blanched area around nasal tube and reposition until blanching disappears. If oral tube is used, maintain neutral position within mouth. Observe color and integrity of gums; if blanched, reposition tube until blanching is relieved.	
	Maintain adequate ventilation and excretion of returned CO_2 from the lungs by monitoring blood gases and regulating ventilatory assistance mechanisms per physician's orders.	Correction of acidosis is essential to maintain homeostasis. Acidosis is powerful pulmonary vasoconstrictor, decreases pulmonary blood flow, and may upset surfactant synthesis. Acidosis dissociates bilirubin from albumin binding sites and predisposes to kernicterus at low bilirubin levels. Acidosis is a central nervous system depressant that depresses respiratory center, which causes increase in CO_2 retention and hypoxia.
	Observe for symptoms of extubation (cyanosis, apnea, respiratory difficulty, bradycardia, no audible breath sounds). Whether accidental or symptomatic of a clogged tube, these conditions warrant *immediate* removal of ineffective tube and respiratory support with bag and mask until reintubation. Insert nasogastric tube (if not present) to decompress stomach.	
	Observe for signs of improvement in respiratory status and ability to have ventilatory support weaned and discontinued: 1. Evaluate blood gas determinations. 2. Observe toleration of lower O_2 concentrations and pressures. 3. Watch for evidence of spontaneous respirations—spontaneous respiratory effort against "set rate" of respirator; ability to assist ventilator by spontaneous respirations.	Criteria for weaning and ultimate discontinuance of ventilator: 1. Normal blood gas values—especially PaO_2, which is indicative of adequate oxygenation 2. Decrease in ventilation pressures 3. Decrease in O_2 concentrations 4. Increased activity, muscle tone, and efforts at simultaneous respirations

Nursing Care Plan: Respiratory Distress Syndrome (continued)

Nursing Diagnosis and Goals	Nursing Interventions and Actions	Rationale
NURSING DIAGNOSIS: Ineffective airway clearance due to increased secretions and absent or diminished cough and gag reflexes	Observe type, color, and quantity of secretions.	Damage to the ciliated cells as a result of alveolar collapse and necrosis leads to pooling of secretions. Preterm infants have weak chest wall musculature and decreased efficiency of cough reflex. Cough and gag reflexes may be absent due to immaturity.
SUPPORTING DATA: Cyanosis Rhonchi Tachypnea Apnea	When Joey is intubated: 1. Observe type of secretions and ease of removal. 2. Because nasal passages are bypassed, provide humidity and moisture within system and better systemic hydration to avoid drying secretions and decreasing ciliary movement. 3. Change infant's position every 1–2 hr to maintain adequate ventilation, drain lung secretions, and promote skin integrity. 4. Suction to remove secretions (see Procedure 32–3). Check working order of each suction machine and pressure setting so that it will be in working order when needed. Tracheal tube suction should last no longer than 5–10 sec. After each suction attempt, ventilate for a few breaths to reinflate atelectatic areas.	Changes in pulmonary secretions can indicate presence of pulmonary fluid retention or infection. Oxygen is dry gas and therefore irritating to airways. Evaporative water losses from skin and lungs are also decreased in high humidity (50%–65%). Apnea or bradycardia will occur if suction is longer than 15–20 sec. Hypoxic insult with drop in PaO$_2$ occurs during suction efforts. Suction, the application of negative pressure to the airway, decrease pulmonary compliance and tidal volume. Suction creates pulmonary atelectasis.
	Observe and record: 1. Tolerance of neonate to suction procedure—color change, cyanosis or remains pink, cardiac changes, bradycardia, arrhythmia. 2. Length of suctioning time. 3. Amount and type of secretions—thick, clear, bloody, green mucus. 4. Frequency of suction is determined by clinical assessment—amount and type of secretions in relation to frequency of suction. Assess need for chest physiotherapy (CPT) by determining extent of atelectasis, volume of secretions, and infant's stability. Suction after CPT.	Accumulation of humidity or secretions within tracheal tube decreases effective ventilation, increases PCO$_2$, and leads to clotted tube (airway). Maintenance of clear tube is especially important with pressure-cycled ventilators, because increased secretions decrease diameter of tube, increase resistance to gas flow, increase pressure within system (possibly to dangerous levels), and decrease tidal volume delivered. Prevents stasis of secretions and promotes drainage. Frequency of CPT should be individualized since procedure may have adverse side effects such as apnea, bradycardia, or hypoxia.
GOALS: Airway will remain patent. Complications of suctioning will be minimized. No evidence of infection will be present or infection will be controlled.		

Nursing Care Plan: Respiratory Distress Syndrome (continued)

Nursing Diagnosis and Goals	Nursing Interventions and Actions	Rationale
NURSING DIAGNOSIS: Potential alteration in nutrition: less than body requirements related to increased metabolic needs of stressed infant	Maintain IV rate at prescribed level; record type and amount of fluid infused hourly. Use infusion pump. Observe vital signs for signs of too-rapid infusion. Maintain normal urine output (1–3 mL/kg/hr). Maintain specific gravity of urine between 1.006 and 1.012. Take daily weights. Manage route of IV administration. With umbilical catheter: Protect catheter from strain or tension (see Procedure 32–2). Restrain as necessary. Prevent dislodgement of catheter. Always keep catheter and stopcock on top of bed linens so they are easily visible.	Fluids are provided to sick neonate by intravenous route and are calculated to replace sensible and insensible water losses as well as evaporative losses due to tachypnea. Overload of circulatory system by too much or too rapid administration of fluid causes pulmonary edema and cardiac embarrassment that may be fatal. Greater nutritional fluid is required because of energy needed to cope with stress. Stressed infants are predisposed to hypoglycemia because of increased metabolic demands as well as reduced glycogen stores and decreased ability to convert fat and protein to glucose.
SUPPORTING DATA: Hypoglycemia (<40 mg %) Hypocalcemia (<7 mg) Decreased daily weight	Observe for occlusion of vessels by clot and for vasospasm—discoloration of skin, discoloration of toes or feet (blanching or cyanosis). If discoloration occurs, contralateral foot may be wrapped with warm cloth, but this is controversial. Removal of catheter is preferred (Korones 1986). Observe for signs of infection or sepsis: temperature instability, drainage, redness or foul odor from cord, lethargy, irritability, vomiting, poor feeding, hypotonia. Peripheral IV in scalp or extremity vein: Prepare equipment, insert IV in vein, and restrain infant. If vessel chosen is an artery, it pulsates. Place peripheral IV in vein (which doesn't pulsate). Maintain proper placement of IV.	Vasospasm in unwrapped foot will be relieved by treatment, and the discoloration will disappear and toes will be pink. If discoloration persists, clot may be occluding vessel—catheter must be removed, or loss of extremity is possible. Very small arteries may not pulsate and arterial area will blanch if saline is infused. Ability to aspirate blood and/or easily inject small amount of saline indicates patent IV. Infiltration is evaluated by area of edema and redness about site, inability to obtain blood on aspiration, or difficulty in injecting through IV line.
GOALS: Nutritional requirements will be met. No signs of fluid overload or dehydration will be present. No long-term complications of arterial catheterization will be present.	Advance as soon as possible from intravenous to oral feedings. Gavage or nipple feedings are used, and IV is used as supplement (discontinued when oral intake is sufficient) (see Procedure 31–1, p 955). Provide adequate caloric intake: amount of intake, type of formula, route of administration, and need for supplementation of intake by other routes. Observe for hypocalcemia. Observe for hypoglycemia: Dextrostix below 45 mg %, urine screening for glucose.	Calories are essential to prevent catabolism of body proteins and metabolic acidosis due to starvation or inadequate caloric intake. Hypocalcemia and hypoglycemia result from delayed or inadequate caloric intake and stress.

Nursing Care Plan: Respiratory Distress Syndrome (continued)

Nursing Diagnosis and Goals	Nursing Interventions and Actions	Rationale
NURSING DIAGNOSIS: Potential for infection related to invasive procedures **SUPPORTING DATA:** Lethargy Temperature instability Increased respiratory distress Hypotension **GOALS:** Joey will be free of infection or infection will be controlled	See section on sepsis nursing care, p 1062. Pay careful attention to infection control by cleaning and replacing nebulizers/humidifers at least every 24 hr; use sterile tubing and replace every 24 hr; use sterile distilled water.	Decreased lung expansion predisposes to atelectasis and secondary superimposed infections. The warm, moist environment found in Isolettes and with O_2 equipment promotes growth of microorganisms.
NURSING DIAGNOSIS: Potential for injury related to impaired thermoregulatory mechanisms secondary to prematurity **SUPPORTING DATA:** Decreased temperature Lethargy Cyanosis Hypoglycemia Apnea/bradycardia Dextrostix <40 mg %	Observe infant for temperature instability and signs of increased oxygen consumption (need for increased O_2 concentration) and metabolic acidosis. Maintain neutral thermal environment. Use servocontrol to maintain constant temperature regulation. Warm all inspired gases. Place a thermometer in the oxygen hood and document the temperature of the delivered gas with vital signs. Oxyhood and Isolette temperature should be maintained in the infant's neutral thermal range. Place thermometer in-line of ventilatory circuit and maintain inspired gas at 34–35C. Use heat shields for small infants.	Cold stress increases oxygen consumption and promotes pulmonary vasoconstriction. This leads to hypoxia and acidosis, which further depress surfactant production. Cold stress leads to chemical thermogenesis (burning brown fat to maintain body temperature), which increases O_2 needs in an already compromised infant. Cold air/oxygenation blown in face of newborn is source of cold stress and is stimulus for increased consumption of oxygen and increased metabolic rate. Heat shields will prevent heat loss by convection and reduce insensible water losses.
GOALS: Joey will be maintained within neutral thermo environment. Cold stress will be minimized.		
NURSING DIAGNOSIS: Potential alteration in fluid volume associated with disease process, parenteral fluid therapy	Careful monitoring of intake and output is essential. Daily weights (sometimes every 8 hour weights are indicated if renal failure is evident).	Cardiac output is diminished due to hypoxia secondary to ventilation/perfusion abnormalities of RDS. Reduced perfusion of kidneys compromises function and leads to oliguria and acid-base abnormalities. Hypoxia increases renal vascular resistance and lowers glomerular filtration rate. Insensible water losses are decreased by humidified environment.

Nursing Care Plan: Respiratory Distress Syndrome (continued)

Nursing Diagnosis and Goals	Nursing Interventions and Actions	Rationale
SUPPORTING DATA: Abnormal urinary output Abnormal daily weights Symptoms of pulmonary edema Electrolyte imbalance	Monitor serum and urine electrolytes and pH. Calculate fluids to meet maintenance requirements in addition to insensible and sensible losses. Monitor blood pressure and review history to determine presence of hypovolemia. Administer volume expansion as ordered. Humidify inspired gases and maintain high ambient humidity.	Hypovolemia may not be evident until acidosis and hypoxemia are corrected and pulmonary vascular resistance decreases. Functional hypovolemia may occur when fluid leaks from the intravascular compartment because of pulmonary vascular endothelial damage.
	Monitor levels of aminoglycosides with each dose administered.	Drugs that are eliminated solely by renal excretion should be administered in modified dosages or time intervals.
	Document and report signs of pulmonary edema: cyanosis, dyspnea, liver enlargement, and tachycardia.	
GOALS: Fluid balance will be maintained. Complications of hypovolemia/hypervolemia will be minimized.		

Epilogue
Joey continued to improve while on the ventilator and by 60 hours after birth is being weaned from the ventilator. He did not develop the potential complications of pneumothorax or patent ductus arteriosus. His parents are at his bedside most of the day holding his little hands and talking to him. His mother is expressing breast milk regularly. The plan is to start breast milk feedings per gavage and extubate from the ventilator as soon as possible.

Persistent Pulmonary Hypertension of the Newborn

Persistent pulmonary hypertension of the newborn (PPHN) is a serious disorder that may affect near-term, term, or postterm neonates. It has been called persistent fetal circulation (PFC) because the problems that occur are a result of right-to-left (R-L) shunting of blood away from the lungs and through the fetal ductus arteriosus and patent foramen ovale.

The disease was originally described only in newborns who had suffered severe perinatal asphyxia. It has since been associated with several events causing hypoxemia and acidosis: postmaturity syndrome, RDS, MAS, intrapartal asphyxia, pneumonia, Group B streptococcal sepsis, and diaphragmatic hernia. Many fetuses have problems that compromise fetal oxygenation prior to the onset of labor (Fox & Duara 1983).

During pregnancy, the fetal pulmonary vascular resistance (PVR) is high due to the lack of air and collapsed position of the lungs. After the initiation of respiration at birth, the cord is clamped and systemic vascular resistance increases with the removal of the placental vascular bed. Expansion of the lungs opens the pulmonary circulation.

The resulting decrease in the resistance of the pulmonary vasculature encourages flow of blood into the pulmonary vascular bed and initiates the disappearance of the fetal R-L shunt. With oxygenation of the blood, the pulmonary circulation dilates further, the ductus narrows, and within a very short time, the adult circulatory pattern is established.

Depending on the etiology, PPHN is classified as primary or secondary. Primary disease results from vascular changes prior to birth, which causes abnormally high PVR. The small arteries develop in the lung periphery as alveolar development occurs. These arteries, which develop along with the alveoli, are normally free of muscular coats. Muscular development progresses between birth and adolescence until full muscularization is present during adult life. Alveolar hypoxia in utero, regardless of the cause, can stimulate precocious muscularization (Perkin & Anas 1984). This early abnormal reconstruction of the arteries results in increased PVR, which interrupts the normal sequence of events that take place with the onset of respiration.

Secondary PPHN occurs when the initial sequences of respiration and change in circulation after birth are interrupted by events that increase the PVR. The increased vascular resistance causes a reversal of the blood flow,

Procedure 32–2 Umbilical Catheterization*

Objective	Nursing Action	Rationale
Assemble equipment	Obtain the following equipment: 1. IV solution and tubing 2. Infusion pump	Regulates infusion.
	3. Umbilical arterial catheter tray	Contains equipment for insertion.
	4. Sterile stopcock	
	5. Solution for skin preparation	Removes bacteria that may be present.
	6. Sterile No. 4-O silk suture and umbilical tape	Ties around umbilical stump.
	7. Sterile umbilical catheter—3½–5 Fr	Inserts in umbilical artery.
	8. Heparinized sterile saline in sterile syringe	Used to flush tubing as necessary.
	9. Sterile gloves	Maintain sterility.
	10. Nonallergic tape	Tape is less irritating to skin.
	11. Spotlight	To visualize field.
Prepare infant	Restrain infant and provide for warmth	Prevents sudden movement. Prevents chilling.
Prepare equipment	Attach tubing to solution and hang on IV standard. Remove all air from tubing and attach to infusion pump. Open umbilical catheter tray and add skin preparation solution, suture, cord ties. Prepare gloves.	Prepares for infusion.
Monitor procedure	The infant is draped, prepped, and catheter is placed Syringe containing heparinized sterile saline is attached to catheter by stopcock. IV tubing is attached to stopcock. Set prescribed rate on infusion pump. Catheter is secured by suture. Secure catheter to infant with nonallergic tape. Obtain abdominal x-ray.	Procedure done by qualified personnel. Check placement of catheter.
Assess infant	Observe the following: 1. Temperature 2. Pulse 3. Respiration 4. Color of legs	Evaluate infant's status.
	Notify physician immediately in case of: 1. Blanching 2. Mottling 3. Cyanosis 4. Coolness of one or both legs	Blood flow to extremities is disrupted.
Maintain newborn records	Record the following: 1. IV—site, type of catheter, solution. 2. Infusion flow rate. 3. Time infusion was started. 4. Infant's response.	Maintain infant's chart.

*Umbilical arterial catheter is used for monitoring arterial pressures, for obtaining arterial blood for blood gas studies, and for infusion in the absence of a venous line.

which opens the fetal shunts. Once this process has begun, it is self-perpetuating: Increased PVR leads to R-L shunting across the ductus, which leads to increased hypoxemia, further increasing the PVR. The cycle is difficult to interrupt, and clinical deterioration is rapid.

MEDICAL THERAPY

The first goal of medical management is early diagnosis of this disorder to halt the progressive worsening of the R-L shunt. Certain diagnostic tests (Fox & Duara 1983) can be used to evaluate the increased PVR and shunting:

1. *Simultaneous preductal and postductal blood gases.* The ductus enters the aorta below the area of the right subclavian and carotid arteries; thus preductal blood samples will have a higher oxygen content than postductal samples in infants with significant R-L shunting. Simultaneous pre- and postductal arterial blood gases demonstrate a 10 percent difference between the two PaO_2 values (>15 torr difference). Pre- and postductal transcutaneous monitors can also demonstrate ductal shunting.

2. *Hyperoxia-hyperventilation test.* Most PPHN infants have a "critical" PCO_2 level at which vasodilation occurs. This PCO_2 level may be less than 20 torr in some infants. Once the critical PCO_2 is reached by manual hyperventilation, the resulting metabolic alkalosis causes pulmonary vasodilation, which reverses the R-L shunt and improves oxygenation. A positive response to the hyperoxia-hyperventilation test is a rise in PaO_2 to greater than 100 torr with hyperventilation. The improved oxygenation can be noted clinically if the infant turns pink. Arterial gases or transcutaneous monitoring can be used to document the increased PaO_2.

3. *Echocardiography.* This procedure will demonstrate R-L shunting and a prolonged ratio of right ventricular ejection period to right ventricular ejection time in infants with PPHN.

4. *Cardiac catheterization.* This test will show normal anatomic structures but R-L shunting of blood at the level of the ductus and foramen ovale. The procedure is extremely traumatic and is usually not necessary to establish a diagnosis in the majority of PPHN infants.

The goal of therapeutic intervention is to lower the PVR and reverse the process of shunting. Maintenance of tissue oxygenation in the presence of R-L shunting presents the greatest therapeutic challenge but is essential to minimize complications.

Initial therapeutic efforts are directed at relieving the precipitating factors, if identified, to reverse the hypertension. In addition, aggressive ventilatory management is undertaken to decrease the PVR and increase oxygenation. Hyperventilation to achieve respiratory alkalosis (pH >7.55) will cause pulmonary vasodilatation, which increases oxygenation. To prevent respiratory interference and achieve hypocarbia, most infants require paralysis with a neuromuscular blocking agent such as pancuronium (Pavulon).

If hyperventilation alone does not lead to a decrease in the PVR, pharmacologic vasodilatation may be attempted by administration of intravenous tolazoline. Since tolazoline also induces systemic vasodilatation, dopamine and/or dobutamine may be required to maintain an adequate cardiac output to maintain the blood pressure.

Oxygenation and ventilation efforts continue until the PaO_2 can be consistently maintained greater than 100 torr. Even when this is achieved, the improvement may be tenuous and reduction of ventilatory support must be made in extremely small increments with intensive surveillance to detect rapid negative responses. Alkalosis and hyperoxia may have to be maintained for several days to avoid sudden return to hypoxemia and increased PVR.

NURSING ASSESSMENT

The nurse assesses for the onset of symptoms, which usually occur in the first 12 to 24 hours of life. Affected newborns exhibit signs of respiratory distress (grunting, nasal flaring, tachypnea), with increased anteroposterior diameter and cyanosis. They typically fail to respond to conventional methods of oxygenation and ventilation. There is significant unexplained hypoxemia in the absence of congenital heart disease. The chest radiograph might show no evidence of pulmonary parenchymal disease (depends on the underlying disease). The hypoxemia and cyanosis associated with PPHN are characteristic of extreme lability. Marked, rapid changes in PaO_2 and color are seen with agitation, stimulation, or therapeutic intervention (suctioning).

NURSING DIAGNOSIS

Nursing diagnoses that may apply to a newborn with PPHN are:

● Alteration in oxygen and carbon dioxide exchange related to airway obstruction

● Alteration in cardiac output related to hypotension

● Ineffective family coping related to life-threatening illness in a term newborn

NURSING GOAL: PREVENTION OF
COMPLICATIONS

Infants with PPHN are critically ill and require experienced, skilled nurses to provide optimal care with minimal manipulaton. Any disturbance may precipitate agitation, which leads to hypoxemia. Therefore goals and priorities of care must be established. If a paralyzing agent is used, nursing care includes monitoring of the newborn's response to artificial oxygenaton and mechanical ventilation. The nurse ensures that the oxygen is delivered in correct amounts and route and records the percentage of oxygen flow. The ventilator settings are checked frequently and recorded every two hours. The nurse carefully suctions the endotracheal tube every two hours or as necessary while assessing the effect of the procedure on the baby's oxygenation and perfusion. The amount and type of secretions are noted. The nurse carefully assesses arterial blood gases and notifies the clinician if the results are out of the acceptable stated range. Transcutaneous monitoring is essential for identification of activities that may compromise the infant's status. (See Table 32–4 for nursing interventions required for transcutaneous monitoring.) Continuous monitoring of vital signs and blood pressure is required, and careful inspection of the skin during positioning is necessary to avoid pressure necrosis.

Pharmacologic vasodilatation may lead to precipitous central hypotension, which must be quickly identified and corrected. The infant must be monitored for other side effects of tolazoline therapy (increased gastric secretion, gastrointestinal bleeding, and oliguria).

With aggressive ventilation, potential for pneumothoraces exists. The nurse can best prevent complications by advanced preparation and close monitoring for signs of compromise. (See discussion of pneumothorax, p 1027, for appropriate nursing interventions.)

NURSING GOAL: PARENT EDUCATION

Many infants suffering PPHR are born at or near term at a time when parents least expect problems—especially life-threatening problems—to occur. The magnitude of the infant's illness and the rapid deterioration may overwhelm them. The nurse should assess their level of understanding and assist them by providing information about their infant's condition in easily understandable terms.

Attachment becomes difficult when the infant responds poorly (as seen by decreased PaO_2) to touching. Parents can be encouraged to talk very softly to their infant since this will usually not compromise the infant's condition. Continuity of nursing care is helpful since it will be less threatening for the parents to relate to a smaller group of nurses (Beachy & Powers 1984).

EVALUATIVE OUTCOME CRITERIA

Nursing care is effective if:

- The risks for development of persistent pulmonary hypertension (PPHN) are identified early, and immediate action is taken to minimize the development of fulminating illness.

- The newborn is free of respiratory distress and establishes effective respiratory function.

- The parents verbalize their concerns about their baby's illness and understand the rationale behind the management of their newborn.

● Care of the Newborn With Complications Due to Respiratory Therapy

Oxygen and mechanical ventilation, while required as therapeutic interventions to reduce hypoxia, hypercarbia, ischemia, and infarction to vital organs, may also have deleterious effects. The concentrations of ambient oxygen administered to the neonate must be titrated according to oxygen tension within arterial blood. Pulmonary air leaks occur in approximately 15 percent of mechanically ventilated neonates. In many cases the air leaks are a consequence of injury due to the disease rather than the mechanical ventilation.

Pulmonary Interstitial Emphysema

Pulmonary interstitial emphysema (PIE) is the accumulation of air in the tissues of the lungs. Extraalveolar air collections are most common with use of positive pressure ventilation. Air collections outside the lung are a function of compliance of the lung and use of increased pressures to ventilate. Overdistention of alveolar air spaces may progress to PIE when rupture occurs and air escapes into the interstitial spaces. Air dissects along perivascular spaces but not into the pleural space or mediastinum. This condition is a precursor of pneumothorax or pneumomediastinum.

Pneumothorax

Pneumothorax, a common complication of respiratory therapy, is an accumulation of air in the thoracic cavity between the parietal and visceral pleura. Pneumothorax occurs when alveoli are overdistended, usually by excessive intraalveolar pressure and rupture; air then leaks into the thoracic cavity. Excessive intraalveolar pressure is a result of stiff, noncompliant lungs and the use of assisted positive pressure ventilation with high inspiratory pressure. Meconium aspiration with subsequent obstruction of the airway and a ball-valve phenomenon produces poor lung compliance and trapping of air in the alveoli. In this situation, pneumothorax is a frequent complication.

Pneumothorax in the newborn causes several physiologic changes: collapse of the lung; compression of the heart and lungs and compromise of venous return to the right heart with mediastinal air; and development of tension in the pleural space. Symptoms of pneumothorax include a sudden unexplained deterioration in the newborn's condition; decreased breath sounds; apnea; bradycardia; cyanosis; increased oxygen requirements; higher PCO_2; decrease in pH; mottled, asymmetric chest expansion; decreased arterial blood pressure; shocklike appearance; and a shift in the apical cardiac impulses to the side opposite the pneumothorax.

X-ray examination is the main method of diagnosing a pneumothorax. Transillumination of the chest can be used when it is not possible to obtain an x-ray series rapidly. Transillumination is the visualization of light transmitted through the air in the affected side of the chest. Follow-up radiographs should always be done to confirm the diagnosis and extent of the pneumothorax.

Pneumothorax is a life-threatening situation for the neonate and demands immediate removal of the accumulated air. The air is aspirated with a syringe attached to an 18-gauge intercath or 23-gauge butterfly needle and inserted into the second or third intercostal space midclavicular line when the newborn is supine. This procedure is done only as an emergency and carries a risk of damaging the myocardium with needle tracks as the air is evacuated. The procedure must be done only by skilled and specifically trained personnel.

For complete resolution of the pneumothorax, a No. 10 Fr thoracotomy tube should be placed appropriately in the chest wall and connected to continuous negative pressure (10–15 cm H_2O) suction with an underwater seal.

Bronchopulmonary Dysplasia

Bronchopulmonary dysplasia (BPD) typically occurs in very compromised LBW infants who require oxygen therapy and assisted mechanical ventilation for the treatment of RDS. It has only rarely been associated with neonatal pneumonia, MAS, PPHN, congenital cardiac disease, and other congenital anomalies. The incidence of BPD is approximately 20 percent, with individual reports ranging widely due to varying methods of grading the severity of the disease (Toce et al 1984). The cause is multifactorial, with oxygen, endotracheal ventilation, barotrauma, mechanical ventilation, patent ductus arteriosus, overhydration, PIE, LGA, and LBW all being implicated.

Infants with BPD show persistent, chronic, pulmonary dysfunction and characteristic radiographic changes. The pulmonary pathology of BPD has been described as four progressive stages according to radiographic findings (Northway et al 1967):

Stage 1 is clinically and radiographically indistinguishable from RDS. Lacking surfactant, the alveoli collapse; the resultant ischemia leads to necrosis of the surrounding tissue and capillaries. The sloughed necrotic material fills the terminal bronchioles causing mucosal and ciliated cell damage.

In Stage 2 radiographs progress to a characteristic "white out" with opacification of lung fields and indistinguishable cardiac borders. These changes are caused by continued sloughing of bronchiolar lining cells and collection of cellular debris in the lumens of the small bronchi. Interstitial edema occurs as the damaged capillaries leak proteins.

During Stage 3 regeneration begins in the lining cells of the bronchioles. Fibrous tissue forms as connective tissue cells proliferate. This leads to distortion and eventual rupture of the alveoli with small amounts of air being trapped in the interstitium. These emphysematous areas surrounded by collapsed alveoli are seen as small cystic light areas on x-ray films. The fibrous tissue also causes distortion of the lymphatic channels and slows the reabsorption of interstitial fluid.

Stage 4 is characterized by hypertrophy of the smooth muscles surrounding the bronchi and bronchioles, which leads to narrowing of the airways. During this period, the mucous-producing cells also hypertrophy, and the increase in mucous production leads to further airway obstruction. Thickening of the pulmonary arteries and capillary membranes leads to narrowing of these vessels, which causes pulmonary hypertension. Cor pulmonale with right ventricular hypertropy and cardiomegaly may occur secondary to the pulmonary hypertension. Radiographs show enlargements of the emphysematous areas.

MEDICAL THERAPY

Prevention of all the factors associated with BPD is not possible. However, optimal physiologic maintenance will minimize the complications. The goals of therapeutic intervention are to provide adequate oxygenation and ventilation, optimal nutrition, and supportive care to ensure adequate rates of growth and development.

Because of the chronic nature of this disease, therapeutic intervention must be individualized to meet the spe-

Table 32–4 Transcutaneous Monitors

Type	Function and rationale	Nursing interventions
TcPO$_2$ Measures oxygen diffusion across the skin. Clark electrode is heated to 43C (preterm) or 44C (term) to warm the skin beneath the electrode and promote diffusion of oxygen across the skin surface. PO$_2$ is measured when oxygen diffuses across the capillary membrane, skin, and electrode membrane (Cohen 1984).	When transcutaneous monitors are properly calibrated and electrodes are appropriately positioned they will provide reliable continuous, noninvasive measurements of PO$_2$, PCO$_2$, and oxygen saturation. Readings vary when skin perfusion is decreased. Reliable as trend monitor. Frequent calibration necessary to overcome mechanical drift. Following membrane change, machine must "warm-up" 1 hour prior to initial calibration; otherwise, after turning it on, it must equilibrate for 30 min prior to calibration. When placed on infant values will be low until skin is heated; approximately 15 min required to stabilize. Second-degree burns are rare but can occur if electrodes remain in place too long. Decreased correlations noted with: older infants (related to skin thickness); infants with low cardiac output (decreased skin perfusion); and with hyperoxic infants. The adhesive that attaches the electrode may abrade the fragile skin of the preterm infant. May be used for both pre- and postductal monitoring of oxygenation for observations of shunting.	Use TcPO$_2$ to monitor trends of oxygenation with routine nursing care procedures. Clean electrode surface to remove electrolyte deposits; change solution and membrane once a week. Allow machine to stabilize before drawing arterial gases; note reading when gases are drawn and use values to correlate. Ensure airtight seal between skin surface and electrode; place electrodes on clean, dry skin on upper chest, abdomen, or inner aspect of thigh; avoid bony prominences. Change skin site and recalibrate at least every 4 hours; inspect skin for burns; if burns occur, use lowest temperature setting and change position of electrode more frequently. Adhesive discs may be cut to a smaller size or skin prep may be used under the adhesive circle only; allow membrane to touch skin surface at center.
TcPCO$_2$ Measures carbon dioxide diffusion across skin. Stowe-Severinghaus electrode is heated to increase blood flow under the electrode. CO$_2$ content is measured when carbon dioxide diffuses across the membrane and changes the pH of the electrolyte creating a change in electrical potential. The change of potential is converted to torr and displayed as TcPCO$_2$ (Monaco et al 1983).	Calibration with stock gases must be performed. TcPCO$_2$ readings are higher than PaCO$_2$ due to: increased solubility of CO$_2$ in blood when temperature increases; increased metabolic production of CO$_2$ in skin cells and tissue when heated; difference between arterial and skin cell CO$_2$ content. Significant mechanical drift noted; poor correlations with extremes of PaCO$_2$	Glass electrode is fragile and must be protected. Carbon dioxide tension measured at the skin is greater than the PaCO$_2$: to convert, divide the reading by 1.6; calculation can be incorporated into calibration of machine so readout will approximate actual PaCO$_2$. Nursing interventions same as for TcPO$_2$.
PULSE OXIMETER Monitors beat-to-beat arterial oxygen saturation. Microprocessor measures saturation by the absorption of red and infrared light as it passes through tissue. Changes in absorption related to blood pulsation through vessel determine saturation and pulse rate (Epstein et al 1985).	Calibration is automatic. Less dependent on perfusion than TcPO$_2$ and TcPCO$_2$; however, functions poorly if peripheral perfusion is decreased due to low cardiac output. Much more rapid response time than TcPO$_2$—offers "real-time" readings Can be located on extremity, digit, or palm of hand leaving chest free; not affected by skin characteristics. Requires understanding of oxyhemoglobin dissociation curve.	Understand and use oxyhemoglobin dissociation curve. Monitor readings and correlate with arterial blood gases. Use disposable cuffs (reusable cuffs allow too much ambient light to enter and readings may be inaccurate).

Table 32–4 Transcutaneous Monitors (continued)

Type	Function and rationale	Nursing interventions
	Pulse oximeter reading of 85%–90% reflects clinically safe range of saturation.	
	Extreme sensitivity to movement; decreases if average of seventh or fourteenth beat is selected rather than beat-to-beat.	
	Poor correlation with extreme hyperoxia.	

cific needs of the infant. Of prime importance is maintenance of adequate gas exchange. At each stage of BPD, pulmonary pathologic changes interfere with adequate oxygenation and normal ventilation. Ventilatory assistance and increased ambient environmental oxygen must be titrated precisely by close monitoring of blood gases to prevent episodic hypoxemia or hyperoxemia and hypercarbia. Antibiotics are indicated for secondary infections. Diuretics and fluid restriction are frequently used to control pulmonary fluid retention and to improve lung function (McCann et al 1985). Electrolyte supplements are used to offset the results of chronic diuretic therapy. Bronchodilators are used to decrease airway resistance and to control bronchospasm. Serial echocardiography is used to monitor cardiac response to the chronic pulmonary disease. Periodic digitalization may be required if cor pulmonale develops.

NURSING ASSESSMENT

At each stage of BPD, the infant exhibits recognizable clinical signs that reflect the pulmonary pathologic changes. Nursing assessment is based on a knowledge of these stages.

In Stage 1, the infant exhibits typical signs of RDS with audible grunting, nasal flaring, and retractions. Due to the extensive alveolar damage, the infant is hypoxic and requires supplemental oxygen and assisted ventilation.

During Stage 2, when the cellular debris fills the lumens of the bronchi and bronchioles, the infant has increased pulmonary secretions that may interfere with extubation. With progression to Stage 3, the alveoli rupture and the capillary membranes thicken. This leads to separation of the capillaries from the alveoli and impairment of oxygen and carbon dioxide exchange. The infant's oxygen dependency becomes apparent and he or she begins to retain carbon dioxide, which prevents extubation. Lymphatic distortion leads to pulmonary interstitial fluid retention and evidence of diffuse rales with auscultation.

The hypertrophy of the bronchiolar smooth muscles characteristic of Stage 4 increases the airway resistance and

the risk of bronchospasm. During this stage infants will manifest bronchospasm by intermittent wheezing respirations, cyanosis, and continued supplemental oxygen requirements. Marked carbon dioxide retention continues to be a problem and ventilator dependency may result. Pulmonary fluid retention and mucous production will be manifested by audible rales and rhonchi, secretions, and chronic cough.

NURSING DIAGNOSIS

Nursing diagnoses that may apply to a baby with BPD include:

● Impaired gas exchange related to chronic retention of carbon dioxide and borderline oxygenation secondary to fibrosis of lungs

● Ineffective airway clearance related to chronic intubation and increased secretion secondary to BPD

● Ineffective parental coping related to prolonged hospitalization and decreased opportunities to hold the baby

NURSING GOAL: MAINTENANCE OF OXYGENATION

The nurse observes carefully any changes in the newborn's oxygenation. Special attention must be given to maintaining the prescribed oxygen concentration during all activities. Since the infant is oxygen dependent, the oxygen level must be maintained, especially during periods of stress, such as when crying; when blood is drawn; while starting an IV; and during an LP, suctioning, chest physiotherapy (CPT), and feeding.

A decrease in the arterial oxygen levels will increase the risk of pulmonary hypertension or cor pulmonale. The nurse obtains blood gases based on the institution's chronic blood gas protocol—for example, every three days, 20 minutes after a permanent change in ambient oxygen concentration (FiO_2), or more frequently if the infant experiences increasing respiratory distress or increasing lethargy.

Postural drainage, CPT, and vibration followed by

suctioning are carried out with close attention to the tolerance of the baby. It is essential to time the care activities with rest periods to avoid fatiguing the infant. The nurse maintains the infant's body temperature as hypothermia or hyperthermia will increase oxygen consumption and may increase oxygen requirements. Positioning on the abdomen helps the baby maintain higher transcutaneous oxygen saturation ($TcPO_2$) and improved ventilation. Providing for adequate nutrition enhances formation of new alveoli and enlargement of the airway diameter.

NURSING GOAL: PREVENTION OF INFECTION

Since the infant with BPD is very susceptible to infection, it is important to discourage anyone with early signs of infectious disease from having contact with the infant. The infant's behavior and vital signs should be monitored for changes that might indicate early developing infection. Changes in color, quantity, or quality of pulmonary secretions are noted and reported. The frequency of CPT and suctioning may need to be increased.

NURSING GOAL: PROVISION OF ADEQUATE NUTRITION

The nurse assists in providing adequate nutrition and monitors the amount of calories the newborn ingests and the energy expended during the feeding process. If possible, at least 90 cal/kg/day should be given to the infant, with increases daily until at least 130 cal/kg/day are taken. As soon as tolerated, a 24-calorie preemie formula is started, especially if the baby is on fluid restriction. More oxygen may be required during the process of feeding, and the least energy consuming feeding method should be used. If the feeding schedule is too stressful, smaller, more frequent feedings may be initiated.

Providing adequate nutritional intake becomes a major nursing task. Infants with BPD frequently experience negative oral sensations due to suctioning and intubation, which can adversely affect their transition to nipple or spoon feeding. In addition, most infants receive numerous, possibly unpalatable, medications with meals. Attempts must be made to include pleasurable activities such as cuddling at mealtime to develop positive associations with appropriate feeding behaviors.

NURSING GOAL: MONITORING OF MEDICATIONS

Bronchodilators, diuretics, electrolyte supplements, and high-calorie supplements may be used in the medical management of the BPD infant. Appropriate timing of administration is essential to maintain adequate blood levels. The nurse must monitor the infant for toxic effects of the medication and adverse effects of the therapy (for example, electrolyte imbalance, such as hypokalemia, and fractures as a result of diuretic therapy).

NURSING GOAL: PROVISION OF SENSORY STIMULATION

Since BPD infants require prolonged hospitalization, the nurse should give special attention to formulating a program of early stimulation activities. Psychomotor delays are seen frequently in these infants and are most likely due in part to prolonged exposure to the hospital environment. Since their tolerance level for activity is limited due to their illness, activities must be individualized for each baby.

NURSING GOAL: PARENT EDUCATION

The birth of a premature infant causes significant stress to the family. When the infant develops BPD and the family becomes aware of the implications of chronic illness and prolonged hospitalization, they may experience despair and find it difficult to cope with this added burden. The nurse can help the family cope by encouraging them to take an active role in their infant's daily activities. Their involvement will help dispel feelings of inadequacy and prepare them to perform the unique tasks necessary to meet their infant's needs (Glass 1985). Prior to discharge, parents must be taught to evaluate their infant's tolerance of activities and to recognize signs of distress due to poor oxygenation, inadequate ventilation, infection, fluid retention, and bronchospasm. The process of learning about the treatment of their infant's BPD can best be accomplished by a program of parent-infant care-taking activities supervised by the nurse while the infant is hospitalized. The chronicity of the disease requires that the parents be taught the essentials of problem recognition so that they can cope with the infant's special problems after discharge.

EVALUATIVE OUTCOME CRITERIA

Nursing care is effective if:

- The parents understand the causes, risks, therapy options, and nursing care involved in the care of their newborn with BPD.

- The parents participate in their newborn's care and show attachment behaviors.

- The parents are able to cope with their frustrations and begin to use outside resources as needed.

Other Pulmonary Complications

Pneumomediastinum is a massive collection of air in the mediastinum, either anterior to the heart or laterally,

Procedure 32–3 Endotracheal Suctioning

Objective	Nursing Action	Rationale
Minimize potential for pulmonary infection through cross-contamination.	Assess respiratory status to determine necessity for suctioning.	Infant should be suctioned only as often as necessary to maintain patent airway and adequate oxygenation.
	Gather all necessary equipment: catheters, suction machine, disposable sterile suction tubing, saline (no preservatives), sterile syringe/needle, and gloves (not powdered). Ensure that gloves, catheters, and liquefying solutions are sterile. Maintain sterile technique throughout entire suctioning procedure.	In healthy individual, lower respiratory tract is free of pathogenic organisms.
	Discard catheter, glove, and saline after each procedure.	Once equipment is moistened and contaminated with body flora and mucus, it becomes a culture bed for noxious organism growth.
	Set wall suction for not more than 80 mm Hg.	Mucosal hemorrhages and tissue invagination occur more frequently when higher pressure is used.
Alleviate partial or total airway obstruction in support of cell oxygenation.	Monitor transcutaneous readings during suctioning procedure and supplement with increased oxygen as needed.	Suctioning physically removes oxygen from airways. In addition, it mechanically occludes airways and therefore diminishes potential for oxygenation. It usually stimulates coughing and increases work of breathing, thereby increasing tissue demand for oxygen.
	Position and immobilize infant.	It is quite difficult to suction alert infant successfully without restraint. An assistant should be employed to ensure effective, atraumatic suctioning in infants.
	Using sterile technique, don sterile glove; hook up appropriate suction catheter; lubricate tip.	"Whistle-tip" catheter should be used for respiratory tract suctioning, because it tends to be less traumatizing to tissues. Catheter size should be no more than ½ the size of lumen to be suctioned in order to minimize hypoxemia due to airway obstruction.
	Place sterile normal saline in a sterile specimen cup or unit dose plastic container.	Prelubrication of catheter is essential to minimize tissue trauma with subsequent obstructive edema.
	If infant is intubated: 1. Disconnect source of oxygenation from newborn just prior to entry of suction catheter.	Suction applied while entering airway increases removal of oxygen from airways.
	2. Assistant should stabilize endotracheal tube while suctioning.	During suctioning, tube can be easily dislodged and increases potential for tissue invagination once catheter tip passes end of tube. Passing the suction catheter more than 1 cm beyond the endotracheal tube risks damaging the carina and creating pneumothoraces (Figure 32–8).
	3. Insert catheter without applied suction into tube the distance from the proximal airway to no more than 1 cm below the end of the endotracheal tube. (This can be determined by noting cm markings on tube or by using calculations for oral-carinal distance.) (Figure 32–9).	

Procedure 32–3 Endotracheal Suctioning (continued)

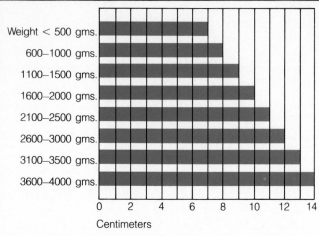

Weight < 500 gms.
600–1000 gms.
1100–1500 gms.
1600–2000 gms.
2100–2500 gms.
2600–3000 gms.
3100–3500 gms.
3600–4000 gms.

0   2   4   6   8   10 12 14
Centimeters

Figure 32–8 Safe length for endotracheal suctioning (From Anderson D, Chandra R: Pneumothorax secondary to perforation of sequential bronchi by suction catheter. *J Pediatr Surg* 1976;11:687)

Note: Measure catheter along appropriate line for weight. Add length E-T tube that is sticking out of mouth. This is the maximum safe distance for insertion of suction catheter through E-T tube.

Objective	Nursing Action	Rationale
	4. Apply suction by placing thumb of assistive hand over vent port or Y-connector (Figure 32–10).	Placing thumb over venting device closes negative pressure system, which allows atmospheric pressure to push secretions and debris into catheter, facilitating their removal.
	5. Slowly withdraw catheter in a pill-rolling rotation.	Rotating catheter in a slow, steady fashion maximizes catheter access to secretions while minimizing potential for tissue invagination.
	6. Clear catheter with sterile saline.	
	7. After each suction attempt, ventilate for a few breaths to reinflate atelectatic areas.	Hypoxia insult with a drop in PaO$_2$ occurs during suction efforts. Suction, the application of negative pressure to the airway, decreases by 50 percent the pulmonary compliance and tidal volume. Suction creates pulmonary atelectasis.
	8. If tenacious secretions are encountered, instill normal saline with syringe (needleless) into tube prior to suctioning.	Instillation of normal saline liquefies and loosens secretions.
	If infant is not intubated: After having failed to get infant to cough voluntarily in effective manner, follow procedure for suctioning intubated infant with these exceptions:	Suctioning to clear airways should be employed only when infant is unable to clear own airways effectively by use of cough reflex. It should be considered a last resort.
	1. Enter airway via nasopharynx, advancing catheter into trachea on inspiration.	Inspiration opens glottis and tends to entrain catheter along with inspired air. Achieving coordination with inspiration is often quite easy with pediatric clients, because they are frequently crying involuntarily during procedure. Instillation of liquefying agents directly into trachea in unintubated infant is not possible. Indirect means must be used.
	2. Attempt to liquefy tenacious secretions by humidification via mist tent, face mask, or hand-held nebulizer.	
Minimize iatrogenic hypoxemia secondary to suctioning.	Suction only when absolutely necessary.	Always assess need for suctioning. There should never be standing orders such as "Suction every hour."

Procedure 32–3   Endotracheal Suctioning (continued)

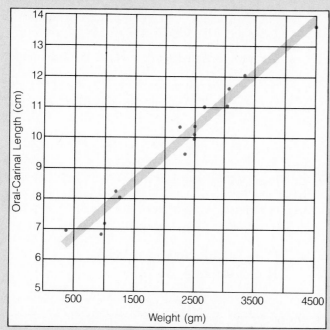

Figure 32–9 *Determining oral-carinal distance.* (From Anderson D, Chandra R: Pneumothorax secondary to perforation of sequential bronchi by suction catheter. *J Pediatr Surg* 1976;11:687)

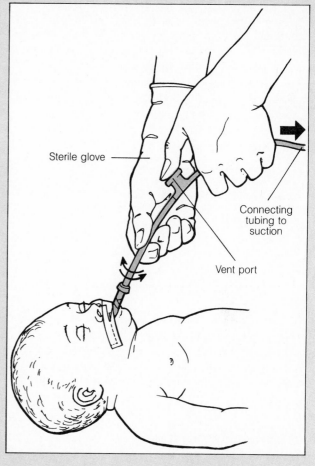

Figure 32–10 *Suctioning with endotracheal tube*

Objective	Nursing Action	Rationale
	Limit each catheter insertion to no more than 10 sec. Reoxygenate newborn (monitoring transcutaneous readings) between each insertion and at conclusion of procedure.	Limiting suction time and frequent reoxygenation counterbalance the mechanical obstruction of airway and removal of available oxygen.
	Remove catheter with suction applied as soon as infant begins to cough.	Holding catheter in airway while infant coughs can deprive infant of needed inspiratory volume at end of cough because of airway obstruction by catheter.
	During procedure, assess infant for signs of bradycardia.	Suctioning can cause vagal response in form of bradycardia, which, if unchecked, can lead to asystole.

compressing mediastinal pleurae. This condition results in compression of the vena cava, tachypnea, cyanosis, and distant or barely audible heart sounds. Air may dissect into the soft tissues of the neck (subcutaneous emphysema).

Pneumopericardium is a collection of air within the pericardial sac with resultant tamponade and diminution of cardiac size.

Pneumoperitoneum is a collection of air in the peritoneal cavity. This condition must be distinguished from a perforated viscera.

● Care of the Newborn With Cold Stress

Cold stress is excessive heat loss resulting in the use of compensatory mechanisms (increased respirations and nonshivering thermogenesis) to maintain core body temperature. Heat loss that results in cold stress occurs in the newborn through the mechanisms of evaporation, convection, conduction, and radiation. (See Chapter 27 for a detailed discussion of thermoregulation.) Heat loss at the time of delivery that leads to cold stress can play a significant role in the severity of RDS and the ultimate outcome for the infant.

The amount of heat lost by an infant depends to a large extent on the actions of the nurse or care giver. Both preterm and SGA newborns are at risk for cold stress because they have decreased adipose tissue, brown fat stores, and glycogen available for metabolism.

As discussed in Chapter 27, the newborn infant's major source of heat production in nonshivering thermogenesis (NST) is brown fat metabolism. The ability of an infant to respond to cold stress by NST is impaired in the presence of several conditions:

- Hypoxemia (PO_2 less than 50)

- Intracranial hemorrhage or any CNS abnormality

- Hypoglycemia (<40 mg %)

When these conditions occur, the infant's temperature should be monitored more closely and the neutral thermal environment conscientiously maintained. The nurse must recognize these conditions and treat them as soon as possible.

The metabolic consequences of cold stress can be devastating and potentially fatal to an infant. Oxygen requirements are raised, glucose use increases, acids are released into the bloodstream, and surfactant production decreases. The effects are graphically depicted in Figure 32–11.

Nursing Assessment

The nurse observes for signs of cold stress. These include increased respirations, decrease in skin temperature, decrease in peripheral perfusion, appearance of hypoglycemia, and the possible development of metabolic acidosis.

Skin temperature assessments are used because initial response to cold stress is vasoconstriction, resulting in a decrease in skin temperature; therefore, monitoring rectal temperature is not satisfactory. A decrease in rectal temperature represents long-standing cold stress with decompensation in the infant's ability to maintain core body temperature.

If a decrease in skin temperature is noted, the nurse determines whether hypoglycemia is present. Hypoglycemia is a result of the metabolic effects of cold stress and is suggested by glucose strip values below 45 mg/mL, tremors, irritability or lethargy, apnea, or seizure activity.

Nursing Goal: Promotion of Thermoregulation

If cold stress occurs, the following nursing interventions should be initiated:

- The newborn is warmed slowly since rapid temperature elevation may cause apnea.

- Skin temperature is monitored every 15 minutes to determine if the infant's temperature is increasing.

- The infant is placed and maintained in a neutral thermal environment.

Nursing Goal: Prevention of Effects of Cold Stress

The presence of anaerobic metabolism is assessed and interventions initiated for the resulting metabolic acidosis. Attempts to burn brown fat increase oxygen consumption, lactic acid levels, and metabolic acidosis. Hypoglycemia may be reversed by adequate glucose intake. See p 1038 for interventions.

● Care of the Newborn With Hypoglycemia

Hypoglycemia is the most common metabolic disorder occurring in IDM, SGA, and preterm AGA newborns. The pathophysiology of hypoglycemia differs for each classification.

AGA preterm infants have not been in utero a sufficient time to store glycogen and fat. Therefore, they have very low glycogen and fat stores and a decreased ability to carry out gluconeogenesis (Fantazia 1984). This situation is further aggravated by increased use of glucose by the tissues (especially the brain and heart) during stress and illness (chilling, asphyxia, sepsis, and RDS). Infants of Class A–C or type I diabetic mothers (diagnosed, suspected, or gestational diabetics) have increased stores of glycogen and fat. However, circulating insulin and insulin responsiveness are higher when compared with other newborns. Because of the cessation of the high in utero glucose loads at birth, the neonate experiences rapid and profound hypoglycemia. The SGA infant has used up glycogen and fat stores because of intrauterine malnutrition and has a blunted hepatic enzymatic response with which to carry out gluconeogenesis. Any newborn who is stressed at birth (from asphyxia or cold) also quickly uses up available glucose stores and becomes hypoglycemic.

Hypoglycemia is defined as a blood glucose below 30 mg/dL in the first 72 hours and below 40 mg/dL after the first three days. It may also be defined as a glucose strip (Dextrostix) result below 45 mg/dL when corroborated with laboratory blood glucose value (see Procedure 32–4).

Medical Therapy

The goal of management includes early identification of hypoglycemia through observation and screening of

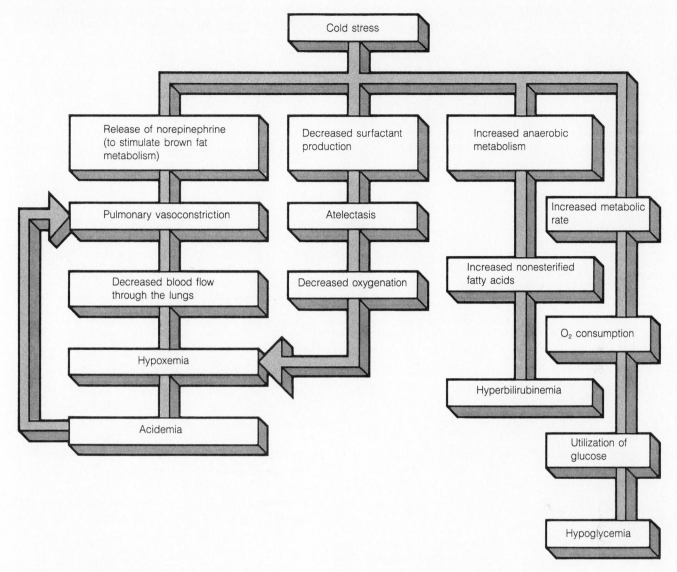

Figure 32–11 Cold stress schematic

newborns at risk. The newborn may be asymptomatic, or any of the following may occur:

- Lethargy, jitteriness

- Poor feeding

- Vomiting

- Pallor

- Apnea, irregular respirations, respiratory distress, cyanosis

- Hypotonia, possible loss of swallowing reflex

- Tremors, jerkiness, seizure activity

- High-pitched cry

Differential diagnosis of an infant with nonspecific hypoglycemic symptoms includes determining if the infant has any of the following:

- CNS disease

- Sepsis

- Metabolic aberrations

- Polycythemia

- Congenital heart disease

- Drug withdrawal

- Temperature instability

- Hypocalcemia

Aggressive treatment is recommended after a single low blood glucose value if the infant manifests any of these symptoms.

Provision of adequate caloric intake is important. Early formula feeding or breast-feeding is one of the major preventive approaches. If early feeding or intravenous glu-

(Text continues on page 1038.)

Procedure 32–4 Glucose Strip Test

Objective	Nursing Action	Rationale
Ensure quick, efficient completion of procedure.	Gather the following equipment: 1. Lancet (do not use needles) 2. Alcohol swabs 3. 2 × 2 sterile gauze squares 4. Small Band-Aid 5. Glucose strips and bottle	All necessary equipment must be ready to ensure that blood sample is collected at time and in manner necessary. Do not use needles because of danger of nicking periosteum. Warm heel for 5–10 sec prior to heel stick with a warm wet towel to facilitate flow of blood.
	Select clear, previously unpunctured site. Clean site by rubbing vigorously with 70 percent isopropyl alcohol swab, followed by dry gauze square. Grasp lower leg and heel so as to impede venous return slightly.	Selection of previously unpunctured site minimizes risk of infection and excessive scar formation. Friction produces local heat, which aids vasodilation. Impeding venous return facilitates extraction of blood sample from puncture site.
Minimize trauma at puncture site.	Dry site completely before lancing.	Alcohol is irritating to injured tissue and may also produce hemolysis.
	With quick piercing motion, puncture lateral heel with blade, being careful not to puncture too deeply. Avoid the darkened areas shown in Figure 32–12. Toes are acceptable sites if necessary.	The lateral heel is the site of choice because it precludes damaging the posterior tibial nerve and artery, plantar artery, and important longitudinally oriented fat pad of the heel, which in later years could impede walking. This is especially important for infant undergoing multiple heel stick procedures. Optimal penetration is 4 mm.

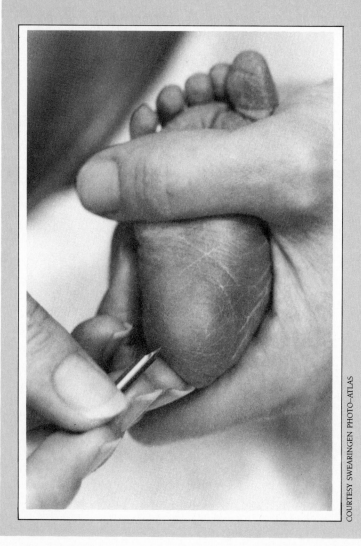

COURTESY SWEARINGEN PHOTO-ATLAS

Figure 32–12 Glucose strip test (heel stick)

Procedure 32–4   Glucose Strip Test (continued)

Objective	Nursing Action	Rationale
Ensure accurate blood sampling.	After puncture has been made, remove first drop of blood with sterile gauze square and proceed to collect subsequent drops of blood onto glucose strip, ensuring that it is a stand-up drop of blood on strip (Figure 32–13).	The first drop is usually discarded because it tends to be minutely diluted with tissue fluid from puncture.

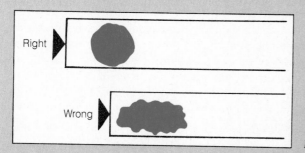

Figure 32–13   Glucose strip drop of blood

| | Wait 60 seconds (apply Band-Aid while waiting), then rinse blood gently from stick under a steady stream of running water (Figure 32–14). Compare immediately against color chart on side of bottle.
Record results on vital signs sheet or on back of graph. Report immediately any findings under 45 mg/dL or over 175 mg/dL. | For accurate results, directions must be followed closely, and reagent strips must be fresh. False low readings may be caused by:
1. Timing.
2. Washing (chemical reaction can be washed off).
3. Squeezing foot, causing tissue fluid dilution. |

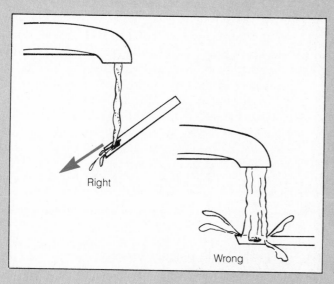

Figure 32–14   Glucose test strip rinse

| Prevent excessive bleeding | Apply folded gauze square to puncture site and secure firmly with bandage.

Check puncture site frequently for first hour after sample | A pressure dressing should be applied to puncture site to stop bleeding.

Active infants sometimes kick or rub their dressings off and can bleed profusely from puncture site, especially if bandage becomes moist or is rubbed excessively against crib sheet. |

cose is started to meet the recommended fluid and caloric needs, the blood glucose is likely to remain above the hypoglycemic level. Intravenous infusions of a dextrose solution (5 percent–10 percent) begun immediately after birth should prevent hypoglycemia. However, in the very small AGA infant infusions of 10 percent dextrose solution may cause hyperglycemia to develop, requiring an alteration in the glucose concentration. Infants require 6 to 10 mg/kg/min of glucose to maintain normal glucose concentrations (Avery & Taeusch 1984). Therefore, an intravenous glucose solution should be calculated based on body weight of the infant, with blood glucose tests to determine adequacy of the infusion treatment.

A rapid infusion of 25 percent to 50 percent dextrose is contraindicated because it may lead to profound rebound hypoglycemia following an initial brief increase. Hypoglycemia resulting from hyperinsulinemia may be helped by administration of long-acting epinephrine. Epinephrine promotes glycogen conversion to glucose; it is also an antiinsulin agent. In more severe cases of hypoglycemia, corticosteroids may be administered. It is thought that steroids enhance gluconeogenesis from noncarbohydrate protein sources (Avery 1987).

The prognosis for untreated hypoglycemia is poor. It may result in permanent, untreatable CNS damage or death.

Nursing Assessment

The objective of assessment is to identify newborns at risk and to screen symptomatic infants. For newborns who are diagnosed as having hypoglycemia, assessment is ongoing with careful monitoring of glucose values. Glucose strips, urine dipsticks, and urine volume (above 1–3 mL/kg/hr) are evaluated frequently for osmotic diuresis and glycosuria.

Nursing Diagnosis

Nursing diagnoses that may apply to the newborn with hypoglycemia are:

- Alteration in nutrition: less than body requirements related to increased glucose use secondary to physiologic stress

- Ineffective breathing pattern related to tachypnea and apnea

- Alteration in comfort related to frequent heel sticks for glucose monitoring

Nursing Goal: Monitoring of Glucose Levels

When caring for a preterm AGA infant, blood glucose levels should be monitored using glucose strips or labo-ratory determinations every four to eight hours for the first day of life, and daily or as necessary thereafter. The IDM should be monitored hourly for the first several hours after birth as this is the time when precipitous falls in glucose are most likely. In the SGA newborn, symptoms usually appear between 24 and 72 hours of age; occasionally they may begin as early as 3 hours of age. Infants who are below the tenth percentile on the intrauterine growth curve should have blood sugar assessments at least every eight hours until 4 days of age or more frequently if any symptoms develop.

Calculation of glucose requirements and maintenance of intravenous glucose will be necessary for any symptomatic infant with low serum glucose levels. Careful attention to glucose monitoring is again required when the transition from intravenous to oral feedings is attempted. Titration of intravenous glucose may be required until the infant is able to take adequate amounts of formula or breast milk to maintain a normal blood sugar level.

Nursing Goal: Decreasing Physiologic Stress

The method of feeding greatly influences glucose and energy requirements. In addition, the therapeutic nursing measure of nonnutritive sucking during gavage feedings has been reported to increase the baby's daily weight gain and lead to earlier nipple feeding and discharge (Field et al 1982, Measel & Anderson 1979). Nonnutritive sucking may also lower activity levels, which allows newborns to conserve their energy stores. Activity can increase energy requirements; crying alone can double the baby's metabolic rate. Establishment and maintenance of a neutral thermal environment has a potent influence on the newborn's metabolism. The nurse pays careful attention to environmental conditions, physical activity, and organization of care and integrates these factors into delivery of nursing care. The nurse identifies any discrepancies between the baby's caloric requirements and received calories and weighs the newborn daily at consistent times, preferably before a feeding. Only then can findings of unusual losses or gains, as well as the pattern of weight gain, be considered reliable.

Evaluative Outcome Criteria

Nursing care is effective if:

- The risk of hypoglycemia is promptly identified, and intervention is started early.

- The newborn's metabolic and physiologic processes are stabilized, and recovery is proceeding without sequelae.

- The parents verbalize their concerns about their baby's health problem and understand the rationale behind management of their newborn.

Research Note

Prolonged hypoglycemia can cause irreversible neurologic damage in the newborn. During pregnancy and labor, the fetal pancreas excretes insulin in response to maternal blood glucose, which readily crosses the placenta. When a maternal hyperglycemia stimulus stops at birth, the newborn continues to produce insulin in a delayed response, which causes neonatal hypoglycemia.

An ex post facto study by Carmen examined the occurrence of neonatal hypoglycemia in relation to intravenous maternal glucose infusions. The study included 62 mother-infant pairs. Of these women 58 had IV glucose infusions in labor. The infants were all healthy term newborns with normal hematocrits. Data including the rate, duration, and amount of glucose given in labor were correlated with a one-hour (NPO) glucose strip value of the baby. Of the babies in this study 43 percent had a serum glucose value of less than 40 mg % and were defined as hypoglycemic.

Carmen found that both an increase in the total grams of glucose given and an increase in the duration of the infusion correlated with decreased newborn serum glucose levels. The most statistically significant parameter was the duration of infusion.

Nurses need to reassess standing orders that include the routine use of glucose infusions in labor. Carmen recommended starting glucose infusions as late in active labor as possible, restricting rates to average less than 10 g/hour when the infusion runs longer than four hours, and providing the nursery staff with information about labor IVs so that they can identify babies at increased risk for hypoglycemia.

Carmen S: Neonatal hypoglycemia in response to maternal glucose infusion before delivery J Obstet Gyncecol Neonat Nurs 1986; 15(July/August):319–323.

● Care of the Newborn With Hypocalcemia

Calcium is transported across the placenta in utero throughout pregnancy and in increasing amounts during the third trimester of pregnancy. This predisposes the infant who is born preterm to have lower serum calcium levels in the neonatal period. Both AGA and SGA preterm infants are at risk for the development of hypocalcemia. This risk is increased in the presence of perinatal asphyxia, trauma, hypotonia, and with the use of bicarbonate in treating acidosis. Infants of diabetic mothers and of mothers with hyperparathyroidism are also at higher risk for hypocalcemia.

Hypocalcemia is a common occurrence in the intrapartally asphyxiated and premature newborn in the first two or three days of life due to a delay in oral feedings, which results in less intestinal absorption of calcium. Hypocalcemia is also associated with the practice of administering low-calcium or calcium-free intravenous fluids.

Serum calcium falls earlier and lower in premature infants than in term infants. The pathogenesis is uncertain, but may be related to parathyroid insufficiency or hypercalcitonemia. While the total serum calcium levels may fall precipitously, ionized calcium levels are relatively spared, which may account for the frequent lack of symptoms. Hypocalcemia in IDMs is probably related to higher serum phosphorus concentrations. Late neonatal hypocalcemia, occurring at the end of the first week of life, usually affects term infants with an uneventful delivery.

Late hypocalcemia is related to administration of milk formulas with relatively high levels of phosphorus in relation to calcium. High levels of phosphorus depress the parathyroid gland, which results in decreased serum calcium (Avery & Taeusch 1984).

Serum calcium levels should be monitored in at-risk newborns. Normal serum calcium levels range from 8.0 to 10.5. mg/dL. Hypocalcemia refers to serum calcium levels less than 7 mg/dL or ionized calcium concentrations less than 3 to 3.5 mg/dL. An ECG measurement of the Q-T interval will assist in the diagnosis.

Medical Therapy

Identification of at-risk and/or symptomatic newborns with screening for hypocalcemia is the first consideration of preventive management.

The symptoms of hypocalcemia are nonspecific and are seen in conjunction with other disorders. The signs and symptoms that may be observed are:

- Apnea
- Cyanotic episodes
- High-pitched cry
- Heightened response to sensory stimuli, twitching, jitteriness
- Seizures (focal or generalized)
- Edema
- Abdominal distention, vomiting

Emergency treatment of symptomatic newborns with intravenous calcium salts will normalize serum concentrations and minimize complications. Initial treatment of symptomatic hypocalcemia is intravenous therapy. Intravenous 10 percent calcium gluconate may be administered as a continuous infusion or in intermittent slow pushes. Intravenous push doses of calcium gluconate should not exceed 2 mL/kg at any one time. Doses may be repeated as necessary three or four times in 24 hours.

Schedules for screening serum calcium levels for various at-risk groups have been recommended and are as follows: IDMs at 6, 12, 24, and 48 hours of age; infants suffering from intrapartal asphyxia at 3, 6, and 12 hours of age; preterm newborns less than 1000 g at 6 hours; and preterm newborns less than 1500 g at 12 hours of age. Healthy preterm newborns greater than 1500 g who are taking milk feedings need not be monitored (Cloherty & Stark 1985).

Maintenance calcium will be given either parenterally or orally. Oral calcium glubionate or calcium gluconate may be used for maintenance. Low-phosphorous milk may be used in the treatment of asymptomatic hypocalcemia.

Treatment for hypocalcemia is usually necessary for only four or five days unless other complications exist. Calcium levels should be monitored every 12 to 24 hours and the dose should be tapered off gradually.

Nursing Assessment

Nursing assessment is aimed at identifying at-risk newborns, monitoring serum calcium levels, and closely observing for symptoms.

Nursing Goal: Safe Administration of Calcium Gluconate

The nurse must be cognizant of several precautions when administering calcium gluconate intravenously.

1. When giving an intravenous push, calcium must be injected very slowly over a period of at least 10 minutes, or no more than 1 mL per minute. The heart rate must be monitored, and if bradycardia or other cardiac arrhythmias occur, the infusion must be discontinued immediately.

2. When calcium is administered as a continuous drip, the heart rate must also be monitored constantly. Calcium must not be mixed with other medications such as phosphate or bicarbonate in the line as the mixture may precipitate.

3. The intravenous site must be observed closely for signs of infiltration, as calcium is very damaging to the tissues. If extravasation at the site of infusion occurs, necrosis and sloughing of the tissue is likely.

4. If the calcium is administered through an umbilical arterial catheter, the tip of the catheter should be far enough from the heart that calcium is not injected directly into the heart. If an umbilical venous catheter is used, the tip must be in the inferior vena cava to avoid necrosis of the liver.

Continued observation and monitoring of serum levels will be required during the transition from intravenous to oral maintenance therapy and again when calcium supplementation is tapered off.

● Care of the Newborn With Jaundice

The most common abnormal physical finding in neonates is *jaundice* (icterus). Jaundice develops from deposit of the yellow pigment, *bilirubin,* in lipid tissues. Unconjugated (indirect) bilirubin is a break-down product derived from hemoglobin that is released from lysed red blood cells and heme pigments found in cell elements (nonerythrocyte bilirubin).

Fetal unconjugated bilirubin is normally cleared by the placenta in utero, so total bilirubin at birth is usually less than 3 mg/dL unless an abnormal hemolytic process has been present. Postnatally, the infant must conjugate bilirubin (convert a lipid-soluble pigment into a water-soluble pigment) in the liver, producing a rise in serum bilirubin in the first days of life.

The rate and amount of conjugation depends on the rate of hemolysis, on the maturity of the liver, and on albumin-binding sites. A normal, healthy, full-term infant's liver is usually mature enough and producing enough glucuronyl transferase that total serum bilirubin levels do not reach pathologic levels (above 12 mg/dL blood).

Serum albumin-binding sites are usually sufficient to meet the normal demands. However, certain conditions tend to decrease the sites available. Fetal or neonatal asphyxia decreases the binding affinity of bilirubin to albumin as acidosis impairs the capacity of albumin to hold bilirubin. Hypothermia and hypoglycemia release free fatty acids that dislocate bilirubin from albumin. Maternal use of sulfa drugs or salicylates interferes with conjugation or interferes with serum albumin-binding sites by competing with bilirubin for these sites.

A number of bacterial and viral infections (cytomegalic inclusion disease, toxoplasmosis, herpes, syphilis) can affect the liver and produce jaundice. *Hyperbilirubinemia* (elevation of bilirubin level) may also result from blood disorders such as polycythemia (twin-to-twin transfusion, large placental transfer of blood), or enclosed hemorrhage (cephalhematoma, bleeding into internal organs, ecchymoses). Increased hemolysis due to conditions such as sepsis, hemolytic disease of the newborn, or an excessive dose of vitamin K may also cause elevated bilirubin levels.

The bilirubin level at which an infant is harmed varies, but at that level the infant may suffer neurologic defects and eventually death. While the mechanism of bilirubin-produced neuronal injury is uncertain, evidence remains that high concentrations of unconjugated bilirubin can be neurotoxic (Avery & Taeusch 1984). Unconjugated bilirubin has a high affinity for extravascular tissue such as fatty tissue (subcutaneous tissue) and the brain. Thus bilirubin not bound to albumin can cross the blood-brain barrier and damage the cells of the CNS and produce kernicterus. *Kernicterus* (meaning "yellow nucleus") refers to the deposition of unconjugated bilirubin in the basal ganglia of the brain and to the symptoms of neurologic damage that follow untreated hyperbilirubinemia. The classic bilirubin encephalopathy of kernicterus most commonly found with blood group incompatibility is virtually unknown today due to aggressive treatment with phototherapy and exchange transfusions.

Kernicterus, usually associated with unconjugated bilirubin levels of over 20 mg/dL in normal term infants and over 10 mg/dL in sick preterm newborns, has been noted at autopsy in both types of babies at lower levels. The risk of kernicterus at lowered bilirubin levels has been associated with asphyxia, acidosis, and low serum albumin levels. Current therapy can reduce the incidence of kernicterus encephalopathy but cannot distinguish all infants who are at risk.

Late complications may include cerebral palsy (de Vries et al 1985), impaired or absent hearing, learning difficulties (Brooten et al 1985), and mental retardation.

Certain prenatal and perinatal factors predispose the newborn to hyperbilirubinemia. During pregnancy, maternal conditions that predispose to neonatal hyperbilirubinemia include hereditary spherocytosis, diabetes, intrauterine infections (TORCH and Gram-negative bacilli) that stimulate production of maternal isoimmune antibodies, and drug ingestion (sulfas, salicylates, novobiocin, diazepam, oxytocin).

A primary cause of hyperbilirubinemia is *hemolytic disease of the newborn* secondary to Rh incompatibility. Thus the woman who is Rh-negative or who has blood type O should be asked about outcomes of any previous pregnancies and her history of blood transfusion. Prenatal amniocentesis with spectrophotographic examination may be indicated in some cases. Cord blood from neonates is evaluated for bilirubin level, which should not exceed 5 mg/dL. Neonates of these mothers are carefully assessed for appearance of jaundice and levels of serum bilirubin.

Isoimmune hemolytic disease, also known as *erythroblastosis fetalis,* occurs after transplacental passage of a maternal antibody that predisposes fetal and neonatal red blood cells to early destruction. Jaundice, anemia, and compensatory erythropoiesis result. Immature red blood cells—erythroblasts—are found in large numbers in the blood; hence the designation erythroblastosis fetalis. *Hydrops fetalis,* the most severe form of erythroblastosis fetalis, occurs when maternal antibodies attach to the Rh antigen of the fetal red blood cells, making them susceptible to destruction by phagocytes. The fetal system responds by increased erythropoiesis within foci in the placenta, extramedullary sites, and hyperplasia of the bone narrow. Rapid

and early destruction of erythrocytes results in a marked increase of immature red blood cells—erythroblasts—that do not have the functional capabilities of mature cells.

If anemia is severe, as seen in hydrops fetalis, cardiomegaly with severe cardiac decompensation and hepatosplenomegaly occur. Severe generalized anasarca and generalized fluid effusion into the pleural cavity (hydrothorax), pericardial sac, and peritoneal cavity (ascites) develop. Jaundice is not present until later because the bili pigments are being excreted through the placenta into the maternal circulation. Severe anemia is also responsible for hemorrhage in pulmonary and other tissues. The hydropic hemolytic disease process is also characterized by hyperplasia of the fetal zone of the adrenal cortex and pancreatic islets. Hyperplasia of the pancreatic islets predisposes the infant to neonatal hypoglycemia similar to that of IDMs. These infants also have increased bleeding tendencies due to associated thrombocytopenia and hypoxic damage to the capillaries. Hydrops is a frequent cause of intrauterine death among infants with Rh disease. In rare cases, the grossly enlarged edemic fetal body and placenta may cause uterine rupture.

ABO incompatibility may result in jaundice, although it rarely results in hemolytic disease severe enough to be clinically diagnosed and treated. Hepatosplenomegaly may be found occasionally in newborns with ABO incompatibility, but hydrops fetalis and stillbirth are rare.

The best treatment for hemolytic disease is prevention. Prenatal identification of the fetus at risk for Rh or ABO incompatibility will allow prompt treatment. See Chapter 19 for discussion of in utero management of this condition.

Certain neonatal conditions predispose to hyperbilirubinemia: polycythemia (central hematocrit 65 percent or more), pyloric stenosis, obstruction or atresia of the biliary duct or of the lower bowel, low-grade urinary tract infection, sepsis, hypothyroidism, enclosed hemorrhage (cephalhematoma, large bruises), asphyxia neonatorum, hypothermia, acidemia, and hypoglycemia. Hepatitis from intrauterine infections or metabolic liver disease elevates the level of conjugated bilirubin.

Neonates born with congenital biliary duct atresia have a poor prognosis; about two-thirds have an inoperable lesion and succumb during the first three years of life. The prognosis for a newborn with hyperbilirubinemia depends on the extent of the hemolytic process and the underlying cause. Severe hemolytic disease results in fetal and early neonatal death from the effects of anemia—cardiac decompensation, edema, ascites, and hydrothorax. Hyperbilirubinemia that is not aggressively treated may lead to kernicterus. The resultant neurologic damage is responsible for death, cerebral palsy, mental retardation, sensory difficulties, or to a lesser degree, perceptual impairment, delayed speech development, hyperactivity, muscle incoordination, or learning difficulties (Klaus & Fanaroff 1986).

Medical Therapy

The goals of medical management are prompt identification of infants at risk for jaundice based on perinatal and neonatal history, laboratory tests to identify the cause of the jaundice, and prompt treatment to prevent the neurologic damage that can result from hyperbilirubinemia.

In the presence of one or more of the predisposing factors, laboratory determination should be made of the maternal and neonatal blood types for Rh or ABO incompatibility. Other necessary laboratory evaluations are Coombs' test, serum bilirubin levels (direct, indirect, and total), hemoglobin, reticulocyte percentage, and white cell count.

Neonatal hyperbilirubinemia of any origin must be considered pathologic (Avery & Taeusch 1984) if any of the following criteria are met:

1. Clinically evident jaundice in the first 24 hours of life

2. Serum bilirubin concentration rising by more than 5 mg/dL per day

3. Total serum bilirubin concentrations exceeding 12.9 mg/dL in term infants or 15 mg/dL in preterm babies (since preterm newborns have less subcutaneous fat, bilirubin may reach higher levels before it is visible)

4. Conjugated bilirubin concentrations greater than 2 mg/dL

5. Persistence of clinical jaundice beyond 7 days in term infants or beyond 14 days in preterm infants

Initial diagnostic procedures are aimed at differentiating jaundice resulting from increased bilirubin production, impaired conjugation or excretion, increased intestinal reabsorption, or a combination of these factors. The Coombs' test is performed to determine whether jaundice is due to hemolytic disease.

If the hemolytic process is due to Rh sensitization, laboratory findings reveal the following: (a) an Rh-positive neonate with a positive Coombs' test; (b) increased erythropoiesis with many immature circulating red blood cells (nucleated blastocysts); (c) anemia, in most cases; (d) elevated levels (5 mg/dL or more) of bilirubin in cord blood; and (e) a reduction in albumin-binding capacity. Maternal data may include an elevated anti-Rh titer and spectrophotometric evidence of fetal hemolytic process.

The Coombs' test can be either indirect or direct. The indirect Coombs' test measures the amount of Rh-positive antibodies in the mother's blood. Rh-positive red blood cells are added to the maternal blood sample. If the mother's serum contains antibodies, the Rh-positive red blood cells will agglutinate (clump) when rabbit immune antiglobulin is added, and the test results are labeled positive.

The direct Coombs' test reveals the presence of antibody-coated (sensitized) Rh-positive red blood cells in the neonate. Rabbit immune antiglobulin is added to the neonatal blood cells specimen. If the neonatal red blood cells agglutinate, they have been coated with maternal antibodies, and the test result is positive.

The direct Coombs' test on the neonate's cells may be negative or mildly positive, but the indirect Coombs' test, when using the neonate's serum on adult red blood cells, may be strongly positive. This finding indicates that the neonate's red blood cells are not coated with the antibody; however, the antibody is present in the neonate's serum.

If the hemolytic process is due to ABO incompatibility, laboratory findings reveal an increase in recticulocytes. The resulting anemia is usually not significant during the neonatal period and is rare later on. The direct Coombs' test may be negative or mildly positive, while the indirect Coombs' test may be strongly positive. Infants with a direct Coombs' positive test have increased incidence of jaundice with bilirubin levels in excess of 10 mg/dL. Increased numbers of spherocytes (spherical, plump, mature erythrocytes) are seen on a peripheral blood smear. Increased numbers of spherocytes are not seen on smears from Rh disease infants.

Regardless of the cause of hyperbilirubinemia, management is directed toward preventing anemia and minimizing the consequences of hyperbilirubinemia.

Treatment has four goals:

- Alleviating the anemia

- Removing maternal antibodies and sensitized erythrocytes

- Increasing serum albumin levels

- Reducing the levels of serum bilirubin

Therapeutic methods of management of hyperbilirubinemia include phototherapy, exchange transfusion, infusion of albumin, and drug therapy. If hemolytic disease is present, it may be treated by phototherapy, exchange transfusion, and drug therapy. When determining the appropriate management of hyperbilirubinemia due to hemolytic disease, the three variables that must be taken into account are the newborn's (1) serum bilirubin level, (2) birth weight, and (3) age in hours. If a neonate has hemolysis with an unconjugated bilirubin level of 14 mg/dL, weighs less than 2500 g (birth weight), and is 24 hours old or less, an exchange transfusion may be the best management. However, if that same neonate is over 24 hours of age, phototherapy may be the treatment of choice to prevent the possible complication of kernicterus (Figure 32–15).

Serum bilirubin mg/dL	Birth weight	<24 hrs.	24–48 hrs.	49–72 hrs.	>72 hrs.
<5	All				
5–9	All	Phototherapy if hemolysis			
10–14	<2500 g	Exchange if hemolysis	Phototherapy		
	>2500 g				Investigate bilirubin > 12 mg
15–19	<2500 g	Exchange		Consider exchange	
	>2500 g			Phototherapy	
20 +	All	Exchange			

☐ Observe   ▨ Investigate jaundice

Figure 32–15   Therapy for isoimmune hemolytic disease in the neonate. Phototherapy is used after any exchange transfusion. If the following conditions are present, treat the neonate as if in the next higher bilirubin category: perinatal asphyxia, respiratory distress, *metabolic acidosis (pH 7.25 or below), hypothermia (temperature below 35C), low serum protein (5 g/dL or less), birth weight less than 1500 g, or signs of clinical or CNS deterioration. (From Avery GB: Neonatology, ed 2. Philadelphia, Lippincott, 1981, p 511)*

PHOTOTHERAPY

Phototherapy may be used alone or in conjunction with exchange transfusion to reduce serum bilirubin levels. Exposure of the neonate to high-intensity light (a bank of fluorescent light bulbs or bulbs in the blue-light spectrum) decreases serum bilirubin levels in the skin. Phototherapy reduces serum bilirubin by facilitating biliary excretion of unconjugated bilirubin. This occurs when light absorbed by the tissue converts unconjugated bilirubin to two isomers called photobilirubin. The photobilirubin moves from the tissues to the blood by a diffusion mechanism. In the blood it is bound to albumin and transported to the liver. It moves into the bile and is excreted into the duodenum for removal with feces without requiring conjugation by the liver (Avery & Taeusch 1984). The photodegradation products formed when light oxidizes bilirubin can be excreted in the urine. Phototherapy plays an important role in preventing a rise in bilirubin levels but does not alter the underlying cause of jaundice, and hemolysis may continue to produce anemia.

It is generally accepted that phototherapy should be started at 4 to 5 mg/dL below the calculated exchange level for each infant. Sick neonates of less than 1000 g should have phototherapy instituted at a bilirubin concentration of 5 mg/dL. Some authors have recommended initiating phototherapy "prophylactically" in the first 24 hours of life in high-risk, very-low-birth-weight infants. However, a recent study (Curtis-Cohen et al 1985) has demonstrated no alteration in the course of hyperbilirubinemia in infants who received prophylactic phototherapy compared with infants in whom phototherapy was begun at a bilirubin concentration of 5 mg/dL. Sick preterm infants who are at least 1500 g should have phototherapy instituted when the bilirubin level is 10 mg/dL. Any neonate with a bilirubin level of 20 mg/dL or above should have an exchange transfusion regardless of weight or age.

EXCHANGE TRANSFUSION

Early or immediate exchange transfusion is indicated in the presence of the following factors:

- Anti-Rh titer of greater than 1:16 in the mother (see Chapter 19)

- Severe hemolytic disease in a previous newborn

- Clinical hemolytic disease of the newborn at birth or within first 24 hours

- Positive direct Coombs' test

- Cord serum of conjugated (direct) bilirubin levels greater than 3.5 mg/dL in the first week

- Serum unconjugated bilirubin levels greater than 20 mg/dL in the first 48 hours

- Hemoglobin less than 12 g/dL

- Infant with hydrops at birth

- Infant at risk of developing kernicterus

Exchange transfusion is used to (a) treat anemia with red blood cells that are not susceptible to maternal antibodies; (b) remove sensitized red blood cells that would be lysed soon (a two-volume exchange removes 85 percent of the infant's red blood cells); (c) remove serum bilirubin; and (d) provide bilirubin-free albumin and increase the binding sites for bilirubin. In Rh incompatibility, fresh (under two days old) group O, Rh-negative whole blood, or packed red blood cells, are chosen. These types of blood contain no A or B antigens or Rh antigens; therefore the maternal antibodies still present in the neonate's blood will not cause hemolysis of the transfused blood. Packed cells are used if the infant is anemic. Citrate-phosphate-dextrose (CPD) blood is preferred because it presents less of an acid load to the infant.

In case of ABO incompatibility, group O with Rh-specific cells and low titers of anti-A and anti-B donor blood is used, not the infant's blood type, since donor blood contains no antigens to further stimulate maternal antibodies.

Every four to eight hours after the transfusion, bilirubin determinations are made. Repeat exchange may be necessary if the serum bilirubin level rises at a rate of 0.5 to 1.0 mg/dL/hr (Avery 1987) or if the bilirubin level exceeds 20 mg/dL. Daily hemoglobin estimates should be obtained until stable, and hemoglobin determinations every two weeks for two months are valuable.

DRUG THERAPY

Phenobarbital is capable of stimulating the liver's production of enzymes that increase conjugation of bilirubin and its excretion. This drug is effective only if given to the pregnant woman over several days prior to two weeks before delivery.

Postnatal drug therapy is of limited value in term infants. It takes three to seven days to show any effect and may take much longer in preterm infants. The use of phenobarbital postnatally for the treatment of hyperbilirubinemia is controversial because the side effects (lethargy with poor feedings) may outweigh its benefits, and preterm newborns may not respond at all.

Other drugs have the capacity to increase conjugation of bilirubin and to keep bilirubin at levels lower than expected. These drugs are too risky to use for the prevention and treatment of neonatal jaundice.

Nursing Assessment

Assessment is aimed at identifying prenatal and perinatal factors that predispose to development of jaundice and identifying jaundice as soon as it is apparent. Clinically, ABO incompatibility presents as jaundice and occasionally hepatosplenomegaly. Hydrops is rare. Hemolytic disease of the newborn is suspected if the placenta is enlarged, if the newborn is edematous with pleural and pericardial effusion plus ascites, if pallor or jaundice is noted during the first 24 to 36 hours, if hemolytic anemia is diagnosed, or if the spleen and liver are enlarged. The nurse carefully notes changes in behavior and observes for evidence of bleeding. If laboratory tests indicate elevated bilirubin levels, the nurse checks the newborn for jaundice about every two hours and records observations.

To check for jaundice, the nurse should blanch the skin over a bony prominence (forehead, nose, or sternum) by pressing firmly with the thumb. After pressure is released, if jaundice is present, the area appears yellow before normal color returns. The nurse should check oral mucosa and the posterior portion of the hard palate and conjunctival sacs for yellow pigmentation in darker-skinned babies. Assessment in daylight gives best results as pink walls and surroundings may mask yellowish tints and yellow light makes differentiation of jaundice difficult. The time of onset of jaundice is recorded and reported. If jaundice appears, careful observation of the increase in depth of color and of the infant's behavior is mandatory.

The newborn's behavior is assessed for neurologic signs of kernicterus, which are rare but may include: hypotonia, diminished reflexes, lethargy, seizures, or opisthotonic posturing.

Nursing Diagnosis

Nursing diagnoses that may apply are included in the Nursing Care Plan beginning on p 1048.

Nursing Goal: Promotion of Effective Phototherapy

Ideally the entire skin surface of the newborn is exposed to the light. Minimal covering is applied over the genitals and buttocks to expose maximum skin surface while protecting the bedding. Phototherapy success is measured every 12 hours or with daily serum bilirubin levels. The lights must be turned off while drawing blood for serum bilirubin levels. Because it is not known if phototherapy injures the delicate eye structures, particularly the retina, the nurse should apply eye patches over the newborn's closed eyes during exposure (Figure 32–16). Phototherapy is discontinued and the eye patches are removed at least once per shift to assess the eyes for the presence of conjunctivitis. Patches are also removed to allow eye contact during feeding (social stimulation) or when parents are visiting (parental attachment).

The irradiance level at the skin determines the effectiveness of the phototherapy. The desired level of irradiance is 5 to 6 microwatts per square centimeter per nanometer. Most phototherapy units will provide this level of irradiance 42 to 45 cm below the lamps. Irradiance levels can be increased slightly as indicated. The nurse can use a photometer to measure and maintain the levels at between 4 and 8.5 microwatts per square centimeter (Avery & Taeusch 1984).

The neonate's temperature is monitored to prevent hyperthermia or hypothermia. The newborn will require additional fluids to compensate for the increased water loss through the skin and loose stools. Loose stools and increased urine output are the results of increased bilirubin excretion. The infant must be observed for signs of dehydration (Braune & Lacey 1983).

A transient bronze discoloration of the skin may occur with phototherapy when the infant has elevated direct serum bilirubin levels or liver disease. As a side effect of phototherapy, some newborns develop a maculopapular rash. In addition to assessing the neonate's skin color for jaundice and bronzing, the nurse examines the skin for developing pressure areas. The neonate should be repositioned at least every two hours to permit the light to reach all skin surfaces, to prevent pressure areas, and to vary the stimulation to the infant. The nurse keeps track of the number of hours each lamp is used so that each can be replaced before its effectiveness is lost.

Nursing Goal: Promotion of Effective Exchange Transfusion

The nurse's responsibilities during exchange transfusion are to: assemble equipment, prepare the baby, assist the physician during the procedure, and maintain a careful record of all events. After the procedure the nurse observes the newborn for complications from the transfusion and clinical signs of hyperbilirubinemia and neurologic damage (Procedure 32–5).

Nursing Goal: Provision of Teaching and Emotional Support to Families

Many parents must face the mother's discharge while the neonate remains in the hospital for treatment of hyperbilirubinemia. The terms *jaundice, hyperbilirubinemia, exchange transfusion,* and *phototherapy* may sound frightening and threatening. Some parents may feel guilty and think they have caused the problem. On occasion, a multidisciplinary team (eg, nurse, obstetrician, pediatrician, clergyman, genetic counselor, psychologist) may collaborate to help the parents cope with the situation. Under stress, parents may not be able to "hear" or understand the physician's first explanations. The nurse must expect that the parents will need explanations repeated and clarified and that they may need help voicing their questions and fears. Eye and tactile contact with the neonate is encouraged. The nurse can coach parents when they visit with the baby. Parents are kept informed of their infant's condition and are encouraged to return to the hospital or telephone at any time so that they can be fully involved in the care of their infant. (See the Nursing Care Plan: Newborn With Jaundice on page 1048.)

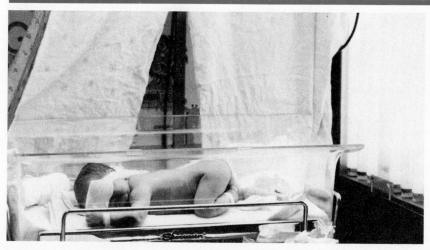

Figure 32–16 Infant receiving phototherapy. The phototherapy light is positioned over the Isolette. To expose as much skin surface as possible, the infant is not dressed. Bilateral eye patches are always in place.

Procedure 32–5 Nursing Responsibilities During Exchange Transfusion*

Objective	Nursing Action	Rationale
Prepare infant.	1. Identify baby.	To prepare correct infant.
	2. Keep newborn NPO for 4 hr preceding exchange transfusion or aspirate stomach.	To decrease chance of regurgitation and aspiration by neonate.
	3. May administer salt-poor albumin (1 g/kg body weight) 1 hr before exchange transfusion.	To increase binding of bilirubin. Do not give to severely anemic or edemic neonate or to neonate with congestive heart failure, because of hazard of hypervolemia.
	4. Assess vital signs.	To provide a baseline.
	5. Position neonate in supine position (Figure 32–17), soft restraints; provide warmth under radiant warmer.	To provide maximum visualization, thermoregulation, and prevent chilling.
	6. Clean abdomen by scrubbing.	To reduce number of bacteria present.
	7. Attach monitor leads to infant.	To assess pulse and respiration.
Prepare equipment.	1. Have resuscitation equipment available (oxygen, oxyhood, 10 percent glucose IV solution and sodium bicarbonate).	To provide life support measures if necessary.
	2. Obtain blood and check it with physician for type, Rh, and age.	To ensure using correct blood.
	3. Attach blood tubing.	To allow infusion.
	4. Apply blood warmer.	To reduce chill.
	5. Open exhange transfusion and umbilical vein trays. Pour prep solution into basins.	To maintain sterility
	6. Prepare gown and gloves for physician.	
Monitor infant status.	Assess pulse, respirations, color, and activity state.	To recognize possible problems and provide data on neonate's response to treatment.
Record blood exchange and medications used.	1. Using blood exchange sheet, record time, amount of blood in, amount of blood out, medications and baby's response, and any other pertinent information.	Donor blood is given at rate of 170 mL/kg of body weight. It replaces 85 percent of infant's own blood.
	2. Inform physician when 100 mL of blood has been used.	Calcium gluconate is given IV after each 100 mL of blood if indicated to decrease cardiac irritability.
Assess neonate response after transfusion.	After the exchange, carefully monitor the following for 24–48 hr: 1. Vital signs 2. Neurologic signs (lethargy, increased irritability, jitteriness, convulsion) 3. Amount and color of urine (hematuria) 4. Presence of edema 5. Signs of necrotizing enterocolitis 6. Infection or hemorrhage at infusion site 7. Signs of increasing jaundice 8. Neurologic signs of kernicterus 9. Calcium, glucose, and bilirubin levels 10. Other complications such as hypokalemia, septicemia, shock, and thrombosis.	To provide information on status of neonate and identification of complications.
Prepare blood samples.	Label tubes and send to laboratory with appropriate laboratory slips.	To follow routines of your institution.
	Retype and cross-match 2 units of blood 2 hours postexchange.	To provide for possible future exchange.

*Exchange transfusion is a therapeutic procedure for hyperbilirubinemia of any etiology.

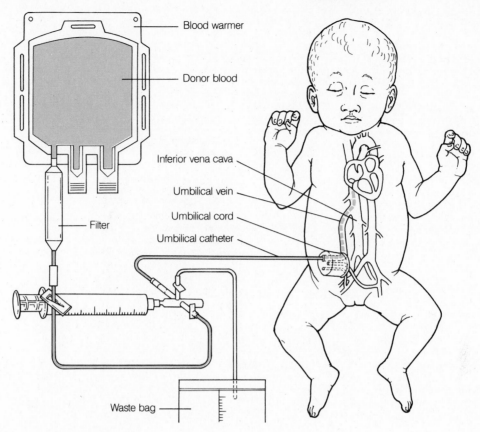

Figure 32–17 Infant receiving exchange transfusion

Labels: Blood warmer / Donor blood / Filter / Waste bag / Inferior vena cava / Umbilical vein / Umbilical cord / Umbilical catheter

● Care of the Newborn With Anemia

Neonatal anemia is often difficult to recognize by clinical evaluation alone. Mean hemoglobin in a full-term newborn is 17 g/dL, slightly higher than in prematures, in whom the mean hemoglobin is 16 g/dL. Infants with hemoglobin values of less than 14 mg/dL (term) and 13 g/dL (preterm) are usually considered anemic. The most common causes of neonatal anemia are blood loss, hemolysis, and impaired red blood cell production.

Blood loss (hypovolemia) occurs in utero from placental bleeding (placenta previa or abruptio placentae). Intrapartal blood loss may be fetomaternal, fetofetal, or the result of umbilical cord bleeding. Birth trauma to abdominal organs or the cranium may produce significant blood loss, and cerebral bleeding may occur due to hypoxia.

Excessive hemolysis of red cells is usually a result of blood group incompatibilities but may be due to infections. The most common cause of impaired red cell production is a deficiency in G-6-PD, which is genetically transmitted. Anemia and jaundice are the presenting signs.

A condition known as *physiologic anemia* exists as a result of the normal gradual drop in hemoglobin for the first 6 to 12 weeks of life. Theoretically, the bone marrow stops production of red blood cells as a response to the elevated oxygenation of extrauterine respirations. When the amount of hemoglobin becomes lower, reaching levels of 10 to 11 g/dL at about 6 to 12 weeks of age, the bone marrow begins production of RBCs again, and the anemia disappears.

Anemia in preterm newborns occurs earlier and reversal by bone marrow is initiated at lower levels of hemoglobin (7–9 g/dL). The preterm baby's hemoglobin reaches a low sooner (4–8 weeks after delivery) than does a term newborn's (6–12 weeks) because preterm red blood cell survival time is shorter compared to the term newborn, because the rate of growth in preterms is relatively rapid, and because a vitamin E deficiency is common in small preterm newborns.

Medical Therapy

The goal of management is early identification and correction of anemia. Hematologic problems can be anticipated based on the obstetric history and clinical manifestations. The age at which anemia is first noted is also of diagnostic value.

Clinically, anemic infants are very pale in the absence of other symptoms of shock and usually have abnormally low red blood cell counts. In acute blood loss, symptoms of shock may be present, such as pallor, low arterial blood

Nursing Care Plan: Newborn With Jaundice

Ellen Harris was born at 34 weeks to a 21-year-old, G 1, P 0, AB 0, O negative mother. She weighed 1660 g and was AGA. Apgars were 7 at one minute and 8 at five minutes. The infant's mother received Rhogam after the delivery. No Rhogam had been given during the pregnancy. Ellen's blood type was A positive with a positive direct Coombs'. Her bilirubin levels at 8 hours of age were 6.0 mg/dL total and 0.9 mg/dL direct. Phototherapy was ordered and started. She has refused most of her breast-feedings and therefore has had only a few stools. She is very lethargic.

Assessment

NURSING HISTORY

Identification of predisposing factors, including:
a. Maternal blood type is O negative.
b. Ellen's blood type is A positive.
c. 34-week-gestation AGA newborn.
   (Preterm newborns tend to have less albumin for bilirubin to bind to.)

PHYSICAL EXAMINATION

a. Jaundice visible at 8 hours of age
b. Hypoactive bowel sounds
c. Decreased stooling
d. Decreased urine output; dark, concentrated
e. Change in behavior: lethargy

LABORATORY EVALUATION

a. Direct positive Coombs'
b. Total bilirubin level—6 mg/dL

ANALYSIS OF NURSING PRIORITIES

1. Monitor for signs of worsening condition.
2. Monitor levels of bilirubin during therapy.
3. Provide adequate hydration.
4. Assess for signs of dehydration.
5. Provide tactile stimulation.
6. Provide parent education.
7. Promote parent-newborn bonding since Ellen must remain in hospital after her mom is discharged.

Nursing Diagnosis and Goals	Nursing Interventions and Actions	Rationale
NURSING DIAGNOSIS: Potential for injury related to jaundice secondary to enterohepatic recirculation of bilirubin **SUPPORTING DATA:** Ellen has jaundice over her face and head primarily. Bilirubin of 6 mg/dL.	Initiate feedings within 4–6 hr after delivery, if possible.	Early feeding in first 4–6 hr tends to discourage high bilirubin levels. Early feeding stimulates bowel activity and passage of bilirubin-containing meconium, thereby eliminating possibility of reabsorption of pigment from intestines.
	Offer Ellen feedings every 3–4 hr.	Adequate hydration facilitates elimination and execretion of bilirubin. Replace fluid losses, due to watery stools, if under phototherapy.
	Give feedings per physician order or protocol.	Increases peristalsis and excretion of bile before it can reenter enterohepatic pathway.
	Administer IV fluids:	IV fluids may be used if baby is dehydrated or in presence of other complications. IV may be started if exchange transfusion is anticipated. Prevents fluid overload.
	1. Monitor flow rate.	
	2. Assess insertion site for evidence of infection.	Identifies infection process.
	Closely assess Ellen's daily patterns to detect notable changes in food ingestion, bowel and urination patterns, sleeping and waking rhythms, irritability.	May indicate signs of worsening condition. Neonate may develop green, watery stools.
	Administer thorough perianal cleansing with each stool or change of perianal protective covering.	Frequent stooling increases risk of skin breakdown.
	Assess Ellen for signs of jaundice.	Observation of jaundice may be initial sign of hyperbilirubinemia.

Nursing Care Plan: Newborn With Jaundice (continued)

Nursing Diagnosis and Goals	Nursing Interventions and Actions	Rationale
	1. Complete assessments in daylight, if possible.	Early detection is affected by nursery environment. Artificial lights (with pink tint) may mask beginning of jaundice.
	2. Observe sclera.	Jaundice may first be noticed as a yellowing of the sclera.
	3. Observe skin color and assess by blanching.	Blanching the skin leaves a yellow color to the skin immediately after pressure is released.
	4. Check oral mucosa, posterior portion of hard palate, and conjunctival sacs for yellow pigmentation in dark-skinned neonates.	Underlying pigment of dark-skinned people may normally appear yellow.
	Keep infant warm.	Action necessary to prevent chill-induced acidosis, a condition that depletes serum albumin-binding sites.
GOALS: Ellen will increase her fluid intake and begin stooling. Any extension of jaundice will be identified. Ellen will not become hypothermic.		
NURSING DIAGNOSIS: Potential for injury related to conjunctivitis, dehydration, and hyperthermia secondary to use of phototherapy.	Maintain treatment modalities.	Method of treatment depends on level of bilirubin, time of onset, and presence of other illness (disease states).
	Phototherapy:	Phototherapy reduces serum bilirubin by facilitating biliary excretion of unconjugated bilirubin. Photo products are largely water soluble, and can be excreted in stool and urine.
SUPPORTING DATA: Ellen is left unclothed with her eyes and genitalia covered while under phototherapy.	Cover Ellen's eyes with eye patches while under phototherapy light.	Protects retina from damage due to high-intensity light.
	Remove Ellen from under phototherapy light and remove eye patches during feedings.	Provides visual stimulation.
	Inspect eyes for conjunctivitis and corneal abrasions.	May be caused by irritation from eye patches.
	Provide minimal coverage only (of diaper area).	Provides maximal exposure. Shielded areas become more jaundiced, so maximum exposure is essential.
	Turn Ellen at regular intervals (eg, every 2 hr).	Provides equal exposure of all skin areas and prevents pressure areas.
	Monitor Ellen's skin and core temperature frequently until temperature is stable.	Hypothermia and hyperthermia are common complications of phototherapy. Hypothermia from exposure to lights, subsequent radiation and convection losses.
	Provide extra fluid intake.	Assures adequate hydration.
	Assess dehydration: 1. Poor skin turgor 2. Depressed fontanelles 3. Sunken eyes 4. Decreased urine output 5. Weight loss 6. Changes in electrolytes	Phototherapy treatment may cause liquid stools and increased insensible water loss, which increases risk of dehydration. As bilirubin levels rise, neonate may become lethargic and more difficult to feed.

Nursing Care Plan: Newborn With Jaundice (continued)

Nursing Diagnosis and Goals	Nursing Interventions and Actions	Rationale
	Observe for bronzing of skin	Bronzing is related to use of phototherapy with increased direct bilirubin levels or liver damage; may last for 2–4 months.
	Check Isolette temperature frequently.	Additional heat from phototherapy lights frequently causes a rise in the Isolette temperature.
	Turn phototherapy lights off when drawing blood for bilirubin levels.	Exposure of blood to phototherapy lights may result in a falsely lowered bilirubin value.
GOAL: Ellen does not encounter eye injury, dehydration, or hyperthermia while under phototherapy.		
NURSING DIAGNOSIS: Potential for neurologic injury related to high levels of unconjugated bilirubin	Observe and report signs of worsening condition (kernicterus): a. Hypotonia, lethargy, poor sucking reflex b. Spasticity and opisthotonus c. Temperature instability d. Gradual appearance of extrapyramidal signs e. Impaired or absent hearing	Deposition of bilirubin in brain leads to development of symptoms. NOTE: Treatment may be more aggressive in presence of neonatal complications such as asphyxia, respiratory distress, metabolic acidosis, hypothermia, low serum protein, sepsis, signs of CNS deterioration (Avery 1987).
SUPPORTING DATA: Ellen's bilirubin might rise above 12 mg/dL, and she may continue to be lethargic and develop seizures.		
GOALS: Ellen is protected from injury resulting from seizures.		
NURSING DIAGNOSIS: Parental anxiety related to having a newborn with jaundice		
SUPPORTING DATA: Ellen's parents expressed worry and asked questions about her welfare and disease process.	Provide explanation of: 1. Infant's condition	Parents may not understand what is happening or why.
	2. Treatment modalities	Physician preference of treatment modalities may vary. Parents may not understand why their newborn is not receiving a treatment that another with the same condition is receiving.
GOALS: Parents will be informed of Ellen's disease process, rationale for treatments, and expected outcome. Ellen's mother will understand the reason for temporary discontinuation of breast-feeding, how to pump her breasts, and how to reinstate breast feeding.	3. Reasons that Mrs Harris may be asked to cease breast-feeding temporarily If breast-feeding is temporarily discontinued, assess Mrs Harris' knowledge of pumping her breasts and provide information and support as needed.	The etiology of breast milk jaundice remains uncertain. The serum bilirubin levels begin to fall within 48 hr after discontinuation of breast-feeding. Opinion of physicians varies regarding the need for discontinuing breast-feeding.
	Assist mother in reestablishment of breast-feeding.	Mother may need support and information to restart breast-feeding.
	Provide tactile stimulation during feeding and diaper changes.	Neonate has normal needs for tactile stimulation.

Nursing Care Plan: Newborn With Jaundice (continued)

Nursing Diagnosis and Goals	Nursing Interventions and Actions	Rationale
	Provide cuddling and eye contact during feedings. Talk to Ellen frequently.	Provides comforting and decreased sensory deprivation.
	Encourage parents to come into nursery for feedings and to touch Ellen.	Presence of equipment may discourage parents from interacting with neonate.
Epilogue		
Ellen is now 3 days old. Her jaundice has not progressed and her bilirubin is less than 10 mg/dL. She is tolerating feedings well and is	more active in her Isolette. Her parents are looking forward to her continued growth and being able to take her home.	

pressure, and a decreasing hematocrit value. The initial laboratory workup should include hemoglobin and hematocrit measurements, reticulocyte count, examination of peripheral blood smear, bilirubin determinations, direct Coombs' test of infant's blood, and examination of maternal blood smear for fetal erythrocytes (Kleihauer-Betke test). Medical management depends on the severity of the anemia and whether blood loss is acute or chronic. The baby should be placed on constant cardiac and respiratory monitoring. Mild or slow chronic anemia may be treated adequately with iron supplements alone or with iron-fortified formulas. Frequent determinations of hemoglobin, hematocrit, and bilirubin levels (in hemolytic disease) are essential. In severe cases of anemia, transfusions are the treatment of choice.

Nursing Assessment

The nurse assesses the newborn for symptoms of anemia (pallor). If the blood loss is acute, the baby may exhibit signs of shock. Continued observations will be necessary to identify physiologic anemia as the preterm newborn grows. Signs of compromise include poor weight gain, tachycardia, tachypnea, and apneic episodes.

Nursing Goal: Promotion of Physical Well-Being

The nurse promptly reports any symptoms indicating anemia or shock. The amount of blood drawn for all laboratory tests should be recorded so that total blood removed can be assessed and replaced by transfusion when necessary. If the newborn exhibits signs of shock, the nurse may need to begin necessary interventions.

● Care of the Newborn With Polycythemia

Polycythemia is a condition in which blood volume and hematocrit values are increased. A common problem in low-risk nurseries, polycythemia affects 2 percent to 17

percent of newborns (Nantze 1985). It is observed more commonly in SGA and full-term infants than in preterm neonates. An infant is considered polycythemic when the central venous hematocrit value is greater then 65 percent to 70 percent, or the venous hemoglobin level is greater than 22 g/dL during the first week of life (Avery 1987).

Several conditions predispose the neonate to polycythemia:

1. At the time of birth an excessive volume of placental blood may transfuse into the infant before the cord is clamped, resulting in a blood volume increase.

2. During gestation an increased amount of blood may cross the placenta to the infant (maternofetal transfusion), resulting in increased blood volume after birth.

3. A twin-to-twin transfusion may occur, in which one twin receives less blood and becomes anemic, and the other twin receives an excess amount of blood and becomes polycythemic.

4. Increased red blood cell production may occur in utero in response to chronic fetal distress in SGA, IDM, or postmature infants and secondary to conditions of PIH and placenta previa.

Other conditions that present with polycythemia are chromosomal anomalies such as trisomy 21, 18, and 13; endocrine disorders such as hypoglycemia and hypocalcemia; and births at altitudes over 5000 feet.

Medical Therapy

The goal of therapy is to reduce the central venous hematocrit to less than 60 percent in symptomatic infants. Treatment of asymptomatic infants is more controversial, but most authorities agree that these newborns benefit from prophylactic exchanges. To decrease the red cell mass, the symptomatic infant receives a partial exchange transfusion in which blood is removed from the infant and replaced millimeter for millimeter with fresh plasma. Supportive treatment of presenting symptoms is required until resolution. This usually occurs spontaneously following the partial exchange transfusion.

Nursing Assessment

The nurse assesses, records, and reports symptoms of polycythemia. The nurse also does an initial screening of the newborn's hematocrit on admission to the nursery.

Many infants are asymptomatic, but as symptoms develop they are related to the increased blood volume, hyperviscosity (thickness) of the blood, and decreased deformability of red blood cells, all of which result in poor perfusion of tissues. The infants have a characteristic plethoric (ruddy) appearance. The most common symptoms observed include:

- Tachycardia and congestive heart failure due to the increased blood volume

- Respiratory distress with grunting, tachypnea, and cyanosis; increased oxygen need; or hemorrhage in respiratory system due to pulmonary venous congestion, edema, and hypoxemia

- Hyperbilirubinemia due to increased numbers of red blood cells hemolysed

- Decrease in peripheral pulses, discoloration of extremities, alteration in activity or neurologic depression, renal vein thrombosis with decreased urine output, hematuria, or proteinuria due to thromboembolism

- Seizures due to decreased perfusion of the brain and increased vascular resistance secondary to sluggish blood flow, which can result in neurologic or developmental problems

Nursing Goal: Promotion of Physical Well-Being

The nurse must observe closely for the signs of distress or change in vital signs during the partial exchange. The nurse must assess carefully for potential complications resulting from the exchange such as transfusion overload (may result in congestive heart failure), irregular cardiac rhythm, bacterial infection, hypovolemia, and anemia.

Nursing Goal: Provision of Teaching and Emotional Support

Parents need specific explanations about polycythemia and its treatment. The newborn needs to be reunited with the parents as soon after the exchange as the baby's status permits.

● Care of the Newborn With Hemorrhagic Disease

Several transient coagulation-mechanism deficiencies normally occur in the first several days of a newborn's life. Foremost among these is a slight decrease in the level of prothrombin, resulting in a prolonged clotting time during the initial week of life. Vitamin K is required for the liver to form prothrombin (factor II) and proconvertin (factor VII) for blood coagulation. Vitamin K, a fat-soluble vitamin, may be obtained from food, but it is usually synthesized by bacteria in the colon, and consequently a dietary source is unnecessary. However, intestinal flora are practically nonexistent in newborns, so they are unable to synthesize vitamin K.

Bleeding due to vitamin K deficiency generally occurs on the second or third day of life, but it may occur earlier in babies of mothers treated with phenytoin sodium (Dilantin) or phenobarbital. These drugs impair vitamin K activity, and bleeding may be seen at birth. Coumarin compounds are vitamin K antagonists that can cross the placenta. Thus the baby exposed to maternal coumarin can also manifest bleeding in the first 24 hours of life. Bleeding may also occur in babies receiving parenteral nutrition without adequate vitamin K additives (1 mg/week).

Bleeding from the nose, umbilical cord, circumcision site, gastrointestinal tract, and scalp, as well as generalized ecchymoses may be seen. Internal hemorrhage may occur.

This disorder can be completely prevented by the prophylactic use of an injection of vitamin K. A dose of 1 mg of AquaMEPHYTON is given as part of newborn care immediately following delivery, and consequently the disease is rarely seen today (see Drug Guide, Chapter 29). Larger doses are contraindicated because they may result in the development of hyperbilirubinemia.

● Care of the Newborn With Congenital Heart Defects

The incidence of congenital heart defects is 7.5 per 1000 live births. They account for one third of the deaths caused by congenital defects in the first year of life. Because accurate diagnosis and surgical treatment are now available, many such deaths can be prevented. It is crucial for the nurse to have comprehensive knowledge of congenital heart disease to detect deviations from normal and to initiate interventions.

Overview of Congenital Heart Defects

Factors that might influence development of congenital heart malformation can be classified as environmental or genetic. Infections of the pregnant woman, such as rubella, coxsackie B, and influenza, have been implicated.

Thalidomide, steroids, alcohol, lithium, and some anticonvulsants have been shown to cause malformations of the heart. Seasonal spraying of pesticides has also been linked to an increase in congenital heart defects.

Infants born with chromosomal abnormalities have a higher incidence of cardiovascular anomalies. Infants with Down syndrome and trisomy 13/15 and 16/18 frequently have heart lesions. Increased incidence and risk of recurrence of specific defects occur in families.

It is customary to divide congenital malformations of the heart into *acyanotic*—those that do not present with cyanosis—and *cyanotic*—those that do present with cyanosis. If an opening exists between the right and left sides of the heart, blood will normally flow from the area of greater pressure (left side) to the area of lesser pressure (right side). This process is referred to as left-to-right shunt and does not produce cyanosis because oxygenated blood is being pumped out to the systemic circulation. If pressure in the right side of the heart, due to obstruction of normal flow, exceeds that in the left side, unoxygenated blood will flow from the right side to the left side of the heart and out into the system. This right-to-left shunt causes cyanosis. If the opening is large, there may be a bidirectional shunt with mixing of blood in both sides of the heart, which also produces cyanosis.

The common cardiac defects seen in the first six days of life are left ventricular outflow obstructions (mitral stenosis, aortic stenosis or atresia), hypoplastic left heart, coarctation of the aorta, patent ductus arteriosus (PDA; the most common defect), transposition of the great vessels, tetralogy of Fallot, and large ventricular septal defect or atrial septal defects (see Figure 32–18). Table 32–5 presents the clinical manifestations and medical/surgical management of these cardiac defects.

Nursing Assessment

The primary goal of the neonatal nurse is early identification of cardiac defects and initiation of referral to the physician. The three most common manifestations of cardiac defect are cyanosis, detectable heart murmur, and congestive heart failure signs (tachycardia, tachypnea, diaphoresis, hepatomegaly, and cardiomegaly).

Nursing assessment of the following signs and symptoms assists in identifying the newborn with a cardiac problem.

1. Tachypnea—reflects increased pulmonary blood flow

2. Dyspnea—caused by increased pulmonary venous pressure and blood flow; can also cause chest retractions, wheezing

3. Color—ashen, gray, or cyanotic

4. Difficulty in feeding—requires many rest periods before finishing even 1 or 2 ounces

5. Diaphoresis—beads of perspiration over the upper lip and forehead; may accompany feeding fatigue

6. Stridor or choking spells

7. Failure to gain weight

8. Heart murmur—may not be heard in left-to-right shunting defects since the pulmonary pressure in the newborn is greater than pressure in the left side of the heart in the early newborn period

9. Hepatomegaly—in right-sided heart failure caused by venous congestion in the liver

10. Tachycardia—pulse over 160, may be as high as 200

11. Cardiac enlargement

Nursing Diagnosis

Nursing diagnoses that may apply to the newborn with a cardiac defect are presented in the Nursing Care Plan, beginning on p 1053.

Nursing Goal: Maintenance of Cardiopulmonary Status

When the baby has dyspnea or cyanosis, oxygen must be given by an oxygen hood, tent, mask, cannula, or oxygen prongs. Mist is often ordered, which requires the use of an oxygen hood or tent. Oxygen administration should always be accompanied by humidity, and the air should be warmed to decrease the drying effects of cold, dry oxygen. Vital signs are carefully monitored for evidence of tachycardia, tachypnea, expiratory grunting, and retractions.

Morphine sulfate, a dose of 0.05 mg/kg of body weight, can be used if the infant is markedly irritable (Graham & Bender 1980). Morphine is thought to decrease peripheral and pulmonary vascular resistance, which results in decreased tachypnea. Infants in congestive heart failure are more comfortable in a semi-Fowler's position.

The nurse provides for rest by administering a sedative as required. Organizing nursing care is a key to decreasing energy requirements and providing periods of rest.

Nursing Goal: Parent Education

After the baby is stabilized and gaining weight, decisions are made about ongoing care and surgical interventions. The parents need careful and complete explanations and the opportunity to take part in decision making. They also require ongoing emotional support.

Table 32-5 Cardiac Defects of the Early Newborn Period

Congenital heart defect	Clinical findings	Medical/surgical management
ACYANOTIC		
Patent Ductus Arteriosus (PDA) ↑ in females, maternal rubella, RDS, <1500 g preterm newborns, high-altitude births	Harsh grade 2–3 machinery murmur upper LSB just beneath clavicle ↑ difference between systolic and diastolic pulse pressure Can lead to right heart failure and pulmonary congestion ↑ LA and LV enlargement, dilated ascending aorta ↑ pulmonary vascularity	Indomethacin—0.2 mg/kg orally (prostaglandin inhibitor) Surgical ligation Use of O_2 therapy and blood transfusion to improve tissue oxygenation and perfusion Fluid restriction and diuretics
Atrial Septal Defect (ASD) ↑ in females and Down syndrome	Initially frequently asymptomatic Systolic murmur 2nd LICS With large ASD, diastolic rumbling murmur LLS border Failure to thrive, URI, poor exercise tolerance	Surgical closure with patch or suture.
Ventricular Septal Defect (VSD) ↑ in males	Initially asymptomatic until end of first month or large enough to cause pulmonary edema Loud, blowing systolic murmur 3rd–4th ICS pulmonary blood flow Right ventricular hypertrophy Rapid respirations, growth failure, feeding difficulties Congestive right heart failure at 6 weeks–2 months of age	Follow medically—some spontaneously close Use of lanoxin and diuretics in CHF Surgical closure with Dacron patch
Coarctation of Aorta	Absent or diminished femoral pulses Increased brachial pulses Late systolic murmur left intrascapular area Systolic BP in lower extremities Enlarged left ventricle Can present in CHF at 7–21 days of life	Surgical resection of narrowed portion of aorta
CYANOTIC		
Tetralogy of Fallot (Most common cyanotic heart defect) Pulmonary stenosis VSD Overriding aorta Right ventricular hypertrophy	May be cyanotic at birth or within first few months of life Harsh systolic murmur LSB Crying or feeding increases cyanosis and respiratory distress X ray: boot-shaped appearance secondary to small pulmonary artery Right ventricular enlargement	Prevention of dehydration and intercurrent infections Alleviation of paroxysmal dyspneic attacks Palliative surgery to increase blood flow to the lungs Corrective surgery—resection of pulmonic stenosis, closure of VSD with Dacron patch
Transposition of Great Vessels (TGA) (↑ females, IDMs, LGAs)	Cyanosis at birth or within 3 days Possible pulmonic stenosis murmur Right ventricular hypertrophy Polycythemia "Egg on its side" x ray	Prostaglandin E to vasodilate ductus to keep it open Initial surgery to create opening between right and left side of heart if none exists Total surgical repair—usually the Mustard procedure
Hypoplastic Left Heart Syndrome	Normal at birth—cyanosis and shocklike congestive heart failure develop within a few hours to days Soft systolic murmur just left of the sternum Diminished pulses Aortic and/or mitral atresia Tiny, thick-walled left ventricle Large, dilated, hypertrophied right ventricle X ray: cardiac enlargement and pulmonary venous congestion	Currently no effective corrective treatment

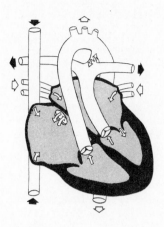

Complete Transposition of Great Vessels

This anomaly is an embryologic defect caused by a straight division of the bulbar trunk without normal spiraling. As a result, the aorta originates from the right ventricle, and the pulmonary artery from the left ventricle. An abnormal communication between the two circulations must be present to sustain life.

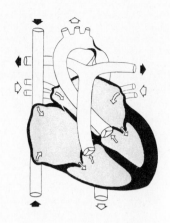

Coarctation of the Aorta

Coarctation of the aorta is characterized by a narrowed aortic lumen. It exists as a preductal or postductal obstruction, depending on the position of the obstruction in relation to the ductus arteriosus. Coarctations exist with great variation in anatomical features. The lesion produces an obstruction to the flow of blood through the aorta causing an increased left ventricular pressure and work load.

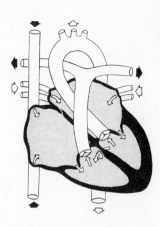

Ventricular Septal Defects

A ventricular septal defect is an abnormal opening between the right and left ventricle. Ventricular septal defects vary in size and may occur in either the membranous or muscular portion of the ventricular septum. Due to higher pressure in the left ventricle, a shunting of blood from the left to right ventricle occurs during systole. If pulmonary vascular resistance produces pulmonary hypertension, the shunt of blood is then reversed from the right to the left ventricle with cyanosis resulting.

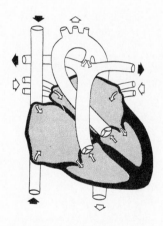

Patent Ductus Arteriosus

The patent ductus arteriosus is a vascular connection that, during fetal life, short circuits the pulmonary vascular bed and directs blood from the pulmonary artery to the aorta. Functional closure of the ductus normally occurs soon after birth. If the ductus remains patent after birth, the direction of blood flow in the ductus is reversed by the higher pressure in the aorta.

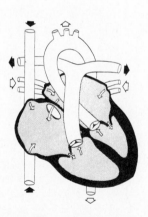

Atrial Septal Defects

An atrial septal defect is an abnormal opening between the right and left atria. Basically, three types of abnormalities result from incorrect development of the atrial septum. An incompetent foramen ovale is the most common defect. The high ostium secundum defect results from abnormal development of the septum secundum. Improper development of the septum primum produces a basal opening known as an ostium primum defect, frequently involving the atrio-ventricular valves. In general, left to right shunting of blood occurs in all atrial septal defects.

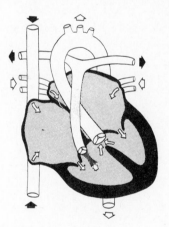

Tetralogy of Fallot

Tetralogy of Fallot is characterized by the combination of four defects: 1) pulmonary stenosis 2) ventricular septal defect 3) overriding aorta 4) hypertrophy of right ventricle. It is the most common defect causing cyanosis in patients surviving beyond two years of age. The severity of symptoms depends on the degree of pulmonary stenosis, the size of the ventricular septal defect, and the degree to which the aorta overrides the septal defect.

Figure 32–18 *Congenital heart abnormalities* (From *Congenital Heart Abnormalities.* Clinical Education Aid no. 7. Ross Laboratories, Columbus, Ohio)

Nursing Care Plan: Newborn With Congenital Heart Defect

Davey Smith is a term, 39 week, AGA newborn born to a 23-year-old G 1, P 0, A+ mother via a normal spontaneous vaginal delivery without complications. A soft and persistent systolic heart murmur was noted at birth. Now at 3 days of age he is found in his crib cyanotic, tachypneic, and generally in distress. On physical assessment the heart murmur is now absent, his heart rate is 190 beat/min, and respirations are at 78 per min. Blood pressure is within normal range.

Chest x ray shows a relatively clear lung field, but the heart is mildly enlarged and has the appearance of an "egg on its side." Now in 100 percent oxygen in a head hood Davey is still cyanotic, and his PO_2 is less than 60. Central venous Hct is 68 mg percent. Starting one day ago, Davey has become dyspneic, tachypneic, and increasingly dusky and has had beads of perspiration over his forehead during feedings.

Assessment	
NURSING HISTORY	PHYSICAL EXAMINATION

NURSING HISTORY

Identification of predisposing factors include:
a. No significant maternal history
b. At birth, soft, persistent heart murmur
c. At 3 days of age, cyanosis, tachypnea, in distress
d. Male child

LABORATORY EVALUATION

a. Hyperoxic test: In 100 percent oxygen PO_2 <60 and cyanotic
b. Hct 68 mg percent
c. X ray: "Egg on its side" with mildly enlarged heart and clear lung fields

PHYSICAL EXAMINATION

a. Respirations 78/min
b. Heart rate 190 beats/min
c. Normal blood pressure
d. Soft systolic heart murmur
e. Beads of perspiration over forehead and dyspnea during feeding
f. Cyanosis

ANALYSIS OF NURSING PRIORITIES

a. Support oxygenation and effective breathing.
b. Provide a neutral thermal environment.
c. Provide for adequate nutrition and fluid needs.
d. Protect from infection.
e. Provide information to the parents regarding oxygen needs and equipment, signs that indicate need for medical assistance, importance of follow-up, home care needs, and long-term care and surgical needs.

Nursing Diagnosis and Goals	Nursing Interventions and Actions	Rationale
NURSING DIAGNOSIS: Alterations in tissue perfusion related to decrease in circulating oxygen	Administer 100 percent oxygen to R/O respiratory distress vs cardiac disorder.	If a right-to-left shunt is present, inspired O_2 will have little or no effect on the presenting sign of cyanosis. If the baby is in respiratory distress, the degree of cyanosis will decrease with the inspired oxygen.
SUPPORTING DATA: Cyanosis of skin, nailbeds, and mucous membranes Tachycardia Tachypnea	Maintain neutral thermal environment.	An inadequate thermal environment will increase oxygen demands thus predisposing the newborn to R–L shunt. Therefore the original cause of cyanosis may be disguised.
	Obtain a cardiorespiratory assessment. Obtain a baseline heart rate and respiratory rate.	Establish baseline data for assessment to R/O cardiac anomalies.
	Obtain blood pressure in all extremities. Palpate peripheral pulses. Auscultate heart sounds to determine if a heart murmur is present.	Absence of femoral pulses may indicate a coarctation of the aorta. Bounding pulses may suggest a patent ductus arteriosus.
	Determine if the liver is >2 cm below the R costal margin. Obtain an initial Hb and Hct.	
GOAL: Caregivers will determine the cause of cyanosis and initiate supportive and/or corrective measures.		

Nursing Care Plan: Newborn With Congenital Heart Defect (continued)

Nursing Diagnosis and Goals	Nursing Interventions and Actions	Rationale
NURSING DIAGNOSIS: Ineffective breathing patterns related to fatigue	Place Davey on abdomen and elevate the head of bed.	Placing Davey on abdomen facilitates optimal chest expansion. Gravity facilitates maximum chest expansion by keeping the diaphragm in its lowest position.
SUPPORTING DATA: Tachypnea Respiratory Rate >60 Dyspnea Increasing irritability	Comfort when crying. Provide ventilatory support per physician order.	Crying increases cyanosis.
GOAL: Caregivers will determine the cause of increasing respirations, provide comfort measures, and decrease fatigue		
NURSING DIAGNOSIS: Alterations in nutrition: less than body requirements related to increased energy expenditure	Provide gavage feeding as needed if Davey tires easily while nipple feeding.	Gavage feeding conserves energy expenditure.
SUPPORTING DATA: Difficulty feeding Trouble coordinating suck and swallow reflex	Give small frequent feedings per physician order.	Small feedings prevent overdistention of stomach and respiratory embarrassment.
Tires easily during feeding Ingests insufficient amount of formula	Give concentrated formula per physician order.	A newborn with a cardiac defect has an increased cardiac work load, which requires a greater expenditure of energy and more calories than a newborn without cardiac problems.
Chokes and becomes dyspneic with feedings Polycythemia	Maintain hydration requirements.	Newborns with cardiac defects tend to have higher Hct due to chronic hypoxemia. Decreased fluid intake aggravates this condition.
	Position in cardiac chair during and after feedings with head and shoulders elevated	Sitting in cardiac chair lessens pressure from stomach on diaphragm.
GOAL: Davey will ingest appropriate calories to gain weight.		
NURSING DIAGNOSIS: Knowledge deficit of parents related to cardiac anomaly and future implications for care	Explain the nature of the defect in simple terms.	
SUPPORTING DATA: Mr and Mrs Smith ask what causes their son's bluish color, and what it means?	Explain the significance of color (if blueness is present). Explain importance of contacting the physician if baby has a cyanotic spell, increasing irritability, or labored breathing or is inconsolable.	Blueness in color is associated with a cyanotic heart lesion. Obtaining medical care immediately alleviates a possibly life-threatening event.
They are anxious about the home care of their child and do not understand medications and their significance.	Teach parents to place baby in the knee-chest position, increase oxygen, and quiet Davey if he has a cyanotic spell.	

Nursing Care Plan: Newborn With Congenital Heart Defect (continued)

Nursing Diagnosis and Goals	Nursing Interventions and Actions	Rationale
	Train Mr and Mrs Smith in CPR technique and maintenance of oxygen and humidification equipment.	Parents need to be prepared for an emergency situation if one should occur at home.
	Teach Davey's parents signs of URIs.	Early treatment of URIs helps prevent further cardiac compromise/stress.
	Make a referral to a home health care agency or the public health nurse for support and follow-up.	Family needs emotional and physical support.
	Explore the parents' support system. Refer to a support group for parents of children with cardiac anomalies.	Parents need to explore and share their feelings with others in similar circumstances.
GOAL: Mr and Mrs Smith will be comfortable in caring for Davey.		

Epilogue

Davey has stabilized and is going home on oxygen and medications. Mr and Mrs Smith have gone to CPR training and received information on home oxygen administration. Davey has successfully undergone a Rashkind balloon septostomy, and his duskiness is diminished.

● Care of the Newborn With Necrotizing Enterocolitis

With recent advances in the field of neonatology, severely ill newborns who would have succumbed a decade ago are now surviving. With this increased survival, a group of newborns are demonstrating a condition called necrotizing enterocolitis (NEC), or necrosis of the bowel, which occurs in the first weeks of life and may cause bowel perforation and ultimately death.

Necrotizing enterocolitis occurs most frequently in newborns weighing less than 1500 g. Onset usually occurs within the first two to three weeks of life, although NEC can be seen as early as the first day of life. Most cases are diagnosed by 1 month of age in all but the most debilitated infants.

The exact cause of NEC is not known, but some predisposing factors are associated with subsequent development of the disease. The current concept is that the etiology is multifocal and involves hypoxemia and intestinal mucosal injury.

An ischemic attack to the intestine may be precipitated by any condition in which systemic shock and hypoxia occur. Such conditions as fetal distress, neonatal shock and asphyxia, low cardiac output syndrome, low Apgar score, RDS, umbilical arterial catheters, infusion of hyperosmolar solution, polycythemia, and prematurity are associated with NEC.

The action of enteric bacteria on the damaged intestine may complicate the process and produce sepsis. Gas formation and possible dissection of air into the portal system are the result of bacterial action. Gram-negative organisms most frequently identified are *E. coli* and *Klebsiella*.

Necrotic lesions may be diffuse involving the stomach in addition to the small and large intestines. Involvement may include isolated areas of small intestine alternating with normal segments or may be restricted to the distal ileum and proximal large bowel. The lesions are characterized by frequent mucosal ulcerations, pseudomembrane formation, and inflammation.

Complications or consequences of necrotizing enterocolitis include:

● Surgical removal of the diseased intestine, leaving insufficient remaining small bowel to support life

● Stenosis of the intestinal tract that develops secondary to NEC or surgery

● Gastrointestinal dysfunction resulting in recurring intolerance to oral feedings, with vomiting, abdominal distention, water-loss diarrhea, and failure to gain weight

● Parenteral hyperalimentation that predisposes to sepsis, thrombosis of major vessels, and metabolic complications such as hyperglycemia, glycosuria, acidosis, osmotic diuresis, dehydration, and hepatic damage (cholestatic jaundice)

● Prolonged hospitalization with separation from parents and possible lack of appropriate developmental stimuli

Medical Therapy

Prevention may not be possible in the compromised, LBW infant. Successful intervention requires early identification and aggressive treatment to decrease the significant morbidity and mortality that accompanies NEC.

Systemic symptoms are those associated with sepsis—temperature instability (often hypothermia), respiratory changes (apnea, labored respirations), cardiovascular collapse, and behavioral changes such as lethargy or irritability. Gastrointestinal symptoms include abdominal distention and tenderness, feeding changes such as vomiting or increased gastric residual (bile-stained), poor feeding, abdominal wall cellulitis (development of an erythematous area on the abdominal wall), and blood (Hematest positive) and reducing substances in the stools.

Clinical findings are corroborated by radiographic findings, which include (a) pneumatosis intestinalis—air in the bowel wall (extraluminal or intramural air bubble and strips); (b) adynamic ileus—a paralytic ileus with stasis; (c) bowel wall thickening and loops of unequal size, bubbly appearance of intestine; and (d) free air—pneumoperitoneum or free air in the portal vein.

Serial anteroposterior and lateral decubitus (or cross-table lateral abdominal) radiographic evaluation is recommended every four to six hours for detection of progression of the disease and determination of complications indicating need for surgical intervention.

Aggressive and early management may avoid the need for surgical intervention. Gastric decompression, fluid and electrolyte replacement, correction of acidosis, maintenance of oxygenation, and parenteral antibiotics are common treatment techniques. Volume expanders such as fresh frozen plasma may be necessary to correct existing hypotension and to improve peripheral perfusion, because large amounts of plasma protein are lost into the gut lumen and peritoneal cavity in the acute phase. Hyperalimentation through a central line (inserted into the superior vena cava) may be indicated.

Recent research (LaGamma et al 1985, Ostertag et al 1986) raises the possibility that dilute formula or breast milk actually affords an advantage rather than increasing the risk of NEC as has been generally accepted in the past. They postulate that gut atrophy and depressed enzyme activity occur when oral nutritional intake is withheld. Thus dilute feedings may protect the immature gut by enhancing normal functional maturation and development of gut flora.

Surgery is indicated at the development of intestinal perforation with pneumoperitoneum, intestinal infarction without perforation, progressive abdominal ascites and/or bowel wall thickening, and clinical deterioration. Even small or subtle changes may indicate rapid progression and worsening of the disease and the need for immediate surgical intervention.

Surgical intervention consists of removal of those areas of bowel that are necrotic or perforated. Intestinal areas of compromised circulation or questionable viability are usually preserved, in hopes of eventual recovery and regeneration. Primary anastomosis is not attempted because of the possibility of connecting areas of ischemic bowel. A gastrostomy is placed to decompress the intestinal tract, and an ostomy is created for drainage until the intestine is reconnected.

Nursing Assessment

Survival of the infant depends on early recognition and treatment and meticulous nursing care. The neonatal nurse providing constant bedside care is often the first person to observe the subtle signs and symptoms of early development of NEC. Recognition of high-risk groups, careful observation for subtle, nonspecific symptoms, and prompt reporting of suspicions promote early, often life-saving treatment.

Nursing Diagnosis

Nursing diagnoses that may apply to the newborn who develops NEC include:

- Alteration in bowel elimination related to ischemic mucous membranes of lower GI tract

- Alteration in tissue perfusion of bowel related to hypoxemia

- Fluid volume deficit related to gastric suctioning secondary to NPO status and abdominal distention

- Alteration of sensory perception related to minimal handling of the newborn

- Ineffective family coping related to possible need for surgery and prolonged hospitalization of newborn

Nursing Goal: Identification of Necrotizing Enterocolitis

The nurse assesses for feeding intolerance, increased gastric residual (undigested formula), and bile-stained emesis; these signs occur because of prolonged gastric emptying. Bowel sounds are hypoactive or absent due to paralytic ileus. The abdominal girth is measured every two to three hours if NEC is suspected. An increase greater than 1 cm in four hours is significant. Abdominal tenderness and the appearance of abdominal wall erythema is evaluated. The nurse routinely checks stools for reducing substances (glucose in the stools). Glucose in the stools occurs in the presence of poor absorption of sugars and may be one of the earliest signs of NEC. Hematest positive stools (blood in the stools) result from ischemia and necrosis of the bowel. Checks for reducing substances and Hematest of the stools is done at least every shift.

Nursing Goal: Promotion of Physical Well-Being

Nursing management consists of supportive therapy and constant observation of the newborn's condition. When the signs of NEC are present, the nurse stops oral feedings to rest the bowel and places or assists in placement of a gastric tube for gastric decompression and drainage. Key nursing care involves maintaining patency of the gastric tube and recording the amount of gastric drainage so that replacement electrolytes and fluids may be given. The nurse monitors the parenteral nutrition infusion and the administration of intravenous antibiotics.

Assessment of vital signs and oxygen concentration, as well as careful observation for development of increasing abdominal girth or worsening clinical condition, is the responsibility of the nursery nurse. Axillary temperatures are taken to decrease rectal mucosa trauma. The baby is handled only minimally to prevent abdominal trauma. Diapers are avoided so that pressure is not placed on the lower abdomen and changes in the abdomen can be observed. The nurse also obtains blood, urine, and stool cultures and assists with a spinal tap for the sepsis workup. Continued monitoring of the baby's status involves obtaining serial x rays and electrolyte and blood gas assessments at least every eight hours. If surgical resection is required, an ostomy will be created temporarily to allow time for the bowel to heal. Meticulous nursing care is required in maintenance of skin integrity around the opening in these debilitated infants (Harrel-Bean & Klell 1983).

Nursing Goal: Early Identification of Complications

Continuous assessment of vital signs is essential to identify impending shock related to peritonitis. The nurse watches for temperature instability, drop in blood pressure, apneic spells, bradycardia, and listlessness. Volume expanders such as fresh frozen plasma are administered as ordered to improve peripheral perfusion and correct hypotension, which is caused by large shifts of plasma protein into the gut lumen and peritoneal cavity.

Nursing Goal: Provision of Support and Education to the Family

Necrotizing enterocolitis may significantly prolong the hospitalization of the infant and further compromise parent-infant attachment. Parents will require full support of the interdisciplinary team to deal with the additional stress of this complication and the consequences of surgical intervention (long-term gastric dysfunction, ostomy). The nurse can facilitate parental education and communication with the many professionals involved in this infant's care.

Parents should be given adequate explanations of treatment modalities and their baby's condition and anticipatory information about the colostomy if surgery is pending. The nurse provides opportunities for the parents to discuss questions and concerns about their baby.

Nursing Goal: Provision of Sensory Stimulation

The nurse can meet the baby's emotional and sensory stimulation needs by stroking the infant's hands and feet and talking to him or her as often as possible when minimal handling is required. When the newborn's condition has improved, provision of visual and auditory stimulation, such as mobiles, windup toys, and music boxes, is important.

Evaluative Outcome Criteria

Nursing care is effective if:

- The newborn is recovering from surgery, tolerates feeding, and has reestablished bowel activity.

- The parents understand the causes, risks, therapy options, and nursing care involved in the care of NEC.

- The parents participate in their newborn's care and show attachment behaviors.

● Care of the Newborn With Infection

Sepsis Neonatorum

Neonates up to 1 month of age are particularly susceptible to infection. Referred to as *sepsis neonatorum,* these infections are caused by organisms that do not cause significant disease in older children. Incidence of severe infection is 0.5 to 2 per 1000 live newborns.

One predisposing factor is prematurity. The general debilitation and underlying illness often associated with prematurity necessitates invasive procedures such as umbilical catheterization, intubation, resuscitation, ventilatory support, and monitoring. Even the full-term infant is susceptible because her or his immunologic system is immature. It lacks the complex factors involved in effective phagocytosis and the ability to localize infection or to respond with a well-defined recognizable inflammatory response.

Maternal antepartal infections such as rubella, toxoplasmosis, cytomegalic inclusion disease, and herpes may cause congenital infections and resulting disorders in the newborn. Intrapartal maternal infections, such as amnionitis and those resulting from premature rupture of membranes and precipitous delivery, are sources of neonatal infection. Passage through the birth canal and contact with the vaginal flora (β-hemolytic streptococci, herpes, listeria, and gonococci) expose the infant to infection. With infection anywhere in the fetus or newborn, the adjacent tissues or organs are very easily penetrated, and the blood-brain barrier is ineffective. Septicemia is more common in males, except for those infections caused by group B β-hemolytic streptococcus.

In the past, Gram-positive organisms (that is, *Staphylococcus aureus* and group A streptococcus pneumococci) were the causative agents of significant neonatal illness. At present, Gram-negative organisms (especially *E. coli,* Aerobacter, *Proteus,* and *Klebsiella*) and the Gram-positive organism β-hemolytic streptococcus are the most common causative agents. Pseudomonas is a common fomite contaminant of ventilatory support and oxygen therapy equipment.

MEDICAL THERAPY

Preventive management is the primary goal of the interdisciplinary team. Hand washing by all who come in contact with the baby is essential. Rooming-in for the initially healthy newborn can cut down on hospital-acquired infections. When sepsis ensues, early identification, appropriate antibiotic therapy, and physiologic support will minimize complications.

Prenatal prevention should include maternal screening for sexually transmitted disease and monitoring of rubella titers in women who are negative. Intrapartally, sterile technique is essential, smears from genital lesions are taken, placenta and amniotic fluid cultures are obtained if amnionitis is suspected and if genital herpes is present toward term, and delivery by cesarean birth may be indicated. Local eye treatment with silver nitrate or an antibiotic ophthalmic ointment is given to all newborns to prevent gonococcal damage.

Infants with a history of possible exposure to infection in utero (for example, PROM more than 24 hours before delivery or questionable maternal history of infection) should have cultures taken as soon after birth as possible. A gastric aspirate and culture of external orifices (such as the ear canal) will reveal the organisms to which the infant was exposed. Cultures are obtained before antibiotic therapy is begun.

1. Two blood cultures are obtained from different peripheral sites. They are taken from a peripheral rather than an umbilical vessel, because catheters have yielded false positives resulting from contamination. The skin is prepared by cleaning with an antiseptic solution, such as one containing iodine, and allowed to dry; the specimen is obtained with a sterile needle/syringe.

2. Spinal fluid culture is obtained following a spinal tap.

3. Urine culture is best obtained from a specimen obtained by a suprapubic bladder aspiration.

4. Skin cultures are obtained of any lesions or drainage from lesions or reddened areas.

5. Nasopharyngeal, rectal, ear canal, and gastric aspirate cultures may be obtained.

Other laboratory investigations include a complete blood count, chest x-ray examination, serology, and Gram stains of cerebrospinal fluid, urine, skin exudate, and umbilicus. White blood count with differential may indicate the presence or absence of sepsis. A level of 30,000 WBC may be normal in the first 24 hours of life, while a low WBC may be indicative of sepsis. A low neutrophil count and a high band count indicate that an infection is present. Stomach aspirate should be sent for culture and smear if a gonococcal infection or amnionitis is suspected. Serum IgM levels are elevated (normal level less than 20 mg/dL) in response to transplacental infections. Counterimmunoelectrophoresis tests for specific bacterial antigens are done if possible. Evidence of congenital infections may be seen on skull x rays for cerebral calcifications (cytomegalovirus, toxoplasmosis), bone x rays (syphilis, cytomegalovirus), and serum-specific IgM levels (rubella). Cytomegalovirus infection is best diagnosed by urine cultures.

Isolation of the causative agent is necessary to obtain the diagnosis of sepsis in a suspected case and to identify the drugs to which the pathogen is susceptible. Because neonatal infection causes high mortality, however, therapy is instituted before results of the septic workup are obtained. A combination of two broad-spectrum antibiotics in large doses is initiated until the culture with sensitivities report is received.

After the pathogen and its sensitivities are determined, appropriate specific antibiotic therapy is begun. Combination of penicillin or ampicillin and aminoglycosides have been used in the past, but new aminoglycoside-resistant enterobacteria and penicillin-resistant staphylococcus necessitate new approaches to antibiotic therapy. The possibility of rotating aminoglycosides has been suggested to prevent development of resistance (McCracken 1985). Use of cephalosporins and in particular, cefotaxime, has emerged as an alternative to aminoglycoside therapy in the treatment of neonatal infections. Duration of therapy varies from 7 to 14 days (Table 32–6). If cultures are negative and symptoms subside, antibiotics may be discontinued after three days. Supportive physiologic care may be required to maintain respiratory, hemodynamic, nutritional, and metabolic homeostasis.

Table 32–6 Neonatal Sepsis Antibiotic Therapy

Drug	Dose	Route	Schedule	Comments
Ampicillin	50–100 mg/kg/day	IM or IV	Every 12 hours* Every 8 hours†	Effective against Gram-positive microorganisms and majority of E. coli strains.
Cefotaxime	100–150 mg/kg/day	IM or IV	Every 12 hours* Every 8 hours†	Active against most major pathogens in infants; effective against aminoglycoside-resistant organisms; achieve CSF bactericidal activity; lack of ototoxicity and nephrotoxicity; wide therapeutic index (levels not required); resistant organisms can develop rapidly if used extensively; ineffective against pseudomonas, listeria.
Gentamicin	5.0–7.5 mg/kg/day	IM or IV	Every 12 hours* Every 8 hours†	Effective against Gram-negative rods and staphylococci; may be used instead of kanamycin against penicillin-resistant staphylococci and E. coli strains and Pseudomonas aeruginosa. May cause ototoxicity and nephrotoxicity. Need to follow serum levels. Must never be given as IV push. Must be given over at least 30–60 min. In presence of oliguria or anuria, dose must be decreased or discontinued. In infant less than 1000 g, dosage interval may be as long as 24 hours. Monitor serum levels before administration of second dose.
Methicillin	50–100 mg/kg/day	IM or IV	Every 12 hours* Every 6–8 hours†	Effective against penicillinase-resistant staphylococci
Nafcillin	50–100 mg/kg/day	IM or IV	Every 12 hours* Every 6 hours†	Effective against penicillinase-resistant staphylococci.
Penicillin G (aqueous crystalline)	50,000–125,000 U/kg/day	IM or IV	Every 12 hours* Every 8 hours†	Initial sepsis therapy effective against most Gram-positive microorganisms except resistant staphylococci; can cause heart block in infants.

*Up to 7 days of age.
†Greater than 7 days of age.

NURSING ASSESSMENT

Symptoms are most often noticed by the nurse during daily care of the neonate rather than during the infant's sporadic contact with the physician. The infant may deteriorate rapidly in the first 12 to 24 hours after birth if β-hemolytic streptococcal infection is present, with signs and symptoms mimicking RDS. On the other hand, the onset of sepsis may be more gradual with more subtle signs and symptoms. The most common symptoms observed include:

1. Subtle behavioral changes—infant "isn't doing well"; is often lethargic or irritable, especially after first 24 hours, and hypotonic. Color changes may include pallor, duskiness, cyanosis, or a "shocky" appearance. Skin is cool and clammy.

2. Temperature instability, manifested by either hypothermia (recognized by a decrease in skin temperature) or hyperthermia (elevation of neonatal skin temperature) necessitating a corresponding increase or decrease in incubator temperature to maintain neutral thermal environment.

3. Poor feeding, evidenced by a decrease in total intake, abdominal distention, vomiting, poor sucking, lack of interest in feeding, and diarrhea.

4. Hyperbilirubinemia.

5. Onset of apnea.

Signs and symptoms may suggest CNS disease (jitteriness, tremors, seizure activity), respiratory system disease (tachypnea, labored respirations, apnea, cyanosis), hematologic disease (jaundice, petechial hemorrhages, hepatosplenomegaly), or gastrointestinal disease (diarrhea, vomiting, bile-stained aspirate, hepatomegaly). A differential diagnosis is necessary because of the similarity of symptoms to other more specific conditions.

NURSING DIAGNOSIS

Nursing diagnoses that may apply to the infant with sepsis neonatorum include:

● Potential for infection related to tachypnea, lethargy, and temperature instability secondary to immature immunologic system

- Fluid volume deficit related to feeding intolerance

- Ineffective family coping related to present illness resulting in prolonged hospital stay

NURSING GOAL: PREVENTION OF INFECTION

In the nursery, environmental control and prevention of acquired infection is the responsibility of the neonatal nurse. The nurse must promote strict hand-washing technique for all who enter the nursery, including nursing colleagues; physicians; laboratory, x-ray, and inhalation technicians; and parents. The nurse must be prepared to assist in the aseptic collection of specimens for laboratory investigations. Scrupulous care of equipment—changing and cleaning of incubators at least every seven days, removal and sterilization of wet equipment every 24 hours, prevention of cross-use of linen and other equipment, periodic cleaning of sinkside equipment such as soap containers, and special care with the open radiant warmers (access without prior hand washing is much easier than with the closed incubator)—will all prevent fomite contamination or contamination through improper hand washing of debilitated, infection-prone newborns. An infected neonate can be effectively isolated in an incubator and receive close observation. Visitation of the nursery area by unnecessary personnel should be discouraged.

NURSING GOAL: PROVISION OF ANTIBIOTIC THERAPY

The nurse administers antibiotics as ordered by the clinician. It is the nurse's responsibility to be knowledgeable about the following:

- The proper dose to be administered, based on the weight of the newborn

- The appropriate route of administration, as some antibiotics cannot be given intravenously

- Admixture incompatibilities since some antibiotics are precipitated by intravenous solutions or by other antibiotics

- Side effects and toxicity

NURSING GOAL: PROMOTION OF PHYSICAL WELL-BEING

In addition to antibiotic therapy, physiologic supportive care is essential in caring for a septic infant. The nurse should:

- Observe for resolution of symptoms or development of other symptoms of sepsis.

- Maintain neutral thermal environment with accurate regulation of humidity and oxygen administration.

- Provide respiratory support: Administer oxygen and observe and monitor respiratory effort.

- Provide cardiovascular support: Observe and monitor pulse and blood pressure; observe for hyperbilirubinemia, anemia, and hemorrhagic symptoms.

- Provide adequate calories, because oral feedings may be discontinued due to increased mucus, abdominal distention, vomiting, and aspiration.

- Provide fluids and electrolytes to maintain homeostasis.

- Detect and treat metabolic disturbances, a common occurrence.

- Observe for the development of hypoglycemia, hyperglycemia, acidosis, hyponatremia, and hypocalcemia.

NURSING GOAL: PROVISION OF SUPPORT AND EDUCATION TO PARENTS

Restriction of parent visits has not been shown to have any effect on the rate of infection and may indeed be harmful for the newborn's psychologic development. With instruction and guidance from the nurse, both parents should be allowed to handle the baby and participate in daily care. Support to the parents is crucial. They need to be informed of the newborn's prognosis as treatment continues and to be involved in care as much as possible. They also need to understand how infection is transmitted.

EVALUATIVE OUTCOME CRITERIA

Nursing care is effective if:

- The risks for development of sepsis are identified early, and immediate action is taken to minimize the development of the illness.

- Appropriate use of aseptic technique protects the newborn from further exposure to illness.

- The baby's symptoms are relieved, and the infection is treated.

- The parents verbalize their concerns about their baby's illness and understand the rationale behind the management of their newborn.

Group B Streptococcus

Group B streptococcus (β-hemolytic streptococcus) has become a leading cause of septicemia in the newborn, and is a major cause of morbidity and mortality in the neonate. Pregnant women who carry group B streptococcus are asymptomatic but harbor the organism in the birth canal, resulting in exposure of the infant to the organism during the birth process. It is estimated that 4 percent to 6 percent of pregnant women have positive cervical cultures, while a larger number have positive vaginal cultures. Approximately 1 percent to 2 percent of neonates are colonized with group B streptococcus but only one in ten of those colonized develops the disease (Korones 1986).

Two clinical disease entities may result from group B streptococcus. One is an early onset form (first week, usually within hours of delivery) of acute septicemia and pneumonia. The other occurs later (one week to three months) presenting as meningitis without respiratory distress. The early form carries a higher mortality risk (approximately 50 percent–80 percent even with appropriate antibiotic therapy) than the later onset form (20 percent–40 percent) (Avery and Taeusch 1984).

In the early onset form of group B streptococcus, the infant appears to be in severe respiratory distress (grunting and cyanosis), may become apneic, and may demonstrate symptoms of shock. There often is meconium-stained amniotic fluid at birth.

The chest x-ray examination may show aspiration pneumonia or may appear similar to that seen in hyaline membrane disease. Early recognition of a group B streptococcal condition is essential to the infant's intact survival, as the course is one of rapid deterioration. Cultures should be done immediately (blood, gastric aspirate, external ear canal, nasopharynx), and antibiotics should be started before results of the cultures are obtained. Antibiotic treatment usually involves aqueous penicillin or ampicillin. Some feel ampicillin combined with gentamicin is superior to ampicillin alone. It is the nurse's responsibility to be alert to all signs and symptoms suggesting sepsis, and to intervene as rapidly as possible when sepsis is suspected. There must be no delay in the administration of antibiotics, as this may determine the infant's ultimate survival.

Syphilis

Because congenital syphilis is difficult to detect at birth, all infants of syphilitic mothers should be screened to determine the necessity of treatment. Diagnostic serologic dilution tests are usually accurate between 3 and 6 months of age. Development and detection of the infant's own antibodies are essential to confirm the diagnosis.

By 3 months of age the congenitally infected infant exhibits the following signs:

- Positive serology; elevated cord serum, immunoglobulin M (IgM)

- Vesicular lesions over palms and soles

- Red rash around mouth and anus; copper-colored rash covering face, palms, and soles

- Hepatosplenomegaly

- Irritability

- Rhinitis (snuffles); fissures at mouth corners and an excoriated upper lip

- Pyrexia

- Painful extremities

- Bone lesions

- Generalized edema, particularly over joints

- Jaundice

- Small for gestational age (SGA) and failure to thrive

The nursing management of these infants and their parents involves careful physical and psychologic care. Drug treatment of choice is penicillin. After proper treatment for 48 hours, the infant should no longer be contagious. Initially, nursing care includes use of isolation techniques. Following treatment, however, general care may ensue.

Gonorrhea

Gonorrhea may be contracted by the fetus during vaginal delivery. Gonorrhea is usually manifested clinically as an eye infection, ophthalmia neonatorum. This is first diagnosed as a conjunctivitis that is indistinguishable from that caused by silver nitrate instillation. However, chemical conjunctivitis disappears within 24 hours, whereas ophthalmia neonatorum becomes more readily apparent in the neonate on the third or fourth postnatal day. Other severe clinical signs are a purulent discharge and ulcerations of the cornea, which can be prevented if treatment is instituted promptly. In some cases, gonorrhea infection may be observed as temperature instability, poor feeding response, and/or hypotonia.

For neonates of all vaginal births, a 1 percent silver nitrate solution or antibiotic ophthalmic ointment is instilled in the conjunctiva of the infant's eyes to prevent infection. Irrigation of the eyes following administration is controversial (see Drug Guide, Chapter 29). Penicillin may also be administered intramuscularly, in lieu of silver nitrate or antibiotic ophthalmic ointment. If allergy to penicillin is suspected, erythromycin or tetracycline may be substituted. If the newborn's eyes are left untreated, partial or complete loss of vision may occur as a result of corneal ulceration.

Herpesvirus

A wide variety of clinical manifestations of herpesvirus hominis (HVH) variety are noted in the newborn. Signs and symptoms are present at birth or by 3 to 4 weeks of age. While most neonatal infections are due to the type 2 agent, approximately 30 percent are due to type 1 strains. The clinical manifestations of infection with type 1 and 2 strains are not significantly different. The disseminated form usually occurs in the first week of life and is associated with DIC, pneumonia, hepatitis with jaundice, hepatosplenomegaly, and neurologic abnormalities. About one-third of affected infants exhibit vesicular skin lesions in small clusters all over the body at birth or several days after. Most cases of localized disease occur in the second week of life. It may affect the central nervous system alone or appear as isolated eye or skin disease.

In the absence of skin lesions, diagnosis is difficult, because the presenting clinical picture resembles septicemia (such as fever or subnormal temperature, respiratory congestion, dyspnea, cough, tachypnea, and tachycardia). It is therefore necessary to obtain cultures from the infant's lesions, throat, conjunctiva, CSF, blood, and urine and to identify the herpesvirus type 2 antibodies in the serum IgM fraction. Positive cultures are observable within 24 to 48 hours.

Preventive therapy may be attempted by cesarean delivery if the mother has recurrent genital infection at the time of delivery and if the membranes are either intact or have been ruptured less than four hours. When neonatal disease is suspected, a definitive diagnosis should be made as rapidly as possible. If diagnosed, the infant should be treated with intravenous vidarabine (Vira-A) or acyclovir (Zovirax). Even with treatment, mortality and sequelae (microcephaly, spasticity, paralysis, seizures, deafness, or blindness) are significant (Hanshaw et al 1985).

Careful hand washing and adequate infection-control methods are essential. Isolation measures should be instituted for all infants born to mothers with genital lesions regardless of the delivery mode. Suspected herpetic infants require gown and glove isolation with linen precautions. Parents need time with their newborns and should be encouraged to touch their babies. Rooming-in should be available for them and the mother is taught appropriate hand-washing procedures. Mothers with active lesions should be taught how to use precautions at home until lesions become inactive (Haggerty 1985).

Monilial Infection (Thrush)

Thrush (oral moniliasis) is caused by the fungus *Candida albicans*, contracted from a yeast-infected vagina during delivery. Clinically, it appears as white plaques distributed on the buccal mucosa, on the tongue, on the gums, inside the cheeks, and even on the lips. As it resembles milk curds, differentiation should be made by using a cotton-tipped applicator gently to attempt to wipe away the patches. If the plaques are thrush, a raw bleeding area beneath them will be exposed. Involvement of the diaper area skin is seen as a bright red, well-demarcated eruption. On occasion, generalized moniliasis may be seen. Lesions are most frequently seen at 5 to 7 days of age. However, infants receiving long-term antibiotic therapy are also susceptible to development of thrush, which may occur at any time during hospitalization.

Care of the neonate infected with *Candida albicans* involves:

1. Maintaining cleanliness of hands, bedding, clothing, diapers, and feeding apparatus, because *Candida albicans* is present in the oral secretions and in the stools. Breast-feeding mothers should be taught to treat their nipples with topical nystatin; otherwise a cycle of reinfection, as well as sore nipples with breakdown of nipple tissue, will occur.

2. Supporting physiologic well-being.

3. Administering drug therapy. Gentian violet (1 percent–2 percent) may be swabbed on oral lesions, usually an hour after feeding, once a day; or nystatin (Mycostatin) is instilled in the oral cavity with a medicine dropper. The mouth should be cleared of milk prior to instillation. It may also be swabbed over the oral mucosa. Topical nystatin is used for skin involvement.

4. Discussing with the parents that gentian violet is a dye and will cause staining of the infant's mouth and possibly the infant's clothing if the saliva is gentian colored. Care must be taken to paint only the lesions since gentian violet is irritating to normal mucosa.

● Care of the Newborn With Congenital Anomalies

The birth of a baby with a congenital defect places both newborn and family at risk. Many congenital anomalies can be life-threatening if not corrected within hours after birth; others are very visible and cause the families emotional distress. Table 32–7 identifies some of the more common anomalies and their early management and nursing care in the neonatal period.

Table 32–7 Congenital Anomalies: Identification and Care in Newborn Period

Congenital anomaly	Nursing assessments	Nursing goals and interventions
Congenital hydrocephalus	Enlarged head Enlarged or full fontanelles Split or widened sutures "Setting sun" eyes Head circumference >90% on growth chart	Assess presence of hydrocephalus: Measure and plot occipital-frontal baseline measurements, then measure head circumference once a day. Check fontanelle for bulging and sutures for widening. Assist with head ultrasound and transillumination. Maintain skin integrity: Change position frequently. Clean skin creases after feeding or vomiting. Use sheepskin pillow under head. Postoperatively, position head off operative site. Watch for signs of infection.
Choanal atresia	Occlusion of posterior nares Cyanosis and retractions at rest Snorting respirations Difficulty breathing during feeding Obstruction by thick mucus	Assess patency of nares: Listen for breath sounds while holding baby's mouth closed and alternately compressing each nostril. Assist with passing feeding tube to confirm diagnosis. Maintain respiratory function: Assist with taping airway in mouth to prevent respiratory distress. Position with head elevated to improve air exchange.
Cleft lip	Unilateral or bilateral visible defect May involve external nares, nasal cartilage, nasal septum, and alveolar process Flattening or depression of midfacial contour (Figure 32–19)	Provide nutrition: Feed with special nipple. Burp frequently (increased tendency to swallow air and reflex vomiting). Clean cleft with sterile water (to prevent crusting on cleft prior to repair). Support parental coping: Assist parents with grief over loss of idealized baby. Encourage verbalization of their feelings about visible defect. Provide role model in interacting with infant. (Parents internalize other's responses to their newborn.)
Cleft palate	Fissure connecting oral and nasal cavity May involve uvula and soft palate May extend forward to nostril involving hard palate and maxillary alveolar ridge Difficulty in sucking Expulsion of formula through nose (Figure 32–19)	Prevent aspiration/infection: Place prone or in side-lying position to facilitate drainage. Suction nasopharyngeal cavity (to prevent aspiration or airway obstruction). During neonatal period, feed in upright position with head and chest tilted slightly backward (to aid swallowing and discourage aspiration). Provide nutrition: Feed with special nipple that fills cleft and allows sucking. Also decreases chance of aspiration through nasal cavity. Clean mouth with water after feedings. Burp after each ounce (tend to swallow large amounts of air). Thicken formula to provide extra calories. Plot weight gain patterns to assess adequacy of diet. Provide parental support: Refer parents to community agencies and support groups. Encourage verbalization of frustrations as feeding process is long and frustrating. Praise all parental efforts. Encourage parents to seek prompt treatment for URI and teach them ways to decrease URI.

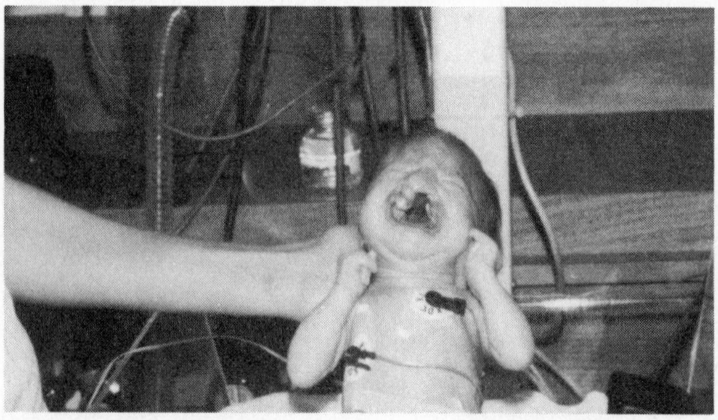

Figure 32–19   Cleft abnormality involving both hard and soft palate and unilateral cleft lip.

Table 32–7 Congenital Anomalies: Identification and Care in Newborn Period (continued)

Congenital anomaly	Nursing assessments	Nursing goals and interventions
Tracheoesophageal fistula (type III)	History of maternal hydramnios Excessive mucous secretions Constant drooling Abdominal distention beginning soon after birth Periodic choking and cyanotic episodes Immediate regurgitation of feeding Clinical symptoms of aspiration pneumonia (tachypnea, retractions, rhonchi, decreased breath sounds, cyanotic spells) Failure to pass nasogastric tube (Figure 32–20)	Maintain respiratory status and prevent aspiration: Withhold feeding until esophageal patency is determined. Quickly assess patency before putting to breast in birth area. Place on low intermittent suction to control saliva and mucus (to prevent aspiration pneumonia). Place in warmed, humidified Isolette (liquefies secretions facilitating removal). Elevate head of bed 20°–40° (to prevent reflux of gastric juices). Keep quiet (crying causes air to pass through fistula and to distend intestines causing respiratory embarrassment). Maintain fluid and electrolyte balance: Give fluids to replace esophageal drainage and maintain hydration. Provide parent education: Explain staged repair—provision of gastrostomy and ligation of fistula, then repair of atresia. Keep parents informed; clarify and reinforce physician's explanations regarding malformation, surgical repair, pre- and postoperative care, and prognosis (knowledge is ego strengthening). Involve parents in care of infant and in planning for future; facilitate touch and eye contact (to dispel feelings of inadequacy, increase self-esteem and self-worth, and promote incorporation of infant into family).

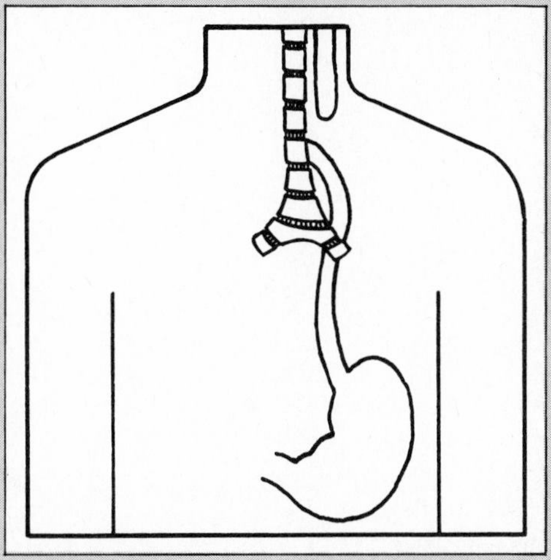

Figure 32–20 The most frequently seen type of congenital tracheo-esophageal fistula and esophageal atresia.

Congenital anomaly	Nursing assessments	Nursing goals and interventions
Diaphragmatic hernia	Difficulty initiating respirations Gasping respirations with nasal flaring and chest retraction Barrel chest and scaphoid abdomen Asymmetrical chest expansion Breath sounds may be absent, usually on left side Heart sounds displaced to right Spasmodic attacks of cyanosis and difficulty in feeding Bowel sounds may be heard in thoracic cavity (Figure 32–21)	Maintain respiratory status: Immediately administer oxygen. Initiate gastric decompression. Place in high semi-Fowler's position (to use gravity to keep abdominal organ's pressure off diaphragm). Turn to affected side to allow unaffected lung expansion. Carry out interventions to alleviate respiratory and metabolic acidosis. Assess for increased secretions around suction tube (denotes possible obstruction). Aspirate and irrigate tube with air or sterile water.
Omphalocele	Herniation of abdominal contents into base of umbilical cord May have an enclosed transparent sac covering	Maintain hydration and temperature: Provide D₅LR and albumin for hypovolemia. Place infant in sterile bag up to above defect. Cover sac with moistened sterile gauze and place plastic wrap over dressing (to prevent rupture of sac and infection). Initiate gastric decompression by insertion of nasogastric tube attached to low suction (to prevent distention of lower bowel and impairment of blood flow). Prevent infection and trauma to defect. Position to prevent trauma to defect. Administer broad-spectrum antibiotics.

Table 32–7 Congenital Anomalies: Identification and Care in Newborn Period (continued)

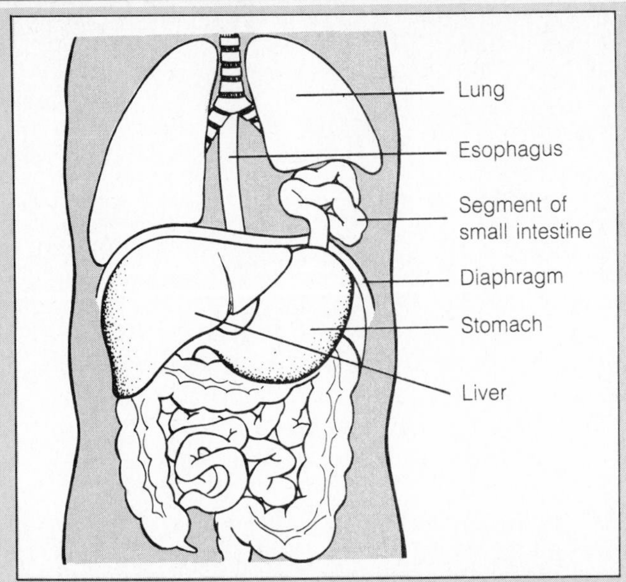

Congenital anomaly	Nursing assessments	Nursing goals and interventions

Figure 32–21 Diaphragmatic hernia. Note compression of the lung by the intestine on the affected side.

Congenital anomaly	Nursing assessments	Nursing goals and interventions
Myelomeningocele	Saclike cyst containing meninges, spinal cord, and nerve roots in thoracic and/or lumbar area (Figure 32–22) Myelomeningocele directly connects to subarachnoid space so hydrocephalus often associated No response or varying response to sensation below level of sac May have constant dribbling of urine Incontinence or retention of stool Anal opening may be flaccid	Prevent trauma and infection: Position on abdomen or on side and restrain (to prevent pressure and trauma to sac). Meticulously clean buttocks and genitals after each voiding and defecation (to prevent contamination of sac and decrease possibility of infection). May put protective covering over sac (to prevent rupture and drying). Observe sac for oozing of fluid or pus. Credé bladder as ordered (to prevent urinary stasis). Assess amount of sensation and movement below defect. Observe for complications: Obtain occipital-frontal circumference baseline measurements, then measure head circumference once a day (to detect hydrocephalus). Check fontanelle for bulging.
Imperforate anus, congenital dislocated hip, and clubfoot	See discussion in Chapter 28	Identify defect and initiate appropriate referral early.

● Care of the Newborn With Inborn Errors of Metabolism

Inborn errors of metabolism are a group of hereditary disorders that are transmitted by mutant genes and result in an enzyme defect that blocks a metabolic pathway and leads to an accumulation of metabolites that are toxic to the infant. Most of the disorders are transmitted by an autosomal recessive gene, requiring two heterozygous parents to produce a homozygous infant with the disorder. Heterozygous parents of some inborn errors of metabolism disorders can be identified by special tests, and some inborn errors of metabolism can be detected in utero.

The detection of many inborn errors of metabolism is now accomplished neonatally through newborn screening programs. These programs principally test for disorders associated with mental retardation.

Phenylketonuria (PKU) is the most common of the amino acid disorders. Newborn screenings have set its incidence at about 1 in 1500 live births (Ampola 1982). The highest incidence is noted in white populations from northern Europe and the United States. It is rarely observed in African, Jewish, or Japanese people.

Phenylalanine is an essential amino acid used by the body for growth, and in the normal individual any excess is converted to tyrosine. The newborn with PKU lacks this converting ability, which results in an accumulation of phenylalanine in the blood. Phenylalanine produces two abnormal metabolites, phenylpyruvic acid and phenylacetic acid, which are eliminated in the urine producing a musty odor. Excessive accumulation of phenylalanine and its abnormal metabolites in the brain tissue leads to progressive mental retardation.

Maple syrup urine disease (MSUD) is an inborn error of metabolism and, when untreated, is a rapidly progressing and often fatal disease caused by an enzymatic defect in the metabolism of the branched chain amino acids leucine, isoleucine, and valine.

Homocystinuria is a disorder caused by a deficiency of the enzyme cystathionine B synthase, which produces a block in the normal conversion of methionine to cystine.

Galactosemia is an inborn error of carbohydrate metabolism in which the body is unable to use the sugars galactose and lactose. Enzyme pathways in liver cells normally convert galactose and lactose to glucose. In galactosemia, one step in that conversion pathway is absent, either because of the lack of the enzyme galactose 1-phosphate uridyl transferase, or because of the lack of the enzyme galactokinase. High levels of unusable galactose circulate in the blood, which causes cataracts, brain damage, and hepatomegaly (Smith 1980).

Another disorder frequently included in mandatory newborn screening blood tests is *congenital hypothyroidism*. An inborn enzymatic defect, lack of maternal dietary iodine, or maternal ingestion of drugs that depress or destroy thyroid tissue can cause congenital hypothyroidism.

The incidence of metabolic errors is relatively low, but for affected infants and their families these disorders pose a threat to survival and frequently require lifelong treatment.

Medical Therapy

A blood test (called the Guthrie blood test) for PKU is required of all newborns by law in most states. The Guthrie test, done before discharge, is a simple screening tool that uses a drop of blood collected from a heel stick and placed on filter paper. The Guthrie test should be done at least 24 hours, but preferably 72 hours, after the initiation of feedings containing the usual amounts of breast milk or formula. Phenylalanine is found in milk, so its metabolites begin to build up in the PKU baby once milk feedings are initiated.

High-risk newborns should be receiving a 60 percent milk intake with no more than 40 percent of their total intake coming from nonprotein intravenous fluids. The PKU testing of high-risk newborns should be deferred for at least 48 hours after hyperalimentation is initiated. Hospitals and birthing centers frequently discharge mother and infant 24 to 48 hours after delivery. It is vital that the parents understand the need for the screening procedure, and a follow-up check is necessary to confirm that the test was done.

Because it is possible to do the testing on an infant with PKU before the phenylalanine concentration rises and thus miss the diagnosis, some states routinely request a repeat test at 10 to 14 days. When the Guthrie blood test is performed early, during the first three to four days of life, a phenylalanine blood level of about 4 to 6 mg/dL is considered a presumptive positive; but only 1 in 20 to 30

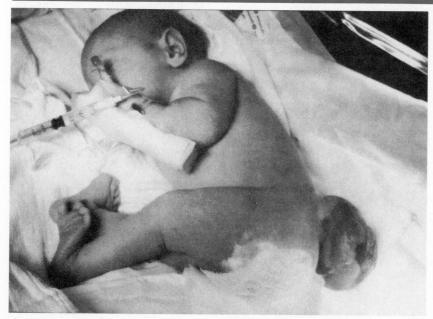

Figure 32–22   Newborn with lumbar meningocele. (Courtesy of Dr Paul Winchester)

CONTEMPORARY DILEMMA

When the Newborn Isn't Perfect

The issue of who is responsible and what should be done for a child with a congenital anomaly or severe handicap has recently been raised. What is the impact on the child and/or the family at the time of the birth and in the future? Severe disability in a newborn also raises questions of evaluating the distress the newborn is going through or will suffer during a lifetime.

A legal term being introduced is "wrongful life" or "wrongful birth" cases. A wrongful life case is a lawsuit brought by a child with a birth defect, which alleges that the physician failed to advise the parents of the risk of birth defects or failed to perform tests that would have indicated the presence or likelihood of birth defects. In addition the suit claims that because the child's parents were deprived of medical information to make an informed choice, the mother conceived and carried to term a child suffering from birth defects. A wrongful birth case is identical to a wrongful life case, with the exception that it is usually brought by the parents rather than the child. Courts have recognized wrongful birth cases over the past decade but have been perplexed by the wrongful life claims because of the traditional view that the involved handicapped child is arguing that he or she would have been better off not being born rather than being born with a birth defect. The courts were unwilling to "weigh the value of life with impairments against the nonexistence of life itself." The courts are now addressing these cases with the focus on the child's right to be compensated for injuries caused by the physician's negligence. This dilemma has prompted philosophical, ethical, moral, legal, and economic questions. The questions and concerns that are being raised include:

- How does one measure the emotional impact of the birth of a severely disabled infant?

- Is not being born preferable to being born with a serious handicap or birth defect?

- Who or what determines quality of life?

- Is a certain quality of life guaranteed?

- What is the social and economic impact on the child and family over the lifetime of the child born with a birth defect/severe handicap?

infants with this level are true positives (Wasserman & Gromisch 1981).

Some states simultaneously test all hospitalized newborns for MSUD, homocystinuria, and PKU during the first three to four days of life. Diagnosis of MSUD is made by analyzing blood levels of leucine, isoleucine, and valine. Confirmation of the diagnosis depends on blood assay for the enzyme oxidative decarboxylase.

In several states newborn screening includes an enzyme assay for galactose 1-phosphate uridyl transferase; this test, however, does not detect galactosemia if it is caused by a deficiency of the enzyme galactokinase.

For hypothyroidism, immediate and appropriate thyroid replacement therapy is established based on newborn screening and laboratory data. Frequently premature infants of less than 30 weeks' gestation have low T_4 or TSH values when compared with normal values of term infants. This may reflect the premature's inability for thyroid binding. Management includes frequent laboratory monitoring and adjustment of thyroid medication to accommodate growth and development of the child. With adequate treatment, children remain free of symptoms, but if the condition is untreated, stunted growth and mental retardation occur.

Nursing Assessment

The clinical picture of a PKU baby involves a normal appearing newborn, most often with blond hair, blue eyes, and fair complexion. Decreased pigmentation may be related to the competition between phenylalanine and tyrosine for the available enzyme, tyrosinase. Tyrosine is needed for the formation of melanin pigment and the hormones epinephrine and thyroxin. Without treatment, the infant fails to thrive, and develops vomiting and eczematous rashes. By about 6 months of age, the infant exhibits behaviors indicative of mental retardation and other CNS involvement, including seizures and abnormal EEG patterns.

Newborns with MSUD have feeding problems and neurologic signs (seizures, spasticity, opisthotonus) during the first week of life. A maple syrup odor of the urine is noted and, when ferric chloride is added to the urine, its color changes to gray-green.

Homocystinuria varies in its presentation, but the more common characteristics are skeletal abnormalities, dislocation of ocular lenses, intravascular thromboses, and mental retardation. Abnormalities occur because of the toxic effects of the accumulation of methionine and the metabolite homocystine in the blood.

Clinical manifestations of galactosemia include vomiting, diarrhea, hepatosplenomegaly, jaundice, and mental retardation. The condition is frequently associated with anemia, sepsis, and cataracts in the neonatal period. Except for cataracts and mental retardation, these findings are reversible when galactose is excluded from the diet. Mental retardation can be prevented by early diagnosis and careful dietary management.

A large tongue, umbilical hernia, cool and mottled skin, low hairline, hypotonia, and large fontanelles are frequently associated with congenital hypothyroidism. Early symptoms include prolonged neonatal jaundice, poor feeding, constipation, low-pitched cry, poor weight gain, inactivity, and delayed motor development.

Nursing Diagnosis

Nursing diagnoses that may apply to the newborn with an inborn error of metabolism are:

- Knowledge deficit related to special dietary management required secondary to inborn error of metabolism

- Ineffective family coping related to parental guilt secondary to hereditary nature of disease

Nursing Goal: Newborn Screening

Newborn screening for several inborn errors of metabolism is mandatory in many states. It is the nurse's responsibility to obtain the heel stick blood on the filter paper prior to discharge of the baby. The first filter paper test screens for PKU, homocystinuria, MSUD, galactosemia, and sickle cell anemia. A second blood specimen is usually required at 7 to 14 days after birth, but the nurse must remember that this second blood specimen tests only for PKU.

Some clinicians have the parents perform a diaper test for PKU. At about 6 weeks of age, the parent should take a freshly wet diaper and press the prepared test stick against the wet area. They note the color of the test stick, record the color on the prepared sheet, and mail the form back to the physician. A green color reaction is positive and indicates probable PKU.

Nursing Goal: Parent Education—Dietary Management

Nursing responsibilities include prompt and appropriate dietary management of the newborn with an inborn error of metabolism. Once identified, an afflicted PKU infant can be treated by a special diet that limits ingestion of phenylalanine. Special formulas low in phenylalanine,

such as Lofenalac, are available. Special food lists are helpful for parents of a PKU child. If treatment is begun before 3 months of age, CNS damage can be minimized.

Controversy exists about when, if ever, the special diet should be terminated. Because of the rigidity and severe limitations of the low phenylalanine diet, many clinicians terminate the special diet at 6 years of age. Brain size does not dramatically increase after age 6, but myelination continues actively through adolescence and to some extent possibly through 40 years of age. The effect of high phenylalanine levels on continued development of the brain after 6 years is not known (Schuett et al 1980).

Female children with PKU are now living longer and may bear children. There is a 95 percent risk of producing a child with mental retardation if the mother with PKU is not on a low-phenylalanine diet during pregnancy. It is recommended that the woman reinstate her low phenylalanine diet a few months before becoming pregnant (Mathews & Smith 1979).

Dietary management of MSUD must be initiated immediately with a formula that is low in the branched-chain amino acids leucine, isoleucine, and valine (Sarett 1979).

Infants with homocystinuria are managed on a diet that is low in methionine but supplemented with cystine and pyridoxine (vitamin B_6). With early diagnosis and careful management, mental retardation may be prevented.

Galactosemia is treated by the use of a galactose-free formula, such as Nutramigen (a protein hydrolysate process formula), a meat-base formula, or a soybean formula. As the infant grows, parents must be educated not only to avoid giving their child milk and milk products but also to read all labels carefully and avoid any foods containing dry milk products.

Parents of affected newborns should be referred to support groups. The nurse should also ensure that parents are informed about centers that can provide them with information about biochemical genetics and dietary management.

Evaluative Outcome Criteria

Nursing care is effective if:

- The risk of inborn errors of metabolism is promptly identified, and early intervention is initiated.

- The parents verbalize their concerns about their baby's health problems, long-term care needs, and potential outcomes.

- The parents are aware of available community health resources and use them as indicated.

Care of the Family of a Newborn With a Complication

Adaptation of the Family

The birth of a baby with a defect or disorder is a traumatic event with the potential for either total disruption or growth of the involved family. Throughout the pregnancy both parents, together and separately, have felt excitement, experienced thoughts of acceptance, and pictured what their newborn would look like. Both parents have wished for a perfect baby and feared a damaged, unhealthy one. Each parent and family member must accept and adjust when the fantasized fears become a reality.

Grieving for the loss of the hoped-for perfect child is necessary before the development of a positive relationship to the existing child can begin. Grief is expressed as shock and disbelief, denial of reality, anger toward self and others, guilt, blame, and concern for the future. Self-esteem and feelings of self-worth are jeopardized.

Fear, separation, and grief begin at the time of delivery when the newborn requires immediate resuscitation or special treatment. Instead of being handed to its mother, the newborn is given to a nurse or a pediatrician who rushes it to a special care area. The joyful cries of "It's a boy!" or "It's a girl!" are absent; there is only the mother's pleading question, "What's wrong with my baby?" If no answer is given to the mother, she frequently fantasizes the worst and assumes that the baby is dead. It is extremely important for the mother's health and the mother-infant relationship that some immediate answer be given to the parents. Honest, simple, and positive facts can be shared: "Your baby is alive"; "Your baby is a girl"; "Your baby has a strong heartbeat but needs some help with breathing"; "Your baby is alive but needs some special care right now"; "The pediatrician is helping your baby now and will talk with you soon." The information that nurses share with parents must always be honest data that nurses can observe and document. Nurses should not make promises that they cannot fulfill and should refrain from offering empty reassurances that everything will be all right.

The period of waiting between suspicion and confirmation of abnormality or dysfunction is a very anxious one for parents because it is difficult, if not impossible, to begin attachment to the infant if the newborn's future is questionable. During the "not knowing period," parents need support and acknowledgment that this is an anxious time and must be kept informed about efforts to gather additional data and maintain the infant's livelihood. Helfer and Kempe (1976) recommend that both parents be told about the problem at the same time, with the baby present. An honest discussion of the problem and anticipatory management at the earliest possible time by health professionals help the parents (a) maintain trust in the physician and nurse, (b) appreciate the reality of the situation by dispel-

ling fantasy and misconception, (c) begin the grieving process, and (d) mobilize internal and external support.

Nurses need to be aware that anger is a universal response and that it is best directed outward, because holding it in check requires great energy, which is diverted away from grieving and physical recovery from pregnancy and giving birth. Anger may be directed unjustifiably at the physician and/or nurse, at the food, at nursing care, or at hospital regulations and routines. Anger with the baby is rarely demonstrated by parents and can precipitate guilt feelings.

A heightened concern for self may be misinterpreted by health professionals as rejection of the newborn. Both parents need time and understanding to deal with their own feelings before they can direct concern toward the baby. In a short span of time, the parent is confronted with the loss of the idealized child, the need to accept a child

Research Note

Previous studies investigating the effects of neonatal intensive care units on parents demonstrate that parents are most anxious about their infants at birth and at the time of discharge. The intent of a care-by-parent unit (CBPU) is to minimize the discharge anxiety by providing parents with an opportunity to learn care-taking skills while living in the hospital with their infants just prior to discharge. The nursing staff will role model required parent behaviors and teach parents required skills in the CBPU. Consolvo evaluated 14 mothers to determine whether the CBPU did, in fact, decrease discharge anxiety.

The researchers administered a State-Trait Anxiety Inventory to mothers prior to admission to the CBPU and prior to discharge. The questionnaire included four situations to evaluate changes in both state anxiety (how the subject feels at a particular moment) and trait anxiety (individual susceptibility to anxiety). The results of the inventory demonstrated a significant decrease in anxiety in response to one situation related to illness. There was no significant difference in trait anxiety or for responses to the other three situations.

This research suggests the need for further study using a larger randomized sample with a control group and evaluation of fathers' as well as mothers' anxiety. If CBPUs are shown to decrease anxiety or to increase parent competence, consideration of a CBPU experience should be a routine part of each NICU infant's discharge planning.

Consolvo CA: Relieving parent anxiety in the care-by-parent unit. J Obstet Gynecol Neonat Nurs 1986;15(March/April):154–159.

who deviates from normal, and a sense of personal failure. In addition, the new mother may be suffering from fatigue and sleep deprivation from her pregnancy and labor and from discomforts arising from cesarean delivery, episiotomy, inability to void, hemorrhoids, and afterpains. In the postpartal period concern for self and dependency are normal events.

In their sensitive and vulnerable state, parents are acutely perceptive of others' responses and reactions (particularly nonverbal) to the child. Parents can be expected to identify with the responses of others. Therefore, it is imperative that medical and nursing staff be fully aware of their feelings and come to terms with those feelings so that they are comfortable and at ease with the child and the grieving family. Professional support and comfort fill the emotional bank account from which parents can draw to nurture the child and themselves so that each can develop to full potential.

Nurses may feel uncomfortable not knowing what to say to parents or may fear confronting their own feelings as well as those of the parents. Each nurse must work out personal reactions with instructors, peers, clergy, parents, or significant others. It is helpful to have a stockpile of therapeutic questions and statements to initiate meaningful dialogue with parents. Opening statements can be as follows: "You must be wondering what could have caused this"; "Are you thinking you (or someone else) may have done something?"; "How can I help?"; "Go ahead and cry. It's worth crying about"; or "Are you wondering how you are going to manage?" Avoid statements such as "It could have been worse"; "It's God's will"; "You have other children"; "You are still young and can have more"; and "I understand how you feel." *This* child is important *now*.

Some nurses find relief for themselves or a means of escape from painful circumstances by overzealous and unrealistic reassurance that "everything will be all right" and by avoidance of the newborn and family. Many medical and nursing staff take refuge in technical jargon and involvement in the technical aspects of the mother's care rather than taking time to talk about the situation. These approaches confuse the parents at a time when they need most to be understood and to understand.

Nurses show concern and support by planning time to spend with the parents, by being psychologically as well as physically present, by encouraging open discussion and grieving, by repetitious explanations (as necessary), by providing privacy as needed, and by encouraging contact with the newborn. Identification and clarification of feelings and fears decrease distortions in perception, thinking, and feelings. Nurses invest the child with value in the eyes of the parents when they provide meticulous care to the newborn, talk and coo (especially in the face-to-face position) while holding or providing care to the newborn, refer to the child by gender or name, and relate the newborn's activities ("He

took a whole ounce of formula"; "She burped so loud that . . ."; "He took hold of the blanket and just wouldn't let go"; "He voided all over the doctor"). Nurses should note the "normal" characteristics and capabilities of each newborn as well as the newborn's needs.

Cues that the parents are ready to become involved with the child's care or planning for the future include their reference to the baby as "she" or "he" or by name and their questioning as to amount of feeding taken, appearance today, and the like.

Many physicians show parents "before" and "after" photographs of conditions requiring surgical intervention. Parents also may benefit from meeting other parents who have faced the same problem through a parental support group or organization that is specific to that problem. Specialists (plastic surgeons, perinatal clinical nurse specialists, neurosurgeons, orthopedists, oral surgeons, dentists, and rehabilitation therapists) can be reassuring and supportive of parents in their short- and long-term goals. However, these types of interventions must be carefully timed to the readiness of the parents.

Mothers may feel inadequate or guilty when they do not feel motherly toward their baby. One mother, looking at her child born with an severe cleft lip and palate, said, "God help me. I can't stand looking at her. I wish she wasn't mine. What a horrid thing to say, but I can't . . . I just can't." She could not bring herself to hold or touch the infant prior to cleft lip repair. She needed considerable assistance to talk of these feelings in a nonjudgmental and accepting atmosphere before she was able to hold the infant after surgery. She proceeded to learn to feed her daughter (whose cleft palate was not yet repaired) and become very "motherly" before the infant was discharged. Her husband, fortunately, facilitated the whole process by his continued love for and acceptance of his wife throughout the experience.

Occasionally a mother may become overprotective and overoptimistic shortly after the baby's birth. The nurse should accept her behavior but continue to remind her that it is okay and natural to feel disappointment, a sense of failure, helplessness, or anger. The overprotectiveness and overoptimism are defense mechanisms. To deny the negative feelings only entrenches them further, delays their resolution, and delays realistic planning.

> I watched her breathe every precious breath on the respirator. I saw her covered with wires and tubes. I kept watch. She was special to me and I would tell her over and over, "Daddy is here. Daddy loves you." The three days she lived were hell—not knowing if she would make it, uncertain about what plans we should make. Somehow I thought she would live; I was hopeful. When she died, at least I was there with her. The grief was unbearable. But there was also a sense of relief. The uncertainty, the waiting were finally over. (*When Pregnancy Fails*)

Developmental Consequences

The baby who is born prematurely, is ill, or has a malformation or disorder is at risk in emotional and intellectual, as well as physical, development. The risk is directly proportional to the seriousness of the problem and the length of treatment. For example, resolution of a meconium plug syndrome during the expected hospital stay, allowing the infant to be discharged with the mother, is not expected to alter the child's developmental course. However, the physical appearance, immediate and repeated surgeries, and complex rehabilitation problems of exstrophy of the bladder or meningomyelocele preclude a normal developmental course for the child.

Medical, surgical, and technical advances in recent years have been responsible for salvaging increasing numbers of preterm and ill neonates. The necessary physical separation of family and child and the tremendous emotional and financial burden have adversely affected the parent-child relationship. A considerable percentage of these children have been rescued only to be emotionally or physically battered by the parents. The most recent trend in many hospitals is to involve the parents with the neonate early, repeatedly, and over protracted periods of time. Early and continued involvement may only mean opportunities to look at or stroke the baby. Later, when the mother's and baby's conditions warrant it, the mother participates in her baby's care (to the extent she is willing) and in planning for the future. This type of involvement facilitates early bonding, attachment, and emotional investment. The parents need a sense of personal success, self-worth, self-esteem, and confidence from knowledge that they can cope with the situation. This atmosphere aids the baby as well—the child may escape battering and may instead be assisted toward self-actualization (Figure 32–23).

Mothers of newborns who are gravely ill are often unable to chance an emotional investment in their child. These mothers need assistance in perceiving the cues and hearing the words that indicate the baby is going to survive. They need time and support to establish a positive relationship with the newborn. A mother who is unable to develop maternal feelings may reject the baby or overcompensate because of underlying guilt feelings; in either case an unproductive relationship may develop. The child may then be further handicapped by inability to relate well to others and by seeing the world as unsatisfying and painful.

The parents must have a clear picture of the reality of the handicap and the types of developmental hurdles ahead. Unexpected behaviors and responses from the baby due to his or her defect or disorder can be upsetting and frightening. For example, parents find it difficult to cope with a baby's lack of motor or social responsiveness and tend to interpret the lack as a form of rejection. The parents may in return respond with rejection, and an unfortunate cycle is begun.

Figure 32–23 Parents and children thrive when parents have realistic expectations of the child's longterm developmental needs.

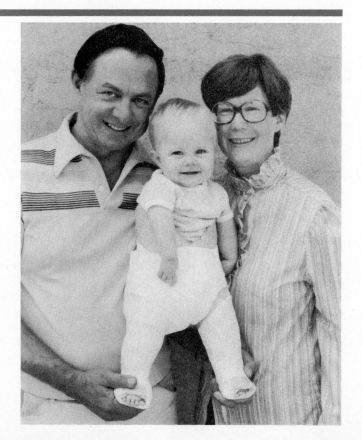

The demands of care of the child and disputes regarding management or behavior stress family relationships. One or more members of the family may make a scapegoat of the child. Another may become the youngster's champion to the exclusion of others. One or the other spouse may feel pushed aside or denied attention and thus may withdraw or leave the family unit. Parents or siblings may feel that their own needs (schooling, material goods, freedom of movement) are being set aside while all assets (financial and other) go to support the one child's needs.

The entire multidisciplinary team may need to pool their resources and expertise to help parents of children born with defects or disorders so that both parents and children can thrive.

KEY CONCEPTS

The sick neonate—whether preterm, term, or post-term—must be managed within narrow physiologic parameters.

These parameters (respiratory and thermal regulation) will maintain physiologic homeostasis and prevent introduction of iatrogenic stress to the already stressed infant.

Maintenance of this physiologic environment must begin immediately, because lost ground is difficult or impossible to recover.

The nursing care of the neonate with special problems involves the understanding of normal physiology, the pathophysiology of the disease process, clinical manifestations, and supportive or corrective therapies. Only with this theoretical background can the nurse make appropriate observations concerning responses to therapy and development of complications.

Neonates communicate needs only by their behavior; the neonatal nurse, through objective observations and evaluations, interprets this behavior into meaningful information about the infant's condition.

The nurse is the facilitator for interdisciplinary communication with the parents, identifying their understanding of their infant's care and their needs for emotional support.

Newborn conditions that commonly present with respiratory distress and require oxygen and ventilatory assistance are hyaline membrane disease, meconium aspiration syndrome, transient tachypnea of the newborn, and persistent pulmonary hypertension of the newborn.

Cold stress sets up the chain of physiologic events of hypoglycemia, pulmonary vasoconstriction, hyperbilirubinemia, respiratory distress, and metabolic acidosis. Nurses are responsible for early detection and initiation of treatment for hypoglycemia.

Cardiac defects are a significant cause of morbidity and mortality in the newborn period. Early identification and nursing and medical care of the cardiac newborn is essential to the improved outcome of these infants. Care of the cardiac newborn is directed toward lessening the work load of the heart and decreasing oxygen and energy consumption.

Differentiation between pathologic and physiologic jaundice is the key to early and successful intervention.

Nursing assessment of the septic newborn involves identification of very subtle clinical signs that are also seen in other clinical disease states.

Inborn errors of metabolism such as galactosemia, PKU, homocystinuria, and maple syrup urine disease are usually a part of a newborn screening program designed to prevent mental retardation through dietary management and medication.

REFERENCES

Ampola MG: *Metabolic Diseases in Pediatric Practice.* Boston, Little, Brown, 1982.

Avery GB: *Neonatology: Pathophysiology and Management of the Newborn.* Philadelphia, Lippincott, 1987.

Avery ME, Taeusch HW (eds): *Schaffer's Diseases of the Newborn.* Philadelphia, Saunders, 1984.

Baskett TF, et al: Antepartum fetal assessment using a fetal biophysical profile score. *Am J Obstet Gynecol* 1984;148:630.

Beachy P, Powers LK: Nursing care of the infant with persistent pulmonary hypertension of the newborn. *Clin Perinatol* 1984;11:681.

Berkowitz RL, et al: *Handbook for Prescribing Medications During Pregnancy.* Boston, Little, Brown, 1981.

Borg S, Lasker J: *When Pregnancy Fails.* Boston, Beacon Press, 1981.

Bowen LW, et al: Maternal-fetal pH difference and fetal scalp pH as predictors of neonatal outcome. *Obstet Gynecol* 1986;67:487.

Braune KW, Lacey L: Common hematologic problems of the immediate newborn period. *J Obstet Gynecol Neonat Nurs* 1983;12(suppl):19s.

Brooten D, et al: Breast-milk jaundice. *J Obstet Gynecol Neonat Nurs* 1985;14:220.

Carlo WA, et al: Decrease in airway pressure during high frequency jet ventilation in infants with respiratory distress syndrome. *J Pediatr* 1984;104:101.

Cloherty JP, **Stark** AR (eds): *Manual of Neonatal Care.* Boston, Little, Brown, 1985.

Cohen MA: Transcutaneous oxygen monitoring for sick neonates. *Am J Mat Child Nurs* 1984;9:324.

Curtis-Cohen M, et al: Randomized trial of prophylactic phototherapy in the infant with very low birth weight. *J Pediatr* 1985;107:121.

deVries LS, et al: Relationship of serum bilirubin levels to ototoxicity and deafness in high-risk low-birth-weight infants. *Pediatrics* 1985;76:351.

Epstein MF, et al: Estimation of $PaCO_2$ by two noninvasive methods in the critically ill newborn infant. *J Pediatr* 1985;106:282.

Fantazia D: Neonatal hypoglycemia. *J Obstet Gynecol Neonat Nurs* 1984;13:297.

Field T, et al: Nonnutritive sucking during tube feedings: Effects on preterm neonates in an intensive care unit. *Pediatrics* 1982;70(3):381.

Fox WW, **Duara** S. Persistent pulmonary hypertension in the neonate: Diagnosis and management. *J Pediatr* 1983;103:505.

Glass SM: Nursing care of the neonate with bronchopulmonary dysplasia. *NAACOG Update Series* 1985;3:5.

Graham TP, **Bender** HW: Preoperative diagnosis and management of infants with critical congenital heart disease. *Ann Thoracic Surg* 1980;29(3):272.

Haggerty L: TORCH: A literature review and implications for practice. *J Obstet Gynecol Neonat Nurs* 1985;14:124.

Hallman M, et al: Exogenous human surfactant for treatment of severe respiratory distress syndrome: A randomized prospective clinical trial. *J Pediatr* 1985;106:963.

Hanshaw JB, et al (eds): *Viral Diseases of the Fetus and Newborn.* Philadelphia, Saunders, 1985.

Harrel-Bean HA, **Klell** CA: Neonatal ostomies. *J Obstet Gynecol Neonat Nurs* 1983;12(suppl):69s.

Helfer RE, **Kempe** CH: *Child Abuse and Neglect: The Family and the Community.* Cambridge, Mass, Ballinger, 1976.

Klaus MH, **Fanaroff** AA: *Care of the High-Risk Neonate.* Philadelphia, Saunders, 1986.

Korones SB: *High-Risk Newborn Infants: The Basis for Intensive Nursing Care,* ed 2. St Louis, Mosby, 1986.

LaGamma EF, et al: Failure of delayed oral feedings to prevent necrotizing enterocolitis. *Am J Dis Child* 1985;139:385.

Mathews A, **Smith** A: Presentation at NAACOG Conference on Genetics, Colorado Springs, Colorado, October 1979.

McCann EM, et al: Controlled trial of furosemide therapy in infants with chronic lung disease. *J Pediatr* 1985;106:957.

McCracken GH: Use of third-generation cephalosporins for treatment of neonatal infections. *Am J Dis Child* 1985;139:1079.

Measel CP, **Anderson** GC: Nonnutritive sucking during tube feedings: Effect upon clinical course in premature infants. *J Obstet Gynecol Neonat Nurs* 1979;8:265.

Monaco F, et al: Calibration of a heated transcutaneous carbon dioxide electrode to reflect arterial carbon dioxide. *Am Rev Respir Dis* 1983;127:322.

Nantze D: Hyperviscosity-polycythemia syndrome. *Neonatal Netw* 1985;4(October):8.

Northway WH, et al: Pulmonary disease following respiratory therapy of hyaline membrane disease: Bronchopulmonary dysplasia. *N Engl J Med* 1967;276:357.

Nugent J: Acute respiratory care of the newborn. *J Obstet Gynecol Neonat Nurs* 1983;12(suppl):31s.

Ostertag SG, et al: Early enteral feeding does not affect the incidence of necrotizing enterocolitis. *Pediatrics* 1986;77:275.

Perkin RM, **Anas** NG: Pulmonary hypertension in pediatric patients. *J Pediatr* 1984;105:511.

Sarett HP: *Products for Dietary Management of Inborn Errors of Metabolism and Other Special Feeding Problems.* Evansville, Ind, Mead Johnson, 1979.

Schuett VE, et al. Diet discontinuation policies and practices of PKU clinics in the United States. *Am J Pub Health* 1980;70(5):498.

Smith EJ: Galactosemia: an inborn error of metabolism. *Nurse Pract* 1980;5(March/April):8.

Toce SS, et al: Clinical and roentgenographic scoring systems for assessing bronchopulmonary dysplasia. *Am J Dis Child* 1984;138:581.

Wasserman E, **Gromisch** DS: *Survey of Clinical Pediatrics,* ed 7. New York, McGraw-Hill, 1981.

ADDITIONAL READINGS

Budreau G, **Kleiber** C: Nursing management of the infant with an intraoral appliance. *J Obstet Gynecol Neonat Nurs* 1987;16(January/February):23.

Canty TG: Esophageal atresia and tracheoesophageal fistula: Aspects of respiratory care. *P/N* 1986;10(4):42.

Campbell VG: Covergowns for newborn infection control? *Am J Mat Child Nurs* 1987;12(January/February):54.

Collins JE: Rational respiratory therapy of newborns. *P/N* 1987;11(March/April):23.

Daily DK: Home oxygen therapy for infants with bronchopulmonary dysplasia: Growth and development. *P/N* 1987;11(May/June):26.

Danaher RR: Complete congenital heart block. *Neonatal Netw* 1987;5(February):19.

Dortch E, **Spottiswoode** P: New light on phototherapy: Home use. *Neonatal Netw* 1986;4(February):30.

Filston HC, **Isant** RJ: *The Surgical Neonate*, ed 2. Norwalk, Conn, Appleton-Century-Crofts, 1985.

Gaffney SE, **Salinger** L: Group B streptococcus: The pregnant woman and her neonate. *J Obstet Gynecol Neonat Nurs* 1987;16(March/April):91.

Gennaro S: Anxiety and problem-solving ability in mothers of premature infants. *J Obstet Gynecol Neonat Nurs* 1986; 15:160.

Gerraughty AB, **Younge** LJ: ECHMO: The artifical lung for gravely ill newborns. *Am J Nurs* 1987;87(May):655a.

Grasso S, **Roversi** GD: Oversized infant of diabetic mother: Its cause and prevention. *J Perinatal Med* 1987; 15:73.

Gregory SEB: Air leaks syndrome. *Neonatal Netw* 1987; 5(April):40.

Harrison LL, **Twardosz** S: Teaching mothers about their preterm infants. *J Obstet Gynecol Neonat Nurs* 1986;15: 165.

Higgins SS, **Kashani** IA: The cyanotic child: Heart defects and parental learning needs. *Am J Mat Child Nurs* 1986;11:259.

Hurst JD, **Stullenbarger** B: Implementation of a self-care approach in a pediatric interdisciplinary phenylketonuria (PKU) clinic. *J Pediatr Nurs* 1986;1(3):159.

Jose JH, et al: Perinatal aspiration syndrome: Current concepts. *P/N* 1986;10(November/December):22.

Landier WC, **Barrell** ML, **Styffe** EJ: How to administer blood components to children. *Am J Mat Child Nurs* 1987;12(May/June):178.

Loper-Hunter D: Bilirubin and the neonate. *Neonatal Netw* 1983;1(June):20.

Mattson D, **O'Connor** M: Transilluminator assistance in neonatal venipuncture. *Neonatal Netw* 1986;5(August): 38.

Mitchell C, **Rutherford** PA: The fragile survivor. *Am J Nurs* 1987;87(May):603.

Pate CMH: Care of the family following the birth of an infant with cleft lip and/or palate. *Neonatal Netw* 1987;5(June):30.

Sawyer SF, et al: Improving survival in the treatment of congenital diaphragmatic hernia. *Ann Thoracic Surg* 1986;41(1):75.

Weibley TT, et al: Gavage tube insertion in the premature infant. *Am J Mat Child Nurs* 1987;12(January/February):24.

Wood AF: Sequelae of perinatal asphyxia. *Neonatal Netw* 1987;5(April):21.

Thirty years ago the delivery of our first son went easily, but my husband failed to show up for visiting hours the next day. When he did come, he asked me to walk to the nurses' lounge. I was so excited about the baby that it didn't seem strange to be going there. When we were alone, he gently told me that our baby was "mongoloid." What an ugly word! Suddenly it felt as if torrents of black spiders were pouring over me. We cried together. A few days later we took our son home and began the long and tender process of parenting a Down syndrome child. It came to us with great clarity at the beginning that none of us has the right to expect our children to be more perfect reflections of ourselves. Each is an individual with a life to be lived to the fullest of its own possibilities. In thirty years we have seen a sense of humor, a love of music, and a loving disposition characterize the son some would call disabled.

The Postpartal Period

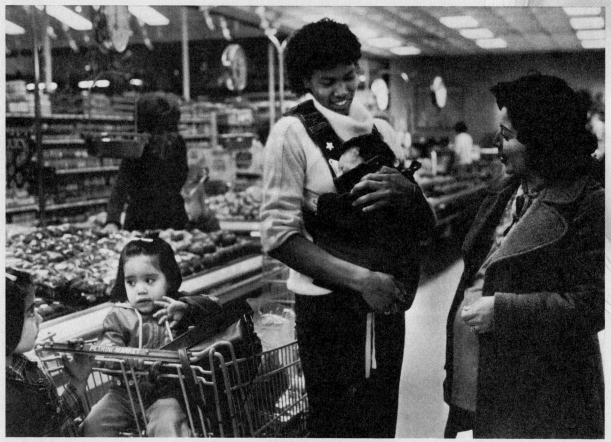

A single black mother with a month-old baby in a pouch chats with a 9-months-pregnant Hispanic woman, whose other children look on.

Part Seven

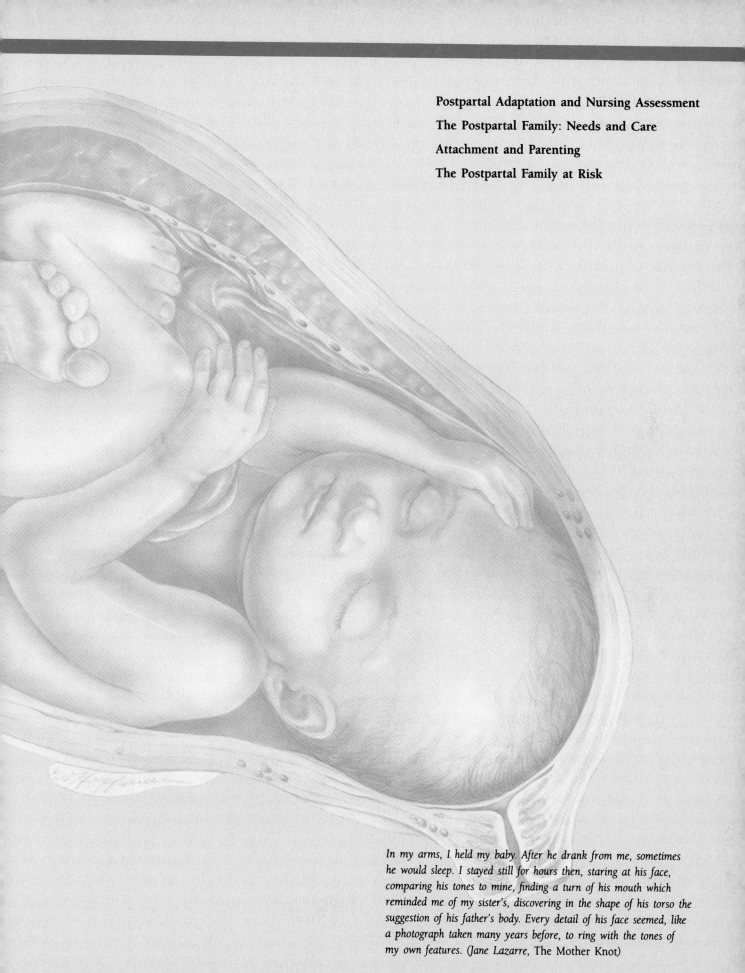

Postpartal Adaptation and Nursing Assessment

The Postpartal Family: Needs and Care

Attachment and Parenting

The Postpartal Family at Risk

*In my arms, I held my baby. After he drank from me, sometimes
he would sleep. I stayed still for hours then, staring at his face,
comparing his tones to mine, finding a turn of his mouth which
reminded me of my sister's, discovering in the shape of his torso the
suggestion of his father's body. Every detail of his face seemed, like
a photograph taken many years before, to ring with the tones of
my own features. (Jane Lazarre, The Mother Knot)*

Postpartal Adaptation and Nursing Assessment

Postpartal Physical Adaptations
Reproductive Organs
Abdomen
Lactation
Gastrointestinal System
Urinary Tract
Vital Signs
Blood Values
Weight Loss
Postpartal Chill
Postpartal Diaphoresis
Afterpains

Postpartal Psychologic Adaptations
Cultural Influences
Development of Attachment
Postpartal Nursing Assessment
Risk Factors
Physical Assessment
Psychologic Assessment

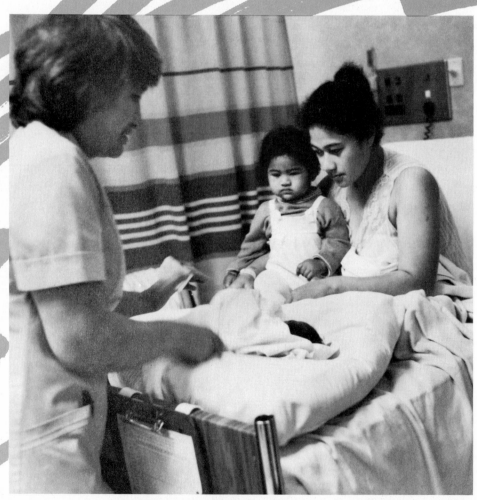

In Wellington, New Zealand, a Maori nurse offers information to a young Maori mother who is about to leave the hospital with her toddler and 3-day-old baby.

Chapter Thirty-Three

- Summarize the physical and psychologic adaptations that occur postpartally as a woman's body returns to its prepregnant state.
- Relate the physiologic changes that occur postpartally to an appropriate nursing assessment.
- Discuss nursing assessment of the psychologic changes that occur in the childbearing woman during the postpartal period.

The *puerperium* (postpartum) is the period of time during which the body adjusts, both physically and psychologically, to the process of childbearing. It begins immediately after delivery and proceeds for approximately six weeks or until the body has completed its adjustment and has returned to a near prepregnant state. Some have referred to the puerperium as "the fourth trimester," and whereas the time span does not necessarily cover three months, this terminology demonstrates the idea of continuity.

The postpartum period does not occur in isolation; it is influenced significantly by the processes that have preceded it. During pregnancy the body adjusted gradually to the physical changes, but now it is forced to respond more rapidly. The method of delivery and circumstances associated with the delivery alter the speed with which the body reacts. Changes in body image and assumption of new roles often influence the outcome and ultimate adaptation to childbearing.

To apply the nursing process successfully when caring for women during the postpartal period, the nurse must first have a clear understanding of the physiologic and psychologic adaptations that occur during this time. This knowledge facilitates early recognition of abnormal findings and subsequent intervention. Explaining to the family the changes that occur also facilitates their adjustment postpartally.

This chapter first describes the physical and psychologic changes that occur postpartally. Using this information as a base, the second portion of the chapter focuses on a thorough postpartal assessment.

• Postpartal Physical Adaptations

The anatomic and physiologic processes of the puerperium involve the reproductive organs and other major body systems.

Reproductive Organs

INVOLUTION OF UTERUS

Immediately following the expulsion of the placenta, the uterus contracts firmly to the size of a large grapefruit, reducing uterine size by over one-half. The fundus can be located by observation and palpation approximately halfway between the symphysis pubis and the umbilicus and is situated in the midline (Figure 33–1). The walls of the contracted uterus are in close proximity and each is 4 to 5 cm thick. Within a few hours after delivery the fundus of the uterus rises to the level of the umbilicus or one finger breadth (1.0 cm) above the umbilicus. If the uterus is higher than one finger breadth or is deviated from the midline and is boggy, the most probable cause of its displacement is a distended urinary bladder. Because the uterine ligaments are still stretched, the uterus can easily be moved by the full bladder.

The uterus remains at the level of the umbilicus for about a day and then on each succeeding postpartal day descends into the pelvis approximately one fingerbreadth. This descent occurs so rapidly that within ten days to two weeks the uterus is again a pelvic organ and cannot be palpated abdominally. If the woman is breast-feeding, the release of oxytocin from the posterior pituitary, which is a response to suckling, may cause the uterus to descend more rapidly into the pelvis.

Barring complications such as infection or retained placental fragments, the uterus approximates the nonpregnant size by four to six weeks. Changes in the weight of the uterus are equally dramatic. Although it weighs 1000 to 1200 g at term, the uterus decreases to 500 g at one week, 300 g at two weeks, and 100 g after the third week (Pritchard et al 1985).

With the dramatic decrease in the levels of circulatory estrogen and progesterone following placental separation, the uterine cells atrophy, and the hyperplasia of pregnancy begins to reverse. Proteolytic enzymes are released, and macrophages migrate to the uterus to promote autolysis (self-digestion). Protein material in the uterine wall is broken down and absorbed. Thus the process is basically one of cell size reduction rather than a radical

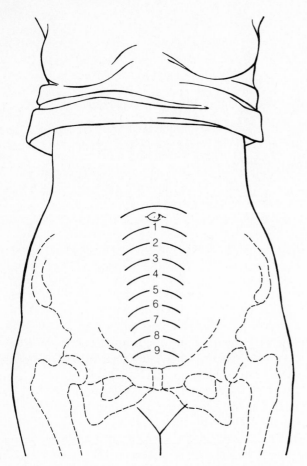

Figure 33–1 Involution of the uterus. The height of the fundus decreases about one fingerbreadth (approximately 1 cm) each day.

decrease in cell number. The term *involution* is used to describe the rapid reduction in size and the return of the uterus to a condition similar to its nulliparous state.

Following separation of the placenta, the decidua of the uterus is irregular, jagged, and varied in thickness. The spongy layer of the decidua is cast off as lochia, and the basal layer of the decidua remains in the uterus to become differentiated into two layers within the first 48 to 72 hours after delivery. The outermost layer becomes necrotic and is sloughed off in the lochia. The layer closest to the myometrium contains the fundi of the uterine endometrial glands, and these glands lay the foundation for the new endometrium. Except at the placental site, the endometrium is formed by the proliferation of the fundi of the endometrial glands and of the stroma from the interglandular connective tissue (Pritchard et al 1985). This process is completed in approximately three weeks.

Involution of the placental site is a similar process but takes up to six weeks for completion. Following separation, the placental site contracts to an area 8 to 9 cm in diameter that appears raised and irregular. Bleeding from the larger uterine vessels is controlled by compression of the retracted uterine muscle fibers. The placental site con-

sists of multiple thrombosed vascular sinusoids that are treated by the body as any other vascular clot. Some of these vessels are eventually obliterated and replaced by new vessels with smaller lumens.

Rather than forming a fibrous scar in the decidua, the placental site heals by a process of exfoliation. This process consists of the undermining of the site by the growth of the endometrial tissue both from the margins of the site and from the fundi of the endometrial glands left in the basal layer of the site. The infarcted superficial tissue then becomes necrotic and is sloughed off.

Exfoliation is one of the most important aspects of involution in an otherwise unremarkable postpartal course for two reasons:

1. If the healing of the placental site left a fibrous scar, the area available for future implantation would be limited, as would the number of possible pregnancies.

2. Failure of the placental site to undergo normal involution may cause late puerperal (delayed postpartum) hemorrhage or subinvolution, which is characterized by persistent lochia, failure of the uterus to decrease in size progressively, lack of uterine tone, and painless fresh bleeding.

Factors that retard uterine involution are prolonged labor, anesthesia or excessive analgesia, difficult delivery, grandmultiparity, a full bladder, incomplete expulsion of the products of conception, and infection. Some factors that enhance involution include an uncomplicated labor and delivery, complete expulsion of the products of conception, breast-feeding, and early ambulation.

LOCHIA

One of the most unique capabilities of the uterus is its ability to rid itself of the debris remaining after delivery. This discharge is termed *lochia* and is classified according to its appearance and contents. *Lochia rubra* takes its name from the dark red color of the discharge. It occurs for the first two to three days and contains epithelial cells, erythrocytes, leukocytes, shreds of the decidua, and occasionally fetal meconium, lanugo, and vernix caseosa. Lochia should not contain large clots; if it does, the cause should be discovered without delay. *Lochia serosa* follows from approximately the third until the tenth day. It is characterized by a pinkish to brownish color and serosanguineous consistency. It is composed of serous exudate (hence the name), shreds of degenerating decidua, erythrocytes, leukocytes, cervical mucus, and numerous microorganisms.

The blood cell component decreases gradually, and a creamy or yellowish discharge persists for an additional week or two. This final discharge is termed *lochia alba* and is composed primarily of leukocytes; large, irregular round or spindle-shaped mononucleated decidual cells; both flat and cylindrical epithelial cells; fat; cervical mucus; cholesterol crystals; and bacteria. When the lochia stops, the cervix is considered closed, and chances of infection ascending from the vagina to the uterus decrease.

Like menstrual discharge, lochia has a musty, stale odor that is not offensive. Microorganisms are always present in the vaginal lochia, and by the second day following delivery the uterus is contaminated with the vaginal bacteria. Researchers speculate that infection does not develop because the organisms involved are relatively nonvirulent. In addition, by the time the bacteria reach the raw, exposed surface of the uterus the process of granulation has begun, forming a protective barrier. Any foul smell to the lochia or used peri-pad suggests infection and the need for prompt assessment.

The volume of lochia discharge during the first week postpartally is approximately 240 to 270 mL (8 to 9 oz) and the volume decreases gradually. Discharge is heavier in the morning than at night because lochia tends to pool in the vagina and uterus when the woman is recumbent and is discharged when she arises. The amount of lochia may also be increased by exertion or breast-feeding.

Evaluation of lochia is necessary not only to determine the presence of hemorrhage but also to assess uterine involution. The type, amount, and consistency of lochia determine the state of healing of the placental site, and a progressive change from bright red at delivery to dark red to pink to white/clear discharge should be observed. Persistent discharge of lochia rubra or a return to lochia rubra indicates subinvolution or late postpartal hemorrhage (see Chapter 36).

Caution should be exercised in the evaluation of bleeding immediately after delivery. The continuous seepage of blood is more consistent with cervical or vaginal lacerations and may be effectively diagnosed when the bleeding is evaluated in conjunction with the consistency of the uterus. Lacerations should be suspected if the uterus is firm, of expected size, and if no clots can be expressed.

CERVICAL CHANGES

Following delivery the cervix is spongy, flabby, and formless and may appear bruised. The external os has a markedly irregular outline suggestive of multiple small lacerations. The os closes slowly. It admits two fingers for a few days following delivery, but by the end of the first week only a fingertip opening remains.

The shape of the external os is permanently changed following the first childbearing. The characteristic dimple-like os of the nullipara changes to the lateral slit (fish mouth) os of the multipara. After significant cervical laceration or several lacerations, the cervix may appear lopsided.

VAGINAL CHANGES

Following delivery the vagina appears edematous and may be bruised. Small superficial lacerations may be evident, and the rugae have been obliterated. The apparent bruising of the vagina is due to pelvic congestion, and resolution takes place rapidly following the birth. The hymen, torn and jagged, heals irregularly, leaving small tags called the *carunculae myrtiformes*.

The size of the vagina decreases and vaginal rugae begin to return by three weeks. This facilitates the gradual return to smaller, although not nulliparous, dimensions. Tone and contractability of the vaginal orifice may be improved by perineal tightening exercises (Kegel's exercises), which may begin soon after delivery and should be incorporated into the exercise regimen. The labia majora and labia minora are flabbier in the woman who has borne a child than in the nullipara.

PERINEAL CHANGES

During the early postpartal period the soft tissue in and around the perineum may appear edematous with some bruising. If an episiotomy or laceration is present, the edges should be approximated. Occasionally ecchymosis occurs, and this may delay healing.

RECURRENCE OF OVULATION AND MENSTRUATION

It has been generally thought that menstruation recurs in non–breast-feeding women within six to eight weeks after delivery. However, it has been demonstrated that only about 40 percent of non–breast-feeding women resume menstruation in six weeks. About 65 percent resume menstruation by the end of 12 weeks, and 90 percent within 24 weeks after delivery. At 12 weeks after delivery only about 45 percent of lactating women are menstruating. Approximately 50 percent of nonnursing mothers ovulate during the first cycle, while 80 percent of the nursing mothers have one or more anovulatory cycles before the first ovulatory one. Research has suggested ovarian, pituitary, and possibly hypothalamic suppression as potential causes of the characteristic infertility of nursing mothers. Currently, however, the exact mechanisms producing this effect remain unclear (Easterling & Herbert 1986).

Abdomen

The uterine ligaments (notably the round and broad ligaments) are stretched and require time to recover. The abdominal wall itself has also been stretched and will appear loose and somewhat flabby for a time. With exercise, abdominal muscle tone will improve greatly within two to three months. In the grandmultipara, the woman in which overdistention of the abdomen has occurred, or the woman with poor muscle tone before pregnancy, the abdomen may fail to regain good tone and may remain flabby. *Diastasis recti* is a separation of the rectus abdominis muscles, which may occur with pregnancy, especially in women with poor abdominal muscle tone. In the event of diastasis, part of the abdominal wall has no muscular support but is formed only by skin, subcutaneous fat, attenuated fascia, and peritoneum. Diastasis recti and poor muscle tone respond well to abdominal exercises. Improvement also depends on the physical condition of the mother, the total number of pregnancies, and the type and amount of physical exercise. Exercise may begin immediately after a vaginal delivery and within a few weeks following a cesarean delivery. See page 1106 for a discussion of postpartal exercises. If rectus muscle tone is not regained, adequate support may be lacking for future pregnancies. This may result in a pendulous abdomen and increased maternal backache.

The striae (stretch marks), which occurred as a result of stretching and rupture of the elastic fibers of the skin, are red to purple at delivery. These gradually fade and after a time appear as silver or white streaks but never completely disappear.

Lactation

During pregnancy, the breasts develop in preparation for lactation as a result of the influence of both estrogen and progesterone. After delivery, the interplay of maternal hormones leads to the establishment of milk production. This process is described in detail in the section on breastfeeding (p 927).

Gastrointestinal System

Hunger following delivery is common, and the mother may enjoy a light meal. Frequently she is quite thirsty and will drink large amounts of fluid as soon as she is permitted to do so. She may continue to drink large amounts of fluid to replace fluid lost during labor.

The bowel tends to be sluggish after delivery due to the lingering effects of progesterone, decreased muscle tone in the intestine, and decreased intraabdominal pressure. The practice of omitting solid food during labor may cause a delay in the first bowel movement.

The pain from an episiotomy, any lacerations, and hemorrhoids may lead the woman to delay elimination for fear of increasing the pain or tearing her stitches. In most instances the initial bowel movement is not uncomfortable. However, refusing or delaying the bowel movement may cause constipation and more discomfort when elimination finally occurs.

Fluids and solid foods are delayed for the woman who delivered by cesarean until peristalsis is returned. Clear liquids are generally begun by the day after surgery

(first postoperative day), and the diet is advanced to solid food by the second or third postoperative day. The woman may experience some discomfort from flatulence initially. This is relieved by early ambulation and the use of antiflatulent medications. It may take a few days for the bowel to regain its tone. Constipation is avoided to prevent pressure on sutures, which could increase discomfort.

The nurse can help the postpartal woman reestablish her normal bowel elimination pattern by promoting early and frequent ambulation, encouraging adequate fluid intake, and providing fresh fruits and fiber in the woman's diet. The cesarean birth mother and the woman who had a difficult delivery may benefit from stool softeners. Stool softeners increase the bulk and moisture in the fecal material and promote more comfortable and complete evacuation. In some cases it may be necessary to administer an enema or suppository to promote elimination.

Urinary Tract

Increased bladder capacity, swelling and bruising of the tissues around the urethra, decreased sensation of bladder filling, and inability to void in the recumbent position put the puerperal woman at risk for overdistention, incomplete emptying, and buildup of residual urine. In addition, women who have had conductive anesthesia have inhibited neural functioning of the bladder and are more susceptible to bladder complications.

Urinary output increases during the early postpartal period (first 12 to 24 hours) due to puerperal diuresis. The kidneys must eliminate an estimated 2000 to 3000 mL of extracellular fluid associated with a normal pregnancy. With PIH, hypertension, and diabetes, an even greater fluid retention is experienced, and postpartal diuresis is increased accordingly.

Bladder elimination presents an immediate problem. If stasis exists, chances increase for urinary tract infection because of bacteriuria and the presence of dilated ureters and renal pelves, which persist for about six weeks after delivery. A full bladder may also increase the tendency of relaxation of the uterus by displacing the uterus and interfering with its contractility, leading to hemorrhage.

Hematuria, resulting from bladder trauma, may occasionally occur after delivery, but the presence of lochia may mask this sign. If hematuria occurs in the second or third postpartal week, there may be a bladder infection. Acetone may be present in the urine of diabetics or of women with prolonged labor and dehydration. Proteinuria may occur during the first week following delivery. However, since proteinuria may be associated with an infectious process (cystitis, pyelitis), it should be further evaluated. A urine specimen contaminated with lochia may be the cause of proteinuria, so any specimen should be obtained as a midstream or a catheterized specimen. To prevent lochial contamination, some agencies have the woman hold gauze pads over her vaginal opening while she voids. The woman with preeclampsia may demonstrate proteinuria for a week or more following delivery.

Vital Signs

During the postpartal period, with the exception of the first 24 hours, the woman should be afebrile. A temperature of 100.4F (38C) may occur after delivery as a result of the exertion and dehydration of labor. Infection must be considered in the woman with a temperature of 100.4F or above on any two of the first ten pospartal days, excluding the first 24 hours, if the temperature is taken at least four times per day.

Blood pressure readings should remain stable and normal following delivery. A decrease may indicate physiologic readjustment to decreased intrapelvic pressure, or it may be related to uterine hemorrhage. Blood pressure elevations, especially when accompanied by headache, suggest preeclampsia, and the woman should be evaluated further.

Puerperal bradycardia with rates of 50 to 70 beats per minute commonly occurs during the first six to ten days of the postpartal period. It may be related to decreased cardiac strain, the decreased vascular bed following delivery, contraction of the uterus, and increased stroke volume. Tachycardia occurs less frequently and is related to increased blood loss or difficult, prolonged labor and delivery.

Blood Values

The blood values should return to the prepregnant state by the end of the postpartal period. Pregnancy-associated activation of coagulation factors may continue for variable amounts of time. This condition, in conjunction with trauma, immobility, or sepsis, predisposes the woman to development of thromboembolism. Plasma fibrinogen is maintained at pregnancy levels for a week, accounting for the higher sedimentation rate observed in the early postpartum period.

Other hemodynamic changes include leukocytosis with elevated white blood counts of 15,000 to 20,000, primarily due to an increased number of granulocytes. Eosinophils are rarely found, and lymphocytes may be reduced.

Blood loss averages 200 to 500 mL with a vaginal delivery and 700 to 1000 mL with cesarean birth. Hemoglobin and erythrocyte values vary during the early puerperium, but they should approximate or exceed prelabor values within two to six weeks as normal concentrations are reached. As extracellular fluid is excreted, hemoconcentration occurs, with a concomitant rise in hematocrit. A drop in values indicates an abnormal blood loss. The following is a convenient rule of thumb: A 4-point drop in hematocrit equals 1 pint of blood loss.

Weight Loss

An initial weight loss of 10 to 12 lb occurs as a result of the delivery of infant, placenta, and amniotic fluid. Puerperal diuresis accounts for the loss of an additional 5 lb during the early puerperium. By the sixth to eighth week after delivery, the woman has returned to approximately her prepregnant weight if she has gained the average 22 to 28 lb.

Postpartal Chill

Frequently the mother experiences a shaking chill immediately after delivery, which may be related to a neurologic response or to vasomotor changes. If not followed by fever, it is clinically innocuous but uncomfortable for the woman. It is the practice in many agencies to cover the woman with warmed bath blankets to alleviate the chill. The mother may also find a warm beverage helpful. Later in the puerperium, chills and fever indicate infection and require further evaluation.

Postpartal Diaphoresis

The elimination of excess fluid and waste products via the skin during the puerperium greatly increases perspiration. Diaphoretic episodes frequently occur at night, and the woman may awaken drenched with perspiration. The practice of covering the mattress with a protective plastic pad also contributes to the woman's discomfort. This perspiration is not significant clinically, but the mother should be protected from chilling. The plastic mattress pad should be covered with both a pad and a sheet to decrease skin contact, and the bed linens and gown should be changed if diaphoresis occurs. Comfort is also enhanced with a daily shower.

Afterpains

Afterpains occur more commonly in multiparas than in primiparas and are caused by intermittent uterine contractions. Although the uterus of the primipara usually remains consistently contracted, the lost tone of the multiparous uterus results in alternate contraction and relaxation. This phenomenon also occurs if the uterus has been markedly distended, as with multiple pregnancies or hydramnios, or if clots or placental fragments were retained. These afterpains may cause the mother severe discomfort for two to three days following delivery. The administration of oxytocic agents stimulates uterine contraction and increases the discomfort of the afterpains. Because oxytocin is released when the infant suckles, breastfeeding also increases the severity of the afterpains. Some women obtain relief by lying on the abdomen with a pillow placed under it to apply abdominal pressure; others prefer rocking in a rocking chair. The nursing mother may find it helpful to take a mild analgesic approximately one hour before feeding her infant. Since the drug will pass into the mother's milk, it is important to use a mild and safe analgesic. An analgesic is also helpful at bedtime if the afterpains interfere with the mother's rest.

● Postpartal Psychologic Adaptations

The postpartal period is a time of readjustment and adaptation for the entire childbearing family, but especially for the mother. The woman experiences a variety of responses as she adjusts to a new family member, postpartum discomforts, changes in her body image, and the reality that she is no longer pregnant. One young mother described her responses well:

I feel like it's the day after Christmas. Of course I'm relieved that everything went well and I have a fine baby, but I feel so let down. I waited and planned for all this; I had an image of what my delivery would be like, and everything was just a little different. I just figured that as soon as I delivered I would feel fine. Why didn't someone tell me I would still be sore; the pain didn't magically disappear! When I was pregnant everyone treated me as though I was a little fragile. Men held doors for me, grocery baggers insisted on loading my groceries; even in rest rooms women told me to go to the head of the line because they remembered being pregnant and having to go to the bathroom. Now when people call or visit all they talk about is the baby. I don't think I'm really jealous, but I do miss the attention. You know, during this past day I've started to realize that my life will never, ever be the same again. No matter what happens, I will never again be the woman I was. I've always wanted to be a mother; I think I'll like being a mother; but I'm not really sure how to do it. Isn't that strange?

During the first day or two following delivery the woman tends to be passive and somewhat dependent. The new mother follows suggestions, is hesitant about making decisions, and is still rather preoccupied with her needs. She may have a great need to talk about her perceptions of her labor and delivery. This helps her work through the process, sort out the reality from her fantasized experience, and clarify anything that she did not understand.

During this time food and sleep are major focuses for her. The woman is physically exhausted from the stress of birth and requires increased rest. However, meals are eagerly awaited, and food-related discussions are common. During this time the woman is talkative but passive. In Rubin's early work (1961) she labeled this the *taking-in* period.

After the new mother has had time to relive her experiences, adjust to her new life, rest, and recover from childbirth, she is ready to resume control of her life. Initially this phase involves control of her bodily functions.

She is concerned about her bowel and bladder elimination. If she is breast-feeding she is concerned about the quality of her milk and her ability to nurse her child successfully. She requires frequent reassurance that she is doing well. This desire to succeed is also apparent in concerns about her ability to be a "good" mother. If the baby is sleepy during a feeding or spits up, the mother may view it as a personal failure. The nurse who is extremely proficient in handling the child may arouse feelings of inadequacy, which can be exhausting and demoralizing for the mother. Rubin (1961) referred to this as the *taking-hold* period.

The postpartum period is characterized by mood swings and emotional lability. Depression and weepiness are common. Other symptoms may include anorexia, tearfulness, difficulty in sleeping, and a "let down" feeling. This depression can occur during hospitalization, but the practice of discharging women early makes it likely that the depression will occur at home. Rubin (1984) suggests that the depression, often referred to as the "postpartum blues," follows a roller coaster pattern, occurring on the third, fifth, and seventh days following delivery. Another study (Kendall et al 1984) found that the fifth day postpartum was the peak day for depression. Psychologic adjustment and hormonal changes are both thought to be causal factors, although fatigue, discomfort, and stimulation overload or deprivation may also play a part.

Postpartally the woman must adjust to a changed body image. Often women, especially primiparas, are surprised and rather dismayed to discover that they do not return to their prepregnant weight and shape as soon as the baby is born. For the woman who had expected to leave the hospital in prepregnancy clothes, this may be a tremendous shock. Women often express dissatisfaction about their appearance and concern with the return of their weight and figure to normal. Multiparas tend to be more positive about their appearance postpartally than primiparas. This may be because the multipara's previous experience has prepared her for the fact that the body does not immediately return to a prepregnant state. It may also be due to the fact that the multipara is focused more on getting enough sleep and time to rest (Strang & Sullivan 1985).

The psychologic outcomes of the postpartal period are far more positive when the parents have access to a support network. During the postpartum period the new mother often desires increased support. She may obtain this support in different ways. Women and their partners often find that family relationships become increasingly important, and the attention that their infant receives from family members is a source of satisfaction to the new parents (Belsky & Rovine 1984). In many cases the ties to the woman's family become especially good. Many fathers report that their relationships with their in-laws become far more positive and supportive (Cronenwett 1985). On the other hand, the increased family interaction can be a source of stress, especially for the new mother, who tends to have more contact with the families.

Childbearing couples often change their social network somewhat following the birth of their child. Once the new parents have made the transition to parenthood, they both tend to have more contact with other parents of small children (Belsky & Rovine 1984). For the woman, interaction with coworkers often declines postpartally, but contact with friends increases. Thus, the woman maintains the size of her network support group but alters it to meet the changes that have occurred in her life-style. Cronenwett (1985) suggests that "socially competent people react to life transitions that negatively affect certain network ties by replacing lost members with new, more compatible relationships. Changes in the network should not necessarily be equated, then, with a net loss of support" (p 351).

Perhaps the greatest concern involves women and their partners who have no family available and no friends to form a social network. Isolation at a time when the woman feels an increased need for support can result in tremendous stress and is often a contributing factor in situations of child neglect or abuse.

A prime focus of research in recent years has been maternal role attainment. *Maternal role attainment* is the process by which a woman learns mothering behaviors and becomes comfortable with her identity as a mother. The formation of a maternal identity indicates that the woman has attained the maternal role. Formation of a maternal identity occurs with each child a woman bears. As the mother grows to know this child and forms a relationship with her or him, the mother's maternal identity gradually, systematically evolves and she "binds in" to the infant (Rubin 1984).

Maternal role attainment occurs in four stages (Mercer 1985):

1. The *anticipatory stage* occurs during pregnancy. The woman looks to role models, especially her own mother, for examples of how to mother.

2. The *formal stage* begins when the child is born. The woman is still influenced by the guidance of others and tries to act as she believes others expect her to act.

3. The *informal stage* begins when the mother begins to make her own choices about mothering. The woman beings to develop her own style of mothering and finds ways of functioning that work well for her.

4. The *personal stage* is the final stage of maternal role attainment. When the woman reaches this stage, she is comfortable with the notion of herself as "mother."

In most cases maternal role attainment occurs within three to ten months following delivery. Social support, the woman's age and personality traits, the temperament of her infant, and the family's socioeconomic status all influence the woman's success in attaining the maternal role.

An area of interesting research involves a comparison of primiparas and multiparas with regard to maternal role attainment. One study (Walker et al 1986a) suggests that for primiparas, "forming the new relationship to their babies and gaining self-confidence in the parenting role appear interdependent" (p 71). For multiparas, on the other hand, a mother's confidence in her care-giving role was not necessarily related to her relationship with her infant (Walker et al 1986b).

The postpartum woman faces a number of challenges as she adjusts to her new role. For many women, finding time for themselves is one of the greatest challenges. It is often difficult for the new mother to find time to read a book, talk to her partner, or even eat a meal without interruption! Women also report feelings of incompetence because they have not mastered all aspects of the mothering role. Often they are unsure of what to do in a given situation. The next greatest challenge involves fatigue due to sleep deprivation. The demands of nighttime care are tremendously draining, especially if she has other children at home. One challenge faced by the new mother involves the feeling of responsibility that having a child brings. Women experience a sense of lost freedom, an awareness that they will never again be quite as carefree as they were before becoming mothers. Finally mothers cite the infant's behavior as a problem, especially when the child is about 8 months old. Stranger anxiety may be developing, the infant may begin crawling and getting into things, teething may cause fussiness, and the baby's tendency to put everything in his or her mouth requires constant vigilance by the parent (Mercer 1985).

All too often postpartum nurses are unaware of the long-term adjustments and stresses that the childbearing family faces as its members adjust to new and different roles. Nurses can help by providing anticipatory guidance about the realities of being a mother. Agencies should have literature available for reference at home. Ongoing parenting groups also give parents an opportunity to discuss problems and become comfortable in new roles.

● Cultural Influences

Many cultures emphasize certain postpartal routines or rituals for mother and baby. These are frequently designed to restore harmony or the hot-cold balance of the body. For Mexican Americans, black Americans, and Orientals, cold must be avoided after delivery. This prohibition includes cold air, wind, and all water (even if heated). Dietary changes also reflect the need to avoid cold foods and restore the balance between hot and cold (Horn 1981).

The diet of the Mexican American reflects this concern about hot-cold balances. Chamomile tea, chicken soup, and corn gruel are offered in the first days. Fruits, vegetables, pork, chili, garlic, beans, and chocolate are avoided (Clark 1978). A Chinese mother may drink chicken soup that contains pigs' knuckles, vinegar, ginger, and peanuts. The vinegar in the soup helps transfer tricalcium phosphate from the bone of the pigs' knuckles into the broth, so the soup helps meet the mother's calcium requirements. The Chinese mother may also be served specially prepared noodles during a traditional celebration on the third day after delivery. This food helps her recovery process and increases lactation (Clark 1978).

The Hmong woman from Laos wants the head of the bed elevated following delivery. This may be accomplished by offering a large pillow or by demonstrating the use of the electric bed so that the woman can elevate her head. The Hmong also stress the need for warmth following childbirth. The woman must be kept warm and given only warm beverages to drink. In keeping with cultural tradition, most Hmong women prefer a diet of poached or stewed chicken served with its broth, rice, and coarsely ground black pepper (LaDu 1985). Korean mothers may prefer a traditional diet of seaweed (tangle) soup and rice, although some may choose to eat both the traditional diet and a more nutritionally balanced diet (Choi 1986).

The black American new mother is offered chicken soup and sassafras tea in the early weeks to aid healing. Liver and hog chitterlings are restricted (liver has a high blood-producing function and is believed to increase lochial flow). Onions and alcohol are avoided because they affect breast milk. The mother may have a two- to six-week period of confinement. Showers, tub baths, and shampoos are restricted during the "sick time" while the lochia flows.

The Mexican American family is concerned with a balance of humors during the postpartal period. The new mother remains in bed for 3 days, begins to walk about her home after 8 days, and may go outside after 15 days. She is helped at home by family members. She avoids bathing for 15 days and carefully covers her head, body, and feet to avoid cold air because she believes that it may cause mastitis, a sudden infection (*pasmo*), a distended belly, frigidity, or sterility. A binder is worn about the abdomen and perineum to protect the body from cold (Clark 1978).

The Vietnamese are also concerned about hot-cold imbalances; consequently the new mother remains inside for 30 days and may not wash her hair or bathe. She also wears heavy clothing and avoids all drafts.

A variety of traditions and rituals also exist in American Indian and other cultural groups. The nurse caring for a mother during the postpartal period carefully assesses the family's beliefs and practices and adapts to them whenever possible. Family members can be encouraged to bring in preferred food and drink and some modifications in client care may be made to follow traditional beliefs.

The extended family frequently plays an essential role during the puerperium. The grandmother is often the primary helper to the mother and newborn. She brings wisdom and experience, allowing the new mother time to rest as well as giving her ready access to someone who can help with problems and concerns as they arise. It is imperative to include members who have authority in the family. Visiting rules may be waived to allow family members or a tribal medicine man access to the mother and newborn. These practices show respect, and the nurse may gain an ally in the care of the mother and baby, especially if the mother follows the advice of her cultural mentor. Often younger members of a specific cultural group have been acculturated by the dominant culture (American, Canadian, etc) and no longer follow traditional practices. In other instances they follow some practices but not others. Nurses can work for a blending of behaviors—the old and the new—to meet the goals of all concerned.

● Development of Attachment

During the postpartal period the parents begin to develop close bonds with their new infant. This process of attachment has been the focus of significant research in the past several years. It is described in depth in Chapter 35.

● Postpartal Nursing Assessment

Comprehensive care is based on a thorough assessment, with identification of individual needs or potential problems.

Risk Factors

The emphasis on ongoing assessment and client education during the puerperium is designed to meet the needs of the childbearing family and to detect and treat possible complications. Table 33–1 identifies factors that may place the new mother at risk during the postpartal period. The nurse uses this knowledge during the assessment and is particularly alert for possible complications that may occur in an individual because of identified risk factors.

Physical Assesssment

Several principles should be remembered in preparing for and completing the assessment of the postpartal woman.

1. As in any assessment, the nurse selects the time that will provide the most accurate data. Palpating the fundus when the woman has a full bladder will not result in a true indication of involution. Thus it is important to have the woman void before beginning the assessment.

Table 33–1   Postpartal High-Risk Factors

Factors	Maternal implications
Preeclampsia-eclampsia	↑ Blood pressure
	↑ CNS irritability
	↑ Need for bedrest → ↑ risk thrombophlebitis
Diabetes	Need for insulin regulation
	Episodes of hypoglycemia or hyperglycemia
	↓ Healing
Cardiac disease	↑ Maternal exhaustion
Cesarean birth	↑ Healing needs
	↑ Pain from incision
	↑ Risk of infection
	↑ Length of hospitalization
Overdistention of uterus (multiple gestation, hydramnios)	↑ Risk of hemorrhage
	↑ Risk of anemia
	↑ Stretching of abdominal muscles
	↑ Incidence and severity of afterpains
Abruptio placentae—placenta previa	Hemorrhage → anemia
	↓ Uterine contractility after delivery → ↑ infection risk
Precipitous labor (<3 hours)	↑ Risk of lacerations to birth canal → hemorrhage
Prolonged labor	Exhaustion
	↑ Risk of hemorrhage
	Nutritional and fluid depletion
	↑ Bladder atony and/or trauma
Difficult delivery	Exhaustion
	↑ Risk of perineal lacerations
	↑ Risk of hematomas
	↑ Risk of hemorrhage → anemia
Extended period of time in stirrups at delivery	↑ Risk of thrombophlebitis
Retained placenta	↑ Risk of hemorrhage
	↑ Risk of infection

2. An explanation of the purpose of regular assessment should be given to the woman.

3. The woman should be as relaxed as possible, and the procedures should be accomplished as gently and smoothly as possible to avoid unnecessary discomfort. Examining the mother who is experiencing afterpains only intensifies her pain, increases tension of muscles, and possibly necessitates medicinal relief.

4. The data obtained during the assessment should be recorded and reported clearly.

A sample assessment form (Figure 33–2) has been included to assist the nursing student in organizing and charting the postpartal physical assessment. Staff nurses may want to devise a similar format as part of the woman's hospital chart to assure continuity and quality of care. Nurses' notes would then concentrate on aspects of care: specific interventions to meet assessed needs; maternal-infant attachment and parenting behaviors; and teaching activities and return demonstrations.

While the nurse is performing the physical assessment, she should also be teaching the client. Assessing the breast provides an optimal time to discuss milk formation, the letdown reflex, and breast self-examination. Mothers are very receptive to instruction on postpartal abdominal tightening exercises when the nurse assesses the woman's fundal height and diastasis. The assessment also provides an excellent time to teach her about the body's physical and anatomic changes postpartally as well as danger signs to report. A Postpartum Physical Assessment Guide can be found on page 1091.

BREASTS

Beginning with the breasts, the nurse should first assess the fit and support provided by the bra. A properly fitting bra provides support to the breasts, thereby promoting maternal comfort. It also helps maintain the shape of the breasts by limiting undue stretching of connective tissue and ligaments during engorgement. If the mother is breast-feeding, the straps of the bra should be cloth, not elastic, and they should be easily adjustable. The back should be wide and should have at least three rows of hooks to adjust for fit. Underwires are not necessary unless the breast is large (C cup or larger). Traditional nursing bras have a fixed inner cup and a separate half cup or flap that can be unhooked to allow for breast-feeding while continuing to support the breast. Some companies have designed the nursing flap to open and close with a plastic snap or with Velcro rather than the traditional loop and hook. Some women find the snap or Velcro much easier and quicker to operate.

Although one brand should not be recommended, several brands of bras can be purchased by the hospital

PART SEVEN

NAME _____

ROOM _____

FEEDING METHOD _____

DATE _____

POSTPARTUM DAY _____

1. BREASTS

   a. General appearance _____

   b. Nipples _____

2. DIASTASIS Rectus abdominis

   a. Length (cm) _____

   b. Width (cm) _____

3. FUNDUS

   a. Height in finger breadths in relationship to

     umbilicus _____

   b. Position _____

   c. Tenderness _____

     (1) with touch _____

     (2) constant _____

4. LOCHIA

   a. Amount _____

   b. Color _____

   c. Consistency _____

   d. Odor _____

5. PERINEUM

   a. Intact _____

   b. Episiotomy _____

     (1) type _____

     (2) healing _____

       (a) REEDA scale _____

   c. Hygiene _____

6. CVA TENDERNESS _____

7. HOMAN'S SIGN _____

   a. Superficial varicosities _____

8. BOWEL AND BLADDER HABITS _____

_____

9. SLEEP PATTERNS _____

_____

10. PSYCHOLOGIC ADAPTATION _____

_____

11. NUTRITIONAL INTAKE _____

_____

12. ADJUSTMENT TO INFANT _____

_____

13. EVALUATION _____

_____

Figure 33–2 Postpartal physical assessment form

and made available as demonstrators so the woman can compare the benefits of one bra against another before investing in a brand and finding out that she would have preferred another had she known about it. Some women prefer a standard bra that hooks in front, and if the breast is not heavy this is acceptable. It is wise for mothers to purchase a nursing bra with a cup a size too large. The breast increases in size with milk production, and a bra that fits well during pregnancy will be too tight during lactation.

Once the bra has been assessed, it should be removed to examine the breasts. First the nurse notes the size and shape of the breasts and any abnormalities, reddened areas, or engorgement. One breast is usually slightly larger than the other. Next the nurse palpates the breasts lightly, checking for heat, edema, engorgement, and caking (swelling of the lobules due to a blockage of the duct), which usually begins in the upper outer quadrant. The mother should be asked whether she has any areas of tenderness or pain; if so, those areas should be examined carefully. The nipples are checked for fissures, cracks and soreness. If the mother says she has problems with inverted nipples, her nipples may also be checked for erectility. This check

is done by asking the woman to place her thumb and first finger on each side of the nipple and gently pull the nipple out from the breast. When released, the nipple and areola should show some signs of erectility. It may be necessary to perform this procedure several times before results are produced. If the baby is nursing well, this assessment may be omitted.

The nursing mother needs to be reminded to keep the nipples supple by using unscented lanolin-based creams (unless she has a wool allergy), and to keep them well cleaned, avoiding a buildup of secretions that could irritate the nipples (see discussion of nipple care, p 934). The nonnursing mother should be assessed for evidence of breast discomfort and appropriate measures taken if necessary (see discussion of lactation suppression in the non-nursing mother, p 1103).

ABDOMEN AND FUNDUS

Having the woman void before doing the assessment assures that a full bladder is not causing any uterine atony; if atony is present, other causes must be investigated.

Postpartum Physical Assessment Guide

Assess/normal findings	Alterations and possible causes*	Nursing responses to data†
VITAL SIGNS		
Blood pressure: Should remain consistent with baseline BP during pregnancy	High BP (PIH, essential hypertension, renal disease, anxiety) Drop in BP (may be normal; uterine hemorrhage)	Evaluate history of preexisting disorders and check for other signs of PIH Assess for other signs of hemorrhage.
Pulse: 50–90 beats/min May be bradycardia of 50–70 beats/min	Tachycardia (difficult labor and delivery, hemorrhage)	Evaluate for other signs of hemorrhage.
Respirations: 16–24/min	Marked tachypnea (respiratory disease)	Assess for other signs of respiratory disease.
Temperature: 36.2–38C (98–100.4F)	After first 24 hr, temperature of 38C (100.4F) or above suggests infection	Assess for other signs of infection; notify physician.
LUNGS		
All lobes clear to percussion and auscultation	High diaphragm (atelectasis or paralysis) Adventitious sounds (infection, reactive airway disease [RAD])	Refer to physician.
BREASTS		
General appearance: Smooth, even pigmentation, changes of pregnancy still apparent; one may appear larger	Reddened area (mastitis)	Assess further for signs of infection.
Palpation: Depending on postpartal day—may be soft, filling, full or engorged	Palpable mass (caked breast, mastitis) Engorgement (venous stasis) Tenderness, heat, edema (engorgement, caked breast, mastitis)	Assess for other signs of infection: if blocked duct consider heat, massage, position change for breast-feeding. See interventions for engorement on pp. 934. Assess for further signs. Report mastitis to physician.
Nipples: Supple, pigmented, intact; become erect when stimulated	Fissures, cracks, soreness (problems with breast-feeding), not erectile with stimulation (inverted nipples)	Reassess technique; recommend appropriate interventions. See p. 934 for appropriate interventions for nursing mothers.
ABDOMEN		
Musculature: Abdomen may be soft, have a "doughy" texture; rectus muscle intact	Separation in musculature (diastasis rectus)	Evaluate size of diastasis; teach appropriate exercises for decreasing the separation.
Fundus: Firm, midline; following appropriate schedule of involution Cesarean birth woman—assess fundus for firmness gently	Boggy (full bladder, uterine bleeding)	Massage until firm; assess bladder and have woman void; attempt to express clots when firm. If bogginess remains or recurs, report to physician.
May be tender when palpated	Constant tenderness (infection)	Assess for evidence of endometritis.
Distention: Cesarean birth women should have no distention or only slight distention. Bowel sounds present by 1st or 2nd postoperative day	Absent bowel sounds, marked distention (decreased or absent peristalsis, paralytic ileus)	Encourage ambulation, obtain order for antiflatulent; report to physician.
LOCHIA		
Scant to moderate amount, earthy odor; no clots	Large amount, clots (hemorrhage) Foul-smelling lochia (infection)	Assess for firmness, express additional clots; begin peri-pad count. Assess for other signs of infection; report to physician.
Normal progression: First 1–3 days—rubra Days 3–10—serosa (Alba seldom seen in hospital)	Failure to progress normally or return to rubra from serosa (subinvolution)	Report to physician.
PERINEUM		
Slight edema and bruising in intact perineum	Marked fullness, bruising, pain (vulvar hematoma)	Assess size; apply ice glove; report to physician.

*Possible causes of alterations are placed in parentheses.
†This column provides guidelines for further assessment and initial nursing actions.

Postpartum Physical Assessment Guide (continued)

Assess/normal findings	Alterations and possible causes*	Nursing responses to data†
PERINEUM (continued)		
Episiotomy: No redness, edema, ecchymosis, discharge, edges well-approximated (REEDA)	Redness, edema, ecchymosis, discharge, or gaping stitches (infection)	Encourage sitz baths, review perineal care, appropriate wiping techniques.
Hemorrhoids: None present; if present, should be small and nontender	Full, tender, inflamed hemorrhoids.	Encourage sitz baths, side-lying position; tucks pads, anesthetic ointments, manual replacement of hemorrhoids; stool softeners, increased fluid intake.
CVA TENDERNESS		
None	Present (kidney infection)	Assess for other symptoms of UTI; obtain clean catch urine; report to physician.
LOWER EXTREMITIES		
No varices or only superficial ones on inspection. No pain with palpation; negative Homan's sign	Positive findings (thrombophlebitis)	Report to physician.
Patellar reflexes 1+ to 2+.	Reflexes 3+ or 4+ (PIH)	
ELIMINATION		
Urinary output: Voiding in sufficient quantities at least every 4–6 hr; bladder not palpable	Inability to void (urinary retention) Symptoms of urgency, frequency, dysuria (UTI)	Employ nursing interventions to promote voiding; if not successful obtain order for catheterization. Report symptoms of UTI to physician.
Bowel elimination: Should have normal bowel movement by second or third day after delivery	Inability to pass feces (constipation due to fear of pain from episiotomy, hemorrhoids, perineal trauma)	Encourage fluids, ambulation, roughage in diet; sitz baths to promote healing of perineum; obtain order for stool softener.

*Possible causes of alterations are placed in parentheses.
†This column provides guidelines for further assessment and initial nursing actions.

The nurse assesses fundal height by determining the relationship of the fundus to the umbilicus. Because of the relaxation of the abdominal wall, the uterus is usually palpable except in obese women. The nurse also notes whether the fundus is in the midline or displaced to either side of the abdomen. The most common cause of displacement is a full bladder. Usually the nurse ascertains tone when first palpating the fundus (see Procedure 33–1).

Following delivery the uterus should be palpated every 15 minutes for one hour, then every 30 minutes for one hour, then every hour for two hours, and then once every eight hours to maintain firm consistency and to evaluate the rate of involution of the uterus. The woman is instructed and encouraged to massage the uterus gently at intervals to enhance uterine contraction.

The vaginally delivered woman presents little difficulty for palpation of the uterus, but modifications are required for cesarean birth mothers. Abdominal dressings often make it difficult to determine the position of the fundus. If a vertical skin incision is made, firmness and position are determined by gently palpating on each side of the incision. With the cesarean birth woman, it is essential to observe the amount of lochia to assess for relaxation of the uterus.

A well-contracted uterus feels as firm as the uterus does during a strong labor contraction. If handled gently, the uterus should not be overly tender. Excessive pain during postpartal examination should alert the nurse to possible genital tract infection. If the uterus is not firm, the nurse should gently massage the fundus with the fingertips of the examining hand, then assess the results. If the uterus becomes firm, the chart should read "Uterus: boggy → firm c̄ light massage." A good habit for the nurse to develop during the postpartal examination is to have the woman lie flat on her back with her head on a pillow and legs flexed. Then the nurse can release the perineal pad to observe the results of uterine massage based on the amount of expelled blood. Occasionally, oxytocic agents such as IV Pitocin, ergonovine maleate (Ergotrate) and methylergonovine maleate (Methergine) are administered postpartally to maintain uterine contraction and prevent hemorrhage (see Drug Guide–Methylergonovine Maleate (Methergine), p 1094).

The boggy uterus that does not contract with light, gentle massage may need more vigorous massage. The amount and character of any expelled blood obtained while massaging the fundus is assessed. When a woman has postpartal uterine atony, the nurse should:

Procedure 33–1   Assessing the Fundus

Objective	Nursing Action	Rationle
Prepare woman.	Explain procedure; have the woman void; position woman flat in bed with head comfortably positioned on a pillow; if the procedure is uncomfortable, woman may flex legs.	Having the woman void assures that a full bladder is not causing any uterine atony. Having the woman flat prevents false high assessment of fundal height. Flexing the legs relaxes the adominal muscles. The uterus may be tender if frequent massage has been necessary.
Determine uterine firmness.	Gently place one hand on the lower segment of the uterus; using the side of the other hand, palpate the abdomen until the top of the fundus is located. Determine whether the fundus is firm. If it is not firm, massage until firm.	Provides support for the uterus. Providing a larger surface for palpation is less uncomfortable for the woman. A firm fundus indicates that the muscles are contracted and bleeding will not occur.
Determine the height of the fundus.	Measure the height of the fundus in fingerbreadths. If the fundal height is more than one fingerbreadth in either direction, use additional fingers (see Figure 33–3).	Fundal height gives information about the progress of involution.
Ascertain position.	Determine whether fundus is deviated from the midline.	Fundus may be deviated when bladder is full.
Record findings.	Fundal height is recorded in fingerbreadths; example: 2 FB ↓ U; 1 FB ↑ U. If massage had been necessary it could be recorded as: Uterus: boggy → firm c̄ light massage	Allows for consistency of reporting among caregivers.

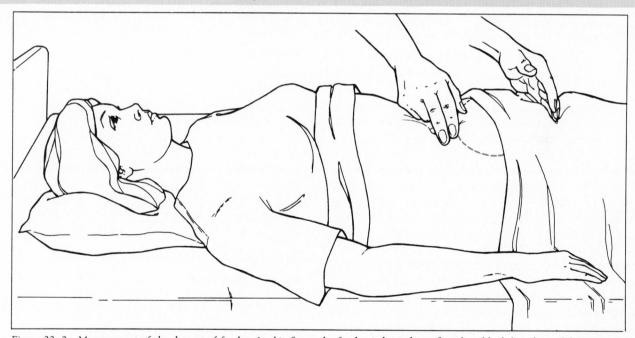

Figure 33–3   Measurement of the descent of fundus. In this figure the fundus is located two fingerbreadths below the umbilicus.

1. Reevaluate for full bladder; if the bladder is full, have the woman void.

2. Question the woman on her bleeding history since delivery or last examination. How heavy does her flow seem? Has she passed any clots? How frequently has she changed pads?

3. For the nursing mother, put the newborn to the mother's breast to stimulate oxytocin production.

4. Reassess the fundus; if the fundus is still boggy, alert the certified nurse-midwife or physician.

In some agencies the nurse assesses for diastasis recti following the uterine assessment and before assessing the lochia. The separation in the rectus abdominis muscles is

Drug Guide   Methylergonovine Maleate (Methergine)

Overview of Obstetric Action

Methylergonovine maleate is an ergot alkaloid that stimulates smooth muscle tissue. Because the smooth muscle of the uterus is especially sensitive to this drug, it is used postpartally to stimulate the uterus to contract. This contraction clamps off uterine blood vessels and prevents hemorrhage. In addition, the drug has a vasoconstrictive effect on all blood vessels, especially the larger arteries. This may result in hypertension, particularly in a woman whose blood pressure is already elevated.

Route, Dosage, and Frequency
Methergine has a rapid onset of action and may be given intramuscularly, orally, or intravenously.

Usual IM dose: 0.2 mg following delivery of the placenta. The dose may be repeated every 2–4 hours if necessary.

Usual oral dose: 0.2 mg every 4 hours (six doses).

Usual IV dose: Because the adverse effects of Methergine are far more severe with IV administration, this route is seldom used. If Methergine is given intravenously, the rate should *not* exceed 0.2 mg/min and the client's blood pressure should be monitored continuously.

Maternal Contraindications
Pregnancy, induction of labor, hepatic or renal disease, threatened spontaneous abortion, uterine sepsis, cardiac disease, hypertension, and obliterative vascular disease contraindicate this drug's use (Loebl & Spratto 1983).

Maternal Side Effects
Hypertension (particularly when administered IV), nausea, vomiting, headache, bradycardia, dizziness, tinnitus, abdominal cramps, palpitations, dyspnea, chest pain, and allergic reactions may be noted.

Effects on Fetus/Neonate
Because Methergine has a long duration of action and can thus produce tetanic contractions, it should never be used during pregnancy as it may result in fetal trauma or death.

Nursing Considerations

1. Monitor fundal height and consistency and the amount and character of the lochia.
2. Assess the blood pressure before administration.
3. Observe for adverse effects or symptoms of ergot toxicity.

evaluated according to its length and width. The student nurse should use a tape measure that measures in centimeters; the skilled practitioner can accurately estimate the distance visually. (A disposable paper tape measure like the one used in the nursery for measuring newborns is preferred.) The separation is palpated first just below the umbilicus, and the width is ascertained. Then the separation is palpated for length toward the symphysis pubis and toward the xiphoid process. If palpation is difficult due to abdominal relaxation, the woman is asked to lift her head unassisted by the nurse. This action contracts the rectus muscles and more clearly defines their edges.

Methods of charting these results vary from institution to institution. Some prefer recording the diastasis measured from the umbilicus down and then from the umbilicus up:

Diastasis: U ↓ 4 cm by 1 cm
          U ↑ 2 cm by 1 cm

Others prefer recording the entire length:

Diastasis: 6 cm by 1 cm

Either method is acceptable.

In the woman who has had a cesarean birth, the abdominal incision should be inspected for evidence of separation and for any signs of infection, including drainage, foul odor, or redness.

LOCHIA

The next aspect to be evaluated is the lochia, which is assessed for character, amount, odor, and the presence of clots. During the first one to three days the lochia should be dark red, similar in appearance to menstrual flow (lochia rubra). A few small clots are normal and occur as a result of blood pooling in the vagina. However, the passage of numerous or large clots is abnormal, and the cause should immediately be investigated. After two to three days the lochia appears more pinkish-brownish or serous (lochia serosa).

Lochia should never exceed a moderate amount, such as four to eight perineal pads daily, with an average of six. However, because this is influenced by an individual woman's pad-changing practices, she should be questioned about the length of time the current pad has been in use, and whether any clots were passed prior to this examination, such as during voiding. If heavy bleeding is reported but not seen, the woman is asked to put on a clean perineal pad and is reassessed in one hour. Usually the flow is moderate, but the woman, who is comparing it to menstrual flow, may consider it heavy. If clots are reported but not seen, the woman is asked to save all pads with clots or not to flush the toilet if clots were expelled during urination. Clots and heavy bleeding may be caused by uterine atony or retained placental fragments and require further assessment. Because of the evacuation of the uterine cavity during cesarean delivery, women with such surgery have less lochia after the first 24 hours than mothers who delivery vaginally. Therefore, amounts of lochia that would be normal in vaginally delivered women are suspect in women who have undergone cesarean delivery.

Agencies vary in the terminology and criteria they use when assessing the quantity of lochia. Jacobson (1985) offers a uniform approach to the assessment of the quantity of lochia. She uses four categories to identify amount—scant, light, moderate, and heavy (Figure 33–4)—within a one-hour period. This approach provides guidelines in the absence of existing criteria. In situations where a more accurate assessment of blood loss is needed, the perineal pads can be weighed. When pads are weighed, 1 gm is considered equivalent to 1 mL blood.

The odor of the lochia may be fleshy but is nonoffensive and never foul. If foul odor is present, so is an infection.

The amount of lochia is charted first, followed by character. For example:

● Lochia: moderate amount rubra

● Lochia: small rubra/serosa

● Lochia: scant/serosa

PERINEUM

The perineum is inspected with the woman lying in a Sims' position, with the top leg positioned over the bot-

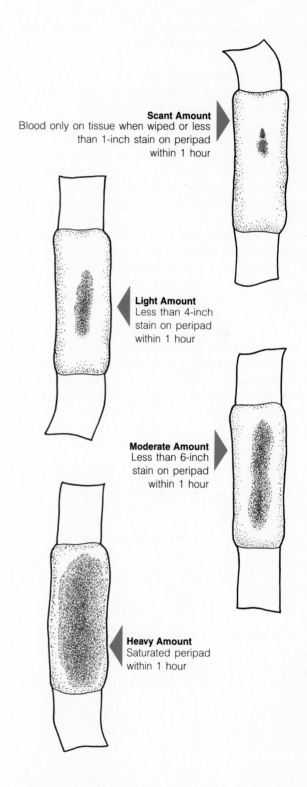

Scant Amount
Blood only on tissue when wiped or less than 1-inch stain on peripad within 1 hour

Light Amount
Less than 4-inch stain on peripad within 1 hour

Moderate Amount
Less than 6-inch stain on peripad within 1 hour

Heavy Amount
Saturated peripad within 1 hour

Figure 33–4 Suggested guideline for assessing lochia volume. (From Jacobson H: A standard for assessing lochia volume. *Am J Mat Child Nurs* 1985;10(May/June):175.)

tom leg. Either side is acceptable. The buttock is lifted to expose the perineum and anus (Figure 33–5). If the perineum has not been incised, it is charted as "Perineum: intact." If an episiotomy was performed or a laceration needed suturing, the wound is assessed.

Davidson (1974) has developed a method of evaluating the episiotomy by identifying five components that indicate the state of healing. The REEDA method allows for a systematic evaluation of the episiotomy for Redness, Edema, Ecchymosis, Discharge, and Approximation (see Table 36–3). The incision should be approximated, only slightly tender, and may have some edema from the time it is repaired to 12 to 24 hours later. After 24 hours some edema may still be present, but the skin edges should be "glued" together so that gentle pressure does not separate them. Gentle palpation should elicit minimal tenderness, and there should be no hardened areas suggesting infection. The perineum may be somewhat edematous even if no episiotomy was performed, but marked swelling may indicate hematoma formation and requires further assessment. These observations provide good evidence that the episiotomy/laceration is healing normally. Ecchymosis interferes with normal healing, as does infection.

The nurse should next assess the state of any hemorrhoids present around the anus for size, number, and pain or tenderness. The following are examples of charting for this portion of the postpartal assessment:

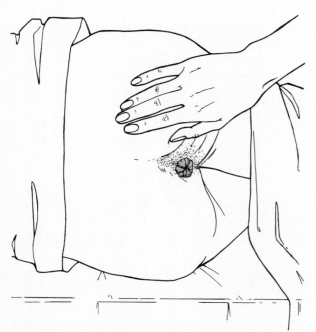

Figure 33–5 Intact perineum with hemorrhoids. Note how the examiner's hand raises the upper buttocks to expose the anal area fully.

- Perineum: intact, no hemorrhoids

- Perineum: episiotomy—skin edges approximated, slight edema; two medium-sized nontender hemorrhoids

- Perineum: laceration—nontender, nonedematous, well approximated; three large, swollen, painful hemorrhoids

LOWER EXTREMITIES

Fewer than 1 percent of all postpartal clients develop thrombophlebitis and thromboembolic disease (Easterling & Herbert 1986). Women who are at increased risk in the postpartal period are those with high parity, previous history of venous thrombosis, dehydration, a traumatic delivery, postpartal hemorrhage, sepsis, delivery by cesarean, and those who have received synthetic estrogens to suppress lactation.

If thrombophlebitis occurs, the most likely site will be the woman's legs. To evaluate the woman, her legs should be stretched out straight and should be relaxed. The foot is then grasped and sharply dorsiflexed. No discomfort or pain should be present. If pain is elicited, the nurse-midwife or physician is notified that the woman has a positive Homan's sign. The pain is caused by inflammation of the vessel. The legs are also evaluated for edema. This may be done by comparing both legs, since usually only one leg is involved. Any areas of redness, tenderness, and increased skin temperature should also be noted.

Women demonstrating signs of deep venous thrombosis, or those considered at high risk because of pelvic surgery or a history of venous thromboembolitic problems, require further evaluation. (See Chapter 36 for additional discussion.) Early ambulation is an important aspect in the prevention of thrombophlebitis. Most women are able to be up shortly after delivery. The cesarean birth mother requires range of motion exercises until she is ambulating more freely.

VITAL SIGNS

Alterations in vital signs may indicate complications, so they are assessed at regular intervals. Blood pressure may be altered slightly as the blood volume peaks immediately after delivery, but this should not present significant problems for the woman. Conversely, blood pressure may drop as a result of blood loss.

The pulse rate may be low during the immediate postpartal period, but this is no cause for alarm. Rates of 50 to 60 beats/min are not unusual as the body attempts to adapt to the decreased pressures intraabdominally as well as to the reduction of the vascular bed with the contraction of the uterus. Pulse rates return to prepregnant norms very quickly unless complications arise.

Temperature elevations may be a sign of infection but must be carefully evaluated. The normal process of wound healing, as well as dehydration and breast engorgement, may also increase body temperature. Temperature elevation (to less than 100.4F or 38C) from normal processes should last for only a few days and should not be associated with other clinical manifestations of infection.

Maternal risk for infections increases with the rise in invasive techniques for diagnosing and treating high-risk pregnancies, such as amniocentesis and fetal blood sampling. It is essential to evaluate temperature elevations in light of other symptomatology, as well as history, to identify factors, such as premature rupture of membranes or prolonged labor, that might increase the incidence of infections in the genital tract.

NUTRITIONAL STATUS

Determination of postpartal nutritional status is based primarily on information provided by the mother and on direct assessment. This is discussed in more detail in Chapter 17.

ELIMINATION

During the hours after delivery the nurse carefully monitors a new mother's bladder status. A boggy uterus, a displaced uterus, or a palpable bladder are signs of urinary distention and require nursing intervention.

The postpartal woman should be encouraged to void every two to four hours. A careful monitoring of intake and output should be maintained, and the bladder should be assessed for distention until the woman demonstrates complete emptying of the bladder with each voiding. The nurse may employ techniques to facilitate voiding, such as helping the woman out of bed to void or pouring warm water on the perineum to promote relaxation.

Spirits of peppermint may be poured into the bedpan (*never* directly onto the urethra or perineum) to encourage voiding. Often the vapors help relax the sphincter so that voiding results. Catheterization should be a "last resort" after all nursing measures have failed. Catheterization is required if the bladder is distended and the woman cannot void or if no voiding has occurred within four to six hours. Nurses must be alert for the problem of urinary retention with overflow. In this case the woman voids small amounts (usually less than 100 mL) frequently but never actually empties the distended bladder. Catheterization is often necessary in such a situation. When the catheter is removed, accurate measuring of the amount of urine is essential until voiding is no longer a problem. The cesarean birth woman may have an indwelling catheter inserted prophylactically.

The same considerations should be made in evaluating bladder emptying once the catheter is removed.

During the physical assessment, the nurse elicits information of a subjective nature from the woman regarding the adequacy of her fluid intake, whether she feels she is emptying her bladder completely when she voids, and any signs of urinary tract infection she may be experiencing. The nurse asks specifically about signs such as urgency, frequency, and dysuria. These data are then used to determine whether all factors are normal or whether additional evaluation is indicated. Many agencies have a policy requiring that a woman's first two voidings following delivery be measured to ensure that the woman is emptying her bladder completely. A normal voiding is at least 100 mL and preferably more.

The nurse also obtains information about the new mother's intestinal elimination and any concerns she may have about it. Many mothers fear that the first bowel movement will be painful and possibly even damaging if an episiotomy has been done. Information must be provided about ways of keeping the stool soft to avoid discomfort and constipation. Often a frank discussion with the nurse does much to alleviate a new mother's anxieties about this subject.

REST AND SLEEP STATUS

As part of the postpartal assessment, the nurse evaluates the amount of rest a new mother is getting. If the woman reports difficulty sleeping at night, the cause should be determined. If it is simply the strange hospital environment, a warm drink, backrub, or mild sedative may prove helpful. Appropriate nursing measures are indicated if the woman is bothered by normal postpartal discomforts such as afterpains, diaphoresis, episiotomy, or hemorrhoidal pain. A daily rest period should be encouraged, and hospital activities should be scheduled to allow time for napping.

Psychologic Assessment

Adequate assessment of the mother's psychologic adjustment is an integral part of postpartal evaluation. This assessment focuses on the mother's general attitude, feelings of competence, available support systems, and caregiving skills. It also evaluates her fatigue level, sense of satisfaction, and ability to accomplish her developmental tasks.

Often fatigue is a significant factor in a new mother's apparent disinterest in her newborn. Frequently the woman is so tired from a long labor and delivery that everything seems to be an effort. To avoid inadvertently classifying a very tired mother as one with a potential bonding problem, the nurse should do the psychologic assessment on more than one occasion. After a nap the new mother is often far more receptive to her infant and her surroundings.

Some new mothers have little or no experience with infants and may feel totally overwhelmed. Women may show these feelings by asking questions and reading all available material or by becoming passive and quiet because they simply cannot deal with their feelings of inadequacy. Unless a nurse questions the woman about her plans and previous experience in a supportive, nonjudgmental way, one might conclude that the woman was disinterested, withdrawn, or depressed. Problem clues might include excessive continued fatigue, marked depression, excessive preoccupation with physical status and/or discomfort, evidence of low self-esteem, lack of support systems, marital problems, inability to care for or nurture the newborn, and current family crises (such as illness, unemployment, and so on). These characteristics frequently indicate a potential for maladaptive parenting, which may lead to child abuse or neglect (physical, emotional, intellectual) and cannot be ignored. Public health nurses or other available community resources may provide greatly needed assistance and may alleviate potentially dangerous situations.

KEY CONCEPTS

The uterus involutes rapidly, primarily through a reduction in cell size.

Involution is assessed by measuring fundal height. The fundus is at the level of the umbilicus within a few hours after delivery and should decrease by approximately one fingerbreadth per day.

The placental site heals by a process of exfoliation, so no scar formation occurs.

Lochia progresses from rubra to serosa to alba and is assessed in terms of type, quantity, and characteristics.

The abdomen may be flabby initially. Diastasis recti should be measured.

Constipation may develop postpartally due to decreased tone, limited diet, and denial of the urge to defecate due to fear of pain.

Decreased bladder sensitivity, increased capacity, and postpartal diuresis may lead to problems with bladder elimination. Frequent assessment and prompt intervention are indicated. A fundus that is boggy but does not respond to massage, is higher than expected, or deviates to the side usually indicates a full bladder.

Postpartally a healthy woman should be normotensive and afebrile. Bradycardia is common.

Postpartally the WBC is often elevated. Activation of clotting factors predisposes the woman to thrombus formation.

The REEDA scale provides criteria for evaluating the episiotomy or a cesarean incision.

Psychological adaptations are traditionally described as taking-in and taking-hold.

Postpartal cultural practices are often based on a belief in a balance between hot and cold.

Postpartal assessment should be completed in a systematic way, usually cephalocaudally. It provides a tremendous opportunity for informal client teaching.

REFERENCES

Belsky J, Rovine M: Social-network contact, family support, and the transition to parenthood. *J Marriage Fam* 1984;46:455.

Choi EC: Unique aspects of Korean-American mothers. *J Obstet Gynecol Neonat Nurs* 1986;15(September/October):394.

Clark AL: *Culture, Childbearing, and Health Professionals.* Philadelphia, Davis, 1978.

Cronenwett LR: Parental network structure and perceived support after birth of first child. *Nurs Res* 1985;34 (November/December):347.

Davidson N: REEDA: Evaluating postpartum healing. *J Nurse-Midwife* 1974;9(2):6.

Easterling WE, Herbert WNP: The puerperium, in Danforth DN, Scott JR (eds): *Obstetrics and Gynecology,* ed 5. Philadelphia, Lippincott, 1986.

Horn BM: Cultural concepts and postpartal care. *Nurs Health Care* 1981;2:516.

Jacobson H: A standard for assessing lochia volume. *Am J Mat Child Nurs* 1985;10(May/June):174.

Kendell RE, et al: Day-to-day mood changes after childbirth: Further data. *Br J Psychiatry* 1984;145:620.

LaDu Eb: Childbirth care for Hmong families. *Am J Mat Child Nurs* 1985;10(November/December):382.

Loebl S, Spratto G: *The Nurse's Drug Handbook,* ed 3. New York, Wiley, 1983.

Mercer RT: The process of maternal role attainment over the first year. *Nurs Res* 1985;34(July/August):198.

Pritchard JA, MacDonald PC, Gant NF: *Williams Obstetrics,* ed 17. New York, Appleton-Century-Crofts, 1985.

Rubin R: *Maternal Identity and the Maternal Experience.* New York, Springer Publishing, 1984.

Rubin R: Puerperal change. *Nurs Outlook* 1961;9:753.

Strang VR, Sullivan PL: Body image attitudes during pregnancy and the postpartum period. *J Obstet Gynecol Neonat Nurs* 1985;14(July/August):332.

Walker LO, et al: Maternal role attainment and identity in the postpartum period: Stability and change. *Nurs Res* 1986a;35(March/April):68.

Walker LO, et al: Mothering behavior and maternal role attainment during the postpartum period. *Nurs Res* 1986b;35(November/December):352.

ADDITIONAL READINGS

Brouse SH: Effect of gender role identity on patterns of feminine and self-concept scores from late pregnancy to early postpartum. *ANS* 1985;7(April):32.

Choi ESC, **Hamilton** RK: The effects of culture on mother-infant interaction. *J Obstet Gynecol Neonat Nurs* 1986;15(May/June):256.

Ferguson H: Planning letter-perfect postpartum care. *Nurs '87* 1987;17(May):50.

Hans A: Postpartum assessment: The psychological component. *J Obstet Gynecol Neonat Nurs* 1986;15(January/February):49.

Leuschen MP, et al: Comparative evaluation of antepartum and postpartum platelet function in smokers and non-smokers. *Am J Obstet Gynecol* 1986;155(December):1276.

Majewski JL: Conflicts, satisfactions, and attitudes during transition to the maternal role. *Nurs Res* 1986;35(January/February):10.

Mercer RT: The relationship of developmental variables to maternal behavior. *Res Nurs Health* 1986;9:25.

Reyes FI, et al: Postpartum disappearance of chorionic gonadotropin from the maternal and neonatal circulations. *Am J Obstet Gynecol* 1985;153:486.

Rutledge DL, **Pridham** KF: Postpartum mothers' perceptions of competence for infant care. *J Obstet Gynecol Neonat Nurs* 1987;16(May/June):185.

Walz BL, **Rich** OJ: Maternal tasks of taking-on a second child in the postpartum period. *Am J Mat Child Nurs* 1983;12(Fall):125.

I had heard about the negatives—the fatigue, the loneliness, loss of self. But nobody told me about the wonderful parts: holding my baby close to me, seeing her first smile, watching her grow and become more responsive day by day. How can I describe the way I felt when she stroked my breast while nursing, or looked into my eyes or arched her eyebrows like an opera singer? This was the deepest connection I'd felt to anybody. Sometimes the intensity almost frightened me. For the first time I cared about somebody else more than myself, and I would do anything to nurture and protect her. (The New Our Bodies, Ourselves)

The Postpartal Family: Needs and Care

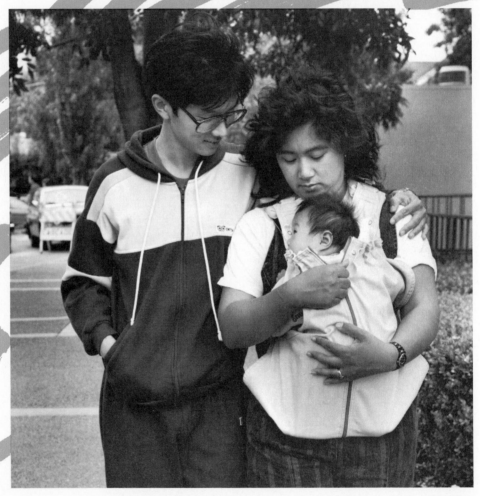

These Chinese-American parents, both university students, take their 3-month-old daughter for a walk.

Chapter Thirty-Four

OBJECTIVES

- **Relate the use of nursing diagnoses to the findings of the "normal" postpartum assessment and analysis.**
- **Delineate nursing responsibilities for client education during the early postpartum period.**
- **Discuss appropriate nursing interventions to meet identified nursing goals for the childbearing family.**
- **Compare the nursing needs of a woman who experienced a cesarean delivery with the needs of a woman who delivered vaginally.**
- **Summarize the nursing needs of the childbearing adolescent during the postpartum period.**
- **Describe possible approaches to follow-up nursing care for the childbearing family.**

Certain premises form the basis of effective nursing care during the postpartal period.

- The best postpartal care is family centered and disrupts the family unit as little as possible. This approach uses the family's resources to support an early and smooth adjustment to the newborn by all family members.

- Knowledge of the range of normal physiologic and psychologic adaptations occurring during the postpartal period allows the nurse to recognize alterations and initiate interventions early. Communicating information about postpartal adaptations to the family facilitates their adjustment to their situation.

- Nursing care is aimed at accomplishing specific goals that ultimately meet individual needs. These goals are formulated after careful assessment and consideration of factors that could influence the outcome of care.

This chapter describes how the nurse can use the nursing process effectively to plan and provide care. Specific nursing responses to the mother's physical needs and the family's psychosocial needs are described at length.

Using the Nursing Process During the Postpartal Period

Often standardized nursing care plans provide the written guidelines for a nurse's action during the postpartal period. Each family is different, however, and the nurse may need to modify interventions to meet a family's needs. Whether a predetermined care plan exists or not, using the nursing process can help the nurse individualize the approach to families and determine priorities.

Nursing Assessment

The postpartal assessment focuses on three interrelated areas of concern—the mother's physical changes and psychological adjustments, the educational needs of the parents, and the family's adjustment to the newest member. During the postpartal assessment, the nurse identifies the strengths of the woman or family as well as actual and potential problems that may influence maternal or family well-being. Ultimately, the assessment findings influence the plan of care.

The assessment period can also be used as a forum for client education. For example, as the postpartal nurse identifies physical changes in the mother, he or she explains to the woman and her partner. As the nurse assesses the parents' skill in handling the new baby, he or she offers information or provides demonstrations that will enhance the parents' competence.

Analysis and Nursing Diagnosis

For most postpartal women, physical recovery goes smoothly and is considered a healthy process. Because of this perception, it is all too common for care givers to think that the woman and her family have no "real" needs and thus that no care plan is needed. Nothing could be further from the truth. Every member of the family has needs, although they may not be obvious, especially if they are psychologic or educational.

The postpartal family's needs, which should be identified during assessment, are the basis for developing nursing diagnoses. Once a nursing diagnosis is made and recorded, systematic action, as delineated in a nursing care plan, can be taken to meet the identified need.

Many nurses have suggested that nursing diagnoses are difficult to make in a wellness setting because of their emphasis on "problems." Stolte (1986) suggests that in some cases resorting to the identification of potential problems may create an artificial situation. She advocates an approach that enables the nurse to identify strengths (called "positive diagnoses") as well as needs or problems. One possible "positive nursing diagnosis" is "Progressive acquisition of maternal role behaviors related to seeking and gaining experience in child care" (p 14). This type of diagnosis focuses on a woman's strength while permitting the nurse to take action to foster further progress in a specific area.

Many agencies that use nursing diagnoses prefer to use the NANDA list exclusively. Consequently, physiologic alterations form the basis of many postpartal diagnoses. Examples of such diagnoses are:

- Alteration in bowel elimination: constipation related to fear of tearing stitches and/or pain.

- Alteration in patterns of urinary elimination related to dysuria.

As primary client educator, the nurse will frequently use the nursing diagnosis "knowledge deficit" when working with postpartal women. Another key nursing diagnosis for the postpartal nurse may be "alteration in parenting related to impaired parent-infant attachment (bonding)." The nursing diagnosis that is most applicable for the couple with an ill or preterm infant may be "alterations in family processes related to an ill family member."

Nursing Plan and Intervention

Many women remain on a postpartum unit for only a short time, so it is often feasible to assign a woman's care to the same nurse. However, time off and shift changes still make it imperative to develop and record a specific care plan. Implementation of the plan by all personnel caring for the postpartal woman promotes consistency, progress in client education, and more effective ongoing assessment and evaluation. An important component of nursing care is client teaching, which is given high priority by many agencies. Sophisticated, detailed forms and guidelines are often available to assist in health teaching. Such tools are a useful adjunct but cannot take the place of the nurse's client-specific plan.

Evaluation

Nursing evaluation on the postpartum unit enables the nurse to refine or modify the care plan based on its effectiveness and/or changes in the woman's status. Evaluation tends to be the most overlooked step of the nursing process, yet the nurse cannot provide quality care without determining whether interventions have been effective.

● Care of the Family During the Postpartal Period

To provide effective care, the nurse must first establish specific goals. The following are common nursing goals for postpartal women:

- To promote comfort and relieve pain

- To promote rest and graded activity

- To promote maternal psychologic well-being

- To provide effective parent education

- To provide anticipatory guidance about sexual activity and family planning

- To promote successful infant feeding

- To enhance parent-infant attachment

- To prepare the family for discharge

Chapter 35 is devoted to the goal of parent-infant attachment, and Chapter 30 addresses infant feeding. Family planning is discussed in Chapter 8. The other postpartum nursing goals are discussed in this chapter.

Nursing Goal: Promotion of Comfort and Relief of Pain

The postpartal woman often experiences varying degrees of pain. Potential sources of discomfort include engorged breasts; an edematous perineum; an episiotomy, laceration, or extension; engorged hemorrhoids; or the development of a hematoma. Hematomas not only cause pain but also are a source of blood loss not as evident as overt bleeding.

Ice packs may be applied to the perineum during the first few hours after delivery, especially if there is a third- or fourth-degree laceration. Ice is effective in reducing edema and also relieves discomfort because of its numbing effect. Chemical ice bags or a disposable glove filled with ice and secured at the wrist with a rubber band may be used. The ice pack is covered with an absorbent pad or wash cloth to avoid an ice burn on the woman's perineum.

After the first few hours have passed, perineal discomfort may be relieved by a variety of approaches, including routine perineal care, sitz baths, heat lamps, topical application of anesthetic ointments or sprays, and administration of analgesics. The woman may also find it helpful to tighten her buttocks before sitting to avoid direct trauma to the perineum. For similar reasons lateral positions may be more comfortable.

Afterpains are common postpartally, especially in multiparous and breast-feeding women. Explaining the cause of the afterpains is an important nursing intervention. Women find that different positions help ease the discomfort. For instance, a woman may lie prone with a pillow placed under her abdomen or she may choose to rock in a rocking chair. For greatest relief, analgesics are administered before the pain is too intense. For breast-feeding mothers, a mild analgesic administered an hour before feeding will promote comfort and enhance maternal-infant interaction.

Discomfort may also be caused by immobility. The woman who has been in stirrups for any length of time may experience muscular aches from the extreme position. It is not unusual for women to experience joint pains and muscular pain in both arms and legs, depending on the effort they exerted during the second stage of labor.

Breast engorgement may be a source of pain for the postpartal woman. Specific nursing interventions for the bottle-feeding mother are discussed in the following section. Nursing interventions for the breast-feeding mother with engorgement are discussed in Chapter 30.

Nurses should be alert to nonverbal as well as verbal manifestations of pain and should intervene with appropriate measures. The physical response to pain may be influenced by the level of fatigue, cultural background, possible lack of acceptance of the pregnancy and new baby, or other situational crises, which trigger psychologic crises that will ultimately affect the family's adjustment. The first approach to pain relief may not be medication; changing positions, providing comfort measures such as a backrub or warm drink, or encouraging the woman to ventilate her feelings in an atmosphere of acceptance are often sufficient. Drugs should be available if other measures fail.

SUPPRESSION OF LACTATION IN THE NONNURSING MOTHER

Suppression of lactation may be accomplished through drug therapy and mechanical inhibition. The most frequently used medication is bromocriptine mesylate (Parlodel), a nonhormonal ergot derivative that inhibits pro-

Research Note

Wong and Stepp-Gilbert compared the effectiveness of a nonpharmaceutical lactation suppressant method to a lactation suppressant drug therapy for non-breast-feeding mothers.

A convenience sample of postpartum women were followed from the immediate postpartum period for 16 days postpartum to elicit data including whether the assigned methods were followed and if they were effective. The 17 women in the nonpharmaceutical group followed a protocol initiated within six hours of delivery of a tight bra or binder, ice packs over the axillary breast areas for 15 to 20 minutes QID, and no breast stimulation. The drug group used Parlodel 2.5 mg BID for 14 days.

The researchers found that most subjects in both groups experienced the lactation process to some degree. The drug group had significantly less engorgement, milk leakage, and discomfort 4 days postpartum, but the lactation process was prolonged until the ninth to sixteenth days. The protocol group had more engorgement, milk leakage, and discomfort on day 4 but the lactation process was completed before day 16.

Nurses can teach this protocol to clients concerned about side effects of drug suppression to minimize engorgement, and should provide information describing the benefits and disadvantages of both methods to all non-breast-feeding clients.

Wong S, Stepp-Gilbert E: Lactation suppression: Nonpharmaceutical versus pharmaceutical method. J Obstet Gynecol Neonat Nurs 1985;14(July/August):302–310.

lactin secretion. It is taken twice a day for two to three weeks. Because its primary side effect is hypotension, it is begun after a new mother's vital signs have stabilized (see Drug Guide–Bromocriptine, p 1104). Successful suppression of lactation has also been reported following the administration of a single intramuscular injection of a long-acting form of bromocriptine (Peters et al 1986).

In the past, estrogen-based medications such as estradiol valerate and chlorotrianisene were used for lactation suppression. Because these drugs are associated with an increased incidence of thromboembolic disease and venous thrombosis, they are rarely, if ever, used in current practice.

Because bromocriptine is expensive and not always completely successful in suppressing lactation, mechanical methods of lactation suppression are becoming increasingly popular. Although signs of engorgement do not usually occur until the second or third postpartum day, prevention of engorgement is best accomplished by beginning non-pharmaceutical methods of lactation suppression as soon as possible after delivery. Ideally this involves having the

Drug Guide Bromocriptine (Parlodel)

Overview of Obstetric Action

Bromocriptine is a dopamine agonist that acts to suppress lactation by stimulating the production of prolactin-in-hibiting factor at the hypothalamic level. This results in decreased secretion of prolactin by the pituitary gland. The drug may also directly inhibit the pituitary by preventing the release of prolactin from the hormone-producing cells (Foster 1982). When administered postpartally it helps suppress milk production and decrease breast leakage and pain. It may also be used for suppression after lactation has already begun.

Route, Dosage, and Frequency
The usual dose is 2.5 mg orally two times per day. The total daily dose generally does not exceed 7.5 mg. The medication is usually taken for 2–3 weeks. Research regarding the efficacy of parenteral administration suggests that a single intramuscular dose of a microencapsulated form of bromocriptine may be effective in suppressing lactation when administered following delivery. This would be useful following obstetric surgery or for women experiencing severe vomiting (Peters et al 1986).

Maternal Contraindications
Maternal hypotension, desire to breast-feed, pregnancy.

Maternal Side Effects
Hypotension is the primary side effect. To prevent problems associated with hypotension, administration should be delayed until the new mother's vital signs are stable. Other side effects include nausea, headache, dizziness, and occasionally faintness and vomiting.

Nursing Considerations

Administration should be delayed until maternal blood pressure is stable. Blood pressure should be carefully monitored if bromocriptine is administered concurrently with any antihypertensives. Taking bromocriptine with meals may help decrease the possibility of nausea. Early resumption of ovulation has occurred in women taking bromocriptine; the woman should be informed of this and receive information about contraceptives (Foster 1982).

---

woman begin wearing a supportive, well-fitting bra within six hours after delivery. The bra is worn continuously until lactation is suppressed (usually about five days) and is removed only for showers (Wong & Stepp-Gilbert 1985). The bra provides support and eases the discomfort that can occur with tension on the breasts because of fullness. A snug breast binder may be used if the woman does not have a bra available or if she finds the binder more comfortable. Ice packs should be applied over the axillary area of each breast for 20 minutes four times daily. This, too, should be begun soon after delivery. Ice is also useful in relieving discomfort if engorgement occurs.

The mother is advised to avoid any stimulation of her breasts by her baby, herself, breast pumps, or her sexual partner until the sensation of fullness has passed (usually about one week). Such stimulation will increase milk production and delay the suppression process. Heat is avoided for the same reason, and the mother is encouraged to let shower water flow over her back rather than her breasts. Suppression takes only a few days in most cases, but small amounts of milk may be produced up to a month after delivery.

EDUCATION FOR SELF-CARE

Perineal care should be encouraged after each elimination to clean the perineum and promote comfort. Some agencies provide "peri-bottles," which the woman fills with warm water that is squirted over the perineum following elimination. She should be instructed to cleanse from front to back to prevent contamination of the vulva from the anal area. Other agencies have wall-mounted surgigators with soap cartridges to cleanse the perineum. The steady stream of warm, soapy water they provide is especially effective for cleaning. When toilet tissue is used, the woman will be more comfortable if she uses a blotting motion. She is also instructed to apply the perineal pad from front to back to prevent contamination from the anal area.

Sitz baths are particularly useful if the perineum has been severely traumatized, as moist heat not only increases circulation to promote healing but also relaxes the tissue to promote comfort and decrease edema.

When assisting a woman into a sitz bath, the nurse should be certain the water temperature is comfortable. Most women find a temperature of 105F comfortable, al-

Research Note

Ramler and Roberts compared warm and cold sitz baths for relieving episiotomy pain. Theoretically the warm sitz bath causes vasodilatation and increased circulation, thereby promoting healing and relieving pain. Cold sitz baths cause an initial vasoconstriction that decreases bleeding, hematoma formation, and edema and has a local anesthetic effect.

The 40 subjects were used as their own controls, with 20 taking a cold sitz bath first, followed six hours later by a warm sitz bath. The other 20 took the warm bath first, then the cold. All baths were taken in the second 24 hours following delivery and at least three hours after any pain medication was taken. The subjects rated their pain before and immediately following the bath and half an hour and one hour after the bath.

The pain scores indicated that the relief provided by a cold sitz bath is greater after the bath but of no longer duration than that of the warm bath. Of the subjects, 20 preferred the cold bath, 10 preferred the warm bath, and 10 had no preference. It is significant to note that 119 subjects refused to participate in the study, and many of these said that they would not take a cold sitz regardless of pain. Perhaps explanations by the nurse could increase clients' acceptance of this apparently effective technique.

Ramler, D Roberts J: A comparison of cold and warm sitz baths for reflief of postpartum perineal pain. J Obstet Gynecol Neonat Nurs 1986;15(November/December):471–474.

though new research suggests that cool sitz baths may be even more effective. They, too, are soothing and cleansing, while the cool temperature helps relieve edema and decrease pain (Ramler & Roberts 1986).

While in a sitz tub, the woman may wear a hospital gown and drape it over the edge of the tub. This keeps her upper body from becoming chilled and provides privacy. The woman should have a call light available that she knows how to use. Often the position and warmth of a sitz bath can make a woman become faint; the nurse should check on her frequently. Once the woman is familiar with the use of the sitz bath, she should be encouraged to use it as frequently as she wishes, generally for about 20 minutes three or four times a day. Many agencies are now using disposable sitz baths that fit inside the toilet. These are convenient for the woman to use as often as she wishes both in the hospital and when she goes home.

Dry heat in the form of heat lamps is sometimes used. The perineum should be cleaned to prevent drying of secretions on the perineum. Heat lamps generally are used for 20 minutes two or three times daily. The heat source should be placed at least 18 inches from the perineum to avoid burns.

Topical anesthetics such as Dermoplast Aerosol Spray or Nupercainal ointment may be used to relieve perineal discomfort. The woman is advised to apply the anesthetic following a sitz bath or perineal care. Because of the danger of tissue burns she must be cautioned not to apply anesthetic before using a heat lamp.

Some mothers experience hemorrhoidal pain after delivery. Relief measures include the use of sitz baths two to three times per day and anesthetic ointments, rectal suppositories, or witch hazel pads applied directly to the anal area. The woman may be taught to digitally replace external hemorrhoids in her rectum (see Chapter 16, p 382). She may also find it helpful to maintain a side-lying or prone position when possible and to avoid prolonged sitting. The mother is encouraged to maintain an adequate fluid intake, and to take stool softeners or laxatives to ensure greater comfort with bowel movements. The hemorrhoids usually disappear a few weeks after delivery if the woman did not have them prior to this pregnancy.

Personal hygiene measures are essential to promote comfort during the postpartal period. Diaphoresis occurs as the body attempts to dispose of the extra fluid retained during pregnancy. Thus a daily shower is very refreshing for the woman and should be strongly encouraged unless cultural beliefs prohibit bathing in the first few days after delivery. Women who have remained NPO (having nothing by mouth) for any length of time require mouth care. Assisting the woman with these basic needs helps her feel more comfortable.

During the puerperium the woman is frequently thirsty as she recovers from delivery and experiences postpartal diuresis. Most mothers enjoy a pitcher of cold water within easy reach. On the other hand, women from some cultures may prefer tepid water. Many women also enjoy milk or fruit juice, and it should be readily available for them.

Nursing Goal: Promotion of Rest and Graded Activity

Following delivery some women feel exhausted and in need of rest. Other women are euphoric and full of psychic energy immediately after delivery, ready to retell their experience of birth repeatedly. The nurse must be astute in evaluating individual needs, always with the goal of providing opportunities for rest. If rest is achieved while in the hospital, there is a greater likelihood that the woman will arrange such opportunities at home, adjusting her schedule to meet this important need. The nurse can provide time for the excited, euphoric woman to air her feelings and then can encourage a period of rest.

Physical fatigue often influences many other adjustments and functions with the new mother. It may also reduce milk flow, thereby increasing problems with breastfeeding. The mother requires energy to make the psychologic adjustments to a new infant and to assume new roles. She makes these adjustments more smoothly when she gets adequate rest.

Certain essential nursing activities such as taking vital signs and assessing the fundus must be done frequently to assess the woman's condition; however, they may create an environment of constant activity, making rest a luxury and not a routine. The nurse may encourage rest by organizing activities to avoid frequent interruptions for the woman. If the new mother chooses, rest times may be provided before encounters with the newborn if rooming-in is not used.

Early ambulation is encouraged postpartally. Activity aids in promoting psychologic well-being and also in reducing the incidence of complications such as constipation and thrombus formation.

The nurse assists the woman the first few times she gets up during the early postpartal period. Fatigue, effects of medications, loss of blood, and possibly even lack of food intake may cause dizziness or faintness when the woman stands up. Because this may be a problem during the woman's first shower, the nurse should remain in the room, check the woman frequently, and have a chair close by in case she becomes faint. Dizziness may be aggravated by standing still and by the warmth of the water, so it is best to keep the first shower somewhat brief. Many postpartal units tape ammonia inhalants to the bathroom door for use in case of fainting. During this first shower the nurse instructs the woman in the use of the emergency call button in the bathroom; if she becomes faint during a future shower, she can call for assistance.

EDUCATION FOR SELF-CARE

○ *POSTPARTAL EXERCISES* The woman is encouraged to begin simple exercises while in the hospital and continue them at home. She is advised that increased lochia or pain means she should reevaluate her activity and make necessary alterations. Most agencies provide a booklet describing suggested postpartal activities. (Exercise routines vary for women undergoing tubal ligation following delivery or for cesarean birth clients.) See Figure 34–1 for a description of some common exercises.

○ *RESUMPTION OF ACTIVITIES* Activity may increase gradually after discharge. The new mother should avoid heavy lifting, excessive stair climbing, and strenuous activity. One or two daily naps are essential and are most easily achieved if the mother sleeps when her baby does.

Some mothers find it easier to remember to avoid overdoing if they wear a robe and gown for the first few days. By the second week at home, light housekeeping may be resumed. Although it is customary to delay returning to work for six weeks, most women are physically able to resume practically all activities by four to five weeks. Delaying returning to work until after the final postpartal examination will minimize the possibility of problems.

Nursing Goal: Promotion of Maternal Psychologic Well-Being

The birth of a child, with the role changes and increased responsibilities it produces, is a time of emotional stress for the new mother. This stress is increased by the tremendous physiologic changes as her body adjusts to a nonpregnant state. During the early postpartal days mood swings are common, and some women become tearful at the slightest provocation.

At first the mother may repeatedly discuss her experiences in labor and delivery. This allows her to integrate her experiences. If she feels that she did not cope well with labor, she may have feelings of inadequacy. If the woman has given birth in a birthing center, she will have the same nurse postpartally. This nurse can provide reassurance if the woman did cope well or opportunities for the woman to discuss her perceptions of childbirth if her coping skills were not particularly effective.

If a new mother is transferred to a postpartum unit, it is helpful if the labor nurse includes information on the woman's coping abilities. In this way the postpartum nurse can provide appropriate reassurance or opportunities for the new mother to talk. Open discussion of feelings is only possible if the nurse has established a warm, supportive relationship with the woman. Follow-up visits from the nurse who assisted her in labor and delivery provide additional opportunities for the mother to relive her experiences and come to terms with them.

During the postpartal period, the mother must adjust to the loss of her fantasized child and accept the child she has borne. This may be more difficult if the child is not of the desired sex or if she or he has birth defects. It is important for postpartum nurses to accept a variety of maternal responses and not expect that all mothers are happy, loving, and excited. Such preconceived notions may limit the nurse's ability to recognize the needs of women who have different initial responses.

Immediately following the delivery the mother is focused on bodily concerns, and teaching may not be totally effective. Because early discharge is common, however, classes and information should be offered, and printed handouts provided for reference as questions arise at home.

Following the initial dependent period, the mother becomes very concerned about her ability to be a successful parent. Skillful intervention by the nurse, with constant reassurance that the client is a successful mother, is vital. During this time the mother is most receptive to teaching, and tactful instruction and demonstration assist her in mothering effectively. The nurse must carefully avoid "taking over" the infant. By functioning as an advisor and allowing the mother to perform the actual care, the nurse demonstrates confidence in the mother's skill and ability, which in turn increases the mother's self-confidence about her effectiveness as a parent.

Some mothers may express concern over their seeming inability to make simple decisions or act decisively during the early postpartal period. They may require reassurance that this behavior is normal and will last only a brief time.

The depression, weepiness, and "let down feeling" that characterize the postpartum blues are often a surprise for the new mother. She and her family often require reassurance that these feelings are normal and an explanation about why they occur. It is vital to provide a supportive environment that permits the mother to cry without feeling guilty. Her privacy should be protected, but the nurse should indicate interest if the woman feels a need to talk. In rare instances initial depression leads to a pathologic condition known as postpartum psychosis (see Chapter 36).

I had my first son several years ago before rooming-in was popular. Postpartally I was in a four-bed room. As a maternity nurse myself, I found it interesting to watch how other nurses interacted with patients. One nursery nurse was especially tactless and at one time or another reduced all three of my roommates to tears. To one she said, "Your baby has cried almost continuously since the last feeding. Try to get him to eat better this time." My roommate was breast-feeding, and cried because she felt like a failure. To another the nurse said, "Boy, your baby really is a little baldy." This roommate cried because her baby was "ugly." To the third the nurse said, "Your baby sure needs lessons in manners. He sprayed all over when I changed him!" I think the nurse was trying to joke but my roommate was in a tizzy thinking her baby would be neglected because of his "rudeness." It's amazing how such little, tactless comments can hurt when a woman's emotions are so topsy-turvy. I didn't need a comment from her to set me off. I shed buckets of tears when my son had to stay in the hospital two extra days because of jaundice. I thought I would never feel in control again!

Nursing Goal: Provision of Parent Education

Meeting the educational needs of the new mother and her family is one of the primary challenges facing the postpartum nurse. Effective education provides the childbearing family with sufficient knowledge to meet many of their own health needs and seek assistance if necessary.

Formal schooling cannot be considered the primary criterion for assessing learning needs. It is far too easy to assume that the woman with limited education has nu-

merous needs when, in fact, she may be very comfortable with her new role and responsibilities. By the same token, the concerns of a highly educated new mother may be overlooked either because the nurse assumes that she already has the information or because a nurse with less education finds her intimidating.

Each woman has educational needs that vary based on age, background, experience, and expectations. The steps of the nursing process provide a useful tool for identifying and meeting educational needs following delivery.

Educational assessment may be accomplished in several ways. Simple observation—how a mother handles her infant, the food she selects—may provide useful information, as do listening, questioning, and sensitivity to nonverbal clues. What areas concern the new mother? Does she seem to have misinformation or confused information? What does she already know that the nurse can build on?

Open-ended questions require a several-word reply and provide far more data for the nurse to use in the assessment than a question requiring a simple "yes" or "no." For example, asking "What plans have you made for handling things when you get home?" will elicit a more detailed response than, "Will someone be available to help you at home?"

To assess learning needs some agencies provide a client handout listing the most frequently identified areas of concern for new mothers. The mother checks those that apply to her or writes in concerns not included.

In many educational settings, planning primarily involves the development of objectives that clarify what is to be taught and describe how the learner will demonstrate achievement of each objective. In planned postpartal classes, objectives are predetermined and generalized to meet the needs of most of the participants. Even in nonstructured, individualized situations, however, objectives can be indentified by the nurse—"Mrs Warren, when we are finished, you will be able to demonstrate the procedure for manually expressing your breast milk and describe appropriate methods of storing it."

The educational method chosen to implement the objectives varies. Agencies with many clients and limited staff may rely heavily on structured classes while smaller units may provide more individualized instruction. Because more effective learning occurs when there is sensory involvement and active participation, television and movies (sight and hearing) are more helpful than lecture (hearing only), and demonstration-return demonstration (sight, touch, hearing, and possibly smell and taste) is even more effective (Bille 1981).

Postpartal units use a variety of approaches—scheduled classes or demonstrations, handouts, group discussions, movies, videotapes, and individual interaction. Some agencies have access to a television channel and can show instructional films at scheduled times during the day. Women should have pencils and paper provided to jot

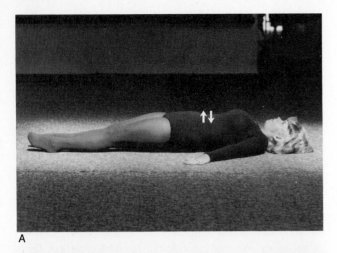

A

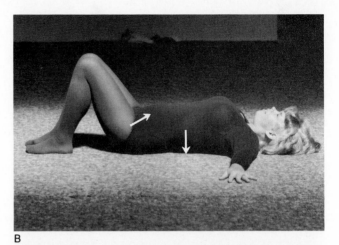

B

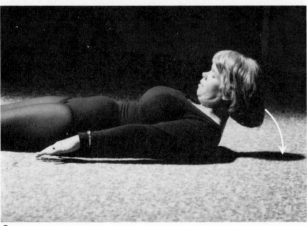

C

Figure 34–1　Postpartal exercises. Begin with five repetitions two or three times daily and gradually increase to ten repetitions. First day: A Abdominal breathing. Lying supine, inhale deeply using the abdominal muscles. The abdomen should expand. Then exhale slowly through pursed lips, tightening the abdominal muscles. B Pelvic rocking. Lying supine with arms at sides, knees bent, and feet flat, tighten abdomen and buttocks and attempt to flatten back on

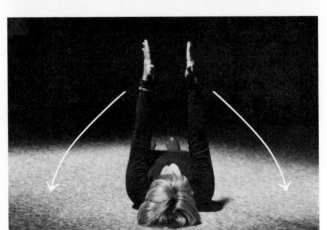

D

floor. Hold for a count of ten, then arch the back, causing the pelvis to "rock." On second day add: C Chin to chest. Lying supine with no pillow and legs straight, raise head and attempt to touch chin to chest. Slowly lower head. D Arm raises. Lying supine with arms extended at 90° angle from body, raise arms so they are perpendicular to the floor. Lower slowly. On fourth day add: E Knee rolls. Lying supine with knees bent, feet flat, and arms

down questions that arise as they view the material. Afterward nurses are available to clarify material or answer any questions about the content.

Timing is important in implementing educational activities. The new mother is more receptive to teaching after the first 24 to 48 hours when she is ready to assume responsibility for her own care and that of her newborn. However, many women are discharged in the early, dependent phase. Because of this, teaching should be done, and handouts should be provided for future reference. New fathers are more likely to attend sessions planned for them if they are scheduled in the evening after visiting hours. If material is planned for siblings, late afternoon teaching, after school or naps, might be most effective.

Demonstration-return demonstration techniques offer opportunities for an individual to practice in a supervised

situation. If principles are emphasized rather than simply encouraging the mimicking of techniques, transfer of the learning to the home situation is facilitated.

Teaching should not be limited to "how to" activities, however. Anticipatory guidance is essential in assisting the family to cope with role changes and the realities of a new baby. Small group discussions provide a chance for the new parents to talk about fears and expectations. Questions may arise regarding sexuality, contraception, child care, and even the grief work associated with relinquishing the fantasized infant in order to accept the actual one.

Information is also essential for individuals with specialized educational needs—the mother who had a cesarean delivery, the adolescent mother, the parents of infants with congenital anomalies, and so on. They may feel overwhelmed, have difficult feelings to work through, and not

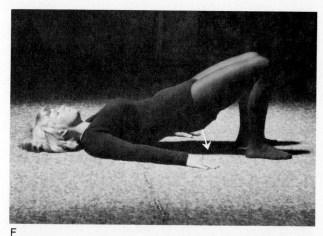

E

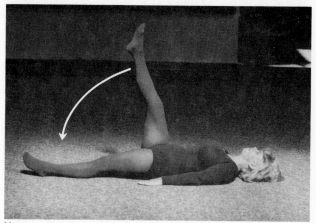

F

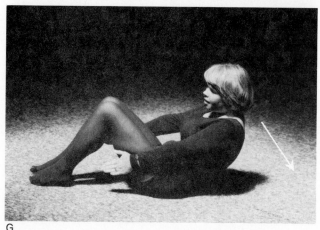

G

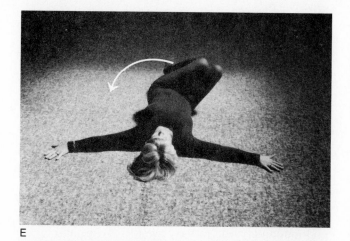

H

extended to the side, roll knees slowly to one side, keeping shoulders flat. Return to original position and roll to opposite side. F Buttocks lift. Lying supine with arms at sides, knees bent, and feet flat, slowly raise the buttocks and arch the back. Return slowly to starting position. On sixth day add: G Abdominal tighteners. Lying supine with knees bent and feet flat, slowly raise head toward knees. Extend arms along either side of knees. Return slowly to

original position. H Knee to abdomen. Lying supine with arms at sides, bend one knee and thigh until foot touches buttocks. Straighten leg and lower it slowly. Repeat with other leg. After two to three weeks, more strenuous exercises such as sit-ups and side leg raises may be added as tolerated. Kegel exercises, begun antepartally, should be done many times daily during postpartum to restore vaginal and perineal tone.

even realize what it is they need to know. Nurses who are attuned to these individual problems can begin providing guidance as soon as possible.

If the family is aware of role changes and common problems, they can anticipate possible behaviors and their origin. They are then better able to cope and less likely to evaluate expected occurrences as abnormal. Education also provides an opportunity to develop sensitivities to new modes of communication that are often required among family members.

Methods for evaluating learning vary according to the objectives and teaching methods. Return demonstrations, question-and-answer sessions, and even programmed instruction are opportunities for evaluating learning, as are formal evaluation tools.

Evaluation of attitudinal or less concrete learning is

more difficult. For example, a mother's ability to express her frustrations over an unanticipated cesarean delivery or a new mother's decision to delay for several weeks a family dinner originally scheduled for the first weekend after she arrives home, may be the nurse's only clues that learning has occurred. Follow-up phone calls after discharge may provide additional evaluative information and continue the helping process as the nurse assesses the family's current educational status and begins planning accordingly.

Nursing Goal: Promotion of Family Wellness

A satisfactory maternity experience may have a positive impact on the entire family. The new or expanding family that receives appropriate information and has adequate time to interact with its newest member in a supportive environment will feel more comfortable and secure at home.

MOTHER-BABY UNITS

In the past, newborns were typically separated from their parents immediately after birth. Today most facilities encourage parents to spend time with their infants. Some facilities offer the option of *mother-baby units* (Other titles used to describe this concept include mother-baby primary nursing, mother-infant nursing, combined care, and family-centered maternity care [Watters, 1985]). A mother-baby unit is based on the concept that mother and infant will both benefit from time spent together, so the infant remains at the mother's bedside and both are cared for by the same nurse. Some agencies call this option *rooming-in*. In other facilities the rooming-in policy varies slightly in that nursery personnel remain responsible for the child at the mother's bedside, while postpartum staff care for the mother.

Mother-baby units provide continuous opportunities for the mother to become acquainted with and learn how to care for her baby. Watters (1985) believes that although agencies may vary slightly in their approach to the concept with regard to staff assignments, visiting hours, and other factors, in all cases this approach helps ensure continuity, improved care, and personal satisfaction for the nurse providing the care.

In a mother-baby unit, the newborn's crib is placed near the mother's bed where she can see her baby easily. The crib should be a self-contained unit stocked with items the mother might require in providing care. A bulb syringe for suctioning the mouth or nares should always be accessible and the mother should be familiar with its use.

Mothers are frequently very tired after delivery, so the responsibility for providing total infant care could be overwhelming. The mother-baby policy must be flexible enough to permit the mother to return the baby to the nursery if she finds it necessary because of fatigue or physical discomfort. Some mothers, fearing staff criticism, may be hesitant to do this and may need encouragement from the nurse. The woman with children at home may require additional rest, and a modified approach may best meet her needs. For example, the baby may return to the central nursery at night, allowing the mother more time for uninterrupted rest.

The mother-baby unit is conducive to a self-demand feeding schedule for both breast-feeding and bottle-feeding infants. The lactating mother may find it especially beneficial to be able to nurse her child every 1½ to 3 hours if necessary.

Many agencies have unlimited visiting hours for the father. Fathers, after washing their hands, are able to care for their infant in a mother-baby unit. These opportunities to hold and care for the child promote paternal self-confidence and foster paternal attachment.

SIBLING VISITATION

Sibling visitation helps meet the needs of both the siblings and their mother. A visit to the hospital reassures children that their mother is well and still loves them. It also provides an opportunity for the children to become familiar with the new baby. For the mother the pangs of separation are lessened as she interacts with her children and introduces them to the newest family member.

Most agencies now recognize the importance of providing siblings with opportunities to see their mother and meet the infant during the early postpartal period (Figure 34–2). Approaches to this issue vary from specified visiting hours for siblings to unlimited visiting privileges.

EDUCATION FOR SELF-CARE

Although the parents have prepared the child for the presence of a new brother or sister, the actual arrival of the infant requires some adjustments. If the woman gives birth in a birthing center, her children may be present for the delivery. They then have an opportunity to spend time with their new sibling and their parents. They may even remain throughout the woman's hospitalization, especially if it is brief, and all go home as a family.

For the mother who is returning home to small children, it is often helpful to have the father carry the new baby inside. This practice keeps the mother's arms free to hug and hold her older children. She thereby reaffirms her love for them before introducing them to their new sibling. Many mothers have found that bringing a doll home with them for the older child is helpful. The child cares for the doll alongside his or her parents, thereby identifying with the parent. This identification helps decrease anger and the need to regress for attention.

If parents feel that bringing a doll home is not appropriate, they may substitute a small present from the new infant to his or her sibling. A carefully chosen gift conveys to the older child that he or she is special, too.

Often older children enjoy working with the parents to care for the newborn. Involvement in care helps the older child develop a sense of closeness to the baby. It also helps the child learn acceptable behavior toward the newborn, feel a sense of accomplishment, and develop tenderness and caring—qualities that are appropriate for both males and females. With constant supervision and assistance as necessary, even very young children can hold the baby or a bottle during feeding. Breast-feeding mothers may allow siblings to help give the new infant an occasional bottle of water.

Regression is a common occurrence even when siblings have been well prepared. The nurse can provide anticipatory guidance so that parents do not become overly upset if their previously toilet-trained child begins to have accidents or requests a bottle to feed from.

Regardless of age, an older sibling needs reassurance that he or she is still special to the parents, a truly loved and valued family member. Parents may be advised to remember to show signs of affection for their older child. Words of love and praise coupled with hugs and kisses are very important. So, too, is special parent-child time. Both parents should spend quality time in a one-to-one experience with each of their older children. This may require some careful planning, but its worth cannot be overestimated. It confirms the parents' love for the child and often helps the child accept the new baby. The nurse and parents can come up with numerous ways unique to their own environment and life-styles to show the older child or children that they are important and have their own places in the family.

It is inevitable that at one time or another an older child will try to hurt the baby (or will hurt the baby unintentionally, not knowing his or her own strength or the effect of hitting). Parents are guided to respond by saying "We all get angry sometimes, and being angry is ok. Hurt-

ing is not ok. I won't let you hurt (the baby) just as I won't let someone else hurt you."

The child, especially one of the opposite sex from the newborn, will raise queries about the appearance of the genitals as compared to his or her own. A simple explanation, such as, "That's what little girls (boys) look like," is often sufficient.

Nursing Goal: Anticipatory Guidance About Sexual Activity and Family Planning

RESUMPTION OF SEXUAL ACTIVITY

Nursing interventions in the postpartal period acknowledge that the parent is also a sexual being. Couples were formerly discouraged from engaging in sexual intercourse until six weeks postpartum. Currently the couple is advised to abstain from intercourse until the episiotomy is healed and the lochial flow has stopped (usually by the end of the third week).

The woman's partner can test for vaginal tenderness by inserting one clean finger (lubricated with a water-based compound such as K-Y jelly) into the vaginal orifice. If no tenderness is experienced, two fingers may be inserted. If this illicits no tenderness, the vaginal vault is almost certainly healed. Because the vaginal vault is still "dry" (hormone-poor), some form of lubrication (K-Y jelly or contraceptive foam) may be necessary during intercourse. The

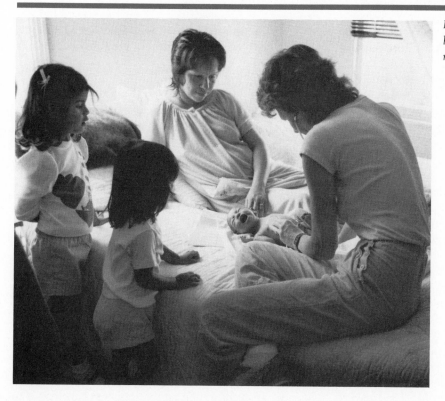

Figure 34–2 The sisters of this newborn became acquainted with the new family member during a nursing assessment.

female-superior or side-by-side positions for coitus may be preferable because they enable the woman to control the depth of penile penetration.

Breast-feeding couples need to be forewarned that, during orgasm, milk may spout from the nipples due to the release of oxytocin with sexual excitement and/or orgasm. Some couples find this pleasurable or amusing; other couples choose to have the woman wear a bra during sex. Nursing the baby prior to sexual activity may also decrease this.

Other factors may inhibit satisfactory sexual experience: The baby's crying may "spoil the mood"; the woman's changed body may be unattractive to some men and women; and maternal sleep deprivation may interfere with a mutually satisfying experience. Couples may also be frustrated if there are changes in the woman's physiologic response to sexual stimulation. These changes are due to hormonal changes and may persist for several months. Many couples report that even four months following delivery, they continue to experience a decline in sexual activity due to lingering discomfort in the woman (often related to episiotomy pain), fatigue, decreased physical strength, and dissatisfaction with personal appearance (Fischman et al 1986).

EDUCATION FOR SELF-CARE

Anticipatory guidance during the prenatal and postnatal period can forewarn the couple of these eventualities and of their temporary nature. Anticipatory guidance is enhanced if the couple can discuss their feelings and reactions as they are experienced. Postpartal discussion groups reassure and support couples.

Couples can be encouraged to express their affection and love through kissing, holding, and talking. Because the man's level of desire does not show the same decrease as the woman's, he requires forewarning that he may experience a decrease in sexual intercourse for up to a year following delivery (Fischman et al 1986).

○   *CONTRACEPTION*   Because many couples resume sexual activity before the postpartal examination, family-planning information should be made available before discharge. A couple's decision to use a contraceptive is often motivated by a desire to gain control over the number of children they will conceive or determine the spacing of future children. In choosing a specific method, consistency of use outweighs the absolute reliability of a given method. Risk factors and contraindications of the various methods must be identified by the nurse to help the couple select a contraceptive method that has practical application and is compatible with the couple's health and physical needs.

Often different methods of contraception are appropriate at different times in the couple's life. Thus they should have a clear understanding of the methods available

to them so that they can make an appropriate choice. The currently available contraceptive methods are discussed in detail in Chapter 8.

Nursing Goal: Preparation for Discharge

Ideally, preparation for discharge begins from the moment a woman enters the hospital or birthing center to deliver her baby. Nursing efforts should be directed toward assessing the couple's knowledge, expectations, and beliefs and then providing anticipatory guidance and teaching accordingly. Because many women remain hospitalized for such a brief time postpartally, it is vital for postpartum nurses to approach health teaching and education for self-care in a systematic way. Most agencies have developed flow sheets such as the one in Figure 34–3. The use of such a tool helps nurses complete teaching and identify any areas of knowledge deficit so that follow-up teaching can be planned.

Before the actual discharge the nurse should spend time with the couple to determine if they have any last-minute questions. In general, discharge teaching should include at least the following information:

1. The woman should contact her care giver if she develops any of the signs of possible complications:

   • Sudden persistent or spiking fever

   • Change in the character of the lochia—foul smell, return to bright red bleeding, excessive amount

   • Evidence of mastitis, such as breast tenderness, reddened areas, malaise

   • Evidence of thrombophlebitis, such as calf pain, tenderness, redness

   • Evidence of urinary tract infection, such as urgency, frequency, burning on urination

   • Continued severe or incapacitating postpartal depression

   • Evidence of infection in an incision (either episiotomy or cesarean), such as redness, edema, bruising, discharge, or lack of approximation

2. The woman should review the literature she has received that explains recommended postpartum exercises, the need for adequate rest, the need to avoid overexertion initially, and the recommendation to abstain from sexual intercourse until lochia has ceased. The woman may take either a tub bath or shower and may continue sitz baths at home if she desires.

3. The woman should be given the phone numbers of the postpartum unit and nursery and encouraged to call if she has any questions, no matter how simple.

4. The woman should receive information on local agencies and/or support groups, such as La Leche League and Mothers of Twins, that might be of particular assistance to her.

5. Both breast-feeding and bottle-feeding mothers should receive information geared to their specific nutritional needs. They should also be told to continue their vitamin and iron supplements until their postpartal examination.

6. The woman should have a scheduled appointment for her postpartal examination and for her infant's first well-baby examination before they are discharged.

7. The mother should clearly understand the correct procedure for obtaining copies of her infant's birth certificate.

8. The new parents should be able to provide basic care for their infants and should know when to anticipate that the cord will fall off; when the infant can have a tub bath; when the infant will need his or her first immunizations; and so on. They should also be comfortable feeding and handling the baby, and should be aware of basic safety considerations including the need to use a car seat whenever the infant is in a car.

9. The parents should also be aware of signs and symptoms in the infant that indicate possible problems and who they should contact about them (see p 910).

The nurse can also use this final period to reassure the couple of their ability to be successful parents. She can stress the infant's need to feel loved and secure. She can also urge parents to talk to each other and work together to solve any problems that may arise.

Nursing care is successful if:

● The woman experiences minor discomfort at most and has a clear understanding of measures she can employ to enhance her comfort.

● The woman is able to verbalize the need for adequate rest and has developed a plan (with the support of her family) to begin graded activity.

● The woman has had an opportunity to discuss her perceptions of her childbearing experience with an empathetic nurse and has some anticipatory knowledge of potential mood changes and emotions she may experience.

● The chosen infant feeding method is successful and the parents seem able to care for their child.

● There is evidence of positive parent-infant attachment.

● The couple clearly understand the available family planning methods and have chosen an option they find suitable for them.

● The woman clearly understands the discharge information she was given and is able to state the actions she will take if any complications develop.

● Care of the Postpartal Family After Cesarean Birth

After a cesarean birth the new mother has postpartal needs similar to those of her counterparts who delivered vaginally. Because she has undergone major abdominal surgery, however, the woman also has nursing care needs similar to those of other surgical clients.

Nursing Goal: Promotion of Maternal Physical Well-Being

The chances of pulmonary infection are increased due to immobility after the use of narcotics and sedatives, and because of the altered immune response in postoperative clients. For this reason, the woman is encouraged to cough and deep breathe every two to four hours while awake for the first few days following cesarean delivery. This procedure may be uncomfortable because it stretches the incisional area. Optimal results are more likely if coughing and deep breathing are done after pain medication has been given and while the abdominal incision is splinted with a pillow. The woman should take several deep breaths, then take another and cough at the end of inspiration.

Leg exercises are carried out every 15 minutes in conjunction with the postpartal check in the recovery room. The exercises should be continued every two hours throughout the first day or two until the woman is ambulatory. The leg exercises indicate when the woman has recovered from the anesthesia, increase circulation, and aid in the improvement of abdominal motility by tightening abdominal muscles.

By the second or third day the cesarean birth mother is usually receptive to learning how to care for herself and her infant. Special emphasis should be given to home management. She should be encouraged to let others assume responsibility for housekeeping and cooking. Fatigue not only prolongs recovery but also interferes with breast-feeding and mother-infant interaction. Demonstration of proper body mechanics in getting out of bed without the use of a side rail and ways of caring for the infant that prevent strain and torsion on the incision are also indicated.

The cesarean delivery woman usually does extremely well postoperatively. If delivery was accompanied by spinal anesthesia, the side effects of general anesthesia are avoided. Even after general anesthesia, however, most

Patient Name:

Medical Record Number:

(addressograph stamp)

STANFORD UNIVERSITY HOSPITAL
Stanford University Medical Center
Stanford, California 94305

TEACHING FLOW SHEET AND DISCHARGE PLANNING
INFANT CARE AND POSTPARTUM

Para_____ DD_____ Fdg _____ Other_____

KNOWLEDGE AND SKILLS TO BE TAUGHT	INSTRUCTIONS/ INITIALS		PATIENT/AND OR SIGNIFICANT OTHER VERBALIZES AND/OR DEMONSTRATES UNDERSTANDING		POST-TEACHING COMMENTS/FOLLOW-UP
	Verbal	Demon.	Return Demon.	Assessment	
OBSERVING BABY					
1. General Appearance			xxxx		
2. Senses		xxxx	xxxx		
3. Protective Reflexes		xxxx	xxxx		
4. Vital Signs -including Temp. Taking					
5. Circulation		xxxx	xxxx		
6. Rashes		xxxx	xxxx		
7. Reflexes of Newborn			xxxx		
8. Stool Cycle		xxxx	xxxx		
9. Emotional Needs		xxxx	xxxx		
BATHING BABY					
1. Shampoo					
2. Bath					
DIAPERING WRAPPING HOLDING BABY					
1. Cradle					
2. Football					
FEEDING					
1. Schedule		xxxx			
2. Reflexes					
3. Bottle					
4. Breast		xxxx			
5. Bubble or Burp					
LAYETTE-LISTS OF SUGGESTIONS		xxxx	xxxx		
PERI-CARE					
1. Hospital (e.g., Sitz Bath)		xxxx			
2. Home		xxxx			
3. Episiotomy		xxxx			
BREAST CARE					
1. If Breast Feeding		xxxx			
2. If Not Breast Feeding		xxxx			
LOCHIAL CHANGES		xxxx	xxxx		
UTERINE INVOLUTION		xxxx	xxxx		
BLADDER FUNCTION		xxxx	xxxx		
AFTERCONTRACTIONS		xxxx	xxxx		
REST		xxxx	xxxx		
DIET		xxxx	xxxx		
EARLY AMBULATION ADVANTAGES		xxxx	xxxx		

Assessment Code: V - Verbalizes concept accurately
                     D - Demonstrates concept safely
                     C - Confidence building needed (V and D accomplished)
                     R - Repeat, Redemonstrate, Remind
                     O - Offered, but refused teaching
               N/A - Not Applicable

Patient Name:

Medical Record Number:

(addressograph stamp)

STANFORD UNIVERSITY HOSPITAL
Stanford University Medical Center
Stanford, California 94305

TEACHING FLOW SHEET AND DISCHARGE PLANNING
INFANT CARE AND POSTPARTUM

KNOWLEDGE AND SKILLS TO BE TAUGHT	INSTRUCTIONS/ INITIALS		PATIENT / AND OR SIGNIFICANT OTHER VERBALIZES AND /OR DEMONSTRATES UNDERSTANDING		POST TEACHING COMMENTS / FOLLOW–UP
	Verbal	Demon.	Return Demon.	Assessment	
FAMILY PLANNING INFORMATION					
EMOTIONAL CHANGES FOR NEW PARENTS		xxxx	xxxx		
OTHER CHILDREN AT HOME		xxxx	xxxx		
BODY MECHANICS AND EXERCISES					
OTHER					

The content of each item with added detail is listed in the Master Teaching Guide.

Assessment Code: V - Verbalizes concept accurately
                       D - Demonstrates concept safely
                       C - Confidence building needed (V and D accomplished)
                       R - Repeat, Redemonstrate, Remind
                       O - Offered, but refused teaching
                       N/A - Not Applicable

DISCHARGE PLANNING

Public Health Referral: (All Clinic patients must have a referral)

Written _____

Sent _____

Follow-Up Appointment Made:

Clinic Appt. - Mother _____

Clinic Appt. - Baby _____

Private M.D. Appt. _____

Social Worker Consult _____

Other follow-up:

Home Assistance _____

Child Protective Services _____

_____ _____

_____ _____

Figure 34–3 A teaching flow sheet and discharge planning guide helps focus health teaching. (Courtesy of Stanford University Hospital, Stanford, California)

women are ambulating by the day after the surgery. Usually by the second or third postpartal day the incision can be covered with plastic wrap so the woman can shower, which seems to provide a mental as well as physical lift. If staples have been used, the incision is sometimes left open to the air and showering is permitted without covering it. Most women are discharged by the fourth or fifth postoperative day, although some go home as early as the third day after delivery.

Nursing Goal: Promotion of Comfort and Relief of Pain

Monitoring and management of the woman's pain is carried out during the postpartum period. Sources of pain include incisional pain, gas pain, referred shoulder pain, periodic uterine contractions (afterbirth pains), and pain from voiding, defecation, or constipation. Incisional and afterbirth pains are most intense during the immediate postpartum period and decrease in intensity and frequency with time.

Nursing interventions are oriented toward preventing or alleviating pain or helping the woman cope with pain. The nurse should undertake the following measures:

- Administer analgesics as needed, especially during the first 24 to 72 hours. Their use will improve the woman's outlook and enable her to be more mobile and active.

- Offer comfort through proper positioning, backrubs, oral care, and the reduction of noxious stimuli such as noise and unpleasant odors.

- Encourage the presence of significant others, including the newborn. This practice provides distraction from the painful sensations and helps reduce the woman's fear and anxiety.

- Encourage the use of breathing, relaxation, and distraction (for example, stimulation of cutaneous tissue) techniques taught in childbirth preparation class.

Some agencies also use transcutaneous electrical nerve stimulation therapy (TENS) following a cesarean delivery to provide pain relief without the use of frequent medication (Frink & Chally 1984).

Discomfort resulting from the accumulation of gas in the intestines usually reaches its peak on the third postoperative day. It is a normal physiologic phenomena resulting from (a) exposure of intestines to air; (b) slowing of gastrointestinal motility due to anesthesia and narcotics with subsequent increase in peristalsis; (c) material previously in the gastrointestinal tract contributing to gas formation; and (d) uncoordinated bowel activity. Measures to

prevent or minimize gas pains include leg exercises, abdominal tightening, ambulation, avoiding carbonated or very hot or cold beverages, avoiding the use of straws, and providing a high-protein, semisolid diet for the first 24 to 48 hours.

The woman may find it helpful to lie prone or on her left side. Lying on the left side allows gas to rise from the descending colon to the sigmoid colon so that it can be expelled more readily. Other women report that a rocking chair helps them obtain relief. Medical interventions for gas pain include the use of antiflatulents (such as Mylicon), suppositories, and enemas.

Preventive measures to avoid pain secondary to constipation include encouraging fluids and administering a stool softener or mild cathartic.

The nurse can be quite instrumental in minimizing discomfort and promoting success and satisfaction as the mother assumes the activities of her new role. Especially for the mother who has intravenous lines in place, instruction and assistance in assuming comfortable positions when holding and/or breast-feeding the infant will do much to increase her sense of competence and comfort. Sitting in a chair or tailor fashion in bed, leaning slightly forward with the infant propped on a pillow in her lap will prevent irritation to the incision. Another preferred position for breast-feeding during the first postoperative days is lying on the side with the newborn positioned along the mother's body.

Nursing Goal: Facilitation of Parent-Infant Attachment

Several factors associated with cesarean birth can promote or inhibit the participation, reciprocal feedback, and synchrony that the mother and infant bring to the initial discovery period. Contributing factors that can make the attachment process more difficult include the physical condition of the mother and her newborn and maternal reactions to separation, stress, anesthesia, and other drugs.

The mother and newborn may be separated after birth because of hospital routines, prematurity, or neonatal morbidity. Healthy babies born by uncomplicated cesarean delivery are not more fragile than their vaginal route counterparts. More agencies are beginning to provide time for the family together in the operating room if the mother's and newborn's conditions permit. However, some agencies still automatically place cesarean newborns in the high-risk nursery for a time.

A mother may feel joy that her infant has been delivered successfully, but she may also react with some hostility toward the infant whose birth necessitated a major assault on her body with its subsequent discomforts. Signs of depression, anger, or withdrawal may indicate a grief response to the loss of the fantasized vaginal birth experience. Fathers as well as mothers may experience feelings of "missing out," guilt that the surgery was the result of something they did "wrong," and even jealousy toward another couple who had a vaginal delivery. The couple may also feel guilty that they are considering their personal needs and not simply the welfare of the infant. Leach and Sproule (1984) point out that the concern of the parents to act in the best interests of their child does not negate their own sense of grief for the loss they experienced.

The nurse can support the parents in a variety of ways. Initially nurses must work through their own feelings about cesarean birth. The nurse who considers a vaginal birth "normal" and refers to it as such, indicates that a cesarean birth is, therefore, "abnormal" rather than simply an alternative method of delivery. By the same token, referring to a woman as "the section" turns her into an object. Thus language and terminology, though seemingly insignificant, can convey to the couple negative messages about their cesarean birth experience.

The nurse should offer positive support to the couple. The cesarean birth couple needs the opportunity to tell their story repeatedly to work through their feelings. As an empathetic listener the nurse can provide factual information about their situation and support whatever effective coping behaviors the couple have in dealing with surgery and the postpartal recovery period. The nurse should provide the parents with choices by allowing them to participate in decision making about the options available to them (for example, participating in rooming-in).

The perception of and reactions to a cesarean birth experience depend on how the woman defines that experience. Her reality is what she perceives it to be. If the woman's attitude is more positive than negative, successful resolution of subsequent stressful events is more likely. Because the definition of events is transitory in nature, the possibility of change and growth is present. Often the mothering role is perceived as an extension of the childbearing role, and inability to fulfill expected childbearing behavior (vaginal birth) may lead to parental feelings of role failure and frustration. The nurse can help families alter their negative definitions of cesarean birth, and bolster and encourage positive perceptions.

● **Care of the Adolescent on the Postpartal Unit**

The adolescent may have special postpartal needs, depending on her level of maturity, support systems, and cultural background. The nurse needs to assess maternal-infant interaction, roles of support people, plans for discharge, knowledge of childrearing, and plans for follow-up care. It is imperative to have a community health service be in touch with the young woman shortly after discharge.

Nursing Goal: Anticipatory Guidance About Contraception

Contraception counseling is an important part of teaching. As previously discussed, the incidence of repeat pregnancies during adolescence is high and the younger the adolescent, the more likely she is to become pregnant again. Often the young woman tells the nurse that she does not plan on engaging in sex again. This denial mechanism is unrealistic, and the nurse must help the young woman realize this. The nurse should make sure that the woman has some method of birth control available to her, and that she understands ovulation and fertility in relation to her menstrual cycle. This is an excellent opportunity for sex education.

Nursing Goal: Promotion of Parenting Skills

The nurse has many opportunities for teaching the adolescent about the newborn in the postpartal unit. It is important to remember that the nurse serves as a role model; therefore, the manner in which she handles the newborn greatly influences the young mother. The father should be included in as much of the teaching as possible.

A newborn physical exam done at the client's bedside accomplishes several goals. The mother has immediate feedback about the newborn's health; she is able to observe the many facets of her baby and sees the proper manner in which to handle the infant. The nurse can teach as the examination progresses, giving the new mother information about the fontanelles, cradle cap, shampooing the newborn's hair, and so on. The nurse might also use this time to teach the young mother about infant stimulation techniques. Because adolescent mothers tend to concentrate their interactions in the physical domain, they need to comprehend the importance of verbal, visual, and auditory stimulation for newborns as well.

Performing an examination at the bedside also gives the adolescent permission to explore her newborn, which she may have been hesitant to do. A Brazelton neonatal assessment (see Chapter 28) will help the client understand her newborn's response to stimuli, a key factor in the client's response to the individuality of her newborn once she goes home. Parents who have some idea of what to expect from their infants will be less frustrated with the newborn's behavior.

The adolescent mother appreciates positive feedback about her fine newborn and her developing maternal responses. This praise and encouragement will increase her confidence and self-esteem.

Group classes for adolescent mothers should include infant care skills, information about growth and development, infant feeding, well-baby care, and danger signals in the ill newborn. An excellent way to incorporate neurologic

THE ROAD NOT TAKEN

A teenage mother's courageous decision reminds her nurse of an earlier time, a remote road, and a different choice.

As I walked along the corridor, I heard a soft voice call, "Nurse!" Once inside room 5622, I saw a delicately pretty teenager holding, rather awkwardly, a squirming newborn. In one hand she clutched a bottle with a little less than half an ounce of formula gone.

"He won't eat. What am I doing wrong?"

Ann Marie wasn't my patient, but who could walk away from that innocent first-time mother's plea? To avoid further chipping away at what little confidence any new mother—especially one so young—may have, I usually avoid "taking over" and efficiently feeding the infant.

"Some newborns need a little extra encouragement at first. Others are just stubborn and refuse to eat until they're good and ready. Let's try to find out which type this little guy is.

"First, we'll make sure nothing else is bothering him. Why don't you see if he needs to have his diaper changed?"

Solemnly, Ann Marie confessed, "I'm sorry. I don't know how."

I shot a quick glance at the bassinet card. Baby Boy E was two days old. In our family-centered maternity unit, teaching is a high priority. As soon as a mother is up to it, we teach her the basics of infant care. Most mothers are well on their way before the day is over. How did Ann Marie slip through the cracks?

More than that was out of sync here. The room was too dark for 10 A.M. I saw no flowers, no cards, no baby toys. From the look of things, Ann Marie had even made her own bed. And why did I feel so drawn to her?

I helped her change the baby's diaper, and with a little coaxing and a few simple "tricks of the trade," I got him to take a little more formula for his mom. Then, hoping to pick up a few more clues, I headed for the nurses' station.

As soon as I reached for Ann Marie's chart, "information" came at me from all sides.

"How could that sweet young girl put that beautiful baby up for adoption?"

"Well, the father walked away from her when she was only five months pregnant. Maybe that's why."

"But she's 19, and she's got her mother to help her. And it's not that difficult to raise a baby by yourself *these days*." (This from a mother of two with a working husband and a home of their own.)

"She loves that baby. Why else would she want it in the room with her all the time? Mark my words: She'll keep it. A baby belongs with its *natural* mother."

I've never been hit by a tidal wave, but at that moment I thought I knew something about what it must feel like. So that's why no one is teaching her anything, and that's why no one goes near her—except Sister Cecelia, the Catholic nun from the children's home where the adoption had been arranged.

But that wasn't all. You see, I was in Ann Marie's shoes once. Nineteen, pregnant, alone—and seeing, as Robert Frost did, "Two roads diverged in a yellow wood. . . ." All that the philosophers at the nurses' station know is that I have a teenager that anyone would be proud of. But only I know at what cost—to me and to her.

What they also don't know is that I've learned a little about why people adopt babies. Years of infer-

(continued)

development and stimulation for newborns is to teach the mothers how to make a few simple toys, such as mobiles and wall hangings.

Lunch groups can be organized around discussions of topics that interest adolescents. These are ideal times to explore the young mothers' ideas about cuddling and rocking their newborns, ways to handle crying, misbehavior, and "spoiling." The nurse can correct misconceptions. Jarrett (1982) found that young mothers were deficient in their knowledge and expectations of their newborns. In her study, nearly half of the adolescents expected their infants to be toilet trained by less than 12 months of age; three-quarters of her sample expected obedient behavior before 12 months. These findings demonstrate the need for education regarding growth and development.

Ideally, teenage mothers should visit adolescent clinics where mother and newborn are assessed for several years after birth. In this way, classes on parenting, vocational guidance, and school attendance can be followed closely. School systems' classes for young mothers are an excellent way of helping adolescents finish school and learn how to parent at the same time.

● **Care of the Woman With an Unwanted Pregnancy**

Sometimes a pregnancy is unwanted. The expectant woman may be an adolescent, unmarried, or economically

THE ROAD NOT TAKEN (continued)

tility, perinatal loss, unrequited love for children—each makes an adoptive couple go to extraordinary lengths to get what others take for granted.

All I saw at that moment was a very brave girl about to make some childless couple's dream come true—and not because she doesn't love her baby, but because she does, probably far more than her critics could imagine.

Minutes later, Sister Cecelia came to visit. Before she went in to see Ann Marie, I talked to her about how adoptions are currently "handled." (Few babies are adopted from our hospital these days, but I do recall a few adoptions years ago, when it was taboo even to let the mother *see* the baby, let alone care for it herself.)

Sister explained that their philosophy includes support for all parties involved, including the biological mother. By giving her the opportunity to care for her baby, she can work through any feelings of doubt she may have. She can give her baby something—a little of herself, a name for the birth record, perhaps some clothing. She has something to keep and to treasure—some memories, a few photographs, a bassinet card. She has time to think and to be sure, with the help of a supportive, nonjudgmental person, that her decision is not so much "best" (because no one really knows that), but that it is the decision that

she alone makes unselfishly out of her love for her baby.

I, too, love my child, and still feel good when someone says, "you've done such a great job with her" or "I don't know how you do it" or "She's a real credit to you." I don't regret my decision. But had there been a Sister Ceclia by my side, perhaps my daughter would now be a credit to someone else—perhaps not.

Being with Ann Marie was easy for me. Ironically, she was my patient the following day—the day she was to leave the hospital with her mother, her baby, and Sister Cecelia (to whom she would give the baby later that day). We talked about many things—about children, about school, about traveling. I taught her how to care for herself after discharge, and I helped her dress the baby. I wheeled her downstairs with the baby in her arms. Then it was time to say good-bye.

All I said was, "I wish I had words to tell you how very brave I think you are." Tears streamed down her cheeks, and down mine. She thanked me. Then she left the hospital without so much as an inkling of what we might have shared—had either of us chosen the other road.

(Reprinted with permission from the *American Journal of Nursing*—Janowski 1987.)

---

restricted. She may dislike children or the idea of being a mother. She may feel that she is not emotionally ready for the responsibilities of parenthood. Her partner may disapprove of the pregnancy. These and many other reasons may cause the woman to continue to reject the idea of her pregnancy. An emotional crisis arises as she attempts to resolve the problem. She may choose to have an abortion, to carry the fetus to term and keep the baby, or to have the baby and relinquish it for adoption.

Many mothers who choose to give their infants up for adoption are young and/or unmarried. More young women choose to keep the child than to give it up, however. Approximately two-thirds of children born out of wedlock are raised by their mothers alone.

The decision of a mother to relinquish her infant is an extremely difficult one. Harvey (1977) reports that there are social pressures against giving up one's child. Some women may want to prove to themselves that they can manage on their own by keeping their infants.

The mother who chooses to let her child be adopted usually experiences intense ambivalence. These feelings may heighten just before delivery and upon seeing her baby. After childbirth, the mother will need to complete a grieving process to work through her loss.

Nursing Goal: Provision of Support to the Woman Relinquishing Her Infant

The woman with an unwanted pregnancy must make the difficult decision: whether to have the child or have an abortion. If she decides to complete the pregnancy, she must decide whether to keep the baby. During this difficult time, the expectant woman may look to others, such as the nurse, for help in making these decisions. The woman should be given information rather than direct advice during this time and should be allowed to discuss her situation and work through the problem.

The mother who decides to relinquish the child usually has made considerable adjustments in her life-style to give birth to this child. She may not have told friends and relatives about the pregnancy and so lacks an extended support system. During the prenatal period, the nurse can help her by encouraging her to express her grief, loneliness, guilt, and other feelings.

When the relinquishing mother is admitted to the maternity unit, the staff should be informed about the mother's decision to relinquish the infant. Any special requests for delivery should be respected, and the woman should be encouraged to express her emotions (Harvey

Postpartal Physical Assessment Guide:
Two Weeks and Six Weeks After Delivery

Assess/normal findings	Alterations and possible causes*	Nursing reponses to data†
VITAL SIGNS		
Blood pressure: Return to normal pre-pregnant level	Elevated blood pressure (anxiety, essential hypertension, renal disease)	Review history, evaluate normal baseline; refer to physician if necessary.
Pulse: 60–90 beats/min (or prepregnant normal rate)	Increased pulse rate (excitement, anxiety, cardiac disorders)	Count pulse for full minute, note irregularities; marked tachycardia or beat irregularities require additional assessment and possible physician referral.
Respirations: 16–24/min	Marked tachypnea or abnormal patterns (respiratory disorders)	Evaluate for respiratory disease; refer to physician if necessary
Temperature: 36.2C–37.6C (98F–99.6F)	Increased temperature (infection)	Assess for signs and symptoms of infection or disease state.
WEIGHT		
2 weeks: probable weight loss of 14–20+ lb	Little or no weight loss (fluid retention, subinvolution, poor dietary habits)	Evaluate dietary habits and nutritional state; review blood pressure to evaluate fluid retention or blood losses.
6 weeks: returning to normal prepregnant weight	Retained weight (poor dietary habits)	Determine amount of daily exercise. Refer to dietitian if necessary for dietary counseling.
	Extreme weight loss (excessive dieting)	Discuss appropriate diets; refer to dietitian if necessary.
BREASTS		
Nonnursing: 2 weeks: may have mild tenderness; small amount of milk may be expressed; breasts returning to prepregnant size 6 weeks: soft, with no tenderness; return to prepregnant size	Some engorgement (incomplete suppression of lactation) Redness; marked tenderness (mastitis) Palpable mass (tumor)	Engorgement usually seen only when no medication has been given to suppress lactation; advise client to wear a supportive, well-fitted bra, avoid hot showers, etc. (see p 935); evaluate for signs and symptoms of mastitis (rare in nonnursing mothers).
Nursing: Full, with prominent nipples; lactation established	Cracked, fissured nipples (feeding problems) Redness, marked tenderness, or even abscess formation (mastitis) Palpable mass (full milk duct, tumor)	Counsel about nipple care (see p 933). Evaluate client condition, evidence of fever; refer to physician for initiation of antibiotic therapy, if indicated. Opinion varies as to value of breast examination for nursing mothers; some feel a nursing mother should examine her breasts monthly, after feeding, when breasts are empty; if palpable mass is felt, refer to physician for further evaluation. For breast inflammation instruct the mother to: 1. Keep breast empty by frequent feeding. 2. Rest when possible. 3. Take aspirin for pain. 4. Force fluids. If symptoms persist for more than 24 hours, instruct her to call her physician.

*Possible causes of alterations are place in parentheses.
†This column provides guidelines for further assessment and initial nursing interventions.

Postpartal Physical Assessment Guide:
Two Weeks and Six Weeks After Delivery (continued)

Assess/normal findings	Alterations and possible causes*	Nursing reponses to data†
ABDOMINAL MUSCULATURE		
2 weeks: improved firmness; although "bread dough" consistency is not unusual, especially in multipara Striae pink and obvious Cesarean incision healing	Marked diastasis recti (relaxation of muscles) Drainage, redness, tenderness, pain, edema (infection)	Evaluate exercise level; provide information on appropriate exercise program. Evaluate for infection; refer to physician if necessary.
6 weeks: muscle tone continues to improve; striae may be beginning to fade, may not achieve a silvery appearance for several more weeks; linea nigra fading		
ELIMINATION PATTERN		
Urinary tract:		
Return to prepregnant urinary elimination routine	Urinary incontinence, especially when lifting, coughing, laughing, and so on (urethral trauma, cystocele) Pain or burning when voiding, urgency and/or frequency, pus or WBC in urine, pathogenic organisms in culture (urinary tract infection)	Assess for cystocele; instruct in appropriate muscle tightening exercises; refer to physician. Evaluate for urinary tract infection; obtain clean-catch urine; refer to physician for treatment if indicated.
Routine urinalysis within normal limits (proteinuria disappeared)	Sugar or ketone in urine—may be some lactose present in urine of breast-feeding mothers (diabetes)	Evaluate diet; assess for signs and symptoms of diabetes; refer to physician.
Bowel habits:		
2 weeks: may still be some discomfort with defecation, especially if client had severe hemorrhoids or 3–4° extension	Severe constipation or pain when defecating (trauma or hemorrhoids)	Discuss dietary patterns; encourage fluid, adequate roughage. Continue use of stool softener if necessary to prevent pain associated with straining; continue sitz baths, periods of rest for severe hemorrhoids; assess healing of episiotomy and/or lacerations; severe constipation may require administration of laxatives, stool softeners, and an enema.
6 weeks: return to normal prepregnancy bowel elimination	Marked constipation	See above.
	Fecal incontinence or constipation (rectocele)	Assess for evidence of rectocele; instruct in muscle tightening exercises; refer to physician.
REPRODUCTIVE TRACT		
Lochia:		
2 weeks: lochia alba, scant amounts, fleshy odor	Foul odor, excessive in amount (infection) Return to lochia rubra or persistence of lochia rubra or serosa	Assess for evidence of infection and/or subinvolution; culture lochia; refer to physician.
6 weeks: no lochia, or return to normal menstruation pattern	See above	See above.
Pelvic examination:		
2 weeks: uterus no longer palpable abdominally; external os closed; uterine muscles still somewhat lax and uterus may be displaced; introitus of vagina still lacking tone—gapes when intraabdominal pressure is increased by coughing or straining Episiotomy and/or lacerations healing; no signs of infection	External cervical os open, uterus not decreasing appropriately (subinvolution, infection) Evidence of redness, tenderness, poor tissue approximation in episiotomy and/or laceration (wound infection)	Assess for evidence of subinvolution and/or infection; refer to physician if indicated.

*Possible causes of alterations are place in parentheses.
†This column provides guidelines for further assessment and initial nursing interventions.

Postpartal Physical Assessment Guide: Two Weeks and Six Weeks After Delivery (continued)

Assess/normal findings	Alterations and possible causes*	Nursing reponses to data†
6 weeks: almost returned to prepregnant size with almost completely restored muscle tone Cervix completely closed with only transverse slit apparent Good return of muscle tone to pelvic floor	Continued flow of lochia, some opening of cervical os, failure to decrease appropriately in size (subinvolution) Marked relaxation of pelvic floor muscles (uterine prolapse)	Assess for evidence of subinvolution and/or infection; refer to physician for further evaluation and for dilatation and curettage if necessary. Assess for evidence of uterine prolapse; discuss appropriate perineal exercises; refer to physician if indicated.
Papanicolaou test: Negative	Test results show atypical cells	Refer to physician for further evaluation and treatment.
HEMOGLOBIN AND HEMATOCRIT LEVELS		
6 weeks: Hb at least 12 g/dL Hct 37% ± 5%	Hb < 12 g/dL Hct 32% or less (anemia)	Assess nutritional status, begin (or continue) supplemental iron; for marked anemia (Hb 9 g/dL) additional assessment and/or physician referral may be necessary.

*Possible causes of alterations are placed in parentheses.
†This column provides guidelines for further assessment and initial nursing interventions.

1977). After the delivery the mother should be allowed access to the infant; she will decide whether she wants to see the newborn. Seeing the newborn often facilitates the grieving process. When the mother sees her baby, she may feel strong attachment and love. The nurse needs to assure the woman that these feelings do not mean that her decision to relinquish the child is a wrong one; relinquishment is often a painful act of love (Arms 1984). Postpartal nursing management also includes arranging ongoing care for the relinquishing mother.

Nursing Goal: Promotion of Acceptance When Woman Denies Pregnancy

Initial denial of pregnancy by women usually moves into acceptance of the pregnant state. Occasionally, however, a nurse may encounter a woman who denies she is pregnant even as she is admitted to the maternity unit. It may seem impossible that a woman who is so obviously pregnant could maintain this delusion. Because of this denial, the woman has not sought prenatal care. Preparation for the birth experience may be incomplete, and the mother and infant may be at risk.

The nurse must establish a trusting relationship with this woman. While building rapport with the woman, the nurse should gently guide the woman to accept reality.

Nursing Goal: Promotion of Family Wellness

In the event that a woman decides to keep an unwanted child, the nurse should be aware of the potential for parenting problems. Families with unwanted children are more crisis prone than others, although in many cases, parents grow to love their child after attachment occurs. The nurse should be ready to initiate crisis strategies or make appropriate referrals as the need arises.

● Follow-up Care of the Postpartum Family

The first several postpartal weeks have been termed *the fourth trimester* to stress the idea of continuity as the family adjusts to having a new member and as the woman's body returns to a prepregnant state. During this period the woman must accomplish certain physical and developmental tasks (Gruis 1977):

● Restoring physical condition

● Developing competence in caring for and meeting the needs of her infant

● Establishing a relationship with her new child

● Adapting to altered life-styles and family structure resulting from the addition of a new member

The new mother and her family may have an inadequate or incorrect understanding of what to expect during the early postpartal weeks. She may be concerned with restoring her figure and surprised because of continuing physical discomfort from sore breasts, episiotomy, or hemorrhoids. Fatigue is perhaps her greatest yet most underestimated problem during the early weeks. This may be

Postpartal Psychologic Assessment Guide

Assess/normal findings	Alterations and possible causes*	Nursing response to data†
ATTACHMENT		
Attachment demonstrated by soothing, cuddling, and talking to infant; appropriate feeding techniques; eye-to-eye contact; calling infant by name.	Failure to attach is demonstrated by lack of behaviors associated with bonding process, calling infant by nickname that promotes ridicule, inadequate infant weight gain, infant dirty, hygienic measures are not being maintained, severe diaper rash, failure to obtain adequate supplies to provide infant care (malattachment).	Provide counseling; refer to public health nurse for continued home visits.
ADJUSTMENT TO PARENTAL ROLE		
Parents are coping with new roles in terms of division of labor, financial status, communication, readjustment of sexual relations, and adjusting to new daily tasks.	Parents are unable to adjust to new roles (immaturity, inadequate education and preparation, ineffective communication patterns, inadequate support, current family crisis).	Provide counseling; refer to parent groups.
EDUCATION		
Mother understands self-care measures.	Mother demonstrates inadequate knowledge of self-care (inadequate education).	Provide education and counseling.
Parents are knowledgeable regarding infant care.	Parents demonstrate inadequate knowledge of infant care (inadequate education).	
Siblings are adjusting to new baby.	Excessive sibling rivalry is evident.	
Parents have chosen a method of contraception.	Birth control method has not been chosen.	

*Possible causes of alterations are placed in parentheses.
†This column provides guidelines for further assessment and initial nursing interventions.

aggravated if she has no extended family support or if there are other young children at home.

Developing skill and confidence in caring for an infant may be especially anxiety provoking for a new mother. As she struggles to establish a mutually acceptable pattern with her baby, small unanticipated concerns may seem monumental. The woman may begin to feel inadequate and, if she lacks support systems, isolated.

Nurses in some agencies are making home visits a few days after discharge to provide follow-up teaching and care. Many obstetricians and nurse practitioners now routinely see all postpartal women one to two weeks after delivery in addition to the routine six-week checkup. Others are advocating that the traditional six-week exam be rescheduled to four weeks postpartally (McKay & Mahan 1985). This extra visit provides an opportunity for physical assessment as well as assessment of the mother's psychologic and informational needs.

Nursing Assessments

Assessments are performed at two weeks and six weeks after birth. The routine physical assessment focuses on the woman's general appearance, breasts, reproductive tract, bladder and bowel elimination, and any specific problems or complaints (see the accompanying Postpartal Physical Assessment Guide). In addition, conversation is used to determine nutrition patterns, fatigue level, family adjustment, and psychologic status of the mother (see the Postpartal Psychologic Assessment Guide on p 1120). Any problems with child care are explored, and referral to a pediatric nurse practitioner or pediatrician is made if needed. Available community resources, including Public Health Department follow-up visits, are mentioned when appropriate. Family planning is discussed to answer any questions the couple may have about the birth control method they have chosen.

In ideal situations a family approach involving the father, infant, and possibly other siblings would permit a total evaluation and provide an opportunity for all family members to ask questions and express concerns. In addition, disturbed family patterns might be more readily diagnosed so that therapy could be instituted to prevent future problems of neglect or abuse.

POSTPARTUM FOLLOW-UP GUIDE
General Information and Significant History

Date _____

Mother's Name _____

Address _____

Phone _____

Marital Status _____ Para _____ Gravida _____ Age _____

Education _____ Employment _____

Prenatal Care _____ Childbirth Education _____

Name(s) of Significant Other(s) _____

Primary Nurse _____

Obstetric Physician _____

Pediatric Physician _____

Other _____

Describe initial postpartum follow-up contact:
(telephone, home visit, clinic)
Significant Personal History:

Significant Antepartal History:
Significant Family History:

Assessment		Intervention	Evaluation	Follow-up
Maternal	**Self-care**	**Maternal**		
Physiologic	Nutrition	Discomfort		
Breasts	Basic four tid plus	Rest		
Engorgement	Fluids	Medication		
Nipples	Vitamins	Nutrition		
Other	Rest/nocturnal	Fluids		
Perineum	Naps	Exercise		
Episiotomy	Breasts	Breasts		
Lacerations	Nipple care	Nipple care		
Hemorrhoids	Massage	Clothing		
Eliminations	Self breast exam	Hygiene		
Bladder	Perineum	Technique		
Bowel	Episiotomy care	Perineum		
Cesarean incision	Hygiene regimen	Hygiene		
Appearance	Rx of pain	Treatment regimen		
Drainage	Sexuality	Sexuality		
Care and cleansing	Vaginal rest	Family planning		
Discomforts and	Family planning	Resumption of intercourse		
concerns	Exercise			
	Appropriate to			
	puerperium			
	Postpartum exercise			
	regimen			
	Mobilization of supports	Using support system		
	Family	Exploring supports		
	Friends	Strategies to use support		
	Other assistance	Handling unwelcome interference		
Maternal role-taking				
Expectations		Coping strategies		
Labor and birth (length, pain, support, etc.)		Adaptability		
Related to newborn (gender, appearance, size)		Information seeking		
Related to mothering (fantasy/reality, ability, etc.)		Increased flexibility		
Experience		Reorganizing		
Previous mothering		Expanding and use supports		
Preparation for parenthood		Bibliotherapy recommended		
Confidence/competence		reading		
Infant feeding				
Infant comforting				
Care and hygiene				
Infant bath				
Umbilical care				
Circumcision care				
Diapering and perineal care				
Verbal identifying		Parent-Infant Interaction		
Name _____ (s/he, it)		Infant states		
Describes infant behaviors, cues, and rhythms		Infant behavioral characteristics		
		Specific cues (hunger,		
		fatigue, distress, etc.)		
Verbal expression of affection "_____"		Sensory stimulation		
Physical expressions of affection (en face,		Contingent caregiving		
positioning, caress, kiss, etc.)				
Infant		Essentials of infant care		
Physiologic		Feeding		
Physical assessment:		Method		
Via report _____		Frequency		
(source and circumstance)		Duration		
Via exam _____				

Figure 34–4 Sample health assessment form to be completed by the nurse on all the members of the childbearing family (Used with permission of NAACOG)

Assessment	Intervention	Evaluation	Follow-up

Vital Signs
  Temp
  Pulse
  Respirations
Color
  Jaundice
  Cyanosis
Skin
  Rashes
  Ecchymosis
  Inflammation
Eyes
Fontanelles
Central nervous system
  Reflexes observed/reported
Genitals
Elimination
  Bladder (frequency, color)
  Bowel (frequency, color, consistency)
Nutrition
  Feeding (method, frequency, quantity, satiation)
Hygiene
  Bathing (method, frequency, safety)
  Umbilicus
  Circumcision
  Perineal cleansing
  Diapering regimen
Sleep/activity patterns
  Sleep/wake pattern (typical 24-hour)
  Irritability
  Consolability (methods and effectiveness)
  Self-comforting (methods and effectiveness)
  Cuddliness
  Responsiveness to caregiver
    Visual
    Auditory
    Smile
  Clarity of cues
	Pre-feeding infant care
	  Satiation cues
	  Bubbling
	Hygiene
	  Bathing
	    Method
	    Safety
	    Organization
	  Eyes
	  Ears
	  Umbilicus
	  Perineum
	    Genitals
	    Diapering
	
	Knowledge of development needs
	Knowledge regarding safety and
	  signs of illness		

Father
Involvement
  Past Experience
  Preparation for this birth
  Style of involvement during pregnant/birth
  Involvement postpartum
  Support to mother (psychological/practical)
  Participation in care of siblings
Self-Care
  Rest
  Nutrition
	Expectations and reality
	  Exploring expectations and
	    myths
	  Identifying primary stressors
	
	Parent growth and development
	
	Importance of father in care of
	  mother and infant		

Father role-taking
  Expectations vs. reality
  Participation in infant care
    Feeding
    Diapering
    Bathing
    Comforting
    Entertaining
	Common stressors of fourth
	  trimester
	
	Crisis balancing factors
	
	Discuss smoking, alcohol, and
	  medications related to
	  breastfeeding		

Siblings
  Age(s)
  Gender(s)
  Preparation
  Expectations
  Initial responses to mother/parents
  Initial responses to infant
  Participation in infant care
  Parent actions to support siblings
  Role of extended family/friends
	Siblings
	  Needs and fears related to
	    new baby
	  Age appropriate regression
	  Strategies for meeting
	    sibling special needs
	  Books for sibling		

Nursing Goal: Promotion of Family Wellness

A trend toward early discharge following delivery has evolved over the past few years, and many women and their newborns leave the hospital or birthing center within 6 to 48 hours following delivery. Proponents cite decreased cost, less exposure of mother and baby to iatrogenic infection, enhanced parent-infant attachment, and decreased disruption of family life as advantages of this practice. However, this practice does raise questions about possible health risks if follow-up care is not provided. In a study of 925 families that were discharged early, Jansson (1985) reported that on home visits, common maternal problems included breast-feeding difficulties, transitory depression, fatigue, pain, and potential attachment problems. The most common problems for the infant included jaundice and inadequate breast-feeding. In most cases the nurse was able to resolve the problem using established protocols; in some cases a telephone consultation with a nurse-midwife or physician was necessary, while some cases required that the woman be seen at the health care agency.

Follow-up care for the postpartal family may be accomplished by home visits, postpartal classes, or follow-up phone calls. In some areas self-help support groups for new mothers are also available (Gosha & Brucker 1986).

Home visits are becoming increasingly popular. Many HMOs, group practices, and nurse-midwives have included home visits as part of their maternity care package. Home visits have long been part of the care provided to high-risk clients by community health nurses. A home visit should include a health assessment of the mother and baby in addition to the completion of necessary teaching or other nursing interventions. A subsequent visit can be scheduled if necessary. Figure 34–4 is a sample form the nurse can complete about the childbearing family when making a home visit.

Postpartal classes are becoming more common as caregivers recognize the continuing needs of the childbearing family. A series of structured classes may focus on topics such as parenting, postpartal exercise, or nutrition, or there may be loosely structured group sessions that address concerns of mothers as they arise. Such classes offer chances for the new mother to socialize, share her concerns, and receive encouragement. Because babysitting arrangements may be difficult or expensive, it is desirable to provide child care for newborns and siblings; in some instances, infants remain with mothers in the class.

KEY CONCEPTS

Nursing diagnoses can be used effectively in caring for women postpartally.

Postpartum discomfort may be due to a variety of factors, including engorged breasts, an edematous perineum, an episiotomy or extension, engorged hemorrhoids, or hematoma formation.

Various self-care approaches are helpful in promoting comfort.

Lactation suppression may be accomplished by mechanical techniques or by administering the medication bromocriptine. Because of the increased risk of thrombus formation, estrogen-based medications are rarely used.

The new mother requires opportunities to discuss her childbirth experience with an empathetic listener.

The first day or two following delivery is marked by maternal behaviors that are more dependent and comfort oriented. Then the woman becomes more independent and ready to assume responsibility.

Mother-baby units provide the childbearing family with opportunities to interact with their new member during the first hours and days of life. This enables the family to develop some confidence and skill in a "safe" environment.

Sexual intercourse may resume once the episiotomy has healed and lochia has stopped. Couples should be forewarned of possible changes; for example, the vagina may be "dry," the level of desire may be influenced by fatigue, or the woman's breasts may leak milk during orgasm.

The couple's decision regarding contraception should be made voluntarily, with full knowledge of options, advantages, disadvantages, and side effects of all the forms of birth control.

Prior to discharge the couple should be given any information necessary for the woman to provide appropriate self-care. They should have a beginning skill in caring for their newborn and should be familiar with warning signs of possible complications for mother or baby. Printed information is valuable in helping couples deal with questions that may arise at home.

Following cesarean birth a woman has the nursing care needs of a surgical client in addition to her needs as a postpartum client. She may also require assistance in working through her feelings if the cesarean delivery was unexpected.

Postpartally the nurse evaluates the adolescent mother in terms of her level of maturity, available support systems, cultural background, and existing knowledge and then plans care accordingly.

Because of the trend toward early discharge, follow-up care is more important than ever. Many approaches are used, especially home visits and telephone follow-up.

REFERENCES

Arms S: *To Love and Let Go*. New York, Knopf, 1984.

Bille DA: *Practical Approaches to Patient Teaching*. Boston, Little, Brown, 1981.

Fischman SH, et al: Changes in sexual relationships in postpartum couples. *J Obstet Gynecol Neonat Nurs* 1986;15(January/February):58.

Foster S: Bromocriptine: Suppressing lactation. *Am J Mat Child Nurs* 1982;7(March/April):99.

Frink BB, **Chally** P: Managing pain responses to cesarean childbirth. *Am J Mat Child Nurs* 1984;9(July/August):270.

Gosha J, **Brucker** MC: A self-help group for new mothers: An evaluation. *Am J Mat Child Nurs* 1986;11(January/February):20.

Gruis M: Beyond maternity: Postpartum concerns of mothers. *Am J Mat Child Nurs* 1977;2(May/June):182.

Harvey K: Caring perceptively for the relinquishing mother. *Am J Mat Child Nurs* 1977;2(January/February):24.

Jansson P: Early postpartum discharge. *Am J Nurs* 1985; 85(May):547.

Janowski MJ: The road not taken. *Am J Nurs* 1987; 87(March):334.

Jarrett GE: Childbearing patterns of young mothers: expectations, knowledge and practices. *Am J Mat Child Nurs* 1982;7(March/April):119.

Leach L, **Sproule** V: Meeting the challenge of cesarean births. *J Obstet Gynecol Neonat Nurs* 1984;13(May/June):191.

McKay S, **Mahan** CS: Ways to upgrade postpartal care. *Contemp OB/GYN* 1985;27(November):63.

Moss JR: Concerns of multiparas on the third postpartum day. *J Obstet Gynecol Neonat Nurs* 1981;10(November/December):421.

Niebyl JR, et al: The effect of chlorotrianisene as postpartum lactation suppression on blood coagulation factors. *Am J Obstet Gynecol* 1979;134:518.

Peters F, et al: Inhibition of lactation by a long-acting bromocriptine. *Obstet Gynecol* 1986;67:82.

Ramler D, **Roberts** J: A comparison of cold and warm sitz baths for relief of postpartum perineal pain. *J Obstet Gynecol Neonat Nurs* 1986;15(November/December):471.

Stolte KM: Nursing diagnosis and the childbearing woman. *Am J Mat Child Nurs* 1986;11(January/February):13.

Taylor C: Cultural aspects of human sexuality, in **Barnard** MU, **Clancy** BJ, **Krantz** KE (eds): *Sexuality for Health Professionals*. Philadelphia, Saunders, 1978.

Watters NE: Combined mother-infant nursing care. *J Obstet Gynecol Neonat Nurs* 1985;14(November/December):478.

Wong S, **Stepp-Gilbert** E: Lactation suppression: Non-pharmaceutical versus pharmaceutical method. *J Obstet Gynecol Neonat Nurs* 1985;14(July/August):302.

ADDITIONAL READINGS

Bates B: Imagery and symbolism in the birth practices of traditional cultures. *Birth* 1985;12(Spring):29.

Bull M, **Lawrence** D: Mother's use of knowledge during the first postpartum weeks. *J Obstet Gynecol Neonat Nurs* 1985;14(July/August):315.

Ellis DJ, **Hewat** RJ: Mother's postpartum perceptions of spousal relationships. *J Obstet Gynecol Neonat Nurs* 1985;14(March/April):140.

Fawcett J, et al: Spouses' body image changes during and after pregnancy: A replication and extension. *Nurs Res* 1986;35(July/August):220.

Hiser PL: Concerns of multiparas during the second postpartum week. *J Obstet Gynecol Neonat Nurs* 1987;16(May/June):195.

Jankowski H, **Wells** SM: Self-administered medications for obstetric patients. *Am J Mat Child Nurs* 1987;12(May/June):199.

Keefe MR: Comparison of neonatal nighttime sleep-awake patterns in nursery versus rooming-in environments. *Nurs Res* 1987;36(May/June):140.

Lee PA: Health beliefs of pregnant and postpartum Hmong women. *West J Nurs Res* 1986;8(1):83.

Lewis P: The discharge of mothers by midwives. *Midwives Chron* 1987;100(January):16.

Sandelowski M, **Bustamante** R: Cesarean birth outside the natural childbirth culture. *Res Nurs Health* 1986;9:81.

Smith LF: New-parent teaching in the ambulatory care setting. *Am J Mat Child Nurs* 1986;11(July/August):256.

Vezeau TM, **Hallsten** DA: Making the transition to mother-baby care. *Am J Mat Child Nurs* 1987;12(May/June):193.

Waryas FS, **Luebbers** WB: A cluster system for maternity care. *Am J Mat Child Nurs* 1986;11(March/April):98.

Not long ago my husband, my sons, and I sat out on the deck enjoying a summer evening and reminiscing. We talked about earlier camping trips, family vacations, and Christmas festivities. Suddenly my nine year old said, "It's fun talking about the olden days, isn't it!" My husband and I laughed but we realized our son was saying something important about the experiences that a family shares, about the memories we build together. I remember so clearly the day I brought my firstborn home from the hospital. My husband dropped me off and then had to return to work. I sat in the living room with my new son and tried to envision the future. How would this small person change our lives? I know now that, though it is sometimes frustrating to be a parent, it is infinitely enriching, too. Our boys have brought great meaning to our lives. When we talk about the "olden days" I realize how many memories we have as a family and how many more we will build in the years to come.

Attachment

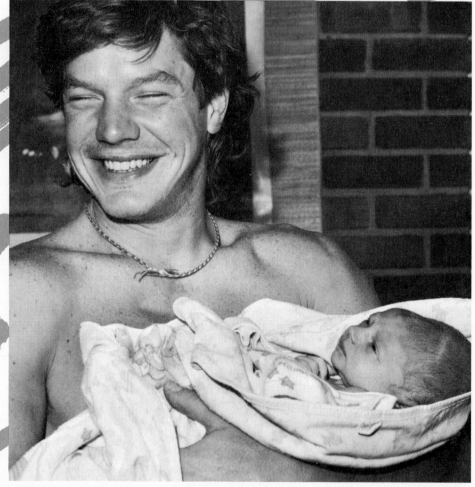

The birth of a father!

Chapter Thirty-Five

OBJECTIVES

- **Describe the attachment process, including the phases of maternal-infant interaction.**
- **Contrast three theories of attachment.**
- **Compare the factors influencing the first maternal-infant interaction.**
- **Contrast the factors affecting family member interactions with the infant.**
- **Explain the types of questions used for evaluating the maternal-infant relationship.**
- **Categorize complications that can affect the maternal-infant attachment process.**
- **Summarize research approaches to enhance attachment.**
- **Select methods the nurse can use to facilitate a positive attachment process.**

There has been a great deal of research on attachment in recent years. The goals of the research have been to describe, operationally define, and relate attachment to cognitive and social outcomes; to support or refute psychologic theories; and to determine public child-care policy.

The early literature on attachment related primarily to the infant's tie to her or his mother, which was understood to occur in the second half of the first year of life when the infant was capable of recognizing the mother. This literature was derived in part from experience with maternally deprived infants. More recently, and motivated in part by disorders and failures in mothering, researchers have investigated the attachment of mothers to infants.

The importance of attachment of fathers and siblings is in the early stages of exploration. Most recently, attachment to the fetus has also received attention.

This chapter begins by exploring the nature, theories, and operation of attachment. Having established this knowledge base, the chapter concludes by discussing nursing assessment and interventions related to attachment.

Nature of Attachment

Attachments are enduring bonds or relationships of affection between persons. Affectional ties exist in families between parents, between parents and their children, and between siblings.

Attachment originally referred to a child's tie to his or her mother, although it was recognized that the tie was to a mother figure, a primary care giver, who was usually, although not necessarily, the biologic mother. Attachment may now refer to an infant's tie to a parent or a parent's tie to the child. The essence of infant attachment is organization and patterning of behavior that results in feelings of closeness to the attachment figure. Elements of this behavior are clinging, crying, smiling, sucking, following, and eye-to-eye contact.

Bonding is a "rapid process of mother-infant attachment" that occurs at or soon after birth (Svejda et al 1980, p 788). Bonding is influenced by such factors as early contact and breast-feeding. However, the terms *attachment* and *bonding* are often used interchangeably.

Theories of Attachment

Attachment is viewed from three major perspectives: psychoanalytic, ethological, and learning theories.

From a psychoanalytic perspective, attachment is explained by instinctual responses and object relations. Attachment is innate, an instinctual drive. The mother is the object of the drive. Fathers are important as support for the mother, but attachment with anyone other than the mother is thought to interfere with and be detrimental to the child's development. Other attachments will follow once attachment to the mother is assured. The quality of later attachments depends on the quality of attachment to the mother.

Within an ethological framework, attachment consists of species specific behaviors. Examples of such behaviors are ducklings imprinting on the first moving object seen after hatching, primates clinging when alarmed, and cats licking newborn kittens to stimulate respiratory and gastrointestinal functioning. Sucking, clinging, crying, smiling, and following are attachment behaviors promoting proximity in the human species.

According to learning theorists, attachment is formed through secondary drives. The mother meets her infant's needs and the infant associates need satisfaction, comfort, and love with her.

Questions about the origin of attachment, behaviors denoting attachment, and interventions to promote attachment may differ depending on the theoretical perspective taken.

● What the Mother Brings to the First Interaction

Prenatal Influences

A mother has a specific genetic makeup of intelligence, personality and temperament, body structure, physical health, and biochemical/hormonal status (Sugarman 1977). Each of these factors influences the environment the mother can provide for the fetus and newborn and affects her ability to relate well to her child. Her cultural and ethnic background will influence her attitudes, behaviors, and practices related to pregnancy and childbirth. Her experiences in infancy and childhood, the mothering she received, and her exposure to appropriate role models will shape her own mothering practices.

The mother's current developmental level and relationships with significant others will provide the foundation for the developing relationship with her fetus and the newborn. Often she will "rework" the relationship with her own mother and develop a closer relationship to her mother as a result.

Family readiness for pregnancy is crucial for providing an environment in which attachment to the fetus and newborn can occur. The optimum environment is created when the baby is planned and wanted, and the family has the necessary resources to provide for the infant.

Present Pregnancy

Each mother brings to her first visual contact with her newborn her reactions to that particular pregnancy, from conception through birth. A variety of factors may influence her response to the pregnancy and the baby: whether the pregnancy was planned and a baby wanted (Perry 1983), complications she experienced in pregnancy, and the support she received from family and friends (Cranley 1981b). Life events essentially unrelated to her pregnant condition may have enhanced a woman's response to pregnancy or depleted the energy reserves and coping ability necessary to pregnancy adjustments. Stress

during pregnancy can interfere with attachment but support from family and others can offset some of the adverse effects of such stress (Cranley 1981b).

By the time of expected delivery, each mother has developed an emotional orientation of some kind toward the fetus. This attachment is based on a tactile-kinesthetic awareness combined with fantasy images and perceptions. For many women, an emotional bond to the fetus develops soon after conception and deepens during pregnancy (Leifer 1980). By the third trimester, significant attachment has occurred (Cranley 1981a, Stainton 1985). Fathers, too, become attached to the fetus (Weaver & Cranley 1983).

Events such as hearing the fetal heart or visualizing the fetus on a screen through sonography affect the mother's perception of her fetus (Kohn et al 1980) and appear to increase her feelings of attachment. However, knowledge of whether the fetus is male or female does not affect attachment (Grace 1984).

Leifer (1977) found that women who did not plan to become pregnant or who conceived for reasons of status or security were frequently among those who had minimal feelings of closeness to the fetus throughout the pregnancy. Those who felt well adjusted in their marriage and emotionally ready to have a baby were able to develop strong affectionate feelings.

● What the Newborn Brings to the First Interaction

Each partner in an interpersonal interaction contributes in some way to the process. In years past, the newborn's influence on the beginning mother-infant relationship was ignored. More recently, research on the capacities of newborns and very young neonates has shown that they are indeed active partners in the exchange and take part in shaping their own human environment from the moment of birth. Newborns do this by virtue of who they are and what they do—their appearance and behavior.

Appearance

At the moment of birth certain information about the newborn's external appearance is available. Each characteristic may have a special meaning for the parents as it relates to their hopes, fears, and expectations. The relatively obvious things are usually noted first: sex, size, shape, color, and presence or absence of abnormality or injury. The eyes are a particularly important feature (Trevathan 1983).

Behaviors

The newborn has, and may demonstrate at birth, certain functional behaviors, such as crying, sucking, eliminating, looking, listening, and startling. In the very first days of life, the infant selectively attends to the human face, prefers the human voice over other sounds, and becomes quiet and alert when picked up and held over the shoulder (Goren et al 1975).

In addition to having behaviors in common with other neonates, each newborn, like the parent, is already a unique combination of genetic potential and life experience. The newborn's life experience is shorter and more limited in scope, of course, but it can have a powerful effect on observable behavior.

The past history and present personality of each mother and father combine with the characteristics and behavior of their infant to influence the quality and direction of the parental relationship. Unique individuals are blending into an equally unique interactional system that changes with time as the actors change and grow.

● The Setting

The physical environment, human environment, and condition of the mother and newborn at first contact may influence the opportunities for interaction.

Physical Environment

Delivery may occur in a variety of settings. The most frequent setting by far is a maternity unit in a hospital. The physical surroundings are, in all probability, relatively strange to the woman as she moves from the admitting area to the labor room; delivery room, recovery area, and her room in the postpartal unit.

She may encounter a variety of unfamiliar equipment and procedures. Noise levels are often high. Food is usually withheld until after delivery. The strain and concomitant psychic stress of frequent accommodations to the physical environment can interfere with the progress of labor and delivery and with the comfort of mother-infant interaction. In addition, the parents may be separated from the newborn.

An increasing number of women are deciding to give birth in their homes. This setting differs from the conventional hospital in that the physical environment is stable, familiar, and optimal for allowing the parents control of the environment and activities surrounding the birth. The infant remains with the parents and the family has time together in a familiar environment. In most instances of home birth, the mother-to-be has taken the major responsibility for selecting, furnishing, and equipping the birth environment.

Consumer and professional efforts to increase the comfort of hospital births while decreasing the risks sometimes associated with home birth have produced an intermediate type of setting: hospital-independent birth centers or hospital birthing rooms. These facilities are more home-like in appearance and do not require moves from one area to another during the progression from labor through early recovery. The newborn remains with the parents in this setting. Many institutions are also offering an early discharge program for families with support at home.

Human Environment

Labor and birth usually occur in a social setting. Very few women express the wish to be alone during childbirth; most respond with distress to the idea of abandonment at such a time. Hospitals generally provide for fairly constant nursing supervision of women in active labor, in the course of delivery, and in the early hours after birth. Usually, however, there is a different caretaker present in each phase of the childbearing activities. This requires the woman to relate to a variety of nurses—each with advice, expectations, and attitudes—at a very vulnerable time.

Most agencies have changed routines to permit the father or other significant persons to be present during and after labor and delivery. This practice increases the possibility that a woman will have the support of one trusted person for the whole childbirth experience. The quality of support available from professionals or laypersons varies considerably according to their clinical and psychosocial skills. There are indications that a woman's perceptions of her physical care and emotional support and her reactions to the nonhuman elements of the environment can influence her mothering responses. One study (Sosa et al 1980) revealed that with the presence of a support person, labor was shorter, there were fewer complications, and the mothers spent more time awake. They talked, stroked, and smiled at the first contact with their infants more than the mothers who labored alone.

Condition of the Interactors

When the postbirth conditions are optimal, mother and newborn are ready to relate effectively to each other and to benefit from the interaction. The mother is emotionally high and alert, primed for maternal responsiveness by her hormonal state. The newborn is in a quiet, alert state, capable of attending to the mother's face and voice. However, several common conditions diminish or divert the mother's physical and psychologic energies. Fatigue, pain, cold, hunger, and thirst are frequently reported by mothers after delivery. Not uncommonly, the postpartal mother experiences a spell of uncontrollable shaking of the legs. The mother may also have received medication for relaxation and pain relief and may be encumbered in her movements by intravenous tubing.

Certain conditions may also lower the newborn's potential for human interaction. In addition to the physiologic adaptations immediately necessary for extrauterine existence, physical maturity, nutritional adequacy, neurologic intactness, bodily discomfort, extremes of temperature, and levels of analgesic and anesthetic agents have all been related to the infant's behavioral responses in the first hours of life—and later. Prophylactic eye treatments interfere with newborns' ability to keep their eyes open and focused on the mother's face. Generally speaking, any situation, condition, or stimulus that detracts from the energy either partner can direct toward attending to the other diminishes the probability of optimal interaction between the two.

● **Mother-Infant Interactions**

Introductory Phase

Observers of very early mother-newborn interactions in hospital settings have presented evidence that a fairly regular pattern of maternal behaviors is exhibited at first contact with the normal newborn (Rubin 1963, Klaus et al 1970). In a progression of touching activities, the mother proceeds from fingertip exploration of the newborn's extremities toward palmar contact with the larger body areas and finally to enfolding the infant with the whole hand and arms. The time taken to accomplish these steps varies from minutes to days, depending, it appears, on the timing of the first contact, the clothing barriers present, and the physical condition of the baby. There also may be ethnic or cultural differences in patterns of interaction. Maternal excitement and elation tend to increase during the time of the initial meeting (Figure 35–1). The mother also increases the proportion of time spent in the *en face* position (Figure 35–2). She arranges herself or the newborn to facilitate direct face-to-face and eye-to-eye contact. The majority of women cradle their infant in their left arm (Trevathan 1982). There is an intense interest in having the infant's eyes open. When the eyes are open, the mother characteristically greets the newborn and talks in high-pitched tones to her or him.

Clinical observations indicate that behaviors differ somewhat in unconventional delivery situations. Home birth and LeBoyer deliveries seem to speed up the behaviors described. Often after a home birth the mother turns almost immediately to pick up and hold the newborn and to rub the infant's cheek with her fingertip. The newborn is often offered the breast before the placenta is expelled. In a delivery patterned after the LeBoyer method, the mother, and sometimes the father, is encouraged to gently massage the infant's whole body while waiting for the placenta to be delivered.

In most instances the mother relies on her senses of sight, touch, and hearing in getting to know what her baby is really like. She tends also to respond verbally to any sounds emitted by the newborn, such as cries, coughs, sneezes, and grunts. Mothers are able to distinguish their infant's odor (Porter et al 1983a), and the sense of smell

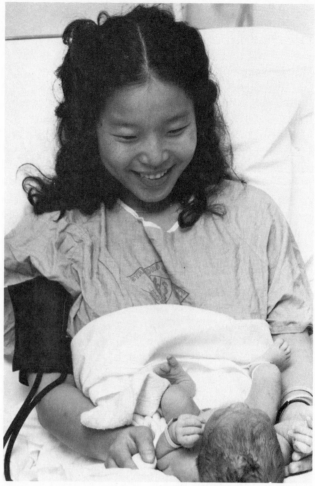

Figure 35–1   *A new mother interacts with her infant.*

may be involved in the acquaintance process (Porter et al 1983b).

While interacting with the newborn, the mother is undergoing her own emotional reactions to the labor and birth and to the baby as she perceives her or him. Sometimes direct comments and nonverbal cues clearly reflect her emotions; sometimes the mother reports only later on her feelings at the time. An expression of "I can't believe it" and a feeling of emotional distance from the newborn are quite common: "I felt he was a stranger." On the other hand, feelings of connectedness between the newborn and the rest of the family can be expressed in positive or negative terms: "He's got your cute nose, Daddy" or "Oh, no! She looks just like the first one, and she was an impossible baby." A mother's facial expressions or the frequency and content of her questions may demonstrate concerns about the infant's general condition or normality, especially if her pregnancy was complicated or if a previously delivered baby was not normal.

There are differences among individuals in the intensity of feeling and in the mode of expression of feelings. For example, intense pleasure may be shown in smiles or in tears. In general, extremely negative feelings are predictive of later problems in the mother-infant relationship.

During the initial mother-newborn interaction the neonate, too, is continuously communicating. Elements of the newborn's appearance and behavior may be perceived by the mother as if they represented intentionality and interpersonal dialogue, and they do influence her responses. The newborn's size says to the mother, "You nourished me well—you did a good job." Individual features say, "I am a part of you, or of my father. I belong with you." Even the time of birth can be read as a message: "I'm cooperative—or uncooperative." The intensity, timing, configuration, and other elements of the newborn's observable activity, however reflexive, are regularly responded to as a very personal communication from the baby to the mother.

Unless care is taken to effect a gentle birth, a number of noxious stimuli impinge on the senses of the newly born neonate. The stimuli may include suctioning, bright lights, cool air, and noise. The infant usually responds by crying. In fact, newborns are typically stimulated to cry to reassure the caretakers that they are well and normal, although the

advisability of this practice has been questioned (Gill et al 1984). When newborns no longer need to concentrate most of their energy in physical and physiologic response to the immediate crisis of birth, they are able to lie quietly with their eyes open, looking about, moving occasionally, making sucking motions, possibly attempting to get hand to mouth. Placed near the mother, the baby appears to focus briefly on her face and to attend to her voice repeatedly in the first moments. When their mother is talking and babies are attending, they are likely to move arms, legs, fingers, or eyelids in an exact synchrony with their mother's minute voice changes (Condon & Sander 1974).

The significant behavioral cues that shape the interaction at the first and subsequent contacts and factors that influence the mother and infant are illustrated in Figure 35–3.

Facilitation of this apparent readiness to relate to each other may increase maternal responsiveness to the newborn's needs (Lozoff et al 1977). In a number of related studies, some groups of mothers were given earlier and/or more extended contact with their newborn than was the routine for control groups of similar mothers and then were observed in later interactions with their newborns. Mothers allowed earlier contact and/or increased in-hospital contact smiled more at their infants, showed more face-to-face behavior, and were quicker to use soothing and comforting behaviors when their infants exhibited distress. They appeared to enjoy subsequent contact with their infants more than the control group of mothers did. Differences between the groups were still observable two years later. However, other studies have found that extra contact makes no difference in maternal behaviors (Curry 1982, Campbell & Taylor 1980) or that the differences were apparent only in those mothers who were lacking in support (Anisfeld & Lipper 1983).

Acquaintance Phase

During the introductory contact after birth, the mother gathers a certain amount of information about her baby. This learning about the partner is the first step in any interpersonal acquaintance. From the remarks, questions, and activities of a new mother in the earliest postpartal days, it is apparent that she is applying herself to the task of getting acquainted with her newborn. She wants to know what kind of newborn she is taking into her family system and what the infant's reaction to her is. She is also consciously involved in clarifying the nature of her own developing feelings toward the newborn. In part she is becoming acquainted with herself as the mother of this particular infant. Gottlieb (1978) described a discovery process in which a mother *identifies* the infant as her own, pointing out what the infant looks like and what the baby can do. Next she *relates* the behavior or appearance to someone or something familiar: "Her nose is just like her daddy's." A

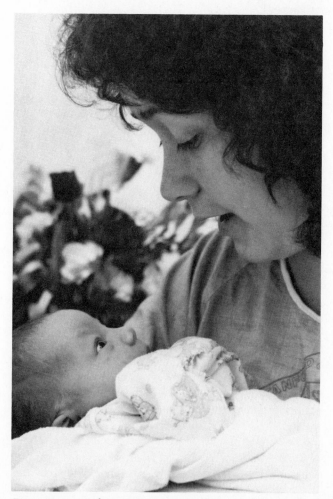

Figure 35–2 En face *position*

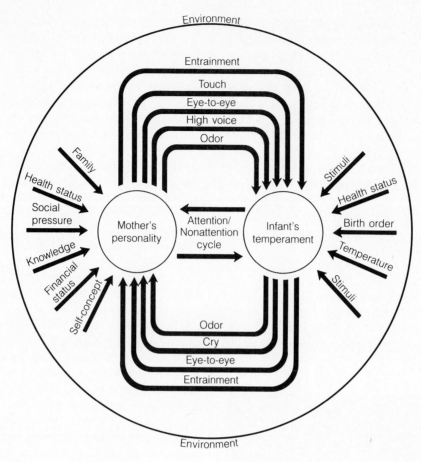

Figure 35–3   Reciprocity system

third step in the process is *interpreting* or giving meaning to the infant's behavior or appearance: "Look at that face, he's going to be a feisty one!"

There is some indication that the degree to which a mother develops feelings of affectionate closeness or attachment to the fetus before birth is generally predictive of the course of maternal feelings toward the newborn immediately after birth and in the acquaintance phase (Leifer 1977). Minimal closeness before birth seems to lead to less enjoyment of the newborn, less responsiveness to needs, and less empathy when the infant is in distress. Women who feel an intense attachment and interaction before birth appear to pick up the relationship at that level after delivery and to develop increased feelings of closeness in the acquaintance phase. They eagerly respond to the newborn's needs and are gratified by the newborn's apparent well-being. In addition, they are likely to be more successful at initiating and maintaining breast-feeding than are minimally attached mothers. Liking the infant at the start apparently contributes to the woman's understanding of her newborn as an individual with unique needs and adds to her willingness to respond to those needs. The positive

orientation at the beginning of contact probably also influences the woman toward a positive perception of her newborn's attitude toward her as a mother. It helps her believe that her baby appreciates her.

The newborn plays an important part in determining the outcome of the acquaintance phase of the mother-infant relationship. If the infant is relatively well organized in responding to the usual caretaking stimuli and is regular in biologic rhythms, she or he tends to be easy to understand. If the infant gives clear behavioral cues about needs, his or her responses to mothering will be predictable. Such predictability makes a mother feel effective and competent—a pleasant feeling. If the newborn responds to motherly ministrations with a predominantly positive mood rather than with irritability, and if he or she has relatively long periods of being quietly awake and attentive, the infant is pleasant to be near and to interact with. Other behaviors that make an infant more attractive to caretakers are smiling, grasping a finger, nursing eagerly, cuddling, and being easy to console.

The newborn is also becoming acquainted with his or her mother. Newborns gather what information they can

Research Note

Blank explored early psychophysiologic mother-infant interactions with the hypothesis that a mother's perception of her infant's physiologic and contact tenderness needs and her anxiety are related to changes in infant satiety, anxiety, and feeding behavior.

Perception of tenderness needs were assessed in 65 healthy, bottle-feeding, low-income mothers. Maternal anxiety was evaluated before and after infant feeding. Infant serum glucose was used to assess satiety and serum cortisol to assess infant anxiety. The amount of formula taken at the feeding was noted as a measure of feeding behavior.

Results showed that mild maternal anxiety was associated with increased maternal discrimination of infant tenderness needs. Mild maternal anxiety at feeding time was associated with increased formula intake and decreased postfeeding infant cortisol (increased feeling of security). Extremely low maternal anxiety around feeding time was associated with decreased formula intake and increased postfeeding cortisol (decreased security). Blank pointed out that extremely low maternal anxiety may pose a real threat to an infant. Nurses need to include both an assessment of anxiety and observations of mother-infant interactions in their care of the postpartum client.

Blank DM: Relating mothers anxiety and perception to infant satiety, anxiety, and feeding behavior. Nurs Res 1986;35(November/ December):347–351.

about their new world. They attend to sights, sounds, tastes, and smells, and experience different tactile and kinesthetic sensations. Within a few days after birth, infants show signs of recognizing recurrent situations and responding to changes in routine.

Phase of Mutual Regulation

In the performance of the necessary tasks of newborn care, such as feeding, bathing, and comforting, the new mother develops some awareness that there is a degree of discrepancy between her wishes and needs and her baby's needs and desires. This awareness ushers in a phase of mutual regulation of behaviors. The degree of control to be exerted by each partner in the interpersonal adjustment is an issue in the early postpartal weeks. Maternal goals related to the resolution of this issue of control are, of course, variable, both among different mothers and in the same mother at different times. In some mother-infant

pairs, the maternal goal is primarily to change the infant to meet the mother's needs. In other pairs it is quite apparent that the mother's intent is primarily to interpret correctly and to gratify completely all of her newborn's needs. Either of those approaches is likely to result in relational disturbances, the degree of distress and tension depending to a large extent on the newborn's reactions to the maternal behaviors used to reach the goal. For example, the mother who wishes to adjust her baby rather than adjust to him or her will have a smoother postpartal course if she is blessed with a highly adaptive infant who is positive in mood. The mother who is intent on meeting every need of her child at the same moment it arises will meet with failure very quickly if the newborn is unpredictable, is irregular in daily rhythms, and presents behavioral cues that are difficult to interpret.

The ideal solution to the control issue would be somewhere between the two extremes. A mother who realizes that she is a person with her own needs will be less vulnerable to the buildup of anger, frustration, anxiety, and guilt. In all but the most ideal situations, each partner must undergo disappointments, and each must at some time subordinate his or her own needs to the needs of the other. The most important consideration is that each should obtain a good measure of enjoyment from the ongoing interactions.

Generally speaking, enjoyment is enhanced during the early months if the infant is sufficiently organized to make clear her or his needs and if the mother's personality allows her to let the infant lead the interaction. Mutual maternal-infant regulation is never instantaneous; it is a process that continues to some degree throughout infancy and childhood. Fortunately, there appears to be a tendency toward improved organization of behavior in the newborn period and an increasing ability to nurture in the mother during the same time.

It is during the mutual adjustment phase that negative maternal feelings are likely to surface or intensify. Because "everyone knows that mothers love their babies," these negative feelings often go unexpressed and are allowed to build up. If they are expressed, the response of friends, relatives, or health care personnel is often to deny the feeling to the mother: "You don't mean that"; "You can't feel that way"; "Your baby is not ugly, he is beautiful." Some negative feelings are normal in the first few days following delivery, and the nurse should be supportive when the mother vocalizes these feelings.

When mutual regulation arrives at the point where both partners have achieved a predominance of enjoyment in each other's company, it is usually obvious to an observer that the relationship is good. It may be said that reciprocity has been achieved. A high degree of reciprocity is characteristic of successful mutual regulation.

Reciprocity

Reciprocity within a mother-infant system may be described as an interactional cycle that occurs simultaneously between the mother and the infant (Brazelton et al 1974). It involves mutual cuing behaviors, expectancy, rhythmicity, and synchrony. There are intimations of reciprocity in the early hours of life. The mother and her infant respond to each other's cues. They develop rhythms in interaction that form the basis for communication (Censullo et al 1985). During several weeks of interactive continuity, they establish a pattern of behavior in which they mesh with each other. When this meshing or synchrony is attained, the mother and infant perform a reciprocal dance of cyclical attention and nonattention. Brazelton and his colleagues have studied this reciprocal process in the laboratory and have carefully analyzed the component parts. They have described five phases of the cycle: (1) initiation, (2) orientation, (3) acceleration, (4) deceleration, and (5) turning away. The first two phases establish the partner's expectations regarding the interaction. Both mother and infant use clusters of behaviors as the interaction develops. Feedback between partners enables them to modulate their behaviors. Sensitivity and adjustment by the mother allows the infant to maintain a homeostatic state and to develop an expanding attention cycle. The infant may begin to develop recognizable patterns of behavior by about 2 weeks of age, and it is often well established by 6 weeks.

If the observer is aware of what to look for, the segments of an interactional cycle can be described as they are observed. The following is a hypothetical example of an interactional period, as it is likely to appear when things are going well:

Initiation: The infant is held on the mother's knee, facing her. He looks toward her with a relaxed expression and makes slow movements with his arms and hands.

Orientation: As the infant makes eye contact with his mother, his eyes brighten and become alert, and he turns his whole body toward her, extending arms and legs in her direction. He reaches toward the mother.

State of attention: The mother smiles and talks to the infant, and he responds by smiling, moving his arms and legs in pedaling motions, cooing, and making other sounds. The eyes alternately become alert and dull as he responds to the smiles and words of his mother. The limbs move rhythmically, in time with the mother's voice. There is a constant slow smooth reaching and circular movement occurring as the tension within the infant's body rises and falls. The infant assumes the look of expectancy.

Acceleration: The infant continues to move, to wave his hands and feet about, and to increase his smiling activity. His eyes are bright and alert. He strains toward his mother in the intensity of the interaction, all the time watching her and cuing to her smile. For the most part, the body movement is smooth, but there may be occasional jerkiness.

Peak of excitement: As the infant becomes wholly involved in the interaction, his movements may become jerky and intense. He brings his hand to his mouth and tries to insert his thumb while still smiling and cooing. The other hand clutches his thigh and he leans forward to his mother as she continues to smile at him. As he endeavors to reach forward, his back arches and his body tends to twist toward one side.

Deceleration: The excitement begins to pass and the infant's movements slow. There is a gradual decrease in body movement, the bright look dims, the eyes become dull, and the lids appear to droop. The smiles fade, and vocalization decreases. Suddenly the infant yawns and begins to suck his thumb as he leans away from his mother. His hands drop to his lap with the fingers widespread, and he appears to be relaxing.

Withdrawal or turning away: The infant's activity slows down almost completely. He slumps against his mother's hands with his body half turned away from her. His eyes are dull and focused in the direction of an object to the side. There is a faint smile on his face. The mother stops smiling and talking to the infant. She just sits holding him quietly, waiting for his next cue. The mother briefly raises her head and glances beyond the infant. This prompts a reaction in the infant. He looks toward his mother, smiles briefly, and looks away again, then turns back to the mother, ready to resume another period of interaction.

The responsibility for monitoring cues and for sensitively initiating or maintaining the interaction rests primarily with the mother. The infant uses the nonattention time to recover from the tension of interaction, to organize behavior, and to process what has been taken in during the attentive periods.

The development of reciprocity between a mother and her infant is evidence of the bond or attachment that has formed between them. It enables the mother to let go of the infant she knew as a fetus during pregnancy. A new relationship now develops with an individual who has a unique character and who evokes a response entirely different from the fantasy response of pregnancy. When reciprocity is synchronous, the interaction between mother and infant is mutually gratifying and is sought and initiated by both partners. Pleasure and delight develop in each other's company, and there is mutual development of love and growth.

Reciprocity may take weeks to develop, and it usually requires sensitive stimuli from both actors. As infants become more organized in their behavior and as senses develop, they are able to give positive feedback to their mothers. As they transmit the appearance of listening, they follow voice and movements, and respond with intentionality to the mother as an individual whom they recognize and seek to communicate with. In cases in which either the mother or the newborn is sick and the initial acquaintance is delayed, a concomitant delay in the development of reciprocity is likely.

Overstimulation or inappropriate stimulation by the mother may interfere with the synchrony of the interaction. In the resultant asynchrony, the mother may be in the attention phase of the reciprocal process when the infant is in the nonattention phase. This asynchrony can lead to frustration on the part of either partner or both and may lead to a disharmonious relationship as both become established in their interactional patterns. In extreme instances mother and infant may cease to communicate with each other.

Infants vary in their strategies for dealing with an overload of stimulation. Four types of reaction have been described in infants responding to unpleasant and inappropriately timed stimuli (Brazelton et al 1974): active physical withdrawal, rejection, decreased sensitivity, and communication of distress. An infant can move away from the source of stimulation, can push the stimulus away, can lapse into drowsiness or sleep, or can fuss and cry. Some of these strategies, if they become characteristic of an infant's behavior, are easier to live with than others; they interact with a mother's expectations and her personality.

The nurse may have the opportunity to observe reciprocity developing between a mother and her newborn in the early weeks of life. If nurses recognize the appearance of asynchrony, they may be able to initiate intervention before the asynchronous behaviors become firmly established.

Attachment

The ultimate goals of nursing care in the maternity cycle are the continuation of life and the enhancement of the quality of that life in terms of physical and mental health. There is reason to believe that a state of mutual attachment or an enduring emotional bond between a parent (or parent surrogate) and an infant is essential to the infant's optimum health. A new mother's feelings of closeness or attachment to her infant also seem to have a positive effect on her own continued personal growth. The same is probably true of a new father. Therefore, the facilitation of parent-infant attachment is a significant goal to pursue.

Attachment is a bond of affection and, as such, is invisible. Behavioral cues must be observed for indications of the presence or absence of the bond. Researchers have used a variety of behaviors as indicators of attachment. In the immediate newborn period, smiling at the infant and addressing him or her by name or in affectionate terms; kissing, touching, and enfolding the infant close to the body; cradling the infant in the left arm and assuming the *en face* position; making positive comments about the appearance and behavior of the infant; finding family resemblances; and expressing positive feelings to the spouse are important behaviors. Later, expressions of enjoying caring for the infant, feeling the infant belongs to the parents, thinking about the infant when away from him or her, making warm comments about the infant, and responding appropriately to infant cues indicate that the parent has developed a bond with the infant.

The maternal role includes both emotional and physical tasks. The emotional component includes qualities that enable the mother to feel warmth, affection, attachment, protectiveness, and devotion to the child. The physical tasks include the knowledge and skill to provide care for the infant, that is, to feed, diaper, bathe, and provide a safe environment.

Whether and how soon a parent displays behaviors indicating attachment depend on many factors; the process is believed to be facilitated by a warm, supportive environment.

Attachment Behaviors in the Adolescent Mother

Adolescents demonstrate attachment behaviors toward their infants (Feller et al 1983), although differences in attachment behaviors have been observed in adolescent mothers compared with older mothers. Adolescent mothers had fewer complications during pregnancy and birth but reported being more scared during labor and having a poorer perception of the experience than older mothers. These perceptions were related to later mothering behaviors in teenagers (Mercer 1985). Avant (1981) found that young mothers were more anxious and had lower attachment scores than older mothers. The younger the adolescent, the less likely she is to display typical adult maternal behaviors of touching, synchrony with her newborn, vocalization, and proximity of mother and newborn (McAnarney et al 1979). It also appears that the most important areas of interaction in the early postpartal period for the adolescent are physical and motor. These mothers appear to be more attuned to these behaviors than to auditory and visual interaction.

Strong ego functioning, as demonstrated by the mother's ability to adapt to pregnancy and to plan for her future, appears to affect the mother's interaction with her newborn. The response of the newborn is also critical. Infants who are healthy are more likely to affect the relationship positively. Adolescents may have problems with parenting because they tend to have less realistic expectations of what an infant can do at a given age. In addition, cognitively immature adolescents may not foresee the consequences of their actions. Neglectful parenting may become a problem. However, many adolescent mothers live with their mothers, who provide support during pregnancy and provide a significant proportion of the care of the infant.

With these considerations in mind the nurse must be attentive to the early maternal-infant interaction, use appropriate modeling and teaching techniques, include the adolescent's mother when appropriate, and refer adolescent mothers for follow-up care when indicated.

● Father-Infant Interactions

The father was traditionally seen only as a source of support for the pregnant woman. He contributed to the growth and development of his newborn indirectly by nurturing and supporting his partner through the pregnancy and the early postpartal weeks. As fathers became more involved in the pregnancy and birth experience, researchers began to study their experiences and feelings about the fetus and newborn.

The majority of fathers demonstrate attachment behaviors toward the fetus; that is, they talk to the fetus, refer to it by name, enjoy watching their wives' abdomens move as the fetus moves, think about the baby, and show other similar behaviors (Weaver & Cranley 1983). A father's attachment to the fetus is more likely to occur when the marital relationship is strong. Fathers who identify with the pregnancy by having physical symptoms similar to pregnancy symptoms also have higher attachment scores (Weaver & Cranley 1983).

A father experiences feelings toward his newborn that are similar to the mother's feelings of attachment. In the past the significance of any psychologic response called fatherliness was minimized. It was implied that, because the man did not have deep physiologic roots of fatherliness, his feelings were somehow of less importance than the mother's and were weaker and longer in developing. Evidence is increasing that a father does have a strong attraction to his newborn and highly positive emotional reactions to first contact. The first hours after delivery appear to be significant in the development of the father-mother-infant bond.

The pregnancy and birth experience is important for fathers as well as mothers. When fathers are involved in pregnancy through a close marital relationship, they have a more positive report of the delivery and new baby (Nicholson et al 1983). A positive birth experience also leads to greater levels of attachment in fathers (Peterson et al 1979).

Greenberg and Morris (1974) noted the reactions of first-time fathers to early contact with their newborns. They used the term *engrossment* to label characteristics of the effect of the newborn on the father—his sense of absorption, preoccupation, and interest in the infant.

Some researchers have found that early contact influences bonding in fathers (Bowen & Miller 1980); others have found no differences related to early contact in the newborn period (Toney 1983) but some effects later. For example, Perry (1983) introduced fathers to their newborn infants by having fathers elicit behavioral responses from the infants and found no differences in perception at either 10 or 30 days after delivery. However, Jones (1981) found that early contact fathers exhibited more nonverbal behavior at one month; that is, they held the infants more.

Research Note

Ventura examined parent coping in relation to infant temperament and parent psychologic responses. The study included 47 mothers and 47 fathers of 2- to 3-month-old infants, who responded to a questionnaire about coping, individual and family functioning, stress events, and infant temperament. The parents and infants were all healthy, and the mothers experienced a normal prenatal and intrapartum course.

Mothers and fathers reported similar helpfulness of coping behaviors, but depression and anxiety were more common for fathers. Mothers found social support and self-development more helpful coping behaviors than did fathers. Mothers who perceived a positive infant response to soothing techniques coped by seeking social support; maintaining family integrity; and being religious, thankful, and content more often than mothers who perceived their infants differently. Fathers who perceived their infants as easily soothed more often coped by being more responsible. Fathers who perceived their infants as fearful and distressed by limitations were more often anxious and depressed and were less likely to use coping behaviors of social support and being responsible.

Ventura's study indicated that optimal family coping involves couples' actions directed at anticipating and managing family tasks. The postpartum nurse needs to consider the mother, the father, and the unique temperament of the baby when providing anticipatory guidance to families to maximize adaptive responses in parents.

Ventura JN: Parent coping: a replication. Nurs Res 1986;35(March/April):77–80.

The emotional reaction to the first sight of the newborn and to later contacts is very positive. The intensity of his feelings may come as a surprise to the new father. The involvement with his newborn can draw a man's time and energy away from the ongoing couple relationship. The man who has been encouraged to support his partner in her new mothering role may feel some guilt about preoccupation with the baby, and the woman may feel ignored or excluded from a significant relationship. It seems likely that couples who shared experiences, relationships, and material things before the birth will also be able to share their infant's attention and the responsibilities of parenting.

When the new father initiates interaction, the newborn responds (Figure 35–4). As with the mother-newborn interaction, the newborn contributes his or her part. The infant cries and moves, indicating aliveness and well-being. Spontaneous and reflexive movements and grimaces are emitted and the father responds by voice and touch. From the beginning, the father's interactive behaviors are different from the mother's, and these differences are perceptible to the infant. A father's odor, voice pitch, appearance, and touch qualities are all different from a mother's. In a face-to-face "play situation," a mother tends to use her hands to enfold and enclose her baby's body and limbs with gentle molding and smoothing motions, whereas the father punctuates his conversation with finger pokes and more exaggerated changes in facial expression, which act to increase the baby's excitement level. Observers have noted differences in an infant's responses to interaction with mother or father as early as two weeks after birth.

Mothers, too, appear to notice a difference. Often in the early weeks, when asked if they play with the baby, mothers say, "No, but my husband does." It seems as if one function of the father-infant interaction is to further acquaint the mother with her baby's range of possible behaviors in the context of a shared relationship.

It might be helpful if, during the pregnancy, nurses explain the potential for engrossment of the father after birth. If both parents are aware that each has needs at this time, they may be better able to support each other's growing relationship to this new family member. To make nursing goals appropriate and intervention effective, more knowledge is needed about the long-term effects of different levels of direct paternal involvement on the quality of the father-child relationship and other family relationships.

● Siblings and Others

Little is known about the components of bonding between the newborn and his or her siblings. Most parents endeavor to prepare their children for the advent of a new baby. Many hospitals are beginning to include sibling classes to help children learn about newborns and become

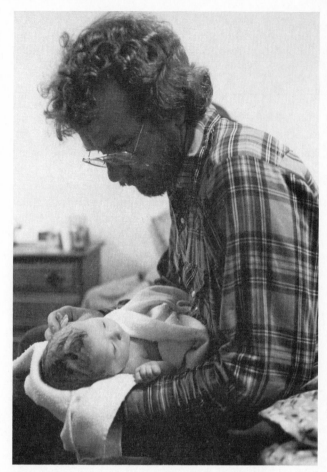

Figure 35–4   A bond develops between father and infant

involved in the socialization of the new member into the family. The type and extent of the preparation may depend on the age of the children and the type of relationships that exist in the home. If the new baby is seen as nonthreatening to the relationships the children have with their parents, there will probably be less disruption, and the new baby will be accepted without serious problems.

Common reactions of a child to the birth of a sibling are negative behaviors toward the mother, withdrawal, sleeping problems, aggressiveness, changes in toileting, and increased attention-seeking (Field & Reite 1984).

The conventional view of the bonding or attachment process has been that the infant was capable of forming only one bond at a time and that this bond should be to the mother. Bowlby (1958) called this tie *monotropy*. More recent work with infants has shown that they are capable of maintaining a number of attachments. These attachments may include siblings, grandparents, aunts, and uncles. Some infants were found to be capable of forming attachments with five or more people simultaneously without loss of quality. The social setting and personalities of the individuals appear to be significant factors in permitting the development of multiple attachments. The advent of open visiting hours and rooming-in permits siblings and grandparents to participate in the attachment process of the newborn's life.

Attachment With Adopted Children

Attachment with adopted children occurs even though many factors thought to be important in the attachment process, such as early contact, may not be possible. Smith and Sherwen (1984) identified factors that adoptive mothers described as aiding the process. These factors included physical contact, such as touching, kissing, or feeding, and shared activities. Factors that interfered were negative behaviors of the child and rejection by the (older) child. More problems seemed to occur when the child was over the age of four when the placement occurred. Some mothers mentioned lack of energy and resources and conflicts in roles, factors that also affect maternal role taking in biologic mothers. As with biologic mothers, the support system of partner, relatives, and friends was very important.

The quality of attachment in adoptive mother-infant pairs is no different from that in nonadoptive situations, at least in middle class families (Singer et al 1985). Early contact does not seem to be necessary for attachment to develop. It appears that a warm, supportive environment with competent and confident parents promotes the formation of affectional bonds.

In some situations, adoptive parents are permitted to be present at delivery and to experience early contact and provide initial care. Some hospitals are allowing adoptive parents to room-in and receive instruction and practice in infant care under supervision of hospital staff. In other situations, the child may be older and may have developed a relationship with another care giver. In these situations, the adoptive parents need assistance and support to allow time for the acquaintance process to occur, to become sensitive to each other's cues, and to develop reciprocity. With appropriate adjustments for time of placement, similar assessments of attachment and interventions to promote attachment can be used in adoptive and biologic families.

Attachment With Severely Handicapped Children

An anomaly in the infant may affect the attachment process. Because reciprocity is an important part of the process of attachment, the process is at risk when one of the interactors is unable to perform her or his role. When a mother interacts with a nonhandicapped child, the more the child smiles, looks, or vocalizes, the more responsive the mother becomes. When the child is blind, deaf, or mentally retarded, the mother must adapt her interactive

behaviors. However, she may not know how to compensate for the child's deficits and may need instruction and role modeling. This is especially true of severely retarded children.

Blacher (1984) found that severely handicapped children do exhibit attachment behaviors and that the children studied showed a range in behavior. She suggested ways to promote attachment in families with handicapped children. The parents' sensitivity to subtle cues could be enhanced. For example, a head turn or ceasing self-stimulatory behavior may be the child's way of recognizing the mother or father. Parents may be either positively or negatively unrealistic about the child's capabilities. Parents can be helped to think realistically about the child's abilities and to respond to the child's signals. Because attachment does occur with severely handicapped children, consideration may be given to the implications of separation when recommending placement of such children. When neither parental attachment nor ability of the child to form an attachment exists, placement of the child outside the home is more likely to be an acceptable appropriate option. When the parents choose to keep the child at home, professionals should help foster attachment.

Assessment and Interventions in Mother-Infant Relationships

Nurses come into professional contact with women and their families at any point in the maternity cycle in public health offices, hospitals, doctor's offices, child protection centers, or in childbirth education classes. Facilitating a mother-infant relationship is usually only one of a number of concurrently operating goals of health care. Much can be done during the performance of other nursing tasks to support the development of maternal attachment.

More often than not, a maternity or public health nurse is concerned with the care of a specific woman and her baby at a given point in time. The nurse can draw on general knowledge of norms, averages, and risk factors, but must apply what is pertinent from that store of information to a mother with a specific history and personality, in a relationship with a specific infant, and within a specific environment. It is well known that individuals classified as high risk are sometimes able to cope effectively with whatever risks are involved and to relate affectionately to a particular newborn. It also happens that what appears to be a perfect image of a potential mother can be shattered by unpredictable events occurring after the image was drawn.

Effective evaluation of a mother-infant relationship requires a broad understanding of a mother and newborn pair as it exists within a family and a wider social setting. The manner in which the nurse carries out an evaluation of a mother-newborn relationship can be concurrently diagnostic, preventive, and therapeutic. While interacting with a maternity client, the nurse can assess her ability to trust people and to enjoy relationships, her skills in communication, and her feeling tone. At the same time the nurse can purposefully work to develop a mutually trusting relationship and an increase in maternal self-esteem and self-confidence. Through direct interaction, the nurse can also make use of his or her modeling potential. He or she can actively demonstrate forms of nurturing, communicating, and problem solving that can be unconsciously picked up and imitated or consciously studied and tested by the mother. When feelings are expressed, the nurse can accept them nonjudgmentally. This practice enables the owner of the feelings to accept them and perhaps to examine and understand them. It also encourages the further expression of feelings. As the nurse reaches tentative conclusions about facts and feelings in the evaluation of a mother-infant relationship, it is often appropriate to share ideas with the mother, both because the mother is a source of validation of the nurse's observation and because being included in the process of assessment can be ego-enhancing for the mother. Some mothers can be very accurate in predicting their own postpartal adjustment and the quality of their support network.

Assessment of Early Attachment

If attachment is accepted as a desired outcome of nursing care, a nurse in any of the various postpartal settings can periodically observe and note progress toward attachment. The following questions can be addressed in the course of nurse-client interaction:

1. *Is the mother attracted to her newborn?* Does she seek face-to-face contact and eye contact? Is she actively reaching out or only passively holding her newborn? Has she progressed from fingertip touch to palmar contact to enfolding the infant close to her body? Is attraction increasing or decreasing? If the mother does not exhibit increasing attraction, why not? Do the reasons lie primarily within her, the baby, or the environment?

2. *Is the mother inclined to nurture her infant?* Is she progressing in her interactions with her infant? Has she selected a rooming-in arrangement if it is available?

3. *Does the mother act consistently?* Is she developing a consistent and predictable approach to the care of her infant? Does she tend to respond to the same situation in the same way from day to day? If not, is the source of unpredictability within her or her infant?

4. *Is her mothering intelligently carried out?* Does she seek information and evaluate it objectively? Does she develop solutions based on adequate knowledge of valid data? How did she prepare herself for the parenting role? Does she evaluate the effectiveness of her maternal care and make appropriate adjustment?

5. *Is she sensitive to the newborn's needs as they arise?* How quickly does she interpret her infant's behavior and react to cues? Does she respond when the baby cries or fusses? Does she seem happy and satisfied with the infant's responses to her efforts? Is she pleased with feeding behaviors? How much of this ability and willingness to respond is related to the baby's nature and how much to her own?

6. *Does she seem pleased with her baby's appearance and sex?* Is she experiencing pleasure in interaction with her infant? What times are the most and least enjoyable? What interferes with the enjoyment? Does she speak to the baby frequently and affectionately? Does she call him or her by name? Does she point out family traits or characteristics she sees in the newborn?

7. *Are there any cultural factors that might modify the mother's response?* For instance, is it customary for the grandmother to assume most of the child-care responsibilities while the mother recovers from childbirth?

When these questions are addressed and the facts have been assembled by the nurse, the nurse's intuitive feelings and formal background of knowledge should combine to answer three more questions: Is there a problem in attachment? What is the problem? What is its source? Each nurse can then devise a creative approach to the problem as it presents itself in the context of a unique developing mother-infant relationship.

Assessment of attachment behaviors has become increasingly important in light of current theories that correlate malattachment with an increased incidence of parenting problems, failure to thrive, and child neglect or abuse. When assessing attachment behaviors, the nurse should be careful not to generalize or give too much importance to any one factor. Adaptive behavior may vary from one situation to the next. Cultural factors such as decreased eye contact should also be considered. All cultures may not recognize or value the same behaviors that members of the Western culture value.

Assessment of the mother-infant (or father-infant) interaction should be made on various occasions to avoid attaching too much significance to one behavior on a given occasion. Some behaviors that may indicate a maladaptive attachment process include refusal by the mother to see her newborn, failure to progress from fingertip to palm when holding or exploring the infant, making no attempt to establish eye-to-eye contact, inability to choose a name, or choosing a name that is so unusual that it imples hostility or ridicule (such as "Jim Beam," "Spirits," "Tornado," or the like).

An attachment assessment form is reproduced in Figure 35–5. It provides for recording observations during the prenatal period through six weeks of life. Those involved in care of the family can become aware of potential problems and provide interventions to enhance attachment.

Guidelines for Intervention

Actions that minimize mental distress and physical discomfort or maximize feelings of well-being and pleasure have the potential of enhancing the quality of mother-infant interaction. Following are some suggested objectives and ways of achieving them:

1. Determine the childbearing and childrearing goals of the infant's mother and father and use them wherever possible in planning nursing care for the family. This includes giving the parents choices about their labor and delivery experience and their initial time with their new infant.

2. Arrange the health care setting so that individual nurse-client professional relationships can be developed and maintained throughout a pregnancy and during the first months of mother-infant adaptation. A consistent care giver during the mother's prenatal experience allows a comfortable trusting relationship to develop in which the mother feels free to express concerns, ask questions, and explore choices. In the hospital a primary nurse can develop rapport and assess the mother's strengths and needs.

3. Enhance the couple's relationship and increase their communication capacity during the pregnancy. A feeling of closeness and personal satisfaction often results when the father plays an active role in the labor and delivery process by acting as the woman's coach and support person. Comfort with such a role will develop most easily if the parents attend prenatal classes. As they learn about pregnancy and delivery, anxiety decreases.

4. Use anticipatory guidance from conception through the postpartal period to prepare the parents for expected problems of adjustment. Prenatal classes often focus on possible problems a new family might encounter. In addition, literature on a variety of concerns, from feeding to sibling rivalry to infant stimulation, helps the new parents cope. If such information is available in the hospital and at the office or clinic, parents can choose according to their need.

5. Include parents in any nursing intervention planning and evaluation. Give choices whenever possible.

6. Remove barriers to voluntary contact among family members and the infant. This may be accomplished by providing time in the first hour after delivery for the new family to become acquainted with as much privacy as possible. Warmth may be maintained by placing the infant against the mother's bare chest and covering both with a warmed blanket. When the father is holding his new daughter or son, the baby may be wrapped in two or three warmed blankets. Postponing eye prophylaxis facilitates eye contact between parents and their newborn. Sibling attendance at the birth or sibling visits also play a role in integrating the newest family member.

7. Initiate and support measures to alleviate parental fatigue.

8. Help parents to identify, understand, and accept both positive and negative feelings related to the overall parenting experience.

9. Support and assist parents in determining the personality and unique needs of their infant. Whenever possible rooming-in should be available. This practice gives the mother a chance to learn her infant's normal patterns and develop confidence in caring for him or her. It also allows the father more uninterrupted time with his infant in the first days of life. If mother and baby are doing well and if help is available for the mother at home, early discharge permits the family to begin establishing their life together.

The following are specific strategies to promote the role of the father in pregnancy and childbirth (Kunst-Wilson & Cronenwett 1981):

1. Include the father in all prenatal visits.

2. Encourage his participation in prenatal and parenting classes.

3. Provide educational material depicting active, involved fathers.

4. Address concerns of fathers related to childbirth and infant care.

5. Have a prenatal session for fathers only, with involved fathers as discussion leaders.

6. Encourage discussion of changes in role and parenting issues.

7. Facilitate the father's presence at labor and delivery and provide support for the role he wishes.

8. Encourage the father to hold his newborn.

9. Allow the parents to have time alone with their infant after delivery.

10. Give the father the opportunity to room-in with the mother.

ATTACHMENT ASSESSMENT FORM

NAME _____ AGE _____ MARITAL STATUS: Single _____ Married _____ Separated _____
GRAVIDA _____ PARA _____ AB _____ DELIVERY DATE _____
EXPECTED DATE OF CONFINEMENT _____ METHOD OF FEEDING _____
SUMMARY OF LABOR AND DELIVERY (anesthesia, complications, presence of a supportive person):
_____

DIRECTIONS: *This form is provided to systematically assess and record the components of the attachment process based on information obtained from available records, observations, and interviews with the parent(s) and other health care providers.*

PRENATAL PERIOD   YES   NO

Planned the pregnancy _____ _____
COMMENTS _____

Confirmed the pregnancy _____ _____
COMMENTS _____

Accepted the pregnancy _____ _____
COMMENTS _____

Received early prenatal care _____ _____
COMMENTS _____

Described fetal movement _____ _____
COMMENTS _____

Personalized the fetus _____ _____
COMMENTS _____

Asked what the fetus was like in utero _____ _____
COMMENTS _____

Attended prenatal classes _____ _____
COMMENTS _____

Planned for infant's needs _____ _____
COMMENTS _____

Thought of possible names _____ _____
COMMENTS _____

Client in good health _____ _____
COMMENTS _____

Father of infant involved _____ _____
COMMENTS _____

AREAS OF CONCERN _____

FIRST POSTPARTUM DAY (*From birth through first day*)   YES   NO

Calls infant by name _____ _____
COMMENTS _____

Describes infant in affectionate terms _____ _____
COMMENTS _____

Offers positive comments about infant's physi- _____ _____
cal appearance
COMMENTS _____

Finds family resemblances _____ _____
COMMENTS _____

Looks and reaches out to infant _____ _____
COMMENTS _____

Hugs and touches infants _____ _____
COMMENTS _____

Kisses infant _____ _____
COMMENTS _____

Smiles at infant _____ _____
COMMENTS _____

Expresses positive emotional feelings to in- _____ _____
fant's father or significant other
COMMENTS _____

Experiences average discomfort _____ _____
COMMENTS _____

Welcomes visitors _____ _____
COMMENTS _____

AREAS OF CONCERN _____

DELIVERY PERIOD (*Birth through 4 hours*)   *Yes*   *No*

Accepts sex of infant _____ _____
COMMENTS _____

Calls infant by name _____ _____
COMMENTS _____

Calls infant by affectionate terms _____ _____
COMMENTS _____

Comments on beauty of infant _____ _____
COMMENTS _____

Realistically appraises the physical appearance _____ _____
of the infant
COMMENTS _____

Looks and reaches out to infant _____ _____
COMMENTS _____

Touches infant _____ _____
COMMENTS _____

Smiles at infant _____ _____
COMMENTS _____

AREAS OF CONCERN: _____

POSTPARTUM PERIOD (*From second day to 6 weeks*)   YES   NO

Want to be near infant _____ _____
COMMENTS _____

Enjoys caring for infant _____ _____
COMMENTS _____

Holds infant close _____ _____
COMMENTS _____

Feels infant belongs to her _____ _____
COMMENTS _____

Feels infant notices her _____ _____
COMMENTS _____

When away, thinks about infant _____ _____
COMMENTS _____

Verbalizes warm comments about infant _____ _____
COMMENTS _____

Recuperates with little difficulty _____ _____
COMMENTS _____

Responds sensitively and appropriately to _____ _____
infant
COMMENTS _____

AREAS OF CONCERN: _____

Figure 35–5 Attachment assessment form with provision for continuity from the prenatal period through delivery and the first postpartum day to six weeks postpartum (From Early Parent-Infant Relationships. National Foundation/March of Dimes, 1978, p 74.)

11. Encourage the father's participation in feeding, holding, and diapering the infant.

12. Include the father in well-baby checks.

13. Provide postpartum classes that include both parents.

14. Facilitate discussion of difficulties in sharing responsibilities for infant care.

15. Encourage formation of parent support groups.

Research Approaches to Enhance Attachment

The importance of attachment is widely recognized as are the adverse effects that may result when attachment does not occur. Researchers attempting to increase attachment have used a variety of strategies with varying degrees of success.

Carter-Jessop (1981) used a prenatal intervention in which she instructed the mothers to feel the fetal parts; become aware of fetal activity and how they affected it; and rub, stroke, and massage their abdomen over the baby daily. Mothers in the experimental group had more maternal behaviors in the postpartum period than mothers who did not focus on the fetus in the same way.

Carson and Virden (1984) tested the Carter-Jessop intervention in a sample of low-income primiparas and multiparas from a multiethnic population. In this sample, the intervention did not affect maternal behaviors postpartum.

Common interventions to enhance attachment in the early newborn period include acquaintance strategies, early contact, and skin-to-skin contact.

Dean, Morgan, and Towle (1982) used a 20-minute teaching session to acquaint the parents with their infant in order to decrease anxiety that might interfere with attachment. They demonstrated reflexes, hearing, and sight and explained normal variations of the newborn that were present in the infant. They found that experimental group mothers had lower anxiety scores.

Anisfeld and Lipper (1983) used an extra contact condition in which the infants spent 45 to 60 minutes skin-to-skin with the mother in the delivery and recovery rooms. The extra contact mothers had higher affectionate contact scores than the routine contact mothers. The treatment was equally effective for multiparas and primiparas. For mothers with low social support, extra contact was particularly valuable.

Curry (1979) compared early contact with a clothed infant with early contact with a naked baby. No differences were observed in maternal attachment behaviors.

DeChateau and Wiberg (1977) provided 15 minutes of contact soon after delivery. Early contact mothers of male infants held their infants more at 36 hours, kissed and looked *en face* at three months, and displayed more affection at one year. There were no differences between early contact and late contact for primiparous mothers at 36 hours.

Jones (1981) compared fathers who held their infants in the delivery room with fathers who did not hold their infants in that first hour. The only difference observed was that at 30 days, the fathers who held their infants in the delivery room interacted more nonverbally. Nonverbal behaviors included such items as eye-to-eye contact, smiling, kissing, and touching.

Toney (1983) offered fathers the opportunity to hold their infants for ten minutes in the first hour after delivery. She found no differences in frequency of bonding behaviors.

From this sampling of studies, it is evident that there are no definitive answers about the importance of early contact, or skin-to-skin contact, or how to enhance attachment. Formation of the attachment bond depends on numerous factors, and the bond may be enhanced by the sensitive approach of a health care provider in a humanistic environment in which parental preferences are given prime consideration.

● Complications in Maternal-Infant Attachment

The mother who experienced a high-risk labor and delivery or who has complications in the immediate postpartal period has an increased risk of encountering difficulties in attachment. She is more likely to have had medications, analgesia, or anesthesia during the intrapartal period, which may influence early interaction with her newborn. In the immediate postpartal period she may be more likely to receive medications or analgesics or to face problems that limit her energy. Complications involving the mother or infant may necessitate separation during the critical early stages of attachment. Although these are only a few of the factors that may be present, they may be significant if they interfere with the bonding or attachment process.

When the mother is ill, she may have to work through her own ambivalence about the illness and the infant's role as the possible cause of the illness. Mothers may express this anxiety in many ways. Three expressions that nurses frequently encounter are: (a) clearly blaming the infant (pregnancy) for the illness; (b) blaming herself and the infant, especially when the pregnancy was unplanned or unwanted; and (c) blaming the infant and infant's father, as if a conspiracy existed to cause the illness.

Occasionally mothers who are aware of the bonding process become very concerned if for reasons such as illness of the baby or themselves they are deprived of postpartal contact. This concern itself can become a crisis for the parents, and to avoid a self-fulfilling prophecy the nurse can assure the couple that strong bonding can occur even when separation is necessary.

Malattachment

During the past 20 years a body of evidence has grown that clearly demonstrates that the most common element in the lives of parents who neglect or abuse their children is a "lack of empathic mothering" in their own lives (Steele and Pollack 1968). This phrase describes inadequate responses of the caretaker to the infant, frequently beginning in the perinatal period and related to poorly developed maternal-infant attachment or insufficient bonding (Helfer & Kempe 1976). Because of this finding, attention has been given to the promotion of adequate parent-infant bonding to prevent malattachment and its related sequelae. Factors that may retard the formation of maternal-infant attachment include "an abnormal pregnancy, an abnormal labor or delivery, neonatal separation, other separation in the first six months, illnesses in the infant during the first year of life, and illnesses in the mother during the first year of life" (Helfer & Kempe 1976, p 29).

In the prenatal period, warning signs that may indicate lack of acceptance of the pregnancy and a potential for malattachment include: negative maternal self-perception, excessive mood swings or emotional withdrawal, failure to respond to quickening, excessive maternal preoccupation with appearance, numerous physical complaints, and failure to prepare for the infant during the last trimester (Helfer & Kempe 1976).

At delivery, signs of maladaptive responses may include lack of interest in seeing the newborn; withdrawal, sadness, or disappointment; negative comments such as "She's such an ugly thing"; or expressions of marked disappointment when told of the infant's sex. When shown the infant, the mother may avoid looking at the child or may regard the child without expression. She may decline to hold the infant, or if she does agree to do so, she may not touch or stroke the infant's face or extremities. The mother may also avoid asking questions or talking to the infant and may suddenly decide she does not want to breast-feed (Johnson 1979).

During the early postpartal period, evidence of maladaptive mothering may include limited handling of or smiling at the infant, lack of preparation or questions about infant needs and care, and failure to snuggle the newborn to her neck and face. The mother may also describe her infant negatively or use animal characteristics in a hostile manner when referring to the infant: "He looks just like a withered old monkey to me!"

The father, too, may exhibit signs of malattachment to his infant. Examples of maladaptive paternal behaviors include inattentiveness and indifference toward the child, rough, unrelaxed handling, and tense, rigid posture. The father may also choose inappropriate types of play and exhibit no protective behavior toward his child (Johnson 1979).

When maladaptive behaviors are identified, various interventions can be used. A team approach involving all nursing shifts is advised. Any positive behaviors are communicated so that each staff member can continue to offer support and stimulate further development of such strengths.

Hospital practices should be examined for factors that may inhibit or exaggerate the maladaptive behaviors. Hospital practices such as strict adherence to four-hour feedings, discouraging the mother from unwrapping and looking at her newborn, or prolonged separation, although far less common today, may create a problem for some mothers.

The mother needs a supportive, understanding person she can interact with as she works through her feelings about her baby. At times, in the presence of severe emotional disorders, a referral to a psychologist or psychiatrist may be necessary. Referral to community agencies such as the Public Health Department is advised so that follow-up care can be established.

The referral should be accompanied by a summary of the hospital course, the identified strengths and maladaptive behaviors, the educational process that was accomplished in the hospital, and the mother's response. Personal or telephone contact may be maintained after discharge so that the mother can continue to have contact with a supportive person with whom she is already acquainted. The mother should be encouraged to call the postpartal unit or newborn nursery if she has questions.

When the Newborn Is Hospitalized

Disorders in attachment may occur after separation due to prolonged hospitalization of the infant. Many mothers and fathers appear to be close to their infants and nurture them in a normal, adaptive way, despite separation. When disorders do occur, the mother's affective state and the father's role are critical components (Herzog 1979).

When bonding problems develop, the mother's affective state may sometimes become progressively pathological. Mothers report postpartum depression, sadness, crying, irritability, and difficulty sleeping. It is unclear whether the bonding problems are the cause or the effect of the mother's state.

Two components of the father's attachment to the infant can interfere with the mother's ability to overcome the effects of separation. The father may compete with the mother in the care and nurturing of the infant, or he may disengage and withdraw from the situation. In either case, the mother is left without the support she needs. It is possible that when a mother is separated from her infant, she

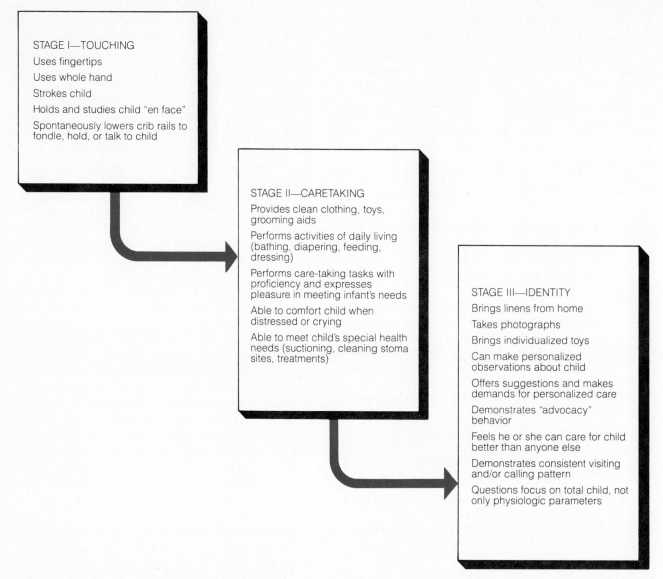

STAGE I—TOUCHING
Uses fingertips
Uses whole hand
Strokes child
Holds and studies child "en face"
Spontaneously lowers crib rails to fondle, hold, or talk to child

STAGE II—CARETAKING
Provides clean clothing, toys, grooming aids
Performs activities of daily living (bathing, diapering, feeding, dressing)
Performs care-taking tasks with proficiency and expresses pleasure in meeting infant's needs
Able to comfort child when distressed or crying
Able to meet child's special health needs (suctioning, cleaning stoma sites, treatments)

STAGE III—IDENTITY
Brings linens from home
Takes photographs
Brings individualized toys
Can make personalized observations about child
Offers suggestions and makes demands for personalized care
Demonstrates "advocacy" behavior
Feels he or she can care for child better than anyone else
Demonstrates consistent visiting and/or calling pattern
Questions focus on total child, not only physiologic parameters

Figure 35-6   Stages of parenting behavior toward an infant in intensive care (From Shraeder BD: Attachment and parenting despite lengthy intensive care. *Am J Mat Child Nurs* 1980;5(January/February):38)

needs extra nurturing in order to provide the necessary nurturing for the infant. Thus it may be that an important role for the father is to nurture his wife so that she can nurture the infant.

NURSING GOAL: PROMOTING ATTACHMENT WHEN THE NEWBORN IS HOSPITALIZED

When infants require lengthy intensive care, special efforts by the nurse may facilitate attachment. It is important that parents believe that the child "belongs" to them rather than to the medical team. They should be encouraged to participate in care and to give suggestions about that care. Schraeder (1980, p 38) suggests establishing a care plan and including specific nursing diagnoses such as "alteration in the parent-child relationship" or "impairment of the parent-infant bond." Nursing interventions are then established according to the stages of parenting behaviors outlined in Figure 35-6. For example, if the mother entered the nursery, lowered the crib rail, and established an *en face* position while talking to the infant, she would be ready to move into stage II. If there is a specific problem, with the feeding schedule or technique, for example, the parents might be encouraged to work with the nurses to help establish the care plan.

Jenkins and Tock (1986) describe sending an informative letter to the parents "from the baby" on a weekly basis to promote proximity. The letter describes the competencies of the infant and behaviors such as "I like to open my eyes when I eat, but I get so tired that I soon close them" (p 34).

During the postpartal period, continued family interaction should be encouraged through supportive staff, liberal visiting policies, and educational offerings for both father and mother. Staff should be trained in assessment techniques and alert for evidence of malattachment, so that appropriate interventions may be initiated. If necessary, referrals to the community health nurse or social services may provide the ongoing assistance needed. Telephone hotlines may provide a useful resource for a frustrated or worried parent, as may classes or parents' groups during the early weeks after delivery.

KEY CONCEPTS

Attachments are enduring affectional bonds.

When attachment does not occur, there are significant negative consequences.

The three major views of attachment are psychoanalytic, ethological, and learning theories.

A mother's genetic makeup and background influences the environment she can provide for the fetus and newborn.

Attachment to the fetus develops during pregnancy.

The infant is a significant partner in the attachment interaction.

The childbirth setting is important in creating an environment for early parent-infant interaction.

Mother-infant interaction proceeds through phases: introductory, acquaintance, mutual regulation, reciprocity and rhythmicity, and attachment.

Attachment behaviors may differ in adolescent mothers.

Fathers, siblings, and others also become attached to the fetus and newborn.

Attachment occurs with adopted children and with handicapped children.

Attachment can be systematically assessed.

Interventions can facilitate attachment.

Complications in parent-infant attachment can occur because of maternal illness or hospitalization of the infant.

REFERENCES

Anisfeld E, Lipper E: Early contact, social support, and mother-infant bonding. *Pediatrics* 1983;72:79.

Avant KC: Anxiety as a potential factor affecting maternal attachment. *J Obstet Gynecol Neonat Nurs* 1981;6:416.

Blacher J: Attachment and severely handicapped children: Implications for intervention. *J Dev Behav Pediatr* 1984;5:178.

Bowen SM, Miller BC: Paternal attachment behavior as related to presence at delivery and preparenthood classes: A pilot study. *Nurs Res* 1980;29:307.

Bowlby J: The nature of the child's tie to his mother. *Int J Psychoanal* 1958;39:350.

Brazelton TB, et al: The origins of reciprocity: The early mother-infant interaction, in Lewis M, Rosenblum LA (eds): *The Effect of the Infant on Its Caregiver.* New York, Wiley, 1974.

Campbell SB, Taylor PM: Bonding and attachment: Theoretical perspectives and empirical findings. Presented at International Conference on Infant Studies, New Haven, Connecticut, April 11–13, 1980.

Carson K, Virden S: Can prenatal teaching promote maternal attachment? Practicing nurses test Carter-Jessop's prenatal attachment intervention. *Health Care Women Int* 1984;5:355.

Carter-Jessop L: Promoting maternal attachment through prenatal intervention. *Am J Mat Child Nurs* 1981;6:107.

Censullo M, Lester B, Hoffman J: Rhythmic patterning in mother-newborn interaction. *Nurs Res* 1985;34:342.

Condon WS, Sander LW: Synchrony demonstrated between movements of the neonate and adult speech. *Child Dev* 1974;45:456.

Cranley MS: Development of a tool for the measurement of maternal attachment during pregnancy. *Nurs Res* 1981a;30:281.

Cranley MS: Roots of attachment: The relationship of parents with their unborn. *Birth Defects* 1981b;17:59.

Curry MA: Contact during the first hour with the wrapped or naked newborn: Effect on maternal attachment behaviors at 36 hours and 3 months. *Birth and Family J* 1979;6:227.

Curry MA: Maternal attachment behavior and the mother's self-concept: The effect of early skin-to-skin contact. *Nurs Res* 1982;31:73.

Dean PG, Morgan P, Towle JM: Making baby's acquaintance: A unique attachment strategy. *Am J Mat Child Nurs* 1982;7:37.

de Chateau P, Wiberg B: Long-term effect on mother-infant behavior of extra contact during the first hour postpartum. *Acta Paediatr Scand* 1977;66:137.

Feller CM, et al: Assessment of adolescent mother-infant attachment. *Issues Health Care Women* 1983;4:237.

Field T, Reite M: Children's responses to separation from mother during the birth of another child. *Child Dev* 1984;55:1308.

Gill NE, White MA, Anderson GC: Transitional newborn infants in a hospital nursery: From first oral cue to first sustained cry. *Nurs Res* 1984;33:213.

Goren CC, et al: Visual following and pattern discrimination of facelike stimuli by newborn infants. *Pediatrics* 1975;56:544.

Gottlieb L: Maternal attachment in primiparas. *J Obstet Gynecol Neonat Nurs* 1978;7:39.

Grace JT: Does a mother's knowledge of fetal gender affect attachment? *Am J Mat Child Nurs* 1984;9:42.

Greenberg M, **Morris** N: Engrossment: The newborn's impact upon the father. *Am J Orthopsychiatry* 1974;44:520.

Helfer RE, **Kempe** CH: *Child Abuse and Neglect.* Cambridge, Mass, Ballinger, 1976.

Herzog JM: Disturbances in parenting high-risk infants: Clinical impressions and hypotheses, in **Field** TM, et al (eds): *Infants Born at Risk.* New York, S.P. Medical and Scientific Books, 1979.

Jenkins RL, **Tock** MKS: Helping parents bond to their premature infant. *Am J Mat Child Nurs* 1986;11:32.

Johnson SH: *High Risk Parenting: Nursing Assessment and Strategies for the Family at Risk.* Philadelphia, Lippincott, 1979.

Jones C: Father to infant attachment: Effects of early contact and characteristics of the infant. *Res Nurs Health* 1981;4:193.

Klaus MH, et al: Human maternal behavior at first contact with her young. *Pediatrics* 1970;46:187.

Kohn CL, **Nelson** A, **Weiner** S: Gravidas' response to real-time ultrasound fetal image. *J Obstet Gynecol Neonat Nurs* 1980;9:77.

Korner AF, **Thoman** EB: Visual alertness in neonates as evoked by maternal care. *J Exp Child Psychol* 1970;10:67.

Kunst-Wilson W, **Cronenwett** L: Nursing care for the emerging family: Promoting paternal behavior. *Res Nurs Health* 1981;4:201.

Leifer M: Psychological changes accompanying pregnancy and motherhood. *Genet Psychol Monogr* 1977;95:55.

Leifer M: Pregnancy. *Signs* 1980;5:754.

Lozoff B, et al: The mother-newborn relationship: Limits of adaptability. *J Pediatr* 1977;91:1.

McAnarney ER, **Lawrence** RA, **Aten** MJ: Premature parenthood: A preliminary report of adolescent mother-infant interaction. *Pediatr Res* 1979;13:327.

McFarlane A: Olfaction in the development of social preferences in the human neonate, in *Parent-Infant Interaction,* Ciba Foundation Symposium 33, New York, Elsevier, 1975.

Mercer RT: Relationship of the birth experience to later mothering behaviors. *J Nurse-Midwife* 1985;30:204.

Milne LS, **Rich** OJ: Cognitive and affective aspects of the responses of pregnant women to sonography. *Matern Child Nurs J* 1981;10:15.

Nicholson J, et al: Outcomes of father involvement in pregnancy and birth. *Birth* 1983;10:5.

Perry S: Parents' perceptions of their newborn following structured interactions. *Nurs Res* 1983;32:208.

Peterson GH, **Mehl** LE, **Leiderman** PH: The role of some birth-related variables in father attachment. *Am J Orthopsychiatry* 1979;49:330.

Porter RH, **Cernoch** JM, **McLaughlin** FJ: Maternal recognition of neonates through olfactory cues. *Physiol Behav* 1983a;30:151.

Porter RH, **Cernoch** JM, **Perry** S: The importance of odors in maternal-infant interactions. *Matern Child Nurs J* 1983b;12:147.

Robson KS: The role of eye-to-eye contact in maternal-infant attachment. *J Child Psychol Psychiat* 1967;8:13.

Rubin R: Maternal touch. *Nurs Outlook* 1963;11:828.

Schraeder BD: Attachment and parenting despite lengthy intensive care. *Am J Mat Child Nurs* 1980;11:32.

Singer LM, et al: Mother-infant attachment in adoptive families. *Child Dev* 1985;56:1543.

Smith DW, **Sherwen** LN: The bonding process of mothers and adopted children. *Top Clin Nurs* 1984;6:38.

Sosa R, et al: The effect of a supportive companion on perinatal problems, length of labor, and mother-infant interaction. *N Engl J Med* 1980;303:597.

Stainton MC: The fetus: A growing member of the family. *Fam Relations* 1985;34:321.

Steele B, **Pollock** C: A psychiatric study of parents who abuse infants and small children, in **Helfer** R, **Kempe** CH (eds): *The Battered Child.* Chicago, University of Chicago Press, 1968.

Sugarman M: Paranatal influences on maternal-infant attachment. *Am J Orthopsychiatry* 1977;47:407.

Svejda MJ, **Campos** JJ, **Emde** RN: Mother-infant "bonding": Failure to generalize. *Child Dev* 1980;51:775.

Toney L: The effects of holding the newborn at delivery on paternal bonding. *Nurs Res* 1983;32:16.

Trevathan WR: Maternal lateral preference at first contact with her newborn infant. *Birth* 1982;9:85.

Trevathan WR: Maternal "en face" orientation during the first hour after birth. *Am J Orthopsychiatry* 1983;53:92.

Weaver RH, **Cranley** MS: An exploration of paternal-fetal attachment behavior. *Nurs Res* 1983;32:68.

ADDITIONAL READINGS

Humenick SS, **Bugen** LA: Parenting roles: Expectation versus reality. *Am J Mat Child Nurs* 1987;12(January/February):36.

Janowski MJ: The road not taken . . . teenage mother's courageous decision. *Am J Nurs* 1987;87(March):334.

Jones LC, **Lenz** ER: Father-newborn interaction: Effects of social competence and infant state. *Nurs Res* 1986;35(May/June):149.

Karraker KH: Adult attention to infants in a newborn nursery. *Nurs Res* 1986:35(November/December):358.

Leander D, et al: Parental response to the birth of a high-risk neonate: Dynamics and management. *Phys Occup Ther Pediatr* 1986;6(Fall/Winter):205.

Sommerfield DP, et al: Do health professionals agree on the parenting potential of pregnant women? *Soc Sci Med* 1987;24(3):285.

Zuskar DM: The psychological impact of prenatal diagnosis of fetal abnormality: Strategies for investigation and intervention. *Women Health* 1987;12(1):91.

It's one of those "grass-is-greener" things—I envied, sometimes even hated Sam when he went out to work. I don't know what I was imagining—that he hung around talking, went out to lunch, did interesting things. One time he was watching me bathe Annie in the sink. He asked if he could do it—he stood there, soaping her back over and over like he couldn't get enough of it, and he talked about how he hated to leave us in the morning and how he worried he would be closed out, left looking in at what she and I had together. (The New Our Bodies, Ourselves)

The Postpartal Family at Risk

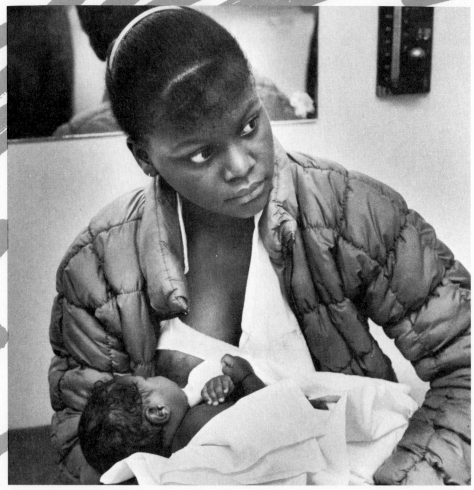

A single mother still in her teens nurses her week-old son while waiting to see a pediatrician at a clinic.

Chapter Thirty-Six

OBJECTIVES

- **List the causes and summarize appropriate nursing interventions for hemorrhage during the postpartal period.**
- **Compare the causative factors, pathophysiology, and nursing interventions of different puerperal infections.**
- **Discuss causative factors, pathophysiology, and nursing interventions for thromboembolic disease of the puerperium.**
- **Contrast puerperal cystitis and pyelonephritis and their implications for maternal nursing care.**
- **Differentiate disorders of the breast and complications of lactation.**
- **Identify the possible precipitating factors associated with puerperal psychiatric disorders.**

A tendency exists to view the puerperium as the smooth, uneventful time that follows the anticipation of pregnancy and the excitement and work of labor and delivery—and often it is. However, the nurse must be aware of problems that may develop postpartally and their implications for the childbearing family.

This chapter deals with the broad area of maternal complications during the puerperium. It emphasizes application of the nursing process to meet the needs of the woman experiencing such complications.

● Using the Nursing Process With Women at Risk During the Postpartal Period

When providing care to the childbearing woman during the postpartal period, the nurse uses the nursing process to make ongoing assessments and detect, as early as possible, the development of any complications. When a potential problem is noted, the nurse analyzes the data; formulates appropriate nursing diagnoses; and develops, implements, and evaluates a plan of care. Often the care will be provided in a collaborative way as the nurse works with other members of the health care team.

Nursing Assessment

Because complications can develop early in the postpartal period (for example, hemorrhage, PIH, or bladder distention) or later (endometritis, thrombophlebitis), the postpartal nurse should make ongoing assessment a major priority. Such assessment is especially important because the nurse is often the first person to detect a developing complication. If a complication does develop, assessment remains important to determine the effectiveness of therapy and to detect any signs that the problem is worsening.

Analysis and Nursing Diagnosis

The nurse analyzes the information gained from assessment and formulates appropriate nursing diagnoses. If, for example, the nurse is caring for a woman who complains of dysuria, the nurse first reviews the woman's history. The nurse learns that the woman was catheterized twice during labor for bladder distention and was also catheterized during the third hour after delivery. The woman reports that she does not feel that she is fully emptying her bladder. The nurse cannot palpate the bladder suprapubically. The woman has no CVA tenderness but her temperature is 100.8F. She is unable to produce another urine specimen so the nurse offers her additional fluids. The nurse then formulates the nursing diagnosis, "alteration in urinary elimination related to dysuria secondary to possible bladder infection."

Nursing Plan and Implementation

Once the data have been analyzed and the diagnosis established, the nurse develops and implements a care plan. In the case of the woman with dysuria, the nurse notifies the physician that the woman may be developing cystitis and obtains an order for a clean-catch urine for culture. The nurse will explain what is occurring to the woman and may administer a mild analgesic, or obtain an order for an antispasmodic if he or she believes the woman is also experiencing bladder spasms.

Evaluation

The nurse evaluates the effectiveness of the plan of care. For example, in the preceding situation the woman was relieved to learn that the nurse took her problem seriously. After receiving the antispasmodic, the woman was able to provide a clean-catch urine specimen, which revealed that the woman did have cystitis. Antibiotic therapy was begun. The nurse concluded that the plan had been effective thus far, but discussions with the woman revealed that a new nursing diagnosis was necessary: knowledge deficit related to a lack of understanding of self-care measures to help prevent UTI. The nurse then began planning an approach to meet this identified need.

Thus the process is cyclic, building on assessment, logical analysis, and well-planned and implemented intervention, followed by evaluation and modification as necessary.

● Care of the Woman With Postpartal Hemorrhage

Puerperal hemorrhage has been divided into early and late postpartal hemorrhage. Early postpartal hemorrhage (or immediate postpartal hemorrhage) occurs when blood loss is greater than 500 mL in the first 24 hours after delivery. Late postpartal hemorrhage (delayed postpartal hemorrhage) occurs after the first 24 hours. Because of the tendency to underestimate the amount of blood lost during delivery, this figure is probably not especially accurate as a guide. Perhaps a more reliable determinant is based on a clinical assessment of excessive blood loss (usually far more than 500 mL) (Visscher & Visscher 1982).

Early Postpartal Hemorrhage

The main causes of early postpartal hemorrhage are uterine atony, lacerations of the genital tract, and retained placenta or placental fragments. Certain factors predispose to hemorrhage: (a) overdistention of the uterus due to hydramnios, a large infant, or multiple gestation; (b) grand multiparity; (c) use of anesthetic agents (especially halothane) to relax the uterus; (d) trauma due to obstetric procedures such as midforceps delivery, intrauterine manipulation, or forceps rotation; (e) a prolonged labor or a very rapid labor; (f) use of oxytocin to induce or to augment labor; (g) uterine infection; and (h) maternal malnutrition, anemia, PIH, or history of hemorrhage.

In most cases the clinician can predict when a woman is at risk for hemorrhage. The key to successful management is prevention. Prevention begins with adequate nutrition, good prenatal care, and early diagnosis and management of any complications that may arise. Traumatic procedures should be avoided, and delivery should take place in a facility that has blood immediately available. Any woman at risk should be typed and cross-matched for blood and have intravenous lines in place. Excellent labor management and delivery technique is imperative.

Uterine atony and retained placenta are discussed in this section. Lacerations are considered in Chapter 25.

UTERINE ATONY

Relaxation of the uterus (or insufficient contractions) following delivery can frequently be anticipated in the presence of (a) overdistention of the uterus that occurs with multiple fetuses, macrosomic fetus, or hydramnios; (b) dysfunctional labor that has already indicated the uterus is contracting in an abnormal pattern; (c) oxytocin stimulation or augmentation during labor; and (d) the use of anesthesia that produces uterine relaxation. Hemorrhage from uterine atony may be slow and steady rather than sudden and massive. The blood may escape the vagina or collect in the uterus. Because of the increased blood volume associated with pregnancy changes in maternal blood pressure and pulse may not occur until blood loss has been significant.

After delivery of the placenta, the fundus should be palpated to assure that it is firm and well contracted. If it is not firm, vigorous massage should be instituted until the uterus contracts. Oxytocics (Pitocin, Methergine, or Ergotrate) may be given. If the bleeding persists, the physician undertakes bimanual uterine compression, which consists of using one gloved hand to massage the uterine fundus externally while the other gloved hand is inserted into the vagina and the closed fist is pressed against the uterus (Figure 36–1A). With this procedure the uterus is com-

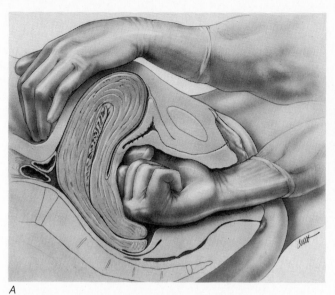
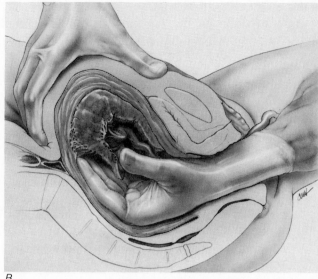

A
B

Figure 36–1   A Manual compression of the uterus and massage with the abdominal hand usually will effectively control hemorrhage from uterine atony.   B Manual removal of placenta. The fingers are alternately abducted, adducted, and advanced until the placenta is completely detached. (Adapted from Pritchard JA, MacDonald PC, Gant NF: Williams Obstetrics, 17 ed. Norwalk, Conn. Appleton-Century-Crofts, 1985.)

pressed and massaged and hemorrhage from uterine atony can usually be controlled. If an intravenous line is not already infusing, one should be established with oxytocin (Pitocin) added at a rapid rate. Blood transfusions may be ordered. Oxygen at 6 to 10 L/min is given by face mask. The physician manually checks the uterine cavity for retained placental fragments and also inspects the cervix and vagina for lacerations. The combination of bimanual compression, oxytocics, and blood transfusion is usually effective in treating uterine atony. If the atony does not respond to these measures, 15-methyl prostaglandin $F_{2\alpha}$ (Prostin 15M) may be administered intramuscularly. This synthetic prostaglandin generally stimulates powerful, sustained contractions. The dose (250 micrograms) may be repeated within 90 minutes, or more as necessary (Few 1987). The side effects, such as nausea, vomiting, and diarrhea, are unpleasant and are often treated with medication. Other side effects include fever, flushing, and elevated diastolic blood pressure. If, despite these measures, bleeding persists, other causes such as placenta accreta or cervical laceration should be considered (Few 1987). The fundus should be assessed frequently for the next few hours to see that it remains contracted.

RETAINED PLACENTA

Hemorrhage may occur after the delivery of the newborn but before delivery of the placenta. In this instance, the physician observes the firmness of the fundus and administers fundal massage if needed. When the placenta is

ready to separate, expression (delivery) of the placenta is enhanced by massaging the fundus. If signs of placental separation have not occurred, the physician manually removes the placenta by inserting a gloved hand into the uterus and placing the fingers at the placental margin. Then the placenta is gently separated from the uterine wall. During this procedure, the other hand remains on the uterine fundus, externally (Figure 36–1B). After delivery of the placenta, the consistency of the fundus is assessed. If it is boggy and bleeding continues, the interventions for uterine atony are performed.

Late Postpartal Hemorrhage

Late postpartal hemorrhage is most frequently caused by retained placental fragments. Hemorrhage from this cause may occur in the hours following the fourth stage of labor or may not develop for a day or two. Placental fragments are occasionally retained for a week or longer. In such cases, they may become necrosed, fibrin may be deposited, and the fragments form a so-called placental polyp (Easterling & Herbert 1986). Brisk bleeding may occur if the "polyp" becomes detached.

MEDICAL THERAPY

To prevent late postpartum hemorrhage from retained placental fragments, the placenta should be inspected after delivery for evidence of missing pieces or cotyledons. The membranes should be inspected for absent sections or for vessels that traverse from the edge of the placenta outward along the membranes, which may indicate placenta succenturiate and a retained lobe. The uterine cavity may also be checked for retained placental fragments or membranes.

Often a boggy uterus postpartally is the first indicator of late postpartal hemorrhage. The most commonly employed intervention is a continuous intravenous infusion of fluids and oxytocin. If the woman is normotensive, methylergonovine or ergonovine may be used. (Typical dosage is methylergonovine 0.2 mg every 4 hours × 6 doses.) If this treatment is not effective or if a placental fragment is retained for several days, curettage is usually indicated, together with the administration of antibiotics to prevent puerperal infection.

NURSING ASSESSMENT

Careful and ongoing assessment of the woman during labor and delivery and evaluation of her prenatal history will help identify factors that put the woman at risk for postpartal hemorrhage.

Periodic assessment for evidence of bleeding is a major nursing responsibility during the postpartal period. The experienced nurse realizes that after the fourth stage of labor most hemorrhage is caused by retained cotyledons, retained fetal membranes, or subnormal or abnormal involution of the placental site (discussed on p 1156).

Careful observation and documentation of vaginal bleeding (often by way of pad count or weighing of the perineal pad) is important if medical intervention is to be undertaken. A boggy uterus that does not stay contracted without constant massage is atonic, whereas a uterus that does not involute appropriately needs to be investigated for possible retained placental tissue and infection.

NURSING DIAGNOSIS

Nursing diagnoses that may apply when a woman experiences postpartal hemorrhage include:

- Knowledge deficit related to a lack of understanding of the signs of delayed postpartal hemorrhage

- Alteration in cardiac output: decreased: fatigue secondary to blood loss postpartally

NURSING GOAL: EFFECTIVE ASSESSMENT AND INTERVENTION TO ENSURE CLIENT WELL-BEING

Regular assessment of fundal height and firmness will alert the nurse to the possible development or recurrence of hemorrhage. The nurse massages a boggy uterus until it is firm and, if it appears larger than anticipated, attempts to express clots. If the woman seems to have a slow, steady,

free flow of blood the nurse begins weighing the perineal pads and monitors the woman's vital signs closely.

If medications such as methylergonovine maleate are begun, the nurse administers them and evaluates their effectiveness.

Because blood loss may cause anemia, the nurse assesses for evidence of pallor or fatigue, and reviews the results of the hematocrit determination. The nurse also encourages the woman to obtain adequate rest and helps her plan activities so that rest is possible.

NURSING GOAL: MANAGEMENT OF HEMORRHAGE

The nurse begins the intravenous infusions and blood transfusions ordered. Oxygen is administered by face mask at 6 to 10 L/min. The woman's blood pressure and pulse are monitored approximately every five minutes. The fundus should be assessed frequently for the next few hours to see that it remains contracted. Intravenous oxytocin will probably be continued for a period of hours. The urinary output should be assessed to determine the adequacy of fluid replacement.

NURSING GOAL: FACILITATION OF PARENT-INFANT ATTACHMENT

Because of the fatigue associated with blood loss, the mother may find it difficult to care for her infant. The nurse can often find ways to promote infant attachment while being cognizant of the health needs of the mother. The mother may require additional assistance in caring for her infant. If she has IVs, even carrying the newborn may be awkward. For the mother who feels compelled to do as much as possible, the nurse may also "give permission" to the mother to return her infant to the nursery so she can have adequate periods of uninterrupted rest. The nurse may also work with the woman's partner and family to find ways to help the mother cope.

NURSING GOAL: EDUCATION FOR SELF-CARE

Due to current trends, the mother may be discharged any time after four hours postdelivery. Because hemorrhage may develop after discharge, she and her family or support persons should receive clear, preferably written, explanations of the normal postpartal course of readjustment, including changes in the lochia and fundus and signs of abnormal bleeding. Instruction for the prevention of bleeding should include fundal massage, ways to assess the fundus for height and consistency, and inspection of the episiotomy and lacerations, if present. The woman should receive instruction in perineal care. The woman and her family are advised to contact their care giver if any of the following occur: excessive or bright red bleeding, a boggy fundus that does not respond to massage, abnormal clots, leukorrhea, high temperature, or any unusual pelvic or rectal discomfort or backache.

EVALUATIVE OUTCOME CRITERIA

Anticipated outcomes of nursing care include the following:

- Signs of postpartal hemorrhage are detected quickly and managed effectively.

- Maternal infant attachment is maintained successfully.

- The woman is able to identify abnormal changes that might occur following discharge and understands the importance of notifying her caregiver if they develop.

Hematomas

Hematomas often occur as a result of injury to a blood vessel without noticeable trauma to the superficial tissue. They may occur following spontaneous as well as forceps deliveries. Hematomas frequently develop in the lower genital tract, especially the vagina or vulva. The soft tissue in the area offers no resistance, and hematomas containing 250 to 500 mL of blood may develop rapidly. Within the vagina, the lateral wall, especially in the area of the ischial spines, is a common site of hematoma formation. Hematomas may also develop in the upper portion of the vagina or may occur upward into the broad ligament.

MEDICAL THERAPY

Small vulvar hematomas may be treated with the application of ice packs and continued observation. Large hematomas generally require surgical intervention to evacuate the clot and achieve hemostasis. General anesthesia is usually required, and if the hematoma is not accessible vaginally, a laparotomy must be performed. Antibiotics and transfusions may also be indicated.

Continuous assessment of the vaginal bleeding is required after surgery. If the hematoma was of the vulva or perineum, the nurse should check for recurrence.

NURSING ASSESSMENT

Often the first clue that a hematoma is forming is the woman's complaints of severe vulvar pain (pain that seems out of proportion or excessive), usually from her "stitches," or of severe rectal pressure. On examination, the large hematoma appears as a unilateral tense, fluctuant bulging mass at the introitus or encompassing the labia majora. The hematoma may not be as apparent as described

here, so the observant nurse checks for unilateral bluish or reddish discoloration of skin of the perineum and buttocks. The area feels firm and is painful to the touch. The nurse should estimate the size of the hematoma carefully with the first assessment to better estimate increases in size and the potential blood loss.

Hematomas can develop in the upper portion of the vagina. In this case, besides pain the woman may have difficulty voiding because of pressure on the urethra or meatus. Diagnosis is comfirmed through careful vaginal examination.

Hematomas that occur upward into the broad ligament may be more difficult to detect. The woman may complain of severe lateral uterine pain, flank pain, or abdominal distention. Occasionally the hematoma can be discovered with high rectal examination or with abdominal palpation although these procedures may be quite uncomfortable for the woman. If the bleeding continues, signs of anemia may be noted.

Signs and symptoms of shock in the presence of a well-contracted uterus and no visible vaginal blood loss may also alert the nurse to the possibility of a hematoma.

NURSING DIAGNOSIS

Nursing diagnoses that may apply when a woman develops a hematoma postpartally include:

- Potential for injury related to tissue damage secondary to prolonged pressure from a large vaginal hematoma

- Alteration in comfort: acute pain related to tissue trauma secondary to hematoma formation

NURSING GOAL: PROMOTION OF COMFORT

If delivery required the use of forceps or a vacuum extractor, or if it was traumatic because of the infant's size or position, the postpartal nurse can promote comfort and decrease the possibility of hematoma formation by applying an ice pack to the woman's perineum during the first hour after delivery.

The discomfort experienced by a woman who develops a hematoma cannot be overlooked. In addition to the treatment measures instituted to prevent hematoma formation, sitz baths will aid fluid absorption once the bleeding has stopped or been controlled and will promote comfort, as will the judicious use of analgesics.

EVALUATIVE OUTCOME CRITERIA

Anticipated outcomes of nursing care include:

- Hematoma formation is to be avoided; if it does occur, it is detected quickly and managed successfully.

- The woman's discomfort is relieved effectively.

- Tissue damage is avoided or minimized.

Subinvolution

Subinvolution of the uterus occurs when the uterus fails to follow the normal pattern of involution but instead remains enlarged. Retained placental fragments or infection are the most frequent causes of subinvolution. With subinvolution the fundus is higher in the abdomen than expected. In addition, lochia often fails to progress from rubra to serosa to alba. Lochia may remain rubra or return to rubra several days postpartum. Leukorrhea and backache may occur if infection is the cause. Subinvolution is most commonly diagnosed during the routine postpartal examination at four to six weeks. The woman may relate a history of irregular or excessive bleeding, or describe the symptoms listed previously. Diagnosis is made when an enlarged, softer-than-normal uterus is palpated with bimanual examination. Treatment involves oral administration of methylergonovine (Methergine) 0.2 mg every 3 to 4 hours for 24 to 48 hours. When metritis is present, antibiotics are also administered. If this treatment is not effective or if the cause is believed to be retained placental fragments, curettage is indicated (Pritchard et al 1985).

● Care of the Woman With a Reproductive Tract Infection

The reproductive tract may be the site of an infection associated with childbirth that can occur any time from delivery to ten days postpartum. The most common infection is metritis/endometritis and is limited to the uterine cavity. However, infection can spread by way of the lymphatics and blood vessels to become a progressive disease resulting in peritonitis or pelvic cellulitis. The woman's prognosis is directly related to the stage of the disease at the time of diagnosis, the invading organism, and the woman's state of health and ability to resist the disease state.

Because infection accounts for a large percentage of postpartal morbidity, it is useful to remember the definition of puerperal morbidity published by the Joint Committee on Maternal Welfare:

> Temperature of 100.4°F (38.0°C) or higher, the temperature to occur on any two of the first ten postpartum days, exclusive of the first 24 hours, and to be taken by mouth by a standard technique at least four times a day.

However, recent studies indicate that the definition's exclusion of the first 24 hours may not be completely accurate (Danforth & Scott 1986).

Antibiotic therapy alone has not caused the decrease in morbidity and mortality that is seen today. Aseptic technique, fewer traumatic operative deliveries, a better understanding of labor dystocia, improved surgical intervention, and a population that is generally at less risk from malnutrition and chronic debilitative disease have also contributed to this reduction.

The vagina and cervix of approximately 70 percent of all healthy pregnant women contain pathogenic bacteria that, alone or in combination, are sufficiently virulent to cause extensive infections. Why the organisms do not cause infection during pregnancy is not altogether clear; however, recent studies indicate that more than the presence of a pathogen in the woman's genital tract is necessary for infection to begin.

The uterus is essentially a sterile cavity prior to rupture of the fetal membranes. Once membranes rupture, vaginal microorganisms may ascend to the uterus so that within 24 hours after rupture, chorioamnionitis can be histologically demonstrated in about 50 percent of women (Vorherr 1982). Thus prolonged rupture of the membranes is a major factor in the development of infection postpartally. Also, the placental site, episiotomy, lacerations, abrasions, and any operative incisions are all potential portals for bacterial entrance and growth. Hematomas are easily infected and enhance the possibility of sepsis. Tissue that has been compromised through trauma is less able to marshal the necessary forces to combat infection. Other factors predisposing the woman to infection include frequent vaginal examinations, lapses in aseptic technique, anemia, intrauterine manipulation, hemorrhage, lacerations of the reproductive tract, cesarean delivery, retained placental fragments, and faulty perineal care.

Infectious Agents

AEROBIC BACTERIAL INFECTIONS

The most common aerobic bacteria found in women with postpartal infection are group B beta hemolytic streptococci and *Escherichia coli*. *E. coli* may be introduced as a result of contamination of the vulva or reproductive tract from feces during labor and delivery. Though it occurs less frequently, group A beta hemolytic streptococcus is responsible for an especially virulent infection. It may be transmitted from the skin or nasopharynx of the woman herself, or more probably from an external source such as personnel or equipment. Because it is highly contagious, it presents a serious problem for hospital personnel (Vorherr 1982). Other aerobic bacteria implicated in puerperal infections include klebsiella, *Proteus mirabilis*, pseudomonas,

Staphylococcus aureus, and *Neisseria gonorrhoeae* (Eschenbach & Wager 1980).

ANAEROBIC BACTERIAL INFECTIONS

After delivery the amniotic fluid, blood, lochia, and decreased numbers of lactobacilli present in the reproductive tract have a neutralizing effect. The pH of the vagina changes from acid to alkaline, which is suitable for the growth of aerobic organisms. Then, approximately 48 hours after delivery, acid end-products accumulate as a result of necrosis of endometrial and placental remnants and the intrauterine environment becomes more favorable to anaerobic organisms. Consequently, approximately 70 percent of puerperal infections are caused by anaerobes (Vorherr 1982). The most common anaerobes involved include bacteroides (all species), peptostreptococcus, peptococcus, and *Clostridium perfringens.*

Types of Infections

LOCALIZED INFECTIONS

A less severe complication of the puerperium is the localized infection of the episiotomy or of lacerations to the perineum, vagina, or vulva. Wound infection of the abdominal incision site following cesarean delivery is also possible. The skin edges become reddened, edematous, firm, and tender. The skin edges then separate, and purulent material, sometimes mixed with sanguineous liquid, drains from the wound. The woman may complain of localized pain and dysuria and may have a low-grade fever (less than 101F or 38.3C). If the wound abscesses or is unable to drain, high temperature and chills may result.

METRITIS

After delivery of the placenta, the placental site provides an excellent culture medium for bacterial growth. The site (in the contracted uterus) is a 4 cm round, dark red, elevated area with a nodular surface composed of numerous veins, many of which become occluded due to clot formation. The remaining portion of the decidua is also susceptible to pathogenic bacteria because of its thinness (approximately 2 mm) and its hypervascularity. The cervix may also present a bacterial breeding ground because of the multiple small lacerations attending normal labor and spontaneous delivery.

The pathogens deposited at the cervix during vaginal examination and those already present invade the decidua and eventually involve the entire mucosa. If the infection is confined to the surface of the mucosa, this area will become necrotic and be sloughed off within 3 to 5 days.

In this instance the discharge is scant (or profuse), bloody, and foul smelling.

The first 24 to 48 hours of the infectious process may be accompanied by a temperature no higher than 38.3C to 38.9C (101F to 102F) and a white blood count that remains in the normal range. As the infection develops further signs become apparent. In more severe cases, symptoms may include uterine tenderness and jagged, irregular temperature elevation, usually between 38.3C (101F) and 40C (104F). Tachycardia, chills, and evidence of subinvolution may be noted. Foul-smelling lochia generally is cited as a classic sign of endometritis, but in the case of infection with beta hemolytic streptococcus, the lochia may be scant and odorless (Pritchard et al 1985).

SALPINGITIS AND OOPHORITIS

Occasionally, bacteria may spread into the lumen of the fallopian tubes, producing infection in the tubes and ovaries. Most often caused by a gonorrheal infection, such infection generally becomes apparent between 9 and 15 days postpartally. Symptoms include bilateral (or unilateral) lower abdominal pain, high temperature, and tachycardia. If tubal closure results, sterility may ensue (Vorherr 1982).

PELVIC CELLULITIS (PARAMETRITIS) AND PERITONITIS

Pelvic cellulitis (parametritis) refers to infection involving the connective tissue of the broad ligament and, in more severe forms, the connective tissue of all the pelvic structures. It is generally spread by way of the lymphatics in the uterine wall, but may also occur if pathogenic organisms invade a cervical laceration that extends upward into the connective tissue of the broad ligament. This laceration then serves as a direct pathway that allows the pathogens already in the cervix to spread into the pelvis. *Peritonitis* refers to infection involving the peritoneum.

A pelvic abscess may form in the case of puerperal peritonitis and most commonly is found in the uterine ligaments, cul-de-sac of Douglas, and the subdiaphragmatic space. Pelvic cellulitis may be a secondary result of pelvic vein thrombophlebitis. This condition occurs when the clot becomes infected and the wall of the vein breaks down from necrosis, spilling the infection into the connective tissues of the pelvis.

As the course of pelvic cellulitis advances, a mass of exudate develops along the base of the broad ligament that may push the uterus toward the opposite wall (if the infection is unilateral), where it will become fixed. If the exudate spreads into the rectocervical septum, a firm mass develops behind the cervix instead. The abscess that results should be drained or resolved through appropriate antibiotic therapy to avoid rupture of the abscess into the peritoneal cavity and development of a possibly fatal peritonitis.

A woman suffering from parametritis may demonstrate a variety of symptoms, including marked high temperature (102F–104F or 38.9C–40C), chills, malaise, lethargy, abdominal pain, subinvolution of the uterus, tachycardia, and local and referred rebound tenderness. If peritonitis develops, the woman will be acutely ill with severe pain, marked anxiety, high fever, rapid, shallow respirations, pronounced tachycardia, excessive thirst, abdominal distention, nausea, and vomiting.

Medical Therapy

Diagnosis of the infection site and causative pathogen is accomplished by careful history and complete physical examination, blood work, cultures of the lochia (although this may be of limited value since multiple organisms are usually present), and urinalysis to rule out urinary tract infection. When a localized infection develops it is treated with antibiotic creams, sitz baths, and analgesics as necessary for pain relief. If an abscess has developed or a stitch site is infected, the suture is removed and the area is allowed to drain.

Metritis is treated by the administration of antibiotics. The route and dosage are determined by the severity of the infection. Severe infection warrants the administration of parenteral antibiotics. Careful monitoring is also necessary to prevent the development of a more serious infection.

Parametritis and peritonitis are treated with intravenous antibiotics. Broad spectrum antibiotics effective against the most commonly occurring causative organisms are chosen initially pending the results of culture and sensitivity reports. If multiple organisms are present, the approach to antibiotic therapy remains empirical. If no improvement is observed, the antibiotic is changed.

The development of an abscess is frequently heralded by the presence of a palpable mass and may be confirmed with ultrasound. An abscess usually requires incision and drainage to avoid rupture into the peritoneal cavity and the possible development of peritonitis. Following drainage of the abscess, the cavity may be packed with iodoform gauze to promote drainage and facilitate healing.

The woman with a severe systemic infection is acutely ill and may require care in an intensive care unit. Supportive therapy will include maintenance of adequate hydration with intravenous fluids, analgesics, ongoing assessment of the infection, and possibly continuous nasogastric suctioning if paralytic ileus develops.

Nursing Assessment

The woman's perineum should be inspected at least twice daily for signs of early developing infection. The REEDA scale helps the nurse remember to consider redness, edema, ecchymosis, discharge, and approximation (see Table 36–1).

Fever, malaise, abdominal pain, foul-smelling lochia, tachycardia, and other signs of infection should be noted and reported immediately so that treatment can be instituted.

Nursing Diagnosis

For nursing diagnoses that might apply, see the Nursing Care Plan on p 1160.

Nursing Goal: Prevention of Infection

The nurse caring for a woman during the postpartal period is responsible for teaching the woman self-care mea-

Table 36–1 REEDA Scale Used to Evaluate Healing

Points	Redness	Edema	Ecchymosis	Discharge	Approximation
0	None	None	None	None	Closed
1	Within 0.25 cm of incision bilaterally	Perineal, less than 1 cm from incision	Within 0.25 cm bilaterally or 0.5 cm unilaterally	Serum	Skin separation 3 mm or less
2	Within 0.5 cm of incision bilaterally	Perineal and/or vulvar, between 1 to 2 cm from incision	Between 0.25 to 1 cm bilaterally or between 0.5 to 2 cm unilaterally	Serosanguineous	Skin and subcutaneous fat separation
3	Beyond 0.5 cm of incision bilaterally	Perineal and/or vulvar, greater than 2 cm from incision	Greater than 1 cm bilaterally or 2 cm unilaterally	Bloody purulent	Skin, subcutaneous fat, and fascial layer separation
Score:	_____	_____	_____	_____	Total _____

From Davidson N: REEDA: Evaluating postpartum healing. *J Nurse-Midwife* 1974;19:7.

sures that are helpful in preventing infection. The woman should understand the importance of careful perineal care, hygiene practices to prevent bacterial contamination of the perineum (such as wiping from front to back and changing the perineal pad after going to the bathroom), and thorough handwashing. The nurse can also encourage sitz baths, which are cleansing and promote healing. Adequate fluid intake coupled with a diet high in protein and vitamin C, which are necessary to promote wound healing, also helps prevent infection.

Nursing Goal: Provision of Effective Care

If the woman is seriously ill, ongoing assessment of urine specific gravity and intake and output are necessary. The nurse also carefully administers antibiotics as ordered and regulates the intravenous fluids. Careful ongoing assessment of the woman's condition is vital to detect subtle changes in her health status. The nurse also recognizes the woman's comfort needs related to hygiene, positioning, oral hygiene, and pain relief.

Promoting maternal-infant attachment can be difficult with the seriously ill woman. The nurse may provide pictures of the infant and keep the mother informed of the infant's well-being. If she feels up to it, the new mother will also benefit from brief visits with her child.

Nursing Goal: Preparation for Discharge

The woman with a puerperal infection needs assistance when she is discharged from the hospital. If the family cannot provide this home assistance, a referral to the community homemakers' service is needed. The community health/visiting nurse service can also be contacted as soon as puerperal infection is diagnosed so that the nurse can meet with the woman for a family and home assessment and development of a home care plan. The community health nurse is aware of the community resources available to assist the woman and planning with her and her family before discharge will assure continuity of care after discharge.

The family needs instruction in the care of a newborn, including feeding, bathing, cord care, immunizations, and significant observations that should be reported. A well-baby appointment should be scheduled. Breast-feeding mothers should be instructed to inspect the infant's mouth for signs of thrush and to report the finding to their physician.

The mother should be instructed regarding activity, rest, medications, diet, and signs and symptoms of complications, and she should be scheduled for a return medical examination.

Evaluative Outcome Criteria

Anticipated outcomes of nursing care include the following:

- The infection is quickly identified and treated successfully without further complications.

- The woman understands the infection and the purpose of therapy; she cooperates with any ongoing antibiotic therapy if indicated following discharge.

- Maternal-infant attachment is maintained.

● Care of the Woman With Thromboembolic Disease

Thromboembolic disease occurs in approximately 1 percent of vaginally delivered women and in 2 percent to 10 percent of women undergoing cesarean birth (Vorherr 1982). Although the disease may also occur antepartally, it is generally considered a postpartal complication. *Venous thrombosis* refers to thrombus formation in a superficial or deep vein with the accompanying risk that a portion of the clot might break off and result in pulmonary embolism. When the thrombus is formed in response to inflammation in the vein wall, it is termed *thrombophlebitis*. In this type of thrombosis the clot tends to be more firmly attached and therefore is less likely to result in embolism. In *noninflammatory venous thrombosis* (also called phlebothrombosis) the clot tends to be more loosely attached and the risk of embolism is greater. The main factors responsible for this type of thrombosis are venous stasis, vascular anoxia, and endothelial damage (Vorherr 1982).

Factors contributing directly to the development of thromboembolic disease postpartally include (a) increased amounts of certain blood clotting factors; (b) postpartal thrombocytosis (increased quantity of circulating platelets) and their increased adhesiveness; (c) release of thromboplastin substances from the tissue of the decidua, placenta, and fetal membranes; and (d) increased amounts of fibrinolysis inhibitors. Predisposing factors are (a) obesity, increased maternal age, and high parity; (b) anesthesia and surgery with possible vessel trauma and venous stasis due to prolonged inactivity; (c) previous history of venous thrombosis; (d) maternal anemia, hypothermia, or heart disease; and (e) use of estrogen for suppression of lactation.

Superficial Leg Vein Disease

Superficial thrombophlebitis is far more common postpartally than during pregnancy. Often the clot involves the saphenous veins. This disorder is more common in women with preexisting varices, although it is not limited to these women. Symptoms usually become apparent about the third or fourth postpartal day: tenderness in a portion

Nursing Care Plan: Puerperal Infection

Kerry Lewis is a 19-year-old Gr 1 P 1 who delivered 36 hours ago after a 6-hour labor with a prolonged second stage that ended with a forceps rotation and delivery of an 8 lb 15 oz baby boy. The placenta was manually removed after an estimated blood loss of 900 mL. At admission Ms Lewis's hemoglobin was 11.1 g. She is breast-feeding her infant.

Assessment

HISTORY

Factors predisposing to infection include:
a. Anemia
b. Prolonged labor
c. Use of forceps
d. Hemorrhage
e. Soft tissue trauma

PHYSICAL EXAMINATION

a. Temperature of 101.8F (38.8C)
b. Client anorexic and lethargic
c. Complains of chills (3 blankets on bed)
d. Pulse 102, respirations 22
e. Complains of marked tenderness with abdominal palpation
f. Lochia brownish and foul-smelling

LABORATORY EVALUATION

White blood count 19,400/mm³
Urinalysis negative for nitrates, blood. Urine culture negative.
Intrauterine culture—not obtained

ANALYSIS OF NURSING PRIORITIES

1. Continue assessment of signs of endometritis and response to antibiotics.
2. Observe for evidence of progressive infection.
3. Implement measures to promote comfort.
4. Provide ongoing information and explanation to Ms Lewis and her family regarding her condition.
5. Foster parent-infant bonding.

Nursing Diagnosis and Goals	Nursing Interventions	Rationale
NURSING DIAGNOSIS: Potential for injury related to spread of infection. **SUPPORTING DATA:** Fever, chills, malaise, tachycardia Abnormal lochia Ms Lewis states, "I feel just terrible and my uterus seems so tender."	Observe, record, and report evidence of change in Kerry's status: a. Monitor vital signs. b. Assess lochia. c. Assess systemic signs such as anorexia, malaise, urine output, degree of discomfort. Administer antibiotics as ordered. Prevent spread of infection through: a. Careful handwashing technique by staff, woman, and visitors b. Appropriate disposal of infected materials such as absorbent pads, perineal pads, and contaminated linens	Metritis produces characteristic signs and symptoms. Should the metritis progress to parametritis these signs would become more pronounced. Antibiotic therapy is the treatment of choice for metritis. Contaminated organisms may be spread in a variety of ways.
GOAL: Ms Lewis' condition will improve following administration of antibiotics. **NURSING DIAGNOSIS:** Alteration in comfort: acute pain related to uterine tenderness and malaise secondary to metritis **SUPPORTING DATA:** Ms Lewis is crying and complaining of discomfort.	Promote comfort through: 1. Adequate periods of rest 2. Emotional support 3. Judicious use of antibiotics 4. Maintenance of cleanliness and warmth 5. Maintenance of semi-Fowler position	Semi-Fowler position promotes comfort and helps prevent spread of infection.
GOAL: Ms Lewis will be comfortable and free of pain so she is able to rest well.		

Nursing Care Plan: Puerperal Infection (continued)

Nursing Diagnosis and Goals	Nursing Interventions	Rationale
NURSING DIAGNOSIS: Knowledge deficit related to lack of understanding of metritis and its treatment. **SUPPORTING DATA:** Stated, "I just don't understand how I got this. Will the antibiotics get rid of it?"	Provide information regarding predisposing factors, signs and symptoms, and treatment. Discuss with Kerry the value of a nutritious diet in promoting healing. Review hygiene practices such as correct wiping after voiding, handwashing, etc, to prevent the spread of infection. Discuss home care routines following postpartal infection.	Women have the right and responsibility to be actively involved in their own health care to the extent that they are able. To be an active participant the woman needs appropriate information.
GOAL: Ms Lewis will be able to discuss her condition and its treatment.		
NURSING DIAGNOSIS: Alteration in parenting related to delayed parent-infant attachment secondary to the client's malaise **SUPPORTING DATA:** IV in right hand (Kerry is right-handed) Stated, "I feel as though I hardly know my baby."	Provide opportunities for the mother to see and hold her infant. Assist mother in caring for her infant while the IV is in place. Encourage mother to feed her infant when she feels able, and assist her in doing so. Newborn: Assess breast-feeding infant's mouth for signs of thrush, which is a common side effect of antibiotics ingested by infant in mother's milk. Treatment should be initiated but breast-feeding need not be stopped. Encourage partner/support person/family to become involved in care of Kerry and her newborn.	Success at feeding infant generally enhances the woman's outlook, encourages mother-infant interaction, and prevents woman from dwelling on herself to exclusion of infant. Breast-feeding is not affected by metritis and should be encouraged. Some institutions still insist on separation of the mother and infant if an infection is present; the mother must be instructed in pumping her breasts (if breast-feeding) and will need support during this separation. Thrush, a monilial infection caused by *Candida albicans*, often occurs when normal oral flora are destroyed by antibiotic therapy.
GOAL: Ms Lewis will feel comfortable with her infant and will begin to bond with him.		

Epilogue

Kerry Lewis remained on IV antibiotics for 3 days and was then changed to oral antibiotics. Her condition improved rapidly on the medication and with this improvement, her spirits lifted. She and her partner attended newborn care classes. Her milk came in on her third hospital day and she was quite excited about the vigorous way in which her young son nursed. Her partner had taken leave from work to help her at home, and both were looking forward to the time together with their newborn.

of the vein, some local heat and redness, absent or low-grade fever, and occasionally slight elevation of the pulse. Treatment involves application of local heat, elevation of the affected limb, bed rest and analgesics, and the use of elastic support hose. Anticoagulants are usually not necessary unless complications develop. In most cases pulmonary embolism is extremely rare. Occasionally the involved veins have incompetent valves, and as a result, the problem may spread to the deeper leg veins, such as the femoral vein.

Deep Leg Vein Disease

Deep venous thrombosis is more frequently seen in women with a history of thrombosis. Certain obstetric complications such as hydramnios, preeclampsia, and operative delivery are associated with an increased incidence. The disease generally occurs unilaterally; in 75 percent of affected women the left leg is the site (Vorherr 1982).

Clinical manifestations may include edema of the ankle and leg, and an initial low-grade fever often followed by high temperature and chills. Depending on the vein involved, the woman may complain of pain in the popliteal and lateral tibial areas (popliteal vein), entire lower leg and foot (anterior and posterior tibial veins), inguinal tender-

ness (femoral vein), or pain in the lower abdomen (iliofemoral vein). The Homan's sign (Figure 36–2) may or may not be positive, but pain often results from calf pressure. Because of reflex arterial spasm, sometimes the limb is pale and cool to the touch—the so-called milk leg or *phlegmasia alba dolens*—and peripheral pulses may be decreased.

MEDICAL THERAPY

The goal of medical managment is prompt diagnosis and treatment to avoid complications. Because cases are seldom clear-cut, diagnosis involves a variety of approaches, such as client history and physical examination, occlusive cuff impedence plethysmography, Doppler ultrasonography, and contrast venography. In questionable cases, contrast venography provides the most accurate diagnosis of deep venous thrombosis. Unfortunately, venography is not practical for multiple examinations or prospective screening and may itself induce phlebitis.

Treatment involves the administration of intravenous heparin, using an infusion pump to permit continuous, accurate infusion of medication. Bed rest is required, and analgesics are given as necessary to relieve discomfort. If fever is present, deep thrombophlebitis is suspected and the woman is also given antibiotic therapy. In most cases thrombectomy is not necessary.

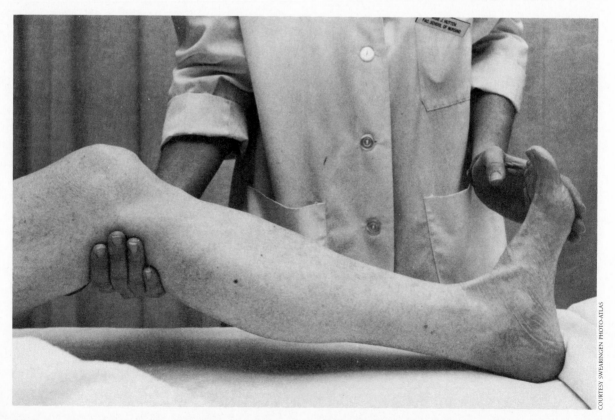

Figure 36–2 Homan's sign. With the client's knee flexed to decrease the risk of embolization, the nurse dorsiflexes the client's foot. Pain in the foot or leg is a positive Homan's sign.

Once the symptoms have subsided (usually in several days), the woman may begin ambulation while wearing elastic support stockings. At this point, anticoagulant therapy is usually changed to sodium warfarin, which the woman continues on for two to six months at home. While on warfarin, prothrombin times are assessed periodically to maintain correct dosage levels.

NURSING ASSESSMENT

The nurse carefully assesses any woman whose history indicates the presence of factors that would predispose her to the development of thrombophlebitis. In addition, as part of regular postpartal assessment the nurse is alert to any complaints by a woman of pain in the leg, inguinal area, or lower abdomen because such pain may indicate deep vein thrombosis. The nurse also assesses the woman's legs for evidence of edema, temperature change, or pain with palpation.

NURSING DIAGNOSIS

Nursing diagnoses that may apply to a postpartal woman with thrombophlebitis are found in the Nursing Care Plan on p 1166.

NURSING GOAL: PREVENTION OF THROMBOPHLEBITIS

Because trauma is often a factor in the development of thrombophlebitis, the nurse avoids keeping the woman's legs elevated in stirrups for prolonged periods. If stirrups are used, they are comfortably padded and adjusted to provide correct support. Early ambulation is encouraged following delivery, and the use of the knee gatch on the bed is avoided. Women confined to bed following a cesarean delivery are encouraged to do regular leg exercises to promote venous return.

NURSING GOAL: PROMOTION OF EFFECTIVE THERAPY

Once the diagnosis is made, the nurse maintains the heparin therapy, provides for appropriate comfort measures, and monitors the woman closely for signs of pulmonary embolism. The nurse also assesses for evidence of bleeding related to heparin and keeps the antagonist for heparin, protamine sulfate, readily available.

NURSING GOAL: EDUCATION FOR SELF-CARE

The nurse is actively involved in education and in preparation of the woman for discharge. The woman is instructed to avoid prolonged standing or sitting because they contribute to venous stasis. She is also instructed to avoid crossing her legs because of the pressure this exerts.

Walking promotes venous return and thus is a suitable activity.

Women who are discharged on warfarin require careful teaching. They must understand the purpose of the medication and be alert to signs of hemorrhage such as bleeding gums, epistaxis, petechiae or ecchymosis, or evidence of blood in the urine or stool. Since careful monitoring is important, the woman should clearly understand the need to keep scheduled appointments for prothrombin time assessment. Because aspirin and nonsteroidal antiinflammatory drugs increase anticoagulant activity, they should be avoided. In fact, the woman should check for possible medication interaction before taking any medication while she is on warfarin. A woman may also elect to carry a Medic Alert card stating that she is on warfarin. In addition she should have vitamin K available in case bleeding occurs. Warfarin is excreted in the breast milk and thus may present problems for breast-feeding mothers. If the woman feels strongly about nursing she may be maintained at home on low doses of subcutaneous heparin since heparin is not excreted in breast milk.

EVALUATIVE OUTCOME CRITERIA

Anticipated outcomes of nursing care include the following:

- If thrombophlebitis develops, it is detected quickly and managed successfully without further complications.

- At discharge the woman is able to explain the purpose, dosage regimen, and necessary precautions associated with any prescribed medications such as anticoagulants.

- The woman can discuss self-care measures and ongoing therapies (such as the use of elastic stockings) that are indicated.

- The woman has bonded successfully with her newborn and is able to care for her or him effectively.

Pulmonary Embolism

A sudden onset of dyspnea accompanied by sweating; pallor; cyanosis; confusion; systemic hypotension; cough, with or without hemoptysis; tachycardia; shortness of breath; fever; and increased jugular pressure may indicate pulmonary embolism. Chest pain that mimics cardiac ischemia, coupled with the woman's verbalized fear of imminent death and complaint of pressure in the bowel and rectum, should alert the nurse to the extensive size of the embolus. A friction rub and evidence of atelectasis may be noted upon auscultation. A gallop (heart) rhythm may be present even if respiratory inspiration is normal, although smaller emboli may present with only transient syncope, tightness of the chest, or unexplained pyrexia.

Even x-ray films and ECG changes and laboratory data are not always reliable. If a case of pulmonary embolism is suspected, prompt treatment should begin even in the absence of corroborative data. If the embolism is small and heparin therapy is begun quickly, the chance of survival is excellent. However, when a large thrombus occludes a major pulmonary vessel, death may occur before therapy can even begin.

Therapy involves the administration of a variety of intravenous medications, such as meperidine hydrochloride to relieve the pain, lidocaine to correct any arrhythmias, and drugs such as papaverine hydrochloride and aminophylline to reduce spasms of the bronchi and coronary and pulmonary vessels (Vorherr 1982). Oxygen is administered and heparin infusion is begun. In severe cases an embolectomy may be necessary, although fibrinolytic therapy with medications (such as streptokinase) that lyse clots may be tried first.

● Care of the Woman With a Urinary Tract Infection

The postpartal woman is at increased risk of developing urinary tract problems due to the normal postpartal diuresis, increased bladder capacity, decreased bladder sensitivity from stretching and/or trauma, and possible inhibited neural control of the bladder following the use of general or regional anesthesia.

Emptying the bladder is vital. Women who have not sufficiently recovered from the effects of anesthesia cannot void spontaneously, and catheterization is necessary.

Retention of residual urine, bacteria introduced at the time of catheterization, and a bladder traumatized by delivery combine to provide an excellent environment for the development of cystitis.

Overdistention

Overdistention occurs postpartally when, as a result of the predisposing factors previously identified, the woman is unable to empty her bladder.

MEDICAL THERAPY

Overdistention, if discovered in the recovery room, is often managed by draining the bladder with a straight catheter as a one-time measure. If the overdistention recurs or is diagnosed later in the postpartal period, an indwelling catheter is generally ordered for 24 hours.

NURSING ASSESSMENT

The overdistended bladder appears as a large mass, reaching sometimes to the umbilicus and displacing the uterine fundus upward. There is increased vaginal bleeding, the fundus is boggy, and the woman may complain of cramping as the uterus attempts to contract.

NURSING DIAGNOSIS

Nursing diagnoses that may apply when a woman has difficulties due to overdistention include:

- Potential for infection related to urinary stasis secondary to overdistention
- Alteration in patterns of urinary elimination related to overdistention

NURSING GOAL: PREVENTION OF OVERDISTENTION

Diligent monitoring of the bladder during the recovery period and preventive health measures greatly reduce the number of women who need to be treated for overdistention of the bladder. Encouraging the mother to void spontaneously and assisting her to use the toilet, if possible, or the bedpan if she has received conductive anesthesia, prevent overdistention in most cases.

NURSING GOAL: SAFE, EFFECTIVE CATHETERIZATION IF NECESSARY

If catheterization becomes necessary, meticulous aseptic technique should be employed during catheter insertion.

As previously mentioned, the vagina and vulva are traumatized to some degree by vaginal delivery, and edema is common. If forceps have been used (a frequent adjunct to conductive anesthesia), the trauma is greater, and edema, especially of the vestibule, is marked. This edema may obscure the urinary meatus, and the nurse needs to be extremely careful in cleansing the vulva and inserting the catheter. It is imperative to discard a catheter that has inadvertently been introduced into the vagina and thus contaminated. Catheterization, an uncomfortable procedure at any time, is generally painful during the puerperium due to the trauma and edema of the tissue. Therefore, the nurse should be especially careful, considerate, and gentle not only in inserting the catheter but also in handling and cleaning the perineal area.

If the amount of urine siphoned from the bladder reaches 900 to 1000 mL, the catheter should be clamped, the Foley balloon inflated, and the catheter attached firmly to the woman's leg. The physician should be notified, and the procedure, including the woman's vital signs before and after the procedure and her responses, should carefully be charted. After an hour, the catheter may be unclamped and placed on gravity drainage. By following this technique, the bladder is protected, and rapid intraabdominal decompression is avoided. When the indwelling catheter is removed, a urine sample is often sent to the laboratory. The tip of the catheter may also be removed and sent for culture.

Cystitis

In 73 percent to 90 percent of the cases of postpartal cystitis and pyelonephritis *E. coli* has been demonstrated to be the causative agent. Aerobacter, *Proteus,* klebsiella, pseudomonas, and *Staphylococcus* are responsible for most of the remainder (Vorherr 1982). In the vast majority of cases the infection ascends the urinary tract from the urethra to the bladder and then to the kidneys because vesiculoureteral reflux forces contaminated urine into the renal pelvis.

MEDICAL THERAPY

When cystitis is suspected in the puerperium, a clean-catch midstream urine sample is obtained for microscopic examination, culture, and sensitivity tests. A catheterized specimen is avoided when possible because of the increased risk of infection. When the bacterial concentration is greater than 100,000 microorganisms per milliliter of fresh urine, infection is generally present; counts between 10,000 and 100,000 are suggestive, particularly if clinical symptoms are noted.

Treatment is theoretically delayed until urine culture and sensitivity reports are available. In the clinical setting, however, antibiotic therapy is often initiated using one of the short-acting sulfonamides, nitrofurantoin (Macrodantin), or, in the case of sulfa allergy, ampicillin. The antibiotic is begun immediately and can be changed if indicated by the results of the sensitivity report (Pritchard et al 1985). Antispasmodics may be given to relieve discomfort.

Pyelonephritis

Pyelonephritis is an inflammation of the renal pelvis that is usually the result of infection. In most cases the infection has ascended from the lower urinary tract. It occurs more commonly on the right, although both kidneys may be affected. If untreated, the renal cortex may be damaged and kidney function impaired.

MEDICAL THERAPY

When pyelonephritis is diagnosed, antibiotic therapy is begun immediately. If sensitivity reports so indicate, the antibiotic can be changed as needed. Bed rest and careful monitoring of intake and output are necessary to detect the development of bacterial shock. Fluids are encouraged; if nausea and vomiting are severe, however, fluids are administered intravenously. Antispasmodics and analgesics are given to relieve discomfort. The woman usually continues to take antibiotics for two to four weeks after clinical and bacteriologic response. A routine clean-catch urine culture should be obtained two weeks after completion of therapy and then periodically for the next two years.

Continuation of breast-feeding during therapy is acceptable and is limited only by the degree of the mother's malaise and clinical discomfort. For the breast-feeding mother the antibiotic chosen should be selected carefully to avoid problems for the infant via the milk.

NURSING ASSESSMENT

Symptoms of cystitis (bladder inflammation) often appear two to three days after delivery. The initial symptoms of cystitis may include frequency, urgency, dysuria, and nocturia. Hematuria and suprapubic pain may also be present. A slightly elevated temperature may occur, but systemic symptoms are often absent.

When a urinary tract infection (UTI) progresses to pyelonephritis, systemic symptoms usually occur, and the woman becomes acutely ill. Symptoms include chills, high fever, flank pain (unilateral or bilateral), nausea, and vomiting, in addition to all the signs of lower UTI. Costovertebral pain also may be elicited. Urine culture and sensitivity are obtained to identify the causative organism.

NURSING DIAGNOSIS

Nursing diagnoses that may apply if a woman develops a UTI postpartally include:

- Alteration in comfort: acute pain related to dysuria secondary to cystitis

- Knowledge deficit related to a lack of understanding of the potential long-term effects of pyelonephritis

- Knowledge deficit related to a lack of understanding of self-care measures to prevent UTI

NURSING GOAL: PREVENTION OF URINARY TRACT INFECTION

As with other conditions, the nurse plays an important role in preventing the development of UTI. Nursing

Nursing Care Plan: Puerperal Thrombophlebitis

Candy Wartner is a 39-year-old Gr 5 P 5 who gained 41 lb with her current pregnancy. Her records indicate than she had a history of excessive weight gain with her previous pregnancies and had also developed venous thrombosis with her third pregnancy. She had a ce- sarean delivery three days ago due to fetal distress. This morning she complained of pain in the right calf. Her nurse noted that it was edematous and tender to palpation. A positive Homan's sign was elicited. Pedal pulses on the right were diminished.

Assessment

HISTORY

Predisposing factors include:
1. Increased maternal age
2. Obesity
3. Increased parity
4. Previous history of venous thrombosis
5. Operative delivery

PHYSICAL EXAMINATION

1. Positive Homan's sign
2. Tenderness and pain in affected area
3. Edema in affected extremity
4. Diminished peripheral pulses

LABORATORY EVALUATION

1. Doppler ultrasonography demonstrates increased circumference of affected leg.
2. Venography confirms diagnosis of thrombophlebitis.

ANALYSIS OF NURSING PRIORITIES

1. Perform frequent assessments to monitor course of condition, woman's response to therapy, and the possible development of complications.
2. Provide appropriate ongoing nursing care and necessary emergency care if complications arise.
3. Maintain maternal-infant interactions.
4. Provide information and answer questions about the cause of the condition, the treatment regime, medications, need for continued medical supervision, and ways to avoid circulatory stasis.

Nursing Diagnosis and Goals	Nursing Interventions	Rationale
NURSING DIAGNOSIS: Alteration in tissue perfusion: peripheral: pain	Assess, record and report signs of thrombophlebitis. Maintain bed rest and warm, moist soaks as ordered.	Bed rest is ordered to decrease possibility that portion of clot will dislodge and result in pulmonary embolism. Warmth promotes blood flow to affected area.

SUPPORTING DATA:
Tenderness and pain in right calf
Edema in right lower leg
Positive Homan's sign
Diminished pedal pulses on right
	Administer analgesics for relief of pain per physician order.
	
	Administer intravenous heparin as ordered, by continuous intravenous drip, heparin lock, or subcutaneously, including:
	1. Monitor IV or heparin lock site for signs of infiltration.
	2. Obtain Lee White clotting times per physician order and review prior to administering heparin.
	3. Observe for signs of anticoagulant overdose with resultant bleeding, including:
	  a. Hematuria
	  b. Epistaxis
	  c. Ecchymosis
	  d. Bleeding gums
	4. Provide protamine sulfate, per physician order, to combat bleeding problems related to heparin overdose.
	
	5. Monitor and report any signs of pulmonary embolism.
	
	6. Initiate or support any emergency treatment.
	7. Initiate progressive ambulation following the acute phase; provide properly fitting elastic stockings prior to ambulation.
		Heparin does not dissolve clot but is administered to prevent further clotting. It is safe for breast-feeding mothers because heparin is not excreted in mother's milk.
		
		Protamine sulfate is heparin antagonist, given intravenously, which is almost immediately effective in counteracting bleeding complications caused by heparin overdose.
		
		Pulmonary embolism is a major complication of thrombophlebitis. Signs and symptoms may occur suddenly and require immediate emergency treatment; prognosis is related to size and location of embolism .
		
		Elastic stockings or "Teds" help prevent pooling of venous blood in lower extremities.

Nursing Care Plan: Puerperal Thrombophlebitis (continued)

Nursing Diagnosis and Goals	Nursing Interventions	Rationale
GOAL: Mrs Wartner's presenting signs and symptoms are relieved and her pain is controlled.	8. Obtain prothrombin time (PT) and review prior to beginning warfarin. Repeat periodically per physician order.	PT is the test most commonly used to monitor the blood of clients receiving warfarin.
NURSING DIAGNOSIS: Potential alteration in parenting related to decreased maternal-infant interaction secondary to bedrest and IVs **SUPPORTING DATA:** On strict bedrest IV infusion in left hand States "How will I ever get to know my baby when I'm so limited?" **GOAL:** Mrs Wartner is able to develop bonds of attachment with her infant.	Maintain mother-infant attachment when mother is on bedrest: 1. Provide frequent contacts for mother and infant; modified rooming-in possible if crib placed close to mother's bed and nurse checks often to help mother lift or move infant. 2. Encourage mother to continue feeding infant (Candy is bottle feeding).	Evidence indicates that first few days of life may be crucial to development of maternal-infant bonds, and separation during this period should be avoided.
NURSING DIAGNOSIS: Alteration in family processes related to an ill family member **SUPPORTING DATA:** While Mrs Wartner is hospitalized, her husband and oldest daughter are caring for the family. Candy states, "I feel so guilty not being home to take care of things." **GOAL:** Mrs Wartner will express the assurance that her family misses her but is coping effectively.	1. Encourage Mrs Wartner to discuss her concerns with her husband. 2. Encourage husband or friend to bring other children to hospital to visit mother and meet new sibling. 3. Contact social services if indicated to obtain additional assistance for family. 4. Encourage husband to bring family pictures and notes from other children. Encourage phone calls.	Illness of any family member impacts the entire family. This is especially pronounced when the family situation is such at that the mother is the nurturer and she is absent. Family members attempt to continue their own roles while also assuming the roles of the missing member. This can result in crisis.
NURSING DIAGNOSIS: Knowledge deficit related to the thrombophlebitis, its treatment, preventive measures, and the medication, warfarin **SUPPORTING DATA:** Mrs Wartner stated, "The doctor said I have to take precautions at home but I don't really know what he means."	1. Discuss ways of avoiding circulatory stasis such as avoiding prolonged standing or sitting; avoiding crossing her legs. 2. Review need to wear support stockings and to plan for rest periods with her legs elevated. 3. Discuss the use of warfarin, its side effects, possible interactions with other medications, and need to have dosage assessed through periodic checks of the prothrombin time.	Such discussion is essential to help the woman understand the condition, her medication and its implications. She must have a clear understanding to be able to provide effective self-care.

Nursing Care Plan: Puerperal Thrombophlebitis (continued)

Nursing Diagnosis and Goals	Nursing Interventions	Rationale

SUPPORTING DATA:
 	
GOAL:
·Mrs Wartner will describe her condition, activities she should avoid, and its long-term implications. She will be able to explain the purpose of her warfarin and the precautions she should take while on it.
	4. Discuss signs of bleeding including:
	  a. Hematuria
	  b. Epistaxis
	  c. Ecchymosis
	  d. Bleeding gums	

Epilogue	
Mrs Wartner was discharged after 12 days in the hospital. Her husband was not able to take more time off from work, but her mother came to stay for two weeks. Mrs Wartner remained on warfarin for nine weeks. During that time she had weekly prothrombin times and, under the supervision of a dietitian, began on a weight reduction diet.	Her older children were eager to help their mother and worked well with the new baby. Mrs Wartner reported to the nurse at her postpartum checkup that things had been "rough," but that the family seemed closer than ever since her illness.

actions to prevent overdistention help avoid the problem of stasis. If catheterization becomes necessary, scrupulous aseptic technique is essential.

Regular, complete bladder emptying, instruction on proper wiping techniques to avoid fecal contamination of the meatus, coupled with good perineal care and frequent changing of the perineal pads all decrease chances of infection. The woman with pyelonephritis must understand the importance of follow-up care after discharge to prevent recurrence or further complications.

NURSING GOAL: EDUCATION FOR SELF-CARE

The postpartal woman should be advised to continue the techniques discussed above following discharge. She is also advised to maintain a good fluid intake and to empty her bladder whenever she feels the urge to void, but at least every two to four hours while awake. She can also void following sexual intercourse to wash any contaminants from the vicinity of the meatus. It is also advisable for the woman to wear underwear with a cotton crotch to facilitate air circulation.

A woman diagnosed with pyelonephritis must understand the potential seriousness of the condition and be urged to monitor herself for any symptoms of UTI.

EVALUATIVE OUTCOME CRITERIA

Anticipated outcomes of nursing care include the following:

- Signs of urinary tract infection are detected quickly and the condition is treated successfully.

- The woman incorporates self-care measures to prevent the recurrence of UTI as part of her personal hygiene routine.

- The woman cooperates with any long-term therapy or follow-up.

- Maternal-infant attachment is maintained and the woman is able to care for her newborn effectively.

● Care of the Woman With Mastitis

Mastitis refers to an inflammation of the breast generally caused by *Staphylococcus aureus* and primarily seen in breast-feeding mothers. Because symptoms seldom occur before the second to fourth week postpartally, nurses often are not fully aware of how uncomfortable and acutely ill the woman may be.

The infection usually begins when bacteria invade the breast tissue. Often the tissue has been traumatized in some way (fissured or cracked nipples, overdistention, manipulation, or milk stasis) and is especially susceptible to pathogenic invasion. The most common source of the bacteria is the infant's nose and throat, although other sources include the hands of the mother or hospital personnel or the woman's circulating blood.

Medical Therapy

Diagnosis is usually based on the symptoms, physical examination, and a culture and sensitivity of the breast milk. Treatment involves the administration of appropriate antibiotics, use of analgesics to ease discomfort, and local application of heat. Opinion varies about the advisability of continuing breast-feeding. In the past, hospital epidemics of staphylococcus were more prevalent, and cessation of nursing was advocated to prevent a vicious cycle of reinfection as the infant consumed infected milk. Current nursery practices and the trend toward early discharge have resulted in far fewer hospital-related infections.

Current literature suggests that the mother should continue to nurse while infected to prevent milk stasis and engorgement, both of which are associated with increased risk of infection and the development of abscess (Niebyl 1985, Danforth & Scott 1986). However, some agencies prefer to have the mother cease nursing while acutely ill and pump her breasts to prevent engorgement. Breast-feeding is resumed after the mother is afebrile and receiving antibiotics.

Occasionally the process of mastitis may continue and a frank abscess develops. The mother's milk and any drainage from the nipple should be cultured and antibiotic therapy instituted. In addition, it is usually necessary to incise surgically and drain the abscessed area. If multiple abscesses are present, multiple incisions will be necessary, usually under general anesthesia. After incision and drainage, the area is packed with sterile gauze. The packing is gradually decreased to permit proper healing.

Often the breast is covered with a sterile surgical dressing and access to the breast is temporarily inhibited, making breast-feeding impossible. If possible, the dressing should be applied so that the woman can continue to breast-feed or pump her breast thereby avoiding engorgement. Once the dressings, drains, and packing have been removed and the incisions are healing well, careful breast-feeding may resume, closely supervised by the experienced nurse.

Nursing Assessment

Once the infection develops, the woman may have a high temperature, chills, tachycardia, and headache. The breasts may be very tender, have a reddened and warm area, feel firm to the touch, or show areas of lumpiness (Figure 36–3).

Nursing Diagnosis

Nursing diagnoses that may apply to the woman with mastitis include:

- Knowledge deficit related to appropriate breast-feeding practices

- Alterations in comfort: acute pain related to the development of mastitis

Nursing Goal: Prevention of Mastitis

Meticulous hand-washing by all personnel is the primary measure in preventing epidemic nursery infections and subsequent maternal mastitis. Prompt attention to mothers who have blocked milk ducts eliminates the stagnant milk as a growth medium for bacteria. Frequent breast-feeding of the infant usually prevents mastitis. If the mother finds that one area of her breast feels distended (caked), she can rotate the position of her infant for nursing, manually express milk remaining in the breast after nursing (or use a nontraumatic breast pump), or massage the caked area toward the nipple as the infant nurses.

Nursing Goal: Education for Self-Care

The nurse should stress to the breast-feeding woman the importance of adequate breast and nipple care to prevent the development of cracks and fissures, a common portal for bacterial entry. The mother should be aware of the importance of preventing engorgement and of emptying her breasts to prevent stasis. Since mastitis tends to develop following discharge it is useful to include information about signs and symptoms in the discharge information. If symptoms develop, the woman should contact her care giver immediately because prompt treatment plays a role in preventing the more serious problem of abscess formation.

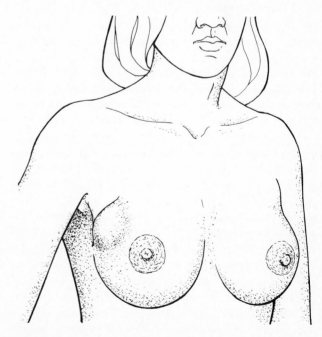

Figure 36–3   Mastitis. Erythema and swelling are present in the upper outer quadrant of the breast. Axillary lymph nodes are enlarged and tender.

Evaluative Outcome Criteria

Anticipated outcomes of nursing care include the following:

- The woman's mastitis is detected early and treated successfully.

- The woman can continue breastfeeding if she chooses.

- The woman understands self-care measures she can employ to prevent the recurrence of the mastitis.

● Care of the Woman With a Postpartal Psychiatric Disorder

Many different types of psychiatric problems may be encountered in the puerperium but only rarely is the disorder serious. Approximately 70 percent to 80 percent of women experience a transient depression during the first week, most commonly on the third postpartal day (Danforth & Scott 1986). This transient depression is usually accompanied by tearfulness and is a self-limiting, brief episode.

The DSM-III (Diagnostic and Statistical Manual III) does not have a definitive heading for postpartum psychosis per se. In some instances the clinical picture will meet the criteria for Schizophreniform Disorder, Paranoid Disorder, Affective Disorder, or Organic Mental Disorder. If not, it is included under 298.20, Atypical Psychosis.

When psychiatric illness occurs after delivery, one or several of the following signs are usually present: depression, delusions, confusion, mania, delirium, hallucinations, anxiety, and sexual dysfunction. Occasionally, violent behavior forms part of the clinical picture; sometimes this violence is directed against the infant. Approximately 1 in 1000 term pregnancies is followed by psychiatric problems sufficiently severe to require hospitalization (Hamilton 1982).

Depression is the most common type of psychiatric disorder seen after childbirth. Depression may be triggered by a variety of factors including (a) unwanted or unplanned pregnancy, (b) unfaithful partner, (c) recent loss of a support person or close friend, (d) worries about the health of the fetus or the newborn, (e) sexual rejection by the partner during pregnancy, (f) separated or single marital status, and (g) major or severe illness of another child (Mozley 1985). It tends to peak about six weeks postdelivery, although symptoms may arise earlier, for example, feelings of failure, self-accusatory thoughts, depression, and exhaustion. Suicidal thinking may be present, which poses a true danger to the woman. Treatment is generally directed at relief of symptoms, and hospitalization may be indicated if the woman seems capable of harming herself.

Postpartal schizophrenic reactions may have an earlier onset—usually by the tenth day, although they may occur earlier. This disorder is manifested by delusional thinking, flight of ideas, and gross distortion of reality, often accompanied by agitation. Although the behavior of these women may seem especially bizarre, if correctly treated their prognosis is excellent (Hamilton 1982).

In some women postpartal psychosis has a more subtle onset and may be characterized by increasing hostility and anger, fearfulness, anxiety, and aversion to sexual activity. Unfortunately, this type of disturbance frequently culminates in an act of violence, such as child abuse.

It is important to consider contributing factors to postpartal psychiatric disorders, because one-fourth of women with a history of postpartal mental illness experience recurrence after a subsequent pregnancy. Contributing factors include (a) a chronic history of inability to deal with life's crises without decompensating; (b) a traumatic relationship with the woman's own mother, especially during childhood; (c) self-defensive or conflicting motives for the pregnancy itself; (d) external variables such as prolonged infertility prior to pregnancy, physical complications during pregnancy or labor and delivery, problems or abnormalities with the infant; (e) concomitant life stresses, such as poverty, a recent family member's death, or home or job change (Barglow 1982).

Medical Therapy

Treatment of mild postpartal psychiatric disorders usually is achieved on an outpatient basis, although medication or hospitalization is indicated in some cases. If the mother appears to have rejected her infant, it is never wise to compel her to care for her or him, as this forces the women to deal with feelings of guilt, shame, and hostility that may overwhelm her and endanger the infant.

Nursing Assessment

The nurse observes the woman for signs of depression, which may be manifested by tearfulness, exhaustion, and statements indicating feelings of failure and self-accusation. Behavior and verbalizations that are bizarre or seem to indicate a potential for violence against herself or others, including the infant, should be reported as soon as possible for further evaluation.

Nursing Diagnosis

Possible nursing diagnoses that may apply to a woman with a postpartum psychiatric disorder include:

- Ineffective individual coping related to postpartum depression

● Potential alteration in bonding related to child neglect secondary to postpartum psychosis

Nursing Goal: Detection of Potential Psychiatric Problems

Although a history of psychiatric problems is not always indicative of current problems, the nurse should be aware of any previous or current emotional problems. In providing daily care the nurse is often the first to note patterns of behavior that suggest possible depression or other psychiatric problems.

If care givers have any doubts about the woman's stability, a referral may be made to the public health service so that follow-up care is possible. In this way problems can be identified before they become major obstacles to the woman's or her infant's emotional health.

Evaluative Outcome Criteria

Anticipated outcomes of nursing care include the following:

● Signs of potential postpartal disorders are detected quickly and therapy is implemented.

● The newborn is cared for effectively by the father or another support person until the mother is able to do so.

KEY CONCEPTS

The main causes of early postpartal hemorrhage are uterine atony, lacerations of the vagina and cervix, and retained placental fragments.

The most common postpartal infection is metritis, which is limited to the uterine cavity.

Thromboembolic disease originating in the veins of the leg, thigh, or pelvis may occur in the antepartum or postpartum periods and carries with it the potential for creating a pulmonary embolus.

A postpartal woman is at increased risk for developing urinary tract problems due to normal postpartal diuresis, increased bladder capacity, decreased bladder sensitivity from stretching and/or trauma, and, possibly, inhibited neural control of the bladder following the use of anesthetic agents.

Mastitis is an inflammation of the breast caused by _Staphylococcus aureus_ and is primarily seen in breastfeeding women. Symptoms seldom occur before the second to fourth postpartal week.

Although many different types of psychiatric problems may be encountered in the postpartal period, depression is the most common. Episodes occur frequently in the week after delivery and are typically transient.

The normal puerperium is a dynamic period during which major changes must take place. When nurses are keenly aware of these normal physiologic and psychologic changes, they can quickly assess when deviations occur in the involutional process. These deviations place additional stress on the body, creating a risk situation for the mother that necessitates immediate intervention and evaluation.

REFERENCES

Barglow P: Postpartum mental illness: detection and treatment, in **Sciarra** JJ (ed): *Gynecology and Obstetrics*. Philadelphia, Harper & Row, 1982, vol 2.

Danforth DN, **Scott** JR (eds): *Obstetrics and Gynecology,* ed 5. Philadelphia, Harper & Row, 1986.

Easterling WE, **Herbert** WNP: The puerperium, in **Danforth** DN, **Scott** JR (eds): *Obstetrics and Gynecology,* ed 5. Philadelphia, Harper & Row, 1986.

Eschenbach D, **Wager** G: Puerperal infections. *Clin Obstet Gynecol* 1980;23(4):1003.

Few BJ: Prostaglandin F_2 for treating severe postpartum hemorrhage. *Am J Mat Child Nurs* 1987;12(May/June):169.

Hamilton JA: Puerperal psychoses, in **Sciarra** JJ (ed): *Gynecology and Obstetrics*. Philadelphia, Harper & Row, 1982, vol 2.

Mozley P: Predicting postpartum depression. *Contemp OB/GYN* 1985;5(May):173.

Niebyl JR: When the nursing mother has mastitis. *Contemp OB/GYN* 1985;26(July):31.

Pritchard JA, **MacDonald** PC, **Gant** NF: *Williams Obstetrics,* ed 17. New York, Appleton-Century-Crofts, 1985.

Visscher HC, **Visscher** RD: Early and late postpartum hemorrhage, in **Sciarra** JJ (ed): *Gynecology and Obstetrics*. Philadelphia, Harper & Row, 1982, vol 2.

Vorherr H: Puerperium: Maternal involutional changes—management of puerperal problems and complications, in **Sciarra** JJ (ed): *Gynecology and Obstetrics*. Philadelphia, Harper & Row, 1982, vol 2.

ADDITIONAL READINGS

Duff P: Diagnosing and treating post-C/S endometritis. *Contemp OB/GYN* 1987;29(March):129.

Fagnant RJ, **Monif** GRG: Septic pelvic thrombophlebitis. *Contemp OB/GYN* 1987;29(February):129.

Gjerdingen DK, et al: Postpartum mental and physical problems. How common are they? *Postgrad Med* 1986;80(December):133.

Hillard PA: Postpartum hemorrhage. *Parents* 1987; 62(January):104.

Low-dose heparin and postoperative wound hematoma. *Nurs Drug Alert* 1987;11(February):11.

Soper DE, et al: Abbreviated antibiotic therapy for the treatment of postpartum endometritis. *Obstet Gynecol* 1987;69(January):127.

Zuckerman BS, et al: Maternal depression: A concern for pediatricians. *Pediatrics* 1987;79(January):110.

We are surviving. Just. Why don't they give Croix de Guerre to people who can go without more than two hours total daily sleep for five weeks? I thought babies ate at six-ten-two-six-ten-two—mine does. He also eats at five-seven-nine-eleven and four-eight-twelve. I am getting rather used to going around with my breasts hanging out. They are either drying from the last feed or getting ready for the next one. But the love—I never knew, never imagined that I would love him like this. This incredible feeling of boundless, endless love—a wish to protect his innocence from ever being hurt or wounded or scratched. And that awful, horrible, mad feeling in the first week that you'll never be able to keep anything so precious and so vulnerable alive. (The New Our Bodies, Ourselves)

Appendices

Common Abbreviations in Maternal-Newborn and Women's Health Nursing

ABC	Alternative birthing center *or* airway, breathing, circulation	C/S	Cesarean section or C-section
Accel	Acceleration of fetal heart rate	CST	Contraction stress test
AC	Abdominal circumference	CT	Computerized tomography
ACTH	Adrenocorticotrophic hormone	CVA	Costovertebral angle
AFAFP	Amniotic fluid alpha fetoprotein	CVP	Central venous pressure
AFP	α-fetoprotein	CVS	Chorionic villus sampling
AFV	Amniotic fluid volume	D&C	Dilatation and curettage
AGA	Average for gestational age	decels	deceleration of fetal heart rate
AID or AIH	Artificial insemination donor (H designates mate is donor)	DFMR	Daily fetal movement response
		DIC	Disseminated intravascular coagulation
AIDS	Acquired Immune Deficiency Syndrome	dil	dilatation
ARBOW	Artificial rupture of bag of waters	DM	Diabetes mellitus
AROM	Artificial rupture of membranes	DRG	Diagnostic related groups
BAT	Brown adipose tissue (brown fat)	DTR	Deep tendon reflexes
BBT	Basal body temperature	ECHMO	Extracorporal membrane oxygenator
BL	Baseline (fetal heart rate baseline)	EDC	Estimated date of confinement
BMR	Basal metabolic rate	EDD	Estimated date of delivery
BOW	Bag of waters	EFM	Electronic fetal monitoring
BP	Blood pressure	EFW	Estimated fetal weight
BPD	Biparietal diameter *or* Bronchopulmonary dysplasia	ELF	Elective low forceps
		epis	Episiotomy
BPM	Beats per minute	FAD	Fetal activity diary
BSE	Breast self examination	FAS	Fetal alcohol syndrome
BSST	Breast self-stimulation test	FBD	Fibrocystic breast disease
CC	Chest circumference *or* Cord compression	FBM	Fetal breathing movements
cc	cubic centimeter	FBS	Fetal blood sample *or* fasting blood sugar test
CDC	Centers for Disease Control	FECG	Fetal electrocardiogram
C-H	Crown-to-heel length	FFA	Free fatty acids
CHF	Congestive heart failure	FHR	Fetal heart rate
CID	Cytomegalic inclusion disease	FHT	Fetal heart tones
CMV	Cytomegalovirus	FL	Femur length
cm	centimeter	FM	Fetal movement
CNM	Certified nurse-midwife	FMAC	Fetal movement acceleration test
CNS	Central nervous system	FMD	Fetal movement diary
CPAP	Continuous positive airway pressure	FMR	Fetal movement record
CPD	Cephalopelvic disproportion *or* Citrate-phosphate-dextrose	FPG	Fasting plasma glucose test
		FRC	Female reproductive cycle
		FSH	Follicle-stimulating hormone
CPR	Cardiopulmonary resuscitation	FSHRH	Follicle-stimulating hormone-releasing hormone
CRL	Crown-rump length	FSI	Foam stability index

G or grav	Gravida	multip	Multipara
GDM	Gestational diabetes mellitus	NANDA	North American Nursing Diagnosis Association
GFR	Glomerular filtration rate	NEC	Necrotizing enterocolitis
GI	Gastrointestinal	NGU	Nongonococcal urethritis
GnRF	Gonadotrophin-releasing factor	NIDDM	Noninsulin-dependent diabetes mellitus (Type II)
GnRH	Gonadotrophin-releasing hormone		
GTPAL	Gravida, term, preterm, abortion, living children; a system of recording maternity history	NIH	National Institutes of Health
		NP	Nurse practitioner
GYN	Gynecology	NPO	Nothing by mouth
HA	Head-abdominal rates	NSCST	Nipple stimulation contraction stress test
HAI	Hemagglutination-inhibition test	NST	Nonstress test or nonshivering thermogenesis
HC	Head compression	NTD	Neural tube defects
hCG	Human chorionic gonadotrophin	NSVD	Normal sterile vaginal delivery
hCS	Human chorionic somatomammotrophin (same as hPL)	OA	Occiput anterior
		OB	Obstetrics
HMD	Hyaline membrane disease	OCT	Oxytocin challenge test
hMG	Human menopausal gonadotrophin	OF	Occipitofrontal diameter of fetal head
hPL	Human placental lactogen	OFC	Occipitofrontal circumference
HVH	Herpes virus hominis	OGTT	Oral glucose tolerance test
ICS	Intercostal space	OM	Occipitomental (diameter)
IDDM	Insulin-dependent diabetes mellitus (Type I)	OP	Occiput posterior
IDM	Infant of a diabetic mother	p	Para
IGT	Impaired glucose tolerance	Pap smear	Papanicolaou smear
IGTT	Intravenous glucose tolerance test	PBI	Protein-bound iodine
IPG	Impedance phlebography	PDA	Patent ductus arteriosus
IUD	Intrauterine device	PEEP	Positive end-expiratory pressure
IUFD	Intrauterine fetal death	PG	Phosphatidyglycerol or Prostaglandin
IUGR	Intrauterine growth retardation	PI	Phosphatidylinositol
JCAH	Joint Commission on the Accreditation of Hospitals	PID	Pelvic inflammatory disease
		PIH	Pregnancy-induced hypertension
LADA	Left-acromion-dorsal-anterior	Pit	Pitocin
LADP	Left-acromion-dorsal-posterior	PKU	Phenylketonuria
LBW	Low birth weight	PMI	Point of maximal impulse
LDR	Labor, delivery and recovery room	PPHN	Persistent pulmonary hypertension
LGA	Large for gestational age	Preemie	Premature infant
LH	Luteinizing hormone	Primip	Primapara
LHRH	Luteinizing hormone-releasing hormone	PROM	Premature rupture of membranes
LMA	Left-mentum-anterior	PTT	Partial thromboplastin test
LML	Left mediolateral episiotomy	PUBS	Percutaneous umbilical blood sampling
LMP	Last menstrual period or Left-mentum-posterior	RADA	Right-acromion-dorsal-anterior
		RADP	Right-acromion-dorsal-posterior
LMT	Left-mentum-transverse	REEDA	Redness, edema, ecchymosis, discharge (or drainage), approximation (a system for recording wound healing)
LOA	Left-occiput-anterior		
LOF	Low outlet forceps		
LOP	Left-occiput-posterior		
LOT	Left-occiput-transverse	RDA	Recommended dietary allowance
L/S	Lecithin/sphingomyelin ratio	RDS	Respiratory distress syndrome
LSA	Left-sacrum-anterior	REM	Rapid eye movements
LSP	Left-sacrum-posterior	RIA	Radioimmune assay
LST	Left-sacrum-transverse	RLF	Retrolental fibroplasia
MAS	Meconium aspiration syndrome or Movement alarm signal	ROA	Right-occiput-anterior
		ROP	Right-occiput-posterior
MCT	Medium chain triglycerides	ROP	Retinopathy of prematurity
mec	Meconium	ROM	Rupture of membranes
mec st	Meconium stain	ROT	Right-occiput-transverse
M & I	Maternity and Infant Care Projects	RMA	Right-mentum-anterior
ML	Midline (episiotomy)	RMP	Right-mentum-posterior
MLE	Midline echo	RMT	Right-mentum-transverse
MRI	Magnetic resonance imaging	RRA	Radioreceptor assay
MSAFP	Maternal serum alpha fetoprotein	RSA	Right-sacrum-anterior
MUGB	4-methylumbelliferyl quanidinobenzoate	RSP	Right-sacrum-posterior

RST	Right-sacrum-transverse	TORCH	Toxoplasmosis, rubella, cytomegalovirus, herpesvirus hominis type 2
SET	Surrogate embryo transfer		
SFD	Small for dates	TSS	Toxic shock syndrome
SGA	Small for gestational age	ū	umbilicus
SIDS	Sudden infant death syndrome	u/a	urinalysis
SOAP	Subjective data, objective data, analysis, plan	UA	Uterine activity
SOB	Suboccipitobregmatic diameter	UAC	Umbilical artery catheter
SMB	Submentobregmatic diameter	UAU	Uterine activity units
SRBOW	Spontaneous rupture of the bag of waters	UC	Uterine contraction
SROM	Spontaneous rupture of the membranes	UPI	Uteroplacental insufficiency
STD	Sexually transmitted disease	U/S	Ultrasound
STH	Somatotrophic hormone	UTI	Urinary tract infection
STS	Serologic test for syphilis	VBAC	Vaginal birth after cesarean
SVE	Sterile vaginal exam	VDRL	Venereal Disease Research Laboratories
TC	Thoracic circumference	WBC	White blood cell
TCM	Transcutaneous monitoring	WIC	Supplemental food program for Women, Infants, and Children
TNZ	Thermal neutral zone		

Appendix B

The Pregnant Patient's Bill of Rights*

The Pregnant Patient has the right to participate in decisions involving her well-being and that of her unborn child, unless there is a clearcut medical emergency that prevents her participation. In addition to the rights set forth in the American Hospital Association's "Patient's Bill of Rights," the Pregnant Patient, because she represents TWO patients rather than one, should be recognized as having the additional rights listed below.

1. *The Pregnant Patient has the right*, prior to the administration of any drug or procedure, to be informed by the health professional caring for her of any potential direct or indirect effects, risks or hazards to herself or her unborn or newborn infant which may result from the use of a drug or procedure prescribed for or administered to her during pregnancy, labor, birth or lactation.

2. *The Pregnant Patient has the right*, prior to the proposed therapy, to be informed, not only of the benefits, risks and hazards of the proposed therapy but also of known alternative therapy, such as available childbirth education classes which could help to prepare the Pregnant Patient physically and mentally to cope with the discomfort or stress of pregnancy and the experience of childbirth, thereby reducing or eliminating her need for drugs and obstetric intervention. She should be offered such information early in her pregnancy in order that she may make a reasoned decision.

3. *The Pregnant Patient has the right*, prior to the administration of any drug, to be informed by the health professional who is prescribing or administering the drug to her that any drug which she receives during pregnancy, labor and birth, no matter how or when the drug is taken or administered, may adversely affect her unborn baby, directly or indirectly, and that there is no drug or chemical which has been proven safe for the unborn child.

4. *The Pregnant Patient has the right* if cesarean birth is anticipated, to be informed prior to the administration of any drug, and preferably prior to her hospitalization, that minimizing her and, in turn, her baby's intake of nonessential preoperative medicine will benefit her baby.

5. *The Pregnant Patient has the right*, prior to the administration of a drug or procedure, to be informed of the areas of uncertainty if there is NO properly controlled follow-up research which has established the safety of the drug or procedure with regard to its direct and/or indirect effects on the physiological, mental and neurological development of the child exposed, via the mother, to the drug or procedure during pregnancy, labor, birth or lactation—(this would apply to virtually all drugs and the vast majority of obstetric procedures).

6. *The Pregnant Patient has the right*, prior to the administration of any drug, to be informed of the brand name and generic name of the drug in order that she may advise the health professional of any past adverse reaction to the drug.

7. *The Pregnant Patient has the right* to determine for herself, without pressure from her attendant, whether she will accept the risks inherent in the proposed therapy or refuse a drug or procedure.

8. *The Pregnant Patient has the right* to know the name and qualifications of the individual administering a medication or procedure to her during labor or birth.

Prepared by Doris Haire, Chair, Committee on Health Law and Regulation, International Childbirth Education Association, Inc., Rochester, N.Y.

9. *The Pregnant Patient has the right* to be informed, prior to the administration of any procedure, whether that procedure is being administered to her for her or her baby's benefit (medically indicated) or as an elective procedure (for convenience, teaching purposes or research).

10. *The Pregnant Patient has the right* to be accompanied during the stress of labor and birth by someone she cares for, and to whom she looks for emotional comfort and encouragement.

11. *The Pregnant Patient has the right* after appropriate medical consultation to choose a position for labor and for birth which is least stressful to her baby and to herself.

12. *The Obstetric Patient has the right* to have her baby cared for at her bedside if her baby is normal, and to feed her baby according to her baby's needs rather than according to the hospital regimen.

13. *The Obstetric Patient has the right* to be informed in writing of the name of the person who actually delivered her baby and the professional qualifications of that person. This information should also be on the birth certificate.

14. *The Obstetric Patient has the right* to be informed if there is any known or indicated aspect of her or her baby's care or condition which may cause her or her baby later difficulty or problems.

15. *The Obstetric Patient has the right* to have her and her baby's hospital medical records complete, accurate and legible and to have their records, including Nurses' Notes, retained by the hospital until the child reaches at least the age of majority, or to have the records offered to her before they are destroyed.

16. *The Obstetric Patient*, both during and after her hospital stay, has the right to have access to her complete hospital medical records, including Nurses' Notes, and to receive a copy upon payment of a reasonable fee and without incurring the expense of retaining an attorney.

It is the obstetric patient and her baby, not the health professional, who must sustain any trauma or injury resulting from the use of a drug or obstetric procedure. The observation of the rights listed above will not only permit the obstetric patient to participate in the decisions involving her and her baby's health care, but will help to protect the health professional and the hospital against litigation arising from resentment or misunderstanding on the part of the mother.

Appendix C

The Pregnant Patient's Responsibilities

In addition to understanding her rights the Pregnant Patient should also understand that she too has certain responsibilities. The Pregnant Patient's responsibilities include the following:

1. The Pregnant Patient is responsible for learning about the physical and psychological process of labor, birth and postpartum recovery. The better informed expectant parents are the better they will be able to participate in decisions concerning the planning of their care.

2. The Pregnant Patient is responsible for learning what comprises good prenatal and intranatal care and for making an effort to obtain the best care possible.

3. Expectant parents are responsible for knowing about those hospital policies and regulations which will affect their birth and postpartum experience.

4. The Pregnant Patient is responsible for arranging for a companion or support person (husband, mother, sister, friend, etc.) who will share in her plans for birth and who will accompany her during her labor and birth experience.

5. The Pregnant Patient is responsible for making her preferences known clearly to the health professionals involved in her care in a courteous and cooperative manner and for making mutually agreed-upon arrangements regarding maternity care alternatives with her physician and hospital in advance of labor.

6. Expectant parents are responsible for listening to their chosen physician or midwife with an open mind, just as they expect him or her to listen openly to them.

7. Once they have agreed to a course of health care, expectant parents are responsible, to the best of their ability, for seeing that the program is carried out in consultation with others with whom they have made the agreement.

8. The Pregnant Patient is responsible for obtaining information in advance regarding the approximate cost of her obstetric and hospital care.

9. The Pregnant Patient who intends to change her physician or hospital is responsible for notifying all concerned, well in advance of the birth if possible, and for informing both of her reasons for changing.

10. In all their interactions with medical and nursing personnel, the expectant parents should behave toward those caring for them with the same respect and consideration they themselves would like.

11. During the mother's hospital stay the mother is responsible for learning about her and her baby's continuing care after discharge from the hospital.

12. After birth, the parents should put into writing constructive comments and feelings of satisfaction and/or dissatisfaction with the care (nursing, medical and personal) they received. Good service to families in the future will be facilitated by those parents who take the time and responsibility to write letters expressing their feelings about the maternity care they received.

United Nations Declaration of the Rights of the Child

Preamble

Whereas the peoples of the United Nations have, in the Charter, reaffirmed their faith in fundamental human rights, and in the dignity and worth of the human person, and have determined to promote social progress and better standards of life in larger freedom,

Whereas the United Nations has, in the Universal Declaration of Human Rights, proclaimed that everyone is entitled to all the rights and freedoms set forth therein, without distinction of any kind, such as race, colour, sex, language, religion, political or other opinion, national or social origin, property, birth or other status,

Whereas the child, by reason of his physical and mental immaturity, needs special safeguards and care, including appropriate legal protection, before as well as after birth,

Whereas the need for such special safeguards has been stated in the Geneva Declaration of the Rights of the Child of 1924, and recognized in the Universal Declaration of Human Rights and in the statutes of specialized agencies and international organizations concerned with the welfare of children,

Whereas mankind owes to the child the best it has to give,

Now therefore,

The General Assembly

Proclaims this Declaration of the Rights of the Child to the end that he may have a happy childhood and enjoy for his own good and for the good of society the rights and freedoms herein set forth, and calls upon parents, upon men and women as individuals, and upon voluntary organizations, local authorities and national Governments to recognize these rights and strive for their observance by legislative and other measures progressively taken in accordance with the following principles:

Principle 1

The child shall enjoy all the rights set forth in this Declaration. Every child, without any exception whatsoever, shall be entitled to these rights, without distinction or discrimination on account of race, colour, sex, language, religion, political or other opinion, national or social origin, property, birth or other status, whether of himself or of his family.

Principle 2

The child shall enjoy special protection, and shall be given opportunities and facilities, by law and by other means, to enable him to develop physically, mentally, morally, spiritually and socially in a healthy and normal manner and in conditions of freedom and dignity. In the enactment of laws for this purpose, the best interests of the child shall be the paramount consideration.

Principle 3

The child shall be entitled from his birth to a name and a nationality.

Principle 4

The child shall enjoy the benefits of social security. He shall be entitled to grow and develop in health; to this end, special care and protection shall be provided both to him and to his mother, including adequate pre-natal and post-natal care. The child shall have the right to adequate nutrition, housing, recreation and medical services.

Principle 5

The child who is physically, mentally or socially handicapped shall be given the special treatment, education and care required by his particular condition.

Principle 6

The child, for the full and harmonious development of his personality, needs love and understanding. He shall, whenever possible, grow up in the care and under the responsibility of his parents, and, in any case, in an atmosphere of affection and of moral and material security; a child of tender years shall not, save in exceptional circumstances, be separated from his mother. Society and the public authorities shall have the duty to extend particular care to children without a family and to those without adequate means of support. Payment of State and other assistance towards the maintenance of children of large families is desirable.

Principle 7

The child is entitled to receive education, which shall be free and compulsory, at least in the elementary stages. He shall be given an education which will promote his general culture, and enable him, on a basis of equal opportunity, to develop his abilities, his individual judgement, and his sense of moral and social responsibility, and to become a useful member of society.

The best interests of the child shall be the guiding principle of those responsible for his education and guidance; that responsibility lies in the first place with his parents.

The child shall have full opportunity for play and recreation, which should be directed to the same purposes as education; society and the public authorities shall endeavour to promote the enjoyment of this right.

Principle 8

The child shall in all circumstances be among the first to receive protection and relief.

Principle 9

The child shall be protected against all forms of neglect, cruelty and exploitation. He shall not be the subject of traffic, in any form.

The child shall not be admitted to employment before an appropriate minimum age; he shall in no case be caused or permitted to engage in any occupation or employment which would prejudice his health or education, or interfere with his physical, mental or moral development.

Principle 10

The child shall be protected from practices which may foster racial, religious and any other form of discrimination. He shall be brought up in a spirit of understanding, tolerance, friendship among peoples, peace and universal brotherhood and in full consciousness that his energy and talents should be devoted to the service of his fellow men.

Adopted by the General Assembly of the United Nations, November 20, 1959.

Appendix E

NAACOG's Standards for Obstetric, Gynecologic, and Neonatal Nursing

• I: NURSING PRACTICE

STANDARD: Comprehensive obstetric, gynecologic, and neonatal (OGN) nursing care is provided to the individual, family, and community within the framework of the nursing process.

INTERPRETATION: The nurse is responsible for decisions and actions within the domain of nursing practice. Comprehensive nursing care includes assisting the person to meet physical, psychosocial, spiritual, and developmental needs. Systematic use of the nursing process which encompasses assessment, nursing diagnosis, planning, implementation, and evaluation will meet the patient's needs. Individualized nursing care is best achieved by collaboration with patient, family, and other members of the health-care team. Complete and accurate documentation of all nursing care and patient response is essential for continuity of care and for meeting legal requirements. The nurse must promote a safe and therapeutic environment for the individual, family, and community.

• II: HEALTH EDUCATION

STANDARD: Health education for the individual, family, and community is an integral part of obstetric, gynecologic, and neonatal nursing practice.

INTERPRETATION: The nurse is responsible for providing pertinent information to the individual, family, and community so they may participate in and share responsibility for their own health promotion, maintenance, and restorative care. The nurse plans, implements, and evaluates health education based on principles of teaching and learning. To enhance health care and promote continuity of health education, the nurse uses the educational resources within the community and collaborates with other health-care providers.

Health education should be documented and evaluated. Evaluation is based on individualized goals and set criteria.

• III: POLICIES AND PROCEDURES

STANDARD: The delivery of obstetric, gynecologic, and neonatal nursing care is based on written policies and procedures.

INTERPRETATION: Policies and procedures define the boundaries of nursing practice within the health-care setting and indicate the qualifications of personnel authorized to perform OGN nursing procedures. The qualifications may include educational preparation and/or certification. The policies and procedures should be in accordance with the philosophy of the agency, state nurse practice act, governmental regulations, and other applicable standards or regulations.

A multidisciplinary framework should be used in writing policies and procedures. Policies and procedures should be evaluated on an ongoing basis and revised as necessary. The policies and procedures should be readily accessible to the health-care providers within the health-care setting.

• IV: PROFESSIONAL RESPONSIBILITY AND ACCOUNTABILITY

STANDARD: The obstetric, gynecologic, and neonatal nurse is responsible and accountable for maintaining knowledge and competency in individual nursing practice and for being aware of professional issues.

INTERPRETATION: Maintaining both the knowledge and skills required to achieve excellence in OGN nursing is incumbent upon the nurse. The nurse should be cognizant of changing concepts, trends, and scientific advances in OGN care. Updating knowledge and skills is achievable through formal education, professional continuing education, and the use of or participation in nursing research. Knowledge of specialty nursing can be recognized through certification.

The nurse should be aware of governmental policies and legislation affecting health care and nursing practice. Participating in legislative and regulatory processes is appropriate for the nurse.

Responsibilities defined in written position descriptions and performance demonstrated by the OGN nurse should be regularly evaluated and documented. In addition, criteria for the evaluation of OGN nursing practice should be drawn from applicable statutes, the ethics of the profession, and current standards of practice.

● V: PERSONNEL

STANDARD: Obstetric, gynecologic, and neonatal nursing staff are provided to meet patient care needs.

INTERPRETATION: The obstetric, gynecologic, and neonatal nursing management determines the staff required for the provision of individualized nursing care commensurate with demonstrated patient needs, appropriate nursing interventions, qualifications of available nursing personnel, and other factors which must be considered. These factors may include nursing care needs; number of deliveries; number and types of surgical procedures; average inpatient census; volume of ambulatory patients; percentage of high-risk patients; educational, emotional, and economic needs of the patients; provision for staff continuing education; medical staff coverage; ancillary services available; size and design of facilities; responsibilities of nursing staff; and ongoing research.

Personnel in each OGN unit should be directed by a registered nurse with educational preparation and clinical experience in the specific OGN area of practice. This nurse is responsible for management of nursing care and supervision of nursing personnel.

When nursing, medical, or other specialty students are assigned to the unit for clinical experience, their roles and responsibilities should be clearly defined in writing. Nursing students should not be included in the unit's staffing plan.

Written position descriptions which identify standards of performance for OGN nurses should be developed and used in periodic personnel evaluations. Documentation should reflect each nurse's participation in orientation and verify knowledge and expertise in those skills required for OGN nursing practice. Orientation and evaluation of personnel for whom the registered nurse is held accountable should be documented as well.

Written policies for the reassignment of OGN nursing personnel should exist to accommodate both increases and decreases of inpatient days and ambulatory visits. The policies should include a contingency plan for staffing during peak activity periods.

Evaluation of Fetal Weight and Maturity by Ultrasonic Measurement of Biparietal Diameter*

Biaparietal Diameter (cm)	Grams	Weight Pounds	Ounces	Weeks of Gestation	Biaparietal Diameter (cm)	Grams	Weight Pounds	Ounces	Weeks of Gestation
1.0	NA	NA		9	6.0	660.4	1	8	25.5
1.1	NA	NA		9	6.1	737.6	1	10	26.0
1.2	NA	NA		9.5	6.2	814.8	1	13	26.0
1.3	NA	NA		10.0	6.3	892.1	2		26.5
1.4	NA	NA		10.0	6.4	969.3	2	2	27.0
1.5	NA	NA		10.5	6.5	1046.5	2	5	27.0
1.6	NA	NA		11.0	6.6	1123.7	2	8	27.5
1.7	NA	NA		11.0	6.7	1200.9	2	10	28.0
1.8	NA	NA		11.5	6.8	1278.2	2	13	28.0
1.9	NA	NA		12.0	6.9	1355.4	3		28.5
2.0	NA	NA		12.0	7.0	1432.6	3	3	29.0
2.1	NA	NA		12.5	7.1	1509.8	3	5	29.0
2.2	NA	NA		13.0	7.2	1587.0	3	8	29.5
2.3	NA	NA		13.0	7.3	1664.3	3	11	29.5
2.4	NA	NA		13.5	7.4	1741.5	3	14	30.0
2.5	NA	NA		14.0	7.5	1818.7	4		30.5
2.6	NA	NA		14.0	7.6	1895.9	4	3	30.8
2.7	NA	NA		14.5	7.7	1973.1	4	5	31.0
2.8	NA	NA		15.0	7.8	2050.4	4	8	31.7
2.9	NA	NA		15.0	7.9	2127.6	4	11	32.0
3.0	NA	NA		15.5	8.0	2204.8	4	14	32.7
3.1	NA	NA		16.0	8.1	2282.0	5		33.0
3.2	NA	NA		16.0	8.2	2359.2	5	3	33.6
3.3	NA	NA		16.5	8.3	2436.5	5	6	34.0
3.4	NA	NA		17.0	8.4	2513.7	5	8	34.6
3.5	NA	NA		17.0	8.5	2590.9	5	11	35.0
3.6	NA	NA		17.5	8.6	2668.1	5	14	35.5
3.7	NA	NA		18.0	8.7	2745.3	6		36.0
3.8	NA	NA		18.0	8.8	2822.6	6	3	36.5
3.9	NA	NA		18.5	8.9	2899.8	6	6	37.0
4.0	NA	NA		19.0	9.0	2977.0	6	8	37.4
4.1	NA	NA		19.0	9.1	3054.2	6	11	38.0
4.2	NA	NA		19.5	9.2	3131.4	6	14	38.4
4.3	NA	NA		20.0	9.3	3208.7	7	2	39.0
4.4	NA	NA		20.0	9.4	3285.9	7	3	39.0
4.5	NA	NA		20.5	9.5	3363.1	7	6	39.8
4.6	NA	NA		21.0	9.6	3440.3	7	10	40.0
4.7	NA	NA		21.0	9.7	3517.5	7	11	40.8
4.8	NA	NA		21.5	9.8	3594.8	7	14	41.0
4.9	NA	NA		22.0	9.9	3672.0	8	2	41.7
5.0	NA	NA		22.0	10.0	3749.2	8	3	NA
5.1	NA	NA		22.5	10.1	3826.5	8	6	NA
5.2	42.6		2	23.0	10.2	3903.6	8	10	NA
5.3	119.9		5	23.0	10.3	3980.9	8	13	NA
5.4	197.1		6	23.5	10.4	4058.1	8	14	NA
5.5	274.3		10	24.0	10.5	4135.3	9	2	NA
5.6	351.5		13	24.0	10.6	4212.5	9	5	NA
5.7	428.7		14	24.5					
5.8	514.9	1	2	25.0					
5.9	583.2	1	5	25.0					

* Data from Hellman and Kobayashi.

Cervical Dilatation Assessment Aid

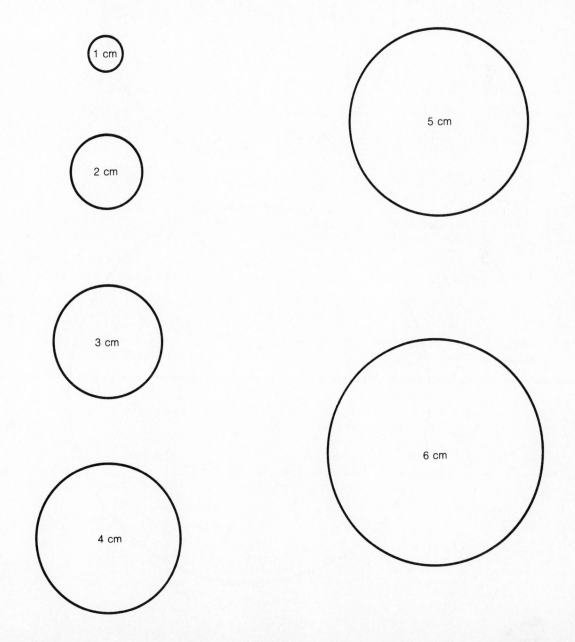

Cervical Dilatation Assessment Aid (continued)

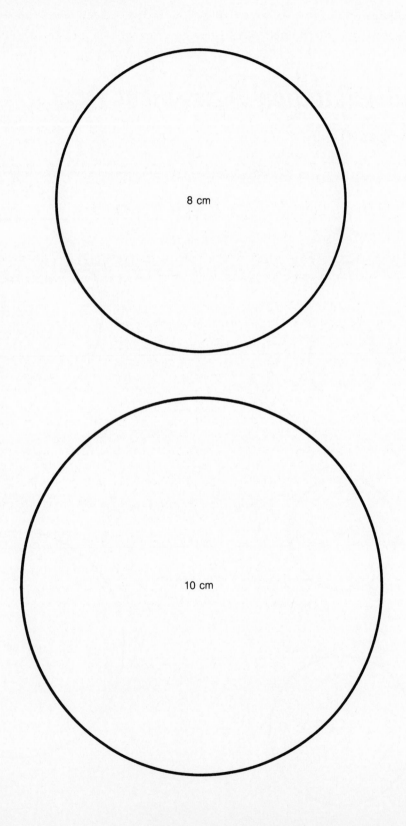

Appendix H

Clinical Estimation of Gestational Age

Clinical estimation of gestational age. (Courtesy Mead Johnson Laboratories, Evansville, Ind.)

▶ **Examination First Hours**

CLINICAL ESTIMATION OF GESTATIONAL AGE
An Approximation Based on Published Data*

PHYSICAL FINDINGS		WEEKS GESTATION (20–48)
VERNIX		APPEARS → COVERS BODY, THICK LAYER → ON BACK, SCALP, IN CREASES → SCANT, IN CREASES → NO VERNIX
BREAST TISSUE AND AREOLA		AREOLA & NIPPLE BARELY VISIBLE NO PALPABLE BREAST TISSUE → AREOLA RAISED → 1-2 MM NODULE → 3-5 MM → 5-6 MM → 7-10 MM → ?12 MM
EAR	FORM	FLAT, SHAPELESS → BEGINNING INCURVING SUPERIOR → INCURVING UPPER 2/3 PINNAE → WELL-DEFINED INCURVING TO LOBE
	CARTILAGE	PINNA SOFT, STAYS FOLDED → CARTILAGE SCANT RETURNS SLOWLY FROM FOLDING → THIN CARTILAGE SPRINGS BACK FROM FOLDING → PINNA FIRM, REMAINS ERECT FROM HEAD
SOLE CREASES		SMOOTH SOLES 1" CREASES → 1-2 ANTERIOR CREASES → 2-3 ANTERIOR CREASES → CREASES ANTERIOR 2/3 SOLE → CREASES INVOLVING HEEL → DEEPER CREASES OVER ENTIRE SOLE
SKIN	THICKNESS & APPEARANCE	THIN, TRANSLUCENT SKIN, PLETHORIC, VENULES OVER ABDOMEN EDEMA → SMOOTH THICKER NO EDEMA → PINK → FEW VESSELS → SOME DESQUAMATION PALE PINK → THICK, PALE, DESQUAMATION OVER ENTIRE BODY
	NAIL PLATES	AP-PEAR → NAILS TO FINGER TIPS → NAILS EXTEND WELL BEYOND FINGER TIPS
HAIR		APPEARS ON HEAD → EYE BROWS & LASHES → FINE, WOOLLY, BUNCHES OUT FROM HEAD → SILKY, SINGLE STRANDS LAYS FLAT → RECEDING HAIRLINE OR LOSS OF BABY HAIR SHORT, FINE UNDERNEATH
LANUGO		AP-PEARS → COVERS ENTIRE BODY → VANISHES FROM FACE → PRESENT ON SHOULDERS → NO LANUGO
GENITALIA	TESTES	TESTES PALPABLE IN INGUINAL CANAL → IN UPPER SCROTUM → IN LOWER SCROTUM
	SCROTUM	FEW RUGAE → RUGAE, ANTERIOR PORTION → RUGAE COVER → PENDULOUS
	LABIA & CLITORIS	PROMINENT CLITORIS LABIA MAJORA SMALL WIDELY SEPARATED → LABIA MAJORA LARGER NEARLY COVERED CLITORIS → LABIA MINORA & CLITORIS COVERED
SKULL FIRMNESS		BONES ARE SOFT → SOFT TO 1" FROM ANTERIOR FONTANELLE → SPONGY AT EDGES OF FONTANELLE CENTER FIRM → BONES HARD SUTURES EASILY DISPLACED → BONES HARD, CANNOT BE DISPLACED
POSTURE	RESTING	HYPOTONIC LATERAL DECUBITUS → HYPOTONIC → BEGINNING FLEXION THIGH → STRONGER HIP FLEXION → FROG-LIKE → FLEXION ALL LIMBS → HYPERTONIC → VERY HYPERTONIC
	RECOIL · LEG	NO RECOIL → PARTIAL RECOIL → PROMPT RECOIL
	ARM	NO RECOIL → BEGIN FLEXION NO RECOIL → PROMPT RECOIL MAY BE INHIBITED → PROMPT RECOIL AFTER 30" INHIBITION

Weeks scale: 20 21 22 23 24 25 26 27 28 29 30 31 32 33 34 35 36 37 38 39 40 41 42 43 44 45 46 47 48

*Brazie JV and Lubchenco LO. *The estimation of gestational age chart.* In Kempe, Silver and O'Brien. *Current Pediatric Diagnosis and Treatment,* ed 3. Los Altos, Calif: Lange Medical Publications, 1974, ch 4.

Appendix I

Classification of Newborns (Both Sexes) by Intrauterine Growth and Gestational Age[1,2]

NAME _____ DATE OF BIRTH _____ BIRTH WEIGHT _____

HOSPITAL NO. _____ DATE OF EXAM _____ LENGTH _____

RACE _____ SEX _____ HEAD CIRC. _____

GESTATIONAL AGE _____

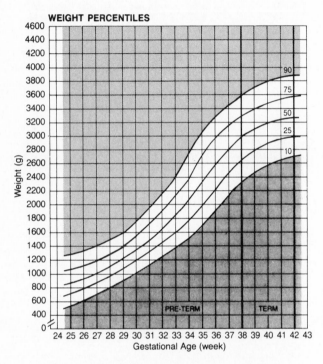

WEIGHT PERCENTILES

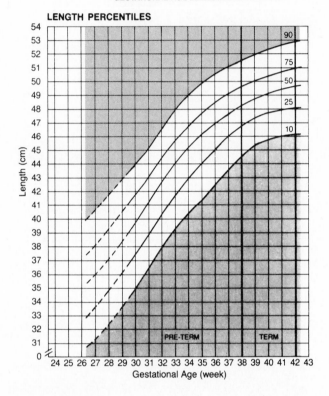

LENGTH PERCENTILES

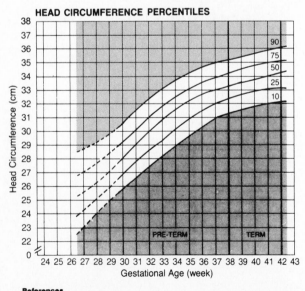

HEAD CIRCUMFERENCE PERCENTILES

CLASSIFICATION OF INFANT*	Weight	Length	Head Circ.
Large for Gestational Age (LGA) (>90th percentile)			
Appropriate for Gestational Age (AGA) (10th to 90th percentile)			
Small for Gestational Age (SGA) (<10th percentile)			

*Place an "X" in the appropriate box (LGA, AGA or SGA) for weight, for length and for head circumference.

References
1. Battaglia FC, Lubchenco LO: A practical classification of newborn infants by weight and gestational age. J Pediatr 71:159-163, 1967.
2. Lubchenco LO, Hansman C, Boyd E: Intrauterine growth in length and head circumference as estimated from live births at gestational ages from 26 to 42 weeks. Pediatrics 37:403-408, 1966.

Actions and Effects of Selected Drugs During Breast-Feeding*

Antimicrobials

Ampicillin: Skin rash, candidiasis; diarrhea

Chloramphenicol: Possible bone marrow suppression; Gray syndrome; refusal of breast

Methacycline: Possible inhibition of bone growth; may cause discoloration of the teeth; use should be avoided

Sulfonamides: May cause hyperbilirubinemia; use contraindicated until infant over 1 month old

Penicillin: Possible allergic response; candidiasis

Metronidazole (Flagyl): Possible neurologic disorders or blood dyscrasias; delay breast-feeding for 12 to 24 hours after last dose

Aminoglycosides: May cause ototoxicity or nephrotoxicity if given for more than two weeks

Tetracycline: Long-term use and large doses should be avoided; may cause tooth staining or inhibition of bone growth

Anticoagulants

Coumarin derivatives (Warfarin): May cause bleeding problems; should be discontinued in mother or breast-feeding temporarily halted if infant to have surgery

Heparin: Relatively safe to use; check PTT

Phenindione (Hedulin): Passes easily into breast milk; neonate may have increased pro time and PTT

Anticholinergics

Atropine: May cause hyperthermia in the newborn; may decrease maternal milk supply

Antihistamines
May cause decreased milk supply; infant may become drowsy, irritable, or have tachycardia

Antimetabolites
Unknown, probably long-term anti-DNA effect on the infant; potentially very toxic

Antithyroids

Thiouracil: Contraindicated during lactation; may cause goiter or agranulocytosis

Bronchodilators

Aminophylline: May cause insomnia or irritability in the infant

Cardiovascular

Propranolol (Inderal): May cause hypoglycemia; possibility of other blocking effects

Quinidine: May cause arrhythmias in infant

Reserpine (Serpasil): Nasal stuffiness, lethargy, or diarrhea in infant

Caffeine
Excessive consumption may cause jitteriness

Corticosteroids
Adrenal suppression may occur with long-term administration of doses greater than 10 mg/day.

Hormones

Androgens: Suppress lactation

Oral contraceptives: Decrease milk supply; may alter milk composition; may cause gynecomastia in male infants

Thyroid hormones: May mask hypothyroidism

Heavy metals

Gold: Potentially toxic

Mercury: Excreted in the milk and hazardous to infant

Laxatives

Cascara: May cause diarrhea in infant

Milk of magnesia: Relatively safe

Phenolphthalein: May cause diarrhea in infant

Narcotic analgesics

Codeine: Accumulation may lead to neonatal depression

Meperidine: May lead to neonatal depression

Morphine: Long-term use may cause newborn addiction

*Based on data from Hill WC: Drugs contraindicated during pregnancy and lactation. *Medical Times* 1987; 115(June):132. Riordan J: *A Practical Guide to Breastfeeding.* St. Louis: Mosby, 1983, pp 140–145. Spencer RT, et al: *Clinical Pharmacology and Nursing Management,* 2nd ed. Philadelphia: Lippincott, 1986, p 1016.

Narcotic analgesics

Codeine: Accumulation may lead to neonatal depression

Meperidine: May lead to neonatal depression

Morphine: Long-term use may cause newborn addiction

Nonnarcotic analgesics

Salicylates: Safe after first week of life

Acetaminophen: Relatively safe for short-term analgesia

Propoxyphene (Darvon): May cause sleepiness and poor nursing in infant

Radioactive materials for testing

Gallium citrate (^{67}G): Insignificant amount excreted in breast milk; no nursing for 2 weeks

Iodine: Contraindicated; may affect infant's thyroid gland

$^{125}I:$ Discontinue nursing for 48 hours

$^{131}I:$ Nursing should be discontinued until excretion is no longer significant; after a test dose, nursing may be resumed after 24 to 36 hours; after a treatment dose, nursing may be resumed after 2 to 3 weeks

$^{99}Technetium:$ Discontinue nursing for 48 hours (half-life = 6 hours)

Sedatives/Tranquilizers

Diazepam (Valium): May accumulate to high levels; may increase neonatal jaundice; may cause sedation

Lithium carbonate: Contraindicated; may cause neonatal flaccidity and hypotonia

Chlordiazepoxide (Librium): Use with caution after infant one week old

Barbiturates May produce sedation

Phenothiazines: May produce sedation

Appendix K

Conversions and Equivalents

Temperature Conversion

(Fahrenheit temperature − 32) × 5/9 = Celsius temperature
(Celsius temperature × 9/5) + 32 = Fahrenheit temperature

Selected Conversions to Metric Measures

Known value	Multiply by	To find
inches	2.54	centimeters
ounces	28	grams
pounds	454	grams
pounds	0.45	kilograms

Selected Conversions from Metric Measures

Known value	Multiply by	To find
centimeters	0.4	inches
grams	0.035	ounces
grams	0.0022	pounds
kilograms	2.2	pounds

Conversion of Pounds and Ounces to Grams

| | | | | | | | Ounces | | | | | | | | | |
S	0	1	2	3	4	5	6	7	8	9	10	11	12	13	14	15
0	—	28	57	85	113	142	170	198	227	255	283	312	340	369	397	425
1	454	482	510	539	567	595	624	652	680	709	737	765	794	822	850	879
2	907	936	964	992	1021	1049	1077	1106	1134	1162	1191	1219	1247	1276	1304	1332
3	1361	1389	1417	1446	1474	1503	1531	1559	1588	1616	1644	1673	1701	1729	1758	1786
4	1814	1843	1871	1899	1928	1956	1984	2013	2041	2070	2098	2126	2155	2183	2211	2240
5	2268	2296	2325	2353	2381	2410	2438	2466	2495	2523	2551	2580	2608	2637	2665	2693
6	2722	2750	2778	2807	2835	2863	2892	2920	2948	2977	3005	3033	3062	3090	3118	3147
7	3175	3203	3232	3260	3289	3317	3345	3374	3402	3430	3459	3487	3515	3544	3572	3600
8	3629	3657	3685	3714	3742	3770	3799	3827	3856	3884	3912	3941	3969	3997	4026	4054
9	4082	4111	4139	4167	4196	4224	4252	4281	4309	4337	4366	4394	4423	4451	4479	4508
10	4536	4564	4593	4621	4649	4678	4706	4734	4763	4791	4819	4848	4876	4904	4933	4961
11	4990	5018	5046	5075	5103	5131	5160	5188	5216	5245	5273	5301	5330	5358	5386	5415
12	5443	5471	5500	5528	5557	5585	5613	5642	5670	5698	5727	5755	5783	5812	5840	5868
13	5897	5925	5953	5982	6010	6038	6067	6095	6123	6152	6180	6209	6237	6265	6294	6322
14	6350	6379	6407	6435	6464	6492	6520	6549	6577	6605	6634	6662	6690	6719	6747	6776
15	6804	6832	6860	6889	6917	6945	6973	7002	7030	7059	7087	7115	7144	7172	7201	7228
16	7257	7286	7313	7342	7371	7399	7427	7456	7484	7512	7541	7569	7597	7626	7654	7682
17	7711	7739	7768	7796	7824	7853	7881	7909	7938	7966	7994	8023	8051	8079	8108	8136
18	8165	8192	8221	8249	8278	8306	8335	8363	8391	8420	8448	8476	8504	8533	8561	8590
19	8618	8646	8675	8703	8731	8760	8788	8816	8845	8873	8902	8930	8958	8987	9015	9043
20	9072	9100	9128	9157	9185	9213	9242	9270	9298	9327	9355	9383	9412	9440	9469	9497
21	9525	9554	9582	9610	9639	9667	9695	9724	9752	9780	9809	9837	9865	9894	9922	9950
22	9979	10007	10036	10064	10092	10120	10149	10177	10206	10234	10262	10291	10319	10347	10376	10404

Pounds

Appendix L

North American Nursing Diagnosis Association Approved Nursing Diagnoses, April 1986*

Activity Intolerance (Specify level)
Activity Intolerance, Potential
Adjustment, Impaired
Airway Clearance, Ineffective
Anxiety
Body Temperature, Potential Alteration in
Bowel Elimination, Alteration in: Constipation
Bowel Elimination, Alteration in: Diarrhea
Bowel Elimination, Alteration in: Incontinence
Breathing Pattern, Ineffective
Cardiac Output, Alteration in: Decreased
Comfort, Alteration in: Pain
Comfort, Alteration in: Chronic Pain
Communication, Impaired Verbal
Coping, Ineffective Individual
Coping, Ineffective Family: Compromised
Coping, Ineffective Family: Disabling
Coping, Family: Potential for Growth
Diversional Activity Deficit
Family Processes, Alteration in
Fear (Specify)
Fluid Volume Deficit, Actual
Fluid Volume Deficit, Potential
Fluid Volume, Alteration in: Excess
Gas Exchange, Impaired
Grieving, Anticipatory
Grieving, Dysfunctional
Growth and Development, Altered
Health Maintenance, Alteration in
Home Maintenance Management, Impaired
Hopelessness
Hyperthermia
Hypothermia
Incontinence, Functional
Incontinence, Reflex
Incontinence, Stress
Incontinence, Total
Incontinence, Urge
Infection, Potential for
Injury, Potential for (Poisoning, Potential for; Suffocation, Potential for; Trauma, Potential for)

Knowledge Deficit (Specify)
Mobility, Impaired Physical
Neglect, Unilateral
Noncompliance (Specify)
Nutrition, Alteration in: Less than Body Requirements
Nutrition, Alteration in: More than Body Requirements
Nutrition, Alteration in: Potential for More than Body Requirements
Oral Mucous Membrane, Alteration in
Parenting, Alteration in: Actual
Parenting, Alteration in: Potential
Post-trauma Response
Powerlessness
Rape Trauma Syndrome
Rape Trauma Syndrome: Compounded
Rape Trauma Syndrome: Silent Reaction
Self-Care Deficit (Bathing/Hygiene, Feeding, Dressing/Grooming, Toileting)
Self-Concept Disturbance (Disturbance in Body Image, Personal Identity, Self-Esteem, Role Performance)
Sensory Perceptual Alteration: Visual, Auditory, Kinesthetic, Gustatory, Tactile, Olfactory
Sexual Dysfunction
Sexuality Patterns, Altered
Skin Integrity, Impairment of: Actual
Skin Integrity, Impairment of: Potential
Sleep Pattern Disturbance
Social Interaction, Impaired
Social Isolation
Spiritual Distress (Distress of the Human Spirit)
Swallowing, Impaired
Thermoregulation, Ineffective
Thought Processes, Alteration in
Tissue Integrity, Impaired
Tissue Perfusion, Alteration in (Cerebral, Cardiopulmonary, Renal, Gastrointestinal, Peripheral)
Urinary Elimination, Alteration in Patterns
Urinary Retention
Violence, Potential for (self-directed or directed at others)

*Definitions, defining characteristics, and related factors are included in McLane, A. (Ed.). (1987). *Classification of nursing diagnoses: Proceedings of the seventh conference.* St. Louis: Mosby.

Glossary

abdominal delivery see *cesarean delivery*.

abdominal effleurage gentle stroking used in massage.

abdominal gestation pregnancy within the abdominal cavity but outside the uterus.

abdominal hysterectomy surgical removal of the uterus through an incision in the abdominal wall.

abortion loss of pregnancy before the fetus is viable outside the uterus; miscarriage.

abruptio placentae partial or total premature separation of a normally implanted placenta.

abstinence refraining voluntarily, especially from indulgence in food, alcoholic beverages, or sexual intercourse.

acceleration periodic increase in the baseline fetal heart rate.

acini cells secretory cells in the human breast that create milk from nutrients in the bloodstream.

acme peak or highest point; time of greatest intensity (of a uterine contraction).

acrocyanosis cyanosis of the extremities.

active acquired immunity formation of antibodies by the pregnant woman in response to illness or immunization.

adduct to draw toward the main axis of the body.

adenomyoma tumor that affects the glandular and smooth muscle tissue, such as the muscles of the uterus.

adnexa adjoining or accessory parts of a structure, such as the uterine adnexa: the ovaries and fallopian tubes.

adolescence period of human development initiated by puberty and ending with the attainment of young adulthood.

afibrinogenemia absence of or decrease in fibrinogen in the blood plasma, so that the blood does not coagulate. This condition may be acquired or congenital, and it may result from such obstetric complications as abruptio placentae and retention of a dead fetus.

afterbirth placenta and membranes expelled after the delivery of the infant, during the third stage of labor; also called *secundines*.

afterpains cramplike pains due to contractions of the uterus that occur after childbirth. They are more common in multiparas, tend to be most severe during nursing, and last two to three days.

agalactia absence or failure of the secretion of breast milk.

AIDS autoimmune deficiency syndrome; a sexually transmitted viral disease that so far has proved fatal in 100 percent of cases.

alae nasi nostrils.

albinism a congenital absence of normal skin pigmentation.

albuminuria readily detectable amounts of albumin in the urine.

allantois tubular diverticulum of the posterior part of the embryo's yolk sac that passes into the body stalk. The allantoic blood vessels develop into the umbilical vein and paired umbilical arteries.

allele one of a series of alternate genes at the same locus; one form of a gene.

alveolus a saclike cavity.

ambient surrounding; that which is around us.

amblyopia reduced vision that is not caused by visible changes in the eye or by refractive error.

amenorrhea suppression or absence of menstruation.

amniocentesis removal of amniotic fluid by insertion of a needle into the amniotic sac; amniotic fluid is used to assess fetal health or maturity.

amniography x-ray examination of the amniotic sac following the injection of a radiopaque dye into the amniotic fluid.

amnion the inner of the two membranes that form the sac containing the fetus and the amniotic fluid.

amnionitis infection of the amniotic fluid.

amnioscopy visualization of the amniotic fluid through the membranes with an amnioscope in order to identify meconium staining of the amniotic fluid.

amniotic relating or pertaining to the amnion.

amniotic fluid the liquid surrounding the fetus in utero. It absorbs shocks, permits fetal movement, and prevents heat loss.

amniotic fluid embolus   amniotic fluid that has leaked into the chorionic plate and entered the maternal circulation.

amniotic sac   the bag or sac formed by the amnion that contains the fetus.

amniotomy   the artificial rupturing of the amniotic membrane.

ampulla   the outer two-thirds of the fallopian tube; fertilization of the ovum by a spermatozoon usually occurs here.

anaerobic catabolism   the breakdown of organized substances into simple compounds in the absence of free oxygen, with the release of energy.

analgesic   drug that relieves pain and does not cause unconsciousness.

androgen   substance producing male characteristics, such as the male hormone testosterone.

android pelvis   male-type pelvis.

anencephaly   congenital deformity in which the cerebrum, cerebellum, and flat bones of the skull are absent.

anesthesia   partial or complete loss of sensation with or without loss of consciousness.

anomaly   a malformation; an organ or structure that is abnormal in position, structure, or form.

anovular menstrual period   cyclic uterine bleeding that is not preceded by ovulation.

anoxia   deficiency of oxygen.

antenatal   before birth.

antepartal   before the onset of labor.

antepartal education   programs teaching childbirth preparation.

antepartum   time between conception and the onset of labor; usually used to describe the period during which a woman is pregnant.

anterior   pertaining to the front.

anterior fontanelle   diamond-shaped area between the two frontal and two parietal bones just above the newborn's forehead.

anteroposterior repair   surgical reconstruction of the upper and lower walls of the vagina to correct relaxed tissue.

anthropoid pelvis   pelvis in which the anteroposterior diameter is equal to or greater than the transverse diameter.

antibody   a specific protein substance developed by the body in response to specific antigens in order to restrict or destroy them.

antigen   a substance formed within the body or introduced into it that induces the formation of antibodies.

antitoxin   an antibody that is capable of neutralizing a specific toxin and that is produced by the body in response to the presence of the toxin.

Apert syndrome   an autosomal dominant disorder characterized by mental deficiency, irregular craniosynostosis, high full forehead and flat occiput, flat facies, hypertelorism, narrow palate, and syndactyly.

Apgar score   a scoring system used to evaluate newborns at 1 minute and 5 minutes after delivery. The total score is achieved by assessing five signs: heart rate, respiratory effort, muscle tone, reflex irritability, and color. Each of the signs is assigned a score of 0, 1, or 2. The highest possible score is 10.

apnea   a condition that occurs when respirations cease for more than 20 seconds, with generalized cyanosis.

areola   pigmented ring surrounding the nipple of the breast.

Arnold-Chiari malformation   a condition in which the inferior poles of the cerebellar hemispheres and the medulla protrude and may herniate through the foramen magnum. It is one of the causes of hydrocephaly, and is usually accompanied by spina bifida or meningomyelocele.

AROM   artificial rupture of (amniotic) membranes through use of a device such as an amnihook or allis forceps.

articulation   connection of bones in the skeleton; joint.

artificial insemination   introduction of viable semen into the vagina by artificial means for the purpose of impregnation.

Aschheim-Zondek test   a test for pregnancy in which the woman's urine is injected subcutaneously into a mouse. After five days, the animal is killed and its ovaries examined. Enlarged ovaries and maturing follicles indicate pregnancy.

asphyxia   a condition caused by a decreased amount of oxygen or an excess amount of carbon dioxide in the body.

aspiration syndrome   a condition that occurs with fetal hypoxia: the anal sphincter relaxes and meconium is expelled; reflex gasping movements draw meconium and other particulate matter contained in the amniotic fluid into the bronchial tree, thereby obstructing air flow after birth.

asynclitism   an oblique presentation of the fetal head; the pelvic planes and those of the fetal head are not parallel.

atelectasis   a condition in which the lungs of the fetus remain unexpanded at birth; it involves alveolar collapse. It may be either partial or complete.

atony   lack of normal muscle tone.

atresia   congenital absence or pathologic closure of a normal anatomic opening. See *choanal atresia; esophageal atresia.*

attitude   attitude of the fetus refers to the relationship of the fetal parts to each other.

auscultation   process of listening for sounds produced within the body in order to detect abnormal conditions.

autoimmune deficiency syndrome   see *AIDS.*

autosome   a chromosome that is not a sex chromosome.

axis   a line, real or imaginary, that a part revolves around or that runs through the center of the body.

azoospermic   absence of spermatozoa in the semen.

bacterial vaginosis   a bacterial infection of the vagina, formerly called *Gardnerella vaginalis* or *Hemophilus vaginalis,* characterized by a foul-smelling, grayish vaginal discharge that exhibits a characteristic fishy odor when 10 percent potassium hydroxide (KOH) is added. Microscopic examination of a vaginal wet prep reveals the presence of "clue cells" (vaginal epithelial cells coated with gram-negative organisms).

bag of waters   the membrane containing the amniotic fluid and the fetus (BOW).

balanced translocation   rearrangement of chromosomal material in which a piece of one chromosome is broken off and joined to another chromosome. An individual with a balanced translocation has the normal amount of genetic material but it is arranged abnormally, making the individual at risk for producing offspring with chromosmal abnormalities.

ballottement a technique of palpation to detect or examine a floating object in the body. In obstetrics, the fetus, when pushed, floats away and then returns to touch the examiner's fingers.

Bandl's ring a thickened ridge of uterine musculature between the upper and lower segments that occurs following a mechanically obstructed labor, with the lower segment thinning abnormally.

Barr body deeply staining chromatin mass located against the inner surface of the cell nucleus. It is found only in normal females; also called *sex chromatin*.

Bartholin's glands two small mucous glands situated on each side of the vaginal orifice that secrete small amounts of mucus during coitus.

basal body temperature (BBT) the lowest waking temperature.

baseline rate the average fetal heart rate observed during a 10-minute period of monitoring.

baseline variability changes in the fetal heart rate that result from the interplay between the sympathetic and the parasympathetic nervous systems.

battledore placenta placenta in which the umbilical cord is inserted on the periphery rather than centrally.

Beckwith syndrome syndrome of unknown etiology, characterized by macroglossia, omphalocele, macrosomia, ear creases, neonatal polycythemia, diastasis recti, and cryptorchidism.

bicornate uterus anomalous uterus resulting from incomplete union of the müllerian ducts. May be double or single with two horns.

bilirubin orange or yellowish pigment in bile; a breakdown product of hemoglobin that is carried by the blood to the liver, where it is chemically changed and excreted in the bile or is conjugated and excreted in the stools.

bimanual palpation examination of the pelvic organs by placing one hand on the abdomen and one or two fingers of the other hand into the vagina.

biopsy excision of a small piece of tissue for microscopic examination and diagnosis.

birth rate number of live birth per 1000 population.

birth center a setting for labor and delivery that emphasizes a family-centered approach rather than obstetric technology and treatment.

birth stool a small wooden chair that a woman may sit on during labor and delivery.

birthing room a room for labor and delivery with a relaxed atmosphere.

Bishop score a prelabor scoring system to assist in predicting whether an induction of labor may be successful. The total score is achieved by assessing five components: cervical dilatation, cervical effacement, cervical consistency, cervical position, and fetal station. Each of the components is assigned a score of zero to three, and the highest possible score is 13.

blastocyst the inner solid mass of cells within the morula.

blastoderm germinal membrane of the ovum.

bleeding diathesis predisposition to abnormal blood clotting.

bloody show pink-tinged mucous secretions resulting from rupture of small capillaries as the cervix effaces and dilates.

brachial palsy partial or complete paralysis of portions of the arm resulting from trauma to the brachial plexus during a difficult delivery.

bradycardia slow heart rate.

Bradley method partner-coached natural childbirth.

Braxton Hicks contractions intermittent painless contractions of the uterus that may occur every 10 to 20 minutes. They occur more frequently toward the end of pregnancy and are sometimes mistaken for true labor signs.

Brazleton's neonatal behavioral assessment a brief examination used to identify the infant's behavioral states and responses.

breast milk jaundice yellowing of the infant's skin caused by pregnanediol in the mother's milk. Pregnanediol inhibits glucuronyl transferase, the enzyme necessary for the conjugation of bilirubin.

breech presentation a delivery in which the buttocks and/ or feet are presented instead of the head.

bregma juncture of the coronal and sagittal sutures of the skull; the area of the anterior fontanelle of the fetus; the brow.

brim the edge of the superior strait of the true pelvis; the inlet.

broad ligament the ligament extending from the lateral margins of the uterus to the pelvic wall; keeps the uterus centrally placed and provides stability within the pelvic cavity.

bronchopulmonary dysplasia (BPD) chronic pulmonary disease of multifactorial etiology characterized initially by alveolar and bronchial necrosis, which results in bronchial metaplasia and interstitial fibrosis. Appears in x-ray films as generalized small, radiolucent cysts within the lungs.

brown adipose tissue (BAT) fat deposits in neonates that provide greater heat-generating activity than ordinary fat. Found around the kidneys, adrenals, and neck; between the scapulas; and behind the sternum; also called brown fat.

Brudzinski's sign in the presence of meningitis, bending the patient's neck produces flexion of the patient's lower extremities.

café-au-lait spots light brown (coffee with cream) marks that appear on the body. The presence of more than six such spots may be accompanied by a neurologic disorder.

caked breasts accumulation of milk in the secreting ducts of the breast after delivery; see also *engorgement*.

Candida albicans a fungus that causes infections such as moniliasis and thrush.

caput the head; the occiput of the fetal head, which appears at the vaginal introitus prior to delivery of the head.

caput succedaneum swelling or edema occurring in or under the fetal scalp during labor.

cardinal ligaments the chief uterine supports, suspending the uterus from the side walls of the true pelvis.

cardinal movements of labor   the positional changes of the fetus as it moves through the birth canal during labor and delivery. The positional changes are descent, flexion, internal rotation, extension, restitution, and external rotation.

cardiopulmonary adaptation   adaptation of the neonate's cardiovascular and respiratory systems to life outside the womb.

carrier   (1) an individual possessing an abnormal gene or chromosome who manifests no outward signs but who can pass on the abnormality to offspring. (2) A person who harbors a specific pathogenic organism in the absence of identifiable disease and is capable of spreading the disease to others.

caramenia   menses.

catarrhal symptoms   symptoms associated with inflammation of the mucous membranes, causing redness and mucoid drainage.

caudal block   regional anesthesia used in childbirth in which the anesthetic agent is injected into the caudal area of the spinal canal through the sacral hiatus, affecting the caudal nerve roots and thereby providing anesthesia to the cervix, vagina, and perineum.

caul   membranes or portions of the amnion covering the fetal head during delivery.

centimeter   unit of measurement used to describe cervical dilatation. Used interchangeably with "fingers" (one "finger" equals 2 cm).

cephalhematoma   subcutaneous swelling containing blood found on the head of an infant several days after delivery, which usually disappears within a few weeks to two months.

cephalic   pertaining to the head.

cephalic presentation   delivery in which the fetal head is presenting against the cervix.

cephalopelvic disproportion (CPD)   a condition in which the fetal head is of such a shape or size, or in such a position, that it cannot pass through the maternal pelvis.

certified nurse-midwife   see *midwife*.

cervical cap   a cup-shaped device placed over the cervix to prevent pregnancy.

cervical cauterization   destruction of the superficial tissue of the cervix by heat, electric current, or freezing.

cervical conization   excision of a cone-shaped section of tissue from the endocervix.

cervical dilatation   process in which the cervical os and the cervical canal widen from less than a centimeter to approximately 10 cm, allowing delivery of the fetus.

cervical erosion   chronic irritation or infection that causes an alteration in the epithelium of the cervix.

cervical esophagostomy   surgical formation of an opening from the esophagus to the neck.

cervical os   the small opening of the cervix that dilates during the first stage of labor. See also *external os; internal os*.

cervical polyp   a small tumor or a stem or pedicle attached to the inside of the cervix.

cervical stenosis   narrowing of the canal between the body of the uterus and the cervical os.

cervicitis   infection of the cervix.

cervix   the "neck" between the external os and the body of the uterus. The lower end of the cervix extends into the vagina.

cesarean delivery   delivery of the fetus by means of an incision into the abdominal wall and the uterus; also called *abdominal delivery*.

cesarean hysterectomy   surgical removal of the uterus immediately after cesarean delivery.

Chadwick's sign   violet bluish color of the vaginal mucous membrane caused by increased vascularity; visible from about the fourth week of pregnancy.

change of life   see *climacteric*.

chignon   a raised area on the vertex of the fetal head as a result of the negative pressure exerted on this area with the use of a vacuum extractor during delivery.

childbed fever   see *puerperal sepsis*.

chloasma   brownish pigmentation over the bridge of the nose and the cheeks during pregnancy and in some women who are taking oral contraceptives. Also called *mask of pregnancy*.

choanal atresia   complete obstruction of the posterior nares by membranous or bony tissue.

chorioamnionitis   an inflammation of the amniotic membranes stimulated by organisms in the amniotic fluid, which then becomes infiltrated with polymorphonuclear leukocytes.

chorioepithelioma   carcinoma of the chorion, with rapid malignant proliferation of the epithelium of the chorionic villi.

chorion   the fetal membrane closest to the intrauterine wall that gives rise to the placenta and continues as the outer membrane surrounding the amnion.

chorionic villi   threadlike projections growing in tufts on the external chorionic surface that project into the maternal uterine sinuses; they help form the placenta and secrete human chorionic gonadotropin (HCG).

chromatids   the two longitudinal halves of each chromosome.

chromosomes   the threadlike structures within the nucleus of a cell that carry the genes.

cilia   hairlike processes that project from epithelial cells and that serve to propel mucus, pus, and dust particles.

circumcision   surgical removal of the prepuce (foreskin) of the penis.

circumoral cyanosis   bluish appearance around the mouth.

circumvallate placenta   a placenta with a thick white fibrous ring around the edge.

cleavage   rapid mitotic division of the zygote; cells produced are called blastomeres.

cleft palate   incomplete closure of the roof of the mouth, producing a passageway between the mouth and nasal cavity. May be unilateral or bilateral, complete or incomplete.

client advocacy   an approach to client care in which the nurse educates and supports the client and protects the client's rights.

climacteric   period marking the cessation of menstruation and the end of a woman's reproductive abilities; the body undergoes significant physiologic and psychologic changes. Also called *change of life* or *menopause*.

clitoris female organ homologous to the male penis; a small oval body of erectile tissue situated at the anterior junction of the vulva.

clubfoot see *talipes equinovarus*.

coccyx a small bone at the base of the spinal column.

cold stress excessive heat loss resulting in compensatory mechanisms (increased respirations and nonshivering thermogenesis) to maintain core body temperature.

colostrum secretion from the breast before the onset of true lactation; contains mainly serum and white blood corpuscles. It has a high protein content, provides some immune properties, and cleanses the neonate's intestinal tract of mucus and meconium.

colpectomy surgical excision of the vagina.

colpotomy incision into the wall of the vagina.

complementary feeding additional feeding given to the infant if still hungry after breast-feeding.

complete dilatation occurs when the cervix is sufficiently dilated for the infant to pass through; usually 10 cm (five "fingers").

conception union of male sperm and female ovum; fertilization.

conceptional age the number of complete weeks since the moment of conception. Because the moment of conception is almost impossible to determine, conceptional age is estimated at 2 weeks less than gestational age.

condom a rubber sheath that covers the penis to prevent conception or disease.

condyloma wartlike growth of skin, usually seen on the external genitals or anus. There are two types, a pointed variety and a broad, flat form usually found with syphilis.

congenital present at birth.

conjoined twins twins attached to each other, either at one small part of the body or in varying degrees up to complete sharing of the body with two heads. One twin may be small and underdeveloped, attached to the other twin parasitically.

conduction loss of heat to a cooler surface by direct skin contact.

conjugate important diameter of the pelvis, measured from the center of the promontory of the sacrum to the back of the symphysis pubis. The diagonal conjugate is measured and the true conjugate is estimated.

conjugate vera the true conjugate, which extends from the middle of the sacral promontory to the middle of the pubic crest.

conjunctivitis inflammation of the mucous membrane lining the eyelids.

consanguinity blood relationship by descent from a common ancestor.

contraception the prevention of conception or impregnation.

contraceptive sponge a small pillow-shaped polyurethane sponge with a concave cupped area on one side, designed to fit over the cervix to prevent pregnancy.

contraction tightening and shortening of the uterine muscles during labor, causing effacement and dilatation of the cervix; contributes to the downward and outward descent of the fetus.

convection loss of heat from the warm body surface to cooler air currents.

contraction stress test a method for assessing the reaction of the fetus to the stress of uterine contractions. This test may be utilized when contractions are occurring spontaneously or when contractions are artificially induced by OCT (oxytocin challenge test) or BSST (breast self-stimulation test).

Coombs' test a test for antiglobulins in the red cells. The indirect test determines the presence of Rh-positive antibodies in maternal blood; the direct test determines the presence of maternal Rh-positive antibodies in fetal cord blood.

copulation sexual intercourse; coitus.

Cornelia DeLange syndrome characterized by micromelia, a down-turning upper lip, short stature, mental retardation, microbrachycephaly, bushy eyebrows, long curly eyelashes, high-arched palate, micrognathia, hirsutism, and simian crease; its etiology remains unknown.

cornua the elongated portions of the uterus where the fallopian tubes open.

corona radiata a ring of elongated cells surrounding the zona pellucida.

corpus the upper two-thirds of the uterus.

corpus luteum a small yellow body that develops within a ruptured ovarian follicle; it secretes progesterone in the second half of the menstrual cycle and atrophies about three days before the beginning of menstrual flow. If pregnancy occurs, the corpus luteum continues to produce progesterone until the placenta takes over this function.

cotyledon one of the rounded portions into which the placenta's uterine surface is divided, consisting of a mass of villi, fetal vessels, and an intervillous space.

couvade in some cultures, the male's observance of certain rituals and taboos to signify the transition to fatherhood.

Couvelaire uterus purplish discoloration and boardlike rigidity of the uterus caused by accumulation of blood in the interstitial myometrium of the uterus from premature separation and subsequent hemorrhage of the placenta.

cradle cap an oily, yellowish crust that may appear on the newborn's scalp and that is caused by excessive secretion of the sebaceous glands in the scalp; also called *seborrhea dermatus*.

craniosynostosis premature closure of cranial sutures.

Credé's maneuver the obsolete method of expelling the placenta by downward manual pressure on the uterus through the abdominal wall.

cretinism condition caused by congenital lack of thyroid gland secretion; characteristics include arrested physical and mental development.

cri-du-chat syndrome chromosomal disorder characterized by microcephaly, downward slant of palpebral fissures, catlike cry, low birth weight, mental deficiency, hypotonia, and simian crease. Caused by partial deletion of the short arm of chromosome number 5.

Crouzon syndrome an autosomal dominant disorder of variable expression characterized by premature craniosynostosis, maxillary hypoplasia, and shallow orbits.

crowning appearance of the presenting fetal part at the vaginal orifice during labor.

CST   see *contraction stress test.*

cul-de-sac of Douglas   retrouterine pouch formed by an extension of the peritoneal cavity that lies between the rectum and the posterior wall of the uterus.

culture   the ideas, customs, traditions, arts, and so on of a particular group of people.

curettage   removal of the contents of the uterus by scraping of the endometrial lining with a currette to obtain specimens for diagnostic purposes, or following an abortion.

cutis marmorate   purplish discoloration of skin on exposure to cold. A transient vasomotor response occurring primarily over the extremities of the infant; occasionally seen in an infant in respiratory distress.

cystocele   hernia of the bladder. Injury to the vesicovaginal fascia during delivery may allow herniation of the bladder into the vagina.

deceleration   periodic decrease in the baseline fetal heart rate.

decidua   endometrium or mucous membrane lining of the uterus in pregnancy that is shed after delivery.

decidual basalis   the part of the decidua that unites with the chorion to form the placenta. It is shed in lochial discharge after delivery.

decidua capsularis   the part of the decidua surrounding the chorionic sac.

decidua vera (parietalis)   nonplacental decidua lining the uretus.

decrement   decrease or stage of decline, as of a contraction.

deletion   in genetics, the loss of a chromosomal segment.

delivery   expulsion of the infant with placenta and membranes from the woman at birth.

deoxyribonucleic acid (DNA)   intracellular complex protein carrying genetic information; consists of two purines (adenine and guanine) and two pyrimidines (thymine and cytosine).

dermatoglyphics   study of the surface markings and skin ridge patterns on fingers, toes, palms of hands, and soles of feet; useful in identification and in genetic studies.

descriptive statistics   statistics that report facts in a concise and easily retrievable way.

desquamation   shedding of the epithelial cells of the epidermis.

diagonal conjugate   distance from the lower posterior border of the symphysis pubis to the sacral promontory; may be obtained by manual measurement.

diaphragm   a flexible disk that covers the cervix to prevent pregnancy.

diaphragmatic hernia   failure of the diaphragm to fuse, resulting in protrusion of the abdominal contents through the diaphragm into the thoracic cavity; may be congenital or traumatic.

diastasis recti abdominis   separation of the recti abdominis muscles along the median line. In women, it is seen with repeated childbirths or multiple gestations. In the newborn, it is usually caused by incomplete development.

diathesis   hereditary predisposition to some abnormality or disease. See also *bleeding diathesis.*

DIC   disseminated intravascular coagulation. May also be called *consumption coagulopathy.*

dilatation of the cervix   expansion of the external os from an opening a few millimeters in size to an opening large enough to allow the passage of the infant.

dilatation and curettage (D and C)   stretching of the cervical canal to permit passage of a curette, which is used to scrape the endometrium to empty the uterine contents or to obtain tissue for examination.

dilatational phase of labor   phase in which active cervical dilatation takes place.

diploid number of chromosomes   containing a set of maternal and a set of paternal chromosomes; in humans, the diploid number of chromosomes is 46.

discordance   discrepancy in size (or other indicators) between twins.

disparate twins   twins that are different from one another, as in weight or appearance; most likely fraternal twins.

dizygotic twins   fetuses that develop from two fertilized ova; also called *fraternal twins.*

Döderlein bacillus   gram-positive bacterium found in normal vaginal secretions.

dominant gene   a gene that is expressed in the heterozygous state. In a dominant disorder the mutant gene overshadows the normal gene.

Down syndrome   an abnormality resulting from the presence of an extra chromosome number 21(trisomy 21); characteristics include mental retardation and altered physical appearance. Formerly called Mongolism or Mongoloid idiocy.

drug-addicted infant   the newborn of an alcoholic or drug-addicted woman.

dry labor   lay term referring to labor in which the amniotic fluid has already escaped. In reality, there is no such thing as "dry labor."

ductus arteriosus   a communication channel between the main pulmonary artery and the aorta of the fetus. It is obliterated after birth by a rising PO_2 and changes in intravascular pressure in the presence of normal pulmonary functioning. It normally becomes a ligament after birth but sometimes remains patent (patent ductus arteriosus), a treatable condition.

ductus venosus   a fetal blood vessel that carries oxygenated blood between the umbilical vein and the inferior vena cava, bypassing the liver; it becomes a ligament after birth.

Duncan's mechanism   occurs when the maternal surface of the placenta presents upon delivery rather than the shiny fetal surface.

duration   the time length of each contraction, measured from the beginning of the increment to the completion of the decrement.

ecchymosis   bleeding into tissue caused by direct trauma, serious infection, and bleeding diathesis.

eclampsia   a major complication of pregnancy. Its cause is unknown; it occurs more often in the primigravida and is accompanied by elevated blood pressure, albuminuria, oliguria, tonic and clonic convulsions, and coma. It may occur during pregnancy (usually after the twentieth week of gestation) or within 48 hours after delivery.

ectoderm outer layer of cells in the developing embryo that give rise to the skin, nails, and hair.

ectopic in an abnormal position.

ectopic pregnancy implantation of the fertilized ovum outside the uterine cavity; common sites are the abdomen, fallopian tubes, and ovaries; also called *oocyesis*.

EDD estimated date of delivery.

effacement thinning and shortening of the cervix that occurs late in pregnancy or during labor.

ejaculation expulsion of the seminal fluids from the penis.

Ellis-Van Creveld syndrome autosomal recessive syndrome characterized by small stature with disproportionally short extremities, polydactyly of fingers and/or toes, hypoplastic nails, and short upper lip. One half the patients also have a cardiac defect.

embolus undissolved matter present in a blood vessel brought there by the blood or lymph current; may be solid, liquid, or gaseous.

embryo the early stage of development of the young of any organism. In humans the embryonic period is from about two to eight weeks of gestation, and is characterized by cellular differentiation and predominantly hyperplastic growth.

endocervical pertaining to the interior of the canal of the cervix of the uterus.

endocrine glands glands that secrete special substances (hormones) that regulate body functions.

endoderm the inner layer of cells in the developing embryo that give rise to internal organs such as the intestines.

endometriosis ectopic endometrium located outside the uterus in the pelvic cavity. Symptoms may include pelvic pain or pressure, dysmenorrhea, dispareunia, abnormal bleeding from the uterus or rectum, and sterility.

endometritis infection of the endometrium.

endometrium the mucous membrane that lines the inner surface of the uterus.

en face an assumed position in which one person looks at another and maintains his or her face in the same vertical plane as that of the other.

engagement the entrance of the fetal presenting part into the superior pelvic strait and the beginning of the descent through the pelvic canal.

engorgement vascular congestion or distention. In obstetrics, the swelling of breast tissue brought about by an increase in blood and lymph supply to the breast, preceding true lactation.

engrossment characteristic sense of absorption, preoccupation, and interest in the infant demonstrated by fathers during early contact with their infants.

enzygotic developed from one fertilized ovum.

epicanthus a fold of skin that extends from the top of the nose to the median end of the eyebrow, covering the inner canthus.

epidural block regional anesthesia effective through the first and second stages of labor.

episiotomy incision of the perineum to facilitate delivery and to avoid laceration of the perineum.

epispadias congenital opening of the urethra on the dorsum of the penis, or opening by separation of the labia minora and a fissure of the clitoris (rare).

Epstein's pearls small, white blebs found along the gum margins and at the junction of the hard and soft palates; commonly seen in the newborn as a normal manifestation.

Erb's Duchenne palsy paralysis of the arm and chest wall as a result of a birth injury to the brachial plexus or a subsequent injury to the fifth and sixth cervical nerves.

erythema toxicum innocuous pink papular rash of unknown cause with superimposed vesicles; it appears within 24 to 48 hours after birth and resolves spontaneously within a few days.

erythroblastosis fetalis hemolytic disease of the newborn characterized by anemia, jaundice, enlargement of the liver and spleen, and generalized edema. Caused by isoimmunization due to Rh incompatibility or ABO incompatibility.

esophageal atresia a malformation in which the esophagus ends in a blind pouch or narrows into a thin cord, failing to form a passage to the stomach.

estrangement in obstetrics, a condition that occurs when a mother is diverted from establishing a normal relationship with her newborn because of separation caused by illness or preterm birth.

estriol metabolic product of estrone and estradiol found in the urine of pregnant women.

estrogens the hormones estradiol and estrone, produced by the ovary.

eugenics the science that deals with the improvement of the human race through control of genetic factors.

euthenics the science that deals with the improvement of the human race through control of environmental factors.

evaporation loss of heat incurred when water on the skin surface is converted to a vapor.

exanthem any eruption of the skin; frequently accompanies infectious diseases.

exchange transfusion the replacement of 70 percent to 80 percent of circulating blood by withdrawing the recipient's blood and injecting a donor's blood in equal amounts, for the purpose of preventing the accumulation of bilirubin or other byproducts of hemolysis in the blood.

exotoxin a toxin produced by microorganisms and excreted into the surrounding medium.

expiratory grunt a sign of respiratory distress indicative of the newborn's attempt to hold air in the alveoli for better gaseous exchange.

expressivity the extent to which a gene is expressed in an individual.

expulsive contractions labor contractions that are effective in contracting the uterine muscle; characteristic of the second stage of labor.

exstrophy of the bladder exposure and eversion of the posterior and lateral walls of the bladder and trigone because of failure of the anterior wall and symphysis pubis to unite.

external os   the opening between the cervix and the vagina.

extrauterine   occurring outside the uterus.

extrauterine pregnancy   ectopic pregnancy in which the fertilized ovum implants outside the uterus.

facial nerve palsy   distortion of the face caused by a lesion of the facial nerve, resulting in peripheral facial paralysis.

facies   pertaining to the appearance or expression of the face; certain congenital syndromes typically present with a specific facial appearance.

failure to thrive (FTT)   term used to describe an infant or child whose growth and development pattern falls below the norms for his or her age.

fallopian tubes   tubes that extend from the lateral angle of the uterus and terminate near the ovary; they serve as a passageway for the ovum from the ovary to the uterus and for the spermatozoa from the uterus toward the ovary. Also called *oviducts* and *uterine tubes*.

false labor   contractions of the uterus, regular or irregular, that may be strong enough to be interpreted as true labor but that do not dilate the cervix.

false pelvis   the portion of the pelvis above the linea terminalis; its primary function is to support the weight of the enlarged pregnant uterus.

familial   the presence of a trait or disorder in more than one member of a family; not necessarily inherited.

family   a group of people united by marriage, blood, or adoption, residing in the same household, maintaining a common culture, and interacting with each other on the basis of their roles within the group. See also *nuclear family* and *traditional family*.

family-centered care   an approach to health care based on the concept that a hospital can provide professional services to mothers, fathers, and infants in a homelike environment that would enhance the integrity of the family unit.

fecundation   impregnation; fertilization.

female reproductive cycle (FRC)   the monthly rhythmic changes in sexually mature females.

ferning   formation of a palm-leaf pattern by the crystallization of cervical mucus as it dries at midmenstrual cycle. Helpful in determining time of ovulation. Observed via microscopic examination of a thin layer of cervical mucus on a glass slide. This pattern is also observed when amniotic fluid is allowed to air dry on a slide and is a useful and quick test to determine whether amniotic membranes have ruptured.

fertility   ability to reproduce.

fertility awareness methods   natural family planning.

fertility rate   number of births per 1000 women aged 15 to 44 in a given population per year.

fertilization   impregnation of an ovum by a spermatozoon.

fetal   pertaining or related to the fetus.

fetal alcohol syndrome (FAS)   syndrome caused by maternal alcohol ingestion and characterized by microcephaly, intrauterine growth retardation, short palpebral fissures, and maxillary hypoplasia.

fetal alveoli   terminal pulmonary sacs that in fetal life are filled with fluid that is a transudate of fetal plasma.

fetal death   death of the developing fetus after 20 weeks' gestation. Also called *fetal demise*.

fetal blood sampling   blood sample drawn from the fetal scalp (or from the fetus in breech position) to evaluate the acid-base status of the fetus.

fetal bradycardia   a fetal heart rate less than 120 beats/minute during a 10-minute period of continuous monitoring.

fetal distress   evidence that the fetus is in jeopardy, such as a change in fetal activity or heart rate.

fetal heart rate (FHR)   the number of times the fetal heart beats per minute; normal range is 120 to 160 beats per minute.

fetal heart tones (FHTs)   the fetal heartbeat as heard through the mother's abdominal wall.

fetal position   relationship of the landmark on the presenting fetal part to the front, sides, or back of the maternal pelvis.

fetal presentation   the fetal body part that enters the maternal pelvis first. The three possible presentations are cephalic, shoulder, or breech.

fetal tachycardia   a fetal heart rate of 160 beats/minute or more during a 10-minute period of continuous monitoring.

fetoscope   an adaptation of a stethoscope that facilitates auscultation of the fetal heart rate.

fetoscopy   a technique for directly observing the fetus and obtaining a sample of fetal blood or skin.

fetotoxic   destructive or poisonous to the fetus.

fetus   the child in utero from about the seventh to ninth week of gestation until birth.

fibroid   see *leiomyoma*.

fimbria   any structure resembling a fringe; the fringelike extremity of the fallopian tubes.

first stage of labor   period of time extending from the onset of regular contractions to the complete dilatation of the cervix.

fissure   an open crack or groove in tissue.

fistula   an abnormal tubelike passage that forms between two normal cavities or to a free surface; may be congenital or caused by trauma, abscesses, or inflammatory processes.

flaccid   flabby, relaxed; absent or defective muscle tone.

flaring of nostrils   widening of nostrils during inspiration in the presence of air hunger; a sign of respiratory distress.

flexion   in obstetrics, a situation that occurs when resistance to the descent of the infant down the birth canal causes its head to flex, or bend, the chin approaching the chest, thus reducing the diameter of the presenting part.

follicle   a small secretory cavity or sac.

follicle-stimulating hormone (FSH)   hormone produced by the anterior pituitary during the first half of the menstrual cycle, stimulating development of the graafian follicle.

fontanelle   in the fetus, an unossified space or soft spot consisting of a strong band of connective tissue lying between the cranial bones of the skull.

footling   a breech presentation in which one or both feet present.

foramen ovale   septal opening between the atria of the fetal heart. Normally, the opening closes shortly after birth; if it remains open, it can be repaired surgically.

forceps obstetric instruments occasionally used to aid in delivery.

foreskin loose skin covering the end of the penis or clitoris; prepuce.

fornix a body with a vaultlike or arched shape.

fornix of the vagina the anterior and posterior spaces into which the upper vagina is divided; formed by the protrusion of the cervix into the vagina.

fourchette transverse fold of mucous membranes at the posterior angle of the vagina that connects the posterior ends of the labia minora.

fraternal twins see *dizygotic twins.*

fremitus vibratory tremors felt through the chest wall by palpation.

frenulum thin ridge of tissue extending from the floor of the mouth to the inferior surface of the tongue along its midline.

frequency the time between the beginning of one contraction and the beginning of the next contraction.

Friedman graph a method of describing and recording labor progress.

Friedman's test a modification of the Aschheim-Zondek pregnancy test in which the woman's urine is injected into a mature, unmated female rabbit. After two days, the rabbit's ovaries are examined; the presence of fresh corpora lutea or hemorrhagic corpora constitutes a positive test.

fundus the upper portion of the uterus between the fallopian tubes.

funic souffle hissing sound synchronous with the fetal heartbeat and considered to be produced in the umbilical cord.

funis a cordlike structure, such as the umbilical cord.

galactorrhea excessive secretion of milk.

gamete a mature germ cell; an egg or sperm.

gametogenesis the process by which germ cells are produced.

gargoylism a hereditary condition, associated with Hurler syndrome, characterized by deformed limbs and hands and grotesque facies, with thickening of the lips, nostrils, and ears.

gastroschisis congenital herniation of the bowel or other abdominal viscera through an extraumbilical defect in the abdominal wall, with no external covering membrane.

gastrula the stage in early embryonic development that follows the blastula.

gavage feeding by means of a tube passed into the stomach.

gene smallest unit of inheritance; genes are located on the chromosomes.

genetic compound a situation in which an individual has two different mutant alleles at a given locus.

genetic heterogeneity a situation that occurs when a trait or disease can be caused by gene pairs located at different loci but presenting a similar clinical picture.

genetics the science that deals with the genetic transmission of characteristics from parents to offspring.

genotype the genetic composition of an individual.

gestation period of intrauterine development from conception through birth; pregnancy.

gestational age the number of complete weeks of fetal development, calculated from the first day of the last normal menstrual cycle.

gestational age assessment tools systems used to evaluate the newborn's external physical characteristics and neurologic and/or neuromuscular development to accurately determine gestational age. These replace or supplement the traditional calculation from the mother's last menstrual period.

glycosuria presence of glucose in the urine.

gonad sex gland; the ovaries in the female and the testes in the male.

gonadotropin a hormone that stimulates the sex glands.

Goodell's sign softening of the cervix that occurs during the second month of pregnancy.

graafian follicle the ovarian cyst containing the ripe ovum; it secretes estrogens.

gravid pregnant.

gravida a pregnant woman.

gynecoid pelvis typical female pelvis in which the inlet is round instead of oval.

gynecology study of the diseases of the female, especially of the genital, urinary, and rectal organs and the breasts.

habitus physical appearance indicating a tendency or predisposition to disease or abnormal conditions.

haploid number of chromosomes half the diploid number of chromosomes. In humans, there are 23 chromosomes, the haploid number, in each germ cell.

harlequin sign a rare color change that occurs between the longitudinal halves of the newborn's body, such that the dependent half is noticeably pinker than the superior half when the newborn is placed on one side; it is of no pathologic significance.

Hegar's sign a softening of the lower uterine segment found upon palpation in the second or third month of pregnancy.

hematoma a swelling or collection of blood in the tissues; a bruise or blood tumor.

hemizygous having only one allele for a given trait instead of a pair.

hemoconcentration increase in the number of red blood cells resulting from a decrease in plasma volume or from increased erythropoiesis.

hemorrhagic disease of newborn hemorrhaging during the first few days of life caused by inadequate supply of prothrombin or by a delay in the production of vitamin K.

hemorrhoids varicose veins of the rectum; may be external or internal.

hereditary able to be passed from one generation to the next through the gametes of the parents.

herpesvirus a family of viruses characterized by the development of clusters of small vesicles. The infection is recurring and is frequently found about the lips and nares; a genital form also exists that is primarily sexually transmitted.

heterozygous   a genotypic situation in which two different alleles occur at a given locus on a pair of homologous chromosomes.

high risk   having an increased possibility of suffering harm, damage, loss, or death.

hirsutism   excessive growth of hair or growth of hair in unusual places.

Homan's sign   pain in the calf when the foot is passively dorsiflexed; an early sign of phlebothrombosis of the deep veins of the calf.

homiothermic   warm-blooded.

homologous   similar in origin or structure but not necessarily in function.

homologous chromosomes   a matched pair of chromosomes.

homozygous   a genotypic situation in which two similar genes occur at a given locus on homologous chromosomes.

hormone   a substance produced in an organ or gland and conveyed by the blood to another part of the body in order to exert an effect.

human chorionic gonadotropin (HCG)   a hormone produced by the chorionic villi and found in the urine of pregnant women; also called *prolan*.

human placental lactogen (HPL)   a hormone synthesized by the syncytiotrophoblast that functions as an insulin antagonist and promotes lipolysis to increase the amounts of circulating free fatty acids available for maternal metabolic use.

Hurler syndrome   lipochondrodystrophy.

hyaline membrane disease   respiratory disease of the newborn characterized by interference with ventilation at the alveolar level, thought to be caused by the presence of fibrinoid deposits lining the alveolar ducts. Also called *respiratory distress syndrome (RDS)*.

hydatidiform mole   degenerative process in chorionic villi, giving rise to multiple cysts and rapid growth of the uterus with hemorrhage.

hydramnios   an excess of amniotic fluid, leading to overdistention of the uterus. Frequently seen in diabetic pregnant women, even if there is no coexisting fetal anomaly. Also called *polyhydramnios*.

hydrocele   accumulation of serous fluid in a saclike cavity, especially in the sac that surrounds the testicle, causing the scrotum to swell.

hydrocephalus   increased accumulation of cerebrospinal fluid within the ventricles of the brain, resulting from interference with normal circulation and absorption of the fluid and especially from destruction of the foramens of Magendie and Lushka; caused by congenital anomalies, infection, injury, or brain tumors.

hydrops fetalis   see *erythroblastosis fetalis*.

hymen   membranous fold that normally partially covers the entrance to the vagina.

hymenal tag   normally occurring redundant hymenal tissue that protrudes from the floor of the female newborn's vagina; disappears spontaneously a few weeks after birth.

hyperbilirubinemia   excessive amount of bilirubin in the blood; indicative of hemolytic processes due to blood incompatibility, intrauterine infection, septicemia, neonatal renal infection, and other disorders.

hypercapnia   an increased amount of carbon dioxide in the blood; acts as a respiratory depressant.

hypercholesterolemia   excessive amount of cholesterol in the blood.

hyperemesis gravdarum   excessive vomiting during pregnancy, leading to dehydration and starvation.

hyperlipidemia   excessive amount of fat in the blood.

hypermagnesemia   excessive amount of magnesium in the blood.

hyperplasia   excessive increase of normal cells in the tissue arrangement of an organ.

hypertelorism   abnormal width between two paired organs.

hypertrophy   increase or enlargement in size of existing cells; usually applies to any increase in size as a result of functional activity.

hypnoreflexogenous method   a combination of hypnosis and conditioned reflexes used during childbirth.

hypocalcemia   abnormally low level of serum calcium levels.

hypofibrinogenemia   lowered levels of fibrinogen in the blood.

hypogalactic   pertaining to deficient secretion of milk.

hypogastric arteries   branches of the right and left iliac arteries that carry deoxygenated blood from the fetus through the umbilical cord (where they are known as umbilical arteries) to the placenta.

hypoglycemia   abnormally low level of sugar in the blood.

hypomagnesemia   abnormally low amount of magnesium in the blood.

hypospadias   abnormal congenital positioning of the male urethra on the undersurface of the penis, or a urethral opening into the vagina.

hypotensive drugs   drugs that lower blood pressure.

hypovolemic shock   a condition in which the patient exhibits lowered blood pressure and increased pulse rate; caused by a decrease in the volume of circulating blood in the body.

hypoxemia   insufficient oxygenation of the blood, resulting in metabolic acidosis.

hypoxia   insufficient availability of oxygen to meet body tissue metabolic needs.

hysterectomy   surgical removal of the uterus. See also *abdominal hysterectomy, panhysterectomy, subtotal hysterectomy,* and *total hysterectomy*.

icterus neonatorum   jaundice in the newborn.

idiopathic respiratory distress syndrome   see *hyaline membrane disease*.

iliopectineal line   bony ridge on the inner surface of the ilium and pubis, dividing the true and false pelves.

immature infant   considerably underdeveloped newborn weighing less than 1134 g (2½ lb) at birth.

imperforate anus   congenital closure of the anal opening, usually by a membranous septum; may be associated with a fistulous tract.

impetigo   a skin disease caused by streptococci or staphylococci and characterized by pustules.

implantation   embedding of the fertilized ovum in the uterine mucosa six or seven days after fertilization; also called *nidation*.

impotence   inability of the male to perform sexual intercourse.

impregnate   to make pregnant or to fertilize.

inborn error of metabolism   a hereditary deficiency of a specific enzyme needed for normal metabolism of specific chemicals.

incompetent cervix   a mechanical defect in the cervix that makes it unable to remain closed throughout a pregnancy; produces dilatation and effacement leading to abortion, usually during the second trimester or early third trimester.

increment   increase or addition; to build up, as of a contraction.

incubation   (1) care of a preterm infant in an incubator; (2) the development of an impregnated ovum; (3) interval between exposure to an infection and the appearance of the first symptoms.

incubator   apparatus in which the temperature can be regulated; used for preterm infants.

induction of labor   the process of causing or initiating labor by use of medication or surgical rupture of membranes.

inertia   inactivity or sluggishness; absence or weakness of uterine contractions during labor.

infant   child under one year of age.

infant death rate   number of deaths of infants under one year of age per 1000 live births in a given population per year.

infant of a diabetic mother (IDM)   at-risk infant born to a woman previously diagnosed as diabetic, or who develops symptoms of diabetes during pregnancy.

inferential statistics   statistics that allow an investigator to draw conclusions about what is happening between two or more variables in a population and to suggest or refute causal relationships between them.

infertility   diminished ability to conceive.

infiltration   process of a substance being passed into or being deposited within a tissue, such as a local anesthetic drug.

informed consent   a legal concept that protects a person's rights to autonomy and self-determination by specifying that no action may be taken without that person's prior understanding and freely given consent.

infundibulopelvic ligament   ligament that suspends and supports the ovaries.

inlet   passage leading to a cavity.

inlet of the pelvis   upper opening into the pelvic cavity.

innominate bone   the hip bone, ilium, ischium, and pubis.

intensity   the strength of a uterine contraction during acme.

internal os   an inside mouth or opening; the opening between the cervix and the uterus.

interspinous diameter   a transverse diameter of the pelvis that is the distance between the ischial spines. Also referred to as *bi-ischial diameter*.

intervillous spaces   irregular spaces in the maternal portion of the placenta that are filled with maternal blood, serving as sites of maternal–fetal gas, nutrient, and waste exchange.

intrapartum   the time from the onset of true labor until the delivery of the infant and placenta.

intrathecal   within the subarachnoid space.

intrauterine device (IUD)   small metal or plastic form that is placed in the uterus to prevent implantation of a fertilized ovum.

intrauterine growth retardation (IUGR)   fetal undergrowth due to any etiology, such as intrauterine infection, deficient nutrient supply, or congenital malformation.

introitus   opening or entrance into a cavity or canal, such as the vagina.

intromission   insertion of one part into another, such as insertion of the penis into the vagina.

in utero   within the uterus.

inversion of the uterus   a condition in which the fundus of the uterus protrudes through the cervix and sometimes through the vaginal introitus; may occur immediately postpartum as a result of too vigorous placental expression while the placenta is still fixed in the uterus.

involution   rolling or turning inward; the reduction in size of the uterus following delivery.

ischial spines   prominences that arise near the junction of the ilium and ischium and jut into the pelvic cavity; used as a reference point during labor to evaluate the descent of the fetal head into the birth canal.

ischium   lower portion of the hip bone.

isthmus   the straight, narrow part of the fallopian tube with a thick muscular wall and an opening (lumen) 2–3 mm in diameter; the site of tubal ligation. Also a constriction in the uterus that is located above the cervix and below the corpus.

IUD   see *intrauterine device*.

IUGR   see *intrauterine growth retardation*.

jaundice   yellow pigmentation of body tissues caused by the presence of bile pigments. See also *pathologic jaundice*; *physiologic jaundice*.

karyotype   the set of chromosomes arranged in a standard order.

Kegel's exercises   perineal muscle tightening that strengthens the pubococcygeus muscle and increases its tone.

kernicterus   an encephalopathy caused by deposition of unconjugated bilirubin in brain cells; may result in impaired brain function or death.

Kernig's sign   nuchal rigidity; stiffness of the neck.

Klinefelter syndrome   a chromosomal abnormality caused by the presence of an extra X chromosome in the male; characteristics include tall stature, sparse pubic and facial hair, gynecomastia, small firm testes, and absence of spermatogenesis.

labia   external folds of skin on either side of the vulva.

labia majora   the larger outer folds of skin on either side of the vulva.

labia minora   the smaller inner folds of skin on either side of the vulva.

labor   the process by which the fetus is expelled from the maternal uterus; also called *childbirth, confinement,* or *parturition.*

laceration   in obstetrics, a tear in the perineum, vagina, or cervix as a result of stretching of the tissues during childbirth.

lactation   process of producing and supplying breast milk.

lactiferous ducts   tiny tubes within the breast that conduct milk from the acini cells to the nipple.

lactogenic hormone   hormone produced by the anterior pituitary to promote growth of breast tissue and to stimulate the production of milk.

lacto-ovovegetarians   vegetarians who include milk, dairy products, and eggs in their diets, and occasionally fish, poultry, and liver.

lactose intolerance   a condition in which an individual has difficulty digesting milk and milk products.

lactosuria   excretion of lactose in the urine during late pregnancy and lactation.

lactovegetarians   vegetarians who include dairy products but no eggs in their diets.

Lamaze method   a method of childbirth preparation, also known as *psychoprophylaxis.*

lambdoidal suture   line forming the base of the triangular posterior fontanelle, separating the occipital bone from the two parietal bones.

lanugo   fine, downy hair found on all body parts of the fetus, with the exception of the palms of the hands and the soles of the feet, after 20 weeks' gestation.

large for gestational age (LGA)   excessive growth of a fetus in relation to the gestational time period.

last menstrual period (LMP)   the last normal menstrual period experienced by the mother prior to pregnancy; sometimes used to calculate the infant's gestational age.

lay midwife   a person who gives care during the prenatal, labor and delivery, and postpartal periods. Education varies from apprenticeship to self-teaching to short-term programs. Skills may be passed from one midwife to another.

LBW   see *low-birth-weight infant.*

Leboyer method   birthing technique that eases the newborn's transition to extrauterine life wherein lights in the delivery room are dimmed and noise is kept to a minimum.

leiomyoma   a benign tumor of the uterus, composed primarily of smooth muscle and connective tissue. Also referred to as a *myoma* or a *fibroid.*

Leopold's maneuvers   series of four maneuvers designed to provide a systematic approach whereby the examiner may determine fetal presentation and position.

letdown reflex   pattern of stimulation, hormone release, and resulting muscle contraction that forces milk into the lactiferous ducts, making it available to the infant; milk ejection reflex.

leukorrhea   mucous discharge from the vagina or cervical canal that may be normal or pathologic, as in the presence of infection.

lie   relationship of the long axis of the fetus and the long axis of the pregnant woman. The fetal lie may be longitudinal, transverse, or oblique.

ligation   suturing or tying shut, as in the suturing closed of the fallopian tubes to prevent pregnancy (*tubal ligation*).

lightening   moving of the fetus and uterus downward into the pelvic cavity; engagement.

linea nigra   the line of darker pigmentation extending from the umbilicus to the pubis noted in some women during the later months of pregnancy.

linkage   occurs when genes for different traits are located near one another on the same chromosome.

lithotomy position   position in which the client lies on her back with thighs drawn up toward her chest and with her knees flexed and abducted.

local infiltration   injection of an anesthetic agent into the subcutaneous tissue in a fanlike pattern.

lochia   maternal discharge of blood, mucus, and tissue from the uterus; may last for several weeks after birth.

lochia alba   white vaginal discharge that follows lochia serosa and that lasts from about the tenth to the twenty-first day after delivery.

lochia rubra   red, blood-tinged vaginal discharge that occurs following delivery and lasts two to four days.

lochia serosa   pink, serous, and blood-tinged vaginal discharge that follows lochia rubra and lasts until the seventh to tenth day after delivery.

locus   the position that a gene occupies on a chromosome.

low-birth-weight (LBW) infant   an infant weight 2500 g or less at birth independent of gestational age assessments.

L/S ratio   the ratio of the phospholipids lecithin and sphingomyelin produced by the fetal lungs; useful in assessing fetal lung maturity.

lunar month   a 28-day cycle corresponding to the phases of the moon. A normal pregnancy lasts 10 lunar months.

lung compliance   degree of distensibility of the lung's elastic tissues.

lutein cells   yellow ovarian cells involved in the formation of the corpus luteum.

luteinizing hormone (LH)   anterior pituitary hormone responsible for stimulating ovulation and for development of the corpus luteum.

luteotropin (LTH)   lactogenic hormone; prolactin.

lysis of adhesions   surgical procedure to release organs tied together by bands of tissue.

lysozyme   enzyme with antiseptic properties, found in blood cells, saliva, sweat, tears, and breast milk.

maceration   wasting away, degeneration, or breaking down of fetal skin, as seen with postterm infants or a fetus retained in the uterus after its death.

macroglossia   hypertrophy of the tongue, as in infants with Down syndrome, or a tongue too large for present oral cavity development, as seen in some preterm neonates.

macrosomia   condition seen in neonates of large body size and high birth weight, as those born of prediabetic and diabetic mothers.

macule   a flat, discolored skin lesion smaller than 1 cm.

malpresentation   a presentation of the fetus into the birth canal that is not "normal," that is, brow, face, shoulder, or breech presentation.

mammary glands   compound glandular elements of the breast that in the female secrete milk to nourish the infant.

maple syrup urine disease   a genetic disorder resulting in the failure to metabolize the amino acids leucine, valine, and isoleucine. The name is derived from the characteristic odor of the urine, and the disease is marked by progressive mental deterioration.

Marfan syndrome   an inherited disorder characterized by abnormally long, thin extremities, spidery fingers and toes, defects of the spine and chest, and congenital heart disease.

mask of pregnancy   see *chloasma*.

mastalgia   breast pain or tenderness.

mastitis   inflammation of the breast.

maternal mortality   number of maternal deaths from any cause during the pregnancy cycle per 100,000 live births.

maturation   in reproduction, the process of cell division that reduces the number of chromosomes in the sperm and ova to one half the number carried in the somatic cells of the species.

meatus   external opening for a passageway to an internal organ, such as the urethral meatus.

mechanism   process by which results are obtained, as in labor and delivery of a fetus.

meconium   dark green or black material present in the large intestine of a full-term infant; the first stools passed by the newborn.

meconium aspiration syndrome (MAS)   respiratory disease of term, postterm, and SGA newborns caused by inhalation of meconium or meconium-stained amniotic fluid into the lungs; characterized by mild to severe respiratory distress, hyperexpansion of the chest, hyperinflated alveoli, and secondary atelectasis.

meconium-stained fluid   amniotic fluid that contains meconium because fetal distress has caused increased intestinal activity and relaxing of the fetus's anal sphincter.

meiosis   the process of cell division that occurs in the maturation of sperm and ova that decreases their number of chromosomes by one half.

membrane   thin, pliable layer of tissue that covers an organ or that divides structures, as in the amnion and chorion surrounding the fetus.

menarche   beginning of menstrual and reproductive function in the female.

Mendelian inheritance   a major category of inheritance whereby a trait is determined by a pair of genes on homologous chromosomes; also called *single gene inheritance*.

meningomyelocele   a defect in the spinal column with resulting protrusion of the spinal cord and membranes.

menopause   see *climacteric*.

menorrhagia   excessive or profuse menstrual flow.

menstrual cycle   cyclic buildup of the uterine lining, ovulation, and sloughing of the lining occurring approximately every 28 days in nonpregnant females.

menstruation (menses)   shedding of the uterine lining at the end of the menstrual cycle, resulting in a bloody discharge from the vagina.

mentum   the chin.

mesoderm   the intermediate layer of germ cells in the embryo that give rise to connective tissue, bone marrow, muscles, blood, lymphoid tissue, and epithelial tissue.

metrorrhagia   abnormal uterine bleeding occurring at irregular intervals.

microcephalic   having an abnormally small head in relation to total body size.

micrognathia   abnormally small lower jaw.

midwife   see *lay midwife; nurse-midwife*.

migration   in obstetrics, movement of the ovum from the ovary down the fallopian tube to the uterus.

milia   tiny white papules appearing on the face of a neonate as a result of unopened sebaceous glands; they disappear spontaneously within a few weeks.

milk-leg   phlebitis and thrombosis of the femoral vein, resulting in venous obstruction and edema of the affected leg.

miscarriage   see *spontaneous abortion*.

mitleiden   a phenomenon in which expectant fathers develop symptoms similar to those of the pregnant woman: weight gain, nausea, and various aches and pains.

mitochondria   slender filament or granular component of cytoplasm in which oxidative reactions occur that provide the cell with energy.

mitosis   process of cell division whereby both daughter cells have the same number and pattern of chromosomes as the original cell.

modeling   the process of teaching behaviors through role playing or having the client talk with a person who has mastered a similar crisis.

molding   shaping of the fetal head by overlapping of the cranial bones to facilitate movement through the birth canal during labor.

Mongolian spot   dark, flat pigmentation of the lower back and buttocks noted at birth in some infants; usually disappears by the time the child reaches school age.

Mongolism   see *Down syndrome*.

moniliasis   yeastlike fungus infection caused by *Candida albicans*.

monosomy   the presence of only a single chromosome of a homologous pair.

monozygotic twins   two fetuses that develop from a single divided fertilized ovum; identical twins.

mons pubis   mound of subcutaneous fatty tissue covering the anterior portion of the symphysis pubis.

mons veneris   fleshy tissue over the symphysis pubis of the female from which hair develops at puberty.

Montgomery's glands   small nodules located around the nipples that enlarge during pregnancy and lactation.

morbidity   incidence of diseased persons in relation to a specific population.

morning sickness   nausea and vomiting occurring during the first trimester of pregnancy; may occur at any time during the day.

Moro reflex   flexion of the newborn's thighs and knees accompanied by fingers that fan, then clench, as the arms are simultaneously thrown out and then brought together, as though embracing something. This reflex can be elicited by startling the newborn with a sudden noise or movement; also called the *startle reflex.*

mortality   incidence of deaths in relation to a specific population.

morula   developmental stage of the fertilized ovum in which there is a solid mass of cells.

mosaic   an individual who has two or more cell lines different from each other in chromosome number or morphology; generally, some cells are normal while others contain chromosomal aberrations.

mottling   discoloration of the skin in irregular areas; may be seen with chilling, poor perfusion, or hypoxia.

mucous plug   a collection of thick mucus that blocks the cervical canal during pregnancy; also called *operculum.*

multigravida   female who has been pregnant more than once.

multipara   female who has had more than one pregnancy in which the fetus was viable.

multiple pregnancy   more than one fetus in the uterus at the same time.

mutagen   an environmental agent, either physical, chemical, or biologic, capable of inducing mutation.

mutation   change or alteration in gene or chromosome structure that may be transmitted to offspring.

myometrium   uterine muscular structure.

nadir   the lowest point.

Nägele's rule   a method of determining the estimated date of delivery (EDD): after obtaining the first day of the last menstrual period, one subtracts 3 months and adds 7 days.

natal   relating to birth.

natural childbirth   prepared childbirth, in which the couple attends a prenatal education program and learns exercises and breathing patterns that are used during labor and childbirth.

navel   area of the abdomen where the umbilical cord emerged from the fetus; the *umbilicus.*

neonatal mortality rate   number of deaths of infants in the first 28 days of life per 1000 live births.

neonate   infant from birth through the first 28 days of life.

neonatology   the specialty that focuses on the management of high-risk conditions of the newborn.

neurofibromatosis syndrome   autosomal dominant syndrome characterized by café-au-lait spots, freckling in the axilla, and subcutaneous dysplastic tumors that may appear along the nerves or in the meninges or eye.

nevus   mole, blemish, or mark.

nevus cavernosus   a blemish or mark that may be either well circumscribed and elevated or may have poorly defined

borders and that is composed of large venous channels; the overlying skin has a red-blue discoloration. The nevus enlarges when the infant cries or strains.

nevus flammeus   large port-wine stain.

nevus vasculosus   "strawberry mark"; raised, clearly delineated, dark red, rough-surfaced birth mark commonly found in the head region.

newborn screening tests   tests that detect inborn errors of metabolism that, if left untreated, cause mental retardation and physical handicaps.

nidation   see *implantation.*

nipple   a protrusion about 0.5 to 1.3 cm in diameter in the center of each mature breast.

nondisjunction   failure of separation of paired chromosomes during cell division.

nonstress test (NST)   an assessment method by which the reaction (or response) of the fetal heart rate to fetal movement is evaluated.

nuclear family   a family group consisting of one or more adults and one or more children.

nulligravida   a female who has never been pregnant.

nullipara   a female who has not delivered a viable fetus.

nurse-midwife   a certified nurse-midwife (CNM) is an RN who has received special training and education in the care of the family during childbearing and the prenatal, labor and delivery, and postpartal periods. After a period of formal education, the nurse-midwife takes a certification test to become a CNM.

nursing diagnosis   a two-part statement that includes the health problem and related etiology.

nystagmus   involuntary rhythmic oscillation of the eyeball in any direction.

obstetric conjugate   distance from the middle of the sacral promontory to an area approximately 1 cm below the pubic crest.

obstetrics   the branch of medicine concerned with the care of women during pregnancy, childbirth, and the postpartal period.

occiput   posterior part of the skull.

ocular hypertelorism   abnormal width between the eyes.

oligohydramnios   decreased amount of amniotic fluid, which may indicate a fetal urinary tract defect.

oliguria   decrease in urine secretion by the kidney (100–400 mL/24 hr).

omphalic   concerning the umbilicus.

omphalitis   infection of the umbilicus.

omphalocele   congenital herniation or protrusion of the abdominal contents into the base of the umbilicus.

oocyesis   see *ectopic pregnancy.*

oogenesis   process during fetal life whereby the ovary produces oogenia, cells that become primitive ovarian eggs.

oophorectomy   surgical removal of the ovary.

oophoritis   infection of the ovaries.

operculum   see *mucous plug.*

ophthalmia neonatorum   purulent infection of the eyes or conjunctiva of the newborn, usually caused by gonococci.

opisthotonis backward flexion of the head and feet due to tetanic spasm.

oral contraceptives "birth control pills" that work by inhibiting the release of an ovum and by maintaining a type of mucus that is hostile to sperm.

orifice normal outlet of a body cavity.

Ortolani's maneuver a manual procedure performed to rule out the possibility of congenital hip dysplasia.

ossification conversion into bone.

osteogenesis imperfecta a dominant inherited disease characterized by blue sclerae and hypoplasia of osteoid tissue and collagen, which results in bone fractures with slight trauma.

outlet dystocia inadequate pelvic size, causing the fetal head to be pushed backward toward the coccyx, making extension of the head difficult.

ovarian ligaments ligaments that anchor the lower pole of the ovary to the cornua of the uterus.

ovary female sex gland in which the ova are formed and in which estrogen and progesterone are produced. Normally there are two ovaries, located in the lower abdomen on each side of uterus.

oviducts see *fallopian tubes.*

ovulation normal process of discharging a mature ovum from an ovary approximately 14 days prior to the onset of menses.

ovum female reproductive cell; egg.

oxygen toxicity excessive levels of oxygen therapy that result in pathologic changes in tissue.

oxytocics drugs that accelerate childbirth and lessen postnatal hemorrhage by stimulating uterine contractions.

oxytocin hormone normally produced by the posterior pituitary, responsible for stimulation of uterine contractions and the release of milk into the lactiferous ducts.

oxytocin challenge test (OCT) also called the contraction stress test (CST), the test is designed to evaluate the circulatory and respiratory status of the fetoplacental unit to determine the ability of the fetus to withstand the stress of labor. While externally monitoring uterine contractions and FHR, oxytocin is administered to stimulate contractions. The FHR pattern is then assessed for evidence of a late deceleration pattern. The test is negative when there are three consecutive contractions in a 10-minute period without late deceleration.

palpation use of fingers or hands to manually determine the characteristics of tissues or organs; see also *bimanual palpation.*

palsy loss of or decreased ability to initiate or control muscle movement; paralysis.

panhysterectomy removal of the entire uterus, the ovaries, and the fallopian tubes.

Papanicolaou (Pap) smear procedure to detect the presence of cancer of the uterus by microscopic examination of cells gently scraped from the cervix.

papule a small, raised, sharply circumscribed lesion less than 1 cm in diameter that may be colored or flesh tone.

para a woman who has borne offspring who reached the age of viability.

parabiotic syndrome anomaly occurring in a small percentage of identical twins, in which one twin is anemic and the second suffers polycythemia as a result of a fetofetal blood transfer via placental vascular anastomoses.

paracervical block a local anesthetic agent injected transvaginally adjacent to the outer rim of the cervix.

parametritis inflammation of the parametrial layer of the uterus.

parametrium layer of muscle and connective tissue extending between the broad ligaments and surrounding the uterus.

parity the condition of having borne offspring who had attained the age of viability.

parturient pertaining to the act of childbirth.

parturition the process of giving birth.

passive acquired immunity transferral of antibodies (IgG) from the mother to the fetus in utero.

pathologic jaundice jaundice that occurs within 24 hours of birth, secondary to an abnormal condition such as ABO-Rh incompatibility.

patulous open widely or spread apart.

pedigree a graphic picture using symbols representing an individual's family tree.

pelvic pertaining to the pelvis.

pelvic axis imaginary curved line that passes through the centers of all the anteroposterior diameters of the pelvis.

pelvic cavity bony portion of the birth passages; a curved canal with a longer posterior than anterior wall.

pelvic cellulitis infection involving the connective tissue of the broad ligament or, in severe cases, the connective tissue of all the pelvic structures.

pelvic diaphragm part of the pelvic floor composed of deep fascia and the levator ani and the coccygeal muscles.

pelvic inlet upper border of the true pelvis.

pelvic outlet lower border of the true pelvis.

pelvic phase of labor the deceleration phase, in which active descent occurs.

pelvimeter an instrument for measuring the diameters and capacities of the pelvis.

pelvis the lower portion of the trunk of the body bounded by the hip bones, coccyx, and sacrum.

penis the male organ of copulation and reproduction.

perforation of the uterus a hole made in the uterus.

perimetrium the outermost layer of the corpus of the uterus; also known as the *serosal layer.*

perinatal mortality rate the number of neonatal and fetal deaths per 1000 live births.

perinatal period the time frame extending from the twenty-eighth week past conception to the twenty-eighth day past birth.

perinatologist a physician specializing in fetal and neonatal care.

perinatology the medical specialty concerned with the diagnosis and treatment of high-risk conditions of the pregnant woman and her fetus.

perineal body wedge-shaped mass of fibromuscular tissue found between the lower part of the vagina and the anal canal.

perineorrhaphy suturing of the perineum, usually performed following a laceration.

perineotomy a surgical incision through the perineum.

perineum the area of tissue between the anus and scrotum in the male or between the anus and vagina in the female.

periodic breathing sporadic episodes of apnea, not associated with cyanosis, that last for about 10 seconds and commonly occur in preterm infants.

periods of reactivity predictable patterns of neonate behavior during the first several hours after birth.

peritoneum a serous membrane that lines the abdomino-pelvic walls.

persistent fetal circulation see *persistent pulmonary hypertension.*

persistent pulmonary hypertention a neonatal syndrome secondary to pulmonary hypertension; seen in preterm infants but more common in term and postterm newborns; characterized by cyanosis, tachypnea, and acidemia.

pessary a device inserted into the body to support an organ or structure, such as a pessary inserted into the vagina to support the uterus.

petechiae pinpoint, raised, round, purplish-red spots caused by minute capillary hemorrhage.

phenotype the whole physical, biochemical, and physiologic makeup of an individual as determined both genetically and environmentally.

phenylalanine a naturally occurring amino acid essential for optimal growth and nitrogen balance in humans.

phenylketonuria (PKU) a recessive hereditary metabolic error that causes the buildup of phenylalanine, leading to mental retardation, brain damage, light pigmentation, and other characteristics. It can be treated with a low-phenylalanine diet.

phimosis abnormal tightness of the foreskin so that it cannot be retracted over the glans; analogous to tightening of the clitoral hood.

phlebitis inflammation of a vein.

phlebothrombosis presence of a clot within a vein without associated symptoms of vein inflammation.

phlegmasia alba dolens postpartal ileofemoral thrombosis (milk-leg).

phocomelia absence of or incomplete formation and development of arms, forearms, thighs, and legs. Hands and feet are present but may be abnormally developed.

phototherapy the treatment of jaundice by exposure to light.

physiologic pertaining to normal or expected functioning of a body or organ.

physiologic anemia of infancy a harmless condition in which the hemoglobin level drops in the first 6 to 12 weeks after birth, then reverts to normal levels.

physiologic jaundice a harmless condition caused by the normal reduction of red blood cells, occurring 48 or more hours after birth, peaking at the fifth to seventh day, and disappearing between the seventh to tenth day.

pica the eating of substances not ordinarily considered edible or to have nutritive value.

Pierre-Robin syndrome a syndrome characterized by mandibular hypoplasia that occurs prior to the ninth week of embryologic development. The mandibular hypoplasia results in micrognathia, glossoptosis, and possibly a cleft in the soft palate. The infant's mandible generally catches up to normal growth by 12 to 24 months of age.

pigeon chest a chest deformity in which the sternum is prominent; transverse diameters may be shortened.

PIH pregnancy-induced hypertension; see *preeclampsia.*

pilonidal cyst a hair-containing cavity in the sacrococcygeal area.

placenta specialized disk-shaped organ that connects the fetus to the uterine wall for gas and nutrient exchange; also called *afterbirth.*

placenta accreta partial or complete absence of the decidua basalis and abnormal adherence of the placenta to the uterine wall.

placenta previa abnormal implantation of the placenta in the lower uterine segment. Classification of type is based on proximity to the cervical os: *total*—completely covers the os; *partial*—covers a portion of the os; *marginal*—in close proximity to the os.

placental pertaining to the placenta.

placental dysfunction placental insufficiency; the placenta fails to meet fetal requirements.

placental dystocia difficulty in the delivery of the placenta.

placental souffle soft blowing sounds produced by blood coursing through the placenta; it has the same rate as the maternal pulse.

platypelloid pelvis an unusually wide pelvis, having a flattened oval transverse shape and a shortened anteroposterior diameter.

plethora a reddened florid complexion, usually caused by an excessive amount of blood in the area.

pneumomediastinum accidental or diagnostically introduced air or gas into the mediastinal area, which could lead to pneumothorax, pneumopericardium, or pneumoperitoneum.

pneumothorax air within the chest cavity between the lung tissue and chest wall, creating a positive pressure space instead of negative pressure.

podalic version a technique designed to produce a change in fetal position or polarity in order to convert an abnormal presentation to a breech presentation.

polar body a small cell resulting from the meiotic division of the mature oocyte.

polycythemia an abnormal increase in the number of total red blood cells in the body's circulation.

polydactyly a developmental anomaly characterized by more than five digits on the hands or feet.

polygenic determined by the action of more than one gene.

polyhydramnios see *hydramnios.*

polymorphous pertaining to lesions in various stages of change.

popliteal angle the angle formed at the knee when the thigh of the supine infant is flexed on the chest and the leg is extended by pressure behind the ankle.

position attitude or posture assumed to achieve comfort or purpose.

positive signs of pregnancy indications that confirm the presence of pregnancy.

posterior back or dorsal surface of a body or body part.

posterior fontanelle small triangular area between the occipital and parietal bones of the skull; generally closes by 8 to 12 weeks of life.

postmature infant a newborn that is overly developed or that is more than 42 gestational weeks of age.

postnatal occurring after birth.

postnatal period period from 28 days following birth to 11 months of age.

postpartal hemorrhage a loss of blood of greater than 500 mL following delivery. The hemorrhage is classified as *early* or *immediate* if it occurs within the first 24 hours and *late* or *delayed* after the first 24 hours.

postpartum after childbirth or delivery.

postterm infant any infant delivered after 42 weeks' gestation.

postterm labor labor that occurs after 42 weeks of gestation.

precipitous delivery (1) unduly rapid progression of labor; (2) a delivery in which no physician is in attendance.

precipitous labor labor lasting less than three hours.

precocious teeth small unrooted teeth found in the newborn.

preeclampsia toxemia of pregnancy, characterized by hypertension, albuminuria, and edema. See also *eclampsia*.

preembryonic stage the first 14 days of human development; also called *stage of the ovum*.

pregnancy the condition of having a developing embryo or fetus in the body after fertilization of the female egg by the male sperm.

pregnancy-induced hypertension (PIH) a hypertensive disorder including preeclampsia and eclampsia as conditions, characterized by the three cardinal signs of hypertension, edema, and proteinuria.

premature infant see *preterm infant*.

premonitory serving as a warning.

prenatal before birth.

prep shaving of the pubic area.

preparatory phase of labor the latent phase of labor.

prepuce a covering or fold of skin.

presentation the fetal body part that enters the maternal pelvis first. The three possible presentations are cephalic, shoulder, or breech.

presenting part the fetal part present in or on the cervical os.

pressure edema accumulation of excessive fluid, primarily in the lower extremities. In obstetrics, it is caused by pressure of the pregnant uterus on the larger veins.

presumptive signs of pregnancy symptoms that suggest but do not confirm pregnancy, such as cessation of menses, quickening, Chadwick's sign, and morning sickness.

preterm infant any infant born before 38 weeks' gestation.

preterm labor labor occurring between 20 and 38 weeks of pregnancy.

priapism persistent abnormal erection of the penis, usually occurring without sexual desire and accompanied by pain and tenderness.

primigravida a woman who is pregnant for the first time.

primipara a woman who has given birth to her first child (past the point of viability), whether or not that child is living or was alive at birth.

primordial original or primitive, being the simplest form of development.

probable signs of pregnancy manifestations that strongly suggest the likelihood of pregnancy, such as a positive pregnancy test, enlarging abdomen, and positive Goodell's, Hegar's, and Braxton Hicks signs.

progesterone a hormone produced by the corpus luteum, adrenal cortex, and placenta whose function it is to stimulate proliferation of the endometrium to facilitate growth of the embryo.

projectile vomiting emesis that appears to have been propelled out of the mouth by extreme force.

prolactin a hormone secreted by the anterior pituitary that stimulates and sustains lactation in mammals.

prolapsed cord umbilical cord that becomes trapped in the vagina before the fetus is delivered.

prolonged labor labor lasting more than 24 hours.

promontory of the sacrum projecting eminence or process of the sacrum corresponding to the junction of the sacrum and L5.

prophylactic pertaining to a preventive measure or to a measure used to ward off a disease or event.

proteinuria the presence of an excessive amount of serum protein in the urine.

pseudocyesis a condition in which the woman has symptoms of pregnancy but in which hormonal pregnancy tests are negative; false pregnancy.

pseudomenstruation blood-tinged mucus from the vagina in the newborn female infant; caused by withdrawal of maternal hormones that were present during pregnancy.

pseudopregnancy see *pseudocyesis*.

psychoprophylaxis psychophysical training aimed at preparing the expectant parents to cope with the processes of labor and to avoid concentration on the discomforts associated with childbirth.

pytalism excessive salivation.

puberty the period of time during which the secondary sexual characteristics develop and the ability to procreate is attained.

pubic pertaining to the pubes or pubis.

pudendal block injection of an anesthetizing agent at the pudendal nerve to produce numbness of the external genitals and the lower one-third of the vagina, to facilitate childbirth and permit episiotomy if necessary.

pudendum the external genitals of humans.

puerperal morbidity a maternal temperature of 100.4F (38.0C) or higher on any two of the first 10 postpartal days, excluding the first 24 hours. The temperature is to be taken by mouth at least four times per day.

puerperal sepsis infection of the reproductive organs caused by unsterile childbirth conditions; also called *childbed fever* and *puerperal fever.*

puerperium the period after completion of the third stage of labor until involution of the uterus is complete, usually six weeks.

pustule a small, raised, sharply circumscribed lesion less than 1 cm in size filled with purulent material.

quickening the first fetal movements felt by the pregnant woman, usually between 16 and 18 weeks' gestation.

radiation heat loss incurred when heat transfers to cooler surfaces and objects not in direct contact with the body.

rales an abnormal respiratory sound heard usually with the aid of a stethoscope; caused by air passing through fluid in the alveoli and terminal bronchioles.

RDS see *hyaline membrane disease.*

Read method natural childbirth preparation centered on eliminating the fear-tension-pain syndrome.

recessive trait a trait that is expressed only when no dominant genes are present.

reciprocal inhibition the principle that it is impossible to feel relaxed and tense at the same time; the basis for relaxation techniques.

recoil to spring back; to return to a starting point; for example, to return to a position of flexion after involuntary extension.

recommended dietary allowances (RDA) government-recommended allowances of various vitamins, minerals, and other nutrients.

rectocele herniation of part of the rectum into the vagina.

reflex an involuntary response.

regional anesthesia injection of local anesthetic agents so that they come into direct contact with nervous tissue.

relaxin a water-soluble protein secreted by the corpus luteum that causes relaxation of the symphysis and cervical dilatation.

residual related to that which is remaining as a residue; for example, formula and gastric secretions present in an infant's stomach prior to the next feeding.

residual urine urine left in the bladder after voiding.

respiratory distress syndrome see *hyaline membrane disease.*

restitution in obstetrics, turning the fetal presenting part either right or left after it has fully exited the birth canal so that the spine is once again in a straight line.

resuscitation restoration of life or consciousness by means of artificial respiration and cardiac massage.

retained placenta placenta that fails to be expelled after childbirth because of adherence or incarceration.

retraction to be drawn up or back.

retroflexion of the uterus the bending back of the body of the uterus toward the cervix, resulting in a sharp angle at the point of bending.

retrolental fibroplasia formation of fibrotic tissue behind the lens; associated with retinal detachment and arrested eye growth, seen with hypoxemia in preterm infants.

retroversion of the uterus the turning backward of the entire uterus in relation to the pelvic area.

Rh factor antigens present on the surface of blood cells that make the blood cell incompatible with blood cells that do not have the antigen.

RhoGAM an anti-Rh (D) gamma-globulin given after delivery to an Rh-negative mother of an Rh-positive fetus or child. Prevents the development of permanent active immunity to the Rh antigen.

rhonchi coarse, abnormal auscultatory sounds made by the passage of air over mucous plugs.

rhythm method the timing of sexual intercourse to avoid the fertile time associated with ovulation.

ribonucleic acid (RNA) the complex protein responsible for transferring genetic information within a cell.

ripe being in a state of optimal readiness or consistency.

risk factors any findings that suggest the pregnancy may have a negative outcome, either for the woman or her unborn child.

role a cluster of interpersonal behaviors, attitudes, and activities associated with an individual in a certain situation or position.

ROM rupture of (amniotic) membranes. Rupture may be PROM (premature), SROM (spontaneous), or AROM (artificial). Some clinicians may use the abbreviation RBOW (rupture of bag of waters).

rooming-in unit a hospital unit where the infant can reside in the same room with the mother after delivery and during their postpartal stay.

rooting reflex an infant's tendency to turn the head and open the lips to suck when one side of the mouth or cheek is touched.

rotation turning of the fetal head as it follows the pelvic curves during childbirth.

round ligaments ligaments that arise from the side of the uterus near the fallopian tube insertion to help the broad ligament keep the uterus in place.

Rubin's test tubal insufflation with a gas, usually carbon dioxide, to test the patency of the tubes or to clear small obstructions.

rugae transverse ridges of mucous membranes lining the vagina, which allow the vagina to stretch during the descent of the fetal head.

sacral promontory a projection into the pelvic cavity on the anterior upper portion of the sacrum; serves as an obstetric guide in determining pelvic measurements.

sacroiliac the joints or articulation between the sacrum and ilium and their associated ligaments.

sacrum five fused vertebrae that form a triangle of bone just beneath the lumbar vertebrae and between the hip bones.

saddle block anesthesia sensory and motor anesthesia of the buttocks, perineum, and inner aspects of the thighs, produced by spinal or intrathecal injection of an anesthetic agent at approximately L3–L5.

sagittal suture a band of connective tissue that separates the parietal bones and extends anteriorly and posteriorly.

salpingitis infection of the fallopian tubes.

scalines eczema on the cheeks, behind the ears, and on the popliteal and antecubital areas.

Scanzoni's maneuver rotation of the presenting fetal head from a posterior position to an anterior position through double forceps application.

scaphoid abdomen abdomen with a sunken interior wall, giving it a small, empty appearance.

scarf sign the position of the elbow when the hand of a supine infant is drawn across to the other shoulder until it meets resistance.

Schultze's mechanism delivery of the placenta with the shiny or fetal surface presenting first.

sclerema patchy or generalized progressive hardening of subcutaneous fat in infants; lesions are cold, yellow, and very firm.

sebaceous glands oil-secreting glands in the skin.

seborrhea dermatus see *cradle cap*.

secondary areola increased area of pigmentation surrounding the areola that occurs during pregnancy as a result of hormonal influences; it becomes apparent at about the third month.

second stage of labor stage lasting from complete dilatation of the cervix to expulsion of the fetus.

secundines see *afterbirth*.

segmentation the process of division of the fertilized ovum into many cells before differentiation into layers.

semen thick whitish fluid ejaculated by the male during orgasm and containing the spermatozoa and their nutrients.

sensitization initial exposure to a substance that results in an immune response.

septic abortion a serious uterine infection that occurs most commonly after an abortion performed by an unskilled person outside an appropriate facility.

sex chromatin see *Barr body*.

sex chromosomes the X and Y chromosomes, which are responsible for sex determination.

sex-limited trait a characteristic that is expressed in only one sex.

sex-linked trait a characteristic that is determined by genes on the X chromosome.

sexually transmitted disease (STD) refers to diseases ordinarily transmitted by direct sexual contact with an infected individual.

show a pinkish mucous discharge from the vagina that may occur a few hours to a few days prior to the onset of labor.

simian line a single palmar crease frequently found in children with Down syndrome.

single gene inheritance see *Mendelian inheritance*.

singleton pregnancy with a single fetus.

sinusoidal pattern a wave form of fetal heart rate where long-term variability is present but there is no short-term variability.

small for gestational age (SGA) inadequate weight or growth for gestational age; birth weight below the tenth percentile.

sole creases lines caused by folds covering the underpart of the foot. The distribution and number of creases contribute to determining gestational age.

souffle a soft blowing sound made by blood turbulence in the vessels.

spermatogenesis the process by which mature spermatozoa are formed, during which the number of chromosomes is halved.

spermatozoa mature sperm cells of the male animal, produced by the testes.

spermicides a variety of creams, foam, jellies, and suppositories, inserted into the vagina prior to intercourse, which destroy sperm or neutralize any vaginal secretions and thereby immobilize sperm.

sphincter muscle a ringlike band of muscle fibers that constricts or closes a passage or orifice.

spina bifida occulta a defect in the vertebrae of the spinal column without protrusion of neural components; may be completely asymptomatic.

spinal block injection of a local anesthetic agent directly into the spinal fluid in the spinal canal to provide anesthesia for vaginal delivery and cesarean birth.

spinnbarkeit describes the elasticity of the cervical mucus that is present at ovulation.

spontaneous abortion abortion that occurs naturally; also called *miscarriage*.

square window the angle formed at the wrist when the infant's hand is flexed toward the ventral forearm.

SROM spontaneous rupture of (amniotic) membranes.

startle reflex see *Moro reflex*.

station relationship of the presenting fetal part to an imaginary line drawn between the pelvic ischial spines.

steepled palate high palate that rises to an angle instead of the more normal round shape.

sterility inability to conceive or to produce offspring.

stillbirth the delivery of a dead infant.

strabismus an eye condition in which the visual axis does not converge on a desired object; incoordinate action of the extrinsic ocular muscles.

striae gravidarum stretch marks; shiny reddish lines that appear on the abdomen, breasts, thighs, and buttocks of pregnant women as a result of stretching the skin.

Sturge-Weber syndrome syndrome of unknown etiology characterized by flat facial hemangiomata and meningeal hemangiomata with seizures.

subinvolution failure of a part to return to its normal size after functional enlargement, such as failure of the uterus to return to normal size after pregnancy.

subluxation incomplete or partial dislocation.

subtotal hysterectomy removal of the fundus and body of the uterus, leaving the cervical stump.

succedaneum see *caput succedaneum*.

sucking reflex the infant's tendency to suck on any object placed in the mouth.

superfecundation successful fertilization of two or more ova during the same menstrual cycle as the result of more than one act of intercourse.

superfetation fertilization and development of an ovum while a developing fetus is already in the uterus.

supernumerary nipples excess number of nipples, varying from small pink spots to normal size and pigmentation, usually present along an imaginary line from midclavicle to groin.

surfactant a surface-active mixture of lipoproteins secreted in the alveoli and air passages that reduces surface tension of pulmonary fluids and contributes to the elasticity of pulmonary tissue.

suture (1) fibrous connection of opposed joint surfaces, as in the skull. (2) The uniting of edges of a wound.

symphysis pubis fibrocartilaginous joint between the pelvic bones in the midline.

synclitism when the biparietal diameter of the fetal head is parallel to the planes of the maternal pelvis.

syndactyly malformation of the fingers or toes in which there may be webbing or complete fusion of two or more digits.

tachycardia abnormally rapid heart rate.

tachypnea excessively rapid respirations.

talipes equinovarus congenital defect of the foot with changes in the ligament and tendons consisting chiefly of contractures and anomalous insertions. The forefoot is adducted and supine and there is inversion of the heel and fixed plantar flexion of the foot. Also known as *clubfoot.*

Tay-Sachs disease a genetic disorder transmitted as an autosomal recessive that occurs primarily among Ashkenazi Jews. The disease produces progressive neurologic damage and is fatal within 18 months to 2 years. No known treatment exists, but the condition can be diagnosed with amniocentesis.

telangiectatic nevi (stork bites) small clusters of pink-red spots appearing on the nape of the neck and around the eyes of infants; localized areas of capillary dilatation.

teratogens nongenetic factors that can produce malformations of the fetus.

term infant a live born infant at 38 to 42 weeks' gestation.

testes the male gonads, in which sperm and testosterone are produced.

testosterone the male hormone; responsible for the development of secondary male characteristics.

tetralogy of Fallot a combination of four congenital anomalies that together make up a specific cardiac syndrome.

therapeutic abortion medically induced termination of pregnancy when a malformed fetus is suspected or when the woman's health is in jeopardy.

thermal neutral zone (TNZ) an environment that provides for minimal heat loss or expenditure.

thermogenesis the production of heat, especially within the body.

third stage of labor the time from delivery of the fetus to complete expulsion of the placenta.

threatened abortion a condition in which discharge of the fertilized ovum is threatened by bleeding from the vagina; may be accompanied by cervical dilatation.

thromboembolus thrombotic material or clot carried by the bloodstream from one site to another vessel, causing obstruction.

thrombophlebitis inflammation of a vein associated with thrombus formation.

thrush a fungus infection of the oral mucous membranes caused by *Candida albicans.* Most often seen in infants; characterized by white plaques in the mouth.

tocodynamometer external device that can be used to estimate uterine contraction pressures during labor.

tongue tie abnormally short frenulum of the tongue that limits its motion.

tonic neck reflex postural reflex seen in the newborn. When the supine infant's head is turned to one side, the arm and leg on that side extend while the extremities on the opposite side flex; also called the *fencing position.*

TORCH an acronym used to describe a group of infections that represent potentially severe problems during pregnancy. TO = toxoplasmosis, R = rubella, C = cytomegalovirus, H = herpesvirus.

torticollis contracted neck muscles, producing a twisting and contraction of the head toward the affected side; wryneck.

total hysterectomy removal of the entire uterus, including the cervix, leaving the ovaries and fallopian tubes.

toxemia a group of pathologic conditions, essentially metabolic disturbances, occurring in pregnant women and manifested by preeclampsia and eclampsia.

tracheoesophageal fistula a congenital anomaly in which there is a communication between the trachea and the esophagus.

traditional family a family type that draws its strength from the autocratic and authoritarian patriarchal line.

transient tachypnea of the newborn a respiratory condition theorized to be caused by excess lung fluid production or failure to remove normal (fetal) lung fluid; characterized by signs of respiratory distress, reduced air entry, and mild hypercarbia. Usually does not require assisted ventilation, and newborns are well in two to five days.

transition the period during labor when the cervix becomes approximately 8 cm dilated, contractions are very strong, and the laboring woman may feel that she cannot go on.

translocation the occurrence of a chromosome segment at an abnormal site.

transverse diameter the largest diameter of the pelvic inlet; helps determine the shape of the inlet.

transverse lie a lie in which the fetus is positioned crosswise in the uterus.

Treacher-Collins syndrome mandibulofacial dysostosis.

Trichomonas vaginalis a parasitic protozoan that may cause inflammation of the vagina, characterized by itching and burning of vulvar tissue and by white, frothy discharge.

trimester three months, or one-third of the gestational time for pregnancy.

trisomy the presence of three homologous chromosomes rather than the normal two.

trophoblast the outer layer of the blastoderm that will eventually establish the nutrient relationship with the uterine endometrium.

true pelvis the portion that lies below the linea terminalis, made up of the inlet, cavity, and outlet.

tubal ligation see *ligation.*

Turner syndrome a number of anomalies that occur when a female has only one X chromosome; characteristics include short stature, little sexual differentiation, webbing of the neck with a low posterior hairline, and congenital cardiac anomalies.

twins two offspring produced by the same pregnancy. See also *dizygotic twins; monozygotic twins.*

type II respiratory distress syndrome see *transient tachypnea of the newborn.*

ultrasound high-frequency sound waves that may be directed, through the use of a transducer, into the maternal abdomen. The ultrasonic sound waves reflected by the underlying structures of varying densities allow various maternal and fetal tissues, bones, and fluids to be identified.

umbilical cord the structure connecting the placenta to the umbilicus of the fetus and through which nutrients from the woman are exchanged for wastes from the fetus.

umbilical vasculitis inflammation of the umbilical cord and its contents.

umbilicus see *navel.*

urachus a canal connecting the fetal bladder with the allantois; at birth, it collapses and becomes mostly fibrotic, forming the median umbilical ligament.

urinary meatus external opening of the urethra.

uterine souffle a soft sound made by the blood within the arteries of a gravid uterus.

uterine tetany prolonged or continuous uterine contractions.

uterine tubes see *fallopian tubes.*

uterosacral ligaments ligaments that provide support for the uterus and cervix at the level of the ischial spines.

uterus the hollow muscular organ in which the fertilized ovum is implanted and in which the developing fetus is nourished until birth.

vagina the musculomembranous tube or passageway located between the external genitals and the uterus of the female.

valgus bent outward.

variable expressivity the differences in severity of a trait produced by the same gene in different individuals.

varicose veins permanently distended veins.

vasectomy surgical removal of a portion of the vas deferens (ductus deferens) to produce infertility.

vegan a "pure" vegetarian; one who consumes no food from animal sources.

vena caval syndrome symptoms of dizziness, pallor, and clamminess resulting from lowering blood pressure when the pregnant woman lies supine and the enlarging uterus presses on the vena cava; also known as *supine hypotensive syndrome.*

venereal disease (VD) see *sexually transmitted disease.*

venous referring to veins or to unoxygenated blood.

vernix caseosa a protective cheeselike whitish substance made up of sebum and desquamated epithelial cells that is present on the fetal skin.

version a change of position, usually to alter the presenting fetal part and facilitate delivery.

vertex the top or crown of the head.

vesical blastoderm a stage in the development of the mammalian embryo consisting of a hollow sphere of cells enclosing a cavity.

vesicular composed of or relating to small saclike structures filled with fluid.

vestibule a space or cavity at the entrance to a canal.

viable capable of living.

villi short vascular processes or protrusions appearing on some membranes. See also *chorionic villi.*

vulva the external structure of the female genitals, lying below the mons veneris.

vulvectomy surgical removal of the vulva.

Waardenburg syndrome a congenital syndrome transmitted as an autosomal recessive trait and characterized by cochlear deafness, wide bridge of the nose, lateral displacement of the medial canthi, confluent eyebrows, eyes of different colors, white eyelashes, white forelock, and leukodermia.

wet lung see *transient tachypnea of the newborn.*

Wharton's jelly yellow-white gelatinous material surrounding the vessels of the umbilical cord.

witch's milk whitish secretion from the infant's mammary glands; it lasts for approximately seven days after delivery and is caused by the influence of the mother's hormones.

womb see *uterus.*

xanthoma yellow-white plaque on the skin as a result of lipid deposition.

X chromosome female sex chromosome.

X linkage genes located on the X chromosome.

Y chromosome male sex chromosome.

zona pellucida transparent inner layer surrounding an ovum.

zygote a fertilized egg.

Resource Directory

This Resource Directory lists associations, support groups, and other organizations that can provide information or other assistance to maternal-newborn nurses and their clients. The resources are organized by topic, usually with brief descriptions of their services. Since many of these organizations have branches or chapters throughout North America, we recommend that you refer to your telephone directory for the location of the local branch.

● GENERAL INFORMATION RESOURCES

National Center for Health Statistics (NCHS)
(produces vital and health statistics for the United States)
Scientific and Technical Information Branch
Department of Health and Human Services
3700 East-West Highway
Room 1-57
Hyattsville, MD 20782
(301) 436-8500

National Health Information Clearinghouse
(provides information on health organizations)
P.O. Box 1133
Washington, DC 20013-1133
(800) 336-4797; in Virginia, call collect (703) 522-2590

National Institute of Child Health and Human Development (NICHD)
National Institutes of Health
9000 Rockville Pike
Bldg 31, Room 2A32
Bethesda, MD 20892
(301) 496-4000

National Library of Medicine (NLM)
(collects and disseminates biomedical information; publishes indexes of journal and research literature related to biomedical fields)
Public Information Office
8600 Rockville Pike
Bethesda, MD 20894
(301) 496-6308

National Technical Information Service (NTIS)
(source of specialized social, scientific, business, and economic information, mostly originated or sponsored by federal agencies)
Department of Commerce
5285 Port Royal Road
Springfield, VA 22161
(703) 487-4600

Public Health Service
200 Independence Avenue, SW
Washington, DC 20201
(202) 245-6867

● ONLINE COMPUTER SERVICES

BRS Information Technologies
1200 Route 7
Latham, NY 12110
(800) 833-4707; (518) 583-1161

DIALOG Information Services, Inc.
3460 Hillview Avenue
Palo Alto, CA 94304
(800) 982-5838; (800) 227-1927; (415) 858-2700

National Library of Medicine
MEDLARS Management Section
Bldg 38A, Room 4N-421
8600 Rockville Pike
Bethesda, MD 20894
(800) 638-8480; (301) 496-6193

● RESOURCES BY TOPIC

Abortion

National Abortion Federation
(provides information and referral for abortion services)
900 Pennsylvania, SE
Washington, DC 20003
Consumer Information Hotline: (800) 772-9100

National Abortion Rights Action League
(*pro-choice political action group*)
1101 14th Street, NW
Washington, DC 20005
(202) 371-0779

National Right to Life Committee
(*pro-life political action group*)
419 7th Street, NW
Suite 402
Washington, DC 20004
(202) 626-8800

Planned Parenthood Federation of America
810 Seventh Avenue
New York, NY 10019
(212) 541-7800
See also Family Planning

Adoption

AASK (Aid to the Adoption of Special Kids)
(*provides assistance to families who adopt older and handicapped
    children*)
3530 Grand Avenue
Oakland, CA 94610
(415) 451-1748

Adoptees' Liberty Movement Association (ALMA) Society
(*provides assistance for adopted children to locate natural parents
    and for natural parents to locate relinquished children*)
P.O. Box 154
Washington Bridge Station
New York, NY 10033
(212) 581-1568

Child Welfare League
67 Irving Place
New York, NY 10003
(212) 254-7410

Permanent Families for Children
(*provides information about adoption, especially of children with
    special needs*)
4 41st, NW
Washington, DC 20001
(202) 638-2952

AIDS (Acquired Immune Deficiency Syndrome)

AIDS Medical Foundation
10 East 13th Street, Suite LD
New York, NY 10003
(212) 206-0670

Shanti Project
(*provides counseling and assistance to individuals with AIDS*)
890 Hayes Street
San Francisco, CA 94117
(415) 558-9644
See also Sexually Transmitted Diseases

Alcohol Abuse

Al-Anon/Alateen
P.O. 862
Midtown Station
New York, NY 10018
(212) 254-7230

Alcoholics Anonymous
P.O. Box 459
Grand Central Station
New York, NY 10017
(212) 686-1100

National Clearinghouse for Alcohol Information
P.O. Box 2345
Rockville, MD 20852
(301) 468-2600

Women For Sobriety, Inc.
(*support group for women with drinking problem*)
P.O. Box 618
Quakertown, PA 18951
(215) 536-8026

Birth Control

See Family Planning

Birth Defects

American Cleft Palate Association
(*provides information about cleft palates and cleft palate centers
    and parent support groups*)
331 Salk Hall
Pittsburgh, PA 15261
(412) 681-9620

Cystic Fibrosis Foundation
1655 Tullie Circle
Suite 111
Atlanta, GA 30329
(404) 325-6973

Institutes for the Achievement of Human Potential
(*resource for parents with brain-injured children*)
8801 Stenton Avenue
Philadelphia, PA 19118
(215) 233-2050

March of Dimes Birth Defects Foundation
Public Health Education Foundation
1275 Mamaroneck Avenue
White Plains, NY 10605
(914) 428-7100

Sibling Information Network
(*resource for professionals and parents who deal with siblings of
    handicapped children*)
249 Glenbrook Road, U-64
University of Connecticut
Storrs, CT 06268
(203) 486-3783

Spina Bifida Association of America
(*provides information and support to parents of infants with neural
tube defects*)
1700 Rockville Pike
Suite 540
Rockville, MD 20852
(800) 621-3141
See also Down Syndrome; Genetic Disorders; Sickle Cell
Anemia

Breast Cancer

Reach to Recovery
(*support program for women who have undergone mastectomies as
a result of breast cancer*)
American Cancer Society
90 Park Avenue
New York, NY 10016
(212) 736-3030
See also Cancer

Breast Feeding

Health Education Associates
(*provides continuing education programs for health professionals on
breast-feeding management*)
211 South Easton Road
Glenside, PA 19038
(215) 576-8071

La Leche League International
(*provides information about breast feeding and support for breast-
feeding mothers*)
9616 Minneapolis Avenue
Franklin, IL 60131
(312) 455-7730

Lact-Aid
(*provides services, literature, and supplies to promote breast-
feeding*)
P.O. Box 1066
Athens, TN 37303
(615) 744-9090
See also Childbirth; Infant Health; Maternal Health

Cancer

American Cancer Society
90 Park Avenue
New York, NY 10016
(212) 736-3030

Cancer Information Service
(*supplies cancer information to general public*)
National Cancer Institute
9000 Rockville Pike
Bethesda, MD 20892
(800) 4-CANCER
See also Breast Cancer; DES Exposure; Smoking

Cesarean Birth

Cesarean Prevention Clarion (periodical)
P.O. Box 152
Syracuse, NY 13210
(315) 424-1942

C/SEC, Inc. (Cesarean/Support Education and Concern)
(*provides information about cesarean birth*)
22 Forest Road
Framingham, MA 01701
(617) 877-8266

VBAC (Vaginal Birth After Cesarean)
10 Great Plain Terrace
Needham, MA 01292

Child Abuse

**C. Henry Kempe National Center for Prevention and
Treatment of Child Abuse and Neglect**
(*publishes a newsletter with information on prevention and
treatment of child abuse*)
University of Colorado Medical Center
Department of Pediatrics
1205 Oneida Street
Denver, CO 80220
(303) 321-3963

National Center on Child Abuse
Office of Child Development
P.O. Box 1182
Washington, DC 20013
(703) 821-2086

**National Committee for Prevention of Child Abuse
(NCPCA)**
(*provides literature on child abuse prevention programs*)
332 South Michigan Avenue
Suite 950
Chicago, IL 60604
(312) 663-3520

Parents Anonymous
(*self-help organization for abusive parents*)
2810 Artesia Blvd.
Redondo Beach, CA 90278
(800) 421-0353; in California (800) 352-0386
See also Missing and Runaway Children; Sexual Abuse and
Assault

Child Health and Development

Canadian Institute of Child Health
410 Laurier Avenue
Suite 803
West Ottawa, Ont. K1R 7T6

**National Center for Education in Maternal and Child
Health**
38th and R Streets, NW
Washington, DC 20007
(202) 625-8400

National Institute of Child Health and Human Development
National Institutes of Health
9000 Rockville Pike
Bldg. 31, Room 2A32
Bethesda, MD 20205
(301) 496-4000

Family Resource Clearinghouse
Child Development Center
Box 85
Metropolitan State College
1006 11th Street
Denver, CO 80204
(303) 556-8362
See also Infant Health

Childbirth

American Foundation for Maternal and Child Health, Inc.
(conducts research on the perinatal period)
30 Beekman Place
New York, NY 10022
(212) 759-5510

Birth: Issues in Prenatal Care and Education (quarterly
journal)
   (publisher also provides directory of instructional materials for
   childbirth educators)
110 El Camino Real
Berkeley,, CA 94705
(415) 658-5099

International Childbirth Education Association
P.O. Box 20048
Minneapolis, MN 55420

Maternity Center Association
(freestanding birth center that provides information and advocacy
   functions)
48 East 92nd Street
New York, NY 10028
(212) 369-7300

**National Association of Parents and Professionals for Safe
   Alternatives in Childbirth**
(provides information and support for alternatives in birth
   experiences)
P.O. Box 267
Marble Hill, MO 63764
(314) 238-2010

National Association of Childbearing Centers
(organization that provides information and suggests guidelines for
   birth centers)
Box 1, Route 1
Perkiomenville, PA 18074
(215) 234-8068

Family Resource Clearinghouse
Box 85
Metropolitan State College
1006 11th Street
Denver, CO 80204
(303) 556-8362
See also Cesarean Birth; Childbirth Education/Preparation;
   Home Birth

Childbirth Education/Preparation

American Academy of Husband-Coached Childbirth
(provides information on the Bradley method of childbirth)
P.O. Box 5224
Sherman Oaks, CA 91413
(818) 788-6662

American Society for Psychoprophylaxis in Obstetrics
(provides information about the Lamaze method of childbirth)
1840 Wilson Blvd.
Suite 204
Arlington, VA 22201
(703) 524-7802

Childbirth Graphics, Ltd.
(provides audiovisual and other types of teaching aids for childbirth
   education)
1210 Culver Rd.
Rochester, NY 14609
(716) 482-7940

Read Natural Childbirth Foundation, Inc.
(provides information about the Dick-Read method of childbirth)
P.O. 956
San Rafael, CA 94915
(415) 456-8462
See also Cesarean Birth; Childbirth; Home Birth

Circumcision

American Academy of Pediatrics
(report on circumcision available for a minimal fee)
P.O. Box 927
Elk Grove, IL 60009-0927
(312) 869-9327

Congenital Disorders/Defects

See Birth Defects; Genetic Disorders

Consumer Information

Auto Safety Hotline
(for consumer complaints about auto safety and child safety seats
   and requests for information on recalls)
U.S. Department of Transportation
National Highway Traffic Safety Administration
Washington, DC 20590
(800) 424-9393; in DC (202) 426-0123

Consumer Information Catalog
(catalog of publications for consumers developed by federal agencies)
Pueblo, CO 81009

Consumer Information Center (CIC)
(distributes publications for consumers developed by federal
   agencies)
18th and E Streets, NW
Washington, DC 20405
(202) 566-1794

Consumer Product Safety Commission
Washington, DC 20207
(800) 638-CPSC

Consumers Union
(*tests quality and safety of consumer products; publishes magazine*
  Consumer Reports)
256 Washington Street
Mount Vernon, NY 10553
(914) 667-9400

Council of Better Business Bureaus
1515 Wilson Blvd.
Arlington, VA 22209
(703) 276-0100

Food and Drug Administration (FDA)
Office of Consumer Affairs
Public Inquiries
5600 Fishers Lane (HFE-88)
Rockville, MD 20857
(301) 443-3170
See also Self-Care

Contraception

See Family Planning

Counseling Services

Family Service Association of America
(*organization of local family counseling agencies throughout North
  America*)
11700 Westlake Park Drive
Milwaukee, WI 53224
(414) 359-2111

Women in Transition (WIT)
(*provides counseling information and referrals for women in distress
  and transition because of divorce, widowhood, and separation*)
112 South 16th Street
Philadelphia, PA 19102
(215) 922-7500

DES (Diethylstilbestrol) Exposure

Department DES
(*provides information to DES mothers and daughters*)
National Cancer Institute
Office of Cancer Communications
Bldg. 31, Room 10A19
Bethesda, MD 20892
(800) 4-CANCER

DES Action/National
(*support group for persons exposed to DES*)
Long Island Jewish Hospital–Hillside Medical Center
New Hyde Park, NY 11040
(516) 775-3450
See also Cancer; Women's Health

Diabetes

National American Diabetes Association
1660 Duke Street
Alexandria, VA 22314
(703) 549-1500

Juvenile Diabetes Foundation International Hotline
(800) 223-1138; in New York (212) 889-7575

National Diabetes Information Clearinghouse
Box: NDIC
Besthesda, MD 20892
(301) 468-2162

Down Syndrome

National Association for Down's Syndrome (NADS)
(*provides information about Down syndrome*)
1800 Dempster
Park Ridge, IL 60068-1146
(312) 823-7550

National Down's Syndrome Society Hotline
141 Fifth Avenue
New York, NY 10010
(800) 221-4602; in New York (212) 764-3070
See also Birth Defects; Genetic Disorders

Drug Abuse

Cocaine Anonymous
See white pages of telephone directory for local chapter

CokEnders
See white pages of telephone directory for local chapter

Fair Oaks Psychiatric Hospital
(*provides counseling and names of treatment centers*)
Summit, NJ
(800) COCAINE

National Clearinghouse for Drug Abuse Information
P.O. Box 416
Dept. DQ
Kensington, MD 20795
(800) 638-2045; in Maryland (800) 492-6605

Eating Disorders

National Anorexic Aid Society, Inc.
P.O. Box 29461
Columbus OH 43229
(614) 436-1112
See also Nutrition

Endometriosis

Endometriosis Association
238 West Wisconsin Avenue
P.O. Box 92187
Milwaukee, WI 53202
(414) 962-8972

Environmental Hazards

Center for Devices and Radiological Health
Food and Drug Administration
5600 Fishers Lane
Room 1505
Rockville, MD 20857
(301) 443-3285

Environmental Protection Agency (EPA)
Public Information Center
Room PM 211-B
401 M Street, SW
Washington, DC 20460
(202) 382-7550

Hazardous Waste Hotline
(800) 424-9346

National Institute of Environmental Health Sciences
P.O. Box 12233
Research Triangle Park, NC 27709
(919) 541-3345
See also Occupational Health

Family

Displaced Homemakers Network
(national advocacy group for women over 35 who have lost their
primary means of support through death, divorce, or disabling of
spouse)
1411 K Street, NW
Suite 930
Washington, DC 20005
(202) 628-6767

Equal Rights for Fathers
P.O. Box 90042
San Jose, CA 95109-3042
(415) 848-2323

Family Research in Health Care
(researches family problems in health care settings)
National Council on Family Relations
1910 W. County Road B.
Suite 147
St. Paul, MN 55113
(612) 633-6933

Family Service Association of America
(provides counseling and assistance to families)
11700 Westlake Park Drive
Milwaukee, WI 53223
(414) 359-2111

Parenthood After Thirty
(provides information and programs for professionals and
individuals who have delayed childbearing)
451 Vermont
Berkeley, CA 94707
(415) 524-6635

Parents Without Partners
(support group for single parents)
8807 Colesville Road
Silver Spring, MD 20910
(301) 588-9354

Stepfamily Association of America
(provides information and publishes quarterly newsletter)
602 E. Joppa Road
Baltimore, MD 21204
(301) 823-7570

Family Planning

Association of Voluntary Sterilization, Inc. (AVS)
(provides information on sterilization and referral service)
122 E. 42nd
New York, NY 10168
(212) 351-2500

Couple to Couple League International, Inc. (CCL)
(teaches natural family planning techniques; publishes manual on
the symptothermal method, The Art of Natural Family
Planning)
P.O. Box 111184
Cincinnati, OH 45211
(513) 661-7612

Planned Parenthood Federation of America
810 Seventh Avenue
New York, NY 10019
(212) 541-7800

National Clearinghouse for Family Planning Information
P.O. Box 10716
Rockville, MD 20850
(703) 558-4990

Food and Nutrition

See Nutrition

Genetic Disorders

National Clearinghouse for Human Genetic Disease
(provides information about inherited diseases; publishes directory of
genetic counseling services)
National Center for Education in Maternal and Child Health
38th and R Streets, NW
Washington, DC 20057
(202) 625-8400
See also Birth Defects; Down Syndrome

Hazardous Wastes

See Environmental Hazards

Hearing-Impaired Children

Amercan Society for Deaf People
(provides education and support to parents of hearing-impaired
children)
814 Thayer Avenue
Silver Springs, MD 20910
(301) 585-5400

Heart Disease

American Heart Association
7320 Greenville Avenue
Dallas, TX 75231
(214) 750-5300

Heart Information Center
National Heart Institute
U.S. Public Health Service
9000 Rockville Pike
Bldg 31, Room 4A21
Bethesda, MD 20892

Home Birth

Association for Childbirth at Home, International
P.O. Box 39498
Los Angeles, CA 90039
(213) 667-0839
See also Childbirth

Infant Death

Compassionate Friends
(self-help group for those who have experienced the death of an infant)
P.O. Box 1347
Oak Brook, IL 60521
(312) 990-0010

SHARE (Source of Help in Airing and Resolving Experiences)
(support group for parents who have suffered loss of newborn baby)
c/o St. John's Hospital
800 E. Carpenter Street
Springfield, IL 62769
(217) 544-6464
See also Sudden Infant Death Syndrome

Infant Health

American Foundation for Maternal and Child Health
(clearinghouse for research on the perinatal period)
300 Beekman Place
New York, NY 10022
(212) 759-5510

American Red Cross
(offers classes to prepare expectant parents for care and nurturing of infant)
17th and E Streets
Washington, DC 20006
(202) 737-8300

National Center for Clinical Infant Programs
(promotes optimum development and mental health for infants and their families)
733 15th Street, NW
Suite 912
Washington, DC 20005
(202) 347-0308
See also Child Health

Infant Nutrition

Beech-Nut Nutrition Hotline
(800) 523-6633; in Pennsylvania (800) 492-2384

Infertility

American Fertility Foundation
2131 Magnolia Avenue
Suite 201
Birmingham, Al 35256
(205) 251-9764

Fertility Research Foundation (FRF)
(provides medical and consultation services for infertile couples; publishes journals, Fertility Review *and* Infertility*)*
1430 Second Avenue
Suite 103
New York, NY 10021
(212) 744-5500

Resolve, Inc.
5 Water Street
Arlington, MA 02174
(617) 643-2424

Test-tube Fertilization
Eastern Virginia Medical School
Norfolk General Hospital
The Howard and Georgeanna Jones Institute for Reproductive Medicine
825 Fairfax Avenue
Norfolk, VA 23507

Intrauterine Procedures

National Institute for Child Health and Human Development
National Institutes of Health
9000 Rockville Pike
Bldg. 31, Room 2A32
Bethesda, MD 20205
(301) 496-4000

Legal Concerns

Health Law Project
(group that studies legal aspects of medicine)
University of Pennsylvania
School of Law
3400 Chestnut Street
Philadelphia, PA 19104-6204
(215) 898-7483

National Center on Women and Family Law
(collects information about family law and women's health issues)
799 Broadway
Room 402
New York, NY 10003
(212) 674-8200

Reproductive Freedom Project
American Civil Liberties Union
132 West 43rd Street
New York, NY 10036

Maternal Health

Maternal Health Society
Box 46563, Station G
Vancouver, B.C. V6R 4G8

National Center for Education in Maternal and Child Health
38th and R Streets, NW
Washington, DC 20057
(202) 625-8400
See also Childbirth; Pregnancy; Women's Health

Medical Organizations

American Academy of Family Physicians
1740 West 92nd Street
Kansas City, MO 64114
(816) 333-9700

American Academy of Pediatrics
P.O. Box 927
Elk Grove, IL 60009-0927
(312) 869-9327

American College of Obstetricians and Gynecologists
600 Maryland Avenue, SW
Suite 300 East
Washington, DC 20024
(202) 638-5577

American Medical Association
535 North Dearborn Street
Chicago, IL 60610
(312) 645-5000

Society of Obstetricians and Gynaecologists of Canada
14 Prince Arthur Avenue
Suite 109
Toronto, Ont. M5R 1A9

Medications (Prescription and Over-the-Counter)

Food and Drug Administration (FDA)
Office of Consumer Affairs
Public Inquiries
5600 Fishers Lane (HFE-88)
Rockville, MD 20857
(301) 344-3719
See also Consumer Information

Midwifery

The Farm
(offers lay midwifery program; published midwifery handbook,
   Spiritual Midwifery; publishes periodical The Birth Gazette)
P.O. 34A
Summertown, TN 38483
(615) 964-3574
See also Nurse-Midwifery

Missing and Runaway Children

Adam Walsh Child Resource Center
1876 N. University Drive
Suite 306
Fort Lauderdale, FL 33322
(305) 475-4847

Childfind
P.O. Box 277
New Paltz, NY 12561
(800) 426-5678; (914) 255-1848

Runaway Hotline
(800) 231-6946; in Texas (800) 392-3352

Multiple Birth

Center for the Study of Multiple Birth
333 East Superior Street
Suite 463-5
Chicago, IL 60611
(312) 266-9093

National Organization of Mothers of Twins Clubs, Inc.
12404 Princess Jeanne, NE
Albuquerque, NM 87112
(505) 275-0955

Nurse-Midwifery

American College of Nurse Midwives
1522 K Street, NW
Suite 1120
Washington, DC 20005
(202) 347-5445

Journal of Nurse-Midwifery (periodical)
Elsevier Science Publishing Co., Inc.
52 Vanderbilt Avenue
New York, NY 10017

Midwives Alliance of North America
(organization of nurse and lay midwives in the United States and
   Canada)
c/o Concord Midwifery Service
30 South Main Street
Concord, NH 03301
(603) 225-9586

Nursing Organizations

American Nurses Association
1101 14th Street, NW
Suite 200
Washington, DC 20005
(202) 789-1800

Canadian Nurses Association
50 The Driveway
Ottawa, Ont. K2P 1E2

Nurses Association of the American College of Obstetricians and Gynecologists (NAACOG)
600 Maryland Avenue, SW
Washington, DC 20024
(202) 638-5577

National League for Nursing (NLN)
Ten Columbus Circle
New York, NY 10019
(212) 582-1022
See also Nurse-Midwifery

Nutrition

American Institute of Nutrition
9650 Rockville Pike
Bethesda, MD 20814
(301) 530-7050

Food and Drug Administration (FDA)
Office of Consumer Affairs
Public Inquiries
5600 Fishers Lane (HFE-88)
Rockville, MD 20857
(301) 443-3170

Obesity

See Nutrition; Weight Control

Occupational Health

Clearinghouse for Occupational Safety and Health Information
National Institute for Occupational Safety and Health
4676 Columbia Parkway
Cincinnati, OH 45226
(513) 533-8236

Women's Occupational Health Resource Center
(provides public education services and maintains an extensive research library)
School of Public Health
Columbia Univeristy
701 West 168th Street
New York, NY 10032
(212) 305-2500

Pregnancy

COPE (Coping with the Overall Pregnancy/Parenting Experience)
37 Clarendon Street
Boston, MA 02116
(617) 357-5588
See also Childbirth; Family Planning; Maternal Health; Women's Health

Premenstrual Syndrome

Premenstrual Syndrome Action
(provides information to public and health professionals about PMS)
P.O. 16292
Irving, CA 92713
(714) 854-4407
See also Women's Health

Preterm Infants

Parents of Prematures
(publishes directory listing support groups for parents of preterm infants; offers information on how to start a local support group and breast-feeding preterm infants)
c/o Houston Organization for Parent Education, Inc.
2990 Richmond
Suite 204
Houston, TX 77098
(713) 524-3089

Rape

See telephone directory for local Rape Centers

Women Against Rape
P.O. Box 02084
Columbus, OH 43202
(614) 291-9751
See also Sexual Abuse and Assault

Self-Care

Medical Self-Care Magazine (periodical)
P.O. Box 1000
Point Reyes, CA 94956
(415) 663-8462

National Self-Help Clearinghouse
(provides information about self-help groups)
33 West 42nd Street
New York, NY 10036
(212) 840-1259

Self-Help Institute
(provides information about self-help groups)
1600 Dodge Avenue
Suite 5122
Evanston, IL 60201
(312) 328-0470

Tel-Med Health Information Service
(provides taped messages on health concerns)
See white pages of telephone directory for listing

Sex Education

Center for Population Options
(develops programs and material to educate teenagers on sex and sexual responsibility)
1012 14th Street, NW
Suite 1200
Washington, DC 20005
(202) 347-5700

Planned Parenthood Federation of America
810 Seventh Avenue
New York, NY 10019
(212) 541-7800
See also Family Planning

Sexual Abuse and Assault

Child Assault Prevention (CAP) Project
Women Against Rape
P.O. Box 02084
Columbus OH 43202
(614) 291-9751

National Committee for Prevention of Child Abuse
332 S. Michigan Avenue
Suite 950
Chicago, IL 60604
(312) 663-3520

Women Against Violence Against Women (WAVAW)
(aims to eliminate sexual violence in the media)
543 North Fairfax Avenue
Los Angeles, CA 90036

Victims Anonymous
(support group for victims of sexual or physical abuse)
9514-9 Reseda Blvd., #607
Northridge, CA 91324
(818) 993-1139
See also Child Abuse; Rape

Sexually Transmitted Diseases

Center for Prevention Services
Centers for Disease Control
1600 Clifton Road, N.E.
Atlanta, GA 30333
(404) 329-1819

Herpes Resource Center
Box 100
Palo Alto, CA 94302
(415) 321-5134

V.D. National Hotline
(800) 227-8922
See also AIDS; Sex Education

Sickle Cell Anemia

Center for Sickle Cell Disease
2121 Georgia Avenue, NW
Washington, DC 20059
(202) 636-7930

Smoking

The following organizations provide information about the effects of smoking as well as how to quit smoking. See the white pages of telephone directory for local chapters.

American Cancer Society
90 Park Avenue
New York, NY 10016
(212) 736-3030

American Heart Association
7320 Greenville Avenue
Dallas, TX 75231
(214) 750-5300

American Lung Association
1740 Broadway
New York, NY 10019
(212) 315-8700

Sudden Infant Death Syndrome (SIDS)

National Sudden Infant Death Syndrome Foundation
(provides information and referrals for families who have lost an infant because of SIDS)
2320 Glenview Road
Glenview, IL 60025
(312) 657-8080
See also Infant Death

Toxic Shock Syndrome

Centers for Disease Control
1600 Clifton Road, NE
Atlanta, GA 30333
(404) 329-3286

Toxic Substances

See Environmental Hazards

Weight Control

The following groups provide information about weight control and support for their members. See the white pages of telephone directory for local chapters.

Overeaters Anonymous
4025 Spencer Street
Suite 203
Torrance, CA 90503
(213) 542-8363

TOPS (Take Off Pounds Sensibly)
P.O. Box 07489
4575 S. Fifth Street
Milwaukee, WI 53207
(414) 482-4620

Weight Watchers International, Inc.
Jericho Atrium
500 North Broadway
Jericho, NY 11753-2196
(516) 939-0400
See also Nutrition

Women's Health

Boston Women's Health Book Collective
(publishes Our Bodies, Ourselves, a well-known book on women's health)
47 Nichols Avenue
Watertown, MA 02172
(617) 924-0271

Coalition for the Medical Rights of Women (CMRW)
(consumer organization that publishes booklets on prenatal concerns)
2845 24th Street
San Francisco, CA 94114
(415) 826-4401

National Action Forum for Older Women at Stony Brook: A Center for the Health and Housing Concerns of Women over 40
(promotes an improved quality of life for women in midlife and older; publishes a newsletter, Forum)
State University of New York
School of Allied Health Professions
Health Sciences Center
Stony Brook, NY 11794
(516) 246-2989

National Women's Health Network
(provides information about and is involved in legislative action for women's health issues)
224 Seventh Street, SE
Washington, DC 20003
(202) 543-9222

Women's Sports Foundation
(provides information about women's sports, physical fitness, and related topics)
(800) 227-3988
See also Childbirth; Family Planning; Maternal Health; Occupational Health

Credits

Epigrams and Featured Quotations

Armstrong, Penny, and Feldman, Sheryl. *A Midwife's Story*. New York: Arbor House, 1986.

Bacall, Lauren. *By Myself*. New York: Alfred A. Knopf, 1978.

Baldwin, Rahima and Palmarini, Terra. *Pregnant Feelings*. Berkeley, CA: Celestial Arts, 1986.

Borg, Susan and Lasker, Judith. *When Pregnancy Fails*. Boston: Beacon Press, 1981.

Boston Women's Health Book Collective, Inc. *The New Our Bodies, Ourselves*. New York: Random House, 1985.

Boston Women's Health Book Collective, Inc. *Ourselves and Our Children*. New York: Random House, 1978.

Danziger, Dennis. *Daddy: The Diary of an Expectant Father*. Tucson, AZ: The Body Press, 1987.

Drabble, Margaret. *The Millstone*. New York: William Morrow, 1966.

Drabble, Margaret. "With All My Love, (Signed) Mama." *The New York Times*. Quoted in Emerson, Sally, ed. *A Celebration of Babies*. New York: Dutton, 1987.

Emerson, Sally, ed. *A Celebration of Babies*. New York: Dutton, 1987.

Hartigan, Harriette. *Women in Birth*. Rochester, NY: Artemis, 1984.

Hoff, Lee Ann. *People in Crisis: Understanding and Helping*, ed 2. Menlo Park, CA: Addison-Wesley, 1984.

Kenton, Leslie. "All I Ever Wanted Was a Baby." Quoted in Emerson, Sally, ed. *A Celebration of Babies*. New York: Dutton, 1987.

Klaus, Marshall, and Klaus, Phyllis H. *The Amazing Newborn*. Reading, Massachusetts: Addison-Wesley, 1985.

Lazarre, Jane. *The Mother Knot*. Boston: Beacon Press, 1976.

Lederman, Regina. *Psychosocial Adaptation in Pregnancy*. Englewood Cliffs, NJ: Prentice-Hall, 1984.

Ledray, Linda E. *Recovering from Rape*. New York: Henry Holt and Company, 1986.

Lee, Laurie. *Two Women*. Andre Deutsch Ltd. Quoted in Emerson, Sally, ed. *A Celebration of Babies*. New York: Dutton, 1987.

Lessard, Suzannah. "Talk of the Town." *The New Yorker* (August 11, 1980) 22.

Peterson, Gayle, with contributions by Lewis Mehl, M.D. *Birthing Normally: A Personal Growth Approach to Childbirth*. Berkeley, CA: Mind/Body Press, 1981.

Rich, Adrienne. *Of Woman Born*. New York: W.W. Norton, 1976.

Sorel, Nancy Caldwell, ed. *Ever Since Eve: Personal Reflections on Childbirth*. New York: Oxford University Press, 1984.

Photographs

All Part and Chapter opening photographs were taken by Suzanne Arms Wimberley, except the one for Chapter 10, which was taken by Karen Rantzman.

The endsheet photographs were taken by Barbara Miller, Cradle Pictures, Detroit, Michigan. Copyright 1987. Courtesy of Memorial Hospital, Colorado Springs, Colorado.

The origins of the photographs that appear within chapters are either given in the figure captions or are as follows:

Suzanne Arms Wimberley:
Figures 1–1, 3–1, 3–2, 4–1, 4–2, 14–6, 15–4, 15–5, 15–6, 16–1, 16–3, 16–8, 16–9, 16–11, 16–12, 17–3, 18–3, 19–1, 20–15, 21–17, 22–5, 22–8B, 23–1, 23–2, 23–3, 23–4, 23–5, 23–6, 27–8, 28–20, 30–1, 30–2, 30–4, 30–5, 30–6, 31–5, and 34–2.

Jeffry Collins:
Figures 28–4C, 28–5C, 28–6B, 28–12, 28–24, 28–29, 28–30, 29–1, 29–2, 29–3, 29–4, 29–6, 29–10, 32–12, and 36–2.
(These photographs originally appeared in PL Swearingen: *The Addison-Wesley Photo-Atlas of Nursing Procedures* [Addison-Wesley, 1984].)

William Thompson, RN, Limited Horizons
Figures 16–6, 22–8A, 23–10, 29–7, 32–16, 34–1, 35–1, and 35–2.

George B. Fry III
Figures 16–7, 23–9 (the series depicting the birth of twins), and 35–4.

Index

M

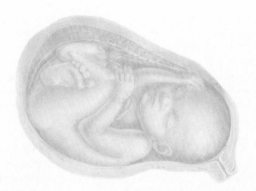

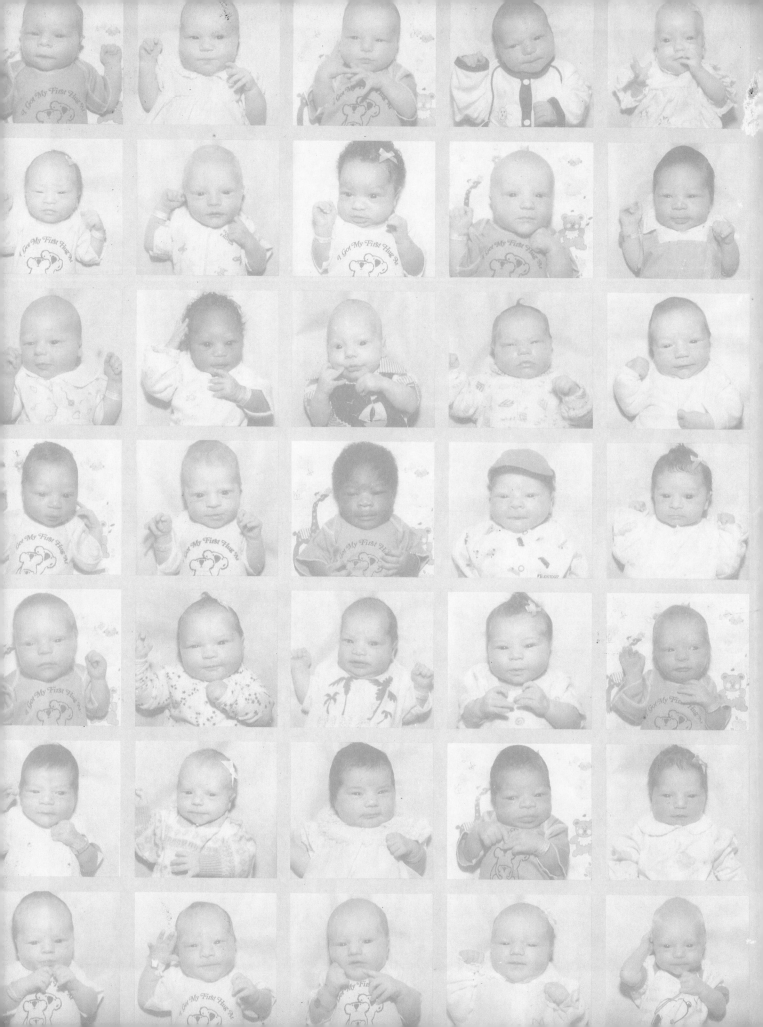